ASTHMA

■ *Volume One* ■

ASTHMA

■ *Volume One* ■

EDITORS

Peter J. Barnes, D.M., D.Sc. F.R.C.P.
Professor and Head
Department of Thoracic Medicine
Imperial College of Medicine at
The National Heart and Lung Institute
London, United Kingdom

Michael M. Grunstein, M.D., Ph.D.
Professor and Chief
Division of Pulmonary Medicine
The Children's Hospital of Philadelphia
University of Pennsylvania School of Medicine
Philadelphia, Pennsylvania

Alan R. Leff, M.D.
Professor and Head
Department of Medicine
Section of Pulmonary and Critical Care
  Medicine
The University of Chicago
Chicago, Illinois

Ann J. Woolcock, M.D., F.R.A.C.P.
Professor of Respiratory Medicine
University of Sydney
Institute of Respiratory Medicine
Royal Prince Alfred Hospital
Sydney, New South Wales
Australia

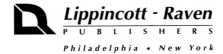
Lippincott - Raven
PUBLISHERS
Philadelphia • New York

Acquisitions Editor: Joyce-Rachel John
Developmental Editor: Judith E. Hummel
Manufacturing Manager: Dennis Teston
Production Manager: Jodi Borgenicht
Production Editor: Raeann Touhey
Cover Designer: Mark Safran
Indexer: Nancy Newman
Compositor: Lippincott–Raven Electronic Production
Printer: Kingsport Press

Printed in the United States of America

9 8 7 6 5 4 3 2 1

Library of Congress Cataloging-in-Publication Data
Asthma / editors, Peter J. Barnes . . . [et al.].
   p.   cm.
  Includes bibliographical references and index.
  ISBN 0-397-51682-7
  1. Asthma.   I. Barnes, Peter J., 1946–   .
  [DNLM: WF 553 A85113 1997]
RC591.A72   1997
616.2′38—dc21
DNLM/DLC
for Library of Congress

Care has been taken to confirm the accuracy of the information presented and to describe generally accepted practices. However, the authors, editors, and publisher are not responsible for errors or omissions or for any consequences from application of the information in this book and make no warranty, express or implied, with respect to the contents of the publication.

The authors, editors, and publisher have exerted every effort to ensure that drug selection and dosage set forth in this text are in accordance with current recommendations and practice at the time of publication. However, in view of ongoing research, changes in government regulations, and the constant flow of information relating to drug therapy and drug reactions, the reader is urged to check the package insert for each drug for any change in indications and dosage and for added warnings and precautions. This is particularly important when the recommended agent is a new or infrequently employed drug.

Some drugs and medical devices presented in this publication have Food and Drug Administration (FDA) clearance for limited use in restricted research settings. It is the responsibility of the health care provider to ascertain the FDA status of each drug or device planned for use in their clinical practice.

Contents

Volume 1

1.   Introduction

2.   Epidemiology

3. Structure, Biology, and Pathology

4. Inflammatory Cells

5. Inflammatory Mediators

6. Target Cells

7. Neural Mechanisms

Volume 2

8.   Inducers and Triggers

9.   Respiratory Physiology

10.   Clinical Assessment

11.   Therapy

12. Management

Contributing Authors

William M. Abraham, Ph.D.
Professor
Department of Medicine
University of Miami School of Medicine
Mount Sinai Medical Center
4300 Alton Road
Miami Beach, Florida 33140

Ian M. Adcock, Ph.D.
Department of Thoracic Medicine
Imperial College School of Medicine at
The National Heart and Lung Institute
Dovehouse Street
London SW3 6LY
United Kingdom

Steven M. Albelda, M.D.
Associate Professor
Department of Medicine
Associate Chief
Pulmonary and Critical Care Division
University of Pennsylvania Medical Center
3600 Spruce Street
Philadelphia, Pennsylvania 19104

Charles G. Alex, M.D.
Associate Professor
Department of Medicine
Division of Pulmonary and Critical Care
  Medicine
Loyola University
Stritch School of Medicine
Department of Veteran's Affairs
Edward Hines Jr. Hospital 111N
Hines, Illinois 60141-5000

Howard L. Alt, M.D.
Department of Psychiatry
Northwestern University Medical School
645 North Michigan Avenue #422
Chicago, Illinois 60611

Gary P. Anderson, Ph.D.
Department of Pharmacology
University of Melbourne
Parkville, Victoria 3052
Australia

Sandra D. Anderson, Ph.D., D.Sc.
Principal Hospital Scientist
Department of Respiratory Medicine
Royal Prince Alfred Hospital
Sydney, New South Wales 2050
Australia

Tony R. Bai, M.D., F.R.A.C.P., F.R.C.P.(C).,
  F.A.C.P., M.B.,Ch.B.
Professor
Department of Medicine
University of British Columbia
Pulmonary Research Laboratory
St. Paul's Hospital
1081 Burrard Street
Vancouver, British Columbia V6Z 1Y6
Canada

Neil C. Barnes, M.D., F.R.C.P.
Department of Respiratory Medicine
The London Chest Hospital
Bonner Road
London E2 9JX
United Kingdom

Peter J. Barnes, D.M., D.Sc.,
  F.R.C.P.
Professor and Head
Department of Thoracic Medicine
Imperial College School of Medicine at
The National Heart and Lung Institute
Dovehouse Street
London SW3 6LY
United Kingdom

David A. Bass, M.D., D.Phil.
Professor of Internal Medicine
Head
Section of Pulmonary and Critical Care Medicine
Bowman Gray School of Medicine
  of Wake Forest University
Medical Center Boulevard
Winston-Salem, North Carolina 27157-1054

Richard Beasley, M.B., Ch.B, M.D.,
  F.R.A.C.P.
Professor
Wellington Asthma Research Group
Department of Medicine
Wellington School of Medicine
Mein Street
Newtown, Wellington
New Zealand

Maria G. Belvisi, BSc., Ph.D.
Lecturer
Department of Thoracic Medicine
Imperial College School of Medicine at
The National Heart and Lung Institute
Dovehouse Street
London SW3 6LY
United Kingdom

I. Leonard Bernstein, M.D.
Clinical Professor
Department of Medicine
Division of Immunology
University of Cincinnati College of
  Medicine
231 Bethesda Avenue
Cincinnati, Ohio 45267-0563

Jonathan A. Bernstein, M.D.
Assistant Professor
Department of Internal Medicine
Division of Allergy/Immunology
University of Cincinnati College of
  Medicine
231 Bethesda Avenue
Cincinnati, Ohio 45267-0563

Judith L. Black, M.B.B.S., Ph.D., F.R.A.C.P.
Associate Professor
National Health and Medical Council Principal
  Research Fellow
Department of Pharmacology
University of Sydney
Sydney, New South Wales 2006
Australia

Eugene R. Bleecker, M.D.
Professor
Department of Medicine
University of Maryland School of Medicine
10 South Pine Street, Suite 800
Baltimore, Maryland 21201

Homer A. Boushey, M.D.
Professor of Medicine
Cardiovascular Research Institute
Asthma Clinical Research Center
University of California at San Francisco
505 Parnassus Avenue
San Francisco, California 94143

Jean J. Bousquet, M.D., Ph.D.
Professor of Medicine
Department of Respiratory Diseases
INSERM U454
Hôpital Arnaud de Villeneuve
371 Avenue Doyen Gaston Giraud
34295-Montpellier-Cedex 5
France

Robert H. Brown, M.D., M.P.H.
Assistant Professor
Departments of Anesthesiology and Critical
  Care Medicine
Division of Physiology, Environmental Health
  Sciences, and Radiology
The Johns Hopkins University
615 North Wolfe Street
Baltimore, Maryland 21205

Susan M. Brugman, M.D.
Associate Professor
Department of Pediatrics
University of Colorado Health Sciences
  Medical Center
Associate Staff Physician
National Jewish Medical and Research Center
1400 Jackson Street
Denver, Colorado 80206

Carl D. Burgess, M.D., M.R.C.P., F.R.A.C.P.
Associate Professor
Department of Clinical Pharmacology
Wellington Asthma Research Group
Department of Medicine
Wellington School of Medicine
Mein Street
Newtown, Wellington
New Zealand

Peter G. J. Burney, M.A., M.D., M.R.C.P., F.F.P.H.H.
Professor
Department of Public Health Medicine
United Medical and Dental School
St. Thomas's Hospital
Lambeth Palace Road
London SE1 7EH
United Kingdom

William W. Busse, M.D.
Professor
Department of Medicine
University of Wisconsin Medical School
600 Highland Avenue
Madison, Wisconsin 53792

Gaetano Caramori, M.D.
Institute of Respiratory Diseases
University of Ferrara
Nuove Cliniche, III Piano
Via Savonarola 9
44100 Ferrara
Italy

George H. Caughey, M.D.
Associate Professor
Department of Medicine
Cardiovascular Research Institute
University of California at San Francisco
90 Medical Center Way
San Francisco, California 94143-0911

Moira M. Chan-Yeung, M.B.B.S., F.R.C.P.C.
Professor
Department of Medicine
Respiratory Division
University of British Columbia
2775 Heather Street
Vancouver, British Columbia V5Z 3J5
Canada

Nicholas Chanarin, B.M., Ch.B., M.R.C.P.
Department of University Medicine
Southampton General Hospital
Tremona Road
Southampton SO16 6YD
United Kingdom

Martin D. Chapman, Ph.D.
Associate Professor
Departments of Medicine and Microbiology
Asthma and Allergic Diseases Center
University of Virginia
Charlottesville, Virginia 22908

Kian Fan Chung, M.D., F.R.C.P.
Reader
Department of Thoracic Medicine
Imperial College School of Medicine at
The National Heart and Lung Institute
Royal Brompton Hospital
Dovehouse Street
London SW3 6LY
United Kingdom

Donald W. Cockcroft, B.S., M.D., F.R.C.P.(C)
Professor
Department of Medicine
Division of Respiratory Medicine
Royal University Hospital
University of Saskatchewan
103 Hospital Drive
Saskatoon, Saskatchewan S7N 0W8
Canada

Matthew J. Colloff, B.Sc., Ph.D.
Senior Research Scientist
Division of Entomology
Commonwealth Scientific Industrial Research
Organization
Black Mountain Laboratories
Clunies Ross Street
Canberra, Australian Capital Territory 2601
Australia

Sandy Cook, Ph.D.
Education Specialist
Department of Medicine
Center for Research in Medical Education and
Health Care
The University of Chicago
5841 South Maryland Avenue
Chicago, Illinois 60637

Jonathan Corne, M.D.
Department of University Medicine
Southampton General Hospital
Tremona Road
Southampton SO16 6YD
United Kingdom

Chris J. Corrigan, M.A., M.Sc., Ph.D., M.R.C.P.
Clinical Senior Lecturer and Honorary
Consultant Physician
Department of Medicine
Charing Cross and Westminister Medical School
University of London
Fulham Palace Road
London W6 8RF
United Kingdom

Manuel G. Cosio, M.D.
Professor of Medicine
Respiratory Division
Royal Victoria Hospital
McGill University
687 Pine Avenue West
Montreal, Quebec H3A 1A1
Canada

**Richard W. Costello, M.B., B.Ch., B.A.O.,
M.R.C.P.I.**
Postdoctoral Fellow
Department of Medicine
Division of Pulmonary and Critical Care
Medicine
The Johns Hopkins University Hospital
615 North Wolfe Street
Baltimore, Maryland 21205

Julian Crane, M.B.B.S., M.R.C.P., F.R.A.C.P.
Associate Professor
Wellington Asthma Research Group
Department of Medicine
Wellington School of Medicine
Mein Street
Newtown, Wellington
New Zealand

Graham K. Crompton, M.B., Ch.B., F.R.C.P.E.
Consultant Physician and Senior Lecturer
Department of Medicine
University of Edinburgh
Teviot Place
Edinburgh EH8 9AG
Scotland

Adnan Custovic, M.D., M.Sc., D.Sc.
Honorary Lecturer
North West Lung Centre
South Manchester University Hospitals
Southmoor Road
Manchester M23 9LT
United Kingdom

Roland Dahl, M.D.
Department of Respiratory Diseases
University Hospital of Århus
DK-8000 Århus
Denmark

Pascal Demdy, M.D.
Department of Respiratory Diseases
INSERM U454
Hôpital Arnaud de Villeneuve
371 Avenue Doyen Gaston Giraud
34295-Montpellier-Cedex 5
France

Gordon Dent, Ph.D.
Research Associate
Center for Pulmonary Medicine and Thoracic
Surgery
Krankenhaus Großhansdorf
Wöhrendamm 80
D-22927 Großhansdorf
Germany

Myrna B. Dolovich, P. ENG.
Associate Clinical Professor
Department of Medicine
McMaster University
Health Sciences Center
1200 Main Street West
Hamilton, Ontario L8N 3Z5
Canada

Jeffrey M. Drazen, M.D.
Chief
Division of Pulmonary and Critical Care
Medicine
Department of Medicine
Brigham and Women's Hospital
Harvard Medical School
75 Francis Street
Boston, Massachusetts 02115

Roger Ellul-Micallef, M.D., Ph.D., F.R.C.P.
Professor and Head
Department of Clinical Pharmacology and
Therapeutics
The University of Malta
Msida MSD 06
Malta

David Evans, Ph.D.
Associate Professor of Public Helath
Department of Pediatrics
Columbia University College of Physicians and
Surgeons
630 West 168th Street
New York, New York 10032-3784

Leonardo Fabbri, M.D.
Associate Professor of Respiratory Medicine
Institute of Respiratory Diseases
University of Ferrara
Nuove Cliniche, III Piano
Via Savonarola 9
44100 Ferrara
Italy

Michelle V. Fannechi, M.D.
Department of Anatomy, Physiology, and Cell
Biology
School of Veterinary Medicine
University of California
Davis, California 95616

Christopher H. Fanta, M.D.
Associate Professor
Department of Medicine
Division of Pulmonary and Critical Care
Medicine
Brigham and Women's Hospital
Harvard Medical School
75 Francis Street
Boston, Massachusetts 02115

Jordan N. Fink, M.D.
Chief
Allergy-Immunology Division
Professor
Department of Medicine
Medical College of Wisconsin
9000 West Wisconsin Avenue
Milwaukee, Wisconsin 53226

Andrew R. Fischer, M.D.
Fellow
Division of Pulmonary and Critical Care
Medicine
Department of Medicine
Brigham and Women's Hospital
Harvard Medical School
75 Francis Street
Boston, Massachusetts 02115

James E. Fish, M.D.
Professor
Department of Medicine
Division of Pulmonary and Critical Care
Medicine
Jefferson Medical College
Thomas Jefferson University
1025 Walnut Street, Room 805
Philadelphia, Pennsylvania 19107

Anthony A. Floreani, M.D.
Assistant Professor
Pulmonary and Critical Care Medicine Section
Department of Internal Medicine
University of Nebraska Medical Center
600 South 42nd Street
Omaha, Nebraska 68198

Allison D. Fryer, Ph.D.
Associate Professor of Physiology
Department of Environmental Health
Science
Division of Physiology
The Johns Hopkins School of Hygiene and
Public Health
The Johns Hopkins University
615 North Wolfe Street
Baltimore, Maryland 21205

Jack Gauldie, Ph.D.
Professor and Chairman
Department of Pathology
McMaster University
1200 Main Street West
Hamilton, Ontario L8N 3Z5
Canada

Erwin W. Gelfand, M.D.
Chairman
Department of Pediatrics
National Jewish Medical and Research Center
1400 Jackson Street
Denver, Colorado 80206

Norma P. Gerard, Ph.D.
Associate Professor
Department of Medicine
Beth Israel Hospital
Harvard Medical School
330 Brookline Avenue
Boston, Massachusetts 02215

James E. Gern, M.D.
Assistant Professor
Department of Pediatrics
Madison Medical School
University of Wisconsin
600 Highland Avenue
Madison, Wisconsin 53792

Peter G. Gibson, M.D., F.R.A.C.P.
Staff Specialist and Clincial Senior
Lecturer
Department of Respiratory Medicine
John Hunter Hospital
Locked Bag 1
Newcastle, New South Wales 2310
Australia

Gerald J. Gleich, M.D.
Professor and Chairman
Department of Immunology
Mayo Clinic and Mayo Foundation
200 First Street Southwest
Rochester, Minnesota 55905

Simon Godfrey, M.D., Ph.D., F.R.C.P.
Professor
Institute of Pulmonology
Hadassah University Hospital
POB 12000
Kiryat Hadassah
Jerusalem 91120
Israel

Roy G. Goldie, B.Sc., Ph.D.
Professor
Department of Pharmacology
University of Western Australia
Nedlands, Western Australia 6907
Australia

Philippe Gosset, Ph.D.
INSERM U416
Institut Pasteur
1, Rue du Professeur Calmette
F-59019 Lille
France

Paul A. Greenberger, M.D.
Professor
Department of Medicine
Division of Allergy/Immunology
Northwestern University Medical School
303 East Chicago Avenue, Suite 207
Chicago, Illinois 60611-3008

Harald Groeben, M.D.
Assistant Professor
Department of Anesthesiology
The Johns Hopkins University
615 North Wolfe Street
Baltimore, Maryland 21205

Nicholas J. Gross, M.D., Ph.D., F.R.C.P.
Department of Medicine and Molecular
*   Biochemistry*
Loyola University
Stritch School of Medicine
Hines Veterans Affairs Hospital
Chicago, Illinois 60141

Michael M. Grunstein, M.D., Ph.D.
Professor and Chief
Division of Pulmonary Medicine
The Children's Hospital of Philadelphia
University of Pennsylvania School of
*   Medicine*
34th Street and Civic Center Boulevard
Philadelphia, Pennsylvania 19104

Hakon Hakonarson, M.D.
Assistant Professor
Department of Pediatrics
The Children's Hospital of Philadelphia
University of Pennsylvania School of Medicine
34th Street and Civic Center Boulevard
Philadelphia, Pennsylvania 19104

Andrew J. Halayko, Ph.D.
Department of Physiology
University of Manitoba
730 William Avenue
Winnepeg, Manitoba R3E 3J7
Canada

Frederick E. Hargreave, M.D.,
*   **F.R.C.P.C.***
Professor
Department of Medicine
McMaster University
St. Joseph's Hospital
50 Charlton Avenue East
Hamilton, Ontario L8N 4A6
Canada

Douglas W. P. Hay, Ph.D.
Associate Director and Head
Department of Pulmonary
*   Pharmacology*
SmithKline Beecham Pharmaceuticals
709 Swedeland Road
King of Prussia, Pennsylvania 19406

Richard G. Hegele, M.D., F.R.C.P.C.,
*   **Ph.D.***
Assistant Professor
Department of Pathology and Laboratory
*   Medicine*
Pulmonary Research Laboratory
University of British Columbia
St. Paul's Hospital
1081 Burrard Street
Vancouver, British Columbia V6Z 1Y6
Canada

Carol A. Hirshman, M.D.
Professor
Departments of Anesthesiology, Environmental
*   Health Sciences and Medicine*
The Johns Hopkins University
Staff Anesthesiologist
Johns Hopkins Hospital
615 North Wolfe Street
Baltimore, Maryland 21205

Mary Beth Hogan, M.D.
Assistant Professor
Department of Pediatrics
West Virginia University School of
*   Medicine*
Morgantown, West Virginia 26506-9214

James C. Hogg, M.D., Ph.D., F.R.C.P.C., F.R.S.C.
Director of Research
Department of Pathology
University of British Columbia
Professor of Research
St. Paul's Hospital
1081 Burrard Street
Vancouver, British Columbia V6Z 1Y6
Canada

Stephen T. Holgate, B.Sc., M.B.B.C., M.D., D.Sc., F.R.C.P.
MRC Clinical Professor of
* Immunopharmacology*
Department of University Medicine
Southampton General Hospital
Tremona Road
Southampton SO16 6YDB
United Kingdom

Patrick G. Holt, Ph.D., F.R.C.Path., D.Sc., M.D.
Professor of Microbiology
Department of Cell Biology
TVW Telethon Institute for Child Health Research
Roberts Road
Subiaco, Western Australia 6008
Australia

Philip W. Ind, M.A., F.R.C.P.
Senior Lecturer
Department of Respiratory Medicine
Royal Postgraduate Medical School
Hammersmith Hospital
Ducane Road
London W12 0HS
United Kingdom

Charles G. Irvin, Ph.D.
Professor
Departments of Medicine, Pediatrics, and
* Pulmonary Physiology*
National Jewish Medical and Research Center
1400 Jackson Street
Denver, Colorado 80206

Elliot Israel, M.D.
Assistant Professor
Department of Medicine
Division of Pulmonary and Critical Care
* Medicine*
Brigham and Women's Hospital
Harvard Medical School
75 Francis Street
Boston, Massachusetts 02115

Pascale Jeannin, Ph.D.
INSERM U416
Institut Pasteur
1, Rue du Professeur Calmette
F-59019 Lille
France

Christine R. Jenkins, M.D.
Institute of Respiratory Medicine
Page Chest Pavilion
Royal Prince Alfred Hospital
Sydney, New South Wales 2050
Australia

Guy F. Joos, M.D., Ph.D.
Professor of Medicine
Department of Respiratory
* Diseases*
University Hospital Ghent
De Pintelaan 185
B-9000 Ghent
Belgium

Rudolf A. Jörres, M.D.
Department of Medicine
Research Laboratory
Krankenhaus Großhansdorf
Zentrum für Pneumologie und
* Thoraxchirurgie*
Wöhrendamm 80
D-22927 Großhansdorf
Germany

Michel Joseph, Ph.D.
Directeur de Recherche au CNRS
Department of Immuno-Allergology
INSERM U416
Institut Pasteur
1, Rue du Professeur Calmette
59019 Lille
France

Elizabeth F. Juniper, M.C.S.P., M.Sc.
Associate Professor
Department of Clinical Epidemiology and
* Biostatistics*
McMaster University
Health Sciences Center
1200 Main Street West
Hamilton, Ontario L8N 3Z5
Canada

Alan K. Kamada, Pharm.D.
Adjoint Assistant Professor
Department of Pharmacy Practice
School of Pharmacy
University of Colorado Health Sciences
  Center
Assistant Professor
Department of Pediatrics
Clinical Pharmacology Division
National Jewish Medical and Research Center
1400 Jackson Street
Denver, Colorado 80206

David A. Kaminsky, M.D.
Assistant Professor
Department of Medicine
Division of Pulmonary Disease and Critical
  Care Medicine
University of Vermont College of Medicine
Fletcher Allen Health Care
Given C-317
Burlington, Vermont 05405

Masayuki Kaneko, M.S.
Basic Research Laboratories
Toray Industries, Inc.
1111 Tebiro
Kamakura, Kanagawa 248
Japan

A. Barry Kay, D.Sc., Ph.D., F.R.C.P.,
  F.R.S.E.
Professor and Honorary Consultant
  Physician
Department of Allergy and Clinical
  Immunology
Imperial College School of Medicine at
The National Heart and Lung Institute
Dovehouse Street
London SW3 6LY
United Kingdom

Jason Kelley, M.D.
Professor
Department of Medicine
University of Vermont College of Medicine
Given C-305
Burlington, Vermont 05405

Gregory G. King, M.B. Ch.B., F.R.A.C.P.
Institute of Respiratory Medicine
Page Chest Pavilion
Royal Prince Alfred Hospital
Sydney, New South Wales 2050
Australia

Johan C. Kips, M.D., Ph.D.
Associate Professor of Medicine
Department of Respiratory Diseases
University Hospital Ghent
De Pintelann 185
B-9000 Ghent
Belgium

Hirohito Kita, M.D.
Assistant Professor
Department of Immunology
Mayo Clinic and Mayo Foundation
200 First Street Southwest
Rochester, Minnesota 55905

Jane Q. Koenig, Ph.D.
Professor
Department of Environmental Health
University of Washington
Seattle, Washington 98195-7234

Onn Min Kon, M.D.
Research Fellow
Department of Allergy and Clinical
  Immunology
Imperial College of Science, Technology, and
  Medicine at
The National Heart and Lung Institute
Dovehouse Street
London SW3 6LY
United Kingdom

Michael I. Kotlikoff, V.M.D., Ph.D.
Professor and Chairman
Department of Animal Biology
School of Veterinary Medicine
University of Pennsylvania
3800 Spruce Street
Philadelphia, Pennsylvania 19104-6046

Monica Kraft, M.D.
Assistant Professor
Department of Medicine
University of Colorado Health Sciences Center
Pulmonary Division
National Jewish Medical and Research Center
1400 Jackson Street
Denver, Colorado 80206

Viswanath P. Kurup, Ph.D.
Professor
Department of Medicine
Allergy-Immunology Center
Medical College of Wisconsin
Veterans Administration Medical Center
5000 West National Avenue
Milwaukee, Wisconsin 53295

Annika Laitinen, M.D., Ph.D.
Assistant Professor
Institute of Biomedicine
Department of Anatomy
University of Helsinki
P.O. Box 9
Siltavuorenpenger 20 A
FIN-00014 Helsinki
Finland

Lauri A. Laitinen, M.D., Ph.D.
Professor of Pulmonary Medicine
Department of Medicine
University Central Hospital
Haartmanninkatu 4
SF-00290 Helsinki
Finland

Gary L. Larsen, M.D.
Professor and Head
Section of Pediatric Pulmonary Medicine
University of Colorado School of Medicine
Senior Faculty Member
Department of Pediatrics
National Jewish Medical and Research Center
1400 Jackson Street
Denver, Colorado 80206

Philippe Lassalle, M.D.
INSERM U416
Institut Pasteur
1, Rue du Professeur Calmette
F-59019 Lille
France

Alan R. Leff, M.D.
Professor and Head
Department of Medicine
Section of Pulmonary and Critical Care Medicine
The University of Chicago
5841 South Maryland Avenue
Chicago, Illinois 60637

Robert F. Lemanske, Jr., M.D.
Professor
Department of Pediatrics and Medicine
University of Wisconsin Hospitals
600 Highland Avenue
Madison, Wisconsin 53792

Richard J. Lemen, M.D.
Professor
Department of Pediatrics
University of Arizona
1501 North Campbell Avenue
Tucson, Arizona 85724-5073

Peter N. Le Souëf, M.D., M.R.C.P., F.R.A.C.P.
Associate Professor
University Department of Pediatrics
University of Western Australia
Head
Department of Respiratory Medicine
Princess Margaret Hospitals for Children
Perth, Western Australia 6001
Australia

Donald Y.M. Leung, M.D., Ph.D.
Professor and Head
Department of Pediatric Allergy/Immunology
National Jewish Medical and Research Center
1400 Jackson Street
Denver, Colorado 80206

Stewart J. Levine, M.D.
Department of Critical Care Medicine
Clinical Center
National Institutes of Health
Building 10, Room 7-D-43
Bethesda, Maryland 20892

Lawrence M. Lichtenstein M.D., Ph.D.
Professor
Department of Medicine
Division of Clinical Immunology
The Johns Hopkins University School of
  Medicine
The Johns Hopkins Asthma and Allergy Center
5501 Hopkins Bayview Circle
Baltimore, Maryland 21224

Stephen B. Liggett, M.D.
Professor of Medicine, Molecular Genetics and
  Pharmacology
Department of Internal Medicine
University of Cincinnati College of Medicine
231 Bethesda Avenue
Cincinnati, Ohio 45267-0564

Kaiser G. Lim, M.D.
Department of Medicine
Beth Israel Deaconess Medical Center
Harvard Medical School
Boston, Massachusetts 02215

Mark C. Liu, M.D.
Associate Professor
Department of Medicine
The Johns Hopkins University School of
  Medicine
The Johns Hopkins Asthma and Allergy Center
5501 Hopkins Bayview Circle
Baltimore, Maryland 21224

Claes-Göran A. Löfdahl, M.D., Ph.D.
Professor
Department of Respiratory Medicine
Lund University Hospital
S-221 85 Lund
Sweden

Mara S. Ludwig, M.D.
Associate Professor
Department of Medicine
Royal Victoria Hospital
McGill University
3626 St. Urbain Street
Montreal, Quebec H2X 2P2
Canada

Piero Maestrelli, M.D.
Assistant Professor and Senior Lecturer
Institute of Occupational Diseases
University of Padua
Via Facciolati 71
35127 Padua
Italy

Helgo Magnussen, M.D.
Professor
Department of Medicine
Research Laboratory
Krankenhaus Großhansdorf
Zentrum für Pneumologie und Thoraxchirurgie
Wöhrendamm 80
D-22927 Großhansdorf
Germany

Jean-Luc Malo, M.D.
Professor
Department of Chest Medicine
Sacré-Couer Hospital
University of Montreal
5400 Gouin Boulevard West
Montreal, Quebec H4J 1C5
Canada

Diana L. Marquardt, M.D.
Associate Professor
Department of Medicine
University of California at San Diego
9500 Gilman Drive
La Jolla, California 92093-0635

James G. Martin, M.D.
Professor
Department of Medicine
Meakins-Christie Laboratories
McGill University
3626 St. Urbain Street
Montreal, Quebec H2X 2P2
Canada

Richard J. Martin, M.D.
Professor
Department of Medicine
University of Colorado; and
Head
Pulmonary Division
National Jewish Medical and Research
*   Center*
1400 Jackson Street
Denver, Colorado 80206

Fernando D. Martinez, M.D.
Professor of Pediatrics
Respiratory Sciences Center
College of Medicine
University of Arizona
1501 North Campbell Avenue
Tucson, Arizona 85724-5030

Helen Mawhinney, M.D., F.R.C.P.
Assistant Clinical Professor
Department of Medicine
University of California at
*   Los Angeles*
Allergy Research Foundation
11620 Wilshire Boulevard, Suite 201
Los Angeles, California 90025

E. Regis McFadden, Jr., M.D.
Arglye J. Beams Professor
Department of Medicine; and
Director
Division of Pulmonary and Critical Care
*   Medicine*
University Hospitals of Cleveland
11100 Euclid Avenue
Cleveland, Ohio 44106-5067

Wylie L. McNabb, Ed.D.
Associate Professor of Clinical Medicine
Department of Medicine
Center for Research in Medical Education
*   and Health Care*
The University of Chicago
5841 South Maryland Avenue
Chicago, Illinois 60637

Hemalini Mehta, M.D.
Fellow
Department of Allergy/Immunology
University of Wisconsin Hospitals and
*   Clinics*
600 Highland Avenue
Madison, Wisconsin 53792

Robert B. Mellins, M.D.
Professor
Department of Pediatrics
Columbia University College of Physicians and
*   Surgeons*
630 West 168th Street
New York, New York 10032-3784

François-B. Michel, M.D.
Professor of Pulmonary Medicine
Department of Respiratory Diseases
INSERM U454
Hôpital Arnaud de Villeneuve
371 Avenue Doyen Gaston Giraud
34295 Montpellier Cedex 5
France

Richard W. Mitchell, Ph.D.
Research Associate and Associate Professor
Pulmonary and Critical Care Medicine Section
Division of the Biological Sciences
The University of Chicago
5841 South Maryland Avenue
Chicago, Illinois 60637

Wayne A. Mitzner, Ph.D.
Professor and Director
Department of Environmental Health
*   Sciences*
Division of Physiology
The Johns Hopkins University
School of Hygiene and Public Health
615 North Wolfe Street
Baltimore, Maryland 21205

David A. Mrazek, M.D., F.R.C.Psych.
Chairman
Department of Psychiatry and Behavioral
*   Sciences*
Children's National Medical Center
111 Michigan Avenue Northwest
Washington, District of Columbia 20010-2970

Richard K. Murray, M.D.
Senior Medical Director
Merck and Company, Inc.
P.O. Box 4, WP53B-3PA
Sumneytown Pike and Broad Street
West Point, Pennsylvania 19486
Clinical Assistant Professor
Department of Medicine
The University of Pennsylvania
34th Street and Civic Center Boulevard
Philadelphia, Pennsylvania 19104

Niels Mygind, M.D.
Associate Professor
Department of Respiratory Diseases
University Hospital of Århus
DK-8000 Århus
Denmark

Jay A. Nadel, M.D.
Professor
Departments of Medicine and Physiology
Cardiovascular Research Institute
University of California at San Francisco
3rd and Parnassus Avenue
San Francisco, California 94143-0130

Harold S. Nelson, M.D.
Senior Staff Physician
Department of Medicine
National Jewish Medical and Research Center
1400 Jackson Street
Denver, Colorado 80206

Stephen P. Newman, Ph.D., F.Inst.P.
Chief Scientist
Pharmaceutical Profiles Ltd.
2 Faraday Building
Highfields Science Park
Nottingham NG7 2QP
United Kingdom

Carole Ober, Ph.D.
Associate Professor
Department of Obstetrics and
*   Gynecology*
The University of Chicago
5841 South Maryland Avenue
Chicago, Illinois 60637-1470

Paul M. O'Byrne, M.B., F.R.C.P.
Professor
Department of Medicine
Health Sciences Center
McMaster University
1200 Main Street West
Hamilton, Ontario L8N 3Z5
Canada

Mitsushi Okazawa, M.D., Ph.D.
Assistant Professor
Departments of Pathology and Laboratory
*   Medicine*
University of British Columbia
St. Paul's Hospital
1081 Burrard Street
Vancouver, British Columbia V6Z 1Y6
Canada

Clive P. Page, B.Sc., Ph.D.
Professor of Pharmacology
Sackler Institute of Pulmonary Pharmacology
King's College
University of London
Manresa Road
London SW3 6LX
United Kingdom

Reynold A. Panettieri, Jr., M.D.
Associate Professor
Department of Medicine
Pulmonary and Critical Care Division
University of Pennsylvania Medical Center
3400 Spruce Street
Philadelphia, Pennsylvania 19104-4283

Peter D. Paré, M.D.C.M., F.R.C.P.
Professor
Department of Medicine
University of British Columbia
St. Paul's Hospital
1081 Burrard Street
Vancouver, British Columbia V6Z 1Y6
Canada

Romain A. Pauwels, M.D., Ph.D.
Professor
Department of Respiratory Diseases
University Hospital Ghent
De Pintelaan 185
B-9000 Ghent
Belgium

Neil E. Pearce, B.Sc., Dip.Sci., Dip.CRS., Ph.D.
Associate Professor
Wellington Asthma Research Group
Department of Medicine
Wellington School of Medicine
Mein Street
Newtown, Wellington
New Zealand

Jennifer K. Peat, Ph.D.
Senior Lecturer
Department of Medicine
University of Sydney
Sydney, New South Wales 2006
Australia

Søren Pedersen, M.D.
Department of Pediatrics
Kolding Hospital
Skovvangen 2-8
DK-6000 Kolding
Denmark

Carl G. A. Persson, Ph.D.
Professor
Department of Clinical Pharmacology
University Hospital of Lund
Lund S-221 85
Sweden

Stephen P. Peters, M.D., Ph.D.
Professor
Department of Medicine
Associate Director
Division of Pulmonary and Critical Care Medicine
Jefferson Medical College
Thomas Jefferson University
805 College Building
1025 Walnut Street
Philadelphia, Pennsylvania 19107

Marco Piatella, M.D.
Resident
Institute of Respiratory Diseases
University of Ferrara
Nuove Cliniche, III Piano
Via Savonarola 9
44100 Ferrara
Italy

Joseph M. Pilewski, M.D.
Assistant Professor
Department of Medicine
University of Pittsburgh Medical Center
3550 Terrace Street
Pittsburgh, Pennsylvania 15261

Emilio Pizzichini, M.D.
Professor
Department of Internal Medicine
Universidade Federal de Santa Catarina
Campus Universitario, Trinidade
Florianopolis, Santa Caterina 88.010-970
Brazil

Marcia M. M. Pizzichini, M.D.
Professor
Department of Internal Medicine
Universidade Federal de Santa Catarina
Campus Universitario, Trinidade
Florianopolis, Santa Caterina 88.010-970
Brazil

Thomas A. E. Platts-Mills, M.D., Ph.D.
Professor of Medicine and Microbiology
Department of Internal Medicine
Asthma Center
University of Virginia
MR-4 Building
Charlottesville, Virginia 22908

Charles G. Plopper, Ph.D.
Professor of Cell Biology
Department of Anatomy, Physiology and Cell
*   Biology*
School of Veterinary Medicine
University of California
Davis, California 95616

Albert J. Polito, M.D.
Fellow in Pulmonary and Critical Care
*   Medicine*
Department of Medicine
The Johns Hopkins University School of
*   Medicine*
720 Rutland Avenue
Baltimore, Maryland 21205

Dirkje S. Postma, M.D.
Department of Pulmonology
University Hospital Groningen
Oostersingel 59
9713 EZ Groningen
The Netherlands

David Proud, Ph.D.
Professor
Department of Medicine
Johns Hopkins University School of
*   Medicine*
Johns Hopkins Asthma and Allergy Center
5501 Hopkins Bayview Circle
Baltimore, Maryland 21224

Klaus F. Rabe, M.D.
Associate Professor
Center for Pulmonary Medicine and Thoracic
*   Surgery*
Krankenhaus Großhansdorf
Wöhrendamm 80
D-22927 Großhansdorf
Germany

Stephen I. Rennard, M.D.
Professor of Medicine
Pulmonary and Critical Care Medicine
*   Section*
Department of Internal Medicine
University of Nebraska Medical Center
600 South 42nd Street
Omaha, Nebraska 68198

Margerita M. Riccio
Research Fellow
Sandoz Research Institute
London SW3 6LY
United Kingdom

Richard A. Robbins, M.D.
Professor and Vice Chairman
Department of Medicine and Physiology
Louisiana State University Medical Center
Associate Chief for Research and
*   Development*
Overton Brooks Veterans Affairs Medical
*   Center*
510 East Stoner Avenue
Shreveport, Louisiana 71101

Clive R. Roberts, B.A., M.A., Ph.D.
Assistant Professor
Department of Medicine
University of British Columbia
St. Paul's Hospital
1081 Burrard Street
Vancouver, British Columbia V6Z 1Y6
Canada

William R. Roche, M.Sc., M.D.,
**   M.R.C.Path., F.F.Path.R.C.P.I.**
Senior Lecturer and Consultant
Department of University Pathology
Southampton General Hospital
Tremona Road
Southampton SO16 6YD
United Kingdom

Marina Saetta, M.D.
Assistant Professor of Medicine
Institute of Occupational Medicine
University of Padua
Via Facciolati 71
Padua 35127
Italy

Cheryl M. Salome, B.Sc.
Research Fellow
Department of Medicine
University of Sydney
Sydney, New South Wales 2006
Australia

Nicholas Saltos, M.B.B.S., F.R.A.C.P.,
**   F.R.C.P., F.R.C.P.I., F.C.C.P.**
Senior Staff Specialist and Senior Clinical
*   Lecturer*
Department of Respiratory Medicine
John Hunter Hospital
New Castle University
New Lambton
Newcastle, New South Wales 2305
Australia

Bengt O. Sarnstrand, Ph.D.
Associate Professor
Department of Pharmacology
Astra Draco AB
S-221 00 Lund
Sweden

Michael Schatz, M.D.
Clinical Professor
Department of Medicine
University of California at San Diego
*   School of Medicine*
Department of Allergy
Kaiser-Permanente Medical Center
7060 Clairemont Mesa Boulevard
San Diego, California 92111

Robert P. Schleimer, Ph.D.
Professor
Department of Medicine
Division of Clinical Immunology
The Johns Hopkins University School of
*   Medicine*
5501 Hopkins Bayview Circle
Baltimore, Maryland 21224

Craig M. Schramm, M.D.
Assistant Professor of Pediatrics
Pediatric Pulmonary Division
University of Connecticut Health Center
Connecticut Children's Medical Center
282 Washington Street
Hartford, Connecticut 06106

John T. Schroeder, Ph.D.
Professor
Department of Medicine
Division of Clinical Immunology
The Johns Hopkins University School of
*   Medicine*
The Johns Hopkins Asthma and Allergy Center
5501 Hopkins Bayview Circle
Baltimore, Maryland 21224

Lawrence B. Schwartz, M.D., Ph.D.
Charles and Evelyn Thomas Professor of
*   Medicine*
Department of Internal Medicine
Virginia Commonwealth University
Richmond, Virginia 23233

Lisa M. Schwiebert, Ph.D.
Instructor
Department of Medicine
Division of Clinical Immunology
The Johns Hopkins University
The Johns Hopkins Asthma and Allergy Center
5501 Hopkins Bayview Circle
Baltimore, Maryland 21224

Malcolm R. Sears, M.B., Ch.B., F.R.A.C.P.,
**   F.R.C.P.(C)**
Professor
Department of Medicine
Firestone Regional Chest and Allergy Unit
St. Joseph's Hospital
McMaster University
25 Charlton Avenue East
Hamilton, Ontario L8N 4A6
Canada

James H. Shelhamer, M.D.
Deputy Chief
Department of Critical Care Medicine
Clinical Center
National Institutes of Health
Building 10, Room 7-D-43
Bethesda, Maryland 20892

Yuji Shimizu, M.D., Ph.D.
Research Advisor
First Department of Internal Medicine
Gunma University School of Medicine
3-39-15 Showa-Machi
Maebashi, Gunma 371
Japan

Michael Silverman, M.D., F.R.C.P.
Professor
Department of Child Health
Clinical Sciences Building
Leicester Royal Infirmary
Leicester, LE2 7LX
United Kingdom

Patricia J. Sime, M.B., Ch.B., M.R.C.P.
Parker B. Francis Pulmonary Research Fellow
Department of Pathology
McMaster University
1200 Main Street West
Hamilton, Ontario L8N 3Z5
Canada

James R. Snapper, M.D.
Professor
Department of Medicine
Center for Lung Research
Vanderbilt University School of Medicine
1161 21st Avenue South
Nashville, Tennessee 37232-2650

Julian Solway, M.D.
Professor of Medicine and Pediatrics
Department of Medicine
Section of Pulmonary and Critical Care Medicine
The University of Chicago
5841 South Maryland Avenue
Chicago, Illinois 60637

Joseph D. Spahn, M.D.
Assistant Professor
Department of Pedatric Allergy/Immunology
University of Colorado School of Medicine
Staff Physician
National Jewish Medical and Research Center
1400 Jackson Street
Denver, Colorado 80206

Sheldon L. Spector, M.D
Clinical Professor
Department of Medicine
University of California at Los Angeles
Director
Allergy Research Foundation
11620 Wilshire Boulevard, Suite 201
Los Angeles, California 90025

Cristiana Stellato, M.D., Ph.D.
Visiting Professor
Department of Medicine
Division of Clinical Immunology
The Johns Hopkins University
The Johns Hopkins Asthma and Allergy Center
5501 Hopkins Bayview Circle
Baltimore, Maryland 21224

Newman L. Stephens, M.D., F.R.C.P.
Professor
Department of Physiology
University of Manitoba
730 William Avenue
Winnepeg, Manitoba R3E 3J7
Canada

Peter J. Sterk, M.D., Ph.D.
Professor of Medicine
Department of Pulmonary Diseases
Leiden University Medical Center
Albinusdreef 2
P.O. Box 9600
NL-2300 RC Leiden
The Netherlands

Donald D. Stevenson, M.D.
Chairman Emeritus
Department of Medicine
Scripps Clinic and Research Foundation
10666 North Torrey Pines Road
La Jolla, California 92037

Geoffrey A. Stewart, B.Sc., Ph.D.
Senior Lecturer
Department of Microbiology
University of Western Australia
Nedlands
Perth, Western Australia 6907
Australia

Judith A. St. George, Ph.D.
Associate Scientific Director
Genzyme Corporation
1 Mountain Road
Framingham, Massachusetts 01701-9322

Mary E. Strek, M.D.
Assistant Professor
Department of Medicine
Section of Pulmonary and Critical Care
* Medicine*
The University of Chicago
5841 South Maryland
Chicago, Illinois 60637

Sean D. Sullivan, Ph.D.
Assistant Professor
Department of Pharmacy and Health
* Services*
University of Washington
School of Pharmacy
H-375 Health Sciences Center
Box 375630
Seattle, Washington 98195

Stanley J. Szefler, M.D.
Professor
Departments of Pediatrics and Pharmacology
University of Colorado Health Sciences Center
Helen Wohlberg and Herman Lambert Chair in
* Pharmacokinetics*
Director
Department of Clinical Pharmacology
National Jewish Medical and Research Center
1400 Jackson Street
Denver, Colorado 80206

Shahriyar Tavakoli, M.D.
Department of Critical Care Medicine
Clinical Center
National Institutes of Health
Building 10, Room 7-D-43
Bethesda, Maryland 20892

Martin J. Tobin, M.D.
Professor
Department of Medicine
Division of Pulmonary and Critical Care
* Medicine*
Loyola University
Stritch School of Medicine
Department of Veterans Affairs
Edward Hines, Jr. Hospital
Hines, Illinois 60141-5000

Galen B. Toews, M.D.
Professor
Department of Internal Medicine
University of Michigan Medical Center
1500 East Medical Center Drive
Ann Arbor, Michigan 48109-0360

André-Bernard Tonnel, M.D.
Professor
Department of Respiratory Medicine
Calmette Hospital
INSERM U416
Institut Pasteur
1, Rue du Professeur Calmette
F-59019 Lille
France

John H. Toogood, M.D., F.R.C.P.C.
Professor
Department of Medicine
Division of Clinical Immunology and Allergy
London Health Sciences Center
800 Commissioners Road, East
London, Ontario N6A 4G5
Canada

Theodore J. Torphy, Ph.D.
Group Director
Departments of Immunopharmacology and
*   Pulmonary Pharmacology*
SmithKline Beecham Pharmaceuticals
709 Swedeland Road
King of Prussia, Pennsylvania 19406

Euan R. Tovey, Ph.D.
Research Fellow
Department of Medicine
University of Sydney
Institute of Respiratory Medicine
Royal Prince Alfred Hospital
Sydney, New South Wales 2050
Australia

Guy M. Tremblay, Ph.D.
Research Associate
Centre de Recherche
Université Laval
Laval Hospital
2725 Chemin Sainte-Foy
Sainte-Foy, Quebec G1V 4G5
Canada

Debra J. Turner, B.Sc.(Hons), Ph.D.
Department of Physiology
University of Western Australia
Nedlands, Western Australia 6907
Australia

Bradley J. Undem, Ph.D.
Associate Professor
Department of Medicine
The Johns Hopkins University
5501 Hopkins Bayview Circle
Baltimore, Maryland 21224

Donata A. Vercelli, M.D.
Chief
Molecular Immunoregulation Unit
San Raffaele Scientific Institute
Via Olgettina 60
20132 Milano
Italy

Ismo T. Virtanen, M.D.
Professor
Institute of Biomedicine
Department of Anatomy
University of Helsinki
P.O. Box 9
Siltavuorenpenger 20 A
FIN-00014 Helsinki
Finland

Elizabeth M. Wagner, Ph.D.
Associate Professor of Medicine
Division of Pulmonary and Critical Care
*   Medicine*
The Johns Hopkins University
5501 Hopkins Bayview Circle
Baltimore, Maryland 21224

Peter D. Wagner, M.D.
Professor
Departments of Medicine and Bioengineering
University of California at San Diego
9500 Gilman Drive
La Jolla, California 92093-0623

Christoph Walker, Ph.D.
Department of Respiratory Diseases
Novartis Pharma Inc.
CH-4002 Basel
Switzerland

Jizhong Wang, Ph.D.
Clinical Systems Analyst
Department of Information Services
St. Boniface General Hospital
730 Tache Avenue
Winnipeg, Manitoba R3E 3J7
Canada

Adam Wanner, M.D.
Joseph Weintraub Professor of Medicine
Chief
Division of Pulmonary and Critical Care
Medicine
University of Miami School of Medicine
1600 Northwest 10th Avenue
Miami, Florida 33101

Peter A. Ward, M.D.
Godfrey D. Stobbe Professor and
Chairman
Department of Pathology
The University of Michigan
1301 Catherine Road
Ann Arbor, Michigan 48109-0602

Edward L. Warren, M.D.
Assistant Professor
Department of Medicine
Division of Pulmonary and Critical Care
Medicine
University Hospitals of Cleveland
11100 Euclid Avenue
Cleveland, Ohio 44106-5067

Paula L. Watson, M.D.
Lung Associates
1895 Floyd Street
Sarasota, Florida 34239

Kevin B. Weiss, M.D., M.P.H.
Associate Professor
Department of Medicine
Director
Center for Health Services Research
Rush Primary Care Institute
Rush Presbyterian-St. Luke's Medical
Center
1653 West Congress Parkway
Chicago, Illinois 60612

Scott T. Weiss, M.D., M.S.
Associate Professor
Department of Medicine
Harvard Medical School
Director
Division of Respiratory and Environmental
Epidemiology
Channing Laboratory
Brigham and Women's Hospital
180 Longwood Avenue
Boston, Massachusetts 02115

Peter F. Weller, M.D.
Professor
Department of Medicine
Beth Israel Hospital
Harvard Medical School
330 Brookline Avenue
Boston, Massachusetts 02215

Lisa M. Wheatley, M.D.
Assistant Professor
Department of Internal Medicine
Division of Allergy and Clinical Immunology
University of Virginia Health Sciences Center
Charlottesville, Virginia 22908

Steven R. White, M.D.
Associate Professor
Department of Medicine
Section of Pulmonary and Critical Care Medicine
Division of Biological Sciences
The University of Chicago
5841 South Maryland Avenue
Chicago, Illinois 60637

Barry Wiggs, Ph.D.
Department of Medicine
University of British Columbia
St. Paul's Hospital
1081 Burrard Street
Vancouver, British Columbia V6Z 1Y6
Canada

Jan-Åke V. Wihl, M.D., Ph.D.
Associate Professor
Department of Otorhinolaryngology
Malmö General Hospital
S-20502 Malmö
Sweden

Ann J. Woolcock, M.D., F.R.A.C.P.
Professor of Respiratory Medicine
University of Sydney
Institute of Respiratory Medicine
Royal Prince Alfred Hospital
Sydney, New South Wales 2050
Australia

Reen Wu, Ph.D.
Professor
Division of Pulmonary and Critical Care
Medicine
School of Medicine and School of Veterinary
Medicine
California Regional Primate Research Center
University of California
Davis, California 95616

Zhou Xing, M.D., Ph.D.
Assistant Professor
Department of Pathology
McMaster University
1200 Main Street West
Hamilton, Ontario L8N 3Z5
Canada

Nan-Shan Zhong, M.D.
Professor
Department of Medicine
Guangzhou Medical College
Guangzhou Institute of Respiratory
* Disease*
151 Yan Jiang Road
Guangzhou City, Guangdong Province 510120
People's Republic of China

Irwin Ziment, M.D.
Professor and Medical Director
Department of Medicine
Olive View / University of California at
* Los Angeles Medical Center*
14445 Olive View Drive
Sylmar, California 91342-1495

Jonathan B. Zuckerman, M.D.
Instructor
Department of Medicine
Division of Pulmonary and Critical Care
* Medicine*
Hospital of the University of
* Pennsylvania*
3600 Spruce Street
Philadelphia, Pennsylvania 19104-4283

Foreword

Asthma, as a combination of signs and symptoms, has been recognized since antiquity. Over the centuries, many disease entities and syndromes were included under this rubric, but were later eliminated as the definition became more precise due to improved understanding of the pathobiology of asthma. In the latter half of the twentieth century, hyperresponsiveness to nonspecific stimuli, reversibility of obstruction, either spontaneously or in response to therapy, and evidence of inflammation of the airways have been incorporated into the definition to provide more precision. Despite such progress, major questions remain: is it a disease of a single cause amenable to a unique solution adhering to the principles of parsimony, or does it remain a syndrome with many possible etiologies, pathobiological sequences, diverse morphologies, and even heterogeneous clinical and epidemiological manifestations? The latter is closest to the truth, as demonstrated in this volume.

What, then, is this condition called asthma? Is it a disorder of the immune system involving lymphocytes and immunoglobulin E? Is it is disorder of smooth muscle involving hypertrophy, hyperplasia, and alteration in the biochemistry and biophysics of this tissue? Is it a dysfunction of the airway epithelium characterized by failure to provide an effective barrier and by the underproduction of dilator substances? Is it an inflammatory process involving cells of both the granulocytic and monocytic series and their mediators/cytokines? Is it caused by secretory cells that produce increased quantities of mucus and the associated failure to eliminate such secretions? Is it a condition of neural tissues and their production of a series of neuropeptides that amplify inflammation and cause smooth muscle constriction? Is it caused by an infectious agent as the instigating factor? Is it an entity that is caused (or precipitated by) environmental exposures (macro or micro)? Is it a genetic aberration even beyond that of atopy? The answers to these questions will be yes, to some degree and in some circumstances.

Asthma affects approximately 6% of the population, causes major morbidity with days lost from work or school, and causes heavy use of health care resources. It is the most common chronic affliction of childhood and the leading cause of hospitalization in the pediatric age group. Thus, asthma surely deserves the increased attention it has received in recent years. This volume presents the rich harvest of information, discoveries, insights, and new questions that have been reaped from intensified research efforts.

The increasing incidence, prevalence, and mortality from asthma in many parts of the world are perplexing to the many who have contributed so meaningfully to the improved and expanded understanding of the epidemiology and pathobiology of this common clinical syndrome and to its increasingly precise and targeted therapies. This lack of conquest only emphasizes the challenges that still face all of us who, at the bench, in the clinic, or in the field, wish to understand, treat, and ameliorate asthma—thereby suduing a worthy foe. A worthy foe it is indeed. As Piet Hein stated in one of his *Grooks*:

> A problem worthy of attack
> Shows its worth by hitting back (1).

Certainly the reductionists have been frequent victims of such "hitting back," since many single hypotheses have been largely unsupportable (i.e., the null hypothesis could not be rejected). In a sense, perhaps we are still trying to drop a procrustean mold on a protean syndrome with common manifestations, but with many underlying mechanisms and provocative stimuli working in various combinations leading to what we recognize as asthma. The many factors—environmental, immunological, morphological, physiological, neural, cellular, and molecular—that must still be identified, categorized, and evaluated daunt us all, but stimulate us to continue seeking a cogent synthesis of many plausible possibilities into an understanding of the entity, or entities, to which this volume is so able and stimulatingly devoted.

The editors and contributors to this book comprise the unquestioned leaders in current scientific investigation related to asthma and provide impressive breadth and depth of discovery and inquiry that set forth the challenges for at least the next decade. Synthesizing and winnowing the many ideas and insights into a cogent picture of what we call asthma are the challenges set forth.

Frustration will beset those who would demand a certain and lucid synthesis. The rewards will come to those who see, accept, and deal with the many challenges and apparent contradictions provided herein. Those perspicacious readers will inherit current and past wisdom, and will likely contribute to the discoveries of the future.

Roland H. Ingram, Jr., M.D.
Martha West Looney Professor of Medicine
Chief, Department of Pulmonary and Critical Care Medicine
The Emory University School of Medicine
Atlanta, Georgia

REFERENCE

1. Hein, P. *Grooks* 1. Garden City, New Jersey: Doubleday and Company, 1969;2.

Preface

Asthma is the most common chronic disease in industrialized nations, and there is every indication that its prevalence is increasing throughout the world. This disease accounts for a large proportion of health care spending and loss of time from school and work. Because of the financial repercussions, asthma is increasingly attracting the attention of a wide spectrum of health care professionals and government officials.

Over the last decade, we have seen major advances in understanding the mechanisms of asthma and great improvements in its management. However, there remain many important unanswered questions about this complex and medically-challenging disease. Why is asthma more prevalent throughout the world? How and why does this disease become persistent in adults? Do different types of asthma exist and what are their causes? These fundamental questions highlight the need for further research at all investigative levels.

In recent years, the number of studies published on asthma and related diseases has increased exponentially, so that it is almost impossible to keep up to date with the rapid progress in the field. These developments are the basis for *Asthma*, which attempts to address comprehensively and integrate current information related to the pathobiology and clinical aspects of asthma. This book was conceived to provide its broad-based readership of health professionals and scientists with a comprehensive overview of the entire field of asthma, as envisioned from the unique perspectives of international authorities in the field. To achieve this overall objective, the book was written by scientists and clinicians who are widely recognized for their important contributions to the science and medicine of asthma, and who are actively engaged in basic or applied research on these topics. The chapters range from the basic science of the pro-inflammatory processes implicated in the pathobiology of asthma to the practical issues pertaining to current day-to-day management of the disease in both adults and children. Accordingly, *Asthma* is divided into a number of relevant thematic basic science and applied/clinical sections. Within each section, each chapter contributes to the overall theme of the section. Collectively, the chapters are aimed at providing a comprehensive current overview of the subject matter, and are extensively referenced.

Since the fields of research in various aspects of the biology of asthma are rapidly developing, it is expected that certain differences of opinion may exist between authors, and that opposing views may be held by equally accomplished investigators. We have taken the position that such differences in opinion among experts in the field are inherent to any rapidly changing field. Therefore, we intentionally allowed for any potential differences of opinion to provide the reader with a more comprehensive overview of the subject matter, and allow the reader to develop his own judgment on the perspectives for any given controversial issue. By encompassing every contemporary aspect of this complex disease, it is anticipated that this textbook will prove to be a major resource for all clinicians involved in asthma care, for academics involved in teaching about the disease, and for investigators pursuing research in the field of airway biology and asthma.

Peter J. Barnes, D.M., D.Sc., F.R.C.P.
Michael M. Grunstein, M.D., Ph.D.
Alan R. Leff, M.D.
Ann J. Woolcock, M.D., F.R.A.C.P.

Acknowledgments

We would like to thank all of our authors for adhering to the tight deadlines. We would also like to thank Lippincott–Raven Publishers for all of their support and encouragement during the preparation of *Asthma*. Special thanks is due to our assistants, Carolyn Green, Nancy Trojan, Margaret Brown, and Victoria Keena-Richter, who provided invaluable help in author contact and editing assistance.

▪ 1 ▪

Introduction

Asthma, edited by P.J. Barnes, M.M. Grunstein, A.R. Leff, and A.J. Woolcock. Lippincott–Raven Publishers, Philadelphia © 1997.

▪ 1 ▪

Overview

Ann J. Woolcock and Peter J. Barnes

In this book we have attempted to bring together the current understanding of asthma: its causes, pathology, clinical features, treatment, and management. All the chapters are written by people who are experts in their field and each chapter is extensively referenced to provide source material for those interested in the various aspects of the disease.

Knowledge about asthma can be divided into a number of subjects as illustrated in Figure 1. Genetic and environmental factors are covered in the section on Epidemiology. Airway inflammation is covered by the sections on Structure, Biology, Pathology, Inflammatory Cells, Inflammatory Mediators, Target Cells, and Neural Mechanisms. Airway narrowing is covered by the sections on Inducers and Triggers and Respiratory Physiology. Symptoms is covered by the section on Clinical Assessment. Management is covered by the sections on Therapy and Management. Outcome does not have a section since little is known about the natural history of the disease. The ways in which the boxes in Figure 1 are linked are largely unknown.

WHAT IS ASTHMA?

In spite of the immense amount of material presented here, we do not know the answer to this question. Our poor understanding of the causes, natural history, and airway behavior in this disease have led us to use the word "asthma" in a number of different ways—to describe symptoms, to describe exacerbations, and to describe the underlying abnormalities in the airways. This loose use of the word asthma causes confusion, and many patients and clinicians fail to appreciate that, frequently, it is a chronic, life-long disease. Asthma is a clinical syndrome that describes a set of symptoms. The cause(s) of asthma remains unknown (1).

Since we do not know what asthma is, we do not know if it is best thought of as a single disease of the airways which varies with severity or if it is better thought of as abnormal behavior of the airways in which they narrow excessively as a result of several factors acting singly or together to produce the narrowing and, therefore, the symptoms. As the chapters of this book have come together it seems increasingly likely that asthma is best thought of as abnormal behavior of the airways and, probably, of the smooth muscle. The dominant hypothesis for the abnormal behavior of the airways is that inflammation, orchestrated by the cytokines of t-helper (TH) 2 cells (interleukin [IL]-4, IL-5 and IL-13), thickens all layers of the airway wall, and the whole length of the airway. The inflammation causes excessive amounts of mediators which cause contraction of the smooth muscle and the thickened airways to narrow, and/or close. However, there may well be other ways in which the symptoms of asthma can be produced. Some examples: viral infections in infants with relatively small diameter airways; breathing without stretching the airways in the presence of methacholine;

A.J. Woolcock: Institute of Respiratory Medicine, Page Chest Pavilion, Royal Prince Alfred Hospital, Camperdown, New South Wales 2050 Australia.
P.J. Barnes: Department of Thoracic Medicine, Imperial College School of Medicine at The National Heart and Lung Institute, London, SW3 6LY United Kingdom.

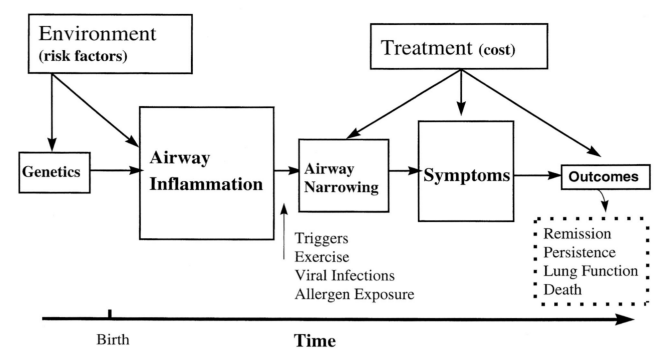

FIG. 1. The sequence of events in asthma that are covered by the sections of this book are illustrated in this figure. In general, the size of the box is proportionally representative of the current knowledge of the subjects in each of the boxes. The greatest amount is known about airway inflammation. However, an overall understanding of asthma is lacking because of insufficient data about how the boxes are linked. To rectify this, the following questions need to be answered: How do environmental factors act with genetic predisposition to cause airway inflammation? How does this cause airway narrowing? How does airway narrowing cause symptoms? and What are the outcomes of treatment?

beta blocking drugs used by people who need beta stimulation to keep smooth muscle relaxed; and inhaling cold dry air under conditions of hyperventilation for long periods, as in cross-country skiers in Scandinavia (2,3). Although most asthmatics are allergic and have a family history of the disease, we do not know the exact mechanisms involved in an individual who wheezes.

WHAT DO WE KNOW ABOUT ASTHMA?

Epidemiologic studies show that wheezing illness in children is increasing in most countries, but differences exist between populations within and between countries. Examination of the risk factors for asthma suggests that the increasing prevalence of the disease in children is related to the loss of a protective factor or factors that previously prevented allergic children (those with specific immunoglobulin (Ig)E to common inhaled allergens) from developing asthma, rather than to the introduction of a new environmental hazard. It is fashionable to blame environmental air pollution for the rising prevalence of the disease. Pollution, especially with sulphur dioxide, can cause wheezing, but there is no direct evidence for air pollution as a cause of the disease in the airways. We do

know that only some allergic children develop asthma, that genetic factors are involved as is the amount of allergen to which the allergic children are exposed, so that reducing the load can prevent asthma or reduce the severity of disease in those who have it.

A great deal is known about airway inflammation in asthma, as can be seen from the dominance of these sections (more than 61 chapters). Figure 2 summarizes the basic aspects of airway inflammation in asthma including the inflammatory cells, mediators, target cells, and neural mechanisms involved. Although there is much to learn about the mechanisms of inflammation, its nature and the way it responds to corticosteroids are still better known than many of the other areas contained in the boxes shown in Figure 1.

We do not understand how inflammation leads to the symptoms of asthma. Inflammation increases the responsiveness of the airways, making them more likely to narrow in response to environmental triggers, but inflammation may directly lead to symptoms, such as cough and chest tightness, through activation of sensitized sensory nerve endings. Why the same degree of airway narrowing measured by forced expiration tests may lead to widely differing degrees of symptoms in different asthmatic patients is largely unknown.

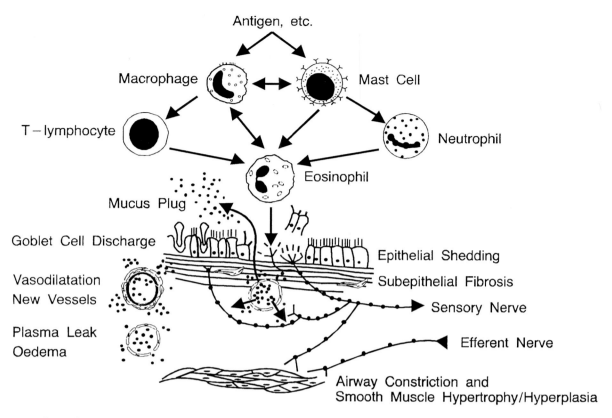

FIG. 2. Some of the essential mechanisms of airway inflammation present in asthma illustrate the fact that many factors are involved in the inflammatory processes of asthma.

We do not know why inflammation in asthma becomes persistent. Although continued exposure to allergen is important, asthma may persist even in the absence of allergen exposure, as illustrated by patients with occupational asthma who may continue to have disease despite complete avoidance of sensitizing agents (4). Lung transplantation studies have provided unexpected results. Two patients who developed asthma after transplantation with lungs from asthmatic patients are reported (despite immunosuppression with cyclosporin A and glucocorticoids). Conversely, two patients with severe asthma who received a lung transplantation from normal donors did not redevelop asthma (5). This suggests that there is a local airway mechanism driving asthmatic inflammation, although more patients need to be studied to establish this.

WHAT ARE THE CONTROVERSIAL ISSUES?

What is the Role of Infections?

One of the issues is the role of infections. In some studies, respiratory infection in early childhood appears to be a risk factor which is independent of the atopic (allergic) status of the child (6). However, the lack of severe infections, especially bacterial and parasitic infections, may be a possible cause of the increasing prevalence and association of the disease with affluence (7). Viral infections definitely trigger exacerbations and are probably the leading cause of exacerbations throughout life. Some viruses, such as respiratory syncytial virus and rhinovirus, seem to be more important than others in causing asthmatic exacerbations (8–11). So far there is no hard evidence that viral infections are responsible for the onset of asthma in a nonasthmatic person. However, other diseases of unknown origin, such as juvenile diabetes and peptic ulceration, have been proved to have an infectious basis.

Other infections may be protective against asthma. African children who have had measles in early childhood are less likely to develop atopy, perhaps indicating that early infection may switch the immune system to be protective (TH1 vs. TH2 driven) (12). The inflammation in asthma is very similar to the host defense mounted against worms and parasites, and there is some evidence that worm infections provide some protection against the development of asthma (13).

How Important are Genetic Factors?

A second controversy relates to the genetic basis of the disease. It seems likely that atopy (the ability to make specific IgE to inhaled allergens) will prove to be linked to a gene or genes; in some populations, over 60% of the population are allergic and the number of allergic people in the population appears to be increasing (14,15). However, in the majority of young adult populations the prevalence of allergic people is about 40% (16). The number of allergic people who develop asthma varies from a few percent in children in China to almost one-half in children in Australia (15,17). There could be many genetically determined factors which, in the presence of allergy and the inhalation of allergens, could make the airways narrow excessively. These include breathing at a lower than normal lung volume; altered responsiveness of β-receptors on the airway smooth muscle; altered contractile properties of the airway smooth muscle; and excessive amounts of TH2 cytokines and lack of anti-inflammatory mechanisms, such as the cytokine IL-10. Because asthma is increasing globally, since genetic dissection of complex traits is difficult and environmental factors are changing rapidly, it may be some time before the genetic factors that predispose an allergic person to airway narrowing are known (18). It seems likely that the genetic determinants in those with severe disease may be revealed in the near future. This is important because those with severe disease have the most disruptions to their lives and use the most medical resources.

How Should We Classify Asthma?

The classification of asthma will remain a problem until more is known about the disease. However, the nature of the disease in people who have no evidence of atopy, as measured by skin tests or serum IgE specific to common aero allergens, continues to be controversial. These so called "intrinsic asthmatics" are more common in adults and it may be that their allergic state cannot be documented, but, alternatively, they may have a different cause for their symptoms. There is some evidence that patients with intrinsic asthma may produce IgE locally, and, indeed, the pathology of intrinsic asthma is identical to that of allergic asthma (19). The natural history of the disease in allergic and nonallergic asthmatics has not been studied.

What is the Role of IgE?

The role of IgE in asthma is controversial. In one study the levels of IgE have been shown to correlate with asthma in populations free from parasites (20). In addition, IgE may affect the behavior of the smooth muscle, since in sensitized animals contraction is altered, and in passively sensitized human smooth muscle, the contractile responses are changed (21,22). It is not clear if IgE

has an effect in its own right or if it acts by releasing mediators from mast cells situated in or near the airway smooth muscle (1,23).

Why Does Asthma Differ in Severity Between Patients?

We have little understanding of why the disease differs in severity so much between patients. This does not appear to be explained entirely by allergen exposure levels or differences in treatment. Why some patients have episodic asthma that requires only occasional bronchodilators, whereas others have continuous and life-threatening symptoms only controlled on a large does of glucocorticoids, is unknown. It is likely that genetic factors are important and determine the intensity of the inflammatory response and the responsiveness of asthma to different treatments. There is now increasing evidence that gene polymorphisms may determine the severity of other inflammatory diseases, such as inflammatory bowel disease and rheumatoid arthritis (24). Polymorphisms of the β2-adrenergic receptor gene have been related to disease severity and clinical manifestation of asthma (25,26). It is likely that the severity of asthma and response to treatment with drugs, such as glucocorticoids, will be determined by multiple gene polymorphism. It is also likely that in the future it may be possible to predict disease outcome and response to different specific therapies, when this information is known. This may be important in concentrating resources on individuals in whom there are likely to be problems.

How Should Asthma Best Be Managed?

The whole area of management remains controversial and has led to a mania in the production of management guideline. Almost all countries have one or more national guidelines. They have arisen because there is no proven best method to treat the disease in its various forms and severities in different age groups. There is a complete lack of data from controlled trials of various forms of treatment in random populations over periods of 5 years. Indeed, there is a lack of data about the natural history of the disease and its outcome, with and without well-controlled treatment. This lack of information, together with the multiplicity of drugs available (often with extravagant claims for their effectiveness), has led to the development of consensus guidelines for management (27–29). Until these trials are done little progress will be made. It is of interest that global studies have been done for diabetes and the guidelines for treating that disease are much more firmly established (30). In asthma we have multiple guidelines based on consensus, but not on data. Although the global guidelines use the word "strategy," they describe the understanding of the disease and knowledge about short-term treatment. A strategy to deal with the disease in global terms is absent.

WHY IS THE DISEASE SO POORLY UNDERSTOOD?

When thinking about the reasons for not being able to answer the question "What is asthma?" a number of other questions arise. Has there been insufficient research? Are the wrong questions being asked? Is it a truly complex abnormality with many different forms and causes? What parts of this book are likely to be included in a future edition, in, say, 50 years time? Will the book be larger or smaller? It seems likely that the clinical features of the disease will be the same but, hopefully, much more will be known about its causes and, therefore, the ways of preventing it, or of gaining a lasting remission.

HOW COULD MORE EFFECTIVE PROGRESS BE MADE?

Forming a Global Strategy

Although asthma is becoming a global problem, at present there is no single international organization that targets asthma. Until now, the World Health Organization has been concerned mainly with the health of developing countries where infectious diseases are far more important than asthma as a health problem. However, as infections decrease and more antibiotics are used, it is likely that asthma will emerge as a problem in developing countries. An international organization is needed that can form a global strategy for asthma with the aims of prevention, documentation of the prevalence and mortality from the disease, and undertaking long-term trials with both pharmacologic and nonpharmacologic interventions. These have been carried out for other diseases, but, at present, no organizational structure exists for asthma.

Defining the Important Questions

Although a few small meetings have attempted to define the important questions, a concerted effort is needed from the leading scientists involved with the areas shown in the boxes in Figure 1 (1,31,32). World meetings of asthma are planned for the future and these offer one opportunity for clinicians, scientists, epidemiologists, and public health planners to meet. From such meetings it might be possible to form a group that can make a consensus of the ways in which the boxes in Figure 1 can be linked. In the meantime, this book attempts to provide state of the art knowledge about asthma as we currently understand it.

REFERENCES

1. Woolcock AJ, Barnes PJ. Asthma—the important questions 3. Report of a workshop held in Paros, Greece June 1995— Introduction. *Am J Respir Crit Care Med* 1996;153(6 Suppl):S1.
2. Skloot G, Permutt S, Togias A. Pathophysiology of asthma: reduced airway-parenchyma interdependence, not smooth muscle hyperresponsiveness. *Am J Resp Crit Care Med* 1994;149:A585.
3. Larsson K, Ohlsen P, Larsson L, Malmberg P, Rydstrom P-O, Ulriksen H. High prevalence of asthma in cross country skiers. *BMJ* 1993; 307:1326–1329.
4. Chan-Yeung M, Malo J-L. Occupational asthma. *N Engl J Med* 1995; 333:107–112.
5. Corris PA, Dark JH. Aetiology of asthma: lessons from lung transplantation. *Lancet* 1993;341:1369–1371.
6. Peat JK, Toelle B, Salome CM, Woolcock AJ. Predictive nature of bronchial responsiveness and respiratory symptoms in a one year cohort study of Sydney schoolchildren. *Eur Respir J* 1993;6:662–669.
7. Woolcock AJ. Is asthma a disease of affluence? In: Seymour W, ed. *Horizons in medicine*, vol 1. London: Blackwell Scientific Publications, 1994:42–50.
8. Castleman WL, Sorkness RL, Lemanske RF, McAllister PK. Viral bronchiolitis during early life induces increased numbers of bronchiolar mast cells and airway hyperresponsiveness. *Am J Pathol* 1990;137: 821–831.
9. Garofalo R, Kimpen JLL, Welliver RC, Ogra PL. Eosinophil degranulation in the respiratory tract during naturally acquired respiratory syncytial virus infection. *J Pediatr* 1992;120:28–32.
10. Duff AL, Pomeranz ES, Gelber LE, et al. Risk factors for acute wheezing in infants and children: viruses, passive smoke, and IgE antibodies to inhalant allergens. *Pediatrics* 1993;92(4):535–540.
11. Calhoun WJ, Dick EC, Schwartz LB, Busse WB. A common cold virus, rhinovirus 16, potentiates airway inflammation following segmental antigen bronchoprovocation in allergic subjects. *J Clin Invest* 1995;147.
12. Shaheen SO, Aaby P, Hall AJ. Measles and atopy in Guinea-Bissau. *Lancet* 1996;347:1369–1371.
13. Lynch NR, Hagel I, Perez M, Di Prisco MC, Lopez R, Alvarez N. Effect of anthelmintic treatment on the allergic reactivity of children in a tropical slum. *J Allergy Clin Immunol* 1993;92:404–411.
14. Barbee RA, Kaltenborn W, Lebowitz MD, Burrows B. Longitudinal changes in allergen skin test reactivity in a community population sample. *J Allergy Clin Immunol* 1987;79:16–24.
15. Leung R, Ho P. Asthma, allergy, and atopy in three south-east Asian populations. *Thorax* 1994;49:1205–1210.
16. Woolcock AJ, Peat JK. Evidence for the increase in asthma world-wide. In: Ciba Foundation Symposium 206. *The rising trends in asthma.* Chichester: Wiley, 1997;206:122–136.
17. Peat JK, Toelle B, Gray L, et al. Prevalence and severity of childhood asthma and allergic sensitisation in seven climatic regions of New South Wales. *Med J Aust* 1995;163:22–26.
18. Lander ES, Schork J. Genetic dissection of complex traits. *Science* 1994;265:2037–2048.
19. Humbert M, Grant JA, Tabora-Barata L. High affinity IgE receptor (FC$_\epsilon$RI) - bearing cells in bronchial biopsies from atopic and nonatopic asthma. *Am J Respir Crit Care Med* 1996;153:1931–1937.
20. Burrows B, Martinez FD, Halonen M, Barbee RA, Cline MG. Association of asthma with serum IgE levels and skin-test reactivity to allergens. *N Engl J Med* 1989;320:271–277.
21. Stephens NL, Halayko A, Jiang H. Normalization of contractile parameters in canine airway smooth muscle: morphological and biochemical. *Can J Physiol Pharmacol* 1992;70:635–644.
22. Black JL, Marthan R, Armour CL, Johnson PR. Sensitization alters contractile responses and calcium influx in human airway smooth muscle. *J Allergy Clin Immunol* 1989;84:440–447.
23. Mitchell RW, Ruhlmann E, Magnussen H, Leff AR, Rabe KF. Passive sensitization of human bronchi arguments smooth muscle shortening velocity and capacity. *Am J Physiol* 1994;267:L218–L222.
24. Wilson AG, Duff GW. Genetic traits in common diseases. *BMJ* 1995; 310:1482–1483.
25. Hall IP, Wheatley A, Wilding P, Liggett SB. Association of Glu 27 b2-adrenoceptor polymorphism with lower airway reactivity in asthmatic subjects. *Lancet* 1995;345:1213–1214.
26. Turki J, Park J, Green S, Martin R, Liggett SB. Genetic polymorphism of the β2-adrenergic receptor in nocturnal and non-nocturnal asthma:

evidence that Gly 16 correlates with the nocturnal phenotype. *J Clin Invest* 1995;95:1635–1641.

27. Woolcock A, Rubinfeld AR, Seale JP, et al. Thoracic society of Australia and New Zealand. Asthma management plan, 1989. *Med J Aust* 1989;151(11–12):650–653.

28. National Institute of Health. Guidelines for the diagnosis and management of asthma. US Department of Health and Human Services, 1991.

29. National Heart Lung and Blood Institute. *Global strategy for asthma management and prevention NHLBI/WHO workshop report.* National Institutes of Health, 1995.

30. Chisholm DJ. The diabetes control and complications trial(DCCT). A milestone in diabetes management. *Med J Aust* 1993;159:721–723.

31. Woolcock AJ. State of the Art: Asthma—what are the important experiments? *Am Rev Respir Dis* 1988;138:730–744.

32. Woolcock AJ, Barnes PJ. Asthma—the important questions, part 2. *Am Rev Respir Dis* 1992;146(Suppl 5):1351–1366.

Asthma, edited by P.J. Barnes, M.M. Grunstein,
A.R. Leff, and A.J. Woolcock.
Lippincott–Raven Publishers, Philadelphia © 1997.

▪ 2 ▪

History of Asthma

Roger Ellul-Micallef

FROM EGYPT TO ROME

Bronchial asthma, like epilepsy, has attracted a great deal of attention since time immemorial because it often presents itself in such a dramatic manner (1). This condition has been identified in ancient Egyptian and Hebrew writings. Of the eight Egyptian medical papyri, only the Ebers papyrus (ca. 1550 B.C.) sheds light on the Egyptian view of respiratory diseases (2). It contains hardly any descriptions of specific diseases but lists remedies to treat symptoms, for example, cough, wheezing, and expectoration. Ebell (3) identifies in it a number of remedies that it is claimed were used to treat asthma. Perhaps one of the earliest recorded prescriptions used in the treatment of this condition was made up of figs, sebestin, grapes, sycamore fruit, frankincense, cumin, fruit of juniper, wine, goose grease, and sweet beer. An extract of henbane (*Hyoscyamus*) was also at times placed on a heated brick and its emanations inhaled. Far less palatable appears to have been the use of excreta from camels or crocodiles.

The history of medical ideas of the ancient people of Israel must be sought among their religious laws compiled in the Mishnah and commented upon in the Talmud, both being repositories of thousands of years of Jewish wisdom. The Mishnaic text of the Babylonian Talmud contains the phrase "rûah kezarit ba' ah alaw," which may be freely translated as, "a short breath causes departure." Danby (4) claimed that this referred to tetanus, whereas Epstein (5), probably more correctly, maintained that asthma was the condition involved.

The word *asthma* is derived directly from the Greek ασθμα, meaning a short-drawn breath, panting, or labored breathing. Various medical historians have attempted to trace the earliest references made to this condition. In their eagerness, they have at times failed to appreciate that the term "asthma" has often been used to denote a degree of severity of breathlessness and not a specific illness.

The term used by Homer to describe painful or difficult breathing had acquired a more clinical connotation by the time of Hippocrates. In the Hippocratic corpus of medical writings, asthma is referred to nine times, but it remains a term for a clinical symptom (6). In his essay on the influence of climate on health, Hippocrates (7) states that children are liable to convulsions and asthma, both being regarded as divine visitations. Hippocrates also noted the possibility that asthma could be an inherited condition. Asthma was believed to be brought about by an imbalance of the humors (a cacochymia) that caused a flow of the evil humor, pituita, or phlegm, thought to arise in the pituitary gland, from where it passed, via the cribriform plate, into the nasal cavities and the lungs. It is perhaps apt to point out that, at the time, Hippocrates thought that air was cooled and distributed throughout the body by the blood vessels, which acted as air conduits. The oldest medical document, after the Hippocratic corpus, is *De Medicina*, compiled by Aulus Cornelius Celsus (8), arguably the greatest of the Latin medical writers. Celsus's classification of diseases presenting with shortness of breath into three classes, depending on the degree of difficult respiration, remained popular well into the Middle Ages: "When the difficulty of breathing is moderate and not suffocating it is called dyspnoea, when it is more vehement so that the breathing is more sonorous and wheez-

R. Ellul-Micallef: Department of Clinical Pharmacology and Therapeutics, University of Malta, Msida MSD 06 Malta.

ing, it constitutes asthma; when the breathing can only take place in an upright position it is termed orthopnoea." Celsus suggested a remedy for asthma that was to persist into the 17th century: "It is not a foolish idea that the lung of a fox should be dried and powdered.... or that the lung of that animal, as fresh as possible, roasted without touching iron in cooking, should be eaten."

The first recognizable clinical description of an asthmatic paroxysm was provided by Aretaeus (9), a Greek physician born in Cappadocia, a Roman province in Asia Minor. His teachings remained in oblivion until a Greek manuscript of his work was discovered. This was translated into Latin and printed in Venice in 1552. Aretaeus noted that the term "asthma" was being employed in a general sense, merely as a symptom, but went on to classify asthma as a disease, emphasizing the wheezing, the dry, often unproductive cough, and the inability to sleep in a prone position. "The disease called orthopnoia," wrote Aretaeus, "is also called asthma because those who have paroxysms pant for breath (*Asthmainousi*)." His clinical description is easily the best account of the condition in ancient times: "They eagerly go into the open air, since no house sufficeth for their respiration; they breathe standing, as if desiring to draw in all the air which they possibly can inhale; and, in their want of air, they also open the mouth as if thus to enjoy the more of it... cough incessant and laborious, expectoration small, thin, cold, resembling the efflorescence of foam... and if these symptoms increase, they sometimes produce suffocation, after the form of epilepsy."

Galen of Pergamus, considered to be the greatest clinician after Hippocrates, advanced a system, based on the Hippocratic doctrine of the "humors," which held undisputed sway for well over a thousand years until challenged by Paracelsus (10). Although he is considered to be the first experimental physiologist, his serious anatomic and physiologic errors had a profound negative influence for centuries. Among these was his contention that the brain communicated directly with the nasopharynx through the ethmoid, which "permitted respiration of the brain" and through which were discharged the "excrements" of the brain. This mistaken theory was finally disproved by Schneider in 1660 (11). Galen believed that asthma was caused by thick viscid humors in the lungs and thought that it resulted from "a lack of room in the cavities of the lungs." Unfortunately, Galen did not appear to consider asthma as a separate condition, as Aretaeus had done before him, although he did try to reproduce it in animals by severing the intercostal muscles, the intercostal nerves, and the cervical spinal cord (12). He thought that asthma was a more severe form of dyspnea, although he appreciated the frequent, sudden, and violent spasmodic respiration during asthmatic attacks. He prescribed attenuant and detergent medicines, forbidding all things hot or cold, as well as astringents, as these might thicken the humors, and tried purging the nostrils. He recommended vinegar and

oxymel of squills and doubted the usefulness of millipedes, though the latter were still to be found in most formularies centuries later. Galen thought that opiates were harmful in asthma, because they cooled too much and thereby thickened the humors. Poppy, mandrake, hemlock, henbane, and fleabane were therefore not to be used in asthma. Caelius Aurelianus, an African doctor born in Numidia and who practised in Rome around the beginning of the 5th century A.D., left us the most complete account of the Methodist school. He is said to have been the first to describe nocturnal asthma. Aurelianus, too, appeared to differentiate asthma from related conditions presenting with breathlessness (13).

The next work of major medical significance after Galen's was that of Paulus Aegineta, a 7th century Byzantine doctor who practised mainly in Alexandria and whose seven books on medicine owe a great deal to the works of Galen, Aetius, and Oribasius (14). His concept of asthma, however, was similar to that of Galen: "Those who breathe thick without fever, like those who run fast, are said to be asthmatic, that is to say, to pant for breath; and from their being obliged to keep the chest erect for fear of being suffocated, they are called orthopnoic. The affection arises from thick and viscid humours becoming infarcted in the bronchial cells of the lungs.... The indication of cure in asthmatic complaints is to consume the viscid and thick humour by attenuant and detergent medicines." For this purpose, Paulus used vinegar of squills, cow parsnip, mustard, and round birthwort taken internally, as well as the external applications of figs, honey, wax, iris, and barley. Bleeding, emetics, and clysters were also recommended.

THE TIME OF THE ARABS

The Muslim invasion of the Middle East and North Africa in the 7th century A.D. resulted in an assimilation, on the part of the Arabs, of significant elements of the Hellenistic culture then prevailing in the conquered lands. In general, Arab physicians followed the teachings of Hippocrates, Celsus, Galen, and Dioscorides without ever questioning them. Among the great physicians who wrote in Arabic was the Persian, Abu-Bakr Muhammad ibn-Zakariyya ar-Rhazi (15,16). Better known in the West as Rhazes, he was born in Rayy, close to Teheran. He was another prolific writer whose two best known books are the *Kitāb al-Hāwì (Liber Continens)*, an encyclopedia of medicine containing many case histories, and the *Kitāb al-Mansùrì (Liber Almansoris)*, where diseases are arranged "a capite usque ad calcem." On the subject of asthma, he quotes both Mesuë and Galen, and contradicts the latter's claim on the efficacy of owls' blood: "I say that owls' blood is not to be given, for I have seen it administered and it was useless" (17).

Abù-Ali al-Husayn ibn-Abd-Allãh ibn-Sinã, known as Avicenna in the West, was called by the Arabs "el Sheik el Reis" (the prince of physicians) (18). His main medical work is the *Kitâb al-Qânùn (Canon)* (19). Avicenna thought that asthma and epilepsy were related conditions and referred to asthma as "caducus pulmonum." This idea lingered on for a long time, and attacks of asthma were still referred to as fits well into the 17th century. Arsenic preparations administered both by inhalation and in pill form were used by a number of Arab physicians, including ar-Rhazi, ibn Mesuë, Yohannan bar Seraphyon, and ibn Sinã. Ar-Rhazi used arsenic to treat a number of medical conditions, including leprosy and asthma: "nec non asthmati, si vel cum illo suffimigatio aut epithema fiant." Ibn-Sinã concurred with ar-Rhazi, recommending it together with a hydromel (a mixture of water and honey) for a number of conditions that included pulmonary suppuration, persistent cough, and hemoptysis; in pill form for asthma; and in a clyster for hemorrhoids! ("Datur quoque in potionibus cum hydromele ad pulmones suppuratos et tussim antiquam sputumque sanguinis et saniei, quandoque etiam in pillulis contra asthma et in clysteribus, contra haemorrhoides ani" [20,21].)

Perhaps the member of this group best known for his writing on asthma is the great Jewish physician and philosopher, Abù-Imrãn Mùsã ibn Ubayd-Allah ibn-Maymùn (22). He was known in the Latin West as Maimonides and to the Jews as Rambam (from the acronym Rabbi Moses ben Maimon). Forced to leave Cordova, he fled to Morocco, where he learned medicine in Fez, and finally settled in Fostat, near Cairo, as Saladin's court physician. Here he served Saladin's son, al-Malik al-Afdal Nùr-ad-Din Alì, as his personal physician. Saladin's son suffered from bronchial asthma and melancholia, and asked Maimonides whether it was advisable for him to move from Alexandria to Cairo. In reply, Maimonides in 1190 wrote what is probably the first extensive treatise on asthma, "Maqãla fi al-Rabw," in which he points out that asthma should be treated according to the various causes that bring it about. He did recommend a change from the humid air of Alexandria to the dry atmosphere of Cairo. This discourse on asthma is prefaced humbly by the statement "I have no magic cure to report; all I have in mind is a rational conduct of life." He advised the patient on hygiene, recommended medicines, and the best diet to follow. In cases of acute asthma, he suggested chicken soup if the patient was afebrile and sweetened barley porridge if the patient had fever. He believed that chicken soup assisted in the expectoration of phlegm (23,24). The use of chicken soup has persisted as a folk remedy for respiratory disorders down to the present time.

MEDIEVAL MEDICINE

Many of the Arabic translations, which had preserved, almost with reverence, the classic works of antiquity, at times with the addition of significant new contributions to knowledge, were translated into Latin and, from around the 11th century onward, had a profound influence on the intellectual life of Europe in the High Middle Ages. The amount of documentation relating to medicine in Europe prior to the 11th century is meager. At this time, theurgic therapy, or a cult of faith healing, was predominant during a period of monastic medicine. The great medical center at Salerno was well established by the middle of the 11th century and reached its greatest splendor in the following century. Here, Judeo-Arabic medical doctrine was introduced and grafted upon Western European culture. Among the better known superintendents of the Medical School of Salerno was Nicolas de Salerno (25), who, in the beginning of the 12th century, is said to have compiled an antidotarium. It was the first formulary and one of the first medical books to be printed (Venice, 1471), and was regularly consulted for centuries. The compilers of the first London *Pharmacopeia*, published in 1618 (26), drew heavily on this antidotarium as well as the "Grabadin" of Mesuë. Among the remedies of Salernitanus for asthma, two were translated from the *Dispensatory Made by the College of Physicians* by Nicholas Culpeper (27). One is an electuary (*Species Electuarii Diamargariton Frigidi*) having among its components "the seeds of Purslain, white Poppies, Endive, Sorrel, Citrons; the three sorts of Sanders, Lignum, Aloes, Ginger; the flowers of Red Roses, Water Lillies, Bugloss, Violets; the berries of Mirtle, the bone of a Stag's heart, Ivory, Roman Doronicum, Cinnamon... both sorts of Corral... Pearls, Amber greece, Camphire, Musk." These were made into a powder, "according to art." This multi-item prescription was reportedly "restorative in consumptions, to help such as are in hectick feavers, to restore strength lost, to help coughs, Asthmaes...." Another no less complex electuary (Pleres Arconticon) was thought to be "exceedingly good for sad, melancholy, lumpish, pensive, grieving, vexing, pining, sobbing, fearful, careful spirits... and succours such as are troubled with Asthmaes, or other cold afflictions of the lungues."

There are no learned Anglo-Saxon medical treatises, but three Leechbooks written at Winchester in the vernacular, around 950 A.D., have survived. The first two of these Leechbooks belonged to the physician Bald and are mainly concerned with therapeutics. Sections 15 to 18 of the First Leechbook deal with respiratory diseases (lungen-àdl). Asthma was referred to as "on hyra brósten nearuwe" ("nearuwe" meaning "narrowed"). The First Leechbook suggests two "salves" for lungen-ádl (lung disease), the first containing brooklime ("hleomac") and goose dung; the second had golden lungwort as its main component (28).

In 13th century England, John Gaddesden (29) wrote a four-volume work on medicine: the *Rosa Anglica Medicinae*. It makes no scientific contributions but describes a number of remedies that, against a backdrop of scholastic speculation, are riddled with mysticism, charms, and superstitions typical of his times. For asthma, John Anglus prescribed "the Lungs of a Fox, two Drams, in Aqua Mellis" and says it is "Medicina sublimes et experta in Asthmate." In English medical literature, the Greek word *asthma* made an appearance as "asma" or "asmy" in the 14th century, was written as "asthma" in the 16th century, and as "astma" in the 17th century. It is first traceable to a 1397 English translation made by John Trevisa of the popular encyclopedia *De Proprietatibus Rerum* (30). This encyclopedia was written around 1240 by Bartolomaeus Anglicus, "de ordine fratrum minorum." This Franciscan friar is said to have studied at Salerno and, in his work, gave a clear picture of life and learning during the 13th century. Trevisa's translation was edited by Wynkyn de Worde and published in 1491 (31). It was one of the finest and earliest books to be printed in England. It is, in fact, the seventh book of *De Proprietatibus* that treats of the human body and its ailments. Trevisa translated Bartolomaeus's references to asthma as "dyffyculte and hardness of brethynge hight Asma" ("hight" is old English for "called").

THE RENAISSANCE

The scientific revolution of the Renaissance burst the bonds that tied scientific thought to Aristotelian physics. Philippus Aureolus Theophrastus Bombastus von Hohenheim, better known as Paracelsus, helped in the breaking off with accepted medieval medical dogma and brought to an end the unquestioned teachings of Galen and ibn Sinã by publicly burning their books in Basel. He is looked upon as the founder of chemical pharmacology and therapeutics. The true influence, however, that Paracelsus may have had on the progress of medicine is difficult to assess. His writings on asthma, unfortunately, only added to the general confusion then still surrounding this condition. In his two short commentaries entitled "De Asthmate" (32), Paracelsus claimed that bronchial asthma could be cured only by liquid (chemical) preparations and not by simple herbs ("Per liquorem pulmonariae curator asthma non per herbam"). His remedies included the distillation of crude tartar in spirit of wine, "tartarum contusum in alcool vini"; "vinum essatum," wine containing herbal extracts; and "vinum de Melissa," considered of great benefit in asthma ("valde magnum in Asthmate"). For Paracelsus, "ultima cura est Sulphure"; sulfur was the drug that would ultimately dry up the phlegm in the asthmatic lung when all else had failed (33).

The year 1552 marks what has perhaps been the most famous consultation for asthma recorded in the annals of medical history. Gerolamo Cardano, Professor of Medicine at the University of Pavia, was asked to travel all the way to Scotland to treat John Hamilton, Archbishop of St. Andrew's, whose asthmatic condition had been steadily deteriorating over the previous 10 years. Cardano was then the most celebrated physician in Europe and also en-

joyed a great reputation as a mathematician. The Archbishop was the brother of the Earl of Arran, who, at the time, was Regent of Scotland, as Mary Stuart was still a minor (34,35).

Cardano is perhaps the most colorful physician to write about asthma. His autobiography, *De Vita Propria Liber* (1575), relates his various vicissitudes (36). He was obviously influenced by Maimonides's treatise on asthma. He must have believed that asthma was incurable but that it could be relieved by a proper regimen. He wrote a "consilium" detailing the necessary treatment, containing frequent references to Galen. His clinical notes on the case and his advice to the Archbishop cover over 20 folio pages. Cardano's conclusions are often based on faulty pathophysiologic assumptions that were prevalent at the time. It was thought that "vapors" and fluids rose from the lungs to the brain, where they were drawn by the rarified atmosphere present there. The "vapors" were said to be exhaled through the skin, but the fluids in time became thick and by their increased weight descended through the trachea back to the lungs, where their viscosity caused irritation.

At clinical conferences attended by Cardano in Paris, on his way to Edinburgh, a controversy had arisen as to whether the condition of the Archbishop's brain was "cold" or "hot." The Parisian physicians had held that it was "cold," and therefore they had insisted that he keep a brazier of burning peat or charcoal wherever he might be, including in his carriage! He was denied fresh air and was allowed only very hot foods and mulled wines. Such a regimen could only have led to a further irritation of his airways. Cardano, on the other hand, insisted that it was "hot," perhaps because he saw the utter failure of whatever had been prescribed before. He immediately switched over to a completely opposite regimen that was equally empirical but that fortunately improved the Archbishop's condition. He decided that the cause of Hamilton's asthma was the high temperature of the brain and therefore decided to purge the head and the body. To this end, the Archbishop was prescribed a precipitate of elaterium in goat's milk and an ointment consisting of ship's tar, mustard, euphorbium, honey of Anathardus, and blister fly, which he had to apply to his skull. Furthermore, he had to wash his head in warm water to which ashes had been added, and this was to be followed by a cold shower and mild massage with cool dry cloths. Definitely less trying was the compound of peaches and sugar of violets that had to be washed down with the milk of a well-nourished ass. The Archbishop was also given a strict work timetable which directed that he should go to bed at eight and secure 10 h of continuous sleep. Probably, even more than from the regular daily routine, Hamilton must have derived benefit from being allowed fresh air, thus escaping the smoky and stuffy rooms and, most importantly, being forbidden to sleep on a feather mattress. Cardano probably did not make any direct connection between feathers and the Archbishop's asthma, although this case is often cited as the first example of allergen avoidance. He simply thought that the feather mattress "heats the spine and causes matter straightaway to ascend to the brain." His approach to the treatment of asthma was a holistic one, giving attention to all aspects of daily life. Following this regimen, the Archbishop grew rapidly better, and Cardano was allowed to leave Edinburgh after having spent 75 days with his patient (37).

Perhaps the most interesting figure of Renaissance medicine is the physician from Brussels, Jean Baptiste van Helmont. A disciple of Paracelsus, he is also regarded as having made important contributions to the liberation of medical concepts from the ancient dogma of Galen, but, like his master, had also many of the same fantastic notions. He is regarded as the forerunner of the iatrochemical school, though his chemistry was markedly tinged with alchemy. He wrote extensively and authoritatively on asthma, being the first asthmatic to do so. His posthumous masterpiece bore the title of *Ortus Medicinae, id est Initia Physicae Inaudita: Progressus Medicinae novus* (38) and was published in 1648 by his son. He clearly stated that in asthma "nothing rains down from the Head in to the Wind-pipe, or Lungs," and that "whatsoever the Cough casts forth, that is made in the Pipes of the Lungs through their proper vice." This was contrary to what was generally accepted in his time. He further took cudgels against this theory of defluxion in another book, *Delirementa Catarrhi* or *The Incongruities, Impossibilities, and Absurdities couched under the vulgar Opinion of Defluxions* (39). In trying to explain the underlying cause of asthma, van Helmont unfortunately draws upon his mystical jargon: "The Asthma therefore in this is like to the Falling-evil [epilepsy], the which, although it doth not strike the mind, doth not contract the sinews, or step up swoonings; yet it sleepeth in some seat; whence at length it defiling the archaeus with a certain contagion, if it doth not contract the Sinews, yet at least wise, it doth the Lungs." He goes on to state, "We may lawfully therefore, by a Philosophical Liberty, name an Asthma the falling-Sickness of the lungs: Indeed its Nest is in the Duumvirate;.... That falling-Sickness of the Lungs is made by a Poyson, which by its property doth affect the lungs, no otherwise than as a Cantarides doth the Instruments of the Urine." The duumvirate of the body, according to van Helmont, was formed by the spleen and stomach, the former presiding over the abdomen, sexual, and other organs, with the latter presiding over sleep, waking, folly, and other functions. This similarity between asthma and epilepsy had originally been described by ibn Sin and referred to as "caducus pulmonum."

Van Helmont has left us some of the most vivid descriptions of asthmatic patients to be found in the medical literature. Perhaps the earliest identified causes of asthma are those that triggered off the condition in "a certain monk of the order of St. Francis" who "is busied in pulling down Houses or Temples. And forthwith as oft as any place is Swept, or the Wind doth otherwise stir up the Dust, he presently falls down, being almost choaked." This monk also had attacks when "he eateth Fishes fried with Oyl" for "he presently falls down, being deprived of Breathing," so as that "he is scarce distinguished from a strangled man" (40).

THE BEGINNING OF SCIENTIFIC MEDICINE: THE 17TH AND 18TH CENTURIES

In the 17th century, medical theorizing followed two different "physiological" schools of thought, the iatromathematical (iatromechanical) and the iatrochemical. The protagonists of the iatrochemical school, who thought that all vital phenomena were chemical in essence, included Thomas Willis, who excelled in the clinical description of various conditions and also made significant anatomic discoveries. He is perhaps best known for his research into the nervous system, in which he was assisted by Richard Lower. Willis is well known to all students of anatomy, having described the arterial arrangement at the base of the brain, which still carries his name: the circle of Willis. He is also credited with the discovery of the presence of sugar in diabetic urine. Thomas Willis wrote what is perhaps the first relatively scientific account on asthma. In his introductory paragraph to his chapter "De Asthmate," originally published in *Pharmaceutice rationalis Sive diatriba de medicamentorum operationibus in humano corpore* in 1674 (41), there is, highlighted in the margin, the phrase, "Asthma morbus maxime terribilis."

Willis (42) distinguished between an asthma that was "mere pneumonicum" (purely pneumonic) where "omnino à ductibus aeriferis obstructis, aut non satis patentibus procedens" (all airways are obstructed and not sufficiently patent) from one that was "mere convulsivum" (purely convulsive), the latter being nervous in origin "sine magna Bronchiorum obstructione, aut compressione" (without any marked bronchial obstruction or compression) and simply due to "cramps of the moving fibres of the bronchia and of the vessels of the lung, the diaphragm and muscles of the breast." This seems to be the first reference to asthma being caused by bronchospasm. In the case of pneumonic asthma, according to Willis, bronchial obstruction could result from thick and viscid humors, purulent matter, extravasated blood, abscess, hard tumor, or even stones that are implanted in the airways. Willis thought that it could also arise from a swelling of the bronchial walls and obstruction from without.

He pointed out that there could also be a third type, "mixtum," and this occurred "quando utraeque partes in vitio conspirant." He claimed that although asthma "is sometimes simple from the beginning," that is, either pneumonic or convulsive, after some time, when the con-

dition deteriorates, "it may be concluded that every invet-
erate Asthma to be a mixt affection, stirr'd up by the default partly of the Lungs ill fram'd, and partly by default
of the Nerves and nervous fibres appertaining to the
breathing parts." Willis (43) believed that whatever
makes the blood boil or rise into an effervescence, such
as a violent motion of the body (exercise) or anger, or excessive outside cold or heat, "vini potus, Venus" (strong
wine and sex), or indeed "meriis Lecti calor" (the mere
heat of the bed) would cause an attack of asthma. He
seemed to be aware of nocturnal asthma and thought that
it could be explained by the overheating of the blood by
the bedclothes, which caused "more plentiful sucking of
air." He advised these patients to sleep on a chair. From
detailed Latin notes that John Locke kept of Willis's lectures on therapeutics, it transpires that the medicinal use
of sulfur was one of his favorite remedies for chest complaints (44). Besides prescribing beer with wormwood
("cervisie cum absinthio") as a morning drink, Willis was
perhaps the first to use coffee in treating asthma, suggesting as an alternative 15 drops of tartarizate elixir in
coffee prepared with sage ("Elixiris proprietatis Tarta-
rizati gutt. xv cum haustu Coffee ex decocto salvie
parari"). These two remedies would relieve the patient
from "paroxysmi Asthmatici de solita ferocia...."

A Treatise of the Asthma, the first monograph on
asthma in English, was written by John Floyer (45), himself an asthmatic, and published in London in 1698. He
dedicated it to his friend, the physician Dr. Phineas
Fowke. In his dedication, he wrote, "I have assigned the
immediate cause of the Asthma, to the Straitness, Compression or Constriction of the Bronchia. If the Asthma
be but partially described, and a false Hypothesis built on
that Description, the Practice answering that is very Im-
pertinent or injurious." He described asthma as "a laborious Respiration, with lifting up the Shoulders, and
Wheezing, from the Compression, Obstruction, or Coarc-
tation of some Branches of the Bronchia, and some lobes
of the Bladders of the Lungs." He classified asthma into
two types: "periodic" and "continued." According to him,
periodic asthma occurred "when the Muscles labour
much for Inspiration and Expiration thro' some Obstruction, or compression of the Bronchia, etc. we properly
call this a Difficulty of Breath, but if this Difficulty be by
the Constriction of the Bronchia, 'tis properly the Periodic Asthma. And if the constriction be great, it is with
Wheezing; but if less, the Wheeziness is not so evident."

The continued asthma depended on "the Compression
of the Vein, and Bronchia, and Bladders of the Lungs or
Nerves" and was supposed to result from a number of
conditions, which included "a dropsie in the Breast, an
Empyema, Inflammatory Tumour, or Abscess or large Tu-
berculum, a Polypus in the Pneumonic Vessels, Stones
bred in the Trachea, a Tumour of the Thymus, straining
the Lungs by Running and by a Windy Tumour of the
Lungs, as it happens in broken-winded Horses" (emphy-

sema). These are obviously causes that could have conceivably given rise to breathlessness and perhaps, at
times, wheezing, but not to asthma as defined today.

Floyer ranged himself against "Chymists, the Empyri-
cal and the Mechanical doctors," that is, the iatro-
chemists, the empiricists, and the iatrophysicists, and was
all in favor of Hippocrates and Galen. He stated that he
was of the opinion that "most of the diseases incurable by
the Modern Practice,.... were oftener cured by the Old
Methods, which have difus'd and neglected upon the account of pure Chymical Medicines,...." John Floyer referred to his own attacks of nocturnal asthma: "I have
omitted to mention this, that my Fits never seize me but
in the Night, and then awake me with a Heaviness, and so
grow worse and worse immediately." Although he was
not correct in working out the pathophysiology of nocturnal asthma, his graphic clinical description of it is difficult to better: "At first waking, about one or two of the
Clock in the Night, the Fit of the Asthma more evidently
begins, the Breath is very slow, but after a little time,
more strait; the Diaphragme seems stiff, and tied or
drawn up by the Mediastinum.... The Asthmatic is immediately necessitated to rise out of his Bed, and sit in an
erect Posture...." He also recognized the various factors
associated with this condition: heredity, exercise, weather
and seasons, atmospheric pollution, tobacco smoking,
certain occupations, infection, personal idiosyncracies,
and "the passions" (emotions), as well as dietary factors.

Many of Floyer's recommendations on diet where similar to those of Maimonides and Willis. He advocated
avoiding a "mucilaginous" diet and forbade his asthmatics the consumption of fish, legumes, and milk, since he
believed that these items thickened the phlegm. His therapeutic advice did not differ very much from that of his
predecessors. He was a strong advocate of purging and
also thought that "by many Blisters apply'd to the Arms
and Legs and Shoulders, which may discharge a Serum
from the Nerves," one could "cure the Asthma Fit." He
was almost obsessed with the value of cold bathing and
recommended it both in his treatise on asthma as well as
in his previously published book on the use and abuse of
bathing (46).

Medicine in the 18th century has been described by
Fielding Garrison (47) to have been "as dull and sober-
sided as that of the Arabic period." Apart from a few original spirits (like Ramazzini, Boerhaave, Hales, Morgagni,
the Hunters, and Jenner), it was essentially the age of the-
orists (Stahl, Hoffmann, Cullen, Barthez, and Brown) and
of the system makers. Classification in medicine came
into vogue with Linnaeus and reached its apex with Albrecht von Haller. Perhaps the best piece of physiologic
work in this century was carried out in the field of respiration. The identification of the various gases in the atmosphere was a major contribution. Carbon dioxide was
discovered by Joseph Black (1757), hydrogen by Henry
Cavendish (1766), nitrogen by Daniel Rutherford (1772),

and oxygen independently by Joseph Priestley and Karl W. Scheele (1774).

Benardino Ramazzini studied in Parma, where he qualified in 1659. He was, first, professor of medicine at the University of Modena and, later, at the University of Padua. He is recognized as the father of occupational medicine. He published his observations as *De Morbis Artificium Diatriba* (48). Early in the 18th century, Ramazzini drew attention to the irritant effect of organic dusts among grain workers in causing both shortness of breath and an urticarial reaction, detailing the pulmonary consequences of many trades and professions. He described cases of asthma in handlers of old mattresses and dusty old clothes—both probably infested with the house dust mite. In the chapters on the diseases of "Starch Makers," "Bakers" and "Millers," "Sifters and Meters of Corn," "Horse-coursers," "Grooms and Post Riders," and workers who "Pick or Hatchel, Flax, Hemp and Silk," he provided graphic descriptions of cases of occupational asthma.

The nervous system became better understood and appreciated during this century, mainly through the efforts of such workers as Morgagni, von Haller, and Robert Whyth. As a consequence of this, a novel medical system developed that was based on the "irritability" and "sympathy" of the muscles and nerves. William Cullen, considered by many to have been second only to Boerhaave, went so far as to state that most diseases were caused by either too much or too little nervous "tone," a pathologic condition that he called a "neurosis." Cullen, in his *Synopsis Nosologiae Methodicae* (49), considered "neuroses" as afflictions of sense and motion that were unaccompanied by pyrexia and for which no localized defect was immediately apparent. These conditions were therefore considered to be "functional" as opposed to "structural" in nature. Included in this new category were hysteria, tetanus, colic, epilepsy, and asthma. He defined asthma as "a difficulty of breathing, returning at intervals, with a sense of straitness in the breast, respiration performed with a wheezing noise at the beginning of a paroxysm, a distressing cough, sometimes more, but towards the end easy and free, often with a copious discharge of phlegm." Cullen's model of the neuroses was to persist well into the 19th century. In discussing asthma, in his successful textbook *First Lines of the Practice of Physic* (50), Cullen argued that the term referring to this condition should be applied in a restrictive and specific manner to one definite disease. As precipitating causes, he listed heat, cold, passions of the mind, particular odors, and irritations of smoke and dust. Cullen was among the first to realize and emphasize the seriousness of this condition: "The asthma, though often threatening immediate death, seldom occasions it, and many persons have lived under this disease. In many cases, however, it does prove fatal; sometimes very quickly and perhaps always at length" (51).

In the same year in which Cullen published in Edinburgh, his *Synopsis Nosologiae Methodicae*, John Millar, another Scottish physician, published his *Observations on the Asthma and on the Hooping Cough* in London (52). In his book, he described the natural history of asthma in children, but unfortunately, at times, confused asthma with croup; the latter was for a long time referred to as "asthma Millari."

Toward the end of the 18th century, Robert Bree wrote perhaps one of the more authoritative books on the subject of asthma. He too "suffered from the tyranny of asthma" and in 1793 had such a severe attack that it made him seek temporary retirement from his profession. His book, *A Practical Inquiry into Disordered Respiration, Distinguishing the Species of Convulsive Asthma, Their Causes and Indications of Cure* (53), according to Munk (54), "embodied the numerous experiments in his own case, gave a more full and complete view of asthma and dyspnoea than had hitherto appeared, and laid down some important therapeutic rules, the practical value of which has been universally acknowledged." He was among the first to try using the inhalation of "factitious gases" (oxygen and carbon dioxide), whose use had been introduced by Thomas Beddoes (55) at his Pneumatic Institute in Bristol.

THE 19TH CENTURY

The medicine of the first half of the 19th century was, with a few notable exceptions, merely a simple extension of the stationary, oftentimes sterile, theorizing of the preceding century. Up to 1850, and perhaps even for some decades after, most of the advancements in medicine were made by French physicians. Toward the end of the 18th century, Paul Varnier (56) described the ability of the normal bronchi to contract in a paper entitled "Sur l'Irritabilité des Poumons," published in 1779. A few years later, Franz Daniel Reisseisen (57) of Strasbourg showed that the bronchial wall contained a distinct layer of muscle that, when it contracted, resulted in a constriction of the bronchial airways. In 1819, Krimer (58) demonstrated that stimulation of the vagus nerve resulted in bronchoconstriction. Following Reisseisen's anatomic study of the bronchial musculature, a number of other fundamental papers appeared reviewing its structure (59). Reisseisen had pointed out that the airway smooth muscle is arranged in such an architectural manner as to allow for the easy adaptation of the rhythmic changes in airway dimensions that he considered an integral part of breathing. Toldt (60) provided one of the earliest, more detailed descriptions of the muscle component of the bronchi. He described the muscle fibers as being arranged in a latticelike form (Gitterförmige), dispelling earlier descriptions of it as forming a completely closed muscular tube.

The great French clinician, Réné T. H. Laënnec (61), contributed to the further clarification of the nature and diagnosis of asthma through the use of the stethoscope, which he invented in 1816. In the first edition of his classic book, *Traité de l'Auscultation Médiate*, his definition of asthma—"Le mot asthma signifie proprement difficulté de réspirer"—was no great improvement on what had previously been published. In his second edition (1826), however, having in the meantime seen a French translation of Reisseisen's work, he was convinced that bronchospasm was an essential feature of asthma. Laënnec wrote, "On conçoit très bien que la contraction spasmodique de ces fibres puisse être portée assez loin poir étrangler les conduits aériens et empêcher la pénétration de l'air dans une grande partie des poumons." He believed that the contraction of the bronchial smooth muscle fibers could be carried to the point of strangling the air passages, preventing the entry of air into a large part of the lung. Laënnec believed the mechanism of the disease to consist of a nervous stimulation causing a spasm of the bronchioles, which is associated with a specific asthmatic catarrh. Laënnec's clinical concept of bronchospasm was later further confirmed experimentally by a number of workers, including Charles J. B. Williams (62), François Achille Longet (63), and Alfred Willem Volkmann (64). The last described a dramatic experiment in which stimulation of the vagus nerves in dead animals resulted in an expiration strong enough to blow out a candle. In 1854, Max Anton Wintrich (65), a professor at Erlangen, repeated the experiments of Longet and Volkmann but obtained negative results. He then put forward the theory that asthma was the result of tonic spasm of the diaphragm. George Budd (66) was also unable to produce bronchial contraction in rabbits. Wintrich's theory was criticized by Biermer, Einthoven (67), and Beer, who, on repeating the experiment of Longet and Volkmann, produced not only constriction of the bronchi but also distension of the lungs.

On the other side of the Atlantic, John Eberle (68), in his popular book *A Treatise on the Practice of Medicine* (1830), reviewed what was then known about asthma and listed atmospheric conditions, inhalation of "offensive vapors," and dietary indiscretions as precipitating factors. Charles Turner Thackrah wrote one of the classic works on occupational medicine. In discussing coffee roasters, he stated that when these workers have been at this job for a number of years they often become asthmatic (69). Thackrah was aware that Laënnec had managed to define and differentiate asthma from other conditions that are characterized by breathlessness, but confessed that he himself was still using the term somewhat loosely. Among the occupations he listed with which asthma was associated were those of feather dressers, corn millers, malsters, snuff makers, flax spinners, some dressers of cloth, rag sorters, willyers, miners, grinders, masons, machine workers, and workers in certain kinds of wood.

The author of one of the best 19th-century books on asthma was Henry Hyde Salter (70). Probably because he was an asthmatic, his special research interest was focused on this condition. He published various papers on asthma and, finally, putting together his many experiences, even personal ones, wrote his magnum opus, *On Asthma: Its Pathology and Treatment*. Salter defined asthma as "paroxysmal dyspnoea of a peculiar character, generally periodic with intervals of healthy respiration between the attacks." He knew that it was "not an uncommon disease" and that "it is one of the direst suffering; the horrors of the asthmatic paroxysm far exceed any acute bodily pain; the sense of impending suffocation, the agonizing struggle for the breath of life, are so terrible, that they cannot even be witnessed without sharing in the sufferer's distress." No other description has better conveyed the asthmatic patient's plight.

He was aware of the hereditary nature of this condition and gave an account of asthma, present in three generations, that was triggered by being in the vicinity of different animals. Similarly, he appreciated the role that emotional disturbances could play in asthma. He believed asthma to be a form of "perverted nervous action" and to be, "exclusively, a nervous disease." Salter classified asthma into two main types: idiopathic, uncomplicated, or *spasmodic*; and symptomatic, complicated, or *organic*. Although the concept of allergy had not yet been introduced, Salter was among the first to point out that animal and vegetable emanations could precipitate an asthmatic attack. He listed among these emanations those of cats, rabbits, horses, wild beasts, guinea pigs, dogs, cattle, hay, and grass. He considered the mechanism by which these emanations cause asthma to be of a nervous reflex nature.

Salter wrongly assumed that inflammation of the respiratory mucus membrane had no role to play in the sudden onset of dyspnea: "To produce such dyspnoea, the inflammation must be intense...." He went on to discuss the various ways in which the bronchial tubes could be narrowed, explaining that as the reason why asthmatic breathing "is accompanied with a shrill sibilant whistle." He believed that the "sibilus of asthma" could not be produced by a "plug of tenacious mucus sticking to the side of the tube...." and because it was transient, it could likewise not be caused by a "vascular tumidity of the mucus membrane...." He therefore concluded that, "by evidence as certain as sight," in asthma, "bronchial spasm must and does exist" and that "no other conceivable supposition will explain the phenomena."

In spite of his otherwise amazing powers of observation and deduction, his theorizing cannot always be considered to have been inspired. He emphasized that "few cases could be found of true spasmodic asthma in which the disease is uninfluenced by the state of the digestive organs, while in a very large number it is entirely under their control." In these cases, he thought, bronchospasm was induced by reflex stimulation via the pneumogastric nerve and by "contaminate" blood, that is, blood-carrying substances that it had picked up from the alimentary canal. Salter listed a number of food items that, "either from their being peculiarly offensive when materially present in the lungs" or by being "specially irritating to the gastric portion of the vagus' could give rise to asthmatic attacks." Salter was certain that "sleep favours asthma." He carefully observed the effects of avoiding sleep, of posture during sleep, and of eating before sleep. He advised his patient to get out of bed at the very onset of an attack; realizing that this may be difficult, he emphasized, "but he *must* do it." Salter knew that asthma was not only "superlatively distressing" but also that, when it came to treatment, it was "peculiarly and proverbially intractable." He admitted that "the remedies for asthma" are "of very irregular and uncertain operation." Salter knew only too well that "vague and erroneous notions" about asthma were entertained by many of his contemporaries. He adduced "the possible absence of appreciable organic change, as shown by postmortem examination, in cases where the disease has not been of long standing" as evidence in favor of a nervous etiology. Salter, too, had his own incorrect views. He held that "asthma never kills; at least I have never seen a case in which a paroxysm proved fatal." Salter believed that "if asthma kills, it always does so by producing organic changes in the heart or lungs, or both" and it is "on this tendency to the generation of organic disease that the gravity of asthma depends." Having tried to be as comprehensive as possible in writing about this condition, he was, however, honest enough to declare that there were "questions that in the present state of our knowledge it would be difficult or impossible to answer." He then focused on the phenomenon of bronchial hyperresponsiveness, which was to occupy the research interest of many investigators in the field of respiratory medicine: "It is clear that the vice in asthma consists, not in the production of any special irritant, but in the irritability of the part irritated."

Armand Trousseau (71), one of the foremost French clinicians of his time, stated "to have myself been long subject to asthma, and my fits used to return about three o'clock in the morning." He considered asthma to be a "capricious" nervous disorder ("véritable nérvose de l'appareil pulmonaire"). He defined what he termed "idiopathic asthma" as a common condition that, according to him, was, however, rarely seen in hospitals; that occurred in the absence of a demonstrable organic lesion; and that presented itself as paroxysms of dyspnea and oppression. He presented a vivid description of a patient with nocturnal asthma who is awakened by a sudden attack: "Thus, an individual in perfect health goes to bed feeling as well as usual, and drops off quietly to sleep, but after an hour or two, he is suddenly awakened by a most distressing attack of dyspnoea. He feels as though his chest were constricted and compressed, and has a sense of considerable distress; he breathes with difficulty, and his inspiration is accompanied by a laryngotracheal whistling sound. The dyspnoea and sense of anxiety increasing, he sits up, rests on his hands, with his arms put back while his face is turgid, occasionally livid, red, or bluish, his eyes prominent, and his skin bedewed with perspiration. He is soon obliged to jump off his bed, and if the room in which he sleeps be not very lofty, he hastens to throw his window open in search of air. Fresh air, playing freely about, relieves him. Yet the fit lasts one or two hours or more, and then terminates." Other patients with nocturnal asthma fared worse for they may have been "obliged to sleep in the most varied and sometimes the queerest attitudes. Sometimes, he can only find sleep by kneeling on his bed and resting his head on his knees, or by spending the night in an armchair, or by propping himself up in bed in the sitting posture; sometimes again, he can only sleep standing, resting on a piece of furniture or on the mantelpiece." He gave a number of thumbnail sketches of patients whose asthma was triggered by various causes. Trousseau continued to use traditional remedies such as "a large flying blister to be applied to the whole chest immediately," "ipecacuanha, given at the onset in emetic doses," "Belladonna or atropia, followed on the ensuing days by the administration of spirits of turpentine...." In his own case, he even used tobacco, as Salter had done: "I am not an habitual smoker, but I then had a cigar, and took a few puffs; in eight or ten minutes the paroxysm was over." He also prescribed stramonium leaves, fumigating with them the rooms where the asthmatic patient lay and also getting the patient to smoke them. He was aware of the early history and use of *Datura* species in traditional Indian medical practice and how General Gent on his return from Madras introduced the preparation to Dr. Sims of Edinburgh. The preparation used by Gent, which had been administered to him by Dr. Anderson, the physician general at Madras, consisted of the dried and pulverized roots of *Datura ferox.* Trousseau knew that Sims had found that *Datura stramonium* was an equally good substitute. He claimed that "of all the remedies which have been tried in asthma, stramonium generally answers best." He pointed out, however, that not all asthmatics were relieved and, in particular, "habitual tobacco-smokers often derive no benefit from it." Possibly this was because such patients were not asthmatics but bronchitics. Trousseau also administered arsenic cigarettes and recommended the inhalation of the fumes of burning niter paper.

In his opinion, asthma was "a special and complete disorder, a manifestation, a peculiar form of a general complaint, having very variable local expressions, sometimes giving rise to paroxysms of dyspnoea, of oppression at the chest, to a curious kind of coryza, and to peculiar catarrhal attacks....." Unfortunately he also had a number of mistaken ideas, believing that "eczematous eruptions, rheumatism, gout, haemorrhoids, hemicrania, and fits of the gravel" were complaints that could replace asthma and could be replaced by it in turn. He also believed in a close association between tuberculosis and asthma—possibly because both conditions were then so frequent. Trousseau asserted that "tubercular individuals may, therefore, give birth to asthmatic children, and, on the other hand, asthmatic subjects may have tubercular children." Strangely enough, Trousseau did not only consider asthma not to be potentially life threatening, ("asthma n'est pas fatale"), but went even further and described it as the certificate of a long life ("le brevet de longue vie")!

During the last three decades of the 19th century, the microscopic examination of the sputum of asthmatic patients revealed the presence of characteristic pointed, octahedral crystals and also of spirals. In 1853, Jean Charcot, the great neurologist at the Salpétrière Hospital in Paris, together with his colleague Charles-Phillippe Robin (72), reported finding characteristic crystals in the blood and spleen of a leukemic patient and in the sputum of a bronchitic woman. In 1860, Charcot, together with his friend Edmé Felix Vulpian (73), published a more detailed study of the crystals. It ought to be pointed out that Charcot never associated these crystals with asthma. It is thought that these crystals had actually been first observed by Friedrich Albert Zenker (74) in 1851, but he did not publish his findings until 1870. Other workers, including August Foerster (75) and Peter Harting (76), reported seeing them in the sputum of bronchitic patients. In 1870, Ernest von Leyden (77), together with his assistant Max Jaffe, were the first to see these crystals in the sputum of an asthmatic patient. The following year, Leyden announced his finding at a medical meeting and published his first report in *Virchow's Archives* in 1872; a more detailed description was presented 14 years later. These crystals came to be termed Charcot–Leyden crystals and for some time were thought to be the cause of the asthmatic attack, possibly by exerting a local mechanical irritant effect on the bronchial mucosa, which in turn reflexly produced bronchospasm. Leyden tried, unsuccessfully, to reproduce asthma by introducing powdered glass into the airway of animals. Salter had included an illustration in his book of "corpuscles" seen in asthmatic sputum, among which were objects that looked like crystals, but he did not identify them. The "corpuscles" were probably eosinophils, which were first described and termed "eosinophilen leukocythen" by Paul Ehrlich (78) in 1879, when he introduced eosin in his technique for the differential staining of leukocytes. De Jong and Romieu (79), in 1923, were among the first to suggest a close relationship between Charcot–Leyden crystals and eosinophils, maintaining that their numbers increased in proportion to the number of eosinophils undergoing degeneration.

Heinrich Curschmann (80), while at Hamburg, discovered and described spiral mucoid casts in asthmatic sputum, which he claimed were the cause of asthma, contesting Leyden's views about the causation of this condition. Curschmann contended that the crystals might be a degenerate form of the spirals. He continued to study them, and they were eventually linked to his name. In 1883, he published a more detailed study of them in relation to the sputum of a variant of asthma that he called "bronchiolitis exudativa" (81). Curschmann realized that these spirals were merely the expectorated mucus casts, formed from inspissated mucus secretions originating in the smaller bronchioles. Sir William Osler (82), in his great textbook *The Principle and Practice of Medicine*, described two forms of the spirals: one was "simply a twisted, spirally arranged mucin, in which are entangled leucocytes, the majority of which are eosinophiles," and a second, "more peculiar" type consisted of "a tightly coiled skein of mucil fibrils with a few scattered cells," in the center of which "is a filament of extraordinary clearness and translucency...." He agreed with Curschmann that they were "doubtless formed in the finer bronchioles and constitute the product of an acute bronchiolitis." He confessed that "it is difficult to explain their spiral nature" and that he did not know of any observations upon the air currents produced by the bronchial ciliated epithelial lining. Osler thought that the flow of these currents could be a rotatory one and that this, combined with bronchospasm, would result in the mucus being "compelled to assume a spiral form." Osler pointed out that these spirals "occur in all instances of true bronchial asthma in the early period of the attack." Curschmann spirals, which often contain eosinophils and crystals, are now known to consist chiefly of glycoprotein. No longer do the crystals or the spirals have any significant diagnostic importance.

Another cell that was subsequently found to be involved in the pathology of asthma is the mast cell. Although Friedrich Daniel von Recklinghausen (83) described the presence of granular cells in connective tissue in 1863, the first definite description of mast cells is also generally attributed to Paul Ehrlich (84). In 1877, while still a medical student and 2 years before his identification of the eosinophil, he described the staining of mast cell granules with certain basic dyes. He coined the term "metachromasia" for the modification in color that occurs when these aniline dyes bind to mast cell granules.

William Osler's medical textbook was the most authoritative source used for medical teaching for quite a number of years. His discussion on asthma was, however, somewhat brief. He, too, observed the similarity of hay fever and asthma and remarked, quoting Sir Andrew Clark, that "these diseases have the same origin and differ only in site." Osler defined asthma as "a neurotic affection, characterized by hyperaemia and turgescence of the mucosa of the smaller bronchial tubes and a peculiar exudate of mucin." He agreed with Eberle on the probable reflex nature of this condition. Unfortunately, his use of the adjective "neurotic" left, in the eyes of the uninformed, a stigma attached to sufferers from asthma that persists even today, though very probably he used the adjective in the sense of neurologic. Osler insisted that the term "asthma" should be used strictly in the context of bronchial asthma. Strangely enough, even this outstanding clinician accepted the prevailing views in his day that asthma could be induced "indirectly, too, by reflex influences, from stomach, intestines or genital organs" and that "flatulence" and "passage of a large quantity of urine" were premonitory sensations. He realized that, besides bronchial smooth muscle contraction and hypertrophy, already emphasized by Salter and Trousseau, mucosal edema and airway mucus also made significant contributions to airflow obstruction: "The hyperaemia and swelling of the mucosa and the extremely viscid, tenacious mucus explain well the hindrance to inspiration and expiration and also the quality of the rales." Osler contributed to the myth that asthma was never fatal, claiming that "death during the attack is unknown." He did, however, emphasize that the asthmatic attack "demands immediate and prompt treatment." His treatment consisted of the usual range of "sedative antispasmodics" such as belladonna, henbane, stramonium, and lobelia, sometimes administered as cigarettes. In addition, he also recommended "Perles of nitrite of amyl" broken "on the handkerchief" and "a dose of spirits of chloroform in hot whisky." Unlike Salter, Osler was of the opinion that "more permanent relief is given by the hypodermic injection of morphia or of morphia and cocaine combined." Osler considered that "the use of compressed air in the pneumatic cabinet" was also beneficial, as were oxygen inhalations. His favorite prophylactic was iodide of potassium, which he gave in a dose of 10 to 20 grains, three times a day. He did not allow his patients to eat any carbohydrates because he believed that these produced flatulence that, in turn, induced attacks. Coffee was also thought to be a more suitable drink than tea, but he did not list it as a remedy.

THE MODERN ERA

The rapid significant developments in science in general, and in medicine in particular, during the present century have obviously been reflected also in the advances made in the understanding and treatment of asthma. Charles Robert Richet, Professor of Physiology in Paris, while working with Paul Portier (85), described, in 1902, the phenomenon of "anaphylaxis." They based their findings on experiments carried out in dogs, using injections of extracts of Portuguese man-of-war and later of the tentacles of sea anemones (*Actina*). In 1905, Clemens von Pirquet, of Berlin, together with Bela Schick (86), described a similar phenomenon in patients who had received single or repeated injections of horse serum. In the following year, von Pirquet (87) suggested that the term anaphylaxis should not be used any longer because it was inaccurate, since no diminution in protection was involved. He coined the term "allergy," from the Greek "allos" (meaning "other"), implying a changed state and indicating the altered reaction to a foreign substance after previous sensitization. In 1906, Alfred Wolff-Eisner (88) suggested that hay fever was an anaphylactic phenomenon taking place in the conjunctiva. He showed that practically all of his 90 asthmatic patients reacted positively to a pollen suspension introduced in the eye. Early pioneers in this field, including François Magendie, Simon Flexner, Theobald Smith, Maurice Arthus, Richard Otto, John Auer, and Paul A. Lewis, rapidly advanced our knowledge in this field.

John Auer and Paul A. Lewis (89), working in Samuel James Meltzer's laboratory, were to play especially important roles. Their studies establishing that bronchiolar stenosis was the principle manifestation of anaphylaxis in the guinea pig were published in 1910. In their paper, they stated that "immediate anaphylactic death in guinea pigs is caused by asphyxia: cessation of respiration is secondary to this asphyxia." They indicated that the asphyxia was "apparently produced by a tetanic contraction of the smooth muscles of the bronchioles, which occludes their lumen gradually, so that finally no air enters or leaves the lungs, in spite of violent respiratory efforts, and the animal is strangulated." That same year, Meltzer (90), influenced by the findings of his two young colleagues, presented a paper at the 25th meeting of the Association of American Physicians, where he suggested that the asthmatic paroxysm was a manifestation of anaphylaxis.

The anaphylactic or non-nervous origin of asthma resulted in a period of exploratory skin testing. In 1911, Leonard Noon (91), of St. Mary's Hospital in London, introduced specific allergy skin testing, using an extract of grass pollen. Diagnosis of hypersensitivity soon led to attempts at specific desensitization, a method of treatment in which Noon, John Freeman (92), in London, and Robert Anderson Cooke (93), in the United States, became pioneers. In 1918, Isaac Chandler Walker (94), a Boston physician, realized that not all asthmatic patients showed prominent skin hypersensitivity. He proposed a classification of asthma based on skin-test responses and introduced the terms "intrinsic" and "extrinsic," depending on whether there were negative or positive skin responses.

Maximilian A. Ramirez (95), in 1919, made an observation which suggested that dermal reactivity and hypersensitivity might both be induced by substances that he called "anaphylactic or reaction bodies" present in the blood. In a very short paper, he described how a 35-year-old Greek waiter became passively sensitized to "horse dandruff" following a "blood transfusion for primary anaemia" and suffered his first asthmatic attack on going for "a carriage ride in Central Park." Ramirez later classified asthma into "allergic exudative" and "nonallergic spastic" types. Carl Prausnitz and Heinz Küstner (96) performed their classic experiment of passively sensitizing human skin and were the first to show the transmissibility of the immediate anaphylactic reaction in 1921 at the Institute of Hygiene, University of Breslau. A. F. Coca and R. A. Cooke (97), in 1923, introduced the term "atopy" to describe a hypersensitivity to allergens that was dependent upon a hereditary predisposition to acquire such a hypersensitivity and that was mediated by a sensitizing agent. This sensitizing agent (antibody) capable of mediating immediate hypersensitivity reactions was called "reagin" by A. F. Coca and E. Grove (98) in 1925. Not until the late 1960s was the real nature of reagin revealed through the discovery of a unique myeloma protein, representing a new immunoglobulin class: IgND. These studies were carried out by S. G. O. Johannson and H. Bennich (99) in Sweden. Johannson (100) reported finding raised levels of IgND in asthma. Further work by this group and, independently, by Kimshige Ishizaka and Teruko Ishizaka (101), from the Children's Asthma Research Institute in Denver, Colorado, elucidated the biological properties of IgND and laid the foundation for the identification of the fifth immunoglobulin class—IgE— in 1968 (102). At the same time, Wide and his colleagues (103) developed the radioallergosorbent test (RAST) for measuring IgE antibodies *in vitro*.

As soon as asthma became recognized to have an allergic basis, research took on a new dimension, with investigators searching for offending allergens, which included pollen grains, fungal spores, and chemicals, as well as drugs. Wilhelm Storm van Leeuwen (104), having shown that both pollen grains as well as mold spores were common allergens, suggested enclosing asthmatic patients in an allergen-proof chamber or exposing them to high altitudes, where such allergens are rare. He is probably the first to have studied aspirin-induced asthma. In 1928, he challenged 100 asthmatics with aspirin and provoked a pulmonary reaction in 16 (105). In the same year, Dekker (106) first implicated a mite as a clinically significant allergen in asthma. It was not until 1967, however, that the group from the University of Leiden, led by M. I. A. Spieksma and R. Voorhorst (107), identified the house dust mite, *Dermatophagoides pteronyssinus*, as the allergen in house dust.

Histamine was implicated in the pathogenesis of allergic diseases by Henry Hallett Dale and Patrick Laidlaw (108), who studied its physiologic effects, shortly after the identification of its structure by Adolf Windaus and Karl Vogt (109) in 1907. Dale and Laidlaw, later both knighted, showed its ability to mimic the features of ana-phylaxis in animals after its intravenous infusion. Soma Weiss (1898–1942) and his colleagues (110), in 1928, re-produced the clinical features of asthma, but not the anaphlyactic shock seen in animals, when they injected histamine intravenously in asthmatic patients. Their find-ings were extended almost 20 years later by John J. Curry (111), who demonstrated that both inhaled and parenteral histamine could induce a fall in vital capacity in asthmat-ics but not in nonasthmatic subjects. Some time later, Schild and co-workers (112), in the Department of Phar-macology at University College in London, showed that when human asthmatic lung was exposed to specific anti-gen *in vitro*, bronchoconstriction was associated with his-tamine release.

Other lipid mediators also started being studied, in-cluding a slow-reacting smooth muscle-stimulating sub-stance in anaphylaxis (SRS-A). In the 1960s and 1970s, various groups of workers identified and isolated the var-ious oxygenated derivatives of cell membrane arachi-donic acid. These eicosanoids were shown to include a whole range of prostaglandins, leukotrienes, thrombox-ane, and platelet-activating factor. Bronchial provocation tests began to be used increasingly at this time to deter-mine airway hyperresponsiveness. Challenge of the bronchi with inhaled allergen was first reported by F. A. Stevens (113) in 1934. In 1941, Dautrebande and Philpott (114) showed that the inhalation of an aerosol of carba-chol produced a bronchoconstriction resembling asthma. Three years later, Robert Tiffeneau and Maurice Beau-vallet (115) proposed that tests employing an acetyl-choline aerosol could be employed to determine the severity of respiratory impairment. These French workers were among the first to explore and measure hyperre-sponsiveness. F. C. Lowell and I. W. Schiller (116) demonstrated, in 1947, a fall in vital capacity in asthmatic patients after exposure to aerosolized pollen extracts. Herbert Herxheimer (117) used such pharmacologic agents as histamine and methylcholine, as well as house dust, in his studies and helped develop the technique of bronchial challenge testing, being the first to distinguish between immediate and late asthmatic responses. Later, Jack Pepys and his group (118) from the Brompton Hos-pital stirred the present interest in the late-onset response with their studies involving industrial enzymes and *As-pergillus fumigatus*.

Soon after Ehrlich's initial description of the eosinophil, it became apparent that the cell was intimately associated with asthma. In 1908, A. G. Ellis (119) described the as-sociation of blood and tissue eosinophilia in the lungs of a patient who died of asthma. The first detailed account of both the macroscopic and microscopic postmortem ap-pearances of the lungs in asthma were published by H. L. Huber and K. K. Koessler (120) in 1922. This classic pa-per describes in detail the clinical and pathologic findings in six cases of asthma, and contains many hand-painted color illustrations of the microscopic appearances. They also reviewed the previously reported 15 cases of asth-matic deaths in which a microscopic examination had been performed. I. G. MacDonald (121), in 1933, was among the first to give an account of the heavy eosinophilic infiltration of the airway walls that was de-tected in histopathologic studies of bronchial tissue taken from patients who had died of asthma. B. S. Cardell and R. S. B. Pearson (122) emphasized the finding of mucus plugging of the bronchi, infiltration of bronchial walls by eosinophils, and thickening of the basement membrane in the postmortems they carried out in fatal cases of asthma. M. S. Dunnill, G. R. Massarella, and J. A. Anderson (123), in 1969, measured the increase in the smooth muscle con-tent of asthmatic airways, and S. Hosain (124), in 1973, showed that this increase in muscle mass is mainly the re-sult of hyperplasia, but that hypertrophy of individual muscle fibers may also contribute to it.

The development of modern drug therapy for the treat-ment of asthma deserves at least a chapter all to itself. This century has witnessed an unprecedented scientific approach to the management of this condition as its pathogenesis and underlying inflammatory nature have become unraveled. The therapeutics of this period reflect the advances made in the basic medical sciences. Anti-cholinergic drugs are probably the oldest single class of pharmacologic agents used in asthma. The first specific mention of *Datura* species in the treatment of asthma was in the *Yogaratnakara* from 17th-century India (125). In 1833, Philipp Lorenz Geiger and Hermann Hesse (126) isolated the active alkaloid atropine ("DATURINE") from *Datura stramonium*, but it was not till 1941 that an objective assessment of its effects in bronchial asthma was carried out by L. Dautreband and colleagues (127), who demonstrated that atropine had a bronchodilating ef-fect and thought that it was particularly useful in treating those patients who had excessive bronchial mucus. In 1959, Herxheimer (128) showed that the smoking of cig-arettes containing atropine sulfate resulted in an increase in vital capacity. The contemporary use of anticholiner-gics in treating bronchial asthma is attributable to the de-velopment of such quaternary anticholinergic agents as ipratropium bromide.

The Chinese have used the herb Ma Huang empirically for various ailments for some 5,000 years. Its chief active principle was isolated in crystalline form in 1887 by the Japanese physician Nagayoshi Nagai (129) and named ephedrine. Ku Kuei Chen and Carl Frederic Schmidt (130) investigated the alkaloid in greater detail. For a long time, it proved to be a popular and effective treatment for asthma. The discovery of adrenaline in the adrenal medulla in 1856 by Edme Felix Alfred Vulpian (131); the demonstration in 1895 by George Oliver and Edward Sharpey-Schäfer (132) that the extract from the adrenal gland was a powerful blood pressure-elevating substance; its isolation in 1901 independently by Jôkichi Takamine

(133) and by Thomas Bell Aldrich (134); and its synthesis in 1904 by Friedrich Stoltz (135), started a new era in the treatment of asthma. In 1900, Solomon Solis-Cohen (136), Professor of Medicine in Philadelphia, was the first to use the relatively crude "adrenal substance" in hay fever and asthma. He wrote, "I believe that we have in this substance a decided addition to therapeutic resources....," commenting finally, "What the active agent is and how much or how little of that active agent is absorbed, I must leave to laboratory students to determine." In 1903, Jesse J. M. Bullowa and David Kaplan (137) reported the first successful use of this drug in the treatment of asthma. Adrenaline could only be administered parenterally, and Percy Camps (138), a physician at Guy's Hospital in London, was the first to try using it by inhalation in 1929. Isoprenaline was synthesized in 1940 by H. Konzett (139), but only became widely available in pressured aerosol form in the early 1960s and was soon associated with the rise in mortality from asthma in Great Britain in the 1960s and soon withdrawn. Until R. P. Ahlquist's classic paper (140), adrenergic receptors were initially regarded as either excitatory or inhibitory. In 1948, Ahlquist showed that there were two classes of receptor, which could be differentiated by their responsiveness to a range of sympathomimetic amines and that, whether effects proved to be stimulating or not, depended upon the tissue being studied. Ahlquist thus distinguished between α- and β-adrenergic receptors. The β-receptors were further subdivided into two classes—β_1 and β_2, by A. M. Lands and his co-workers (141) in 1967. Their seminal work paved the way for the development of the potent selective β_2-adrenergic drugs we use today. The effect of Salbutamol was described in animals in 1968, and a number of clinical trials followed and were reported on in 1969. Terbutaline sulfate, introduced in the early 1970s, was shown to have a similar action profile as Salbutamol. Interest has recently centered around the development of longer-acting β_2-adrenoreceptor agonists such as formeterol and salmeterol, as well as the pro-drug bambuterol.

Theophylline (dimethyl xanthine) was isolated from cocoa (*Theobromine cacao*) in 1888 by the German, Nobel prize winner Albrecht Kossil (142). A soluble derivative, theophylline ethylenediamine (aminophylline), that could be administered parenterally was produced by P. Dessauer (143) in 1908. The bronchodilator activity of this group of drugs (methylxanthines) was first demonstrated in 1921 in the United States by David Israel Macht and Giu Ting (144), and theophylline was first used therapeutically in asthma a year later by Samson Hirsch (145) in Frankfurt. G. R. Hermann and M. B. Aynesworth (146), and J. A. Greene and co-workers (147), were the first to use aminophylline successfully in "status asthmaticus" and in "bronchial obstruction in cardiac failure" in 1937.

Following the isolation in crystalline form of cortisone, originally termed compound E, from the adrenal cortex, by Edward Kendall (148) in his laboratory at the Mayo Clinic in December 1933, the further characterization of the structure and the synthesis and understanding of the mode of action of glucocorticoids proved to be a slow process. This was mainly because of the initial need to handle large amounts of starting material and because of the limited technology then available. Cortisone was first used clinically in patients with rheumatoid arthritis, in a study carried out by Philip Hench (149) in 1949. Bordley and his co-workers (150) reported using ACTH in the treatment of acute severe asthma, whereas Harvier's group (151) published their findings on the use of this hormone in chronic asthma. It soon became apparent that ACTH offered no advantages over glucocorticoids, even in children, where it had been thought to cause less stunting of growth, and soon fell out of use. In 1950, two separate clinical studies on the effects of cortisone in bronchial asthma were published by Haydon Carryer and co-workers (152) and by Randolph and Rollins (153). Soon after the introduction of prednisone and prednisolone, under the names of metacortandracin and metacortandrolone, by Herzog's group (154) in 1955, Barach et al. (155) showed their therapeutic value in asthma, pointing out their decreased mineralocorticoid effects. In 1955, hydrocortisone was first administered intravenously to asthmatic patients by Burrage and Irwin (156). In an attempt to potentiate the anti-inflammatory effects and diminish unwanted systemic effects, a number of other glucocorticoids have been subsequently synthesized and studied. These include methylprednisolone, dexamethasone, cloprednol, and triamcinolone. None appear to have any marked advantages over prednisolone, which remains the standard oral preparation. Since the introduction of these drugs in the therapy of asthma, there has been no lack of controversy as to their usefulness, the indications for their use, doses required to control severe asthma, and their modes of action as well as the sites at which they are presumed to exert such actions. In 1956, in a multicenter trial conducted by the Medical Research Council (157,158) in Great Britain, it was concluded that glucocorticoids had no long-term value in chronic asthma but were useful in acute asthma. Although the positive role of these drugs in the treatment of chronic asthma was soon established, doubts about their usefulness in acute asthma have been expressed from time to time.

As glucocorticoids became more readily available, they rapidly gained a prominent role in the management of a wide variety of clinical conditions. There followed a quick appreciation of their serious side effects and potential hazards. Because of this, efforts were made, as early as 1950, to deliver them locally to the airways. Among the first attempts was that by Reeder and Mackay (159), who employed nebulized cortisone in the treatment of cases of bacterial pneumonia. A year later, in 1951, M. L. Gelfland (160) used cortisone as an aerosol suspended in saline to treat asthma. Subsequently, several attempts were made at administering inhaled hydrocortisone as a powder or as a solution to both adults and children suffering from asthma. They generally met with very limited success because the doses that were required for clinical effectiveness resulted in systemic side effects. As the search continued for more active glucocorticoids, dexamethasone phosphate became available and was soon tried in asthma. It, too, however, proved disappointing because it was found to be absorbed and to be systemically active when inhaled. The breakthrough came with the development of the topically active glucocorticoids, betamethasone valerate and beclomethasone dipropionate, in the United Kingdom. They were the first inhaled glucorticoids to achieve clinical success in the management of asthma and to be devoid of any significant side effects. Two independent studies were published in 1972 by Tim Clark (161) and Harry Morrow Brown (162). Other compounds became available later and include triamcinolone acetonide, flunisolide, budesonide, and flucatisone. The first objective study reporting improvement in lung function in asthmatics following glucocorticoid administration appeared in 1974 (163). Further studies soon followed, both from the same group from Edinburgh and Malta as well as from other workers (164). The modes of action of glucocorticoids in asthma are being determined, and these drugs are now firmly established as the most important anti-inflammatory agents in the management of this condition.

Among the pharmacologic agents used for the treatment of asthma, disodium cromoglycate was unique, at the time of its discovery, in being the only drug with no bronchodilating action and with a mainly prophylactic mode of action. This drug, a cromone, was derived from khellin. It had been known for centuries that the fruit of the wild Eastern Mediterranean plant "Ammi visnaga" (*Umbelliferae*), known to the Arabs as "khella," possessed the property of relaxing the muscle spasm in renal colic and was also a diuretic. K. Samaan and his co-workers (165) were the first to report that its active principle, khellin, has a direct relaxant action on visceral smooth muscle and coronary arteries and they later studied its pharmacology in greater detail. Further interest was aroused by the finding reported by G. V. Anrep and his associates (166) in 1947 that the drug caused a selective and marked increase in coronary blood flow. Other investigators soon became interested in the chemical and pharmacologic properties of khellin and its congeners, as well as in its clinical use in angina pectoris and bronchial asthma. The chemistry and physiologic actions of these compounds were later extensively reviewed by C. P. Huttrer and E. Dale (167). Khellin, however, was found to possess marked emetic properties when taken orally. In 1956, Roger Altounyan (168), himself an asthmatic, joined a team of pharmaceutical research workers who were investigating several synthesized derivatives of khellin. Altounyan evaluated a number of these compounds on himself, using antigen challenge techniques,

because he doubted that animal testing was the best model for asthma pharmacology. In January 1965, FPL 670, later called disodium cromoglycate, was synthesized, tested, and found to offer the best protection against antigen-induced airway obstruction. The first report on its action as a specific inhibitor of reaginic antibody–antigen mechanisms appeared in *Nature* in 1967 (169). It soon came to be regarded as a classic mast cell-stabilizing agent. This is no longer considered to be its main effect, and it is now thought that its other multiple pharmacologic effects account for its clinical prophylactic activity. Following the introduction of disodium cromoglycate, various workers tried to introduce an oral mast cell-stabilizing agent. The drug ketotifen was launched with claims that it possessed such an activity in the late 1970s. The last drug with mast cell effects to be introduced was nedocromil sodium in the mid-1980s. It has been shown to possess a similar range of activities in various test systems as disodium cromoglycate and appears to be even more powerful in some of them.

Never as now, in the history of bronchial asthma, has so much knowledge been accumulated about this condition. No physicians, in any other age, have had at their disposal the pharmacologic means that can effectively prevent, as well as rapidly treat, bronchial asthma. May I be allowed to quote Armand Trousseau (67) one final time: "How often, gentlemen, has it not happened that very learned, intelligent and attentive physicians have seen, without discerning them, disorders which another more careful and a better observer, perhaps more fortunate also, and better served by circumstances, has discovered and recognised afterwards!" Further education of the patient and the physician should ultimately result in a far more favorable outcome than that obtained presently.

REFERENCES

1. Ellul-Micallef R. Asthma: a look at the past. *Br J Dis Chest* 1976; 70:112–116.
2. Ebers G. *Das hermetische buch uber die arzneimittel der alten aegypter.* Leipzig: Henrichs, 1875.
3. Ebell B. *The papyrus ebers.* Copenhagen: Levin Munksgaard, 1937.
4. Danby H. *The mishnah.* Oxford: Oxford University Press, 1933.
5. Epstein I. *The babylonian talmud.* London: Soncino, 1935.
6. Adams F, trans. *The genuine works of Hippocrates.* Baltimore: Williams and Wilkins, 1939.
7. Hippocrates. Airs, waters, places. In: Chadwick J, Mann WN, eds. *The medical works of Hippocrates.* Oxford: Blackwell Scientific, 1950; 90–111.
8. Celsus A. *De medicina,* 3 vols. Spencer WG, trans. London: Heinmann, 1935–1938.
9. Adams F, trans. *The extant works of Aretaeus, the Cappodocian.* London: Sydenham Society, 1856.
10. Galen C. *Oeuvres anatomiques physiologiques et médicales de Galien.* Daremberg Ch, trans. Paris: Baillière, 1856.
11. Schneider CV. *Liber primum de catarrhis* Wittenburg: T Mevii and E Schumacheri, 1660.
12. Marock G. *Die geschichte des bronchialasthmas.* Kleviert: Quankenbüch, 1934.
13. Caelius A. *De morbis acutis et chronicis.* Drabkin IE, trans. Chicago: University of Chicago, 1950.

14. Adams F, trans. *The seven books of Paulus Aegineta,* vol 1. London: Sydenham Society, 1844.
15. Ar-Rhazi M. *Kitab al-Häwi fit-tibb (Continens).* Hyderabad: Deccan, 1955–1971.
16. Meyerhof M. Thirty-three clinical observations by Rhazes (circa 900 AD). *Isis* 1935;23:321–372.
17. Withington ET. *Medical history from the earliest times.* London, 1873.
18. Gohlman WE. *The life of ibn Sina: a critical edition and annotated translation.* New York: Albany, 1974.
19. Ibn-Sina A. *Kitab al-Qänün fit-tibb,* 2 vols. Rome, 1593.
20. Avicenna. *Liber canonis.* Di Cremona G, trans. Mediolani: P de Lavagna, 1473.
21. Gruner OC. *A treatise on the canon of medicine of Avicenna.* London: Luzac, 1930.
22. Maimonides M. *The medical writings of Moses Maimonides: treatise on asthma.* Muntner S, ed. Philadelphia: JB Lippincott, 1963.
23. Muntner S. Maimonides' treatise on asthma. *Dis Chest* 1968;54:128–132.
24. Rosner F. Moses Maimonides' treatise on asthma. *Thorax* 1981;36:245–251.
25. Salernitanus N. *Antidotarium.* Venice: N Jensen, 1471.
26. *Pharmacopeia londinensis: opera medicorum collegii londinensis.* London: John Marriott, 1618.
27. Culpeper N. *A physical directory or a translation of the dispensatory made by the College of Physicians of London,* 2nd ed. London: Peter Cole, 1650.
28. Bonser W. *Medical background of Anglo-Saxon England.* London: Wellcome Historical Medical Library, 1963.
29. Gaddesden J. *Rosa anglica practica medicinae a capite ad pedes.* Pavia: JA Berretta, 1492.
30. Bartolomaeus A. *De proprietatibus rerum.* London: T Bertheleti, 1535.
31. Trevisa J, trans. *Bartolomeu de proprietatibus re.* Westminster: W de Worde, 1495.
32. Hohenheim PTB von (Paracelsus). *Aureoli opera.* Strasbourg: Lazari Zerners, 1603.
33. Hester J, trans. *Paracelsus: the key of philosophie.* London: Valentine Simmes, 1596.
34. Morley H. *The life of Girolamo Cardano of Milan, physician,* 2 vols. London: Chapman and Hall, 1854.
35. Cardano G. *The book of my life [De vita propria liber].* Stoner J, trans. London: JM Dent and Sons, 1931.
36. Wykes A. *Doctor Cardano: physician extraordinary.* London: Muller, 1969.
37. Cardano G. *Opera omnia Hieronymi Cardani: mediolanensis,* 10 vols. Lyons: Spon, 1663.
38. Helmont JB van. *Ortus medicinae, id est initia physicae inaudita.* Amstelodami: Elzevivium, 1648.
39. Helmont JB van. *Delirementa catarrhi: or the incongruities, impossibilities, and absurdities, couched under the vulgar opinion of defluxions.* London: William Lee, 1650.
40. Helmont JB van. *Oriatrike or physick refined.* London: L Lyoyd, 1662.
41. Willis T. *Pharmaceutice rationalis sive diatriba de medicamentorum operationibus in humano corpore.* London: Robertum Scott, 1674.
42. Willis T. *The London practice of physick or the whole practical part of physick contained in the works of Dr Willis (Faithfully made English by Eugenius).* London: Basset and Crooke, 1685.
43. Willis T. *Opera omnia,* 2 vols. Geneva: Samuelem de Tournes, 1680.
44. Dewhurst K. *John Locke: physician and philosopher.* London: Wellcome Historical Medical Library, 1963.
45. Floyer J. *A treatise of the asthma.* London: R Wilkin, 1698.
46. Floyer J. *An enquiry into the right use and abuses of the hot, cold and temperate baths in England.* London: R Clavell, 1697.
47. Garrison FH. *An introduction to the history of medicine,* 4th ed. Philadelphia: WB Saunders, 1963.
48. Ramazzini B. *De morbis artificium diatriba.* Mutinae: A Capponi, 1700.
49. Cullen W. *Synopsis nosologiae methodicae.* Edinburgh: G Creech, 1769.
50. Cullen W. *First lines of the practice of physic.* Edinburgh: W Creech, 1777.
51. Cullen W. *The works,* 2 vols. Edinburgh: W Blackwood, 1827.
52. Millar J. *Observations on the asthma and on the hooping cough.* London: T Cadel, 1769.
53. Bree R. *A practical enquiry into disordered respiration, distinguishing the species of convulsive asthma.* London: R Phillips, 1797.
54. Munk W. *The roll of the College of Physicians of London,* 2nd ed. London: The College, 1878.
55. Beddoes T. *Considerations on the medicinal use of factitious airs, and on the manner of obtaining them in large quantities. Part 1.* Bristol: Bulgin and Rosser, 1794.
56. Varnier P. Sur l'irritabalitè des poumons. *Mem Soc R Med* 1779;1:392.
57. Reisseisen FD. *Über den Bau der Lungen.* Berlin: Rucker, 1822.
58. Krimer W. *Untersuchungen über die nächste Ursache des Hustens mit Beziehung aus die Lehren vom Athemholen und vom Croup.* Liepzig: Carl Cnobloch, 1819.
59. Ellul-Micallef R. Airway smooth muscle in health and in asthma. *Br J Dis Chest* 1973;67:107–113.
60. Toldt C. *Lehrbuch der Gewelbelehre.* Stuttgart, 1888.
61. Laënnec RTH. *Traité de l'auscultation médiate.* Paris: Brosson and Chaudé, 1819 (2nd ed, 1826).
62. Williams CJB. Experiences sur la contractilité des poumons et des bronches. *Gaz Med (Paris)* 1841;9:517–519.
63. Longet FA. Recherches expérimentales sur la nature des mouvements intrinsèques du poumon et sur une nouvelle cause de l'emphysème pulmonaire. *C R Acad Sci (Paris)* 1842;55:500–503.
64. Volkmann AW. *Nervenphysiologie: Handwörkerbuch der Physiologie,* vol 2. Braunschweig: Wagner, 1844.
65. Wintrich MA. Einleitung zur Darstellung der Krankheiten der Respirationsorgane. In: Virchow R, ed. *Handbuch der speziellen Pathologie und Therapie,* vol 5. Erlangen, 1854.
66. Budd G. Remarks on emphysema of the lungs. *Med Chir Trans* (2nd ser) 1840;23:27–32.
67. Einthoven W. Ueber die Wirkung der Bronchialmunkskel, nach einer neuen Methode untersuch, und über Asthma Nervosum. *Arch Ges Physiol* 1892;51:367–371.
68. Eberle J. *Treatise on the practice of medicine,* vol 2. Philadelphia: J Grigg, 1830.
69. Meiklejohn A. *The life, work and times of Charles Turner Thackrah, surgeon and apothecary of Leeds.* Edinburgh: E and S Livingstone, 1957.
70. Salter HH. *On asthma, its pathology and treatment.* London: Churchill, 1860.
71. Trousseau A. *Lectures on clinical medicine,* vol 1. London: New Sydenham Society, 1868.
72. Charcot JM, Robin C-P. Observations de leucocythemie. *C R Soc Biol (Paris)* 1853;5:44–46.
73. Charcot JM, Vulpian EF. Note sur les cristaux particuliers trouvés dans le sang et les viscères d'un sujet leucemique. *Gaz Med (Paris)* 1860;755–757.
74. Zenker FA. Charcotsche Kristalle im Blut und Gewebe Leukämischer und in den Sputis. *Dtsch Arch Klin Med* 1870;18:125–128.
75. Foerster A. *Atlas der mikroskopischen pathologischen Anatomie.* Leipzig: Voss, 1854.
76. Harting P. *Das Mikroskope.* Braunschweig: Vieweg und Son, 1859.
77. Leyden E von. Zur Kentniss des Bronchialasthmas. *Virchows Arch [A]* 1872;54:324–344.
78. Ehrlich P. Beitrage Zur Kentniss der granulirten Bindegewebszellen und der eosinophilen Leukocythen. *Arch Anat Physiol* 1879;166–169.
79. De Jong SI, Romieu M. Cristaux de Charcot-Leyden et éosinophiles. *Bull Mem Soc Med Hop (Paris)* 1923;47:55–58.
80. Curschmann H. Über die Bedeutung der Leyden'schen Krystalle für die Lehre von Asthma Bronchiale. *Verh Dtsch Ges Inn Med* 1882;1:191–201.
81. Curschmann H. Über Bronchiolitis Exsudativa und ihr Verhältnis zum Asthma Nervosum. *Dtsch Arch Klin Med (Leipzig)* 1883;32:1–34.
82. Osler W. *The principles and practice of medicine.* Edinburgh: YJ Pentland, 1892.
83. Recklinghausen FD von. Ueber Eiter- und Bindegewebskörperchen. *Virchows Arch [A]* 1863;28:157–197.
84. Ehrlich P. Beiträge zur Kenntnis der Anilinfärbungen und ihrer Verwendung in der mikroskopischen Technik. *Arch Mikrosk Anat* 1877;13:263–277.
85. Portier P, Richet CH. De l'action anaphylactique de certain venins. *C R Soc Biol (Paris)* 1902;54:170–172.
86. Pirquet C von, Schick B. *Die Serumkrankheit.* Vienna: F Deuticke, 1905.
87. Pirquet C von. Klinische Studien über Vakzination und Vakzinale Allergie. *Munch Med Wochenschr* 1906;53:1457–1458.
88. Wolff-Eisner A. *Das Heufieber: sein Wesen und seine Behandlung.* Münich: JF Lehman, 1906.

89. Auer J, Lewis PA. The physiology of the immediate reaction of anaphylaxis in the guinea pig. *J Exp Med* 1910;12:151–175.
90. Meltzer SJ. Bronchial asthma as a phenomenon of anaphylaxis. *JAMA* 1910;55:1021–1024.
91. Noon L. Prophylactic inoculation against hayfever. *Lancet* 1911;1:1572–1573.
92. Freeman J. Further observations on the treatment of hayfever by hypodermic injections of pollen vaccine. *Lancet* 1911;2:814–817.
93. Cooke RA. The treatment of hayfever by active immunisation. *Laryngoscope* 1918;23:108–110.
94. Walker IC. A clinical study of 400 patients with bronchial asthma. *Boston Med Surg J* 1918;179:288–295.
95. Ramirez MA. Horse asthma following blood transfusion. *JAMA* 1919;73:984.
96. Prausnitz C, Küstner H. Studien über die Ueberempfindlichkeit. *Zbl Bkt* 1921;86:160–169.
97. Coca AF, Cooke RA. On the classification of the phenomena of hypersensitiveness. *J Immunol* 1923;8:163–182.
98. Coca AF, Grove E. Studies in hypersensitiveness. XIII. A study of atopic reagins. *J Immunol* 1925;10:445–448.
99. Johannson SGO, Bennich H. Studies on a new class of human immunoglobulins: immunological properties. In: Killander J, ed. *Gammaglobulins: structure and control of biosynthesis.* Stockholm: Almqvist and Wiksell, 1967.
100. Johannson SGO. Raised levels of a new immunoglobulin class (IgND) in asthma. *Lancet* 1967;2:951–954.
101. Ishizaka K, Ishizaka T. Identification of gamma-E antibodies as a carrier of reaginic activity. *J Immunol* 1967;99:1187–1198.
102. Editorial. Reagin and IgE. *Lancet* 1968;1:1131.
103. Wide L, Bennich H, Johannson SGO. Diagnosis of allergy by an invitro test for allergic antibodies. *Lancet* 1967;2:1105–1109.
104. Storm van Leeuwen W. *Allergic diseases: diagnosis and treatment of bronchial asthma, hayfever and other allergic diseases.* Philadelphia: JB Lippincott, 1925.
105. Storm van Leeuwen W. Pathognomonische Bedeutung der ueber Empfindlichkeit gegen Aspirin bei Asthmatiker. *Munch Med Wochenschr* 1928;37:1588–1594.
106. Dekker H. Asthma und Milben. *Munch Med Wochenschr* 1928;75:515–517.
107. Voorhorst R, Spieksma FTM, Varekamp K, Lenpen MJ, Lykema AW. The house dust mite (*Dermatophagoides pteronyssinus*) and the allergens it produces. *J Allergy* 1967;39:325–339.
108. Dale HH, Laidlaw P. The physiological function of beta-iminoazolylethylamine. *J Physiol (Lond)* 1910;41:318–344.
109. Windaus A, Vogt K. Synthese des Imidazolyläthylamins. *Berl Dtsch Chem Ges* 1907;40:3691–3695.
110. Weiss S, Robb CP, Ellis HL. The systemic effects of histamine in man. *Arch Intern Med* 1932;49:360–396.
111. Curry JJ. The action of histamine on the respiratory tract in normal and asthmatic subjects. *J Clin Invest* 1946;25:785–791.
112. Schild HO, Hawkins DF, Mongar JL, Herxheimer H. Reactions of isolated human asthmatic lung and bronchial tissue to a specific antigen: histamine release and muscular contraction. *Lancet* 1951;2:376–382.
113. Stevens FA. A comparison of pulmonary and dermal sensitivity to inhaled substances. *J Allergy* 193;5:285–287.
114. Dautrebande L, Philpott E. Crise d'asthma expérimental par aérosols de carbaminoylcholine chez l'homme traité par dispersat de phenylaminopropane. *Presse Med* 1941;49:942–944.
115. Tiffeneau R, Beauvallet M. Broncho-constriction par aérosols acétylcholinques: test pour la mesure de l'insuffisance respiratoire. *Bull Soc Med Hop (Paris)* 1945;61:107–110.
116. Lowell FC, Schiller IW. Measurement of changes in vital capacity as a means of detecting pulmonary reactions to inhaled aerosolized allergenic extracts in asthmatic subjects. *J Allergy* 1947;19:100–104.
117. Herxheimer H. The late bronchial reaction in induced asthma. *Int Arch Allergy* 1952;3:323–326.
118. Pepys J. Inhalation challenge tests in asthma. *N Engl J Med* 1975;293:758–762.
119. Ellis AG. The pathologic anatomy of bronchial asthma. *Am J Med Sci* 1908;136:407–410.
120. Huber HL, Koessler KK. The pathology of bronchial asthma. *Arch Intern Med* 1922;30:687–760.
121. MacDonald IG. The local and constitutional pathology of bronchial asthma. *Ann Intern Med* 1933;6:253–256.
122. Cardell BS, Pearson RSB. Death in asthmatics. *Thorax* 1959;14:341–352.
123. Dunnill MS, Massarella GR, Anderson JA. A comparison of the quantitative anatomy of the bronchi in normal subjects and in status asthmaticus, in chronic bronchitis and in emphysema. *Thorax* 1969;24:176–181.
124. Hosain S. Quantitative measurement of bronchial muscle in man with asthma. *Am Rev Respir Dis* 1973;107:99–103.
125. Kashikar CG. *Yogaratnakara* Chowkhamba Sanskrit series. Varanasi, 1955.
126. Geiger PL, Hesse H. Darstellung des Atropins. *Ann Pharm (Heidelberg)* 1833;5143–5181.
127. Dautrebande L, Lovejoy FW Jr, McCredie RM. New studies on aerosols. XVIII. Effects of atropine microaerosols on the airway resistance in man. *Arch Int Pharmacodyn Ther* 1962;139:198–205.
128. Herxheimer H. Atropine cigarettes in asthma and emphysema. *BMJ* 1959;2:167–168.
129. Nagai N. Ephedrin. *Pharm Ztg* 1887;32:700–702.
130. Chen KK, Schmidt CF. The action of ephedrine: the active principle of the Chinese drug Ma Huang. *J Pharmacol Exp Ther* 1924;24:339–357.
131. Vulpian EFA. Note sur quelques réactions propres à la substance des capsules surrénales. *C R Acad Sci (Paris)* 1856;43:663–665.
132. Oliver G, Sharpey-Schäfer E. The physiological action of extract of the suprarenal capsules. *J Physiol (Lond)* 1895;18:230–276.
133. Takamine J. The blood-pressure-raising principle of the supra-renal glands. *Ther Gaz* 1901;17:221–224.
134. Aldrich TB. A preliminary report on the active principle of the suprarenal gland. *Am J Physiol* 1901;5:457–461.
135. Stoltz F. Über adrenaline und alkylaminoacetobenzcatechin. *Berl Dtsch Chem Ges* 1904;37:4149–4154.
136. Solis-Cohen S. The use of adrenal substances in the treatment of asthma. *JAMA* 1900;34:1164–1166.
137. Bullowa JJM, Kaplan D. On the hypodermic use of adrenaline chloride in the treatment of asthmatic attacks. *Med News (NY)* 1903;783–787.
138. Camps PWL. A note on the inhalation treatment of asthma. *Guys Hosp Rep* 1929;79:496–498.
139. Konzett H. Neue broncholytisch hochwirksame Körper der Adrenalinreihe. *N S Arch Exp Pathol Pharmakol* 1940;197:27–32.
140. Ahlquist RP. A study of the adrenoreceptors. *Am J Physiol* 1948;153:586–599.
141. Lands AM, Arnold A, McAuliff JA, Luduena FP, Brown JG. Differentiation of receptor systems activated by sympathomimetic amines. *Nature* 1967;214:597–599.
142. Kossil A. Über eine neue base auf den pflanzenreich. *Berl Dtsch Chem Ges* 1888;21:2164.
143. Dessauer P. Euphyllin, ein neues diuretikum. *Ther Mon* 1908;22:401–403.
144. Macht DI, Ting G. A study of anti-spasmodic drugs on the bronchus. *Pharmacol Exp Ther* 1921;18:373–398.
145. Hirsch S. Klinischer und experimenteller beitrag zur krampflösenden wirkung der purin derivate. *Klin Wochenschr* 1922;1:615–618.
146. Hermann GR, Aynesworth MB. Successful treatment of persistent extreme dyspnoea "status asthmaticus": use of theophylline ethylene diamine intravenously. (1938, classical article) *J Lab Clin Med* 1990;115:512–525.
147. Greene JA, Paul WD, Faller AE. The action of theophylline with ethylene diamine on intrathecal and venous pressures in cardiac failure and on bronchial obstruction in cardiac failure and in bronchial asthma. *JAMA* 1937;109:1712–1715.
148. Kendall EC. A physiologic and chemical investigation of the suprarenal cortex. *J Biol Chem* 1936;114:57–58.
149. Hench P. The effect of a hormone of the adrenal cortex (compound E) and of pituitary ACTH on rheumatoid arthritis. *Proc Mayo Clin* 1949;24:181–197.
150. Bordley JE, Carey RA, Harvey AM, et al. Preliminary observations on the effect of adrenocorticotropic hormone (ACTH) in allergic diseases. *Bull Johns Hopkins Hosp* 1949;85:396–398.
151. Harvier P, Coste F, Turiaf J, Delbarre F, Basset G, Caramanian P. Le traitement par l'ACTH de l'etat de mal asthmatique prolongé. *Bull Mem Soc Med Hop (Paris)* 1950;66:1438–1451.
152. Carryer HM, Koelsche GA, Prickman LE, Maytum CK, Lake CF, Williams HL. Effects of cortisone on bronchial asthma and hay fever

occurring in subjects sensitive to ragweed pollen. *J Allergy* 1950; 21:282–295.

153. Randolph TG, Rollins JP. Effects of cortisone on bronchial asthma. *J Allergy* 1950;21:288–293.

154. Herzog HL, Nobile A, Tolksdorf S, et al. New anti-arthritic steroids. *Science* 955;121:176.

155. Barach AL, Bickerman HA, Beck GJ. Clinical and physiological studies on the use of metacortandracin in respiratory disease. 1. Bronchial asthma. *Dis Chest* 1955;27:515–520.

156. Burrage WS, Irwin JW. Hydrocortisone in the therapy of asthma. *Ann NY Acad Sci* 1955;66:377–382.

157. Medical Research Council. Controlled trial of effects of cortisone acetate in chronic asthma. *Lancet* 1956;2:798–803.

158. Medical Research Council. Controlled trial of effects of cortisone in status asthmaticus. *Lancet* 1956;2:803–806.

159. Reeder WH, Mackay GS. Nebulized cortisone in bacterial pneumonia. *Dis Chest* 1950;18:528–534.

160. Gelfland ML. Action of cortisone by aerosol method in the treatment of bronchial asthma. *N Engl J Med* 1951;245:293–296.

161. Clark TJH. Effect of beclomethasone dipropionate delivered by aerosol in patients with asthma. *Lancet* 1972;1:1361–1364.

162. Morrow Brown H, Storey G, George WHS. Beclomethasone dipropionate: a new steroid aerosol for the treatment of allergic asthma. *BMJ* 1972;1:585–590.

163. Ellul-Micallef R, Borthwick RC, McHardy GJR. The time course of response to prednisolone in chronic bronchial asthma. *Clin Sci Mol Med* 1974;47:105–117.

164. Ellul-Micallef R. Glucocorticoids. In: Barnes PJ, Rodger IW, Thomson NC, eds. *Asthma: basic mechanisms and clinical management,* 2nd ed. London: Academic, 1992.

165. Samaan K, Hossein AM, Fahim I. The response of the heart to visammin and to khellin. *J Pharm Pharmacol* 1949;1:538–544.

166. Anrep GV, Barsoum GS, Kenway MR, Misrahy G. Therapeutic uses of khellin. *Lancet* 1947;1:557–558.

167. Huttrer CP, Dale E. The chemistry and physiological action of khellin and related products. *Chem Rev* 1951;48:543–579.

168. Altounyan REL. Inhibition of experimental asthma by a new compound, disodium cromoglycate, "Intal." *Acta Allergol* 1967;22:487–489.

169. Cox JSG. Disodium cromoglycate (FPL 670) ("Intal"): a specific inhibitor of reaginic antibody–antigen mechanisms. *Nature* 1967;216:1328–1329.

Asthma, edited by P.J. Barnes, M.M. Grunstein,
A.R. Leff, and A.J. Woolcock.
Lippincott–Raven Publishers, Philadelphia © 1997.

▪ 3 ▪

Definitions and Clinical Classification

Ann J. Woolcock

Practical Definition Asthma	**Classification** Types of Asthma Other Classifications

The fundamental abnormalities in asthma remain unknown so no formal definition is possible. The first mention of the word *asthma* in Greek appears in the *Iliad* of Homer and is said to derive from the verb to "exhale with the mouth open, to pant" (1). The term appears in the ancient Greek literature and was first used as a diagnosis of abnormality by Hippocrates of Kos (1).

The use of the word and descriptions of asthma, with suggestions about the nature of the fundamental abnormality, are traced in the previous chapter on history. The first person to write about asthma in terms of a definition was Floyer in 1698 (2). It was recognized by Salter more than 100 years ago that increased airway irritability is a basic abnormality in people with asthma (3). In 1946 Curry defined this irritability in terms of changes in the vital capacity in response to inhaled histamine (4); in 1958 Tiffeneau (5) suggested that the fundamental abnormality in patients with asthma is "excitability" of the bronchial smooth muscle. The first systematic attempt to define asthma was at the Ciba Symposium held in 1958 to define and classify the diseases related to emphysema (6). At that meeting asthma was defined as "the condition of subjects with widespread narrowing of the bronchial airways, which changes its severity over short periods of time, either spontaneously or under treatment, and is not due to cardiovascular disease." In 1971 another consensus attempt was made to define asthma and the conclusion reached at that meeting is shown in the Table 1 (7). Table 1 lists most of the definitions that have been used between 1971 and 1995. They reflect the difficulty that respirologists have in finding a universal definition of

asthma, because of our poor understanding of its causes, its natural history, and its pathology. The 1995 Global Initiative for Asthma's (GINA) definition of asthma is especially cumbersome (8).

After the Ciba Symposium in 1958, the definition was modified by the American Thoracic Society (19,20) in 1962 to include the phrase "characterized by increased responsiveness of the trachea and bronchi to various stimuli." This definition is unsatisfactory because it avoids the issue of whether a single definable disease, with a unique pathogenesis and pathology, exists within the syndrome of diseases with the clinical label of asthma. The problem is further aggravated by the use of the terms "seasonal allergic asthma," "pollen asthma." "exercise-induced asthma," "nocturnal asthma," and "occupational asthma," all of which appear frequently in the literature, usually without a precise definition and with the implication that asthma can be defined and classified in relation to the cause or nature of the episodes of airway narrowing.

In recent years the importance of airway inflammation and the associated airway hyperresponsiveness (AHR) has been widely recognized (21,22). It is still too early to define asthma in terms of a characteristic form of inflammation found on biopsy, because inflammation is also found in some people without symptoms (23). Nor can asthma be defined in terms of responses to histamine or methacholine challenge because abnormal responses are found in individuals without symptoms (24,25) and AHR is present in other diseases, especially chronic obstructive pulmonary disease (COPD) (26,27). Also, attacks of airway narrowing can result from exposure to allergens in people who do not have AHR (28). Moreover, airway responsiveness may be normal in the patients with asthmatic symptoms (29,30), probably indicating episodic

A. J. Woolcock: Institute of Respiratory Medicine, Page Chest Pavilion, Royal Prince Alfred Hospital, Camperdown, New South Wales 2050 Australia.

TABLE 1. *Definitions of asthma 1959–1995*

Year	Author	Ref type	Definition	Reference
1959	Fletcher CM, et al	Symposium (CIBA Guest)	"At present the diagnoses 'chronic bronchitis,' 'asthma,' and 'emphysema' are used without any general agreement about the clinical conditions to which they refer…"	(9)
1961	WHO	Report	"Asthma refers to the condition of subjects with widespread narrowing of the bronchial airways, which changes its severity over short periods of time either spontaneously or under treatment, and is not due to cardiovascular disease."	(10)
1962	Meneely GR, et al	Report ATS	"Asthma is a disease characterized by an increased responsiveness of the trachea and bronchi to various stimuli and manifested by a widespread narrowing of the airways that changes in severity either spontaneously or as a result of therapy."	(11)
1971	Scadding JG	Book section (CIBA study group)	"The word 'asthma' is most commonly used to refer to a disorder of function widely variable dyspnea due to variations in resistance to gas flow in the pulmonary airways. Asthma alone should imply no more than the presence of this functional disturbance."	(12)
1975	Crofton J, Douglas A	Book chapter	"The term 'bronchial asthma,' often used unqualified as 'asthma,' is employed to describe recurrent, generalized airways obstruction that, at least in the early stages is paroxysmal and reversible."	(13)
1983	Scadding JG	Book chapter	"Asthma is a disease characterized by wide variations over short periods of time in resistance to flow in intrapulmonary airways."	(14)
1987	Woolcock AJ	Book chapter	"Asthma is defined as bronchial hyperresponsiveness together with intermittent symptoms of wheezing, chest tightness, or cough. Symptoms in the last 12 months distinguish 'current' from 'past' asthma."	(15)
1991	US NIH	Expert Panel Report	"Asthma is a lung disease with the following characteristics: (1) airway obstruction that is reversible (but not completely so in some subjects) either spontaneously or with treatment (2) airway inflammation and (3) increased airway responsiveness to a variety of stimuli."	(16)
1992	US NIH	International Guidelines	"Asthma is a chronic inflammatory disorder of the airways in which many cells play a role, including mast cells and eosinophils. In susceptible individuals this inflammation causes symptoms that are usually associated with widespread but variable airflow obstruction that is often reversible either spontaneously or with treatment, and causes an associated increase in airway responsiveness to a variety of stimuli."	(17)
1994	Woolcock AJ	Book chapter	"Asthma is a disease of the airways that makes the airways prone to narrow too much and too easily in response to a wide variety of provoking stimuli."	(18)
1995	NIH, NHLBI	Global Initiative for Asthma (GINA)	"Asthma is a chronic inflammatory disorder of the airways in which many cells play a role, in particular mast cells, eosinophils, and T lymphocytes. In susceptible individuals this inflammation causes recurrent episodes of wheezing, breathlessness, chest tightness, and cough, particularly at night and/or in the early morning. These symptoms are usually associated with widespread but variable airflow limitation that is at least partly reversible either spontaneously or with treatment. The inflammation also causes an associated increase in airway responsiveness to a variety of stimuli."	(8)

asthma. Nevertheless, it is clear that most patients with persistent asthma, as defined below, have characteristic pathologic changes and abnormal airway behavior that can be demonstrated as an abnormal response to inhaled histamine or methacholine (31). Thus, it is clear that a specific definition of asthma, in terms of a single measurable abnormality, is not yet possible. Definitions are, however, essential for epidemiologic studies that compare populations and for laboratory and chemical studies that assess the effects of pharmacologic and nonpharmacologic interventions. Failure to agree on definitions and to give details of patients studied when describing research has greatly hampered progress in understanding this disease. The "practical" definitions included here are suggested in the light of present knowledge and will change as understanding of the disease increases.

PRACTICAL DEFINITIONS

In this chapter, the word *asthma* refers to the underlying abnormality in the airway walls. The term "airway narrowing" refers to episodes in which the airways narrow for short periods of time and cause symptoms of wheeze, chest tightness, and breathlessness, and the term "exacerbation" refers to episodes of airway narrowing that last for hours or days and are difficult to reverse. "Acute asthma" is an ambiguous term that gives no indication of the nature of the underlying disease and is not used in this chapter.

Asthma

Clinical

A disease of the airways that makes the airway prone to narrow too much and too easily in response to a variety of provoking stimuli that have no such effect in nonasthmatic subjects.

Pathologic

A disease of the airways characterized by chronic inflammation with infiltration of lymphocytes, eosinophils, and mast cells, with epithelial desquamation, and thickening and disorganization of the tissues of the airway wall including the basement membrane.

Airway Hyperresponsiveness

An abnormality of the airways that allows them to narrow too much and too easily in response to a provoking stimulus. In practice, it is defined as the provoking dose or concentration (PD_{20} or PC_{20}) of an inhaled substance that causes a 20% change in lung function.

Atopy (Allergy)

The production of abnormal amounts of immunoglobulin E (IgE) antibodies in response to contact with aeroallergens. The terms "atopy," "atopic state," and "allergy" are used interchangeably. Atopy can be demonstrated easily by skin prick tests using common aeroallergens. It can also be demonstrated by RAST tests. Increased serum IgE, caused by ingested substances and parasites, without IgE specific to aeroallergens, is not atopy.

Allergen

A substance that, when inhaled or ingested, leads to the production of specific IgE antibodies. Most allergens are inhaled and referred to as aeroallergens, whereas only a few ingested substances appear to elicit IgE responses that last beyond infancy. Recently the World Health Organization (WHO) has published a nomenclature for allergens (32).

CLASSIFICATION

Types of Asthma

Table 2 shows a suggested classification of asthma based on symptoms, bronchodilator use, baseline lung function, and airway responsiveness. Many people experience wheezing or tightness in the chest at some time in their lives. Not all of them have the same phenotype and the presence of abnormal airway responsiveness between episodes of symptoms is the crucial factor in this classification because its presence determines the need for treatment with inhaled corticosteroids between episodes. Airway responsiveness can be determined by either a measurement of AHR or indirectly by peak expiratory flow (PEF) variability measured on waking for a week. (30).

Persistent Asthma

A disease characterized by frequent symptoms plus chronic abnormality of the airways as demonstrated by an abnormal dose-response curve to histamine or methacholine and/or increased variability of daily peak flow readings. This form of asthma appears to be incurable, al-

TABLE 2. *Suggested classification of asthma*[a]

	Symptoms	Bronchodilator required for symptoms	Baseline lung function (FEV_1) (After BD)	Airway Responsiveness (By challenge or PEF variability)
Persistent asthma	Frequent	Regularly	>80% pred.	Increased—mild—severe
Obstructed asthma	Frequent	Regularly	<80% pred.	Increased—mild—severe
Episodic asthma	Intermittent	Intermittently	Normal, unchanged	Normal
Asthma in remission	Past but none > 12 months	None > 12 months	Normal, unchanged	Increased—mild
Potential asthma	None, ever	Never	Normal, unchanged	Increased—mild—moderate
Trivial wheeze	Intermittent, mild	No	Normal, unchanged	Normal

[a]Based on symptoms, lung function, and airway responsiveness in symptom-free interval (before treatment with inhaled corticosteroids).

though some children become asymptomatic during adolescence and may be regarded as having "asthma in remission." The pathologic changes of this form of asthma are described below.

In population studies in which the individual is seen only once, the presence of an abnormal dose-response curve to methacholine or histamine plus wheeze in the previous 12 months is classified as "current asthma" (33). In longitudinal studies most individuals with "current asthma" are found to have "persistent asthma."

Obstructed Asthma

This is a form of persistent asthma with evidence of airflow limitation that persists after maximal treatment with bronchodilators and oral corticosteroids. The pathologic changes responsible for the airflow limitation are not known.

Episodic Asthma

In this form of asthma, periodic episodes of the symptoms of airway narrowing occur at intervals and are of sufficient severity to require treatment, but there is no detectable abnormality of airway function between the episodes. Episodic asthma is common in individuals who have attacks of airway narrowing during the pollen season. It is sometimes seen early in the course of occupational asthma and has been described in nonallergic individuals (29). The pathologic changes have not been described.

Asthma in Remission

An individual with a past history of persistent asthma who has had neither symptoms nor taken therapy for the last 12 months. Such individuals usually have some degree of persisting AHR (34).

Potential Asthma

An individual who has AHR, usually in the moderate range, but has no symptoms of asthma. Identified during surveys, some, particularly those who are atopic, may develop asthma at a later time (35). Those who develop symptoms appear not to have different histologic changes in the airways from those who remain symptom free (36).

Trivial Wheeze

An individual, without AHR, who has episodes of wheezing that are mild or short lived and do not require treatment. All measures of airway function are normal.

Other Classifications

On the basis of the atopic status or the occurrence of a sensitizing agent at work, other classifications are also used.

Extrinsic (Atopic) Asthma

Asthma (of any of the above classifications) occurring in an atopic individual. Atopic individuals with persistent asthma can have symptoms produced by a variety of provoking agents other than allergens.

Occupational Asthma

Asthma caused by a sensitizing substance at the workplace. The symptoms and airway narrowing are demonstrated by provocation with the specific substance. It may be episodic or persistent. This subject is discussed in detail in Chapter 85.

Intrinsic Asthma

Asthma occurring in an individual without evidence of atopy. The disease often begins in adult life, there are no differences in pathology or in response to treatment with corticosteroids between intrinsic and extrinsic asthma, and some workers suggest that all asthma may, in fact, be extrinsic (37).

Is Asthma a Single Disease?

Recent experiments show that the symptoms of asthma, together with decreased expiratory volumes, can be produced in normal individuals by certain maneuvers, suggesting that the symptoms and reduced expiratory volumes are due to altered behavior of the bronchial smooth muscle (38,39). Altered behavior of bronchial smooth muscle could potentially be caused by many situations, but the most common appears to result from chronic allergic inflammation, either due to bronchoconstricting mediators released from inflammatory cells in the airways that are attracted and orchestrated by TH_2 cells or to the presence of IgE or a combination. In other individuals without a history of asthma, beta-blocking drugs can cause asthma. Clearly asthma, in terms of symptoms, is not one disease, because wheezing can be caused by a number of situations independent of a chronic inflammatory process. Furthermore, a number of causal agents including allergens, occupational sensitizers, and chronic exposure to cold dry air can lead to persistent disease.

This then raises the question: "should we use the term 'asthma' to describe symptoms, to describe attacks of airway narrowing, and to describe an inflammatory disease?" As Hargreave pointed out (40), we use the word asthma loosely. Attempts to use it more precisely have been met with the rejoinder that "but everyone knows the difference between 'acute' and 'chronic' asthma." However, there would be advantages to having a new set of words to describe (a) symptoms of airway narrowing/inflammation, (b) the various circumstances that lead to symptoms (e.g., wheezing with viral infections, episodic symptoms associated with exposure to pollens and the symptoms produced by exercise), and (c) the different abnormalities of the airway wall (usually thought to be inflammatory) that we now call "asthma" and that probably are induced by a variety of mechanisms, including responses to aeroallergens, responses to occupational sensitizers, responses to constant exposure to cold dry air, and perhaps genetic abnormalities that alter the function of bronchial smooth muscle.

CONCLUSIONS

Until we understand more about the nature of the abnormalities that lead to wheezing, care should be taken in the use of the word "asthma" and a qualification made to indicate the sense in which the word is used. Asthma should continue to be regarded as an "altered state of breathing," as described by Hippocrates. The most satisfactory definition is "a state of the airways that causes them to narrow excessively in response to provoking stimuli that normally have no such effect."

REFERENCES

1. Marketos SG, Ballas CN. Bronchial asthma in the medical literature of Greek antiquity. *J Asthma* 1982;19(4):263–269.
2. Floyer J. *A treatise of the asthma*. London: R Wilkin, 1698.
3. Salter HH. *On asthma: its pathology and treatment*. New York: W. Wood and Company, 1882;284–285.
4. Curry JJ. The action of histamine on the respiratory tract in normal and asthmatic subjects. *J Clin Invest* 1946;25:785–791.
5. Tiffeneau R. L'hyperexcitabilite des terminaisons sensitives pulmonaires de l'asthmatique. *Presse Med* 1958;66:1250–1252.
6. Unknown. Terminology, definitions and classifications of chronic pulmonary emphysema and related conditions. A report of the conclusions of a Ciba Guest Symposium. *Thorax* 1959;14:286–299.
7. Porter R, Birch J, eds. *Identification of asthma*. Edinburgh: Churchill Livingstone, 1971.
8. *Global Initiative for Asthma. Global Strategy for Asthma Management and Prevention NHLBI/WHO Workshop Report*. National Institutes of Health, National Heart, Lung, and Blood Institute. 1995.
9. Fletcher CM, Gilson JG, Hugh-Jones P, Scadding JG. Terminology, definitions and classification of chronic pulmonary emphysema and related conditions. A report of the conclusions of a Ciba guest symposium. *Thorax* 1959;14:286–299.
10. WHO. *Chronic cor pulmonale: report of an expert committee*. World Health Organization Technical report series. WHO, 1961.
11. Meneely GR, Renzetti AD, Steele JD, Wyatt JP, Harris HW. Chronic bronchitis, asthma and pulmonary emphysema. A statement by the committee on diagnostic standards for nontuberculosis respiratory disease. *Am Rev Respir Dis* 1962;85:762–768.
12. Porter R, Birch J, eds. General discussion. In: Porter R, Birch J, eds.
13. *Identification of asthma*. Edinburgh: Churchill Livingstone, 1971; 13–34. Ciba Foundation Study Group; vol 38.
13. Crofton J, Douglas A. *Bronchial asthma. Respiratory diseases*. Oxford: Blackwell Scientific, 1975.
14. Scadding JG. Definition and clinical categories of asthma. In: Clark TJH, Godfrey S, ed. *Asthma*. London: Chapman and Hall, 1983; 13–21.
15. Woolcock AJ. Asthma. In: Wetherall DJ, Ledingham JGG, Warrell DA, eds. *Oxford textbook of respiratory medicine*, 2nd ed. Oxford: Oxford University Press, 1987;15.75–15.83.
16. *Executive summary: guidelines for the diagnosis and management of asthma*. National Asthma Education Program Expert Panel Report. U.S. Department of Health and Human Services, Public Health Service National Institutes of Health, 1991.
17. *International consensus report on diagnosis and management of asthma*. U.S. Department of Health and Human Services, Public Health Services National Institute of Health, 1992.
18. Woolcock AJ. Asthma. In: Murray JF, Nadel J, eds. *Textbook of respiratory medicine*. Philadelphia: Saunders, 1994;1288–1330.
19. American Thoracic Society. Chronic bronchitis, asthma and pulmonary emphysema. *Thorax* 1960;15:762–768.
20. American Thoracic Society. Medical section of the National Tuberculosis Association. Chronic bronchitis, asthma, and pulmonary emphysema. A statement by the Committee on Diagnostic Standards for Nontuberculous Disease. *Am Rev Respir Dis* 1962;85:762–768.
21. Hargreave FE, Juniper EF, Ryan G, et al. Clinical significance of nonspecific airway hyperreactivity. In: Hargreave FE, eds. *Airway reactivity. Mechanisms and clinical relevance*. Missussauga, Ontario: Astra Pharmaceuticals Canada Ltd., 1980;216–221.
22. Nadel JA, Holtzman MJ. Regulation of airway responsiveness and secretion: role of inflammation. In: Kay AB, Austen KF, Lichtenstein LM, eds. *Asthma: physiology, immunopathology, and treatment*. London: Academic Press, 1984;129–155.
23. Holgate ST, Roche W, Djukanovic R, Wilson J, Brutten K, Howarth P. The need for a pathological classification of asthma. *Eur Respir J* 1991;4(suppl 13):113S–122S.
24. Townley RG, Dennis M, Itkin IH. Comparative action of acetyl-beta-methacholine, histamine, and pollen antigens in subjects with hay fever and patients with bronchial asthma. *J Allergy* 1965;36:121–137.
25. Britton WJ, Woolcock AJ, Peat JK, Sedgwick CJ, Lloyd DM, Leeder SR. Prevalence of bronchial hyperresponsiveness in children: the relationship between asthma and skin reactivity to allergens in two communities. *Int J Epidemiol* 1986;15:202–209.
26. Klein RC, Salvaggio JE. Nonspecificity of the bronchoconstricting effect of histamine and acetyl-beta-methylcholine in patients with obstructive airways disease. *J Allergy* 1966;37:158–168.
27. Yan K, Salome CM, Woolcock AJ. Prevalence and nature of bronchial hyperresponsiveness in subjects with chronic obstructive pulmonary disease. *Am Rev Respir Dis* 1985;132:25–29.
28. Permutt S, Rosenthal RR, Norman PS, Menkes HA. Bronchial challenge in ragweed-sensitive patients. In: Lichtenstein LM, Austen, KF, eds. *Asthma: physiology, immunopharmacology and treatment*. New York: Academic Press, 1977;265–281.
29. Stanescu DC, Frans A. Bronchial asthma without increased airway reactivity. *Eur J Respir Dis* 1982;63:5–12.
30. Woolcock AJ, Barnes PJ. Asthma—the important questions, part 2. *Am Rev Respir Dis* 1992;146(suppl 5):1351–1366.
31. Laitinen LA, Heino M, Laitinen A, Kava T, Haahtela T. Damage of the airway epithelium and bronchial reactivity in patients with asthma. *Am Rev Respir Dis* 1985;131:599–606.
32. King TP, Hoffman D, Lowenstein H, Marsh DG, Platts-Mills TAE. Allergen nomenclature (reprinted from *Bulletin of the World Health Organization* 1994;72:798–806). *J Allergy Clin Immunol* 1995;96: 5–14.
33. Toelle BG, Peat JK, Salome CM, Mellis CM, Woolcock AJ. Towards a definition of asthma for epidemiology. *Am Rev Respir Dis* 1992;146: 633–637.
34. Townley RG, Ryo UY, Kolotkin BM, Kang B. Bronchial sensitivity to methacholine in current and former asthmatic and allergic rhinitis patients and control subjects. *J Allergy Clin Immunol* 1975;56: 429–442.
35. Hopp RJ, Townley RG, Biven RE, Bewtra AK, Nair NM. The presence of airway reactivity before the development of asthma. *Am Rev Respir Dis* 1990;141:2–8.

36. Laprise C, Boulet M, Laviolette M, Boulet L-P. Long-term stability of physiological and histological parameters in subjects with asymptomatic airway hyperresponsiveness(AAHR). *Am J Respir Crit Care Med* 1996;153:A876.

37. Saetta M, Di Stefano A, Maestrelli P, et al. Airway mucosal inflammation in occupational asthma induced by toluene diisocyanate(TDI). *Am Rev Respir Dis* 1992;145:160–168.

38. Ding DJ, Martin JG, Macklem PT. Effects of lung volume on maximal methacholine-induced bronchoconstriction in normal humans. *J Appl Physiol* 1987;63:1324–1330.

39. Skloot G, Permutt S, Togias A. Pathophysiology of asthma: reduced airway-parenchyma interdependence, not smooth muscle hyperresponsiveness. *Am J Respir Crit Care Med* 1994;149:A585.

40. Dolovich J, Hargreave FE, O'Byrne P, Ruhno J, Newhouse MT. Asthma terminology: troubles in wordland. *Am Rev Respir Dis* 1986;134(5): 1102.

■ 2 ■

Epidemiology

Asthma, edited by P.J. Barnes, M.M. Grunstein, A.R. Leff, and A.J. Woolcock.
Lippincott–Raven Publishers, Philadelphia © 1997.

▪ 4 ▪

Epidemiologic Trends

Peter G. J. Burney

| Changes in Prevalence of Asthma | Changes in the Use of Health Services |
| Changes in the Prevalence of Atopy | Changes in Mortality |

Assessing the direction and strength of trends across time depends on the use of historical data, which have inevitable limitations. However, although the historical record is open to question in ways that contemporary surveys are not, there is accumulating evidence that asthma has increased in prevalence in a wide number of settings over the last few decades, at least. The causes for the increase are as yet unresolved, but they seem likely to be related, in part, to at least a contemporary increase in the prevalence of atopy as reflected in less well-documented increases in other atopic diseases and in rare studies of changes in sensitization to common aeroallergens. Any trends in prevalence need to be taken into account when interpreting trends in mortality and use of services.

CHANGES IN PREVALENCE OF ASTHMA

Two features are required of studies designed to examine changes in the prevalence of asthma over time. The first is that the definition of asthma remains constant over the time of the study, and that the history is elicited in the same way. The definition of asthma is still unsettled and small changes in the definition may lead to very large differences in the estimated prevalence of the condition. Table 1 shows the prevalence of a number of symptoms related to asthma from a single prevalence study (1). It is clear that the criterion for deciding on the presence of asthma could have a pronounced effect on the estimated prevalence. The second feature is that the population under study remains the same. No study can fully satisfy this criterion since either the individuals that make up the population must change or

the population must get older. However, large changes in the population brought about by migration will clearly lead to problems in deciding whether any change in prevalence was due to secular changes, independent of changes brought about by migration.

Furthermore, it is desirable that the studies are not based on the definition of asthma as a clinical entity. This is because, as will be discussed later, it is likely that the criteria for diagnosing asthma have changed over the course of time. Changes in the prevalence of diagnosed asthma are possibly of some interest in themselves but cannot be taken to imply a change in the prevalence of disease.

Table 2 gives the results from a number of studies which have estimated the prevalence of asthma or asthmalike symptoms in the same population at different times (2–24). Most studies are based on only two points in time and are for this reason, taken individually, inherently unreliable. Any one of the comparisons relying on this design is open to major bias from any difference in

P.G.J. Burney: Department of Public Health Medicine, United Medical and Dental School, St. Thomas's Hospital, London SE1 7EH United Kingdom.

TABLE 1. *12-month period prevalence of reported symptoms and conditions among young adults aged 20 to 44 years in 3 East Anglian towns*

Symptom	Percent Prevalence (95% confidence interval)
Woken by cough	28.2 (27.3–29.1)
Hay fever or nasal allergies	27.8 (26.9–28.7)
Wheeze	25.1 (24.2–26.0)
Woken in the morning with chest tightness	18.0 (17.4–18.7)
Wheeze without a cold	17.6 (16.8–18.4)
Wheeze with breathlessness	13.8 (13.1–14.5)
Woken at night by an attack of breathlessness	8.1 (7.5–8.6)
Attack of asthma	5.1 (4.7–5.6)

TABLE 2. *Prevalence of asthma or asthma-like symptoms in population studies on more than one occasion.*

Definition	Population group	Town, Country	Period	Number surveyed	Prevalence (%)	Annual increase (%)	Reference
Asthma or wheezing	Schoolchildren aged 5, 6,15, and 16 years	Birmingham, England	1956–1957	49,273	1.8		Morrison Smith (2)
			1968–1969	20,958	5.4	9.3	
			1974–1975	10,171	6.3	2.	
Wheeze	Schoolchildren aged 8–13 years	Aberdeen, Scotland	1964	2,743	10.4		Ninan and Russell (3)
			1989	3,942	19.8	2.6	
Episodes of shortness of breath					5.4		
					10.2	2.6	
Asthma					4.1		
					10.2	3.6	
Wheeze or asthma	Schoolchildren aged 7 years	Melbourne, Australia	1964		19.1		Robertson et al.(4)
			1990		46.0	3.4	
Diagnosed asthma	Recruits aged 18 years	Finland, National	1966	ns	0.29		Haahtela et al. (5)
			1989	ns	1.78	7.9	
Asthma assessed by nurses or medical students	Schoolchildren aged 4–5 years	Geneva, Switzerland	1968	4,781	1.7		Varonier et al.(6)
			1981	3,270	2.0	1.3	
	Schoolchildren aged 14–15 years	Geneva, Switzerland	1968	2,451	1.9		
			1981	3,500	2.8	3.0	
Self-reported asthma	University students	Paris, France	1968	ns	3.3		Perdrizet et al. (7)
			1982	ns	5.4	3.5	
Asthma reported by parents	Schoolchildren aged 11–13 years	Lower Hutt, New Zealand	1969	952	7.1		Mitchell (8)
			1982	858	13.5	4.9	
Diagnosed asthma	Recruits aged 18 years	Sweden, National	1971		1.9		Åberg (9)
			1981		2.8	3.9	
Wheeze past 12 months	Schoolchildren aged 12 years	Caerphilly, South Wales	1973	818	9.8		Burr et al. (10)
			1988	965	15.2	2.9	
Wheeze most days /nights, last 12 months	Schoolchildren aged 5–11 years	England, National	1973	3,318	ns	boys 4.3	Burney et al. (11)
			1986	3,483	ns	girls 6.1	
Occasional wheeze last 12 months						boys 1.0 girls 1.7	
Asthma attack last 12 months						boys 6.9 girls 12.8	
Asthma as described to parents	Schoolchildren aged 7–15 years	Taipei, Taiwan	1974	23,678	1.3		Hsieh and Shen (12)
			1985	147,373	5.1	12.4	
Wheeze or asthma	Schoolchildren aged 12–18 years	Hawke's Bay, New Zealand	1975	715	26.2		Shaw et al. (13)
			1989	435	34.0	1.9	
Self-reported asthma	General, all ages	Norway, National	1975	11,014	1.4		Magnus et al. (14)
			1985	10,576	2.4	5.6	
	0–6 years		1975	1,132	1.1		
			1985	983	2.0	5.8	
	7–15 years		1975	1,710	1.5		
			1985	1,497	2.4	4.7	
	16–24 years		1975	1,337	0.7		
			1985	1,301	1.9	9.9	
	25–44 years		1975	2,628	1.0		
			1985	3,097	1.7	5.2	
	45–66 years		1975	2,941	1.9		
			1985	2,283	2.9	4.6	
	67 + years		1975	1,266	2.0		
			1985	1,415	3.7	6.6	
Doctor diagnosed asthma	Population aged 12–18 years	Finland, National	1977–1979	4,335	1.0		Rimpelä et al. (15)
			1991	3,059	2.8	8.2	
Wheeze	Schoolchildren	Croydon, England	1978		9.6		Anderson et al. (16)
			1991		11.4	1.3	
Self-reported asthma	General 0–4 years	United States, National	1981	4,083	2.8		Weitzman et al. (17)
			1988	4,949	2.9	0.5	
	5–11 years		1981	5,659	3.6		
			1988	6,641	5.0	4.8	
	12–17 years		1981	5,482	2.8		
			1988	5,521	4.5	7.0	
Wheeze	General aged 18–55 years	Busselton, Australia	1981		17.5		Peat et al. (18)
			1990		28.8	5.7	
Self-reported asthma	General aged 18–55 years	Busselton, Australia	1981		9.0		
			1990		16.3	6.8	

TABLE 2. *(Continued)*

Definition	Population group	Town, Country	Period	Number surveyed	Prevalence (%)	Annual increase (%)	Reference
Wheezing	Schoolchildren aged 7–12 years	Oslo, Norway	1981	1,772	9.2		Skjønberg et al. (19)
			1993	4,521	10.7	1.3	
Attacks of breathlessness					3.3		
					7.1	6.6	
Diagnosed asthma					3.4		
					8.0	7.4	
Wheeze	Schoolchildren aged 8–10 years	Belmont	1982	718	10.4		Peat et al. (20)
			1992	873	27.6	10.2	
Wheeze	Schoolchildren aged 8–10 years	Wagga Wagga	1982	769	15.5		
			1992	795	23.1	4.1	
Wheeze most days /nights, last 12 months	Schoolboys aged 5–11 years	Scotland	1982		4.7		Rona et al. (21)
			1992		4.9	0.4	
	Schoolgirls aged 5–11 years		1982		2.6		
			1992		3.3	2.4	
Occasional wheeze last 12 months	Schoolboys aged 5—11 years	Scotland	1982		14.6		
			1992		18.6	2.5	
	Schoolgirls aged 5–11 years		1982		9.0		
			1992		11.3	2.3	
Asthma attach last 12 months	Schoolboys aged 5–11 years	Scotland	1982		3.9		
			1992		10.3	10.2	
	Schoolgirls aged 5–11 years		1982		2.1		
			1992		5.9	10.9	
Wheeze most days / nights, last 12 months	Schoolboys aged 5–11 years	England	1982		3.2		
			1992		4.4	3.2	
	Schoolgirls aged 5–11 years		1982		2.6		
			1992		3.6	3.3	
Occasional wheeze last 12 months	Schoolboys aged 5–11 years	England	1982		12.6		
			1992		19.0	4.2	
	Schoolgirls aged 5–11 years		1982		9.5		
			1992		13.5	3.6	
Asthma attack last 12 months	Schoolboys aged 5–11 years	England	1982		4.2		
			1992		11.8	10.9	
	Schoolgirls aged 5–11 years		1982		2.7		
			1992		7.0	10.0	
Wheezy breathing (cumulative prevalence)	Schoolchildren aged 5–18 years	South Australia	1984	1,032	24.1		Crockett et al. (22)
			1992		36.2	5.2	
Self-reported asthma	Adults selected ages 35–66 years	Norrbotton, Sweden	1986	5,698	5.7		Lundbäck et al. (23)
			1992	5,617	6.7	2.7	
Attacks of breathlessness			1986	5,698	10.9		
			1992	5,617	13.5	3.6	
Wheeze			1986	5,698	12.2		
			1992	5,617	11.5	–1.0	
Doctor assessed asthma	Recruits ages 17–18 years	Israel, National	ns	134,863	1.7		Laor et al. (24)
			ns	144,491	2.2	10.0	
			ns	163,832	4.4	26.3	

methods used or on any intercurrent event that might influence responses, such as an epidemic of respiratory disease just prior to one of the surveys. If such an event were to have occurred and to have influenced people's memories of respiratory disease, the estimate given might have been either higher or lower than that recorded. Nevertheless, though the estimated increases over time are variable, they are remarkable in that all but one of the estimates given here are positive. Moreover, the studies that have given estimates based on more than two points in time are in agreement and are unlikely to be accounted for by unpredictable variations due to such temporary phenomena, particularly in the case of the national study of health and

growth in England 1973 to 1986, which is based on 8 identical surveys over a period of 13 years (11). Care should nevertheless be taken before putting great weight on the findings of any single study and the comparison of rates between studies is probably unsafe.

The studies include studies of reported asthma and studies of symptom prevalence. Where both have been estimated as in Busselton, Australia, and the National Study of Health and Growth the studies of asthma estimate larger increases than studies of symptoms (11,18, 21). This may imply that a greater readiness to diagnose asthma is a factor in the increase in estimates of asthma prevalence.

The prevalence of diagnosed asthma in 1981, according to Weitzman's (17) analysis of the National Health Interview Survey in the United States, was higher in African Americans, in those of low socio-economic status, and in those of low birth weight, but rose more rapidly in the following 7 years among Caucasian children, in those not from low income families, and in those with birthweights over 2,500 g. The increase in England between 1973 and 1986 was more marked in relatively persistent wheeze than in occasional wheeze, though this was not the case when assessed later in the same study between 1982 and 1992 in either England or Scotland (11,21). On the other hand, national data from the United States and a study of children in Croydon, South London, suggested that the disability among those with a diagnosis of asthma had declined in the intervening period (16,17). This possibly indicates that the definition of asthma had changed to include milder subjects in the meantime, or that the management of asthma had improved.

A few studies have attempted to collect evidence of changes in physiological function to further test the view that the changes represent a true change in pathology, and not simply a change in reporting either of disease or of symptoms. Burr et al. (10) reported an increase, though not a significant increase, in the prevalence of bronchial hyperresponsiveness in response to exercise in his study of Welsh schoolchildren. Peat et al. (20) reported a similar and significant increase in the response to histamine in children in Australia. In contrast, Peat et al. (18) did not show an increase in responsiveness in adults living in Busselton, despite showing an increase in the prevalence of wheeze. All these studies are based on measurements at only two points in time and, so, are open to the problems of interpretation discussed earlier. However, the evidence suggests, at least for children, that the increases in reported symptoms are accompanied by pathophysiological changes.

It is important to attempt some understanding of the nature of the increase that has occurred. In particular it is important to know whether the increase is long-term or short-term, and, hence, whether the increase might be expected to be reversed quickly. It is also important to assess to what extent the changes in use of services and mortality have been influenced by changes in prevalence.

Changes in prevalence might come about in one of two ways. On the one hand, there might be changes (for instance in levels of air pollution) which would have an acute effect on the susceptible population at any age, increasing the probability that they would be asthmatic at the time of exposure. This type of effect is sometimes described as a "period effect." Alternatively, changes might occur at only one time in a person's life, but remain fixed within that particular "birth cohort" so that the risk of disease remains consistently increased or decreased thereafter. This might be because of an irreversible change in that person, or because of a persistent change in exposure (as for instance if someone took up cigarette smoking early in life). This type of effect is sometimes described as a "cohort effect."

Evidence for the view that there has been a cohort effect in the changing pattern of asthma comes from one study from the United States. This showed that the increase in the incidence (new cases) of asthma in a population in Rochester, Minnesota, was confined to the 1 to 14-year-old age group between the 1960s and the 1980s (25). Incidence rates did not increase outside this age group. Taken together with our knowledge of the persistence of asthma into later life, these findings make it plausible that the changes in asthma are a cohort effect taking place early in life.

CHANGES IN THE PREVALENCE OF ATOPY

There is evidence that the other atopic conditions, hay fever and eczema, have also increased in prevalence at the same time, but this evidence is less abundant. Some of this evidence comes from the same studies that have already been described, though even among these the evidence is not as consistent as for asthma and wheezy conditions (3,10). Skjørnberg et al. (19), for instance, reported a decline in the prevalence of hay fever and a significant decline in the prevalence of urticaria among girls in Oslo between 1981 and 1993, though both conditions increased among boys, hay fever significantly so. Almost all of the evidence is based on self-reported hay fever and eczema. This again raises problems of interpretation but attempts to derive questionnaires and other instruments for the measurement of the prevalence of these conditions are a more recent enterprise than the design of respiratory symptoms questions. The most plentiful evidence for an increase is in the case of eczema, in which case there have been studies documenting increases over time. These include studies from Denmark and comparisons from national studies in the United Kingdom of children born in 1946, 1958, and 1970 (26,27). The evidence, as it stands, is strongly suggestive of a general increase in atopic disease. It is highly likely that this explains the greater part at least of the increase in asthma.

Objective evidence of an increase in sensitivity to aeroallergens comes from reports of skin test surveys of populations in Tucson and London, though Peat et al. (20) found an increase in hyperresponsiveness and respiratory symptoms in children without any increase in skin test sensitivity (28,29). The view that sensitivity to aeroallergens has been increasing across a wide range of places is, however, supported further by two reports that the prevalence of specific immunoglobuling (Ig)E antibodies against common aeroallergens has been increasing. One study from Switzerland has shown this increase in a series of studies of local schoolchildren (30). The other shows the same changes for Japanese schoolgirls (31).

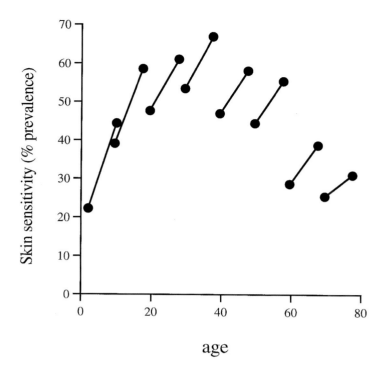

FIG. 1. Longitudinal changes in skin sensitivity (any response greater than control) in cohort of 1,333 subjects living in Tucson, by age over an 8-year period.

Both surveys show that the increased prevalence in atopy is not dominated by any particular allergen, but is due to a general increase in the prevalence of sensitivity to many local allergens. This is an important observation in searching for an explanation for the increase. It at least suggests that the explanation is unlikely to be increased exposure to a single allergen, and probably rules out exposure to allergen as the critical event triggering the increased prevalence.

There is little evidence on which to assess whether the increase in atopy has been a cohort effect or a period effect. However, plotting the data from Barbee et al. (28) (Fig. 1) suggests that the rate of increase in sensitization has been more rapid in succeeding generations, implying a possible cohort effect. In interpreting these data in this way, however, it should be borne in mind that a) the data represent only two measurements eight years apart, b) the standardization of skin tests is difficult, and c) the allergens were local allergens and the substantial in-migration of possibly allergic subjects might have affected the results.

CHANGES IN THE USE OF HEALTH SERVICES

It might be expected that the increase in prevalence might, in turn, lead to further changes. Because of the strong tie between a person's acknowledgment of having asthma and that person's use of asthma treatments, it would be expected to follow that the proportion of the population receiving treatment for asthma may have increased. This has indeed been documented in a number of countries, including the United Kingdom, the United States (Michigan), and Canada (Manitoba) (32–34). This has also been reflected in increasing sales of asthma medications (35,36). Changes in terminology do not appear to explain these changes, at least in the British data (37).

In addition, there also seems to have been a major increase in hospital admissions due to asthma. This has been of concern to those who pay for health services. Again, this increase has been documented in a wide range of countries including England and Wales, New Zealand, the United States, Australia, Canada, and Greece (Athens) (38–47). The reasons for the increase are not altogether clear.

In England, hospital admission statistics have been collected since 1958 and it is possible to follow changes in admission rates since that time. Figure 2 gives the data for males plotted by the year of hospital admission. There is a small increase in admission rates in the 1960s in all age groups, superimposed on a major increase that is most marked in the youngest age group, the 0 to 4 year olds. This pattern has been used to suggest that the problem is related to specific age groups. However, if the data are plotted by age and year of birth, rather than by age and date of admission, a different pattern of disease emerges. In this case (Fig. 3), with the exception of the oldest age group, the 45 to 64 year olds, the age groups overlie each other. This suggests that age is less important than the year of birth. The older age group has a markedly

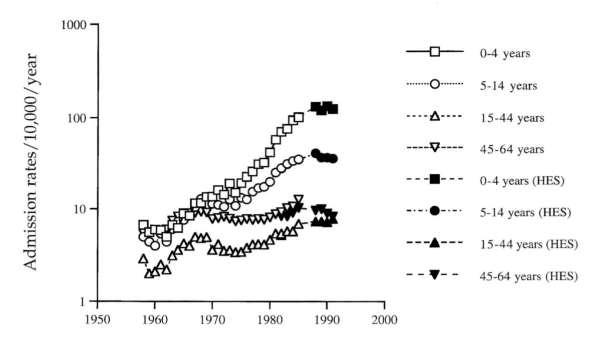

FIG. 2. Male asthma admissions in England 1958 to 1992 by year of admission. HES, health examination survey.

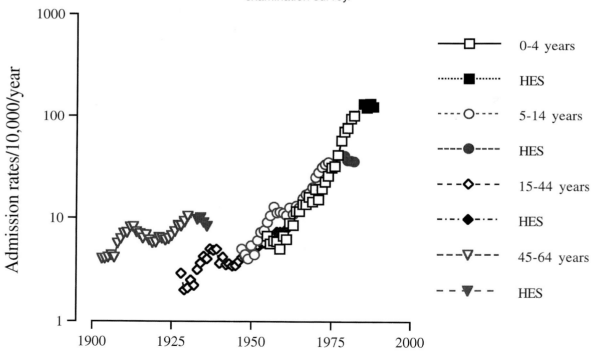

FIG. 3. Male asthma admissions in England 1958 to 1992 by year of birth. HES, health examination survey.

greater admission rate than the other age groups and this may be related to the increased prevalence of fixed airway obstruction and cigarette-induced airway damage.

Interpreting this pattern of increase is not straightforward because it is not possible to partition linear trends over time into cohort and period effects. However, a cohort effect in which succeeding generations have an increased risk of admission that is evident early in life and remains with them at least into early middle age, explains both the period and age effects, and may, therefore, be preferred as the simplest explanation. This could be an effect of early health service experience laying down a pattern of health service use that persists into later life; but it is also compatible with an increasing prevalence of disease in succeeding cohorts. Taking the data displayed in Figure 3, the estimated annual percentage increase in admission rates for succeeding birth cohorts aged 0 to 44 years in the years 1958 to 1988 was 5%. This is well within the range of estimates of increases in disease given in Table 2. There does not seem to be any strong incentive to look for other explanations for the trends over the majority of the period for which we have records.

However, the data for females are more complex (Figs. 4 and 5). In this case, the trends for the two youngest age groups again overlie each other when plotted by year of birth. However, the young adult age group, the 15 to 44

year olds, have an admission rate that parallels that of the two younger age groups but is higher in all cohorts. This fact could indicate that age is an important modifier of risk in women in this group, even though it seems to have no effect in men. In turn, it could also suggest an influence of female sex hormones in increasing the admission rate to hospitals. Other differences in risk between men and women of this age group should not be ignored; but they seem unlikely to be great enough or constant enough to explain such a marked difference between the groups.

In other data sets the interpretation is more difficult. In Saskatchewan, for instance, there has been an increase in admission rates among the Native North American population (48). Figures 6 and 7 show these rises plotted both by date of admission and date of birth. The plot of admission rates against date of birth suggests that trends in 0 to 4 year olds and 15 to 34 year olds could be explained by a common trend by date of birth; but in this case, the 5 to 14 year olds appear to have a significantly lower admission rate. This explanation is not as clearly superior to alternative explanations, and it would be equally plausible to suggest that there had been a relatively consistent increase for each of the age groups, which would be compatible with a common period effect.

In the light of an increasing admissions rate of 5% per annum, a figure compatible with estimates of increases in

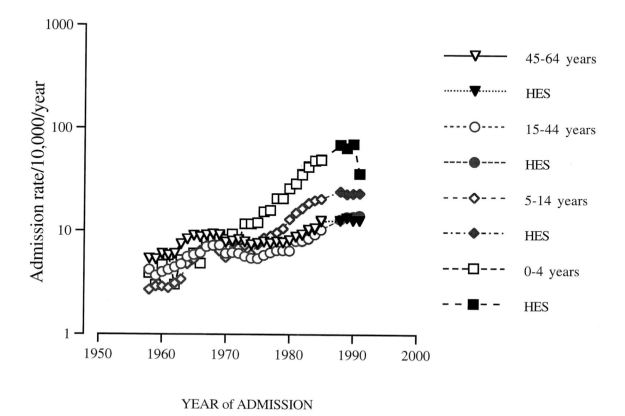

YEAR of ADMISSION

FIG. 4. Female asthma admissions in England 1958 to 1992 by year of admission. HES, health examination survey.

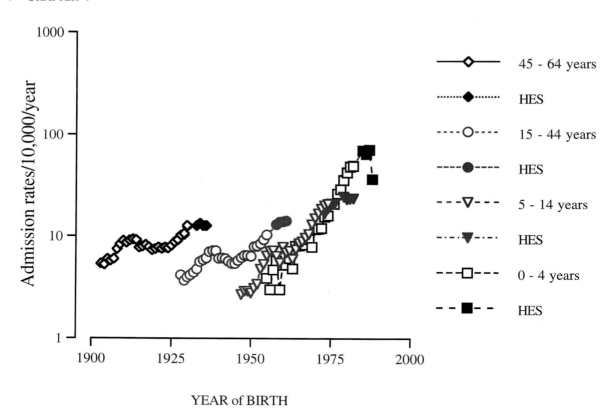

FIG. 5. Female asthma admissions in England 1958 to 1992 by year of birth. HES, health examination survey.

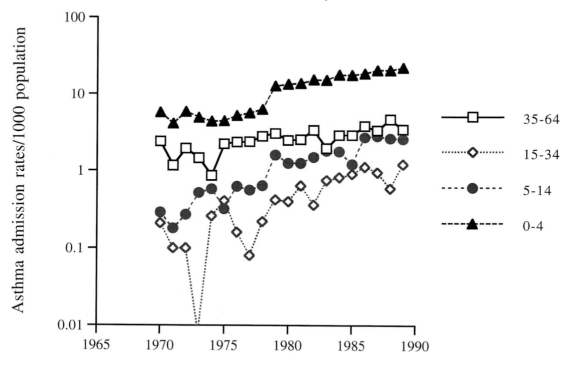

FIG. 6. Admission rates for Saskatchewan Indians 1970 to 1989 by age group and year of admission.

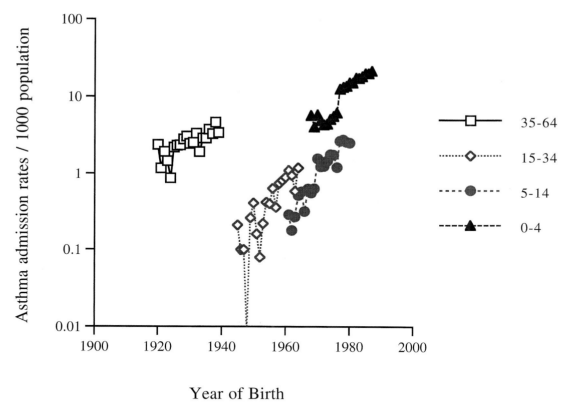

FIG. 7. Admission rates for Saskatchewan Indians 1970 to 1989 by age group and year of birth.

disease over this period of time, it might be asked why any other explanation need be sought than that higher prevalence led directly to a proportional increase in admissions. However, the explanation is not as simple. There are countries such as Finland where admission rates have remained steady in spite of evidence of increasing prevalence (5,15,49). Conversely, there have been areas such as Croydon where an increase in admissions of approximately 5% per annum has been observed, but an increase in wheeze of only 1% per annum (50). In addition to this there is clear evidence that factors other than the prevalence of disease influence admission rates (51,52).

The effect of changes in the use of diagnostic terms on reported admission rates has been disputed, but admission rates do not seem to have been strongly affected by changes in the severity of those admitted. One New Zealand study has even suggested that the threshold of admission had increased (39,44,45,53). Increased re-admission rates have been found to explain part or all of the increase in some studies, but not in others (39,49,54). In England it has been suggested that the trend could in part be explained by an increasing trend for patients to seek emergency care directly from the hospital (39,50,54).

Exceptions to the general trend of increasing admissions have been reported from Italy, Finland (where increases were confined to the elderly and accounted for by increased readmissions), and the Netherlands, where ad-

mission rates for asthma declined throughout the 1980s except among the 0 to 4 year olds, where there was an increase (49,55,56). In recent years there has been at least some evidence for a decline, or at least a slowing down of the increase in use of services in the United States, and, more recently, in England and Wales (43,57,58). In a study of hospitalizations in Portland, Oregon, the reduction in admissions was shown to occur, despite a continuing increase in episodes of asthma (57). In the United Kingdom, interpretation of the changing trend has been complicated by changes in the way that statistics are collected, but they have occurred at a time of increasing pressures on the health services to find alternatives to the admission of patients into hospitals.

CHANGES IN MORTALITY

Trends in mortality have also been a cause of concern. Between the mid-1970s and the mid-1980s, a number of countries experienced an increase in mortality in 5 to 34 year olds, a group often selected to monitor asthma mortality, as being the least likely to include other causes of death (59–65). In some studies this increase was more marked among males than females (60,63). Figure 8 shows the changes in mortality rates for all causes and for asthma by age groups from 5 to 64 years old in the European Community between the periods 1974 to 1978 and 1980 to 1984 (66). The greatest increase in asthma mortality is in those aged 15 to 24 years, among whom it increased at 5.6% per annum. However, changes in asthma mortality were positive in all age groups except the youngest (5 to 14 year olds), where mortality was constant, and the 35 to 44 year olds, where it fell by 0.5% per annum. This is in marked contrast to the changes in mortality rates from all causes which fell for all these age groups at between 1% and 2% per annum with the exception of the 25 to 34 year olds where mortality was falling by only 0.02% per annum. Most of these increases levelled off again or began to fall in the early and mid-1980s, first in New Zealand and then in other countries such as England and Wales. Rates continued to increase in France to the end of the 1980s (65).

Though widespread, these changes during the 1970s and 1980s have not been universal. Japan and Finland saw general downward trends in asthma mortality between the early 1970s and early 1980s; Canada experienced a stable mortality rate during the 1980s, despite an increasing hospitalization rate. Spain has seen a long-term decline in asthma mortality rates (46,62,67).

Mortality rates among 5 to 34 year olds have been much more stable over the century as a whole. In some countries there was a very large, but short-lived, increase

in mortality in the 1960s, though the generally much smaller increase in mortality in the late 1970s and early 1980s was more marked than the 1960's epidemic in New Zealand (62,68). These sudden increases were seen in most age groups at the same time, though not to the same extent. This suggests that they were due to some event that affected mortality fairly directly. The causes of these increases are the subject of Chapter 5. However, the epidemic in the 1960s was associated with the sale of high-dose isoproterenol inhalers, though an association with sales of low-dose inhalers was less clearly established (68).

Mortality data show a more complex pattern than admission rates, although, overall, the changes have been less remarkable over the century. More formal analysis of the data from England and Wales shows that some of this change is due to changes between generations and that the direction of change is for succeeding generations to have successively greater risks of death from asthma (69). These accelerating risks, however, have been counterbalanced by period effects which have tended, with the exception of the major increases in the 1960s and 1970s to 1980s, to have an opposite effect. Such a pattern of changes would be expected where asthma prevalence was increasing, but where other changes, perhaps improvements in treatment, have had a generally favorable effect.

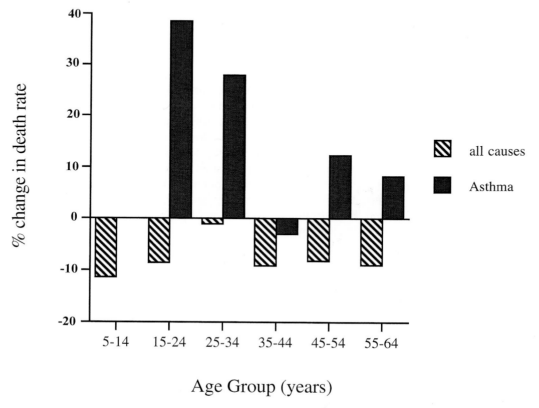

FIG. 8. Changes in mortality in the European Community between 1974 to 1978 and 1980 to 1984.

TABLE 3. *Relative mortality (95% confidence interval) in patients with asthma by date of issue of life insurance policies according to the Medical Impairment Study*

Date of Issue of Policies	1885-1908	1909-1927	1952-1976
Asthma at examination or one attack in the last 5 years	1.19 (0.95–1.43)	1.47 (1.21–1.73)	
Two or more attacks in the last 5 years	1.25 (1.06–1.44)	1.59 (1.42–1.96)	
All Asthma	1.21 (1.07–1.35)	1.54 (1.40–1.68)	1.26 (1.21–1.31)

The same analyses suggest that the most recent changes in deaths imply lower mortality rates in the cohorts born in more recent years.

An important exception to these observations has been reported from Spain where there is a cohort effect but it has been in the opposite direction, reducing mortality rates for asthma in successive generations (67). Here the mortality rates have been declining at least since the early 1970s, in contrast to the trends in neighboring France (65,70).

Direct evidence of changes in case-fatality is difficult to find. Although there is some evidence from the statistics of the life insurance companies, the interpretation of these does depend on assumptions relating to the kind of lives assured at different periods (71). Nevertheless, the historical record, mostly from the United States, suggests that the case fatality rates have been fairly even across the century. It should be noted that there was no major increase in mortality in the United States in the 1960s as there was in some other countries. Table 3 shows the relative risk of death in those whose lives were insured at different periods if asthma was identified in the medical examination prior to issuing the policy. Case fatality would not be expected to be effected by simple changes in prevalence of disease. However, case fatality would be affected by changes in the severity of disease, including artefact changes resulting from the reclassification of the condition to include milder cases (a change that would not be expected by itself to alter mortality rates for the disease), and by changes in treatment. Bearing in mind that the figures quoted here will also be affected by the types of people having their lives insured (which will have had an unpredictable effect), there is little evidence from this source for the improvement of the life expectancy of patients with asthma over the first three quarters of the current century. This is not an entirely surprising conclusion. The major excess of deaths among patients with asthma is predominantly in the later years of life.

CONCLUSIONS

There is good evidence that the prevalence of wheezy illness has been increasing over the last couple of decades at least, and from indirect evidence we may assume that this has been happening from the early part of the century at least in those countries with high prevalence rates. It appears that this has been accompanied for the most part by changes in the prevalence of other atopic conditions and in the prevalence of sensitivity to common aeroallergens. It would be natural to conclude that much of the increase was secondary to this change in the prevalence of atopy. However, it is likely that other factors are also involved and these would have to explain the changes in Australia. The increase in admission to hospitals with asthma has been at approximately the same rate as the increase in the prevalence of disease and, although there is good reason to believe that hospital admission rates are affected by both health service factors and local prevalence rates (51,52). The recent change in admission rates with a slowing down in the increase may, however, be due to health service pressure on costs and, in particular, financial pressure to reduce the use of in-patient facilities (57,58). The major changes in mortality during the latter part of the 20th century probably have little to do with changes in prevalence. It is likely, though, that mortality rates have been affected by changes in prevalence, and this may be what is implied by the weak cohort effects found in mortality trends. The changes in prevalence that have almost certainly occurred make it difficult to assess any long-term changes in the case fatality of the disease. Although some evidence exists from life insurance studies, mostly in the United States, suggesting that these have been relatively constant over the century, their interpretation is difficult.

Although the changes reported here are widespread, it should not be assumed that they have been universal. There is good reason to suppose that those who believe that they have a problem are more likely to study it than those who do not believe that there is a problem. Only a more systematic estimate of trends would allow generalizations to be made about such changes. The question of whether the same upward trends in prevalence are continuing is difficult to answer without continuing monitoring of trends in prevalence in the same populations over a number of years.

REFERENCES

1. Jarvis D, Lai E, Luczynska C, Chinn S, Burney P. Prevalence of asthma and asthmalike symptoms in young adults living in three East Anglian towns. *Br J General Practice* 1994;44:493–497.

2. Morrison Smith J. The prevalence of asthma and wheezing in children. *Br J Dis Chest* 1976;70:73–77.

3. Ninan TK, Russell G. Respiratory symptoms and atopy in Aberdeen schoolchildren: evidence from two surveys 25 years apart. *BMJ* 1992; 304:873–875.

4. Robertson CF, Heycock E, Bishop J, Nolan T, Olinsky A, Phelan PD. Prevalence of asthma in Melbourne schoolchildren: changes over 26 years. *BMJ* 1991;302:1116–1118.

5. Haahtela T, Linholm H, Björksten F, Koskenvuo K, Laitinen LA. Prevalence of asthma in Finnish young men. *BMJ* 1990;301:266–268.

6. Varonier HS, de Haller J, Schopfer C. Prévalence de l'allergie chez les enfants et les adolescents. *Helv Pediatr Acta* 1984;39:129–136.

7. Perdrizet S, Neukirch F, Cooreman J, Liard R. Prevalence of asthma in adolescents in various parts of France and its relationship to respiratory allergic manifestations. *Chest* 1987;91:104S–106S.

8. Mitchell EA. Increasing prevalence of asthma in children. *NZ Med J* 1983;96:463–464.

9. Åberg N. Asthma and allergic rhinitis in Swedish conscripts. *Clin Exp Allergy* 1989;19:59–63.

10. Burr ML, Butland BK, King S, Vaughan Williams E. Changes in asthma prevalence: two surveys 15 years apart. *Arch Dis Child* 1989; 64:1452–1456.

11. Burney PGJ, Chinn S, Rona R. Has the prevalence of asthma increased in children? Evidence from the national study of health and growth 1973-1986. *BMJ* 1990;300:1306–1310.

12. Hsieh K, Shen J. Prevalence of childhood asthma in Taipei, Taiwan and other Asian Pacific countries. *J Asthma* 1988;25:73–82.

13. Shaw RA, Crane J, O'Donnell TV, Porteous LE, Coleman ED. Increasing asthma prevalence in a rural New Zealand adolescent population: 1975-89. *Arch Dis Child* 1990;65:1319–1323.

14. Magnus P, Kongerud J, Bakke JV. Har vi en astmaepidemi? *Tidsskr Nor Lægeforen* 1991;111:972–975.

15. Rimpelä AH, Savonius B, Rimpelä KK, Haahtela T. Asthma and allergic rhinitis among Finnish adolescents in 1977-1991. *Scand J Soc Med* 1995;23:60–65.

16. Anderson HR, Butland BK, Strachan DP. Trends in prevalence and severity of chioldhood asthma. *BMJ* 1994;308:1600–1604.

17. Weitzman M, Gortmaker SL, Sobol AM, Perrin JM. Recent trends in the prevalence and severity of childhood asthma. *JAMA* 1992;268: 2673–2677.

18. Peat JK, Haby M, Spijker J, Berry G, Woolcock AJ. Prevalence of asthma in adults in Busselton, Western Australia. *BMJ* 1992;305:1326–1329.

19. Skjønsberg O, Clench-Aas J, Leegaard J, Skarpaas I, Giæver P, Bartonova A, Moseng J. Prevalence of bronchial asthma in schoolchildren in Oslo, Norway. Comparison of data obtained in 1993 and 1981. *Allergy* 1995;50:806–810.

20. Peat JK, van den Berg RH, Green WF, Mellis CM, Leeder SR, Woolcock AJ. Changing prevalence of asthma in Australian children. *BMJ* 1994;308:1591–1596.

21. Rona RJ, Chinn S, Burney PGJ. Trends in the prevalence of asthma in Scottish and English primary school children 1982–1992. *Thorax* 1995;50:992–993.

22. Crockett A, Cranston J, Alpers J. The changing prevalence of asthma like symptoms in South Australian rural schoolchildren. *J Pediatr Child Health* 1995;31:213–217.

23. Lundbäck B, Stjernberg N, Jönsson A-C, Lindström M, Jönsson E, Forsberg B, Nyström L, Rosenhall L. The prevalence of asthma and respiratory symptoms is still increasing. Report from the obstructive lung disease in Northern Sweden study. In: Lundbäck B. *Asthma, chronic bronchitis, and respiratory symptoms: prevalence and important determinants. The obstructive lung disease in northern Sweden study.* Umeå University Medical Dissertations. New Series 387.

24. Laor A, Cohen L, Danon YL. Effects of time, sex, ethnic origin, and area of residence on prevalence of asthma in Israeli adolescents. *BMJ* 1993;307:841–844.

25. Yunginger JW, Reed CE, O'Connell EJ, Melton LJ, O'Fallon WM, Silverstein MD. A community based study of the epidemiolgy of asthma: incidence rates 1964-83. *Am Rev Respir Dis* 1992;146:888–894.

26. Schultz Larsen F, Holm N, Henningsen K. Atopic dermatitis, a genetic-epidemiologic study in a population based twin sample. *J Am Acad Dermatol* 1986;15:487–494.

27. Taylor B, Wadsworth M, Wadsworth J, Peckham C. Changes in the reported prevalence of childhood eczema since the 1939–1945 war. *Lancet* 1984;ii:1255–1257.

28. Barbee R, Kaltenhorn W, Lebowitz M, Burrows B. Longitudinal chnages in allergen skin test reactivity in a community population sample. *J Allergy Clin Immunol* 1987;79:16–24.

29. Sibbald B, Rink E, D'Souza M. Is the prevalence of atopy increasing? *Br J General Practice* 1990;40:338–340.

30. Gassner M. Immunologische-allergologische Reactionen unter veranderten Unweltbedungingen. *Schweitz Rundsch Med Prax* 1992;81: 426–430.

31. Nakagomi T, Itaya H, Tominaga T, Yamaki M, Hisamatsu S-I, Nakagomi O. Is atopy increasing? (letter) *Lancet* 1994;343:121–122.

32. Fleming D, Crombie D. Prevalence of asthma and hayfever in England and Wales. *BMJ* 1987;294:279–283.

33. Gerstman B, Bosco L, Tomita D, Gross T, Shaw M. Prevalence and treatment of asthma in the Michigan Medicaid patient population younger than 45 years, 1980-1986. *J Allergy Clin Immunol* 1989;83: 1032–1039.

34. Manfreda J, Becker AB, Wang P-Z, Roos L, Anthonsen N. Trends in physician diagnosed asthma prevalence in Manitoba between 1980 and 1990. *Chest* 1993;103:151–157.

35. Keating G, Mitchell E, Jackson R, Beaglehole R, Rea H. Trends in sales of drugs for asthma in New Zealand, Australia and the United Kingdom 1975-81. *BMJ* 1984;289:348–351.

36. Department of Health. Asthma: an epidemiological overview. Central Health Monitoring Unit Epidemiological Overview Series. London, HMSO, 1995.

37. Ayres JG, Noah ND, Fleming DM. Incidence of episodes of acute asthma and acute cronchitis in general practice 1976-87. *Br J Gen Pract* 1993;43:361–364.

38. Mitchell E. International trends in hospital admission rates for asthma. *Arch Dis Child* 1985;60:376–378.

39. Anderson HR, Bailey P, West S. Trends in the hospital care of acute childhood asthma 1970-1978: a regional study. *BMJ* 1980;281: 1191–1194.

40. Alderson M. Trends in morbidity and mortality from asthma. *Population Trends* 1987;49:18–23.

41. Anderson HR. Increase of hospital admissions for childhood asthma: trends in referral, severity and readmissions from 1970 to 1985 in a health region of the United Kingdom. *Thorax* 1989;44:614–619.

42. Jackson R, Mitchell E. Trends in hospital admission rates and drug treatment for asthma in New Zealand. *NZ Med J* 1983;96:728–730.

43. Halfon N, Newacheck P. Trends in the hospitalisation of acute childhood asthma, 1970-1984. *Am J Public Health* 1986;76:1308–1311.

44. Carman P, Landau L. Increased paediatric admission with asthma in Western Australia—a problem of diagnosis. *Med J Aust* 1990;152: 23–26.

45. Kun HY, Oates RK, Mellis CM. Hospital admissions and attendences for asthma—a true increase? *Med J Aust* 1993;159:312–313.

46. Wilkins K and Mao Y. Trends in rates of admission to hospital and death from asthma among children and young adults in Canada during the 1980s. *Can Med Assoc J* 1993;148:185–190.

47. Priftis K, Anagnostakis J, Harokopos E, Orfanou I, Petraki M, Saxoni-Papageorgiou P. Time trends and seasonal variation in hopsital admissions for childhood asthma in the Athens regions of Greece: 1978–1988. *Thorax* 1993;48:1168–1169.

48. Sentilselvan A, Habbick B. Increased asthma hospitalisations among registered Indian children and adults in Saskatchewan, 1970-1989. *J Clin Epidemiol* 1995;48:1277–1283.

49. Keistinen T, Tuuponen T, Kivelä S-L. Asthma related hospital treatment in Finland, 1972-86. *Thorax* 1993;48:44–47.

50. Strachan D, Anderson HR. Trends in hospital admission rates for asthma in children. *BMJ* 1992;304:819–820.

51. Burney P, Papacosta AO, Withey C, Colley J, Holland WW. Hospital admission rates and the prevalence of asthma symptoms in 20 local authority districts. *Thorax* 1991;46:574–579.

52. Connett G, Warde C, Wooler E, Lenney W. Audit strategies to reduce hospital admissions for acute asthma. *Arch Dis Child* 1993;69:202–205.

53. Dawson K. The severity of asthma in children admitted to hospital: a 20 year review. *N Z Med J* 1987;100:520–521.

54. Storr J, Barrell E, Lenney W. Rising asthma admissions and self-referral. *Arch Dis Child* 1988;63:774–779.

55. Fasoli M, La Vecchia C, Formigaro M, Repetto R. Trends in hospital admissions for asthma in Lombardy, Italy, 1976–1986. *J Epidemiol Community Health* 1992;46:171–172.

56. Wever A, Wever-Hess J. Trends en de frequentie van zeikenhuisopname

Medicine (10), Osler states that death during an acute attack of asthma is unknown. He clearly describes severe attacks of asthma, attacks that today we would consider life threatening and likely to lead to death without medical intervention. Despite these pronouncements, examination of mortality statistics from the 1860s in England and Wales (11) and from the early 1900s in Australia (12) and New Zealand (13) shows that deaths from asthma were officially recorded. In the United Kingdom, mortality for both men and women fell between 1867 and the beginning of the 1900s, although for the great majority of this period rates were below 1/100,000 in the 5- to 34-year-old age group. The greater mortality among males during this period has been attributed to the deleterious effects of the industrial conditions in which men worked (11). What is striking in all three countries is the stability of rates well below 1/100,000 between 1910 and 1940 (Fig. 1).

Early Treatments

In 1901 Takamine and Aldrich independently isolated the hormone adrenaline (14,15) and in 1903 it was first used successfully to treat severe asthma (16). In 1907 adrenaline was shown to relax muscle in isolated tracheal preparations (17). By 1920 enthusiasm for adrenaline by injection was at its height and by 1929 adrenaline was being used by inhalation (18). Ephedrine, which had been an ingredient of traditional Chinese remedies since antiquity, became an increasingly popular treatment in the 1920s, providing sustained bronchodilatation by mouth (19). The stimulant properties of both tea and coffee had been appreciated for centuries but the airway effects of the principle active ingredient of coffee, caffeine, were not demonstrated until 1912 (20). The first use of theophylline in the treatment of asthma was by rectal suppository in 1922 (21). The 1930s saw the widespread introduction of the methyl xanthines. In 1937 the successful use of aminophylline intravenously (22) opened the way for theophylline as the cornerstone of the acute management of severe asthma. In the 1940s the synthetic β-receptor agonist, isoprenaline, was introduced and for the next 20 years was the principal inhaled treatment for asthma (23).

Increasing Awareness of Asthma Mortality

Interestingly, by the ninth edition of Sir William Osler's textbook, published in 1923 after his death (in the first revision by Thomas McCrae), the didactic statement concerning death during an attack of asthma is omitted (24). It would appear that death during severe asthma was rare at the beginning of this century and for that reason alone was unlikely to have been observed. By the 1930s the situation was changing. Witts in 1936 noted that whereas death during an acute attack was unusual, it was not as unusual as had been taught, especially during prolonged status asthmaticus, unrelieved by adrenaline or ephedrine (25). In 1948 Coope echoed the same caution (26). In reflecting on this in the United States in the 1960s, Alexander noted an increase in mortality from 2.5/100,000 in 1937 to 4.5/100,000 in 1950, declining however to 2.8/100,000 by 1959 (27).

A rising trend in mortality in the 5- to 34-year-old age group was also noted in the United Kingdom from the early 1940s (11). Similar increases have also been recorded in New Zealand and Australia (12,13). These increases in mortality occurred during the same period in which aminophylline and isoprenaline were introduced and increasingly used in the treatment of asthma. Although there is no evidence that there was any link between these therapeutic advances and asthma mortality, in the light of recent events these observations represent an interesting prologue.

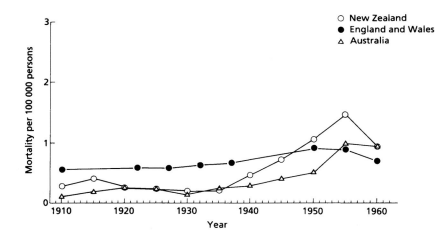

FIG. 1. Asthma mortality (per 100,000) in persons aged 5–34 years in New Zealand, Australia, and England and Wales, 1910–1960. (Adapted from Speizer F, Doll R. A century of asthma deaths in young people. *Br Med J* 1968;3:245–246; and Baumann A, Lee S. Trends in asthma mortality in Australia, 1911–1986 (Letter). *Med J Aust* 1990;153:366; and Beasley R, Smith K, Pearce N, Crane J, Burgess C, Culling C. Trends in asthma mortality in New Zealand, 1908–1986. *Med J Aust* 1990; 152:570–573.)

In 1953 Williams examined mortality in England and Wales between 1938 and 1949 and showed an average mortality of 2,931 deaths per year, a rate of 7/100,000 for all ages, accounting for 0.6% of all deaths during that period. For 1949, 96% of deaths occurred in those over the age of 25 years. In his own practice most deaths were among severe asthmatics of long standing with many previous episodes of status asthmaticus. He also observed a clear seasonal pattern to mortality, increasing in winter, which he attributed to colds and respiratory infections precipitating severe asthma (28).

THE 1960s

Isoprenaline in Metered Dose Inhalers

The early 1960s saw the introduction of the metered dose inhaler containing isoprenaline and powered by freons (29). This preparation was capable of delivering a reproducible dose of aerosol to the airways and was viewed as a major therapeutic advance. Not long after their widespread introduction and availability over the counter, the first reports of sudden and sometimes unexpected deaths among patients using them. McManis reported three deaths appeared in patients with status asthmaticus after injections of adrenaline given after treatment with isoprenaline (30). In the United Kingdom, Greenberg and Pines reported 12 deaths in which excessive use of aerosols containing isoprenaline, adrenaline, or orciprenaline had been documented before death (31). These observations were soon followed by evidence that asthma mortality had increased abruptly in some countries, the most striking increase being observed in New Zealand (Fig. 2)

An Epidemic of Asthma Mortality

In 1967, in response to the concern over treatment-related deaths, Speizer, Doll, and Heaf reviewed international trends in asthma mortality between 1951 and 1964 in 19 countries (1). The study was a landmark and the first to recognize and deal with many of the problems associated with such investigations. The authors showed that there had been a sharp decline in mortality between 1957 and 1959, which they attributed to the introduction of the seventh revision of the ICD coding in 1958. This revision removed the bronchitis and asthma association, previously classified as asthma. The epidemic rise in asthma mortality had occurred during the 7th ICD classification period.

They also showed wide international variation in crude mortality from 1.1 to 9.7 per 100,000. Part of this variation they attributed to differences in diagnostic fashion. They focused on three age groups: 10- to 14-year, 5- to 34-year, and 35- to 64-year-olds. This was partly because the increase had affected the younger age groups and partly because asthma may be confused with other causes of death with increasing age. By comparing trends for different respiratory disorders in England and Wales, they were able to show that this increase was not a change in diagnostic fashion as the rise in asthma mortality had not been associated with a corresponding decline in deaths from pneumonia, acute or chronic bronchitis, or chronic respiratory diseases. The changes were striking, beginning abruptly in 1960, with mortality increasing threefold for the 5- to 34-year-olds between 1959 and 1966.

The authors concluded that these data represented a real increase in mortality and were not an artifact of coding or diagnostic change. The paper was a watershed in

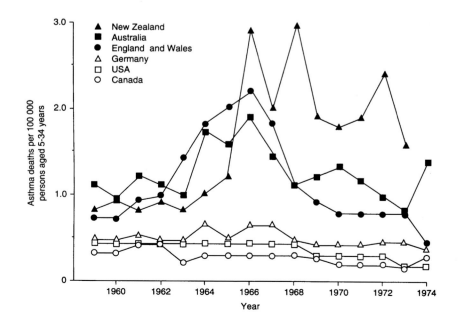

FIG. 2. Asthma mortality (per 100,000) in persons aged 5–34 years in New Zealand, Australia, England and Wales, Germany, United States, and Canada, 1960–1974. (Adapted from Jackson R, Sears MR, Beaglehole R, Rea HH. International trends in asthma mortality: 1970 to 1985. *Chest* 1988;94(5):914–918.)

the examination of asthma mortality and studies since have usually followed their approach.

Associations Between Aerosol Sales and Trends in Mortality

A year later, Inman and Adelstein examined these trends in asthma mortality in the United Kingdom, relating them to the rise and fall in sales of bronchodilator aerosols and in particular those containing isoprenaline. They concluded that the excess deaths were most likely due to excessive self-medication and that the equally abrupt decline in mortality was most likely due to warnings issued by the Committee for Safety of Drugs in June 1967 and the restriction of over-the-counter sales in December 1968 (32). The epidemic declined as abruptly as it had begun and before further epidemiologic studies could be undertaken.

Biologic plausibility for the association between β-agonist aerosols and death came from a number of animal studies that showed adverse cardiac effects of isoprenaline and orciprenaline. Lockett demonstrated a marked increase in sensitivity to isoprenaline and orciprenaline in the fatigued cat heart with arrest in asystole (33). Collins et al. demonstrated a similar increase in sensitivity in dogs when given isoprenaline under conditions of hypoxemia (34). Animal studies of freon aerosol propellants also showed cardiotoxicity but only at levels far in excess of clinical exposure (35).

By the end of the 1960s considerable circumstantial evidence implicated bronchodilator aerosols in the epidemic. A large increase in mortality in a number of countries had occurred in young asthmatic patients, disturbing a century of relatively stable asthma mortality statistics (11). The changes coincided with the rise and fall in sales of a new form of therapy that had been available without prescription. The impact had been most pronounced among young patients at an age when they began to take responsibility for their own asthma management. Warnings issued by health authorities and restrictions placed on the sales of bronchodilator aerosols in some countries, including the United Kingdom, were associated with a sudden decline in mortality to pre-epidemic levels (32).

THE 1970s

Review, Anomalies, and Reinterpretation of the Epidemic

The 1970s saw considerable review and debate of asthma mortality and the epidemic. Fraser et al. undertook a regional case study of series of deaths in young people in the United Kingdom to explore the circumstances surrounding death in asthmatics who died between 1968 and 1969. They investigated the deaths of 52 young persons and concluded that although all had severe asthma, death was unexpected and sudden in 80% of cases, in most because the severity of the attack had not been appreciated. In a third of the cases in which information was available, there was evidence that suggested excessive inhalation of bronchodilators had occurred. No other potentially contributory factors were observed (36).

Further review of the epidemic revealed two apparent anomalies in the hypothesis that treatment and bronchodilator aerosols, in particular, might be responsible. First, in Australia, where mortality had increased and declined abruptly, the time trends for declining mortality and isoprenaline sales did not appear to coincide (37). Second, other countries in which isoprenaline was available, and in particular the United States, had not experienced any significant increase in mortality (1). These two anomalies together with the inherent weakness of ecological associations and the natural difficulty in accepting that a major advance in asthma management might be deleterious, led during the 1970s to a process of reinterpretation based on review of the previous data (38). It was suggested that asthma severity had generally been underestimated and deaths were more likely to be associated with under rather than over treatment (39). By 1979 this process had led to a significant shift in opinion concerning the 1960s epidemic. A *Lancet* editorial argued that there was a growing realization that pressurized aerosols were not the main culprit and that attention had turned to the occasional failure of clinicians to treat asthma attacks promptly and adequately (40). The introduction of more selective β 2–specific agonists and the trend toward the end of the 1970s of using them on a regular basis (41), without any further reports of epidemics of mortality, further supported the argument that therapy was not implicated. Although these arguments were to some extent justified, particularly those relating to under-recognition of asthma severity, they entirely failed to explain why mortality had increased and decreased so abruptly and why some countries had suddenly experienced an under-recognition of asthma severity and others had not. This process of reinterpretation was to become important because it almost certainly influenced thinking in relation to the second epidemic in New Zealand in the 1980s.

An explanation for the apparently random geographical distribution of the epidemics was provided in 1978 by Stolley, who noted that there was a much closer association between epidemics of deaths and the availability and sales of high-dose preparations of isoprenaline (up to five times the standard dose). Thus, in eight countries where high-dose isoprenaline was licensed, six had experienced sudden increases in mortality (England and Wales, Ireland, Scotland, Australia, New Zealand, and Norway). In the Netherlands and Belgium the introduction of the high-dose preparation had been late and sales volumes were low. No epidemics had been recorded in countries that had not licensed the high-dose formulation of isoprenaline (42). No other plausible hypothesis has been put forward that would explain the timing and distribution of this epidemic.

In Australia, Gandevia reported that the relationship between sales of isoprenaline aerosols and mortality did not fit. He showed that mortality among 5- to 54-year-olds had risen and fallen between 1963 and 1968 but sales of isoprenaline had continued progressively (37). In 1976, Campbell again reviewed the relationship between sales of aerosols and mortality in Australia, and concluded that in the four most populace states, the correlation between deaths and mortality was very close between 1961 and 1966, but not thereafter. He attributed the later lack of correlation of sales with deaths to the repeated warnings issued both officially and unofficially in Australia (43). The first warning by McManis in 1964 focused on the combination of adrenaline and isoprenaline, but from 1965 a number of specific warnings about overuse of bronchodilator aerosols were issued by the Australian Health Department and further warnings appeared after publication of Speizer's study in the United Kingdom.

Thus, these two apparent anomalies, one of geographic distribution, the other of ecological association, had received explanations but not until almost a decade after the epidemic, when mortality had long since declined. The opinions that these anomalies had helped to generate were largely retained.

THE 1980s

Second Epidemic in New Zealand

As the concerns surrounding asthma mortality in the late 1960s and the reviews of the 1970s swung the balance of opinion away from an association with asthma treatment (38), mortality again rose abruptly in New Zealand (44). Because these changes have now been studied in more detail than any other, these events will be detailed. In many ways the events in the early 1980s in New Zealand were a rerun of those 15 years earlier in the United Kingdom.

A sudden increase in asthma deaths began in New Zealand in 1976, although it was not recognized until 1981 when Wilson et al. reported a cluster of deaths in Auckland, many of which were sudden and unexpected. These were essentially a collection of case reports and a brief review of mortality in Auckland. In their report, Wilson et al. suggested that one possible cause might be the combined use of both β-agonist aerosols and long-acting theophylline preparations (recently introduced to New Zealand) and both used extensively (45).

Subsequently, Jackson et al. (44) reviewed international trends in asthma mortality among 5- to 34-year-olds, from 1959 to 1979 in six countries, three of which, New Zealand, Australia, and England and Wales, had experienced the previous epidemic. On this occasion, the authors confirmed an epidemic confined to New Zealand and again they considered the same potentially spurious explanations for an increase in mortality. The authors concluded that the large increase in mortality in New Zealand could not be explained by changes in ICD coding, diagnostic fashion, or inaccurate death certification. The most likely explanation was an increased case fatality related to asthma management. The changes were even more striking than the previous epidemic in the 1960s, with mortality in New Zealand increasing to four times the rate in Australia or England and Wales (Fig. 3).

National Case Study of Asthma Deaths

In August 1981 an asthma task force convened by the New Zealand Medical Research Council commenced a 2-year national survey of asthma deaths in persons under 70

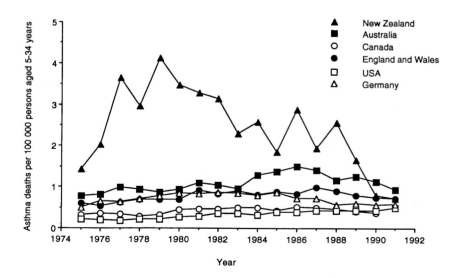

FIG. 3. Asthma mortality (per 100,000) in persons aged 5–34 years in New Zealand, Australia, Canada, England and Wales, United States, and Germany, 1974–1992. (Adapted from Jackson R, Sears MR, Beaglehole R, Rea HH. International trends in asthma mortality: 1970 to 1985. *Chest* 1988;94(5):914–918.)

years of age. This survey was modeled on a previous case survey in the United Kingdom (46) and unfortunately did not include a control group, an omission that led inevitably to difficulties in discussing specific risk factors for asthma mortality (47).

This study was published in 1985 and confirmed that the increase in asthma deaths was real. The study suggested a number of factors that had likely contributed to asthma deaths: inadequate assessment of asthma severity and inappropriate drug therapy including underuse of corticosteroids and over-reliance on β-agonists. In many cases there was delay both in seeking and in providing medical care. A lack of follow-up after treatment of acute attacks was also observed. A major problem with these results was that there was no adequate explanation for why any of these factors should have suddenly changed between 1976 and 1977. From individual reports from family members and in some cases medical practitioners, the authors concluded that there was little evidence of excessive use of bronchodilator drugs before death; in fact such use was suggested in only 9 of 271 cases.

The report emphasized problems of underuse of effective treatment, particularly oral and inhaled steroids, and that this was a considerably greater problem than the overuse of β-agonists. This was unlikely to be an explanation for the epidemic, as a large increase in sales of inhaled steroids occurred during the late 1970s and 1980s.

Subsequent reviews of these data by the same authors led to contradictory statements concerning the role of bronchodilator therapy with suggestions that most patients had repeatedly used their inhaled bronchodilators, and in some cases home nebulizers, to administer inappropriately large doses of β-agonists (48).

In retrospect, the lack of focus on therapy as a possible cause of the epidemic is surprising. However, in its historical context the reasons are apparent. After the confirmation of an epidemic in New Zealand, Keating et al. published a paper comparing sales of asthma medications in Australia, the United Kingdom, and New Zealand from 1975 to 1981. This study showed a marked increase in sales in all three countries, but most marked for all medications in New Zealand. In particular, the study showed a steep increase in drug sales between 1979 and 1980, some 3 years after the start of the epidemic, and was most striking for inhaled bronchodilators (49).

This study influenced approaches to the further investigation of the epidemic suggesting as it did that the increase in sales of asthma treatment was an appropriate response to some change in the natural history of asthma in New Zealand. Further examination of the timing of this increase revealed that it coincided with changes to prescribing advice for β-agonists, in particular with recommendations that β-agonists be given regularly rather than as required (50). A small case-controlled study was undertaken on the Auckland portion of the data and subsequently published by Rea et al. (51). This study compared cases who had died with both hospital and community controls. The study identified risk factors for asthma mortality (see later) but did not examine asthma treatment.

International Trends—Fact or Artifact

Although the changes in New Zealand were striking and had been confirmed by a detailed 2-year national survey, the initial study by Jackson had also revealed a small upward trend in mortality in other countries (44). This observation and the confirmation of a further epidemic in New Zealand prompted investigation of time trends elsewhere. In the United Kingdom Burney estimated an increase in mortality of 50% in the 5- to 34-year-old age group between 1974 and 1984, predominantly among males (52). This period included the 1979 revision of the ICD coding. When the data were re-examined for the period 1979–1989, entirely within the 9th revision much of the rising trend disappeared (53). Most studies have suggested that in the 5- to 34-year-old age group this revision accounts for only a small increase, but the period of study may be important. In a further analysis of deaths in the United Kingdom over a longer time period, between 1931 and 1985, Burney suggested that death was independently associated with both birth date and date of death, suggesting a birth cohort effect, and an effect of factors at the time of death (54).

In 1988 Sly observed an increase in asthma mortality in the United States between 1978 and 1984 (55), and then in 1990 Weiss et al. confirmed this trend and showed that much of the increase in the United States was being driven by large increases in particular urban locations (56). Further studies, for example in Philadelphia, suggested that the increases were most pronounced in areas with poor socioeconomic circumstances and high in minority populations (57). In Sweden mortality among young adults rose 5% for the period 1973–1988 compared with 1952–1972. Most of this increase occurred in the 15- to 24-year-old age group. The authors noted an increased tendency for sudden and unexpected death among supposedly mild asthmatics (58).

In 1988 Jackson reviewed mortality trends in more detail for 5- to 34-year-olds in 14 countries between 1970 and 1985. Excluding New Zealand, he noted a sixfold variation in mortality and observed that 11 countries had a higher average mortality in 1982–1984 than 1979–1981, and in six of these the increase was 20% or more. There was no evidence that the 9th revision of the ICD, introduced in 1979, had materially influenced these changes (5). Bridge coding exercises in the United Kingdom (52) and New Zealand (5) in this age group suggested that no more than a 6% and 2.4% increase, respectively, would be expected from the change to the 9th ICD revision.

The authors concluded that part of the increase in mortality could have been explained by diagnostic transfer. In

England and Wales and in the United States the increase in asthma mortality coincided with a decline in all respiratory mortality. In the United States, however, a further breakdown of the respiratory category revealed an increase in all forms of obstructive respiratory deaths. As this is the category to which asthma is most likely to be transferred, in the United States this appears an unlikely explanation (5).

The large variation between countries noted in this study and previously in the 1960s in part is likely to be related to accuracy of death certification. In a study designed to examine this, Burney has suggested that both genuine differences in nosology and differences in accuracy, especially ambiguous cases, may have a significant impact on mortality rates (6).

Most of these studies have tended to show an increase in asthma mortality over the last 30 years. For the reasons discussed previously, there is a need to be cautious in interpreting these data given the potential for ICD coding effects and changes in diagnostic fashion over long time periods. Although it may not be conclusive that mortality has in fact increased, there is no evidence that it has declined, and this in itself is surprising. As Burney has pointed out, asthma is eminently amenable to treatment, and mortality from many such diseases has declined. This paradoxical situation could arise if asthma treatment carried both benefit and risk, mortality being a product of their balance (52).

By the end of the 1980s, a second real epidemic of deaths had been identified, confined to New Zealand, and studies from many countries had suggested an upward trend in asthma mortality. The reasons for these changes were unclear.

FENOTEROL HYPOTHESIS

Circumstantial Evidence Suggesting an Hypothesis

Inevitably the sudden increase in mortality prompted an examination of the sales of specific β-agonists and their association with increasing mortality. Fenoterol was introduced to New Zealand in April 1976 at the commencement of the epidemic. Further inquiry revealed that fenoterol had achieved 30% of the market share for β-agonist inhalers in New Zealand within 3 years, compared with less than 5% in most other countries. The per capita use was higher than anywhere else in the world (59). Compared with salbutamol, fenoterol was approximately twice as potent on a weight basis, but despite that, it was dispensed in a 200 μg per puff preparation compared with 100 μg per puff for salbutamol. Although the recommendations for fenoterol dosage were one puff, it transpired that most asthma patients were in fact using two puffs at a time, as they had always done with salbutamol (60).

These observations led to an examination of the extrapulmonary effects of salbutamol and fenoterol with isoprenaline in volunteers. This study suggested that inhalation of fenoterol caused greater inotropic and chronotropic effects than salbutamol, with the magnitude of the changes due to fenoterol being very similar to those from isoprenaline (61). This similarity between fenoterol and isoprenaline resulted from the accumulative effect of fenoterol being longer acting than isoprenaline, rather than greater potency.

Last, a further report from the Asthma Task Force on a subgroup of 75 patients who had died and who also had home nebulizers had shown a greater proportion of deaths among patients prescribed fenoterol for nebulization than would have been predicted from the market share (62). Even in the first report from Wilson of the cluster of deaths in Auckland, fenoterol featured in 60% of the sudden deaths while having only 30% of the market share (45).

Thus, a picture incriminating fenoterol emerged from this circumstantial data, reminiscent of the isoprenaline forte hypothesis in the 1960s. A potent high-dose bronchodilator with greater cardiovascular effects than other β-agonists had been introduced and widely used coincident with a sudden increase in mortality. This evidence suggested the need to study fenoterol in more detail. This time it was possible to undertake the more definitive case-controlled studies that had been denied those examining the 1960s epidemic.

Case-control Studies

These observations led to three case-control studies to investigate the possible role of fenoterol in this epidemic. The first study included all deaths in the 5- to 45-year-old age group during 1981–1983 and controls selected from patients hospitalized for nonfatal asthma (63). The only treatment consistently associated with a significantly increased risk of death was fenoterol. The possibility that these increased risks were the result of selective prescribing to more severe asthmatics (i.e., confounding by severity) was investigated by examining subgroups defined by markers of chronic asthma severity. In these subgroups the relative risk of death in those using fenoterol was markedly increased, ranging from 2.2 to 13.3 in the most severe subgroup.

These findings largely excluded the possibility that the association between fenoterol and asthma death was due to confounding by severity as in this situation the fenoterol relative risk would have decreased, as the analysis was increasingly restricted to the most severe subgroups. In view of the widespread use of fenoterol in New Zealand, there was little reason to suspect that fenoterol was being prescribed selectively to the most severe patients. Further analysis of this and subsequent studies have failed to show evidence of confounding by asthma severity among the population of asthmatics used in these studies (64).

A second case-controlled study was undertaken to address a major criticism of the first study, that the source of data on prescribed medication was different for cases and controls (65). In this second study, in which all prescribing information came from hospital records, similar relative risks for fenoterol were found. A third case-controlled study was undertaken for deaths between 1981 and 1987 using two control groups in response to further criticism of appropriate control selection (66). Fenoterol was again associated with an increased risk of death with either control group, the control group suggested by critics in fact yielding higher relative risks.

The Saskatchewan Epidemiology Project

The New Zealand studies led to considerable debate, and in response Boehringer Ingelheim funded a series of studies in Canada (the Saskatchewan Asthma Epidemiology Project) specifically designed (67) to examine critically the New Zealand findings. This study examined 44 asthma deaths and 233 controls in the province of Saskatchewan during 1980 to 1987 (68). The Saskatchewan study was similar in many respects to the New Zealand studies and used the same severity markers. When the data were analyzed in the same way as the New Zealand stud-

ies, the fenoterol relative risk was 5.3, and the salbutamol relative risk 1.0 (Table 2). Almost half the deaths having been prescribed fenoterol compared with 16% of the controls. Thus, the risk of death associated with fenoterol was stronger than the risk found in New Zealand when the studies were analyzed in an identical manner.

The authors interpreted the findings as reflecting a class effect of β-agonists, but conceded that the study showed that fenoterol was more hazardous than other β-agonists in the dose in which it was marketed. The accompanying editorial in the *New England Journal of Medicine* concluded that there was enough doubt about the safety of fenoterol to avoid it altogether (69); Hensley (a member of the Scientific Advisory Board of the study) also noted that the Saskatchewan findings supported the New Zealand findings and that "the weight of evidence and availability of alternative medication should lead to a recommendation that fenoterol not be used to treat asthma" (70). Thus, four case-controlled studies, three in New Zealand and one in Canada, had shown an increased risk of death associated with the prescription of a high-dose formulation of fenoterol by metered dose inhaler.

Effect of Restrictions on Fenoterol Prescribing

It has been possible to observe the effects of warnings about the use of fenoterol and restrictions placed on fenoterol sales by the New Zealand Department of Health

TABLE 2. *Studies of fenoterol and asthma deaths*

	Second New Zealand study	Third New Zealand study[a]	Saskatchewan study
Study period	1977–1981	1981–1987	1980–1987
Study base	Patients with a hospital admission for asthma in previous year	Patients with a hospital admission for asthma in previous year	Patients with 10 different asthma prescriptions during 1978–1987
Study design	Nested case-controlled study	Nested case-controlled study	Nested case-controlled study
Matching for severity?	Yes	Yes	No
Source of drug information	Routine hospital records	Routine hospital records	Routine prescription records
Main exposure information	Prescribed[b] medication	Prescribed[b] medication	Dispensed medication
Additional information	Nil	Nil	Number of units per month
Information on use?	No	No	No
Severity markers	Hospital admissions, oral steroids, 3+ categories of drugs	Hospital admissions, oral steroids, 3+ categories of drugs	Hospital admissions, oral steroids, 3+ categories of drugs
Odds ratios			
Fenoterol	2.0	2.1	5.3
Salbutamol	0.7	0.6	1.0
Both drugs	3.2	4.5	4.4
Fenoterol only	1.9	2.0	3.7
Salbutamol only[c]	1.0	1.0	1.0
Neither	1.1	1.2	0.3

[a]Findings using control group A.
[b]Prescribed medication is synonymous with dispensed medication because prescribed β-agonists were free during the study period.
[c]Reference category.

(71). From 1983 to 1988 mortality in the 5- to 34-year-old age group had averaged 2.3/100,000 and was 2.2/100,000 in the first 6 months of 1989. In April 1989 warnings were issued by the Department of Health concerning the safety of fenoterol, with a suggestion that alternatives be used. In the second 6 months of 1989 mortality had fallen to 1.1/100,000 and has subsequently fallen further (Fig. 4), after the withdrawal of fenoterol from the Druf Tariff in 1990. This dramatic change coincided with a reduction in fenoterol sales while total β-agonist sales remained unchanged.

Individual Versus Class Effect of β-agonists

In some countries trends in asthma mortality suggested a gradual increase since the early 1970s although, as discussed earlier, these trends are less easily confirmed than those associated with epidemics. These trends were apparent in a number of countries where fenoterol was either unavailable, such as the United States, or sold in very small volumes, such as the United Kingdom (59).

In 1990 Sears et al. published the results of a crossover study comparing regular versus on-demand fenoterol in patients with mild to moderate asthma (72). Asthma control was significantly worse during the period of regular fenoterol treatment. This study generated considerable debate and, while providing a further potential mechanism to explain the New Zealand epidemic, also raised two important questions: Were these findings peculiar to fenoterol, or applicable to all β-agonists; and could they explain the gradual international trend in asthma mortality? The answer to these questions remains unclear.

However, a recent study by Chapman et al. (73) with salbutamol rather than fenoterol suggests that chronic effects from different β-agonists may be different. Chapman studied 341 patients in a 4-week crossover trial, comparing 200 μg salbutamol four times daily for 2 weeks with salbutamol as required. Using criteria similar to Sears, symptom control was identical in 70 patients, but in the remainder, control was achieved more often with regular salbutamol. However, the patients in the salbutamol study were more severe and in this group on-demand and regular treatment may result in similar doses of β-agonist being received.

The Saskatchewan study group has also suggested a class effect of β-agonists on asthma mortality, most recently with the publication of their cohort analysis (74). The associations found in this study have been criticized on a number of counts. The findings are based on the questionable comparison of groups using either fenoterol or salbutamol with very small numbers being prescribed neither drug and in some cases no β-agonists (75). The claim for a class effect therefore rests on the strong and unlikely assumption that there was no difference in asthma severity between patients who were, or were not, prescribed β-agonists.

This issue is relevant to the gradual increase in mortality but not to the issue of epidemics. As Tattersfield has noted, both epidemics have been associated with use of high-dose preparations of β-agonist drugs with less β 2 selectivity, and both have improved when the drugs were withdrawn (76). It seems unlikely that epidemiologic data will answer the question of a class effect of β-agonists on asthma mortality; as Barrett and Strom have pointed out, epidemiologic study designs will forever be limited because treatment decisions may be influenced by disease severity and prognosis. It seems equally unlikely that large multicenter randomized controlled trials comparing regular versus as required β-agonist use with asthma death will ever be undertaken given the expense and the rarity of asthma deaths (77).

STUDIES OF OTHER RISK FACTORS FOR ASTHMA MORTALITY

Although most analytical epidemiologic studies of asthma deaths have focused on pharmacologic risk factors, several case-controlled studies have examined associations between markers of asthma severity and the risk of death. These associations are important because

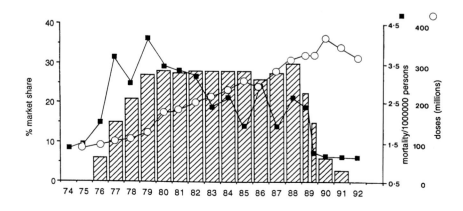

FIG. 4. Total β-agonist sales (doses × 10⁶) fenoterol market share (percentage) and asthma mortality (per 100,000 persons aged 5–34 years) in New Zealand 1974–1992. (■) is asthma mortality per 100,000 persons aged 5- to 34-years. (○) is total β-agonist sales (doses × 10⁶).

greater asthma severity is likely to be related to poor management, and may explain some of the findings of greater asthma mortality in some communities. Recognition of these markers helps to identify asthmatics at increased risk of death. Such markers have, as we have seen, also been used to examine the issue of confounding by severity in studies of asthma mortality.

Four studies have examined the association between markers of asthma severity and risk of asthma death in adults (Table 3) (51,68,78,79). These have involved three markers of chronic asthma severity: a) a hospital admission during the previous 12 months; b) prescription of three or more categories of asthma drugs; and c) prescription of oral corticosteroids. All three markers of chronic asthma severity were associated with an increased risk of subsequent death. This was particularly true for the marker "a hospital admission for asthma in the previous 12 months," and the occurrence of multiple hospital admissions for asthma in the previous 12 months carried a greatly increased risk of asthma death. The marker "three or more categories of prescribed asthma drugs" was also strongly associated with deaths and readmissions. The evidence was more equivocal for the marker "prescribed oral corticosteroids," which had only a weak association with subsequent risk of death in the

New Zealand study, but showed a stronger association with death in the studies in Perth and Saskatchewan. The equivocal findings may be because this class of drugs may be beneficial in the severe group of patients to whom it is prescribed; thus, it may identify a high-risk group of patients, whose risk is in turn lowered by its use.

Two of these studies have also examined the association between acute severity markers and risk of death in a subsequent asthma attack (78,79). In both studies, a $PaCO_2$ of 45 mm Hg was associated with a fourfold risk of subsequent death, and in one study a PEFR of less than 100 L/min was associated with an approximately twofold risk of subsequent death. The use of markers of acute asthma severity is difficult because of the poor quality and paucity of available data. Nevertheless, it would appear that a PEFR of less than 100 L/min or a $PaCO_2$ of 45 mm Hg are markers of an increased risk of death in a subsequent attack of asthma. These two factors are essentially markers of a near-fatal attack.

On the basis of these studies, it is possible to outline a crude index of asthma severity. For example, Rea et al. (51) have previously proposed a severity index based on a combination of empirical and clinical observations: asthma was defined as moderate if the patient had been frequently prevented from working, often woke at night,

TABLE 3. *Case-controlled studies of markers of chronic and acute asthma severity and subsequent risk of death*

	Rea et al. (51)		Ryan et al. (78)		Crane et al. (79)		Spitzer et al. (68)	
Location	Auckland		Perth		New Zealand		Saskatchewan	
Time period	1981–1982		1976–1980		1981–1987		1980–1987	
Study base	Asthmatics		Asthmatics with recent hospital admission		Asthmatics with recent hospital admission		Asthmatics with 10+ prescriptions in 1978–1987	
Period at risk	1+ years		2–6 years		1 year		1–8 years	
Deaths	44		186		39[a]		44	
Controls	44		452		263		233	
	OR	(95% CI)	OR	(95% CI)	OR	(95% CI)	OR	(95% CI)
Chronic severity markers								
Three or more categories of asthma drugs	3.0	1.0–11	—	—	1.7	0.9–3.3	—	—
Oral corticosteroids	—	—	2.3	1.6–3.3	1.3	0.6–2.8	3.1	1.5–6.5
Admission in previous 12 months	16.0	2.5–666	—	—	3.5	1.8–6.9	—	—
5+ admissions in previous 12 months	—	—	—	—	8.8	1.2–56	—	—
A&E visit in previous 12 months	8.5	2.0–76	—	—	—	—	—	—
Acute severity markers								
$PaCO_2$ 45	—	—	1.9	1.1–3.1	4.0	0.9–21	—	—
$PaO_2<60$	—	—	1.2	0.7–1.9	—	—	—	—
$FEV_1<1.0$	—	—	0.8[b]	0.3–1.9	1.5	0.1–34	—	—
FVC<40% pred	—	—	1.6	0.8–3.0	—	—	—	—
PEFR<100 L/min	—	—	—	—	1.9	0.7–5.4	—	—
$K+<3.5$ mmol/L	—	—	—	—	0.4	0.1–1.5	—	—

[a]Cases and controls who were prescribed fenoterol were excluded.
[b]$FEV_1<40\%$ predicted.
OR, odds ratio; CI, confidence interval; A&E, accident and emergency department.

or needed to visit the doctor urgently because of asthma once or twice in the last year (or any combination of these); patients were classified as having severe asthma if there had been one or more hospital admissions or three or more urgent general practitioner or accident and emergency departments visits in the previous 12 months. When the four studies are considered together, the category of severe asthma can be further divided into a subgroup of patients with very severe asthma comprising those severe asthmatics (according to the classification of Rea et al.) who have had three or more admissions in the previous 12 months or who have had a near-fatal attack in the previous 12 months.

Several of these studies have also examined characteristics of the asthmatic that may be associated with an increased risk of death. In particular, Rea et al. have noted that the risk of asthma death in adults is associated with psychosocial problems and other psychological characteristics of the patient, as well as the underlying severity of the asthma. Similarly, Ryan et al. and Crane et al. have noted an association between asthma deaths and prescription of psychotropic drugs, which is a marker for the existence of psychosocial problems. Strunk et al. (80) have reached similar conclusions in a small study in children that found that various psychosocial factors such as conflicts between the patient's parents and hospital staff regarding medical management, depressive symptoms, and disregard of asthma symptoms were associated with an increased risk of asthma death.

CONCLUSIONS

The epidemiology of asthma mortality over the last 30 years has been characterized by two patterns, a gradual increase and two discrete epidemics, and particular interest has centered on the possible role of asthma treatment in both these trends. Just as for the individual, a fatal outcome will be the combination of many adverse factors, so the trends in mortality within communities will represent the sum of many positive and negative influences.

For the gradual rise in mortality, these factors include a spurious increase from changes in diagnostic fashion and coding practices, a reflection of increasing asthma prevalence and severity and asthma treatment itself. As has been illustrated by some of the epidemiologic studies, current asthma treatment with bronchodilators may be increasing severity and hence mortality while the focus on anti-inflammatory therapy with topical and systemic corticosteroids may be reducing severity and hence mortality.

However, the most striking feature of the last 30 years has been the epidemics of deaths, in the 1960s and again in the 1970s and 1980s in New Zealand. The evidence linking these epidemics directly to the widespread use of two high-dose, less selective β-agonists, isoprenaline and fenoterol, respectively, appears to these authors at least, convincing. To date there are no alternative hypotheses to explain both these epidemics.

Although the data implicating therapy in asthma mortality is likely to remain controversial for the foreseeable future, it would seem prudent to take heed of the lessons from the last 30 years to reduce real or potential risk factors to a minimum. In addition to the current focus on asthma education and the use of adequate doses of topical anti-inflammatory therapy, using β-agonists to relieve symptoms and avoiding isoprenaline and fenoterol altogether would seem sensible.

ACKNOWLEDGMENTS

Neil Pearce and Julian Crane are supported by senior research fellowships and the Wellington Asthma Research Group is supported by a program grant from the Health Research Council of New Zealand. The authors would like to thank Denise Fabian for expert assistance in the preparation of this manuscript.

REFERENCES

1. Speizer F, Doll R, Heaf P. Observations on recent increases in mortality from asthma. *Br Med J* 1968;i:335–339.
2. Sears M, Rea H, de Boer G, et al. Accuracy of certification of deaths due to asthma: a national study. *Am J Epidemiol* 1986;124:1004–1011.
3. Jackson R. A century of asthma mortality. In: Beasley R, Pearce N, eds. *The role of β-agonist therapy in asthma mortality*. New York: CRC Press, 1993;29–47.
4. Lambert P. Oral theophylline and fatal asthma (letter). *Lancet* 1981;ii:200–201.
5. Jackson R, Sears MR, Beaglehole R, Rea HH. International trends in asthma mortality: 1970 to 1985. *Chest* 1988;94:914–918.
6. Burney PG. The effect of death certification practice on recorded national asthma mortality rates. *Rev Epidemiol Sante Publ* 1989;37:385–389.
7. Laennec R. *A treatise on the diseases of the chest and on mediate auscultation*, 2nd ed. London: 1827.
8. Adams F. *The extant works of Aretaeus, the Cappadocian*. London: The Sydenham Society, 1856.
9. van Helmont J. *Oriatrike, or a physic refined*. London: Lodowich LLoyd, 1662.
10. Osler W. *The principles and practice of medicine*, 4th ed. Edinburgh: Pentland, 1901.
11. Speizer F, Doll R. A century of asthma deaths in young people. *Br Med J* 1968;3:245–246.
12. Baumann A, Lee S. Trends in asthma mortality in Australia, 1911–1986 (Letter). *Med J Aust* 1990;153:366.
13. Beasley R, Smith K, Pearce N, Crane J, Burgess C, Culling C. Trends in asthma mortality in New Zealand, 1908–1986. *Med J Aust* 1990;152:570–573.
14. Aldrich T. A preliminary report on the active principle of the suprarenal gland. *Am J Physiol* 1901;5:457.
15. Takamine J. The blood-pressure raising principle of the supra-renal glands. *Therap Gaz* 1901;17:221.
16. Bullowa J, Kaplan D. On the hypodermic use of adrenalin chloride in the treatment of asthmatic attacks. *Medical News* (NY) 1903;83:787.
17. Kahn R. Zur Physiologie der Trachea. *Arch Physiol* 1907:398.
18. Camps P. A note on the inhalation treatment of asthma. *Guy's Hosp Rep* 1929;79:496.
19. Chen K, Schmidt C. The action of ephedrine, the active principle of the Chinese drug Ma Huang. *J Pharmacol Exp Ther* 1924;24:339–357.
20. Trendelenburg P. Physiologische und pharmakologische Untersuchun-

gen an der isolierten Bronkialmuskulatur. *Arch Exp Pathol Pharmakol* 1912;69:79.

21. Hirsch S. Klinischer und experimenteller Beitrag zur krampflosenden Wirkung der Purin Derivative. *Klin Wochenschrift* 1922;1:615.

22. Greene J, Paul W, Faller A. The action of theophylline with ethylenediamine on intrathecal and venous pressures in cardiac failure and on bronchial obstruction in cardiac failure. *JAMA* 1937;109:1712.

23. Brewis R. Introduction. In: Brewis R, ed. *Classic papers in asthma*, vol 2. London: Science Press Ltd, 1991:11.

24. Osler W. *The principles and practice of medicine*, 9th ed. Edinburgh: Pentland, 1923.

25. Witts L. Prognosis in Asthma. *Lancet* 1936;i:273–274.

26. Coope R. *Diseases of the chest*, 2nd ed. Edinburgh: E and S Livingstone Edinburgh, 1948.

27. Alexander H. A historical account of death from asthma. *J Allergy* 1963;34:305–313.

28. Williams D. Deaths from asthma in England and Wales. *Thorax* 1953;8:137–140.

29. Ganderton D, Jones T. *Drug delivery to the respiratory tract*. Chichester: Ellis Horwood, 1987.

30. McManis A. Adrenaline and isoprenaline: a warning. *Med J Aust* 1964;2:76.

31. Greenberg M, Pines A. Pressurized aerosols and asthma (letter). *Br Med J* 1967;i:563.

32. Inman W, Adelstein A. Rise and fall of asthma mortality in England and Wales in relation to use of pressurized aerosols. *Lancet* 1969;ii:279–285.

33. Lockett M. Dangerous effects of isoprenaline in myocardial failure. *Lancet* 1965;ii:104–106.

34. Collins J, McDevitt D, Shanks R, Swanton J. The cardiotoxicity of isoprenaline during hypoxia. *Br J Pharmacol* 1969;36:35–45.

35. Anonymous. Fluorocarbon aerosol propellants. *Lancet* 1975;i:1073–1074.

36. Fraser P, Doll R. Geographical variations in the epidemic of asthma deaths. *Br J Prev Soc Med* 1971;2534–2536.

37. Gandevia B. Pressurized sympathomimetic aerosols and their lack of relationship to asthma mortality in Australia. *Med J Aust* 1973;1:273–277.

38. Pearce N, Crane J, Burgess C, Jackson R, Beasley R. β-agonists and asthma mortality: déjà vu. *Clin Exp Allergy* 1991;21:401–410.

39. Read J. The reported increase in mortality from asthma: a clinico-functional analysis. *Med J Aust* 1968;21:879–884.

40. Editorial. Fatal asthma. *Lancet* 1979;ii:337–338.

41. Sears M, Taylor D. The β 2 agonist controversy. Observations, explanations and relationships to asthma epidemiology. *Pharmacoepidemiology* 1994;11:259–283.

42. Stolley PD. Why the United States was spared an epidemic of deaths due to asthma. *Am Rev Respir Dis* 1972;105:883–890.

43. Campbell A. Mortality from asthma and bronchodilator aerosols. *Med J Aust* 1976;i:386–391.

44. Jackson R, Beaglehole R, Rea H, Sutherland D. Mortality from asthma a new epidemic in New Zealand. *Br Med J* 1982;285:771–774.

45. Wilson J, Sutherland D, Thomas A. Has the change to β- agonists combined with oral theophylline increased cases of fatal asthma? *Lancet* 1981;1:235–237.

46. British Thoracic Association. Death from asthma in two regions of England. *Br Med J* 1982;285:1251–1255.

47. Sears M, Rea H, Fenwick J, Gillies A, Holst P, O Donnell T, RPG. R. Asthma mortality in New Zealand: a two year national study. *NZ Med J* 1985;98:271–275.

48. Sears MR, Beaglehole R. Asthma morbidity and mortality: New Zealand. *J Allergy Clin Immunol* 1987;80:383–388.

49. Keating G, Mitchell E, Jackson R, Rea H. Trends in sales of drugs for asthma in New Zealand, Australia, and the United Kingdom. *Br Med J* 1984;289:348–351.

50. Crane J. β-agonists and asthma mortality a perspective. In: Beasley R, Pearce N, eds. *The role of β-agonist therapy in asthma mortality*. New York: CRC Press, 1993;243–256.

51. Rea H, Scragg R, Jackson R. A case-control study of deaths from asthma. *Thorax* 1986;41:833–839.

52. Burney P. Asthma mortality in England and Wales: evidence for a further increase, 1974–1984. *Lancet* 1986;1:323–326.

53. Anderson HR, Strachan DP. Asthma mortality in England and Wales, 1979–89. *Lancet* 1991;337:8753. (letter)

54. Burney P. Asthma deaths in England and Wales 1931–85: evidence for a true increase in asthma mortality. *J Epidemiol Commun Health* 1988;42:316–320.

55. Sly RM. Mortality from asthma, 1979–1984. *J Allergy Clin Immunol* 1988;82:705–717.

56. Weiss KB, Wagener DK. Geographic variations in US asthma mortality: small-area analyses of excess mortality, 1981–1985. *Am J Epidemiol* 1990;132(suppl)1:S107–S115

57. Lang D, Polansky M. Patterns of asthma mortality in Philadelphia from 1969 to 1991. *N Engl J Med* 1994;331:1542–1546.

58. Foucard T, Graff-Lonnevig V. Asthma mortality rate in Swedish children and young adults 1973–88. *Allergy* 1994;49:616–619.

59. Beasley R, Crane J, Burgess C, Pearce N, Jackson R. Fenoterol and severe asthma mortality (letter). *NZ Med J* 1989;102: 294–295.

60. Windom H, Burgess C, Crane J, Pearce N, Kwong T, Beasley R. The self-administration of inhaled β-agonist drugs during severe asthma. *NZ Med J* 1990;103:205–207.

61. Crane J, Burgess C, Beasley R. Cardiovascular and hypokalaemic effects of inhaled salbutamol, fenoterol, and isoprenaline. *Thorax* 1989;44:136–140.

62. Sears MR, Rea HH, Fenwick J, Gillies AJ, Holst PE, O'Donnell TV, Rothwell RP. 75 deaths in asthmatics prescribed home nebulisers. *Br Med J Clin Res Ed* 1987;294:477–480.

63. Crane J, Pearce N, Flatt A, Burgess C, Jackson R, Kwong T, Ball M, Beasley R. Prescribed fenoterol and death from asthma in New Zealand, 1981–83: case control study. *Lancet* 1989;139:917–922.

64. Beasley R, Burgess C, Pearce N, Grainger J, Crane J. Confounding by severity does not explain the association between fenoterol and asthma death. *Clin Exp Allergy* 1994;24:660–668.

65. Pearce N, Grainger J, Atkinson M, Crane J, Burgess C, Culling C, Windom H, Beasley R. Fenoterol and death from asthma in New Zealand, 1977–1981: a new case-control design. *J Clin Res Pharmacoepidemiol* 1990;4:142–143 (abst).

66. Grainger J, Woodman K, Pearce N, Crane J, Burgess C, Keane A, Beasley R. Prescribed fenoterol and death from asthma in New Zealand, 1981–7: a further case-control study. *Thorax* 1991;46:105–111.

67. Horwitz R, Spitzer W, Buist S, Cockcroft D, Ernst P, Habbick B. Clinical complexity and epidemiologic uncertainty in case-control research: fenoterol and asthma management. *Chest* 1991;100:1586–1591.

68. Spitzer WO, Suissa S, Ernst P, et al. The use of β-agonists and the risk of death and near death from asthma. *N Engl J Med* 1992;326:501–506.

69. Burrows B, Lebowitz MD. The β-agonist dilemma (editorial). *N Engl J Med* 1992;326:560–561.

70. Hensley MJ. Fenoterol and death from asthma (letter). *Med J Aust* 1992;156:12.

71. Pearce N, Beasley R, Crane J, Burgess C, Jackson R. End of the New Zealand asthma mortality epidemic. *Lancet* 1995;345:41–44.

72. Sears MR, Taylor DR, Print CG, Lake DC, Li QQ, Flannery EM, Yates DM, Lucas MK, Herbison GP. Regular inhaled β-agonist treatment in bronchial asthma. *Lancet* 1990;336:1391–1396.

73. Chapman K, Kesten S, Szalai J. Regular vs as-needed inhaled salbutamol in asthma control. *Lancet* 1994;343:1379–1382.

74. Suissa S, Ernst P, Boivin J, Horwitz R, Habbick B, Cockcroft D. A cohort analysis of excess mortality in asthma and the use of inhaled β-agonists. *Am J Respir Crit Care Med* 1994;149:604–610.

75. Pearce N, Crane J, Burgess C, Beasley R. The association between β-agonist use and death from asthma (letter). *JAMA* 1994;271:822–823.

76. Tattersfield A. Use of β 2 agonists in asthma: much ado about nothing? Still cause for concern. *Br Med J* 1994;309:794–795.

77. Barrett T, Strom B. Inhaled β-adrenergic receptor agonists in asthma: more harm than good? *Am J Respir Crit Care Med* 1995;151:574–577.

78. Ryan G, Musk AW, Perera DM, Stock H, Knight JL, Hobbs MS. Risk factors for death in patients admitted to hospital with asthma: a follow-up study. *Aust NZ J Med* 1991;21:681–685.

79. Crane J, Pearce N, Burgess C, Woodman K, Robson B, Beasley R. Markers of risk of asthma death or readmission in the 12 months following a hospital admission for asthma. *Int J Epidemiol* 1992;21:737–744.

80. Strunk R, Mrazek D, Fuhrmann G, LaBreque J. Physiologic and psychological characteristics associated with deaths due to asthma in childhood. *JAMA* 1985;254:1193–1198.

Asthma, edited by P.J. Barnes, M.M. Grunstein,
A.R. Leff, and A.J. Woolcock.
Lippincott–Raven Publishers, Philadelphia © 1997.

▪ 6 ▪

Ethnic Differences

Cheryl M. Salome and Ann J. Woolcock

Between Countries	Canada/Greenland
Within Countries	United States of America
New Zealand	China and Chinese in Other Countries
Fiji	Israel
United Kingdom	Singapore

Studies of differences in the prevalence, natural history, severity, and mortality due to asthma in ethnic groups can be used to define the risks of disease and thus to improve the understanding of the etiology of the disease. The definition of ethnicity is difficult, fluid, and imprecise. Senior and Bhopal (1) have suggested that it implies one or more of the following: shared origins or social background, shared culture or traditions, and a common language or religious tradition. They conclude that epidemiologic reports "should state explicitly how (ethnic group) classifications were made."

Ethnicity is sometimes used as a synonym for race. Race is considered to be biologically determined, people with a common set of physical characteristics, usually skin color. This common phenotype is often taken to indicate a common genotype, and a degree of genetic homogeneity, thus suggesting a biologic basis for disease resistance or susceptibility. However, this idea has been invalidated by genetic studies that show that differences between racial groups are small compared with the amount of genetic variation within a local population (2). The genes that determine the physical characteristics, which are commonly used to define racial groups, are not necessarily associated with those that determine disease susceptibility. Because the definition of race is extremely

imprecise, it is widely agreed that race is of little use in explaining the determinants of disease prevalence or severity (1,3). Using ethnic rather than racial backgrounds to define populations acknowledges that there may be differences in culture and lifestyle as well as in genetic composition.

Given the difficulties of accurately defining ethnicity, the assessment of results from studies that have examined ethnic differences in disease must be tempered by an awareness of their limitations. Ideally, observations of differences between ethnic groups should include detailed examination of the relative importance of environmental, lifestyle, cultural and genetic influences (1), and should form the basis for subsequent development of testable hypotheses concerning the etiology of disease.

One of the problems of comparing epidemiologic studies of asthma is that the definition of asthma is inconsistent. For epidemiologic studies, the presence of airway hyperresponsiveness (AHR) plus recent respiratory symptoms remains the gold standard (4,5). Few studies include a measure of AHR and most report the prevalence of recent wheeze. Recent attempts to standardize questionnaires has meant that many studies now report responses to standard questions about symptoms. Several studies have also incorporated a video questionnaire to overcome bias due to language or cultural differences in the understanding of the term "wheeze" (6). In other studies, translation and back-translation techniques have been used to develop comparable questionnaires in a number of different languages (7). In this chapter we discuss the ethnic differences in asthma between and within countries.

C. M. Salome: Department of Medicine, University of Sydney, Sydney, New South Wales 2006 Australia.

A. J. Woolcock: Institute of Respiratory Medicine, Page Chest Pavilion, Royal Prince Alfred Hospital, Camperdown 2050 Australia.

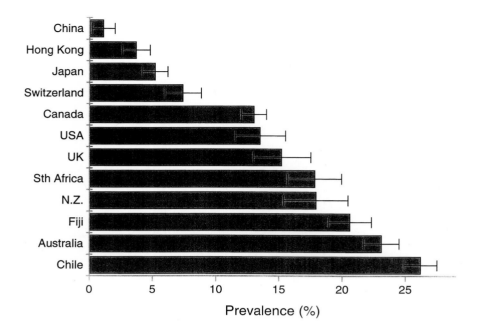

FIG. 1. Prevalence (and 95% confidence intervals) of recent wheeze, i.e., wheeze in the last 12 months, in children living in 12 different countries.

BETWEEN COUNTRIES

Figure 1 shows the prevalence of wheeze in the last 12 months in 7- to 11-year-old children living in 12 countries (7–13). Some of the differences are no doubt due to methodologic differences, but the variations are sufficiently great to suggest that some populations are at greater risk than others. Nevertheless, it is difficult to separate variations in risk due to ethnic factors from those due to geographic factors. The prevalence of recent wheeze was similar in children in Australia, New Zealand, and South Africa, countries that probably meet the criteria for a common ethnicity. In China and Japan, recent wheeze is uncommon, whereas the prevalence is intermediate in Canada, the United States, and the United Kingdom. The five countries with the highest prevalence of recent wheeze are all in the southern hemisphere.

WITHIN COUNTRIES

New Zealand

Ethnic differences in the prevalence and severity of asthma have been extensively studied in New Zealand, where both hospital admissions (14) and deaths (15) due to asthma are higher in Maori and Pacific Islanders than in Europeans. A number of studies have been undertaken to determine if these differences in morbidity and mortality reflect differences in the prevalence or severity of the disease in these groups (16–19). In these studies, ethnicity was defined in terms of self-reported ethnic affiliation, rather than any biologic or genetic marker. Subjects

(or their parents) were asked to nominate their ethnic origin by selecting from among Maori, Pacific Island Polynesian, European, or others. Studies of blood groups indicate that there has been considerable interracial mixing in New Zealand (20), but perceived ethnicity remains a strong determinant of health status and health service utilization (14).

Figure 2 shows the prevalence of wheeze during the last 12 months obtained from four studies (16–19). In Pacific Islanders, the prevalence of recent wheeze is no greater than that in Europeans but, among Maori, wheezing appears to be more common than in the other two groups. This difference is not reflected in differences in the prevalence of AHR. In children, the prevalence of AHR to histamine was significantly higher in Europeans (20.2%) than in Maori (13.2%) or Pacific Islanders (8.7%) ($p<0.001$ in both cases) (16) whereas in adolescents the prevalence of AHR to methacholine did not differ significantly between Maori (14.5%) and non-Maori (14.2%) (18). Differences in the prevalence of recent wheezing in the adolescent group disappeared after adjustment for current smoking (18). Among adults, the difference in prevalence of recent wheeze could be accounted for by the fact that symptoms tended to increase with age in Maori while declining with age in the non-Maori population (19). This suggests that the natural history of wheezing illness in Maori may differ from that in non-Maori. It is possible that continuing exposure to tobacco smoke results in greater nonallergic bronchial symptoms in both adolescent and adult Maori. Studies are currently underway to measure AHR and atopy in a subsample of this population and will help to elucidate the nature of wheezing illness in adult Maori.

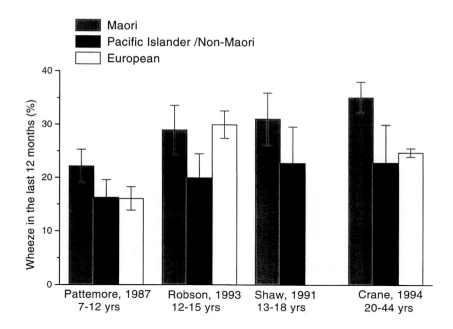

FIG. 2. Prevalence of recent wheeze in Maori, Pacific Islanders, and Europeans measured in four studies from New Zealand. In the study by Shaw et al. (6), data from Pacific Islanders and Europeans were combined into a single non-Maori group.

It seems likely that high levels of morbidity and mortality from asthma among Pacific Islanders and Maori are not accounted for by differences in prevalence. To determine if differences in the nature of the disease or its severity could be responsible, Mitchell (21) studied asthmatic children, aged 0 to 14 years, admitted to Auckland hospital. The study showed that, after adjustment for socioeconomic status, there was no evidence for any differences in the nature or severity of asthma in Polynesian, Maori, or European children admitted to the hospital, although Polynesian children were more likely to have been in the hospital before and were less likely to have taken asthma medication in the 24 hours before admission. The most striking differences, however, were in the medication prescribed at the time of discharge. Prophylactic therapy (inhaled or systemic corticosteroids, cromoglycate or ketotifen) was prescribed for 26% of Europeans, 17% of Maori, and only 5% of Pacific Islanders on discharge from the first admission and for 59% of Europeans, 41% of Maori, and 38% of Pacific Islanders if there had been previous admissions. Mitchell concluded that there are ethnic differences in the medical management of the disease that cannot be accounted for by socioeconomic status.

Fiji

In Fiji there are two main ethnic groups: the indigenous Melanesian Fijians and the Fiji Indians, descendants of indentured laborers who arrived in Fiji in the late 19th century. National hospital admission data for respiratory illness in 5- to 14-year-old children showed that between 1985 and 1989, admissions for asthma were three times higher in Indian children than in Melanesian Fijian children (22). However, during the same period, Fijian children had more than threefold higher admission rates for pneumonia and other respiratory infections, including influenza, tuberculosis, and bronchiectasis.

Flynn has reported two studies (7,23) of urban and rural children that have examined the reasons for these differences in admission rates. In these studies, the questionnaires underwent repeated translation and back-translation to ensure that comparable idiomatic English, Fijian, and Hindi versions were obtained. Ethnicity in the children was defined on the basis of the ethnicity of both parents, but no information was given on how ethnicity was defined in the parents.

In urban children, in Suva, a study of respiratory symptoms (see Fig. 3) showed that the prevalence of recent wheeze was identical in both Fijians and Indians (20.6%), but productive cough was significantly more common in Fijians than Indians (29% vs. 17%) ($p < 0.0001$) (7). The prevalence of AHR to histamine in Indian children was double that in Fijians (30% vs. 15%), but the prevalence of atopy was similar (38% vs. 36%). Current asthma, defined as AHR plus recent wheeze, was nearly three times higher in Indian children than Fijian children (11.3% vs. 4%) (7).

In rural children (23), as in the urban populations, the prevalence of recent wheeze was similar in Indians (19.4%) and Fijians (19.8%), but frequent episodes of wheeze (>4/year) were more common among Indian children (8.9%) than among Fijians (2.9%). The prevalence of productive cough remained higher in rural Fijians than in Indians (35.8% vs. 23.9%).

Environmental factors may explain some of the differences in symptoms between the two groups. Three envi-

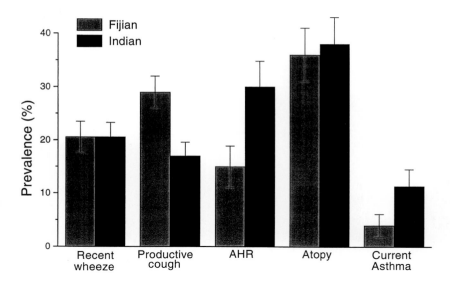

FIG. 3. Prevalence of recent wheeze, productive morning cough, airway hyperresponsiveness to histamine (AHR), atopy (a positive skin prick test), and current asthma (AHR; recent wheeze) in Fijian and Indian children living in Suva, Fiji. (Data from Flynn MGL. Respiratory symptoms, bronchial responsiveness, and atopy in Fijian and Indian children. *Am J Respir Crit Care Med* 1994; 150:415–420.)

ronmental factors significantly associated with productive cough were also associated with ethnicity. Fijians had more smokers in the home, more domestic crowding, and cooked more commonly with kerosene. The presence of a smoker in the home was associated with wheeze in the last 12 months in urban children but not in the rural population. However, the cause of the increased frequency of wheezing and prevalence of AHR among Indian children in this population is not known, and it is not clear if environmental factors play a role. These studies suggest that the threefold higher hospital admissions for asthma in Indian children reflects the threefold higher prevalence of current asthma in Indian children.

United Kingdom

In the United Kingdom, hospital admission rates for asthma appear to be higher in Asians, principally from Indian and Pakistani ethnic groups, than in Europeans (24, 25). There have been few community-based studies, using standard definitions of asthma, comparing the prevalence of asthma in these ethnic groups. However, two studies of primary schoolchildren suggest that the increased hospitalization rates are not due to differences in prevalence (26,27). In Southampton, the prevalence of "wheeze in the last 12 months" was higher in European (19.6%) than Asian children (11.9%) (26), whereas in South London there was no significant difference (15% vs. 17%, respectively) (27). Both studies used English language questionnaires for most subjects, but translations of questionnaires may have been misleading in any case, because there is no comparable term for wheeze in Punjabi, Bengali, or Urdu (26). Ethnicity in these studies was defined by nominated racial affiliation (26) or classified by the investigator on appearance (27).

Morrison-Smith and Cooper (28) suggest that ethnic differences in hospitalization rates for asthma in the United Kingdom are largely explained by differences in environmental conditions. In a population of children attending an asthma clinic in Birmingham, they have shown that, regardless of race, children born in England have a higher risk of developing asthma within the first 4 years of life than those born abroad. Furthermore, although there was no difference between ethnic groups in the clinical severity of asthma in children attending this clinic, Asian children were admitted to the hospital significantly more often than white children ($p < 0.001$).

Canada/Greenland

In 1974, Herxheimer observed that asthma was extremely rare, if not nonexistent, among Eskimo or Inuit people of Greenland and northern Canada (29). A further study (30) suggested that not only were the Inuit less susceptible to asthma, but they also had a lower prevalence of coronary heart disease, psoriasis, and rheumatoid arthritis, leading to a speculation that a diet high in marine lipids may be an important protective factor. However, until recently, there were no studies in which standard methods for defining and measuring asthma were used to compare the prevalence of asthma in Inuit with that in control populations. Hemmelgarn et al. (31) have now undertaken such a study in 5- to 15-year-old schoolchildren, comparing a small Inuit community with Montreal children, using both a standard questionnaire and measures of AHR and atopy. Their preliminary findings suggest that the Inuit have a higher prevalence of both wheeze in the last 12 months (7.7% vs. 3.2%) and AHR to exercise (19.5% vs. 8.8%), but lower levels of atopy (8.6% vs. 34%). Studies are currently underway in other

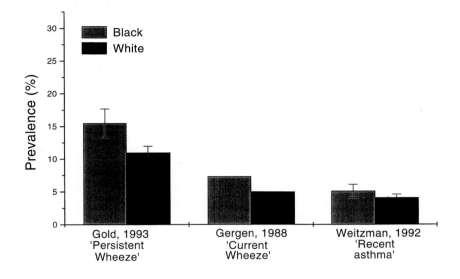

FIG. 4. Prevalence of asthma-related symptoms in three studies in black children and white children from the United States.

communities to confirm these preliminary findings. The striking feature of this study is that the prevalence of both wheeze and AHR in Montreal children appears remarkably low, compared with other "European" children around the world. However, this low prevalence of wheeze was not found in other studies of Canadian children (13).

United States of America

In the United States, a recent review described the phenomenon of "inner-city" asthma, where morbidity and mortality due to asthma seems to be increased in impoverished inner city neighborhoods (32). Because these neighborhoods are inhabited by a disproportionately nonwhite population, it is not clear whether the increased risk is associated with ethnicity, socioeconomic status, or physical environment. Both mortality (33,34) and hospitalizations (34,35) due to asthma are 3 to 5 times greater in blacks than whites, but it is not clear if differences in morbidity and mortality reflect true differences in prevalence. Figure 4 shows data from three large population studies of children that have measured responses to a range of questions about asthma related symptoms (12,

36,37). Although most have asked about wheeze, the questions were not standardized, making it difficult to compare the findings. The data suggest that, even after adjusting for socioeconomic status, there is a small excess of wheezing among black children, but these differences are not sufficient to account for the large disparity in hospital admissions and deaths due to asthma. Recent studies suggest that socioeconomic status is a more powerful risk factor than is ethnicity for hospital admissions or deaths due to asthma (32). In U.S. soldiers it was found that morbidity and mortality related to asthma does not differ significantly between blacks and whites (38), suggesting that apparent ethnic differences in susceptibility may be abolished by standardized living conditions and environmental exposures.

China and Chinese in Other Countries

Studies within China suggest that the prevalence of both asthma and allergic illness is relatively low (10,39). There has been widespread migration of ethnic Chinese during the last century, resulting in large local populations in a number of countries outside China. Table 1 shows data from cross-sectional studies in Chinese sub-

TABLE 1. *Prevalence (%) of asthma and allergic illness in Chinese children at different sites in the Asian region*

Site	Year of study	Age range	Asthma ever	Recent wheeze	Rhinitis	Atopy[a]
Hong Kong (42)	1985	7–13	1.3	—	—	—
Guangzhou (10)	1987	11–17	2.4	2.8	—	34
Taipei (41)	1991	7–15	5.8	—	20.7	—
San Bu, China (40)	1992	11–20	1.6	1.1	2.1	49.0
Hong Kong (40)	1992	11–20	6.6	3.7	15.7	57.7
Borneo (40)	1992	11–20	3.3	4.9	11.2	63.9

[a]Atopy = 1 skin test ≥3 mm wheal.

jects within the Asian region (10,40–42) that show that, although there are variations between sites, the prevalence of asthma and recent wheeze is much lower than that found in most western countries (see Fig. 1). The sites covered in these studies vary widely in socioeconomic profile, environmental air pollutants, and the degree to which traditional lifestyle and health practices are maintained, suggesting that these are not major factors in the low prevalence.

There have been few studies in which the prevalence of asthma and atopy have been compared in Chinese and non-Chinese people living in the same geographic region. However, one such study was undertaken by Leung et al. in Melbourne, Australia (43). In this study, subjects were identified by random selection from the Melbourne telephone book, based on 33 distinct surnames of ethnic Chinese background. The study group included both an immigrant group, born outside Australia, and a nonimmigrant, Australian-born group. More than 80% of the Chinese born outside Australia originated from Hong Kong, Malaysia, or Vietnam, and the median length of stay in Australia at the time of study was 6.0 years, (range 0.1–42.5 years). Control non-Asian subjects were also selected from the phone book. Data were obtained by telephone interview, conducted wherever possible in the native language of the respondent. A random subsample of each group underwent skin prick tests.

Figure 5 shows the results of this study, compared with data from a group of Chinese schoolchildren studied in Hong Kong (40). The prevalence of recent wheeze in children is greater in Chinese immigrants to Australia than in Chinese living in Hong Kong. Selection bias, in terms of those people who are likely to migrate, and differences in the method of administration of the questionnaire, may account for some differences in prevalence. This study shows that Australian-born Chinese do not dif-

fer from their non-Chinese counterparts in the prevalence of recent wheeze or asthma, which suggests that the low prevalence of asthma in Chinese is due to environmental factors rather than to any intrinsic ethnic difference in susceptibility. The risk of both hay fever and asthma in the immigrant group was strongly associated with length of stay in Australia, suggesting that exposure to factors local to the Australian environment were responsible for the increasing prevalence of allergic illness.

The high prevalence of atopy among Chinese, both in Asia and in Australia, in these studies is surprising. The prevalence of atopy in the non-Asian control group was comparable with data from other studies in Australia (44). The findings are not supported by those of Zhong et al. (10), who measured the prevalence of atopy in a random population of Chinese adolescents at 34% (Table 1). However, a study of allergic patients in California, which included a small number (54) of Californian-born Chinese, suggested that Chinese patients were more likely to be allergic to grass pollens than Caucasian patients (45).

Israel

In Israel, compulsory universal military service has allowed the collection of health data from a very large random sample of young men and women aged 17 to 18 years. Laor et al. (46) reported data from 443,186 conscripts (59% male), in whom ethnic origin was defined by the place of birth of either the conscript, their father, or their grandfather. Asthma was defined on the basis of a previous diagnosis and/or symptoms in the last 3 years, and was confirmed in each case by a physical examination and lung function tests at rest and after exercise. The study suggests that asthma is more prevalent among conscripts of Western origin (European, American, or South

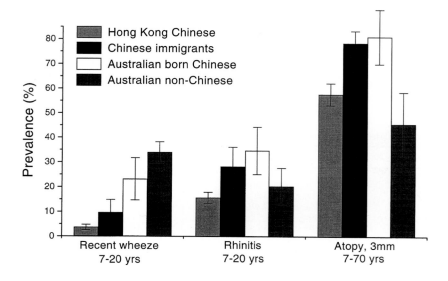

FIG. 5. Prevalence of recent wheeze, rhinitis, and atopy in subjects living in Hong Kong and Melbourne, Australia.

African) (3.6%) than among those of Israeli (2.3%), Asian (2.5%), or North African (1.7%) origin. However, data from this and other studies (47,48) show that differences in the prevalence of asthma are also associated with area of residence, suggesting that local environmental factors play an important role.

Singapore

This small island has provided an ideal situation in which three different ethnic groups (Chinese, Indian, and Malay) can be compared. Both adults and children have been studied (49) and the results show higher levels of asthma in Indians and Malays than in the Chinese that could not be accounted for by smoking or by atopy. A similar finding was obtained in Malaysia by Ross et al. in 1984 (50). Although it is tempting to attribute the lower prevalence in Chinese to genetic differences, it is likely that the ethnic differences dictate differences in lifestyle and that environmental factors, including furnishings and diet, may account for the differences. This area of the world provides an ideal place for an ongoing study of the risk factors for asthma, especially as it seems likely that the prevalence is increasing.

CONCLUSIONS

The studies outlined in this chapter have classified people into groups on the basis of some perceived ethnic affiliation, nominated either by the subject, the investigator, or the attending doctor. Ethnicity, defined in this way, is a complex mixture of environmental, lifestyle, cultural, and genetic factors, all of which could influence the health of the individual. Despite the limitations of such a definition, it is possible to draw some conclusions about ethnic differences in asthma.

Ethnic affiliation is clearly a determinant of asthma related morbidity and mortality in a number of countries where the data show that hospital admissions and deaths due to asthma are higher in some groups, especially black groups in the United States and Maori in New Zealand. The reasons for these differences are complex and not fully understood. In most cases the differences in morbidity and mortality are greater than can be accounted for by differences in the prevalence or severity of the disease. The differences are associated with socioeconomic status, and it is often difficult to distinguish the individual contributions of ethnicity and socioeconomic status to health status. In the United States, in particular, socioeconomic status is an important determinant of access to appropriate medical care. In some countries, such as New Zealand and the United Kingdom, medical management of asthma in one ethnic group differs from that received by other groups, regardless of socioeconomic status or disease severity. These differences have important impli-

cations for the interpretation of perceived differences and for the planning and delivery of health services.

There is some evidence for slight differences in the prevalence of asthma between ethnic groups, but it seems likely that these differences are due to environmental factors rather than to any intrinsic differences in biologic susceptibility. Although data that evaluate the risk factors associated with asthma in different ethnic groups are not available, the evidence points to lifestyle and environmental exposures playing a major role in determining the risk of asthma. In general, the more affluent the group the more prevalent the asthma, although blacks in the inner cities of the United States are an exception. Because of the lack of well controlled studies it is not clear whether they have more asthma, but the disease appears to be more severe. In addition, the studies suggest that delivery of health care can play an important role in the degree to which the disease is controlled in individuals with asthma.

REFERENCES

1. Senior PA, Bhopal R. Ethnicity as a variable in epidemiological research. *Br Med J* 1994;309:327–30.
2. Jones JS. How different are human races? *Nature* 1981;293:188–90.
3. Huth EJ. Identifying ethnicity in medical papers. *Ann Intern Med* 1995; 122:619–621.
4. Toelle BG, Peat JK, Salome CM, Mellis CM, Woolcock AJ. Toward a definition of asthma for epidemiology. *Am Rev Respir Dis* 1992;146: 633–637.
5. Sterk PJ, Fabbri LM, Quanjer PH, et al. Airway responsiveness: standardized challenge testing with pharmacological, physical and sensitizing stimuli in adults. *Eur Respir J* 1993;suppl:53–83.
6. Shaw R, Woodman K, Ayson M, et al. Measuring the prevalence of bronchial hyper-responsiveness in children. *Int J Epidemiol* 1995;24: 597–602.
7. Flynn MGL. Respiratory symptoms, bronchial responsiveness, and atopy in Fijian and Indian children. *Am J Respir Crit Care Med* 1994; 150:415–420.
8. Burr ML, Limb ES, Andrae S, Barry DMJ, Nagel F. Childhood asthma in four countries: a comparative survey. *Int J Epidemiol* 1994;23:341–347.
9. Robertson CF, Bishop J, Sennhauser FH, Mallol J. International comparison of asthma prevalence in children: Australia, Switzerland, Chile. *Pediatr Pulmonol* 1993;16:219–226.
10. Zhong NS, Chen RC, O-yang M, Wu JY, Fu WX, Shi LJ. Bronchial hyperresponsiveness in young students of southern China: relation to respiratory symptoms, diagnosed asthma, and risk factors. *Thorax* 1990; 45:860–865.
11. Leung R, Bishop J, Robertson CF. Prevalence of asthma and wheeze in Hong Kong schoolchildren: an international comparative study. *Eur Respir J* 1994;7:2046–2049.
12. Gold DR, Rotnitzky A, Damokosh AI, et al. Race and gender differences in respiratory illness prevalence and their relationship to environmental exposures in children 7 to 14 years of age. *Am Rev Respir Dis* 1993;148:10–18.
13. Dales RE, Raizenne M, El-Saadany S, Brook J, Burnett R. Prevalence of childhood asthma across Canada. *J Epidemiol* 1994;23:775–781.
14. Mitchell EA, Borman A. Demographic characteristics of asthma admissions to hospital. *NZ Med J* 1986;99:576–579.
15. Sears MR, Rea HH, Fenwick J, et al. Deaths from asthma in New Zealand. *Arch Dis Child* 1986;61:6–10.
16. Pattemore PK, Asher MI, Harrison AC, Mitchell EA, Rea HH, Stewart AW. Ethnic differences in prevalence of asthma symptoms and bronchial hyperresponsiveness in New Zealand schoolchildren. *Thorax* 1989;44:168–176.
17. Robson B, Woodman K, Burgess C, et al. Prevalence of asthma symp-

toms among adolescents in the Wellington region, by area and ethnicity. *NZ Med J* 1993;106:239–241.

18. Shaw RA, Crane J, O'Donnell TV. Asthma symptoms, bronchial hyperresponsiveness and atopy in a Maori and European adolescent population. *NZ Med J* 1991;104:175–179.

19. Crane J, Lewis S, Slater T, et al. The self reported prevalence of asthma symptoms among New Zealanders. *NZ Med J* 1994;107:417–421.

20. Woodfield DG, Simpson LA, Seber GA, McInerney PJ. Blood groups and other genetic markers in New Zealand Europeans and Maoris. *Ann Hum Biol* 1987;14:29–37.

21. Mitchell EA. Racial inequalities in childhood asthma. *Soc Sci Med* 1991;32:831–836.

22. Flynn MGL. Hospital admission rates for asthma and pneumonia in Fijian and Indian children. *J Pediatr Child Health* 1994;30:19–22.

23. Flynn MGL. Respiratory symptoms of rural Fijian and Indian children in Fiji. *Thorax* 1994;49:1201–1204.

24. Myers P, Ormerod LP. Increased asthma admission rates in Asian patients: Blackburn 1987. *Respir Med* 1992;86:297–300.

25. Jackson SHD, Bannan LT, Beevers DG. Ethnic differences in respiratory disease. *Postgrad Med J* 1981;57:777–778.

26. Pararajasingam CD, Sittampalam L, Damani P, Pattemore PK, Holgate ST. Comparison of the prevalence of asthma among Asian and European children in Southampton. *Thorax* 1992;47:529–532.

27. Johnston IDA, Bland JM, Anderson HR. Ethnic variation in respiratory morbidity and lung function in childhood. *Thorax* 1987;42:542–548.

28. Morrison-Smith J, Cooper SM. Asthma and atopic disease in immigrants from Asia and the West Indies. *Postgrad Med J* 1981;57:774–776.

29. Herxheimer H, Shaefer O. Asthma in Canadian Eskimos (letter). *N Engl J Med* 1974;291:1419.

30. Kromann N, Green A. Epidemiological studies in the Upernavik district, Greenland. Incidence of some chronic diseases 1950–1974. *Acta Medica Scandinavica* 1980;208:401–406.

31. Hemmelgarn B, Loozen E, Saralegui S, Chatwood S, Ernst P. Airways hyperresponsiveness and atopy: a comparison of Inuit and Montreal schoolchildren. *Canadian Respir J* 1995;2:92–96.

32. Weiss KB, Crain EF. Inner-city asthma. The epidemiology of an emerging US public health concern. *Chest* 1992;101(suppl 6):362S–367S.

33. Schenker MB, Gold EB, Lopez RL, Beaumont JJ. Asthma mortality in California, 1960–1989. Demographic patterns and occupational associations. *Am Rev Respir Dis* 1993;147:1454–1460.

34. Carr W, Zeitel L, Weiss K. Variations in asthma hospitalizations and deaths in New York city. *Am J Pub Health* 1992;82:59–65.

35. Gerstman BB, Bosco LA, Tomita DK, Gross TP, Shaw MM. Prevalence and treatment of asthma in the Michigan Medicaid patient population younger than 45 years, 1980–1986. *J Allergy Clin Immunol* 1989;83:1032–1039.

36. Gergen PJ, Mullally DI, Evans R. National survey of prevalence of asthma among children in the United States, 1976 to 1980. *Pediatrics* 1988;81:1–7.

37. Weitzman M, Gortmaker SL, Sobol AM, Perrin JM. Recent trends in the prevalence and severity of childhood asthma. *JAMA* 1992;268:2673–2677.

38. Ward DL. An international comparison of asthma morbidity and mortality in US soldiers, 1984 to 1988. *Chest* 1992;101:613–620.

39. Leung R, Jenkins M. Asthma, allergy and atopy in southern Chinese schoolchildren. *Clin Exp Allergy* 1994;24:353–358.

40. Leung R, Ho P. Asthma, allergy, and atopy in three south-east Asian populations. *Thorax* 1994;49:1205–1210.

41. Hsieh KH, Tsai YT. Increasing prevalence of childhood allergic disease in Taipei, Taiwan, and the outcome. *Prog Allergy Clin Immunol* 1991;2:223–225.

42. Koo LC, Ho JH-C, Matsuki H, Shimizu H, Mori T, Tominaga S. A comparison of the pevalence of respiratory illnesses among nonsmoking mothers and their children in Japan and Hong Kong. *Am Rev Respir Dis* 1988;138:290–295.

43. Leung R, Carlin JB, Burdon JGW, Czarny D. Asthma, allergy and atopy in Asian immigrants in Melbourne. *Med J Aust* 1994;161:418–425.

44. Peat JK, Toelle B, Gray L, et al. Prevalence and severity of childhood asthma and allergic sensitisation in seven climatic regions of New South Wales. *Med J Aust* 1995;163:22–26.

45. Kaufman HS, Kelly PT, Modin GW. Antigen recognition in Chinese and Caucasians. *Ann Allergy* 1984;53:135–137.

46. Laor A, Cohen L, Danon YL. Effects of time, sex, ethnic origin, and area of residence on prevalence of asthma in Israeli adolescents. *Brit Med J* 1993;307:841–844.

47. Amir J, Horev Z, Jaber L, Varsano I. Prevalence of asthma in Israeli school children. A comparative study of Jewish and Arab population. *Isr J Med Sci* 1992;28:789–792.

48. Auerbach I, Springer C, Godfrey S. Total population survey of the frequency and severity of asthma in 17 year old boys in an urban area in Israel. *Thorax* 1993;48:139–141.

49. Ng TP, Hui KP, Tan WC. Prevalence of asthma and risk factors among Chinese, Malay and Indian adults in Singapore. *Thorax* 1994;49:347–351.

50. Ross I. Bronchial asthma in Malaysia. *Br J Dis Chest* 1984;78:369–375.

Asthma, edited by P.J. Barnes, M.M. Grunstein,
A.R. Leff, and A.J. Woolcock.
Lippincott–Raven Publishers, Philadelphia © 1997.

▪ 7 ▪

Risk Factors

Immunoglobulin E and Atopy

Skin Test Criteria for Atopy
"Intrinsic"and "Extrinsic" Asthma, and Relation to
    Serum IgE
Correlations Between Skin Tests and Bronchial
    Responsiveness to Inhaled Allergen
Allergens Associated with Asthma
Can Adult Asthma Develop in the Absence of Atopy?
Relationship Between Serum IgE, Clinical Asthma,
    and Airway Responsiveness in Children
Correlations of Airway Responsiveness with Atopy
    Detected by Skin Testing
Influence of the Degree of Atopy on Asthma and
    Airway Responsiveness

Relationship Between Serum IgE or Skin Tests,
    Clinical Asthma, and Airway Responsiveness
    in Adults
Influence of Atopy on Development of New Adult
    Asthma
Influence of Atopy on Persistence of Childhood
    Asthma
Effect of Atopy on Emergency Room Presentations
    with Acute Asthma
Influence of Smoking on IgE and Atopy
Differences in Epidemiology of Asthma and Atopy in
    Different Ethnic Groups and Different Regions
Is Increasing Asthma Linked with Increasing Atopy?

A clinical link between allergy and asthma has long been recognized, especially in children (1). Many children with asthma manifest other clinical features of atopy including eczema and rhinitis (2–4) especially in early childhood (5), have a family history of allergic disease (3,4,6), and have positive skin tests (1–3,5,7,8) or elevated serum immunoglobulin E (IgE) levels (2,9,10). Likewise, asthma is common among atopic children, e.g., 76% of children attending a dermatology clinic with atopic dermatitis reported wheezing compared with 12% of controls (11). The severity of asthma and the persistence of wheezing into later childhood are both strongly related to atopy (1, 12,13). Wheezing children with diagnosed hay fever or eczema were four times as likely to have persistent wheezing to age 20 years than wheezing children without

these diagnoses (12). Atopic sensitization has also been shown to relate to airway hyperresponsiveness (AHR), a physiologic characteristic of asthma (8,14–18). In children, not only does allergy substantially increase the likelihood of the presence of AHR (15,16), but also the degree of AHR is closely related to the degree of atopy (17,18).

Atopy is also common among adults with asthma. In a British community study, 178 of 198 adult asthmatics 18 to 50 years old had at least one positive skin test when tested to house dust mite, grass, or cat (19). House dust mite responses were positive in 74.7%, grass in 72.7%, and cat in 57.0%. In the United States, the prevalence of asthma in 6- to 24-year-olds surveyed in the National Health and Nutrition Study 1976–1980 (NHANES II) increased with the increasing number of positive skin tests (odds ratio 3.5 for one positive test, and 4.2 for two or more positive tests) (20). Asthma was specifically associated with skin test sensitivity to house dust (odds ratio 2.9) and *Alternaria* (odds ratio 5.1).

    M. R. Sears: Department of Medicine, Firestone Regional Chest and Allergy Unit, St. Joseph's Hospital, McMaster University, Hamilton, Ontario L8N 4A6 Canada.

SKIN TEST CRITERIA FOR ATOPY

Skin testing for allergy has gradually evolved from the use of crude extracts of plants and animal danders to a semiquantitative science using standardized allergens that are well characterized and purified (21). Methods of performing skin tests can be standardized and compared (22–26). However, there remains a degree of uncertainty as to the size of a skin test response that should be interpreted as indicating sensitization. Studies have used responses of 1 mm (27–29), 2 mm (15,30,31), 2 mm and at least half the size of the histamine weal (6), 3 mm (8,32–34), 4 mm (35–38), and even 5 mm (39) weal diameter (related to weal response to a negative control substance) to categorize a subject as atopic. Another study has used erythema to define atopy (20). Still other studies have used intradermal tests, making comparisons between studies even more uncertain (40,41). Meinert et al. found considerable differences in estimations of prevalences and incidences of allergic sensitization of children in Germany, due in part to observer bias, and recommended using the ratio of allergen weal size to histamine weal as the most appropriate definition of atopy (42), to overcome another observed problem of increasing weal size on repeated tests at yearly intervals. It appears that even small weal sizes of 1 mm to important allergens such as house dust mite and cat indicate sensitization that has relevance to epidemiologic studies (43), whereas larger weal responses are more significantly related to clinically relevant trigger factors for asthma.

"INTRINSIC" AND "EXTRINSIC" ASTHMA, AND RELATION TO SERUM IGE

Rackemann suggested in 1918 that asthma be classified as "intrinsic" (nonatopic) and "extrinsic" (atopic) (44). "Extrinsic" asthma is usual in children (1–3,5,7,8,30,45), but many adults and some children have negative skin tests (24,45,46). Danish children with "intrinsic" asthma (no reactivity to common allergens but serum IgE may have been above levels found in healthy children) were reported to show more hyperinflation, more hospital admissions due to asthma and/or pneumonia, more elevated serum IgG and IgM, a higher likelihood of bacterial airway infection, and more progression of their disease despite treatment with corticosteroids (45). In other studies, however, groups of asthmatics selected as atopic (three or more positive skin tests) or nonatopic (no positive skin tests) did not differ greatly in most of the clinical features of their asthma, although the definition of atopy (1-mm weal) may have influenced this finding (27). The prevalence of asthma in siblings of "intrinsic" (8.0%) and "extrinsic" (6.8%) asthmatics in France was similar, suggesting similar genetic influences (47). Burrows et al. seriously challenged the concept of "intrinsic"

asthma by reporting that, even in skin test negative adults, the prevalence of asthma was closely related to the serum IgE level standardized for age and sex (48). No asthma was present in those with the lowest IgE levels, whereas the log odds ratio for asthma increased linearly with the serum IgE level after controlling for possible confounders and the degree of reactivity to skin tests.

In 1966, Ishizaka et al. reported that immediate "reaginic" hypersensitivity was due to IgE (49). Shortly thereafter, the relationship between IgE and atopic disease in both children and adults was established. In a study of 6- to 17-year-old children in Australia, serum IgE levels in subjects with asthma, wheezy bronchitis, cough and sputum, eczema, or hay fever were significantly higher than levels in control children (50). In Melbourne children, the mean serum IgE was highest in those with the most severe asthma, both at age 10 (1,309 ng/ml) and age 14 (2,163 ng/ml) (1). Many subsequent studies have confirmed these early studies correlating asthma with IgE, both in children and in adults.

CORRELATIONS BETWEEN SKIN TESTS AND BRONCHIAL RESPONSIVENESS TO INHALED ALLERGEN

Rosenthal et al. reported that responses to skin tests and to airway challenge with ragweed were correlated in a quantitative fashion (51), but that these did not correlate well with clinical asthma. They suggested that inhaled allergen challenge was more specific for IgE antibody in the airway than for "asthma" expressed as its usual phenotype. Extending these findings, Bryant and colleagues showed highly significant correlation coefficients between the serum level of allergen-specific IgE and the degree of airway responsiveness to that allergen. The results with IgE were even stronger than the results correlating skin testing with airway response to allergen (52). Overall, 85% of those with an elevated serum level of IgE specific for an allergen had a positive airway challenge to that allergen, compared with 2% of those with serum IgE levels in the negative range.

ALLERGENS ASSOCIATED WITH ASTHMA

Over the last two decades, the strength of relationships between specific allergens detected by IgE or skin testing and asthma has become more precisely defined. Although the strength of results varies somewhat between different regions (because of prevalence of specific allergens), the most frequent positive skin test or specific IgE antibody related to asthma is sensitivity to house dust mite (*Dermatophagoides pteronyssinus* or *D. farinae*) (20,30,53–60). In a birth cohort of 1,037 New Zealand children followed from age 3 to 21 years, the relative risk for asthma symptoms of mite-sensitive children was 1.94

[95% confidence interval (CI) 1.29, 2.92], for AHR was 4.45 (2.69, 7.36) and for concurrent symptoms and AHR was 6.71 (1.21, 13.38) (all $p<0.05$) (31). Somewhat less striking, but highly relevant, relative risks were associated with cat dander (odds ratio for symptoms 2.27 (1.20, 4.30), for AHR 2.66 (1.42, 4.98) and for the combination 4.19 (2.11, 8.31). To a lesser extent other furred animals (61) and molds, especially alternaria (20), have been related to asthma. Although skin test sensitivity to grass pollen is common among children and adults, its relationship to asthma is much less important than house dust mite or cat (31,43,54), although grass pollen allergy does relate strongly to allergic rhinitis or hay fever (20,43).

More recently, especially in inner city areas of the United States, cockroach allergy has been commonly identified as common among those presenting to emergency rooms with severe asthma (62), and among those referred for specialist assessment of asthma, in whom cockroach sensitivity was noted in 48% (compared with house dust 76%, ragweed 45%, cat 40%, and dust mite 24%) (55).

CAN ADULT ASTHMA DEVELOP IN THE ABSENCE OF ATOPY?

In a sentinel study, Burrows and colleagues investigated the association of asthma or allergic rhinitis as self-reported by 2,657 persons aged 6 to 95 years in Tucson, Arizona with serum IgE and skin test reactivity to allergen (48). They found that, irrespective of age or atopic status by skin test, the prevalence of asthma was closely related with serum IgE levels standardized for age and sex. Regardless of age, no asthma was reported by 177 subjects with IgE levels >1.46 SD below the mean for their age and sex, whereas the log odds ratio increased linearly with serum IgE levels after controlling for skin test reactivity and possible confounders. (Fig. 1). The prevalence of self-reported asthma was 37.3% among subjects with IgE Z scores of 2.0 or more. The relationship between the prevalence of reported asthma and ranges of serum IgE Z scores are shown in Fig. 2. Allergic rhinitis, on the other hand, was closely related to skin tests independently of IgE level. From these epidemiologic findings, Burrows et al. concluded that asthma is almost always associated with an IgE-related reaction, suggesting that virtually all asthma has an allergic basis, even if atopy is not detected by skin testing. However, one criticism made of the study was that the majority of the five skin test allergens used (house dust, grass, tree mix, weed mix, mould mix) may have been more likely to detect allergies pertinent to rhinitis than to asthma.

It has been suggested that the association between asthma and IgE may mean that the inflammatory mechanism of asthma may itself increase IgE, e.g., by release of interleukin-4 from T lymphocytes, so that the association may be secondary rather than causal (63,64). The provocative agent for such an effect is unknown.

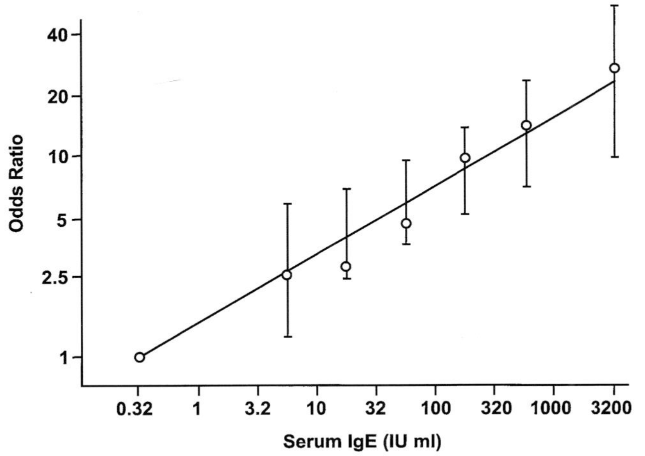

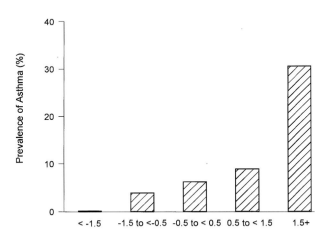

FIG. 1. Odds ratio (log scale) for Tucson subjects having asthma at seven levels of the total serum IgE concentration, after correction for age, sex, smoking habits, and skin test index in a logistic analysis. The *solid line*, representing the risk of asthma, is a weighted least-squares linear regression model fitted to the odds ratio at each log IgE level. The *vertical lines* are 95% confidence intervals around the regression for each odds ratio. (From Burrows B, Martinez FD, Halonen M, Barbee RA, Cline MG. Association of asthma with serum IgE levels and skin-test reactivity to allergens. *New Engl J Med* 1989; 320:271–277.)

FIG. 2. Prevalence of asthma in relation to IgE Z scores, standardized for age and sex, in the 1,662 Tucson persons with completely negative allergy skin tests to house dust, grass, tree mix, weed mix, and mould mix. The trend for prevalence to increase with increasing Z scores was highly significant ($p<0.0001$). (From Burrows B, Martinez FD, Halonen M, Barbee RA, Cline MG. Association of asthma with serum IgE levels and skin-test reactivity to allergens. *New Engl J Med* 1989; 320:271–277.)

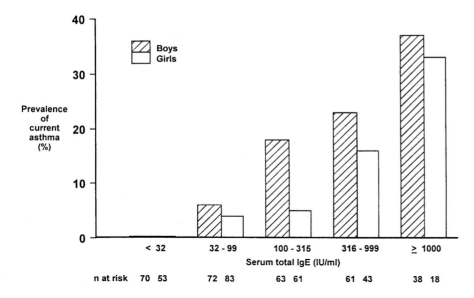

FIG. 3. Relation between serum total IgE and diagnosed current asthma in 11-year-old New Zealand children, by gender. The trend to increased prevalence as IgE increases is highly significant ($p<0.0001$) for boys, girls, and combined genders. (From Sears MR, Burrows B, Flannery EM, Herbison GP, Hewitt CJ, Holdaway MD. Relation between airway responsiveness and serum IgE in children with asthma and in apparently normal children. *N Engl J Med* 1991; 325:1067–1071.)

RELATIONSHIP BETWEEN SERUM IGE, CLINICAL ASTHMA, AND AIRWAY RESPONSIVENESS IN CHILDREN

In the previously described birth cohort of New Zealand children, the presence of physician-diagnosed asthma reported at age 11 strongly correlated with serum total IgE, both in boys and girls (10) (Fig. 3). As in adults, there were no reported cases of diagnosed asthma among those with the lowest level of serum IgE (below 32 units/L), and an increasing prevalence of asthma as IgE level increased.

Those with no history of wheezing had the lowest geometric mean serum IgE level (83.9 IU/ml, 95% CI 72.8, 96.8), whereas those with previously diagnosed asthma no longer current had intermediate levels [169.8 (89.1, 323.6)] and those with current asthma had the highest levels [456.6 (351.0, 617.6), $p<0.0001$].

There was also a clear relationship between total serum IgE and the presence of methacholine responsiveness in this New Zealand cohort (10), not only among children with wheezing symptoms or a diagnosis of asthma, but also among children who denied any respiratory symptoms (Fig. 4) AHR was not found in any asymptomatic child whose serum IgE was less than 32 IU/ml. However, both the prevalence and degree of AHR increased as the level of serum IgE increased ($p<0.001$). This suggested that serum IgE was causally related to AHR even without clinical expression of airway disease.

When AHR was expressed as a dose-response slope of the decline in forced expiratory volume in one second (FEV_1) during methacholine challenge in this cohort, a relationship between airway responsiveness and baseline lung function was seen only in those with at least moderately increased levels of serum IgE (65). Once serum IgE, reported asthma, and baseline lung function were taken

into account, other diagnoses and symptoms contributed relatively little to prediction of AHR, suggesting that IgE is a critical factor in the development of AHR in childhood.

The time when IgE levels become predictive of asthma is not clearly defined. The Tucson pediatric asthma study group found no relationship between cord blood IgE and a diagnosis of asthma or rhinitis by age 6 years, but serum IgE measured at 9 months was significantly related to subsequent development of asthma by age 6 years, sug-

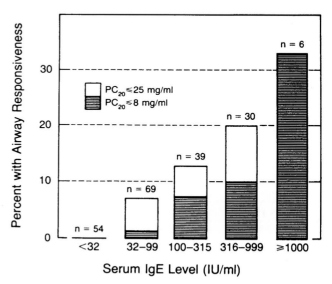

FIG. 4. Proportion of 11-year-old New Zealand children with no reported history of asthma, wheezing, hay fever, or eczema who had airway responsiveness to methacholine, according to serum IgE level. *p* for trend <0.001. (From Sears MR, Burrows B, Flannery EM, Herbison GP, Hewitt CJ, Holdaway MD. Relation between airway responsiveness and serum IgE in children with asthma and in apparently normal children. *N Engl J Med* 1991; 325:1067–1071.)

gesting that early allergic sensitization is important in the development of asthma (66).

Not all studies have found correlations between total serum IgE and characteristics of asthma. Takeda et al. found no correlation between airway responsiveness and serum IgE levels in a small study of 47 asthmatic children, or between airway responsiveness and RAST titers to *D. farinae* (67). They suggested that, although AHR and atopy both relate to asthma, the magnitude of allergic sensitization (as measured by IgE) did not influence the degree of AHR. However, large epidemiologic studies do support a substantive association between serum IgE, the clinical diagnosis of asthma, and the detection of airway responsiveness in children.

CORRELATIONS OF AIRWAY RESPONSIVENESS WITH ATOPY DETECTED BY SKIN TESTING

Although asthma in childhood can be related to total and specific serum IgE levels, there have been many more studies relating development of asthma and AHR to skin test responsiveness to allergens. Peat and colleagues studied 2,363 Australian children in Wagga Wagga (inland New South Wales) and Belmont (coastal), where the dominant allergens were respectively grasses and house dust mite, and concluded that within each population, the type of allergen to which the individual was sensitized, the quantity of aeroallergen present in the environment, and the degree of atopy as measured by the number and size of skin reactions were all factors that interact to increase the likelihood of airway responsiveness (16). Atopic children in both areas had an increased risk of having airway responsiveness, and to a lesser extent respiratory symptoms, diagnosed asthma and hay fever. The risk of airway responsiveness was further increased in children atopic to both pollens and house dust mites; in Wagga Wagga, the odds ratio was 7.5 (95% CI 5.2, 10.6) compared with 2.5 (1.4, 4.1) if only mite sensitive, and 3.3 (2.5, 4.3) if only pollen sensitive. Children with a high atopic score (derived from the number and size of the skin test reactions to four allergen groups tested) had a higher likelihood of AHR (Fig. 5) (16).

Clifford et al. found a highly significant association between airway responsiveness to methacholine and atopy in 7- to 11-year-old Southampton children, independent of symptoms and age group (68,69). In a subsequent longitudinal study of respiratory symptoms and airway responsiveness in 7- to 8-year-old Southampton children, atopy to *D. pteronyssinus*, cat fur, and/or mixed grass pollen was associated with a lower FEV$_1$, increased prevalence of airway responsiveness, greater day-to-day and between-day variation in peak flow rate, and greater severity of respiratory symptoms compared with the absence of atopy (30).

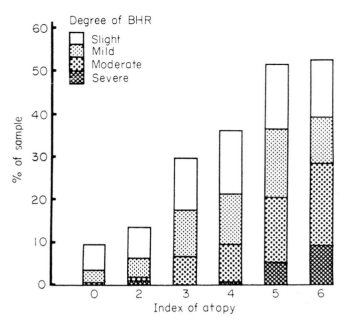

FIG. 5. Relationship in Australian children between degree of AHR and degree of atopy expressed as an index derived from the number of allergen groups to which children were reactive and the size of the reaction. (From Peat JK, Britton WJ, Salome CM, Woolcock AJ. Bronchial hyperresponsiveness in two populations of Australian schoolchildren. III. Effect of exposure to environmental allergens. *Clin Allergy* 1987; 17:291–300.)

In the birth cohort of New Zealand children, a strong relationship was found between skin test sensitivity to house dust mite and to cat allergen measured at age 13 years, and development of both wheezing symptoms and AHR to methacholine (31). Relative risks for wheezing, airway responsiveness, or the combination were not increased by grass sensitivity, despite this being the most common positive skin test, but sensitization to mite and/or to cat increased relative risks for development of wheezing symptoms (1.94 and 2.27, respectively), AHR (4.45 and 2.66, respectively), and for the combination of these features (6.71 and 4.19, respectively). Sensitivity to grass pollen was highly predictive of hay fever but not asthma (43).

INFLUENCE OF THE DEGREE OF ATOPY ON ASTHMA AND AIRWAY RESPONSIVENESS

In the New Zealand cohort, the prevalence of current asthma increased with increasing number of positive skin tests. Only 4.1% of those with no positive skin tests reported asthma, but 9.1%, 11.4%, 32.8%, and 40.5%, respectively, of those with 1, 2, 3 or 4 or more positive skin tests reported asthma (*p* for trend = 0.0000) (43). There was a highly significant trend to increased prevalence of

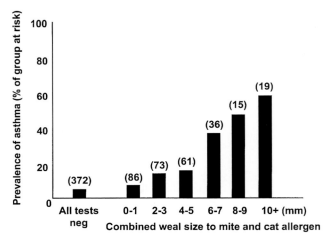

FIG. 6. Prevalence of diagnosed asthma in 13-year-old New Zealand children, by magnitude of skin test weal diameters to house dust mite and cat allergen (number in parentheses = number at risk). (From Sears MR, Burrows B, Flannery EM, Herbison GP, Holdaway MD. Atopy in childhood. I. Gender and allergen related risks for development of hay fever and asthma. *Clin Exp Allergy* 1993; 23:941–948.)

asthma with increasing degree of sensitization to mite and cat allergen as measured by increasing combined weal size to these allergens (Fig. 6) (43). Similarly, the prevalence of AHR to methacholine progressively increased as the combined weal size to mite and cat allergen increased (Fig. 7) (17).

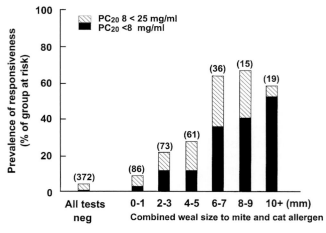

FIG. 7. Prevalence of airway responsiveness to methacholine in 13-year-old New Zealand children, by magnitude of skin test weal diameters to house dust mite and cat allergen (number in parentheses = number at risk). Measurable airway responsiveness (▨, $PC_{20} \leq 25$ mg/ml) and hyperresponsiveness (■, $PC_{20} \leq 8$ mg/mL). (From Sears MR, Burrows B, Herbison GP, Holdaway MD, Flannery EM. Atopy in childhood. II. Relationship to airway responsiveness, hay fever and asthma. *Clin Exp Allergy* 1993; 23:949–956.)

RELATIONSHIP BETWEEN SERUM IGE OR SKIN TESTS, CLINICAL ASTHMA, AND AIRWAY RESPONSIVENESS IN ADULTS

An early study of airway responsiveness and atopy in adults in Western Australia found a strong relationship between airway responsiveness to histamine, respiratory symptoms, atopy as determined by skin prick tests, smoking, and abnormal lung function ($p<0.001$) (70). Two thirds of those with $PD_{20} <2.5$ μmol histamine had one or more positive skin tests, and more than half had four or more positive tests (severe atopy).

In a longitudinal study of Tucson adults, the occurrence of wheeze in the absence of colds (suggesting asthma) was associated with both smoking and skin test reactivity. The prevalence of wheeze was higher among skin test–positive ex-smokers and nonsmokers than among those who were skin test negative (71). There was a suggestion in these data of an effect of serum IgE on the prevalence of wheeze.

Among 20- to 44-year-old adults surveyed in Australia as part of the European Community Respiratory Health Survey, wheezing when exposed to animals, feathers or dust (odds ratio 15.1), or to plants or pollen (odds ratio 9.6) were significantly associated with asthma in the last 12 months (72). In this population, atopy was present in 86.3% of persons with current asthma (odds ratio 6.4) and was strongly associated (odds ratios 3.1 to 8.7) with symptoms of nocturnal dyspnea, current wheeze, wheeze on exposure to trees, grass, flowers, or pollen, or when near animals, feathers, or dust (73).

Boston adults participating in the Normative Aging study were screened to exclude all with asthma and other chronic lung disease at the inception of the cohort, and then followed longitudinally for development of new symptoms. The prevalence of new asthma, cough and sputum production, and hay fever all increased with age-adjusted total serum IgE concentration, this relationship being strongest for new asthma. (39)

INFLUENCE OF ATOPY ON DEVELOPMENT OF NEW ADULT ASTHMA

In a study of college students followed up 23 years later, the risk of developing adult asthma was 10.5% among those who as students had reported rhinitis, compared with 3.6% among those not reporting rhinitis ($p<0.002$) (74). Similarly, adult asthma developed in 10.6% of individuals with positive skin tests as students, compared with 3.2% incidence in those with previously negative skin tests (p<0.001). Likewise, in a longitudinal study in rural Manitoba, atopic adults (as determined by skin tests or serum IgE) were more likely than nonatopics to develop new respiratory symptoms and physician-diagnosed asthma during a 12-year follow-up period (75).

In a U.S. study, atopic persons suspected of having asthma but with a negative methacholine challenge were more likely to develop later asthma than nonatopic persons during a 10-year follow-up period (76).

INFLUENCE OF ATOPY ON PERSISTENCE OF CHILDHOOD ASTHMA

In an early longitudinal study of childhood asthma, McNicol and Williams followed Melbourne children from 7 to 14 years of age, and noted that those with the greatest severity of asthma, and the most persistent asthma, were much more likely to have positive skin tests to rye grass allergen and house dust mite allergen, as well as a higher mean blood eosinophil count (1). These children also had higher serum IgE levels, and a higher prevalence of eczema, urticaria, and hay fever. Longer term follow-up of this cohort showed that at age 28 years, hay fever was common in all groups, but increased from 25% in the control group to 67% in the group with the most severe persistent asthma (28). IgE levels, peripheral blood eosinophil counts, and skin reactions were all significantly higher in those with more severe asthma than in the control group. These persons showed a progressive increase across the severity classes, which were, respectively, wheezers with no symptoms in the last 3 years, wheezers with no wheeze in the last 3 months, wheeze less than once per week in the last 3 months, and wheeze more than once per week in the last 3 months. IgE levels increased across these classes from <100 to >400 mg/ml, average skin reaction from <1.0 mm to >2.5 mm, house dust and cat reaction from 0.5 to >2 mm for each, and rye grass reaction from <2 mm to >5 mm. Serum IgE levels in those with persistent asthma were higher at age 28 years than at age 21 years.

A longitudinal study of 66 Italian infants with early wheezing showed that children who had persistent wheezing continuously or intermittently after 3 years of age were almost all (27 of 29) reactive to one or more allergens (77). However, 22 of the 37 infants who were not persistently wheezing also had a positive skin test response. Serum levels of total IgE were significantly higher in the group with persistent wheezing ($p<0.001$). Only 3 of the 37 infants who did not persistently wheeze had specific IgE antibodies at the initial investigation, and none developed specific IgE during the follow-up period, whereas among the 29 infants who had persistent wheezing at 3 years, 13 initially had specific IgE antibodies and 7 more developed these during follow-up.

Among 80 Swedish children with wheezy bronchitis followed prospectively for 12 years, most (54%) had ceased to wheeze before the age of 3 years, but 28% had persistent asthma (78). Of these, 59% had developed allergy compared with 10% of those who had stopped wheezing.

Martinez et al. followed 1,246 newborns in Tucson, Arizona to age 6 years, and found that those with early onset of a wheezing disorder that did not persist to age 6 years did not have elevated serum IgE levels or skin test reactivity (but were more likely to have mothers who smoked), whereas children with persistent wheezing at age 6 years were more likely to have mothers with asthma ($p<0.001$), and to have elevated serum IgE levels in the first year of life ($p<0.01$) and at age 6 ($p<0.0001$) (79).

EFFECT OF ATOPY ON EMERGENCY ROOM PRESENTATIONS WITH ACUTE ASTHMA

Among patients below age 50 years presenting to the emergency room of the University of Virginia Hospital, IgE antibody to dust mites, cockroach, cat dander, and grass and ragweed pollens were four times more likely to occur among persons with acute severe asthma than among control persons with any diagnosis other than shortness of breath (80). The prevalence of IgE antibodies to different allergens demonstrated significant seasonal and socioeconomic differences, suggesting that the associated risk is related to the degree of exposure to allergens. Among children attending an Atlanta hospital for asthma, 69% had IgE antibodies to house dust mite, cat, or cockroach compared with 27% of controls ($p<0.001$) (62). A combination of sensitization and significant exposure to the relevant antigen was present in 21 of 35 children with asthma, compared with 3 of 22 controls (odds ratio 9.5, $p<0.001$). In this population, black children were exposed to higher levels of mite and cockroach allergen.

INFLUENCE OF SMOKING ON IGE AND ATOPY

Several factors may influence the relationship between serum IgE, positive skin test, and asthma, including smoking. *In utero* cigarette smoking appears to have no influence on cord blood IgE, but there is an association between environmental tobacco smoke exposure and total serum IgE levels in children (14). In a study of 4,990 Swedish children, those living in a damp house with parents who smoked had the highest prevalence and relative risk for airway responsiveness and allergic asthma prevalences (23.5% and 11.6%, respectively, relative risks 2.8 and 2.5, respectively) (81). These data suggest that environmental pollutants may act synergistically to increase airway reactivity and allergy, especially in children with a family history of asthma.

Sherrill et al., examining both children and adults in the longitudinal Tucson Epidemiological Study of Airways Obstructive Disease, found a significant relationship between the number of cigarettes smoked and IgE level (82). Persons with skin test reactivity had statistically significant higher levels of total serum IgE than persons without skin test reactivity, independent of their smoking status. However, IgE levels of current smokers did not decrease with age at the same rate as nonsmokers, and so they have elevated levels throughout adulthood. The mechanism for the elevation of IgE with smoking is not known, but the significant dose-response relationship is suggestive of a causal association. Whereas earlier studies have demonstrated higher IgE levels among smokers than nonsmokers, this study was the first to demonstrate relationship between the amounts smoked and the level of IgE (82).

DIFFERENCES IN EPIDEMIOLOGY OF ASTHMA AND ATOPY IN DIFFERENT ETHNIC GROUPS AND DIFFERENT REGIONS

Significant differences in asthma and atopy have been noted between races living in the same environment. In the Unites States, black children have higher rates of respiratory illness including wheeze and asthma (83), and slightly greater skin test reactivity (23.2% vs. 19.8% in whites in the NHANES II study) (84). Important predictors of positive skin test among children in the United States were age, urban residence, and poverty status, and in white children sex was also important (84). In a later study (NHANES III), skin test reactivity was greatest in non-Hispanic blacks especially to cockroaches, alternaria, and pollens, but there was no difference in reactivity to cat and house dust mite among the ethnic groups (85). Among rural adolescents in New Zealand, atopy is more common among Maoris than non-Maoris (37.7% vs. 26.9%) (38). Maoris also had more symptoms of asthma, although this difference disappeared when allowance was made for smoking.

The same ethnic group moved to a new environment may develop a different level of atopy to those remaining in the old environment. Asians migrating to Australia develop higher prevalences of sensitization to major allergens than do native-born Australians, with higher prevalences of hay fever and asthma increasing significantly with length of stay in Australia (86). It has been suggested that this increase in asthma and allergic disease may relate not only to allergen exposure, but also to other factors such as diet (86). Living in urban areas appears to increase the prevalence of sensitization to allergens compared with rural dwellers (87,88). This difference is affected by factors other than pollution, as Polish children living in areas of increased pollution had less atopy than children living in urban areas of Sweden (88).

Further information on regional differences in atopy will be available when the European Community Respiratory Health Study is completed (89). However, regional variation even within countries results in substantial differences in clinical presentation of asthma. Allergen levels and positive skin prick tests varied between humid coastal and dry inland regions in Australia, with greater mite sensitization on the coast and alternaria sensitization inland (90). In each region, the allergen to which there was the greatest prevalence of sensitization also resulted in the highest odds ratio for current asthma. Odds ratios for current asthma in children sensitized to house dust mite were 21.3 by the coast and 2.7 inland, and in children sensitized to alternaria 3.4 by the coast and 5.6 inland.

IS INCREASING ASTHMA LINKED WITH INCREASING ATOPY?

Many studies confirm that the true prevalence of asthma is increasing (91–97). One reason for this is likely to be increased atopy (92,96) and especially house dust mite allergy. House dust mites were previously regarded as absent in sub-Arctic regions, e.g., in Scandinavia, but have been found there in increasing prevalence in recent studies (98,99) perhaps because of changes in house construction (100–102).

A closely related reason is increased exposure to allergens. Among 8-to 10-year-old Australian children studied at an interval of 10 years, the prevalence of wheezing in the last 12 months and of airway responsiveness to histamine increased 1.4 to twofold, but the prevalence of atopy documented by skin tests remained unchanged (103). Importantly, in that study, the numbers of house dust mites in domestic dust increased fivefold, and so whereas the overall prevalence of atopy may not have changed, the exposure to house dust allergen is likely to have increased, which may be the factor accounting for increased asthmatic symptoms. Similarly, adults in Western Australia were surveyed in 1981 and 1990, during which the prevalence of hay fever and asthma increased while the prevalence of atopy did not change (104). This suggests an increased exposure to allergen rather than an increased susceptibility to sensitization was responsible for the increased prevalence of symptoms.

Local increases in asthma have been associated with a local increase in a specific allergen exposure, e.g., importation of mesquite trees in Kuwait (105), use of blankets increasing house dust mites in Papua New Guinea (106,107), exposure to the green nimiti midge in Sudan (108), and exposure to soya bean dust in Barcelona (109).

It has been suggested that increased atopy may relate to early viral infections that can be associated with increased IgE, but Cogswell et al. followed a group of 92 British children with one atopic parent, and found more infections (3.6/year) among those not developing atopy than among those who did (3.0/year) tending to negate this hypothesis (29).

Changes in family size may be a factor in the increased likelihood of atopy. Strachan showed that the more older siblings there were, the lower was the probability of an atopic diagnosis (110). Similarly, von Mutius et al. found the prevalence of atopic sensitization decreased linearly with an increasing number of siblings (32). Hence, the trend to smaller families could have significantly influenced the prevalence of atopy, although direct evidence for this is not available.

Increased smoking may influence the prevalence of atopy. Burrows found higher total IgE in smokers than nonsmokers, although they had fewer skin test reactions (111). Smokers had greater persistence of IgE, whereas ex-smokers showed a fall in serum IgE after stopping smoking. Confirmation of Burrows' findings has come from four studies (112–115), but two other studies did not find a relationship between IgE and smoking (116,117). Maternal smoking may increase cord serum IgE levels in infants and increase the risk of subsequent allergy (118). Maternal smoking has increased, and so this may be another factor increasing atopy, and therefore asthma, in children (119,120).

Migration to other countries has almost invariably been associated with an increase in atopy. Two clear examples of this are the movement of Tokelauan Islanders to New Zealand (121,122) and Asian immigrants to Australia (86). This suggests that a change of environmental exposure increases the level of atopy, although many of these individuals remain asymptomatic.

Atopy may have increased over time without necessarily being explained by any of these mechanisms. In Japan, studies in 13- to 14-year-old girls showed IgE antibodies to one or more allergens in 21.4% in 1978, 25.0% in 1981, 35.5% in 1985, and 39.4% in 1991, with significant increases in prevalence of antibodies to grasses, house dust, and Japanese cedar ($p<0.01$) (123).

In Italy, the prevalence of atopy to at least one skin test increased in 9-year-old children from 24.7% to 42.4% over an interval of 9 years from 1983 to 1992, and in 13-year-olds from 30.0% to 42.2% over 5 years from 1987 to 1992 (124). Interestingly, the weal diameter to histamine control also increased over this period, suggesting a greater capacity to respond to histamine or to histamine-releasing substances. The prevalence of asthma in these populations increased from 12.2% to 15.0%, and airway responsiveness to carbachol from 35% to 49%. Hence, there was in this population a more substantial increase in the prevalence of atopy than of asthma.

CONCLUSIONS

There is a clear relationship between atopy as determined by skin test sensitivity or by total or specific serum IgE, and the clinical syndrome of asthma both in children and in adults. There are sufficient data to relate the presence of airway responsiveness to methacholine or histamine to atopy, both in symptomatic and in asymptomatic persons. The nature of the allergen to which sensitization has occurred, the degree of sensitivity, and the magnitude of exposure to that allergen are highly relevant in this re-

spect. The persistence of childhood asthma and the development of new asthma are strongly related to atopy. The increasing prevalence of asthma is at least in part explained by increasing atopy, or increased exposure to allergens.

ACKNOWLEDGMENT

I am grateful to Dr. Benjamin Burrows for his review of this chapter and his encouragement in the study of allergic factors in relation to the epidemiology of asthma, and to Mrs. Pearl Davis for preparation of this manuscript.

REFERENCES

1. McNichol KN, Williams HE. Spectrum of asthma in children—II, allergic components. *Br Med J* 1973;4:12–16.
2. Loftus BG, Price JF. Clinical and immunological characteristics of pre-school asthma. *Clin Allergy* 1986;16:251–257.
3. Tuchinda M, Habananananda S, Vareenil J, Srimaruta N, Piromrat K. Asthma in Thai children: a study of 2,000 cases. *Ann Allergy* 1987;59:207–211.
4. Sherman CB, Tosteson TD, Tager IB, Speizer FE, Weiss ST. Early childhood predictors of asthma. *Am J Epidem* 1990;132:83–95.
5. Suoniemi I, Bjorksten F, Haahtela T. Dependence of immediate hypersensitivity in the adolescent period on factors encountered in infancy. *Allergy* 1981;32:263–268.
6. Frischer T, Kuehr J, Meinert R, Karmaus W, Urbanek R. Risk factors for childhood asthma and recurrent wheezy bronchitis. *Eur J Pediatr* 1993;152:771–775.
7. Zimmerman B, Feanny S. Reisman J, Hak H, Rashed N, McLaughlin FJ, Levison H. Allergy in asthma. I. The dose relationship of allergy to severity of childhood asthma. *J Allergy Clin Immunol* 1988;87:63–70.
8. Peat JK, Woolcock AJ. Sensitivity to common allergens: relation to respiratory symptoms and bronchial hyperresponsiveness in children from three different climatic areas of Australia. *Clin Exp Allergy* 1992;21:573–581.
9. Stempel DA, Clyde WA, Henderson FW, Collier AM. Serum IgE levels and the clinical expression of respiratory illness. *J Pediatrics* 1980;97:185–190.
10. Sears MR, Burrows B, Flannery EM, Herbison GP, Hewitt CJ, Holdaway MD. Relation between airway responsiveness and serum IgE in children with asthma and in apparently normal children. *N Engl J Med* 1991;325:1067–1071.
11. Salob SP, Atherton DJ. Prevalence of respiratory symptoms in children with atopic dermatitis attending pediatric dermatology clinics. *Pediatrics* 1993;91:8–12.
12. Giles GG, Lickiss N. Gibson HB, Shaw K. Respiratory symptoms in Tasmanian adolescents: a followup of the 1961 birth cohort. *Aust NZ J Med* 1984;14:631–637.
13. Dave NK, Hopp RJ, Biven RE, Degan J, Bewtra AK, Townley RG. Persistence of increased nonspecific bronchial reactivity in allergic children and adolescents. *J Allergy Clin Immunol* 1990;86:147–153.
14. Weiss ST, Sparrow D, O'Connor GT. The interrelationship among allergy, airways responsiveness, and asthma. *J Asthma* 1993;30:329–349.
15. Peat JK, Britton WJ, Salome CM, Woolcock AJ. Bronchial hyperresponsiveness in two populations of Australian schoolchildren. II. Relative importance of associated factors. *Clin Allergy* 1987;17:283–290.
16. Peat JK, Britton WJ, Salome CM, Woolcock AJ. Bronchial hyperresponsiveness in two populations of Australian schoolchildren. III. Effect of exposure to environmental allergens. *Clin Allergy* 1987;17:291–300.
17. Sears MR, Burrows B, Herbison GP, Holdaway MD, Flannery EM. Atopy in childhood. II. Relationship to airway responsiveness, hay fever and asthma. *Clin Exp Allergy* 1993;23:949–956.
18. Sears MR, Burrows B, Herbison GP, Flannery EM, Holdaway MD.

Atopy in childhood. III. Relationship with pulmonary function and airway responsiveness. *Clin Exp Allergy* 1993;23:957–963.

19. Corne J, Smith S, Schreiber J, Holgate ST. Prevalence of atopy in asthma. *Lancet* 1994;344:344–345.

20. Gergen PJ, Turkeltaub PC. The association of individual allergen reactivity with respiratory disease in a national sample: data from the second National Health and Nutritional Examination Survey, 1976–80 (NHANES II). *J Allergy Clin Immunol* 1992;90:579–588.

21. WHO/IUS Allergen Nomenclature Subcomittee World Health Organization, Geneva, Switzerland. Allergen nomenclature. *Clin Exp Allergy* 1995;25:27–37.

22. Grater WC, Dockhorn R, Boggs P, Don RL. Report of the American College of Allergists' Committee on standardization of allergenic extracts. *Ann Allergy* 1982;49:49–54.

23. Berkowitz RB, Tinkelman DG, Lutz C, Crummie A, Smith K. Evaluation of the multi-test device for immediate hypersensitivity skin testing. *J Allergy Clin Immunol* 1992;90:979–985.

24. Aas K. Allergic asthma in childhood. *Arch Dis Child* 1969; 44:1–10.

25. Lockey R, Lichenstein L, Bloach K, et al. The use of *in vitro* tests for IgE antibody in the specific diagnosis of IgE-mediated disorders and in the formulation of allergen immunotherapy. *J Allergy Clin Immunol* 1992;90:263–267.

26. Bousquet J, Michel FB. Precision of prick and puncture tests. *J Allergy Clin Immunol* 1992;90:870–872.

27. Research Committee of the British Thoracic and Tuberculosis Association. Skin tests and clinical features of asthma. *Br J Dis Chest* 1975; 69:125–135.

28. Kelly WJW, Hudson I, Phelan PD, Pain MCF, Olinsky A. Atopy in subjects with asthma followed to the age of 28 years. *J Allergy Clin Immunol* 1990;85:548–557.

29. Cogswell JJ, Halliday DF, Alexander JR. Respiratory infections in the first year of life in children at risk of developing atopy. *Br Med J* 1982;2845:1011–1013.

30. Clough JB, Williams JD, Holgate ST. Effect of atopy on the natural history of symptoms, peak expiratory flow, and bronchial responsiveness in 7- and 8-year-old children with cough and wheeze. *Am Rev Respir Dis* 1991;143:755–760.

31. Sears MR, Herbison GP, Holdaway MD, Hewitt CJ, Flannery EM, Silva PA. The relative risks of sensitivity to grass pollen, house dust mite and cat dander in the development of childhood asthma. *Clin Exp Allergy* 1989;19:419–424.

32. von Mutius E, Martinez FD, Fritzsch C, Nicolai T, Reitmeir P, Thiemann H-H. Skin test reactivity and number of siblings. *Br Med J* 1994;308:692–695.

33. Peat JK, Tovey E, Gray EJ, Mellis CM, Woolcock AJ. Asthma severity and morbidity in a population sample of Sydney schoolchildren: part II—importance of house dust mite allergens. *Aust NZ J Med* 1994;24:270–276.

34. Norman E, Rosenhall L, Nystrom L, Jonsson E, Stjernberg N. Prevalence of positive skin prick tests, allergic asthma, and rhinoconjunctivitis in teenagers in northern Sweden. *Allergy* 1994;49:808–815.

35. Peat JK, Salome CM, Woolcock AJ. Longitudinal changes in atopy during a 4-year period: relation to bronchial hyperresponsiveness and respiratory symptoms in a population sample of Australian children. *J Allergy Clin Immunol* 1990;85:65–74.

36. Crane J, O'Donnell TV, Prior IA, Waite DA. The relationship between atopy, bronchial hyperresponsiveness, and a family history of asthma: a cross-sectional study of migrant Tokelauan children in New Zealand. *J Allergy Clin Immunol* 1989;84:768–772.

37. Sporik R, Ingram JM, Price W, Sussman JH, Housinger RW, Platts-Mills TAE. Association of asthma with serum IgE and skin test reactivity to allergens among children living at high altitude. Tickling the dragon's breath. *Am J Respir Crit Care Med* 1995;151:1388–1392.

38. Shaw RA, Crane J, O'Donnell TV. Asthma symptoms, bronchial hyperresponsiveness and atopy in a Maori and European adolescent population. *NZ Med J* 1991;104:175–179.

39. Tollerud DJ, O'Connor GT, Sparrow D, Weiss ST. Asthma, hay fever, and phlegm production associated with distinct patterns of allergy skin test reactivity, eosinophilia, and serum IgE levels. *Am Rev Respir Dis* 1991;144:776–781.

40. Brand PLP, Kerstjens HAM, Jansen HM, Kauffman HF, de Monchy JGR and Dutch CNSLD Study Group. Interpretation of skin tests to house dust mite and relationship to other allergy parameters in patients with asthma and chronic obstructive pulmonary disease. *J Allergy Clin Immunol* 1993;91:560–70.

41. Roorda RJ, Gerritsen J, vanAalderen WMC, Knol K. Skin reactivity and eosinophil count in relation to the outcome of childhood asthma. *Eur Respir J* 1993;6:509–516.

42. Meinert R, Frischer T, Karmaus W, Kuehr J. Influence of skin prick test criteria on estimation of prevalence and incidence of allergic sensitization in children. *Allergy* 1994;49:526–532.

43. Sears MR, Burrows B, Flannery EM, Herbison GP, Holdaway MD. Atopy in childhood. I. Gender and allergen related risks for development of hay fever and asthma. *Clin Exp Allergy* 1993; 23:941–948.

44. Rackermann FM. A clinical study of one hundred and fifty cases of bronchial asthma. *Arch Intern Med* 1918;22:517–552.

45. Ostergaard PAA. Non-IgE-mediated asthma in children. *Acta Paediatr Scand* 1985;74:713–719.

46. Grieco MH. Pathogenesis of bronchial asthma. In: Gupta S, Good RA, eds. *Cellular, molecular and clinical aspects of allergic disorders.* New York: Plenum Medical Book Co, 1979; 417–467.

47. Pirson F, Charpin D, Sansonetti M. et al. Is intrinsic asthma a hereditary disease? *Allergy* 1991;46:367–371.

48. Burrows B, Martinez FD, Halonen M, Barbee RA, Cline MG. Association of asthma with serum IgE levels and skin-test reactivity to allergens. *New Engl J Med* 1989;320:271–277.

49. Ishizaka K, Ishizaka T, Hornbrook MM. Physico-chemical properties of human reaginic antibody. IV. Presence of a unique immunoglobulin as a carrier of reaginic activity. *J Immunol* 1966;97:75.

50. Turner KJ, Rosman DL, O'Mahony J. Prevalence and familial association of atopic disease and its relationship to serum IgE levels in 1,061 school children and their families. *Int Arch Allergy* 1974;47:650–664.

51. Rosenthal RR, Bruce CA, Lichtenstein LM, Norman PS. The role of inhalation challenge. *Int Arch Allergy Appl Immunol* 1975;49:89–94.

52. Bryant DH, Burns MW, Lazarus L. The correlation between skin tests, bronchial provocation tests and the serum level of IgE specific for common allergens in patients with asthma. *Clin Allergy* 1975;5:145–157.

53. Green WF, Woolcock AJ, Stuckey M, Sedgwick C, Leeder SR. House dust mites and skin tests in different Australian localities. *Aust NZ J Med* 1986;16:639–643.

54. Ferrante E, Corbo GM, Valente S, Ciappi G. Associations between atopy, asthma history, respiratory function and non-specific bronchial hyperresponsiveness in unselected young asthmatics. *Respiration* 1992;59:169–172.

55. Kang BC, Johnson J, Veres-Thorner C. Atopic profile of inner-city asthma with a comparative analysis on the cockroach sensitive and ragweed sensitive subgroups. *J Allergy Clin Immunol* 1993;93:802–811.

56. Sporik R, Chapman MD, Platts-Mills TAE. House dust mite exposure as a cause of asthma. *Clin Exp Allergy* 1992;22:897–906.

57. Kagamimori S, Naruse Y, Watanabe M, Nohara S, Okada A. An epidemiological study on total and specific IgE levels in Japanese schoolchildren. *Clin Allergy* 1982;12:561–568.

58. Platts-Mills TAE, de Weck AL. Dust mite allergens and asthma - a worldwide problem. *J Allergy Clin Immunol* 1989;83:416–427.

59. Frischer T, Meinert R, Karmaus W, Urbanek R, Kuehr J. Relationship between atopy and frequent bronchial response to exercise in school children. *Pediatr Pulmonol* 1994;17:320–325.

60. Kuehr J, Frischer T, Meinert R, et al. Sensitization to mite allergens is a risk factor for early and late onset of asthma and for persistence of asthmatic signs in children. *J Allergy Clin Immunol* 1995;95:655–662.

61. Kjellman B, Pettersson R. The problem of furred pets in childhood atopic disease. *Allergy* 1983;38:65–73.

62. Call RS, Smith TF, Morris E, Chapman MD, Platts-Mills TAE. Risk factors for asthma in inner city children. *J Pediatrics* 1992;121:862–866.

63. Rolla G, Bucca C. Asthma and serum levels of IgE. *N Engl J Med* 1989;320:1696–1697.

64. Burrows B, Martinez FD, Cline MG, Lebowitz MD. The relationship between parental and children's serum IgE and asthma. *Am J Respir Crit Care Med* 1995;152:1497–1500.

65. Burrows B, Sears MR, Flannery EM, Herbison GP, Holdaway MD. Relationships of bronchial responsiveness assessed by methacholine to serum IgE, lung function, symptoms and diagnoses in 11-year-old New Zealand children. *J Allergy Clin Immunol* 1992;90:376–385.

66. Halonen M, Stern DA, Wright AL, Taussig LM, Martinez FD. Active asthma and rhinitis at age six in relation to serum IgE levels at birth, nine months and six years. *Am J Respir Crit Care Med* 1994;149:A911.

67. Takeda K, Shibasaki M, Takita H. Relation between bronchial responsiveness to methacholine and levels of IgE antibody against dermatophagoides farinae and serum IgE in asthmatic children. *Clin Exp Allergy* 1993;23:450–454.

68. Clifford RD, Radford M, Howell JB, Holgate ST. Prevalence of atopy and range of bronchial response to methacholine in 7 and 11 year old schoolchildren. *Arch Dis Child* 1989;64:1126–1132.

69. Clifford RD, Howell JB, Radford M, Holgate ST. Associations between respiratory symptoms, bronchial response to methacholine, and atopy in two age groups of schoolchildren. *Arch Dis Child* 1989;64:1133–1139.

70. Woolcock AJ, Peat JK, Salome CM, et al. Prevalence of bronchial hyperresponsiveness and asthma in a rural adult population. *Thorax* 1987;42:361–368.

71. Barbee RA, Halonen M, Kaltenborn WT, Burrows B. A longitudinal study of respiratory symptoms in a community population sample. Correlations with smoking, allergen skin-test reactivity, and serum IgE. *Chest* 1991;99:20–26.

72. Kutin JJ, Abramson M, Raven J, et al. Risk factors for asthma in young adults: jobs, allergens and parents. *Aust NZ J Med* 1994;24:449.

73. Abramson M, Kutin J, Raven J, et al. Risk factors for atopy in young adults. *Aust NZ J Med* 1994;24:474.

74. Settipane RJ, Hagy GW, Settipane GA. Development of new asthma and allergic rhinitis in a 23–year follow-up of college students. *J Allergy Clin Immunol* 1991;87:232.

75. Erzen D, Warren CPW, Manfreda J. Atopy and the development of respiratory symptoms. *Eur Respir J* 1994;7:254S.

76. Puolijoki H, Impivaara O, Liippo K, Tala E. Later development of asthma in patients with a negative methacholine inhalation challenge examined for suspected asthma. *Lung* 1992;170:235–241.

77. Businco L, Frediani T, Lucarelli S, Finocchi M, Puddu M, Businco E. A prospective study of wheezing infants: clinical and immunological results. *Ann Allergy* 1979;43:120–122.

78. Foucard T, Sjoberg O. A prospective 12 year followup study of children with wheezy bronchitis. *Acta Paediatr Scand* 1984;73:577–583.

79. Martinez FD, Wright AL, Taussig LM. et al. Asthma and wheezing in the first six years of life. *N Engl J Med* 1995;332:133–138.

80. Pollart SM, Chapman MD, Fiocco GP, Rose G, Platts-Mills TAE. Epidemiology of acute asthma: IgE antibodies to common inhalant allergens as a risk factor for emergency room visits. *J Allergy Clin Immunol* 1989;83:875–882.

81. Andrae S, Axelson O, Bjorksten B, Fredriksson M, Kjellman N-IM. Symptoms of bronchial hyperreactivity and asthma in relation to environmental factors. *Arch Dis Child* 1988;63:473–478.

82. Sherill DL, Halonen M, Burrows B. Relationships between total serum IgE, atopy, and smoking: a twenty year follow-up analysis. *J Allergy Clin Immunol* 1994;954–962.

83. Gold DR, Rotnitzky A, Dasmokosh AI, et al. Race and gender differences in respiratory illness prevalence and their relationship to environmental exposures in children 7 to 14 years of age. *Am Rev Respir Dis* 1993;148:10–18.

84. Gergen PJ, Turkeltaub PC, Kovar MR. The prevalence of allergic skin test reactivity to eight common aeroallergens in the U.S. population: results from the Second National Health and Nutrition Examination Survey. *J Allergy Clin Immunol* 1987;80:669–679.

85. Bang KM, Gergen PJ, Turkeltaub PC. Skin test reactivity in a US national sample: results from phase I of the Third National Health and Nutrition Examination Survey. *J Allergy Clin Immunol* 1993;91:308.

86. Leung R. Asthma, allergy and atopy in South-East Asian immigrants in Australia. *Aust NZ J Med* 1994;24:255–257.

87. Poysa L, Korppi M, Pietikainen M, Remes K, Juntunen-Backman K. Asthma, allergic rhinitis and atopic eczema in Finnish children and adolescents. *Allergy* 1991;46:161–165.

88. Braback L, Breborowicz A, Dreborg S, Knutsson A, Pieklik H, Bjorksten B. Atopic sensitization and respiratory symptoms among Polish and Swedish school children. *Clin Exp Allergy* 1994; 24:826–835.

89. Burney P. Asthma prevalence and risk factors. In: Vuylsteek K, Hallen M, eds. *Epidemiology*. Amsterdam: IOS Press, 1994.

90. Peat JK, Tovey E, Mellis CM, Leeder SR, Woolcock AJ. Importance of house dust mite and alternaria allergens in childhood asthma: an epidemiological study in two climatic regions in Australia. *Clin Exp Allergy* 1993;23:812–820.

91. Norman E, Rosenhall, L Nystrom L, Bergstrom E, Stjernberg N. High prevalence of asthma and related symptoms in teenagers in Northern Sweden. *Eur Respir J* 1993;6:834–839.

92. Burney, PGJ, Bousquet J. Evidence for an increase in atopic disease and possible causes. *Clin Exp Allergy* 1993;23:484–492.

93. Burney PGJ, Chinn S, Rona RJ. Has the prevalence of asthma increased in children? Evidence from the national study of health and growth 1973–86. *Br Med J* 1990;300:1306–1310.

94. Aberg N. Asthma and allergic rhinitis in Swedish conscripts. *Clin Exp Allergy* 1989;19:59–63.

95. Aberg N, Engstrom I, Lindberg U. Allergic diseases in Swedish schoolchildren. *Acta Paediatr Scand* 1989;78:246–252.

96. Ninan TK, Russell G. Respiratory symptoms and atopy in Aberdeen school children: evidence from two surveys 25 years apart. *Br Med J* 1992;304:873–875.

97. Fleming DM, Crombie DL. Prevalence of asthma and hay fever in England and Wales. *Br Med J* 1987;294:279–283.

98. Munir AKM, Einarsson R, Kjellman N-IM, Bjorksten B. Mite (Der p 1, Der f I) and cat (Fel d I) allergens in homes of babies with a family history of allergy. *Allergy* 1993;48:158–163.

99. Wickman M, Nordvall SL, Pershagen G, Sundell J, Schwartz B. House dust mite sensitization in children and residential characteristics in a temperate region. *J Allergy Clin Immunol* 1991;88:89–95.

100. Harving H, Korsgaard J, Dahl R. Clinical efficacy of reduction in house-dust mite exposure in specially designed, mechanically ventilated "healthy" homes. *Allergy* 1994;49:866–870.

101. Wjst M, Heinrich J, Liu P, et al. Indoor factors and IgE levels in children. *Allergy* 1994;49:766–771.

102. Munir AKM, Bjorksten B, Einarsson R, et al. Mite allergens in relation to home conditions and sensitization of asthmatic children from three climatic regions. *Allergy* 1995;50:55–64.

103. Peat JK, van den Berg RH, Green WF, Mellis CM, Leeder SR, Woolcock AJ. Changing prevalence of asthma in Australian children. *Br Med J* 1994;308:1591–1596.

104. Peat JK, Haby M, Spijker J, Berry G, Woolcock AJ. Prevalence of asthma in adults in Busselton, Western Australia. *Br Med J* 1992;305:1326–1329.

105. Ellul-Micallef R, Al-Ali S. The spectrum of bronchial asthma in Kuwait. *Clin Allergy* 1984;14:509–517.

106. Turner KJ, Dowse GK, Stewart GA, Alpers MP, Woolcock AJ. Prevalence of asthma in the South Fore people of the Okapa District of Papua New Guinea. Features associated with a recent dramatic increase. *Int Arch Allergy Appl Immunol* 1985;77:158–162.

107. Dowse GK, Turner KJ, Stewart GA, Alpers MP, Woolcock AJ. The association between dermatophagoides mites and the increasing prevalence of asthma in village communities within the Papua New Guinea highlands. *J Allergy Clin Immunol* 1985;75:75–83.

108. Kay AB, Maclean U, Wilkinson AH, GadElRab MO. The prevalence of asthma and rhinitis in a Sudanese community seasonally exposed to a potent airborne allergen (the "green nimitti" midge, *cladotanytarsus lewisi*). *J Allergy Clin Immunol* 1983;71:345–352.

109. Anto JM, Sunyer J, Rodriques-Roisin R, Suarez-Cervera M, Vazquez L and the Toxicoepidemiological Committee. Community outbreaks of asthma associated with inhalation of soybean dust. *N Engl J Med* 1989;320:1271–1273.

110. Strachan DP. Hay fever, hygiene, and household size. *Br Med J* 1989; 299:1259–1260.

111. Burrows B, Halonen M, Barbee RA, Lebowitz MD. The relationship of serum immunoglobulin E to cigarette smoking. *Am Rev Respir Dis* 1981;124:523–525.

112. Warren CPW, Holford-Strevens V, Wong C, Manfreda J. The relationship between smoking and total immunoglobulin E levels. *J Allergy Clin Immunol* 1982;69:370–375.

113. Zetterstrom O, Osterman K, Machado L. Johansson SGO. Another smoking hazard: raised serum IgE concentration and increased risk of occupational allergy. *Br Med J* 1981;283:1215–1217.

114. Bahna SL, Heinder DC, Myhre BA. Immunoglobulin E pattern in cigarette smokers. *Allergy* 1983;38:57–64.

115. Vollmer WM, Buist AS, Johnson LR, McCamant LE, Halonen M. Relationship between serum IgE and cross-sectional and longitudinal FEV$_1$ in two cohort studies. *Chest* 1986;90:416–423.

116. Taylor RG, Gross E, Joyce H, Holland F, Pride NB. Smoking, allergy, and the differential white blood cell count. *Thorax* 1985;40:17–22.

117. Freidhoff LR, Meyers DA, Marsh DG. A genetic-epidemiologic study of human immune responsiveness to allergens in an industrial population. II. The associations among skin sensitivity, total serum IgE,

age, sex, and the reporting of allergies in a stratified random sample. *J Allergy Clin Immunol* 1984;73:490–499.

118. Magnusson CGM. Maternal smoking influences cord serum IgE and IgD levels and increases the risk for subsequent infant allergy. *J Allergy Clin Immunol* 1986;78:898–904.

119. Pierce JP, Fiore MC, Novotny TE, Hatziandreu EJ, Davis RM. Trends in cigarette smoking in the United States. Educational differences are increasing. *JAMA* 1989;261:56–60.

120. Fielding JE. Smoking and women. Tragedy of the majority. *N Engl J Med* 1989;317:1323–1325.

121. Waite DA, Eyles EF, Tonkin SL, O'Donnell TV. Asthma prevalence in Tokelauun childen in two environments. *Clin Allergy* 1980;10:71–75.

122. Crane J, O'Donnell TV, Prior IAM, Waite DA. Symptoms of asthma, methacholine airway responsiveness and atopy in migrant Tokelauan children. *NZ Med J* 1989;102:36–38.

123. Nakagomi T, Itaya H, Tominaga T, Yamaki M, Hisamatsu S, Nakagoma O. Is atopy increasing? *Lancet* 1994;343:121–122.

124. Ronchetti R, Bonci E, Macri F, et al. Prevalance of bronchial reactivity and allergen skin prick test positivity in Italian school children: increase over 9 years. *Eur Respir J* 1994;7:480s.

Asthma, edited by P.J. Barnes, M.M. Grunstein, A.R. Leff, and A.J. Woolcock.
Lippincott–Raven Publishers, Philadelphia © 1997.

▪ 8 ▪

Indoor Allergens as a Risk Factor for Asthma

Adnan Custovic and Martin D. Chapman

HISTORY

The earliest written report of a respiratory disorder characterized by wheezing (probably asthma) can be found in the ancient Chinese text *Nei Chung Su Wen* (*Cannon of Internal Medicine*) dating from the 26th century B.C. (1). The origin of the word "asthma" is Greek, meaning "wind" or "to blow." Ancient Greek physicians recognized the disorder, and the earliest description of asthma in Western literature is attributed to Aretaeus the Cappadocian, who, in the second century A.D., wrote: "If from running, gymnastic exercises, or any other work, the breathing becomes difficult, it is called asthma" (2). Interestingly, Aretaeus considered the disease to be ". . . coldness and humidity of the spirit . . ." (2). It is now realized that the humidity of the environment, rather than that of a spirit, can contribute to the development of asthma through its favorable effect on the house dust mite population growth in modern domestic dwellings. Among the first to associate environmental factors and respiratory disease was German physician Georgius

Agricola (1494–1555), who recognized occupational pulmonary disease caused by dust in miners (3). Italian physician Gerolamo Cardano (1501–1576) went one step further and used environmental control to treat asthma in what can now be considered as the first recorded (and successful) example of allergen avoidance (4). Such was Cardano's reputation that he was summoned to Scotland by John Hamilton, Archbishop of St. Andrews, who, as a primate of Scotland and brother of the Regent, was a powerful and important figure. In a prolonged consideration of the case lasting several months, Cardano made a recommendation that the Archbishop should get rid of his feather bedding. This was followed by a "miraculous" remission of his intractable asthma. Flemish physician Jan Baptista van Helmont (1577–1644), an asthma sufferer himself, realized that symptoms could be caused by inhalation of airborne dust, describing vividly an asthma attack in one of his patients, a monk (". . . as oft as the space is swept or the wind doth otherwise stir up the dust, he presently falls down being almost choked . . .") (5). The most influential text on asthma written in the 19th century was Henry Salter's book *On Asthma: It's Pathology and Treatment,* in which he wrongly considered asthma to be primarily a psychologic disease. However, Salter (1823–1871) also realized that asthma attacks can be initiated by ". . . stroking a cat, sleeping on a feather pillow or passing a poultry shop . . ." (6).

A. Custovic: North West Lung Centre, South Manchester University Hospitals, Manchester M23 9LT United Kingdom.

M. D. Chapman: Departments of Medicine and Microbiology, Asthma and Allergic Diseases Center, University of Virginia, Charlottesville, Virginia 22908.

The awareness of the importance of inhaled substances was furthered by the recognition of hay fever and the lower respiratory symptoms sometimes associated with this disease. Interestingly, it was again an asthma sufferer, English physician John Bostock (1773–1846), who provided us with a classic description of seasonal rhinitis and asthma ("To the sneezing are added a further sensation of tightness of the chest, and difficulty of breathing, with a general irritation of fauces and trachea") (7). Charles Blackley (1820–1900), yet another allergy sufferer, proved conclusively that pollen is a cause of hay fever. In his still widely admired book *Experimental Researches on the Cause and Nature of Catarrhus Aestivus (Hay-Fever or Hay-Asthma)*, he wrote: "I have shown that the peculiar and distinctive action of pollen is seen in the oedema which is produced in the cellular tissue of any part to which it is applied. This I believe is the true cause of the dyspnoea of hay-asthma, and I am also inclined to think that when all the phenomena of ordinary asthma have been thoroughly investigated a similar condition will be found to be the cause of dyspnoea in the latter disease also" (8). The idea of allergen exposure as a cause of asthma was born in Blackley's visionary work.

The 20th century brought much better understanding of the pathophysiology of asthma and other allergic disorders. The term "allergy" was introduced in 1906 by the Austrian pediatrician Clemens von Pirquet (1874–1967), originating from "allos" (other), suggesting a deviation from the normal state. About the same time, different investigators, some of them familiar with Blackley's work, were identifying pollen as an allergen causing hay fever, and animal dander and house dust as other important triggers of allergic symptoms. Leonard Noon (1878–1913) and John Freeman (1877–1962) started with administration of pollen-derived extracts in the treatment of seasonal allergic rhinitis, establishing the principles of immunotherapy (9). Fascinating research was going on into genetics and pathophysiology of the allergic disease. Robert Cooke (1880–1960) reported positive family history of allergy in 48% of patients with allergic disease (10), introducing the concept of the importance of genetics in allergic disease (described in Chapter 11). Increasing knowledge of the mediators of inflammation and the discovery of mechanisms underlying the early and late phase inflammatory response contributed to a better understanding of allergic response. In 1921, Kern reported that most patients with asthma show weal and flare reaction after skin testing with extracts of dust from their own homes (11). Storm van Leeuwen (1882–1933) created a "climate" chamber in Holland in 1927, in an attempt to recreate the environment of the high-altitude sanatoria that were already known to be the places to benefit asthma sufferers, and demonstrated that the asthmatic patients improved if moved from their homes into the chamber (12).

About three centuries after Van Helmont's observations on the importance of inhaled dust in triggering asthma attacks, mites of the family *Pyroglyphidae* were established as the single most important source of allergens in house dust (13). In 1967 Ishizaka et al. discovered that weal and flare reactions were mediated by immunoglobulin E (IgE) antibodies (14). Roger Altounyan (1922–1987) described in 1970 an increase in nonspecific bronchial hyperreactivity (BHR) in patients with seasonal asthma during the pollen season, which returned to normal when pollen counts were low (15). Cockroft et al. demonstrated that nonspecific BHR increased after allergen bronchial provocation and that this increase correlated with late reaction (16), indicating that the relationship between allergens and BHR probably involve airway inflammation. Asthma is now considered to be a chronic inflammatory airway disease, and the specific role of inflammatory cells and mediators is being elucidated.

The second half of the 20th century has witnessed another important phenomenon: an increase in asthma prevalence. At the end of the century we are facing a paradox: despite better and more powerful asthma medication than ever before, the prevalence and severity of the disease is on the increase throughout the world (17–26). Asthma is now the most common chronic disease in childhood. In the search for the explanation of the observed time trend in asthma prevalence, environmental factors have received deserved attention. Among many different environmental influences (e.g., viral infections, passive smoking, air pollution), indoor allergens, particularly those of house dust mites and domestic pets (cats and dogs), are recognized as a major risk factor for asthma worldwide.

Much of the current understanding of the crucial role of indoor allergens in asthma derived initially from immunochemical studies on the identification and analysis of allergen molecules.

MOLECULAR BIOLOGY OF INDOOR ALLERGENS

Most allergens are low-molecular-weight (5–50 kDa) water-soluble proteins or glycoproteins, which rapidly penetrate through mucosal membranes and may facilitate the immediate symptoms seen in allergic patients. Apart from these general properties, allergens are a diverse group of proteins, without as yet any known structural feature that could be associated with their ability to stimulate IgE antibody production.

Purification of allergens derived from pollens, house dust mites, animal dander, insects, and fungi is essential for structural and immunologic studies investigating why these molecules readily induce IgE antibody formation, whereas protein antigens from other sources (e.g., bacteria, viruses) usually do not. Some inhalant allergens are so immunogenic that they induce humoral and cellular responses in up to 30% of the population after remarkably low-dose natural exposure (only 1 µg of mite or pollen allergen per year) (27). The isolation of house dust mite, cat, dog, and cockroach allergens allowed the biochemical properties of these allergens to be defined. The usage of the purified allergens for skin testing and serum IgE antibody assays enabled their allergenic properties to be established.

Furthermore, the production of monoclonal antibodies (mAb) has provided reliable and consistent markers for specific allergens. This has led to improved purification procedures and the development of allergen detection tests. Since the application of molecular cloning techniques in the late 1980s, more than 20 indoor allergens have been sequenced, in addition to a similar number of grass, weed, tree pollen, and venom allergens (28–30). As a result of this extensive scientific effort, allergens now constitute one of the most clearly defined groups of molecules in biomedical research.

Allergen Cloning and Sequencing Strategies

A list of indoor allergens that fulfill the World Health Organization (WHO)/International Union of Immunolog-ical Societies (IUIS) allergen nomenclature guidelines is shown in Table 1. A note on nomenclature: the Allergen Nomenclature subcommittee of the IUIS devised a systematic nomenclature that designates allergens using the first three letters of the genus, followed by a single letter for the species and a number to indicate the chronologic order in which the allergen was isolated (31). Many of the listed allergens were originally defined on the basis of the biochemical and allergenic properties of the natural allergen, e.g., the Group 1 and Group 2 *Dermatophagoides* allergens and Fel d 1. In these cases, the availability of partial protein sequences facilitated the determination of the complete nucleotide sequence using either complementary DNA (cDNA) cloning or polymerase chain reaction (PCR)–based techniques. Recently, however, the most common strategy employed is to screen cDNA expression libraries with human IgE antibodies and to sequence clones that show a high prevalence of IgE antibody binding. This approach is particularly useful where there are little or no pre-existing data on the allergen, as it allows nucleotide and amino acid sequence to be rapidly obtained.

It is important to consider several approaches to allergen cloning and sequencing. For example, two allergens have recently been cloned directly from a cockroach

TABLE 1. *Structural and functional properties of indoor allergens*

Source	Allergen[a]	MW	Function	Sequence[b]
House dust mite:				
Dermatophagoides spp.	Group 1	25 kDa	Cysteine protease	cDNA
	Group 2	14 kDa	Epididymal protein	cDNA
	Group 3	25 kDa	Serine protease	cDNA
	Der p 4	~60 kDa	Amylase	Protein
	Der p 5	14 kDa	Unknown	cDNA
	Der p 6	25 kDa	Chymotrypsin	Protein
	Group 7	22–28 kDa	Unknown	cDNA
Euroglyphus maynei	Eur m 1	25 kDa	Cysteine protease	PCR
Blomia tropicalis	Blo t 5	14 kDa	Unknown	cDNA
Lepidoglyphus destructor	Lep d 2	14 kDa	Epididymal protein	None
Mammals:				
Felis domesticus	Fel d 1	36 kDa	(Uteroglobin)	PCR
Canis familiaris	Can f 1	25 kDa	Calycin	cDNA
Mus musculus	Mus m 1	19 kDa	Calycins, pheromone	cDNA
Rattus norvegicus	Rat n 1	19 kDa	Binding proteins	cDNA
Cockroach:				
Blattella germanica	Bla g 1	20–25 kDa	Unknown	None
	Bla g 2	36 kDa	Aspartic protease	cDNA
	Bla g 4	21 kDa	Calycin	cDNA
	Bla g 5	22 kDa	Glutathione transferase	cDNA
	Bla g 5	18 kDa	Troponin	cDNA
Periplaneta americana	Per a 1	20–25 kDa	Unknown	None
	Per a 3	72–78 kDa	Unknown	None
Fungi:				
Aspergillus fumigatus	Asp f 1	18 kDa	Cytotoxin (mitogillin)	cDNA

[a]New nomenclature proposed by the WHO/IUIS subcommittee. (From King TP, Hoffman D, Lowenstein H, Marsh DG, Platts Mills TAE, Thomas WR. Allergen nomenclature. *Int Arch Allergy Immunol* 1994; 105: 224–233.)

[b]Method given for full sequence determination, where available. However, protein sequences are incomplete; usually N-terminal or internal peptide sequences have been determined.

(*Blattella germanica*) cDNA library by screening with IgE antibodies (Bla g 4, Bla g 5) (32). Another major cockroach allergen, Bla g 2, was cloned by screening the library with high-titer murine polyclonal IgG antibody. N-terminal and internal protein sequences matched the nucleotide sequence of the full length Bla g 2 cDNA clone, and provided further useful markers for confirming the sequence (33). The major cat allergen, Fel d 1, comprises two separate protein chains and provides an example of an allergen that could not be cloned from cDNA. The sequencing in this case was accomplished from the protein (>95%) and completed by PCR (34). Ultimately, whatever sequencing strategy is adopted, the allergenic importance of the protein has to be established by skin testing, serum IgE assays, or histamine release studies. If the recombinant allergen is to be used for diagnostic or treatment purposes, it is essential to compare quantitatively the reactivity of natural and recombinant allergens.

Homology searches of nucleotide and amino acid sequence data bases have allowed the biologic function of many allergens to be established. If no significant homology exists, the allergen function usually remains unknown. When the protein family for which an allergen belongs is known, then three-dimensional allergen structure can sometimes be predicted on the basis of known x-ray crystal structures. For example, the German cockroach allergen, Bla g 4, is a calycin (or lipocalin) and several proteins of known tertiary structure, including two major allergens, β-lactoglobulin and mouse and rat urinary proteins, belong to this family (35,36). The calycin family contains two well defined groups of 16- to 28-kDa proteins: the lipocalins and the fatty-acid binding proteins (36). From the allergy point of view, the lipocalins are more relevant, as they are predominantly extracellular proteins often found in external secretion. The tertiary structure of calycins have a folding pattern consisting predominantly of extended β-pleated sheets in a barrel structure, containing the binding site for hydrophobic ligand. Using homology-based modeling techniques, it has been possible to construct two three-dimensional models for Bla g 4, and these models can be used to design further structural experiments. Crystallographic studies of the mouse urinary allergen have shown that it is calycin that functions as a pheromone binding protein (35). There is good evidence that cockroach allergens are secreted or excreted and, by analogy, it is also possible that Bla g 4 has a pheromone binding function. Several other important allergens belong to the calycin family, including the major dog allergens Can f 1 and Can f 2, and horse allergen Equ c 1. Structural studies can indicate the biologic function of particular allergens, and in turn knowledge of the biology of allergens may lead to novel approaches to controlling their production.

Recombinant Allergens/Peptides in Diagnosis and Treatment

Breakthroughs in allergen biotechnology mean that it is now possible to consider using these reagents for diagnosis and treatment of allergic disease. The rationale for using recombinant allergens for diagnosis is that expression systems are capable of producing one or two highly purified and homogeneous allergens in practically unlimited supply. From the clinician's point of view, diagnosis by skin testing or serum IgE assays would be based on one or two well defined allergens, rather than a heterogeneous protein mixture. Clearly, this approach relies on the fact that recombinant allergens have comparable immunologic reactivity to the natural protein. Recombinant grass or tree pollen allergens retain their antigenic properties, and the potential for diagnostic use for these allergens looks promising (37,38). Recombinant mite Group 2 allergens show comparable IgE reactivity to the natural allergens on skin testing, serum IgE assays, and histamine release (39,40). However, recombinant mite Group 1 allergens produced in bacteria of yeast are not as immunoreactive as the natural allergen (41). For Fel d 1, the situation is more complex because of its structure (the molecule comprises two polypeptide chains and N-linked carbohydrate), and the recombinant chains do not contain all the epitopes that are present on native Fel d 1 (42,43). Nonetheless, recent protein refolding studies indicate that it is possible to bring the two recombinant Fel d 1 chains together in a fully immunoreactive form (44). Recombinant birch pollen allergens (Bet v 1 and Bet v 2) have recently been introduced for *in vitro* diagnostic procedures, and the rapid progression in biotechnology suggests that within a few years recombinant allergens will be available for most common allergen sources.

There are several applications of molecular biology in new treatment strategies. Traditional extracts for immunotherapy using natural allergen extracts could progressively be replaced with a cocktail of a few selected recombinant allergens. Perhaps a more exciting prospect has emerged from work both on molecular biology and on T-cell responses to allergens: a development of novel immunotherapies based on the downregulation of T-cell responses using synthetic peptides directed against known T-cell epitopes to "desensitize" T cells. The Fel d 1 recombinant peptide is currently undergoing clinical trials (45).

METHODS OF ASSESSING ALLERGEN EXPOSURE

Allergens present in house dust are among the most common environmental antigens to which humans are naturally exposed. They can comprise up to 20% of the protein in house dust extracts (46). Standardized methods

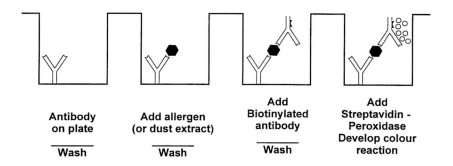

Antibody on plate ——— **Wash**

Add allergen (or dust extract) ——— **Wash**

Add Biotinylated antibody ——— **Wash**

Add Streptavidin - Peroxidase Develop colour reaction

FIG. 1. Monoclonal antibody-based ELISA for allergens.

for measuring indoor allergen exposure are essential for assessing the relationship between exposure and sensitization and the degree of exposure associated with provocation of asthmatic symptoms.

Measurement of Exposure to Mite Allergens

There are three generally accepted methods of estimating exposure to dust mite allergens: mite counts, assays of specific mite allergens, and measurement of guanine (47). Mite counts have been shown to be a good index of exposure, but the technique is time consuming and requires a considerable acarologic expertise. Furthermore, mite counts do not necessarily reflect the level of mite allergens, as allergen levels in house dust can remain high for several months after the fall in mite numbers (48). A semiquantitative assay for guanine (Acarex test) may provide a useful screening test in clinical practice for the assessment of presence of mites (49). In research studies, mAb-based assays are the most widely used method for assessing allergen exposure.

Immunoassays have had a major impact on many areas of biomedical research. They have been developed for a wide range of antigenic substances; are sensitive, specific, reproducible; and can give quantitative measurement of a given antigen in absolute units (e.g., ng or µg of protein). Over the past decade immunoassays for measuring dust mite, cat, dog, cockroach, rodent, and some fungal allergens have been developed. This technology has been used to compare allergen levels in reservoir dust samples from the homes of patients with asthma and other atopic disorders, to analyze the effect of different avoidance procedures on the allergen levels in homes, and to investigate the particle size distribution and concentration of airborne allergens. As a result of these studies it has been possible to propose thresholds for allergen levels that are clinically important and to achieve a better understanding of the dose-response relationship between asthma and indoor allergen exposure.

The principle of the two-site enzyme-linked immunosorbent assay (ELISA) is shown on Fig. 1. Microtiter wells are coated with mAb (e.g., to mite or other allergen)

and incubated for 1 hour with several dilutions of the extract with the unknown quantity of the particular allergen. The mAb on plate then binds the allergen in question, and bound allergen is detected using a biotinylated second mAb directed against a nonoverlapping epitope. Streptavidin peroxidase and a suitable chromogenic substrate is used for the detection of the second mAb. The concentration of specific allergen in the extract is proportional to the intensity of color that develops. The assay results are interpolated from the control curve constructed using the doubling dilutions of a reference allergen preparation.

Environmental Allergen Measurement

Immunoassays currently in use for the measurement of indoor allergens are summarized in Table 2 (46,50–61). ELISA assays are technically straightforward and can be used for testing large numbers of samples, thus making them ideal for large-scale epidemiologic studies and clinical trials. Allergens are usually measured in dust samples collected by vacuuming dust reservoirs (carpet, mattress, bedding, and upholstered furniture) for a

TABLE 2. *Indoor allergen measurement by mAb ELISA*

Allergen	Capture[a] mAb	Second[b] antibody	Reference standards
Der p 1	5H8	4C1	NIBSC 82/518, UVA 93/03
Der f 1	6A8	4C1	CBER E1-Df, UVA 93/02
Group 2	1D8	7A1	CBER E1-Df or Dp; UVA 92/01, 92/02
Fel d 1	6F9	3E4	CBER Cat E5
Can f 1	Cf-1b	Rabbit IgG ab	NIBSC 84/685
Bla g 1	10A6	Rabbit IgG ab	UVA 93/04
Bla g 2	7C11	8F4	UVA 93/04
Asp f 1	4A6	Rabbit IgG ab	Affinity purified Asp f 1

[a]Used as 50% ammonium sulfate fractions of ascites and coated on microtiter plates at 1 µg/well.

[b]Biotinylated mAb used at ~20 ng/well. Rabbit secondary antibodies are detected using peroxidase-labeled polyclonal goat antirabbit IgG.

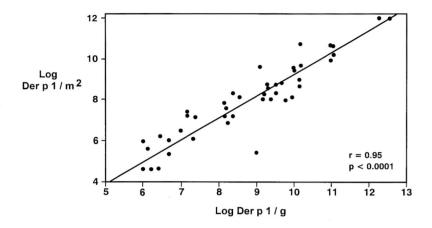

FIG. 2. Correlation of mite allergens Der p 1 expressed as recoverable allergen per unit area against allergen per unit weight in 53 mattress samples of dust. (From Custovic A, Taggart SCO, Niven RM, Woodcock A. Evaluating exposure to mite allergens. *J Allergy Clin Immunol* 1995;96:134–135.)

standardized period of time (2–5 min/m^2) (47). Results of reservoir samples are usually expressed as allergen per unit weight (e.g., μg Der p 1/g of dust) (28,47). It has been suggested that recoverable allergen per unit area is a better "index" of exposure (62). This was particularly advocated for the trials of mite control that involve killing mites followed by repeated vacuuming to remove dead mites and allergen pool, or when mite control involves addition of certain chemicals (e.g., acaricides) (63). However, the recovery is influenced by a number of factors (flow rate of the vacuum cleaner used for sample collection, technique of the collector, cleaning regime in the house where sampling is taking place) (64). Furthermore, there is a good quantitative correlation between the results expressed as recoverable allergen per unit weight and per unit area (Fig. 2) (65). Expressing results per unit weight is easier to standardize and sieving dust makes it easier to compare samples collected at different sites. Most studies have used this method and it is therefore easy to compare data between different trials. For these reasons, allergen concentration per unit weight (μg/g) is recommended as the primary measure of allergen exposure (28). Expressing the results per unit area could be useful in certain circumstances, particularly in trials where size of the dust reservoir is changed by intervention. Levels of allergens in settled dust vary greatly from house to house. Domestic allergens (mite, cat, dog) can be found not only in domestic dwellings, but also in the indoor environment of different public places and public transport (Fig. 3) (66).

Airborne Allergen: Particle Sizing

Airborne sampling is widely used in the assessment of occupational exposure and, as this is probably the primary route of exposure, it might be considered more representative as a measure of inhaled allergen than allergen levels in the reservoir dust. However, as yet airborne sampling has serious limitations as a method for mea-

surement of exposure to house dust mite allergens, because without disturbance mite allergen concentrations are generally below the detection limits of the assays (28,65,67).

Airborne allergen levels are critically dependent on disturbance (28,47,65,67). The particle size distribution of the airborne allergen is highly relevant to the way sensitization occurs and the clinical presentation of asthma. Several studies have therefore evaluated the airborne levels and compared airborne characteristics of different allergens (55,68–74). A number of different devices have been used to determine particle size of indoor allergens including Cascade impactors (Casella, Andersen) and Impingers. The major difference between the two is that the impactor collects particles on a solid surface and the impinger collects them on water. Using the cascade impactor, de Blay et al. compared the airborne concentration and particle size of dust mite (Group 1 and Group 2) and cat allergen before, during, and after disturbance (68). The study demonstrated that both Group 1 and Group 2 mite allergens were airborne only during disturbance and fell rapidly after disturbance. Dramatic differences were found in the airborne behavior between mite and cat allergens, as a significant proportion of Fel d 1 was associated with small particles (<5 μ) (Fig. 4). The particle size distribution of major dog allergen Can f 1 has recently been determined using an Andersen sampler (Fig. 5) (74). As in the case of cat allergen, most dog allergen is contained on relatively large particles (>10 μ), and there is a smaller proportion (~20%) associated with small particles (<5 μ), which may be more relevant in term of symptoms. This could explain differences between the clinical presentation of mite-sensitive asthmatics and those who are sensitized to pets. Mite-allergic patients are usually unaware of the relationship between allergen exposure at home and asthma symptoms, and even a carefully taken allergy history can not unequivocally implicate mites as a cause of symptoms. On the other hand, cat- or dog-allergic patients often develop symptoms within minutes of entering a home with a cat

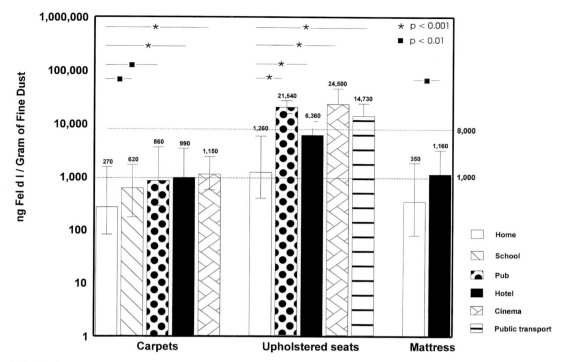

FIG. 3. Geometric means and ranges for Fel d 1 levels (ng/g of fine dust) from different sampling sites in domestic households, public buildings, and public transport. (From Custovic A, Taggart SCO, Woodcock A. House dust mite and cat allergen in different indoor environments. *Clin Exp Allergy* 1994;24: 1164–1168.)

or a dog, or simply by stroking an animal. Aerodynamic properties of indoor allergens are shown in Table 3. Knowledge of the sources of allergens, their airborne characteristics, and particle size distribution are therefore essential both for understanding the development and clinical presentation of asthma, and for the design of successful strategies to reduce the personal exposure and disease severity.

ALLERGEN EXPOSURE AS A CAUSE OF ASTHMA

Development of the techniques for measuring the exposure to allergens enabled a series of epidemiologic studies looking into a relationship between allergens and asthma to be undertaken in different parts of the world. Initially, most of these studies related to house dust mite

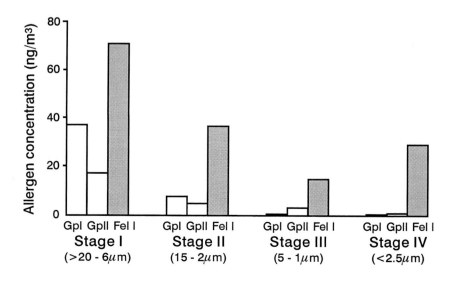

FIG. 4. Airborne mite- and cat-allergen levels (in ng/m³) on cascade-impactor stages during disturbance. Values are the mean levels for 30-min sampling (15 min of disturbance and 15 mins after disturbance) in seven houses. (From De Blay F, Heymann PW, Chapman MD, Platts-Mills TAE. Airborne dust mite allergens: comparison of Group II mite allergens with Group I mite allergen and cat allergen Fel d I. *J Allergy Clin Immunol* 1991; 88:919–926.)

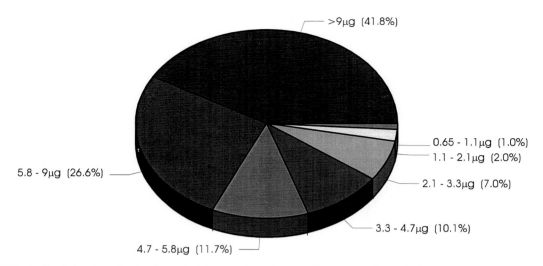

FIG. 5. Particle size distribution of airborne dog allergen (in percents) on Andersen sampler stages. Values are the mean levels for 8-hr sampling in the absence of disturbance in 10 houses. (From Custovic A, Green RM, Fletcher A, Smith A, Pickering CAC, Chapman MD, Woodcock A. Aerodynamic properties of the major dog allergen, Can f 1: distribution in homes, concentration, and particle size of the allergen in the air. *Am J Respir Crit Care Med* [*in press*].)

TABLE 3. *Comparison of the aerodynamic properties of the indoor allergens*[a]

Allergen	Airborne allergen (ng/m3)		Particle size
	Undisturbed	Disturbed (20–40 min)	
Mite:			
Group 1	<0.2	20–90	10–40 μm
Group 2	<0.2	13–26	>10 μm (80%)
Cat:			
Fel d 1[c]	6–17	117–212	>5 μm (75%)
			<3 μm (25%)
Dog:			
Can f 1[c]	1–80	69–416	>5 μm (80%)
			<5 μm (20%)
Cockroach:			
Bla g 1[b]	<0.01	9	>10 μm
Bla g 2[b]	<0.02	2	>10 μm

[a]Mean data from studies carried out 1990–1995. (From Luczynska CM, Li Y, Chapman MD, Platts-Mills TAE. Airborne concentrations and particle size distribution of allergen derived from domestic cats *(Felis domesticus)*: measurement using cascade impactor, liquid impinger and a two site monoclonal antibody assay for *Fel d I. Am Rev Respir Dis* 1990;141:361–367; De Blay F, Heymann PW, Chapman MD, Platts-Mills TAE. Airborne dust mite allergens: comparison of Group II mite allergens with Group I mite allergen and cat allergen *Fel d I. J Allergy Clin Immunol* 1991;88:919–926; Chapman MD, Vailes LD, Hayden ML, Platts-Mills TAE, Arruda LK. Cockroach allergens and their role in asthma. In: Kay AB, ed. *Allergy and allergic disease.* Oxford: Blackwells Scientific Publishing, 1996 (*in press*); Price JA, Pollack I, Little SA, Longbottom JL, Warner JO. Measurement of airborne mite antigen in homes of asthmatic children. *Lancet* 1990; 336:895–897; Custovic A, Green R, Fletcher, et al. Aerodynamic properties of the major dog allergen, Can f 1: distribution in homes, concentration, and particle size of allergen in the air. *Am J Respir Crit Care Med* (*in press*).)

allergens and asthma. This was due in part to mites being the most important source of allergens in temperate climates and partly because two site mAb ELISA to Group 1 mite allergens was the first to be developed. Recently, however, evidence has been mounting on the role of other indoor allergens in the development and maintenance of asthmatic symptoms. However, for other allergens it is impossible to distinguish between the effects of exposure on sensitization and on the expression of asthma. There is now strong evidence that sensitization and exposure to indoor allergens is a primary cause of asthma.

Criteria for Causality

In 1965 Sir Austin Bradford Hill postulated criteria necessary to demonstrate that an association represents a causal relationship (Table 4) (75). In 1992 Richard Sporik applied Hill's criteria to the association between house dust mites and asthma, strongly indicating causality (76). In each of the subsequent sections the evidence that in-

TABLE 4. *Hill's criteria for causality*

1. The strength of association is large (Association)
2. Repeated observations in different populations have consistent findings (Consistency)
3. A cause leads to a specific effect (Specificity)
4. A cause precedes an effect (Temporality)
5. There is a dose-response gradient (Biological gradient)
6. There is experimental evidence (Experiment)
7. There are analogous explanations (Analogy)
8. The mechanism is biologically plausible (Plausibility and coherence)

door allergens are a *cause* of asthma and fulfill Hill's criteria will be critically reviewed.

The Strength of Association is Large

Epidemiologic studies have consistently shown that that up to 85% of patients with asthma are skin prick–sensitive to house dust mites, as compared with only 5% to 30% in the general population. These highly significant differences, observed in studies from all over the world, leave little doubt that sensitivity to dust mites is a risk factor for asthma (47,77–85). It was conclusively shown that the strongest predictor of asthma is sensitization to indoor allergens (reviewed in Table 5). As the development of IgE-mediated hypersensitivity requires allergen exposure, it can be expected that in the areas with low exposure to certain allergens, the prevalence of sensitization to that particular allergen will be low as well.

Allergen Exposure, Sensitization, and Asthma

Testing the hypothesis of a cause and effect relationship between exposure to dust mite allergens and asthma, Charpin et al. compared the prevalence of asthma and positive skin test to mites in subjects living in the Alps (Briancon) and those living at sea level (Martigues) (82). The prevalence of mite allergy in adults was found to be fourfold higher in those living in Martigues (44.5%) compared with Briancon (10%). In a later study conducted by the same authors, a similar pattern of sensitization was found in schoolchildren (83). Mite allergen level in mattresses was found to be much lower in the Alps (0.36 µg/g of dust) than at sea level (15.8 µg/g of dust). The authors suggested that living in a mite-free environment reduces the risk of sensitization and development of respiratory symptoms.

In another comparison of the relationship between mite allergen exposure and asthma, Peat et al. compared two population samples of Australian children living in Lismore (a hot, humid, coastal region) to Moree/Narrabri (a hot, dry inland region) (84). Der p 1 levels were much higher at the coast (83 vs. 11.2 µg/g), but prevalence of mite sensitivity was similar in both regions (28.6 vs. 26.4%). However, BHR in children sensitized to mites was more severe in coastal children. The authors concluded that high mite levels in a humid coastal region significantly increase bronchial responsiveness in sensitized

TABLE 5. *Sensitization and exposure to indoor allergens as a risk factor for asthma, 1989–1995*

Authors	Geographic location	Allergens	Odds ratio/significance
High altitude studies			
Sporik et al., 1995 (86); Ingram, 1995 (87)	Los Alamos, New Mexico, USA	Cat and dog	6.2[b]; $p<0.001$[a]
Charpin et al., 1991; 1988 (83,82)	Martigues and Briancon, France	Mite	$p<0.02$[a]
Population studies			
Arruda et al., 1991 (124)	Sao Paulo, Brazil	Mite	$p<0.001$[a]
Peat et al., 1991–1995 (81,84,85,160,180)	Coastal and inland Australia	Mite; cat and dog	2.7–20.9[a]; 2.4–4[a]
Lau et al., 1989 (132)	Germany	Mite	5–11[c]
Price et al., 1990 (123)	London, UK	Mite	$p<0.01$[c]
Wickman et al., 1991; 1993 (91,92)	Stockholm, Sweden	Mite	4.9[a]; 25.7[b]
Kuehr et al., 1992–1995 (89,128,129)	South-western Germany	Mite, "animal dander"	2.2–4[a]; 2.6–3.6[a]; 2.8[b]
Custovic et al., 1996 (122)	Manchester, UK	Mite	$p<0.01$[b]
Emergency room studies			
Gelber et al., 1993 (118)	Wilmington, USA	Mite, cat, cockroach	6.2–16.3[b]; $p<0.001$[a]
Call et al., 1992 (93)	Atlanta, USA	Mite, cat, cockroach	9.5[b]; $p<0.001$[a]
Duff et al., 1993 (167)	Charlottesville, Virginia, USA	Mite	4.5[a]
Sporik et al., 1993 (116)	Poole, UK	Mite and cat	$p<0.001$[a]; $p<0.001$[b]
Pollart et al., 1989 (117)	Charlottesville, Virginia, USA	Mite, cat, cockroach	$p<0.001$[a]
Prospective studies			
Arshad et al., 1992 (147); Hide 1994 (148)	Isle of Wight, UK	Mite; cat	6.1[c]; $p<0.01$[c]; 16.1[c]
Sporik et al., 1990 (112)	Poole, UK	Mite	19.7[a]; 4.8[b]
Sears et al., 1989 (80)	Dunedin, New Zealand	Mite, cat, dog	6.7, 4.2, 3.7[a]
Arshad et al., 1992 (90)	Isle of Wight, UK	Mite, cat	3.2[a]; $p=0.002$[a]

[a]Sensitization (IgE antibodies) alone.
[b]Sensitization and exposure.
[c]Exposure as a risk factor for sensitization.

TABLE 6. *House dust mite allergen levels in dust collected from beds in 6 regions of NSW, Australia*

	Lismore	Belmont	Sydney	Moree	Wagga Wagga	Broken Hill
Der p 1 (µg/g)	47.80	36.50	22.50	6.50	1.40	0.70
% above 10 µg/g	92.60	88.70	80.90	45.70	15.60	3.70

Data courtesy of Dr. Jennifer Peat, Department of Medicine, University of Sydney.

children. Peat et al. conducted a series of epidemiologic studies comparing regions in Australia that differed in asthma admission rates for children (suggesting a difference in prevalence) and in climatic conditions (suggesting a difference in exposure to mite allergens). In six regions of New South Wales, schoolchildren were assessed for the presence of respiratory symptoms, nonspecific BHR, sensitization to common allergens, and exposure to Der p 1. From what has been said before, it does not come as a surprise that exposure to mite allergens was much higher in humid coastal regions (Lismore, Belmont, and Sydney) than in the drier inland regions (Moree, Wagga Wagga, and Broken Hill) (Table 6). In regions with high mite allergen exposure, more children were skin test–positive to mites and those who were sensitized to mites were at significant risk for having current asthma. The prevalence of sensitization to indoor allergens (mite, cat, and cockroach) and odds ratio for children having asthma is shown in Table 7. These data confirm that there is a dose-response relationship between exposure to indoor allergens and the risk of asthma, and that this association is very strong. After adjusting for sensitization to other allergens, the risk of mite-sensitized children having asthma approximately doubled with every doubling of Der p 1 level (85).

A recent study in Los Alamos, New Mexico, United States, highlights the importance of exposure and sensitization to cat and dog allergens. The town is at a high altitude (~2,200 m) and in a dry area. Sporik et al. investigated the prevalence of asthma, pattern of sensitization, and exposure to indoor allergens in a group of schoolchildren (86). The mite allergen concentration was very low, but the striking characteristic of the town was the large number of households (77%) with a cat or a dog. The strongest associated risk for asthma was cat sensitization. The low prevalence of mite and cockroach sensitization reflected low levels of exposure. In a further study of the same population Ingram et al. found that the combination of sensitization and increased exposure for both cat and dog showed a strong correlation with asthma (Table 8) (87). These results strongly suggest that in the areas with high levels of cat and dog allergen in the homes, asthma will be associated with sensitization to these allergens.

In the areas of high prevalence of mite sensitization, duration of exposure to domestic animals was found to be a significant determinant of sensitization (88). Kuehr et al. reported that former, but not current, cat ownership was significantly related to sensitization to cat dander (89). Similarly, Arshad et al. found that positive skin tests to cat dander were more prevalent in infants who were exposed to cats and dogs (90). Clearly, exposure to allergens is essential for sensitization to occur. Wickman et al. reported that even in the areas with low mite allergen exposure (Stockholm, Sweden), there was a close association between mite sensitization and asthma (odds ratio 4.9) (91). In a further study of factors favoring sensitization to mite, positive skin tests and the presence of specific serum IgE antibodies to mites were found to be strongly associated with the presence of domestic mites in mattress and floor dust (i.e., exposure to mites) (92).

A recent study suggested that in the inner-city areas with a high proportion of cockroach-infested houses, sen-

TABLE 7. *Prevalence of sensitization to dust mite, cat and dog allergens and odds ratio (OR) for children having current asthma in the presence of sensitization to one allergen and adjusted for sensitization to the other allergens*

	Lismore	Belmont	Sydney	Moree	Wagga Wagga	Broken Hill
Mite allergy (%)	21.40	20.40	25.60	14.90	11.20	11.70
Current asthma—OR	20.9[a]	16.5[a]	7.7[a]	3.1[a]	2.7[a]	3.7[a]
Cat allergy (%)	5.10	4.70	4.00	4.20	4.30	5.20
Ever owned cat (%)	—	—	—	57.90	46.20	54.50
Cat in the home (%)	37.20	26.80	25.10	26.90	22.10	28.70
Current asthma—OR	4.5[a]	1.6 (NS)	1.4 (NS)	2.5[a]	2.8[a]	2.4[a]
Cockroach allergy (%)	11.30	11.80	11.40	13.60	4.90	8.10
Current asthma—OR	1.1 (NS)	1.2 (NS)	1.6 (NS)	0.9 (NS)	1.5 (NS)	0.5 (NS)

[a]Significant at p<0.05.
NS, nonsignificant.
Data courtesy of Dr. Jennifer Peat, Department of Medicine, University of Sydney.

TABLE 8. *Prevalence of IgE Antibody to Indoor Allergans[a] Among Middle School Children in Los Alamos, New Mexico, United States of America*

	Symptomatic			
	BHR +ve (n=21)	BHR −ve (n=36)	Controls (n=54)	p value[b]
Dust mite	1 (5%)	6 (17%)	2 (4%)	0.38
Dog	14 (67%)	7 (19%)	8 (15%)	<0.0001
Cat	13 (62%)	10 (28%)	9 (17%)	<0.001
Cockroach	0 (0%)	0 (0%)	1 (2%)	0.35
Rus. thistle	10 (48%)	10 (28%)	12 (22%)	0.05
Rye grass	6 (29%)	9 (25%)	22 (41%)	0.19

[a]Prevalence of >40 RAST units or CAP > grade II.
[b]Significance assessed by Chi-square tests for trends.

sitization to cockroach allergens was common, highlighting the importance of these allergens as a risk factor for asthma (93). High prevalence of cockroach sensitization (up to 70%) was found among asthmatic patients in several United States cities (94–100). Cockroaches have been reported to be an important cause of asthma in the other parts of the world, including South-East Asia, Central America, India, South Africa, and most recently Europe (101–105). In Strasbourg, cockroach-sensitive patients with asthma were found to have high levels of cockroach allergens in their houses (105). Cockroach sensitization is not confined to inner-city populations, but occurs wherever substandard housing or apartment buildings sustain cockroach infestation (106).

Primary Sensitization

It is important to differentiate primary sensitization to an allergen from symptoms caused by ongoing allergen exposure in a subject already sensitized. Early infancy has been identified as a critical period for primary sensitization to occur. Evidence to support this view comes from studies relating atopy to month of birth. Children born just before the Birch pollen season in Scandinavia have a higher risk of sensitization to Birch pollen than those born after the season (107). Similar observations were made in relation to house dust mite exposure received by children born in the autumn, when mite numbers tend to be higher than at other times of the year (108). Exposure to cats and dogs in early infancy is associated with specific IgE sensitization and allergic disease later in childhood (109,110). The importance of early exposure to mite allergen in primary sensitization has been defined in recent studies. Household exposure to elevated levels of Der p 1 in amounts greater than 2 µg/g of dust in carpets and bedding during infancy is associated with increased prevalence of positive skin tests and increased concentrations of IgE specific to house dust mite by the age of 5 years in children of atopic parents (111). In ad-

dition, in a cohort of 68 children prospectively followed from birth until the age of 11 years, Sporik et al. found that exposure to Der p 1 level greater than 10 µg/g of household dust measured in infancy was associated with a 4.8-fold relative risk of developing atopic asthma at the age of 11 years (112). Mite sensitization at age 11 years was associated with a 19.7 odds ratio for having asthma, confirming strength of the association in a prospective study. Furthermore, exposure to high allergen levels at the age of 1 year was inversely related to the age of onset of asthma in mite-sensitive children.

Sensitization to an allergen can occur at any age (76). The predisposed infants, though, appear to be more susceptible to development of sensitization than older individuals, suggesting that exposure has different effects at different ages (112,113).

Allergen Exposure and Asthma Symptoms

Prevalence rates are only one way of measuring the magnitude and dimension of a particular disease. Severity and clinical activity also provide an important measure of the impact of the disease on patients' lives, on the health care system, and on the quantity of medical care that an individual patient requires. In the case of asthma, several studies have suggested that these features may be related to allergen exposure (48,114,115). A study on the exposure to mite allergen and pediatric hospital admissions has shown that most children admitted to the hospital with exacerbation of asthma were both sensitized and exposed to mite allergen and also suggested that continued exposure to higher concentrations of mite allergen may be associated with the risk of readmission (116). Sensitization to mites, cat, and cockroach was found to be a significant risk factor for acute asthma in patients admitted to the hospital emergency department in Charlottesville, Virginia (117). A case-controlled study on patients presenting to an emergency room in Wilmington confirmed a strong relationship between sensitization to indoor allergens and acute asthma (118). The data, however, did not establish or refute a quantitative relationship between current exposure and the risk of acute asthma among sensitized individuals. Results of the emergency room studies are summarized in Table 5. In one of the first studies relating dust mites and asthma, visits to the hospital by mite-sensitive asthmatic subjects correlated with mite growth curves in their homes (13). After a controlled or seasonal exposure to allergens, sensitized subjects experience an increase in BHR (16,119). Exposure to *Alternaria* allergen has been shown to be a risk factor for sudden respiratory arrest in asthmatics (120). Van der Heide et al. reported that seasonal changes in exposure to mite allergens affect the level of airway hyperresponsiveness in mite allergic asthmatics, and suggested that even relatively small changes in al-

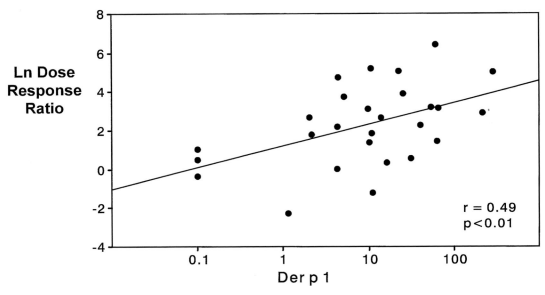

FIG. 6. Correlation between mite allergen exposure in bed and BHR (expressed in dose-response ratio). (From Custovic A, Taggart SCO, Francis HC, Chapman MD, Woodcock A. Exposure to house dust mite allergens and the clinical activity of asthma. *J Allergy Clin Immunol* 1996;98:64–72.)

lergen exposure may influence the degree of airway reactivity (121). It has recently been shown that in a group of mite-sensitive asthmatics, after controlling for the effects of possible confounding factors (smoking, viral infections, and the effects of other allergens) the severity of asthma (measured by BHR, peak flow variability, and pulmonary function) is related to exposure to mite allergens in the bed (Fig. 6) (122).

Repeated Observations in Different Populations have Consistent Findings

"Has the association been repeatedly observed by different persons, in different places, circumstances and times" (75). Studies from many countries have demonstrated an increased prevalence of immediate hypersensitivity in patients with asthma. Similar findings have been reported in the United Kingdom (78,90,112,116,122, 123), Europe (82,83,88,89,91), the United States (86,87, 93–100,117,118), South America (124), Australia (81, 84,85), New Zealand (77,80), Asia (101), and Africa (104), making the issue of indoor allergens and asthma a worldwide problem (Table 5). Most studies have reported high prevalence of mite allergy among patients with asthma compared with control subjects, whereas negative studies came from the areas of low mite exposure (reviewed in the Report of the First International Workshop on Mite Allergens and Asthma, 47). Characteristics of exposure strongly influence the pattern of sensitization in different areas (82–87), indicating that it is important to understand the local climatic and housing conditions to

identify the principal causes of asthma in any particular area.

A Cause Leads to a Specific Effect

"Is the association limited to particular group of individuals and particular disease" (75). All attempts to implicate exposure and sensitization to indoor allergens in the etiology of other disorders have failed [e.g., sudden infant death syndrome (125) and Kawasaki disease (126)], and it is only in asthma that there is strong evidence of association that demonstrates characteristics of causality. Wickman et al. found a strong association between asthma and mite sensitization, but no association in the case of allergic rhinitis and atopic dermatitis (91). Immediate hypersensitivity to common allergens has not been related to any lung disease other than asthma (30,49).

A Cause Precedes an Effect

Probably the best example of exposure to indoor allergen (mite) leading to the increase in the prevalence of asthma (with sensitization likely to be an intermediate phase) was reported from Papua, New Guinea (127). Asthma there was a rare, almost nonexistent disease, with a prevalence of 0.1% until the early 1970s. This was followed by a striking increase in prevalence to 7.3% over several years. More than 90% of these patients showed hypersensitivity to mites. The likely explanation of this "asthma epidemic" is the introduction of blankets that were subsequently found to contain large number of dust mites (>1,000 mites/g of dust). These blankets were a perfect microhabitat for mite population growth in houses that were otherwise lacking the suitable places for mite survival. Furthermore, adult men used the blankets for wrapping in during sleep, and ~90% of the asthmatics (again predominantly men) reported that asthma symptoms were preceded by the acquisition of blankets. In the previously mentioned prospective study from Poole (U.K.), 92% of children with asthma were exposed to a high level of mite allergens in the first year of life (112). Kuehr et al. in Germany followed a cohort of children for 3 years investigating risk factors for sensitization and asthma symptoms and recently reported that sensitization to mite allergens antedated the onset of asthma symptoms (128). Levels of mite allergens in this cohort show significant association with the incidence of specific sensitization (129). Similarly, Ohman et al. found that the presence of mite-specific IgE antibodies preceded the onset of wheezing in adults (130). It is interesting that sensitization to pollens in young adults was identified as a risk factor for developing seasonal allergic rhinitis later on (131).

There is a Dose-response Gradient

"The clear dose-response relationship . . . puts the case of causality in a clearer light" (75). How can we explain the fact that although there was a significant difference in mite allergen level between the previously mentioned study of two areas in Australia (84), the prevalence of sensitization was very much the same? At the same time, prevalence of skin test sensitivity to mites was significantly lower in the French Alps than at sea level (82,83). The explanation probably lies in the fact that in Australia even in areas with low exposure, this level was sufficiently high to exceed the threshold for sensitization for predisposed individuals, i.e., all those who were predisposed were exposed to a sufficient level of mite allergens and therefore developed sensitization. In Briancon, however, low allergen exposure was insufficient to induce sensitization in susceptible individuals and therefore a much lower prevalence of sensitization was found. This suggests the existence of a quantitative relationship between the allergen exposure and sensitization, i.e., the higher the exposure, the larger the proportion of exposed individuals who become sensitized. One of the first studies relating house dust mites to asthma suggested that the level of 100 mites/g of dust was significant (13). Since then, a number of reports from different parts of the world demonstrated a dose-response relationship between allergen exposure at home, sensitization, and asthma. The First International Workshop on Mite Allergens and Asthma thus proposed two provisional threshold levels for mite allergens that represent risk for sensitization and asthma: more than 2 µg Group 1 mite allergen/g dust (equivalent to 100 mites/g) was regarded as repre-

senting risk for the development of IgE antibody and asthma, and a higher level of 10 µg Group 1 mite allergen/g dust (equivalent to 500 mites/g) was regarded as a risk for an acute attack of asthma (47). Several studies have confirmed the provisional threshold for sensitization. Lau et al. demonstrated a strong correlation between sensitization to mites and the mite allergen exposure, suggesting that threshold concentration of ≥2 µg/g should be regarded as a high risk, and a concentration ≥10 µg/g as a very high risk for specific mite sensitization (Table 5) (132). Likewise, Kuehr et al. reported that in primary schoolchildren already sensitized to allergens other than mites, exposure to levels above 2 µg/g Group 1 mite allergen represents a significant risk for mite sensitization, and suggested this level to be regarded as a minimal avoidance target for primary prevention of asthma (129). The U.S. Institute of Medicine Report on the Health Effects of Indoor Allergens analyzed the dose-response relationship between exposure and sensitization using the data from several studies, and reported a significant positive correlation between cumulative exposure to dust mite allergen and the risk of allergic sensitization (Fig. 7) (133). A dose-response relationship between mite allergen exposure and BHR in asthmatic patients already sensitized to mites has been reported (122,134,135). It is likely, however, that the relationship between exposure and asthma symptoms in sensitized individuals is much more complex than in the case of exposure and sensitization (76,93,116,118). Some sensitized patients will react to a very low dose of allergen, whereas in the others the level required to cause symptoms will be much higher than the one that induced sensitization (136). Thus, the level of 10 µg Group 1 allergen/g dust is a level commonly associated with symptoms, but is not a threshold value. For allergens other than mites, it is difficult to establish the threshold levels and to distinguish the effect of exposure on sensitization from the effect on asthma symptoms. In some inner-city areas of the United States, cat ownership among the African American community is unusual. The levels of Fel d 1 in the homes are low (usually ≤1 µg/g dust), as is the prevalence of sensitization to cat, thus providing a good example of low exposure (118). At the same time, asthma symptoms in cat-allergic patients commonly occur in homes with cats, more than 95% of which contain ≥8 µg Fel d 1/g dust. Thus, it is possible to propose a provisional threshold level that represents the risk for cat sensitization as ≥1 µg Fel d 1/g dust, and a level of ≥8 µg Fel d 1/g of dust can be considered as level at which most cat-allergic patients will experience symptoms (118). Ingram et al. indicated that for dog allergen 2 µg and 10 µg Can f 1/g dust have the same significance as the threshold levels for cat allergen of 1 µg and 8 µg Fel d 1/g dust, respectively (87). Cat and dog allergen can be detected in homes without pets and in the number of public places, suggesting that the exposure is possibly best defined as "community exposure." The

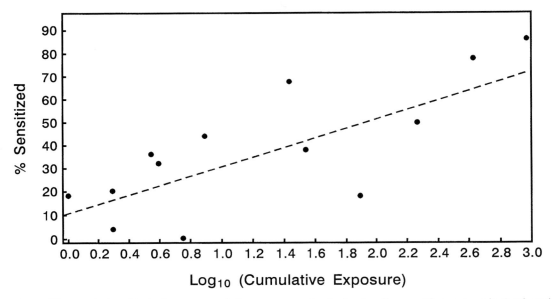

FIG. 7. Direct relationship between cumulative exposure to dust mite allergen (Group 1 µg/g dust) and sensation. (From Pope AM, Patterson R, Burge H, eds. *Indoor allergens. Assessing and controling adverse health effects.* Washington, DC: National Academy Press, 1993; Lau S, Falkenhorst G, Weber A, Werthmann I, Lind P, Buettner-Goetz P, Wahn U. High mite-allergen exposure increases the risk of sensitization in atopic children and young adults. *J Allergy Clin Immunol* 1989;84:718–725; Sporik R, Holgate S, Platts-Mills TAE, Cogswell J. Exposure to house dust mite allergen (Der p l) and the development of asthma in childhood. *N Engl J Med* 1990;323:502–507; Charpin D, Birnbaum J, Haddi E, et al. Altitude and allergy to house dust mites. *Am Rev Respir Dis* 1991;143:983–986; and Price JA, Pollock I, Little SA, Longbottom JL, Warner JO. Measurement of airborne mite antigen in homes of asthmatic children. *Lancet* 1990; 336:895–897. Calculated by C. Rice, Cincinnati.)

provisional threshold representing the risk for sensitization to cockroach allergen has been estimated as 2U of Bla g 2/g dust (93) (Table 9).

There is Experimental Evidence

If allergen exposure is an important risk factor for asthma, then reducing patients' exposure should improve their asthma control. Two kinds of studies have demonstrated the effectiveness of allergen reduction in the treatment of asthma: those in which patients were removed

TABLE 9. *Proposed threshold values for indoor allergens*

	Exposure leading to:	
	IgE sensitization	Allergic symptoms
Dust mite:		
Group 1 allergen	2 µ/g	10 µg/g[a]
Mite counts	>100 mites/g	>500 mites/g[a]
Guanine	>0.9 mg/g	>3.0 mg/g
Cat: Fel d 1	>1 µg/g	>8 µg/g[a]
Dog: Can f 1	>2 µg/g	>10 µg/g[a]
Cockroach: Bla g 2	>2 units/g	?

[a]A level above which individuals who are going to develop symptoms will do so. This level increases the risk of acute asthma, but is not a threshold value.

from their homes and those in which measures aiming at the reduction in allergen levels were applied in patients' houses.

Mite-sensitive children with asthma taken from their homes in Holland to the mite-free environment of Davos in Switzerland had a progressive reduction in nonspecific bronchial hyperreactivity over a period of 1 year (137, 138). Similarly, a progressive reduction in symptoms occurred when asthmatic children were removed from their homes in the north of Italy and admitted to the residential home at Misurina in the Italian Alps, 1,756 m above sea level (139). In further studies at Misurina, Piacentini et al. reported a significant decrease in mite antigen–induced basophil histamine release, mite-specific serum IgE level, and methacholine BHR in 20 asthmatic children, with reversal of this trend after 15 days of allergen exposure at sea level (140), and Peroni et al. demonstrated significant reduction in total and mite-specific serum IgE after 3 and 9 months at Misurina, with a significant increase 3 months after returning home (141). This study also reported a decrease in late allergen-induced bronchial reaction after 6 and 9 months at Misurina, with an enhancement of BHR by mite allergen–specific bronchial challenge. These results indicate that allergen avoidance leads to a decrease of airway inflammation with consequent improvement in nonspecific BHR and symptoms and that re-exposure results in a rapid relapse (141). Attempts to create mite allergen–free conditions at lower altitudes by admitting adult patients in the "allergen-free" environment of a hospital room resulted in the improvement in BHR and reduction in treatment requirements (142). Three months after discharge, the BHR had increased and more medication was needed for the control of symptoms.

The task of creating an allergen-free environment in patients' homes has proven to be a difficult one (76). There are conflicting data on the effectiveness of allergen avoidance carried out in houses, primarily because the early studies used measures that were not aggressive enough to reduce exposure and consequently failed to show beneficial effect (143). Once sufficiently aggressive measures were used and follow-up was long enough, the improvement in asthma symptoms, reduction in the medication use, and decrease in bronchial reactivity both in children and adults were convincingly demonstrated (144–146).

Hide et al. looked into the effect of avoidance of mite allergens and certain foods from birth onward on the development of atopy and asthma. The results indicated that eczema and episodic wheezing might be prevented (147, 148). Even though the reduction in Der p 1 level in the active group was relatively modest (to approximately 6 μg/g), a significant reduction in sensitization to mites was observed (149).

The results of studies using bronchial challenge with allergens represent an important indicator of the mechanisms involved under conditions of natural exposure. It has been shown that allergen bronchial challenge increases the number of circulating eosinophils, basophils, and their progenitor cells (150), the number of eosinophils in bronchoalveolar lavage fluid (151), and the expression of ICAM-1 in epithelium (152).

The results of *in vitro* studies offer an insight into the possible mechanisms involved. *D. pteronyssinus*–specific T-cell clones from atopic individuals were found to resemble closely murine TH2 cells by secreting substantial interleukin (IL)-4, IL-5, and IL-6 and minimal IFN-γ, whereas nonatopic T-cell clones resembled murine TH1 cells by secreting substantial IFN-γ, little IL-5, and no IL-4 (153). Furthermore, the atopics' TH2-like clones provided help for IgE production. Warner et al. have recently demonstrated that cord blood T cells of infants who subsequently develop atopic dermatitis or asthma when stimulated with food (milk and egg proteins) and/or inhalant allergens show proliferative response with lower IFN-γ production and detectable IL-4 mRNA expression, indicating a possible mechanism for the early expression of atopic phenotype (154).

There are Analogous Explanations

Patients with seasonal asthma who are sensitized to pollens experience exacerbation of symptoms when the pollen count is >300 grains/cm^2 (155), which is analogous to the symptoms that occur in sensitized patients with perennial asthma when exposed to the high levels of an offending allergen. Some patients develop asthma after exposure and immunologic sensitization to a number of chemical agents at their workplace, primarily but not exclusively in the industrial setting. More than 150 chemical agents have been reported to cause asthma (156), and the treatment of choice is removal from the workplace where the exposure occurred, resembling the exposure, sensitization, and development of asthma symptoms and allergen avoidance in asthmatics sensitized to indoor allergens. Longitudinal studies of workers exposed to some of the sensitizers indicated that the highest incidence of sensitization occurred within 2 years of first employment, with concomitant cigarette smoking increasing the risk of sensitization (157).

The Mechanism is Biologically Plausible

The development of asthma can be considered to consist of several distinct but closely related phases (Fig. 8) (28,64,76,158). The first phase is development of IgE-mediated sensitization influenced by hereditary factors (innate ability to develop persistent IgE antibody responses) and environmental factors (exposure to allergens). Without an innate ability to respond, even exposure to a large quantity of allergens will not have any effect. On the other hand, if a genetically predisposed individual is exposed to a certain level of allergen, IgE-mediated hypersensitivity can occur, with the prevalence of sensitization depending on the level of exposure. It is likely that with sufficient exposure the probability of sensitization becomes almost an inevitability (76). Sensitization is an asymptomatic process, and it is likely that there is a simple dose-response relationship between exposure and sensitization (i.e., the higher the exposure to the offending allergen, the higher percentage of children exposed will become sensitized). The next phase in asthma development occurs if sensitized individuals continue to be exposed to the offending allergens. In this case they are at risk of developing airway inflammation and BHR, which are the key features of asthma. Established BHR is usually associated with symptoms, although a few individuals will have increased airway reactivity even without symptoms. In the presence of inflammation and BHR, airways become more susceptible to a number of triggers. In this phase, a number of specific (i.e., allergen-causing sensitization) and more often nonspecific factors such as viral infections, cold air, exercise, passive smoke, and pharmacologic agents (e.g., histamine and methacholine) can trigger airway obstruction and asthmatic symptoms. It is possible that sensitization and the development of airway inflammation and BHR are under separate genetic control (i.e., exposure increases the risk of sensitization

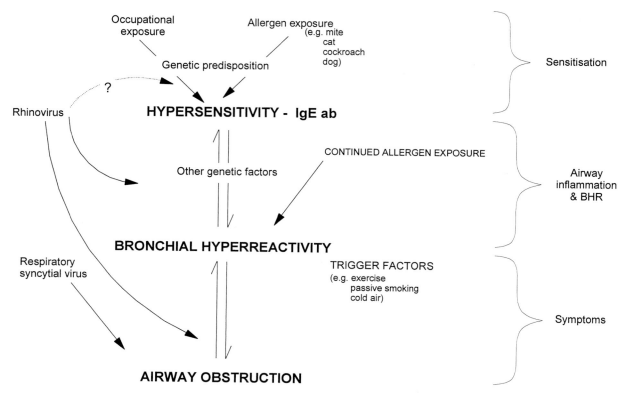

FIG. 8. Etiology of asthma and bronchial reactivity. Modification of figure by Prof. T.A.E. Platts-Mills, Asthma and Allergy Diseases Center, Charlottesville, Virginia.

in predisposed individuals, and continued exposure of those sensitized who are genetically predisposed increases the risk of symptomatic asthma) (159). This is a somewhat simplified model of asthma development, and it is probable that a number of other factors are involved (e.g., viruses, passive tobacco smoke, etc.).

Can understanding of the mechanisms involved in asthma development help us explain the phenomenon of increasing asthma prevalence? Peat et al. recently reported a dramatic increase in asthma prevalence between 1982 and 1992 in two populations of Australian children living in different climatic regions (160). The increase in airway reactivity occurred mostly in children sensitized to common allergens; the number of dust mites in their homes increased fivefold during the same period of time. The authors speculated that it is therefore possible that the allergen exposure has increased from being above the threshold for sensitization to being above the threshold for increased airway reactivity, or that a susceptibility of population has increased as a result of some other change in lifestyle (160), and possibly changes in diet (161). A number of other factors have been implicated in the increasing prevalence of allergy worldwide, including improved diagnostic tools and increased awareness, decreased immune stimulation, decreasing family size, improved standards of hygiene with fewer infections, increasing age of mothers, lower infestation with parasites,

etc. This important question, however, is still awaiting an answer.

OTHER CONTRIBUTORY FACTORS

Increased levels of tobacco smoke exposure, both *in utero* and after delivery, has been shown to cause wheeze in infancy and clinically significant asthma and reduced pulmonary function later in childhood (see Chapter 82) (162–164).

Viral respiratory tract infections can cause acute exacerbation of wheeze in childhood, with respiratory syncitial virus (RSV) being predominant in infancy and rhinovirus and adenovirus becoming increasingly important in older children (for review see ref 165; also see Chapter 83). Human rhinoviruses (HRV) were associated with up to 60% of asthma exacerbations in children (166). In a case-controlled study, Duff et al. investigated infants and children treated in the emergency room for acute wheezing and found a different pattern for those before than over 2 years of age. Wheezy infants had a high rate of viral infections (predominantly RSV—odds ratio 8.2) and a low prevalence of IgE antibody to inhalant allergens, whereas in children after 2 years of age sensitization to inhalant allergens became most important (odds ratio 4.5), with viruses (predominantly HRV) remaining a significant risk (odds ratio 3.7) (167). The combination of IgE antibody and virus was the most significant risk factor after the age of 2 years (odds ratio 10.6), which suggests synergism between these factors. A recent study demonstrated that atopic persons have greater severity of cold symptoms after inoculation with HRV 16 than nonatopic individuals, indicating that atopic patients may be more susceptible to develop severe symptoms (168). Calhoun et al. have recently shown that upper respiratory HRV infection in allergic persons potentiates allergen-specific rather than nonspecific airway inflammation, and that this can persist for at least 1 month after inoculation, suggesting that one of the mechanisms involved in worsening asthma symptoms is an accentuation of allergic responses that may increase airway inflammation (169). However, as yet it has not been conclusively shown that viral infection alone can induce asthma without inherited predisposition such as atopy (165,170).

There is an increasing concern over the effects of indoor and outdoor air pollution on respiratory health, particularly asthma (see Chapters 80 and 81). Air pollution has been implicated as a risk for asthma in two ways: a) as a facilitator of sensitization by decreasing the allergen threshold values for IgE sensitization, thus increasing the asthma prevalence, and b) as a trigger of asthma symptoms, possibly by enhancing the airway response to allergens, thus increasing morbidity of already established asthma (171). There is a growing evidence for the latter option. Nitrogen dioxide (NO_2) alone (172) and in combination with sulfur dioxide (SO_2) (173) has been recently found to enhance the bronchoconstrictive airway response of mild asthmatics to inhaled mite allergen without itself causing any bronchoconstriction in control exposures. Molfino et al. found that ozone enhances airway responses to ragweed and grass pollens (174). Ozone exposure was also indicated as having both an intrinsic inflammatory action and a priming effect on mite allergen–induced responses in the nose of dust mite–sensitive patients with perennial asthma (175). However, there is little evidence to suggest that air pollution has more than an adjuvant effect. Samet et al. have prospectively followed more than 1,200 infants for 18 months and found that exposure to indoor NO_2 from gas cooking stoves does not increase the risk of wheeze (176). There is some experimental evidence in mice to suggest that intraperitoneal diesel exhaust particulates stimulate production of IgE to ovalbumin or Japanese cedar pollen (177). Intranasal administration of particulate matter collected by airborne sampling near a motorway enhances the IgE antibody production in mice (178), or increases IgE antibody expression in humans (179). It is not clear, though, how these experiments in laboratory animals relate to humans. It is possible that natural exposure to diesel particulates may increase the expression of hay fever.

Asthma, however, is associated with sensitization to indoor allergens and there is no convincing evidence that air pollution can facilitate sensitization to these agents.

CONCLUSIONS

People in the developed countries spend more than 90% of their time indoors, and an additional 5% in transport (133), and it is likely that this trend will continue. Therefore, it is not surprising that the indoor environment is attracting increasing attention. Considerable changes have occurred in the lifestyle and housing in Western societies over the last 40 years that were paralleled with an increase in asthma prevalence, focusing scientific efforts on the role of exposure to indoor allergens. The strongest predictor of both chronic symptoms and acute exacerbation of asthma is sensitization to indoor allergens (reviewed in Table 5). The association between sensitization and exposure to indoor allergens and asthma is such that "we can pass from this observed association to a verdict of causation" (75). There is a dose-response relationship between sensitization of genetically predisposed individuals and exposure to the relevant indoor allergen, thus making it possible to propose threshold levels for exposure that represent a risk for sensitization. The quantitative relationship between exposure and symptoms in patients already sensitized is more complex because of a number of possible confounding factors (e.g., other allergens, viruses, asthma medication). Allergen avoidance is recommended in the treatment of established asthma but it has to be allergen specific.

If the increase in exposure to indoor allergens has contributed to the observed increase in asthma prevalence, the important issue in the long run is whether asthma can be prevented by allergen avoidance in infants at high risk of developing allergic disease.

REFERENCES

1. Nei Ching Su Wen. *The yellow emperor's classic of internal medicine.* Baltimore: Williams and Wilkins, 1949.
2. Adams F, ed. *The extant works of Aretaeus the Cappadocian.* London: Sydenham Society, 1856.
3. Georgius Agricola. Treatise of mining. Estelle S, Simons B, eds. *Ancestors of allergy.* New York: Global Medical Communications Ltd., 1994.
4. Dana CL. The story of a great consultation. *Ann Med Hist* 1921; 13: 122.
5. Feather IH, Warner JA, Holgate ST, Thompson PJ, Stewart GA. Cohabiting with domestic mites. *Thorax* 1993;48:5–9.
6. Salter HH. *On asthma; its pathology and treatment.* London: 1860.
7. Bostock J. A case of periodical affection of the eye and chest. *Read,* March 10, 1819.
8. Blackley CH. *Experimental researches on the causes and nature of cattharus aestivus (hay-fever or hay-asthma).* London: Bailliere, Tindal and Cox, 1873. Reprint. Dawson's of Pall Mall, 1959.
9. Freeman J. Dangers and dissapointments of hay-fever desensitisation. *Int Arch Allergy* 1955;6:197–202.
10. Cooke RA, Van der Veer A Jr. Human sensitisation. *J Immunol* 1916;1:201–205.

11. Kern RA. Dust sensitization in bronchial asthma. *Med Clin North Am* 1921;5:751–758.
12. Storm van Leeuwen W, Einthoven W, Kremer W. The allergen proof chamber in the treatment of bronchial asthma and other respiratory diseases. *Lancet* 1927;1:1287–1289.
13. Voorhorst R, Spieksma FThM, Varekamp H, Leupen MJ, Lyklema AW. The house dust mite (*Dermatophagoides pteronyssinus*) and the allergens in produces: identity with the house dust allergen. *J Allergy Clin Immunol* 1967;39:325–339.
14. Ishizaka K, Ishizaka T, Hornbrook MM. Allergen-binding activity of gamma-E, gamma-G and gamma-A antibodies in sera from atopic patients. *In vitro* measurement of reaginic antibody. *J Immunol* 1967;98:490–501.
15. Altounyan REC. Changes in histamine and atropine-responsiveness as a guide to diagnosis and evaluation of therapy in obstructive airway disease. In: Pepys J, Frankland AW, eds. *Disodium chromoglycate in allergic airway disease.* London: Butterworth, 1970;47–53.
16. Cockroft DW, Ruffin RE, Dolovitch J, Hargreave FE. Allergen-induced increase in airway reactivity. *Clin Allergy* 1977;7:503–513.
17. Gergen PJ, Weiss KB. The increasing problem of asthma in the United States. *Am Rev Respir Dis* 1992;146:823–824.
18. Burney P, Chinn S, Rona RJ. Has the prevalence of asthma increased in children? Evidence from the national study of health and growth 1973–86. *BMJ* 1990;300:1306–1310.
19. Robertson CF, Heycock E, Bishop J, Nolan T, Olinski A, Phelan P. Prevalence of asthma in Melbourne schoolchildren:changes over 26 years. *BMJ* 1991;302:1116–1118.
20. Shaw RA, Crane J, O'Donnell TV, Porteous LE, Coleman ED. Increasing asthma prevalence in a rural New Zealand adolescent population: 1975–1989. *Arch Dis Child* 1990;65:1319–1323.
21. Haahtela T, Lindholm H, Bjorksten F, Koskenvuo K, Laitinen LA. Prevalence of asthma in Finnish young men. *BMJ* 1990;301:266–268.
22. Burr ML, Limb ES, Andrae S, Barry DMJ, Nagel F. Childhood asthma in four countries: a comparative survey. *Int J Epidemiol* 1994;23:341–347.
23. Robertson CF, Bishop J, Sennhauser FH, Mallol J. International comparison of asthma prevalence in children: Australia, Switzerland, Chile. *Pediatr Pulmol* 1993;16:219–226.
24. Nishima S. A study of the prevalence of bronchial asthma in school children in western districts of Japan: comparison between the studies in 1982 and 1992 with the same methods and same districts. *Arerugi* 1993;42:192–204.
25. Leung R, Jenkins M. Asthma, allergy and atopy in southern Chinese school students. *Clin Exp Allergy* 1994;24:353–358.
26. Luyt DK, Burton PR, Simpson H. Epidemiological study of wheeze, doctor diagnosed asthma and cough in pre-school children in Leicestershire. *BMJ* 1993;306:1386–1390.
27. Chapman MD. Purification of allergens. *Curr Opin Immunol* 1989;1:647–653.
28. Platts-Mills TAE, Thomas WR, Aalberse RC, Vervloet D, Chapman MD. Dust mite allergens and asthma: report of a second international workshop. *J Allergy Clin Immunol* 1992;89:1046–1060.
29. Thomas WR. Mite allergens groups I–VII. A catalogue of enzymes. *Clin Exp Allergy* 1993;23:350–353.
30. Kraft D, Sehon A, eds. *Molecular biology and immunology of allergens.* Boca Raton, Fla: CRC Press, 1993.
31. King TP, Hoffman D, Lowenstein H, Marsh DG, Platts-Mills TAE, Thomas WR. Allergen nomenclature. *Int Arch Allergy Immunol* 1994;105:224–233.
32. Arruda LK, Vailes LD, Hayden ML, Benjamin DC, Chapman MD. Cloning of cockroach allergen, Bla g 4, identifies ligand binding proteins (or calycins) as a cause of IgE antibody responses. *J Biol Chem* 1995;270:31196–201.
33. Arruda LK, Vailes LD, Mann BJ, Shannon J, Fox JW, Vedvick TS, Hayden ML, Chapman MD. Molecular cloning of a major cockroach (*Blatella germanica*) allergen, Bla g 2: sequence homology to the aspartic proteases. *J Biol Chem* 1995;270:19563–19568.
34. Morganstern J, Griffith IJ, Brauer AJ, Rogers BL, Bond JF, Chapman MD, Kuo M. Amino acid sequence of Fel d 1, the major allergen of domestic cat: protein sequence analysis and cDNA cloning. *Proc Natl Acad Sci* 1991;88:9690–9694.
35. Bocskei Z, Groom CR, Flower DR, Wright CE, Phillips SEV, Cavaggioni A, Findlay JBC, North ACT. Pheromone binding to two rodent urinary proteins revealed by x-ray crystallography. *Nature* 1992;360:186–188.
36. Flower DR, North ACT, Attwood TK. Structure and sequence relationship in the lipocalins and related proteins. *Prot Sci* 1993;2:753–761.
37. Valenta R, Sperr WR, Ferreira F, et al. Induction of specific histamine release from basophils with purified natural and recombinant birch pollen allergens. *J Allergy Clin Immunol* 1993;91:88–97.
38. Ferreira FD, Hoffman-Sommergruber K, Breitender H, Pettenburger K, Ebner C, Sommergruber W et al. Purification and characterisation of recombinant Bet V 1, the major birch pollen allergen. *J Biol Chem* 1993;268:19574–19580.
39. Chua KY, Dilworth RJ, Thomas WR. Expression of *Dermatophagoides pteronyssinus* allergen, Der p II, in *Escherichia coli* and binding studies with human IgE. *Int Arch Allergy Appl Immunol* 1990;91:124–129.
40. Yuuki T, Okumara Y, Ando T, et al. Synthesis of biologically active recombinant Der f II. *Int Arch Allergy Appl Immunol* 1991;94:354–356.
41. Chua KY, Parminder KK, Thomas WR, Vaughan PR, Macreadie IG. High frequency IgE binding to the Der p 1 allergen expressed in yeast. *J Allergy Clin Immunol* 1992;89:95–102.
42. Bond JF, Brauer AW, Segal DB, Nault AK, Rogers BL, Kuo MC. Native and recombinant Fel d 1 as probes into the relationship of allergen structure to human IgE immunoreactivity. *Mol Immunol* 1993;30:1529–1541.
43. Slunt JB, Rogers BL, Chapman MD. IgE antibodies to recombinant forms of Fel d 1: dichotomy between fluid-phase and solid-phase binding studies. *J Allergy Clin Immunol* 1995;95:1221–8.
44. Keating KM, Segal DB, Craig S, et al. Enhanced immunoreactivity and preferential heterodimer formation of reassociated Fel d I chains. *Mol Immunol* 1995;32:287–293.
45. Norman PS, Ohman JL, Long AA, et al. Early clinical experience with T cell reactive peptides from cat allergen Fel d I. *J Allergy Clin Immunol* 1994;93:231.
46. Chapman MD, Aalberse RC, Brown MJ, Platts-Mills TAE. Monoclonal antibodies to the major feline allergen Fel d I. II: single step affinity purification of Fel d I, N terminal sequence analysis and development of a sensitive two site immunoassay to assess Fel d I exposure. *J Immunol* 1988;140:812–818.
47. Platts-Mills TAE, de Weck AL. Dust mite allergens and asthma—a worldwide problem. *J Allergy Clin Immunol* 1989;83:416–427.
48. Tovey ER, Chapman MD, Wells CW, Platts-Mills TAE. The distribution of dust mite allergen in the houses of patients with asthma. *Am Rev Respir Dis* 1981;124:630–635.
49. Chapman MD. Guanine—an adequate index of mite exposure? *Allergy* 1993;48:301–302.
50. Heyman PW, Chapman MD, Fox JW, Aalberse RC, Platts-Mills TAE. Antigenic and structural analyses of Group II allergens (Der p II and Der f II) from house dust mite (*Dermatophagoides spp.*). *J Allergy Clin Immunol* 1989;83:1055–1067.
51. Ovsyannikova IG, Vailes L, Li Y, Hayman PW, Chapman MD. Monoclonal antibodies to Group II *Dermatophagoides spp.* allergens: murine immune response, epitope analysis, and development of a two-site ELISA. *J Allergy Clin Immunol* 1994;94:537–546.
52. Luczynska CM, Arruda LK, Platts-Mills TAE, Miller JD, Lopez M, Chapman MD. A two site monoclonal antibody ELISA for the quantification of the major *Dermatophagoides spp.* allergens, Der p I and Der f I. *J Immunol Methods* 1989;118:227–235.
53. Pollart SM, Mullins DE, Vailes LD, Sutherland WM, Chapman MD. Identification, quantitation and purification of cockroach allergens using monoclonal antibodies. *J Allergy Clin Immunol* 1991;87:511–521.
54. Pollart SM, Smith TF, Morris EC, Platts-Mills TAE, Chapman MD. Environmental exposure to cockroach allergens: analysis using a monoclonal antibody-based enzyme immunoassay. *J Allergy Clin Immunol* 1991;87:505–510.
55. De Blay F, Chapman MD, Platts-Mills TAE. Airborne cat allergen Fel d I: environmental control with cat *in situ*. *Am Rev Respir Dis* 1991;143:1334–1339.
56. Yasueda H, Mita H, Yui Y, Shida T. Measurement of allergen associated with house dust mite allergy I. Development of sensitive radioimmunoassays for the two groups of *Dermatophagoides* mite allergens, Der p I and Der p II. *Int Arch Allergy Appl Immunol* 1990;90:182–189.
57. Lind P. Enzyme linked immunosorbent assay for determination of major excrement allergens of house dust mite species *D. pteronyssinus, D. Farinae* and *D. Microceras*. *Allergy* 1986;41:442–451.

58. DeGroot H, Goei KGH, van Swieten P, Aalberse RC. Affinity purification of a major and minor allergen from dog extract: serologic activity of affinity purified Can f I and of Can f I depleted extract. *J Allergy Clin Immunol* 1991;87:1056–1065.

59. DeGroot H, van Swieten P, Lind P, Aalberse RC. Monoclonal antibodies to the major feline allergen Fel d I. I. Biologic activity of affinity purified Fel d I and of Fel d I depleted extracts. *J Allergy Clin Immunol* 1988;82:778–786.

60. Schou C, Hansen GN, Lintner T, Lowenstein H. Assay for the major dpg allergen, Can f I: investigation of house dust samples and commercial dog extracts. *J Allergy Clin Immunol* 1991;88:847–853.

61. Lombardero M, Carreira J, Duffort O. Monoclonal antibody based radioimmunoassay for the quantitation of the major cat allergen (Fel d I or Cat-1). *J Immunol Methods* 1988;108:71–76.

62. Collof MJ, Ayres J, Carswell F, et al. The control of allergens of dust mites and domestic pets:a position paper. *Clin Exp Allergy* 1992;22 (suppl 2):1–28.

63. Colloff MJ. Practical and theoretical aspects of the ecology of house dust mites (*Acari: Pyroglyphidae*) in relation to the study of mite-mediated allergy. *Rev Med Veterin Entomol* 1991;79:611–629.

64. Platts-Mills TAE, Hayden ML, Woodfolk JA, Call RS, Sporik R. House dust mite avoidance regimens for the treatment of asthma. In: David TJ, ed. *Recent advances in paediatrics 13*. Edinburgh, United Kingdom: Churchill Livingstone, 1995;45–58.

65. Custovic A, Taggart SCO, Niven RM, Woodcock AJ. Evaluating exposure to mite allergens. *J Allergy Clin Immunol* 1995;96:134–135.

66. Custovic A, Taggart SCO, Woodcock A. House dust mite and cat allergen in different indoor environments. *Clin Exp Allergy* 1994;24: 1164–1168.

67. Sporik R, Chapman M, Platts-Mills T. Airborne mite antigen. *Lancet* 1990;336:1507–1508 (letter).

68. De Blay F, Heymann PW, Chapman MD, Platts-Mills TAE. Airborne dust mite allergens: comparison of Group II mite allergens with Group I mite allergen and cat allergen Fel d I. *J Allergy Clin Immunol* 1991;88:919–926.

69. Sakaguchi M, Inouye S, Yasueda H, Tatehisa I, Yoshizawa S, Shida T. Measurement of allergen associated with house dust mite allergy. II. Concentrations of airborne mite allergens (Der I and Der II) in the house. *Int Arch Allergy Appl Immunol* 1990;90:190–193.

70. Van Metre TE, Marsh DG, Adkinson NF, et al. Dose of cat (Felis domesticus) allergen 1 (Fel d I) that induces asthma. *J Allergy Clin Immunol* 1986;78:72–75.

71. Swanson MC, Campbell AR, Klauck MJ, Reed CE. Correlation between levels of mite and cat allergens in settled and airborne dust. *J Allergy Clin Immunol* 1989;83:776–783.

72. Wentz PE, Swanson MC, Reed CE. Variability of cat allergen shedding. *J Allergy Clin Immunol* 1990;85:94–98.

73. Luczynska CM, Li Y, Chapman MD, Platts-Mills TAE. Airborne concentrations and particle size distribution of allergen derived from domestic cats (*Felis domesticus)*: measurement using cascade impactor, liquid impinger and a two site monoclonal antibody assay for Fel d I. *Am Rev Respir Dis* 1990;141:361–367.

74. Custovic A, Green R, Fletcher A, Smith A, Pickering CAC, Chapman MD, Woodcock AJ. Aerodynamic properties of the major dog allergen, Can f 1: distribution in homes, concentration, and particle size of allergen in the air. *Am J Respir Crit Care Med (in press)*.

75. Hill AB. The environment and disease: association or causation? *Proc R Soc Med* 1965;58:295–300.

76. Sporik R, Chapman MD, Platts-Mills TAE. House dust mite exposure as a cause of asthma. *Clin Exp Allergy* 1992;22:897–906.

77. Burrows B, Martinez FD, Halonen M, Barbec RA, Cline MG. Association of asthma with serum IgE levels and skin test reactivity to allergens. *N Engl J Med* 1989;320:271–277.

78. Smith JM, Disney ME, Williams JD, Goels ZA. Clinical significance of skin reactions to mite extracts in children with asthma. *BMJ* 1969;ii:723–726.

79. Di Berardino L, Angrisano A, Gorli L, Catlaneo M, Lodi A. Allergy to house dust and storage mites in children: epidemiologic observation. *Ann Allergy* 1987;59:104–106.

80. Sears MR, Herbison GP, Holdaway MD, Hewitt CJ, Flannery EM, Silva PA. The relative risk of sensitivity to grass pollen, house dust mite and cat dander in the development of childhood asthma. *Clin Exp Allergy* 1989;19:419–424.

81. Peat JK, Tovey E, Gray EJ, Mellis CM, Woolcock AJ. Asthma sever-

82. Charpin D, Kleisbauer JP, Lanteaume A, et al. Asthma and allergy to house dust mites in population living in high altitudes. *Chest* 1988;93: 758–761.

83. Charpin D, Birnbaum J, Haddi E, et al. Altitude and allergy to house dust mites. *Am Rev Respir Dis* 1991;143:983–986.

84. Peat JK, Tovey E, Mellis CM, Leeder SR, Woolcock AJ. Importance of house dust mite and Alternaria allergens in childhood asthma: an epidemiological study in two climatic regions of Australia. *Clin Exp Allergy* 1993;23:812–820.

85. Peat JK, Tovey E. Mellis CM, Woolcock AJ. House-dust mite allergens:an important cause of childhood asthma. *Aust NZ J Med* 1994;24:473.

86. Sporik R, Ingram MJ, Price W, et al. Association of asthma with serum IgE and skin test reactivity to allergens among children living at high altitude: tickling the dragon's breath. *Am J Respir Crit Care Med* 1995;151:1388–1392.

87. Ingram JM, Sporik R, Rose G, Honsinger R, Chapman MD, Platts-Mills TAE. Quantitative assessment of exposure to dog (Can f 1) and cat (Fel d 1) allergens: relation to sensitisation and asthma among children living in Los Alamos, New Mexico. *J Allergy Clin Immunol* 1995;96:449–56.

88. Desjardins A, Benoit C, Ghezzo H, et al. Exposure to domestic animals and risk of immunologic sensitisation in subjects with asthma. *J Allergy Clin Immunol* 1993;91:979–986.

89. Kuehr J, Frischer T, Karmaus W, et al. Early childhood risk factors for sensitisation at school age. *J Allergy Clin Immunol* 1992;90:358–363.

90. Arshad SH, Hide DW. Effect of environmental factors on the development of allergic disorders in infancy. *J Allergy Clin Immunol* 1992;90:235–241.

91. Wickman M, Nordvall SL, Pershagen G, Sundell J, Schwartz B. House dust mite sensitisation in children and residential characteristics in a temperate region. *J Allergy Clin Immunol* 1991;88:89–95.

92. Wickmann M, Nordvall SL, Pershagen G, Korsgaard J, Johansen N. Sensitisation to domestic mites in a cold temperate region. *Am Rev Respir Dis* 1993;148:58–62.

93. Call RS, Smith TF, Morris E, Chapman MD, Platts-Mills TAE. Risk factors for asthma in inner city children. *J Pediatrics* 1992;121:862–866.

94. Kang B. Study on cockroach antigen as a probably causative agent in bronchial asthma. *J Allergy Clin Immunol* 1976;58:357–365.

95. Kang B, Vellody D, Homburger H, Yunginger JW. Cockroach cause of allergic asthma. Its specificity and immunologic profile. *J Allergy Clin Immunol* 1979;63:80–86.

96. Schulaner FA. Sensitivity to the cockroach in three groups of allergic children. *Pediatrics* 1970;45:465–466.

97. Mendoza J, Snyder FD. Cockroach sensitivity in children with bronchial asthma. *Ann Allergy* 1970;28:159–163.

98. Hulett AC, Dockhorn RJ. House dust mite (*D. farinae*) and cockroach allergy in a midwestern population. *Ann Allergy* 1979;42:160–165.

99. Fromer JM, Anderson JA, Yanari S, Bailey JA. Cockroach sensitivity among children: exposure history, skin test, and IgE-radioallergosorbent test reactivity. *J Allergy Clin Immunol* 1980;65:203.

100. Menon P, Menon V, Hilman B, Stankus R, Lehrer SB. Skin test reactivity to whole body and fecal extracts of American (*Periplaneta americana*) and German (*Blattella germanica*) cockroaches in atopic asthmatics. *Ann Allergy* 1991;67:573–577.

101. Thong YH, Omar A, Kok A, Robinson MJ. Skin reactivity to household aeroallergens in children with bronchial asthma. *Sing Med J* 1976;17:90–91.

102. Lan JL, Lee DT, Wu CH, Chang CP, Yeh CL. Cockroach hypersensitivity: preliminary study of allergic cockroach asthma in Taiwan. *J Allergy Clin Immunol* 1988;82:736–740.

103. Tandon N, Maitra S, Saha GK, Modak A, Hati AK. Role of cockroaches in allergy to house dust in Calcutta, India. *Ann Allergy* 1990;64:155–157.

104. Fraser BN. Cockroaches in relation to bronchial asthma in the Durban area. *South Afr Med J* 1979;55:637–639.

105. De Blay F, Kassell O, Chapman MD, Ott M, Verot A, Pauli G. Mise en evidence des allergens majeurs des blattes par test ELISA dans la poussiere domestique. *Presse Med* 1992;21:1685.

106. Chapman MD, Vailes LD, Hayden ML, Platts-Mills TAE, Arruda LK. Cockroach allergens and their role in asthma. In: Kay AB, ed. *Allergy*

and allergic disease. Oxford: Blackwell Scientific Publishers, (*in press*).

107. Bjorksten F, Suoniemi I, Koski V. Neonatal birch pollen contact and subsequent allergy to birch pollen. *Clin Allergy* 1980;10:581–591.

108. Korsgaard J, Dahl R. Sensitivity to house dust mite and grass pollen in adults. Influence of the month of birth. *Clin Allergy* 1983;13;529–536.

109. Warner JA, Little SA, Pollock I, Longbottom JL, Warner JO. The influence of exposure to house dust mite, cat, pollen and allergens in the homes on primary sensitisation in asthma. *Pediatr Allergy Immunol* 1991;1:79–86.

110. Vanto T, Koivikko A. Dog hypersensitivity in asthmatic children. *Acta Paediatr Scand* 1983;72:571–575.

111. Rowntree S, Cogswell JJ, Platts-Mills TAE, et al. Development of IgE and IgG antibodies to food and inhalant allergens in children at risk of atopic disease. *Arch Dis Child* 1985;60:727–735.

112. Sporik R, Holgate S, Platts-Mills TAE, Cogswell J. Exposure to house dust mite allergen (Der p I) and the development of asthma in childhood. *N Engl J Med* 1990;323:502–507.

113. Aalberse RC, Nieuwenhuys EJ, Hey M, Stapel SO. "Horoscope effect" not only for seasonal but also for non-seasonal allergens. *Clin Exp Allergy* 1992;22:1003–1006.

114. Andersen I, Korsgaard J. Asthma and the indoor environment: assessment of health implications of high indoor relative humidity. *Environ Int* 1986;12:121–127.

115. Kivity S. Solomon A. Soferman R. Schwartz Y, Mumcouglu KY, Topilsky M. Mite asthma in childhood: a study of the relationship between exposure to house dust mites and disease activity. *J Allergy Clin Immunol* 1991;91:844–849.

116. Sporik R, Platts-Mills TAE, Cogswell JJ. Exposure to house dust mite allergen of children admitted to hospital with asthma. *Clin Exp Allergy* 1993;23:740–746.

117. Pollart SM, Chapman MD, Fiocco GP, Rose G, Platts-Mills TAE. Epidemiology of acute asthma: IgE antibodies to common inhalant allergens as a risk factor for emergency room visits. *J Allergy Clin Immunol* 1989;83:875–882.

118. Gelber LE, Seltzer LH, Bouzoukis JK, Pollart SM, Chapman MD, Platts-Mills TAE. Sensitisation and exposure to indoor allergens as risk factor for asthma among patients presenting to hospital. *Am Rev Respir Dis* 1993;147:573–578.

119. Aalberse R, Kauffman HF, Koeter GH, Postma DS, De Vries K, De Monchy JGR. Dissimilarity in methacholine and adenosine 5′-monophosphate responsiveness 3 and 24 hours after allergen challenge. *Am Rev Respir Dis* 1991;144:352–357.

120. O'Hallaren MT, Yunginger JW, Offord KP, et al. Exposure to an aeroallergen as a possible precipitating factor in respiratory arrest in young patients with asthma. *N Engl J Med* 1991;324:359–363.

121. Van der Heide S, de Monchy JGR, de Vries K, Bruggink TM, Kauffman HK. Seasonal variation in airway hyperresponsiveness and natural exposure to house dust mite allergens in patients with asthma. *J Allergy Clin Immunol* 1994;93:470–475.

122. Custovic A, Taggart SCO, Francis HC, Chapman MD, Woodcock AJ. Exposure to house dust mite allergens and the clinical activity of asthma. *J Allergy Clin Immunol* 1996;98:64–72.

123. Price JA, Pollock I, Little SA, Longbottom JL, Warner JO. Measurement of airborne mite antigen in homes of asthmatic children. *Lancet* 1990;336:895–897.

124. Arruda LK, Rizzo MC, Chapman MD, et al. Exposure and sensitisation to dust mite allergens among asthmatic children in Sao Paulo, Brazil. *Clin Exp Allergy* 1991;21:433–439.

125. Clark JW, Yunginger JW, Bonnes PA, Ray CG, Saltzstein SL. Serum IgE antibodies in sudden infant death syndrome. *J Periatrics* 1979;95:85–86.

126. Jordan SC, Platts-Mills TAE, Mason W, et al. Lack of evidence for mite–antigen mediated pathogenesis in Kawasaki's disease. *Lancet* 1983;i:931 (letter).

127. Dowse GK, Turner KJ, Stewart GA, Alpers MP, Woolcock AJ. The association between *Dermatophagoides* mites and the increasing prevalence of asthma in village communities within the Papua New Guinea highlands. *J Allergy Clin Immunol* 1985;75:75–83.

128. Kuehr J, Frisher T, Meinert R, et al. Sensitisation to mite allergens is a risk factor for early and late onset of asthma and for persistence of asthmatic signs in children. *J Allergy Clin Immunol* 1995;95:655–662.

129. Kuehr J, Frischer T, Meinert R, et al. Mite allergen exposure is a risk

130. Ohman JL, Sparrow D, MacDonald MR. New onset wheezing in an older male population: evidence of allergen sensitization in a longitudinal study. *J Allergy Clin Immunol* 1993;91:752–757.

131. Hagy GW, Settipane GA. Prognosis of positive allergy skin tests in an asymptomatic population. *J Allergy Clin Immunol* 1971;48:200–211.

132. Lau S, Falkenhorst G, Weber A, Werthmann I, Lind P, Buettner-Goetz P, Wahn U. High mite-allergen exposure increases the risk of sensitization in atopic children and young adults. *J Allergy Clin Immunol* 1989;84:718–725.

133. Pope AM, Patterson R, Burge H, eds. *Indoor allergens. Assessing and controling adverse health effects*. Washington, DC: National Academy Press, 1993.

134. Chur V, Falkenhorst G, Hermannsdoerfer P, Lau S, Wahn U. Studies on the influence of mite allergen exposure and the influence on sensitisation and bronchial hyperreactivity of atopic children. *N Engl Reg Allergy Proc* 1988;9:295.

135. Marks G, Tovey E, Woolcock AJ. In subjects with asthma the concentration of Der p I in beds correlates with the severity of bronchial hyperresponsiveness and symptoms. *Am Rev Respir Dis* 1993;147:A458 (abstr).

136. Platts-Mills TAE, Woodfolk JA, Sporik RB, Chapman MD, Heymann PW. Relevance of indoor allergen measurement and the use of avoidance measures in the treatmant of allergic disease. In: *Postgraduate syllabus and asthma consultant's course*. New York: American Academy of Allergy & Immunology, 1995;111–125.

137. Kerrebijn KF. Endogenous factors in childhood CNSLD: methological aspects in population studies. In: Orie NGM, Van der Lende R, eds. *Bronchitis III*. Assen, The Netherlands: Royal Van Gorcum, 1970;38–48.

138. Platts-Mills TAE, Chapman MD. Dust mites: immunology, allergic disease, and environmental control. *J Allergy Clin Immunol* 1987;80:755–775.

139. Boner AL, Niero E, Antolini I, Valletta EA, Gaburro D. Pulmonary function and bronchial hyperreactivity in asthmatic children with house dust mite allergy during prolonged stay in the Italian Alps (Misurina 1756 m). *Ann Allergy* 1985;54:42–45.

140. Piacentini GL, Martinati L, Fornari A, et al. Antigen avoidance in a mountain environment: influence on basophil releasability in children with allergic asthma. *J Allergy Clin Immunol* 1993;92:644–650.

141. Peroni DG, Boner AL, Vallone G, Antolini I, Warner JO. Effective allergen avoidance at high altitude reduces allergen-induced bronchial hyperresponsiveness. *Am J Respir Crit Care Med* 1994;149:1442–1446.

142. Platts-Mills TAE, Tovey ER, Mitchell EB, Moszoro H, Nock P, Wilkins SR. Reduction of bronchial hyperreactivity during prolonged allergen avoidance. *Lancet* 1982;2:675–678.

143. Burr ML, Dean BV, Merrett TG, Neale E, St Leger AS, Verrier-Jones ER. Effects of anti-mite measures on children with mite sensitive asthma-a controlled trial. *Thorax* 1980;35:506–512.

144. Murray AB, Ferguson AC. Dust-free bedrooms in the treatment of asthmatic children with house dust mite allergy: a controlled trial. *Pediatrics* 1983;71:418–422.

145. Walshaw MJ, Evans CC. Allergen avoidance in house dust mite sensitive adult asthma. *Q J Med* 1986;58:199–215.

146. Ehnert B, Lau-Schadendorf S,, Weber A, Buettner P, Schou C, Wahn U. Reducing domestic exposure to dust mite allergen reduces bronchial hyperreactivity in sensitive children with asthma. *J Allergy Clin Immunol* 1992;90:135–138.

147. Arshad SH, Matthews S, Gant C, Hide DW. Effect of allergen avoidance on development of allergic disorder in infancy. *Lancet* 1992;339:1493–1497.

148. Hide DW, Matthews S, Matthews L, et al. Effect of allergen avoidance in infancy on allergic manifestation at age two years. *J Allergy Clin Immunol* 1994;93:842–846.

149. Hide DW, Hakim EA. A controlled trial of allergen avoidance in infancy for the prevention of allergy in high risk children. In: *Environmental measures in the prevention of allergy*. The UCB Institute of Allergy, Chemin du Foriest, 1994;43–49.

150. Gibson PG, Manning PJ, O'Byrne PM, et al. Allergen induced asthmatic responses. Relationship between increases in airway responsiveness and increase in circulating eosinophils, basophils and their progenitors. *Am Rev Respir Dis* 1991;143:331–335.

151. Diaz M, Gonzales MC, Galleguillos FR, et al. Leukocytes and mediators in bronchoalveolar lavage during allergen-induced late-phase asthmatic reactions. *Am Rev Respir Dis* 1989;139:1383–1389.

152. Fukuda T, Nakajima H, Ando N, et al. Upregulation of intercellular adhesion molecule-1 (ICAM-1) expression on bronchial epithelium in symptomatic asthmatics and following bronchial allergen antigen exposure, ICACI XIV:91 (abstr).

153. Wierenga EA, Snoek M, Bos JD, Jansen HM, Capsenberg ML. Comparison of diversity and function of house dust mite specific T cell lymphocyte clones from atopic and non-atopic donors. *Eur J Immunol* 1990;20:1519–1526.

154. Warner JA, Miles EA, Jones AC, Quint DJ, Colwell BM, Warner JO. Is deficiency of interferon gamma production by allergen triggered cord blood cells a predictor of atopic asthma? *Clin Exp Allergy* 1994;24:423–430.

155. Pollart SM, Reid MJ, Fling JA, Chapman MD, Platts-Mills TAE. Epidemiology of emergency room asthma in northern California: association with IgE antibody to ryegrass pollen. *J Allergy Clin Immunol* 1988;82:224–230.

156. Butcher BT, Bernstein IL, Schwartz HJ. Guidelines for the clinical evaluation of occupational asthma due to small molecular weight chemicals. *J Allergy Clin Immunol* 1989;84:834–838.

157. Venables K, Dally M, Nunn A, et al. Smoking and occupational allergy in workers in a platinum rafinery. *BMJ* 1989;299:939–942.

158. Platts-Mills TAE. Mechanisms of bronchial reactivity: the role of Immunoglobulin E. *Am Rev Respir Dis* 1992;145:S44–S47.

159. Platts-Mills TAE, Ward GW Jr, Sporik R, Gelber LE, Chapman MD, Heymann PW. Epidemiology of the relationship between exposure to indoor allergens and asthma. *Int Arch Allergy Appl Immunol* 1991;94:339–345.

160. Peat JK, van der Berg RH, Green WF, Mellis CM, Leeder SR, Woolcock AJ. Changing prevalence of asthma in Australian children. *BMJ* 1994;308:1591–1596.

161. Seaton A, Godden DJ, Brown K. Increase in asthma: a more toxic environment or a more susceptible population. *Thorax* 1994;49:171.

162. Martinez FD, Cline M, Burrows B. Increased incidence of asthma in children of smoking mothers. *Pediatrics* 1992;89:21–26.

163. Ehrlich R, Kattan M, Godbold J, et al. Childhood asthma and passive smoking. Urinary cotinine as a biomarker of exposure. *Am Rev Respir Dis* 1992;145:594–599.

164. Chilmonczyk BA, Salmun LM, Megathlin KN, et al. Association between exposure to environmental tobacco smoke and exacerbation of asthma in children. *N Engl J Med* 1993;328:1665–1669.

165. Sporik R. Early childhood wheezing. *Curr Opin Pediatr* 1994;6:650–655.

166. Johnston S, Pattemore P, Smith S, et al. The association of viral infections with longitudinal changes in respiratory symptoms and/or peak flow recordings in schoolchildren. *Eur Respir J* 1992;5:109S.

167. Duff AL, Pomeranz ES, Gelber LE, et al. Risk factors for acute wheezing in infants and children: viruses, passive smoke, and IgE antibodies to inhalant allergens. *Pediatrics* 1993;92:535–540.

168. Bardin PG, Fraenkel DJ, Sanderson G, et al. Amplified rhinovirus colds in atopic subjects. *Clin Exp Allergy* 1994;24:457–464.

169. Calhoun WJ, Dick EC, Schwartz LB, Busse WW. A common cold virus, rhinovirus 16, potentiates airway inflammation after segmental antigen bronchoprovocation in allergic subjects. *J Clin Invest* 1994;94:2200–2208.

170. Landau LI. Bronchiolitis and asthma: are they related? *Thorax* 1993;48:293–295.

171. Anto JM, Sunyer J. Nitrogen dioxide and allergic asthma: starting to clarify an obscure association. *Lancet* 1995;345:402–403.

173. Tunnicliffe WS, Burge PS, Ayres JG. Effect of domestic concentrations on hitrogen dioxide on airway responses to inhaled allergen in asthmatic patients. *Lancet* 1994;344:1733–1736.

173. Devalia JL, Rusznack C, Herdman MJ, Trigg CJ, Tarraf H, Davies RJ. Effect of nitrogen dioxide and sulphur dioxide on airway response of mild asthmatic patients to allergen inhalation. *Lancet* 1994;344:1668–1671.

174. Molfino NA, Wright SC, Katz I, et al. Effect of low concentrations of ozone on inhaled allergen responses in asthmatic subjects. *Lancet* 1991;338:199–203.

175. Peden DB, Setzer RW, Devlin RB. Ozone exposure has both a priming effect on allergen-induced responses and an intrinsic inflammatory action in the nasal airways of perennially allergic asthmatics. *Am J Respir Crit Care Med* 1995;151:1336–1345.

176. Samet JM, Lambert WE, Skipper BJ, et al. Nitrogen dioxide and respiratory illness in infants. *Am Rev Respir Dis* 1993;148:1258–1265.

177. Muranaka M, Suzuki S, Koizumi K, et al. Adjuvant activity of diesel-exhaust particulates for the production of IgE antibody in mice. *J Allergy Clin Immunol* 1986;77:616–623.

178. Takafuji S, Suzuki S, Koizumi K, et al. Enhancing effect of suspended particulate matter on the IgE antibody production in mice. *Int Arch Allergy Appl Immunol* 1989;90:1–7.

179. Diaz Sanchez D, Dotson AR, Takenaka H, Saxon A. Diesel exhaust particles induce local IgE production *in vivo* and alter the pattern of IgE massanger RNA isoforms. *J Clin Invest* 1994;94:1417–1425.

180. Peat JK, Tovey ER, Mellis CM, Beloossova E, Woolcock AJ. House dust mite allergens: an important cause of childhood asthma. *Thor Soc News* 1994;June:28–30.

Asthma, edited by P.J. Barnes, M.M. Grunstein, A.R. Leff, and A.J. Woolcock.
Lippincott–Raven Publishers, Philadelphia © 1997.

▪ 9 ▪

Risk Factor

Diet

Scott T. Weiss

Methods of Diet Assessment and Clinical Research
Antioxidants
  Retinol/Beta-Carotene
  Vitamin E
  Vitamin C
  Vitamin B₆
  Selenium/Glutathione Peroxidase

Caffeine
Alcohol
N₃-N₆ Fatty Acids
Urinary Cations, Sodium Potassium, and Magnesium
  Sodium/Potassium
  Magnesium
  Breast Feeding

At the present time, there is great interest in trying to understand the role, if any, of diet in modifying the effect of these environmental exposures on the development and the natural history of asthma. This chapter will consider a variety of dietary constituents thought to influence inflammatory mechanisms, airway responsiveness, level of lung function, or asthma as a syndrome. The biochemical bases for these effects will also be addressed. Finally, the chapter will suggest future directions for research into the role of diet and the development of asthma.

METHODS OF DIET ASSESSMENT AND CLINICAL RESEARCH

Although case-controlled studies have been used to assess diet-disease relationships, there are no case-controlled studies that have examined dietary factors and their relationship to asthma. Case-controlled studies tend to be particularly problematic for dietary research because of recall and selection bias of subjects. This is particularly true, given that there is a range of variation in

diet in Western populations and inevitable error in measuring intake; there are also expected relative risks in most studies of diet, and asthma being relatively small, ranging on the order of 0.5 to 2. Stronger study designs include a prospective cohort study, where problems of recall bias are diminished and disease outcomes can be measured precisely. We will also consider the limited number of randomized controlled trials of diet and asthma outcomes. In interpreting dietary data, we will use the rubric of Bradford Hill (1). We will assess the strength of the association, its consistency across studies, the presence or absence of the dose-response relationship between the nutrient and the asthma outcome, the temporal relationship of the diet exposure to the asthma outcome, biologic plausibility, and the coherence with existing studies. Negative studies on diet and asthma will also receive consideration. There are a variety of reasons for null associations between diet and asthma outcomes that are given in Table 1. Particular attention needs to be paid to the nature of how diet was assessed, the particular population that was studied, and the presence or absence of confounding by other dietary constituents.

A variety of methods have been used to assess the relationship of diet to asthma. These methods are summarized in Table 2. In general, short-term dietary methods have relatively little applicability to a chronic disease such as asthma. These methods are appropriate for short-term di-

---

S.T. Weiss: Department of Medicine, Harvard Medical School; and Division of Respiratory and Environmental Epidemiology, Channing Laboratory, Brigham and Women's Hospital, Boston, Massachusetts 02115.

TABLE 1. *Reasons for lack of association between diet and asthma*

1. No variation in nutrients in population.
2. Variation exists, but only on flat portion of dose-response curve.
3. Imprecise assessment of diet.
4. Low statistical power; small sample size.
5. Negative confounding
6. Latent period not considered.

Adapted from Willett W. *Nutritional epidemiology*. New York: Oxford University Press, 1990;1–396.

etary interventions. Validation of these methods is difficult, although direct observation, weighing the food, use of duplicate meals, and direct comparison of recall and diet record have been used in an attempt to validate these methods. The method that has been most often used by epidemiologists has been the food frequency questionnaire (2). The rationale for this technique is that average long-term diet over months and years is the most important exposure, rather than intake on a few specific days. The basic approach includes a food list and a frequency response section for subjects to report their average intake over some defined period of time (e.g., last 6 months, last year). For a food item to be informative, it must be used reasonably often by an appreciable number of individuals; it must have a substantial content of nutrients of interest; and there must be some variability in the population. A variety of techniques have been used to minimize recall bias on food frequency questionnaires (2). In addition, substantial work has been done to validate food frequency techniques by comparing results with serum levels of specific nutrients. Because of the low relative risks and the degree of error in measuring diet, relatively large sample sizes have been needed to demonstrate associations in epidemiologic studies of diet and disease. One significant problem in most of the existing epidemiologic data and asthma is that sample size remains relatively small in most studies.

ANTIOXIDANTS

Free radicals are reactive chemical species, easily derived from oxygen, that are chemically unstable. Oxygen free radicals are capable of damaging cellular compo-

nents, and, thus, of contributing to inflammation. Chemical oxidants can be derived from cigarette smoke, viral infections, or allergen exposure, the three most important environmental exposures for asthma. Antioxidant vitamins are the first line of defense against oxidant injury. We will consider Vitamin A (retinol), pro Vitamin A (beta carotene), Vitamin C (ascorbic acid), Vitamin E (alphatocopherol), Vitamin B_6 (pyridoxine), and selenium.

Retinol/Beta-Carotene

Both beta-carotene and retinol are essential vitamins. Retinol is required for differentiating epithelia from mucous secretion. Beta carotene is known to have an antioxidant function. Although retinol is toxic if taken in excess doses, beta carotene can be ingested at high doses for long periods without risk of toxicity. In addition to the antioxidant properties, beta carotene retinoids may be important for glycosolation reactions and may actually alter genomic expression within cells. In general, there is a good correlation between food frequency questionnaire estimates of retinol intake and serum retinol levels (3). Cigarette smokers tend to have lower levels of serum beta carotene and dietary beta carotene intake (3). Smokers tend to ingest lower levels of carotene and nonsmokers who are exposed to passive smoke tend to ingest lower levels as well (4). Administration of beta carotene inhibits chemoluminescence and frequencies of sister chromatid exchanges leukocytes from cigarette smokers (5).

To date, there have been no specific studies which have examined either beta carotene or retinol and either one's relationship to asthma outcomes. There has been, however, one study which has examined Vitamin A intake and its relationship to airflow obstruction (6). Morabia and co-workers investigated the relationship of retinol intake as assessed by 24-hour recall, and a food frequency questionnaire and its relationship to airflow obstruction (6). They used data from the first National Health and Nutrition Examination Survey (NHANES I). Airflow obstruction was defined as a forced expiratory volume in one second (FEV_1)/forced vital capacity (FVC) ratio ≤ 65% of predicted. They employed a case-controlled design in which controls were subjects with FEV_1/FVC ratio > 65% of predicted. The investigators found a significant

TABLE 2. *Questionnaire methods for assessing relationship of diet to asthma*

	Sources of Error	Reproducibility	Validity	Limitations
Short-Term				
24-Hour Recall	Recall Bias	High	High	Short-Term
3- to 7-Day Diet Record	Recall/Response Bias	High	Moderate	Short-Term
Long-Term				
Food Frequency Questionnaire	Recall Bias	Moderate	Moderate	Long-Term

Adapted from Willett W. Nutritional Epidemiology. New York: Oxford University Press, 1990;1–396.

relationship between reduced retinol intake and an increased level of airflow obstruction. The analysis tended to be confirmed by an analysis of foods. The relationship appeared stronger among Caucasians and smokers. No attempt was made to examine asthma in this study, nor were other nutrients besides retinol assessed. No association with beta carotene was observed.

Vitamin E

Vitamin E (alphatocopherol) is found in vegetable oils (soybean, corn, cottonseed, saffron). The dietary requirement is linked to dietary intake of polyunsaturated fatty acids, particularly linoleic acids (7). Vitamin E is a fat-soluble antioxidant which prevents free radical attack on polyunsaturated fatty acids and other membrane lipids. Vitamin C assists in maintaining Vitamin E in its reduced form; thus, it is difficult to separate the antioxidant effects of Vitamin C and Vitamin E. Vitamin E protects the lung against oxidant injury in animal models (8). Cigarette smokers have increased dietary intake of Vitamin E (9). In addition, cigarette smokers show increased oxidative metabolism to Vitamin E relative to nonsmokers. Miedema et al. (10) examined the relationship between diet and the development of chronic nonspecific lung disease (CNSLD), asthma, bronchitis, and emphysema in a 25-year prospective study in Zutphen, The Netherlands, from 1960 to 1988. These investigators found no relationship between Vitamin E and the occurrence of CNSLD. Troisi et al. (11) examined the relationship of Vitamin E intake to the development of adult-onset asthma among 77,866 nurses aged 34 to 68. This was a prospective study of adult-onset asthma in which the diagnosis of asthma was validated by chart review. The authors noted nearly a 50% reduction in asthma incidence when comparing women in the highest quintile of Vitamin E intake to those women in the lowest quintile. When supplements were considered, a positive association between use of Vitamin E and asthma incidence was noted, although this appeared to be due to women at high risk of asthma initiating use of vitamins prior to diagnosis. Finally, Britton and co-workers (12) examined the relationship of Vitamin E to FEV and FVC in a sample of 2,633 subjects aged 18 to 70 in the vicinity of Nottingham, England. The subjects with Vitamin E intake one standard deviation above the mean had 20 mL higher FEV and 23 mL higher FVC. However, when Vitamin C intake was considered, this effect no longer was statistically significant. This may have been due to the fact that Vitamin C and Vitamin E intakes were significantly correlated (r=0.29, p=0.001). This study was cross-sectional and did not consider any asthma-specific outcomes, such as airway responsiveness, asthma, or atopy.

In summary, relatively little data exist on Vitamin E and any asthma-related outcomes. Taken together, the papers by Troisi and Britton do suggest that Vitamin E may have an impact on asthma, but that smaller studies will have trouble differentiating this effect from Vitamin C, since the two vitamins function together.

Vitamin C

Vitamin C is a water-soluble free radical scavenger of singlet oxygen, superoxide antion, and peroxyl free radicals (13,14). Vitamin C also functions as a co-enzyme in the biosynthesis collagen, and, thus, may contribute to lung repair (14). Vitamin C may also play a role in immune function. It is transported into neutrophils and lymphocytes (15,16). A variety of studies have demonstrated that serum Vitamin C levels are lower in cigarette smokers than in nonsmokers (17). This effect appears to be a result of both decreased intake as well as increased metabolism (18,19). The correlation between serum Vitamin C levels and Vitamin C intake as assessed by a food frequency questionnaire is on the order of 0.4 (20). A variety of acute studies in asthmatic patients have demonstrated modest decreases in airway reactivity and improvement in pulmonary function. The negative studies have tended to use smaller doses of Vitamin C. No studies have examined serum levels or outcomes other than airway responsiveness or spirometry. The epidemiologic data are also consistent. Two studies have not measured Vitamin C directly, but have examined intake of fresh fruit and vegetables. The Zutphen Study found that fruit and vegetable intake is inversely related to the collective incidence of asthma, bronchitis, and emphysema, higher fruit and vegetable intake being associated with approximately a 25% reduction in obstructive airway disease risk (odds ratio 0.73, 95% confidence interval 0.53 to 0.99) (10). No specific effect of Vitamin C was found. Strachan et al. (21) studied a random population in the United Kingdom and found that subjects who consumed low levels of fresh fruits had an FEV_1 80 mL lower on average than those who were regular consumers.

Three studies have assessed the relationship of Vitamin C intake to wheeze or asthma. Schwartz and Weiss (22) found an inverse association between serum Vitamin C levels, but not intake measured by 24-hour recall and the prevalence of wheeze within the past year. These data are from NHANES II (22). The investigators found a 30% decrease in wheeze (odds ratio and 95% confidence interval 0.71, 0.858 to 0.88), for a 2-standard deviation increase in Vitamin C adjusting for age, gender, race, socioeconomic status, cigarette smoking, and total energy intake. Troisi et al. (11) examined the effect of Vitamin C intake on the subsequent development of asthma among women in the Nurses Health Study. They found no relationship between Vitamin C intake and the development of asthma in adult women. This one study that found no relationship looked at food frequency data and asthma as the outcome. At least this raises the question as to whether misclassification accounts for the lack of the association in the Nurses Health Study data.

A series of small case-controlled studies have examined serum levels of Vitamin C in asthma patients and controls (Table 3, refs 23-32). Solousi (33) performed a case-controlled study with 62 asthma patients and 57 controls and found ascorbic-acid levels in the asthma patients lower plasma and white blood cells. These studies, by virtue of their design, are unable to address the question of whether the low plasma Vitamin C levels are the cause or the consequence of airway inflammation.

With regard to lung function outcomes, Schwartz and Weiss (34) found a relationship between low levels of Vitamin C assessed by 24-hour recall and a food frequency questionnaire and lower levels of FEV_1 in subjects in NHANES I (34). This positive correlation is such that the difference between the first and the third tertile in terms of Vitamin C intake was associated with an approximately 20 mL difference in FEV_1. These findings were confirmed by Britton et al. (12) in the Nottingham cohort. Britton estimated that a one-standard deviation decrease in Vitamin C was approximately equivalent to the adverse effects of five packyears of cigarette smoking on FEV_1. These papers adjusted for age, gender, cigarette smoking, total calories Vitamin E intake, race, and socioeconomic status. To date, there are no longitudinal studies on the relationship of Vitamin C intake and decline in lung function, nor are there studies that have examined more specific asthma-related outcomes, such as airway reactivity.

In summary, of all antioxidant vitamins, the data linking Vitamin C with respiratory outcomes seem strongest. Short-term clinical trials in asthma patients, in general, show modest effects on lung function and airway responsiveness. The relationship to lung function is consistent in cross-sectional epidemiologic studies. There are, however, no data conclusively linking Vitamin C levels to asthma onset.

Vitamin B$_6$

Vitamin B_6 (Pyridoxine) is found in cereals, bread, whole grain, liver, spinach, bananas, fish, poultry, meats, nuts, potatoes, green leafy vegetables, and avocados. It is a co-enzyme for enzymes involved in the metabolism of amino acids and fatty acids and converting tryptophane to niacin. At least one study utilizing a case-controlled design found that asthmatics have lower levels of Vitamin B_6 compared to normal controls (35).

Selenium/Glutathione Peroxidase

The trace element selenium is an essential co-enzyme for the functioning of the glutathione peroxidase enzyme system. This antioxidant system scavenges free radicals, at least during inflammation. Selenium also functions as a co-factor enhancing the effect of Vitamin E (36). Selenium may also be important in modulating the inflammatory effects of leukotrienes produced by metabolism of arachidonic acid (36).

Flatt and co-workers (37) compared blood and plasma selenium and glutathione peroxidase activity in 56 adult asthmatic patients and 59 nonasthmatic control patients in New Zealand. When compared to the control subjects, the asthmatic patients had lower values of whole blood

TABLE 3. *Acute Studies of Vitamin C in Asthma*

Authors	Population	Dose	Outcome	Comments
Mohsenin et al. 1983 (23)	14 asthmatics	1 gram single dose	34% decrease in airway reactivity to methacholine	hours
Ogilvy et al. 1981 (24)	6 normals	1 gram single dose	35% decrease in airway reactivity to highest dose	hours
Zuskin et al. 1973 (25)	17 normals	500 mg single dose	significant decrease in airway responsiveness to histamine	hours
Ting et al. 1983 (26)	20 asthmatics	500 mg, 1 gram just prior to spirometry	no effect on FEV_1	3 days
Malo et al. 1986 (27)	16 asthmatics	2 grams single dose	no effect on FEV_1 or PC_{20} methacholine	4 days
Schachter et al. 1982 (28)	12 asthmatics	500 mg	improved FVC; improved exercise challenge	2 days
Hunt 1938 (29)	25 asthmatics		no effect	
Bucca et al. 1989 (30)	7 healthy subjects 7 heavy smokers	2 grams	acute decrease in airway responsiveness in smokers	1 hour
Anderson et al. 1980 (31)	10 asthmatic children	1 gram/day, 6 months	decreased IgE; improved cellular and immune functions	
Anderson et al. 1983 (32)	16 asthmatic children	1 gram/day	no effect on exercise-induced bronchospasm, improvement in leukocyte function	

FEV_1, forced expiratory volume in one second; FVC, forced vital capacity; IgE, immunoglobulin E.

selenium and glutathione peroxidase. There was a 1.9-and 5.8-fold increased risk of asthma in subjects with the lowest range of blood selenium and glutathione peroxidase activity, respectively (95% confidence interval 0.6 to 5.6 for selenium and 1.6 to 21.2 for glutathione peroxidase). Levels seemed to be lowest in patients and control subjects who were nonatopic. Hasselmark et al. (38) measured serum levels of glutathione peroxidase and selenium in 20 adult patients with intrinsic asthma and 20 control subjects. Glutathione levels, and not selenium levels, were significantly lower in asthma patients than in controls. These investigators subsequently performed a randomized controlled trial of selenium supplementation (39). Twenty-four adult intrinsic asthmatics were randomized to either supplementation with 100 micrograms of selenium or placebo for 14 weeks. Selenium levels increased in the treatment group and there was subjective symptomatic improvement, but no objective change in lung function.

Bibi and co-workers (40) examined serum glutathione peroxidase levels in 56 asthmatic children. Children with acute attacks of asthma were found to have lower levels than asymptomatic patients. Selenium levels were not examined.

Pearson et al. (41) studied selenium and glutathione peroxidase levels in 18 aspirin-sensitive asthmatic subjects, 18 nonasthmatic aspirin-tolerant controls, and 18 asthmatic subjects who were aspirin-tolerant. Aspirin-tolerant asthmatics had higher selenium values than aspirin-sensitive asthmatics or healthy controls. There was a correlation between serum selenium concentration and plasma glutathione peroxidase enzyme activity in all groups, but the correlation was lowest in the aspirin-sensitive asthmatics, suggesting that glutathione peroxidase activity is a function of both availability of selenium and, as yet, unidentified factors.

Stone and colleagues (42) studied plasma, whole blood, and platelet selenium and whole blood and platelet glutathione peroxidase activity in 49 adult asthma patients and 76 healthy controls. Asthma patients had lower selenium measurements in whole blood (odds ration 3.54) or plasma (odds ration 5.08), but platelet levels and glutathione peroxidase levels were not different in cases and controls. These data are consistent with the hypothesis that selenium deficiency is related to asthma occurrence. However, all data are currently from case-controlled studies of prevalent cases; thus, the temporal relationship between selenium levels and asthma occurrence is unknown.

Shaw et al. (43) studied risk factors for asthma occurrence among 708 Kawaeran school children aged 8 to 13 years in New Zealand. In a subset of these children, selenium levels were measured 8 years previously. Asthmatic children were more likely to have lower levels of selenium than normal children (odds ratio 3.1, 95% confidence intervals 0.9 to 11.8). This analysis controlled for gender, age, family history of asthma, environmental tobacco smoke exposure, and atopy.

In summary, there are several case-controlled studies linking serum selenium levels to asthma occurrence. Though subject to potential recall bias (the usual problem with case-controlled studies), this seems unlikely as exposure is objectively measured with serum levels. Taken together, these studies provide reasonably strong support for a relationship between selenium and asthma. The studies do not establish whether selenium deficiency antedates and predicts asthma onset.

Caffeine

Caffeine is perhaps the oldest dietary therapy for asthma, dating back to the Greeks. Caffeine exerts its pharmacologic effects for antagonism of adonosive receptors. Some believe that this may be mediated by methylxanthine effects, such as its inhibition of phosphodiesterase. Both of these mechanisms would result in bronchodilation of airway smooth muscle. Caffeine is absorbed orally and reaches its peak plasma levels about half an hour after its ingestion. It is excreted by the kidney.

There have been seven acute studies of the effect of caffeine in asthma (44–50) (Table 4). All studies involved adult asthmatic subjects and ranged in size from 7 to 23 subjects. The dose of caffeine given ranged from 0.2 to 10 mg/kg, the equivalent of approximately 3 cups of coffee. All studies evaluated respiratory outcomes at between 1 and 3 hours after coffee ingestion when bronchodilutation should be maximal. Four studies examined spirometry and three studies examined airway responsiveness. The results of these three studies with airway responsiveness data are interesting in that the studies found significant increases in FEV_1 that were maximal at 1.5 hours and approximated 40% of the effect (200 mg dose of aminophyllin) (46,47,50). In contrast, the effects on airway responsiveness were minimal. One study found no effect on carbachol challenge; the other two studies found a slight increase in PC_{20} to histamine. These results are consistent in that caffeine is likely to have a bronchodilator effect which would increase pulmonary function but may have no effect or change on underlying airway inflammation.

Epidemiologic data have also been obtained. Pagano (51) examined data from the 1983 Italian National Health Survey on 72,284 individuals over the age of 15, randomly selected within a strata of geographic area, place of residence, and household size in order to be representative of the Italian population. These studies evaluated cross-sectionally the relationship of coffee drinking to asthma risk. Compared with subjects who did not drink coffee, the age and gender adjusted relative risks were 0.95 for 1 cup of coffee, 0.77 for 2 cups of coffee, and 0.72 for 3 or more cups of coffee per day. The universal

TABLE 4. *Acute studies of caffeine in asthma*

Study	Subjects	Dose of caffeine	Outcome	Remarks
Gong 1986 (44)	9 asthmatic subjects, double blind, randomized crossover	dose response to . 2, 2.5, 5.6, 7.2 mg/kg on different days; 200 mg aminophylline on separate day	spirometry, specific conductors, peak increase in FEV_1 at 45 minutes post maximum dose of caffeine	maximum caffeine dose 40% of aminophylline dose
Bukowskyj 1987 (45)	8 asthmatic subjects, randomized, double blind crossover	placebo or 5 mg/kg of caffeine; blood caffeine levels up to 8 mg	spirometry, peak increase at 1.5 hours	
Collacone 1990 (46)	10 adult asthmatics, randomized, double blind crossover	placebo vs. 5 mg/kg of caffeine; blood caffeine levels 105 minutes past ingestion	PC_{20} histamine after caffeine = 2.65 mg/ml; not significantly different	caffeine decreased airway responsiveness minimally; no correlation with caffeine levels
Crivelli 1986 (47)	7 adult asthmatics, randomized, double blind	placebo vs. 6 mg/kg of caffeine	carbachol inhalation challenge	no effect of caffeine on airway responsiveness
Becker 1994 (48)	23 asthmatic subjects aged 8 to 18, randomized, double blind	10 mg/kg caffeine (n=13) vs. 5 mg/kg theophylline (n=10); blood levels	spirometry significant improvement from baseline in both groups	caffeine = theophylline
Kivity 1990 (49)	10 adult asthmatics, randomized, double blindcrossover	caffeine two doses 3.5 mg/kg and 7.0 mg/kg vs. placebo	spirometry after exercise; maximal blood levels 2 hours for both	caffeine only effective at higher 7 mg/kg dose
Henderson 1993 (50)	8 adult asthmatics, randomized, double blind	caffeine 5 mg/kg vs. placebo	PC_{20} histamine; caffeine 0.99 mg/mL, placebo 0.53 mg/mL	small but statistically significant effect on PC_{20}

FEV_1, forced expiratory volume in one second.

relationship between coffee drinking and asthma was not significantly affected by age. Schwartz and Weiss (52) also examined the relationship between coffee and asthma occurrence using data from NHANES II. Subjects who drank coffee on a regular basis had a 29% reduction in the odds of having current asthma symptoms (odds ratio 0.71; 95% confidence interval 0.55 to 0.93) when compared with noncoffee drinkers. The effect exhibited a significant dose-response relationship with the number of cups of coffee consumed per day being inversely related to asthma prevalence (Fig. 1). The relationship was independent of age, gender, and cigarette smoking. In summary, there appears to be clear evidence that coffee drinking does have beneficial effects on asthma and asthma symptoms.

Alcohol

Virtually nothing is known about the relationship of alcohol ingestion to asthma. Alcohol can decrease superoxide production from neutrophils, but the relevance of this finding to clinical asthma is unknown (53). Clark and Ayres (54) studied 168 asthmatic outpatients and found that 32% reported that alcohol tended to worsen their symptoms and that they began wheezing when they drank alcoholic beverages. However, another 22% of patients said that alcohol intake actually made their asthma symptoms better. These latter patients were more likely the older subjects with more severe asthma. Deficiencies of this study relate to the lack of a control group and ob-

server bias with regard to symptoms. There is controversy as to whether alcohol acts as a bronchodilator or as a bronchoconstrictor (55). At the present time there is no clear evidence that alcohol intake in moderation has any effect on asthma or airway responsiveness.

N3-N6 Fatty Acids

Horrobin (56) hypothesized that the low prevalence of asthma among Greenland Eskimos was due to their high intake of eicosapentaenoic acid (EPA).

These Omega 3 fatty acids are essential for cell membranes. N_3 and N_6 fatty acids are believed to shunt the eicosinoid production away from the arachidonic acid pathway and toward the prostanoic pathway, thus decreasing the production of bronchoconstrictive leukotrienes (see Chapter 40). *In vitro* studies and studies of small groups of human asthmatic subjects supplemented with doses of EPA show that the generation of leukotrienes by neutrophils and mononuclear leukocytes was decreased by EPA supplements in the diet (57). These results stimulated a small number of short-term clinical trials examining the effect of EPA on asthma. These results are summarized in Table 5 (58–61). Although the doses were quite large, the duration of the studies was relatively short, with only one study being as long as 6 months. No effect was seen in any study of changes in airway responsiveness, symptoms, spirometry, or improvement in seasonal or late-phase reaction symptoms. Empirically, one study was able to demonstrate a

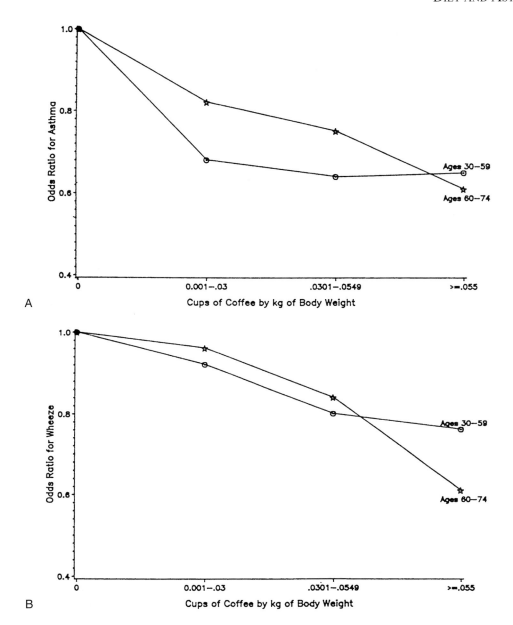

FIG. 1. Odds ratios for the relationship between cups of coffee consumed per kilogram of body weight and the presence of current asthma (**A**) and the frequent wheeze (**B**). Subjects 30 to 59 years old are depicted by open circles and subjects 60 to 74 years old are depicted by stars. (From Schwartz J, Weiss ST. Caffeine intake and asthma symptoms. *Ann Epidemiol* 1992;2:627–635, with permission.)

50% inhibition of leukotriene D4 and D5. Recently Dry and Vincent (62) studied a group of asthmatic patients in which 1 gram of Omega 3 fatty acids was given for one year and found a consistent mild increase in FEV_1 at the end of 9 months.

Schwartz and Weiss (63) reported on the relationship of dietary fish intake to level of pulmonary function in the NHANES I. In this investigation, in which over 30,000 individuals, representative of the United States population, were studied, there was about an 80 mL in FEV_1 difference between subjects who regularly con-

sumed fish vs. those who did not. This analysis controlled for age, race, gender, and smoking, but did not effectively control for social class. In addition, the analysis was cross-sectional; it is unlikely, however, that subjects knew of the fish-pulmonary function association. No specific analysis was done to look at asthmatics.

Two separate studies in Australian children support the protective association of fish oil and asthma. Peat and co-workers (64) included a question about fish intake in one of the four communities studied as part of a general epidemiological survey of asthma risk factors. Regular fish

TABLE 5. *Clinical trials of eicosapentanenoic acid in asthma*

Study	Population	Dose	Duration	Outcome	Comment
Kirsch 1988 (58)	12 asthmatics	Low dose .1g/d; High dose 4.0 g/d	8 weeks	symptoms, spirometry	no effect
Arm 1988 (59)	20 asthmatics	3.2 g/d	10 weeks	neutrophil, fatty acids	50% inhibition of LTB; clinical parameters unchanged
Thien 1993 (60)	37 asthmatics	3.2 g/d	6 months	symptoms, airway responsiveness to histamine	no change in airway responsiveness with allergen season
Thien 1992 (61)	16 atopic subjects	3.2 g	10 weeks	airway responsiveness, late-phase skin reaction	no effect on late-phase skin reaction

LTB, leukotriene B_4.

intake was associated with an 8% prevalence of bronchial hyperresponsiveness (defined as a demonstrable PD_{20} to histamine at 3.9umoles) compared to a 16.2% prevalence in nonfish eaters. This report did not differentiate type of fish intake or adjust for social class. In a subsequent report, however, these investigators utilized a validated food frequency questionnaire on 574 randomly selected children (65). After adjusting for a variety of co-variates children whose parents reported eating fresh oily fish had significantly less asthma (odds ratio 0.26, 95%CI 0.09-0.72, p <0.01).

Recently, Shahar et al. (66) reported on the relationship of N_3 polyunsaturated fatty acids to various parameters of chronic obstructive lung disease. The population studied were 8,960 subjects who had ever smoked cigarettes and who had participated in the atherosclerosis risk in community study (ARIC). These subjects were between the ages of 45 and 64 years of age, and living in four U.S. communities: Forsythe County, Jackson, MI; Minneapolis, MN; and Washington County, MD. The analysis was restricted to cigarette smokers, although no clear justification for why this was done was given in the paper. Both fish consumption and N_3 fatty acid consumption, as determined by a food frequency questionnaire, were related to doctors' diagnoses of emphysema and chronic bronchitis and spirometrically detected chronic obstructive pulmonary disease (COPD). Using any of the three COPD definitions, there seemed to be a consistent dose-response relationship between fish intake and COPD risk. Level of education, pack years of smoking, age, race, gender, height, and weight were all considered in the regression analysis. Compared to the lowest quartile of fish-intake dose, the highest quartile subjects had 0.59 risk of developing COPD (95% confidence interval 0.46 to 0.75).

In summary, current data on the relationship of N_3 and N_6 fatty acids to asthma are unclear. Short-term randomized controlled trials clearly show no effect. One longer term randomized controlled trial in established disease demonstrates a minimal benefit in terms of FEV_1. Population-based studies suggest that fish intake may have a slight effect on FEV_1 level, but it is unclear whether this is simply a function of inadequate control for confounding variables, such as social class and income. Finally, although there is one study which demonstrates the relationship of N_3 fatty acids to COPD, the study eliminated all nonsmokers and focused only on individuals who smoked (66). A full analysis of this cohort data and the relationship of fish oil to COPD is not available. Although biologically plausible and worthy of further study, it appears that fish oil is only one of many dietary factors that may be related to asthma occurrence.

URINARY CATIONS, SODIUM POTASSIUM AND MAGNESIUM

Sodium/Potassium

Sodium and potassium are cations that influence the electrical potential across epithelial cell membranes and, as such, may affect cellular permeability and depolarization. These effects may influence cellular response to inflammation and airway responsiveness, a central feature of asthma.

Few areas in the relationship of diet to asthma are as confusing and as complex as the relationship of sodium and potassium to asthma. These studies are summarized in Table 6. In 1986, Burney (67) hypothesized, on the basis of ecological data, that salt intake might be related to asthma. Following this initial report, Burney conducted an observational study examining urinary sodium excretion and its relationship to inhaled histamine among asthmatic patients, and found a significant relationship (68). This report was followed by a paper by Javaid et al. (69), in which a small number of asthmatic subjects were followed for 1 month in a randomized controlled trial; again, PC_{20} to histamine increased with increased sodium intake. Medici et al. (70) performed a similar study on 14 asthmatics using a randomized controlled trial over a 9-

TABLE 6. *Studies on Na+/K+ and their relationship to asthma/airway reactivity*

Study	Population	Measure of Na/K	Duration	Outcome	Comment
Javaid 1988 (69)	10 asthmatics, 6 male, 4 female	(2) 24-hour urines; only Na average taken; K not examined	1 month	histamine challenge test	significant increase in PC_{20}
Burney 1989 (71)	201 asthmatics, ages 7 to 54	randomized trial of low salt vs. high fiber diet; K not examined	1, 2, 3 months	daily variation	15.6% improvement in diurnal peak flow in low salt group
Medici 1993 (70)	14 asthmatics	randomized trial of salt restriction and salt loading vs. placebo	3, 6, 9 weeks	symptoms, lung function, PD_{20} methacholine	worsening of symptoms with salt loading; no effect on PD_{20}
Pistelli 1993 (75)	2,593 subjects, ages 9 to 16; low asthma prevalence but 38% positive methacholine test	questionnaire about excessive salt use; untimed urine sample in A.M	retrospective	symptoms, PD_{20} methacholine	symptoms related to personal table salt by questionnaire in boys; PD_{20} related to urinary excretion of K
Carey 1993 (72)	22 asthma patients	randomized double blind placebo controlled trial; high vs. low Na diet	5 weeks	symptoms, peak flow, bronchodilator use	improvement in all parameters on low Na
Sparrow 1991 (74)	273 subjects; low asthma prevalence (4%)	24-hour urine Na/K	retrospective	airway responsiveness	no relationship to Na; positive relationship to K, older subjects
Britton 1994 (76)	1,702 adults, aged 18 to 70	24-hour urine Na/K	retrospective	airway responsiveness	no relationship of responsiveness to Na

week period, comparing salt loading to placebo, and found a worsening of symptoms with salt loading, but no effect on PD_{20} to methacholine. Burney et al. (71) subsequently performed a large randomized controlled trial of a low sodium diet vs. a high fiber diet in 201 asthmatics, followed at 1, 2, and 3 months, looking at daily variation in peak flow as the outcome. He found that there was a 15% improvement in diurnal peak flow in the low salt group. It is important to note that all of these studies were performed in asthmatic patients. A similar randomized controlled trial was done by Carey and co-workers (72) in which 22 asthmatic patients were randomized, either to high or low sodium diet, in a double-blind placebo-controlled trial that lasted 5 weeks. Symptoms, peak flow, and bronchodilator use were the outcomes of the study. There was an improvement in all parameters on the low sodium diet. Lieberman and Heimer (73) were the only investigators to find no effects of dietary sodium on asthma severity. They studied 17 adult asthma patients and changed their dietary sodium over a 3-week period and found no relationship to peak flow variables.

In summary, short-term randomized controlled trials consistently demonstrate a relationship between salt intake and a variety of parameters of asthma functioning. The population based data are, however, less convincing. In 1991, Sparrow and co-workers (74) studied 273 subjects in the Normative Aging Study. The mean age of

these subjects was 60 years, and the prevalence of asthma was low. Twenty-four-hour urine sodium potassium was related to methacholine airway responsiveness, and there was no significant relationship for sodium, although there was a positive relationship to an increased airway responsiveness in higher urinary potassium. Pistelli et al. (75) studied 2,593 subjects between the ages of 9 and 16 in Italy. There were questions about personal salt use and untimed A.M. urine sample was obtained. Outcomes were symptoms and PD_{20} to methacholine. Symptoms were related to personal salt use by questionnaire in boys only, and the PD_{20} was not related to salt use, but to urinary excretion of potassium. In 1994, Britton et al. (76) studied 1,702 adults aged 18 to 70 in Nottingham, England, with a 24-hour urine for sodium and potassium. Airway responsiveness to sodium was observed. However, there was a weak relationship between sodium in the urine and skin test reactivity. It is important to consider potential mechanisms by which sodium might be involved in increasing airway responsiveness in asthma.

Tribe and co-workers (77) examined this issue and found that incubation of human leukocytes in serum from men with hyperresponsive airways leads to an increase in intracellular sodium level, probably, in part, through increased sodium influx into cells (77). This influx is independent of sodium chloride co-transport and sodium hydrogen ion exchange. It is also independent of serum IgE and of dietary sodium levels. Dietary sodium, as measured by urinary sodium excretion, had additional independent effects on airway responsiveness in these studies. This study did not measure sodium potassium adenosine triphospherate (ATPase) activity directly and, hence, cannot definitively answer the questions related to mechanisms of this physiologic effect. A series of studies has demonstrated that furosemide is an effective treatment for asthma, again supporting the idea that excess sodium may be an important determinant of airway responsiveness (78).

There is a striking difference in result between the clinical studies and the epidemiologic investigations. It should be noted that a single 24-hour urine is a very insensitive method for reflecting chronic dietary sodium intake. There is substantial within-person variability with regard to sodium intake, and a food frequency questionnaire is not optimal to assess dietary sodium. Low power may also be a problem, since most of the epidemiologic studies are relatively small. Finally, there may be negative confounding by other cationic variables, such as potassium and/or magnesium (see following). Other possible explanations include the fact that bronchial responsiveness has been linked to increased sodium/potassium ATPase activity in animal models, as well as the increased extracellular potassium in smooth muscle contraction (79,80). Control of potassium homeostasis is through the adrenergic system. This control is impaired in asthmatic subjects. High levels of potassium in those subjects with increased airway responsiveness to methacholine may simply reflect this abnormal adrenergic control. This then would be a consequence, rather than a cause, of the problem. Additional complicating factor beside low power and negative confounding is the possibility that other dietary constituents could influence these relationships. Urinary and dietary sodium are known to be linked to dietary fat intake and antioxidant intake may also affect transport of anions across cell membranes.

Magnesium

Magnesium is an essential divalent cation that is responsible for maintenance of electrical potential across cell membranes and, therefore, bronchomotor tone. Additional biologic functions of magnesium include its role as an essential cofactor and ATP requiring enzymes (81). Finally, magnesium is involved in deoxyribonucleic acid (DNA) and ribonucleic acid (RNA) synthesis and replication. On a functional level, magnesium can relax airway smooth muscle *in vitro* (82). Magnesium can also inhibit cholinergic neuromuscular transmission and stabilize mast cell membranes to prevent the release of histamine (83). Excess magnesium will block and magnesium deficiency will potentiate the actions of calcium (84). Magnesium is involved in the physiologic regulation of calcium influx through cell membranes, and, therefore, excess or deficiency will influence sodium and potassium metabolism. Finally, magnesium can influence the stabilization of mast cells and stimulate the generation of prostacyclin and nitric oxide (85–87). Magnesium in the diet is obtained principally from green vegetables, unprocessed grains, and dairy products. Magnesium is leeched from food during the cooking process; therefore, refined or processed foods are likely to be lower in magnesium. Animal studies have suggested that magnesium deficiency may potentiate histamine release in animals exposed to antigen (88).

There are a large number of acute studies that have examined the effect of infused magnesium sulfate ($MgSO_4$) on asthmatic patients. These studies are summarized in Table 7 (89–100). The earliest report was in 1940 when Haury (89) showed that approximately one-half of asthma patients having acute attacks had low serum magnesium levels. There is no statistically significant difference in magnesium levels in subjects with acute attacks between those who had low levels and those who did not. However, two patients did respond dramatically to magnesium infusion. Okayama (101) studied 10 asthmatic patients with mild asthma attacks. He performed a randomized controlled trial in which five patients received 0.5 umol per minute of $MgSO_4$ over 20 minutes. In the time course, changes in spirometry and airway resistance were studied. In another five patients, dose-response curves to $MgSO_4$ were performed. He found that there is a dose-response relationship between infused magnesium and the relief of bronchoconstriction. Maximum responses occurred after 20 minutes, although magnesium concentrations in serum increased over 24 hours. Maximum responses were 117% for FVC and 118% for FEV_1. Symptoms of shortness of breath also improved. Despite these acute effects on physiologic parameters, the role in improving clinical outcomes is less clear. Although most emergency room reports have demonstrated transient benefit from the use of infused magnesium in acute exacerbations of asthma, the magnitude of the change has been relatively small, the benefits have been temporary, and the results have been difficult to separate from the effects of other treatments. Finally, most emergency room studies have failed to demonstrate improvements in differences in hospitalization rates or repeat emergency room visit rates in those given i.v. magnesium in the emergency room. One of the largest studies was a prospective study involving 120 asthmatics in the emergency room who received 2 g of $MgSO_4$ intravenously, in addition to standard therapy. No difference in symptoms or need for hospitalization was observed (95). In a smaller double-blind placebo control trial of 48 asthmatics, Tiffany et al. (96) showed that 2 g of $MgSO_4$ as a bolus or continuous infusion over 4 hours resulted in no significant improvement in FEV_1 or peak flow compared to placebo. Taken together, these acute studies demonstrate

TABLE 7. *Magnesium for acute asthma episodes*

Study	Population	Magnesium dose	Outcome	Comment
Green 1992 (95)	120 adult asthmatics 18 to 65, randomized controlled trial	2 g i.v. plus standard care vs standard care	hospitalization, duration of ER treatment	no significant effects
Tiffany 1993 (96)	48 adult asthmatics , 18 to 60 randomized controlled trial	2 g i.v. plus standard care vs standard. care	PEFR, FEV_1	no significant effect up to 260 minutes
Hoppen 1990 (94)	6 adult asthmatics admitted to hospital, randomized	3 g i.v.	FEV_1	significant improvement
Chande 1992 (97)	10 adult asthmatics 21 to 37 with stable asthma given methacholine than magnesium, randomized	2 g i.v. vs. saline vs. albuterol	FEV_1	magnesium had no effect
Kuitert 1991 (93)	case report, 56-year-old woman	2.46 g i.v. over 20 minutes	↓$PaCO_2$, ↓tidal volume	improved
Haury 1940 (89)	66 asthma patients, 40 normal subjects	magnesium levels in serum	difference in serum levels	no difference
Bloch 1995 (100)	135 adult asthmatics 18 to 65 with acute exacerbation, randomized controlled trial	2 g i.v. vs. placebo	hospital admission rate, FEV_1	decrease in admission, no effect on FEV_1
Rolla 1987 (98)	16 adults and children with asthma 8 to 41, stable patients, randomized controlled trial	2 g i.v. following methacholine vs. saline	FEV_1, change in PD_{20}	significant improvement
Skobaloff 1989 (91)	38 adult asthmatics, randomized controlled trial of treatment in acute exacerbation	1.2 g i.v. plus standard care vs. placebo plus standard care	peak flow, hospital admission	significant improvement in both outcomes
Rolla 1988 (90)	9 asthmatics 12 to 52, stable, randomized controlled trial	inhaled magnesium 0.10-0.80 mmol	FEV_1, methacholine	significant improvement in methacholine challenge
Rolla 1988 (92)	10 adult asthma patients, randomized, double blind crossover	2 g	FEV_1	significant but small improvement in FEV_1
Falkner 1992 (99)	23 asthmatics, 15 controls	none; simply measured serum levels	—	no significant difference

i.v., intravenous; ER, emergency room; PEFR, peak expiratory flow rate; FEV_1, forced expiratory volume in one second; $PaCo_2$, partial pressure of carbon dioxide in arterial gas.

no conclusive benefit to short-term infusion of magnesium in acute asthma attacks or in the emergency room setting. They do confirm that magnesium deficiency might result in long-term effects with regard to asthma outcomes. Bernstein and co-workers performed a randomized placebo-control crossover study of intravenous magnesium for chronic stable asthma. No difference was observed between asthmatic and nonasthmatic subjects with regard to FEV_1, FVC, or forced expiratory flow between 25% and 75% of vital capacity (FEF_{25-75}) (102).

Britton and co-workers (103) investigated the effect of dietary magnesium in their population-based study of diet and asthma (103). They studied 2,633 adults aged 18 to 70 from the general area of Nottingham, England, with a food frequency questionnaire to measure dietary magnesium intake and examined its relationship to FEV_1 airway reactivity to methacholine and self-report of wheeze in the past 12 months. One hundred mg per day or higher magnesium intake was associated with a higher FEV_1 (95% confidence interval 11.9 to 43.5) (Fig. 2), and a reduction in the relative odds of airway hyperresponsiveness of 0.82 (95% confidence intervals 0.72 to 0.93) (Fig. 3). The same 100 mg increase in dietary magnesium was associated with a reduction in wheeze symptoms (odds ratio 0.85, 95% confidence intervals 0.76 to 0.95). These analyses were adjusted for age, gender, height, effects of atopy and cigarette smoking, and caloric intake. Although a cross-sectional study, the consistency of these results is quite striking. In

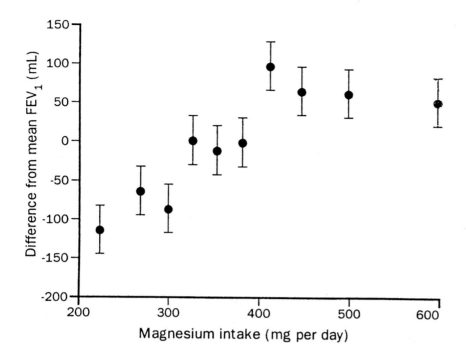

FIG. 2. Mean (SE) difference in FEV$_1$ from the mean expected population value in mL. Adjusted for age, gender, height, skin wheal diameter, and pack-years smoking, by midpoints of deciles of magnesium intake in mg/day. (From Britton J, Pavord I, Wisniewski A, Knox A, Lewis S, Tattersfield A, Weiss S. Dietary magnesium, lung function, wheezing, and airway hyperreactivity in a random adult population. *Lancet* 1994; 344:357–362, with permission.)

other words, not only was dietary magnesium intake associated with a decrease in symptoms, it was also associated with improved lung function and decreased airway reactivity. These findings need to be replicated in a longitudinal study. Britton speculates that the interrelationship of magnesium with potassium and sodium may mean that low levels of dietary magnesium could potentially confound or confuse an interrelationship of sodium or potassium with asthma or airway responsiveness. This hypothesis will require further investigation.

Breast Feeding

Despite multiple studies, the role of breast feeding in the prevention of asthma remains controversial. As many studies reject as support the role of breast feeding in the prevention of atopic sensitization (104). The theoretical benefits of breast milk derive from the transfer of maternal antibody which, thus, protects the infant from bacterial and viral illnesses. Most importantly, infants who are breast fed markedly reduce their ingestion of foreign pro-

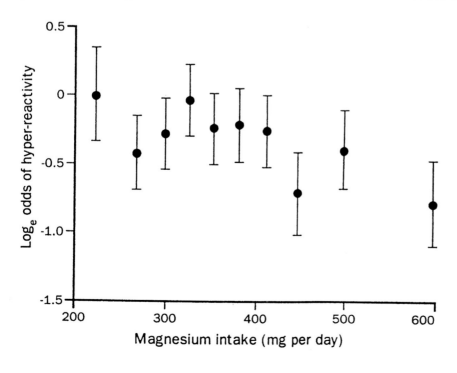

FIG. 3. Natural log odds ratios and standard errors for hyperreactivity to methacholine. Adjusted for age, gender, skin wheal diameter, and pack-years smoking history, by midpoints of declines of magnesium intake. (From Britton J, Pavord I, Wisniewski A, Knox A, Lewis S, Tattersfield A, Weiss S. Dietary magnesium, lung function, wheezing, and airway hyperreactivity in a random adult population. *Lancet* 1994; 344:357–362, with permission.)

teins that may be sensitizing, namely cow's milk. The lack of benefit of breast feeding may relate, in part, to a reconsideration of the relative role and importance of infection in the pathogenesis of asthma in early life, and the recognition that breast milk can be contaminated with foreign proteins via the maternal diet which can be sensitizing to the fetus. In addition to these immunologic issues, controlled trials of breast feeding in allergic sensitization can be criticized for a variety of methodologic reasons including inadequate duration of breast feeding, lack of control of maternal diet, small sample size, inadequate duration, early introduction of solid foods, and inadequate control of other co-variates known to influence sensitization and asthma.

Recent studies suggest that further research on breast feeding and its role in asthma may be beneficial. Wright and co-workers (105) reported on the effect of breast feeding on recurrent wheezing at age 6 years in the Tuscon Birth cohort. A total of 988 children were followed for 6 years, breast feeding was unrelated to serum IgE levels or to skin test reactivity and was protective against wheezing but only in the nonatopic children OR=3.03, 95%CI=1.06 to 8.69). These data suggest that breast feeding may interact with genetic risk in a complex manner. Recently, three clinical trials have examined breast feeding and its influence on the development of allergic disorders of infancy, namely allergy, eczema, and asthma (106–108). The studies followed the children of atopic mothers for a variable length of time from 1 to 2 years. In all studies there was no reduction in the incidence of inhalational allergies or asthma. These studies limited maternal food allergen exposure, controlled for other covariates and had adequate sample size to detect small benefits, thus, eliminating some of the criticisms of earlier studies. Despite the methodologic advantages of these three trials, the results were still negative. Further work will obviously be necessary to determine future directions for research in this area.

CONCLUSIONS

The study of diet as a risk factor and a potential modifier of the effect of other environmental exposures on asthma is in its infancy. To date, the number of large scale epidemiologic investigations is small, most are cross-sectional, and most are focused on adults. It would appear that, based on existing data, the relationship of Vitamin C to asthma and selenium to asthma is on the strongest methodologic ground. What appears to be needed are prospective investigations in children, particularly children between birth and age 10. It is estimated that over one-half of all asthma cases are diagnosed by age 6; therefore, to truly identify the role of dietary factors in the development of asthma would appear to require studies that focus on younger subjects. This will require the use of serum levels to measure exposure or new methodologic developments to assess dietary intake in children, since the food frequency approach has not been validated for children this young. Taken as a whole, the existing data are sufficiently suggestive of important associations, and that this is an area that will demand further investigation in the future.

REFERENCES

1. Hill AB. The environment and disease: association and causation? *Proc R Soc Med* 1965;58:295–300.
2. Barbor TF, Stephens RS, Marlett GA. Verbal report methods in clinical research on alcoholism: response bias and its minimization. *J Studies on Alcohol* 1987;48:410–424.
3. Roidt L, White E, Goodman GE, Wahl PW, Owenn GS, Rollins B, Karkeck JM. Association of food frequency questionnaire estimates of Vitamin A intake with serum Vitamin A levels. *Am J Epidemiol* 1988;128:645–654.
4. Sidney S, Caan BJ, Friedman GD. Intake of carotene in nonsmokers with and without passive smokers in the house. *Am J Epidemiol* 1989;129:1305–1309.
5. Richards GA, Theron AJ, Van Rensburg CSJ, Van Rensburg AJ, Van Der Merwe CA, Kuyl JM, Anderson P. Investigation of the effects of oral administration of Vitamin E and Beta Carotene on the chemiclum in essence responses and the frequency of sister chromatial exchanges in circulating leukocytes from cigarette smokers. *Am J Respir Dis* 1990;142:648–654.
6. Morabia A, Sorenson A, Kumenyika SK, Abbey H, Cohen BH, Chee E. Vitamin A, cigarette smoking, and airway obstruction. *Am J Respir Dis* 1989;140:1312–1313.
7. Bieri JG, Corash L, Hubbard US. Medical uses of Vitamin E. *N Engl J Med* 1983;308:1063–1071.
8. Sato S, Kawakami M, Maeda S, Takishima T. Scanning electron microscopy of the lungs of vitamin E-deficient rats exposed to a low concentration of ozone. *Am Rev Respir Dis* 1976;113:809–821.
9. Fulton M, Thomson M, Elton RA, Brown S, Wood DA, Oliver MF. Cigarette smoking, social class and nutrient intake: relevance to coronary heart disease. *Eur J Clin Nutr* 1988;42:797–803.
10. Miedema I, Feskens EJM, Heederik D, Kromhout D. Dietary determinants of long term incidence of chronic nonspecific lung disease. *Am J Epidemiol* 1993;138:37–45.
11. Troisi RJ, Willet WC, Weiss ST, Trichopoulos D, Rosner B, Speizer FE. A prospective study of diet and adult onset asthma. *Am J Respir Crit Care Med* 1995;151:1401–1408.
12. Britton JR, Pavord ID, Richards KA, et al. Dietary antioxidant vitamin intake and lung function in the general population. *Am J Respir Crit Care Med* 1995;151:1383–1387.
13. Anderson R, Theron AJ, Ras GJ. Regulation by the antioxidants ascorbate, cysteine, and dapsone of the increased extracellular and intracellular generation of reactive oxidants by activated phagocytes from cigarette smokers. *Am Rev Respir Dis* 1987;135:1027–1032.
14. Levine M. New concepts in the biology and biochemistry of ascorbic acid. *N Engl J Med* 1986;314:892–902.
15. Washko P, Rotrosen D, Levine M. Ascorbic acid transport and accumulation in human neutrophils. *J Biol Chem* 1989;204:18996–19002.
16. Bergsten P, Amitai G, Kehrl J, Dhairwal DR, Klein A, Levine M. Millimolar concentrations of ascorbic acid in purified human nonnuclear leukocytes: depletion and reaccumulation. *J Biol Chem* 1990;265:2584–2587.
17. Schechtman G, Byrd JC, Grudow HW. The influence of smoking on Vitamin C status in adults. *Am J Public Health* 1989;79:158–162.
18. Burr ML, Elwood PC, Hole DJ, Hurley RJ, Hughes RE. Plasma and leukocyte ascorbic acid levels in the elderly. *Am J Clin Nutr* 1974;27:144–151.
19. Kallner AB, Hartmann D, Hornig DH. On the requirements of ascorbic acid in man: steady-state turnover and body pool in smokers. *Am J Clin Nutr* 1981;34:1347–1355.
20. Willett WC, Reynolds RD, Cottrell-Hoehner S, Sampson L, Browne ML. Validation of a semiquantitative food frequency questionnaire:

comparison with a 1-year diet record. *J Am Diet Assoc* 1987;87: 43–47.

21. Strachan DP, Cox BD, Erzinclioglu SW, Walters DE, Whichelow MJ. Ventilatory function and winter fresh fruit consumption in a random sample of British adults. *Thorax* 1991;46:624–629.

22. Schwartz J, Weiss ST. Dietary factors and their relationship to respiratory symptoms: NHANESII. *Am J Epidemiol* 1990;132:67–76.

23. Mohsenin V, DuBois AB, Douglas JS. Effect of ascorbic acid on response to methacholine challenge in asthmatic subjects. *Am Rev Respir Dis* 1983;127:143–147.

24. Ogilvy CS, DuBois AB, Douglas JS. Effect of ascorbic acid and indomethacin on the airways of healthy male subjects with and without induced bronchoconstriction. *J Allergy Clin Immunol* 1981;67: 363–369.

25. Zuskin E, Lewis AJ, Bouhays A. Inhibition of histamine induced airway constriction by ascorbic acid. *J Allergy Clin Immunol* 1973; 51:218–226.

26. Ting S, Mansfield LE, Yarborough J. Effects of ascorbic acid on pulmonary functions in mild asthma. *J Asthma* 1983;20:39–42.

27. Malo JL, Cartier A, Pineau L, Archevêque J, Ghezzo H, Martin RR. Lack of effects of asorbic acid on spirometry and airway responsiveness to histamine in subjects with asthma. *J Allergy Clin Immunol* 1986;78:453–458.

28. Schachter EN, Schlesinger A. The attenuation of exercise induced bronchospasm by ascorbic acid. *Ann Allergy* 1982;49:146–151.

29. Hunt HB. Ascorbic acid in bronchial asthma. *B Med J* 1938;1:726.

30. Bucca C, Rolla G, Caria E, Arossa W, Bugioni M. Effects of Vitamin C on airway responsiveness to inhaled histamine in heavy smokers. *Eur Respir J* 1989;2:229–233.

31. Anderson R, Hay I, Van Wyk HA, Theran A. Ascorbic acid in bronchial asthma. *SA Med J* 1983;63:649–652.

32. Anderson R, Hay I, Van Wyk H, Oosthuizen R, Theron A. The effect of ascorbate on cellular humoral immunity in asthmatic children. *S Afr Med J* 1980;58:974–977.

33. Solousi SO, Ojutiku OO, Jessop WJE, Iboko MI. Plasma and white blood cell ascorbic acid concentrations in patients with bronchial asthma. *Chemica Acta* 1979;92:161–166.

34. Schwartz J, Weiss ST. The relationship of dietary vitamin C intake to level of pulmonary function in the First National Health and Nutrition Survey (NHANES I). *Am J Clin Nutr* 1994;59:110–114.

35. Reynolds RD, Natta CL. Depressed plasma pynidoxal phosphate concentrations in adult asthmatics. *Am J Clin Nutr* 1985;41:684–688.

36. Burk RF. Biological activity of selenium. *Ann Rev Nutr* 1983;3: 53–70.

37. Flatt A, Pearce N, Thompson CD, Sears MR, Robinson MF, Beasley R. Reduced selenium in asthmatic subjects in New Zealand. *Thorax* 1989;1990;45:95–99.

38. Hasselmark L. Malmgren R, Unge G, Zetterstrom O. Lowered platelet glutathione peroxidase activity in patients with intrinsic asthma. *Allergy* 1990;45:523–527.

39. Hasselmark L, Malmgren R, Zetterstrom O, Unge G. Selenium supplementation in intrinsic asthma. *Allergy* 1993;48:30–36.

40. Bibi H, Schlesinger M, Tabachnick E, Schwartz Y, Iscovitz H, Iaina A. Erythrocyte glutathione peroxidase activity in asthmatic children. *Ann Allergy* 1988;61:339–340.

41. Pearson DJ, Suarez-Mandez VJ, Day JP, Miller PF. Selenium status in relation to reduced glutathione peroxidase activity in aspirin sensitive asthma. *Clin Exp Allergy* 1991;21:203–208.

42. Stone J, Hinks LJ, Beasley R, Holgate ST, Clayton BA. Reduced selenium status of patients with asthma. *Clin Sci* 1989;77:495–500.

43. Shaw R, Woodman K, Crane J, Moyes C, Kennedy J, Pearce N. Risk factors for asthma symptoms in Kawaeran children. *N Z Med J* 1994; 107:387–391.

44. Gong H, Simmons MS, Tashkin DP, Hui KK, Lee EY. Bronchodilator effects of caffeine in coffee. *Chest* 1986;89:335–342.

45. Bukowskyj M, Nakatsu K. The bronchodilator effect of caffeine in adult asthmatics. *Am Rev Respir Dis* 1987;135:173–175.

46. Collacone A, Bertolo L, Wolkone N, Cohen C, Kreisman H. Effect of caffeine on histamine bronchoprovocation in asthma. *Thorax* 1990; 45:630–632.

47. Crivelli M, Wahlländer A, Jost G, Preisig R, Bachofen H. Effect of dietary caffeine on airway reactivity in asthma. *Respiration* 1986;50: 258–264.

48. Becker AB, Simons KJ, Gillepsie CA, Simons FE. The bronchodila-

tor effects and pharmacokinetics of caffeine in asthma. *N Engl J Med* 1984;310:743–746.

49. Kivity S, Ben Aheron Y, Mon A, Topilsky M. The effect of caffeine on exercise induced bronchoconstriction. *Chest* 1990;97:1083–1085.

50. Henderson JC, O'Connell F, Fuller RW. Decrease of histamine induced bronchoconstriction by caffeine in mild asthma. *Thorax* 1993; 48:824–826.

51. Pagano R, Negri E, Decarli A, LaVecchia C. Coffee drinking and prevalence of asthma. *Chest* 1988;94:386–389.

52. Schwartz J, Weiss ST. Caffeine intake and asthma symptoms. *Ann Epidemiol* 1992;2:627–635.

53. Sadis CW, Christensen RH, Pratt PC, Lynn WS. Neutrophil elastase activity and superoxide production are diminished in neutrophils of alcoholics. *Am Rev Respir Dis* 1990;141:1249–1255.

54. Ayers JG, Clark TJH. Alcohol and asthma. *Br J Dis Chest* 1983; 77:370–375.

55. Gong H, Tashkin DP, Calorese BM. Alcohol induced bronchospasm in an asthmatic patient: evaluation of the mechanism. *Chest* 1981;80: 167–173.

56. Horrobin DF. Low prevalences of coronary heart disease (CHD), boriasis, asthma, and rheumatoid arthritis in Eskimos: are they caused by high dietary intake of eicosapentaenaic acid (EPA), a genetic variation of essential fatty acid (EFA), metabolism, or a combination of both? *Medical Hypotheses* 1987;22:421–428.

57. Payon DG, Wong MY, Chernou-Rogan T, et al. Alterations in human leukocyte function induced by ingestion of eicosapentaenaic acid. *J Clin Immunol* 1986;6:402–410.

58. Kirsch CM, Payan DG, Wong MYS, et al. Effect of eicosapentaenaic acid in asthma. *Clin Allergy* 1988;18:177–187.

59. Arm JP, Horton CE, Mencia-Huerta JM, et al. Effect of dietary supplementation with fish oil lipids on mild asthma. *Thorax* 1988;43:84–92.

60. Thien FCK, Mencia-Huerta JM, Lee TH. Dietary fish oil effects on seasonal hay fever and asthma in pollen sensitive subjects. *Am Rev Respir Dis* 1993;147:1138–1143.

61. Thien FCK, Atkinson BA, Khan A, Mencia-Huerta JM, Lee TH. Effect of dietary fish oil supplementation on the antigen induced late phase response in the skin. *J Allergy Clin Immunol* 1992;89:829–835.

62. Dry J, Vincent D. Interest of fish oil in asthma: results of a one year double blind study. *Int Arch Allergy Appl Immunol* 1991;95:156–157.

63. Schwartz J, Weiss ST. The relationship of dietary fish intake to level of pulmonary function in the First National Health and Nutrition Examination Survey (NHANES I). *Eur Respir J* 1994;7:1821–1824.

64. Peat JK, Salome CM, Woolcock AJ. Factors associated with bronchial hyperresponsiveness in Australian adults and children. *Eur Respir J* 1992;5:921–929.

65. Hodge L, Salome CM, Peat JK, Haby MM, Xuan W, Woolcock AJ. Consumption of oily fish and childhood asthma risk. *Med J Aust* 1996;164:137–140.

66. Shahar E, Folsom AR, Melnick SL, et al. Dietary N-3 polyunsaturated fatty acids and smoking related chronic obstructive pulmonary disease. *N Engl J Med* 1994;331:228–233.

67. Burney PGJ, Britton JR, Chinn S, et al. Response to histamine and 24-hour sodium excretion. *Br Med J Clin Res Ed* 1986;292:1483–1486.

68. Burney PGJ. A diet rich in sodium may potentiate asthma: epidemiological evidence for a new hypothesis. *Chest* 1987;91:1435–1485.

69. Javaid A, Cushley MJ, Bone MF. Effect of dietary salt on bronchial reactivity to histamine in asthma. *BMJ* 1988;297:297–454.

70. Medici TS, Schmidt AZ, Hacki M, Vetter W. Are asthmatics salt sensitive? *Chest* 1993;104:1138–1143.

71. Burney PGJ, Neild JE, Twort CHC, et al. Effect of changing dietary sodium on the airway response to histamine. *Thorax* 1989;44:36–41.

72. Carey OJ, Locke C, Cookson JB. Effect of alterations of dietary sodium on the severity of asthma in men. *Thorax* 1993;48:714–718.

73. Lieberman D, Heimer D. Effects of dietary sodium on the severity of bronchial asthma. *Thorax* 1992;47:360–362.

74. Sparrow D, O'Connor GT, Rosner B, Weiss ST. Methacholine airway responsiveness and 24-hour urine excretion of soidum and potassium. *Am Rev Respir Dis* 1991;144:722–725.

75. Pistelli R, Forastiere F, Corbo GM, et al. Respiratory symptoms and bronchial responsiveness are related to dietary salt intake and urinary potassium excretion in male children. *Eur Respir J* 1993;6:517–522.

76. Britton J, Pavord I, Richards K, et al. Dietary sodium intake and the risk of airway hyperreactivity in a random adult population. *Thorax* 1994;49:875–880.

77. Tribe RM, Barton JR, Poston L, Burney PGJ. Dietary sodium intake and cellular sodium transport. *Am J Respir Crit Care Med* 1994;149:1426–1433.

78. Lockhart A, Slutsky AS. Furosemide and loop diuretics in human asthma. *Chest* 1994;106:244–249.

79. Falliers CJ, Cardosa R, Bone H, Coffey R, Middleton E. Discordant allergic manifestations in monozygotic twins, genetic identity versus clinical and biochemical differences. *J Allergy* 1971;47:209–219.

80. Souhrada JF, Souhrada M. Significance of the sodium pump for airway smooth muscle. *Eur J Respir Dis* 1983;128:196–205.

81. Levine BS, Coburn JW. Magnesium: the mimic/antagonist of calcium. *N Engl J Med* 1984;310:1253–1255.

82. Spivey WH, Skobeloff EM, Levin RM. The effect of magnesium chloride on rabbit bronchial smooth muscle. *Ann Emerg Med* 1990;19:1107–1112.

83. Del Certillo J, Engbeeck L. The nature of the neuromuscular block produced by magnesium. *J Physiol* 1954;124:370–384.

84. Matthew R, Altuma BM. Magnesium and the lungs. *Magnesium* 1988;7:173–187.

85. Bois P. Effect of magnesium deficiency on mast cells and urinary histamine in rats. *Br J Exp Path* 1963;44:151–155.

86. Nadler JL, Goodson S, Rude RK. Evidence that prostacyclin mediates the vascular action of magnesium in humans. *Hypertension* 1987;9:379–383.

87. Kemp PA, Gardine SM, March JE, Bennett T, Rubin PC. The effects of NG-Nitro-L-Arginine methyl ether on regional neurodynamic responses to MgSO4 in conscious rats. *Br J Pharmacol* 1994;111:325–331.

88. Wei W, Franz KB. A synergism of antigen challenge and severe magnesium deficiency on blood and urinary histamine levels in rats. *J Am Coll Nutr* 1990;9:616–622.

89. Haury VG. Blood serum magnesium in bronchial asthma and its treatment by the administration of magnesium sulfate. *J Lab Clin Med* 1940;26:340–341.

90. Rolla G, Bucca C, Caria E, et al. Acute effect of intravenous magnesium sulfate on airway obstruction of asthmatic patients. *Ann Allergy* 1988;61:388–391.

91. Skobaloff EM, Spivey WH, McNamara RM, Greenspan L. Intravenous magnesium sulfate for the treatment of acute asthma in the Emergency Department. *JAMA* 1989;262:1210–1213.

92. Rolla G, Bucca C, Arossa W, Bugiani M. Magnesium alleviates methacholine induced bronchoconstriction in asthmatics. *Magnesium* 1987;6:201–204.

93. Kuitert LM, Kletchko SL. Intravenous magnesium sulfate in acute life threatening asthma. *Ann Emerg Med* 1991;20:1243–1245.

94. Hoppen M, Van Melle L, Impens N, Schandevyl W. Bronchodilating effect of intravenous magnesium sulfate in acute severe bronchial asthma. *Chest* 1990;97:373–376.

95. Green SM, Rothrock SG. Intravenous magnesium for acute asthma: failure to decrease emergency room duration or need for hospitalization. *Ann Emerg Med* 1992;21:260–265.

96. Tiffany BR, Berk WA, Todd IK, White SR. Magnesium bolus or infusion fails to improve expiratory flow in acute asthma exacerbations. *Chest* 1993;104:831–834.

97. Chande VT, Skoner DP. A trial of nebulized magnesium sulfate to reverse bronchospasm in asthmatic patients. *Ann Emerg Med* 1992;21:1111–1115.

98. Rolla G, Bucca C, Caria E. Dose related effect of inhaled magnesium sulfate on histamine bronchial challenge in asthmatics. *Drugs Exp Clin Res* 1988;14:609–612.

99. Faulkner D, Glausen J, Allen M. Serum magnesium levels in asthmatic patients during acute exacerbations of asthma. *Am J Emerg Room* 1992;10:1–3.

100. Bloch H, Silverman R, Manclaire N, Grant S, Jaqminas L, Scharf SM. Intravenous magnesium sulfates as a adjunct in the treatment of acute asthma. *Chest* 1995;107:1576–1581.

101. Okayama H, Aikawa T, Okayama M, Saski H, Wu S, Takishima T. Bronchodilating effect of intravenous magnesium sulfate in bronchial asthma. *JAMA* 1987;257:1076–1078.

102. Bernstein WK, Khastgir T, Khastgir A, et al. Lack of effectiveness of magnesium in chronic stable asthma. *Arch Int Med* 1995;155:271–276.

103. Britton J, Pavord I, Wisniewski A, Knox A, Lewis S, Tattersfield A, Weiss S. Dietary magnesium, lung function, wheezing, and airway hyperreactivity in a random adult population. *Lancet* 1994;344:357–362.

104. Kramer MS. Does Breast feeding help protect against atopic disease? Biology, methodology, and a golden jubilee of controversy. *J Pediatr* 1988;112:181–190.

105. Wright AL, Holberg CJ, Taussig LM, Martinez FD. Relationship of infant feeding to recurrent wheezing at age 6 years. *Arch Pediatr Adolesc Med* 1995;149:758–763.

106. Arshad SH, Hide DW. Effect of environmental factors on the development of allergic disorders in infancy. *J Allergy Clin Immunol* 1992;90:235–241.

107. Faith-Magnusson K, Kjellman N-I M. Development of atopic disease in babies whose mothers were receiving exclusion diet during pregnancy—a randomized study. *J Allergy Clin Immunol* 1987;80:869–875.

108. Zeiger RS, Heller S, Mellon MH, et al. Effect of combined maternal and infant food-allergen avoidance on development of atopy in early infancy: a randomized study. *J Allergy Clin Immunol* 1989;84:72–89.

Asthma, edited by P.J. Barnes, M.M. Grunstein,
A.R. Leff, and A.J. Woolcock.
Lippincott–Raven Publishers, Philadelphia © 1997.

▪ 10 ▪

Risk Factors

Development and Natural History

Fernando D. Martinez

The inception, course, and prognosis of asthma in childhood have been matters of considerable study during the last 40 years. It is now clear that events occurring during the first decade of life may be decisive in triggering the mechanisms responsible for the inception of asthma. Although many issues remain open for debate, significant progress has been made in our understanding of the relation between viral lower respiratory illnesses (LRIs) in early life and the development of asthma; of the different phenotypic expressions of asthma; and of the role of allergies in general and especially of early allergic sensitization on the inception and persistence of asthmatic symptoms and bronchial hyperresponsiveness during childhood.

THE BEGINNINGS OF CHRONIC ASTHMA

Results of longitudinal studies including studies of asthmatics of all ages have conclusively shown that both the inception of asthmatic symptoms and the first diagnosis of asthma occur most frequently during the first years of life (1). It is certainly true that asthma may develop in the workplace in subjects who have no recollection of having had chronic respiratory symptoms prior to their asthma-related job experience. These cases, however, constitute only a small proportion of all asthma patients, and chronic asthma is primarily a disease that begins soon after birth.

As with all diseases for which there is no known cure, knowledge of the factors that determine the first expression of asthma is very important in the design of strategies for the primary prevention of the disease. Studies in twins have demonstrated that as much as 60% of the susceptibility to asthma is inherited (2). But this also means that concordance for asthma in monozygotic twins is far from perfect, and that environmental factors have a strong influence in modulating the phenotypic expression of the disease. It is thus not surprising that so much attention has been paid to the environmental factors that may protect or predispose individuals to the development of asthma during childhood.

Lower Respiratory Illnesses During Infancy and Asthma

Clear evidence suggests that viral LRIs occurring in early life are associated with an increased risk of developing asthma later in life (3). Until recently, however, the factors explaining this association were not well understood. Early studies performed in children who had viral bronchiolitis as infants showed that many of these children had bronchial hyperresponsiveness many years after their original episodes of LRI (4). Studies of lung function in older children and adolescents also consistently demon-

F. D. Martinez: Respiratory Sciences Center, College of Medicine, University of Arizona, Tucson, Arizona 85724-5030.

strated that subjects with a history of LRI in early life had significant deficits in several spirometric parameters, especially those derived from flow-volume loops (5). It was thus suggested that the LRI itself could alter airway development and cause an increased propensity to abnormal responses to environmental stimuli. This conclusion seemed to be supported by several reports by Welliver and co-workers (6), who observed that, in some infants, virus-specific immunoglobulin (Ig) E could be detected in nasal secretions and a correlation was observed between the amount of virus-specific IgE and both the severity of the LRI and the likelihood that wheezing symptoms would persist until the age of 7–8 (7). These results were thus interpreted as suggestive of a causal relation between viral infection and asthma: the viral infection itself could perhaps be the trigger that started the chronic inflammatory changes that are characteristic of asthma. Reports of a temporal relation between viral infections and the inception of allergic symptoms in children (8) seemed to give further credence to this interpretation.

Recent studies have suggested that a different, more complex explanation of these findings may be possible. Several authors (9,10) have now shown that lower levels of lung function predate the development of respiratory symptoms in many children who later developed LRIs. Moreover, it has been shown that two different wheezing phenotypes coexist during the first 3 years of life. Whereas almost one-third of all young children have at least one episode of wheezing LRI before age 3, almost 60% of these children will have no further such episodes by the age of 6 (11). These infants show none of the risk factors known to be associated with chronic asthma later in life and, specifically, show no increased prevalence of markers of an allergic diathesis or of a family history of asthma. However, it is this group of patients (labeled transient early wheezers) that shows lower premorbid lung function when compared with subjects who had no LRIs. It is thus plausible to surmise that LRIs in these children are associated with a mechanical airway obstruction caused by edema or mucus accumulation that may occur in all small children during LRIs (11), but that may reach a critical, "wheezing" level in this particular group of children with a predisposing lung structure. Because airway growth probably surpasses lung growth during the toddler years (12), these subjects usually outgrow their symptoms, although lower levels of lung function may persist in these children many years after their acute LRI (5).

Early-Onset Chronic Asthma

The finding that lower levels of lung function predated the development of wheezing LRIs offered an explanation for the respiratory symptoms occurring in early life in up to 60% of infants and young children who do not seem to be at higher risk for continued wheezing during the tod-

dler and early school years. However, what causes the other 40% of children (that is, those who will still have recurrent wheezing episodes at age 6, labelled persistent wheezers) to have airway obstruction during the same type of viral infections is not well understood. These children start life with levels of lung function that are not significantly different from those of children who will never wheeze and, therefore, a simple "mechanical" influence determining their wheezing episodes is unlikely. Unfortunately, it is not possible to separate these children from those with a good prognosis by using clinical data, and infant pulmonary function tests are not easy to perform and cannot be used to identify single individuals at risk. Indirect data, however, indicate that these children have many of the risk factors known to be associated with childhood asthma: they have a strong family history of asthma, they are predominantly males (up to 60%), they often wheeze apart from colds during the first year of life, and they have a high prevalence of atopic dermatitis and rhinitis (11). Most importantly, they show significantly increased serum IgE levels during the first year of life. All this evidence suggests that these children may be having airway obstruction by a mechanism that is similar to that causing chronic asthma in older children, that is, by a form of chronic airway inflammation associated with and triggered by IgE-mediated reactions. The data by Welliver and co-workers (6,7) show that children who later had persistent wheezing had increased production of virus-specific IgE and increased histamine levels in nasal secretions during viral wheezing LRIs, which can be reinterpreted as providing indirect support for this hypothesis. It is not known, however, if the virus-specific IgE is responsible for triggering the wheezing-associated airway obstruction in these children. Very recent observations from our own laboratories appear to challenge this concept. We observed that persistent wheezers (for example, children who had wheezing LRIs in early life and were still wheezing at a mean age of 6 years) showed a markedly higher IgE response to viral LRIs, as assessed by the total serum IgE level measured during and approximately 1 month after the LRI (F. D. Martinez, unpublished observation). This enhanced IgE response, however, appeared to be multispecific: infants with wheezing LRIs associated with isolation of respiratory syncytial virus (RSV) in their nasal secretions could have virus-specific IgE against RSV or against other viruses such as parainfluenza (M. Halonen, unpublished observation). It is therefore possible that production of virus-specific IgE may be the consequence of a generalized tendency to respond to infection initially, and subsequently to other environmental stimuli such as allergens, with enhanced IgE-mediated immunity.

Interestingly, we also observed significant differences between transient early wheezers and persistent wheezers in the response by circulating eosinophils to acute infection (F. D. Martinez, unpublished observations). Transient early wheezers (and children who had nonwheezing LRIs) showed the expected response to acute viral or bacterial infection (13), i.e., a marked decreased in circulating eosinophils. Persistent wheezers, however, showed no changes in circulating eosinophils. Garofalo et al. (14) had recently reported that both infants with upper respiratory illness due to RSV and those with RSV LRI showed suppressed eosinophil counts during acute infection, although the latter showed less suppression than the former. Our results suggest that children with wheezing LRIs belong to two distinct groups: transient infant wheezers have the same level of suppression of eosinophil counts as children with nonwheezing LRIs, whereas persistent wheezers show no suppression of eosinophil counts.

What causes infection-related eosinopenia is not well understood, but both vascular margination and bone marrow inhibition of eosinophil precursors have been proposed (15). Our data suggested that persistent wheezers have alterations in the control of the number of circulating eosinophils that can be observed as early as during their first wheezing LRI. Garofalo et al. (14) studied concentration of eosinophil cationic protein (ECP) in nasopharyngeal secretions obtained from a group of children with various forms of respiratory illness. ECP is a cytotoxic protein contained in the granules of eosinophils and has been suggested as having a role in the pathogenesis of asthma. These authors found that children with RSV bronchiolitis had significantly higher levels of ECP in nasal secretions than children with RSV upper respiratory tract illnesses, with RSV nonwheezing LRIs or with nonRSV upper respiratory tract illnesses. More recently, Sigurs et al. (16) reported no differences in nasal serum ECP during acute RSV infections between infants who would still have bronchial obstructive symptoms 2 years later and those who would not. Unfortunately, these studies were either cross-sectional (14) or entailed a brief follow-up (16) and, therefore, the proportion of transient early wheezers or persistent wheezers present, as defined by long-term follow-up studies, was not ascertained.

Available data suggest that genetic and environmental factors regulating IgE and eosinophil responses to infection in early life may be crucial in setting up the physiologic environment for the development of chronic asthma. It is likely that many such factors interact in determining such responses, but the fact that both IgE levels and eosinophil function are controlled by cytokines produced by T-helper type (TH)2-like lymphocytes points to the selection process leading to the maturation of this lymphocyte subtype as an important step in the beginnings of asthma.

T-Cell Subtypes and Early Sensitization to Asthma-Related Allergens

It is now widely accepted that mature CD4 T-helper lymphocytes respond to stimuli with different patterns of cytokine production and release, depending on their degree of maturation and on the phenotype they have differentiated into. These differential responses were first observed in mice (17) and have been confirmed in humans (18), although not all T-helper cell types show identical cytokine responses in the two species. It has been established that TH1-like cells produce interferon-γ (IFN-γ) and interleukin 2 (IL-2) and do not produce IL-4 or IL-5, whereas TH2-like cells produce IL-4 and IL-5 but not IFN-γ or IL-2. It is now clear that there is a wide range of T-helper cells producing different cytokines both in circulation and in peripheral tissues (19), but what seems to be important for the pathogenesis of chronic asthma is which of the two main poles (TH1-like or TH2-like) is preferentially activated.

We are only beginning to understand the genetic and environmental factors associated with the preferential selection of TH2-like clones, which seems to be taking place already during the first year of life. It is now well established that approximately 90% of cord blood CD4+ T cells express CD45RA compared with 40 to 60% of the adult counterparts (20). The CD45RA isoform is characteristic of mature naive T cells, and the cells convert to CD45RO after antigenic stimulation. This paucity of mature memory cells may explain in part why neonatal T-cell populations have been found to be deficient in overall cytokine secretion capacity and especially in IFN-γ. The proportion of CD45RO cells in circulation steadily increases during childhood, and adult equivalent frequencies are attained between 15 and 20 years of age (20). Miles et al. (21) showed that the numbers of CD4+ CD45RO+ cells in cord blood were significantly lower among children born to at least one atopic, asthmatic parent and who developed allergic symptoms by the age of 1 year, than among children with the same familiar background but who developed no such symptoms. They interpreted their findings as suggesting either suppression of T-cell activation or lack of antigenic priming in utero in children who would later develop allergies. Holt et al. (22) assessed T-cell function in infants aged 7 to 35 months whose first-degree relatives had a history of atopic disease and compared their results with those of children whose first-degree relatives did not have such a history. They found that those with a family history of allergy had decreased proliferative capacities of progenitor T cells and that individual T-cell clones from a small group of these subjects produced less IFN-γ and IL-4 when stimulated. They concluded that children at risk for the development of allergies in early life had a maturational deficiency in CD4 T-cell function and that variations in the postnatal maturation of T cells may be a contributing factor in the development of different patterns of responsiveness to environmental antigenic stimuli.

Our own longitudinal studies in Tucson, Arizona, have provided evidence that, in children who will later become sensitized to the mold *Alternaria*, peripheral blood mononuclear cells (PBMCs) obtained at a mean age of 9 months, but not at birth, show markedly decreased IFN-γ and IL-2 responses to indirect stimuli (for example, PHA and concanavalin A) than in children who will not become sensitized to these allergens (23). No association was observed, however, between production of these cytokines by PBMCs at age 11 and sensitization to *Alternaria* or any other allergen at age 11, or between cytokine production before age 1 and sensitization to *Alternaria* occurring after age 6 (M. Halonen, unpublished observations). These results are particularly intriguing because the association between allergic sensitization and cytokine responses in the first year of life was very specific for *Alternaria*. In our semiarid region, as in certain areas of inland Australia (24), *Alternaria* is the main allergen associated with asthma, much like house dust-mite allergens are the main risk factors for the development of asthma in more humid regions of the world. Although *Alternaria* is an outdoor allergen, it may become very abundant indoors, particularly in homes where humidification is used for cooling purposes. The data suggest that a process of selection of TH1-like or TH2-like clones probably occurs at very early stages during the development of the T-helper system. A relative scarcity of TH1-like clones may predispose subjects exposed indoors to certain antigens (such as house dust mites or *Alternaria*) to a preferential IgE-mediated, TH2-promoted response, in contrast with the TH1-promoted response to these same antigens that is predominant in nonatopic subjects.

This process of early allergic sensitization appears to be strongly associated with the development of chronic asthma in early life. In elegant studies performed in Australia, Peat et al. (25) showed that subjects who became sensitized to allergens before the age of 8 were several times more likely to develop persistent asthmalike symptoms during childhood than subjects who became sensitized to similar allergens after age 8. Our group confirmed similar trends in subjects living in Tucson, Arizona (F. D. Martinez, unpublished observations). We also observed that subjects who were sensitized to aeroallergens in early life showed skin-test reactivity to more allergens that those who became sensitized later, and also had more persistently positive skin tests and significantly higher serum IgE levels. This is in tune with the observation by Sears and co-workers (26) of a direct relation between number of positive skin tests to which a subject is allergic and risk of having asthmalike symptoms. These data, taken as a whole, strongly suggest that early allergic sensitization is an important risk factor for chronic asthma, and that it is often associated with a multispecific activation of TH2-like clones, which may be associated with a relative paucity of TH1-like clones in subjects who become sensitized to allergens very early in life. This multispecific activation may be an important characteristic of chronic asthma and contrasts with the marked specificity of IgE produced against parasitic infection,

for example, which is usually not associated with allergic symptoms. This multispecific activation may also explain why several studies have now observed that, even among subjects who are skin test negative to common aeroallergens, a significant positive correlation is present between total serum IgE level and the risk of having chronic asthma or asthmalike symptoms (27).

Risk Factors for Decreased Interferon-γ Production by PBMCs

Both genetic and environmental factors are known to control the expression of asthma and allergies, and it is not unreasonable to surmise that this control may be mediated at least in part through a process that leads to a relative paucity of TH1-like clones in circulation during early life. Very few studies are available that address possible hereditary influences on cytokine production by PBMCs. As stated earlier, data by Holt et al. suggest that the maturation process of the T-cell system may be influenced by genetic factors: children of allergic parents show a delayed development of IFN-γ-producing TH1-like clones when compared with controls (22). In our own laboratories, we observed a significant negative correlation between production of both IL-2 and IFN-γ by PBMCs in 9-month-old children and the number of positive skin test reactions to common aeroallergens in their parents (23). The strongest effect was observed when both parents were highly atopic and, in this case, production of cytokines by PBMCs, particularly IFN-γ, was very low. Inheritance of atopy might be mediated by the preferential selection of TH2-like clones in the offspring of atopic subjects.

Our understanding of the environmental factors that may influence the clonal selection process leading to a preponderance of one or the other form of mature T lymphocytes is very limited. There is certainly some evidence from epidemiologic studies of an inverse relation between infections in early life and allergies (28). It has been a long-standing observation that allergies seem to be more frequent and more severe among "Westernized" populations (29) and among populations with a higher standard of living. The hypothesis has been proposed that the timing and/or frequency of infections in early life may influence the type of T-helper cell clones preferentially expanded in response to environmental stimuli (30). Direct data to confirm this hypothesis are still fragmentary. We recently reported (28) strikingly lower levels of total serum IgE and lower prevalence of skin test reactivity to aeroallergens subsequent to rather severe nonwheezing LRIs occurring during the first 3 years of life. IFN-γ production by PBMCs was significantly higher in children who had nonwheezing LRIs in the first 3 years of life than in those who did not. Lynch et al. (31) reported increased prevalence of sensitization to aeroallergens (as assessed by skin test reactivity) after treatment of parasitic infections in a uncontrolled study of extremely poor Venezuelan children. Only one study in experimental animals has tested the relation between infection and IgE responses. Kudlacz et al. (32) sensitized two groups of guinea pigs with ovalbumin aerosols: one group was preinfected with parainfluenza virus type 3 at 7 or 19 days before sensitization, while the other group was left uninfected. The preinfected group showed significantly diminished histamine production by antigen-stimulated lung tissue *in vitro* when compared with the uninfected group. Likewise, preinfected sensitized animals that were challenged with ovalbumin showed no increase in airway reactivity to histamine or increased eosinophil population in bronchoalveolar lavage fluid. Uninfected sensitized animals showed increased airway reactivity and increased eosinophilia response in the bronchoalveolar lavage fluid. Although not conclusive, these data from human and animal studies suggest that infections may modify the nature of the immune reactivity to environmental stimuli.

NATURAL COURSE OF ASTHMA DURING CHILDHOOD AND EARLY ADULT LIFE

In the previous section, the factors determining the initiation and persistence of asthma and asthmalike symptoms during infancy and early childhood were discussed in some detail. Unfortunately, very few studies provide information on the incidence and long-term outcome of chronic asthma and wheezing during the school years. It is therefore not well understood, for example, whether age at initiation of asthma symptoms is an important factor in determining its prognosis, whether the incidence of asthma remains low after the age of 8–10, and what the factors are that determine remission and relapse of asthma during childhood.

Perhaps the most extensive prospective study available is the follow-up of different groups of wheezing children selected at the age of 7 years in Melbourne, Australia, in 1964 (33). This study has several important limitations: information on the first years of life was obtained retrospectively at age 7 and thus may be biased by preferential recall, and the control group included only a very small number of asymptomatic children. However, no other clinical study is available that provides comprehensive follow-up data of wheezy children from birth to the age of 35.

Wheezing Syndromes of the Early School Years

Researchers in the Melbourne study distinguished at least two clinical expressions of asthma during the early school years. In a first group, called infrequent episodic asthma, wheezing episodes were frequently reported by parents to have started after the age of 3, were usually as-

sociated with viral infections, and were rarely troublesome. Of children in this group, 40% to 50% had ceased to have episodes by the age of 10 years, and remission was still occurring during adolescence. Approximately 10% to 20% of children whose symptoms had stopped by the end of the first decade had self-reported relapses during adolescence and early adult life. Very few of these subjects, however, developed persistent asthma as adults. In fact, both level of lung function and prevalence of bronchial responsiveness measured during the adult years were very similar in this group when compared with controls.

Few other comprehensive follow-up studies of asthmalike symptoms from childhood to adult life are available. Recently, results of a recall of adult subjects from Aberdeen, Scotland, who had been assessed for asthma and wheezing as schoolchildren 25 years earlier have become available (34). Three groups of subjects were included: those who had a diagnosis of asthma during childhood (as assessed by a physician), those whose parents reported wheezing only in the presence of a cold, and those who had no respiratory symptoms. When compared with the latter group, subjects who had asthma in childhood were 14 times more likely to wheeze and 7 times more likely to have bronchial hyperresponsiveness to methacholine at age 34–40 years. Subjects who had asthma during childhood were also much more likely to be using asthma medication and had significantly lower levels of lung function. Prognosis for children who were classed as having wheeze only with colds was better than for those who had asthma. Members of this group were more likely to have wheeze at age 34–40 than those who had no symptoms as children, but their symptoms were mild and did not usually interfere with normal life, as was the case for asthmatics. Prevalence of hyperresponsiveness to methacholine was not significantly higher in this group than in controls, and level of lung function was within normal ranges.

These results suggest that a wheezing syndrome probably exists during the early school years that may be different from that affecting children with more severe or persistent asthma symptoms. Wilson et al. (35) have suggested that bronchial responsiveness (as assessed by methacholine or cold-air challenge [CAC]) may not be increased among wheezy children aged 4 to 5 years. They proposed the hypothesis that these children may wheeze by a mechanism other than the airway inflammation that is characteristic of chronic asthma. Unfortunately, this conjecture was based in a small uncontrolled study (35). We recently assessed airway response to CAC in almost 500 6-year-old, unselected children who are part of a long-term study of risk factors for the development of asthma (36). We found a strong association between wheezing in the previous 12 months and a positive response to CAC at age 6 (odds ratio, 2.4; 95% confidence interval, 1.4–4.0). Moreover, response to CAC was strongly and positively associated with skin test reactivity to allergens and with total serum IgE levels. Response to

CAC at age 6 was strongly predictive of subsequent wheezing at age 11, but only among children who were current wheezers at age 6. The data showed that there are at least two groups of wheezing children at age 6: one group (more than one-fourth of all wheezing 6-year-olds) has airway hyperresponsiveness and is usually skin test positive to allergens; most of these patients (up to 84% if they are skin test positive) will still be wheezing by age 11. A second group shows no airway hyperresponsiveness and is usually skin test negative; only 34% of these patients will still be wheezing by age 11 (36).

What causes wheezing in this latter group of children identified as having a good prognosis in data from Melbourne, Aberdeen, and Tucson is difficult to establish. The mechanical factors apparently involved in the pathogenesis of transient infant wheezing do not seem to be at play in this group: mean levels of lung function measured at age 6 (for the Tucson data) or during childhood and early adulthood (for the Aberdeen and Melbourne data) were not significantly different for this group when compared with controls. As stated earlier, the data from Aberdeen and Melbourne suggest that these children have symptoms mainly in relation with respiratory infections, and an alteration might exist in the immune response to infections in these children. Very recent studies performed in the same group of children from Tucson at age 11 discussed earlier have shown that children who wheezed at age 6 but had stopped wheezing by age 11 had, as expected, a prevalence of hyperresponsiveness to methacholine that was not significantly different from that of nonwheezing children. However, this same group of children had significantly increased variability of daily peak flow measurements when compared with children who never wheezed (37). Children who wheezed both at age 6 and at age 11 had both increased peak flow variability and increased prevalence of methacholine responsiveness when compared with controls. A common alteration of control of airway tone might be present in all children who wheeze at age 6. However, only those who show increased response to methacholine or to cold air with associated skin test reactivity and high levels of IgE may have the kind of persistent airway inflammatory process that is characteristic of chronic asthma.

Chronic Asthma

The preceding discussion illustrates the complexity of the clinical expressions of asthma at different ages. It is clear, however, that chronic asthma appears to be associated with a well-defined set of risk factors. Peat et al. (38) showed that children aged 8 to 11 years who presented with current wheeze and bronchial hyperresponsiveness to histamine had more severe symptoms, markedly increased daily variability, continued bronchial hyperresponsiveness, and more atopy during a 1-year follow-up. In the Melbourne study, early onset of symptoms was a characteristic of children who would later have chronic

asthma that persisted during childhood and into adult life (33). In these patients, the most troublesome period was between the ages of 8 and 14, and airway obstruction was reported to occur for months at a time; many of these children were seldom wheeze free. The majority of these children were males, and they were almost always highly hyperresponsive to airway challenges. Only about 5% of these children became wheeze free as adults, although boys seemed to improve more during puberty than girls; 60% continued to have persistent, symptomatic, and troublesome asthma. Lung function levels were significantly lower in these children when compared with those with infrequent episodic asthma or with asymptomatic controls. However, the data suggested no further deterioration in lung function after the age of 7 years.

These data are consistent with those of Merkus et al. (39), who reported that the slope of the growth of lung function during the school years was not significantly different between asthmatic children and nonasthmatic children. Asthmatic children, however, had lower levels of lung function at the start of follow-up in the early school years, much like in the data from Melbourne. In fact, it has been suggested that chronic asthma in adults is not associated with the marked deterioration in lung function that is characteristic of chronic obstructive lung disease associated with smoking (40). This issue is highly controversial, and several studies have shown that bronchial responsiveness is an important risk factor for increased loss of lung function in smokers (41). This controversy is beyond the scope of this chapter. It is important to stress, however, that there is consistent evidence suggesting that most of the more severe deterioration in lung function seen in older children and adults with asthma has already occurred by the early school years. The causes of this deterioration are unknown. The only published study that has assessed lung function levels shortly after birth and then reassessed lung function in early childhood in subjects with asthma-like symptoms has been discussed earlier (11). This study showed that children who would later develop persistent wheezing start life with mean levels of airway function that are within normal ranges. By the age of 6, persistent wheezers had significant deterioration in lung function as compared with children who were free of reported wheeze. It appears that the state of persistent bronchial hyperresponsiveness that is characteristic of chronic asthma may alter lung development, particularly at the period of fastest lung growth, for example, between birth and the age of 7 years. Whether the impairment in lung function observed in these subjects is causally associated with more severe asthma or is otherwise only a marker of asthma severity is unknown.

CONCLUSIONS

Increasing evidence suggests that the roots of most cases of chronic asthma can be found in early life. This evidence supports the concept of chronic asthma as a developmental disease, in which genetic and environmental factors affecting the maturation of the airways and the immune system during childhood create the basis for the airway inflammatory process and altered reactivity to stimuli that are characteristic of chronic asthma. This form of asthma is quite persistent in its clinical expression, and complete remissions during adult life are rare. There are, however, other less severe and less persistent expressions of asthma at all ages. These forms are usually characterized by intermittent wheezing often associated with respiratory infections, but the pathogenesis of this altered reactivity to infection is not well understood and may vary with age.

REFERENCES

1. Barbee RA, Dodge R, Lebowitz ML, Burrows B. The epidemiology of asthma. *Chest* 1985;87(Suppl 1):21S–25S.
2. Duffy DL, Martin NG, Battistutta D, Hoffer JL, Matthews JD. Genetics of asthma and hay fever in Australian twins. *Am Rev Respir Dis* 1990;142:1351–1358.
3. Sherman CB, Tosteson TD, Tager IB, Speizer FE, Weiss ST. Early childhood predictors of asthma. *Am J Epidemiol* 1990;132:83–95.
4. Kattan M, Keens TG, Lapierre JG, Levison H, Bryan AC, Reilly BJ. Pulmonary function abnormalities in symptom-free children after bronchiolitis. *Pediatrics* 1977;59:683–688.
5. Voter KZ, Henry MM, Stewart PW, Henderson FW. Lower respiratory illness in early childhood and lung function and bronchial reactivity in adolescent males. *Am Rev Respir Dis* 1988;137:302–307.
6. Welliver RC, Kaul TN, Ogra PL. The appearance of cell-bound IgE in respiratory-tract epithelium after respiratory-syncytial-virus infection. *N Engl J Med* 1980;303:1198–1202.
7. Welliver RC, Duffy L. The relationship of RSV-specific immunoglobulin E antibody responses in infancy, recurrent wheezing, and pulmonary function at age 7–8 years. *Pediatr Pulmonol* 1993;15:19–27.
8. Frick OL, German DF, Mills J. Development of allergy in children. I. Association with virus infections. *J Allergy Clin Immunol* 1979;63:228–241.
9. Martinez FD, Morgan WJ, Wright AL, Holberg CJ, Taussig LM. Initial airway function is a risk factor for recurrent wheezing respiratory illnesses during the first three years of life. *Am Rev Respir Dis* 1991; 143:312–316.
10. Tager IB, Hanrahan JP, Tosteston TD, et al. Lung function, pre- and post-natal smoke exposure, and wheezing in the first year of life. *Am Rev Respir Dis* 1993;147:811–817.
11. Martinez FD, Wright AL, Taussig LM, et al. Asthma and wheezing in the first six years of life. *N Engl J Med* 1995;332:133–138.
12. Morgan WJ, Martinez FD, Wright AL, Taussig LM. Forced expiratory flow (FEF) tracks from infancy to six years of age. *Am Rev Respir Dis* 1991;143:A508.
13. Wardlaw AJ. Eosinophils in the 1990s: new perspectives on their role in health and disease. *Postgrad Med J* 1994;70:536–552.
14. Garofalo R, Dorris A, Ahlstedt S, Welliver RC. Peripheral blood eosinophil counts and eosinophil cationic protein content of respiratory secretions in bronchiolitis: relationship to severity of disease. *Pediatr Allergy Immunol* 1994;5:111–117.
15. Bass DA. Behavior of eosinophil leukocytes in acute inflammation. II. Eosinophil dynamics during acute inflammation. *J Clin Invest* 1975; 56:870–879.
16. Sigurs N, Bjarnason R, Sigur-Bergsson F. Eosinophil cationic protein in nasal secretion and in serum and myeloperoxidase in serum in respiratory syncytial virus bronchiolitis: relation to asthma and atopy. *Acta Paediatr* 1994;83:1151–1155.
17. Mosmann TR, Cherwinski H, Bond MW, Giedlin MA, Coffman RL. Two types of murine helper T cell clones. I. Definition according to profiles of lymphokine activities and secretory proteins. *J Immunol* 1986; 136:2348–2357.
18. Romagnani S. Human TH1 and TH2 subsets: regulation of differentiation and role in protection and immunopathology. *Int Arch Allergy Immunol* 1992;98:279–285.
19. Kelso A. TH1 and TH2 subsets: paradigms lost? *Immunol Today* 1995; 16:374–379.
20. Holt PG, Nelson DJ. Host defenses and immunology. In: Silverman M, ed. *Childhood asthma and other disorders.* London: Chapman and Hall Medical, 1995;3:67–86.
21. Miles EA, Warner JA, Lane AC, Jones AC, Colwell BM, Warner JO. Altered T lymphocyte phenotype at birth in babies born to atopic parents. *Pediatr Allergy Immunol* 1994;5:202–208.
22. Holt PG, Clough JB, Holt BJ, et al. Genetic "risk" for atopy is associated with delayed postnatal maturation of T-cell competence. *Clin Exp Allergy* 1992;22:1093–1099.
23. Martinez FD, Stern DA, Wright AL, Holberg CJ, Taussig LM, Halonen M. Association of interleukin-2 and interferon-γ production by blood mononuclear cells in infancy with parental allergy skin tests and with subsequent development of atopy. *J Allergy Clin Immunol* 1995;96: 652–660.
24. Peat JK, Toelle BG, Gray EJ, Haby MM, Belousova E, Woolcock AJ. Prevalence and severity of childhood asthma and allergic sensitization in seven climatic regions of New South Wales. *Med J Aust* 1995;163: 22–26.
25. Peat JK, Salome CM, Woolcock AJ. Longitudinal changes in atopy during a 4-year period: relation to bronchial hyperresponsiveness and respiratory symptoms in a population sample of Australian schoolchildren. *J Allergy Clin Immunol* 1990;85:65–74.
26. Sears MR, Herbison GP, Holdaway MD, Hewitt CJ, Flannery EM, Silva PA. The relative risks of sensitivity to grass pollen, house dust mite and cat dander in the development of childhood asthma. *Clin Exp Allergy* 1989;19:419–424.
27. Burrows B, Martinez FD, Halonen M, Barbee R, Cline M. Association of asthma with serum IgE levels and skin-test reactivity to allergens. *N Engl J Med* 1989;320:271–277.
28. Martinez FD, Stern DA, Wright AL, Taussig LM, Halonen M, Group Health Medical Associates. Association of nonwheezing lower respiratory tract illnesses in early life with persistently diminished serum IgE levels. *Thorax* 1995;50:1067–1072.
29. Strachan DP. Hay fever, hygiene, and household size. *BMJ* 1989;299: 1259–1260.
30. Martinez FD. Role of viral infections in the inception of asthma and allergies during childhood: could they be protective? *Thorax* 1994;49: 1189–1191.
31. Lynch NR, Hagel I, Perez M, Di Prisco MC, Lopez R, Alvarez N. Effect of anthelmintic treatment on the allergic reactivity of children in a tropical slum. *J Allergy Clin Immunol* 1993;92:404–411.
32. Kudlacz EM, Knippenberg RW. Parainfluenza virus type-3 infection attenuates the respiratory effects of antigen challenge in sensitized guinea pigs. *Inflamm Res* 1995;44:105–110.
33. Phelan PD, Olinsky A, Oswald H. Asthma: classification, clinical patterns and natural history. *Baillieres Clin Paediatr* 1995;3:307–318.
34. Godden DJ, Ross S, Abdalla M, et al. Outcome of wheeze in childhood: symptoms and pulmonary function 25 years later. *Am J Respir Crit Care Med* 1994;149:106–112.
35. Wilson NM, Bridge P, Silverman M. Bronchial responsiveness and symptoms in 5–6 year old children: a comparison of a direct and indirect challenge. *Thorax* 1995;50:339–345.
36. Lombardi E, Morgan WJ, Wright AL, Stein R, Holberg CJ, Martinez FD. Predictive value of cold air challenge at age 6 for subsequent wheezing at age 11. *Am Rev Respir Crit Care Med* 1996;153: A428(abstr).
37. Stein RT, Holberg CJ, Morgan WJ, Lombardi E, Wright AL, Martinez FD. Determinants of peak flow variability and methacholine responsiveness in children: a prospective study. *Am Rev Respir Crit Care Med* 1996;153:A428(abstr).
38. Peat JK, Toelle BG, Salmone CM, Woolcock AJ. Predictive nature of bronchial responsiveness and respiratory symptoms in a one year cohort study of Sydney schoolchildren. *Eur Respir J* 1993;6:662–669.
39. Merkus PJ, van Essen-Zandvliet EE, Kouwenberg JM, et al. Large lungs after childhood asthma: a case–control study. *Am Rev Respir Dis* 1993;148:1484–1489.
40. Burrows B, Bloom JW, Traver GA, Cline MG. The course and prognosis of different forms of chronic airways obstruction in a sample from the general population. *N Engl J Med* 1987;317:1309–1314.
41. O'Connor GT, Sparrow D, Weiss ST. The role of allergy and nonspecific airway hyperresponsiveness in the pathogenesis of chronic obstructive pulmonary disease: state of the art. *Am Rev Respir Dis* 1989; 140:225–252

Asthma, edited by P.J. Barnes, M.M. Grunstein, A.R. Leff, and A.J. Woolcock.
Lippincott–Raven Publishers, Philadelphia © 1997.

▪ 11 ▪

Genetics of Atopy

Carole Ober

Atopy is a disorder of immunoglobulin E (IgE) antibody response after exposure to ubiquitous, nonpathogenic allergens and is commonly associated with allergic rhinitis (hay fever), atopic dermititis (eczema), and asthma. Laboratory findings in atopic individuals include elevated total serum IgE levels, the presence of antigen-specific IgE antibodies, and skin test reactivity to common allergens. The sensitization to ubiquitous allergens in the lung of atopic individuals and the subsequent cascade of immunologic responses that occurs upon repeat exposure are not completely understood. However, it is clear that the physiological process is complex, involving interactions and signalling between a variety of cell types (Sections 4 and 6), mediators of inflammation (Section 5), and neural mechanisms (Section 7). Thus, it is likely that variations in a potentially large number of genes could underlie inter-individual variability in IgE response to nonpathogenic allergens. This chapter will review genetic studies of atopy and the progress that has been made in identifying genes that may confer susceptibility to atopic disorders. Characteristics of atopic disease related more specifically to asthma (i.e., bronchial hyperresponsiveness) will be reviewed in the following chapter.

ATOPY IS A GENETIC CONDITION

A heritable component to IgE responsiveness has long been recognized due to the familial clustering of atopic diseases, particularly among monozygotic twins (1). More recent studies have demonstrated significant correlations between first-degree relatives (parent-offspring, sib-sib) with respect to total IgE levels and skin-test reactivity, further suggesting that genetic factors influence IgE production (2). Segregation analyses of family data, used to test the fit-specific genetic models, have yielded evidence for a wide variety of genetic models in atopy, including recessive, dominant, co-dominant, polygenic, and maternal inheritance (3,4). These discrepant results are consistent with the hypothesis that more than one genetic locus confers susceptibility to atopy and that alleles at each locus may have different effects (i.e., dominant, recessive, additive). Such genetic heterogeneity can hamper genetic studies by potentially "masking" the effects of susceptibility loci when families with different underlying genetic susceptibilities are pooled for analysis. Thus, it may be particularly difficult to elucidate the effects of specific "atopic" genes in studies of heterogeneous populations, in which different genetic forms of atopy may be segregating in different families. Furthermore, while the effects of genes with relatively large effects (i.e., "major" genes) may be detectable in heterogeneous populations, identifying genes with relatively small effects may only be possible in genetically homogeneous populations, in which a less variable genetic background would allow the detection of the genes with smaller effects. Despite these caveats, recent advances in molecular biology and in the analytic approaches to linkage analysis have resulted in considerable progress in the identification of chromosomal re-

C. Ober: Department of Obstetrics and Gynecology, The University of Chicago, Chicago, Illinois 60637-1470.

gions that influence IgE levels and in providing direct evidence that atopy is a genetic condition.

This chapter will review the methodologic issues related to studying the genetics of complex disorders, the analytic approaches and laboratory techniques that are used to map human disease genes, and the current status of our knowledge about the specific genes that may influence atopic phenotypes.

CONSIDERATIONS IN THE DESIGN OF GENETIC STUDIES OF ATOPY

The search for genes that influence IgE responsiveness is confounded by the complexities of the disorder (Table 1). First, it is likely that many genes influence the atopic phenotype. Such genetic heterogeneity poses the single most important problem in designing studies of complex diseases, such as atopy. Various approaches can be taken to minimize this problem, although it can never be overcome completely. Careful definition of the phenotype can help sort out clinical subtypes of atopy, which may represent different genetic types as well. For example, total IgE production may be under the control of one locus and IgE response to a particular allergen may be under genetic control of a second locus. In this example, considering individuals with either elevated total IgE or specific IgE as "atopic" may mask the effects of the individual loci. On the other hand, if two different loci influence total IgE levels but one gene is the major influence in some families and the second gene is the major influence in

other families, pooling families could obscure the effects of both loci. Because both sets of families are indistinguishable at the level of the phenotype, i.e., elevated total IgE, there would be no reason to study them separately. This problem can be addressed by studying a very large number of families, which will increase the likelihood of sampling a sufficiently large number of families belonging to one or both subsets, thereby increasing the power of the study to detect susceptibility genes, or by studying families from genetically homogeneous populations, which would increase the likelihood that the same genetic locus influences the phenotype (IgE) in all families.

A second complication of genetic studies of atopy is that not all individuals who carry the susceptibility (or at-risk) genotype will be atopic. Penetrance refers to the proportion of individuals with a susceptibility genotype who express the phenotype. With complex diseases, such as atopy, penetrance is never complete (i.e., < 100%) and can explain what appears to be "skipping generations" in pedigrees. Thus, one can never be sure that "unaffected" individuals do not have the at-risk genotype. This problem is often addressed by employing analytical strategies that examine only effected pedigree relatives, most commonly effected sib pairs (5,6). With this approach only individuals expressing the phenotype are included in the analysis and penetrance (or nonpenetrance) is no longer a concern.

Third, not all atopic individuals (even within a single family) will have the same genotype at the susceptibility locus. "Phenocopies" are individuals in whom the ostensibly identical phenotype results from the effects of alleles at different genetic loci or environmental factors.

TABLE 1. *Features of genetic disorders with complex (multifactorial) etiologies*

	Definition	Methodologic Considerations
Genetic Heterogeneity	More than one genetic locus influences the phenotype	1. Careful definition of phenotype 2. Large sample sizes 3. Study genetically homogeneous populations
Penetrance	The proportion of individuals with the susceptibility genotype who express the phenotype	1. Study affected relative pairs only
Phenocopies	Not all relatives with the same phenotype will have the same genotype	1. Limit sample to nuclear or small extended families 2. Study genetically homogeneous populations
Varied Expressivity	Individuals with the same genotype may express different phenotypes	1. Stratify samples by clinical subtypes (requires large samples) 2. Study continuously distributed (quantitative) traits
Environmental Influences	The expression of the phenotype results from an interaction between the genotype and environmental factors	1. Assess relevant environmental variables, when possible 2. Minimize environmental heterogeneity within sample, when possible
Mode of Inheritance Unknown	The underlying genetic model (dominant vs. recessive vs. intermediate) at each locus is not known; the joint effects of alleles at different loci are not known (additive vs. interactive)	1. Use nonparametric linkage analysis (i.e., affected pair methods)

See text for discussion.

For diseases as common as atopy it would not be surprising if more than one susceptibility locus was segregating within a single family. This can be minimized by studying smaller families in which there will be fewer unrelated people who marry into the family and introduce different atopy susceptibility alleles, or by studying genetically homogeneous populations, in which fewer susceptibility loci may be segregating. Exposure to certain environmental factors may also result in phenocopies, such as in cases of occupational asthma.

A further complication is that there is considerable varied expressivity among atopic individuals, even within single families. The variable expression of the atopic phenotype makes it difficult to classify many individuals as affected or unaffected. The expression and severity of atopic parameters, such as total IgE levels or skin test reactivity, will vary with respect to many variables, such as season and age at the time of evaluation, as well as with respect to their co-occurence with asthma, hay fever and eczema. Varied expressivity makes it difficult to determine whether two atopic individuals in the same family who differ with respect to associated features (e.g., one has asthma and one does not) are expressing different manifestations of the same gene or are harboring different genetic susceptibilities. This problem is difficult to reconcile prior to identifying the susceptibility locus. However, in a large sample of families in whom the phenotype has been well-characterized, stratification of subjects with respect to disease expression increases the likelihood of identifying the effects of specific genes. Furthermore, disease-associated measures, such as IgE levels, may be analyzed as continuous (quantitative) variables. With the latter strategy, individuals do not have to be categorized; rather, all individuals with the measure are included in the analysis.

Environmental factors can influence not only the onset but also the severity of atopic disease. Individuals with a susceptibility genotype may not have had sufficient environmental exposures to demonstrate elevated IgE levels or positive skin tests; or individuals with only minor genetic susceptibilities may not have had sufficient repeated exposures to environmental triggers to induce the atopic phenotype. Although one could attempt to study subjects during different seasons and at different ages, it is not possible to control for all of the potential environmental influences. Thus, the genetic model must take into account the effects of unknown environmental factors that could potentially affect the penetrance and expression of the atopic phenotype (Fig. 1)

Lastly, for most diseases with complex, or multi-factorial, etiologies, the underlying genetic model is unknown. The susceptibility alleles may be dominant or recessive and the effects of alleles at different loci may confer risk independent of each other or their effects may be additive or interactive. As a result, nonparametric linkage analysis, such as the affected relative pair methods, may be more appropriate for studying complex diseases (discussed later).

GENETIC APPROACHES TO STUDYING COMPLEX DISEASES

There are two basic approaches for identifying genes that underlie human diseases. The first is called the candidate gene approach because one begins by identifying specific genes whose known function suggests that they could be influencing the atopic phenotype. This approach involves searching for mutations (or deoxyribonucleic acid [DNA] sequence variations) within the

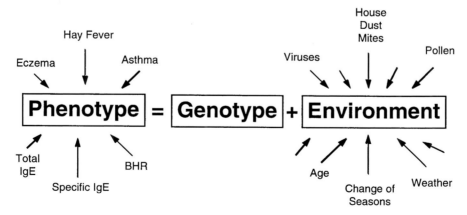

FIG. 1. For multi-factorial, or complex conditions, such as atopy, the phenotype is influenced by interactions between the individual's genetic make-up (genotype) and environmental factors. The atopic phenotype can be assessed by clinical diagnoses, such as eczema, hay fever, or asthma, or by quantitative laboratory measures, such as total serum IgE levels, specific IgE, or bronchial hyperresponsiveness (BHR). Numerous environmental factors can potentially influence the phenotype.

gene itself that are present in individuals with the phenotype but not in unaffected individuals. The limitation of the candidate gene approach is that you are limited to genes of known function, and only a few thousand of the estimated 50,000 to 100,000 human genes are actually known (7). Thus, this approach has been of limited utility in the search for human disease genes; although notable successes of the candidate gene approach have been the discoveries that mutations in the gene-encoding collagen (COL1A1) cause osteogenesis imperfecta type 1 and mutations in the glucokinase gene cause an autosomal-dominant form of noninsulin-dependent diabetes mellitus (NIDDM), called maturity-onset diabetes of the young (or MODY) (8–11). For diseases with complex etiologies, such as atopy, the large number of potential "candidate" genes (Table 2; ref. 12) makes directly screening each candidate gene in atopic individuals an impractical approach.

The second approach is the genome-wide search for disease genes using polymorphic DNA sequences that are spaced throughout the genome, and linkage analysis to identify chromosomal regions that co-segregate with the disease phenotype in families. Once a candidate region is identified through linkage analysis, the disease-causing gene can be identified through positional cloning if there are no candidate genes in the region, or by directly screening candidate genes if there are candidates in the region (13–15). Both approaches have been utilized successfully in studies of mendelian (single gene) disorders after the gene has been localized to specific chromosomal regions by linkage analysis. Examples of the positional cloning approach are the successful cloning of the genes causing cystic fibrosis and Huntington's disease; an example of the candidate gene screening approach is the successful cloning of the gene that causes Marfan syndrome (16–21).

The genome-wide search is an extremely powerful tool that could potentially identify all genes (with detectable effects) that influence a particular phenotype. The recent completion of the first genome-wide search in a complex disorder, insulin-dependent diabetes mellitus (IDDM), has been encouraging (22). In addition to the previously known IDDM susceptibility loci (human leukocyte antigens [HLA] and the insulin gene hypervariable region), three chromosomal regions showed evidence of linkage in two separate samples, suggesting that genes influencing IDDM are located within these regions, although the specific genes have not yet been identified. Such genome-wide searches for genes that influence atopy are currently underway in many laboratories around the world and it is likely that additional atopy susceptibility loci (or candidate regions) will be revealed in the near future.

Although the candidate gene and genome-wide search approaches have been presented as alternative strategies, often they are used in combination. As discussed previously, after linkage to a chromosomal region is found through a genome search, candidate genes in the linked region can be screened for disease-causing mutations. Alternatively, one could limit the genome search to regions that contain candidate genes. With this approach, recently termed the positional candidate gene approach, chromosomal regions that contain known candidate genes are studied using linkage or association studies (discussed later) (14). If the region is linked or associated with the disease in question, then the candidate gene(s) in that region can be screened for mutations. This is a very powerful approach for studying diseases with a large number of candidate genes, such as atopy, because the screening of candidate regions can be accomplished with relative ease, and it is considerably less costly than screening the entire human genome. In fact, to date all of the major findings with respect to atopy

TABLE 2. *Examples of candidate "atopy genes" and their chromosomal locations[a]*

Locus	Gene	Chromosomal Location
FCER1A	Fc-receptor for IgE (α chain)	1q23
ELAM	Endothelial adhesion molecule	1q22-q25
IGK	Immunoglobulin kappa cluster	2p12
IL-2	Interleukin-2	4q26-q27
IL-4	Interleukin-4	5q23-q31
ADRB2R	β2-adrenergic receptor	5q31-q32
MHC	Major histocompatibility complex	6p21.3
TCRG	T-cell receptor, gamma cluster	7p15-p14
ACHE	Acetylcholinesterase	7q22
TCRB	T-cell receptor, beta cluster	7q35
CHRM2	Cholinergic receptor 2	7q35
C5	Complement component 5	9q33
IL-2RA	Interleukin-2 receptor, alpha	10p15-p14
ADRA2R	α2-adrenergic receptor	10q24-26
CALCA	α-calcitonin	11p15.4
LYAM1	Lymphocyte adhesion molecule	11q23-q25
IGF1	Insulinlike growth factor-1	12q23
TCRA	T-cell receptor, alpha	14q11.2
TCRD	T-cell receptor, delta	14q11.2
IGH2	Immunoglobulin heavy chain	14q32.33
CHRM5	Cholinergic receptor 5	15q26
IGF1R	Insulinlike growth factor-1 receptor	15q25-qter
CD11A	Antigen CD11A	16p12.3
CR3A	Complement component receptor	16p11.2
MYH11	Myosin, smooth muscle	16p13.1
PRKCA	Protein kinase C, alpha	17q22-q24
C3	Complement component 3	19p13.3
ICAM1	Intercellular adhesion molecule-1	19p13.2
PLC1	Phospholipase C, gamma	20q12-q13.1
CD18	Antigen CD18	21q22.3
IGK	Immunoglobulin kappa	22q11
IL-2RB	Interleukin-2 receptor, beta	22q13

[a]From Online Mendelian Inheritance of Man, Johns Hopkins University.

genes have utilized this approach. However, the limitation of this approach is the same as that of the traditional candidate gene approach discussed earlier, and the only way to identify all genes that influence a complex phenotype is through a genome-wide search.

THE ANALYTIC TOOLS: ASSOCIATION STUDIES AND LINKAGE ANALYSIS

Association studies compare the frequencies of marker (or candidate susceptibility alleles) between unrelated subjects with the disease and unrelated control (normal) subjects. Significant associations indicate a causal or physiologic relationship between the marker allele and the disease, or linkage disequilibrium between alleles at the disease and marker loci[1]. The latter provides information on the location of the disease locus because linkage disequilibrium will only be detected over relatively small physical or genetic distances (23–25). Association studies yield relative risk estimates and associated alleles may be used to stratify patients into more homogeneous subgroups. The best example of the latter is the use of HLA types to subdivide diabetes mellitus into its two major subforms, IDDM and NIDDM, and to further stratify IDDM patients into autoimmune-mediated and nonautoimmune-mediated IDDM (26).

Association studies may also be particularly useful in inbred or other genetically homogeneous populations. Populations with relatively recent origins and a small number of founders will have fewer independent chromosomes and, presumably, fewer loci contributing to the disease, i.e., less genetic heterogeneity than in outbred populations. In addition, due to the recent origins there will have been relatively fewer meioses since the founding population. Fewer recombinations between homologous chromosomes will preserve larger segments of the founding chromosomes and linkage disequilibrium will be detected over greater physical and genetic distances than in outbred populations. Linkage disequilibrium mapping has proven successful for mapping genes for single gene disorders (27–31).

Linkage disequilibrium mapping may be particularly useful for identifying genes for complex diseases, such as atopy, in inbred populations such as the Amish, Hutterites, and the population living on the island of Tristan de Cunha (32–34).

Although association studies may provide information about the physical location of a disease gene, confirmation of an allele's involvement in disease susceptibility requires family-based linkage studies. Linkage studies are designed to locate (or map) susceptibility loci by examining whether a certain allele at a "marker"

locus is transmitted in families with the disease more than expected by chance alone. If two loci are on separate chromosomes, alleles at these loci would segregate (be inherited) together approximately 25% of the time. For example, the ABO blood group locus is on chromosome 9q34 and the human leukocyte antigen (HLA)-DR locus is on chromosome 6p21. If one parent has type AB blood and the DR2,DR5 genotype at the HLA locus, the offspring of this parent could inherit the A allele at the ABO locus and the DR2 alleles at the HLA-DR locus, the A allele and the DR5 allele, the B allele and the DR2 allele, or the B allele and the DR5 allele (Fig. 2). These four combinations should occur in equal frequencies because the loci are not linked. Because recombination (crossing over) between homologous chromosomes occurs quite commonly during meiosis, most loci on the same chromosome behave as though they are not linked. That is, recombination occurs between the two loci in at least 50% of meioses, and the recombination fraction, or θ, is said to be >0.50. However, the likelihood of recombination gets smaller as the physical distance between two loci gets smaller. Recombination fractions (θ) are estimated from directly observing the inheritance of alleles at two (or more) loci in families (Figure 3); θ <0.50 is evidence for linkage. A centiMorgan (cM) is a measure of linkage, named after the geneticist Thomas Hunt Morgan. Two loci are considered to be 1 cM apart if θ = 1% (i.e., recombination occurs in 1% of meioses) and is approximately equal to 1 million base pairs (equal to 1,000 kilobase [kb] or 1 megabase) of DNA. Note that recombination can only be observed in offspring of individuals who are heterozygous (i.e., carry different alleles on each chromosome) at the disease and the marker loci. In Figure 3, if the affected father in the second generation was homozygous at the marker locus (e.g., genotype 2,2), there would be no information in this family at this locus because all children would inherit allele 2 from the affected father regardless of whether they inherited the mutant or normal allele at the disease locus. Thus, using marker loci at which a high proportion of the population are heterozygotes is a critical component of a successful linkage study.

Statistical tests for determining linkage fall into two broad categories, parametric and nonparametric. The parametric method, called lod score analysis, is the more powerful approach, but requires that a genetic model (including mode of inheritance and penetrances of each genotype) be specified. Because this is rarely known for complex disorders like atopy, nonparametric approaches may be more appropriate in studies of multi-factorial diseases.

The lod score is the log of the likelihood ratio of linkage (θ < 0.5) to nonlinkage ($\theta \geq$ 0.5). A lod score of 3.0 corresponds to an odds of 1,000 to 1 in favor of linkage; therefore, a lod $\geq$ 3.0 is considered to be evidence for

---

[1]Linkage disequilibrium is the nonrandom association of alleles at linked loci in populations. Alleles that are in linkage disequilibrium will appear to be "associated" at the population level.

Parent Genotype
(HLA-DR locus on 6p)
(ABO locus on 9p)

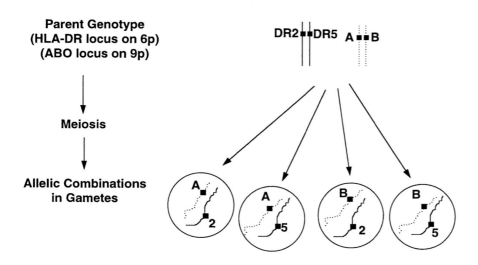

Meiosis

Allelic Combinations
in Gametes

FIG. 2. Alleles at unlinked loci assort independently during meiosis. Alleles at the ABO locus on chromosome 9 (*dotted lines*) and at the HLA-DR locus on chromosome 6 (*solid lines*) will assort independently, resulting in relatively equal proportions (25%) of gametes with each combination of alleles at these two (unlinked) loci. Due to recombination, most loci on the same chromosome also assort independently during meiosis.

linkage. A lod <-2.0 (odds of 100:1 against linkage) is considered to be significant evidence against linkage. Lod scores between -2.0 and 3.0 are inconclusive evidence for or against linkage and require studying additional families before the null hypothesis (no linkage) can be accepted. Lod score analysis was developed for and has been used extensively in studies of single gene disorders, where lod scores of >3 are unlikely to provide

false evidence of linkage (type I error). However, for complex disorders in which the likelihood of type 1 errors may be greater, a lod score of >3.0 is desirable (24). Formal linkage analysis is discussed in detail by Ott (35).

Nonparametric linkage approaches are less powerful for detecting a true linkage but may be more suitable for complex disorders in which the genetic models are un-

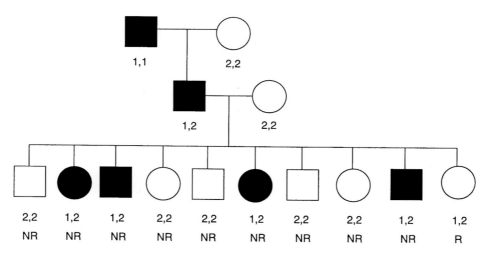

FIG. 3. A dominant condition is segregating in this family; affected individuals are shaded. Genotypes at a linked marker locus are shown below each symbol. The father in generation II inherited both the disease and allele 1 at the marker locus from his father (generation I). If the marker locus and the disease locus were unlinked, approximately 50% of the offspring in generation III would inherit allele 1, regardless of disease status. Because the disease and marker loci are linked, all but one offspring that inherited allele 1 also inherited the disease and all offspring that inherited paternal allele 2 are unaffected. The last affected child in the sibship inherited paternal allele 1 but did not inherit the disease, representing a recombination (R) between the disease locus and the marker locus. The other children are nonrecombinants (NR). Based on information from this family, the recombination fraction (θ) is 0.10 (recombination in 1 of 10 paternal meioses), and the two loci would be estimated to be 10 cM apart (see text for discussion).

known. In fact, this approach may be more powerful for detecting linkage than a lod score analysis in which the wrong model is specified. These methods rely on analyses of relative pairs, most commonly sib pairs (5,6). The assumption underlying the sib pair approach is that two sibs will inherit an allele at a particular locus that is identical-by-descent[2] from their father 25% of the time and from their mother 25% of the time (different probabilities are assigned to other relative pairs depending on their relatedness). Thus, the probability that two sibs will have one allele that is identical-by-descent from either parent is 50%, the probability that they will have two alleles that are identical-by-descent (1 from each parent) is 25% (i.e., genetically identical at the locus), and the probability that they will have no alleles that are identical-by-descent from either parent is 25%.

Sib pairs who are affected by the same disease will presumably have inherited one allele (if the susceptibility allele is a dominant) or two alleles (if the susceptibility allele is a recessive) that are identical-by-descent at the disease locus. If a marker locus is not linked to the disease locus, the affected sib pairs should share 2, 1, or 0 alleles, 25%, 50%, and 25% of the time, respectively (i.e., random expectations). However, if a marker locus is linked to the disease locus (i.e., $\theta < 0.50$), the sibs will share alleles more often than expected. Deviations from the expected proportions of 25%, 50%, 25% in affected sib pairs are evidence for linkage.

Sib pair analysis has the additional advantage over parametric linkage analysis in that one only needs to study affected sib pairs and does not need to include other family members, whereas parametric analyses benefit from studying intact families including unaffected relatives. Therefore, not only is the sampling strategy simpler and less costly in a sib pair design, but the classification of individuals with equivocal phenotypes and issues relating to penetrance can be ignored because these individuals are not included in the sample. Although the power of sib pair analysis to detect linkage is strengthened if genotypes (but not affection status) of the parents are available, this is not required. The simplicity of affected relative pair study design and the lack of knowledge regarding underlying genetic models in complex diseases have made affected sib pair analysis a popular approach for genetic studies of complex disorders (22,32,36,37).

LABORATORY TECHNIQUES

The recent explosion of successful gene mapping studies can be attributed largely to the development, refinement, and automation of the molecular biologic techniques used to identify inter-individual differences in DNA sequences. As mentioned previously, the power of both linkage and association studies is dependent on the ability to distinguish between alleles at homologous loci. A polymorphic locus is a locus at which there is more than one allele present in the population and the frequency of the least common allele occurs on at least 1% of chromosomes. Prior to the discovery of DNA polymorphisms, there were only approximately 50 polymorphic loci in humans that were amenable to linkage analysis. These included the HLA loci, red cell blood groups (e.g., ABO, Rh, MN), serum proteins (e.g., transferrin, immunoglobulin allotypes), and red cell enzymes (e.g., G6PD), to name a few. Therefore, not only was there a paucity of loci available for linkage studies, but with the exception of the HLA loci, most polymorphisms involved a small number of alleles and usually < 50% of individuals in the population were heterozygous for alleles at any one locus. Additionally, determining genotypes at these loci often require fresh cell or serum samples and specialized typing procedures.

DNA, on the other hand, provides an unlimited source of genetic polymorphisms. Because only 5% to 10% of the 3 billion base pairs of DNA comprising a haploid genome contains functional genes, 95% of our DNA can mutate (presumably) without altering gene function. Mutations in noncoding regions of DNA accumulate over evolutionary time, yielding an abundant source of genetic variability in the population. Additional advantages to studying DNA polymorphisms are that DNA does not have to be processed immediately, it can be stored indefinitely, and it can be extracted from very small samples of any tissue containing nucleated cells. Lastly, the techniques utilized for genotyping individuals are routine in many laboratories and have recently become automated (38).

There are two types of DNA polymorphisms that can be used for linkage analysis. Restriction fragment length polymorphisms (RFLPs) were the first type of DNA polymorphism described and usually represent single base-pair (nucleotide) differences between individuals that alter the recognition sequence of bacterial enzymes known as restriction endonucleases (Fig. 4). Because individuals differ at approximately every 1,000 base pairs and there are more than 500 restriction enzymes that recognize unique sequences, there are potentially thousands of RFLPs in the human genome. This fact led Botstein and colleagues (39) to suggest in 1980 that with a complete RFLP map of the human genome we should be able to map all human disease genes. Indeed, RFLP analysis was used to localize many genes, including the genes for Huntington's disease and cystic fibrosis during the first wave of gene-mapping studies in the 1980s; a complete RFLP map of the human genome was completed by 1987 (40–45). Despite the fact that RFLP

---

[2]Alleles that are identical-by-descent (IBD) are idential alleles inherited from a common ancestor; in this example the common ancestors are the parents.

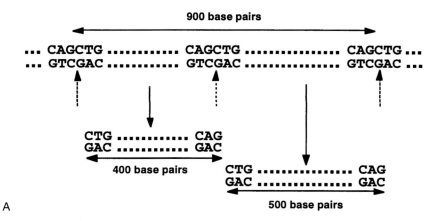

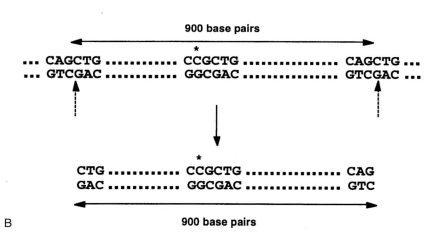

A

B

FIG. 4. A restriction enzyme that recognizes the nucleotide sequence CAGCTG on the forward strand and GTCGAC on the reverse strand (the site of cleavage is shown by hatched arrows), will recognize and cut double-stranded DNA at the three sites shown in Figure 4A. After digestion with this restriction enzyme (*solid arrows*), a 500-base-pair and a 400-base-pair fragment will be generated (**A**). (**B**) A transversion of an adenine (A) to a cytosine (C) (*designated by an asterisk*) within this sequence will eliminate one of the restriction enzyme recognition sites. After digestion with this restriction enzyme, a 900-base-pair fragment will be generated after enzyme digestion. Restriction fragment length polymorphisms (RFLPs) refer to differences between individuals with respect to restriction fragment lengths (400 bp + 500 bp vs. 900 bp in this example).

analysis revolutionized our ability to map disease genes, this approach was limited by the fact that most RFLPs are bi-allelic and heterozygosity levels are usually <50%. In addition, restriction enzymes are costly and the procedures for genotyping individuals are time consuming. Thus, by the early 1990s, the use of RFLPs for linkage analysis had become fairly obsolete, after the discovery of a second type of DNA polymorphism, called short tandem repeat polymorphisms (STRPs).

In addition to inter-individual differences with respect to DNA sequences that give rise to RFLPs, differences also exist with respect to the amount of DNA present in individual genomes. Distributed throughout the genome are sequences of DNA that occur as tandem (head to tail) repeats. Although the sequences themselves are present in every genome at precisely the same chromosomal location or locus, the number of repeats varies from chromosome to chromosome (Fig. 5). The size of the repeated unit also varies from two base

pairs to over a hundred base pairs, and repeated sequences are present at thousands of loci throughout the genome. Larger repeat sequences, called minisatellite DNA, were first described in 1985 (46). When minisatellite DNA at several loci are studied simultaneously they provide a unique DNA fingerprint and these loci are used commonly in forensic medicine, paternity testing, and conservation studies in endangered species (46). Shorter DNA sequences (2-5 base-pair repeats), called microsatellite DNA or STRPs, were first described in 1989 (47). An STRP map of the human genome was completed in 1994, providing mapped markers that are distributed throughout the genome and that can be used for linkage analysis (48). The abundance of STRPs in the human genome allows for the identification of markers that have many alleles (≥5) and high heterozygosity levels (>70%). In addition, STRP genotyping techniques are rapid, relatively inexpensive, and amenable to automation (38).

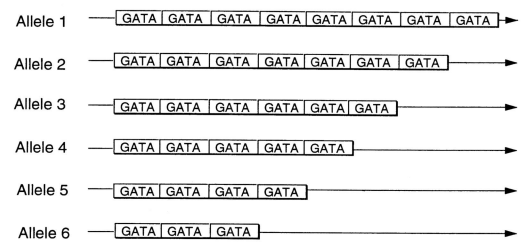

FIG. 5. Short tandem repeat polymorphisms (STRPs). In this example, a four bp repeat (GATA) is tandemly repeated on the chromosome. Different chromosomes in the population will carry different number of repeats, representing different alleles at this locus.

MAPPING ATOPY GENES

Although genome-wide searches to identify genes that influence atopy and atopy-associated phenotypes are currently underway in many laboratories around the world, all genetic studies reported to date have focused on candidate genes or regions. Four chromosomal regions containing candidate genes have been identified that are associated with or linked to atopy in one or more populations. These include HLA genes on chromosome 6p21.3, the high-affinity Fc-receptor for IgE on chromosome 11q13, the T-cell receptor α/δ chain loci on chromosome 14q11.2, and the cytokine gene cluster on chromosome 5q31-33 (4,32,36,37,49–69). Candidate genes that have been specifically excluded by linkage studies in selected populations include the TCR-β locus on chromosome 7q35, the esterase D locus on chromosome 13q14, and the HLA-DP locus on 6p21.3 (37,63,64).

The HLA Complex: Chromosome 6p21.3

HLA-region genes could influence the atopy phenotype in a variety of ways. First, the initial sensitization process begins in the lung when peptides from degraded allergen are presented to T cells by an HLA molecule. Therefore, differences among individuals with respect to HLA alleles could influence antigen binding and presentation or interactions with T cells, and such differences could influence the initial sensitization to allergen. The HLA class II genes, HLA-DR and HLA-DQ, are particularly good candidates because class II genes present peptides to CD4 T cells and elicit the production of antibodies. Although the primary focus of genetic studies has been on the HLA genes per se, this gene-rich region includes many other genes involved in immune reactions, some of which may also influence the atopic phenotype.

Studies of HLA haplotypes in allergic families were the first to explore the role of specific genes (or gene complexes) in atopy. Early investigations in the 1970s focused on families with multiple members with hay fever and examined the segregation of HLA haplotypes (determined by HLA-A and HLA-B locus antigens, at that time called the HL-A first and second locus, respectively) and ragweed hay fever or response to antigen E (AgE) (48–53). AgE was the ragweed pollen antigen that elicited an IgE response in atopic individuals and was measured by skin-test reactivity or IgE-antibody response. (AgE was later renamed *Amb a* I.) The hypothesis proposed by these investigators was that a locus within the HLA complex regulated immune response to antigen E. This hypothetical locus was called IrE and was presumed to be homologous to the Ir genes in the murine H-2 complex, which controls immune response. These studies provided evidence for the nonrandom segregation of HLA haplotypes with ragweed hay fever in the study families, and suggested that a locus segregating within the HLA complex determines ragweed sensitivity (48–53). Interestingly, Blumenthal and colleagues (50) suggested that the hypothetical IrE gene was centromeric to the HLA-B locus, and the order of genes in this region was HLA-A—HLA-B—MLR-S—IrE, where MLR-S was the name given to the locus believed at that time to control the ability to stimulate a mixed lymphocyte response (MLR) (51). It is now known that genetic control of the MLR is not determined by a single locus, but the ability to stimulate lymphocytes in a mixed lymphocyte reaction is determined by the class II HLA loci, particularly by alleles at the HLA-DR locus, which were later shown to influence IgE response to ragweed allergens (discussed later) (54–56,60,61). Although the methodologies employed in these early studies have been criticized, the suggestion that a locus regulating sensitivity to ragweed hay fever is linked to HLA and centromeric to HLA-B was proven correct by later studies (49,50,54,55,60,61,70).

In a series of elegant studies, Marsh and colleagues (54) have demonstrated that the HLA-DR2/Dw2 alleles, DRB1*1501 and DRB1*1502, are associated with the production of IgE antibody to short ragweed pollen allergen, *Amb a* V (formerly called Ra5) (55,60,61). In their first study, they reported that 95% of 38 ragweed allergic subjects with IgE antibodies to *Amb a* V were HLA-Dw2+ as compared with 22% of 139 ragweed allergic subjects without IgE antibodies (P < 0.0001) (54). HLA-Dw2 was strongly correlated with the magnitude of log[IgE Ab] and log[IgG Ab] levels, as demonstrated by multiple regression analysis (P < 0.00001 in two independent samples). Furthermore, the quantitative and qualitative IgG response to ragweed immunotherapy was significantly greater in allergic subjects who were HLA-Dw2+ as compared with allergic subjects who were HLA-Dw2- (P < 0.0001) (55). However, the fact that not all HLA-Dw2+ individuals respond after natural exposure to low doses of inhaled *Amb a* V led the investigators to suggest that a second locus may be necessary to facilitate the response to the antigenic determinant on *Amb a* V in HLA-Dw2+ individuals (55). They speculated that the second locus may be a gene encoding the T-cell receptor (55).

More recent studies by this group using molecular genetic techniques have shown that the IgE response to *Amb a* V is determined by HLA-DR alleles DRB1*1501 (previously called DR2.2) in Caucasians and DRB1*1502 (previously called DR2.12) in Asians, and that the HLA-DQ loci do not contribute to this response (60,61). Using CD4, *Amb a* V-specific T-cell clones and a polyclonal *Amb a* V-reactive T-cell line from DRB1*1501+ individuals, proliferative responses were observed when DRB1*1501 or DRB1*1502 antigen-presenting cells were present, regardless of the HLA-DQ genotype (60). Furthermore, the T-cell responses were eliminated by anti-DR (but not anti-DQ or anti-DP) antibodies, establishing a primary role for the HLA-DR gene products (i.e., DRB1*1501 and DRB1*1502 alleles) in restricting the T-cell recognition of *Amb a* V (60). The DRB1*1501 and DRB1*1502 alleles share an identical amino-acid sequence in the second exon, except for a single amino-acid difference (Gly-Val) at position 86. Thus, the polymorphic residues unique to these two alleles may influence the binding and presentation of *Amb a* V peptides, and the unique amino-acid at position 86 may influence the binding of specific T-cell clones, since DRB1*1502+ cells were not capable of presenting *Amb a* V to DRB1*1501-restricted T cells (60).

In similar, but less fully developed experiments, Marsh's group and others have reported associations between specific HLA-DR types and IgE responses to short ragweed pollen (*Amb a* VI), rye grass (*Lol p* I and *Lol p* II), American feverview pollen (*Parthenium hysteropho-*

rus), birch pollen (*Bet v* I), cat (*Fel d* I), and mold (*Alt a* I) (56–59,62,63). A summary of these results is presented in Table 3. HLA associations were not found with IgE response to house dust mite allergens (*Der p* I and *Der p* II), Timothy grass (*Phl p* V), or dog (*Can f* I) in a single study (63). Furthermore, linkage between the HLA-linked STRP, D6S105, and "atopy" was not detected in Dutch families ascertained through an asthmatic parent (71). In the latter study, atopy was defined as either the presence of ≥1 positive skin tests (≥ 2 mm), a positive radioallergosorbent test (RAST) (≥ 35 RU/mL), or an elevated total serum IgE level.

Collectively these investigations suggest that polymorphic amino-acid sequences in the HLA-DR gene (most likely the second exon of the HLA-DRB1 gene) differentially bind peptides derived from a variety of allergens and influence IgE antibody production. The relative risks associated with HLA-DR alleles (Table 3) are among the highest reported for HLA-associated diseases, suggesting that HLA-DR encodes a major gene influencing IgE response (72). Because different HLA-DR types appear to be associated with response to specific allergens, pooling families with IgE responses or skin test reactivity to a variety of allergens may, in fact, mask the relationship between HLA-DR alleles and atopy, and future association or linkage studies with HLA should consider IgE response or skin test reactivity to single (purified) allergens (71).

The High-Affinity Fc-Receptor for IgE (Fcε RI-β): Chromosome 11q13

The Fc-receptor for IgE is expressed on mast cells and basophils. When specific IgE bound to Fc-receptors on mucosal mast cells encounters inhaled allergen during sec-

TABLE 3. *HLA associations with IgE to specific allergens*

Allergen	Primary Association	Risk	Reference
Amb a V	DR2/Dw2	88.4[a]	54
Amb a VI	DR5	4.4[a]	56
Lol p I	DR3	5.9[a]	57
Lol p II	DR3	2.9[a]	57
Lol p III	DR5	10.3[a]	58
Bet v I	DRw52	3.4[b]	62
Parthenium hysterophorus	DR3	11.3[b]	59
Fel d I	DR1	2.0[c]	63
Alt a I	DR4	1.9[c]	63

[a]Relative risk calculated using Mantel-Haenszel method for multiple samples (72); pooled estimate based on published frequencies in clinic and Westinghouse samples (IgE positive vs. IgE negative allergic subjects)
[b]Relative risk calculated in IgE positive vs. IgE negative allergic subjects
[c]Odds ratio calculated in IgE positive vs. controls

ondary and later exposures, the Fc-receptors aggregate on the cell surface and activate, either directly or indirectly, enzymes in the cell membrane. The subsequent cascade of cellular events causes the mast cell to release various chemicals that are responsible for many allergic symptoms, including the release of histamine and interleukin-4 (IL-4). Thus, genetic variation in the Fc-receptor for IgE could influence allergic responses. The high-affinity $Fc_{\varepsilon}RI$ is composed of three subunits: α, β, and γ. The α and γ subunits are encoded by genes on chromosome 1q23 and the β subunit is encoded by a gene on chromosome 11q13.

The first evidence for linkage to an "atopy" gene was reported by Cookson and colleagues in 1989 (64). In this first study, they ascertained seven English families through members with hay fever or asthma. All family members were categorized as atopic if they met at least one of the following criteria: positive skin prick test to at least one antigen (2 mm greater than a negative control), total serum IgE level greater than 2 standard deviations of the geometric mean of the population, or elevated specific serum IgE to at least one common antigen (≥ 0.35 RAST units/mL). Linkage analysis between an RFLP (locus D11S97; probe pMS.51) on chromosome 11q13 and atopy revealed a maximum lod score of 5.58 at $\theta = 0.105$, suggesting that a gene influencing the atopic phenotype was within 10.5 cM of their linked marker. In a series of subsequent studies, Cookson's group reported that the 11q13 markers confer risk for atopy only when inherited from the mother, confirmed linkage between atopy and maternally-inherited D11S97 in over 150 affected sib pairs, and determined that (in a proportion of families) the risk is due to a single base-pair mutation in the $Fc_{\varepsilon}RI$-β gene (4,65,67). In the latter study, a substitution of a leucine for an isoleucine at position 181 (Leu181) in the fourth transmembrane domain of the receptor was an atopy susceptibility allele if it was maternally, but not paternally inherited. In an independent sample of 60 unrelated English and Welsh families with allergic asthmatic probands, Leu181 was identified in 10 (17%) and was maternally inherited in each case (67). In another sample of 163 unrelated atopic patients, 25 (15%) were Leu181 positive and this mutation was significantly correlated with total serum IgE (P = 0.01) and specific IgE to grass pollen (P = 0.03) (67). The Leu181 allele was detected in 4.2% of individuals in a random population survey of 1,020 Australians in one study, but was not detected in a second study in Australia of 610 individuals who were members of twin pairs ascertained for a history of wheeze or asthma, 198 parents of the twins, or 131 unrelated controls with unknown status with respect to asthma (67,73).

These combined data suggest that in 60% of atopic families studied by the Cookson group, the atopic phenotype co-segregated with maternally inherited 11q13 markers and that Leu181 occurred in 17% of these families. In 40% of families atopy was not linked to 11q13, suggesting that susceptibility to atopy in these families

was determined by alleles at loci that are not linked to 11q13. That the Leu181 mutation was present in only 17% of families with 11q13-linked atopy further suggests that 11q13 genes other than the $Fc_{\varepsilon}RI$-β gene or mutations other than Leu181 in the $Fc_{\varepsilon}RI$-β gene underlie atopy in the majority of these families.

Replication studies of linkage between atopy and 11q markers by other investigators have yielded conflicting results (Table 4). One study from Japan reported evidence for linkage between atopy and the 11q13 marker D11S97 in four families and one study from the Netherlands reported evidence for linkage between atopy and 11q13 markers (PYGM and D11S97) in 26 affected sib pairs (68,69). Interestingly, the latter study did not find evidence for linkage with the $Fc_{\varepsilon}RI$-β gene per se, and found no significant differences in the proportion of maternal and paternal alleles that were shared by affected sib pairs. Like Cookson's results described previously, these results are consistent with a second locus on 11q13 that influences atopy. It should be noted that both studies reporting evidence for linkage with 11q markers used stricter criteria for defining atopy than the criteria used in Cookson's initial report (64,68,69) (Table 4).

Evidence for linkage between atopy and 11q13 was not found in 20 Dutch families, 95 English families, four large Japanese families, nine British families, and three large U.S. midwestern families (71,74,76,77) (Table 4).

In total, these data indicate that a locus on chromosome 11q13 may influence the atopy phenotype in some families. However, evidence for linkage to the $Fc_{\varepsilon}RI$-β gene is limited to a small proportion of the 11q-linked families, raising the possibility that other genes in this region may influence the atopic phenotype.

The α/δ Chains of the T-Cell Receptor (TCR-α/δ): Chromosome 14q11.2

Most TCRs are composed of α- and β-chains, but a small proportion are composed of γ- and δ-chains. γ/δ T cells are present in the respiratory epithelium and may serve as a "first line of defence" against pathogens, as well as protection from IgE-mediated responses to inhaled antigens (78). The TCR β-chain is encoded by genes on chromosome 7q35, the α- and δ-chains are encoded by genes on chromosome 14q11.2, and the γ-chain is encoded by genes on chromosome 7p15-p14.

T cells play an integral role in the allergic response. For example, the production of specific IgE is determined by unique interactions between the TCR and the HLA/peptide complex. In addition, the relative balance between the T helper 1 (TH1) and T helper 2 (TH2) responses may underlie allergic symptoms (78). The TH2 response includes the production of cytokines that signal B cells to mature into antibody-secreting plasma cells (IL-4), regulate eosinophil growth and differentiation (IL-5), cause the proliferation of mast cells (IL-9), and

TABLE 4. *Summary of linkage studies of atopy and loci on chromosome 11q13*

Reference	Study Sample	Atopic Phenotype	Locus	Results
Cookson (64)	7 British families ascertained through members with hay fever or asthma	≥ 1 of the following: a) total IgE > 2 s.d. geom. mean; b) RAST > 3.5 to ≥1 antigen; c) skin prick test > 2 mm to ≥ 1 antigen	D11S97	Lod = 5.58, θ = 0.105
Amelung(71)	26 Dutch sib pairs with asthma	same as Cookson (64)	INT2	Lod < −2.0, θ = 0.12
Hizawa(75)	4 large Japanese families ascertained through asthmatic proband	1 of the following: a) total IgE 2 s.d. geom. mean; b) ≥1 elevated specific IgE titer; c) skin prick test positive to ≥ 1 allergen	D11S97	Lod = −2.63, θ=0
Lymphany (76)	9 British families ascertained through proband with allergy or asthma	≥1 of the following: a) total IgE > 2 s.d. geom. mean; b) RAST score ≥1+; c) skin prick test > 2 mm to ≥ 1 antigen	PYGM INT2	Lod = −9.17, θ = 0.001 Lod = −4.97, θ = 0.001
Rich (77)	3 large midwestern U.S. families including 126 sib pairs	All of the following: a) skin prick test > 5 mm to ≥1 antigen; b) total serum IgE > 87.3 U/mL; c) specific IgE > 0.35 PRU/mL	D11S97	Lod = −2.0, θ = 0.22 Sib pair, P = 0.86
Shirakawa (68)	4 Japanese families ascertained through asthmatic probands	All of the following: a) total IgE > 2 s.d. geom. mean; b) RAST > 3.5 to ≥3 antigen; c) intradermal skin test response > 9 mm to > 3 allergens	D11S97	Lod = 4.88, θ = 0.07
Coleman (74)	95 nuclear families ascertained through 2 first degree relatives with atopic asthma	Same as Cookson (64)	D11S97 PYGM FCREB1	Excluded evidence for linkage with these loci by lod score analysis (lod = −7.8) and in 101 affected sib pairs
Collée (69)	26 Dutch sib pairs with asthma	All of the following: a) ≥2 symptoms by questionnaire; b) specific IgE≥0.35 PRU/mL; c) elevated total serum IgE	D11S97 PYGM FCER1B	P < 0.01 P < 0.01 Not significant

IgE, immunoglobuling E; RAST, radioallergosorben test.

downregulate TH1 response (IL-10). In atopic individuals, the TH2 response may be upregulated resulting in a prolonged IgE response to nonpathogenic allergens.

Only one study has been reported to date that has examined evidence for linkage between specific IgE response to common allergens and the TCR-β (7q35) and TCR-α/δ loci (14q11.2) (37). This study included 410 British and 413 Australian subjects, including a total of 312 sib pairs (although not all sib pairs were positive for every antibody). Serum samples from British subjects were tested for IgE antibodies against six purified antigens and serum samples from Australian subjects were tested for IgE antibodies against three purified antigens. A positive response was the equivalent to 1 RAST unit or greater (37). Genotypes for STRPs in the TCR-β and the TCR-α genes were determined in all subjects and an affected sib pair analysis was conducted.

Alleles at the TCR-β locus were not shared among British and Australian affected sib pairs more often than would be expected by chance (P > 0.10 for each of the five allergen-specific antibodies tested and for total IgE > 70% of the geometric mean in pooled sample). In contrast, sharing of TCR-α alleles was increased in both British and Australian sib pairs (Table 5). In the pooled sample of British and Australian subjects there was significantly more sharing of alleles at the TCR-α locus among sibs with high IgE titers against house dust mites, grass, and cats and with high total IgE (P < 0.02 for each comparison), although when each population was considered separately there was no evidence for linkage with IgE against grass, and total IgE in the British subjects or with IgE against *Der p* II and house dust mites in the Australian subjects (37).

These data are consistent with the hypothesis that genetic variability at the TCR-α/δ loci influences IgE response to specific allergens. However, the numbers of sib pairs with positive titers against each allergen was fairly small, particularly in the British sample where the number of affected sib pairs ranged between seven (grass) to 18 (*Der p* II). In the pooled sample the number of sib

TABLE 5. *Results of sib pair analyses of specific IgE and TCR-α alleles[a,b].*

IgE Phenotype	Number Sib Pairs Sharing			P-value
	0 Alleles	1 Alleles	2 Alleles	
HDM	21	12	8	0.0005
Grass	20	17	11	0.02
IgE >70%	21	16	7	0.002
Der p I	17	8	4	0.0002
Der p II	18	13	5	0.002
Fel d I	14	4	3	0.00006

[a]Data for English and Australian sib pairs are pooled.
[b]From Moffatt MF, Hill MR, Cornélis Schou C, et al. Genetic linkage of T-cell receptor α/δ complex to specific IgE responses. *Lancet* 1994;343:1597–1600.
IgE, immunoglobulin E.

pairs was larger (range = 21 sib pairs with antibodies against *Fel d* I to 48 sib pairs with antibodies against grass), but was still fairly small for most of the comparisons. Furthermore, statistical tests with multiple clinical (IgE) markers increase the likelihood of a type I (false-positive) error, although some of the P-values in the pooled sample would remain significant even after using a correction for multiple comparisons (79). Regardless, these potentially interesting data need to be replicated in other data sets before conclusions can be drawn regarding the role of the TCR-α/δ genes in influencing variability in the atopic phenotype.

The Cytokine Gene Cluster: Chromosome 5q31-33

The cytokine gene cluster on chromosome 5q31-33 contains an abundance of genes that could influence the atopic phenotype (Figure 6). Cytokines in this region are involved in the atopic response by regulating the isotype switch in B cells from IgM to IgE (IL-4, IL-13), the growth and differentiation of mast cells (IL-3, IL-9) and eosinophils (IL-5), the survival of mast cells (IL-10). Other genes in this region include growth factors (granulocyte-macrophage colony-stimulating factor [GM-CSF], fibroblast growth factor A [FGFA]), growth factor receptors (colony-stimulating factor receptor 1 [CSF1R], platelet-derived growth

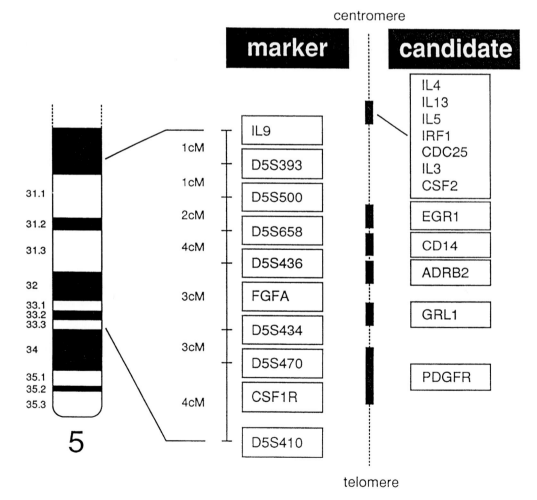

FIG. 6. Relative order of STRPs and approximate location of candidate genes for asthma, BHR, atopy on chromosome 5q. (Modified from Postma DS, Bleeker ER, Amelung PJ, Holroyd KJ, et al. Genetic susceptibility to asthma—bronchial hyperresponsiveness coinherited with a major gene for atopy. *N Engl J Med* 1995;333:894–900.)

factor receptor [PDGFR]), the lymphocyte-specific gluco-corticoid receptor (GRL), and the β₂-adrenergic receptor (ADRB2). Therefore, this region contains genes that are particularly good candidates for genes that may influence atopic phenotypes.

Two studies have reported linkage between total serum IgE and markers on chromosome 5q31-32. In the first study, Marsh and colleagues (32) studied linkage between 5q markers and total and specific IgE levels in 11 large Amish families. The Amish are a reproductive isolate of European origins that lives in farming communities with a relatively uniform environment. Reproductive isolation enhances the likelihood that fewer atopy genes are segregating in the population, while their traditional lifestyle (including the prohibition of smoking) reduces the potential confounding effects of environmental factors (32). A total of 349 sib pairs in the 11 families were genotyped for eight STRPs spanning the region from centromeric to the IL-13 gene in 5q31 to the CSF1R gene in 5q33. Clinical variables included log [total IgE] (adjusted for sex and age), and log [specific IgE] to a composite of 20 airborne allergens and to house dust mites, *Der p* and *Der f*. Antibody measurements were used as quantitative variables in the sib pair analysis.

Five STRPs in the 5q31.1 region provided significant evidence of linkage by sib pair analyses using quantitative log [total IgE]. The most significant evidence for linkage was with IL-4 (P = 0.0069), D5S393 (P = 0.0058) and D5S399 (P = 0.0020) (32). Three loci mapping outside of the 5q31.1 region (D5S404, D5S210, CSF1R) did not show evidence for linkage (P > 0.10). None of the markers showed evidence for linkage with the measurements of specific IgE (P ≥ 0.20). The evidence for linkage with log [total IgE] became more significant when log [multiallergen IgE] was included as a covariate, along with age and sex (34). Furthermore, the evidence for linkage between the 5q31.1 markers and log [total IgE] was greatest in the 128 "nonatopic" sib pairs, whereas there was no evidence for linkage between 5q31.1 markers and log [total IgE] in the 66 sib pairs with specific IgE antibodies. Lod score analysis of these data provided only minimal evidence for linkage (maximum lod score = 1.84 for D5S210 at a θ = 0). Thus, this study suggested a role for genes in the 5q31-33 region influencing total IgE levels, but not IgE response to specific allergens. Marsh and colleagues suggested that the IL-4 gene is the most likely candidate in this region; however, the results of this study do not exclude candidate genes distal to the IL-4 gene.

A second study examined linkage between total IgE levels and genes in the 5q cytokine cluster in 55 Dutch families (36). These families were ascertained through a symptomatic asthmatic proband, who was originally studied between 1962 and 1970 (71,80,81). In recent years, probands and their relatives (spouses, children, grandchildren) have been re-evaluated. This study included 55 families in whom DNA samples were available for ge-netic studies. Linkage analysis with eight 5q STRPs and log[total IgE] was conducted using the sib pair method and lod score analysis. Two of the eight STRPs, D5S393 and CSF1R, were among the STRPs studied in the Amish families described earlier (34).

Significant evidence for linkage was seen with the STRP, D5S436, in sib pair analysis (P=0.003). The flanking markers, D5S393 (proximal) and CSF1R (distal), provided more modest evidence for linkage (P=0.01 and 0.03, respectively) (36). Linkage with these markers became more significant when individuals with total IgE levels > mean ± 3 SD were removed. Lod score analysis further supported linkage with D5S436 (lod = 3.56, Θ = 0.09); lod scores for other markers were < 1.6 (36). These data are consistent with the presence of a gene linked to D5S436 that influences total IgE levels in these families. However, because these families were ascertained through a parent with asthma and many individuals with asthma also have serologic evidence of atopy (82–85), the findings in this study may in fact represent linkage to asthma, as discussed by the investigators (36).

The cytokine gene cluster on chromosome 5q is a large genetic region, spanning over 10,000 kb of DNA and containing numerous genes that could potentially influence the atopic phenotype (34). Based on results of these two studies it is tempting to speculate that genetic susceptibilities to atopy are influenced by at least two genes in this region, one gene at the proximal end of the region linked to the IL-4 gene and a second locus more distal and linked to D5S438 (32,36). The IL-4 gene itself is a likely candidate because this cytokine controls the B-cell isotype switch from IgM to IgE and polymorphisms in the 5'-promotor region of the IL-4 gene have been reported and could influence gene expression (86). The β₂-adrenergic receptor gene, which maps between D5S436 and CSF1R, is a likely candidate in the more distal region. Polymorphisms in this gene are associated with lower airway reactivity (87), which is often associated with elevated IgE levels (82–85,87). Speculations aside, these studies provide intriguing data regarding the role of chromosome 5q genes in atopy and asthma and will no doubt be followed by many additional studies of genes in this region in atopic families.

CONCLUSIONS

Despite the methodologic limitations inherent in genetic studies of complex diseases, significant progress has been made to date in identifying specific genes or chromosomal regions that influence the atopic phenotypes. Using a candidate gene approach, four genetic regions have been shown to be associated with atopy, at least in selected families. Replication of these results is required, however, because the probability of false-positive lod scores may be increased if the incorrect mode of inheritance is specified, and the true mode of inheritance for atopic phenotypes is unknown (24,88). Nonetheless, ongoing studies of the genetics of atopy promise to provide additional evidence for linkage with novel genes or regions or with other known candidate genes. Confirming significant linkage results in independent samples, examining interactions between multiple linked genes, and elucidating the true genetic mechanisms underlying these phenotypes will be a major future challenge to geneticists.

ACKNOWLEDGMENTS

The author is supported by grants HL49596, HD21244, and HD27686.

REFERENCES

1. Meyers DA, Marsh DG. Allergy and asthma. In: King RA, Rotter JI, Motulsky AG, eds. *The genetic basis of common diseases.* New York: Oxford University Press, 1992;130–149.
2. Lebowitz MD, Barbee R, Burrows B. Family concordance of IgE, atopy, and disease. *J Allergy Clin Immunol* 1984;73:259–264.
3. Morton NE. Major loci for atopy? *Clin Exp Allergy* 1992;22:1041–1043.
4. Cookson WOCM, Young RP, Sandford AJ, et al. Maternal inheritance of atopic IgE responsiveness on chromosome 11q. *Lancet* 1992;340: 381–384.
5. Suarez BK, Rice J, Reich T. The generalised sib pair IBD distribution: its use in the detection of linkage. *Ann Hum Genet* 1978;42:87–94.
6. Risch N. Linkage strategies for genetically complex traits. II. The power of affected relative pairs. *Am J Hum Genet* 1990;46:229–241.
7. Fields C, Adams MD, White O, Venter JC. How many genes in the human genome? *Nat Genet* 1994;7:345–346.
8. Prockop DJ, Constantinou CD, Dombrowksi KE, et al. Type I procollagen: the gene-protein system that harbors most of the mutations causing ostiogenesis imperfecta and probably more common heritable disorders of connective tissue. *Am J Med Genet* 1989;34:60–67.
9. Froguel P, Vaxillaire M, Sun F, Velho G, Zouali H, Butel MO. Close linkage of glucokinase locus on chromosome 7p to early-onset non-insulin-dependent diabetes mellitus. *Nature* 1992;356:162–164.
10. Hattersley AT, Turner RC, Permutt MA, et al. Linkage of type 2 diabetes to the glucokinase gene. *Lancet* 1 1992;339:1307–1310.
11. Stoffel M, Patel P, Lo Y-MD, et al. Missense glucokinase mutation in maturity-onset diabetes of the young and mutation screening in late-onset disease. *Nat Genet* 1992;2:153–156.
12. Rashbas J. Online Mendelian inheritance of man. *Trends Genet* 1995;11:291–292.
13. Collins FS. Positional cloning: let's not call it reverse anymore. *Nat Genet* 1992;1:3–6.
14. Collins FS. Positional cloning moves from perditional to traditional. *Nat Genet* 1995;9:347–350
15. Ballabio A. The rise and fall of positional cloning? *Nat Genet* 1993;3: 277–279
16. Rommens JM, Iannuzzi MC, Kerem B, et al. Identification of the cystic fibrosis gene: chromosome walking and jumping. *Science* 1989; 245:1059–1065.
17. Riordan JR, Rommens JM, Kerem B, Kerem B, et al. Identification of the cystic fibrosis gene: cloning and characterization of the complimentary DNA. *Science* 1989; 245:1066–1072.
18. Kerem B, Rommens JM, Buchanan JA, et al. Identification of the cystic fibrosis gene: genetic analysis. *Science* 1989; 245:1073–1080.
19. Huntington's Disease Collaborative Research Group, The. A novel gene containing a trinucleotide repeat that is expanded and unstable in Huntington's disease chromosomes. *Cell* 1993; 971–983.
20. Maslen CL, Corson GM, Maddox BK, Glanville RW, Sakai LY. Partial sequence of a candidate gene for the Marfan syndrome. *Nature* 1991; 352:334–337.
21. Dietz HC, Cutting GR, Pyeritz RE, et al. Marfan syndrome caused by a recurrent de novo missense mutation in the fibrillin gene. *Nature* 1991;353:337–339.
22. Davies JL, Kawaguchi Y, Bennett ST, et al. A genome-wide search for human type 1 diabetes susceptibility genes. *Nature* 1994;371:130–136.
23. de la Chapelle A. Disease gene mapping in isolated human populations: the example of Finland. *Am J Med Genet* 1993;30:857–865.
24. Lander ES, Schork NJ. Genetic dissection of complex traits. *Science* 1994;265:2037–2048.
25. Jorde LB. Linkage disequilibrium as a gene-mapping tool. *Am J Hum Genet* 1994;56:11–14.
26. Rotter JI, Vadheim CM, Rimoin DL. Diabetes mellitus. In: King RA, Rotter JI, Motulsky AG, eds. *The genetic basis of common diseases.* New York: Oxford University Press, 1992;413–481.
27. Hästbacka J, de la Chapelle A, Kaitila I, Sistonen P, Weaver A, Lander E. Linkage disequilbrium mapping in isolated founder populations: diastrophic dysplasia in Finland. *Nat Genet* 1992;2: 204–211.
28. Kestilä M, Männikkö M, Holmberg C, et al. Congenital nephrotic syndrome of the Finnish type maps to the long arm of chromosome 19. *Am J Hum Genet* 1994;54:757–764.
29. Höglund P, Sistonen P, Norio R, et al. Fine mapping of the congenital chloride diarrhea gene by linkage disequilibrium. *Am J Hum Genet* 1995;57:95–102.
30. Puffenberger EG, Kauffman ER, Bolk S, et al. Identity-by-descent and association mapping of a recessive gene for Hirschsprung disease on human chromosome 13q22. *Hum Molec Genet* 1994;3:1217–1225.
31. Houwen RJH, Baharloo S, Blankenship K, Raeymaekers, Juyn J, Sandkuijl LA, Freimer NB. Genome screening by searching for shared segments: mapping a gene for benign recurrent intrahepatic cholestasis. *Nat Genet* 1994;8:380–346.
32. Marsh DG, Neely JD, Breazeale DR, et al. Linkage analysis of IL4 and other chromosome 5q31.1 markers and total serum immunoglobulin E concentrations. *Science* 1994;264:1152–1156.
33. Ober C, Bombard A, Dhaliwal R, Elias S, Fagan J, Laffler T, Martin AO, Rosinsky B. Studies of cystic fibrosis in Hutterite families using linked DNA probes. *Am J Hum Genet* 1987;41:1145–1151.
34. Zamel N, McClean PA, Sandell PR, Siminovitch KA, Slutsky AS. Asthma on Tristan da Cunha: Looking for the genetic link. *Am J Respir Crit Care Med* 1996; 153:190–1906.
35. Ott J. *Analysis of human genetic linkage.* Baltimore: The Johns Hopkins University Press, 1992.
36. Meyers DA, Postma DS, Panhuysen CIM, et al. Evidence for a locus regulating total serum IgE levels map to chromosome 5. *Genomics* 1994; 23:464–470.
37. Moffatt MF, Hill MR, Cornélis Schou C, et al. Genetic linkage of T-cell receptor a/d complex to specific IgE responses. *Lancet* 1994;343: 1597–1600.
38. Schwengel DA, Jedlicka AE, Nanthakumar EJ, Weber JL, Levitt RC. Comparison of fluorescence-based semi-automated genotyping of multiple microsatellite loci with autoradiographic techniques. *Genomics* 1994;22:46–54.
39. Botstein D, White RL, Skolnick M, David RW. Construction of a genetic linkage map in man using restriction fragment length polymorphisms. *Am J Hum Gen* 1980;32:314–331
40. Gusella JF, Wexler NS, Conneally PM, et al. A polymorphic marker genetically linked to Huntington's disease. *Nature* 1983;306:234–238.
41. Eiberg H, Mohr J, Schmiegelow K, Nielsen LS, Williamson R. Linkage relationships of paraoxonase (PON) with other markers: Indication of PON-cystic fibrosis synteny. *Clin Genet* 1985;28:265–271.
42. Tsui L-C, Buchwald M, Barker D, et al. Cystic fibrosis locus defined by a genetically linked polymorphic DNA marker. *Science* 19851230: 1054–1057.
43. Wainwright BJ, Scambler PJ, Schmidtke J, et al. Localization of cystic fibrosis locus to human chromosome 7cen-q22. *Nature* 1985;318: 384–385.
44. White R, Woodward S, Leppert M, et al. A closely linked genetic marker for cystic fibrosis. *Nature* 1985;318:382–384.
45. Donis-Keller H, Green P, Helms C, et al. A genetic linkage map of the human genome. *Cell* 1987;51:319–37.
46. Jeffreys AJ, Wilson V, Thein SL. Hypervariable 'minisatellite' regions in human DNA. *Nature* 1984;314:67–73.
47. Weber JL, May PE. Abundant class of human DNA polymorphisms which can be typed using the polymerase chain reaction. *Am J Hum Genet* 1989;44:388–396.

48. Gyapay G, Morissette J, Vignal A, et al. The 1993-94 Genethon human genetic linkage map. *Nat Genet* 1994;7246–7339.
49. Levine RB, Stember RH, Fotino M. Ragweed hayfever: genetic control and linkage to HL-A haplotypes. *Science* 1972;178:1201–1203.
50. Blumenthal MN, Amos DB, Noreen H, Mendell NR, Yunis EJ. Genetic mapping of Ir locus in man: linkage to second locus of HLA. *Science* 1974;184;1301–1303.
51. Yunis EJ, Amos DB, Blumenthal MN. Genetic mapping of IrE outside of HL-A-MLR-S complex. *Transplant Proc* 1975;VII:49–51.
52. Yoo T-J, Flink RJ, Thompson JS. The relationship between HL-A antigens and lymphocyte response in ragweed allergy. *J Allergy Clin Immunol* 1976;57;25–28.
53. Mendell NR, Blumenthal M, Amos DB, Yunis EJ, Elston RC. Ragweed sensitivity: segregation analysis and linkage to HLA-B. *Cytogenet Cell Genet* 1978;22:330–334.
54. Marsh DG, Hsu SH, Roebber M, et. al. HLA-Dw2: a genetic marker for human immune response to short ragweed pollen allergen Ra5.I. Response resulting primarily from natural antigenic exposure. *J Exp Med* 1982;155:1439–1451.
55. Marsh DG, Meyers DA, Freidhoff LR, et al. HLA-Dw2: a genetic marker for human immune response to short ragweed pollen allergen Ra5.II. Response after ragweed immunotherapy. *J Exp Med* 1982;155: 1452–1463.
56. Marsh DG, Freidhoff LR, Ehrlich-Dautsky E, Bias WB, Roebber M. Immune responsiveness to *Ambrosia artemisiifolia* (short ragweed) pollen allergen Amb a VI (Ra6) is associated with HLA-DR5 in allergic humans. *Immunogenetics* 1987;26:230–236.
57. Freidhoff LR, Ehrlich-Kautsky E, Meyers DA, Ansari AA, Bias WB, Marsh DG. Association of HLA-DR3 with human response to Lol p I and Lol p II allergens in allergic subjects. *Tissue Antigens* 1988;31: 211–219.
58. Ansari AA, Freidhoff LR, Meyers DA, Bias WB, Marsh DG. Human immune responsiveness to Lolium perenne pollen allergen Lol p III (Rye III) is associated with HLA-DR3 and DR5. *Hum Immunol* 1989; 25:59–71.
59. Sriramarao P, Sevlakumar B, Damodaran C, Subba Rao BS, Prakash O, Subba Rao PV. Immediate hypersensitivity to Parthenium hysterophorus. I. Association of HLA antigens and Parthenium rhinitis. *Clin Exp Allergy* 1990;20;555–560.
60. Huang S-K, Zwollo P, Marsh DG. Class II major histocompatibility complex restriction of human T cell responses to short ragweed allergen, Amb a V. *Eur J Immunol* 1991;21:1469–1473.
61. Zwollo P, Ehrlich-Kautsky E, Scharf SJ, Ansari AA, Erlich HA, Marsh DG. Sequencing of HLA-D in responders and nonresponders to short ragweed allergen, Amb a V. *Immunogenetics* 1991;33:141–151.
62. Fischer GF, Pickl WF, Faé I, et al. Association between IgE response against Bet v I, the major allergen of birch pollen, and HLA-DRB alleles. *Hum Immunol* 1992;33:259–265.
63. Young RP, Dekker JW, Wordsworth BP, et al. HLA-DR and HLA-DP genotypes and immunoglobulin E responses to common major allergens. *Clin Exp Allergy* 1994;24:431–439.
64. Cookson WOCM, Sharp PA, Faux JA, Hopkin JM. Linkage between immunoglobulin E responses underlying asthma and rhinitis and chromosome 11q. *Lancet* 1989;i:1292–1295.
65. Young RP, Sharp PA, Lynch JR, et al. Confirmation of genetic linkage between atopic EgE responses and chromosome 11q. *J Med Genet* 1992;29:236–238.
66. Sandford AJ, Shirakawa T, Moffatt MF, et al. Localisation of atopy and β subunit of high-affinity IgE receptor (FcεRI) on chromosome 11q. *Lancet* 1993;341:332–334.
67. Shirakawa T, Li A, Dubowitz M, et al. Association between atopy and variants of the b subunit of the high-affinity immunoglobulin E receptor. *Nat Genet* 1994;7:125–130.
68. Shirakawa T, Morimoto K, Hashimoto T, Furuyama J, Yamamoto M, Takai S. Linkage between IgE responses underlying asthma and rhinitis (Atopy) and chromosome 11q in Japanese families. *Cytogenet Cell Genet* 1991;58:1970–1971.
69. Collée Jm, ten Kate LP, de Vries HG, Kliphuis JW, Bouman K, Scheffer H, Gerritsen J. Allele sharing on chromosome 11q13 in sibs with asthma and atopy. *Lancet* 1993;342:936.
70. Bias WB, Marsh DG. HL-A linked antigen E immune response genes: an unproven hypothesis. *Science* 1975;188:375–377.
71. Amelung PJ, Panhuysen CIM, Postma DS, et al. Atopy and bronchial hyperresponsiveness: exclusion of linkage to markers on chromosomes 11q and 6p. *Clin Exp Allergy* 1992;22:1077–1084.
72. Armitage, P. *Statistical methods in medical research.* Oxford: Blackwell Scientific Publications, 1971.
73. Duffy DL, Healey SC, Chenevix-Trench G, Martin NG, Weger J, Lichter J. Atopy in Australia. *Nat Genet* 1995;10:260.
74. Coleman R, Trembath RC, Harper JI. Chromosome 11q13 and atopy underlying atopic eczema. *Lancet* 1993;341:1121–1122.
75. Hizawa N, Yamaguchi E, Ohe M, Itoh A, Furuya K, Ohnuma N, Kawakami Y. Lack of linkage between atopy and locus 11q13. *Clin Exp Allergy* 1992;22:1065–1069.
76. Lympany P, Welsh KI, Cochrane GM, Kemeny DM, Lee TH. Genetic analysis of the linkage between chromosome 11q and atopy. *Clin Exp Allergy* 1992;22:1085–1092.
77. Rich SS, Roitman-Johnson B, Greenberg B, Roberts S, Blumenthal MN. Genetic analysis of atopy in three large kindreds: no evidence for linkage to D11S97. *Clin Exp Allergy* 1992;22:1070–1076.
78. Holt PG. Immunoprophylaxis of atopy: light at the end of the tunnel? *Immunol Today* 1994;15:484–489.
79. Cochran WC, Snedecor GW. *Statistical methods.* Ames: Iowa State University Press, 1980.
80. Postma DS, De Vries K, Koeter GH, Sluiter HJ. Independent influence of reversibility of airflow obstruction and non-specific hyperreactivity on the long-term course of lung function in chronic airflow obstruction. *Am Rev Respir Dis* 1986;134:276–280.
81. Postma DS, Sluiter HJ. Prognosis of chronic obstructive pulmonary disease: the Dutch experience. *Am Rev Respir Dis* 1989;140:S100–S105.
82. Burrows B, Martinez FD, Halonen M, Barbee RA, Cline MG. Association of asthma with serum IgE levels and skin-test reactivity to allergens. *N Engl J Med* 1989;320:271–277.
83. Clifford RD, Pugsley A, Radford M, Holgate ST. Symptoms, atopy, and bronchial response to methacholine in parents with asthma and their children. *Arch Dis Childhood* 1987;62:66–73.
84. Gergen PJ. The association of allergen skin test reactivity and respiratory disease among whites in the U.S. population. *Arch Intern Med* 1991;151:487–492.
85. Sears M, Burrows B, Flannery EM, Herbison GP, Hewitt CJ, Holdaway MD. Relation between airway responsiveness and serum IgE in children with asthma and in apparently normal children. *N Engl J Med* 1991;325:1067–1071.
86. Borish L, Mascali JJ, Klinnert M, Leppert M, Rosenwasser LJ. SSC polymorphisms in interleukin genes. *Hum Molec Genet* 1994;3:1710.
87. Hall IP, Wheatley A, Wilding P, Liggett SB. Association of glu 27 b2-adrenoceptor polymorphism with lower airway reactivity in asthmatic subjects. *Lancet* 1995;345:1213–1214.
88. Risch N. Genetic linkage: interpreting lod scores. *Science* 1992; 255:803–804.

Asthma, edited by P.J. Barnes, M.M. Grunstein,
A.R. Leff, and A.J. Woolcock.
Lippincott–Raven Publishers, Philadelphia © 1997.

▪ 12 ▪

Genetics of Asthma

Dirkje S. Postma and Eugene R. Bleecker

Finding Genes	**Genetics of Asthma and its Phenotypes**
Problems in Genetic Studies of Asthma: a Complex Trait	Genetics of Atopy
	Genetic Studies on Airways Hyperresponsiveness
Use of Asthma Phenotypes for Genetic Studies of Asthma	**Regulation of the Inflammatory Process in Asthma**

Asthma is a disease characterized by respiratory symptoms such as wheeze and cough, variable airways obstruction, and the presence of airways hyperresponsiveness. A marker of the underlying pathophysiologic abnormality is airway wall inflammation. Atopy is a disorder characterized by prolonged and enhanced immunoglobulin E (IgE) responses to commonly encountered, otherwise innocuous, environmental peptide antigens. Atopy is an important component of allergic asthma, rhinitis, and eczema since allergen exposure triggers immunologic inflammation and associated symptoms. The specific immune response has been thoroughly studied and its overall mechanism has been defined. However, not all individuals with asthma have atopy, showing that the two conditions, though closely related, are not interchangeable. While the genetics of atopy are described in Chapter 11, this chapter will focus on the genetics of asthma and only discuss the hereditary component of atopy as it relates to asthma.

The worldwide prevalence of asthma, as well as its morbidity and mortality, is still increasing. Notwithstanding this observation, there is still no cure for asthma, with current therapy only ameliorating symptoms. Investigators studying the genetics of atopy and asthma, therefore, have set goals to find the responsible gene(s), hoping that these studies will lead to the development of new thera-

pies. The first step has been to confirm the long-lasting hypothesis that asthma and allergies involve interactions between environmental and host factors. Since Cooke and colleagues (1) in 1916 published their systematic study, it has been apparent that these conditions have familial, if not genetic components. In this chapter we will review the recent progress that has been made, suggesting atopy (expressed in different ways) to be linked with specific chromosome regions, specifically 11q and 5q (2–6). Advances in several fields of research have made it possible to start understanding the genetics of complex diseases such as allergy and asthma. These fields include a better understanding of the pathogenesis of asthma and associated allergy by characterization of IgE response, T-cell function, and cytokine regulation. In addition, recent advances in molecular and analytic genetics have made it feasible to study the genetics of complex conditions such as asthma and allergy, which are not inherited in a simple Mendelian fashion.

FINDING GENES

Genes influence every level of biologic organization, from a single cell to an entire population. It seems clear that virtually all diseases have some component of "genetic predisposition," thereby making some individuals more at risk than others to express or develop a disease. It is, however, extremely difficult to find a specific gene responsible for a specific disease. The haploid human genome is composed of approximately 3 billion base pairs of deoxyribonucleic acid (DNA) and is estimated to contain 30,000 to 100,000 genes. The complexity of the

D. S. Postma: Department of Pulmonology, University Hospital Groningen, 9713 EZ Groningen, The Netherlands.

E. R. Bleeker: Department of Medicine, University of Maryland School of Medicine, Baltimore, Maryland 21201.

human genome has been compared to printing of a book. If one copy of one strand of the haploid human genome is printed, it would occupy 340,000 pages. A mutation causing, for instance, sickel cell anemia would represent misprinting one single letter on a page (7). Such a complexity has frustrated the identification of defective genes for many decades. The application of innovative molecular genetic methods coupled with sophisticated new computer generated statistical techniques has made this formidable task a virtual reality.

There are two basic approaches in mapping genes for asthma that need to be considered: complex segregation analysis, followed by linkage analysis using the most parsimonious genetic model identified by this segregation analysis, and linkage analysis using affected pairs of relatives (sib-pairs) without a specified genetic model. Segregation analysis tests the mode of inheritance by using qualitative data, such as serum level of IgE, or quantitative data on the disease, such as presence or absence of hyperresponsiveness. The analysis also includes environmental factors and family structure. It compares the observed number of affected individuals with the expected numbers using various Mendelian modes of inheritance, e.g., recessive, dominant etc. For linkage analysis, DNA marker data are used together with data on the trait and family structure.

Genes that influence the expression of asthma can be searched for by testing simple associations with specific polymorphisms of candidate genes in affected and unaffected individuals. The candidate gene approach is limited by the number of genes known to be related to the pathophysiologic mechanisms that are thought to be important in asthma and allergy. The method depends on the partial functional information about the disease, which is not enough to precisely pinpoint the culprit gene, but sufficient to form a series of educated guesses based on disease pathogenesis, or clues based on chromosomal abnormalities such as deletions or translocations. One such example is the successful demonstration that the dominantly inherited familial cancer syndrome of Li and Fraumenti is due to germline missense mutations in the p53 genes (8). Some examples of candidate genes for atopy and asthma are presented in Table 1.

A second approach is to perform a genome-wide search where polymorphic DNA markers are measured throughout the human genome. These markers may be placed relatively closely (10 cM intervals) or further apart. An important aspect is that the markers should be relatively evenly spaced and may not respresent actual disease genes. Linkage analysis is then performed using marker data and phenotypic characteristics. Both of the approaches usually involve positional cloning techniques, since even for the candidate gene approach polymorphic markers flanking the candidate genes are used for linkage analysis. Positional cloning involves the localization of disease genes to particular chromosomal segments by ge-

TABLE 1. *Candidate genes in asthma*

Candidate Gene	Chromosomal Location	Candidate Gene	Chromosomal Location
TNF receptor 2	1p	IL-9	5q
G-CSF receptor	1p	IL-12-b	5q
VCAM-1	1p	β2 receptor	5q
FcIgE receptor-α	1q	Corticosteroid receptor	5q
FcIgE receptor-γ	1q	HLA system	6p
Selectin E	1q	IL-6	7p
Selectin P	1q	T-cell receptor β	7
IL-10	Chr 1	Fcε receptor	11q
PAF receptor	Chr 1	TNF receptor 1	12q
IL-1	2q	Mast cell GF	12q
IL-5 rec	3p	IFN-γ	12q
IL-12A	3p	T-cell receptor α	14
IL-8	4q	IL-4 receptor	16p
IL-2	4q	Integrin αL	16p
GM-CSF	5q	G-CSF	17q
IL -13	5q	ICAM-2	17q
IL-3	5q	ICAM-1	19p
IL-4	5q	IFN-γ rec 2	21q
IL-5	5q	Integrin-β2	12q

TNF, tumor necrosis factor; IL, interleukin; G-SCF, granulocyte-colony stimulating factor; VCAM, vascular cell adhesion molucule; HLA, human leukocyte antigen system; PAF, platelet-activating factor; IFN, interferon; GM-CSF, granulocyte-macrophage colony-stimulating factor; ICAM, intercellular adhesion molucule.

netic linkage. Genetic linkage (Fig. 1) is assessed by the co-transmission of markers tested on known locations of the chromosome with the phenotype. Linkage is thought to be present with a logarithm of the likelihood ratio (LOD) score of 3. This represents an odds of 1:1000 of having linkage of the gene with the disease. An alternative approach for linkage is to use sib-pair analysis which does not assume a genetic model for inheritance. When linkage is found, the next step is to specifically locate the disease gene from the identified region using fine mapping. Positional cloning has been successful with single gene diseases such as cystic fibrosis, and also with the complex disease of Alzheimers and early-onset breast cancer.

PROBLEMS IN GENETIC STUDIES OF ASTHMA: A COMPLEX TRAIT

A recent publication of Lander and Schork (9) reviews the problems in genetic analyses of complex traits that exist with atopy and asthma and is recommended for more details. It defined the term "complex trait" as "any phenotype that does not exhibit classic Mendelian recessive or dominant inheritance attributable to one single gene locus." Thus, unlike simple, single-gene diseases, complex diseases involve the input of several different, often overlapping sets of genes. These conditions may involve genetic heterogeneity, multi-factorial inheritance, and phenocopies. Penetrance or expression of the trait

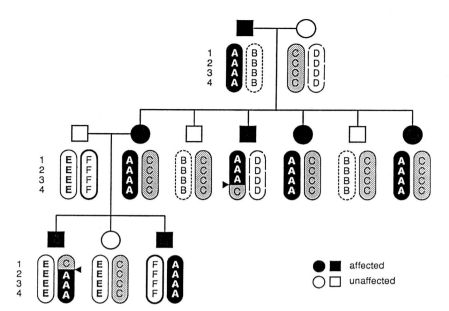

affected ● ■
unaffected ○ □

FIG. 1. Linkage analysis. If *A* is affected gene one can deduce from first offspring (*arrow*) that *C* is not the location.

may be influenced by environmental conditions. Problems in genetic analyses arise when the genotype and phenotype do not simply correspond. This may occur when the same genotype can result in different phenotypes, due to effects of chance, to environmental exposure, to interactions with other genes, or when different genotypes may give rise to the same phenotype. Furthermore, it is often impossible to find a genetic marker that shows perfect cosegregation with a complex trait. This may be due to incomplete penetrance and phenocopy, genetic (or locus) heterogeneity, high frequency of disease-causing alleles, and other transmission mechanisms. Some individuals who inherit a predisposing allele may not manifest the disease (incomplete penetrance), and others who have not inherited the predisposing allele may, nonetheless, develop the disease as a result of random causes (phenocopy). The "disease" genotype at a given locus may, thus, increase the probability of disease, but does not fully determine the outcome. This is an important problem with asthma, where age, allergen exposure, and various other exposures that include the effects of (viral) infections and environmental agents such as cigarette smoke and air pollutants, will affect the expression of the disease. An example is a study in which we followed 189 young adult asthmatic individuals for 25 years. We observed that after 25 years 4% were atopic initially but lost their atopy, whereas another 17% were nonatopic initially but became atopic after 25 years. Furthermore, 11% of these asthmatic individuals were no longer asthmatic after 25 years, i.e., they did not have asthmatic symptoms or hyperresponsiveness to histamine and had near-normal lung function. In this case genetic mapping is hampered by the fact that genetic investigations show the 'atopic' allele to be present in individuals

who do not have the 'atopic' phenotype, just because the course of the expression of atopy in these individuals over time is unknown.

Mutations in any one or several genes may result in identical phenotypes, i.e., when the genes are required for a common biochemical pathway or cellular structure (genetic heterogeneity). One example is retinitis pigmentosa, where mutations in at least 14 different loci may result in retinal degeneration (10,11). Until the genes are mapped, one has no way to know whether two patients suffer from the same disease for different genetic reasons. Genetic heterogeneity may further hinder genetic mapping since chromosomal regions may cosegregate with a disease in some families, but not in others. In contrast, allelic heterogeneity, where multiple disease-causing mutations occur at a single gene, does not interfere with gene mapping. Some traits may require the presence of mutations in multiple genes simultaneously. This is called polygenic inheritance. Polygenic traits do occur in human diseases, e.g., some forms of Hirschsprung disease, where mutations on chromosome 13, 21 and possibly elsewhere are necessary for disease development (12). If polygenic inheritance will occur in atopy or asthma, it will complicate genetic mapping, because no single locus is strictly required to produce a high value for IgE or the clinical expression of asthma.

Finally, problems arise when the disease-causing allele occurs at high frequency in the population. The LOD score will then be low and it will be difficult to pinpoint the linkage with any precision. Atopy is remarkably common. The population prevalence for atopy lies between 20% and 40%, and the prevalence of a positive skin-prick test to house dust or grass pollen in young adults has been found between 40% and 50% in western populations (13,14)

USE OF ASTHMA PHENOTYPES FOR GENETIC STUDIES OF ASTHMA

Asthma is a respiratory disease that is presently characterized by variable airways obstruction, airways inflammation, and hyperresponsiveness. The asthma phenotype is far more difficult and complicated to quantify than, for instance, an atopic phenotype. Since an early description of asthma by Laënnec in 1819, there have been many definitions (see Chapter 3). The well-considered complete descriptions of the asthma syndrome are hardly operational as a standardized method when performing genetic studies and analysing all family members with asthma. In the latter situation, it is often very difficult to distinguish between affected and unaffected family members. There appears to be a large group of individuals who cannot simply be defined as unaffected, since they have some, but not all, of the characteristics of asthma. Therefore, it is attractive to study asthmatic phenotypes in the first place, or eventually to define asthma using a series of logical steps, thus developing an asthma algorithm, e.g., by classifying individuals as definite asthma (all phenotypes present), probable asthma (most phenotypes present), or nonspecified airways disease (one single phenotype present or asthma cannot be distinguished from chronic obstructive lung disease). Despite the complexity in defining asthma, there are a number of closely related phenotypic characteristics that can be used in studies investigating the genetics of asthma. These include allergic parameters (total serum IgE, specific IgE, responses and results of allergy skin testing), airways hyperresponsiveness to various agents, and stimuli and markers of airways inflammation. (These topics are discussed in detail in other chapters.) A recent State of the Art has also summarized both asthma and atopy phenotypes (15).

Airway inflammation is discussed in detail in other chapters. To date, a standardized, well-validated and general applicable parameter of allergic bronchial inflammation has not been identified. The relationship between airway inflammation and the presence and severity of symptoms, peak flow variability or airways hyperresponsiveness is insufficient to validate any of these indirect, noninvasive parameters as a reliable indicator of the degree of airways inflammation. Although current definitions of asthma emphasize the importance of airways inflammation, it is hardly operational to use as a phenotype, because bronchoscopic examinations in several hundreds of family members, as required for genetic analyses, are not feasible. One needs to search for indirect, surrogate, measures of inflammation in asthma. It is plausible that a useful indirect measure is airway hyperresponsiveness, either measured by a directly acting or an indirectly acting stimulus.

Pathophysiologic inflammatory phenotypes of asthma may be the transcriptional dysregulation of T-lymphocyte-derived cytokines. For instance, polymorphisms within the interleukin gene cluster on chromosome 5 have been investigated to identify markers that may link it to transcriptional dysregulation. In this way Borish et al. (16) were able to identify polymorphisms in the 5' promoter region of these genes. This may either reflect base exchanges in genetic elements that directly regulate gene transcription or may be linked to gene dysregulation, thereby contributing to inflammatory changes in the airways.

GENETICS OF ASTHMA AND ITS PHENOTYPES

Several studies have shown an increased frequency of asthma in first-degree relatives of asthmatic subjects, as compared to control subjects, illustrating a familial aggregation of the diseases. Edfors-Lub (17) performed a twin study with 7000 same-sex twins born between 1886 and 1925. The concordance for self-reported asthma was 19% in monozygotic twins and 5% in dizygotic twins, comparable to the 4% prevalence in the whole twin population. Another study of 3800 twin-pairs in Australia supported the suggestion of genetic component to the development of asthma (18). However, other studies have reported no significant differences in self-reported asthma between monozygotic and dizygotic twins. Sibbald and co-workers reported the prevalence of asthma and atopy in families of 77 asthmatic and 87 control children attending a London general practice (19). They found that the prevalence of asthma was higher in first-degree relatives of asthmatic children (13%) than in control children (4%). Furthermore, there was a comparable increased prevalence of asthma in relatives of atopic and nonatopic asthmatics, suggesting that there is a hereditary component to both types of asthma. This finding was supported by Pirson et al. (20), who observed a prevalence of 8% among siblings of intrinsic asthmatic individuals, 7% in those of extrinsic asthmatics, and 4% in control subjects. The similarity between atopic and nonatopic patients in the distributions of asthma among their parents and siblings shows that they may share a common genetic defect if they are hereditary. Family studies by Gerrard and Fergusson (21,22) showed that the prevalence of asthma, hay fever, and eczema in offspring were all higher when parents had one or more of these disorders. However, children were not likely to develop the same type of allergic condition as their parents (Table 2). However, there are as yet no formal segregation or linkage studies available to prove this hypothesis.

TABLE 2. *Significant concordance of various allergic manifestations in children and parents*

Parents	Children		
	asthma	hay fever	eczema
asthma	38.84	0.00	1.74
hay fever	12.88	15.38	4.77
eczema	2.44	0.02	10.41

Genetics of Atopy

Genetics of atopy is discussed fully in Chapter 11 but some aspects are relevant to the genetic study of asthma. Atopy was first investigated in family and twin studies (17,23–30). An intra-pair correlation co-efficient for total serum IgE of 82% in monozygotic twins compared with 52% in dizygotic twins was found in a study of 107 twins, yielding an overall heritability of 61% (23). In addition, it has been shown that the pair-wise concordances for log total serum IgE levels for monozygotic twins raised apart were similar to those for monozygotic twins raised together (24). This suggested a strong genetic control of serum IgE levels. Indeed, several segregation analyses in family studies on the genetics of atopy point to involvement of a major gene for IgE regulation. Different modes of inheritance have been suggested, partly based on the distribution of IgE levels in different families. Gerrard's (25) and Marsh's (31) studies provided evidence for recessive inheritance of high IgE levels with a very frequent "low" IgE gene. Meyers et al. (26) showed evidence for recessive inheritance of a rare "low" IgE gene. There have also been suggestions for co-dominant inheritance and for polygenic control (27,28). Borecki et al. (29) showed that "a single gene effect could influence both IgE production and liability to allergies." A recent study of Martinez and co-workers (32) suggested that total serum IgE levels are controlled by a major autosomal/co-dominant gene. However, there is not a major difference between recessive and co-dominant inheritance because of partial expression of the trait in heterozygotes. Finally, a recent study by Xu et al. showed two unlinked loci regulating IgE levels (33) (see Table 3). Cultural inheritance and other environmental causes of familial correlation may mimic Mendelian transmission, and therefore, no amount of statistical analysis can prove the existence of a major locus (33). There are several factors that could account for these conflicting reports. Genetic heterogeneity may be present, i.e., the association of the same phenotype with the inheritance of different genetic determinants (34). A selection process based on atopic subjects may lead to ascertainment of the bias, and the timing of the IgE measurements

may affect the results as well (30,35). It is well-known that total serum IgE levels can significantly vary in allergic asthmatics after exposure to relevant allergens. It is possible that some studies measure basal levels and others exposed (higher) levels of IgE. It is important to remember that segregation analysis of a quantitative trait such as total serum IgE levels is very dependent on the observed distribution to determine the mode of inheritance. Finally, it is also possible that the results obtained in isolated population groups, such as the Amish, may not be applicable to the general population.

The first report mapping a major gene for atopy to a chromosome has been from Cookson et al. (2), who defined atopy based on positive skin test and/or elevated total serum IgE and/or elevated specific IgE. They first showed a maximum LOD score of 5.58 using an autosomal/ dominant model of inheritance to a DNA marker on 11q. They suggested the presence of at least one major gene for atopy, but several other investigators have been unable to confirm this linkage to 11q; some even excluded this region (36–42). Brereton and co-workers (42) investigated whether genetic heterogeneity might be the cause for the lack of linkage of atopy to 11q (i.e., whether a proportion of families within the group shows evidence of linkage, while the remainder show no evidence of linkage). They could, however, also not find linkage in subsets of families. Only one study reported evidence for linkage to chromosome 11q in sib-pair analysis in nuclear families with two affected children (43). Additional studies by Cookson et al. suggested that the transmission of atopy at chromosome 11q was only detectable through maternal inheritance (4). The authors suggested that this was the reason why other investigators did not find linkage to 11q, since they did not assume maternal inheritance, thereby obscuring linkage. However, other groups have not yet published evidence for maternal inheritance or linkage to 11q. The β-subunit of the high-affinity IgE receptor has been suggested as the candidate gene on 11q and several mutations have been detected (44,45). The authors found a common variant (181Leu) with positive IgE response in a random population. In 60 families with allergic asthma probands, 181Leu was found in 10 (17%), with evidence of maternal inheritance and associated with atopy (45).

Recent studies have reported linkage of a locus for IgE production to chromosome 5q (5,6). Sib-pair analysis showed that sibs with similar serum IgE levels had usually inherited the same copies of chromosome 5q (equal from the mother and father) (6). A sib-pair approach (LOD score 3.56) was used which is not model-dependent, and it was confirmed by the likelihood approach based on the model that was derived from the segregation analysis of total serum IgE. In this model, recessive inheritance of high levels gave a good fit to the data. Given the manner in which these families were ascertained (through a parent with asthma), it was not clear from these results whether

TABLE 3. *Two locus LOD scores for total IgE and D5S436*

	Θ	LOD
General: 2 codominant loci with polygenic component	0.08	4.86
Epistasis: genotypes with 'high' levels: aaBb, aabb	0.08	4.64
Epistasis: genotypes with 'high' levels: AABB, aaBb, aabb	0.09	4.67
Epistasis: genotypes with 'high' levels: aaBb, aabb, Aabb	0.10	1.99
Epistasis: genotypes with 'high' levels: aa—, Aabb	0.10	1.61

IgE, immunoglobulin E.

the evidence from linkage to the total serum IgE level phenotype is actually due to linkage to the asthma phenotype (6). Another interesting possibility is that linkage was observed because of a relationship between high IgE levels and the asthma phenotype. Since all the probands had asthma, the co-segregation observed between their marker alleles and their IgE levels may reflect the presence of a gene important to asthma. Further studies have to show whether this is also the case in allergic families without members with asthma. This region on 5q is an important one (see Fig. 6, Chapter 11) since it contains genes that regulate a large number of factors that are important in the inflammatory process in allergy and asthma: for instance, the interleukin (IL) 4 group of cytokines (IL-4, IL-5, IL-3 and granulocyte–macrophage colony-stimulating factor [GM-CSF]), which have overlapping effects on B cells and stimulate proliferation of granulocytes, macrophages, and eosinophils (46,47). This region is discussed in detail in Chapter 11.

Evidence has been found that a two-loci model fits the inheritance of high serum IgE levels better than a one-locus model (33). This indicates that at least two different loci are required for expression of the atopic phenotype. One locus explains 50% of the variability of the level of total serum IgE, the other 18%. The exact location of these gene(s) in the genome is as yet unknown. Candidate genes are presently thought at chromosome 11, 5, 14, and 6. However, at present different research groups have found linkage at different genes. The complete picture is not yet clear.

Linkage of specific IgE (for house dust mites, cats, dogs, molds and grass pollen) to the T-cell receptor (TCR) α and β gene complexes on chromosome 14 and 7, respectively was observed (48). Linkage in sib-pairs was not observed for TCR-β, but it was for TCR-α in both Australian and English families. This is important since TCR-Vα use may induce IL-4 dominant (TH2) helper T cells, which enhance IgE production (49). Affected sib-pairs showed significant sharing of TCR-α microsatellite alleles from both parents, suggesting that a gene (or genes) in this region also modifies specific IgE responses. It is not yet clear whether this is restricted to specific IgE or a general IgE response. The importance of specific response to allergens (antigen cognate) vs. nonspecific response (noncognate) has been addressed by many investigators as well. In cognate IgE responsiveness, a major histocompatibility complex (MHC) class II molecule (HLA [human leukocyte antigen system]) on an antigen presenting cell presents a processed antigen fragment to the T-cell receptor on a helper TH2 or TH0 cell. By contrast, there is generalized polyclonal upregulation of IgE production in the noncognate response, in which basophils (and possibly other FcεR1+ cells) interact with B cells (Table 4) (50). It has been suggested that noncognate IgE is related to asthma since log total serum IgE appeared to be linearly related to the risk for asthma

TABLE 4. *Immune effector cells bearing Fc receptors for IgE*

High-affinity FcεR	Low-affinity FcεR
mast cells	monocytes
basophils	macrophages
	lymphocytes
	eosinophils
	platelets

IgE, immunoglobulin E.

after adjustment for specific IgE responsiveness (51). In a recent paper Dizier et al. (52) presented their results of formal genetic analyses by segregation analysis, either taking specific response to allergens (either positive RAST or skin test) into account or not. The 234 nuclear families were randomly collected in one Australian town during the winter season when IgE levels are the lowest. Familial transmission of total IgE level was compatible with the segregation of a recessive major gene and residual familial correlation when the specific allergen response was ignored. When corrected for the specific allergen response, the recessive mode of inheritance of IgE was still present, but not the significant familial correlations. This suggests that the gene, which accounted for 28% of the variation in the trait, may be involved in the control of basal IgE production independently of the specific response to allergen.

Several studies have shown that the HLA complex is involved in the specific IgE response, but not in the nonspecific one, and a striking association between the expression of HLA genes and, for instance, pollen allergy has been shown (53). However, conflicting results on the association between the HLA system and asthma have been published, some studies showing evidence of linkage via haplotype sharing other studies suggesting that the HLA system has no role in asthma (54–60). Formal linkage of atopy and asthma to chromosome 6, on which the HLA system is located, has been addressed, but no linkage has yet been reported (39).

Genetic Studies on Airways Hyperresponsiveness

Both studies of families and twins have utilized measures of airways responsiveness to help establish a genetic link to asthma. Family studies have shown that there is an increased prevalence of airway hyperresponsiveness among the relatives of asthmatics compared with nonasthmatic individuals, but a high proportion of those with airway hyperresponsiveness have no clinical symptoms of asthma (61,62). In a twin study Hopp and coworkers (23) showed that hyperresponsiveness to methacholine is under genetic influence with an estimated heritability of 66%. Hopp et al. (63) analyzed data on airway hyperresponsiveness in nuclear families, ascertained by recruitment of an asthmatic proband (ages 6 to 25 years), compared with families without an asthma/allergy history. Probands from both families were excluded from the analysis. The data confirmed their earlier observations for a genetic basis of hyperresponsiveness (64). There appeared to be a bimodal distribution of airways responsiveness, suggesting a single biochemical or phys-

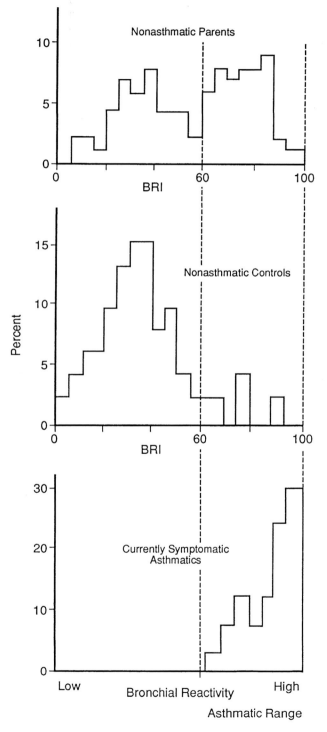

Fig. 2. Bimodal distribution of bronchial reactivity in nonasthmatic parents; unimodal for nonasthmatic controls and asthmatics.

TABLE 5. *Sib-pair analysis for airway hyperresponsiveness (AHR)*

Sib-Pair Analysis for D5S436 for Bronchial Responsiveness to Histamine			
Sibs	No. of Pairs	Mean *	p-Value **
Both AHR-	173	0.55	0.02
1 AHR+, 1AHR-	114	0.390	0.0002
Both AHR+	35	0.64	0.009

*Proportion of alleles that were identical-by-descent
**p value for linear regression—p=0.000002, t=4.7, d.f.=320
AHR, airway hyperresponsiveness.

ical defect (Fig. 2). This bimodal distribution in airway hyperresponsiveness in nonasthmatic parents has been reported by Hopp (65) as well, who demonstrated no significant association between airway hyperresponsiveness and atopic status. This would further suggest that, while IgE influences airway hyperresponsiveness and approximately 30% of the variance in airway hyperresponsiveness is explained by an individual's total serum IgE level, it does not cause it alone (66,67). This is also suggested in a sib-pair analysis in children of probands in 84 Dutch families (Table 5). Probands were ascertained in a hospital-based population and were identified as having asthma 25 years ago by the presence of hyperresponsiveness and symptoms compatible with asthma. There is significant evidence for linkage of hyperresponsiveness in these sib-pairs to chromosome 5q in the vicinity of the interleukin complex known for their importance in IgE regulation and asthma. This linkage was also present when corrected for high serum IgE levels, at least not excluding the possibility that indeed hyperresponsiveness may be genetically determined separately from atopy. Furthermore, linkage of hyperresponsiveness to regions on chromosome 6 and 11 in these families was excluded (39) (Table 6). This first evidence of linkage for airways hy-

TABLE 6. *Results of linkage analysis for AHR*

			Recombination fraction				
Model	0.01	0.05	0.10	0.20	0.30	0.40	Θ when lod<−2.00
Chromosome 11: INT2 Model							
1	−6.92	−3.95	−2.38	−0.93	−0.29	−0.03	0.12
2	−7.28	−4.74	−3.14	−1.50	−0.67	−0.22	0.16
Chromosome 6: D6S105 Model							
1	−10.58	−6.74	−4.37	−1.93	−0.77	−0.21	0.20
2	−5.38	−3.58	−2.38	−1.03	−0.35	−0.04	0.12

Model 1: Dominant
Model 2: Recessive
Model used included weights for the possible classes of 0.80.

perresponsiveness shows how important this area of 5q is in regulation of asthma subphenotypes.

Other investigators did not find a bimodal distribution of hyperresponsiveness in a population of college students (68). Their finding of a unimodal distribution suggests a multi-factorial basis for hyperresponsiveness. This may either mean an important environmental influence, or a polygeneic component. The former is also supported by segregation analysis in the families reported by Townley et al. (69). The bimodal distribution may not be due to segregation at a single autosomal locus. As for atopy, certain environmental stimuli may be required for its expression as the asthma phenotype.

REGULATION OF THE INFLAMMATORY PROCESS IN ASTHMA

The important development showing linkage of IgE and airway hyperresponsiveness to 5q provides insight to understanding the genetic regulation of inflammation in asthma. IgE is a unique immunoglobulin containing an Fc region with very high affinity for mast cells and basophils and lower affinity for T and B lymphocytes, monocytes, and eosinophils. The biologic effect of IgE occurs via bridging of these high-affinity receptors for IgE (Fc$_\varepsilon$R) via the interaction of IgE with allergens which trigger a series of biochemical events that result in the release of preformed mediators from their secretory granules into the extracellular environment and the generation of newly formed lipid metabolites from the mast cell membranes and production of cytokines. This is followed by an influx of eosinophils and CD4-positive lymphocytes. The net result is an intense local inflammatory process with vasodilation, vasculature leakage, mucosal edema, inflammatory exudate, goblet cell secretions, and smooth muscle contraction. The clinical manifestation of a particular atopic reaction depends on the extent and anatomic location of mast cell degranulation. It includes symptoms of itching, nasal blockade, watery secretions, and sneeze or cough, chest tightness, and wheeze, characteristics of hay fever and asthma.

Knowledge of the previously mentioned inflammatory pathway(s) resulting in the asthmatic phenotype has led to hypothesis that regulation of IgE production, eosinophilia, and lymphocyte activation might be important mechanisms for genetic determinations of asthma. Thus, the Fc$_\varepsilon$RI-β is an excellent candidate for an atopy gene. The receptor acts as a trigger for the allergic process, and mast cells are known to release significant amounts of cytokines which can upregulate the IgE response to allergens. Sequencing has now detected two variants in addition to the more usual wild type. Maternal inheritance of both variants was associated with severe atopy in Irish and English families (44). The findings suggest that Fc$_\varepsilon$RI-β is the chromosome 11 atopy gene. Yet, the replication by other investigators has to prove this. Other researchers set out to look at cytokines involved in IgE production and eosinophil survival and activation. This has now been supported by finding linkage of both high serum total IgE levels and airways hyperresponsiveness to chromosome 5q. Studies have shown that atopy is associated with the TH2 subset of CD4+ cells. The development of B cells to IgE-secreting plasma cells is induced by IL-4 and suppressed by IFNγ. In addition, IL-4 has been defined as a "switch factor" for IgE, regulating transcription of the germline Cε gene. Finally, IL-4 also enhances the expression of Fc$_\varepsilon$RII on lymphocytes and monocytes, which can further upregulate IgE production. Some cytokines may further upregulate IL-4-induced IgE synthesis, e.g., IL-5 and IL-6. It is possible that there is a genetic abnormality in this gene, since linkage has been found (see earlier) between high serum IgE levels and chromosome 5.

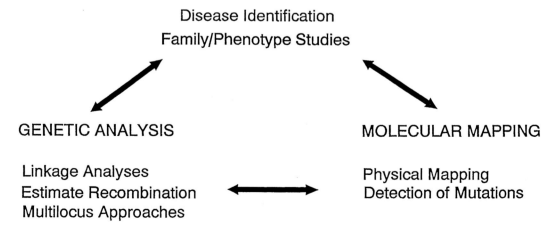

APPROACHES TO POSITIONAL CLONING

Disease Identification
Family/Phenotype Studies

GENETIC ANALYSIS

Linkage Analyses
Estimate Recombination
Multilocus Approaches

MOLECULAR MAPPING

Physical Mapping
Detection of Mutations

FIG. 3. Approach for detecting genes for asthma.

Thus, important accomplishments have been made during the last few years in determining the genetic mechanisms of asthma and allergy. Future studies combining efforts of several different types of investigations (Fig. 3) will employ fine mapping techniques to elucidate the specific gene(s) responsible for the development of asthma. This may ultimately lead to new diagnostic standards and to unraveling some of the basic genetic regulatory mechanisms that result in the susceptibility to asthma.

REFERENCES

1. Cooke RA, Van der Veer A. Human senstization. *J Immunology* 1916;1:201–305.
2. Cookson WOCM, Sharp PA, Faux JA, Hopkin JM. Linkage between immunoglobulin E responses underlying asthma and rhinitis and chromosome 11q. *Lancet* 1989;1:1292–1295.
3. Collee JM, Ten Kate LP, de Vries HG, et al. Allele sharing on chromosomes 11q13 and in sibs with asthma and atopy. *Lancet* 1993;342:936.
4. Cookson WOCM, Young RP, Sandford AJ, et al. Maternal inheritance of atopic IgE responsiveness on chromosome 11q. *Lancet* 1992;340: 381–384.
5. Marsh DG, Neely JD, Breazeale DR, et al. Linkage Analysis of IL4 and other chromosome 5q31.1 markers and total serum immunoglobulin E concentrations. *Science* 1994;264:1152–1156.
6. Meyers DA, Postma DS, Panhuysen CIM, et al. Evidence for a locus regulating total serum IgE levels mapping to chromosome 5. *Genomics* 1994;23:464–470.
7. Beaudet A, Ballabio A. In: Esselbacher K, Braunwald E et al., *eds. Harrison's principle of internal medicine 17th ed.* New York: McGraw Hill Inc., 1994; 349.
8. Collins F. Positional cloning moves from perdition to traditional. Nature Genetics 1995;9: 347.
9. Lander ES, Schork NJ. Genetic dissection of complex traits. *Science* 1994;265:2037–2048.
10. Bleeker-Wagemakers LM, Gal A, Kumar-Singh R et al. Evidence for nonallelic genetic heterogeneity in autosomal recessive retinitis pigmentosa. *Genomics* 1992;14:811–812.
11. Kumar-Singh R, Kenna PF, Farrar GJ, Humphries P. Evidence of further genetic heterogeneity in autosomal dominant retinitis pigmentosa. *Genomics* 1993;15:212–215.
12. Puffenberger EG, Kauffman ER, Bolk S et al. Identity by descent and association mapping of a recessive gene for Hirschprung disease on human chromosome 13q22. *Hum Mol Genet* 1994;3:1217–1225.
13. Cline MG, Buttrows B. Distribution of allergy in a population sample residing in Tucson, Arizona. *Thorax* 1989;44:425–431.
14. Peat JK, Britton WJ, Salome CM, Woolcock AJ. Bronchial hyperresponsiveness in two populations of Australian school children. III Effect of exposure to environmental allergens. *Clin Allergy* 1987;17:271–281.
15. Sandford A, Weir T, Paré P. The Genetics of Asthma. (State of the Art.) *Am J Respir Crit Care Med* 1996;153:1749–1765.
16. Borish L, Mascali JJ, Klinnert M, Leppert M, Rosenwasser LJ. SSC polymorphisms in interleukin genes. *Human Mol Genetics* 1994;3:710.
17. Edfors-Lub M. Allergy in 7000 twin pairs. *Acta Allergol* 1971; 26: 249–285.
18. Duffy DL, Martin NF, Battistutta D, Hoffer JL, Mathews JD. Genetics of asthma and hay fever in Australian twins. *Am Rev Respir Dis* 1990;142:1351–1358.
19. Sibbald B, Horn MEZ, Brain EA et al. Genetic factors in childhood asthma. *Thorax* 1980;35:671–674.
20. Pirson F, Charpin D, Sansonetti M, et al. Is intrinsic asthma a hereditary disease? *Allergy* 1991;46:367–371.
21. Gerrard J, Vickers P, Gerrard C. The familial incidence of allergic disease. *Ann Allergy* 1976;36:10–15.
22. Fergusson D, Horwood L, Shannon F. Parental asthma, parental eczema, and asthma and eczema in early childhood. *J Chron Dis* 1983;36: 517–524.
23. Hopp RJ, Bewtra AK, Watt GD, Nair NM, Townley RG. Genetic analysis of allergic disease in twins. *J Allergy Clin Immunol* 1984; 73:265–270.
24. Blumenthal MN, Bonini S. Immunogenetics of specific immune responses to allergens in twins and families. In: Marsh DG, Blumenthal MN, eds. *Genetic and environmental factors in clinical allergy.* Minneapolis: University of Minnesota Press 1990:132–139.
25. Gerrard JW, Rao DC, Morton NE, A genetic study of immunoglobulin E. *Am J Hum Genet* 1978;30:28–37.
26. Meyers DA, Beaty TH, Freidhoff LR, Marsh DG. Inheritance of serum IgE (basal levels) in man. *Am J Hum Genet* 1987;41:51–62.
27. Meyers DA, Bias WB, Marsh DG. A genetic study of total IgE in the Amish. *Hum Hered* 1982;32:15–23.
28. Hasstedt SJ, Meyers DA, Marsh DG. Inheritance of immunoglobulin E: genetic model fitting. *Am J Hum Genet* 1983;14:61–66.
29. Borecki IB, Rao DC, Lalouel JM, Mc Gue M, Gerrard JW. Demonstration of a common major gene with pleiotropic effects on immuglobulin E levels and allergy. *Genet Epidemio* 1985;2:327–338.
30. Cookson WOCM, Sharp PA, Faux JA, Hopkin JM. Linkage between immunoglobulin E responses underlying asthma and rhinitis and chromosome 11q. *Lancet* 1989;1:1292–1295.
31. Marsh DG, Bias WB, Ishizaka K. Genetic control of basal serum immunoglobulin E level and its effect on specific reaginic sensitivity, *Proc Natl Acad Sci U S A* 1974;71:3588–3592.
32. Martinez FD, Holberg CJ, Halonen M, Morgan WJ, Wright AL, Taussig LM. Evidence for Mendelian inheritance of serum IgE levels in hispanic and non-hispanic white families. *Am J Hum Genet* 1994;55: 555–565.
33. Xu J, Levitt RC, Panhuysen CIM, et al. Evidence for two unlinked loci regulating total serum IgE levels. *Am J Hum Genet* 1995;57:425–430.
34. Elston RC. Segregation analysis. In: Harris H, Hirschhorn K, eds. *Advances in human genetics.* vol 2. New York: Plenum Press, 1981;63–120.
35. Blumenthal MN, Namboodiri KK, Mendell NR, Gleich GJ, Elston RC, Yunis EJ. Genetic transmission of serum IgE levels. *Am J Med Genet* 1981;10:219–228.
36. Lympany P, Welsh K, MacChochrane G, Kemeny DM, Lee TH. Genetic analysis using DNA polymorphism of the linkage between chromosome 11q13 and atopy and bronchial hyperresponsiveness to methacholine. *J All Clin Imm* 1992;89:619–628.
37. Lympany P, Welsh KI, Cochrane GM, Kemeny DM, Lee TH. Genetic analusis of the linkage between chromosome 11q and atopy. *Clin and Exp Allergy* 1992;22:1085–1092.
38. Rich SS, Roitman-Johnson B, Greenberg B, Roberts S, Blumenthal MN. Genetic analysis of atopy in three large kindreds: no evidence of linkage to D11S97. *Clin and Exp Allergy* 1992;22:1070–1076.
39. Amelung PJ, Panhuysen CIM, Postma DS, et al. Atopy and bronchial hyperresponsiveness. Exclusion of linkage to markers on chromosome 11q and 6p. *Clin Exp Allergy* 1992;22:1077–1084.
40. Hizawa N, Yamaguchi E, Ohe M, et al. Lack of linkage between and locus 11q13. *Clin Exp Allergy* 1992;22:1065–1069.
41. Coleman R, Trembath RC, Harper JI. Chromosome 11q13 and atopy underlying atopic eczema. *Lancet* 1993;341:1121–1122.
42. Brereton HM, Ruffin RE, Thompson PJ, Turner DR. Familial atopy in Australian pedigrees: adventitious linkage to chromosome 8 is not confirmed nor is there evidence of linkage to the high affinity IgE receptor. *Clin and Exp Allergy* 1994;24:868–877.
43. Collee JM, Ten Kate LP, de Vries HG, et al. Allele sharing on chromosomes 11q13 and in sibs with asthma and atopy. *Lancet* 1993;342: 936.
44. Sandford AJ, Shirakawa T, Moffatt MF, et al. Localisation of atopy and β subunit of high-affinity IgE receptor (FcεRI) on chromosome 11q. *Lancet* 1993;341:332–336.
45. Shirakawa T, Li A, Dubowitz M, Dekker JM, et al. Association between atopy and variants of the β subunit of the high-affinity immunoglobulin E receptor. *Nature Genetics* 1994;7:125–130.
46. Katz MF, Beer DJ. T lymphocytes and cytokine networks in asthma: Clinical and therapeutic implications. *Adv Int Med* 1993;38:189–221.
47. Kelly J. Cytokines of the lung. *Am Rev Respir Dis* 1991;141:765–788.
48. Moffatt MF, Hill Mr, Cornelis F, et al. Genetic linkage of T-cell receptor α/δ complex to specific IgE responses. *Lancet* 1994;343:1597–1600.
49. Heinzel FP, Sadick MD, Mutha SS, Locksley RM. Production of interferon τ, interleukin-2, interleukin-4, and interleukin-10, by CD4+ lymphocytes *in vivo* during healing and progressive murine leishmaniasis. *Proc Natl Acad Sci U S A* 1991;88:7011–7015.
50. Gauchat J-F, Henchoz S, Mazzel G, et al. Induction of human IgE synthesis in B cells by mast cells and basophils. *Nature* 1993;365: 340–343.

51. Burrows B, Martinez ED, Halonene M, Barbee RA, Cline MG. Association of asthma with serum IgE levels and skin-test reactivity to allergens. *N Engl J Med* 1989;320:271–277.
52. Dizier MH, James AJ, Faux J, et al. Detection of a recessive major gene for high IgE levels acting independently of specific response to allergens. *Genetic Epidemiology* 1995;12:93–105.
53. Marsh DG, Zwollo P, Ansari AA. Towards a total human immune response finger print: the allergy model. In: Said EL, Shami A, Merret TG, eds. *Allergy and molecular biology.* Oxford/New York: Pergamon Press, 1989;65–82.
54. Hafez M, Zedan M, El-Shennawy FA, Abd El-Hafez SA, El-Khyat H. HLA antigens and extrinisic bronchial asthma. *J Asthma* 1984;21:259–263.
55. Wagatsuma Y, Yakura H, Nakayama E, et al. Inheritance af asthma in families and its linkage to HLA haplotypes. *Acta Allergol* 1976;31:455–462.
56. Rachelefsky G, Park MS, Seigal S, Terasaki PJ, Katz R, Saito S. Strong association between β-lymphocyte group-2 specificity and asthma. *Lancet* 1976;2:1042–1044.
57. Turton CWG, Morris L, Buckingham JA, Lawler DS, Turner-Warwick M. Histocompatibility antigens in asthma: population and family studies. *Thorax* 1979;34:670–676.
58. Flaherty DK, Geller M, Surfus JE, Leo GM, Reed CE, Rankin J. HLA antigen frequencies and natural history of *Alternaria*-sensitive and perennial nonallergic asthmatics. *J Allergy Clin Immunol* 1980;66:408–416.
59. Morris MJ, Faux JA, Ting A, Morris PJ, Lane DJ. HLA-A, B and C and HLA-DR antigens in intrinsic and allergic asthma. *Clin Allergy* 1980;10:173–179.
60. Brady RE, Glovsky MM, Opelz G, Terasaki P, Malish DM. The association of an HLA asthma-associated haplotype and immediate hypersensitivity in familial asthma. *J Immunogenet* 1981;8:509–517.
61. Konig P, Godfrey S. Prevalence of exercise-induced bronchial lability in families of children with asthma. *Arch Dis Child* 1973;48:513–518.
62. Clifford RD, Pugsley A, Radford M, Holgate ST. Symptoms, atopy, and bronchial response to methacholine in parents with asthma and their children. *Arch Dis Child* 1978;62:66–73.
63. Hopp RJ, Bewtra AK, Nair NM, Watt GD, Townley RG. Methacholine inhalation challenge studies in a selected population. *Am Rev Respir Dis* 1986;134:994–998.
64. Hopp RJ, Townley RG. Evidence that bronchial reactivity may be inherited. *Pediatr Res* 1985;19(2):248A.
65. Hopp RJ, Bewtra AK, Nair NM, Townley RG. Bronchial reactivity patterns in nonasthmatic parents of asthmatics. *Ann Allergy* 1988;61:184–186.
66. Cockcroft DW, Murdock KY, Berscheid BA. Relationship between atopy and bronchial hyperresponsiveness to histamine in a random population. *Ann Allergy* 1984;53:26–29.
67. Burrows B, Martinez FD, Halonen M, Barbee RA, Cline MG. Association of asthma with serum IgE levels and skintest reactivity to allergens. *N Engl J Med* 1989;320:271–277.
68. Cockroft DW, Berscheid BA, Murdock KY. Unimodel distribution of bronchial responsiveness to inhaled histamine in a random population. *Chest* 1983;83:751–754.
69. Townley RG, Bewtra A, Wilson AF, et al. Segregation analysis of bronchial response to methacholine inhalation challenge in families with and without asthma. *J Allergy Clin Immunol* 1986;77:101–107.

▪ 3 ▪

Structure, Biology, and Pathology

Asthma, edited by P.J. Barnes, M.M. Grunstein,
A.R. Leff, and A.J. Woolcock.
Lippincott–Raven Publishers, Philadelphia © 1997.

▪ 13 ▪

Upper Airways

Hemalini Mehta and William W. Busse

Anatomy/Biology
  Nose
  Paranasal Sinuses
  Oral Cavity
  Pharynx
  Eustachian Tube and Middle Ear

Pathology
  Allergic Rhinitis
  Nonallergic Rhinitis
  Nasal Polyps
  Sinusitis

The upper airways in human beings serve an important role in humidification and warming of the air that we breathe. They also protect the lower airways from pathogens and toxic substances present in the environment.

ANATOMY/BIOLOGY

Nose

Basic Anatomy

The interior of the nose is divided by the nasal septum into two separate cavities. These begin at the nostrils (anterior nares) and are divided by the septum until the posterior nares, where the cavities unite and join the nasopharynx. The vestibule forms the transition zone between the external and internal environment. It is covered by epidermis containing sebaceous glands and hairs (vibrissae), which filter large particulate matter. The nasal vestibules narrow to a slit of 0.3 to 0.4 cm, commonly called the internal ostium or nasal valve, which forms the junction between the vestibule and the main nasal cavity (1). The nasal valve is the narrowest point of the nasal cavity and thus has an important influence on nasal respiration by limiting the rate of inspiratory nasal airflow. It accounts for approximately half the total resistance to respiratory airflow (2).

H. Mehta: Department of Allergy/Immunology, University of Wisconsin Hospitals and Clinics, Madison, Wisconsin 53792.
W. W. Busse: Department of Medicine, University of Wisconsin Medical School, Madison, Wisconsin 53792.

The nasal septum forms the medial wall of the nasal cavity, and the inferior, middle, and superior turbinates make up the lateral wall. The septum consists of an anterior cartilaginous part, which supports the nasal tip, and a posterior bony plate. The nasal turbinates are C-shaped bony structures that contribute to the irregular outline of the nasal cavity and are important to their air-filtering and air-conditioning functions. The superior, middle, and inferior meatus lie inferior to the three turbinates.

1. The inferior meatus, lying between the floor of the nose and the lower turbinate, contains the opening of the nasolacrimal duct lying about 3 cm behind the posterior margin of the nostril (3) (Fig. 1).
2. The middle meatus contains the orifices of the frontal, maxillary, and anterior and middle ethmoidal sinuses (4) (Fig. 1).
3. The superior meatus houses the opening for the posterior ethmoid cells (4).
4. The sphenoid sinus opens high in the nose, near the posterior end of the superior turbinate, and drains into the sphenoethmoidal recess (4) (Fig. 1).

Histology

The vestibule is lined by an internal extension of the skin of the external nose. This includes a stratified squamous epithelium with an underlying dermis containing hair and sebaceous glands. The short, stiff hairs present at the entrance to the nares are extremely sensitive to certain kinds of mechanical stimuli that cause itch, tickle, and sneezing (5). The anterior one third of the nasal cavity is

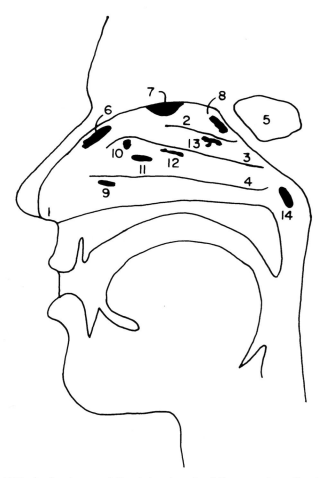

FIG. 1. Anatomy of the lateral wall of the nasal cavity. **1:** Vestibule. **2:** Attachment of superior turbinate. **3:** Attachment of middle turbinate. **4:** Attachment of inferior turbinate. **5:** Sphenoid sinus. **6:** Olfactory sulcus. **7:** Olfactory region. **8:** Sphenoethmoidal recess containing opening for sphenoidal sinus. **9:** Nasolacrimal duct opening. **10:** Frontal sinus ostium. **11:** Maxillary sinus ostium. **12:** Ostia of the anterior and middle ethmoidal cells. **13:** Ostia of the posterior ethmoidal cells. **14:** Eustachian tube opening.

lined with a squamous and transitional epithelium. Just past the nasal valve area on the cartilaginous septum lies Kiesselbach's plexus, a region of wide and long capillary loops (6). This region is a common source of nasal bleeding, especially in children. Most of the nasal mucosa is covered with ciliated pseudostratified columnar epithelium, which is the respiratory epithelium that lines the entire airway up to the bronchi. Olfactory epithelium is found only in the upper part of each nasal cavity and occupies an area of 1.5 cm² (7).

Functions of the nose

The nose participates in three major functions: respiration, filtration, and olfaction.

Respiration

Nasal breathing is more physiologic for human beings. Mouth breathing is used only in demanding conditions such as exercise, voice use, or nasal obstruction to supplement nasal respiration. As the air enters the nasal cavity, vascular engorgement of the turbinates occurs to provide warmth and humidification. The temperature in the nose remains constant at 31 to 34°C, regardless of the external environment (8). Inspired air is humidified to 85% to 95%, and water is withdrawn from expired air to reduce the amount of insensible loss (8). The nasal mucosa is fairly water-tight and usually prevents release of too much water into the atmosphere, thus preventing drying of the mucosa.

Filtration

In addition to humidification and warming of air, the nose also plays a role in filtration. Vibrissae in the nasal vestibule remove particles larger than 15 μ in size (9). This functions as a first line of host defense. The irregular shape of the nasal cavity promotes turbulence and increases the interaction between the airstream and the nasal mucosa. This allows the nose to clear the inspired air of suspended or soluble particles and prevents the inhalation of potentially harmful particles into the lungs. Approximately 85% of particles larger than 4 to 5 μ, such as pollen grains, are filtered out by the nose, whereas only 5% of those less than 1 to 2 μ, such as mold spores, are removed (3). The nasal mucociliary system, composed of cilia and mucus, plays an additional role in filtration. A mucous blanket covers the entire nasal cavity and filters out particles and water-soluble gases such as formaldehyde and sulfur dioxide. Daily mucus production ranges from 1 to 2 liters, most of which is water. Mucociliary transport moves mucus and its contents posteriorly toward the nasopharynx, where it is swallowed. In the anterior portion of the inferior turbinate, however, the mucociliary transport is anterior. Evaluation with scintillation cameras and radiolabeled particles have shown that cilia will transport at a rate of 1 to 20 mm/min; an average of 10 to 20 minutes is necessary to clear inhaled particles from the nasal cavity (10). Nasal mucociliary clearance is increased with exercise or ingestion of hot liquids, and is decreased during sleep (10,11).

Inspired air exposes the nasal cavity to micro-organisms and foreign proteins. Mucosal immunity is therefore provided by several nonspecific and acquired enzymes and factors. Lysozyme, a bacteriolytic enzyme, is selective for certain gram-positive bacteria (12). Lactoferrin, an iron-binding protein, exerts a bacteriostatic effect on certain gram-positive and -negative bacteria as well as *Candida albicans* (13). Immunoglobulins comprise a large percentage of the protein content of mucus. These include IgA, which constitutes the majority of immunoglobulins, as well as IgG, IgM, IgD, and IgE (14).

Olfaction

The sense of smell plays an important role in humans by providing a warning of rotten foods and toxic substances as well as stimulating or depressing the appetite. The olfactory area of the nose is relatively small and lies posterosuperiorly. The groove anterior to the middle turbinate leading to the olfactory area is known as the olfactory cleft (7). The area through which air flows to get to the olfactory cleft is medial and anterior to the lower part of the middle turbinate (15). Changes in this area may affect olfaction because this region may function as a regulator of airflow to the olfactory cleft. Only volatile substances that are soluble in water and lipids can be smelled by humans. These substances penetrate the mucus covering the olfactory mucosa and stimulate bipolar neurons, which converge to form the olfactory nerve that transports the signal to the olfactory cortex. To determine the relationship between nasal obstruction and olfaction, Rous et al. evaluated the olfactory ability of 50 patients with nasal deformities (16). These investigators demonstrated that above a threshold resistance, nasal obstruction resulted in an elevation of the olfactory threshold in the involved nare. Obstruction at the middle turbinate or above, secondary to swelling of the nasal mucosa or bony obstruction, has also clearly been shown to attenuate olfaction (17).

Paranasal Sinuses

The paranasal sinuses consist of four paired cavities that have openings into the nasal passage (Fig. 2). At birth, the ethmoid sinuses, which are located along the medial orbit, are the only sinuses that are well developed. These sinuses extend from the anterior region of the medial orbit to the optic foramen. The ethmoid sinuses are anatomically divided by bony septi into the anterior, middle, and posterior cells. These air-containing cells number 6 to 10 and have a honeycombed appearance. The sinuses communicate with the nasal cavity through small ostia, leading to a slow exchange of air between the nose and the sinuses.

The largest of the sinuses, the maxillary sinuses, are triangular shaped structures that lie lateral to the nasal cavity. The floor of the maxillary sinus, when fully formed, extends below the nasal cavity and sits above the maxilla, close to the lateral maxillary teeth. The superior wall forms the floor of the orbit. The ostium for the maxillary sinus lies in the superior part of the medial wall of the sinus, a position that does not favor spontaneous, gravitational emptying of the cavity. Although radiographically evident in infancy, the maxillary sinuses are not fully developed until age 7 years.

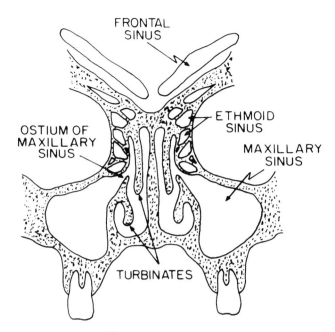

FIG. 2. Paranasal sinuses.

The frontal sinuses begin developing above the orbital rim shortly after birth and finish this process during adolescence. They are radiographically evident between the ages of 3 and 7 years. Frontal sinuses are absent in 3% to 5% of the population.

The sphenoid sinus, the most posterior of the sinuses, is the last to develop, and is not radiographically evident until age 9 years. It lies in the skull base at the junction of the interior and middle cranial fossae in the body of the sphenoid bone. The sphenoids are inferior to the sella turcica and medial to the cavernous sinus.

Histologically, the mucous lining of the paranasal sinuses contains the same ciliated pseudostratified columnar epithelium that is present in the nasal cavity (18). Like the nose, the sinuses are cleared by mucociliary transport. Interestingly, the direction of mucociliary clearance does not change after surgery in which a new anatomic opening has been created for ventilation (19).

The biologic function of the sinuses is incompletely understood. Potential physiologic functions include a) to lessen skull weight, b) to provide resonating chambers for speech, c) to aid in olfaction, d) to provide thermal insulation for the skull and orbit, e) to protect from trauma, f) to provide sound protection for transmission of the sound of one's speech to the ears, and g) to equalize pressure during respiration (20).

Oral Cavity

The oral cavity is bounded anteriorly by the lips, posteriorly by the anterior tonsillar pillar, inferiorly by the floor of the mouth, and superiorly by the hard and soft palates.

Chronic nasal obstruction with secondary oral breathing may lead to a high arched palate. This consequence occurs because the tongue is prevented from modeling the hard palate during growth. The mouth is lined by nonkeratinizing, stratified squamous epithelium and houses the tongue, which is covered by a modified epithelium containing the filiform papillae at the tip, the fungiform papillae at the tip and margins, the foliate papillae on the posterolateral part of the tongue, and the vallate papillae on the dorsum. The sensations of bitter, sweet, sour, and salty arise from special sensory receptors located in the tongue (21). The taste buds require the presence of adequate amounts of saliva for normal function. The oropharynx is involved in mastication, taste, and articulation.

Pharynx

The pharynx is a 12- to 13-cm long muscular tube in the adult divided into three parts: the oropharynx, the nasopharynx, and the hypopharynx (Fig. 3). It functions to transport air, solids, and liquids from the external to the internal environment. Irritation of neurons within the pharynx can induce vagal reflexes that can lead to bradycardia, dysrhythmia, bronchospasm, laryngospasm, apnea, and hiccups. A common irritant for this reflex is acid from gastroesophageal reflux.

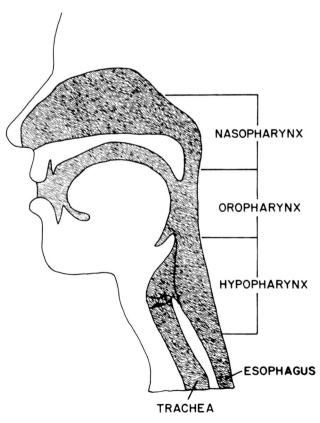

FIG. 3. Pharynx.

Oropharynx

The oropharynx is that portion of the pharynx situated behind the oral cavity, below the palate, and above the level of the epiglottis. It is made up of the anterior pillar (palatoglossus muscle), the posterior pillar (palatopharyngeus muscle), the tonsillar fossae (area between two muscles), and the posterior and lateral pharyngeal walls. The epithelium-covered tonsils are specialized lymph nodes that protect against invading organisms and play a role in local immunity. The oropharynx also includes the valleculae, the base of the tongue, the anterior surface of the soft palate, and the lingual surface of the epiglottis. The oropharynx is lined with nonkeratinizing stratified squamous epithelium.

Nasopharynx

The nasopharynx begins at the choanae, which are the posterior openings of the nasal cavity. The nasopharynx houses the adenoids and the openings of the eustachian tube and sphenoid sinuses. The muscular soft palate sits on the anterior wall of the nasal pharynx and functions to direct the flow of air and food between the oropharynx and nasopharynx. The nasopharynx is lined by respiratory ciliated pseudostratified squamous epithelium.

Hypopharynx

The hypopharynx is bound posteriorly by the posterior pharyngeal wall, laterally by the piriform sinuses, anteriorly by the larynx, and inferiorly by the esophageal inlet. The lining consists of nonkeratinized stratified squamous epithelium. The hypopharynx controls the distribution of food during swallowing by elevating the larynx and pulling the epiglottis over the vocal cords. The reverse sequence allows air to enter the lungs. The lingualar tonsils are present at the base of the tongue.

Eustachian Tube and Middle Ear

The eustachian tube opens into the middle ear space and connects the middle ear space to the nasopharynx. It is initially horizontal at birth and, with growth, gradually changes to an angle of 45°. The tube consists of a mobile, cartilaginous portion (medial two thirds) and a bony portion (lateral one third). The junction between the two parts, called the isthmus, is narrow and usually the site for inflammatory stenosis of the eustachian tube. The eustachian tube is lined with pseudostratified columnar ciliated epithelium, which is continuous with the mucosa of the nasopharynx. It functions mainly to equalize pressure between the middle ear and the nasopharynx. The tensor veli palatini and the levator palatini muscles open the eustachian during swallowing or yawning.

PATHOLOGY

Allergic Rhinitis

Allergic rhinitis, or hay fever, is a common medical problem for the patient and the physician alike. The estimated frequency of allergic rhinitis in the general United States population ranges from 15% to 20%. Allergic rhinitis can begin at any age, but usually appears before age 20 years; most commonly, symptoms occur between the ages of 12 and 15 years. It rarely presents before 18 months of age. Usually an individual requires 2 to 3 years of exposure to the offending allergen before developing symptoms. Although allergic rhinitis shows a male predominance in adolescence, the ratio of males to females equalizes in young adulthood.

Allergic rhinitis may be seasonal or perennial, depending on the sensitizing allergen. Seasonal allergic rhinitis is typically due to pollens from grasses, trees, and weeds. In temperate climates, outdoor molds may contribute to symptoms in all seasons except the winter, when the concentration of spore counts diminishes. In humid climates, however, fungi can cause perennial allergic rhinitis symptoms. Perennial exposure to nonseasonal allergens, such as animal dander and house dust mites, leads to symptoms year-round. Fungi may be important indoor allergens in damp environments. Pollens from weeds, grasses, and trees vary from one geographic location to another. To identify the offending allergen, clinicians must become familiar with the individual plant pollination seasons in his/her area. The seasonal distribution of plant pollens in the midwestern portion of the United States is demonstrated in Fig. 4.

Symptoms of allergic rhinitis consist of paroxysms of sneezing, clear rhinorrhea, nasal pruritis, and nasal obstruction that fluctuates from side to side, as well as in level of intensity. Patients also may complain of red, itchy eyes. With nasal congestion, snoring and mouth breathing may be prevalent. Frequently, allergic individuals will also complain of symptoms of fatigue; the basis to this symptom is not well established.

On physical examination, the conjunctivae show edema and hyperemia. Tearing is usually present. The nasal mucous membranes often will be edematous and pale blue in color with clear, watery secretions. Excessive nasal itching may lead to nose rubbing and the so-called allergic salute, a characteristic gesture of pushing the tip of the nose upward with the palm of the hand. Prolonged nose rubbing in children may lead to the formation of a transverse crease across the bulbar portion of the nose (22). In individuals with severe nasal congestion, the periorbital skin may show allergic "shiners," a darkening of the tissues beneath the eye, usually caused by venous engorgement. Last, on examination of the ears, a middle ear effusion may be detected.

Immunologically, allergic rhinitis is characterized by an IgE-mediated reaction, with release of mediators and recruitment of inflammatory cells. The immune reaction to a sensitizing allergen includes IgE antibody production with its binding firmly to receptors on circulating basophils and tissue mast cells. The cross-linking of at least two IgE molecules by antigen triggers within minutes the secretion of preformed and synthesized mediators from the mast cell and basophil. The mast cell assumes a pivotal role in the immediate phase of the allergic reaction. It releases several inflammatory mediators, such as histamine, prostaglandin D_2, leukotrienes C_4, D_4, and E_4, and kininogens, that are capable of inducing acute symptoms. Histamine is probably the most important of these mediators. It causes vascular engorgement and nasal congestion. Histamine stimulates secretion of mucus through a direct action and increases plasma protein extravasation, causing tissue edema. Finally, by an indirect reflex mechanism, histamine increases glandular secretion (23).

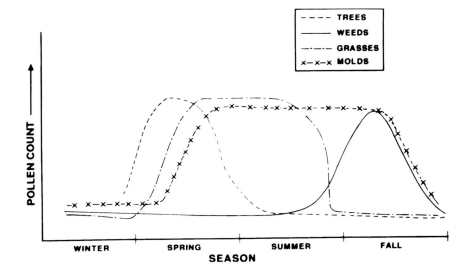

FIG. 4. Seasonal distribution of plant pollens in the Midwestern portion of the United States.

Sneezing also can be provoked by challenging the nasal mucosa directly with histamine (24).

During the allergic immune response, several cytokines are generated, which contribute to the characteristic inflammation observed in both the early- and late-phase responses. These protein molecules are potent inflammatory mediators that are stable and can be generated for prolonged periods. In allergic rhinitis, the mast cell is an important source of these cytokines, including interleukin-4 (IL-4), IL-5, and IL-6 and may contribute to the chronic mucosal inflammation found in this disease (25). In addition, mast cell–derived chemotactic factors may contribute to the recruitment of neutrophils, basophils, and eosinophils to the nasal mucosa (26). These recruited cells account for the appearance of the late-phase response to antigen, which develops 3 to 11 hours after the initial antigen exposure (27). The late-phase allergic response also has been associated with an increase in regional concentrations of IL-1, GM-CSF, IL-5, and IL-6, as recently demonstrated by Sim et al., after nasal allergen challenge in atopic individuals (28). IL-1, produced primarily by monocytes and macrophages, has been shown to be proinflammatory and can activate both eosinophils and neutrophils (29). Both IL-5 and GM-CSF prolong eosinophil survival and prime eosinophils for mediator release (30,31). IL-6 shares several activities with IL-1 and is also an important cofactor in the regulation and secretion of IgE (32).

Recently, a novel new class of small cytokines, called chemokines, (see Chapter 51) named for their chemotactic ability to recruit inflammatory cells, has been identified. This group of proteins activates leukocytes and may serve a role in inflammation. The chemokine, MCP-1, appears to be as effective as a complement component in stimulating exocytosis and histamine release from human basophils (33). RANTES also has been shown to be an effective basophil and eosinophil chemoattractant (34,35). Recent studies have shown that RANTES may also play a role in activation of eosinophils (36). MCP-3 combines both properties and is as effective as MCP-1 in inducing mediator release in basophils and is as effective as RANTES as a chemoattractant (37). All these chemokines may play a key role in the recruitment and activation of eosinophils and basophils and thereby contribute to the late-phase allergic response. The late-phase reaction establishes the chronic nature to allergic rhinitis and primes the nasal tissue. This priming effect decreases the concentration of allergen required to produce allergic symptoms.

The diagnosis of allergic rhinitis is usually straightforward. An accurate, detailed history and a physical examination is helpful in patients who have a temporal association between symptoms and exposure to seasonal allergens. An effective initial screening tool is the presence of eosinophils on a nasal smear. This test, however, is nonspecific and may not show eosinophilia in those individuals with no recent exposure to allergen (38). An increase of total serum IgE concentration may be found in 30% to 40% of patients with allergic rhinitis. This test is of limited value, however, because results vary widely. The presence of specific IgE antibodies to allergens, in contrast, is helpful in establishing a diagnosis. Allergen skin testing using potent preparations with positive and negative controls is the diagnostic procedure of choice for identifying the offending allergen in individual patients. *In vitro* radioimmunoassay tests (RAST) using patient sera and radiolabeled antibody may be employed in very young children, or in individuals with skin dermatitis or unusual rashes, for whom skin testing is not feasible, and in patients who cannot discontinue antihistamines.

The treatment of patients with allergic rhinitis can be divided into three categories: avoidance and environmental control, medications, and immunotherapy (Fig. 5).

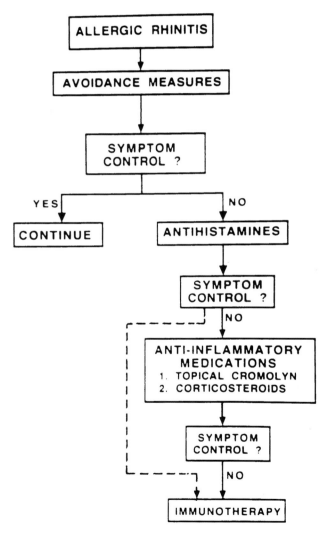

FIG. 5. Allergic rhinitis treatment flow chart. (From Mehta H, Kumar A, Busse WW. Principles of immunotherapy in allergic rhinitis. In: Leff AR, ed. *Pulmonary pharmacology and therapeutics.* New York: McGraw-Hill, 1995:385–392.)

Once specific allergens are identified, avoidance and environmental control should be a part of every patient's therapeutic regimen. Allergen avoidance is the most effective therapy for allergic rhinitis when exposure can be avoided. For those patients with extreme sensitivity to seasonal pollens, exposure can be reduced by remaining indoors and running an air conditioner, both in the house and in automobiles (39). Although effective, this approach has limitations. By contrast, specific control measures for the reduction of indoor allergens, such as house dust mite and animal dander, are practical and effective. Measures to avoid house dust mite exposure include encasing the mattress, pillows, and box spring in occlusive covers; weekly washing of all bedding in hot water; and dehumidification to <50% (40). Removal of reservoirs, such as carpeting, and application of acaricides is recommended if the initial three measures are not effective. Animal allergens may be eliminated by removal of the pet from the environment. For those patients who are resistant to removing their pet from the home, weekly washings may substantially reduce airborne levels of allergen (40). Most common aeroallergens, however, cannot be avoided completely. This is especially true for patients with multiple sensitivities that result in constant exposure to airborne allergens resulting in severe, perennial symptoms.

Because of unavoidable exposures and severe symptoms, medications may be necessary for symptom control. The usual first-line medication for individuals with allergic rhinitis is antihistamines. Both first and second generation antihistamines inhibit the effect of histamine at the target organ. Although they have little effect on nasal congestion, antihistamines are beneficial in reducing sneezing, nasal itching, and rhinorrhea. Traditional first generation H_1-antagonists are sedating but, when given on a regular basis at bedtime, often are tolerated. Second generation, nonsedating antihistamines, such as terfenadine, loratadine, and astemizole, cause less sedation because of their limited penetration of the blood–brain barrier. Topical cromolyn sodium may be effective for patients who do not respond to antihistamines. Intranasal cromolyn sodium, although it prevents the release of certain inflammatory mediators and has few side effects, has little decongestant activity, and does not give prompt symptomatic relief. Topical, intranasal corticosteroids (beclamethasone, budesonide, triamcinolone, flu-

nisolide, and fluticasone) are the most effective medications available for allergic rhinitis. When used for more than 4 to 7 days, these corticosteroid sprays prevent the allergen-provoked pathophysiology of both the early and late phases of allergic rhinitis (41).

Immunotherapy is an effective adjunctive management strategy for allergic rhinitis. It should be considered in the patient whose history demonstrates classic seasonal rhinitis symptoms during two or more consecutive seasons with an inability to control symptoms by avoiding the aeroallergen and/or by use of well tolerated pharmacotherapy (42). Immunotherapy may also be indicated for patients who have had one season of rhinitis with unusually severe symptoms or intolerable side effects from medications.

It has been proposed that immunotherapy for allergic rhinitis may not only improve symptom control, but may also have disease-modifying properties. In this sense, the consideration of immunotherapy is of interest and importance in the treatment of allergic rhinitis.

Nonallergic Rhinitis

Nonallergic rhinitis is more common in adults than children and is characterized by the absence of positive skin prick tests or radioallergosorbent test (RAST) to common allergens. Nonallergic rhinitis is then subdivided into the vasomotor and eosinophilic subgroups. The term "vasomotor rhinitis" has been used to describe patients with nonallergic perennial rhinitis who complain of overresponsiveness of the nose to irritants, emotional factors, odors, and minimal changes in temperature and humidity. Nonallergic rhinitis with eosinophilia (NARES) characterizes those individuals with nonallergic rhinitis whose nasal smears reveal marked eosinophilia (usually 20–25%) during symptomatic periods (43). NARES is responsible for 15% of rhinitis cases seen by physicians (44). Monoret-Vautrin and colleges have suggested that the NARES syndrome is the early phase of the classic triad of nasal polyposis, asthma, and intolerance to aspirin (45). The NARES group of patients is similar to those with allergic rhinitis, except for the absence of an identifiable allergen. Characteristics of allergic and nonallergic rhinitis is displayed in Table 1.

TABLE 1. *Characteristics of allergic and nonallergic rhinitis*

	Allergic rhinitis	Vasomotor rhinitis	NARES syndrome
Affected group	Adults, children	Adults	Adults
History	Congestion, sneezing, pruritis, rhinorrhea	Congestion, rhinorrhea, postnasal drainage	Congestion, sneezing, pruritis, rhinorrhea
Nasal exam	Pale mucosa	Boggy mucosa, hyperemia	Pale mucosa
Skin tests	Positive	Negative	Negative
Therapy	Antihistamines, decongestants, topical corticosteroids	Decongestants, topical corticosteroids, ipratropium	Decongestants, topical corticosteroids

Individuals with nonallergic rhinitis usually experience symptoms of nasal obstruction, rhinorrhea, and postnasal drainage with little pruritis and sneezing. Patients with NARES syndrome, however, have paroxysms of sneezing and nasal itching. On physical examination, the nasal mucosa is boggy and deep red in color with clear secretions. This finding is not present in all individuals, however. Patients with NARES syndrome usually demonstrate a pale mucosa rather than hyperemia. Although the term "vasomotor" implies a vascular component to the disease, this has not clearly been demonstrated. It has been postulated that individuals with vasomotor rhinitis suffer from an imbalance of the autonomic nervous system, and the excessive parasympathetic activation causes the hypersecretion present in this group (46). The cause of NARES syndrome is unknown.

Initial therapy, especially of vasomotor rhinitis, should include avoidance of all recognizable irritant factors. This approach, however, has limitations. For those individuals who cannot avoid the irritant factor(s), medications may be necessary. For the treatment of nonallergic rhinitis, first-line drugs such as oral decongestants often are effective. For those patients with refractory symptoms, intranasal corticosteroids may be tried. Those individuals with NARES syndrome show a strikingly good response to medical therapy with corticosteroids (47). Anticholinergic agents such as ipratropium have also been shown to be effective, especially in patients with vasomotor rhinitis (46). In those individuals with vasomotor rhinitis, it is important to stress that therapy may not cause complete symptom resolution, because treatment of this condition often is difficult and may require multiple medications.

Nasal Polyps

Nasal polyps are benign pedicled masses of nasal or sinus mucosa. These masses usually originate from the ethmoid sinuses, with a few originating from the maxillary or sphenoid sinuses. Polyps usually occur after age 40 years and are more prevalent in men. The appearance of nasal polyps in a child should alert a physician to the possibility of cystic fibrosis. The incidence of nasal polyposis in patients with cystic fibrosis is reported to range from 6% to 48% (48,49). The association of asthma, nasal polyps, and aspirin sensitivity was described by Samter in 1967, and is commonly called the asthma triad, or Samter's syndrome (50). In a large study by Settipane et al., 16.7% of their patients with asthma had nasal polyps (51). Conversely, approximately 70% of 211 patients with nasal polyps had asthma. In an additional study, involving 6,000 patients, only 6.7% of patients with asthma had nasal polyps (52). In a series of 35 patients with clinical and radiographic evidence of nasal polyposis, 9% were noted to have aspirin sensitivity (53). Several authors have debated the role of allergic disease

in nasal polyposis. In a study involving 3,000 atopic individuals, Caplin et al. found that only 0.5% had nasal polyps (54). Using history and skin tests, Drake-Lee et al. found no evidence of an increased incidence of allergic disorders in 200 patients who were admitted for polypectomy (55).

Most patients with nasal polyps complain of nasal congestion and perennial rhinitis. Facial pain, headache, and eustachian tube dysfunction may be common. Anosmia may be present and is usually seen if polyps replace more than 80% of the nasal cavity (53). Paranasal sinusitis is a common complication secondary to obstruction of the ostia. On examination of the nares, polyps appear as transparent, glistening, smooth-walled, grayish yellow masses. Their appearance has been likened to a peeled grape. They are most commonly found in the middle meatus, extend to the nasal cavity, and may protrude into the anterior nares. Polyps are often bilateral, and a unilateral mass should alert the physician to the possibility of a neoplasm. An exception to this are antrochoanal polyps, which usually develop in the first two decades of life, are unilateral, and arise from the maxillary sinus (56). It is not uncommon for antrochoanal polyps to enlarge and obstruct the nasopharynx. This type of polyp comprises 3% to 6% of all polyps (56).

Although the histologic appearance of nasal polyps is heterogeneous, epithelial damage and thickening of the basement membrane are ubiquitous (57,58). On examination of the pathology of nasal polyps, there is an appearance of generalized inflammation. It is fairly well known that nasal polypoid tissue is infiltrated by eosinophils and mast cells (59,60). Histamine concentration also is greater in nasal polyp tissue and fluid compared with that found in normal mucosa, demonstrating possible release of mediators from mast cells (61,62). Stoop et al. have demonstrated a significantly higher number of EG2+ (activation marker) eosinophils in polyp tissue compared with unaffected mucosa from the same patient or that obtained from healthy controls (63). In addition to showing that eosinophils are activated in polyp tissue, this study also indicates that the inflammatory process in the polyp tissue is more severe than the surrounding mucosa. Interestingly, examination of nasal polyps from patients with cystic fibrosis shows little infiltration of eosinophils with a fairly delicate basement membrane (58).

Recent immunologic evaluation by Liu and colleagues examining lymphocyte subtypes in nasal polypoid tissue found significantly greater numbers of CD8 cells compared with CD4 subtypes (64). Recently, proto-oncogenes, c-*myc*, l-*myc*, *fos*, and *jun*, were demonstrated in human nasal polyps using Northern blots and were found to be similar to those found in small cell carcinoma of the lung (65). Further studies need to be done to determine if these findings play a role in why polyps develop and reoccur so frequently. Finally, nasal polyp fluid has demonstrated increased concentrations of IgG, IgM, IgE, and

IgA compared with serum values (59). Despite extensive immunologic investigation of nasal polyposis, the exact pathogenesis of this disease remains undetermined.

Current treatment modalities most often are targeted at the polyp and not the underlying cause because the causes are usually unidentifiable. Topical nasal steroids are essential for the management of nasal polyposis. If polyps do not respond to nasal steroids, a medical polypectomy may be tried with a short burst of oral corticosteroids (prednisone 30 mg daily for 7 days, then 10 mg daily for an additional 7 days). In most situations, this leads to reduction of the polyp mass and allows for greater penetration and effectiveness of intranasal steroids. Treatment of nasal polyps often includes antibiotics for associated bacterial sinusitis. Even if patients strictly adhere to their medication regimen, polyps may persist or reoccur.

Patients with nasal polyps that are refractory to maximal medical therapy are candidates for surgery. Surgery may involve just a single polypectomy or more extensive procedures to remove the actual tissue source of the polyp. Recently a functional endoscopic approach has been increasingly used. In a recent study by Lanza et al., 85% of individuals reported an improvement in symptoms at an 18-month follow-up after endoscopic total sphenoethmoidectomy (66). Levine et al. found that the success after treatment rate was similar regardless of the severity of polyposis, indicating that nasal polyps tend to reoccur (67).

Sinusitis

The paranasal sinuses are protected against infection by lysozymes, secretory immunoglobulins, and an active mucociliary system. A malfunction in this self-cleansing mechanism leads to accumulation and stagnation of mucus with secondary infection by bacteria normally present in the nose and sinuses. The sinuses communicate with the nasal cavity through small ostia leading to a slow exchange of air between the nose and the sinuses. Any obstruction of the ostia also interrupts the cleaning mechanism of the sinuses and leads to retained secretions. This obstruction then causes a change in the composition of the secretions and a decrease in the PO_2 secondary to interruption of air flow into the sinuses (68). The change in gas metabolism within the sinus cavity leads to ciliary and epithelial damage and favors the growth of bacteria. There are several factors that contribute to ostial obstruction, including allergic rhinitis and medications leading to mucosal inflammation and anatomic variations such as septal deviation and nasal polyps. A list of these conditions is displayed in Table 2.

Sinusitis is a common disease, accounting for 16 million physician visits annually (69). Sinus infections are classified arbitrarily as acute (0–3 weeks), subacute (3 weeks to 3 months) and chronic (>3 months). The maxil-

TABLE 2. *Factors predisposing to ostial obstruction and/or sinusitis*

Systemic	Environmental
Cystic fibrosis	Cigarette smoke
Immotile cilia syndrome	Barotrauma
Pregnancy	Mechanical
Hypothyroidism	Polyps
Immunodeficiency	Foreign bodies
Medications	Tumors
OTC topical decongestants	Septal deviation
Antihypertensives	Concha bullosa
Oral contraceptives	Large adenoids
Infectious	Miscellaneous
Tooth infection	Allergic rhinitis
Upper respiratory infection	Nonallergic rhinitis

lary sinuses are the ones most commonly affected in adults, followed by the ethmoid, frontal, and sphenoid sinuses. In children, the ethmoid sinuses are most frequently affected by infection. Common organisms causing acute sinusitis in adults are *Streptococcus pneumoniae* and *Haemophilus influenzae* (70). Children are most commonly infected with *S. pneumoniae, Moraxella catarrhalis,* and *H. influenzae* (71). The organisms involved in acute, subacute, and chronic sinusitis are summarized in Table 3. Studies examining the bacteriology of acute maxillary sinusitis have shown that nasal smears and cultures are usually contaminated and do not reflect the bacterial pathogens present in the sinuses (72). Direct antral puncture or surgical sampling are considered the definitive test. These methods are not used frequently except in cases with antibiotic resistance. Infections with fungi such as *Mucor* and *Aspergillus* also occur (73), and primarily affect immunocompromised hosts. Greenberger and colleagues have also documented allergic *Aspergillus* sinusitis, which occurs in nonimmunocompromised individuals and is felt to be secondary to a hypersensitivity response to the organism (74).

Symptoms of acute sinusitis in the adult usually include facial pain, as well as tooth pain, purulent nasal secretion, fever, nasal congestion, cough, and headache. A

TABLE 3. *Common organisms in sinusitis*

Acute sinusitis	Subacute sinusitis	Chronic sinusitis
Adults		
S. pneumoniae	S. pneumoniae	Anaerobes
H. influenzae	H. influenzae	Staphylococci
Children		
S. pneumoniae	S. pneumoniae	S. pneumoniae
M. catarrhalis	M. catarrhalis	M. catarrhalis
H. influenzae	H. influenzae	H. influenzae
		Severe symptoms
		Anaerobes
		Staphylococci

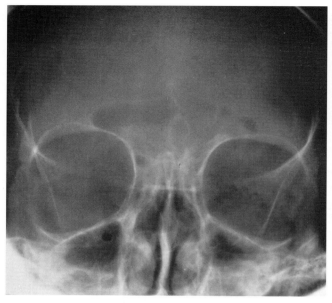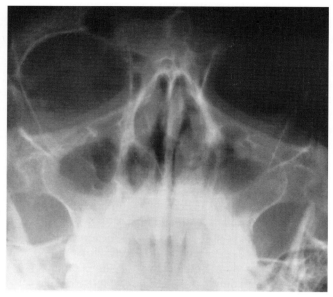

A

B

FIG. 6. Pan sinusitis. **A:** Note left frontal sinus air-fluid level and right frontal sinus opacification. **B:** Left maxillary sinus air-fluid level. Right maxillary sinus with thickened mucosa.

history of facial pain associated with rapid changes in position may also be elicited. Symptoms of sinusitis in children are similar to adults, except that fever and facial pain are not elicited as often. In a study by Wald and colleagues, symptomatic complaints were analyzed in 30 children, ages 1 to 16 years, in whom the diagnosis of acute sinusitis was confirmed by radiographic assessment (75). The most common symptoms were cough (24 of 30 children) and nasal discharge (23 of 30 children). Fever was noted in 9 children, headache in 10, and malodorous breath in 15. It is reasonable to suspect sinusitis in any patient with an upper respiratory tract infection that persists beyond 7 to 10 days. Few symptoms of sinusitis are highly sensitive, except for toothache; however, this is present in only 11% of patients (76). Symptoms of chronic sinusitis may be similar to those of acute sinusitis. However, a patient may complain only of a chronic cough, postnasal drainage, or hoarseness.

On physical exam, palpable tenderness may be present in those individuals with frontal or maxillary sinusitis. This, however, is an unsensitive and nonspecific finding. Examination of the nose with a nasal speculum may demonstrate the presence of purulent drainage. The nasal mucosa is usually inflamed and hyperemic. Cytologic exam of nasal secretions is usually not helpful because many of polymorphonuclear cells are present in both viral upper respiratory infections and sinus infections. The use of transillumination is also not always reliable and requires complete unilateral sinus opacification to be diagnostic (77).

Diagnosis of sinus disease can be aided by the use of radiographs (Fig. 6). There is no single projection that al-

lows all the sinuses to be visualized. The occipitomental view (Waters view) with the head tilted back and the mouth open provides good visualization of the maxillary sinuses. The occipitofrontal view (Caldwell view) with the head tilted forward demonstrates both the ethmoid and frontal sinuses. The sphenoid sinus can best be evaluated on a lateral view. The presence of opacification, airfluid levels, or mucosal thickening more than 5 to 8 mm is strongly associated with a clinical diagnosis of acute sinusitis (78,79). In chronic sinusitis, the findings are less obvious. Air-fluid levels are unusual, and more common signs are mucosal thickening and opacification. Abnormal radiologic findings have been documented in children with viral upper respiratory tract infections up to 2 weeks after symptom resolution (80). Computed tomography (CT) is currently considered the "gold standard," especially for evaluation of chronic inflammation of the paranasal sinuses. CT of the paranasal sinuses in the coronal plane provides excellent visualization of the anatomic and deep structures of the sinuses, including excellent delineation of lesions in the osteomeatal complex (Fig. 7). In a study by Lazar et al., CT scans detected sinus disease in 40% of 45 patients with chronic sinusitis who had normal sinus x-rays (81). In some institutions, a screening CT of the sinuses, with a limited number of views and low-dose radiation exposure, is available (82). It is usually offered at a cost competitive approach with plain film studies.

The treatment of sinusitis should focus on eradication of infection, reduction of inflammation, and restoration of ventilation of the sinuses. Medical treatment of sinusitis includes antibiotic therapy for 14 to 21 days, anal-

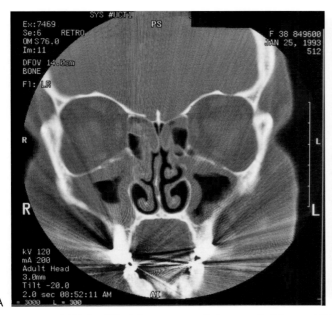 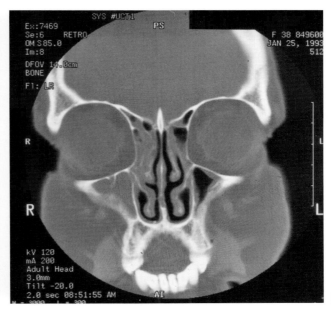

FIG. 7. CT of the paranasal sinuses. **A:** Mucosal thickening of both maxillary sinuses. The right is worse than the left. **B:** Mucosal thickening to a lesser degree is also present in the ethmoid air cells, again right greater than left.

gesics, topical and oral decongestants, and fluids. For treatment failures, a second course of antibiotics may be justified. For those individuals who fail to respond to two consecutive courses of antibiotics, referral to an otolaryngologist for aspiration and culture may be warranted. The underlying cause of inflammation or obstruction must be targeted for medical therapy to be successful and to prevent future episodes of sinusitis. Only if an adequate trial with medical therapy fails should surgery be considered.

The association between sinusitis and asthma is well documented. The plaguing question of whether sinusitis actually causes a worsening of asthma has not been answered. Studies, however, have demonstrated an improvement of asthma after treatment for sinusitis (83–85). Several mechanisms have been proposed to explain this relationship, including pulmonary aspiration of upper airway secretion, aspiration of inflammatory mediators directly into the lungs, and triggering of the naso-sinus-bronchial reflex. Recent studies examining the role of direct aspiration of sinus material into the lungs have shown negative results. Bordin and colleagues, using isotype labeling, could not show aspiration of infected material from the upper airway into the lungs (86). Irvin et al. have postulated, using an animal model that demonstrates airway hyperresponsiveness secondary to induction of sinusitis, that the worsening of asthma due to sinusitis results from the direct passage of inflammatory mediators from the upper to the lower respiratory tract (87). Elicitation of the naso-sinus-bronchial reflex with a secondary increase in responsiveness of the lower air-

ways has been demonstrated in a viral infected animal model and after nasal provocation in humans (88,89). This reflex involves stimulation of receptors in the nose, sinuses, and pharynx, with secondary signal transportation to the medulla. From here the signal travels to the vagal nucleus onto the vagus nerve down to the bronchi, leading to bronchoconstriction (90). However, using rabbits positioned head down, Irvin et al. did not demonstrate bronchoconstriction resulting from the naso-sinus-bronchial reflex despite florid sinus inflammation (87).

REFERENCES

1. Cole P. Upper respiratory airflow. In: Proctor DF, Andersen I, eds. *The nose, upper airway physiology and the atmospheric environment.* Amsterdam: Elsevier Biomedical Press, 1982;163–189.
2. Proctor DF, Adams GK. Physiology and pharmacology of nasal function and mucus secretion. *Pharmacol Ther* 1976;2B:492–.
3. Becker W, Naumann HH, Pfaltz CR. *Ear, nose, and throat diseases: a pocket reference.* New York: Thieme Medical Publishers, Inc., 1994.
4. Graney DO, Baker SR. Nose: anatomy. In: Cummings CW, Fredrickson JM, Harker LA, Krause CJ, Schuller DE, eds. *Otolaryngology-head and neck surgery.* St. Louis: Mosby-Year Book, 1993;631.
5. Eccles R. Nasal airways. In: Busse WW, Holgate ST, eds. *Asthma and rhinitis.* Cambridge: Blackwell Scientific Publication, 1995;73.
6. Langes J. *Clinical anatomy of the nose, nasal cavity and paranasal sinuses.* New York: Thieme Medical Publishers, 1989.
7. Rhys Evans PH. Anatomy of the nose and paranasal sinuses. In: Kerr AG, Groves J, Wright D, eds. *Scott-Brown's otolaryngology.* London: Butterworth & Co, 1987:138.
8. Drake-Lee AB. Physiology of the nose and paranasal sinuses. In: Kerr AG, Groves J, Wright D, eds. *Scott-Brown's otolaryngology.* London: Butterworth & Co, 1987:162.
9. Geurkink N. Nasal anatomy, physiology, and function. *J Allergy Clin Immunol* 1983; 72:123–128.
10. Proctor DF. The mucociliary system. In: Proctor DF, Andersen IB, eds.

The nose, upper airway physiology and the atmospheric environment. Amsterdam: Elsevier Biomedical Press, 1982;245.

11. Bang BG, Bang FB. Nasal mucociliary systems. In: Brain JD, Proctor DF, Reid LM, eds. *Lung biology in health and disease,* vol 5, part I, Respiratory defense mechanisms. New York: Marcel Dekker, 1977; 405.

12. Iacono VJ, MacKay BJ, DiRienzo S, et al. Selective antibacterial properties of lysozyme for oral microorganisms. *Infect Immun* 1980;29: 623.

13. Arnold RR, Cole HF, McGhee JR. A bactericidal effect for human lactoferrin. *Science* 1977;197:263.

14. Widdicombe JG, Wells UM. Airway secretions. In: Proctor DF, Andersen IB, eds. *The nose, upper airway physiology and the atmospheric environment.* Amsterdam: Elsevier Biomedical Press, 1982;215.

15. Leopold DA. The relationship between nasal anatomy and human olfaction. *Laryngoscope* 1988;98:1232.

16. Rous J, Kober F. Influence of one-sided nasal respiratory occlusion on the olfactory threshold values. *Arch Klin Ohren Nasen Kehlkopfheiklk* 1970;196:374.

17. Scott AE. Clinical characteristics of taste & smell disorders. *Ear Nose Throat J* 1989;68:297.

18. Latta JS, Schall RF. The histology of the epithelium of the paranasal sinuses under various conditions. *Ann Otol Rhinol Laryngol* 1934;43:945.

19. Naclerio RM. Embryology, anatomy, and physiology of the upper airway. In: Middleton E, Reed CE, Ellis EF, Adkinson NF, Yunginger JW, Busse WW, eds. *Allergy: principles and practice.* St. Louis: Mosby-Year Book, 1993;740.

20. Drettner B. The paranasal sinuses. In: Procter DF, Andersen IB, eds. *The nose, upper airway physiology and the atmospheric environment.* Amsterdam: Elsevier Biomedical Press, 1982.

21. McBurney D, Gent J. On the nature of taste qualities. *Psychol Bull* 1979;86:151.

22. Myers MA. The "nasal crease": a physical sign of allergic rhinitis, *JAMA* 1960;174:1204.

23. Despot JE. Inflammatory mediators in allergic rhinitis. *Immunol Allergy Clin North Am* 1987;7:37.

24. Doyle WJ. Physiologic responses to intranasal dose-response challenges with histamine, methacholine, bradykinin and prostaglandin in adult volunteers with and without nasal allergy. *J Allergy Clin Immunol* 1990;86:924.

25. Bradding P, Feather IH, Wilson S, Bardin PG, Heusser CH, Holgate ST, Howarth PH. Immunolocalization of cytokines in the nasal mucosa of normal and perennial rhinitic subjects. The mast cell as a source of IL-4, IL-5, and IL-6 in human allergic mucosal inflammtion. *J Immunol* 1993;151:3853.

26. Nagakura T, Onda T, Iikura Y, et al. *In vitro* and *in vivo* antigen-induced release of high-molecular weight neutrophil chemotactic activity from human nasal tissue. *Am J Rhinol* 1988;2:7.

27. Dvoracek JE. Induction of nasal late-phase reactions by insufflation of ragweed-pollen extract. *J Allergy Clin Immunol* 1984;73:363.

28. Sim TC, Grant JA, Hilsmeier KA, Fukuda Y, Alam R. Proinflammatory cytokines in nasal secretions of allergic subjects after antigen challenge. *Am J Respir Crit Care Med* 1994;149(2 pt 1):339.

29. Dinarello CA. Interleukin-1 and its biologically related cytokines. *Adv Immunol* 1989;44:153.

30. Silberstein DS, Owen WF, Gasson JC, et al. Enhancement of human eosinophil cytotoxicity and leukotriene synthesis by biosynthetic (recombinant) granulocyte-macrophage colony-stimulating factor. *J Immunol* 1986;137:3290.

31. Lopez AF, Sanderson CJ, Gamble JR, Campbell HD, Young IG, Vadas MA. Recombinant human interleukin-5 is a selective activator of human eosinophil function. *J Exp Med* 1988;157:219.

32. Borish L, Joseph BZ. Inflammation and the allergic response. *Med Clin North Am* 1992;76:765.

33. Kuna P, Reddigare SR, Rucinski D, Oppenheim JJ, Kaplan AP. Monocyte chemotactic and activating factor is a potent histamine-releasing factor for human basophils. *J Exp Med* 1992;175:489.

34. Kameyoshi A, Dorschner A, Mallet AI, Christophers E, Schroeder JM. Cytokine RANTES released by thrombin-stimulated platelets is a potent attractant for human eosinophils. *J Exp Med* 1992;176:587.

35. Kuna P, Reddigari SR, Schall TJ, Rucinski D, Viksman MY, Kaplan AP. RANTES, a monocyte and T lymphocyte chemotactic cytokine, releases histamine from human basophils. *J Immunol* 1992;149:636.

36. Alam R, Stafford S, Forsythe PA. RANTES is a chemotactic and activating factor for human eosinophils. *J Immunol* 1993;150:3442.

37. Baggiolini M, Dahinden CA. CC chemokines in allergic inflammation. *Immunol Today* 1994;5:127.

38. Zeiger RS. Allergic and non-allergic rhinitis: classification and pathogenesis. Part II. Non-allergic rhinitis. *Am J Rhinol* 1989;3:113.

39. Soloman WR. Exclusion of particulate allergens by window air conditioners. *J Allergy Clin Immunol* 1980;65:305.

40. Platts-Mills TAE. Controlling indoor allergens in patients with asthma. *J Respir Dis* 1992;13:20.

41. Pipkorn U, Proud D, Lichtenstein LM, et al. Inhibition of mediator release in allergic rhinitis by pretreatment with topical glucocorticosteroids. *N Engl J Med* 1987;316:1506.

42. Rocklin RE. Clinical and immunologic aspects of allergen-specific immunotherapy in patients with seasonal allergic rhinitis and/or allergic asthma. *J Allergy Clin Immunol* 1983;72:323.

43. Jacobs RL, Freedman PM, Boswell RN. Nonallergic rhinitis with eosinophilia (NARES syndrome): clinical and immunological presentation. *J Allergy Clin Immunol* 1981;67:253.

44. Monoret-Vautrin DA, Wayoff M, Hsieh V. Non-allergic eosinophilic rhinitis: from clinical diagnosis to pathogenic study. *Ann Otolaryngol Chir Cervicofac* 1988;105:553.

45. Moneret-Vautrin DA, Hsieh V, Wayoff M, Guyot JL, Mouton C, Maria Y. Nonallergic rhinitis with eosinophilia syndrome a precursor of the triad: nasal polyposis, intrinsic asthma, and intolerance to aspirin. *Ann Allergy* 1990;64:513.

46. Dolovich J, Kennedy L, Vickerson F, Kazim F. Control of the hypersecretion of vasomotor rhinitis by topical ipratropium bromide. *J Allergy Clin Immunol* 1987;80:274.

47. Mullarkey MF, Hill JS, Webb DR. Allergic and nonallergic rhinitis: their characterization with attention to the meaning of eosinophilia. *J Allergy Clin Immunol* 1980;65:122.

48. Crockett DM, McGill TJ, Friedman EM, Healy GB, Salkeld LJ. Nasal and paranasal sinus surgery in children with cystic fibrosis. *Ann Otol Rhinol Laryngol* 1987;96:367.

49. Stern RC, Boat TF, Wood RE, Matthews LW, Doershuk CF. Treatment and prognosis of nasal polyps in cystic fibrosis. *Am J Dis Child* 1982;136:1067.

50. Samter M, Beers RF. Concerning the nature of the intolerance to ASA. *J Allergy* 1967;40:281.

51. Settipane GA, Chaffee FH, Klein DE. Aspirin intolerance: a prospective study in an atopic and normal population. *J Allergy Clin Immunol* 1974;53:200.

52. Settipane GA, Chaffee FH. Nasal polyps in asthma with rhinitis: a review of 6037 patients. *J Allergy Clin Immunol* 1977;59:17.

53. Drutman J, Harnsberger HR, Babbel RW, Sonkens JW, Braby D. Sinonasal polyposis: investigation by direct coronal CT. *Neuroradiology* 1991;36:169.

54. Caplin I, Haynes TJ, Spahn J. Are nasal polyps an allergic phenomenon? *Ann Allergy* 1971;29:631.

55. Drake-Lee AB, Lowe D, Swanston A, Grace A. Clinical profile and recurrence of nasal polyps. *J Laryngol Otol* 1984;98:783.

56. Cook PR, Davis WE, McDonald R, McKinsey JP. Antrochoanal polyposis: a review of 33 cases. *Ear Nose Throat J* 1993;72:401.

57. Oppenheimer EH, Rosenstein BJ. Differential pathology of nasal polyps in cystic fibrosis and atopy. *Lab* 1979;40:445.

58. Wladislavosky-Waserman P, Kern EB, Holley KE, Eisenbrey AB, Gleich GJ. Epithelial damage in nasal polyps. *Clin Allergy* 1984;14:241.

59. Chandra RK, Abrol BM. Immunopathology of nasal polypi. *J Laryngol Otol* 1974;84:1019.

60. Stoop AE, Hameleers DMH, van Run PEM, Biewenga J, van der Baan S. Lymphocytes and nonlymphoid cells in the nasal mucosa of patients with nasal polyps and of healthy subjects. *J Allergy Clin Immunol* 1989;84:734.

61. Bumstead RH, El-Ackad T, Smith JM, et al. Histamine, norepinephrine, and serotonin content of nasal polyps. *Laryngoscope* 1984;89: 832.

62. Drake-Lee AB. Histamine and its release from nasal polyps: preliminary communication. *J R Soc Med* 1984;77:120.

63. Stoop AE, van der Heijden HA, Biewenga J, van der Baan S. Eosinophils in nasal polyps and nasal mucosa: an immunohistochemical study. *J Allergy Clin Immunol* 1993;91:616.

64. Liu CM, Shun CT, Hsu MM. Lymphocyte subsets and antigen specific IgE antibody in nasal polyps. *Ann Allergy* 1994;72:19.

65. Emery B, Baraniuk J, Minna J, Lebovics R, Kaliner M. Proto-oncogene expression in human nasal polyposis. *J Allergy Clin Immunol* 1990;95:225.

66. Lanza DC, Kennedy DW. Current concepts in the surgical management of nasal polyposis. *J Allergy Clin Immunol* 1992;90:543.

67. Levine HL. Functional endoscopic sinus surgery: evaluation, surgery, and follow-up of 250 patients. *Laryngoscope* 1990;100:79.

68. Aust R. Measurement of ostial size and oxygen tension in the maxillary sinus. *Rhinology* 1976;14:43.

69. Kennedy DW. First-line management of sinusitis: a national problem? *Otolaryngol Head Neck Surg* 1990;103:847.

70. Gwaltney JM Jr. Sinusitis. In: Mandell GL, Douglas RG, Bennett JE, eds. *Principles and practice of infectious diseases*, 3rd ed. New York: Churchill Livingstone, 1990:510.

71. Wald ER. Microbiology of acute and chronic sinusitis. *Immunol Allergy Clin North Am* 1994;14:31.

72. Hamory BH, Sande MA, Sydnor JA, Seale DL, Gwaltney JM Jr. Etiology and antimicrobial therapy of acute maxillary sinusitis. *J Infect Dis* 1979;139:197.

73. Kavanagh KT, Parham DM, Hughes WT, Chanin LR. Fungal sinusitis in immunocompromised children with neoplasms. *Ann Otol Rhinol Laryngol* 1991;100:331.

74. Katzenstein AL, Sale SR, Greenberger PA. Allergic Aspergillus sinusitis: a newly recognized form of sinusitis. *J Allergy Clin Immunol* 1983;79:89.

75. Wald ER, Milmoe GJ, Bower A, et al. Acute maxillary sinusitis in children. *N Engl J Med* 1981;304:749.

76. Williams JW, Simel DL, Roberts L, Samsa GP. Clinical evaluation of sinusitis-making the diagnosis by history and physical examination. *Ann Intern Med* 1992;117:705.

77. Spector SL, Lotan A, English G, Philpot I. Comparison between transillumination and the roentgenogram in diagnosing paranasal sinus disease. *J Allergy Clin Immunol* 1981;67:22.

78. Evans FO, et al. Sinusitis of the maxillary antrum. *N Engl J Med* 1975;293:735.

79. Wald ER. Acute maxillary sinusitis in children. *N Engl J Med* 1981;304:749.

80. Kovatch AL, Wald ER, Ledesma-Medina J, Chiponis DM, Bedlingfield DM. Maxillary sinus radiographs in children with nonrespiratory complaints. *Pediatrics* 1984;73:306.

81. Lazar RH, Younis RT, Parvey L. Comparison of plain radiographs, coronal CT, and intraoperative findings in children with chronic sinusitis. *Otolaryngol Head Neck Surg* 1992;107:29.

82. Gross GW, McGeady SJ, Kerut T, Ehrlich SM. Limited slice CT in the evaluation of paranasal sinus disease in children. *AJR* 1991;156:367.

83. Friedman R, Ackerman M, Wald E, Cassellmant M, Friday G, Fireman P. Asthma and bacterial sinusitis in children. *J Allergy Clin Immunol* 1984;74:185.

84. Cummings NP, Lere JL, Wood R, Adinoff A. Effect of treatment of sinusitis on asthma and bronchial reactivity: results of a double-blind study. *J Allergy Clin Immunol* 1983;73(suppl):143.

85. Rachelefsky GS, Katz RM, Siegel SC. Chronic sinus disease with associated reactive airways disease in children. *Pediatrics* 1984;73:526.

86. Borden PG, Van Hearden BB, Joubert JR. Absence of pulmonary aspiration of sinus contents in patients with asthma and sinusitis. *J Allergy Clin Immunol* 1990;86:82.

87. Irvin CG. Sinusitis and asthma: an animal model. *J Allergy Clin Immunol* 1992;90:521.

88. Buckner CK, Songsiridej V, Dick EC, Busse WW. *In vitro* and *in vivo* studies on the use of the guinea pig as a model for virus-provoked airway hyperreactivity. *Am Rev Respir Dis* 1985;132:305.

89. Nolte P, Gerber D. On vagal bronchoconstriction in asthmatic patients by nasal irritation. *Eur J Respir Dis* 1983;64:110.

90. Settipane GA. Rhino-sino-bronchial reflex. *Immunol Allergy Prac* 1985;29.

91. Mehta H, Kumar A, Busse WW. Principles of immunotherapy in allergic rhinitis. In: Leff AR, ed. *Pulmonary pharmacology and therapeutics.* New York: McGraw-Hill, 1995:385–392.

Asthma, edited by P.J. Barnes, M.M. Grunstein, A.R. Leff, and A.J. Woolcock.
Lippincott–Raven Publishers, Philadelphia © 1997.

▪ 14 ▪

Normal Airway Structure

Manuel G. Cosio and Marina Saetta

Bronchial System at Birth
Development of the Bronchial Tree to
    Adulthood
Function and Structure of the Fully
    Developed Airways

Function
Morphology
On the Maintenance of Normal Airway Structure
    and Function

BRONCHIAL SYSTEM AT BIRTH

When a child is born, the lung development is far from complete (1–3). Only a small proportion of the alveoli found in an adult lung is present, and the peripheral airways are still being formed. Indeed, in her first law of lung development, Reid (4) states that the development of the conducting airways is complete around the 16th week of gestation, whereas the alveoli develop mainly after birth.

On around the 26th day of gestation, the lungs start to develop in a process that will continue until after the child is born. Table 1 shows the course of this developmental process. The "embryonic" stage (from 26 days to 7 weeks) is characterized by organogenesis and the formation of the major airways, after which the lung development can be divided into five distinct stages: the "pseudoglandular" stage (weeks 5–17), during which the beginnings of a bronchial tree are created; the "canalicular" stage (weeks 16–26), which includes the formation of what will be the lung periphery, the epithelial differentiation, the formation of the air–blood barrier and the first signs of surfactant; the "saccular" stage (weeks 24–38), in which the expansion of the air spaces takes place; the "alveolar" stage, which, as we mentioned above, begins in the last weeks of pregnancy and continues into childhood. A newborn baby born at term could have between 10 and 149 million alveoli, with the average being 55 million (5). Debate is still active concerning both the

starting point and completion of alveolar formation, but certainly most of the 300 million alveoli an average adult can boast are formed postnatally (6). Some authors (7) believe the process ends at 8 years of age, but recent research (8–10) tends to suggest that the process ends earlier than previously thought. Burri (2) proposes the fifth and final "microvascular maturation" stage (from birth to 2–3 years) as a total restructuring of the capillary system and remodeling of the parenchymal septa.

This course of development means that compared with adults', the conducting airways in the newborn baby have a much greater relative volume than that of the gas exchange area. This is a relationship that changes during a child's development (11). Static lung compliance (mainly reflecting the volume of peripheral air spaces) in the newborn baby is smaller per unit of lung weight than in the adult, and gradually increases as the years pass. On the other hand, pulmonary resistance (mainly governed by the diameter of the conducting airways) is high at birth and decreases as the child grows up. This situation mirrors the expansion of the lung peripheral airways and the increase in cross section of the larger airways. However, the increase in static lung compliance after birth is greater than the decrease in total pulmonary resistance, as peripheral air spaces are in a much more rudimentary state of development at birth than the larger airways.

The development of peripheral airways is of great importance in the process of lung maturation. By measuring the conductance of central and peripheral airways in post mortem lungs of persons of various ages, Hogg and co-workers (12) have shown that central conductance did not alter much throughout infancy and childhood, but that peripheral conductance was very low until about 5 years of

M. G. Cosio: Respiratory Division, Royal Victoria Hospital, McGill University, Montreal, Quebec H3A 1A1 Canada.
M. Saetta: Institute of Occupational Medicine, University of Padua, Padua 35127 Italy.

TABLE 1. *Stages of lung development*

Name of Stage	Duration	Characteristics
Embryonic	26th day to 7 weeks	Organogenesis; formation of major airways
Pseudoglandular	5–17 weeks	Formation of bronchial tree; birth of the acinus
Canalicular	16–26 weeks	Formation of the prospective lung periphery; epithelial differentiation; formation of air–blood barrier; appearance of surfactant
Terminal sac (saccular)	24–38 weeks	Expansion of air spaces
Alveolar	36 weeks/birth/to 1–2 years	Alveolization by formation of secondary septa
Microvascular maturation	Birth to 2–3 years?	Remodeling of interalveolar septa and restructuring of the capillary bed

From Burri PH. Postnatal development and growth. In: Crystal RG, West JB, eds. The lung: scientific foundations. New York: *Raven Press*, 1991; Section 4, 1:677–687.

age, at which point it approximated adult levels. The pattern of lung volume increase may explain this phenomenon. In the first 5 years of life, a child's lung air space increases tenfold, mainly because of the multiplication of alveoli. The alveolar diameters remain almost constant, and, peripheral conductance increases only slightly. The remaining two- or threefold increase is primarily due to alveolar expansion; this is accompanied by a sharp increase in peripheral conductance. Hogg found that peripheral resistance in children up to 5 years is disproportionately large.

Other mechanical characteristics of the lung at birth are a relatively low functional residual capacity, which could mean instability of air spaces and terminal airways; large compliance in the tracheobronchial tree, which puts the infant at risk of dynamic airway compression if this is accompanied by low lung recoil resulting from low content of pulmonary elastin and collagen; a compliant chest wall, which may explain partially why children with acute airways obstruction rapidly deteriorate. In fact, the force exerted by the diaphragm cannot effect volume exchange if it is dissipated in distorting the chest wall (13).

The complex nature of lung development in children is reflected in many of the manifestations of pulmonary disease. The mechanical properties are constantly evolving in this period and, consequently, the manifestations of pulmonary disease differ accordingly. In the first years of life, pulmonary disease has an extremely rapid course and carries a high mortality risk, whereas in the older child a similar onset of lung disease would have less drastic effects. For example, for an infant bronchiolitis is often a fatal illness that rarely occurs in the older child or adolescent. Asthma attacks, although no less frequent in the older person, are considerably less severe than when experienced by the infant. Croup is considered a medical emergency that can strike in the first years of life, and is a mere sore throat in later years. Pulmonary involvement of cystic fibrosis can be similarly categorized. This is partly because the infant has small lungs, but other important factors are that the functional residual capacity of this small lung is relatively low and the peripheral airways resistance proportionately very high, and there is an increase in the tendency for the more compliant airways to close and the chest wall to distort. In varying degrees all these contribute to make the infant lung vulnerable.(13)

DEVELOPMENT OF THE BRONCHIAL TREE TO ADULTHOOD

The cartilaginous conducting airways are fully developed at the moment a child is born but most of the peripheral airways and alveoli are still being formed (1). A newborn baby's trachea and bronchi will have grown about three times larger by the time he reaches adulthood (1), and his lung volume will be 25 times greater (about 200 cm³ at birth and 5,000 cm³ for the average adult) (7). The growth of the conductive bronchial tree appears to be steady and strictly proportionate to the child's overall growth pattern, as Hislop and co-workers (14) found as a result of their measurements in children of different ages of the lengths and diameters of the branches on an axial pathway from hilium to periphery. Cudmore et al. (15) reported similar observations, and in addition found that the airway conductance per gram of lung tissue, independently of the stage of development of the child, remains constant throughout the pre-acinar region.

Hogg and co-workers (12) found a uniformity in the growth pattern of the bronchial tree with the exception of the peripheral airways in children <5 years of age, which were found to be disproportionately narrow. This suggested that the peripheral airways developed more slowly in the first years of life. A further differentiation in the stages of lung development was recorded by Zeltner and co-workers (16), who identified a first stage (from birth to about 18 months) in which the compartments involved in the transport of oxygen (air spaces and capillary volume) increased in volume at a disproportionate rate, followed by a second stage (up to adulthood) characterized by an overall even and steady pulmonary growth.

The airways in the fully grown lung are divided into cartilaginous bronchi, membranous bronchioles, and gas exchange ducts (17). The anatomic dead space of the lung comprises mainly the volume of the upper airways and the cartilaginous airways. The gas exchange ducts are the respiratory bronchioles and alveolar ducts, and do not contribute to anatomic dead space. The membranous bronchioles, which are noncartilaginous airways of ≤1 mm diameter, being surrounded by the structural connective lung tissue, enlarge as the lung volume expands (17). Although the bronchioles down to the first gas exchange airways ought to represent about 25% of the anatomic dead space, their contribution to anatomic dead space is minimal because of gas phase diffusion and mechanical mixing in the distal airways resulting from cardiac impulse. The flow of air between alveoli, which permits an equal level of air pressure throughout the lung and prevents localized overinflation, occurs either through the pores of Kohn, which are small holes in the alveolar walls, or through the accessory bronchoalveolar communications of Lambert, which are small channels connecting preterminal bronchioli to neighboring alveoli (18). The former are first seen in the lung at around 6 years of age, the latter at around 8 year of age (19,20).

FUNCTION AND STRUCTURE OF THE FULLY DEVELOPED AIRWAYS

Function

The function of the bronchial tree is to conduct air to the alveolar surface where gas transfer takes place between respired air and gas dissolved in the blood of pulmonary capillaries. The inspired air should be distributed evenly to the alveolar capillary bed with minimal resistance to flow. The conducting zone of the lung includes the trachea, bronchi, and nonalveolated bronchioles in which air cannot diffuse through the well developed wall.

The bronchial tree exhibits a complicated branching pattern expanded from the trachea to the membranous bronchioles. Cumming and associates (21) point out that usually, in nature, the distribution and collection of nutrients requires a branching system and that biologic branching systems show great similarity. For example,

deciduous trees must provide large surface areas of leaves exposed to sunlight so that photosynthesis can proceed with appropriate supplies transported from the ground. Similar circumstances exist in the lung in which a branching system of conducting airways is essential to transport the maximal amount of air with minimal resistance to the respiratory zone.

Data describing the branching structure of the lung derive from Horsfield and Cumming (22), Strahler (23), and Weibel (6). The basic branching pattern of the lung is dichotomous. In any such system the branching may be symmetric (two branches equal in all respects) or asymmetric (variation in the diameter or length of branches in a given generation, or in the number of divisions to the end branches, or a combination of these). The bronchial tree system is one of asymmetric dichotomy (Fig. 1) because there is a variation in both branch diameters and the number of divisions.

Horsfield and Cumming (22) and Strahler (23) proposed counting generations proximally from branches of arbitrary, but uniform, diameter (0.7 mm in their study), a method that reveals a close relationship between the diameter of a branch, the number of distal respiratory bronchioles it supplies, and its generation number. With such a system one can describe accurately the dimensions of the tracheobronchial tree, the number of branches and their length, diameter, and volume (Fig. 1).

Using resin casts of human lungs inflated at a volume of 5 L, Horsfield and Cumming (22) measured the length and the diameter at midpoint of every branch from an arbitrary diameter of 0.7 mm. The number of bronchial branches plotted against their order number showed a linear relation (Fig. 2A) that defined the number of branches of any order. The slope of the line defined the branching ratio. The branching ratio of the bronchial tree (number law or branching law) is obeyed precisely from orders 6 through 15 (order 1 is defined as an airway of 0.7 mm in diameter). Thus, every branch gives rise to 2.8 daughter branches. A similar law is applicable to the diameter of the branching system, decreasing from the largest to the smallest, in strict geometric progression, so that the diameter of any given order is predictable (Fig. 2B) and can be found by divid-

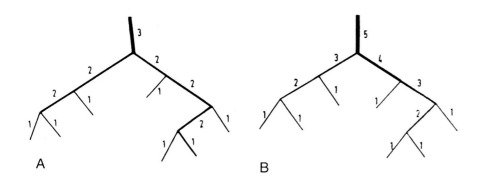

FIG. 1. Asymmetric dichotomy of the bronchial tree. Branching orders defined by the methods of Strahler **(A)** and of Horsfield and Cumming **(B)**. (From Cumming G, Horsfield K, Harding LK, Prowse K. Biological branching systems with special reference to the lung airways. *Bull Physiopathol Resp* 1971; 7:31–40.)

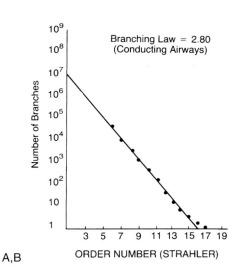
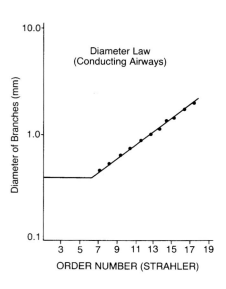

A,B

FIG. 2. Number of branches **(A)** and their diameter **(B)** plotted against their order number. B, Note that orders 1 through 7 undergo no diameter change—diminution in caliber ceases at order 7, chiefly respiratory bronchioles. (From Cumming G, Horsfield K, Harding LK, Prowse K. Biological branching systems with special reference to the lung airways. *Bull Physiopathol Resp* 1971; 7:31–40.)

ing the diameter of its parent by 1.4. However, the diameter law is not applicable throughout the whole airway system and no diminution in airway diameter is seen from order 7 to more distal branches. It could be postulated that there is a functional significance for this change in branching pattern, which occurs at the point at which the movement of gases changes from convective flow to diffusive mixing (21). The diameter of each new generation of airways decreases progressively from the trachea outward. However, the change in caliber is such that the cross-sectional area of the airway lumen steadily increases at successive levels throughout the bronchial system (Fig. 3) (6). This increase is especially marked distal to the origin of the bronchioles where branching is accompanied by practically no decrease in diameter of new generations. The increase in sectional area means that the velocity of air flow must be sharply reduced as the air stream moves peripherally through the airways. Accordingly, patterns of flow (laminar or turbulent) and resistance to air flow differs substantially in central and peripheral airways.

The length of bronchial tree segments also follows a fixed principle: the length of any branch can be found by dividing the parent's length by 1.49. The overall path length from carina to distal respiratory bronchioles ranges from 7.7 to 22.4 cm. The lengths of branches with diameters above 0.7 mm (7.5–21.6 cm) are considerably longer than the ones below 0.7 mm, which range from 0.2 to 0.9 cm. The computed volume of airways from carina to 0.7 mm bronchi (71 mL) added to the volume of the upper airways from the mouth to the carina (80 mL) is almost identical to the anatomic death space calculated by physiologic techniques.

The engineering of the airways also is complicated by variations in the size and angulation of each pair of branches: the branch serving the longer pathway is straight and has a larger cross-sectional area than the smaller, more angulated branch leading to the closer gas exchange units. The asymmetry in pathway lengths has a considerable effect on local resistances to air flow and to the transit times from mouth to gas exchange sites; this arrangement may serve, in part, to equalize the distribution of resistance among the various pathways (24).

During quiet breathing through the mouth, the flow regime in the bronchial tree is almost laminar (25). How-

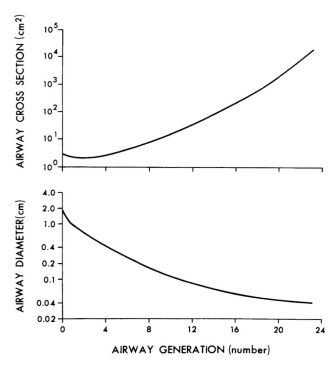

FIG. 3. Average diameter and cross-sectional area of airway segments plotted semilogarithmically against airway generation. The trachea is generation 0, the mainstem bronchi generation 1, etc. (From Weibel ER. *Morphometry of the human lung.* Heidelberg: Springer-Verlag, 1963.)

ever, when breathing through the nose during conditions demanding increased flow rates (like exercise) and through narrowed airways substantial turbulence may occur. As a consequence, a larger proportion of the work of breathing will be utilized to overcome the increased resistance.

The pressure necessary to produce laminar flow through a tube can be calculated by the Poiseuille equation (26) and is directly related to the length of the tube and the viscosity and flow rate of the gas and inversely related to the tube radius to the 4th power.

$$\Delta P = 8 \times Length \times Viscosity \times Flow/\pi \times Radius^4$$

Airway radius is the dominant variable in determining resistance. When the flow regime is laminar, the flow rate is linearly related to pressure. However, with nonlaminar flow regimes, a greater increase in pressure is required to produce a given increment in flow, and the relationship between pressure and flow becomes nonlinear. With nonlaminar regimes gas density also plays a role, resistance decreasing with gases of low density, so that the previous equation will have a new term:

$$\Delta P = (Length \times Viscosity \times \dot{V}) + (Density\, \dot{V}^2)/Radius^4$$

The importance of the added term (Density $\dot{V}^2$) depends on the type of flow regime.

Total airway resistance represents the contribution of the resistance of the various levels of the airway from larynx and large cartilaginous airways down to respiratory bronchioles added in series. The site of major airway resistance has been studied in dogs (27) and human lungs (28) using a retrograde catheter technique to partition the contribution of the large cartilaginous and the small airways less than 2 mm in diameter. These studies revealed that peripheral airway resistance was only a small proportion of the total resistance of the entire tracheobronchial tree. In addition, as lung volume was changed total resistance increased near total lung capacity (TLC) (28). The least resistance in the small airways was related to their large overall cross-sectional areas in the lung periphery. However, other studies, using different techniques to partition central and peripheral resistance, have questioned the original findings of Macklem (27) and Hogg (28) and have shown significantly higher peripheral resistance in normal lungs (29,30). Furthermore, in contrast to the results in previous studies, Van Brabandt et al. and Hoppin et al. found that a) when lung volume was decreased with the vagus nerves intact, the increase in peripheral resistance was at least as great as the increase in central resistance, b) the lung volume dependencies of central and peripheral resistances were not abolished by vagotomy, and c) neither resistance increased systematically at high lung volumes (29,30). These findings are consistent with the behavior of airways where they are examined by tantalum bronchography (31,32) and morphometry (33).

As demonstrated by the Poiseuille equation, airway resistance depends on the number, length, and cross-sectional area of the conducting airways. The number of airways in the normal lung is determined by the pattern of branching established by the 16th week of fetal life. The length of airways varies considerably from person to person depending on age and body size; airway length also varies in an individual depending on the phase of ventilation, lengthening during inspiration as lung volume increases and shortening during expiration. Because resistance to air flow in a given airway changes according to the fourth power of the radius of the airway, the cross-sectional area within the tracheobronchial tree is by far the most variable determinant of airway resistance. The cross-sectional area of any given airway must be determined by the balance between two opposing forces: those tending to distend the walls and those tending to contract the walls, primarily tension of airway smooth muscle and elastic elements. Airways change length and diameter during breathing and in general both dimensions change in proportion to the lung volume; this outward friction is provided either from the attached lung parenchyma, in the case of terminal bronchioles, or from the indirect effects of pleural pressure in the case of intrapulmonary conducting airways. Changes in lung volume above functional residual capacity (FRC) have little effect on airway resistance but between FRC and residual volume (RV) airway resistance increased rapidly and approached infinity at RV. Although it is useful to relate measurements of airway resistance to those of lung volume, the determinant of the relationship between lung volume and airway resistance is the elastic recoil at the given lung volume (34). Changes in the geometry of normal bronchi depend not only on the transmural pressure across their walls, but also on the distensibility of the elements composing the walls. These phenomena are reflected in the diameter-pressure and height-pressure relationships of the airways. The results of these studies fall into two general categories: one in which most of the changes occur at relatively low distending pressures (6–10 cm H_2O) (35) and one in which both length and diameter change continuously over the full range of pressures (31). These discrepant results can be explained by differences in bronchial smooth muscle tone at the time the experiments were conducted (32). When bronchomotor tone is absent, the airways become relatively floppy and distend almost fully at low pressures. By contrast, when tone is present the airways distend more slowly and continuously during inflation. Smooth muscle tone also accounts for the presence and magnitude of hysteresis in the dimensions of the airways as the lungs are inflated. There is little or no hysteresis when bronchomotor tone is absent, and hysteresis progressively develops as tone is augmented (32).

It is of interest that, under apparently normal conditions of airway tone, the percentage change in diameter along the length of intrapulmonary airways is so consistent because the distending pressure differs from one segment to another. The small bronchioles are directly tethered by the lung parenchyma and are thus stretched by the elastic recoil of the lung (33,36), whereas the airways surrounded by a connective tissue sheath are exposed to a pressure that is about the same as pleural pressure at FRC but becomes increasingly more negative during lung inflation (37). Thus, the distensibility of the various segments must differ to offset the differences in distending pressures; this means that bronchi should be stiffer than bronchioles, a prediction for which there is experimental support (38). Airway caliber and, therefore, resistance also is influenced by complex neurohumoral controls. Both intra- and extrathoracic airways respond to changes in lung volumes, as described before, but a portion of the lung volume effect is reflexly mediated and is attenuated by prior administration of atropine (39). In addition, there are active stimuli to both bronchodilation and bronchoconstriction. Airway caliber is under reflex control through afferent lung receptors and efferent autonomic cholinergic, adrenergic, and "purinergic" nerves (see below). Local changes in gas tension—either hypoxia (40) or hypercapnia (41)—can narrow airways. The resultant decrease in ventilation to areas of low PO_2 or PCO_2 represents a compensatory mechanism that serves to promote a match between ventilation and perfusion; as such, it is analogous to, although less important than, hypoxia vasoconstriction.

In patients with lung disease, increased airway resistance is the most common cause of increased work of breathing. The processes that narrow airways and increase resistance may be either acute and reversible or chronic and irreversible. They include changes in the characteristics of the surface material on the airway lumens, reflex and hormonally mediated smooth muscle constriction, degeneration of the supporting structure of both large and small airways, destruction of alveolar attachments, and peripheral airway obstruction by mucous plugging, inflammation, and scarring.

Morphology

The morphology of the trachea bronchi and nonalveolated airways consists of a surface epithelium and subepithelial tissue containing a loose network of fibers, a rich capillary plexus muscle, glands, and unmyelinated nerves. The proportion and type of these elements vary at different levels of the bronchial tree. The morphology of the airways has been reviewed extensively by Fraser (42).

Epithelium

The bulk of the epithelial layer consists of ciliated and secretory cells, either goblet or clara. The ciliated cell is the most abundant cell in normal epithelium (43). Basal, intermediate, lymphoreticular, and neuroendocrine cells are also found in lesser numbers. The epithelium is constantly being renewed, with turnover rates that vary between 7 and 131 days (44). Even more, the response to epithelial injury by reconstitution of the epithelial layer is fast; recovery by 7 days has been shown in animals after experimental injury (45).

Ciliated Cells

Ciliated cells extend from the luminal surface of the airway to the basement membrane. The cells attach firmly to the basement membrane and to one another at the luminal surface by tight junctions. These tight junctions form a physical barrier to most substances, making the epithelial layer fairly impermeable and transport across the epithelium takes place by means of cytoplasmic vesicles (46,47). Transepithelial movement of fluid and electrolytes (41,48) probably is related to the abundant microvilli present in the basal aspects of the epithelium (43,48). Each ciliated cell has approximately 200 cilia on the lumen surface (44,49), measuring 6 μm in the proximal airways and decreasing to 3.6 μm in the bronchioles (50). Numerous short microvilli also can be seen in the cell surface, and they might be involved in the secretion of part of the periciliary mucous layer (51,52). The ciliated cells could play a role in the modulation of local airway inflammation by the secretion of cytokines and granulocyte/macrophage colony stimulating factor (53).

Goblet Cells

Goblet cells represent about 20% to 30% of the epithelial cells in the more proximal airways (43,54) and only occasional goblet cells are seen in the bronchioles (55,56). With chronic airway irritation, they may increase substantially in number in both proximal and distal airways (57,58).

Basal Cells

It is believed widely that basal cells are reserve cells from which the epithelium is normally repopulated (59, 60). They are more abundant in the proximal airways and they gradually diminish in number toward the periphery (61,62). Intermediate cells form a poorly defined layer above the basal cells from which they are derived. These cells show evidence of ciliogenesis and mucous granule accumulation.

Clara Cells

Clara cells, or nonciliated bronchiolar secretory cells, are conspicuous and abundant in bronchioles, comprising most of the epithelium along with the ciliated cells (63–65). It is generally believed that clara cells have a secretory function. They are furnished with a prominent Golgi apparatus, abundant endoplasmic reticulum and mitochondria, and numerous ovoid membrane bound bodies, presumably secretory granules (66–68). Clara cells probably synthesize lipids (65), proteins (65,69), and a surfactant-related glycoprotein (66,70). The most tenable explanation for a secretory role of clara cells is that they contribute their secretions to the extracellular lining of the bronchioles (51,71–73), and this film may have a surface tension–lowering function. Clara cells have other important functions, i.e., they have been shown to contain a low molecular weight protease inhibitor (74) of potential importance for the integrity of the bronchiolar epithelium; clara cells are known to contain enzymes that presumably serve to detoxify inhaled toxic substances (64,65); these cells also have an important progenitor function and after epithelial injury they may differentiate into ciliated cells and alveolar epithelium (75,76).

K cells

K cells, also known as neuroendocrine, amine-containing, or small granule cells, have been described recently in the bronchial epithelium (77–79). They are believed to be similar to the Kultschitsky cell of the gastrointestinal tract (hence K cells) and have been included in the APUD series of cells (amine precursor uptake and decarboxylase system) (80). They are abundant in the epithelium of newborns but much less numerous in adult lungs (81). They are found at all levels of the bronchial tree, although they are more frequent in peripheral than in central airways (44), and they are also found in bronchial glands. Extensive innervation to these cells has been shown (82) by some and little or none by others (44,83). Ultrastructurally, the cytoplasm contains a prominent Golgi apparatus, abundant smooth endoplasmic reticulum, prominent numbers of microtubules and microfilaments, some of them neurofilaments (84), and, most important, neurosecretory granules (44,48,79). As other APUD cells, the epithelial K cells are believed to control other cellular functions by means of a variety of amine-related polypeptide hormones. Although the precise function of these cells in the airways is unknown, it has been suggested they are responsible, at least in part, for local control of airway and vascular function (77). Because it has been shown that these cells increase in number in hypoxic conditions, it is believed that K cells might play a role in the hypoxic responses of the pulmonary vasculature (85,86). It has been proposed that in both the developing and regenerating epithelium, K cells might influence the migration and growth of intraepithelial nerve fibers (87).

Clumps of 10 to 30 K cells have been described in the bronchial, bronchiolar, and even alveolar epithelium of human infants (88) and adults (89) and are recognized as neuroepithelial bodies. The cells in these bodies reach the luminal surface of the airways, and their bases rest on the basement membrane in intimate contact with small nerve fibers (79,90). They have neurosecretory granules containing serotonin and other peptides (91,92). The precise function of the neuroepithelial bodies is not clear (44), and it has been suggested that they function as a mediator of pulmonary and vascular changes with hypoxia (77, 79,91,92).

Submucosa and Lamina Propria

The subepithelial tissue comprises a lamina propria, found between the basement membrane and the muscle and a submucosa. The lamina propria is more prominent in the proximal bronchi than in the distal airways and it consists principally of a capillary network, reticulin fibers, and fairly prominent elastic tissue oriented mainly in a longitudinal direction. The elastic tissue is thick, forming well defined bundles in cartilaginous airways, and extends to the peripheral airways where it can be seen over the whole circumferences of the wall (62). The submucosa contains cartilage, muscle, and other supportive connective tissue elements, the tracheobronchial glands, and various cells related to airway function an defense mechanisms.

The airway cartilage is well formed in horseshoe-shape rings in the trachea and becomes more scarce and irregular in shape in the smaller airways, disappearing in airways 1 to 2 mm in diameter (93). The bronchial cartilages are tethered together by fibroelastic fibers arranged in a longitudinal and oblique direction. These fibers, especially in the smaller airways, join with the elastic tissue of the lamina propria (94–96) and probably help transmit the tensions arising in the lung parenchyma during respiration to the more rigid cartilaginous tissue (95–97).

The smooth muscle in the trachea and large bronchi muscle bridges the posterior opening of the U-shaped cartilages. Muscle can also be found in the anterior portion (97) and in longitudinally oriented muscle fibers and present dorsal to the transverse muscle layer (98). Medium and small bronchi have a proper muscle layer but they do not circumscribe the airway with a band of uniform thickness; rather, the muscles have a helical orientation with fibers spiralling in both directions and criss-crossing in the walls (99). Because of the different arrangement of the fibers, the effect of muscle contraction depends on the location and density of fibers. In the large airways, muscle contraction will oppose the tips of the cartilage. In medium and small bronchi contraction reduces both the caliber and length of the bronchus. Muscle contraction, therefore, leads to greater rigidity in all airways. Airway muscle can undergo hyperplasia in diseases such as asthma and chronic obstructive pulmonary disease (COPD). The development of the hyperplasia is probably related to physical strain (100) and mediated by endothelin (101) and/or other growth factors.

Bronchial glands are one of the characteristic features of the submucosal layer beneath the lamina propria in the trachea and bronchi. Bronchial glands are especially numerous in medium-sized bronchi, less prevalent in smaller bronchi, and absent in bronchioles (102). The glands are connected to the epithelial surface by a ciliated duct. Multiple tubules lined by either mucous or serous cells open into collecting ducts. The ratio of serous to mucous cells is about 0.5 (103). Other constituents of the glands are clear cells, probably lymphocytes, mast cells, occasional Kultschitsky cells, and myoepithelial cells. Myoepithelial cells are located between the basement membranes and epithelial cells and may aid the movement of secretions along the tubules by contracting and squeezing the secretory cells (104). The glands are innervated by unmyelinated nerve fibers that, on the basis of their ultrastructural characteristics, are believed to be parasympathetic efferent nerves (104).

There are morphologic and histochemical differences between mucous and serous cells. The material that reaches the airway lumen, therefore, represents a mixture of the products of both cell types and any chemical reactions that result from the combination. Sulfated mucin and sialo mucin have been shown within the mucous-secreting portions of the gland (105,106); there is also evidence that the mucous secretions have antiprotease properties (107). The nature of the serous cell secretions has not been well established, although they probably secrete a low viscosity substance that might help in flushing out the secretions of the mucous cells (106). The secretions of the serous cells might participate in the defense of the local milieu by the antibacterial properties of lysozyme (108), lactoferrin (109), low molecular weight protease inhibitor (108), and dineric immunoglobulin A (IgA) (110) known to be secreted by these cells.

The factors that control the basal rate of secretions are not well understood. Increased rates of mucous gland secretion can be provoked by vagally mediated reflexes (111,112) and by both beta- and alpha-adrenergic–stimulating influences (112–114). Upon reaching the mucosa, irritants initiate a reflex via the parasympathetic nervous system that causes cough and mucous secretion, suggesting that these two defense mechanisms are linked (113). Production of mucus also is stimulated by inflammatory mediators and histamine, prostaglandins, LTD4, and substance P (113,115–117) have been shown to stimulate effectively the production of mucus.

Cells concerned with airway defense are found scattered in the airway walls. Lymphocytes can be found in the epithelium and subepithelial tissues either singly or in clusters. These clusters, or bronchus-associated lymphoid tissue (118), are found in most lungs by age 5 years (119) and have features similar to normal lymph node tissue

(120). In the peripheral airways, these clusters are less well organized and are called lymphoid aggregates (121). It has been suggested that these lymphoid aggregates are possibly involved in antigen processing and local IgA production (122). Plasma cells are mainly found in the large bronchi, in relation to mucous glands and close to the basement membrane. These are primarily of the IgA type (123). Mast cells are seen throughout the lamina propria and submucosa (124), and in animals have been found to be more numerous in peripheral airways (125). Their function in normal lungs is uncertain, but is possibly related to their two major proteinases, tryptase and chymase.

Airway Innervation

The earlier concepts of innervation of human airways have been undergoing change because of expanded research and have recently been reviewed extensively (126). Histochemical and electron microscopic studies have revealed the presence of acetylcholinesterase-positive nerve fibers and "cholinergic" nerve profiles in the smooth muscle and glands from the lobar bronchi to bronchioles (127–129). Recently, the concept of nerves in human airways has been widened to introduce adrenergic nerves as well that can be found in smooth muscle (sparse) and glands from lobar bronchi to bronchioles (128–130).

Bronchial smooth muscle tone is known to be regulated by acetylcholine via muscarinic receptors (131) and by catecholamines via α- and β-adrenergic receptors (131,132). *In vitro* studies with human bronchial smooth muscle strips have also revealed a third neural system, a nonadrenergic noncholinergic inhibitory regulatory mechanism (131). Vasoactive intestinal peptide (VIP) has been suggested as a possible relaxant of bronchial smooth muscle tone (133), and in this respect, may serve as a neurotransmitter for the nonadrenergic inhibitory system in the human respiratory tract (134). Nerve fibers containing VIP immunoreactivity are found in the smooth muscle, glands, vessels, and microganglia (135). VIP-like immunoreactivity is localized in large granules or vesicles of nerve profiles (136).

The human bronchial epithelium receives terminal fibers from the peribronchial plexus (137–139). In the epithelium axon profiles seem to have two predominant locations: either close to the airway lumen or at the base of the epithelium close to the basement membrane. Nerves near the lumen are found mostly in the larger airways and relatively few are observed in the smaller airways (140). Two populations of axon profiles can be found in the epithelium. The "mitochondrial type"—conforming to the classic morphologic criteria of afferent axonal fibers—are found only at the base of the epithelium (141). The "vesicle type" are found near the airway lumen in central airways and at the base of the epithelium at all airway levels. These axons could be afferent and also efferent to either ciliated or gland cells in the epithelium (141).

Sensory receptors of the airways can be described as those primarily involved in the physiologic control of breathing patterns (slowly adapting pulmonary stretch receptors) and those primarily concerned with changes in pathologic conditions (rapidly adapting irritant and C-fiber receptors) (142).

Neurepithelial bodies also may be receptors with afferent nerves (89,143) responding to changes in the partial pressure of oxygen (144). The concentration and structure of the intraepithelial nerves and APUD cells have been established (140). These cells are in close association with basal intraepithelial nerves.

It is evident that both the quality and quantity of innervation vary so much between human and animal species that results from animal experiments should be interpreted with caution. Therefore, this summary of airways innervation has been based on what is known of the neural elements of human airways.

ON THE MAINTENANCE OF NORMAL AIRWAY STRUCTURE AND FUNCTION

Two structures that envelop the airway, epithelium and the lung parenchyma, actively participate in defending the airway patency and minimize resistance to flow. Beyond that, the epithelium is probably the critical factor preserving the normal airway structure, hence the airway function. How this is accomplished is reviewed briefly here.

Epithelium

The epithelial layer plays an extremely important role in the defense mechanism of the airways, and it does so in various ways (145). Epithelial cells secrete aqueous substances and mucus, and each one is tightly joined to its neighbor, providing an effective barrier for the airway lumen. The ciliated cells, which are the most numerous of the exposed cells in the airway, propel the mucus of the airway lumen backward and outward, helping to expel unwanted debris. The epithelium can repair itself after injury and can become a regulator of other components in the airways such as smooth muscle, vessels, and inflammatory cells. Furthermore, the clara cells contribute to the defenses of the airway by the secretion of a low molecular weight protease inhibitor (79) that may be important in maintaining the integrity of the bronchiolar epithelium. In addition, the presence of cytochrome the P450 mono-oxygenase system suggests that these cells might have a detoxification function (68,69).

Airways in the lung seem to remain open at a transpulmonary pressure of 0. If this should be so, it is somewhat surprising when the small radii of curvature of the bronchioles is considered. Thus, some factor, or factors, appear to be present that stabilize these airways and protect them against closure. According to Macklem et al. surfactant lines and stabilizes bronchioles, protecting them against excessive radius changes with changes in lung volume (146). This surface material is most likely produced by the clara cells, where a surfactant-related glycoprotein within their cytoplasm has been shown (71,76).

Airway permeability is controlled tightly by the epithelium, preserving a relative dryness of the airway lumen that allows the surface lining to protect them from closure. If permeability is altered, plasma exudate immediately fills the interstices between epithelium projections; this exudate could alter the surface tension of the airway lining fluid, which could compromise the airway lumen. Plasma proteins have been shown to inhibit lung-surfactant function by significantly increasing surface tension (147). This has been suggested as a physical mechanism that could increase airway resistance and contribute to airway hyperresponsiveness (147).

To function effectively, the epithelium of the lung needs to be intact. If epithelial cells are damaged, the afferent nerve endings and receptors to irritants normally protected are susceptible to substances that may cause bronchoconstriction and inflammation. Studies on airway tissue show that airway epithelial cells can affect smooth muscle tone (148). Airway smooth muscle is more responsive to various mediators, such as histamine, acetylcholine (148), platelet-activating factor (149), and antigen (150) when the epithelial layer is removed. The bronchodilatatory effects of beta-agonists (151), calcium antagonists (152), and prostaglandins (152) are possibly also modulated by the epithelium, as is the responsiveness of bronchial smooth muscle through the release of a relaxant factor for airway smooth muscle (153).

Airway epithelium can also influence airway inflammation in several ways. It can release chemotactic products for neutrophils (154), lymphocytes (155), and monocytes (156). It also may be capable of interacting with lymphocytes for presenting antigens, as the airway epithelial cells can express major histocompatibility complex class I and class II antigens (157). Another system implicated in airway inflammatory responses, which could be triggered by the alteration of epithelium, is the sensory nerves; this neurogenic inflammation is the result of the release of tachykinins (substance P, neurokinin A, and neurokinin B) by nerve fibers present in the epithelium, smooth muscle, and blood vessels. Mucous secretion, an increase in airway microvascular permeability, exudation of plasma into the airway lumen, (158–161), contraction of smooth muscle *in vitro* (162–164), interaction with mast cells (165,166), chemotaxis and adhesion of neutrophils in the bronchial circulation (167,168), activation of monocytes to release inflammatory cytokines, and degranulation of eosinophils, which could cause further damage to the epithelium, are all consequences of the stimulation of these nerves, which, taken as a whole, are known as neurogenic inflammation. The enzyme-neutral endopeptidase limits the inflammatory effects of tachykinins by degrading them and therefore inactivating them (169). When neutral endopeptidase is prevented from acting, either by the stripping of the epithelial layer or by the specific inhibitors, smooth muscle responses to bronchoconstrictive substances increase (170). When the airway epithelium is lost or altered, the effects of tachykinins are more pronounced, both with respect to the airway smooth muscle and airway mucosa.

Airway-parenchyma Interdependence

In healthy airways the peripheral airway smooth muscle is prevented from shortening by an elastic afterload from the forces of lung elastic recoil (171). This elastic load increases with the lung volume. The theory of interdependence between airway and parenchyma states that the pressure on the external surface of intrapulmonary airways is equal to the sum of the forces applied to the outer surface of the airway by the attached alveolar walls, expressed as a fraction of the external surface area of the airway. In situations of airway inflammation, the airway walls become thicker, the attached alveolar walls shorter, there is a decrease in the forces acting on the airway wall, and there is an increase in the outer airway surface area, all resulting in a decrease in the pressure applied to the airway. Macklem (172) has postulated that the thickening of the airway wall external to the smooth muscle can influence the relationship between smooth muscle contraction and airway narrowing by uncoupling lung elastic recoil forces from the airway smooth muscle, and allowing it to shorten excessively. Another possible consequence of the airway inflammatory process is the destruction of the alveolar supports around the airways (alveolar attachments), which may increase airway narrowing even further because of loss of radial traction forces (36,173).

REFERENCES

1. Burri PH. Development and growth of the human lung. In: Fishman AP, Fisher AB, eds. *Handbook of physiology, the respiratory system, section 3 respiration.* Bethesda: American Physiological Society, 1985, 1;1–46.
2. Burri PH. Postnatal development and growth. In: Crystal RG, West JB, eds. *The lung: scientific foundations.* New York: Raven Press, 1991; Section 4, 1:677–687.
3. Thurlbeck WM. Pre- and postnatal organ development. In: Chernick V, Mellins RN, eds. *Basic mechanisms of paediatric respiratory disease: cellular and integrative.* Philadelphia: Decker Inc, 1991;23–25.
4. Reid L. The embryology of the lung. In: de Renck AVS, Porter S, eds. *Ciba foundation: symposium on development of the lung.* London: Churchill, 1967;109–430.
5. Plopper CG, Thurlbeck WM. Growth, ageing and adaptation. In: Murray JF, Nadel JA, eds. *Textbook of respiratory medicine.* Philadelphia: WB Saunders, 1994;36–49.

6. Weibel ER. *Morphometry of the human lung.* Heidelberg: Springer-Verlag, 1963.
7. Dunnil MS. Postnatal growth of the lung. *Thorax* 1962; 17:329–333.
8. Thurlbeck WM. Postnatal human lung growth. *Thorax* 1982; 37:564–571.
9. Langston C, Kida K, Reed M, Thurlbeck WM. Human lung growth in late gestation and in the neonate. *Am Rev Respir Dis* 1984; 129:607–613.
10. Zeltner TB, Cadniff JH, Gehr P, Pfenninger J, Burri PH. The post-natal development and growth of the human lung. I Morphometry. *Respir Physiol* 1987; 67:247–267.
11. Mortale JP. Physiology of postnatal growth. In: Crystal RG, West JB, eds. *The lung: scientific foundations.* New York: Raven Press, 1991, Section 6, 2:1735–1741.
12. Hogg J, Williams J, Richardson J, Macklem P, Thurlbeck W. Age as a factor in the distribution of lower-airway conductance in the pathologic anatomy of obstructive lung disease. *N Engl J Med* 1970; 282: 1283–1287.
13. Bryan AC, Mansell AL, Levison H. Development of the mechanical properties of the respiratory system. In: Hodson WA, ed. *Development of the lung. Lung biology in health and disease series.* New York: Marcel Dekker, 1977;445–468.
14. Hislop A, Muir DCF, Jacobsen M, Simon G, Reid L. Postnatal growth and function of the pre-acinar airways. *Thorax* 1972; 27:265–274.
15. Cudmore RE, Emery JL, Mithal A. Postnatal growth of bronchi and bronchioles. *Arch Dis Child* 1962; 37:481–484.
16. Zeltner TB, Caduff JH, Gehr P, Pfenninger J, Burri PH. The postnatal development and growth of the human lung. I Morphometry. *Respir Physiol* 1987; 67:247–267.
17. Staub NC, Albertine KH. Anatomy of the lung. In: Murray JF, Nadel JA, eds. *Textbook of respiratory medicine.* Philadelphia: WB Saunders, 1994;3–35.
18. Meyrick B, Reid LM. Ultrastructure of alveolar lining and its development. In: Hosdon WA, ed. *Development of the lung. Lung biology in health and disease series.* New York: Marcel Dekker, 1977;135–214.
19. Boyden EA. Notes on the development of the lung in infancy and early childhood. *Am J Anat* 1967; 121:749–762.
20. Boyden EA. Development of the human lung. In: Kelley VC, ed. *Brenneman's practice of pediatrics, vol 4.* Hagerstown: Harper and Row, 1972.
21. Cumming G, Horsfield K, Harding LK, Prowse K. Biological branching systems with special reference to the lung airways. *Bull Physiopathol Resp* 1971; 7:31–40.
22. Horsfield K, Cumming G. Morphology of the bronchial tree in man. *J Appl Physiol* 1968; 24:373–383.
23. Strahler AN. Equilibrium theory of erosional slopes approached by frequency distribution analysis. *Am J Sci* 1950; 248:673.
24. Horsfield K, Cumming G. Functional consequences of airway morphology. *J Appl Physiol* 1968; 24:384–390.
25. Lisboa C, Ross WRD, Jardim J, Macklem PT. Pulmonary pressure–flow curves measured by a data-averaging circuit. *J Appl Physiol* 1979; 47:621–627.
26. Landau LD, Lifshitz EM. Viscous fluids. In: *Fluid mechanics,* 2nd ed. New York: Pergamon Press, 1987;44–94.
27. Macklem PT, Mead J. Resistance of central and peripheral airways measured by a retrograde catheter. *J Appl Physiol* 1967; 22:395–401.
28. Hogg JC, Macklem PT, Thurlbeck WM. Site and nature of airway obstruction in chronic obstructive lung disease. *N Engl J Med* 1968; 273:1355–1360.
29. Van Brabandt H, Cauberghs M, Verbeken E, Moerman P, Lauweryns JM, de Woestijne KP. Partitioning of pulmonary impedance in excised human and canine lungs. *J Appl Physiol* 1983; 55:1733–1742.
30. Hoppin FG Jr, Green M, Morgan MS. Relationship of central and peripheral airway resistance to lung volume in dogs. *J Appl Physiol* 1978; 44:728–737.
31. Hughes JMB, Hoppin FG Jr, Mead J. Effect of lung inflation on bronchial length and diameter in excised lungs. *J Appl Physiol* 1972; 32: 25–35.
32. Hahn HL, Graf PD, Nadel JA. Effect of vagal tone on airway diameters and on lung volume in anesthetized dogs. *J Appl Physiol* 1976; 41:581–589.
33. Klingele TG, Staub NC. Terminal bronchiole diameter changes with volume in isolated air-filled lobes of cat lung. *J Appl Physiol* 1971; 30:224–227.

34. Stubbs SE, Hyatt RE. Effect of increased lung recoil pressure on maximal expiratory flow in normal subjects. *J Appl Physiol* 1972; 32: 325–331.
35. Hyatt RE, Flath RE. Influence of lung parenchyma on pressure-diameter behavior of dog bronchi. *J Appl Physiol* 1966; 21:1448–1452.
36. Saetta M, Ghezzo H, Kim WD, King M, Angus GE, Wang NS, Cosio MG. Loss of alveolar attachments in smokers: a morphometric correlate of lung function impairment. *Am Rev Respir Dis* 1985; 132:894–900.
37. Inoue H, Inoue C, Hildebrandt J. Vascular and airway pressures, and interstitial edema, affect peribronchial fluid pressure. *J Appl Physiol* 1980; 48:177–185.
38. Wilson AG, Massarella GR, Pride NB. Elastic properties of airways in human lungs post-mortem. *Am Rev Respir Dis* 1974; 110:716–729.
39. Inners CR, Terry PB, Traystman RJ, Menkes HA. Effects of lung volume on collateral and airways resistance in man. *J Appl Physiol* 1979; 46:67–73.
40. Saunders NA, Betts MF, Pengelly LD, Rebuck AS. Changes in lung mechanics induced by acute isocapnic hypoxia. *J Appl Physiol* 1977; 42:413–419.
41. Widdicombe JH, Gashi AA, Basbaum CB, Nathanson IT. Structural changes associated with fluid absorption by dog tracheal epithelium. *Exp Lung Res* 1986; 10:57–69.
42. Fraser RS. The normal chest. In: Fraser RG, Paré JAP, Paré PD, Genereux GP. *Diagnosis of diseases of the chest,* 3rd ed. Philadelphia: WB Saunders, 1988;5–16.
43. Rhodin JAG. The ciliated cell. Ultrastructure and function of the human tracheal mucosa. *Am Rev Respir Dis* 1966; 93:1–15.
44. Breeze RG, Wheeldon EB. The cells of the pulmonary airways. State of the art. *Am Rev Respir Dis* 1977; 116:705–777.
45. Wynne JW, Ramphal R, Hood CL. Tracheal mucosal damage after aspiration. A scanning electron microscope study. *Am Rev Respir Dis* 1981; 124:728–732.
46. Bhalla DK, Crocker TT. Tracheal permeability in rats exposed to ozone. An electron microscopic and autoradiographic analysis of the transport pathway. *Am Rev Respir Dis* 1986; 134:572–579.
47. Richardson J, Bouchard T, Ferguson CC. Uptake and transport of exogenous proteins by respiratory epithelium. *Lab Invest* 1976; 35:307–314.
48. Nathanson I, Nadel JA. Movement of electrolytes and fluid across airways. *Lung* 1984; 162:125–137.
49. Gail DB, Lenfant CJM. State of the art. Cells of the lung: biology and clinical implications. *Am Rev Respir Dis* 1983; 127:366–387.
50. Serafini SM, Michaelson ED. Length and distribution of cilia in human and canine airways. *Bull Eur Physiopathol Resp* 1977; 13: 551–559.
51. Allison AC. Respiratory tract mucus. In: *Ciba foundation symposium 54 (new series).* New York: Excerpta Medica, Elsevier/North–Holland, 1978.
52. Kilburn KH. A hypothesis for pulmonary clearance and its implications. *Am Rev Respir Dis* 1968; 98:449–463.
53. Smith SM, Lee DKP, Lacy J, Coleman DL. Rat tracheal epithelial cells produce granulocyte/macrophage colony-stimulating factor. *Am J Respir Cell; Mol Biol* 1990; 2:59–68.
54. McDowell EM, Barrett LA, Glavin F, Harris CC, Trump BF. The respiratory epithelium. I. Human bronchus. *J Natl Cancer Inst* 1978; 61: 539–549.
55. Ebert RV, Terracio MJ. The bronchiolar epithelium in cigarette smokers. Observations with the scanning electron microscope. *Am Rev Respir Dis* 1975; 111:4–11.
56. Bucher U, Reid L. Development of the mucus–secreting elements in human lung. *Thorax* 1961; 16:207–218.
57. Tos M. Mucous elements in the airways. *Acta Otolaryngol* 1976; 82: 249–251.
58. Lumsden AB, McLean A, Lamb D. Goblet and Clara cells of human distal airways: Evidence for smoking–induced changes in their numbers. *Thorax* 1984; 39:844–849.
59. Lane BP, Gordon R. Regeneration of rat tracheal epithelium after mechanical injury: I. The relationship between mitotic activity and cellular differentiation. *Proc Soc Exp Biol Med* 1974; 145: 1139–1144.
60. Blenkinsopp WK. Proliferation of respiratory tract epithelium in the rat. *Exp Cell Res* 1967; 46:144–154.
61. Jeffery PK, Reid L. New observations of rat airway epithelium: a quantitative and electron microscopic study. *J Anat* 1975; 120:295–320.
62. Monkhouse WS, Whimster WF. An account of the longitudinal mucosal corrugations of the human tracheo–bronchial tree, with observations on those of some animals. *J Anat* 1976; 122:681–695.
63. Kölliker A. Zur Kentniss des Baues der Lunge des Menschen. *Verh Physik Med Ges Wurzburg* 1981; 16:1.
64. Plopper CG. Comparative morphologic features of bronchiolar epithelial cells. The Clara cell. *Am Rev Respir Dis* 1983; 128:S37–S41.
65. Widdicombe JG, Pack RJ. The Clara cell. *Eur J Respir Dis* 1982; 363: 202–220.
66. Cutz E, Conen PE. Ultrastructure and cytochemistry of Clara cells. *Am J Pathol* 1971; 62:127–141.
67. Azzopardi A, Thurlbeck WM. The histochemistry of the nonciliated bronchiolar epithelial cell. *Am Rev Respir Dis* 1969; 99:516–525.
68. Niden AH. Bronchiolar and large alveolar cell in pulmonary phospholipid metabolism. *Science* 1967; 158:1323–1324.
69. Ebert RV, Kronenberg RS, Terracio MJ. Study of the surface secretion of the bronchiole using radioautography, *Am Rev Respir Dis* 1976; 114:567–573.
70. Thurlbeck A, Horsfield K. Branching angles in the bronchial tree related to order of branching. *Resp Physiol* 1980; 41:173–181.
71. Yoneda K. Pilocarpine stimulation of the bronchiolar Clara cell secretion. *Lab Invest* 1977; 37:447–452.
72. Gil J, Weibel ER. Extracellular lining of bronchioles after perfusion–fixation of rat lungs for electron microscopy. *Anat Rec* 1971; 169:185–199.
73. Mahvi D, Bank H, Harley R. Morphology of naphthalene-induced bronchiolar lesion. *Am J Pathol* 1977; 86:558–572.
74. Mooren HWD, Kramps JA, Franken C, Meijer CJ, Dijkman JA. Localisation of low-molecular-weight bronchial protease inhibitor in the peripheral human lung. *Thorax* 1983; 38:180–183.
75. Korhonen LK, Holopainen E, Paavolainen M. Some histochemical characteristics of tracheobronchial tree and pulmonary neoplasms. *Acta Histochem* 1969; 32:57–73.
76. Castleman WL, Dungworth DL, Schwartz LW, Tyler WS. Acute respiratory bronchiolitis. An ultrastructural and autoradiographic study of epithelial cell injury and renewal in rhesus monkeys exposed to ozone. *Am J Pathol* 1980; 98:811–840.
77. Pack RJ, Widdicombe JG. Amine-containing cells of the lung. *Eur J Respir Dis* 1984; 65:559–578.
78. Becker KL, Gazdar AF, eds. *The endocrine lung in health and disease.* Philadelphia: WB Saunders, 1984.
79. Cutz E. Neuroendocrine cells of the lung. An overview of morphologic characteristics and development. *Exp Lung Res* 1982; 3:185–208.
80. Pearse AGE, Takor TT. Embryology of the diffuse neuroendocrine system and its relationship to the common peptides. *Fed Proc* 1979; 38:2288–2294.
81. Gosney JR, Sissons MCJ, O'Malley JA. Quantitative study of endocrine cells immunoreactive for calcitonin in the normal adult human lung. *Thorax* 1985; 40:866–869.
82. Jeffery P, Reid L. Intra-epithelial nerves in normal rat airways: a quantitative electron microscope study. *J Anat* 1973; 114:35–45.
83. Gould VE. The endocrine lung. (Editorial). *Lab Invest* 1983; 48:507–509.
84. Torikata C, Mukai M, Kawakita H, Kageyama K. Neurofilaments of Kultschitsky cells in human lung. *Acta Pathol Jap* 1986; 36:93–104.
85. Keith IM, Will JA. Hypoxia and the neonatal rabbit lung: neuroendocrine cell numbers, 5-HT fluorescence intensity, and the relationship to arterial thickness. *Thorax* 1981; 36:767–773.
86. Taylor W. Pulmonary argyrophil cells at high altitude. *J Pathol* 1977; 122:137–144.
87. Stahlman MT, Gray ME. Ontogeny of neuroendocrine cells in human fetal lung. I. An electron microscopic study. *Lab Invest* 1984; 51:449–463.
88. Lauweryns JM, Peuskens JC. Neuro-epithelial bodies (neuroreceptor or secretory organs?) in human infant bronchial and bronchiolar epithelium. *Anat Rec* 1972; 172:471–481.
89. Lauweryns JM, Goddeeris P. Neuroepithelial bodies in the human child and adult lung. *Am Rev Respir Dis* 1975; 111:469–476.
90. Lauweryns JM, Cokelaere MN, Theunynck P. Neuro-epithelial bodies in the respiratory mucosa of various mammals. A light optical histochemical and ultrastructural investigation. *Z Zellforsch* 1972; 135: 569–592.

91. Lauweryns JM, Cokelaere M, Theunynck P. Serotonin producing neuroepithelial bodies in rabbit respiratory mucosa. *Science* 1973; 180: 410–413.

92. Lauweryns JM, Cokelaere M. Hypoxia-sensitive neuro-epithelial bodies. Intrapulmonary secretory neuroreceptors, modulated by the CNS. *Z Zellforsch* 1973; 145:521–540.

93. Vanpeperstraete F. The cartilaginous skeleton of the bronchial tree. *Adv Anat Embryol Cell Biol* 1974; 48:1–80.

94. von Hayek H. *The human lung.* New York: Hafner Publishing Co, 1960.

95. Krahl VE. Anatomy of the mammalian lung. In: Fenn WO, Rahn H, eds. *Handbook of physiology, section 3, respiration, vol 1.* Washington DC: American Physiological Society, 1964;213–284.

96. Starcher BC. Elastin and the lung. Review article. *Thorax* 1986; 41: 577–585.

97. Hakansson CH, Mercke U, Sonesson B, Toremalm NG. Functional anatomy of the musculature of the trachea. *Acta Morphol Neerl-Scand* 1976; 14:291–297.

98. Wailoo M, Emery JL. Structure of the membranous trachea in children. *Acta Anat* 1980; 106:254–261.

99. Matsuba K, Thurlbeck WM. A morphometric study of bronchial and bronchiolar walls in children. *Am Rev Respir Dis* 1972; 105:908–913.

100. Smith PG, Janiga KE, Bruce MC. Strain increases airway smooth muscle cell proliferation. *Am J Respir Cell Mol Biol* 1994; 10:85–90.

101. Glassberg MK, Ergul A, Wanner A, Puett D. Endothelin-1 promotes mitogenesis in airway smooth muscle cells. *Am J Respir Cell Mol Biol* 1994; 10:316–321.

102. Whimster WF, Lord P, Biles B. Tracheobronchial gland profiles in four segmental airways. *Am Rev Respir Dis* 1984; 129:985–988.

103. De Poitiers W, Lord PW. Biles B, Whimster WF. Bronchial gland histochemistry in lungs removed for cancer. *Thorax* 1980; 35:546–551.

104. Meyrick B, Reid L. Ultrastructure of cells in the human bronchial submucosal glands. *J Anat* 1970; 107:281–299.

105. Lamb D, Reid L. Histochemical types of acidic glycoprotein produced by mucous cells of the tracheobronchial glands in man. *J Pathol* 1969; 98:213–219.

106. Spicer SS, Schulte BA, Chakrin LW. Ultrastructural and histochemical observations of respiratory epithelium and gland. *Exp Lung Res* 1983; 4:137–156.

107. Nadziejko C, Finkelstein I. Inhibition of neutrophil elastase by mucus glycoprotein. *Am J Respir Cell Mol Biol* 1994; 11:103–107.

108. Mooren HWD, Meyer CJLM, Kramps JA, Franken C, Dijkman JH. Ultra-structural localization of the low molecular weight protease inhibitor in human bronchial glands. *J Histochem Cytochem* 1982; 30: 1130–1134.

109. Wiggins J, Hill SL, Stockley RA. Lung secretion sol-phase proteins: comparison of sputum with secretions obtained by direct sampling. *Thorax* 1983; 38:102–107.

110. Brandtzaeg P. Mucosal and glandular distribution of immunoglobulin components: differential localization of free and bound SC in secretory epithelial cells. *J Immun* 1974; 112:1553–1559.

111. Ueki I, German VF, Nadel JA. Micropipette measurement of airway submucosal gland secretion. Autonomic effects. *Am Rev Respir Dis* 1980; 121:351–357.

112. Nadel JA. New approaches to regulation of fluid secretion in airways. *Chest* 1981; 80:849–851.

113. Nadel JA. David B, Phipps RG. Control of mucus secretion and ion transport in airways. *Annu Rev Physiol* 1979; 41:369–381.

114. Phipps RJ, Nadel JA, Davis B. Effect of alpha-adrenergic stimulation on mucus secretion and on ion transport in cat trachea in vitro. *Am Rev Respir Dis* 1980; 121:359–365.

115. Shelhamer JH, Marom Z, Sun F, Bach MK, Kaliner M. The effects of arachnoids and leukotrienes on the release of mucus from human airways. *Chest* 1982; 81:36S–37S.

116. Marom Z, Shelhamer JH, Bach MK, Morton DR, Kaliner M. Slow-reacting substances, leukotrienes C4 and D4, increase the release of mucus from human airways in vitro. *Am Rev Respir Dis* 1982; 126: 449–451.

117. Peatfield AC, Barnes PJ, Bratcher C, Nadel JA, Davis B. Vasoactive intestinal peptide stimulates tracheal submucosal gland secretion in ferret. *Am Rev Respir Dis* 1983; 128:89–93.

118. Bienenstock J, Clancy RL, Perey DYE. Bronchus-associated lymphoid tissue (BALT): its relationship to mucosal immunity. In: Kirk-patrick CH, Reynolds HY, eds. *Immunologic and infectious reactions in the lung.* New York: Marcel Dekker, 1976;29.

119. Emery JL, Dinsdale F. The postnatal development of lymphoreticular aggregates and lymph nodes in infants' lungs. *J Clin Pathol* 1973; 26: 539–545.

120. Heppleston AG, Young AE. Uptake of inert particulate matter by alveolar cells: an ultrastructural study. *J Pathol* 1973; 111:159–164.

121. Kaltreider HB. Expression of immune mechanisms in the lung. *Am Rev Respir Dis* 1976; 113:347–379.

122. Bienenstock J, Befus AD, McDermott M. Mucosal immunity. *Monogr Allergy* 1980; 16:1–18.

123. Soutar CA. Distribution of plasma cells and other cells containing immunoglobulin in the respiratory tract of normal man and class of immunoglobulin contained therein. *Thorax* 1976; 31:158–166.

124. Brinkman GL. The mast cell in normal bronchus and lung. *J Ulstrastruct Res* 1968; 23:115–123.

125. Gold WM, Meyers GL, Dain DS, Miller RL, Bourne HR. Changes in airway mast cells and histamine caused by antigen aerosol in allergic dogs. *J Appl Physiol* 1977; 43:271–275.

126. Kaliner MA, Barnes PJ eds. *The airways. Neural control in health and disease.* New York: Marcel Dekker, 1988.

127. Richardson JB. Nerve supply to the lungs. *Am Rev Respir Dis* 1979; 119:785–802.

128. Partanen M, Laitinen A, Hervonen A, Toivanen M, Laitinen LA. Catecholamine- and acetylcholinesterase-containing nerves in human lower respiratory tract. *Histochemistry* 1982; 76:175–188.

129. Laitinen A, Partenen M, Hervonen A, Laitinen LA. Electron microscopic study of the innervation of the human lower respiratory tract: evidence of adrenergic nerves. *Eur J Respir Dis* 1985; 67:209–215.

130. Pack RJ, Richardson PS. The aminergic innervation of the human bronchus: a light and electron microscopic study. *J Anat* 1984; 138: 493–502.

131. Richardson JB, Beland J. Noradrenergic inhibitory nervous system in human airways. *J Appl Physiol* 1976; 41:764–771.

132. Simonsson BG, Svedmyr M, Skoogh BE, Andersson R, Bergh NP. *In vivo* and *in vitro* studies on alpha-receptors in human airway. Potentiation with bacterial endotoxine. *Scand J Respir Dis* 1972; 53:227–236.

133. Said SI, Kitamura S, Yoshida T, Preskitt J, Hoden LD. Humoral control of airways. *Ann NY Acad Sci* 1974; 221:103–114.

134. Barnes PJ. The third nervous system in the lung: physiology and clinical perspectives. *Thorax* 1984; 39:561–567.

135. Dey RD, Shannon WA Jr, Said S. Localisation of VIP-immunoreactive nerves in airways and pulmonary vessels of dogs, cats, and human subjects. *Cell Tissue Res* 1981; 220:231–238.

136. Laitinen A, Partanen M, Hervonen A, Pelto-Huikko M, Laitinen LA. VIP-like immunoreactive nerves in human respiratory tract. *Histochemistry* 1985; 82:313–319.

137. Larsell G, Dow RS. The innervation of the human lung. *Am J Anat* 1933; 52:125–146.

138. Gaylor JB. The intrinsic nervous mechanism of the human lung. *Brain* 1934; 57:143–160.

139. Pessacq TP. The innervation of the lung of newborn children. *Acta Anat 1971*; 79:93–101.

140. Laitinen A. Ultrastructural organisation of intraepithelial nerves in the human airway tract. *Thorax* 1985; 40:488–492.

141. Laitinen A. Detailed analysis of neural elements in human airways. In: Kaliner MA, Barnes PJ, eds. *The airways. Neural control in health and disease.* New York: Marcel Dekker, 1988;44.

142. Sant'Ambrogio G. Information arising from the tracheobronchial tree of mammals. *Physiol Rev* 1982; 62:531–569.

143. Hung KS, Hertwech MS, Hardy JD, Loosli CG. Ultrastructure of nerves and associated cells in bronchiolar epithelium of the mouse lung. *J Ultrastruct Res* 1973; 43:426–437.

144. Lauweryns JM, Cokelaere M. Intrapulmonary neuro-epithelial bodies: hypoxia sensitive neuro-(chemo) receptors. *Experientia* 1973: 29: 1384–1386.

145. Rennard ST, Beckman JD, Robbins RA. Biology of airway epithelial cells. In: Crystal RG, West JB, eds. *The lung: scientific foundations.* New York: Raven Press, 1991; Section 6, 1:157–167.

146. Mackelm PT, Proctor DF, Hogg JC. The stability of peripheral airways. *Respir Physiol* 1970; 8:191–203.

147. Finkelstein RA, Cosio MG. Disease of the small airways in smokers:

smokers' bronchiolitis. In: Epler GR, ed. *Diseases of the bronchioles.* New York: Raven Press, 1994;115–137.

148. Flavahan NA, Aarthus LL, Rimele TJ, Vanhoutte PM. Respiratory epithelium inhibits bronchial smooth muscle tone. *J Appl Physiol* 1985; 58:834–838.

149. Brunelleschi S, Haye-Legrand I, Labat C, Norel X, Benveniste J, Brink C. Platelet-activating factor acether-induced-relaxation of guinea pig airway muscle: role of prostaglandin E2 and the epithelium. *J Pharmacol Exp Ther* 1987; 243:356–363.

150. Hay DWP, Raeburn D, Farmer SG, Fleniry WW, Fedan JS. Epithelium modulates the reactivity of ovalbumin-sensitized guinea-pig airway smooth muscle. *Life Sci* 1986; 38:2461–2468.

151. Stuart-Smith K, Vanhoutte PM. Heterogeneity in the effects of epithelium removal in the canine bronchial tree. *J Appl Physiol* 1987; 63:2510–2515.

152. Raeburn D, Hay DWP, Robinson VA, Farmer SG, Fleniry WW, Fedan JS. The effect of verapamil is reduced in isolated airway smooth muscle preparations lacking the epithelium. *Life Sci* 1985; 38:809–816.

153. Barnett K, Jacoby DB, Nadel JA, Lazarus SC. The effects of epithelial cells supernatant on contractions of isolated canine tracheal smooth muscle. *Am Rev Respir Dis* 1988; 138:780–783.

154. Shoji S, Ertl R, Rennard SI. Cigarette smoke stimulates release of neutrophil chemotactic activity from cultured bronchial epithelial cells. *Clin Res* 1987; 35:539A.

155. Robbins RA, Shoji S, Linder J, Gossman GL, Allington LA, Klassen LW, Rennard SI. Bronchial epithelial cells release chemotactic activity for lymphocytes. *Am J Physiol* 1989; 257:L109–L115.

156. Koyama S, Rennard SI, Shoji S, Romberger D, Linder J, Ertl R, Robbins RA. Bronchial epithelial cells release chemoattractant activity for monocytes. *Am J Physiol* 1989; 257:L130–L136.

157. Glanville AR, Tazelaar HD, Theodore J, Imoto E, Rouse RV, Baldwin JC, Robin ED. The distribution of MHC class I and II antigens on bronchial epithelium. *Am Rev Respir Dis* 1989; 139: 330–334.

158. Lundberg JM, Saria A, Brodin E, Rosell S, Folkers R. A substance P antagonist inhibits vagally–induced increase in vascular permeability and bronchial smooth muscle contraction in the guinea–pig. *Proc Natl Acad Sci* 1983; 80:1120–1124.

159. Coles SJ, Neill KH, Reid LM. Potent stimulation of glycoprotein secretion in canine trachea by substance P. *J Appl Physiol: Respirat Environ Exercise Physiol* 1984; 57:1323–1327.

160. Rogers DF, Awvdkij B, Barnes PJ. Effects of tachykinins on mucus secretion in human bronchi *in vitro. Eur J Pharmacol* 1989; 174:283–286.

161. McCormack DG, Salonen RO, Barnes PJ. Effect of sensory neuropeptides on canine bronchial and pulmonary vessels *in vitro. Life Sci* 1989; 45:2405–2412.

162. Carstairs JR, Barnes PJ. Autoradiographic mapping of substance P receptors in the lung. *Eur J Pharmacol* 1986; 127:295–296.

163. Martling C–R, Theordorsson–Norheim E, Lundberg JM. Occurrence and effects of multiple tachykinins: substance P, neurokinin A, neuropeptide k in human lower airways. *Life Sci* 1987; 40: 1633–1643.

164. Joos G, Pauwels R, van der Straeten M. Effect of inhaled substance P and neurokinin A on the airways of normal and asthmatic subjects. *Thorax* 1987; 42:779–783.

165. Joos GF, Pauwels RA, van der Straeten ME. The mechanism of tachykinin-induced bronchoconstriction in the rat. *Am Rev Respir Dis* 1988; 137:1038–1044.

166. Joos GF, Pauwels R, van der Straeten ME. The effect of nedocromil sodium on the bronchoconstrictor effect of neurokinin A in subjects with asthma. *J Allergy Clin Immunol* 1989; 83:663–668.

167. McDonald DM. Respiratory tract infections increase susceptibility to neurogenic inflammation in the rat trachea. *Am Rev Respir Dis* 1988; 137:1432–1440.

168. Marasco WA, Showell HJ, Beeker EL. Substance P binds to formylpeptide chemotaxis receptor on the rabbit neutrophil. *Biochem Biophys Res Commun* 1981; 99:1065–1072.

169. Johnson AR, Ashton J, Schultz WW, Erdös EG. Neutral metalloendopeptidases in human lung tissue and cultured cells. *Am Rev Respir Dis* 1985; 132:564–568.

170. Frossard N, Rhoden KJ, Barnes PJ. Influence of epithelium on guinea pig airway responses to tachykinins: role of endopeptidase and cyclooxygenase. *J Pharmacol Exp Ther* 1989; 248:292–298.

171. Gunst SJ, Warner DO, Wilson TA, Hyatt RE. Parenchymal interdependence and airway response to methacholine in excised dog lobes. *J Appl Physiol* 1988; 65:2490–2497.

172. Macklem PT. Factors determining bronchial smooth muscle shortening. *Am Rev Respir Dis* 1991; 143:S47–S48.

173. Anderson AE, Foraker AG. Relative dimensions of bronchioles and parenchymal spaces in lungs from normal subjects and emphysematous patients. *Am J Med* 1962; 32:218–226.

Asthma, edited by P.J. Barnes, M.M. Grunstein,
A.R. Leff, and A.J. Woolcock.
Lippincott–Raven Publishers, Philadelphia © 1997.

▪ 15 ▪

Development of Airways

Charles G. Plopper, Reen Wu, Michelle V. Fannechi, and Judith A. St. George

OVERVIEW OF LUNG DEVELOPMENT

The cellular composition and architectural organization of the distal respiratory system (trachea, bronchi, and lungs) is highly complex at maturity in an adult. Over 40 morphologically distinct cell phenotypes are organized into a highly branched series of tissues surrounding the air passages. This very complex structure begins as an evagination of the undifferentiated epithelium from the foregut into a surrounding mesenchymal bundle. All of the developmental stages associated with the transformation from this simple tubular structure into a highly complex organ system are potentially susceptible to modification by toxic agents. The susceptibility of the lung as a target organ for specific toxicants may be altered by the cellular processes involved in each of these developmental events (see Plopper and Thurlbeck [1] for a detailed review).

A number of aspects of the developmental process need to be considered when the potential pulmonary de-velopmental toxicity of a compound is being evaluated. First, lung development is a multievent process that is not restricted to prenatal life. Although the initial evagination of the tracheobronchial bud begins early in gestation, the majority of lung growth and development occurs postnatally. Second, only a restricted number of maturational events must be complete at birth for successful postpartum survival of an organism. Third, there are three general categories of events occurring throughout the pre- and postnatal periods in which the lung develops: overall growth, branching morphogenesis, and cellular differentiation. The overall size of the lungs and trachea increases in a rather steady progression throughout pre- and postnatal life until body size ceases to increase. The intrapulmonary conducting airway tree also forms by branching morphogenesis, which is initiated by formation of the tracheobronchial bud. The highly complex structure of the gas exchange area also requires an extensive period of branching morphogenesis to form alveolar saccules and ducts. For formation of the interalveolar septa, the process is termed *alveolarization.* Two vascular trees and the capillary beds associated with both the conducting airways and the gas exchange area are formed at the same time as the airway tree. The cells of the airway tree, matrix, and interstitium differentiate at varying rates. Fourth, all of these developmental events occur in combination with a steadily increasing total cell mass.

The impact of disease agents and environmental toxicants on most of the developmental events critical for the successful maturation of the lower respiratory tract are not well understood or well documented. One of the rea-

C. G. Plopper and M. V. Fannechi: Department of Anatomy, Physiology and Cell Biology, School of Veterinary Medicine, University of California, Davis, California 95616.

R. Wu: Division of Pulmonary and Critical Care Medicine, School of Medicine and School of Veterinary Medicine; and California Regional Primate Research Center, University of California, Davis, California 95616.

J. A. St. George: Genzyme Corporation, Framingham, Massachusetts 01701-9322.

sons for this is that the mechanisms regulating the complex series of morphogenetic and differentiational events are only now being identified. Some of the regulatory factors, such as hormones and cytokines, have been recognized, but epithelial-matrix interactions and cell-cell (epithelial-epithelial or epithelial-mesenchymal) interactions are only beginning to become evident. Disease agents can modify developmental events in many ways. For example, exposure to toxins, such as tobacco smoke, can result in a poorly functioning, or inadequate, gas exchange system. Infectious agents also can induce a partially differentiated cell population to develop phenotypes not found in uninjured lung or alter the expression of phenotypes present so they are more resistant to injury.

Development of the lungs in mammals has been divided into a number of stages based primarily on the events occurring in the gas exchange area. Four of these stages are prenatal. In temporal sequence they are embryonic, pseudoglandular, canalicular, and saccular. As can be determined from evaluating the stages in the timing of these stages, summarized by species in Table 1, these events occur over different proportions of the fetal development, and each species is at a different stage of development when parturition occurs.

The embryonic stage is the earliest stage and is characterized by the budding of the future tracheobronchial tree from the foregut. In most species, the embryonic stage includes the formation of the largest conducting airways by branching into the surrounding mesenchyme.

The next stage is the pseudoglandular stage, which involves the continued branching and budding of the bronchial tree. The budding is generally asymmetric dichotomous, which means that one of the two daughter branches is smaller than the other and has a different branch angle from the parent airway. This branching continues until all of the airway generations characteristic of conducting airways in the adult have been formed down to the most distal, or terminal, bronchioles. This stage gets its definition from the fact that all of the tubules are lined by cuboidal to columnar-shaped epithelial cells, containing large amounts of glycogen, which have spread into the surrounding mesenchymal tissue. The vascular tree is absent from the growing lung at this stage.

A number of events occur during the next, or canalicular, stage. The vascular system begins to develop and the mesenchymal tissue between the branches of the airways becomes filled with vascular tissue. The airways that will become the future gas exchange area are formed by continuing branching and budding of the airway tree. As these air spaces continue to branch and expand, contact is made with a rich capillary network whose appearance is associated with thinning of the epithelium lining the more distal aspects of the gas exchange area.

The fourth interuterine stage is the saccular stage, characterized primarily by a dramatic increase in gas exchange surface area and in overall lung volume. There is an increase in the proportion of gas-exchanging air space and a further diminution of the mesenchymal mass between air saccules and vascular tissue.

The size of the normal lung in an adult animal is closely related to individual body size. The alteration of lung growth by toxins can be determined by measurements of wet lung weight or total lung volume. In relation to the body size of the individual, both of these measurements need to be determined either as body weight or some measurement of length, such as crown-rump length. The most reliable of these measurements is a determination of total lung volume, because changes in wet lung weight can be produced by a variety of factors that may not accurately reflect a change in lung growth, including amount of stored blood, presence of interstitial or alveolar edema, or technical problems associated with removal and weighing. Lung volume, as determined by the displacement of lungs fixed at maximum pressure by inflation of fixative through the trachea, has a close logarithmic allometric relationship to body weight in adults (2). Lung growth can be altered either by a decrease in overall size (termed *hypoplasia*) or by an overgrowth in volume (*hypertrophy*). Even though overall lung volume may not be altered by a toxicologic process, shifts in the rate of growth of specific subcompartments are possible. A major concern is the growth of the gas exchange portion of the lung. This can take the form of decreases in the surface or the volume of alveolar air space or the capillary bed, all of which also have allometric relationships to body size in the adult (2). Another factor that could be altered as part of an overall growth process is the relative proportion of the non-gas-exchanging compartments of the lung (the conducting airways and the major pulmonary arteries and veins) in relation to the proportion of

TABLE 1. *Comparative species development of fetal lungs (gestational age in days)*

	Pseudoglandular	Canalicular	Saccular	Term
Rat[a]	16–19 (73–86%)	19–20 (86–91%)	21 (95%)	22
Rabbit[a]	21–24 (65–75%)	24–27 (75–84%)	27 (84%)	32
Primate	57–80 (34–48%)	80–140 (48–84%)	140 (85%)	168
Sheep[a]	95 (60%)	95–120 (60–80%)	120 (80%)	150
Mouse	16 (80%)	18 (90%)	19 (95%)	20
Human[a]	52–112 (18–40%)	112–168 (40–60%)	168 (60%)	280

[a]From Meyrick B, Reid, L. In: Hodson A., ed. *Development of the lung.* New York: Dekker, 1977;135–214.

the lung that is gas exchange area. In most species, the gas exchange area composes approximately 85% of the lung volume in adults. While differentiational and morphogenetic events are occurring, the structures undergoing these changes (epithelial and endothelial cells lining the surfaces) are differentiating and also proliferating to provide an adequate lining of the increasing surface areas produced by overall increases in size. Whether a cytotoxic event that targets a differentiating cell population alters this population's ability to proliferate and adequately populate the increasing surface area is not well known. Overall, growth of the lung represents a change in overall size that involves an increase in volume of specific subcompartments associated with an increase in surface area requiring continued proliferation, even of relatively well-differentiated populations, until overall body growth ceases.

BRANCHING MORPHOGENESIS

Tracheobronchial Airways

Branching morphogenesis is the process by which the tracheobronchial airway tree is formed and organized. The process involves the growth by evagination of epithelial tubes into a mesenchymal matrix. The growth involves not only an increase in size and length of the tubes created by cellular proliferation, but also branching or bifurcation of the tubes as growth continues. This process forms the conducting airways in the early stages of the lung development, produces the basic framework and organization of the gas exchange area (parenchyma), and produces the vascular trees involved in conducting blood to and from the gas exchange area. The growth of the conducting airways, parenchyma, and blood vessels continues into the latest stages of lung development. It has long been recognized that a number of factors are critical in modulating the pattern of branching morphogenesis. The most critical of these appears to be the adjacent mesenchyma. The mesenchyma appears to influence two of the critical factors that drive the budding involved in branching morphogenesis: focal cell proliferation and epithelial cell shape changes (3). These appear to be modulated by rates of deoxyribonucleic acid (DNA) synthesis and expression of cytoskeletal elements, especially microfilaments. Other factors that may regulate and alter this process include extracellular matrix components, specifically fibronectin and laminin (4–7). It is thought that the airway contractions during early lung development may also alter blood formation. This is not the case, however. Altering the calcium channel function appears to downregulate airway-branching activity (8). It appears that some of the balance between proximal conducting airways and alveolar gas exchange area during early branching morphogenesis may be regulated by factors

such as epidermal growth factor, transforming growth factor (TGF)-α, and retinoic acid and its derivatives (9,10). Increasing concentrations of retinoic acid or retinol dramatically downregulate budding and growth of peripheral portions of the tubular branches and apparently enhance expansion and growth of the proximal portions of these branching trees. The end product of this branching morphogenesis of the epithelial portions of the lung and its final growth results in a well-organized tracheobronchial tree whose architecture varies by lung lobe and by species, but is highly consistent in adults of the same species (11). As a consequence, the impact of maternally administered exposure to lung toxins on the early branching of the conducting airway trees and the associated vasculature can be detected by some rather straightforward assessments. To establish whether lung compartmentalization has been altered—that is, whether the proportion of the adult lung occupied by the vasculature and the conducting airways, as opposed to the gas exchange area, has changed—point-counting morphometric approaches that give relatively accurate estimates of the percentage of lung volume occupied by different subcompartments can be used. The reduction in the proportion of the lung that is occupied by the vasculature and the conducting airway system is a strong indicator that exposure has had a negative impact on growth of these structures. Direct counts of the number of branches along defined airway paths and their size (diameter and length) indicate increased branching morphogenesis. These approaches can be done either directly from microdissected fixed lungs (12) or by the use of casts made of conducting airway trees (11).

Characteristics of the vascular tree in the lungs are reasonably complete on a species basis (13). Establishing arterial and venous size, diameter, and wall thickness and the extension of the branching pattern, which can be accomplished at the same time as the airway branching pattern is established, will be highly indicative of modulation of this pattern during early fetal lung development.

Respiratory Bronchioles

The most distal airways, located at the junction between the gas exchange area and tracheobronchial airway tree, form an extensive transitional zone in the human lung. This zone, exceeding three generations of branching in humans, is characterized by intermixing of alveolar epithelium, simple cuboidal epithelium mixed with the pseudostratified cuboidal epithelium (with basal, mucus, and ciliated cells) found in more proximal airways (see Plopper and ten Have-Opbroek [14] for a review). The respiratory bronchioles are extensive (exceeding three generations) in humans, macaques, dogs, cats, and ferrets. In rhesus monkeys, and possibly in other primates, including humans, the two epithelial populations, bronchiolar and alveolar, are distributed on opposite sides of the airway in relation to the position of the pulmonary arteriole (15). A pseudostratified population with ciliated cells lines numerous generations of respiratory bronchioles on the side adjacent to the pulmonary arteriole. The alveolarized areas are surrounded by a simple cuboidal bronchiolar epithelial population on the side opposite the arteriole. In the majority of mammalian species, the bronchiolar epithelium occupies the proximal portion of the transitional bronchiole, and alveolar gas exchange epithelium lines the distal portion. This is the case for mice, hamsters, rats, guinea pigs, rabbits, pigs, sheep, cattle, and horses (16).

The composition of the peribronchiolar region associated with Clara cells includes the presence of smooth muscle adjacent to the basal lamina, extensive collagen interspersed with elastin, and few capillaries. Those capillaries that are present are not closely associated with the epithelial basal lamina. The principal vessel in the area is the pulmonary arteriole. In contrast, the alveolar portions of this transitional zone generally include a substantial capillary bed closely applied to the basal lamina of the alveolar epithelial populations. Although the matrix composition of the alveolar gas exchange portions of the lung have been studied in some detail, the same is not true for the matrix associated with the bronchioles (17).

In fetal animals, where the majority of epithelial cells are poorly differentiated or undifferentiated, the boundary between the epithelium lining presumptive distal conducting airway and that lining future gas exchange regions is relatively easily defined in some species (18–20). The features include differences in epithelial configuration and modifications in the surrounding mesenchymally derived components. Most of these components, including smooth muscle and fibroblastlike cells, appear to mature somewhat more quickly then do the associated epithelium (21,22). The morphogenesis of the respiratory bronchiole during fetal lung development has been studied in detail in only one species: rhesus monkeys (21). The respiratory bronchiole begins as a tube lined by glycogen-filled cuboidal cells intermixed with an occasional ciliated cell. Alveolarization begins in the most proximal aspect of the respiratory bronchiole, at approximately 60% gestation in rhesus monkeys and in humans. The alveolarization appears as a formation of outpocketings into surrounding extracellular matrix. The outpocketings, which are lined by cuboidal epithelium, occur only on the side of the potential respiratory bronchiole opposite the pulmonary arteriole. They begin at the same time that secondary septa are forming in the distal acinus. Outpocketing or alveolarization occurs over a very short period of time (5 days) in rhesus monkeys. As alveolarization progresses from proximal to distal in the potential respiratory bronchiole, the epithelial cells also differentiate. By 67% gestation, ciliated cells are confined to the epithelium adjacent to the pulmonary arteriole, and the cytodifferentiation of the epithelial cells characteristic of alveoli is beginning in the

outpocketings. Contacts between epithelium and underlying fibroblastic cells are observed for a very brief period in regions of respiratory bronchiole development. Epithelium of proximal generations of respiratory bronchiole differentiates earlier than more distal generations, but much later than in the trachea.

Submucosal Glands

The developmental events involved in formation of submucosal glands have been well described for a number of species, including rats (23), opossums (24), ferrets (25), rhesus monkeys (26), and humans (27,28). The sequence of events in humans has been characterized subgrossly (29,30) and histologically (27,28,31,32). The ultrastructure and histochemistry of gland development have been characterized in the most detail in rhesus monkeys (26). In rhesus monkeys, most of the process occurs in the fetus between the end of the pseudoglandular stage and the beginning of the terminal sac stage of development. Gland development implies four phases: (a) the formation of buds by projections of undifferentiated cells from the maturing surface epithelium, (b) the outgrowth and branching of these buds into cylinders of undifferentiated cells, (c) the differentiation of mucus cells in proximal tubules associated with proliferation of tubules and acini and with undifferentiated cells distally, and (d) differentiation of serous cells in peripheral tubules and acini, with continued proliferation in most distal areas. The cells forming gland buds are not basal cells, as first thought, but rather an undifferentiated cell similar to the surface epithelium (Fig. 1) (26). Connective tissue appears to play a role in this process, as evidenced primarily through the presence of cartilage plates in the areas of initial bud formation. Glands appear first at the junction of cartilage plate and smooth muscle, followed by areas over cartilage plates and then in the area over smooth muscle. The secretory cell population differentiates in a centrifugal pattern, with nearly mature cells lining proximal tubules and immature cells in more distal portions. Mucus cells in the proximal portion of the gland develop before serous cells. Glandular mucus cells and serous cells differentiate at different times during development and through a different sequence of events (26).

EPITHELIAL DIFFERENTIATION

Overview

Of the over 40 different cellular phenotypes that have been identified in the lungs of adult mammals, the differentiation of the epithelial cells lining the air passages appears to be the most critical in the successful function of the lung in adults. At least eight of these cell phenotypes line the tracheobronchial conducting airways, including

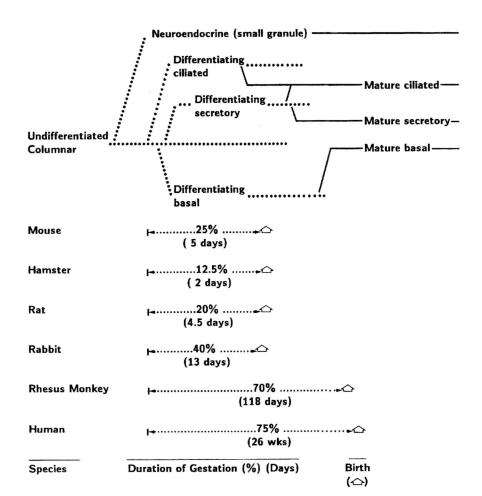

Mouse   ⊢··········25% ··········▷
(5 days)

Hamster   ⊢··········12.5% ········▷
(2 days)

Rat   ⊢··········20% ··········▷
(4.5 days)

Rabbit   ⊢··········40% ··········▷
(13 days)

Rhesus Monkey   ⊢·····················70% ·············▷
(118 days)

Human   ⊢·····················75% ·············▷
(26 wks)

Species	Duration of Gestation (%) (Days)	Birth (▷)

FIG. 1. Pattern of epithelial differentiation in the trachea. Relative time of appearance of different phenotypes in relation to parturition.

ciliated cells, basal cells, mucus goblet cells, serous cells, Clara cells, small mucus granule cells, brush cells, neuroendocrine cells, and a number of undifferentiated or partially differentiated phenotypes that have not been well characterized. The abundance and distribution of these cell types within the conducting airway tree vary by position within the tree and by species. The pattern of differentiation of the tracheal epithelial lining has been characterized for a large number of species (33). The general pattern appears to be the same for most species in terms of which phenotypes are identified earliest during development and which differentiate later (summarized in Fig. 1). The critical difference between differentiation of these epithelial cells during development is the percentage of intrauterine life in which the differentiation occurs. The epithelium of the trachea is the earliest of all the epithelial populations to differentiate. In some species it is relatively differentiated prior to birth, and in other species the majority of the differentiation occurs postnatally. In most species, with the possible exception of ferrets, ciliated cells differentiate first. Nonciliated cells with secretory granules appear next. Basal and small mucus granule cells appear last. There is a polarity in the differentiation of cil-

iated cells in the trachea, with the epithelium over the smooth muscle undergoing ciliogenesis earlier than that on the cartilaginous side. The reverse appears to be true for the nonciliated secretory cells, with secretory granules appearing on the cartilaginous side of the trachea first.

Pattern in Trachea and Bronchi

The ultrastructural features of overall tracheal epithelial differentiation in developing fetuses have been described in rabbits (34), mice (35), hamsters (36,37), and rats (32). In view of the diversity in the airways in different species, small laboratory mammals may not be adequate models for the study of human tracheobronchial epithelium (32). The most extensive study of the development of the mucus cell was performed on the trachea of rhesus monkeys (38) and is reviewed here. Gestation for rhesus monkeys averages 168 days, with the stages of lung development as follows: embryonic period, 21 to 55 days gestational age (DGA); pseudoglandular, 56 to 80 DGA; canalicular, 80 to 130 DGA; and terminal sac, 131 to term (39).

In the youngest fetuses, all cells appear as illustrated in Figure 2A. The cells are columnar and the apices of most of the cells reach the luminal surface. Nuclei have little heterochromatin, and the cytoplasm is filled from base to apex with glycogen. The few organelles present are located in the apex of the cell and included short narrow strands of granular endoplasmic reticulum (GER), small spherical mitochondria, and a small Golgi apparatus located adjacent to the lateral surface of the cell (Fig. 2A). These cells were present in the epithelial lining in the youngest animal in the embryonic stage to the middle of the canalicular phase.

In fetuses near the end of the embryonic period, many cells similar to those at younger ages, but containing larger numbers of apical organelles, are observed. The organelles include spherical mitochondria and increased amounts of GER with dilated cisternae. The cisternae of the Golgi apparatus are dilated and surrounded by enlarged membrane-bound vacuoles, and glycogen is concentrated near the nucleus and intermixed with the organelles. These cells are observed in fetuses up to early in the canalicular stage.

Through most of the pseudoglandular stage, most nonciliated cells had increased numbers of apical membrane-bound secretory granules containing a flocculent matrix, with a small electron-dense spherical core (Fig. 2B).

Most of the remaining cytoplasm is still filled with glycogen. The cytoplasm surrounding the glycogen is more electron dense than in younger ages and occupied more of the apical portion of the cell. The nuclei exhibit prominent nucleoli and small patches of heterochromatin. The mitochondria exhibit noncircular profiles and appeared to be tubular. The amount of GER appears to be the same as in younger ages, but the cisternae were no longer dilated. The Golgi apparatus is surrounded by vacuoles of various sizes. The luminal surface of these cells is covered by long, regular microvilli. In somewhat older animals (late pseudoglandular), the apices of a large proportion of the secretory cells are filled with spherical granules (Fig. 2C). Most of these cells have abundant cytoplasmic glycogen, most of which is basal to the nucleus. Apical to the nucleus, glycogen is interspersed among organelles and granules. The cells appear more fusiform than at younger ages, being wide at the luminal side and narrow at the base (Fig. 2C). In fetuses from midcanalicular stage and older, secretory cells containing cytoplasmic glycogen are rare and, when observed, the glycogen content was minimal. From this time to parturition, only two forms of secretory cells are observed. Both cells have little cytoplasmic glycogen, and the cytoplasm was condensed. There is a distinct variation in the abundance of apical secretory granules in these cells, ranging

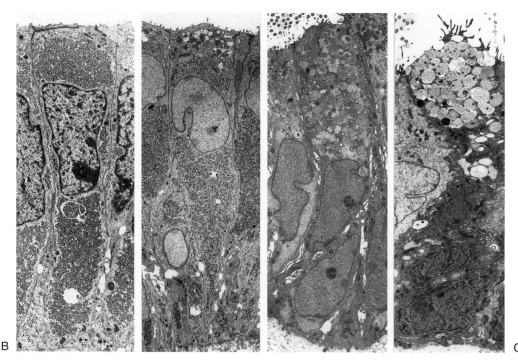

A,B

C,D

FIG. 2. Summary of the pattern of cytodifferentiation of mucus cells in the trachea of the rhesus monkey. **A:** Glycogen-filled (*Gly*) columnar cells; 46-day gestation. **B:** Glycogen-filled columnar cell with tapered base and apical granules; 62-day gestation. **C:** Glycogen-depleted columnar cell with abundant apical granules; 90-day gestation. **D:** Columnar cell filled with dense-cored secretory granules; 141-day gestation.

from very few, in cells with a narrow cytoplasm and few organelles, to cells with an abundance of these granules (Fig. 2D). The cytoplasm of these cells contain small mitochondria and varying amounts of GER. The Golgi apparatus is located on the apical side of the nucleus and showed variable degrees of activity. In cells with more granules (Fig. 2D), the Golgi apparatus is larger, has more cisternal stacks, and has larger and more numerous adjacent vesicles. Long, regular microvilli are a characteristic feature of the surface of the secretory cells. There is considerable variability in the abundance of these cellular forms between 105 days and parturition. In the earlier ages, they are of approximately equal abundance. Near parturition, most of the secretory cells resemble that in Figure 2D. Some of the cells have an even larger percentage of their cytoplasm occupied by granules than illustrated in Figure 2D.

In the postnatal period, most of the secretory cells have an abundance of electron-lucent granules filling their apical cytoplasm. The majority of these granules have small electron-dense cores. A few have large electron-dense biphasic cores, as is observed in the adult. In general, the nucleus and its surrounding cytoplasm are restricted to the basal portion of the cell and the Golgi apparatus, and other organelles occupy a small percentage of the cytoplasm. Through 134 days postparturition, there are, however, a few secretory cells the cytoplasm of which contained abundant organelles and a variable number of secretory granules, as is observed in the late fetal period (Fig. 2D). By 134 days of postnatal age, nearly all of the secretory cells have a configuration similar to that observed in adults. The cytoplasm is filled with electron-lucent secretory granules that appeared to distend the cell's cytoplasm. The nucleus is compressed at the basal portion of the cell, and organelles are minimal. In most cases, the cytoplasmic granules contains a biphasic core. The central part of the core is the most electron-dense portion of the granules.

Tracheobronchial epithelium continually renews itself. To identify the progenitor cell types that are involved in the self-renewal *in vivo*, the traditional approach is to carry out mitotic index and nuclear labeling studies. For the nuclear labeling study, the incorporation of [3H]thymidine or bromdeoxyuridine is used. Using these approaches, most of the data suggest that less than 1% of the epithelial cell population is involved in cell proliferation (40–44). Both basal and secretory cell types are capable of incorporating these nucleotide precursors and mitosis, whereas ciliated cells are considered to be terminally differentiated and incapable of division (45). In fact, only under exceptional circumstances are the ciliated cells of isolated hamster trachea capable of synthesizing DNA, as evidenced by the incorporation of [3H]thymidine (46). Differentiation and proliferation normally are inversely related. Based on this view, a number of investigators (47,48) suggest that it is the basal cell type that

serves as the stem cells, or the progenitor cell type that is involved in normal maintenance as well as in the regeneration and redifferentiation of bronchial epithelium after injury. However, this view is inconsistent with data obtained from the developmental studies and studies of injury/repair results. In the developing tracheas of a number of animal species, including humans and nonhuman primates, basal cells are derived from an undifferentiated columnar epithelium (49). Furthermore, the appearance of the basal cell type in the tracheal surface lining layer occurs after the appearance of ciliated and nonciliated secretory cell types (50). Furthermore, in the growing intrapulmonary airways (51,52), the basal cell type is not found in the smallest airway (49). In the injury models, such as the mechanical and toxic gases exposure model, hyperproliferation is seen in the secretory cell type, but not in the basal cell type (44,53–55). These results point out that it is less likely for the basal cell type to serve as a progenitor cell type that initiates the growth of airway epithelium and the repair of epithelial damage (49).

New experiments in the repopulation of epithelial cells on denuded tracheal grafts have been used to assess the "progenitor" nature of various bronchial epithelial cell types. Denuded tracheal grafts generally are produced by removing the lining epithelial layer by repeated freezing and thawing of tracheal grafts, a technique developed several years ago by Nettesheim and his colleagues (56). Using this technique, combined with the cell separation technique, Hook and his colleagues (57,58) have demonstrated the repopulation of a mucociliary epithelium in the denuded tracheal graft by enriched basal cell population from rabbits and rats. These experiments clearly demonstrate the polypotent nature of the basal cell type. However, there are several deficiencies in these experiments. First of all, the definition of basal cell type is based on the ultrastructural picture and the immunohistochemical stain. It is well known, though, that secretory cells lose their differentiated features upon cell isolation and culturing *in vitro*. The degranulated secretory cells may resemble the basal cell type, and the morphologic tools used in these studies cannot distinguish satisfactorily the basal one from the degranulated secretory cell type in dissociated and isolated cell preparations. Furthermore, for the preparations in these studies, the purity of basal cell type population is only 90%. When Johnson et al. (59) used flow cytometry to isolate basal cells, they found that basal cells from rat trachea had a colony-forming efficiency of 0.6%, whereas secretory cells and unsorted cells had efficiencies of 3.4% and 2.6%, respectively. From these results, the authors concluded that basal cells had less proliferative activity than did secretory cells. It is therefore difficult to conclude from these tracheal graft repopulation studies that basal cell type is the progenitor cell type responsible for the initiation of airway epithelial cell growth and the repair to response to injury.

Regulation in Trachea and Bronchi

Regulation of the maturation of the fetal airway secretory apparatus has not been well examined, so the factors that control development and the mechanisms of these controls are poorly understood. The effects of epidermal growth factor (EGF) on lung development has been examined in rhesus monkeys. EGF treatment *in utero* markedly stimulates the maturation of the tracheal secretory apparatus, including both the tracheal surface and submucosal glands (60). The secretory apparatus is more differentiated in that there are more mucus cells, increased secretory product stored in the epithelium and glands, and increased quantities of secretory product in lavage and amniotic fluid. By contrast, treatment with triamcinalone, a glucocorticoid, induces maturation of the gas exchange area (61), but does not affect the maturation of the secretory apparatus (Table 2).

Although *in vivo* studies have been lacking, substantial data are available on the regulation of microciliary differentiation *in vitro*. There are at least three stages of development of the airway epithelial cell culture system. The development of serum-free hormone-supplemented medium enables a continuous cultivation of various tracheobronchial epithelial cells in culture. Successful completion of this stage allows the second stage of development to incorporate critical factors, such as vitamin A and the collagen gel substratum, for airway epithelial cell differentiation. In the third stage of development, a physiology-relevant culture condition is developed. The development of a biphasic culture system for bronchial epithelial cells is a major advance in the *in vitro* model to study airway epithelial cell physiology and injury and repair.

Tracheobronchial epithelial cells, like many other epithelial cells, lose their differentiated functions upon culturing *in vitro*. However, the loss of differentiated functions—at least in the primary tracheobronchial epithelial culture—is transient. Evidence of transient dedifferentiation comes from two experiments. One is a repopulation study in which cultured cells are replated on denuded tracheal grafts that are carried by immune-deficient mice

(56). It was observed more than 14 years ago that undifferentiated rabbit tracheal epithelial cells maintained long-term in culture are able to repopulate on denuded rat tracheal grafts and form a new mucociliary epithelium (62,63). This result suggests that epithelial cells, despite dedifferentiation in culture, maintain their intrinsic differentiated potential, which eventually is expressed if an appropriate environment is provided. Because of this encouraging result, subsequent developments in optimizing hormonal requirements and the utilization of vitamin A supplement and collagen gel substratum (64,65) for epithelial cultures further enhance the differentiated nature of cultured tracheobronchial epithelial cells. Lee et al. (66) were the first to demonstrate new ciliogenesis in primary hamster tracheal epithelial cultures based on the semiquantitative determination of ciliated population. Subsequently, it was demonstrated that mucus cell differentiation also occurs in hamster tracheal cultures (67). The large molecular weight of secretory glycoproteins secreted by cultured hamster tracheal epithelial cells are linked as *O*-glycosides (67,68). Based on the amino acid and carbohydrate composition analyses of the *in vitro* secretory products as compared with the *in vivo* mucin products purified from sputum and epithelial cell layer, it may be concluded that cultured hamster tracheal epithelial cells are able to secrete authentic mucin (69). Similar results have since been demonstrated in both human (70) and guinea pig (71) tracheobronchial epithelial cultures. These developments further strengthen the notion that a mucociliary epithelium can be achieved in culture if the culture condition is developed properly.

In 1986, Wu et al. (72) developed a Whitcutt chamber to grow airway epithelial cells between air and a liquid medium interface. The development of this chamber was based on the physiologic consideration that airway epithelial cells *in vivo* are usually located between air and a liquid interface. This notion is quite different from the traditional tissue culture technique that tends to culture cells under a medium-immersed condition. Using this chamber, columnarized formation of cultured epithelial cells was observed, and with further development of mucociliary differentiation in culture (73,74). DeJong et al. (75) and Gray et al. (76) recently applied the biphasic culture systems to both human and monkey tracheobronchial epithelial cells and observed the formation of a fully differentiated epithelial cell layer with prominent features of ciliary beating and mucus-secreting granules. However, in contrast to airway epithelial cells derived from rodents, mucociliary differentiation of human and monkey cultures occurs much later (at least 21 days after plating). One of the major problems associated with such a long-term biphasic culture is the drying out on the apical side of cultured epithelial cell layers, despite 100% humidity in the incubator. To avoid such a problem, a trace amount of culture medium is added to the apical side of the culture. The addition of 0.05 mL of culture medium to top of

TABLE 2. *Effect of epidermal growth factor (EGF) and triamcinalone acetonide (TAC) on total glycoconjugate detectable in the trachea of fetal rhesus monkeys*

DGA	Treatment	Total secretory product (mm^3 × 10^3/mm^2) (±1 SD)
128	None	0.48 ± 0.37
150	None	1.36^a ± 0.33
128	EGF	.77^a ± 0.28
150	TAC (1 mg/day)	1.27 ± 1.35
150	TAC (10 mg/day)	0.75 ± 0.34

DGA, days gestational age.
^{a}p < 0.05 compared with 128 DGA control.

an approximately 5-cm^2 surface of a monkey tracheobronchial epithelial culture maintains the culture more than 2 months without any deterioration. Scanning electron microscopy has demonstrated extensive ciliary features on the culture surface, and transmission electron microscopy has demonstrated the formation of abundant mucus-secreting granules and the columnarized features with a two- to four-cell layer. Interestingly, the basal cell layer is compressed and resembles the *in vivo* basal cell type with such features as prominent tonofilament structure and a high nucleus–cytoplasm ratio. By contrast, if excessive medium (for example, 0.5 mL) was added to the apical side of the culture, a condition similar to the traditional immersed culture system, both the compact and columnarized features are reduced. Furthermore, the extent of mucociliary differentiation in such a culture is qualitatively decreased.

Tracheobronchial epithelium is one of the vitamin A-targeted tissues (77–80). The epithelium requires vitamin A for the preservation and induction of the expression of differentiated functions. Keratinizing squamous metaplasia of normal mucociliary epithelium is the primary lesion that occurs in the vitamin A-deficient state. The normal, columnar, mucociliary epithelium becomes underlain with the new, stratified, squamous, keratinizing epithelium; distinctive keratohyaline granules usually can be seen before the development of sheets of keratin. Accompanying these morphologic changes is a reduction in the synthesis of mucus glycoproteins. Both *in vivo* and *in vitro* organ culture studies have shown that the administration of vitamin A or its synthetic derivatives (retinoids) can reverse this phenomenon. At the other extreme, excess vitamin A can even convert stratified skin epithelium in chick embryos to an epithelium containing mucus-secreting granules (81). Thus, it appears that the controls for mucus cell differentiation and squamous metaplasia are inversely linked by vitamin A.

The cell type responsive to vitamin A regulation of squamous cell differentiation and mucus cell differentiation in airway epithelium has not been identified. There are at least two possibilities. One is that both mucus and squamous cells are derived from different cell types and both of them are competing for the same growth environment. The presence of vitamin A alters the growth environment, which favors the proliferation of mucus progenitor cells, while the absence of vitamin A favors the proliferation of the progenitor cell type of squamous cell epithelium. McDowell and colleagues have demonstrated that vitamin A treatment enhances the proliferation of small mucus-granule cell type in primary hamster tracheal epithelial cultures (82–84). However, it has not been demonstrated that vitamin A deficiency leads to enhanced squamous cell proliferation. In a separate study, vitamin A was shown to enhance DNA synthesis of basal cells of keratinocyte cultures (85). In addition, there is no evidence that vitamin A inhibits squamous cell prolifera-

tion. The other possibility is that both mucus and squamous cells are derived from the same cell type, and vitamin A stimulates this uncommitted cell type to express mucus cell phenotypes. There is some evidence to support this explanation. It is not unusual to observe cells with the differentiated features of both mucus cell type (that is, secretory granules) and squamous cell type (that is, tonofilaments). Furthermore, it is known from the *in vivo* injury/repair study that degranulated mucus cells (or an intermediate cell type) are capable of incorporating [^{3}H]thymidine and then differentiating into squamous cell type. A similar phenomenon exists *in vitro* in primary tracheobronchial epithelial cultures immediately after plating. These results support the notion that the progenitor cell types of mucus and squamous epithelia are related and that the differential expression of these phenotypes is regulated by vitamin A.

Cellular Basis of Vitamin A-Dependent Mucus Cell Differentiation in Culture

Vitamin A is very important for expression of mucus differentiated functions in human and monkey tracheobronchial epithelial cells to express mucus differentiated functions. The presence of vitamin A is essential for a continuous maintenance of the integrity of airway epithelium cultured on collagen gel substratum. In the absence of vitamin A supplements, the epithelium deteriorates within 1 to 2 weeks, whereas a multiple cell layer of epithelium can be maintained long term in the vitamin A-supplemented condition. The expression of mucus differentiated cell types in culture depends on vitamin A. To trace the origin of the mucus cell type in culture further, we carried out kinetics studies with pulse and chase of [^{3}H]thymidine labeling. According to the cell kinetics, a majority of mucus cell type in culture is derived from a process of cell differentiation independent from cell proliferation. A mucus cell population capable of DNA synthesis in culture is rare, occurring only during the early period of primary culture. Within 4 to 6 days, a majority of the new mucus cell population is developed from replicative nonmucus cell type after DNA synthesis has ceased. Vitamin A and its derivatives apparently play an essential role in this transformation. Interestingly, this transformation is inhibited by TGF-β_1.

Pattern in Bronchioles

The process of cytodifferentiation of the nonciliated cells of distal bronchioles entails substantial rearrangement, loss, and biogenesis of cellular organelles. Up to late fetal age, terminal bronchioles are lined by simple cuboidal to columnar epithelium composed of glycogen-filled nonciliated cells with few organelles. The shifts in cellular components with time for species in which the predominant cellular constituent in adults is agranular endoplasmic reticulum (AER), such as in mice, hamsters, rats, and rabbits, are summarized in Figure 3. The pattern is essentially similar for these species. What varies from species to species is the timing of these events. The first event is a dramatic loss in cytoplasmic glycogen. In rab-

bits, this drop is from approximately 70% of cytoplasmic volume to less than 10% cytoplasmic volume in adults. A similar substantial loss occurs in rats, hamsters, and mice. In rabbits, this loss begins immediately prior to birth and continues for up to 4 weeks of postnatal age (86). A similar change occurs in mice (87). In rats, the loss of cyto-

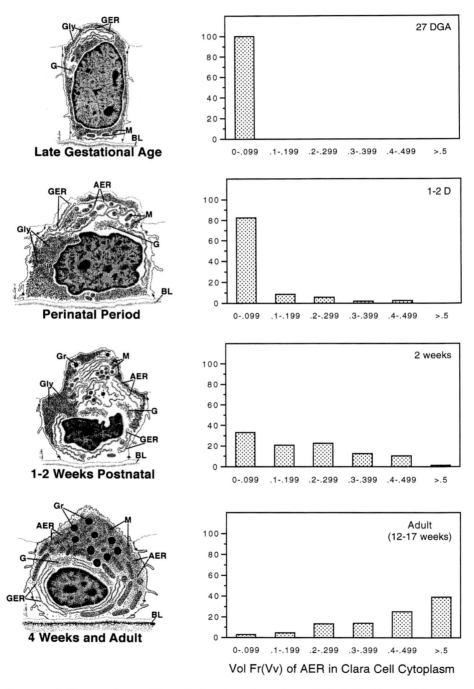

Vol Fr(Vv) of AER in Clara Cell Cytoplasm

FIG. 3. Pattern of Clara cell cytodifferentiation based on the rabbit. **Left:** The cellular composition changes are illustrated. **Right:** The heterogeneity is summarized in the proportion of cytoplasm filled with agranular endoplasmic reticulum (AER) as a percentage of the cell population evaluated. Even in adults, at least 5% of the Clara cell population has little AER (less than 5% of cytoplasmic volume).

plasmic glycogen begins at birth and drops to adult levels within the first week of postnatal life (88). In hamsters, cytoplasmic glycogen is not detectable immediately after birth (89). Associated with the drop in cellular glycogen is a substantial biogenesis of membranous organelles, especially AER (Table 3). Smooth endoplasmic reticulum is not detected in nonciliated cells until immediately prior to birth in rabbits (Fig. 3) (90). At birth, fewer than 20% of the cells contain greater than 10% AER. By 2 weeks, in almost 70% of the nonciliated cells, AER occupies greater than 10% (up to 50%) of the cell volume. The adult configuration is reached at approximately 28 days postnatally in rabbits. In mice, the adult configuration of AER is reached at approximately 3 weeks postnatally (87). Granular endoplasmic reticulum in prenatal animals is approximately twice as abundant in rabbit Clara cells as it is in rats (Fig. 3) (91). The decrease in cellular abundance of GER occurs gradually in rabbits and is still double the adult configuration (2% of cell volume) at 4 weeks postnatally, but in rats the level decreases by 50% immediately postpartum and is at or near the adult configuration (less than 1%) by 10 days postnatally. The situation for rats and mice appears similar to that for rabbits, but for hamsters GER is near the adult configuration immediately postpartum (89,92). Secretory granule appearance also varies by species. The earliest at which secretory granules are detected in the Clara cells of rabbits and mice is within the first week of postnatal life, whereas in rats and hamsters granules are abundant pre-

natally. In rabbits as well as mice, granule abundance resembling adult levels occurs by 21 days postnatally. In rats, granule abundance reaches adult abundance by 7 days postnatally and is at adult configuration immediately postpartum in the hamster. The only species in which Clara cell differentiation has been characterized fully where the adult Clara cell population does not have an abundance of AER is rhesus monkeys (22). In that species, the loss of cytoplasmic glycogen and an increase, rather than a decrease, in GER occurs over a substantial period both prenatally and postnatally. Studies in humans suggest that developmental events for Clara cells are similar to those in rhesus monkeys, but may extend longer than the 6 months to a year (postnatally) required for differentiation of all of the nonciliated cells in terminal respiratory bronchioles of monkeys.

The expression of cytochrome P450 monooxygenases (CYP) in Clara cells during their differentiation has been evaluated in only three species: rabbits, hamsters, and rats (91,93,94). Protein for the NADPH P450 reductase and CYP2B is detected earliest, with the reductase somewhat later than CYP2B in rabbits. CYP4B is detected 2 to 3 days of age later (Table 3). The initial distribution is in the most apical border of a small percentage of the nonciliated cell population. During the period in which the amount of detectable protein increases, the distribution changes in two ways. First, an immunologically detectable protein is found in an increasing proportion of the nonciliated cells as animals become older. Second, the

TABLE 3. *Development of agranular endoplasmic reticulum (AER), P450 reductase, and monooxygenase enzymes in rabbit lung*

Assay	Amount or activity					
	27–28 DGA	1–2 DPN	7 DPN	14 DPN	20 DPN	Adult
	% of adult value					
AER[a,b]	0.2	8.2	8.2	30.1	64.5	100
P450 reductase						
Immunohistochemistry[b,c]	±	+	++	++	++++	++++
Western blot	+	+	++	++	++++	++++
P450 isozyme 2B						
Immunohistochemistry[b]	0	±	+	++	++++	++++
Western blot	0	0	±	+	++++	++++
P450 isozyme 4B						
Immunohistochemistry[b]	0	+	++	++	++++	++++
Western blot	0	±	+	++	+++	++++
Microsomal P450[d]	0	0	20.9	44.5	56.0	100
P450 activity						
Ethoxyresorufin[e]	0	10.8	11.7	14.9	59.3	100
Pentoxyresorufin[f]	0	6.5	8.1	29.9	51.8	100

DGA, days gestational age; DPN, days postnatally.
[a]Average adult cell volume for AER is 43.9 ± 3.5%.
[b]Bronchiolar epithelium.
[c]Symbols indicate staining intensities in relation to adult (++++).
[d]Average adult level of microsomal P450 is 0.575 ± 0.238 nmol/mg of microsomal protein.
[e]Average adult ethoxyresorufin *O*-dealkylase activity is 47.99 ± 14.69 pmol/mg of protein/min.
[f]Average adult pentoxyresorufin *O*-dealkylase activity is 64.07 ± 64.51 pmol/mg of protein/min.

distribution of detectable protein within an individual cell increases from the apex to the base with increasing age. The youngest age at which intracellular protein can be detected immunohistochemically varies substantially within these three species. Protein becomes detectable in hamsters approximately 3 to 4 days prior to birth and reaches the distribution and intensity observed in the adult by 3 days postnatally. CYB4B is not detectable before 1 day postnatally, but is at adult levels shortly thereafter. In rabbits and rats, the timing is somewhat different. NADPH reductase is found initially just prior to birth in rabbits, and CYP2B and 4B are not observed until after birth. All of these proteins have an adult distribution and intensity by 28 days postnatally. In rats, CYP2B, CYP4B, and reductase are detected in the first 2 to 3 days of postnatal life and are apparently at adult densities and distributions by 21 days postnatally. CYP1A1 is not detectable prenatally in rats but can be detected in increasing, but small, amounts until it reaches adult levels at approximately 21 days postnatally. Intracellular expression of protein precedes the appearance and increase in the abundance of AER by 2 to 4 days in each of these species. Activity for these proteins is first detected approximately 2 to 3 days after the protein is immunologically detectable within Clara cells. The activity studies have been done with whole lung homogenates and reflect potential activity from other cell populations as well as from Clara cells. While both the AER abundance and antigenic protein intensity reach the adult configuration in approximately 3 to 4 weeks in rats and rabbits, the activity for these isozymes is still considerably below that for adults. This suggests that the functionality of these proteins continues to increase after the protein density and organelle composition have reached adult levels of expression. Table 2 summarizes the relationship between changes in AER abundance, expression of immunoreactive protein, and microsomal P450 activity for rabbits. The timing for rats is somewhat shifted to the left for postnatal time points and to the right for perinatal ones compared with rabbits.

The pattern of expression of the Clara cell secretory protein is similar to that of the cytochrome P450 monooxygenase system in relation to the appearance of cellular organelles. While there is substantial interspecies variability in the timing of expression, the general pattern is similar, at least for the four species studied in most detail: rats, rabbits, hamsters, and mice (87,90,93,95–98). The protein appears earliest in the central or apical portion of a few cells per bronchiole, and the number of cells in which antigen can be detected increases with increasing age. In hamsters, the secretory protein antigen can be detected in a number of cells by the beginning of the last trimester of pregnancy and reaches the adult configuration in terms of density and number of cells labeled at about 3 to 4 days postnatally. In rats, a small proportion of the cells are labeled prenatally, and the distribution observed in the adult is present at about 7 days postnatally.

This adult configuration occurs between 3 and 4 weeks in rabbits, and the earliest detectable signal in the Clara cells is immediately prior to birth. The timing in mice and rats is similar to that in rabbits. Immunoreactive protein has also been detected in late fetal humans, but when the distribution resembles adults has not been determined. Intracellular expression of the protein follows the changes in GER and is closely related to the first appearance and increase in the abundance of secretory granules. Western blotting of this protein indicates that it is present earlier in lung homogenate than its appearance in bronchiolar Clara cells suggests. This is because secretory cells in proximal airways express the protein much earlier and, in general, are more differentiated in the perinatal period than are secretory cells of bronchioles. In hamsters, the situation is the inverse, with the bronchioles differentiating in this respect prior to the bronchi.

Regulation in Bronchioles

Factors regulating Clara cell differentiation are not well understood. The postnatal nature of the majority of the cytodifferentiation process in most species suggests that it is independent of the hormones associated with pregnancy and parturition. The fact that the timing varies by as much as 2 to 3 weeks in different species would further suggest that the process may be under regulation of a variety of factors that act in different temporal sequences and with different levels of influence in different species. A number of mediators have been shown to stimulate cytodifferentiation of type II alveolar epithelial cells and produce architectural rearrangements of lung connective tissue elements to promote gas exchange, including corticosteroids, thyroid hormone, epidermal growth factor, and cyclic AMP (99). Whether all of these mediators influence Clara cell differentiation is not known. The best studied are the glucocorticoids, especially dexamethasone. Treatment in the perinatal period retards Clara cell differentiation as evidenced by an increase in cytoplasmic glycogen and minimal alterations in organelles in both rats and mice (100,101). Dexamethasone administered either prenatally or immediately postnatally elevates the surfactant protein messenger ribonucleic acid (mRNA) levels in lungs of rats of all ages, producing this elevation in both alveolar type II cells and Clara cells (102). Glucocorticoid administered to pregnant rabbits appears to have a stimulatory effect on the differentiation of secretory potential in fetal Clara cells by elevating the amount of the uteroglobinlike Clara cell secretory protein (103,104). Dexamethasone administered to pregnant rabbits also has a stimulatory effect on the pulmonary cytochrome P450 system in fetuses, based on measurements of whole lung microsomes (105–107). While glycogenolysis is retarded by dexamethasone treatment, glucagon, epinephrine, and 8-bromo-cAMP produce a rapid drop in Clara cell glycogen content (88).

One of the factors that appears to have the most impact on Clara cell differentiation is injury during the developmental period, in which normal differentiation occurs. Normal differentiation is characterized by loss of glycogen and appearance of secretory granules, and by differentiation of Clara cells into ciliated cells, even in the absence of frank injury to either ciliated or Clara cells. Postnatal exposure to compounds that injure the respiratory system retard Clara cell differentiation. Hyperoxia during the early postnatal period inhibits differentiation (Massaro et al., unpublished data; 108,109). Injury by treatment with 4-ipomeanol impedes Clara cell differentiation even for a short term after treatment is discontinued (110). Not only are Clara cells in postnatal animals more susceptible to injury than are Clara cells in adults, but the expression of the P450 system in the posttreatment period is markedly reduced. In rats, exposure to cigarette smoke of either the pregnant mother or the newborn accelerates the appearance of one cytochrome P450 monooxygenase isozyme, CYP1A1, but not CYP2B (94). The increased P450 expression is primarily in the Clara cell population and is not found in either alveolar type II cells or in the vascular endothelium, both targets for inducers in adult animals. Other factors besides postnatal hyperoxia, including maternal undernutrition during the last 5 days of pregnancy, retard Clara cell differentiation, but these effects appear to be reversible with time (88,108–110).

There is considerable indirect evidence to suggest that a number of growth factors, including TGF-α, EGF, basic fibroblast growth factor (FGF), insulinlike growth factors, and platelet-derived growth factor, may play roles in regulating bronchiolar epithelial differentiation (111,112). The EGF receptor (EGFr) has been detected in bronchiolar epithelium throughout pre- and postnatal lung development in rats and prenatal development in lambs (113, 114). EGFr has also been detected in human lung at midgestation (115,116) and has been detected in human and rat fetal lung extracts (113,117). Both ligands of EGFr, as well as TGF-α and EGF, have been detected immunohistochemically in bronchiolar epithelium in a number of species. EGF is barely detectable in bronchiolar epithelium of fetal humans (first and second trimesters), but is present in postnatal human lung (118). EGF has been reported in homogenates of lung from late fetal (21-day gestational age) and adult rats (119), and immunoreactive protein has been detected in bronchiolar epithelium throughout fetal development in rats and mice (120,121). TGF-α has been detected in bronchiolar epithelium of midgestational humans (122). It can be extracted and mRNA can be detected in fetal rat lung homogenates (123). Late fetal (21-day gestational age) and adult rat lung contains EGF (119). TGF-α is found in bronchiolar epithelium of fetal rats (120). Platelet-derived growth factor receptor has also been detected in bronchiolar epithelium during most of the prenatal stages of lung development (115,116). Basic FGF and its receptor are found in bronchiolar epithelium during most of fetal rat lung development (124). Both the FGF receptor and the protein appear to colocalize in the epithelium and adjacent interstitial compartments. There is some suggestion that insulinlike growth factors are involved in aspects of epithelial development in bronchioles (125). These growth factors may play a role in autocrine regulation because both receptors and the proteins themselves appear within the bronchiolar epithelium. They also may play a paracrine role because growth factor protein appears to be distributed to interstitial cell components, fibroblasts, and smooth muscle surrounding bronchiolar epithelium, during various stages of lung development. At present, there is no direct evidence that any of these factors influence bronchiolar epithelial maturation. There is, however, evidence that pharmacological doses of EGF alters branching morphogenesis in mice (126), enhances differentiation of alveolar type II cells in fetal rabbits, monkeys, and sheep (33,127,128) and alters the differentiation of tracheal epithelium in rhesus monkeys (60). Additional study is needed to determine what role any of these growth factors or receptors may play in differentiation of bronchiolar epithelium.

REFERENCES

1. Plopper CG, Thurlbeck WM. Growth, aging and adaptation. In: Murray JF, Nadel JA, eds. *Textbook of respiratory medicine,* vol 1. Philadelphia: WB Saunders, 1994;36–49.
2. Pinkerton KE, Gehr P, Crapo JD. Architecture and cellular composition of the air–blood barrier. In: Parent RA, ed. *Comparative biology of the normal lung.* Boca Raton, FL: CRC, 1992;121–128.
3. Goldin GV, Hindman HM, Wessells NK. The role of cell proliferation and cellular shape change in branching morphogenesis of the embryonic mouse lung: analysis using aphidicolin and cytochalasins. *J Exp Zool* 1984;232:287–296.
4. Roman J, McDonald JA. Expression of fibronectin, the integrin α 5, and α-smooth muscle actin in heart and lung development. *Am J Respir Cell Mol Biol* 1992;6:472–480.
5. Schuger L, Skubitz APN, O'Shea KS, Chang JF, Varani J. Identification of laminin domains involved in branching morphogenesis: effects of anti-laminin monoclonal antibodies on mouse embryonic lung development. *Dev Biol* 1991;146:531–541.
6. Durham PL, Snyder JM. Characterization of α-1, β-1 and γ–1 laminin subunits during rabbit fetal lung development. *Dev Dyn* 1995;203:408–421.
7. Sinkin RA, Sanders RS, Horowitz S, Finkelstein JN, Lomonaco MB. Cell-specific expression of fibronectin in adult and developing rabbit lung. *Pediatr Res* 1995;37:189–195.
8. Roman J. Effects of calcium channel blockade on mammalian lung branching morphogenesis. *Exp Lung Res* 1995;21:489–502.
9. Partanen A. *Current topics in developmental biology.* San Diego: Harcourt Brace Jovanovich, 1990.
10. Cardoso WV, Williams MC, Mitsialis SA, Joyce-Brady M, Rishi AK, Brody JS. Retinoic acid induces changes in the pattern of airway branching and alters epithelial cell differentiation in the developing lung *in vitro. Am J Respir Cell Mol Biol* 1995;12:464–476.
11. McBride JT. Architecture of the tracheobronchial tree. In: Parent RA, ed. *Treatise on pulmonary toxicology:* comparative biology of the normal lung. Boca Raton, FL: CRC, 1991;49–61.
12. Plopper CG. Structural methods for studying bronchiolar epithelial cells. In: Gil J, ed. *Models of lung disease: microscopy and structural methods.* New York: Dekker, 1990;537–559.

13. Kay JM. Blood vessels of the lung. In: Parent PA, ed. *Comparative biology of the normal lung.* Boca Raton, FL: CRC, 1991;163–172.

14. Plopper CG, ten Have-Opbroek AAW. Anatomical and histological classification of the bronchioles. In: Epler GR, ed. *Diseases of the bronchioles.* New York: Raven Press, 1994;15–25.

15. Tyler NK, Plopper CG. Epithelial differentiation of the terminal and respiratory bronchiolar epithelium in the lungs of fetal rhesus monkeys. *Anat Rec* 1989;225:297–309.

16. Plopper CG, Hyde MM. Epithelial cell of bronchioles. In: Parent R., ed. *Comparative biology of the normal lung.* Boca Raton, Florida: CRC, 1992; 85–92.

17. Sannes PL. Basement membrane and extracellular matrix. In: Parent RA, ed. *Comparative biology of the normal lung.* Boca Raton, FL: CRC, 1992;129–144.

18. ten Have-Opbroek AAW. The structural composition of the pulmonary acinus in the mouse. *Anat Embryol* 1986;174:49–57.

19. ten Have-Opbroek AAW. Lung development in the mouse embryo. *Exp Lung Res* 1991;17:111–130.

20. ten Have-Opbroek AAW, Otto-Verberne CJM, Dubbeldam JA, Dykman JH. The proximal border of the human respiratory unit, as shown by scanning and transmission electron microscopy and light microscopical cytochemistry. *Anat Rec* 1991;229:339–354.

21. Tyler NK, Hyde DM, Hendrickx AG, Plopper CG. Morphogenesis of the respiratory bronchiole in rhesus monkey lungs. *Am J Anat* 1988; 182:215–223.

22. Tyler NK, Hyde DM, Hendrickx AG, Plopper CG. Cytodifferentiation of two epithelial populations of the respiratory bronchiole during fetal lung development in the rhesus monkey. *Anat Rec* 1989;225:297–309.

23. Smolich JJ, Stratford BF, Maloney JE, Ritchie BC. New features in the development of the submucosal gland of the respiratory tract. *J Anat* 1978;127:223–238.

24. Krause WJ, Leeson CR. The postnatal development of the respiratory system of the opossum. I. Light and scanning electron microscopy. *Am J Anat* 1973;137:337–354.

25. Leigh MV, Gambling TM, Carson JL, Collier AM, Wood RE, Boat TF. Postnatal development of tracheal surface epithelium and submucosal glands in the ferret. *Exp Lung Res* 1986;10:153–169.

26. Plopper CG, Weir AJ, Nishio SJ, Cranz DL, St. George JA. Tracheal submucosal gland development in the rhesus money, *Macaca mulatta*: ultrastructure and histochemistry. *Anat Embryol* 1986;174:167–178.

27. Thurlbeck WM, Benjamin B, Reid L. Development and distribution of mucus glands in the foetal human trachea. *Br J Dis Chest* 1961;55: 54–64.

28. Bucher U, Reid L. Development of the mucus-secreting elements in human lung. *Thorax* 1976;1961;16:219–225.

29. Tos M. Development of the tracheal glands in man. *Acta Pathol Microbiol Scand* 1966;185:1–30.

30. Tos M. Distribution and situation of the mucus glands in the main bronchus of human fetuses. *Anat Anz* 1968;123:481–485.

31. Lamb D, Reid L. Acidic glycoproteins produced by the mucus cells of the bronchial submucosal glands in the fetus and child: a histochemical autoradiographic study. *Br J Dis Chest* 1972;66:248–253.

32. Jeffery PK, Reid LM. Ultrastructure of airway epithelium and submucosal glad during development. In: Hodson WA, ed. *Development of the lung.* New York: Marcel Dekker, 1977;87–134.

33. Plopper CG, St. George JA, Cardoso W, Wu R, Pinkerton K, Buckpitt AR. Development of airway eipthelium: patterns of expression for markers of differentiation. *Chest* 1992;101(Suppl):2S–5S.

34. Leeson TS. The development of the trachea in the rabbit, with particular reference to its fine structure. *Anat Anz* 1961;110:S214–S223.

35. Kawamata S, Fujita H. Fine structural aspects of the development and aging of the tracheal epithelium of mice. *Arch Histol Jpn* 1983;46: 355–372.

36. Emura M, Mohr U. Morphological studies on the development of tracheal epithelium in the Syrian gold hamster. *Z Versuchstierkd* 1975; 17:14–26.

37. McDowell EM, Newkirk C, Coleman B. Development of hamster tracheal epithelium. I. A quantitative morphologic study in the fetus. *Anat Rec* 1985;213:429–447.

38. Plopper CG, Alley JL, Weir AL. Differentiation of tracheal epithelium during fetal lung maturation in the rhesus monkey *Macaca mulatta.* *Am J Anat* 1986;175:59–71.

39. Boyden EA. The development of the lung in the pig-tail monkey (*Macaca nemestrina* L.). *Anat Rec* 1976;186:15–38.

40. Lane BP, Gordon RE. Regeneration of rat tracheal epithelium after mechanical injury. I. The relationship between mitotic activity and cellular differentiation. *Proc Soc Exp Biol Med* 1974;145:1139–1144.

41. Boren HG, Paradise LJ. Cytokinetics of lung. In: Harris CC, ed. *Pathogenesis and therapy of lung cancer,* vol 10. New York: Marcel Dekker, 1978;369–418.

42. Donnelly HM, Haack DG, Heird CS. Tracheal epithelium: cell kinetics and differentiation in normal rat tissue. *Cell Tissue Kinet* 1982;15: 119–130.

43. Keenan KP, Combs JW, McDowell EM. Regeneration of hamster tracheal epithelium after mechanical injury. *Virchows Arch* [B] 1982;41: 215–229.

44. Evans MJ, Shami SG. Lung cell kinetics. In: Massaro D, ed. *Lung cell biology.* New York: Marcel Dekker, 1989;41:1–31.

45. McDowell EM, Trump BF. Conceptual review: histogenesis of preneoplastic and neoplastic lesions in tracheobronchial epithelium. *Surv Synth Pathol Res* 1984;2:235–279.

46. Rutten AA, Beems RB, Wilmer JW, Feron VJ. Ciliated cells in vitamin A-deprived culture hamster tracheal epithelium to divide. *In Vitro Cell Dev Biol* 1988;24:931–935.

47. Jeffrey PK, Ayers M, Rogers D. The mechanisms and control of bronchial mucus cell hyperplasia. In: Chantler EN, Elder JB, Elstein M, eds. *Mucus in health and disease II.* New York: Plenum, 1982; 399–409.

48. Copra DP. Squamous metaplasia in organ culture of vitamin A-deficient hamster trachea: cytokinetic and ultrastructural alterations. *J Natl Cancer Inst* 1982;69:895–905.

49. Evans MJ, Moller PC. Biology of airway basal cells. *Exp Lung Res* 1991;17:513–531.

50. Plopper CG, St. George J, Pinkerton RE, et al. Tracheobronchial epithelium *in vivo*: composition, differentiation and response to hormones. In: Thomassen DG, Nettesheim P, eds. *Biology, toxicology and carcinogenesis of respiratory epithelium.* New York: Hemisphere, 1990;6–23.

51. Hislop A, Muri DCF, Jacobsen M, Simon G, Reid L. Postnatal growth and function of the pre-acinar airways. *Thorax* 1972;27:265–274.

52. Burrington JD. Tracheal growth and healing. *J Thorac Cadiovasc Surg* 1978;76:453–458.

53. Basbaum C, Jany B. Plasticity in the airway epithelium. *Am J Physiol* 1990;259:L38–L46.

54. Keenan KP, Wilson TS, McDowell EM. Regeneration of hamster tracheal epithelium after mechanical injury. IV. Histochemical, immunocytochemical and ultrastructural studies. *Virchows Arch* [B] 1983;43: 213–240.

55. Johnson NF, Hubbs AF. Epithelial progenitor cells in the rat trachea. *Am J Respir Cell Mol Biol* 1990;3:579–585.

56. Terzaghi M, Nettesheim P, Williams ML. Repopulation of denuded tracheal grafts with normal, preneoplastic, and neoplastic epithelial cell population. *Cancer Res* 1978;38:4546–4553.

57. Inayama Y, Hook GER, Brody AR, et al. The differentiation potential of tracheal basal cells. *Lab Invest* 1988;58:706–717.

58. Inayama Y, Hook GER, Brody AR, Jetten AM, Gray T, Nettesheim P. *In vitro* and *in vivo* growth and differentiation of clones of tracheal basal cells. *Am J Pathol* 1989;134:539–550.

59. Johnson NF, Hubbs AF, Thomassen DG. Epithelial progenitor cells in the rat respiratory tract. In: Thomassen DG, Nettesheim P, eds. *Biology, toxicology and carcinogenesis of respiratory epithelium.* Washington, DC: Hemisphere, 1990;88–98.

60. St. George JA, Read LC, Cranz DL, Tarantal AF, George-Nascimento C, Plopper CG. Effect of epidermal growth factor on the fetal development of the tracheobronchial secretory apparatus in rhesus monkey. *Am J Respir Cell Mol Biol* 1991;4:95–101.

61. Buton TE, Plopper CG. Triamcinolone-induced structural alterations in the development of the lung of the fetal rherus macaque. *Am J Obst Gyn* 1984;148:203–219.

62. Wu R, Groelke JW, Chang LY, Porter ME, Smith D, Nettesheim P. Effects of hormones on the multiplication and differentiation of tracheal epithelial cells in culture. In: Sirbasku D, Sato GH, Pardee A, eds. *Growth of cells in hormonally defined media.* Cold Spring Harbor, NY: Cold Spring Harbor Laboratory, 1982;641–656.

63. Wu R, Smith D. Continuous multiplication of rabbit tracheal epithelial cells in a defined hormone-supplemented medium. *In Vitro* 1982;18:800–812.

64. Wu R. *In vitro* differentiation of airway epithelial cells. In: Schiff LJ,

ed. *In vitro* models of respiratory epithelium. Boca Raton, FL: CRC, 1986;1–26.

65. Robinson CB, Wu R. Culture of conducting airway epithelial cells in serum-free medium. *J Tissue Cult Method* 1991;13:95–102.

66. Lee TC, Wu R, Brody AR, Barrett JC, Nettesheim P. Growth and differentiation of hamster tracheal epithelial cells in culture. *Exp Lung Res* 1983;6:27–45.

67. Wu R, Nolan E, Turner C. Expression of tracheal differentiated functions in a serum-free hormone-supplemented medium. *J Cell Physiol* 1985;125:167–181.

68. Kim KC, Rearick JI, Nettesheim P, Jetten AM. Biochemical characterization of mucin secreted by hamster tracheal epithelial cells in primary culture. *J Biol Chem* 1985;260:4021–4027.

69. Wu R, Plopper CG, Cheng PW. Mucin-like glycoprotein secreted by cultured hamster tracheal epithelial cells: biochemical and immunological characterization. *Biochem J* 1991;277:713–718.

70. Wu R, Martin WR, St. George JA, et al. Expression of mucin synthesis and secretion in human tracheobronchial epithelial cells grown in culture. *Am J Respir Cell Mol Biol* 1990;3:467–478.

71. Adler KB, Cheng PW, Kim KC. Characterization of guinea pig tracheal epithelial cells maintained in biphasic organotypic culture: cellular composition and biochemical analysis of released glycoconjugates. *Am J Respir Cell Mol Biol* 1990;2:145–154.

72. Wu R, Sato GH, Whitcutt JM. Developing differentiated epithelial cell cultures: airway epithelial cells. *Fund Appl Toxicol* 1986;6:680–689.

73. Adler KB, Schwarz JE, Whitcutt MJ, Wu R. A new chamber system for maintaining differentiated guinea pig respiratory epithelial cells between air and liquid phases. *Biotechniques* 1987;5:462–465.

74. Whitcutt MJ, Adler KB, Wu R. A biphasic chamber system for maintaining polarity of differentiation of cultured respiratory tract epithelial cells. *In Vitro Cell Dev Biol* 1988;24:420–428.

75. DeJong PM, Van Strekenburg MAJA, Hesseling SC, et al. Ciliogenesis in human bronchial epithelial cells cultured at the air–liquid interface. *Am J Respir Cell Mol Biol* 1994;10:271–277.

76. Gray TE, Guzman K, Davis CW, Abdullah LH, Nettesheim P. Mucociliary differentiation of serially passaged normal human tracheobronchial epithelial cells. *Am J Respir Cell Mol Biol* 1996;14:104–112.

77. Wolbach SB, Howe PR. Tissue changes following deprivation of fat-soluble A vitamin. *J Exp Med* 1926;42:753–781.

78. Wong YC, Buck RC. An electronic microscopic study of metaplasia of the rat tracheal epithelium in vitamin A deficiency. *Lab Invest* 1971;24:55–66.

79. Harris CC, Silverman T, Jackson F, Boren HG. Proliferation of tracheal epithelial cells in normal and vitamin A-deficient Syrian golden hamsters. *J Natl Cancer Inst* 1973;51:1059–1062.

80. Sporn MI, Clamon GH, Dunlop NJ, Newton DL, Smith JM, Saffiotti U. Activity of vitamin A analogues in cell cultures of mouse epidermis and organ cultures of hamster trachea. *Nature* 1975;253:47–49.

81. Fell HB, Mellanby E. Metaplasia produced in cultures of chick ectoderm by high vitamin A. *J Physiol* 1953;119:470–488.

82. McDowell EM, Ben T, Coleman B, Chang S, Newkirk C, DeLuca LM. Effects of retinoic acid on the growth and morphology of hamster tracheal epithelial cells in primary culture. *Virchows Arch [B]* 1987;54:38–51.

83. DeLuca LM, McDowell EM. Effects of vitamin A status on hamster tracheal epithelium *in vivo* and *in vitro*. *Food Nutr Bull* 1989;11:20–24.

84. McDowell EM, DeSanti AM, Newkirk C, Strum JM. Effects of vitamin A-deficiency and inflammation on the conducting airway epithelium of Syrian golden hamsters. *Virchows Arch [B]* 1990;59:231–242.

85. Kopan R, Fuchs E. The use of retinoic acid to probe the relation between hyperproliferation-associated keratins and cell proliferation in normal and malignant epidermal cells. *J Cell Biol* 1989;109:295–307.

86. Plopper CG, Alley JL, Serabjit-Singh CJ, Philpot RM. Cytodifferentiation of the nonciliated bronchiolar epithelial (Clara) cell during rabbit lung maturation: an ultrastructural and morphometric study. *Am J Anat* 1983;167:329–357.

87. ten Have-Opbroek AAW, DeVries ECP. Clara cell differentiation in the mouse: ultrastructural morphology and cytochemistry for surfactant protein A and Clara cell 10 kD protein. *Microsc Res Tech* 1993;26:400–411.

88. Massaro GD. Nonciliated bronchiolar epithelial (Clara) cells. In: Massaro D, ed. *Lung cell biology*. New York: Marcel Dekker, 1989;81–114.

89. Ito T, Newkirk C, Strum JM, McDowell EM. Modulation of glycogen stores in epithelial cells during airway development in Syrian golden hamsters: a histochemical study comparing concanavalin A binding with the periodic acid–Schiff reaction. *J Histochem Cytochem* 1990;38:691–697.

90. Cardoso W, Stewart LG, Pinkerton KE, et al. Secretory product expression during Clara cell differentiation in the rabbit and rat. *Am J Physiol* 1993;8:L543–L552.

91. Plopper CG, Weir AJ, Morin D, Chang A, Philpot RM, Buckpitt AR. Postnatal changes in the expression and distribution of pulmonary cytochrome P450 monooxygenases during Clara cell differentiation in the rabbit. *Mol Pharmacol* 1993;44:51–61.

92. Strum JM, Singh G, Katyal SL, McDowell EM. Immunochemical localization of Clara cell protein by light and electron microscopy in conducting airways of fetal and neonatal hamster lung. *Anat Rec* 1990;227:77–86.

93. Strum JM, Ito T, Philpot RM, DeSanti AM, McDowell EM. The immunocytochemical detection of cytochrome P-450 monooxygenase in the lungs of fetal, neonatal, and adult hamsters. *Am J Respir Cell Mol Biol* 1990;2:493–501.

94. Ji CM, Plopper CG, Witschi HP, Pinkerton KE. Exposure to sidestream cigarette smoke alters bronchiolar epithelial cell differentiation in the postnatal rat lung. *Am J Respir Cell Mol Biol* 1994;11:312–320.

95. Katyal SL, Singh G, Brown WE, Kennedy AL, Squeglia N, Wong-Chong ML. Clara cell secretory (10 kdaltons) protein: amino acid and cDNA nucleotide sequences, and developmental expression. *Prog Respir Res* 1990;25:29–35.

96. Strum JM, Compton RS, Katyal SL, Singh G. The regulated expression of mRNA for Clara cell protein in the developing airways of the rat, as revealed by tissue *in situ* hybridization. *Tissue Cell* 1992;24:461–471.

97. Singh G, Katyal SL. Secretory proteins of Clara cells and type II cells. In: Parent RA, ed. *Comparative biology of the normal lung.* Boca Raton, FL: CRC, 1992;93–108.

98. Singh G, Katyal SL, Wong-Chong ML. A quantitative assay for a Clara cell-specific protein and its application in the study of development of pulmonary airways in the rat. *Pediatr Res* 1986;20:802–805.

99. Smith BT. Lung maturation in the fetal rat: acceleration by injection of fibroblast–pneumonocyte factor. *Science* 1979;204:1094–1095.

100. Sepulveda J, Velasquez BJ. Study of the influence of NA-872 (Ambroxol) and dexamethasone on the differentiation of Clara cells in albino mice. *Respiration* 1982;43:363–368.

101. Massaro D, Massaro G. Dexamethasone accelerates postnatal alveolar wall thinning and alters wall composition. *Am J Physiol* 1986;251:R218–R224.

102. Phelps DS, Floros J. Dexamethasone *in vivo* raises surfactant protein B mRNA in alveolar and bronchiolar epithelium. *Am J Physiol* 1991;260:L146–L152.

103. Fernandez-Renau D, Lombardero M, Nieto A. Glucocorticoid-dependent uteroglobin synthesis and uteroglobin mRNA levels in rabbit lung explants cultured *in vitro*. *Eur J Biochem* 1984;144:523–527.

104. Lombardero M, Nieto A. Glucocorticoid and developmental regulation of uteroglobin synthesis in rabbit lung. *Biochem J* 1981;200:487–494.

105. Devereux TR, Fouts JR. Effect of pregnancy or treatment with certain steroids on N,N-dimethylaniline demethylation and N-oxidation by rabbit liver or lung microsomes. *Drug Metab Dispos* 1975;3:254–258.

106. Devereux TR, Fouts JR. Effect of dexamethasone treatment on N,N-dimethylaniline demethylation and N-oxidation in pulmonary microsomes from pregnant and fetal rabbits. *Biochem Pharmacol* 1977;27:1007–1008.

107. Fouts JR, Devereux TR. Developmental aspects of hepatic and extrahepatic drug-metabolizing enzyme systems: microsomal enzymes and components in rabbit liver and lung during the first month of life. *J Pharmacol Exp Ther* 1972;183:458–468.

108. Massaro GD, McCoy L, Massaro D. Development of bronchiolar epithelium: time course of response to oxygen and recovery. *Am J Physiol* 1988;254:R755–R760.

109. Massaro GD, Olivier J, Massaro D. Brief perinatal hypoxia impairs postnatal development of the bronchiolar epithelium. *Am J Physiol* 1989;257:L80–L85.

110. Massaro GD, McCoy L, Massaro D. Hyperoxia reversibly suppresses

development of bronchiolar epithelium. *Am J Physiol* 1986;251: R1045–R1050.

111. Jetten AM. Growth and differentiation factors in tracheobronchial epithelium. *Am J Physiol* 1991;260:L361–L373.

112. Kelley J. Cytokines of the lung. *Am Rev Respir Dis* 1990;141: 765–788.

113. Strandjord TP, Clark JG, Madtes DK. Expression of TGF-α, EGF, and EGF receptor in fetal rat lung. *Am J Physiol* 1995;11:L384–L389.

114. Johnson MD, Gray ME, Carpenter G, Pepinsky RB, Stahlman MT. Ontogeny of epidermal growth factor receptor and lipocortin-1 in fetal and neonatal human lungs. *Hum* Pathol 1990;21:182–191.

115. Caniggia I, Liu J, Han R, et al. Fetal lung epithelial cells express receptors for platelet-derived growth factor. *Am J Respir Cell Mol Biol* 1993;9:54–63.

116. Han RNN, Liu J, Tanswell K, Post M. Ontogeny of platelet-derived growth factor receptor in fetal rat lung. *Microsc Res Tech* 1993;26: 381–388.

117. Nexo E, Kryger-Baggesen N. The receptor for epidermal growth factor is present in human fetal kidney, liver and lung. *Regul Pept* 1989;26:1–8.

118. Stahlman MT, Orth DN, Gray ME. Immunocytochemical localization of epidermal growth factor in the developing human respiratory system and in acute and chronic lung disease in the neonate. *Lab Invest* 1989;60:539–547.

119. Raaberg L, Poulsen SS, Nexo E. Epidermal growth factor in the rat lung. *Histochemistry* 1991;95:471–475.

120. Johnson MD, Gray ME, Carpenter G, Pepinsky RB, Sundell H, Stahlman MT. Ontogeny of epidermal growth factor receptor/kinase and of lipocortin-1 in the ovine lung. *Pediatr Res* 1989;25:535–541.

121. Snead ML, Luo W, Oliver P, et al. Localization of epidermal growth factor precursor in tooth and lung during embryonic mouse development. *Dev Biol* 1989;134:420–429.

122. Strandjord TP, Clark JG, Hodson WA, Schmidt RA, Madtes DK. Expression of transforming growth factor-α in mid-gestation human fetal lung. *Am J Respir Cell Mol Biol* 1993;8:266–272.

123. Kida K, Utsuyama M, Takizawa T, Thurlbeck WM. Changes in lung morphologic features and elasticity caused by streptozotocin-induced diabetes mellitus in growing rats. *Am Rev Respir Dis* 1983;128:125–131.

124. Han RNN, Liu J, Tanswell AK, Post M. Expression of basic fibroblast growth factor and receptor: immunolocalization studies in developing rat fetal lung. *Pediatr Res* 1992;31:435–440.

125. Stiles AD, d'Ercole AJ. The insulin-like growth factors and the lung. *Am J Respir Cell Mol Biol* 1990;3:93–100.

126. Warburton D, Seth R, Shum L, et al. Epigenetic role of epidermal growth factor expression and signaling in embryonic mouse lung morphogenesis. *Dev Biol* 1992;149:123–133.

127. Catterton WZ, Escobedo MB, Sexson WR, Gray ME, Sundell HW, Stahlman MT. Effect of epidermal growth factor on lung maturation in fetal rabbits. *Pediatr Res* 1979;13:104–108.

128. Sundell HW, Gray ME, Serenius FS, Escobedo MB, Stahlman MT. Effects of epidermal growth factor on lung maturation in fetal lambs. *Am J Pathol* 1980;100:707–726.

129. Plopper CG, Weir AJ, Nishio SJ, et al. Elevated susceptibility to 4-ipomeanol cytotoxicity in immature Clara cells of neonatal rabbits. *J Phar Exptl Ther* 1994;269:867–88.

130. Meyrick B, Reid L. In: Hodson A, ed. *Development of the lung.* New York: Dekker, 1977;135–214.

Asthma, edited by P.J. Barnes, M.M. Grunstein,
A.R. Leff, and A.J. Woolcock.
Lippincott–Raven Publishers, Philadelphia © 1997.

▪ 16 ▪

Postmortem Pathology

James C. Hogg and Richard G. Hegele

Normal Anatomy	**Functional Consequences of Airway Remodeling in**
Pathologic Anatomy	**Asthma**

In his discussion of asthma in the first edition of his classic textbook of medicine, Osler wrote: "We have no knowledge of the morbid anatomy of true asthma. Death during the [acute] attack is unknown" (1). The notion that asthma was a comparatively benign condition with virtually no mortality prevailed well into this century (2), but reports of unexplained increases in asthma mortality, especially since the mid- to late 1980s, have resulted in a fundamental rethinking of this issue (3–7). Results of epidemiologic studies have suggested that these apparent increases in asthma mortality are not artifacts of diagnosis or classification, and have occurred despite (or perhaps because of) advances in therapy (3,8). Overall, there is considerable interest in elucidating the possible mechanisms of fatal asthma. To provide a comprehensive perspective about the evolution of knowledge concerning the postmortem pathology of asthma, we first discuss the normal anatomy of the tracheobronchial tree and provide an historical review of reports pertaining to the pathologic findings observed in patients who die of asthma.

NORMAL ANATOMY

Some of the important anatomic features of the normal human tracheobronchial tree are summarized in Fig. 1. Examination of the bronchogram (Fig. 1A) shows that it is possible to trace pathways from the trachea to the alve-

oli of different lengths depending on the lung segment in which the airways are located. The quantitative data that support this concept were contributed by Horsfield et al. (9), who showed (Fig. 1B) that the number of generations of airway branching points from the trachea to the lobular airways leading to the alveolar surface varies from 8 to 24, depending on the pathway taken. The airways in these pathways narrow at different rates in relation to their length, and Weibel (10) showed that the small bronchi and bronchioles 2 mm in diameter are spread from the 4th to the 14th generations of airway branching (Fig. 1C) and that the increase in the number of airways in each generation of branching rapidly expands the total cross-sectional area of the airways in the peripheral lung beyond the 2 mm airways (Fig. 1D). These anatomic features optimize the central conducting airways for bulk flow and provide the large cross-sectional area needed for rapid diffusion of O_2 and CO_2 between the conducting airways and the gas-exchanging surface.

As visualized under the light microscope, the structure of the conducting airways can be considered in terms of compartments that have functionally important implications (11). These compartments include the airway epithelium and subepithelial connective tissue (often referred to as "submucosa" or "lamina propria," despite the absence of a separate muscularis mucosa and muscularis propria in the airway wall), the smooth muscle, and the adventitia (12). Bronchi are defined by the presence of a fibrocartilage layer external to the smooth muscle and tubuloalveolar glands that communicate with the airway lumen via ducts. By contrast, membranous bronchioles are airways that lack cartilage in their walls and have no associated alveolated structure; respiratory bronchioles have a mixture of bronchial epithelial and alveolated surface (13). The bronchial epithelial lining consists of pseudostratified, ciliated columnar epithelial cells admixed

J. C. Hogg: Department of Pathology, University of British Columbia; and St. Paul's Hospital, Vancouver, British Columbia V6Z 1Y6 Canada.

R. G. Hegele: Department of Pathology and Laboratory Medicine, Pulmonary Research Laboratory, University of British Columbia; and St. Paul's Hospital, Vancouver, British Columbia V6Z 1Y6 Canada.

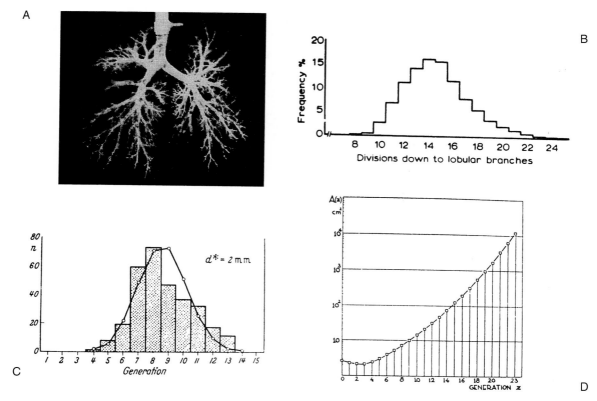

FIG. 1. A: A normal postmortem bronchogram from a 19-year-old man who died suddenly for reasons unrelated to the lung. **B:** Number of divisions down to the lobular branches. (From Horsfield K, Cumming G. Morphology of the bronchial tree in man. *J Appl Physiol* 1968; 24:373–383.) **C:** Generations in which 2-mm airways are located. (From Weibel ER. *Morphometry of the human lung.* New York: Academic Press, 1963.) **D:** Cross-sectional area at each generation. (From ref. Weibel ER. *Morphometry of the human lung.* New York: Academic Press, 1963.) Comparison with C shows that there is a marked increase in cross-sectional area beyond airways that are 2 mm in diameter.

with goblet cells that covers the lumen and extends into the mucous glands. The epithelium gradually becomes cuboidal in the bronchioles and has a reduced number of ciliated cells as the alveolar surface is approached (14). The basal aspect of airway epithelial cells is attached to a thin basement membrane (80–90 nm width) that contains primarily type IV collagen and elastin. By transmission electron microscopy, the thin basement membrane or basal lamina can be distinguished readily from the underlying subepithelial connective tissue, which contains abundant fibrillar collagen and elastic fibers. Quantitative studies (15,16) of the airways summarized in Figure 2 show that the trachea and mainstem bronchi of normal persons consist of approximately 30% cartilage, 15% mucous glands, and 5% smooth muscle, with the remainder taken up by a connective tissue matrix and the bronchial vascular and lymphatic systems. With progression toward the periphery of the bronchial tree, the amount of cartilage and glands decreases, and the percentage of smooth muscle increases from 5% of wall tissue in the central bronchi to about 20% of the total wall thickness in the bronchioles. The degree to which the

smooth muscle surrounds the airway lumen varies according to site, such that the airway smooth muscle is located within the posterior membranous sheath of the trachea and mainstem bronchi but surrounds the entire lumen of the airway in the bronchioles. Consequently, the same degree of muscle shortening has a smaller effect on the caliber of the trachea and central airways than on the distal bronchi and bronchioles (17). The adventitial layer consists of loose bundles of collagen admixed with blood vessels, lymphatics, and nerves. Rather than representing isolated units in space, the conducting airways can interact with the surrounding lung parenchyma, for example through alveolar attachments distributed along the circumference of the adventitia. An important functional property of these alveolar attachments is their ability to limit the amount of airway narrowing to bronchoconstrictor agents particularly at higher lung volumes (18).

The arteries, which supply the bronchial tissue of the left lung, originate from the ventral side of the upper part of the thoracic aorta. The right bronchial arterial supply is more variable in its origin and may arise from the first to third intercostal artery, the right internal

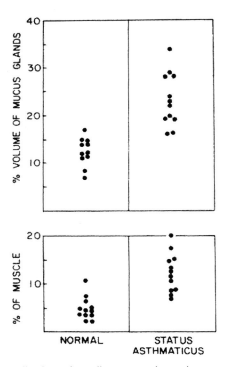

FIG. 2. Distribution of cartilage muscle and mucous glands at each airway generation. Note that the cartilage and mucous glands disappear and that the bronchioles defined by the absence of these elements have the greatest percentage of wall thickness taken up by muscle. (Data replotted from Dunnill MS, Massarella GR, Anderson JA. A quantitative anatomy of the bronchi in normal subjects, in status asthmaticus, in chronic bronchitis and in emphysema. *Thorax* 1969;24:176–179.)

mammary artery, or the right subclavian artery (14,19). Miller's classic anatomic studies (14) showed that two to three arterial branches accompany each of the larger bronchi and that anastomoses between these branches form an arterial plexus that runs at right angles to the muscle layer. Small branches of this plexus penetrate the smooth muscle layer to form a capillary network that has the same long axis as the bronchial tree. These capillaries empty into venous radicals, which form a venous plexus between the airway smooth muscle and the epithelial basement membrane. Short branches extend from this plexus through the muscle layer to form a second plexus of larger vessels along the outer surface of the airway smooth muscle. In some species, this outer plexus contains large venous sinuses that can extend into the submucosal layer of the major bronchi, where there is no smooth muscle between the cartilage and epithelium (20). The venous drainage of the first two or three subdivisions of the bronchial tree is into the azygous and hemiazygous venous systems, such that blood empties into the right atrium of the heart and enters the pulmonary circulation. By contrast, most of the intrapulmonary bronchial venous flow drains into the pulmonary circulation, thereby emptying into the left atrium and entering the systemic circulation (14,19). Airways disease markedly increases the anastomotic flow between pulmonary and bronchial vascular systems, but the degree to which this occurs in asthma has not been adequately studied.

PATHOLOGIC ANATOMY

A classic postmortem finding in patients who have died from status asthmaticus is that the lungs are markedly hyperinflated when the thorax is opened (Fig. 3). This hyperinflation is due to air trapping caused by widespread plugging of the airways that extends from the segmental and subsegmental airways to the smaller bronchi and bronchioles (21). The gross appearance of the cut surface of the asthmatic lung is usually intact and thus contrasts sharply with the parenchymal destruction observed on the cut surface of hyperinflated emphysematous lungs.

Histologic examination of the airways in patients who died of asthma reveals the presence of an inflammatory reaction with extensive remodeling of the airway wall, with relative sparing of the lung parenchyma (Fig. 4). Case reports describing the histopathologic features of asthma appeared in the late 19th century German literature (22,23); these observations were extended by Huber and Koessler's classic paper in 1922 on the pathology of asthma (24). These authors reviewed the existing literature on the pathology of asthma (a total of 15 asthmatic patients in whom descriptions of postmortem pathology were published) and provided histopathologic assessment of an additional six cases. They noted that the postmortem pathology in the lungs of asthmatic patients—in whom the cause of death could be reasonably attributed to asthma—was heterogeneous, but they established some common themes that have since been used as guidelines to distinguish asthma from other conditions. For example, the authors emphasized the presence of intraluminal mucous secretion, airway epithelial desquamation and repair (e.g., goblet cell metaplasia), presence of a thickened, "hyalinized" subepithelial basement membrane [later shown by electron microscopy and immunohistochemistry to consist of increased collagen fibrils and extracellular matrix, rather than thickening of the true basal lamina (25)], and airway inflammatory infiltrates consisting of an admixture of mononuclear cells and eosinophils. In addition, they extended previous descriptions of asthma pathology by commenting that the tenacious plugs filling the airway lumen consisted of an exudate of plasma and inflammatory cells, particularly eosinophils, as well as epithelial cells that have sloughed from the airway surface. Furthermore, in an early attempt at airway morphometry, Huber and Koessler used available technology (i.e., the eyepiece micrometer) to compare external airway diameters and

A

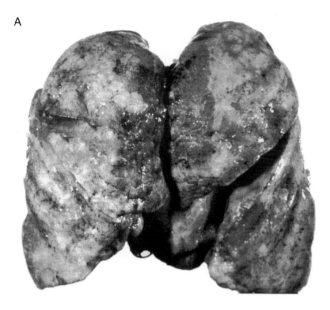

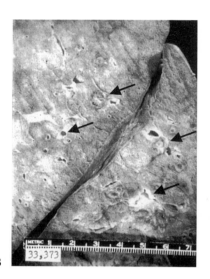

B

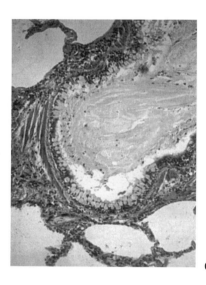

C

FIG. 3. Lungs excised at autopsy in a patient who died from status asthmaticus. **A:** Marked hyperinflation of the lungs as a consequence of air trapping. **B:** Cut surface of the lung in which there is extensive mucous plugging of airways with relatively intact lung parenchyma. **C:** Lung photomicrograph that shows mucous plugging within the lumen of a small bronchiole (H&E staining; magnification ×240).

calculated areas of the airway compartments between their six cases of asthma to seven nonasthmatic control patients. Based on the results of this morphometric evaluation, the authors concluded that in asthmatic patients:

> . . . the actual thickness of the walls of bronchi and bronchioli of more than 0.2 mm outside diameter is increased, as compared with similar structures in nonasthmatic persons. This difference is due to increased thickness of all layers from the epithelium to the outer fibrocartilaginous layer.

In summary, the work of Huber and Koessler represented a landmark in the description of the postmortem pathology of asthma that few subsequent reports have matched.

Over the next several decades, reports (26–33) of the pathologic findings of patients who died of asthma essentially confirmed and extended the original findings of Huber and Koessler to include hundreds of patients. The histopathologic features of asthma were consistent with an inflammatory process involving a mucosal surface (34); however, a major limitation of these studies was their focus on descriptive histopathologic observations, and the paucity of quantitative information resulted in many conclusions being speculative. For example, in his

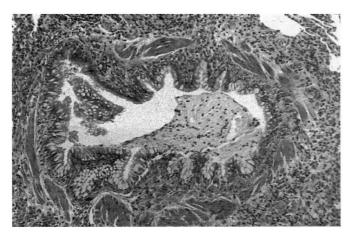

FIG. 4. Lung photomicrograph of a patient who died from status asthmaticus. The airway (*center*) shows the characteristic histopathologic features of asthma, including epithelial necrosis and sloughing in association with intraluminal mucus, apparent thickening of the subepithelial basement membrane, increased smooth muscle, and inflammatory infiltrates through the full thickness of the airway wall (H&E staining; magnification ×120).

assessment of postmortem gross and microscopic pathology of 20 patients who died from status asthmaticus, Dunnill (15) reasoned that the intraluminal mucous plugging, epithelial cell sloughing, and transudation of edema fluid from dilated submucosal capillaries into the lumen were the pertinent pathophysiologic mechanisms contributing to asthma death, whereas acute bronchospasm was not considered to be important because there was no associated crenation of the bronchial mucosa. This concept contrasted sharply with that advanced by pharmacologists who argued that the rapid reversibility of asthmatic attacks must mean that the major abnormality was in airway smooth muscle function. Overall, descriptive studies have provided valuable information for generation of hypotheses about the relative importance of smooth muscle to airway inflammation in fatal asthma, but they cannot provide definitive answers about the exact cause of death.

A long-standing concern to studying the histopathology of asthma was the effect of possible observer bias on interpretations of results, because a trained pathologist cannot be "blinded" to the airway lesions typical of asthma. In the late 1950s and early 1960s, major conceptual and technical advances in the field of stereology provided investigators with a method of quantifying the changes in airway morphometry in asthma and other lung diseases (10,35). The impact of advances in stereology cannot be overemphasized because investigators were able to make a fundamental shift from descriptive to quantitative studies of the histopathology of asthma. For example, Dunnill (36) applied a point-counting technique to assess volume fractions of airway compartments in lung tissue sections obtained from "normal" persons who

died suddenly, in comparison with patients who died from status asthmaticus, chronic bronchitis, or emphysema. The selection of airways for this analysis (i.e., segmental bronchi) was based on anatomic location rather than on airways having a similar internal or external diameter, because of concerns that pathologic lesions such as tissue fibrosis or edema could affect measurements of these diameters and thereby confound statistical comparisons. Dunnill used the point-counting technique to estimate the volume fractions of mucous glands, smooth muscle, cartilage, and "connective tissue" (i.e., every component not included under the other headings) and the results showed that the segmental bronchi of patients who died from status asthmaticus had significantly increased volume fraction of smooth muscle in comparison with the other three groups. In comparison with the "normal" controls, the segmental bronchi had a significantly higher volume fraction of mucous glands and a lower volume fraction of connective tissue. However, Dunnill did not transform the data to estimate the absolute volumes of the various compartments in the lung. As is discussed below, this issue becomes important when comparing results of point counting to subsequent work in which investigators attempted to measure absolute areas of the submucosal, smooth muscle, and adventitial compartments in the airways of asthmatic patients.

Despite the advances made possible by application of morphometric techniques on lung tissue sections from asthmatic patients, it remained unresolved whether the observed changes in airway morphometry were unique to the cases examined or whether similar changes could also be observed in other case series. There also was concern about whether the assumptions inherent in the morphometric techniques themselves could influence interpretations of results. These issues were investigated by Takizawa and Thurlbeck (16), who applied four morphometric methods to the same lung tissue sections of three groups of patients. By application of the point-counting technique to study airway morphometry in asthmatic patients, these investigators confirmed Dunnill's original results, and thereby strengthened the evidence for the changes in airway morphometry being generalized to fatal asthma. However, Takizawa and Thurlbeck also noted that application of other morphometric methods to the same lung tissue sections could produce marked discrepancies in interpretations of results. For example, results of the point-counting technique suggested that the airways of asthmatic patients showed mucous gland enlargement, but application of the Reid index (37) to the same material did not lead to this conclusion. Possible reasons for this apparent discrepancy were discussed, and the advantages and limitations of the various techniques were compared and contrasted. In summary, the work of Takizawa and Thurlbeck represented a further advance in airway morphometry, and there has since been considerable effort in the field of stereology to evaluate experimental designs and techniques in terms of producing statistical alpha errors (i.e., rejecting the null hypothesis when it is true) and beta errors (i.e., accepting the null hypothesis when it is false) (38–41).

Since the 1960s, the increased use of the rigid and subsequently the flexible bronchoscope permitted investigators to obtain bronchial biopsies from living asthmatic patients (42–44). This technical advance provided the opportunity to study differences between the lesions of fatal and nonfatal asthma, including asthma in clinical remission (45). A major contribution of the introduction of bronchial biopsies was that it brought pathologists and physiologists into agreement that airway inflammation was an important factor in the pathogenesis of reversible airflow obstruction and bronchial hyperresponsiveness (46). Coupled with the increased use of bronchoalveolar lavage, investigators have been able to perform increasingly elaborate characterization of inflammatory cells in the lungs of asthmatic patients (47). However, bronchoscopic methods have important limitations in that they do not sample the major site of the airways obstruction in the peripheral airways and only sample the inflammatory response based in the vascular plexus in the subepithelial tissue. Furthermore, bronchial biopsy does not provide information on airway dimensions and bronchoalveolar lavage and cannot localize the source of the inflammatory cells present in the bronchoalveolar lavage (BAL) fluid (see Chapter 18). With the apparent recent increases in asthma mortality, there has been renewed interest in studying autopsy material in patients who die of asthma.

One of the major problems with stereologic analysis of postmortem specimens has been the difficulty in obtaining a reliable estimate of airways size. This problem is the result of the fact that airway diameter depends on lung inflation and postmortem lung volume rarely is measured or controlled. This makes it impossible to relate postmortem measurements of airways size and physiologic measurements of airways function. The realization that the mucosa folds as the airways narrow allowed James et al. (48) to introduce a standard method of measuring airway perimeter that obviates this problem. In a study of airway perimeters and wall areas on serial lung slices that were exposed *in vitro* to either carbachol or theophylline, these investigators showed that the airway internal perimeter (P_i) remained constant during maximum contraction and relaxation. This provided investigators with a reliable standard for airway size that is independent of lung tissue handling or processing and consequently is useful for quantification of absolute perimeters and areas of airway compartments in asthma and in other airway diseases.

Over the last few years, several reports have described changes in airway morphometry in fatal asthma, in which investigators used P_i as an index of airway size (49–51). An important advance provided by these studies is the analysis of lungs from known asthmatic patients who died of nonrespiratory causes, in contrast with early publications of patients dying from status asthmaticus. Taken together, the results of these reports have established that the increased airway wall thickening observed in fatal asthma is related to increased thickness of all compartments of the airway wall and that the submucosal and adventitial thickening is in part related to increased volume of the bronchial microvasculature. However, the number of vessels per unit tissue was the same as observed in patients with nonfatal asthma and in patients with chronic obstructive pulmonary disease (COPD), such that the prominence of the vasculature observed in Figure 5 can probably be attributed to congestion rather than to a disproportionate increase in the number of vessels.

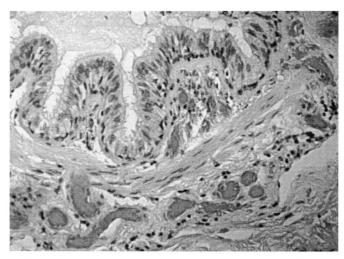

FIG. 5. Lung photomicrograph of a patient who died of asthma. The prominent blood vessels in the subepithelial connective tissue and in the adventitia are the result of vascular congestion rather than a disproportionate increase in the number of blood vessels in the airway wall (H&E staining; magnification ×360).

FUNCTIONAL CONSEQUENCES OF AIRWAY REMODELING IN ASTHMA

The concept that the same degree of smooth muscle shortening will cause greater reduction in airway caliber when the wall is thickened by disease has been suggested by several authors (52,53). Moreno and associates (53) calculated that the thickening of the airway wall caused by asthma would have only a minor effect on the lumen of a fully detailed airway. However, they also showed that when a modest increase in wall thickness was associated with smooth muscle shortening, the two factors acting in series produced an exaggerated encroachment of the wall on the lumen and markedly increased airways resistance. Subsequent studies by James et al. (54) showed that the increase in wall thickness caused smaller bronchi and bronchioles of asthmatic lungs to close when smooth muscle shortening was within the accepted normal range.

Wiggs et al. (55) examined the effects of these postmortem changes on airways function using a computer model. Their analysis showed that maximum stimulation of the smooth muscle caused airways resistance to increase and reach a plateau in the normal lung. This finding is consistent with the observations of Woolcock et al. (56), who reported that the changes in FEV_1 reach a plateau in normal persons who are stimulated maximally by inhaled bronchoconstrictors. However, in asthmatic lungs, stimulation of the airways and shortening of the smooth muscle results in a rapid increase in airways resistance without a plateau. By using the computer simulation to examine the central and peripheral airways separately, they were also able to show the increase occurred primarily in the peripheral airways and was probably due to widespread airways closure. The same model can also account for the rapid reversibility of the airway narrowing because muscle lengthening will rapidly increase airway caliber and decrease airways resistance. The concept that the peripheral airways are the major site of airways obstruction in asthma has now been confirmed by direct measurement in living patients by Yanai et al. (57).

The functional consequences of changes in the mucosa and lumen of the airways of asthmatics have been the most difficult to investigate, but they must be important determinants of airways caliber. In normal lungs, the surface tension in the lumen of the peripheral airways is low because these airways are lined by surfactant (58). Therefore, an exudate of plasma into the lumen as part of the inflammatory process should increase the surface tension and cause the airways to narrow and close; this tendency should be enhanced further by the secretion of mucus on to the airway surface. Lambert et al. (59) were the first to suggest that the normal folding pattern of the bronchial mucosa may also influence airway caliber, and they suggested that the replacement of the multiple mucosal folds in normal airways with fewer larger folds in asthma would reduce the caliber of the airway lumen. Wiggs et al. (60) have recently shown that the folding pattern of the airway is controlled by the relative stiffness of the subepithelial layer to the surrounding airway tissue. This suggests that the changes in the subepithelial connective tissue in the asthmatic airways might play a key role in determining the folding pattern. Many of the problems associated with mucosal function and its effect on airway caliber are currently under active investigational these analyses should lead to a better understanding of airways function in both health and disease.

CONCLUSIONS

In summary, the structural changes observed at postmortem examination in the airways of asthmatic patients are readily explained by an inflammatory process involving tissue with a mucous-secreting surface. The abnormal structure that results from this process can be attributed to the reorganization of the airway tissue components associated with this chronic inflammatory process. The end result is a generalized thickening of all the layers in the airway wall, with changes in the structure and function of the mucosal surface that enhance airways narrowing and closure. These structural changes act in series with airways smooth muscle shortening, and lengthening of the muscle can account for the reversible nature of the airways obstruction. Much remains to be learned about the details of the inflammatory process present in the airways and the abnormalities in both structure and function associated with it. It is also possible that new treatment capabilities will result from the insights gained into these mechanisms.

REFERENCES

1. Osler W. Bronchial asthma. In: *The Principles and Practice of Medicine*, 1st ed. New York: D. Appleton and Co, 1892;497–501.
2. Alexander HC. A historical account of death from asthma. *J Allergy* 1963;34:305–312.
3. Buist AS. Report of a symposium: asthma mortality: trends and determinants. *Am Rev Respir Dis* 1987;136:1037–1039.
4. Jackson B, Sears MR, Beaglehole R, et al. International trends in asthma mortality. *Chest* 1988;94:914–919.
5. Robin ED, Lewiston N. Unexpected, unexplained sudden death in young asthmatic subjects. *Chest* 1989;96:790–793.
6. Zach MS, Karner U. Sudden death in asthma. *Arch Dis Child* 1989;64:1446–1451.
7. Wassenfallen JB, Schaller MD, Feihl F, et al. Sudden asphyxic asthma: a distinct entity? *Am Rev Respir Dis* 1990;142:108–111.
8. Mao Y, Semenciw R, Morrison H, MacWilliam L, Davies J, Wigle D. Increased rates of illness and death from asthma in Canada. *Can Med Assoc J* 1987;137:620–624.
9. Horsfield K, Cumming G. Morphology of the bronchial tree in man. *J Appl Physiol* 1968;24:373–383.
10. Weibel ER. *Morphometry of the human lung.* New York: Academic Press, 1963.
11. Bai A, Eidelman DH, Hogg JC, et al. Proposed nomenclature for quantifying subdivisions of the bronchial wall. *J Appl Physiol* 1994;77:1011–1014.
12. Kuhn CI. Normal anatomy and histology. In: Thurlbeck WM, ed. *Pathology of the lung.* New York: Thieme Medical Publishers, 1988;11–50.
13. Plopper CG, Ten Have-Opbroek AAW. Anatomical and histological classification of the bronchioles. In: Epler GR, ed. *Diseases of the bronchioles.* New York: Raven Press, 1994;15–25.
14. Miller WS. *The lung,* 3rd ed. Springfield, IL: Charles C Thomas, 1943;73–84.
15. Dunnill MS. The pathology of asthma with special reference to changes in the bronchial mucosa. *J Clin Pathol* 1960;13:27–33.
16. Takizawa T, Thurlbeck WM. Muscle and mucous gland size in the major bronchi of patients with chronic bronchitis, asthma and asthmatic bronchitis. *Am Rev Respir Dis* 1971;104:331–336.
17. Wiggs BR, Moreno R, Hogg JC, Hilliam C, Pare PD. A model of the mechanics of airway narrowing. *J Appl Physiol* 1990;69:849–860.
18. Macklem PT. Bronchial hyporesponsiveness. *Chest* 1985;87:158S–159S.
19. Cudkowicz L. *The human bronchial circulation in health and disease.* Baltimore: Williams and Wilkins Company, 1968.
20. Hill P, Goulding D, Webber SE, Widdicombe JG. Blood sinuses in the submucosa of the large airways of sheep. *J Anat* 1989;162:235–247.
21. Rigler LG, Koucky. R. Roentgen studies of pathological physiology of bronchial asthma. *Am J Roetengenol* 1938;39:353–362.
22. Curschmann H. Ueber bronchiolitis exsudativa und ihr verhaltnis zum asthma nervosum. *Dtsch Arch Klin Med* 1882;32:1–34.

23. Leyden E. Ueber bronchial asthma. *Deutsch Militararzatl Ztschr* 1886;15:51.
24. Huber HL, Koessler KK. The pathology of bronchial asthma. *Arch Int Med* 1922;30:689–760.
25. Roche WR, Beasley R, Williams JH, Holgate ST. Subepithelial fibrosis in the bronchi of asthmatics. *Lancet* 1989;i:520–524.
26. Kountz WB, Alexander HL. Death from bronchial asthma. *Arch Pathol* 1928;5:1003–1019.
27. MacDonald IG. The local and constitutional pathology of bronchial asthma. *Ann Internal Med* 1933;6:253–277.
28. Craige B. Fatal bronchial asthma. *Arch Intern Med* 1941;67:399–410.
29. Earle BV. Fatal bronchial asthma. A series of fifteen cases with a review of the literature. *Thorax* 1953;8:195–206.
30. Houston JC, de Navasquez S, Trounce JR. A clinical and pathological study of fatal cases of status asthmaticus. *Thorax* 1953;8:207–213.
31. Cardell BS, Pearson RSB. Death in asthmatics. *Thorax* 1959;14:341–352.
32. Messer J, Peters GA, Bennet WA. Cause of death and pathological findings in 304 cases of bronchial asthma. *Dis Chest* 1960;38:616–624.
33. Richards W, Patrick JR. Death from asthma in children. *Am J Dis Child* 1965;110:4–21.
34. Florey H. The secretion of mucus and inflammation in mucus membranes. In: Florey H, ed. *General pathology*, 3rd edition. London: Lloyd-Luke Medical Books, 1962: 167–196.
35. Dunnill MS. Quantitative methods in the study of pulmonary pathology. *Thorax* 1962;17:320–328.
36. Dunnill MS, Massarella GR, Anderson JA. A comparison of the quantitative anatomy of the bronchi in normal subjects, in status asthmaticus, in chronic bronchitis and in emphysema. *Thorax* 1969;24:176–179.
37. Reid L. Measurement of the bronchial mucous gland layer: A diagnostic yardstick in chronic bronchitis. *Thorax* 1960;15:132–141.
38. Gundersen HJG, Osterby R. Optimizing sampling efficiency of stereological studies in biology: or "Do more less well". *J Microscopy* 1981;121:65–73.
39. Dunnill MS. Some statistical aspects of sampling in morphometry. *Analyt Quantit Cytol Histol* 1985;7:250–255.
40. Weibel ER. Measuring through the microscope: development and evolution of stereological methods. *J Microscopy* 1989;155(pt 3):393–403.
41. Chang L-Y, Mercer RR, Pinkerton KE, Crapo JD. Quantifying lung structure: experimental design and biologic variation in various models of lung injury. *Am Rev Respir Dis* 1991;143:625–634
42. Glynn AA, Michaels L. Bronchial biopsy in chronic bronchitis and asthma. *Thorax* 1960;15:142–153.
43. Cutz E, Levison H, Cooper DM. Ultrastructure of airways in children with asthma. *Histopathology* 1978;2:407–421.
44. Djukanovic R, Wilson JW, Lai CKW, Holgate ST, Howarth PH. The safety aspects of fiberoptic bronchoscopy, bronchoalveolar lavage, and endobronchial biopsy in asthma. *Am Rev Respir Dis* 1991;143:772–777.
45. Foresi A, Bortorelli G, Pesci A, Chetta A, Olivieri D. Inflammatory markers in bronchoalveolar lavage and in bronchial biopsy in asthma during remission. *Chest* 1990;98:528–535.
46. Djukanovic R, Roche WR, Wilson JW, et al. Mucosal inflammation in asthma. *Am Rev Respir Dis* 1990;142:434–457.
47. Robinson DS, Hamid Q, Ying S, et al. Predominant TH2-like bronchoalveolar T-lymphocyte population in atopic asthma. *N Engl J Med* 1992;326:298–304.
48. James AL, Hogg JC, Dunn LA, Pare PD. The use of internal perimeter to compare airway size and to calculate smooth muscle shortening. *Am Rev Respir Dis* 1988;138:136–139.
49. Saetta M, di Stefano A, Rosina C, Thiene G, Fabbri LM. Quantitative structural analysis of peripheral airways and arteries in sudden fatal asthma. *Am J Respir Crit Care Med* 1991;143:138–143.
50. Carroll N, Elliot J, Morton A, James A. The structure of large and small airways in nonfatal and fatal asthma. *Am J Respir Crit Care Med* 1993;147:405–410.
51. Kuwano K, Bosken CH, Pare PD, Bai TR, Wiggs BR, Hogg JC. Small airways dimensions in asthma and in chronic obstructive pulmonary disease. *Am Rev Respir Dis* 1993;148:1220–1225.
52. Friedman BJ. Functional anatomy of the bronchi. *Bull Pathophysiol Respir* 1972;8:545–551.
53. Moreno R, Hogg JC, Pare PD. Mechanics of airway narrowing. *Am Rev Respir Dis* 1986;133:1171–1180.
54. James AL, Pare PD, Hogg JC. The mechanics of airway narrowing in asthma. *Am Rev Respir Dis* 1989;139:242–246.
55. Wiggs BR, Moreno R, James A, Hogg JC, Pare PD. A model of the mechanics of airway narrowing in asthma. In: Kaliner MA, Barnes PJ, Persson KGA, ed. *Asthma: its pathology and treatment.* New York: Marcel Dekker, 1991;73–101.
56. Woolcock AJ, Salome CM, Yan K. The shape of the dose response curve to histamine in asthmatic and normal subjects. *Am Rev Respir Dis* 1984;130:71–75.
57. Yanai M, Sekizawa K, Ohrui T, Sasaki H, Takishima T. Site of airway obstruction in pulmonary disease: direct measurements of intrabronchial pressure. *J Appl Physiol* 1992;72:1016–1023.
58. Macklem PT, Proctor DF, Hogg JC. The stability of peripheral airways. *Respir Physiol* 1970;8:191–203.
59. Lambert R. The role of the bronchial basement membrane and airway collapse. *J Appl Physiol* 1991;71:666–673.
60. Wiggs BR, Hrousis CA, Drazen JM, Kamm RD. The implications of airway wall buckling in asthmatic airways. *Am J Respir Crit Care Med* 1994;149:A585.

Asthma, edited by P.J. Barnes, M.M. Grunstein, A.R. Leff, and A.J. Woolcock. Lippincott–Raven Publishers, Philadelphia © 1997.

▪ 17 ▪

Bronchial Biopsies

Annika Laitinen, Lauri A. Laitinen, and Ismo T. Virtanen

Developments in bronchoscopic, electron microscopic, and immunocytochemical techniques have been essential to the current increase in knowledge of airway pathology in asthmatic patients (1–7). Use of bronchial biopsies has led to considerable achievements in better understanding of the pathologic features of asthma and the underlying mechanisms of airway inflammation, mainly during the last decade. Bronchial biopsy techniques have limitations, however, and can be performed only in specialized centers for asthma patients (8). To conduct quantitative morphologic studies, bronchial biopsy specimens should be taken and processed by standardized methods (8). At the morphologic level, there is the possibility of artifactual destruction of the airway epithelium and mucosa during the procedure, which may confuse the interpretation of pathologic changes. Airway smooth muscle cannot in fact be systematically studied by the biopsy method. In this chapter, we review the studies that have provided information about airway histology and morphology by the bronchial biopsy technique.

INDICATIONS FOR INVESTIGATIVE BRONCHOSCOPY IN ASTHMA

The major scientific indications for investigational bronchoscopy of the tracheobronchial tree in asthmatic subjects are the following: (a) to investigate the morphologic, pathologic, immunologic, biochemical, molecular biologic, and neurobiologic factors important in understanding the pathogenesis and pathophysiology, and the clinical features of asthma; (b) to obtain information that can predict the natural history of asthma; (c) to investigate the effects of acute and chronic therapeutic and pathologic interventions on the morphology, cellular interactions, and biochemical events in the airways; (d) to study airway epithelial function *in situ* (8); and (e) to study cultured cells obtained from biopsies. This list is not entirely inclusive; other indications may exist, especially those based on the most recent research.

SAFETY CONCERNS

Because of the possibility of precipitating acute severe bronchial obstruction during a biopsy on an asthma patient, the following evaluations are recommended before initiating the procedure. A complete medical history and

A. Laitinen and I. T. Virtanen: Institute of Biomedicine, Department of Anatomy, University of Helsinki, FIN-00014 Helsinki, Finland.
L. A. Laitinen: Department of Medicine, University Central Hospital, SF-00290 Helsinki, Finland.

physical examination are essential, including information as to the severity and frequency of asthma attacks, current medications, and specific allergies. The severity and activity of the patient's illness should be ascertained by some assessment of the duration and frequency of acute episodes of asthma, the number and duration of hospitalizations, frequency of nocturnal awakenings, cicardian variations in lung function, medication requirements, or measures of the level of responsiveness to standard bronchoprovocation with metacholine, histamine, exercise, or isocapnic hyperventilation. The history of other coexisting medical conditions should be recorded, with special emphasis on the cardiovascular system. Laboratory data consisting of baseline pulmonary function studies that objectively measure the level of airflow obstruction and arterial oxygen saturation by oximetry are necessary before initiation of the bronchoscopic procedures. Arterial oxygen saturation, cardiac rhythm, and blood pressure always should be monitored during these procedures. Before studying patients with severe airflow obstruction, measurement of arterial blood gases may be indicated in addition to oximetry to exclude the presence of alveolar hypoventilation. In general, patients with asthma who have a history of acute severe respiratory failure with severe episodes of airflow obstruction should not be selected for biopsy studies (8).

Bronchial biopsies should be performed under direct vision. Biopsies or brushings of two to four areas have been performed without difficulty in patients with asthma. No data exist on either the indications for or safety of transbronchial lung biopsies in the investigation of obstructive airway disease, but this procedure is likely to be associated with a higher level of morbidity. The safety of repeat lavages and airway biopsies from different segments of the lung has been established (8). Two such procedures in a 6- to 24-h period have appeared to be well tolerated (9–11).

METHODOLOGIC PROBLEMS RELATED TO BRONCHIAL BIOPSY STUDIES IN ASTHMA

Since asthmatic patients seldom have lung surgery, fresh specimens can in principle be obtained only by bronchoscopy. Bronchoalveolar lavage (BAL) and biopsying the airway mucosa are the main possibilities for obtaining proper samples from the bronchial tree. In asthma, these sources seem to provide complementary information about pathologic processes in the airways in asthma. Spontaneous or induced sputum recently has been studied, as well, as an alternative noninvasive method (see Chapter 12). Biopsy, BAL, and sputum samples represent, however, different airway sites. In addition, information derived from these different techniques is quantitatively and to some extent qualitatively different, involving different processing procedures. Very few

studies have compared these three methods (12), but one of the major advantages of bronchial biopsy specimens in comparison to sputum and BAL is that biopsy samples represent material from the actual site of the disease. Table 1 summarizes some advantages and problems related to bronchial biopsies.

Since obtaining comparable material can be complicated by the different clinical phenotypes of asthma and the duration of the disease, as well as the medication used, careful patient characterization is essential in biopsy studies. Problems causing artifactual destruction of biopsy specimens can be reduced by use of the proper forceps and a proper biopsying technique, by immediate evaluation of the specimen size when it is removed from the forceps, by fast fixation, by orientation before embedding, and by careful further handling of the specimen.

To make studies comparable, the biopsy procedure and analysis should be standardized. The biopsy size that is crucial for further analysis of the specimen varies because of differences in forceps model and size and in biopsying technique. The handling procedure for the biopsy, fixation, cutting, and staining may differ among laboratories. Because of differences in quantitation methods used by different research groups, the inflammatory cell numbers can be counted and expressed in many different ways. The numbers of cells in biopsy specimens have been counted at a depth of 50 to 200 μm beneath the airway epithelium. Results will differ if inflammatory cells are not uniformly dispersed or depth of the biopsy is

TABLE 1. *Some characteristics of biopsy studies in asthma*

Positive
  Biopsy samples represent material from the actual site of the disease, although from a limited area.
  Specimens can be processed by several different methods such as light microscopy, electron microscopy, immunohistochemistry, biochemistry, and cell cultures.
  Quantitative information is available at cellular and histologic levels about tissue components and cellular infiltrates.
  Serial biopsy samples reveal pathophysiologic mechanisms behind the disease.
  Evaluation of changes in cellular and other parameters in drug intervention studies is possible.
Negative
  Small numbers of patients and healthy subjects have been studied, with a lack of reference material for both groups.
  The small size of specimens enables study of only restricted areas of the mucosa, and correlation validation is needed for the airways as a whole.
  Invasive, the method requires systemic and topical medication, and induces some degree of trauma in the airways.
  The method cannot be performed routinely and is difficult to use repeatedly to perform in normal subjects, with special skills required to master the technique properly.

insufficient (see Figs. 1 and 2). Cell counts have been expressed as cells per length of basement membrane (BM), as percentage of cells of 100 cells counted, as percentage of total cell numbers, and as cell numbers per square millimeter of airway mucosa (13–18). Such a diversity of methods in part explains why such differing results regarding cellular infiltrates have been published and makes comparisons between studies difficult.

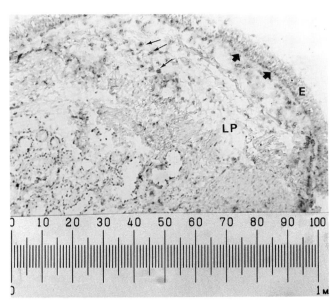

FIG. 2. Bronchial biopsy from a patient with asthma (same method as in Fig. 1). A monoclonal antibody is used to detect CD3+ lymphocytes (some of which are marked with *arrows*). The airway epithelium *(E)* surrounds the specimen. CD3+ lymphocytes are dispersed throughout the lamina propria *(LP)*. In the epithelium, many lymphocytes are located close to the epithelial basement membrane *(arrowheads)*. Scale bar, 1 mm (1,000 μm).

ACHIEVEMENTS WITH BRONCHIAL BIOPSIES IN ASTHMA RESEARCH

Recognition of Pathologic Changes in the Airway Mucosa

Little knowledge exists about the sequence of cellular events during the disease or of possible airway mucosal changes early in asthma. Morphologic studies of bronchial biopsy specimens (2,6,7,15,19,20) have led to the concept of asthma as an inflammatory airway disease.

Inflammation includes an increase in the number of inflammatory cells, cell destruction, edema formation, and an increase in the bronchial blood flow and in extravasation—all representing the outcome of the inflammatory reaction. So far, the primary cause, the site of damage, and mechanisms inducing the inflammatory reaction remain to be elucidated. In asthma, the main structures in the airway mucosa with tissue destruction as revealed by biopsy studies are the airway epithelium (Figs. 3 and 4) and vascular endothelium (Figs. 5 and 6) (1,2,13,16,19,22,23).

Structural Changes in the Airway Epithelium

To evaluate the epithelial structure in the bronchial biopsy specimen requires knowledge of the normal epithelium. The airway epithelium forms an interface be-

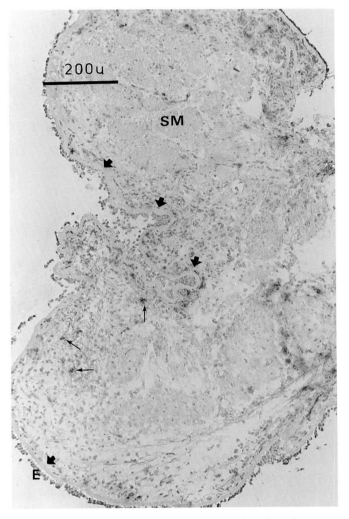

FIG. 1. Light microscopy. The specimen is taken from an asthmatic patient having had the disease for 7 months. Immediately after biopsy, the specimen was fixed in liquid nitrogen and later cut at 6-μm thickness with a cryostat. Alkaline phosphatase anti-alkaline phosphatase staining using a monoclonal antibody (AA1, Dako) against mast cell tryptase was done. The section shows the size obtainable with fiberoptic bronchoscopy technique. Only basal epithelial cells *(E)* are seen around the specimen. The subepithelial basement membrane is clearly visible *(arrowheads)*. The specimen contains many bundles of bronchial smooth muscle *(SM)*. The mast cells *(arrows)* are mainly close to the subepithelial basement membrane and also around the smooth muscle bundles. Scale bar, 200 μm.

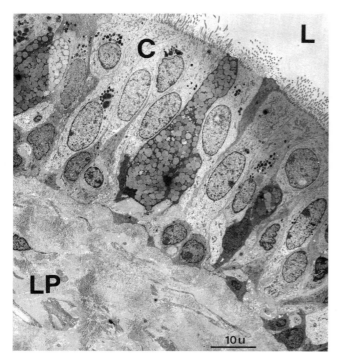

FIG. 3. Low-power transmission electron microscopy. The specimen is taken from the airway mucosa of a normal control subject. The picture shows normal pseudostrafied ciliated columnar epithelium. Most of the epithelial cells reaching the lumen are ciliated and few goblet cells are visible. There are no inflammatory cells in the lamina propria *(LP)*. *L,* airway lumen; *C,* ciliated cell. (Original magnification, ×2,000.) Scale bar, 10 μm. (From Laitinen LA, Laitinen A, Haahtela T. Airway mucosal inflammation even in patients with newly diagnosed asthma. *Am Rev Respir Dis* 1993;147:697–704, with permission.)

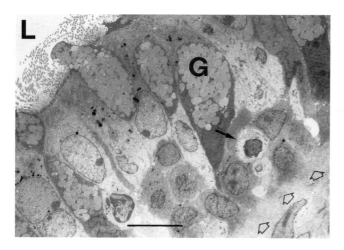

FIG. 4. The specimen is from an asthmatic patient having had the disease for less than 1 year. The airway epithelium exhibits goblet cell hyperplasia, the number of goblet cells *(G)* in the airway epithelium is increased, and the number of ciliated cells is decreased. A highly degranulated mast cell *(arrow)* is located intraepithelially close to the basement membrane *(arrowheads)*. *L,* airway lumen. (Original magnification, ×2,000.) Scale bar, 10 μm.

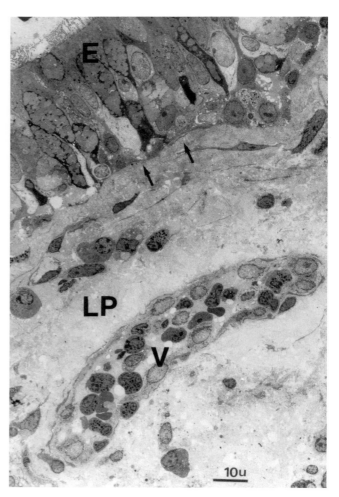

FIG. 5. Inflammatory cells both in the airway epithelium *(E)* and lamina propria *(LP)* in an asthmatic patient. Many eosininophils are visible in a longitudinally cut venule *(V)* close to the subepithelial basement membrane *(arrows)*. Some of the eosinophils are visible adhering to the vessel wall. (Original magnification, ×2,000.) Scale bar, 10 μm.

tween the external and internal environments, protecting against foreign substances such as microorganisms, allergens, and noxious chemicals and against excessive loss of heat and moisture. The defense function of the epithelium is established by a specific cellular organization of epithelial cells and their biochemical properties. The epithelial cells are bound by specific junctions including tight and adhering junctions and desmosomes (Figs. 7 and 8). The presence of ciliated cells in the epithelium is important in mucociliary transport (24,25). Current evidence has, however, implied that interactions between epithelial cells and the subepithelial connective tissue in the mucosa are important for normal homeostatic balance. The health and integrity of the airway epithelium may be important factors regulating the functions of connective tissue cells and the composition of the extracellular matrix (25–28). Recently the role of the airway epithe-

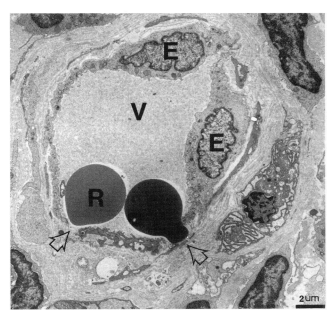

FIG. 6. Asthmatic patient. A postcapillary venule *(V)* in the lamina propria has 1-μm large gaps *(arrowheads)* between endothelial cells *(E)*. Two red blood cells *(R)* are penetrating through the gaps from the lumen to the connective tissue. (Original magnification, ×7,800.) Scale bar, 2 μm.

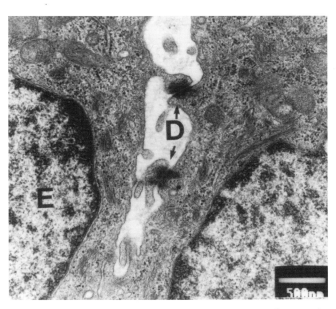

FIG. 7. A specimen from the airway epithelium of an asthmatic patient. The epithelial cells are bound tightly to each other by desmosomes *(D)*. Scale bar, 500 μm.

lium as a potential source of growth factors and agents capable of regulating airway smooth muscle tone has received attention.

Normal respiratory epithelium consists of pseudostratified ciliated columnar epithelium, with ciliated cells outnumbering the goblet cells. In general, no more than two layers of nuclei can be observed, with all of the cells of the epithelium resting on the basal lamina (Fig. 3). The four main cell types most often found in the normal human bronchial epithelium (24,29) are ciliated cells, basal cells, secretory (mucous or goblet) cells, and neurosecretory cells (Kultchitsky cells and amine-containing or APUD [amine precursor uptake decarboxylation] cells). The ciliated, secretory, and some of the neurosecretory cells extend into the lumen. The most numerous cell type in the normal human respiratory epithelium is the ciliated cell, with roughly three to five ciliated cells for every mucous cell (29,30). As many as ten ciliated cells to one goblet cell in the normal human airway epithelium have been described (31). Normal epithelium contains a few lymphocytes and nerve profiles near the lumen and BM. The so-called intermediate cell type referred to in the literature is either a preciliated or presecretory cell according to ultrastructural criteria, although an indeterminate cell type may exist (24,25,29).

In specimens from patients dying of status asthmaticus, it has been difficult to find normal areas of bronchial epithelium. One prominent feature is marked airway edema with shedding of airway columnar epithelial cells.

In many areas, only a layer of basal or reserve cells has been left on the basal lamina (32,33).

The application of endoscopic bronchial biopsy techniques has led to recognition of structural changes in the airway epithelium of asthmatic patients. Evaluated by both light microscopy and electron microscopy (EM), the first studies showed that mild-to-severe asthmatic patients have damaged airway epithelium (2,13,16). In addition to shedding of the columnar epithelial cells, the ciliated cell line has been reported to be the most elaborately affected cell type (1,19,33). Some possible mechanisms behind loss of epithelial integrity and shedding have only recently been elucidated, as described later in this chapter in conjunction with the BM and adhesion to the extracellular matrix.

An important question is the extent to which columnar epithelial cells are lost. The presence of shed epithelial cells in the sputum of asthmatic patients is well described in the form of creola bodies and Curschmann's spirals and has been considered a characteristic feature of asthma, being one of the first features described in airway pathology of asthma (34). In bronchial lavage, asthmatic patients have shown greater numbers of shed epithelial cells in the lavage fluid than do nonasthmatic control subjects (6). Based on histologic evaluations of biopsy specimens, several authors have reported epithelial shedding in the airways of mild-to-severe asthma (1,2,13,16). However, mechanical denudation of the epithelium caused by the biopsy procedure itself as occurs even in control subjects (19) may be difficult to distinguish from actual epithelial shedding caused by the dis-

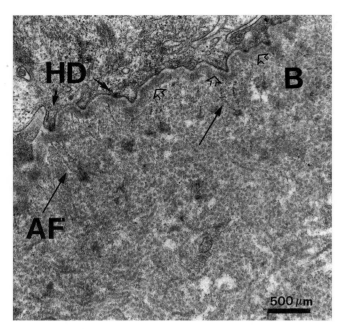

FIG. 8. The basal part of the epithelium. Epithelial cells adhere to the basement membrane *(B)* by hemidesmosomes *(HD).* The *open arrowheads* depict the basal lamina of the basement membrane. The *long thin arrows* show anchoring fibrils *(AF)* consisting of type VII collagen. In the basement membrane, they terminate to anchoring plaques. (Original magnification, ×31,000.) Scale bar, 500 µm.

ease. Unsolved problems with fiberoptic biopsy techniques causing artifactual loss of the epithelium have precluded quantitative assessment of the extent of epithelial shedding (13,35).

It has been difficult to secure evidence of structural epithelial changes other than airway epithelial shedding. Structural changes other than this could be detected when bronchial biopsies from newly diagnosed asthmatics were taken by means of rigid-tube bronchoscopy and studied by EM (18). The method enables the study of airway mucosa with less artifactual loss of the epithelial cells than with the fiberoptic technique. To establish epithelial structure, the number of cells touching the lumen were counted; the most discernible finding was that of goblet cell hyperplasia. The epithelium was made up of a greater than normal ratio of goblet to ciliated cells (Fig. 4).

In another EM study, bronchial biopsy specimens from patients with chronic asthma showed bronchial epithelium having an increased number both of tight junction openings and of widening of the intercellular spaces, a situation correlated with bronchial hyperresponsiveness. With increased density of eosinophils, the incidence of these epithelial parameters increased, suggesting that eosinophils are related to epithelial damage. No direct correlation was detected between lymphocytes and epithelial damage (16).

The Role of the Airway Epithelium in Airway Inflammation

Leukocyte recruitment to the site of inflammation depends on both chemotactic mechanisms and adherence of leukocytes to adhesion receptors on the vascular endothelium. Recent studies have implied that airway epithelial cells are involved in the inflammation of asthma and that the airway epithelium is an important target of the inflammatory process. On the other hand, epithelial cells may orchestrate the recruitment and activation of several different types of inflammatory cells by releasing chemotactic factors with proinflammatory properties and by expressing adhesion molecules (36–43).

Immunohistochemical and cell culture studies have shown that epithelial cells from asthmatics show an enhanced interleukin-8-like activity which is chemotactic for CD4+ T lymphocytes (42). Epithelial cells can express other potent inflammatory cytokines, such as granulocyte-macrophage colony-stimulating factor (GM-CSF), interleukin 6 (IL-6) (39–41), and a newly discovered chemokine monocyte chemoatractant protein 1 (MCP-1) (43), suggesting that they are in an activated state contributing to the inflammatory pathology of asthma. Bronchial epithelial cells can be induced to express IL-1 (36), IL-6, IL-8, GM-CSF, and MCP-1 (39,41) by treatment with IL-1 and tumor necrosis factor produced by activated macrophages. MCP-1 has been detected to be highly expressed on airway epithelial cells in asthmatic patients with a distribution similar to that of GM-CSF (43). That MCP-1 is a chemoattractant and activating agent for monocytes (44) suggests that it may play a role in macrophage recruitment, contributing to accumulation of macrophages in the bronchial epithelium. A paracrine feedback pathway thus may exist between the epithelial cells producing GM-CSF and MCP-1 and macrophages capable of producing IL-1.

Increased intercellular adhesion molecule 1 (ICAM-1) expression in bronchial epithelial cells in asthmatic patients in comparison to that of control subjects and chronic bronchitic patients has been described by Vignola and co-workers (45). Controversial findings have been published by Montefort and co-workers (46). Immunostaining for ICAM-1 was observed in both the epithelium and endothelium, and leukocyte adhesion molecule 1 in the endothelium, with no significant differences between bronchial biopsy specimens from asthmatics and normal volunteers (46).

Changes in Inflammatory Cells and Mediators in the Airway Mucosa in Asthma

Although many studies during the last decade have suggested that asthma is a chronic inflammatory disease characterized by increased mast cells, eosinophils, lymphocytes, and macrophages (3,5–7,14,16,17,47–49), conflicting findings have suggested no statistically significant differences in frequency of mast cells, eosinophils, lymphocytes, and neutrophils detected in the airway mucosa of atopic asthmatics in comparison to healthy controls (13).

Variable numbers of inflammatory cells in the airway mucosa in asthma include such findings as the following: The numbers of eosinophils (6,14,16) and neutrophils (6), but not of mast cells and lymphocytes, were significantly greater in the airway mucosa of mild allergic asthmatic patients (6,14) and in chronic asthmatic patients (16) in comparison to control subjects. Patients with mild atopic asthma exhibited significantly more mast cells in the air-

way mucosa, but no significant differences in the numbers of eosinophils and neutrophils, in comparison to control subjects (4). Airway inflammation characterized by more eosinophils and lymphocytes has been described in mild atopic asthmatics (48,49) and in newly defined asthmatic patients having had the disease for less than 1 year (18). Patients with mild asthma who formed a homogeneous group with respect to duration of asthma showed significant increases in inflammatory cell numbers in the airway mucosa and a clear difference in cell distribution between epithelium and lamina propria. Numbers of mast cells, eosinophils, lymphocytes, and macrophages in the airway epithelium of asthmatic patients were greater than in con-

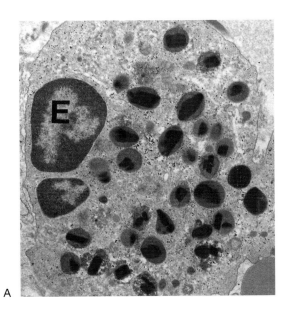
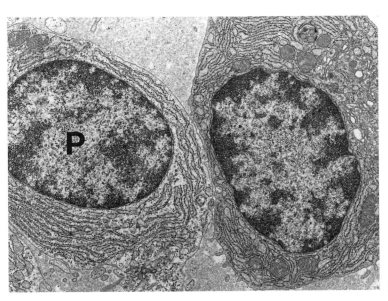
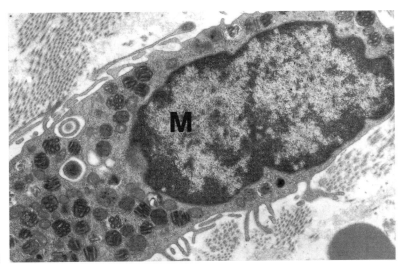
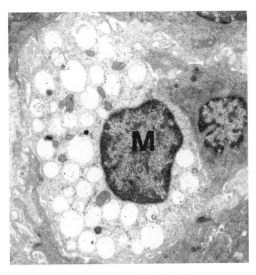

FIG. 9. Specific ultrastructural features of different types of mucosal cells. **A:** An eosinophil *(E)* with granules containing typical crystalloid cores. **B:** The ultrastructure of two plasma cells *(P)*, the cell cytoplasma containing lots of endoplasmic reticulum. **C:** A granulated mast cell *(M)* **(D)** in the airway mucosa of a control subject in comparison to a highly degranulated mast cell *(M)* in the airway epithelium of an asthmatic patient. (Magnification, ×13,000.)

trol subjects. Because the asthmatic patients had more eosinophils, lymphocytes, macrophages, and plasma cells in the lamina propria than did controls (Fig. 9A–D), it was concluded that asthma is an inflammatory process even at a clinically early stage of the disease and that, in asthmatic airways, there are signs of a general inflammatory response caused by more than one cell type (18).

The difference in composition of the cellular infiltrate found in asthma may depend upon several factors. A study comparing patients characterized clinically as having the extrinsic (EA) or intrinsic (IA) type of asthma (17) showed for IA an intense cellular infiltrate containing increased numbers of total lymphocytes (CD45+), CD3+, and CD4+ lymphocytes, CD68+ macrophages, IL-2 receptor-bearing cells (CD25+), total eosinophils (major basic protein), and EG2+ eosinophils in comparison to normal subjects. Similar increases occuring in EA patients in comparison to controls were noted only in the numbers of CD25+ and EG2+ eosinophils. In addition, a relationship was observed between asthma severity and magnitude of the eosinophil infiltrate. Recently, aspirin-sensitive asthmatics were shown to have significantly more mast cells (AA1) and total eosinophils (BMK13), and fewer macrophages (EMB11) in the airway mucosa than did nonaspirin-sensitive asthmatics (non-ASA) (50). The numbers of T lymphocytes (anti-CD3), activated eosinophils (EG2), and neutrophils (NP57) were, however, similar in both groups.

In addition to problems related to patient selection characteristics, purely technical issues may greatly influence quantitation results of biopsy specimens as mentioned earlier.

Clinical Importance of Airway Inflammation

The substantial individual variability in number of mast cells, eosinophils, lymphocytes, and neutrophils in the airway mucosa in asthma offers important clues to disease process. The regular occurrence of mast cells in the airway epithelium, even in mild asthmatics with short disease duration, suggests the importance of these cells in the initial stage of the disease (51). Pesci et al. (47), studying different histochemical characteristics of airway mast cells, suggested that there is progressive mast cell degranulation when mast cells move toward the airway lumen both in asthmatics and in control subjects, but that this degranulation is more evident in asthmatics, and that the number of degranulated mast cells in the airway epithelium is significantly greater in asthmatics than in controls. In both groups, granulated mast cells were absent from the epithelium whereas, in the lamina propria, granulated mast cells formed about one-third of the total in asthmatics and two-thirds of the total mast cells in normal subjects.

An increased eosinophil count has been found both in asthmatics with stable disease and in those with evidence of disease activity (52–54). In bronchial biopsy specimens, an increase in number of eosinophils in the bronchial mucosa has been related to increase in the asthma symptoms (53). Eosinophils thus may contribute to the pathophysiologic process responsible for a change from stable asthma into asthma exacerbation. The presence of a few neutrophils in the airway epithelium is probably a normal phenomenon because neutrophils may be found even in the lavage fluid of normal subjects (6). In a biopsy study of mild asthmatics, neutrophil numbers were actually greater in control specimens (6). Increased numbers of both neutrophils and eosinophils have been associated with late asthmatic response in allergen challenge tests (54). Chronic asthma of long duration in which there is lung function impairment may be associated with epithelial and mucosal neutrophil influx probably reflecting a far-advanced severe stage of the inflammatory process or even infection in the airways.

Basement Membrane and Extracellular Matrix Biopsy Evaluation

The BMs are thin layers of specialized extracellular matrix (ECM) forming a supporting structure on which epithelial cells grow. They not only provide mechanical support, but also influence cell-specific functions (55). At the EM level, the BM can be visualized as consisting of a lamina lucida and a lamina densa, which form the basal lamina, and a lamina reticularis (56). The major molecular components of BMs are collagen type IV, laminins, entactin/nidogen, and proteoglycans (55). These components are expressed in BMs throughout the body. In normal airway mucosa, the lamina reticularis is a rather thin, not very well defined, area, and its composition is not well known (57).

Not much is known about the ECM and BM in the airway mucosa of asthmatic subject (Fig. 10). Some studies have suggested that the subepithelial BM in asthmatics is thickened (13,57). Several other investigators also have described a thickened BM as characteristic of asthma (13, 57,58). It has been proposed that such thickening could be one cause of disease that is becoming more persistent. The components suggested as contributing to the thickening of the BM in asthma are collagen types I, III, V (57, 58), and VII and glycoproteins, fibronectin, and tenascin (59). The significance and reversibility of these changes in asthma remains unknown, but their accumulation may represent an imbalance between the ongoing inflammatory process and remodeling of the airway mucosa.

The Collagens

Collagenous proteins are the major constituents of ECMs. At least 18 different collagen types have been identified that contain at least one collagen triple helix as

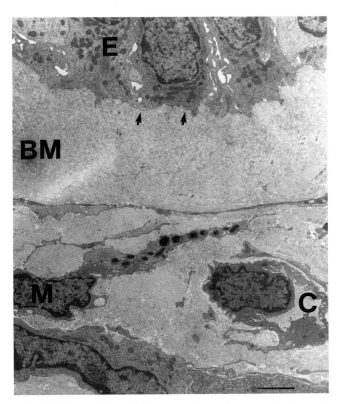

FIG. 10. The thickened basement membrane *(BM)* area in an asthmatic patient. The *arrowheads* depict the basal lamina part of the basement membrane. On the basal lamina are some epithelial *(E)* basal cells. Beneath the basement membrane are a mast cell *(M)* and a capillary *(C)*. (Original magnification, ×7,800.) Scale bar, 2 μm.

a structural motif. After purification of the traditional collagen molecule types I–VIII, use of complementary deoxyribonucleic acid (cDNA)-derived amino acid sequences to obtain their primary structure has enabled identification of the number of proteins with collagenous domains to expand rapidly (60).

Collagen type IV is an important component of the BM and forms networks by self-assembly. Laminin–entactin/nidogen complexes self-associate into less ordered aggregates (55). Laminin and type IV collagen serve as substrates for migration and attachment for epithelial cells (61,62). Roche et al. (57), using polyclonal antisera, showed that in asthma the abnormally dense lamina reticularis beneath the bronchial epithelium is composed of interstitial collagen types I, III, and V and fibronectin and suggested that it is produced by myofibroblasts lying beneath the epithelium (63). No change in the collagen type IV expression was noted (57).

The lamina reticularis contains anchoring fibrils that may connect the BM to the underlying stromal connective tissue. Type VII collagen is the only member of the long-chain collagens and is found solely within anchoring fibrils (64). One end of the collagen type VII is in-

serted into the lamina densa of the subepithelial BM, and the other end is inserted in the stroma within an anchoring plaque containing type IV collagen material (Fig. 8). In the normal human bronchi, type VII collagen detected immunohistochemically was found to be restricted to the BM underlying the epithelium (65). By immunohistochemistry, the staining pattern of the type VII collagen pattern was detected to be broader in the subepithelial BM of asthmatic patients than in that of the control subjects (66).

The Laminins

Among the BM components, special interest has recently been focused on laminins (Lns). The Lns form a family of asymmetric cross-shaped proteins and, according to present nomenclature, contain one α-chain (α1–α5), one β-chain (β1–β3), and one γ-chain (γ1–γ2). The first Ln characterized, Ln-1, was isolated from a murine tumor, and at least 10 different Lns are now known (67). In the adult human bronchi, immunoreactivity against Ln chains α1, β1, and γ1 has been demonstrated in the BM, blood vessels, and smooth muscle cells. Ln α3- and β3-chains are seen in the bronchial BM, the Ln α2-chain occasionally in nerves, and the Ln β2-chain in only smooth muscle cells and blood vessels (68). These studies suggest that bronchial BM contains both Ln-1 and Ln-5, the latter being able to interact with collagen type VII.

Bronchial biopsies have made possible the study of Ln chain distribution in asthmatic airways, and several Ln-binding integrins such as α2β1, α3β1, α6β1, and α6β4 (Fig. 11) have thus been detected on human bronchial epithelial cells (69,70). A recent biopsy study showed no difference in Ln α1 distribution and thickness among the seasonal and chronic asthmatic patients and controls, but the thickness of Ln β2 immunoreactivity in the BM was significantly greater in chronic and occupational asthma than in controls. Interestingly, the Ln α2-chain, which is negative in normal adult airways, stained positive in the BM of occupational and chronic asthma patients, but not in mild asthmatics or control subjects (71). Since the Ln α2- and β2-chains appear to function only during morphogenesis of the lungs (68), some mechanism in the asthmatic process seems to activate the expression of these Ln chains and possibly shift the combination of normally occurring Ln-1 (α1β1γ1) to a different Ln combination. This change could disturb epithelial integrity and binding since the assembly forms of Ln (Ln-2, α2β1γ1; and Ln-4, α2β2γ1) containing the Ln α2-chain normally do not bind to the common Ln integrin receptor integrin α2β1. Thus, increased expression of these Lns in asthma might lead to weakened cellular attachment and loss of epithelial cells. On the other hand, loss of BM attachment and integrin signaling is known to lead to apoptotic death of epithelial cells.

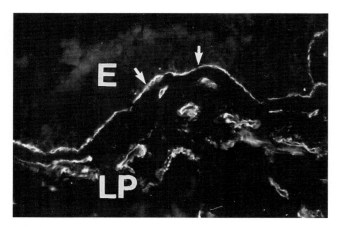

FIG. 11. Indirect immunofluorescence. The monoclonal antibody against integrin α₆-subunit shows its location at the epithelial *(E)* basement membrane border. Also, small blood vessels in the lamina propria *(LP)* show a positive reaction for α₆-integrin subunit. (Original magnification, ×300.)

The laminins are especially interesting for the pathology of asthma, since they also may serve as substrates for the attachment and spread of several inflammatory cells important in asthma, such as monocytes (72), T lymphocytes (73), mast cells (74), and eosinophils (75). Eosinophils have been shown to adhere to ECM components by different receptors such as integrin α6β1 receptor for Ln

(76) and cell surface antigen α4β1 (very late antigen [VLA]-4) for fibronectin (75). The eosinophil–fibronectin interaction has been shown to prolong eosinophil survival (75); the effect of the eosinophil–Ln interaction is not known.

Tenascin and Fibronectin

Tenascin is a large ECM glycoprotein that is highly expressed during embryonic development especially at the epithelial–mesenchymal border (77,78) but, in adult tissues, its expression is mostly downregulated. It reemerges during wound healing and inflammatory processes (77). In bronchial biopsies from asthmatic patients, tenascin expression has been reported to be increased in the BM area in comparison to that of normal subjects (Fig. 12A and B)(59). Reexpression of tenascin may be related to the inflammatory process in the airways or some similar type of mechanisms normally functioning during the embryonic development of the conducting airways. Brewster and co-workers (63) demonstrated in asthma the presence of fibronectin in the abnormally thickened LF beneath the bronchial epithelium. Tenascin and fibronectin have opposite functions in many cell models, tenascin being inhibitory, whereas Fn promotes adhesion, for instance of bronchial epithelial cells (77). Cultured human bronchial epithelial cells produce both of these ECM glycoproteins (79,80).

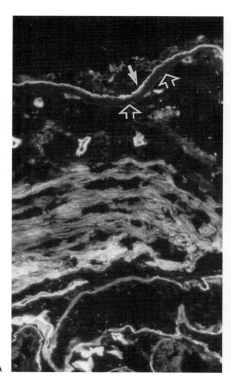
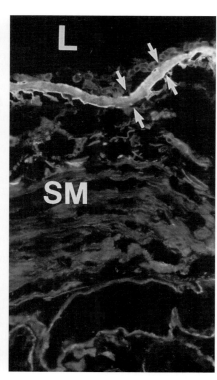

FIG. 12. Indirect immunofluorescence. Asthmatic patient. The specimen has been examined by double-label immunostaining by exposing the specimen first to a monoclonal antibody to tenascin, followed by FITC conjugate, and then to the rabbit antiserum to laminins, followed by the rhodamine isothiocyanate-coupled goat–anti-rabbit IgG antibody. The pictures taken with different filters demonstrate laminin immunoreactivity **(A)** on top of that of tenascin **(B)**. The laminin immunoreactivity is seen as a thin line subepithelially *(white arrowhead)* corresponding to the basal lamina part of the basement membrane. The *open white arrowheads* depict the lower border of the basement membrane. The tenascin immunoreactivity seems to occupy the whole basement membrane area (between *four white arrowheads*). *L,* airway lumen; *SM,* smooth muscle. (Original magnification, ×300.)

BRONCHIAL BIOPSIES AND BRONCHIAL PROVOCATION TESTS

The dynamics of airway responses can be studied by taking bronchial biopsy specimens before and after bronchial provocations. Because the sulfidopeptidyl leukotrienes had been implicated as contributers to the pathophysiology of asthma, Laitinen and co-workers (9) assessed the effects of inhaled leukotriene E₄ (LTE₄) in comparison to those of methacholine provocation on airway mucosal morphology in asthmatic patients. The second specimen was taken 4 h after the provocation, because the airway hyperresponsiveness induced by LTE₄ is at its highest between 4 and 7 h after its inhalation (81). Similar decreases in specific airway conductance were produced with inhalation of methacholine and of LTE₄. Specimens taken 4 h after the LTE₄ provocation showed a marked increase in total eosinophil count and a slight increase in the number of neutrophils in the lamina propria in every patient. Methacholine provocation, however, produced no detectable consistent changes in leukocyte numbers (81). The mechanism by which inhaled LTE₄ caused the recruitment of such large numbers of eosinophils is unclear. Bronchoconstriction per se caused no cellular infiltration, because airflow obstruction provoked by methacholine did not induce leukocytic recruitment. As methacholine is widely used in clinical testing of bronchial hyperresponsiveness, it may be of importance that after methacholine inhalation no changes in common cell parameters occurred. This result should, however, be tested on larger numbers of patients and compared with tissue morphology after histamine diphosphate inhalation. This study emphasized the potential of antisulfidopeptidyl leukotriene drugs as possible "steroid-sparing drugs" (9).

Many recent biopsy studies have focused on the mechanisms by which inflammatory cells are recruited into the airways in asthma. Biopsy specimens have been taken via the fiberoptic bronchoscope in conjunction both with local and with inhalation allergen challenges. One advantage of local segmental challenging is considered to be the possibility of controlling the site of the challenge and also the possibility of using the other bronchus at the same time as the control. The role of adhesion molecules in allergic inflammation has been studied by bronchial biopsy specimens taken in connection with local allergen challenges; these studies have provided evidence that late-phase selective eosinophilia is associated with increased expression of vascular adhesion molecule 1 (VCAM-1). Montefort and co-workers (10) showed an influx of mast cells, neutrophils, eosinophils, and CD3+ lymphocytes into the airway mucosa of atopic asthma 6 h after allergen challenge. These changes were accompanied by increased expression of endothelial ICAM-1 and E-selectin, but not of VCAM-1. The authors suggested that this early influx of inflammatory cells was facilitated by release of preformed cytokines from activated mast cells (10). Similar results were reported by Bentley et al. (11) 24 h after local allergen challenge. A positive correlation was observed between the increased expression of ICAM-1 and VCAM-1 in the epithelium and the eosinophilic infiltrate.

Crimi and co-workers (82) studied the mechanics behind early and late asthmatic responses by taking bronchial biopsy and bronchoalveolar lavage samples from allergic patients with a history of exercise-induced asthma. Bronchial biopsy specimens taken 3 h after a methacholine or an exercise challenge test showed exercise to be associated with mast cell degranulation and with an influx of eosinophils in the airway lumen. The percentage of degranulating mast cells was significantly greater after the exercise than after the metacholine challenge. Similar results were earlier shown in the bronchial mucosa after late-phase asthmatic response to an allergen (83)

BIOPSIES AND CELL CULTURES

For primary epithelial cell cultures, epithelial cells from the trachea or bronchi have been isolated by several methods such as explant cultures, enzymatic dissociation, and bronchial brushings (84–88). Only a few studies (mainly related to mechanisms behind the inflammatory process) have been conducted on cultured bronchial epithelial cells from asthmatics. Bellini and co-workers (42) showed that cultured epithelial cells from asthmatic patients expressed enhanced IL-8 activity for CD4+ lymphocytes. With increased knowledge about extracellular matrix components required for the growth, phenotypic differentiation, and secretory functions of epithelial cells, recognition of primary abnormalities in their functions in asthma could lead to better understanding of the basic mechanisms behind development of asthma.

BIOPSY STUDIES IN THE EVALUATION OF TREATMENT EFFECTS

Morphologic studies of bronchial biopsy specimens provide a reliable assessment of the local conditions at the site of the asthmatic inflammation, as well as a means to study the effects of drug therapy.

Because asthma is now believed to be an inflammatory disease of the airways, there has been an increase in the use of anti-inflammatory drugs, with several open studies conducted on the effects of inhaled corticosteroid treatment on airway mucosa in asthmatic patients. Lundgren and co-workers (21) examined the influence of inhaled corticosteroids on the bronchial mucosa in biopsy samples from six asthmatic patients before and after 10 years of steroids inhaled daily, in comparison with biopsy specimens from six healthy subjects, and demonstrated in samples taken before the treatment that asthmatic patients showed a significant increase in inflammatory cell counts in comparison to those of healthy controls. In all asthma patients, scanning EM showed a reduced coverage by cilia, but no difference in the thickness of the BM or the thickness of the epithelium between asthmatic patients and control subjects. Long-term treatment with inhaled steroids significantly decreased inflammation and reduced epithelial damage, but the patients still retained bronchial hyperreactivity. As at the beginning of the study, no difference appeared in the thickness of the BM between controls and asthmatics treated with inhaled corticosteroids (19). Jeffery and co-workers (89), comparing inhaled budesonide and terbutaline therapy, showed that 4 weeks of treatment of atopic asthmatics with budesonide reduced airway inflammation. The numbers of mast cells and eosinophils in the airway mucosa were reduced, but there was no change in lymphocyte numbers or in the thickness of the lamina reticularis. In another study, six weeks of inhalation therapy with beclometasone diproprionate produced a clinical improvement in asthma associated with a significant reduction in airway epithelial and

mucosal mast cells and eosinophils and submucosal T lymphocytes (90).

In a comparative double-blind study, Laitinen and co-workers (91) demonstrated that after 3 months therapy with inhaled budesonide the reduction of inflammatory cell numbers in the mucosa was associated with restoration of the normal epithelium (Fig. 13A and B). Trigg and co-workers (58) showed in a placebo-controlled study that inhaled beclomethasone-diproprionate therapy for 4 months reduced the number of toluidine-blue-staining mast cells and total and activated eosinophils in biopsy specimens. The GM-CSF expression in the bronchial epithelium was significantly reduced, as was the thickness of type III collagen deposition in the lamina reticularis in the steroid-treated group in comparison to the placebo group. No change in helper or activated helper T cells was detected.

A recent study (59) evaluated the effect of inhaled budesonide treatment on airway subepithelial fibrosis in seasonal asthmatics by immunohistochemistry. During 4 weeks of treatment, the glycoprotein tenascin content in

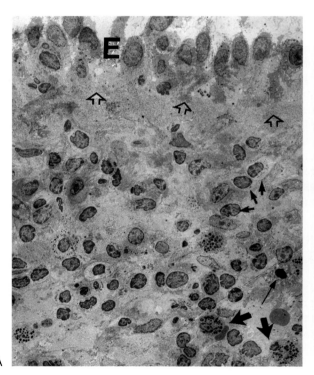 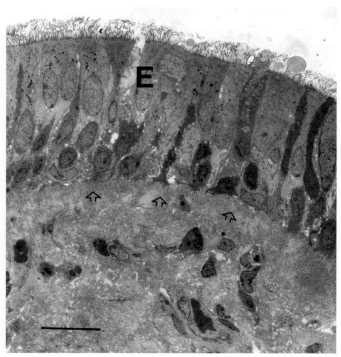

A   B

FIG. 13. Low-power transmission electron microscopy. **A:** Airway mucosa in a biopsy specimen obtained from an asthmatic patient with extrinsic asthma of 9 months. The epithelium is greatly damaged; only basal cells are visible on the basement membrane *(open arrowheads)*. An intense inflammatory reaction with eosinophils *(thick arrowheads)*, lymphocytes *(thin arrowheads)*, and plasma cells and mast cells *(long thin arrow)* is visible in the lamina propria. **B:** Airway of same patient after 3 months of inhaled corticosteroid treatment. A normal epithelium with ciliated cells is restored. The inflammatory cells have disappeared. (Original magnification, ×2,000.) (From Laitinen LA, Laitinen A, Haahtela T. A comparative study of the effects of an inhaled corticosteroid budesonide and beta 2 agonist terbutaline on airway inflammation in newly diagnosed asthma: a randomised double-blind, parallel-group controlled trial. *J Allergy Clin Immunol* 1992;90:32–42, with permission.)

the BM area decreased in the inhaled-steroid group in comparison to the placebo group, but no significant change was measured in the thickness of the collagen band. This suggests that the inflammation, but not the fibrotic process, in the BM is prevented by a short-term inhaled-steroid treatment.

The effects of 16 weeks of treatment with nedocromil sodium, albuterol, and placebo were studied in asthmatic patients by use of bronchial biopsies. There was a reduction in the number of total and activated eosinophils in the bronchial mucosa in the nedocromil-sodium group, but an increase in the albuterol-treated group, resulting in significant morphologic differences between the two treatments (92).

Another immunohistochemical study (93) does not support the concept of nedocromil sodium as a potent anti-inflammatory drug because no superiority of the inhaled-nedocromil-sodium treatment over that of the β_2-adrenergic, albuterol, could be shown at the morphologic level in biopsy specimens taken from chronic asthmatic patients after 4 weeks of treatment. The eosinophil counts in the airway mucosa were not significantly reduced in either group, and they showed no difference between groups, despite a trend toward a decrease with nedocromil sodium and an increase with albuterol.

CONCLUSIONS

Bronchial biopsies have substantially increased our knowledge of pathologic changes in the airways of asthma patients. This information, together with the results of clinical studies, has established asthma to be an inflammatory disease of the airways. This has led to a total change in the treatment of asthma during the last decade: Now the main target of treatment is the airway inflammation, whereas the bronchoconstriction is treated only when necessary (94–98).

ACKNOWLEDGMENTS

The skillful technical assistance of Ms. Pia Rinkinen is acknowledged. The authors are grateful to Carolyn Brimley Norris, Ph.D., for language editing. Preparation of this chapter was supported by a grant from the Finnish Anti-Tuberculosis Association Foundation.

REFERENCES

1. Glynn AA, Michaels L. Bronchial biopsy in chronic bronchitis and asthma. *Thorax* 1960;15:142–153.
2. Laitinen LA, Heino M, Laitinen A, Kava T, Haahtela T. Damage of the airway epithelium and bronchial reactivity in patients with asthma. *Am Rev Respir Dis* 1985;131:599–606.
3. Laitinen LA, Laitinen A. Mucosal inflammation and bronchial hyperreactivity. *Eur Respir J* 1988;1:488–489.
4. Losewicz S, Gomez E, Ferguson H, Davies R. Inflammatory cells in the airways in mild asthma. *BMJ* 1988;297:1515–1516.
5. Reid LM, Gleich GJ, Hogg, Kleinerman J, Laitinen LA. Pathology. In: Holgate ST, ed. *The role of inflammatory processes in airway hyperresponsiveness.* Oxford: Blackwell, 1989;36–79.
6. Beasley R, Roche WR, Roberts JA, Holgate ST. Cellular events in the bronchi in mild asthma and after bronchial provocation. *Am Rev Respir Dis* 1989;139:806–817.
7. Bousquet J, Chanez P, Lacoste JY, et al. Eosinophilic inflammation in asthma. *N Engl J Med* 1990;323:1033–1039.
8. Workshop summary and guidelines: investigative use of bronchoscopy, lavage, and bronchial biopsies in asthma and other airway diseases. *J Allergy Clin Immunol* 1991;38:808–814.
9. Laitinen LA, Laitinen A, Haahtela T, Vilkka V, Spur BW, Lee TH. Leukotriene E₄ and granulocytic infiltration into the asthmatic airways. *Lancet* 1993;341:989–990.
10. Montefort S, Gratziou C, Goulding D, et al. Bronchial biopsy evidence for leukocyte infiltration and and upregulation of leukocyte endothelial cell adhesion molecules 6 hours after local allergen challenge or sensitized asthmatic airway. *J Clin Invest* 1994;93:1411–1421.
11. Bentley AM, Durham SR, Robinson DS, et al. Expression of endothelial and leukocyte adhesion molecules, intercellular adhesion molecule-1, E-selectin, and vascular cell adhesion molecule-1 in the bronchial mucosa in steady state and allergen-induced asthma. *J Allergy Clin Immunol* 1993;92:857–868.
12. Maestrelli P, Saetta M, Di Stefano A, et al. Comparison of leukocyte counts in sputum, bronchial biopsies, and bronchoalveolar lavage. *Am J Respir Crit Care Med* 1995;152:1926–1931.
13. Jeffery PK, Wardlaw AJ, Nelson FC, Collins JV, Kay AB. Bronchial biopsies in asthma: an ultrastructural, quantitative study and correlation with hyperreactivity. *Am Rev Respir Dis* 1989;140:1745–1753.
14. Djukanovic R, Wilson JW, Britten KM, et al. Quantitation of mast cells and eosinophils in the bronchial mucosa of symptomatic atopic asthmatics and healthy control subjects using immunohistochemistry. *Am Rev Respir Dis* 1990;142:863–871.
15. Hamid Q, Azzawi M, Ying S, et al. Expression of mRNA for interleukin-5 in mucosal biopsies from asthma. *J Clin Invest* 1991;87:1541–1546.
16. Ohashi Y, Motojima S, Fukuda T, Makino S. Airway hyperresponsiveness, increased intracellular spaces of bronchial epithelium, and increased infiltration of eosinophils and lymphocytes in bronchial mucosa in asthma. *Am Rev Respir Dis* 1992;145:1469–1476.
17. Bentley AM, Menz G, Storz CHR, et al. Identification of T lymphocytes, macrophages, and activated eosinophils in the bronchial mucosa in intrinsic asthma: relationship to symptoms and bronchial responsiveness. *Am Rev Respir Dis* 1992;146:500–506.
18. Laitinen LA, Laitinen A, Haahtela T. Airway mucosal inflammation even in patients with newly diagnosed asthma. *Am Rev Respir Dis* 1993;147:697–704.
19. Seminario MC, Gleich GJ. The role of eosinophils in the pathogenesis of asthma. *Curr Opin Immunol* 1994;6:860–864.
20. Olivieri D, Foresi A. Airway inflammation in asthma. *Curr Opin Pulmonary Med* 1995;1:31–39.
21. Lundgren R, Söderberg M, Hörstedt, Stenling R. Morphological studies of bronchial mucosal biopsies from asthmatics before and after ten years of treatment with inhaled steroids. *Eur Respir J* 1988;1:883–889.
22. Laitinen A, Laitinen LA. Vascular beds in airways of normal subjects and asthmatics. *Eur Respir J* 1990;3:658s–662s.
23. Laitinen LA, Laitinen A. Histology and electron microscopy. In: Butler J, ed. *The bronchial circulation.* New York: Marcel Dekker, 1992;79–98.
24. McDowell EM, Beals TF. *Biopsy pathology of the bronchi.* Philadelphia: WB Saunders, 1987.
25. Thompson AB, Robbins RA, Romberger DJ, et al. Immunological functions of pulmonary epithelium. *Eur Respir J* 1995;8:127–149.
26. McGowan, SE. Extracellular matrix and the regulation of lung development and repair. *FASEB J* 1992;6:2895–2904.
27. Raghow R. The role of extracellular matrix in post inflammatory wound healing and fibrosis. *FASEB J* 1994;8:823–831.
28. Albelda SM. Endothelial and epithelial cell adhesion molecules. *Am J Respir Cell Mol Biol* 1991;4:195–203
29. Rhodin JAG. *Histology: a text and atlas.* New York: Oxford University Press, 1974;607–645.
30. McDowell EM, Barrett LA, Glavin F, Harris CC, Trump BF. The respiratory epithelium. 1. Human bronchus. *J Natl Cancer Inst* 1978;61:539–554.

31. Söderberg M, Hellström S, Sandström T, Lundgren R, Bergh A. Structural characterization of bronchial mucosal biopsies from healthy volunteers: a light and electron microscopical study. *Eur Respir J* 1990;3: 261–266.

32. Dunnill MS, Massarella GR, Anderson JA. A comparison of the quantitative anatomy of the bronchi in normal subjects, in status asthmaticus, in chronic bronchitis, and in emphysema. *Thorax* 1969;24:176–179.

33. Cutz F, Levison H, Cooper DM. Ultrastructure of the airways in children with asthma. *Histopathology* 1978;2:407–421.

34. Naylor B. The shedding of the mucosa of the bronchial tree in asthma. *Thorax* 1962;17:69–72.

35. Lozewicz S, Wells C, Gomez E, et al. Morphological integrity of the bronchial epithelium in mild asthma. *Thorax* 1990;45:12–15.

36. Mattoli S, Miante S, Calabro F, Mezzeti M, Fasoli A, Allegra L. Bronchial epithelial cells exposed to isocyanates potentiate activation and proliferation of T cells. *Am J Physiol* 190;259:L320–L327.

37. Ackerman V, Marini M, Vittori E, Bellini A, Vassali G, Mattoli S. Detection of cytokines and their cell sources in bronchial biopsy specimens from asthmatic patients: relationship to atopic status, symptoms, and level of airway hyperresponsiveness. *Chest* 1994;105:687–696.

38. Woolley KL, Ädelroth E, Woolley MJ, et al. Interleukin-3 in bronchial biopsies from nonasthmatics and patients with mild and allergen-induced asthma. *Am J Respir Crit Care Med* 1996;153:350–355.

39. Cromwell O, Hamid Q, Corrigan C, et al. Expression and generation of interleukin-8, IL-6 and granulocyte-macrophage colony-stimulating factor by bronchial epithelial cells and enhancement by IL-1β and tumor necrosis factor-α. *Immunology* 1992;77:330–337.

40. Marini M, Vittori E, Hollemborg J, Mattoli S. Expression of the potent inflammatory cytokines, granulocyte–macrophage-colony-stimulating factor and interleukin-6 and interleukin-8, in bronchial epithelial cells of patients with asthma. *J Allergy Clin Immunol* 1992;89:1001–1009.

41. Sousa AR, Poston RN, Lane SJ, Nakhosteen JA, Lee TH. Detection of GM-CSF in asthmatic bronchial epithelium and decrease by inhaled corticosteroids. *Am Rev Respir Dis* 1993;147:1557–1561.

42. Bellini A, Yoshimura H, Vittori E, Marini M, Mattoli S. Bronchial epithelial cells of patients with asthma release chemoattractant factors for T lymphocyte. *J Allergy Clin Immunol* 1993;92:412–424.

43. Sousa AR, Lane SJ, Nakhosreen JA, Yoshimura T, Lee TH, Poston RN. Increased expression of monocyte chemoattractant protein-1 in bronchial tissue from asthmatic subjects. *Am J Respir Cell Mol Biol* 1994; 10:142–147.

44. Rollins BJ, Yoshimura T, Leonard EJ, Pober JS. Cytokine activated human endothelial cells synthesize and secrete a monocyte chemoattractant, MCP-1/JE. *Am J Pathol* 1990;136:1229–1233.

45. Vignola AM, Campbell AM, Chanez P, et al. HLA-DR and ICAM-1 expression on bronchial epithelial cells in asthma and chronic bronchitis. *Am Rev Respir Dis* 1993;148:689–694.

46. Montefort S, Roche WR, Howarth PH, et al. Intercellular adhesion molecule-1 (ICAM-1) and leucocyte adhesion molecule-1 (ELAM-1) expression in the bronchial mucosa of normal and asthmatic subjects. *Eur Respir J* 1992;5:815–823.

47. Pesci A, Foresi A, Bertorelli G, Chetta A, Olivieri D. Histochemical characteristics and degranulation of mast cells in epithelium and lamina propria of bronchial biopsies from asthmatic and normal subjects. *Am Rev Respir Dis* 1993;147:684–689.

48. Azzawi M, Bradley B, Jeffery PK, et al. Identification of activated T lymphocytes and eosinophils in bronchial biopsies in stable asthma. *Am Rev Respir Dis* 1990;142:1407–1413.

49. Bradley B, Azzawi M, Jacobson M, et al. Eosinophils, T lymphocytes, mast cells, neutrophils and macrophages in bronchial biopsies from atopic asthma: comparison with nonatopic asthma and normal controls and relationship to bronchial hyperresponsiveness. *J Allergy Clin Immunol* 1991;88:661–674.

50. Nasser SMS, Pfister R, Christie PE, et al. Inflammatory cell populations in bronchial biopsies from aspirin sensitive asthmatic subjects. *Am J Respir Crit Care Med* 1996;153:90–96.

51. Salvato G. Asthma and mast cells of bronchial connective tissue. *Experientia* 1968;18:330–331.

52. Filley WV, Holley KE, Kephart GM, Gleich GJ. Identification by immunofluorescence of eosinophil MBP in lung biopsies of patients with bronchial asthma. *Lancet* 1982;2:11–16.

53. Laitinen LA, Laitinen A, Heino M, Haahtela T. Eosinophilic airway inflammation during exacerbation of asthma and its treatment with inhaled corticosteroid. *Am Rev Respir Dis* 1991;143:423–427.

54. De Moncy JGR, Kauffman HF, Venge P. Bronchoalveolar eosinophilia during allergen-induced late asthmatic reactions. *Am Rev Respir Dis* 1985;131:373–377.

55. Paulsson M. Basement membrane proteins: structure, assembly and cellular interactions. *Crit Rev Biochem Mol Biol* 1992;27:93–127.

56. Dunsmore SE, Rannels DE. Extracellular matrix biology in the lung. *Am J Physiol* 1996;270:L3–L27.

57. Roche WR, Beasley R, Williams JH, Holgate ST. Subepithelial fibrosis in the bronchi of asthmatics. *Lancet* 1989;1:520–524.

58. Trigg CJ, Manolitsas ND, Wang J, et al. Placebo-controlled immunopathologic study of four months of inhaled corticosteroids in asthma. *Am J Respir Crit Care Med* 1994;150:17–22.

59. Laitinen A, Altraja A, Linden M, et al. Treatment with inhaled budesonide and tenascin expression in bronchial mucosa of allergic asthmatics. *Am J Crit Care Med* 1994;149:A942(abst).

60. Mayne R, Brewton RG. New members of the collagen superfamily. *Curr Opin Cell Biol* 1993;5:883–890.

61. Herbst TJ, McCarthy JB, Tsilibary EC, Furcht LT. Differential effects of laminin, intact type IV collagen, and specific domains of type IV collagen on endothelial cell adhesion and migration. *J Cell Biol* 1988; 106:1365–1373.

62. Rickard KA, Taylor J, Rennard SI, Spurzem JR. Migration of bovine bronchial epithelial cells to extracellular matrix components. *Am J Respir Cell Mol Biol* 1993;8:63–68.

63. Brewster CE, Howarth PH, Djukanovic R, Wilson J, Holgate ST, Roche WR. Myofibroblasts and subepithelial fibrosis in bronchial asthma. *Am J Respir Cell Mol Biol* 1990;3:507–511.

64. Sakai LY, Keene DR, Morris NP, Burgeson RE. Type VII collagen is the major structural component of anchoring fibrils. *J Cell Biol* 1986;103: 1577–1586.

65. Wetzels RHW, Robben HCM, Leight IM, Schaafsma HE, Vooijs GP, Ramaekers FCS. Distribution patterns of type VII collagen in normal and malignant human tissues. *Am J Pathol* 1991;139:451–459.

66. Altraja A, Laitinen A, Kämpe M, et al. Inhaled budesonide has no effect on the distribution of collagen types III and VII in bronchial epithelial basement membrane in allergic asthmatics. *Am J Respir Crit Care Med* 1994;149:A632(abst).

67. Timpl R, Brown JC. The laminins. *Matrix Biol* 1994;14:275–281.

68. Virtanen I, Laitinen A, Tani T, et al. Differential expression of laminins and their integrin receptors in developing and adult human lung. *Am J Respir Cell Mol Biol* 1996;15:184–196.

69. Mette SA, Pilewski J, Buck CA, Albelda SM. Distribution of integrin cell adhesion receptors in normal bronchial epithelial cells and lung cancer cells *in vitro* and *in vivo*. *Am J Respir Cell Mol Biol* 1993;8: 562–572.

70. Shepard D. Identification and characterization of novel airway epithelial integrins. *Am Rev Respir Dis* 1993;148:S38–S42.

71. Altraja A, Laitinen A, Virtanen I, et al. Expression of laminins in the airways of various types of asthmatic patients: a morphometric study. *Am J Respir Cell Mol Biol* 1996;15:482–488.

72. Jiang Y, Zhu JF, Luscinskas FW, Graves DT. MCP-1 stimulated monocyte attachment to laminin is mediated by beta 2-integrins. *Am J Physiol* 1994;267:1112–1118.

73. Hershkovics R, Lider O, Baram D, Reshef T, Miron S, Mekori YA. Inhibition of T cell adhesion to extracellular matrix glycoproteins by histamine: a role for mast cell degranulation products. *J Leukoc Biol* 1994;56:495–501.

74. Walsh LJ, Kaminer MS, Lazarus GS, Lavker RM, Murphy GF. Role of laminin in localization of human dermal mast cells. *Lab Invest* 1991; 65:433–440.

75. Answar AR, Moqbel R, Walsh GM, Kay AB, Wardlaw AJ. Adhesion to fibronectin prolongs eosinophil survival. *J Exp Med* 1993;177:839–843.

76. Georas SN, McIntyre BW, Ebisawa M, et al. Expression of a functional laminin receptor (α6β1, very late activation antigen-6) on human eosinophils. *Blood* 1993;82:2872–2879.

77. Erickson HP. Tenascin-C, tenascin-R and tenascin-X: a family of talented proteins in search of functions. *Curr Opin Cell Biol* 1993;5:869–876.

78. Weinacker A, Ferrando R, Elliot M, Hogg J, Balmes J, Sheppard D. Distribution of integrins αvβ6 and α9β1 and their known ligands, fibronectin and tenascin, in human airways. *Am J Respir Cell Mol Biol* 1995;12:547–557.

79. Härkönen E, Virtanen I, Linnala A, Laitinen LA, Kinnula VK. Modulation of fibronectin and tenascin production in human bronchial ep-

ithelial cells by inflammatory cytokines *in vitro. Am J Respir Cell Mol Biol* 1995;13:109–115.

80. Linnala A, Kinnula V, Laitinen LA, Lehto VP, Virtanen I. Transforming growth factor-β regulates the expression of fibronectin and tenascin in BEAS 2B human bronchial epithelial cells. *Am J Respir Cell Mol Biol* 1995;13:578–585.

81. O'Hickey SP, Hawksworth RJ, Fong CY, Arm JP, Spur BW, Lee TH. Leukotrienes C$_4$, D$_4$ and E$_4$ enchance histamine responsiveness in asthmatic airways. *Am Rev Respir Dis* 1991;144:1053–1057.

82. Crimi E, Balbo A, Milanese M, Miadonna A, Rossi GA, Brusasco V. Airway inflammation and occurrence of delayed bronchoconstriction in exercise-induced asthma. *Am Rev Respir Dis* 1992;146:507–512.

83. Crimi E, Chiaramondia M, Milanese M, Rossi GA, Brusasco V. Increase of mast cell numbers in bronchial mucosa after the late phase asthmatic response to allergen. *Am Rev Respir Dis* 1991;144:1282–1286.

84. Gruenert DC, Finkbeiner WE, Widdicombe JH. Culture and transformation of human airway epithelial cells. *Am J Physiol* 1995;268:L347–L360.

85. De Jong PM, van Sterkenburg MA, Kempenaar JA, Dijkman JH, Ponec M. Serial culturing of human bronchial epithelial cells *in vitro. In Vitro Cell Dev Biol* 1993;29A:379–387.

86. Devalia JL, Sapsford RJ, Wells CW, Richman P, Davies RJ. Culture and comparison of human bronchial and nasal epithelial cells *in vitro. Respir Med* 1990;84:303–312.

87. Van Scott MR, Yankaskas JR, Boucher RC. Culture of airway epithelial cells: research techniques. *Exp Lung Res* 1986;11:75–94.

88. Kelsen SG, Mardini IA, Zhou S, Benovic JL, Higgins NC. A technique to harvest viable tracheobronchial epithelial cells from living human donors. *Am J Respir Cell Mol Biol* 1992;7:66–72.

89. Jeffery PK, Godfrey RW, Ädelroth E, Nelson F, Rogers A, Johansson SA. Effects of treatment on airway inflammation and thickening of basement membrane reticular collagen in asthma: a quantitative light and electron microscopic study. *Am Rev Respir Dis* 1992;145:890–899.

90. Djukanovic R, Wilson JW, Britten KM, et al. Effect of inhaled corticosteroid on airway inflammation and symptoms in asthma. *Am Rev Respir Dis* 1992;145:669–674.

91. Laitinen LA, Laitinen A, Haahtela T. A comparative study of the effects of an inhaled corticosteroid budesonide and beta 2 agonist terbutaline on airway inflammation in newly diagnosed asthma: a randomised double-blind, parallel-group controlled trial. *J Allergy Clin Immunol* 1992;90:32–42.

92. Manolitsas ND, Wang J, Devalia JL, Trigg CJ, McAulay AE, Davies RJ. Regular albuterol, nedocromil sodium and bronchial inflammation in asthma. *Am J Respir Crit Care Med* 1995;151:1925–1930.

93. Altraja A, Laitinen A, Meriste S, et al. Effect of regular nedocromil sodium or albuterol on bronchial inflammation in chronic asthma. *J Allergy Clin Immunol* 1996 (*in press*).

94. Barnes PJ. A new approach to the treatment of asthma. *N Engl J Med* 1989;321:1517–1527.

95. Haahtela T, Järvinen M, Kava T, et al. Comparison of a β$_2$-agonist, terbutaline, with an inhaled corticosteroid, budesonide, in newly detected asthma. *N Engl J Med* 1991;325:388–392.

96. British Thoracic Society. Guidelines for the management of asthma in adults. Statement by the research unit of the Royal Collage of Physicians of London, King's Fund Center, National Asthma Campaign. *BMJ* 1990;142:434–457.

97. Expert panel report guidelines for diagnosis and management of asthma. *J Sch Health* 1991;6:249–250.

98. Jones KP. Guideliness on the management of asthma. (letter) *Thorax* 1993;48:S1–S24.

Asthma, edited by P.J. Barnes, M.M. Grunstein, A.R. Leff, and A.J. Woolcock. Lippincott–Raven Publishers, Philadelphia © 1997.

▪ 18 ▪

Bronchoalveolar Lavage in Studies

Mark C. Liu

The use of bronchoalveolar lavage (BAL) to sample cells and fluids from the lungs of persons with asthma has played a major role in advancing the understanding of asthma as a chronic inflammatory disease of the airways (1,2). Examination of asthmatics under a variety of clinical or experimental conditions has identified cellular, biochemical, or molecular events associated with disease severity, bronchoprovocation, or pharmacologic intervention. Most significantly, BAL studies, coupled with those of airway biopsy, brushings, and induced sputum, have provided solid evidence for a characteristic form of airway inflammation associated with asthma. Even in patients with mild or asymptomatic disease, airway inflammation is present, and appears to involve many of the same cells observed in fatal disease at autopsy, such as eosinophils, basophils, mast cells, and lymphocytes. These inflammatory cells are part of a complex interaction involving both cells recruited from the circulation to the inflamed airway, as well as resident cells in the airway wall. These interactions may ultimately control the degree of airway obstruction and reactivity manifested as

the day-to-day variations in airway function of clinical asthma, but also these interactions may underlie the chronic, structural changes associated with progressive or fatal disease.

Asthma is often associated with underlying atopy and an immunoglobulin E (IgE) response, and many of the inflammatory changes described in asthma resemble the inflammatory response of the atopic individual to allergen exposure. Because of this resemblance, models of allergen challenge by inhalation to the whole lung or by challenge of an isolated airway segment during bronchoscopy have been used to examine mechanisms of inflammation and alterations in airway function that may be relevant to clinical disease. In comparing whole lung with segmental challenge models, the provoked inflammatory changes appear to be qualitatively similar, and depend on allergen dose and distribution as well as individual sensitivity. Nearly identical changes can be elicited in allergic individuals whether or not they have asthma. In general, a more intense inflammatory response occurs with segmental challenge limited to a small portion of the lung than with whole lung challenge, where declines in lung function limit the allergen dose delivered (3). Many of the conclusions regarding mechanisms of inflammation in asthma reviewed in this chapter rely on results from al-

M. C. Liu: Department of Medicine, The Johns Hopkins University School of Medicine, Johns Hopkins Asthma and Allergy Center, Baltimore, Maryland 21224.

lergen challenge models. An assumption implicit in these studies, and unlikely to be completely true, is that asthma represents a chronic, sustained form of the same events that occur after allergen challenge. This caveat applies especially to asthma occurring in the nonatopic individual. Nevertheless, the approach has provided insights into the multiplicity of inflammatory events that may underlie the complex, clinical disease of asthma.

SAFETY OF BRONCHOSCOPY AND BRONCHOALVEOLAR LAVAGE IN ASTHMA

Largely based on clinical experiences with complications from bronchoscopy in patients with asthma or airway reactivity, legitimate concerns were initially raised regarding the use of bronchoscopy exclusively as a research procedure in patients with asthma. Subsequent experience, however, has shown that bronchoscopy with BAL, airway biopsy, or provocations can be performed with safety and acceptable risk provided that careful attention is paid to patient selection, lung function, use of premedications and dosages of local anesthesia, and performance of procedures by experienced personnel in appropriate facilities for monitoring and treatment. In the United States, a workshop sponsored by the National Institutes of Health first established guidelines for bronchoscopy in asthmatic persons in 1985 (4) which was updated and expanded to include bronchial biopsies and provocation procedures in 1991 (5). Similar guidelines were established in Europe (6). In general, patients with mild-to-moderate, stable asthma with an FEV_1 ≥60% of predicted were considered good subjects for bronchoscopy and a variety of studies, including BAL, biopsy, brushings, placement of endobronchial catheters, or airway provocations (4–7). Persons with severe disease and lower levels of pulmonary function were considered at greater risk for complications. To examine this question, van Vyve et al. studied a group of 50 asthmatic and 25 nonasthmatic persons undergoing bronchoscopy with BAL and biopsy without bronchodilator premedication or supplemental oxygen. The lowest FEV_1 was 37% of predicted, and 20% of asthmatic persons had an FEV_1 below 60% of predicted. Decreases of 4% to 5% in oxygen saturation were observed in asthmatics but were not different from normals. FEV_1 decreased from 76% to 55% of predicted in asthmatics, whereas normals decreased from 97% to 80% of predicted. Although the percentage decreases in lung function was significantly greater in asthmatics than normals, there was no relationship between the baseline lung function or asthma severity and the decreased lung function induced by bronchoscopy (8). In a similar study of 20 asthmatics with milder disease premedicated with albuterol, ipratropium, atropine, and midazolam, Djukanovic et al. reported greater decreases in lung function in asthmatics than in nonasthmatics (97% to 75% of predicted FEV_1 vs. 110% to 102%, respectively) and the decrease in

FEV_1 in asthmatics was correlated with bronchial hyperreactivity to methacholine (9). These studies and the general experience with research bronchoscopy in asthma have reinforced the initial impression that even in persons with a broad range of clinical disease severity, airways obstruction, and airways hyperreactivity, the procedure can be performed with acceptable risks and safety provided appropriate precautions are taken. This caution seems especially appropriate because there may be no way to predict which individual will have an adverse reaction to the procedure.

STRENGTHS AND LIMITATIONS OF BRONCHOALVEOLAR LAVAGE USED TO STUDY ASTHMA

Several technical aspects of BAL must be considered in interpreting data derived from this technique (10). The strengths of the technique are that measuring concentrations in BAL fluids may offer the best assessment of the release or accumulation of inflammatory mediators, proteins, lipids, cytokines, or other soluble products. BAL may also be the best technique to recover adequate numbers of inflammatory cells for functional studies and to assess alterations in airway permeability.

The BAL procedure, however, does have significant limitations. The invasive nature of the procedure and the need for medications and local anesthesia may alter airway or cellular functions and limits the ability to perform repeated procedures. BAL samples only a portion of the cells and fluids associated with the epithelial surface of airways, and returns from the airways are usually "contaminated" by a significant contribution derived from alveolar surfaces. Hence, findings from BAL may not reflect changes occurring within the airway or airway tissues most relevant to asthma.

Perhaps the most significant technical problem with BAL, however, is the variable dilution of cells and airway fluids that occurs with the procedure. This dilution factor may vary with the technique of BAL (11) or the presence of disease. Total volumes instilled for BAL have varied from as little as 5 mL up to 400 mL (5); however, investigators have generally used total volumes from 100 to 240 mL of normal saline delivered and recovered in multiple aliquots. Despite attempts to assess dilution using indicators added to BAL fluids such as inulin or methylene blue (12), or endogenous markers such as urea, potassium, or albumin (13–17), each of these markers has limitations, and no method to correct for the dilutional effect of BAL has been widely accepted. At this time, it would appear that the best way to control for this variable is to perform the BAL procedure in a consistent, standardized fashion to minimize systematic errors. Results can then be reported as a quantity per mL of returned fluid, avoiding complicated and often unhelpful manipulations of original measurements. Using a standardized BAL protocol, normative values for cellular and protein constituents of BAL have been published by the BAL Cooperative Study Group with a recommendation that cell numbers be reported as cells per mL of recovered fluid as well as percentage (18).

BAL CYTOLOGY IN ASTHMA

Comparison with Bronchial Biopsy

Comparison of inflammatory cell numbers from BAL and bronchial biopsy reveal marked differences. In normal individuals, about 10 to 20 million cells are recovered from each site of BAL when lavage volume exceeds 100 mL. BAL cell numbers are dominated by macrophages and lymphocytes, comprising 80% to 90% and 10% to 20% of cells recovered, respectively. Eosinophils and neutrophils account for <1% each, and mast cells for <0.5%. Ciliated epithelial cells may also be seen in BAL of nonasthmatic persons; however, their recovery may be due to airway trauma from bronchoscopy itself. By contrast, estimates of total inflammatory cell number in bronchial biopsies range from 400 to 4,000/mm^3 of tissue. Lymphocytes are the predominant inflammatory cell in the airway mucosa, accounting for 60% to 90% of inflammatory cells within the epithelium, and 40% to 80% within the submucosa. Mast cells account for ≤20% and macrophages for <10% of inflammatory cells. Occasionally, large numbers of neutrophils are found in nonasthmatic individuals, but eosinophils are rare. This comparison raises the important, unresolved issue of the relationship between inflammatory events occurring in the airway tissue and BAL compartment. At this time, the techniques are best viewed as providing equally important and complementary information.

MAST CELLS

Mast cells make up a small proportion of cells recovered by BAL, with estimates in nonasthmatic persons ranging from 0.02% to 0.48% (19,20). In asthmatic persons, normal numbers (19,21–24) or increases of two- to sixfold have been reported in atopic (14,20,25–30) as well as nonatopic asthmatics (31). Persons with allergic rhinitis may also have elevated numbers of airway mast cells (27). In several studies, increased mast cell numbers have been inversely correlated with baseline pulmonary function and increased bronchial hyperreactivity (26,28, 29). Mast cells in the BAL and in the airway submucosa are mostly the mucosal type containing tryptase in secretory granules designated MC$_T$, as opposed to the tissue type mast cell containing both tryptase and chymase, designated MC$_{TC}$.

Ongoing mast cell degranulation is present in chronic asthma as evidenced by increased levels of the mast cell mediators histamine and tryptase (22,24,30,32,33), although BAL histamine levels also may be elevated in allergic rhinitic persons without asthma (19,27). *In vitro,* both spontaneous and IgE-mediated release of histamine is enhanced in BAL mast cells of asthmatic versus nonasthmatic persons (28), and spontaneous histamine release is increased in symptomatic versus asymptomatic asthmatics (24).

Lying on and within the airway, mast cells are well positioned to respond to a provocative stimulus. They are the only resident cell in the airway that can interact with allergen via IgE bound to the high affinity receptor, Fc$_\varepsilon$RI, although other cells such as macrophages, eosinophils, lymphocytes, and platelets may also interact with allergens via the low-affinity IgE receptor, Fc$_\varepsilon$RII. With allergen challenge of the airways, the mast cell responds within minutes with release of both preformed mediators such as histamine and tryptase and newly synthesized products such as prostaglandin D$_2$ and the sulfidopeptidyl leukotriene, LTC$_4$ (21,34–39). Indeed, the immediate response to allergen challenge is clearly dominated by products that are identified with the mast cell. These products are potent bronchoconstrictors and may induce alterations in vascular permeability. Mast cell numbers in the bronchial mucosa may also increase after the late-phase response to allergen challenge (40). Besides allergen, other stimuli such as exercise, aspirin, or chemicals may also provoke mast cell degranulation, leading to bronchoconstriction and vascular changes.

Mast cells may further participate in the inflammatory changes in asthma by elaboration of cytokines. In response to IgE-dependent stimuli, mouse mast cell lines have been shown to produce a profile of cytokines including interleukin-3 (IL-3), IL-4, IL-5, and IL-6 similar to the TH2 profile produced by T lymphocytes. Human lung mast cells have been shown to release IL-4 (41), IL-5 (42,43), and IL-13 *in vitro,* and mucosal biopsies of asthmatics have revealed positive staining by immunohistochemistry for IL-4, IL-5, IL-6, and TNF-α in mast cells (44). Further localization of cytokines to mast cell subsets reveals preferential IL-4 expression by MC$_T$ mast cells with predominantly IL-5 and IL-6 expression by the MC$_{TC}$ subset (45).

BASOPHILS

Basophils also possess the Fc$_\varepsilon$RI receptor and are capable of immediate response to allergen. Basophils have previously been reported in the sputum of symptomatic asthmatics (46). Recent studies have demonstrated basophil infiltration of airways in cases of fatal asthma (47) and in bronchial biopsies of patients with asthma (48). During the late response to segmental allergen challenge, large numbers of basophils appear in the BAL fluid, and have been noted in airway tissue (21,49,50). Recently, the basophil has also been identified as a rich source of IL-4 and IL-13, demonstrating both spontaneous release and response to IgE-mediated stimuli (51,52).

MACROPHAGES

Macrophages are the predominant cell recovered by BAL of both nonasthmatic and asthmatic persons. Although most macrophages likely are recovered from alveoli, small volume lavage or lavage of isolated airway segments (53) support macrophage predominance in conducting airways as well as alveoli. Thus, macrophages are well positioned to respond to and regulate inflammation along the airway. Although the prominence of macrophages along the airway surface and their diverse functions strongly implicate macrophages as playing a role in asthma, it is unclear whether that role is one of facilitating inflammatory responses or one of dampening responses. On the one hand, macrophages can perform accessory cell functions by presenting antigen and providing secondary signals, e.g. IL-1, required for differentiation and proliferation of specific lymphocyte responses. These functions may well play a role in sensitizing the airway to respond to further exposures. On the other hand, alveolar macrophages in some systems have been found to be poor antigen-presenting cells, and in the large proportions of macrophages to lymphocytes (5–10:1) found on the airway surface, macrophages may actually suppress lymphocyte responses (54). Hence, the role of the resident macrophage in initiating immune responses is unclear. Adding to this complexity are the findings that blood monocytes may be better antigen-presenting cells than macrophages and may be recruited to sites of inflammation. In addition, dendritic cells are present in the airways and appear to be much more potent antigen-presenting cells than macrophages (55).

Nevertheless, airway macrophages may participate in airway inflammation by multiple mechanisms. Alveolar macrophages express the low-affinity receptor (FcεRII) for IgE (56) and expression appears to be increased in asthmatics (57) compared with normals. Macrophage release of lysosomal enzymes in response to segmental allergen challenge has been demonstrated *in vivo* (58). *In vitro* studies reveal that alveolar macrophages can respond to antigen via IgE to release LTB_4 and LTC_4, PGD_2, superoxide anion, and lysosomal enzymes (59–62). Macrophages also produce other important inflammatory mediators such as platelet-activating factor (PAF), prostaglandin $F_{2\alpha}$, and thromboxane (63,64). These mediators may play important roles in producing bronchoconstriction or causing inflammatory changes, including cell recruitment and altered vascular permeability.

Pro-inflammatory cytokines produced by macrophages include IL-1, TNF-α, IL-6, and granulocyte-macrophage colony-stimulating factor (GM-CSF), which may induce endothelial cell activation, cellular recruitment, and prolonged eosinophil survival. IL-6 and TNF-α may be released by IgE-dependent stimulation (65). Macrophages also elaborate histamine-releasing factors that appear to act on basophils and mast cells via binding to surface IgE (66–68). Hence, macrophages may play a role in perpetuating mast cell activation in asthma and late-phase responses independently from repeated exposures to specific allergen.

EPITHELIUM

Although airway epithelium is not normally a component of BAL, epithelial cells are often recovered in the BAL of asthmatic persons. In some cases, the number of epithelial cells has been correlated with the degree of airway hyperreactivity (29,30,50). Damage to and shedding of the airway epithelium have long been recognized as histologic features of asthma. Clinically, epithelium may be seen in expectorated sputum, and "Creola bodies" described historically as a sputum finding in asthma are clumps of shed epithelial cells (69). Even in mild disease, extensive change and loss of epithelium has been reported (50,70–72), although some of these abnormalities may be due to the fragility of epithelial attachment in asthmatic persons and subsequent loss of epithelium during collection and processing of tissue.

It is clear that the epithelium is not simply a passive barrier and conveyor of mucus but serves important biochemical and immunologic roles. *In vitro* studies demonstrate epithelial-derived relaxing factors such as nitric oxide that may modulate airway contractile responses. Epithelium produces the prostanoids $PGF_{2\alpha}$ and PGE_2 that may produce airway contraction or regulate immune responses (18). In addition, human epithelial cells or cell lines have been shown to release several cytokines such as IL-6, IL-8, tumor necrosis factor (TNF), granulocyte colony-stimulating factor (G-CSF) and GM-CSF. Studies of bronchial epithelial cells from asthmatic and nonasthmatic persons suggest that the epithelium in asthmatics is in an activated state and produces greater amounts of GM-CSF, IL-6, IL-8, and monocyte chemotactic protein-1 (MCP-1) (73–75). The level of GM-CSF in epithelium has been correlated with numbers of eosinophils and bronchial hyperresponsiveness (76). Epithelial cells are also capable of synthesizing the C-C chemokine, RANTES (regulated on activation, normal T cell expressed and secreted), which may play an important role in the specific recruitment of eosinophils, lymphocytes, and basophils to the airway surface. RANTES released into BAL fluids has been reported after segmental allergen challenge, although eosinophil influx was correlated with IL-5 levels and not RANTES (77).

LYMPHOCYTES

Normally, lymphocytes comprise only 10% to 20% of total cells recovered by BAL, but are the predominant cell in airway biopsy specimens. It is unknown whether lymphocytes recovered by BAL are representative of the tissue population or a selected subset of this population. Nearly all lymphocytes in BAL fluids are T lymphocytes (50,78,79). Although the mean ratio of CD4:CD8 T cells is between 1.5 and 2:1 and similar to that found in peripheral blood, the distribution of ratios is often greater in BAL than in blood. The large majority of BAL T cells, in common with other T-cell populations on mucosal surfaces, express the surface marker CD45RO associated with memory T cells that have undergone a previous antigenic stimulus. In contrast, naive T lymphocytes express the surface marker CD45RA and represent the majority of circulating T cells. This difference in T-cell subsets between BAL and blood compartments is consistent with a selective recruitment process or transformation of recruited cells by the airway microenvironment.

In asthma, most studies have demonstrated normal numbers of T lymphocytes in BAL fluids with normal CD4:CD8 ratios, although mild increases in lymphocytes or decreases in CD4:CD8 ratios have been found in some studies (78,80–82). Although most T cells bear the $\alpha\beta$ heterodimer T-cell receptor, $\gamma\delta$ receptor-bearing T cells are present in small numbers in the airways and marked elevations have recently been reported in atopic asthmatics (83).

Although the total number of lymphocytes is most often normal in asthmatics, evidence for T-cell activation has been documented by increases in both acute (IL-2R) and chronic (HLA-DR, VLA-1) markers of cell activation that are increased on T cells of asthmatics compared with normal controls (78,82,84). Activated T cells have been related to disease severity assessed by decreased FEV_1 and increased bronchial hyperreactivity (82), and 24 hours after allergen bronchoprovocation of allergic asthmatics, increased IL-2R (CD25) expression has been found (85).

After allergen challenge, changes in T-cell subpopulations may occur rapidly as one study demonstrated decreased recovery of lymphocytes 10 minutes after segmented allergen challenge. Although both CD4 and CD8 cells were affected, the major effect was on CD4+ cells, resulting in a significant decrease in the CD4:CD8 ratio (86). Six hours after whole lung bronchoprovocation, similar findings have been reported, but only in those asthmatic persons who developed a late-phase response (87). These results are likely to reflect decreases in cell recoveries by BAL related to adherence, rather than real losses of lymphocytes from the epithelium or airway. At later times (18–24 hr) after segmental allergen challenge, clear increases in BAL lymphocytes have been observed and mainly involve increases in the CD4+ and CD45RO+ populations. The adhesion molecule profile on these CD4+ cells, including increased expression of L-selectin, suggest active recruitment of a selected population of T lymphocytes from the circulation (88).

T lymphocytes have long been recognized as critical to the development of immune responses, and recent work in the murine system has identified two types of T-cell clones defined by the profile of cytokines produced. TH1 cells can be characterized by production of IL-2 and IFN-γ and are involved in developing cell-mediated immunity, whereas TH2 cells can be characterized by production of IL-4 and IL-5 and are involved in promoting humoral immunity and IgE responses. Both cell types produce IL-3 and GM-CSF. Whereas such a dichotomy of helper T-cell functions may be less clear in humans than in the mouse, the profile of cytokine production defined by functional T-cell subpopulations appears to play a critical role in regulating immune responses associated with inflammatory disease. Asthma and the inflammatory response to allergen have been associated with a profile of cytokines characteristic of a TH2 response. The cellular sources of these cytokines is certainly not limited to the T lymphocyte, however, as multiple cellular sources for TH2 cytokines have been identified as discussed below.

NEUTROPHILS

There is little evidence to support a central role for the neutrophil in asthma, although an important facilitative role in airway inflammation has not been ruled out. Generally, normal numbers of neutrophils are present in BAL of asthmatics; one such study reported neutrophils correlating with eosinophils, mast cells, and duration of asthma (30). Increased numbers of neutrophils have been demonstrated in other studies (24,82,89). After allergen challenge, an increase in neutrophils may accompany the eosinophil response, although the kinetics of the influx of these two cell types may be different. The neutrophil influx may occur early and disappear within 24 hours whereas the eosinophil influx may take longer to resolve (90).

Neutrophil influx has been observed after inhalation challenge with antigen, ozone, toluene diissocyanate, and plicatic acid, the active principal in western red cedar asthma. In models of allergic inflammation involving segmental challenge, neutrophil influx also accompanies the influx of eosinophils but does not appear to be specific for allergen because significant neutrophil responses may be seen in control sites of saline challenge (21,34). Hence, prior bronchoscopy itself may lead to some degree of airway neutrophilia, although BAL of asthmatic persons may not always lead to diffuse inflammation and neutrophil influx (91).

EOSINOPHILS

Increased numbers of eosinophils is the most characteristic cellular abnormality in BAL associated with asthma. In general, mean percentages in asthma range from 2% to 11% (24,28,82,92). Normal numbers have been reported in persons with mild disease (19,50,79,86), and allergic persons without asthma may also have elevated numbers of eosinophils (19).

Eosinophils in asthma appear to be activated and undergoing chronic degranulation. Bousquet et al. examined 43 patients with chronic asthma representing a wide range of disease severity and found that blood eosinophilia, BAL eosinophilia, and BAL eosinophil cationic protein (ECP) levels correlated with asthma severity (92). In studying groups of mild asthmatic persons with and without symptoms, Wardlaw et al. observed increases in BAL eosinophils and eosinophil major basic protein (MBP) in the symptomatic group. Correlations between these parameters, and bronchial hyperreactivity to methacholine, were found (93). In comparing groups of symptomatic versus asymptomatic asthmatics, Broide et al. reported increased BAL eosinophils and the eosinophil granule products, major basic protein (MBP) and eosinophil-derived neurotoxin (EDN). Walker et al. also observed increased numbers of BAL eosinophils in asthmatic versus nonasthmatic persons, and BAL eosinophilia was correlated with activated CD4+ T lymphocytes expressing the IL-2 receptor, and with decreased FEV_1 and increased methacholine hyperresponsiveness (82). These studies support the eosinophil and its products as playing a central, effector function in the inflammation associated with asthma.

After whole lung allergen challenge, modest increases in BAL eosinophils of severalfold compared with prechallenge control levels are usually found within 4 to 6 hours after challenge and may persist for at least 24 hours (90,94,95). BAL eosinophil responses to segmental challenge may be quite variable and depend on allergen dose. Large increases in total BAL cell numbers with eosinophil percentages averaging 40% to 60% at 20 to 48 hours are commonly observed (21,34,96).

Eosinophils may also participate in asthma and allergic inflammation by production of cytokines. Cytokines that may be produced by eosinophils include IL-1α (97), IL-3 (98), IL-5 (99), IL-6 (100), IL-8 (101), GM-CSF (102), TNF-α (103), MIP1-α (103), TGF-α (104), and TGF-β (105); however, the *in vivo* contribution of eosinophil cytokine production to airway inflammation remains to be determined (106).

PLATELETS

After allergen bronchoprovocation, the release of platelet factor 4 (PF4) into blood has been reported and supports a role for the platelet in asthma (107). The platelet granule products, PF4 and β-thromboglobulin, are also increased in BAL during the late response after segmental allergen challenge (108). These products are members of the C-X-C chemokine family of cytokines and may play a role in cellular recruitment. Further, platelets are a source of histamine releasing factors, PAF, and thromboxane, which may play important roles in inflammation.

MEDIATORS

Histamine

Histamine is produced by the enzymatic decarboxylation of histamine and stored in the granules of mast cells and basophils. Elevations of histamine concentrations in BAL fluids from asthmatics generally range from 3- to more than 10-fold greater than nonasthmatics, thus supporting a role for chronic mast cell activation in asthma (24,32,33,40), although normal levels have also been reported (23). Increased histamine levels may not be specific for asthma, however, because elevations similar to those in asthma have been found in allergic rhinitic patients with no asthma (19,27). In some studies, however, elevated BAL histamine levels have been correlated with the degree of airway obstruction or hyperreactivity (25, 27,30,94,109). After allergen challenge, increased levels of histamine are observed within minutes, and elevations of more than 100-fold have been measured after segmental allergen challenge (21,23). Smaller increases persist up to 48 hours after challenge (21,34).

Tryptase

Elevated or normal levels of tryptase have been reported in asthma and, like histamine, marked increases have been reported within minutes after segmental allergen challenge (23,34), supporting a mast cell source of histamine released during the immediate response because basophils do not contain tryptase. Conversely, the persistence of increased histamine without tryptase in the late antigen response supports a basophil source for histamine (34). The function of tryptase in asthma is unclear, but the enzyme may cleave certain complement proteins and possesses kallikrein-like activity.

Lipid Mediators

In contrast with preformed or granule-associated mediators such as histamine, the lipid mediators, including prostaglandins (PG), leukotrienes (LT), and platelet-activating factors (PAF), are newly synthesized in response to a stimulus (110,111). PG and LT are derived from the metabolism of arachidonic acid released from phospholipids in the cell membrane by the action of phospholipases, such as A_2 or C. Arachidonic acid is metabolized via the cyclo-oxygenase pathway to produce prostanoids PGE_2, PGD_2, $PGF_{2\alpha}$, PGI_2, and thromboxane $(TX)A_2$, whereas metabolism of arachidonic acid via the lipoxygenase pathway results in the formation of hydroxyeicosatetraenoic acids (HETEs) and leukotrienes (LT) B_4, C_4, D_4, and E_4. PAF, 1-0-alkyl-2-acetyl-sn-glycero-3-phosphocholine, is derived from ether-linked phospholipids in the cell membrane whose cleavage results in formation of the immediate precursor, lyso-PAF. The enzyme acetyl transferase converts lyso-PAF to PAF and the enzyme acetyl hydrolase in plasma and leukocytes catabolizes PAF back to lyso-PAF. Production of PAF and arachidonic acid metabolites are often closely linked because a main substrate for phospholipase A_2 is 1-0-alkyl-2-arachidonyl-sn-glycero-3-phosphocholine, whose cleavage results in the formation of both arachidonic acid and lyso-PAF. Because virtually all cells can produce a variety of lipid mediators, this discussion describes the cellular sources of mediators and their actions within the context of those products that have been reported in BAL fluids of asthmatic persons.

Direct evidence for the role of lipid mediators in airway inflammation and asthma has been obtained by analysis of BAL fluids from asthmatic individuals both at baseline and after bronchoprovocation with allergen. Total prostanoids, particularly PGD_2 and its metabolite, 9α, 11β-PGF_2, were increased in mild allergic asthmatics compared with both allergic rhinitic and normal control groups (19). Challenge of the airways of allergic asthmatic persons with antigen instilled via the bronchoscope resulted in release, within minutes, of multiple prostanoids including PGD_2, 9α, 11β-PGF_2, TXB_2 (the stable metabolite of TXA_2), and 6-keto-$PGF_{1\alpha}$ (the stable metabolite of prostacyclin PGI_2) (21,38, 39,89). Quantitatively, these products are dominated by PGD_2 implicating airway mast cells in the immediate response to antigen. However, the presence of other products suggests the involvement of multiple other cell types in the immediate response, including the macrophage that may produce TXB_2 and PGD_2, the platelet that is a rich source of TXB_2, and the endothelial cell that produces PGI_2.

PGD_2 causes contraction of airway smooth muscle *in vitro* and is a potent bronchoconstrictor after inhalation in both normal and asthmatic persons. It is the most potent bronchoconstricting prostanoid with activity 3.5 times that of $PGF_{2\alpha}$ (112) and 30 times that of histamine (113). The metabolite of PGD_2, $9\alpha,11\beta$-PGF_2, is equal in bronchoconstricting potency to PGD_2 (113). TXA_2 is a potent constrictor of airways and vessels and causes platelet aggregation. PGI_2 has opposite effects on airways, vessels, and platelets from TXA_2. PGE_2 is a bronchodilator.

Elevated levels of LTC_4, LTE_4, LTB_4, and 20-OH-LTB_4 have been reported in persons with asthma compared with atopic and normal control groups (38,39,89). Within minutes after segmental allergen challenge of atopic persons, release of LTC_4 has been detected (17,38); however, another report using gas chromatography–mass spectrometry to measure LTs within minutes after segmental allergen challenge failed to detect release of LTB_4 and LTC_4 (39). Persistent elevations of LTC_4 have been reported during the late-phase response (6 hr) after inhalation challenge with allergen (94) and 48 hours after segmental challenge (34).

The sulfidopeptide leukotrienes, LTC_4, D_4, and E_4, previously referred to as slow-reacting substances of anaphylaxis, are bronchoconstrictors that demonstrate a potency up to 3,000-fold greater than histamine or methacholine upon inhalation in humans (114,115). They also enhance mucous secretion and induce edema formation (116,117). LTB_4 is a modest bronchoconstrictor but has potent effects on neutrophil chemotaxis and degranulation.

Potential sources of LTC_4 include lung mast cells, basophils, macrophages, and eosinophils. LTB_4 is produced by mast cells, basophils, macrophages, and neutrophils. Although leukotriene synthesis is generally limited to inflammatory cells, other cells such as platelets and endothelial cells that do not normally produce LTs because of their inability to produce the precursor LTA_4 can produce LTC_4 from exogenous LTA_4 derived from other sources such as the neutrophil (118,119).

Although PAF activity assessed by bioassay has been reported in blood during the late asthmatic response (120) and in BAL of asthmatics (121), measurements based on gas chromatography–mass spectrometry have detected low or undetectable levels of PAF in BAL fluid with no differences found between allergic persons with or without asthma and normal controls (122). Furthermore, increased PAF levels were not demonstrated after segmental allergen challenge at times from 5 minutes to 20 hours. In contrast, high levels of lyso-phospholipids, including hexadecyl-lyso-glycerophosphocholine (i.e., lyso-PAF), palmitoyl-lyso GPC, and myristoyl-lyso-GPC, were measured in BAL fluids and were markedly increased at 20 hours after segmental allergen challenge. The presence of acetylhydrolase and soluble phospholipase A_2 activities in BAL fluids at this time suggests that one reason for the failure to detect PAF *in vitro* is its rapid metabolism because *in vivo* PAF may be produced by many cells including mast cells, macrophages, neutrophils, and endothelial cells (122).

Kinins

Kinins are peptide mediators that can cause vascular permeability and smooth muscle contraction. Kinin inhalation causes bronchospasm in asthmatics, but not in normal individuals (466). Elevated levels of the kinin generating enzyme, tissue kallikrein, and kinin have been found in asthmatic persons (123). After segmental challenge, kinin generation was accompanied by the influx of high molecular weight kininogen substrate and tissue kallikrein activity (124). Some kinin generation was observed within minutes after segmental allergen challenge, but 19 hours after challenge, marked increases in kinins were associated with albumin influx (21).

EOSINOPHIL GRANULE PRODUCTS

Products from the eosinophil granule include major basic protein (MBP), eosinophil-derived neurotoxin (EDN), eosinophil cationic protein (ECP), and eosinophil peroxidase (EPO), which have cytotoxic effects on tissue and cells. Elevations of MBP, ECP, and EDN have been observed in asthmatic versus nonasthmatic persons or in symptomatic versus asymptomatic asthmatics (20,24, 92,125). Clinical asthma severity and decreased FEV$_1$ have been correlated with BAL ECP levels (125). After segmental allergen challenge of allergic persons, all eosinophil granule products are increased during the late response but not during the immediate response (34). After whole lung bronchoprovocation, increased eosinophil products have been associated with late-phase responders (95), but this association was not confirmed in another study (94). The presence of eosinophil granule products indicates that activation and degranulation of eosinophils is associated with the eosinophil influx observed in asthma and allergic inflammation.

ADHESION MOLECULES

A critical initial step in the recruitment of cells to a site of inflammation is the interaction of adhesion molecules on circulating cells with those on vascular endothelium. Adhesion molecules belonging to the family of selectins or integrins may play important roles in the chronic airway inflammation observed in asthma. These molecules include E-selectin, intercellular adhesion molecule-1 (ICAM-1), and vascular cell adhesion molecule-1 (VCAM-1) on the vascular endothelial cell; and their respective ligands, sialyl-Lewis-X for E-selectin, lymphocyte function associated antigen-1 (LFA-1, CD11a/CD18) and macrophage antigen-1 (Mac-1, CD11b/CD18) for ICAM-1, and very late antigen-4 (VLA-4, CD49d/CD29) for VCAM-1.

Recent studies examining the role of adhesion molecules in asthma have been conflicting. In one study, expression of ICAM-1 and E-selectin in bronchial biopsies was the same between normals and mild asthmatic persons. Six weeks of inhaled corticosteroids decreased eosinophils but did not alter ICAM-1 or E-selectin expression (126). The results did not support a role for these adhesion molecules in airway eosinophilia. Twenty-four hours after whole lung allergen challenge, however, VCAM-1 and ICAM-1 expression was observed and correlated with eosinophil infiltration (127). In spontaneous asthma, ICAM-1, VCAM-1, and E-selectin appeared to be actively synthesized by endothelial cells and expression was correlated with eosinophil infiltration (128). Six hours after segmental allergen challenge, increased ICAM-1 and E-selectin expression was associated with leukocyte infiltration. No change in VCAM-1 was observed (129). In a group of 20 patients with allergic asthma, VCAM-1 expression but not E-selectin or ICAM-1 expression correlated with IL-4 levels in BAL fluids and submucosal eosinophils, supporting a role for selective VCAM-1 expression induced by IL-4 in airway eosinophilia (130). These studies suggest complex interactions among adhesion molecules and inflammatory cells may influence leukocyte recruitment.

Indirect evidence for the involvement of adhesion molecules in airway inflammation has been obtained by examination of BAL fluids 20 to 24 hours after segmental allergen challenge of allergic persons with or without asthma in whom increased levels of the soluble forms of E-selectin (131), ICAM-1 (132), and VCAM-1 (133) have been found. The increased concentrations of these adhesion molecules exceeded those that could be attributed to plasma influx alone. Simultaneous examination of adhesion molecule expression on infiltrating eosinophils, neutrophils, and basophils during late-phase inflammation revealed increased expression of β_2 integrins such as CD11b/CD18 and reduced expression of L-selectin compared with blood (131). This altered pattern of adhesion molecule expression may be due to the migration process itself because identical changes occur on eosinophils that have migrated through vascular endothelium *in vitro* (134).

REACTIVE OXYGEN SPECIES (ROS)

Several inflammatory cell types, including macrophages, neutrophils, and eosinophils, are capable of generating reactive oxygen species. These oxidants include superoxide anion, hydroxyl radicals, hydrogen peroxide, singlet oxygen, and hypohalous acids, which may cause cellular injury and alterations in airway function (135,136). Increased generation of ROS has been demonstrated in BAL cells from asthmatics compared with nonasthmatic individuals (137). During nocturnal asthma, spontaneous superoxide anion generation by BAL cells is increased compared with daytime generation, and is inversely correlated with the ratio of morning to evening FEV$_1$ (138). During both the immediate and the late inflammatory response after segmental antigen challenge, enhanced production of ROS, particularly superoxide anion, by BAL cells compared with BAL cells from baseline or saline-challenged controls has been demonstrated (139–141). Alveolar macrophages and eosinophils have been identified as the predominant sources of these ROS, and spontaneous ROS production by BAL cells has been correlated with airway injury assessed by albumin influx during the late response (139). Further evidence for ROS in the inflammation associated with asthma is derived from measures of antioxidants in BAL fluids. Smith et al. reported higher levels of the antioxidant glutathione and normal levels of superoxide dismutase and catalase in BAL fluids of asthmatics versus nonasthmatics, suggesting that higher levels of antioxidants were produced in response to an increased oxidant burden. Higher glutathione levels were correlated with lower reactivity to methacholine (142).

IMMUNOGLOBULINS

Immunoglobulins on the airway surface may be involved in the initiation or prevention of inflammatory responses and elevations have been reported in asthmatics compared with normal control groups. The relative contributions of plasma versus local production of immunoglobulins in the airway have not been clarified. Elevated levels of secretory IgA (sIgA) and lactoferrin reported in asthma suggest increase epithelial cell secretion (143). In a comparison of mild allergic asthmatic, allergic rhinitic, and normal persons, IgA and total IgA in BAL fluids were increased in rhinitics compared with normals with a trend toward an increase in the asthmatics compared to normals. No differences were found in IgG and IgM. Eighty-four percent of total IgA was present as sIgA, supporting local secretory mechanisms (144). IgA has been shown to mediate eosinophil degranulation *in vitro* (145), and increased IgA receptors have been reported on the eosinophils of allergic individuals (146), supporting IgA-mediated mechanisms for eosinophil activation in airway inflammation. Increases of IgM reported in asthmatic compared with normal controls may be related to a combination of local production and plasma exudation (33,147), whereas increases reported in IgG subclasses 1–4 appear to be most likely related to plasma exudation (148).

MARKERS OF AIRWAY PERMEABILITY

Albumin, urea, and fibrinogen are components in blood that have been used as markers of vascular and epithelial permeability because increased concentrations of these substances in BAL fluids suggest plasma exudation. Asthmatics may display increased BAL albumin that decreases with inhaled steroid therapy (149), although other studies did not support increased albumin levels in asthmatics (13,33,150,151). After segmental challenge with allergen, influx of albumin (152) and fibrinogen (153) occurred within minutes, and increased albumin and urea were observed during the late response and have been correlated with levels of histamine and prostanoid mediators, eosinophil influx, and kinin generation (21). Eosinophil and platelet granule products (108) and spontaneous production of superoxide by BAL cells have been correlated with albumin influx into BAL fluid (139).

HYALURONIC ACID

The chronic inflammation associated with asthma is likely to involve airway remodeling, particularly in severe or progressive disease. Thickening of the basement membrane region below the airway epithelium is a histologic feature of asthma, although its functional significance is unknown. By immunohistochemistry, thickening of this region has been characterized as a form of fibrosis because of deposition of collagen types III, V, and fibronectin below the true basement membrane composed of collagen type IV, laminin, and fibronectin (154). This fibrotic component of asthma is associated with the presence of myofibroblasts (155). Hyaluronic acid is a glycosaminoglycan component of the extracellular matrix of the lung. Hyaluronic acid was the only glycosaminoglycan found in the therapeutic BAL of several patients with severe asthma (156) and elevated levels of hyaluronic acid have been correlated with severity of clinical function in asthma (125). These findings are consistent with increased fibroblast activity or destruction of extracellular matrix in asthma.

CYTOKINES

Cytokines are secreted proteins that are involved in virtually every aspect of immune and inflammatory responses, including antigen presentation, development of cell-mediated and humoral immunity, differentiation of precursor cells in bone marrow, adhesion molecule expression, and cell recruitment, infiltration, and activation. Cytokines determine the nature of the inflammatory or immunologic response as well as the effector mechanisms involved in the response. The cytokine network is characterized by redundancy with multiple cellular sources of the same cytokine, broad and overlapping biologic functions of different cytokines, and shared receptor components for cytokines on target cells. In addition, the cytokine profile may depend on the state of cellular activation or differentiation, and cytokines themselves may be able to stimulate their own production from certain cellular sources. Given these complexities, it should be no surprise that observations regarding the cellular sources and the roles of certain cytokines in asthma and allergic inflammation is extremely complex and predominant pathways in disease pathogenesis have yet to be defined.

Using a variety of techniques including immunoassay, assays of biologic activity, immunohistochemistry, *in situ* hybridization (ISH), or reverse transcription–polymerase chain reaction (RT-PCR), cytokine production or gene expression has been examined in asthma or after allergen bronchoprovocation. The cytokines present and elevated in BAL fluids or cells under these conditions include tumor necrosis factor-α (TNF-α), interleukins (IL) 1-6, 8, 13, and 16, soluble IL-2 receptor, GM-CSF, interferon-γ (IFN-γ), transforming growth factor-α (TGF-α), RANTES, and macrophage inflammatory protein-1α (MIP-1α). IL-10 is decreased in asthma compared with normals. Recent reviews of cytokines and their possible roles in inflammation associated with asthma and allergic responses are available (157–159) and the present discussion will be limited to findings from *in vivo* human studies in which BAL studies suggest a role for certain cytokines in regulating the immunologic or inflammatory response.

In a series of studies to examine the role of cytokines in asthma, Robinson et al. reported that BAL cells from atopic asthmatics expressed a TH2-predominant cytokine profile compared with normal controls. By ISH of BAL cells, increased numbers of cells expressing mRNA for

IL-2, IL-3, IL-4, IL-5, and GM-CSF but not IFN-γ were reported. Expression of IL-4 and IL-5 was predominantly in the T-lymphocyte population (160). To examine the relationship between cytokines and clinical measures of asthma severity, BAL cells from patients with symptomatic and asymptomatic asthma were studied by the same technique. Increased numbers of cells positive for IL-3, IL-4, IL-5, and GM-CSF, but not IL-2 or IFN-γ, were found in the symptomatic group compared with those without symptoms, supporting a TH2-predominant cytokine profile. Significant correlations were found between expression of IL-4, IL-5, and GM-CSF, and low FEV₁, bronchial hyperreactivity, and clinical asthma severity (161). Treatment with prednisolone for 2 weeks decreased methacholine hyperresponsiveness that was associated with decreased BAL eosinophils. Cells expressing IL-4 and IL-5 were decreased, whereas those expressing IFN-γ were increased (162). Allergen inhalation resulted in increased CD4 cells expressing CD25 with increases in cells expressing IL-4, IL-5, and GM-CSF, but not IL-3, IL-2, or IFN-γ (85,163). Using immunoassays or bioassays, Walker et al. described different cytokine elevations associated with allergic and nonallergic asthma. IL-4 and IL-5 were increased in the allergic asthmatic group, whereas IL-2 and IL-5 were increased in the nonallergic asthmatic group (78). By immunoassays or bioassays, Broide et al. reported increased levels of TNF, GM-CSF, IL-1β, IL-2, and IL-6, but not IL-1α or IL-4 in BAL fluids from symptomatic versus asymptomatic asthmatics (164).

The preponderant evidence places the TH2-associated cytokines IL-4 and IL-5 in a central role in asthma and allergic inflammation (165). IL-4 induces the isotype switching of B cells to synthesis of IgE (166,167), stimulates T-cell proliferation and differentiation of T lymphocytes into the TH2 phenotype primarily involved with regulating humoral immunity and allergy (168), and specifically enhances the expression of VCAM-1 on endothelial cells that promotes the selective recruitment of eosinophils, basophils, monocytes, and lymphocytes that bear the specific ligand VLA-4 on their surface (169, 170). Allergic inflammation appears to involve specific recruitment of these types of leukocytes from the circulation (21). Although lymphocytes appear to be a predominant source of IL-4, other sources reported in histologic specimens include mast cells examined by immunohistochemistry in bronchial biopsies of asthmatics (44,45), eosinophils in nasal and airway biopsies from asthmatics (171), and basophils (172).

IL-5 is probably the most important cytokine controlling eosinophilopoeisis and promotes the differentiation (173), recruitment (174) activation, and survival of eosinophils (175). However, IL-3, GM-CSF, and IFN-γ also promote eosinophil activation and survival. IL-3 is a mast cell growth factor and can also activate and prolong survival of basophils.

After segmental allergen challenge, levels of GM-CSF in BAL fluids increased during the late response (96, 176). By ISH, lymphocytes were the predominant source with a small contribution from macrophages (96), although later studies also demonstrated GM-CSF and IL-5 expression in eosinophils (177). Virchow et al. demonstrated significant increases in levels of IL-1, IL-2, IL-5, IL-6, IL-8, TNF-α, and GM-CSF, but not IL-4 and IFN-γ, 18 hours after segmental allergen challenge compared with saline challenge or 10 minutes after allergen challenge. IL-5 levels correlated with eosinophil numbers and activated CD4+ T cells expressing CD25 (i.e., IL-2R) suggesting T cell–derived IL-5 as the cause of airway eosinophilia (178). Other studies have demonstrated increased IFN-γ and TNF-α levels in BAL fluids after segmental allergen challenge (179,180). Similar findings associating IL-4, IL-5, or soluble VCAM levels in BAL fluids with airway eosinophilia have also been reported using similar models (34,133,181). Using blocking antibodies against various cytokines, IL-5 has been identified as the major eosinophil-active cytokine in the late response to allergen challenge (182). After segmental allergen challenge, mRNA levels assessed by competitive RT-PCR from BAL cells were markedly increased for IL-4 and IL-5 with no change in IFN-γ. IL-5 mRNA expression was limited to the mononuclear cell fraction, supporting a predominant lymphocyte source (183,184).

In addition to IL-4, IL-5, and the cytokines such as IL-3, GM-CSF, and IFN-γ that activate and prolong survival of eosinophils, each of the cytokines mentioned above has activities that may play important roles in asthma. IL-1 is a monocyte/macrophage product that plays a major role as a lymphocyte activating factor. IL-1 provides a second signal required for T-cell activation and proliferation after T-cell receptor interaction with the antigen-MHC complex on an antigen-presenting cell. In addition to its role in immune responses, IL-1 may play a major proinflammatory role by activating endothelial cells to express adhesion molecules including ICAM, VCAM, and E-selectin involved in leukocyte recruitment. TNF is also a product of mononuclear phagocytes that acts like IL-1 in inducing expression of adhesion molecules in endothelial cells. IL-2 is a major factor involved in the proliferation of T cells that express the high-affinity IL-2 receptor. IL-6 plays a role in B-cell maturation into mature plasma cells capable of immunoglobulin secretion. IL-8 is a member of the C-X-C chemokine family and is one of the most potent chemotactic factors for neutrophils. IFN-γ is the main macrophage-activating cytokine and may be involved in cell recruitment by inducing ICAM-1 expression on endothelial cells. IFN-γ may also inhibit allergic responses by inhibiting of IgE production induced by IL-4 (185).

By competitive RT-PCR, induction of mRNA for IL-13 was demonstrated in BAL cells after segmental challenge of allergic asthmatic individuals, and expression was limited to the mononuclear cell population suggesting a lymphocyte source. Increase in IL-13 immunoreactivity in BAL fluids was also demonstrated (186). IL-13 shares many of the activities of IL-4 on macrophages and B cells, and like IL-4 specifically induces VCAM-1 expression on endothelial cells. Unlike IL-4, however, IL-13 does not have effects on T lymphocytes.

By ISH, expression of TGF-α has been localized predominantly to infiltrating eosinophils during the late response after segmental allergen challenge. Release of TGF-α protein was also demonstrated at this time (187). TGF-α is related to epidermal growth factor and may promote angiogenesis and fibroblast activity.

Recently, IL-10 levels in BAL of allergic asthmatics were found to be significantly lower than normals, supporting the possibility that lack of an intrinsic anti-inflammatory peptide plays a role in asthma (188). IL-10, or cytokine synthesis inhibitory factor, has major down-regulating effects on allergic inflammation by inhibiting IL-4 and IL-5 production, eosinophil survival, and IgE synthesis.

In a recent study of chemotactic activities in BAL fluids 6 hours after antigen challenge of allergic asthmatic persons, the major T-cell chemoattractant appeared to be IL-16 (i.e., lymphocyte chemoattractant factor), a chemotactic factor with specificity for CD4+ T lymphocytes. MIP-1α also contributed to the lymphocyte chemotactic activity in BAL fluids (189).

CONCLUSIONS

Bronchoscopy with BAL has become a widely accepted and powerful tool to examine the airways of asthmatic patients. The procedure can be performed safely with acceptable risk under a wide variety of clinical and experimental conditions; however, its use should be guided by the importance of the scientific questions to be answered. BAL has provided valuable information on the alterations in cell numbers, state of cellular activation, inflammatory mediators, cytokines, and airway permeability that may accompany asthma and allergic inflammation. In fact, much of our understanding of asthma as an inflammatory disease is derived from BAL data. Although BAL has provided insights into the complexity of inflammatory and immunologic mechanisms involved in asthma, the studies have highlighted the variability of findings in patients with apparently similar clinical disease. It should be appreciated that the mechanisms and critical pathways by which airway inflammation are translated into the clinical manifestations of asthma are only beginning to be appreciated. Answers regarding the importance of inflammatory events identified by BAL studies to the pathogenesis of asthma await specific interventions that can be applied in humans to block specific pathways. These limitations should be kept in mind when one attempts to apply insights gained into asthma pathogenesis to the care and treatment of patients.

REFERENCES

1. Smith DL, Deshazo RD. Bronchoalveolar lavage in asthma—an update and perspective. *Am Rev Respir Dis* 1993;148:523–532.
2. Djukanovic R, Roche WR, Wilson JW, et al. Mucosal inflammation in asthma. *Am Rev Respir Dis* 1990;142:434–457.
3. Calhoun WJ, Jarjour NN, Gleich GJ, Stevens CA, Busse WW. Increased airway inflammation with segmental versus aerosol antigen challenge. *Am Rev Respir Dis* 1993;147:1465–1471.
4. National Institutes of Health Workshop Summary—Summary and recommendations of a workshop on the investigative use of fiberoptic bronchoscopy and bronchoalveolar lavage in individuals with asthma. *J Allergy Clin Immunol* 1985;76:145–147.
5. Bleecker ER, McFadden ER, et al. Workshop summary and guidelines: investigative use of bronchoscopy, lavage, and bronchial biopsies in asthma and other airway diseases. *J Allergy Clin Immunol* 1991;88:808–814.
6. European Society of Pneumology Task Group on BAL . Technical recommendations and guidelines for bronchoalveolar lavage (BAL). *Eur Respir J* 1989;2:561–585.
7. Rankin JA, Snyder PE, Schachter EN, Matthay RA. Bronchoalveolar lavage: its safety in subjects with mild asthma. *Chest* 1984;85:723–728.
8. Van Vyve T, Chanez P, Bousquet J, Lacoste J-Y, Michel F-B, Godard P. Safety of bronchoalveolar lavage and bronchial biopsies in patients with asthma of variable severity. *Am Rev Respir Dis* 1992;146:116–121.
9. Djukanovic R, Wilson JW, Lai CKW, Holgate ST, Howarth PH. The safety aspects of fiberoptic bronchoscopy, bronchoalveolar lavage, and endobronchial biopsy in asthma. *Am Rev Respir Dis* 1991;143:772–777.
10. Reynolds HY. Bronchoalveolar lavage. *Am Rev Respir Dis* 1987;135:250–263.
11. Lam S, LeRiche JC, Kijek K, Phillips D. Effect of bronchial lavage volume on cellular and protein recovery. *Chest* 1985;88:856–859.
12. Moller GM, deJong TAW, van der Kwast TH, et al. Immunolocalization of interleukin-4 in eosinophils in the bronchial mucosa of atopic asthmatics. *Am J Respir Cell Mol Biol* 1996;14:439–443.
13. Ward C, Duddridge M, Fenwick J. Evaluation of albumin as a reference marker of dilution in bronchoalveolar lavage fluid from asthmatic and control subjects. *Thorax* 1993;48:513–522.
14. Rennard SI, Basset G, Lecossier D, et al. Estimation of volume of epithelial lining fluid recovered by lavage using urea as a marker of dilution. *J Appl Physiol* 1986;60:532–538.
15. Davis GS, Giancola MS, Costanza MC, Low RB. Analyses of sequential bronchoalveolar lavage samples from healthy human volunteers. *Am Rev Respir Dis* 1982;126:611–616.
16. Reynolds HY, Fulmer JD, Kazmierowski JA, Roberts WC, Frank MM, Crystal RG. Analysis of cellular and protein content of bronchoalveolar lavage fluid from patients with idiopathic pulmonary fibrosis and chronic hypersensitivity pneumonitis. *J Clin Invest* 1977;59:165–175.
17. Marcy TW, Merrill WM, Rankin JA, Reynolds HY. Limitations of using urea to quantify epithelial lining fluid recovery by bronchoalveolar lavage. *Am Rev Respir Dis* 1987;135:1276–1280.
18. Churchill L, Chilton FH, Resau JH, Bascom R, Hubbard WC, Proud D. Cyclooxygenase metabolism of endogenous arachidonic acid by cultured human tracheal epithelial cells. *Am Rev Respir Dis* 1989;140:449–459.
19. Liu MC, Bleecker ER, Lichtenstein LM, et al. Evidence for elevated levels of histamine, prostaglandin D2, and other bronchoconstricting prostaglandins in the airways of subjects with mild asthma. *Am Rev Respir Dis* 1990;142:126–132.
20. Adelroth E, Rosenhall L, Johansson S, Linden M, Venge P. Inflammatory cells and eosinophilic activity in asthmatics investigated by bronchoalveolar lavage. *Am Rev Respir Dis* 1990;142:91–99.
21. Liu MC, Hubbard WC, Proud D, Stealey BA, et al. Immediate and late inflammatory responses to ragweed antigen challenge of the pe-

ripheral airways in allergic asthmatics. *Am Rev Respir Dis* 1991;144:51–58.

22. Gravelyn TR, Pan PM, Eschenbacher WL. Mediator release in an isolated airway segment in subjects with asthma. *Am Rev Respir Dis* 1988;137:641–646.

23. Wenzel SE, Fowler AAIII, Schwartz LB. Activation of pulmonary mast cells by bronchoalveolar allergen challenge: *In vivo* release of histamine and tryptase in atopic subjects with and without asthma. *Am Rev Respir Dis* 1988;137:1002–1008.

24. Broide DH, Gleich GJ, Cuomo AJ, et al. Evidence of ongoing mast cell and eosinophil degranulation in symptomatic asthma airway. *J Allergy Clin Immunol* 1991;88:637–648.

25. Tomioka M, Ida S, Shindoh Y, Ishihara T, Takishima T. Mast cells in bronchoalveolar lumen of patients with bronchial asthma. *Am Rev Respir Dis* 1984;129:1000–1005.

26. Kirby JG, Hargreave FE, Gleich GJ, O'Byrne PM. Bronchoalveolar cell profiles of asthmatic and nonasthmatic subjects. *Am Rev Respir Dis* 1987;136:379–383.

27. Casale TB, Wood D, Richerson HB, Trapp S, Metzger WJ, Zavala D, Hunninghake GW. Elevated bronchoalveolar lavage fluid histamine levels in allergic asthmatics are associated with methacholine bronchial hyperresponsiveness. *J Clin Invest* 1987;79:1197–1203.

28. Flint KC, Leung KBP, Hudspith BN, Brostoff J, Pearce FL, Johnson NMI. Bronchoalveolar mast cells in extrinsic asthma: a mechanism for the initiation of antigen specific bronchoconstriction. *Br Med J* 1985;291:923–926.

29. Wardlaw AJ, Dunette S, Gleich GJ, Collins JV, Kay AB. Eosinophils and mast cells in bronchoalveolar lavage in subjects with mild asthma. *Am Rev Respir Dis* 1988;137:62–69.

30. Foresi A, Bertorelli G, Pesci A, Chetta A, Olivieri D. Inflammatory markers in bronchoalveolar lavage and in bronchial biopsy in asthma during remission. *Chest* 1990;98:528–535.

31. Mattoli S, Mattoso V, Soloperto M, Allegra L, Fasoli A. Cellular and biochemical characteristics of bronchoalveolar lavage fluid in symptomatic non-allergic asthma. *J Allergy Clin Immunol* 1991;87:794–802.

32. Zehr BB, Casale TB, Wood D, Floerchinger C, Richerson HB, Hunninghake GW. Use of segmental airway lavage to obtain relevant mediators from the lungs of asthmatic and control subjects. *Chest* 1989;95:1059–1063.

33. Van Vyve T, Chanez P, Bernard A, et al. Protein content in bronchoalveolar lavage fluid of patients with asthma and control subjects. *J Allergy Clin Immunol* 1995;95:60–68.

34. Sedgwick JB, Calhoun WJ, Gleich GJ, et al. Immediate and late airway response of allergic rhinitis patients to segmental antigen challenge. *Am Rev Respir Dis* 1991;144:1274–1281.

35. Wenzel SE, Fowler AA,III, Schwartz LB. Activation of pulmonary mast cells by bronchoalveolar allergen challenge. *Am Rev Respir Dis* 1988;137:1002–1008.

36. Wenzel SE, Westcott JY, Larsen GL. Bronchoalveolar lavage fluid mediator levels 5 minutes after allergen challenge in atopic subjects with asthma: relationship to the development of late asthmatic responses. *J Allergy Clin Immunol* 1991;87:540–548.

37. Wenzel SE, Larsen GL, Johnston K, Voelkel NF, Westcott JY. Elevated levels of leukotriene C4 in bronchoalveolar lavage fluid from atopic asthmatics after endobronchial allergen challenge. *Am Rev Respir Dis* 1990;142:112–119.

38. Wenzel SE, Westcott JY, Smith HR, Larsen GL. Spectrum of prostanoid release after bronchoalveolar allergen challenge in atopic asthmatics and in control groups: an alteration in the ratio of bronchoconstrictive to bronchoprotective mediators. *Am Rev Respir Dis* 1989;139:450–457.

39. Murray JJ, Tonnel AB, Brash AR, et al. Release of prostaglandin D2 into human airways during acute antigen challenge. *N Engl J Med* 1986;315:800–804.

40. Crimi E, Chiaramondia M, Milanese M, Rossi GA, Brusasco V. Increased numbers of mast cells in bronchial mucosa after the late-phase asthmatic response to allergen. *Am Rev Respir Dis* 1991;144:1282–1286.

41. Bradding P, Feather IH, Howarth PH, et al. Interleukin 4 is localized to and released by human mast cells. *J Exp Med* 1992;176:1381–1386.

42. Jaffe JS, Glaum MC, Raible DG, et al. Human lung mast cell IL–5 gene and protein expression: Temporal analysis of upregulation following IgE-mediated activation. *Am J Respir Cell Mol Biol* 1995;13:665–675.

43. Jaffe JS, Raible DG, Post, et al. Human lung mast cell activation leads to IL-13 mRNA expression and protein release. *Am J Respir Cell Mol Biol* 1996;15:473–481.

44. Bradding P, Roberts JA, Britten KM, et al. Interleukin-4, -5, and -6 and tumor necrosis factor-alpha in normal and asthmatic airways: evidence for the human mast cell as a source of these cytokines. *Am J Respir Cell Mol Biol* 1994;10:471–480.

45. Bradding P, Okayama Y, Howarth PH, Church MK, Holgate ST. Heterogeneity of human mast cells based on cytokine content. *J Immunol* 1995;155:297–307.

46. Kimura I, Tanizaki Y, Saito K, Takahashi K, Ueda N, Sato S. Appearance of basophils in the sputum of patients with bronchial asthma. *Clin Allergy* 1975;1:95–98.

47. Koshino T, Teshima S, Fukushima N, et al. Identification of basophils by immunohistochemistry in the airways of postmortem cases of fatal asthma. *Clin Exp Immunol* 1993;23:919–925.

48. Koshino T, Arai Y, Miyamoto Y, et al. Airway basophil and mast cell density in patients with bronchial asthma: Relationship to bronchial hyperresponsiveness. *J Asthma* 1996;33(2):89–95.

49. Guo C-B, Liu MC, Galli SJ, Bochner BS, Kagey-Sobotka A, Lichtenstein LM. Identification of IgE-bearing cells in the late-phase response to antigen in the lung as basophils. *Am J Respir Cell Mol Biol* 1994;10:384–390.

50. Beasley R, Roche WR, Roberts JA, Holgate ST. Cellular events in the bronchi in mild asthma and after bronchial provocation. *Am Rev Respir Dis* 1989;139:806–817.

51. MacGlashan D, White JM, Huang SK, Ono SJ, Schroeder J, Lichtenstein LM. Secretion of interleukin-4 from human basophils: the relationship between IL-4 mRNA and protein in resting and stimulated basophils. *J Immunol* 1994;152:3006–3016.

52. Li H, Sim TC, Alam R. IL-13 released by and localized in human basophils. *J Immunol* 1996;156:4833–4838.

53. Eschenbacher WL, Gravelyn TR. A technique for isolated airway segment lavage. *Chest* 1992;92:105–109.

54. Liu MC, Proud D, Schleimer RP, Plaut M. Human lung macrophages enhance and inhibit lymphocyte proliferation. *J Immunol* 1984;132:2895–2903.

55. Langhoff E, Steinman RM. Clonal expansion of human T lymphocytes initiated by dendritic cells. *J Exp Med* 1989;169:315–320.

56. Melewicz FM, Kline LE, Cohen AB, Spiegelberg HL. Characterization of Fc receptors for IgE on human alveolar macrophages. *Clin Exp Immunol* 1982;49:374–370.

57. Williams J, Johnson S, Mascali JJ, Smith H, Rosenwasser LJ, Borish L. Regulation of low affinity IgE receptor (CD23) expression on mononuclear phagocytes in normal and asthmatic subjects. *J Immunol* 1992;149:2823–2829.

58. Tonnel AB, Joseph M, Gosset P, Fournier E, Capron A. Stimulation of alveolar macrophages in asthmatic patients after local provocation test. *Lancet* 1983;1:1408.

59. Fuller RW, Morris PK, Richmond R, et al. Immunoglobulin E-dependent stimulation of human alveolar macrophages: significance in type 1 hypersensitivity. *Clin Exp Immunol* 1986;65:416–426.

60. Rankin JA. The contribution of alveolar macrophages to hyperreactive airway disease. *J Allergy Clin Immunol* 1989;83:722–729.

61. Fuller RW. The role of alveolar macrophage in asthma. *Res Med* 1989;83:177–178.

62. Tonnel M, Tonnel AB, Capron A, Voisin C. Enzyme release and superoxide production by human alveolar macrophages stimulated with immunoglobulin E. *Clin Exp Immunol* 1980;40:416–420.

63. MacDermot J, Kelsey CR, Wadell KA, Richmond R, Knight RK, Cole PJ. Synthesis of leukotriene B4 and prostanoids by human alveolar macrophages: analysis by gas chromatography/mass spectrometry. *Prostaglandins* 1984;27:163–179.

64. Arnoux B, Duval D, Benveniste J. Release of platelet activating factor (PAF-acether) from alveolar macrophages by the calcium ionophore A23187 and phagocytosis. *Eur J Clin Invest* 1980;10:437–441.

65. Gosset P, Tsicopoulos A, Wallaert B, Joseph M, Capron A, Tonnel A-B. Tumor necrosis factor alpha and interleukin-6 production by human mononuclear phagocytes from allergic asthmatics after IgE-dependent stimulation. *Am Rev Respir Dis* 1992;146:768–774.

66. Liu MC, Proud D, Lichtenstein LM, MacGlashan DW Jr., et al. Human lung macrophage-derived histamine-releasing activity is due to IgE dependent factors. *J Immunol* 1986;136:2588–2595.

67. MacDonald SM, Lichtenstein LM, Proud D, Plaut M, Naclerio RM, Kagey-Sobotka A. Studies of IgE-dependent histamine releasing factors: heterogeneity of IgE. *J Immunol* 1987;139:506–512.

68. MacDonald SM, Rafnar T, Langdon J, Lawrence LM. Molecular identification of an IgE-dependent histamine-releasing factor. *Science* 1995;269:688–690.

69. Naylor B. The shedding of the mucosa of the bronchial tree in asthma. *Thorax* 1962;17:69–72.

70. Jeffery PK, Wardlaw AJ, Nelson FC, Collins JV, Kay AB. Bronchial biopsies in asthma: an ultrastructural, quantitative study and correlation with hyperreactivity. *Am Rev Respir Dis* 1989;140:1745–1753.

71. Ollerenshaw SL, Woolcock AJ. Characteristics of the inflammation in biopsies from large airways of subjects with asthma and subjects with chronic airflow limitation. *Am Rev Respir Dis* 1992;145:922–927.

72. Laitinen LA, Heino M, Laitinen A, Kava T, Haahtela T. Damage of the airway epithelium and bronchial reactivity in patients with asthma. *Am Rev Respir Dis* 1985;131:599–606.

73. Marini M, Vittori E, Hollemborg J, Mattoli S. Expression of the potent inflammatory cytokines, granulocyte-macrophage-colony-stimulating factor and interleukin-6 and interleukin-8 in bronchial epithelial cells of patients with asthma. *J Allergy Clin Immunol* 1992;89:1001–1009.

74. Sousa AR, Lane SJ, Nakhosteen JA, Yoshimura T, Lee TH, Poston RN. Increased expression of the monocyte chemoattractant protein-1 in bronchial tissue from asthmatic subjects. *Am J Respir Cell Mol Biol* 1994;10:142–147.

75. Sousa AR, Poston RN, Lane SJ, Nakhosteen JA, Lee TH. Detection of GM-CSF in asthmatic bronchial epithelium and decrease by inhaled corticosteroids. *Am Rev Respir Dis* 1993;147:1557–1561.

76. Wang JH, Trigg CJ, Devalia JL, Jordan S, Davies RJ. Effect of inhaled beclomethasone dipropionate on expression of proinflammatory cytokines and activated eosinophils in the bronchial epithelium of patients with mild asthma. *J Allergy Clin Immunol* 1994;94:1025–1034.

77. Sur S, Kita H, Gleich GJ, Chenier TC, Hunt LW. Eosinophil recruitment is associated with IL-5, but not with RANTES, twenty-four hours after allergen challenge. *J Allergy Clin Immunol* 1996;97:1272–1278.

78. Walker C, Bode E, Boer L, Hansel TT, Blaser K, Virchow JC. Allergic and nonallergic asthmatics have distinct patterns of T-cell activation and cytokine production in peripheral blood and bronchoalveolar lavage. *Am Rev Respir Dis* 1992;146:109–115.

79. Poulter LW, Norris A, Power C, Condez A, Schmekel B, Burke C. T-cell dominated inflammatory reactions in the bronchi of asthmatics are not reflected in matched bronchoalveolar lavage specimens. *Eur Respir J* 1992;5:182–189.

80. Kelly C, Ward C, Stenton CS, Bird G, Hendrick DJ, Walters EH. Number and activity of inflammatory cells in bronchoalveolar lavage fluid in asthma and their relation to airway responsiveness. *Thorax* 1988;43:684–692.

81. Kelly CA, Stenton SC, Ward C, Bird G, Hendrick DJ, Walters EH. Lymphocyte subsets in bronchoalveolar lavage fluid obtained from stable asthmatics, and their correlations with bronchial responsiveness. *Clin Exp Allergy* 1988;19:169–175.

82. Walker C, Kaegi MK, Braun P, Blaser K. Activated T cells and eosinophilia in bronchoalveolar lavages from subjects with asthma correlated with disease severity. *J Allergy Clin Immunol* 1991;88:935–942.

83. Spinozzi F, Agea E, Bistoni O, et al. Increased allergen-specific, steroid-sensitive γδT cells in bronchoalveolar lavage fluid from patients with asthma. *Ann Intern Med* 1996;124:223–227.

84. Wilson JW, Djukanovic R, Howard PH, Holgate ST. Lymphocyte activation in bronchoalveolar lavage and peripheral blood in atopic asthma. *Am Rev Respir Dis* 1992;145:958–960.

85. Robinson D, Hamid Q, Bentley A, Ying S, Kay AB, Durham SR. Activation of CD4+ T cells, increased TH2-type cytokine mRNA expression, and eosinophil recruitment in bronchoalveolar lavage after allergen inhalation challenge in patients with atopic asthma. *J Allergy Clin Immunol* 1993;92:313–324.

86. Gratziou C, Carroll M, Walls A, Howarth PH, Holgate ST. Early changes in T lymphocytes recovered by bronchoalveolar lavage after local allergen challenge of asthmatic airways. *Am Rev Respir Dis* 1992;145:1259–1264.

87. Gonzalez MC, Diaz P, Galleguillos FR, Ancic P, Cromwell O, Kay AB. Allergen-induced recruitment of bronchoalveolar helper T-cells (OKT4) and suppressor T-cells (OKT8) in asthma: relative increases in OKT8 cells in single early responders compared with those in late-phase responders. *Am Rev Respir Dis* 1987;136:600–604.

88. Schlosberg M, Bochner BS, Xiao HQ, et al. Adhesion molecule profiles of blood and bronchoalveolar T-lymphocytes after segmental antigen challenge of allergic asthmatic subjects: evidence for active lymphocyte recruitment. *Am J Respir Crit Care Med* 1996;(submitted).

89. Lam S, Al-Majed S, Chan H, Tse K, LeRiche JC, Chan-Yeung M. Differences in mediator release between allergic rhinitis and asthma. *J Allergy Clin Immunol* 1991;87:842–849.

90. Metzger WJ, Richerson HB, Worden K, Monick M, Hunninghake GW. Bronchoalveolar lavage of allergic asthmatic patients following allergen bronchoprovocation. *Chest* 1986;89:477–483.

91. Jarjour NN, Calhoun WJ. Bronchoalveolar lavage in stable asthmatics does not cause pulmonary inflammation. *Am Rev Respir Dis* 1990;142:100–103.

92. Bousquet J, Chanez P, Lacoste JY, et al. Eosinophilic inflammation in asthma. *N Engl J Med* 1990;323:1033–1039.

93. Wardlaw AJ, Dunnette S, Gleich GJ, Collins JV, Kay AB. Eosinopils and mast cells in bronchoalveolar lavage in subjects with mild asthma. *Am Rev Respir Dis* 1988;137:62–69.

94. Diaz P, Gonzalez C, Galleguillos FR, et al. Leukocytes and mediators in bronchoalveolar lavage during allergen-induced late-phase asthmatic reactions. *Am Rev Respir Dis* 1989;139:1383–1389.

95. deMonchy JGR, Kauffman HF, Venge P, et al. Bronchoalveolar eosinophilia during allergen-induced late asthmatic reactions. *Am Rev Respir Dis* 1985;131:373–376.

96. Broide DH, Firestein GS. Endobronchial allergen challenge in asthma. Demonstration of cellular source of granulocyte macrophage colony-stimulating factor by in situ hybridization. *J Clin Invest* 1991;88:1048–1053.

97. del Pozo V, de Andres B, Martin E, et al. Murine eosinophils and IL-1: Alpha IL-1 mRNA detection by *in situ* hybridization. *J Immunol* 1990;144:3117–3122.

98. Kita H, Ohnishi T, Okubo Y, Weiler D, Abrams JS, Gleich GJ. Granulocyte/macrophage colony-stimulating factor and interleukin 3 release from human peripheral blood eosinophils and neutrophils. *J Exp Med* 1991;174:745–748.

99. Desreumaux P, Janin A, Colombel JF, et al. Interleukin 5 messenger RNA expression by eosinophils in the intestinal mucosa of patients with coeliac disease. *J Exp Med* 1992;175:293–296.

100. Hamid Q, Barkans J, Meng Q, et al. Human eosinophils synthesize and secrete interleukin-6, in vitro. *Blood* 1992;80:1496–1501.

101. Braun RK, Franchini M, Erard F, et al. Human peripheral blood eosinophils produce and release interleukin-8 on stimulation with calcium ionophore. *Eur J Immunol* 1993;23:956–960.

102. Moqbel R, Hamid Q, Ying S, et al. Expression of mRNA and immunoreactivity for the granulocyte/macrophage colony-stimulating factor in activated human eosinophils. *J Exp Med* 1991;174:749–752.

103. Costa JJ, Matossian K, Resnick MB, et al. Human eosinophils can express the cytokines tumor necrosis factor-α and macrophage inflammatory protein-1alpha. *J Clin Invest* 1993;91:2673–2684.

104. Wong DTW, Weller PF, Galli SJ, et al. Human eosinophils express transforming growth factor-α. *J Exp Med* 1990;172:673–681.

105. Ohno I, Lea RG, Flanders KC, et al. Eosinophils in chronically inflamed human upper airway tissues express transforming growth factor β-1 gene (TGF-β). *J Clin Invest* 1992;89:1662–1668.

106. Kita H. Editorial—the eosinophil: a cytokine-producing cell? *J Allergy Clin Immunol* 1996;97:889–892.

107. Knauer KA, Lichtenstein LM, Adkinson NF Jr, Fish JE. Platelet activation during antigen-induced airway reactions in asthmatic subjects. *N Engl J Med* 1981;304:1404–1407.

108. Averill FJ, Hubbard WC, Proud D, Gleich GJ, Liu MC. Platelet activation in the lung following antigen challenge in a model of allergic asthma. *Am Rev Respir Dis* 1992;145:571–576.

109. Jarjour NN, Calhoun WJ, Schwartz LB, Busse WW. Elevated bronchoalveolar lavage fluid histamine levels in allergic asthmatics are associated with increased airway obstruction. *Am Rev Respir Dis* 1991;144:83–87.

110. Chilton FH, Lichtenstein LM. Lipid mediators of the allergic reaction. *Chem Immunol* 1990;49:173–205.

111. Henderson WR. The role of leukotrienes in inflammation. *Ann Intern Med* 1994;121:684–697.

112. Hardy CC, Robinson C, Tattersfield AE, Holgate ST. The bronchoconstricting effect of inhaled prostaglandin D2 in normal and asthmatic men. *N Engl J Med* 1984;311:209–213.

113. Beasley CRW, Robinson C, Featherstone RL, et al. 9a, 11B-prostaglandin F2, a novel metabolite of prostaglandin D2 is a potent

contractile agonist of human and guinea pig airways. *J Clin Invest* 1987;79:978–983.

114. Holroyde MC, Altounyan REC, Cole M, Dixon M, Elliott EV. Bronchoconstriction produced in man by leukotrienes C and D. *Lancet* 1981;2:17–18.

115. Griffin M, Weiss JW, Leitch AG, et al. Effects of leukotriene D on the airways in asthma. *N Engl J Med* 1983;308:436–439.

116. Coles SJ, Neill KH, Reid LM, et al. Effect of leukotrienes C4 and D4 on glycoprotein and lysozyme secretion by human bronchial mucosa. *Prostaglandins* 1983;25:155–170.

117. Sofer NA, Lewis RA, Corey EJ, Austen KF. Local effects of synthetic leukotrienes (LTC4, LTD4, LTE4 and LTB4) in human skin. *J Invest Dermatol* 1983;80:115–119.

118. Feinmark SJ, Cannon PJ. Endothelial cell leukotriene C4 synthesis results from intercellular transfer of leukotriene A4 synthesized by polymorphonuclear leukocytes. *J Biol Chem* 1986;261: 16466–16472.

119. Maclouf JA, Murphy RC. Transcellular metabolism of neutrophil-derived leukotriene A4 by human platelets. A potential cellular source of leukotriene C4. *J Biol Chem* 1988;263:174–181.

120. Nakamura T, Morita Y, Kuriyama M, Ishihara K, Ito K, Miyamoto T. Platelet-activating factor in late asthmatic response. *Int Arch Allergy Appl Immun* 1987;82:57–61.

121. Stenton SC, Court EN, Kingston WP, et al. Platelet-activating factor in bronchoalveolar lavage fluid from asthmatic subjects. *Eur Respir J* 1990;3:408–413.

122. Chilton FH, Averill FJ, Hubbard WC, Fonteh AN, Triggiani M, Liu MC. Antigen-induced generation of lyso-phospholipids in human airways. *J Exp Med* 1996;183:2235–2245.

123. Christiansen SC, Proud D, Cochrane CG. Detection of tissue kallikrein in the bronchoalveolar lavage fluids of asthmatic subjects. *J Clin Invest* 1987;79:188–197.

124. Christiansen SC, Proud D, Sarnoff RB, Juergens U, Cochrane CG, Zuraw BL. Elevation of tissue kallikrein and kinin in the airways of asthmatic subjects after endobronchial allergen challenge. *Am Rev Respir Dis* 1992;145:900–905.

125. Bousquet J, Chanez P, Lacoste JY, et al. Indirect evidence of bronchial inflammation assessed by titration of inflammatory mediators in BAL fluid of patients with asthma. *J Allergy Clin Immunol* 1991;88: 649–660.

126. Montefort S, Roche WR, Howarth PH, et al. Intercellular adhesion molecule-1 (ICAM-1) and endothelial leucocyte adhesion molecule-1 (ELAM-1) expression in the bronchial mucosa of normal and asthmatic subjects. *Eur Respir J* 1992;5:815–823.

127. Bentley AM, Durham SR, Robinson DS, et al. Expression of endothelial and leukocyte adhesion molecules intercellular adhesion molecule-1, E-selectin, and vascular cell adhesion molecule-1 in the bronchial mucosa in steady-state and allergen-induced asthma. *J Allergy Clin Immunol* 1993;92:857–868.

128. Ohkawara Y, Yamauchi K, Maruyama N, et al. *In situ* expression of the cell adhesion molecules in bronchial tissues from asthmatics with air flow limitation: *in vivo* evidence of VCAM-1/VLA-4 interaction in selective eosinophil infiltration. *Am J Respir Cell Mol Biol* 1995;12: 4–12.

129. Montefort S, Gratziou C, Goulding D, et al. Bronchial biopsy evidence for leukocyte infiltration and upregulation of leukocyte-endothelial cell adhesion molecules 6 hours after local allergen challenge of sensitized asthmatic airways. *J Clin Invest* 1994;93: 1411–1421.

130. Fukuda T, Fukushima Y, Numao T, et al. Role of interleukin-4 and vascular cell adhesion molecule-1 in selective eosinophil migration into the airways in allergic asthma. *Am J Respir Cell Mol Biol* 1996;14:84–94.

131. Georas SN, Liu MC, Newman W, Beall WD, Stealey BA, Bochner BS. Altered adhesion molecule expression and endothelial activation accompanies the recruitment of human granulocytes to the lung following segmental antigen challenge. *Am Rev Respir Cell Mol Biol* 1992;7:261–269.

132. Takahashi N, Liu MC, Proud D, Yu XY, Hasegawa S, Spannhake EW. Soluble intercellular adhesion molecule-1 (sICAM-1) in bronchoalveolar lavage fluid of allergic subjects following segmental antigen challenge. *Am J Respir Crit Care Med* 1994;150:704–709.

133. Zangrilli JG, Shaver JR, Cirelli RA, et al. sVCAM-1 levels after segmental antigen challenge correlate with eosinophil influx, IL-4 and

134. Ebisawa M, Bochner BS, Georas SN, Schleimer RP. Eosinophil transendothelial migration induced by cytokines I. Role of endothelial and eosinophil adhesion molecules on IL-1-B–induced transendothelial migration. *J Immunol* 1992;149:4021–4028.

135. Freeman BA, Crapo JD. Biology of disease: free radicals and tissue injury. *Lab Invest* 1982;47:412–426.

136. Barnes PJ. Reactive oxygen species and airway inflammation. *Free Radic Biol Med* 1990;9:235–243.

137. Cluzel M, Damon M, Chanez P, et al. Enhanced alveolar cell luminol-dependent chemiluminescence in asthma. *J Allergy Clin Immunol* 1987;80:195–201.

138. Jarjour NN, Busse WW, Calhoun WJ. Enhanced production of oxygen radicals in nocturnal asthma. *Am Rev Respir Dis* 1992;146:905–911.

139. Sanders SP, Zweier JL, Harrison SJ, Trush MA, Rembish SJ, Liu MC. Spontaneous oxygen radical production at sites of antigen challenge in allergic subjects. *Am J Respir Crit Care Med* 1995;151(6):1725–1733.

140. Calhoun WJ, Bush PK. Enhanced reactive oxygen species metabolism of airspace cells and airway inflammation follow antigen challenge in human asthma. *J Allergy Clin Immunol* 1990;86:306–313.

141. Calhoun WJ, Reed HE, Moest DR, Stevens CA. Enhanced superoxide production by alveolar macrophages and air-space cells, airway inflammation, and alveolar macrophage density changes after segmental antigen bronchoprovocation in allergic subjects. *Am Rev Respir Dis* 1992;145:317–325.

142. Smith LJ, Houston M, Anderson J. Increased levels of glutathione in bronchoalveolar lavage fluid from patients with asthma. *Am Rev Respir Dis* 1993;147:1461–1464.

143. van de Graaf EA, Out TA, Kobesen A, Jansen HM. Lactoferrin and secretory IgA in the bronchoalveolar lavage fluid from patients with a stable asthma. *Lung* 1991;169:275–283.

144. Peebles RSJr, Liu MC, Lichtenstein LM, Hamilton RG. IgA, IgG and IgM quantification in bronchoalveolar lavage fluids from allergic rhinitics, allergic asthmatics, and normal subjects by monoclonal antibody-based immunoenzymetric assays. *J Immunol Methods* 1995; 179:77–86.

145. Abu-Ghazaleh , Fujisawa T, Mestecky J, Kyle RA, Gleich GJ. IgA-induced eosinophil degranulation. *J Immunol* 1989;142:2393–2400.

146. Monteiro R, Hostoffer R, Cooper M, Bonner J, Gartland G, Kubagawa H. Definition of immunoglobulin A receptors on eosinophils and their enhanced expression in allergic individuals. *J Clin Invest* 1993;92:1681.

147. Hol BEA, van de Graaf EA, Out TA, Hische EAH, Jansen HM. IgM in the airways of asthma patients. *Int Arch Allergy Appl Immun* 1991;96:12–18.

148. Out TA, van de Graaf EA, van den Berg NJ, Jansen HM. IgG subclasses in bronchoalveolar lavage fluid from patients with asthma. *Scand J Immunol* 1991;33:719–727.

149. van de Graaf EA, Out TA, Roos CM, Jansen HM. Respiratory membrane permeability and bronchial hyperreactivity in patients with stable asthma. *Am Rev Respir Dis* 1991;143:362–368.

150. Lam S, LeRiche JC, Kijek K, Phillips D. Effect of bronchial lavage volume on cellular and protein recovery. *Chest* 1988;6:856–859.

151. Fick R, Metzger W, Richerson H. Increased bronchovascular permeability after allergen exposure in sensitive asthmatics. *J Appl Physiol* 1987;63:1147–1155.

153. Salomonsson P, Gronneberg R, Gilljam H, et al. Bronchial exudation of bulk plasma at allergen challenge in allergic asthma. *Am Rev Respir Dis* 1992;146:1535–1542.

154. Roche WR, Beasley R, Williams JH, Holgate ST. Subepithelial fibrosis in the bronchi of asthmatics. *Lancet* 1989;1:520–524.

155. Brewster CEP, Howarth PH, Djukanovic R, Wilson J, Holgate ST, Roche WR. Myofibroblasts and subepithelial fibrosis in bronchial asthma. *Am J Respir Cell Mol Biol* 1990;3:507–511.

156. Sahu S, Lynn WS. Hyaluronic acid in the pulmonary secretions of patients with asthma. *J Biol Chem* 1978;173:565–568.

157. Borish L, Rosenwasser LJ. Update on cytokines. *J Allergy Clin Immunol* 1996;97:719–734.

158. Schleimer RP, Benenati SV, Friedman B, Bochner BS. Do cytokines play a role in leukocyte recruitment and activation in the lungs? *Am Rev Respir Dis* 1991;143:1169–1174.

159. Kelley J. Cytokines of the lung. *Am Rev Respir Dis* 1990;141: 765–788.

160. Robinson DS, Hamid Q, Ying S, et al. Predominant TH2-like bronchoalveolar T-lymphocyte population in atopic asthma. *N Engl J Med* 1992;326(5):298–304.

161. Robinson DS, Ying S, Bentley AM, Meng Q, North J, Durham SR, Kay AB, Hamid Q. Relationships among numbers of bronchoalveolar lavage cells expressing messenger ribonucleic acid for cytokines, asthma symptoms, and airway methacholine responsiveness in atopic asthma. *J Allergy Clin Immunol* 1993;92:397–403.

162. Robinson D, Hamid Q, Ying S, et al. Prednisolone treatment in asthma is associated with modulation of bronchoalveolar lavage cell interleukin-4, interleukin-5, and interferon-γ cytokine gene expression. *Am Rev Respir Dis* 1993;148:401–406.

163. Kay AB, Ying S, Varney V, et al. Messenger RNA expression of the cytokine gene cluster, IL-3, IL-4, IL-5, and GM-CSF in allergen-induced late-phase reactions in atopic subjects. *J Exp Med* 1991;173:775–778.

164. Broide DH, Lotz M, Cuomo AJ, Coburn DH, Freeman EC, Wasserman SI. Cytokines in symptomatic asthma airways. *J Allergy Clin Immunol* 1992;89:958–967.

165. Del Prete GF, De Carli M, D'Elios MM, et al. Allergen exposure induces the activation of allergen-specific TH2 cells in the airway mucosa of patients with allergic respiratory disorders. *Eur J Immunol* 1993;23:1445–1449.

166. Del Prete G, Maggi E, Parronchi P, et al. IL-4 is an essential factor for the IgE synthesis induced *in vitro* by human T cell clones and their supernatants. *J Immunol* 1988;140:4193–4198.

167. Coffman RL, Seymour BWP, Lebman DA. The role of helper T cell products in mouse B cell differentiation and isotype regulation. *Immunol Rev* 1988;102:5–28.

168. Swain SL, Weinberg AD, English M, Huston G. IL-4 directs the development of Th2-like helper effectors. *J Immunol* 1990;145:3796–3806.

169. Schleimer RP, Sterbinsky SA, Kaiser J, et al. IL-4 induces adherence of human eosinophils and basophils but not neutrophils to endothelium. *J Immunol* 1991;148:1086–1092.

170. Bochner BS, Luscinskas FW, Gimbrone MA Jr, et al. Adhesion of human basophils, eosinophils, and neutrophils to IL-1 activated human vascular endothelial cells: contributions of endothelial cell adhesion molecules. *J Exp Med* 1991;173:1553–1557.

171. Nonaka M, Nonaka R, Woolley K, et al. Distinct immunohistochemical localization of IL-4 in human inflamed airway tissues. *J Immunol* 1995;155:3234–3244.

172. MacGlashan DW, White JM, Huang SK, Ono SJ, Schroeder J, Lichtenstein LM. Secretion of interleukin-4 from human basophils: the relationship between IL-4 mRNA and protein in resting and stimulated basophils. *J Immunol* 1994;152:3006–3016.

173. Clutterbuck EJ, Hirst EMA, Sanderson CJ. Human interleukin-5 (IL-5) regulates the production of eosinophils in human bone marrow cultures: comparison and interaction with IL-1, IL-3, IL-6, and GMCSF. *Blood* 1989;73:1504–1512.

174. Wang JM, Rambaldi A, Biondi A, Chen ZG, Sanderson CJ, Mantovani A. Recombinant human interleukin-5 is a selective eosinophil chemoattractant. *Eur J Immunol* 1989;19:701–705.

175. Lopez AF, Sanderson CJ, Gamble JR, Campbell HD, Young IG, Vadas MA. Recombinant human interleukin-5 is a selective activator of human eosinophil function. *J Exp Med* 1988;167:219–224.

176. Kato M, Liu MC, Stealey BA, et al. Production of granulocyte-macrophage colony-stimulating factor in human airways during allergen-induced late-phase reactions in atopic subjects. *Lymphokine Cytokine Res* 1992;11:287–292.

177. Broide DH, Paine MM, Firestein GS. Eosinophils express interleukin 5 and granulocyte-macrophage colony-stimulating factor in mRNA at sites of allergic inflammation in asthmatics. *J Clin Invest* 1992;90:1414–1424.

178. Virchow J, Walker C, Hafner D, et al. T cells and cytokines in bronchoalveolar lavage fluid after segmental allergen provocation in atopic asthma. *Am J Respir Crit Care Med* 1995;151:960–968.

179. Calhoun WJ, Murphy K, Stevens CA, Jarjour NN, Busse WW. Increased interferon-γ and tumor necrosis factor-α in bronchoalveolar lavage fluid after antigen challenge in allergic subjects. *Am Rev Respir Dis* 1992;145:A638.

180. Cembrzynska-Nowak M, Szklarz E, Inglot AD, Teodorczyk-Injeyan JA. Elevated release of tumor necrosis factor-α and interferon-γ by bronchoalveolar leukocytes from patients with bronchial asthma. *Am Rev Respir Dis* 1993;147:291–295.

181. Dobrina A, Menegazzi R, Carlos TM, et al. Mechanisms of eosinophil adherence to cultured vascular endothelial cells. Eosinophils bind to the cytokine-induced endothelial ligand vascular cell adhesion molecule-1 via the very late activation antigen-4 integrin receptor. *J Clin Invest* 1991;88:20–26.

182. Ohnishi T, Kita H, Weiler S, et al. IL-5 is the predominant eosinophil-active cytokine in the antigen-induced pulmonary late phase reaction. *Am Rev Respir Dis* 1993;147:901–907.

183. Huang SK, Essayan DM, Krishnaswamy G, et al. Detection of allergen- and mitogen-induced human cytokine transcripts using a competitive polymerase chain reaction. *J Immunol Methods* 1994;168:167–181.

184. Liu MC, Xiao HQ, Lichtenstein LM, Huang SK. Prednisone inhibits TH2-type cytokine gene expression at sites of allergen challenge in subjects with allergic asthma. *Am J Respir Crit Care Med* 1994;149:A944.

185. Pene J, Rousset F, Briere F, et al. IgE production by normal human lymphocytes is induced by interleukin-4 and suppressed by interferons alpha and gamma and prostaglandin E2. *Proc Natl Acad Sci* 1988;85:6880–6884.

186. Huang SK, Xiao HQ, Kleine-Tebbe J, Paciotti G, Marsh DG, Lichtenstein LM, Liu MC. IL-13 expression at the sites of allergen challenge in patients with asthma. *J Immunol* 1995;155:2688–2694.

187. Liu MC, Matossian K, Wong DTW, Weller PF, Galli SJ. Expression of mRNA for transforming growth factor-α (TGF-α) by eosinophils at sites of segmental airway challenge with antigen in allergic asthmatic subjects. *Am Rev Respir Dis* 1992;145:A452.

188. Borish L, Aarons A, Rumbyrt J, Cvietusa P, Negri J, Wenzel S. Interleukin—10 regulation in normal subjects and patients with asthma. *J Allergy Clin Immunol* 1996;97:1288–1296.

189. Cruikshank WW, Long A, Tarpy RE, et al. Early identification of interleukin-16 (lymphocyte chemoattractant factor) and macrophage inflammatory protein 1-α (MIP1-α) in bronchoalveolar lavage fluid of antigen-challenged asthmatics. *Am Rev Respir Cell Mol Biol* 1995;13:738–747.

Asthma, edited by P.J. Barnes, M.M. Grunstein,
A.R. Leff, and A.J. Woolcock.
Lippincott–Raven Publishers, Philadelphia © 1997.

▪ 19 ▪

Inflammation

Basic Concepts

Peter A. Ward

Permeability Changes	**Role of Cytokines in the Inflammatory Response**
Endothelial Activation	**Injurious Products of Activated Leukocytes**
Leukocyte Recruitment	

The inflammatory response is a protective mechanism initiated by a variety of conditions, including tissue injury, the presence of infectious agents, and events related to ischemia reperfusion. An inflammatory response protects the tissue and allows for its return to normal function. In some circumstances, such as loss of parenchyma in the case of responses to infectious diseases (e.g., tuberculosis) or ischemic myocardial injury, return to normal function may not be possible, and an array of growth factors comes into play, causing accelerated production of connective tissue matrix and other events that lead to the formation of scar tissue. This chapter describes the current knowledge about mediators involved in the inflammatory response and the manner by which the inflammatory response contributes to tissue injury.

PERMEABILITY CHANGES

Vascular permeability change associated with triggering of an inflammatory response is an active process leading to a transient opening of the tight junctions between endothelial cells and, perhaps also, the rapid endocytic transport of plasma, water, and salt across the cytoplasmic confines of endothelial cells. Obviously, if there is structural damage to the endothelial lining, irreversible permeability may occur, resulting in a prolonged leak of plasma constituents beyond the confines of the vascular compart-

ment. If injury to the endothelium is especially severe, escape of red blood cells (hemorrhage) can also develop. Consideration of the vascular permeability increase in the content of the inflammatory response will be restricted to mediator-induced, transient, and reversible vascular permeability. The transient opening of endothelial tight junctions is assumed to be controlled by mediators that activate contractile elements within endothelial cells and cause lateral shrinking of endothelial cells; this opens the junctional areas. Upon relaxation of these contractile elements, endothelial cells then resume tight junction formations, and the permeability changes are reversed. Only if endothelial cells have been structurally injured is the permeability change likely to be irreversible. Many mediators have been incriminated in permeability changes associated with the acute inflammatory response (1,2). These include vasoactive active amines (histamine, serotonin), peptides such as bradykinin and kinin-related molecules, and lipids such as arachidonate metabolites (eicosanoid products such as prostaglandins and leukotrienes) and the platelet-activating factor, which is a glycerol-based type of lipid with an acetyl group in the C2 position. Except for the vasoactive amines, permeability mediators do not preexist but are synthesized by cells (e.g., eicosanoids) or induced by activation of enzymes that cleave substrates in plasma (as in the case of kinins).

ENDOTHELIAL ACTIVATION

The endothelial lining of blood vessels is not a passive barrier, but is subject to activation processes that can al-

P. A. Ward: Department of Pathology, The University of Michigan, Ann Arbor, Michigan 48109-0602.

ter endothelial function. In addition to the effects of vasopermeability mediators on endothelial cells (as described above), the endothelium (or monolayers of endothelial cells) can be activated by contact with various mediators, causing several possible outcomes. The first is the expression of *adhesion molecules* either through an active protein synthetic process [such as production of intercellular adhesion molecule-1 (ICAM-1), E-selectin, etc.] or by translocation of adhesion-promoting molecules contained in Weible-Palade bodies (granules) of endothelial cells (3–6). A second class of products from activated endothelial cells includes *inflammatory mediators* that, once synthesized by endothelial cells, appear to remain chiefly membrane-bound but, in some cases, may be secreted (7,8). These mediators include platelet-activating factor (PAF) and interleukin-8 (IL-8), which both have the ability to activate neutrophils and monocytes. Under certain conditions, activated endothelial cells also may generate other cytokines such as tumor necrosis factor-α (TNF-α) (8). Accordingly, leukocytes adherent to endothelial cells (by the mechanisms described below) can be activated by their contact with these endothelial-derived mediators. Endothelial cells can produce oxidants that have phlogistic potential, such as *oxygen radicals* (superoxide anion, O_2^-) and nitric oxide ($\cdot$NO) (9,10). $\cdot$NO produced by endothelial cells appears to function as a factor that causes relaxation of subendothelial smooth muscle, thereby regulating vascular tone and blood pressure. Under certain conditions, the simultaneous generation of both $\cdot$NO and O_2^- would lead to formation of toxic radicals, as described below. Activated endothelial cells also can generate a series of *procoagulant factors*, which may be associated with the formation of intravascular thrombi along the endothelial cell surface. These same cells also can express anticoagulants such as tissue plasminogen activator, which has countereffects on the procoagulant products of activated endothelial cells. The balance in the production of these factors by endothelial cells determines if the outcome is proinflammatory or anti-inflammatory.

Regional activation of the endothelium resulting in expression of adhesion molecules, cytokines, and other factors localizes the inflammatory response to an area of injury. In this respect, the endothelium undergoes a modification so that it can promote the inflammatory process only in the context of the area of altered endothelium, thereby restricting the scope of the inflammatory response. Factors such as thrombin, LTB$_4$, C5a, TNF-α, and interleukin-1 (IL-1) can activate the endothelium to bring about expression of various adhesion-promoting molecules. This then sets the stage for adhesion and recruitment of leukocytes into an inflammatory locale. Table 1 shows adhesion-promoting molecules contained either on the surfaces of endothelial cells or leukocytes. The *selectin family* of molecules, which are defined by the presence of an oligosaccharide binding site near the N-terminal region of the se-

TABLE 1. *Adhesion molecules involved in leukocyte-endothelial interactions*

Selectins:	P-, L-, and E
Ig superfamily:	Intercellular adhesion molecule-1 (ICAM-1)
	Vascular cellular adhesion molecule-1 (VCAM-1)
	Platelet-endothelial cell adhesion molecule-1 (PECAM-1)
β1 integrins:	α2β1, etc.
β2 integrins:	CD11a/CD18 (LFA-1)
	CD11b/CD18 (Mac-1)
	CD11c/CD18

lectin molecule, represents an important group of adhesion-promoting molecules in the inflammatory process (4,11–15). There is also evidence that selectins are the first adhesion molecules to be engaged during the inflammatory process. Surface expression of P-selectin is limited to activated platelets and the activated endothelium after translocation and fusion to cytoplasmic granules to the cell membrane, resulting in expression of P-selectin on the surface of the endothelial cell or platelet. When this happens, the P-selectin expressing cell will then bind to another cell containing the "counter-receptor" for P-selectin. Neutrophils and monocytes contain the P-selectin glycoprotein ligand-1 (PSGL-1), which then allows activated platelets to bind to neutrophils and monocytes (thereby enhancing the respiratory burst of the leukocyte and formation of oxidants) and facilitates adhesion of monocytes and neutrophils to the activated endothelium, setting the stage for transmigration. L-selectin is constitutively expressed on virtually all leukocytes. Upon activation, it is usually shed, resulting in a sharp decrease in cell content of L-selectin (5,16). This shedding process appears to be caused by enzymatic cleavage of L-selectin near its transmembrane domain by a chymotrypsin-like enzyme. Cross-linking of L-selectin with antibody will, in some situations, lead to leukocyte activation. To what extent natural "counter-receptors" for L-selectin will do the same is not clear. E-selectin is confined to endothelium and is not constitutively expressed (11). When endothelial cells are activated by contact with cytokines such as TNF-α or IL-1, or when these cells are incubated with bacterial endotoxin (lipopolysaccharide, LPS), gene activation occurs with upregulation of the message for E-selectin (and also ICAM-1). Protein expression then ensues, with E-selectin (and ICAM-1) appearing on the surface of the activated endothelial cell and remaining present for a few hours. Downregulation of expressed E-selectin probably is caused by endocytic removal of surface E-selectin. The "counter-receptors" for the selectins appear to be proteins or lipids, bearing on their surfaces oligosaccharides with the sialyl Lewis^x motif (17,18). In some cases, these oligosaccharides are expressed on mucin-like molecules, although the upregulation and turnover of these counter-receptors are not well understood. Selectins appear to be molecules engaged early in the course of events in the inflammatory response and are required in most instances of leukocyte transmigration (including lymphocyte recirculation) (13, 15,18–20).

The *immunoglobulin superfamily* consists of at least three types of adhesion-promoting molecules, including ICAM-1, vascular cellular adhesion molecule (VCAM-1), and platelet-endothelial cell adhesion molecule-1 (PECAM-1). ICAM-1 is constitutively expressed on endothelial cells but can be upregulated when endothelial cells are activated by cytokines such as TNF-α and IL-1 or with LPS (21). The ICAM-1 counter-receptor on leukocytes includes two molecules in the β2 integrin family, CD11a/CD18 (LFA-1) and CD11b/CD18 (Mac-1, CR3) (see Table 1). ICAM-1 is not limited to endothelial cell expression but, at least in the case of the lung, is also constitutively expressed on type 1 alveolar epithelial cells (22). VCAM-1, whose counter-receptor is VLA-4 (which is present on mononuclear cells and eosinophils), is ordinarily not constitutively expressed on the endothelium but is upregulated, especially upon endothelial cell contact with IL-4 (23–25). VLA-4 also is subject to upregulation on lymphocytes, monocytes, and macrophages by a variety of stimuli. There are suggestions that VCAM-1 can be expressed on bronchial epithelial cells, although this has not been precisely determined. Platelet-endothelial cell adhesion molecule-1 (PECAM-1) is a constitutively expressed adhesion molecule of the immunoglobulin superfamily and is present on the basolateral junctions of endothelial cells, including the intercellular junctional zones (26,27). It appears to be neither upregulated nor downregulated. The receptor for PECAM-1 is not known, although it has been demonstrated that PECAM-1 molecules can associate with one another. Low levels of PECAM-1 have been described on the neutrophil. PECAM-1 is apparently important in facilitating the transmigration of neutrophils through the endothelial barrier, as has been demonstrated both *in vitro* and *in vivo* by the use of PECAM-1 blocking antibodies (28–30). The use of blocking antibodies to PECAM-1 prevents the chemotactic migration of neutrophils across monolayers of endothelial cells and *in vivo* interferes with neutrophil accumulation in experimentally induced peritonitis and alveolitis. Accordingly, PECAM-1 appears to be one in a series of at least three different adhesion molecules that are required for efficient transmigration of leukocytes.

The β1 integrins consist of a large family of heterodimeric molecules containing alpha and beta chains, often with binding activity to motifs containing arginine, glycine and aspartic acid (RGD). β1 integrins appear to have binding properties for many connective tissue matrix molecules and may be important for the movement of leukocytes that have moved beyond the endothelial barrier. The β2 integrins may also play an important role in regulation of connective tissue matrix production.

The β2 integrins consist of at least three heterodimeric molecules, CD11a/CD18 (LFA-1), CD11b/CD18 (Mac-1), and CD11c/CD18 (31–33). The counter-receptor for both LFA-1 and Mac-1 is ICAM-1. LFA-1 also interacts with ICAM-2. There is evidence that Mac-1 (also known as complement receptor 3, CR3) has binding interactions with complement activation products, such as a split product of C3, namely iC3b. Additional factors that bind to these adhesion molecules probably also exist. Relatively little is known about the counter-receptor for CD11c/CD18. Levels of Mac-1 on surfaces of neutrophils can be increased with activation of phagocytic cells, especially neutrophils, because these cells contain a pool of sequestered Mac-1 in secondary granules that normally are present within the cytoplasm (31). Upon activation of neutrophils, granules are translocated to the surface of the cell where they fuse with the cell membrane, resulting in significant increases in Mac-1 expression on the cell surface. Although studies with gene "knock-out" mice suggest that deleted expression in any single vascular adhesion molecule (e.g., L-selectin, ICAM-1, P-selectin) may result in an "adaptation" phenomenon that attenuates the effects on the inflammatory response of a lost component, it is clear that in the case of a genetically determined defect involving CD18 in humans, these individuals are deprived significantly of their ability to mount an inflammatory response and are subject to life-threatening bacterial infections (34).

In general, adhesion molecules play key roles in facilitating not only the recruitment of leukocytes into an inflammatory site, but they are also crucial in facilitating the recirculation of lymphocytes. For instance, in the high endothelial venules (HEV) of lymph nodes, lymphocyte L-selectin interacts with an endothelial counter-receptor, which has been termed *glycoprotein cell adhesion molecule-1* (GlyCAM-1) (35). This molecule is present constitutively on endothelial cells of HEVs and may be subject to upregulation. Endothelial GlyCAM-1 facilitates adhesive interactions between endothelial cells and T cells, such that lymphocyte transmigration occurs into extravascular regions of the lymph node, then into efferent lymphatics, and, finally, back into the blood stream. Blocking of L-selectin or GlyCam-1 causes a build-up of lymphocytes in the blood compartment, which results from their impeded egress from the vascular compartment.

LEUKOCYTE RECRUITMENT

Recruitment of leukocytes into an inflammatory site usually involves at least two general changes. The first involves an alteration (activation) of the endothelium, defined by upregulation of adhesion-promoting molecules that facilitate the binding of leukocytes to the activated endothelium. In addition, leukocytes themselves may undergo within the vascular compartment upregulation by factors such as complement activation products (e.g., C5a), which cause increased Mac-1 expression on neutrophils. This combination of both leukocyte activation, as well as endothelial activation, appears to be the optimal sequence of events that facilitates efficient attachment of leukocytes to the activated endothelium, followed by the transmigration of these cells. It is also important to note that, when leukocytes are treated with certain monoclonal antibodies to subunits of LFA-1 or Mac-1, the binding affinities of the β2 integrins increase substantially and appear to cause intracellular signaling (as reflected by increases in intracellular calcium). Accordingly, it may be that engagement of β2 integrins by their natural ligands leads to signal transduction events in leukocytes, thereby further enhancing their functional responsiveness. This would be the counterpart of "priming" of leukocytes that have come into contact with activated endothelial cells that also contain on their cell surfaces agonists (e.g., IL-8, TNF-α) for leukocytes.

Adhesion-promoting molecules participate in a defined sequence of steps (reviewed in refs. 35–40), the first of which involves selectin engagement with their counter-receptors, resulting in low-affinity binding interactions. These reversible adhesive interactions have, by time-lapse photography, been described as a "rolling" phenomenon of leukocytes along the endothelial surface. Rolling appears to be due to reversible adhesive interactions with endothelial cells. By the use of blocking interventions, L- and P-selectin molecules have been demonstrated to be important in the rolling phenomenon *in vivo*, chiefly in the postcapillary venules. The second interaction in the adhesion-promoting sequence appears to be engagement of β2 integrins with their endothelial cell counter-receptors, such as ICAM-1, leading to high-affinity binding and firm adhesive interactions between leukocytes and endothelial cells. This results in a cessation of lateral motility of leukocytes and their firm binding to the endothelium. A crucial step for transmigration probably requires generation of chemotactic molecules in the extravascular vicinity of the activated endothelium, such that adherent leukocytes can follow a chemotactic gradient as they move through the intercellular junctions and into the interstitial space. Because, as described above, the activated endothelium can also produce mediators such as PAF and IL-8, there is evidence that the adhesive interactions of leukocytes with these products expressed on surfaces of endothelial cells results in stimulation or some type of signal transduction process that "primes" leukocytes as they begin their transmigratory path. As the leukocytes begin to move through the intercellular junction of the endothelium, the third adhesion molecule engagement features PECAM-1 interactions with transmigrating leukocytes. This conclusion is based on the fact that blocking of PECAM-1 *in vitro* (on endothelial monolayers) or *in vivo* results in a much diminished transmigratory response of the adherent leukocytes

(see above). To what extent other adhesion interactions are also involved in these transmigration events remains to be determined.

ROLE OF CYTOKINES IN THE INFLAMMATORY RESPONSE

In general, virtually all cytokines affect the immune response in a variety of different ways, but the focus in this chapter is their role in the inflammatory system. Cytokines, which are products of activated cells, are defined as relatively low molecular weight peptides/proteins (with a molecular mass usually of less than 25 kDa). These molecules can activate other cells and were first described as products from activated lymphocytes. The term "lymphokine" was coined, but it soon became apparent that many other cell types (in addition to lymphocytes) were able to produce these biologically active products. As shown in Table 2, from the standpoint of the inflammatory system, cytokines can be categorized into three areas, depending on their biologic function. The classical *proinflammatory cytokines* include TNF-α and IL-1 (41,42). Cytokines have biologic effects on both leukocytes and endothelial cells. They can stimulate phagocytic cells by engagement of high-affinity cell surface receptors, resulting in induction of chemotactic responses, respiratory burst activity, and enzyme secretion (43,44). Cytokines also can stimulate endothelial cells, causing adhesion-molecule expression (ICAM-1, E-selectin) and generation of mediators such as PAF and IL-8. Another category of cytokines includes the *chemokine group* (IL-8 family of cytokines), which is divided into the α-chemokine and β-chemokine families (see Chapter 51). The structural motifs of the α-chemokine family have a C-X-C structure (cysteine molecules separated by another amino acid), and the β chemokine family have the C-C structure. The term "chemokine" was coined because of the initial observations that members of the IL-8 family of cytokines can cause *in vitro* chemotactic migration of a variety of different types of leukocytes. In general, members of the α-chemokine family are chemotactic for neutrophils, whereas members of the β-chemokine family are chemotactic for monocytes and macrophages (41–52). To a lesser extent, both families of chemokines have chemotactic activity for T cells. The intradermal injection of re-

TABLE 2. *Inflammatory activities of cytokines*

Classic proinflammatory cytokines (TNF-α, IL-1)
Stimulation of phagocytic cells (chemotaxis, respiratory burst, etc.)
Stimulation of endothelial cells
Chemokine (IL-8) family (α and β chemokines)
Anti-inflammatory cytokines (IL-4, IL-10, etc.)
Proinflammatory cytokines (TNF-α, IL-1)

combinant chemokines causes leukocyte accumulation at the site of injection, supporting the view that chemokines facilitate recruitment of leukocytes (46–53). Although it has been concluded that the major biologic effects of chemokines result from their chemotactic activity, chemokines have other important biologic effects. For example, MIP-1α, which is a β-chemokine, regulates lung macrophage production of TNF-α and IL-1, suggesting that, to some extent, chemokines have autocrine stimulatory activity for phagocytic cells (54). *In vivo* blocking of MIP-1α in the lung inflammatory model of IgG immune complex–induced injury is protective by blocking accumulation of neutrophils. However, the defect in neutrophil accumulation appears to be due to greatly diminished lung production of TNF-α, which, accordingly, causes greatly reduced vascular upregulation of ICAM-1. *In vivo* blocking of MIP-1α in the lung inflammatory model of IgG immune complex–induced injury is protective by blocking accumulation of neutrophils. Diminished lung production of TNF-α would lead to greatly reduced vascular upregulation of ICAM-1. The third category of cytokines affecting the inflammatory response is the emerging group of *"regulatory cytokines,"* which have anti-inflammatory activities (55–59). Cytokines in this category include IL-4, IL-10, and, perhaps, IL-12 and IL-13. IL-10 was initially described as the "cytokine synthesis inhibitory factor" (57). Some of these cytokines (IL-4, IL-10) also have additional suppressive activities, such as reducing expression of inducible nitric oxide synthase (58). When used *in vivo,* the anti-inflammatory cytokines (IL-4 and IL-10) have powerful effects in blocking inflammatory responses in experimental animals. For instance, small (ng) concentrations of either IL-4 or IL-10 will suppress lung inflammatory responses to intrapulmonary deposition of IgG immune complexes (59). These effects have been shown to be linked to suppressed production in lung of TNF-α, which is required for *in vivo* upregulation of endothelial adhesion molecules (ICAM-1, E-selectin). Because of the potent anti-inflammatory effects of IL-4 and IL-10, these cytokines are considered to be candidates for blocking of inflammatory reactions in humans, including those associated with allograft rejection. Another cytokine-related product of activated phagocytic cells with regulatory effects on the inflammatory system is the IL-1 receptor antagonist, which is produced after the initial expression by simulated phagocytic cells of TNF-α and IL-1. The IL-1 receptor antagonist has a moderate degree of homology with IL-1 and binds to the IL-1 receptor in a non–signal-transducing manner. It therefore appears to be an important regulator of the inflammatory system and counters the effects of biologically released IL-1 (60,61). Other macrophage products with anti-inflammatory activities are soluble receptors, including soluble TNF-α receptor-1 and soluble IL-1 receptor, which are released by activated phagocytic cells and act like antibodies with relatively high binding affinity for soluble cytokines and have pro-

tective effects *in vivo* in certain types of inflammatory injury (62,63). Accordingly, these soluble receptors prevent cytokine binding to cell-associated receptors. Clearly, cytokines have a broad range of activities. They bind with high affinity to receptors, inducing signal transduction events in receptor-bearing cells, whereas other such cytokines regulate the cytokine network. Understanding the network of cytokine interactions should lead to a better understanding of the inflammatory response.

INJURIOUS PRODUCTS OF ACTIVATED LEUKOCYTES

When leukocytes have been recruited to an inflammatory site, they release oxidants, proteases, and biosynthetically generated products (such as growth factors and cytokines). In the context of understanding how the inflammatory response may lead to injury, oxidant pathways of leukocytes often are activated (as described in Fig. 1). The NADPH oxidase pathway features an enzyme that is assembled on the cell membrane of the phagocytic cell by fusion of at least two cytoplasmic factors with cell membrane–associated components (reviewed in ref. 2). The assembled oxidase, as the name implies, uses NADPH as substrate to bring about progressive single electron transfer to molecular oxygen, with the first product being a radical, superoxide anion (O_2^-). O_2^- itself seems to be rather nontoxic, but its further reduction or its interaction with ·NO can cause generation of tissue-damaging oxidants. The addition of a second electron generates hydrogen peroxide which, in the presence of myeloperoxidase released from neutrophils, produces hypochlorous acid (HOCl), which is a powerful oxidant. HOCl can also activate metalloproteinases such as collagenases and gelatase, which exist in precursor forms in tissues. The addition of a third electron in this scheme converts hydrogen peroxide to the hydroxyl radical, an exceedingly reactive species. This electron transfer requires the presence of a transition metal such as reduced iron or copper. The final addition of an electron (to the hydroxyl radical) results in the formation of the fully oxidized form of oxygen, water. The NADPH oxidase pathway appears to be important in bacterial killing. In humans with chronic granulomatous disease of childhood, a defect in NADPH oxidase results in a high susceptibility to bacterial infections (64). Because of several different genetically determined defects in components of the oxidase in humans, the clinical presentation of these patients may vary, depending on which subunit of the oxidase is affected.

A second pathway of cell activation that leads to oxidant production in phagocytic cells involves induction of inducible nitric oxide synthase (iNOS), which interacts with L-arginine to produce nitric oxide (·NO) and citrulline (Fig. 1). ·NO causes smooth muscle relaxation, especially in vas-

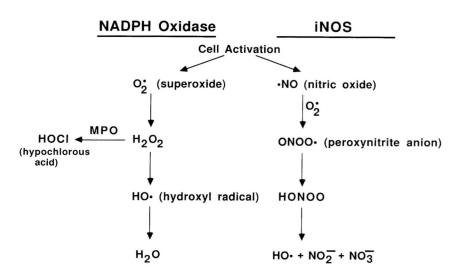

FIG. 1. Oxidant-generating pathways in activated phagocytic cells.

cular walls. ·NO alone appears to be relatively nontoxic. It can reduce adhesiveness of leukocytes to activated endothelial cells, thereby acting as an inflammatory regulator (65). The interaction of ·NO with $O_2·$ results in a reactive intermediate, peroxynitrite anion (ONOO·), which is highly reactive with thiols and other oxidizable groups (66). Nitrosylation of tyrosines (resulting in nitrotyrosine) can serve as a marker of ·NO production in ischemia-reperfusion conditions and other inflammatory responses. Peroxynitrite anion, when protonated, can be converted to the hydroxyl radical. Decay products of this system include nitrite (NO_2^-) and nitrate (NO_3^-), which serve as quantitative markers of ·NO production. There is evidence that ·NO production by phagocytic cells is associated with the killing of ingested parasites (such as trypanosomes and mycobacterial species), but release from activated phagocytic cells of ·NO, especially if $O_2·$ also is being produced (through the assembled NADPH oxidase on the surface of the phagocytic cell), potentially sets the stage for tissue damage by production of ONOO· (67,68).

A second group of toxic products from activated leukocytes includes proteases, which are released from granule-bound sources. In the case of macrophages, biosynthesis of these enzymes also occurs. The best known examples of these are the serine proteases, which include elastase and cathepsin B (reviewed in ref. 69). These proteases can attack a number of substrates in tissues and are regulated by their natural inhibitor, α-protease inhibitor. The loss of regulation of these proteases resulting from genetically determined defects of α-1 protease inhibitor is associated with the development of familial emphysema. It is assumed that loss of this inhibitory activity causes the body to be deprived of its major regulator of serine proteases, for which leukocytic elastase is the most important example. Products of tobacco combustion cause significant oxidative inactivation of α1-protease inhibitor in lung, which may be relevant to a higher inci-

dence of pulmonary emphysema in smokers. The other group of proteases released from activated phagocytic cells (especially macrophages) includes the metalloproteinases such as collagenases, cysteine proteases, etc. (70–72). These are powerful enzymes that can degrade connective tissue matrices and, like the serine proteases, are regulated by the presence of natural occurring inhibitors, tissue inhibitors of metalloproteases (TIMPs). The complex array of products from activated leukocytes, including both oxidants and proteases, leads to tissue damage as a result of triggering of the inflammatory response. Understanding in greater detail the pathways and the points at which these pathways can be intercepted may lead to more effective anti-inflammatory approaches for humans.

REFERENCES

1. Antone JC, Ward PA. Inflammation. In: Rubin E, Farber J, eds. *Pathology*, 2nd ed. Philadelphia: JB Lippincott, 1994;32–66.
2. Gallin JI, Goldstein IM, Snyderman R, eds. *Inflammation: basic principles and clinical correlates*, 2nd ed. New York: Raven Press, 1992.
3. McEver RP. Leukocyte–endothelial cell interactions. *Curr Opin Cell Biol* 1992;4:840–849.
4. Bevilacqua MP. Endothelial-leukocyte adhesion molecules. *Annu Rev Immunol* 1993;767–804.
5. Geng J-G, Bevilacqua MP, Moore KL, et al. Rapid neutrophil adhesion to activated endothelium mediated by GMP-140. *Nature* 1990;343:757–760.
6. Rothlein R, Barton RW, Winquist R. The role of intercellular molecule-1 (ICAM-1) in the inflammatory response. In: *Cellular and molecular mechanisms of inflammation*. Orlando: Academic Press, 1994;71–80.
7. Sanders WE, Wilson RW, Ballantyne CM, Beaudet AL. Molecular cloning and analysis of an *in vivo* expresion of murine P-selectin. *Blood* 1992;795–800.
8. Zimmerman GA, Lorant D, McIntyre TM, et al. Juxtacrine intercellular signaling: another way to do it. *Am J Respir Cell Mol Biol* 1993;9:573–577.
9. Murphy HS, Shayman JA, Till GO, et al. Superoxide responses of endothelial cells to C5α and TNFα: divergent signal transduction pathways. *Am J Physiol* 1992;263:L51–L59.
10. Ignarro LJ, Byrns RE, Buga GM, Wood KS. Endothelium-derived relaxing factor from pulmonary artery and vein possesses pharmacologic

and chemical properties identical to those of nitric oxide radical. *Circ Res* 1987;61:866–879.

11. Bevilacqua MP, Stengelin S, Gimbrone MA Jr, Seed B. Endothelial leukocyte adhesion molecule 1: an inducible receptor for neutrophils related to complement regulatory proteins and lectins. *Science* 1989; 243:1160–1165.

12. Bevilacqua MP, Pober JS, Mendrick DL, Cotran RS, Gimbrone MA Jr. Identifiction of an inducible endothelial-leukocyte adhesion molecule. *Proc Natl Acad Sci USA* 1987;84:9238–9242.

13. Lasky LA. Selectins: interpreters of cell-specific carbohydrate information during inflammation. *Science* 1992;258:964–969.

14. McEver RP, Beckstead JH, Moore KL, Marshall-Carlson L, Bainton DF. GMP-140, a platelet a-granule membrane protein, is also synthesized by vascular endothelial cells and is localized in Weibel-Palade bodies. *J Clin Invest* 1989;84:92–99.

15. Vestweber D. Selectins: cell surface lectins which mediate the binding of leukocytes to endothelial cells. *Semin Cell Biol* 1992;3:211–220.

16. Tedder TF, Penta AC, Levine HB, Freedman AS. Expression of the human leukocyte adhesion molecule, LAM-1: identity with the TQ1 and Leu-8 differentiation antigens. *J Immunol* 1990;144:532–540.

17. Smith CW. Molecular determinants of neutrophil adhesion. *Am J Respir Cell Mol Biol* 1990;2:487–489.

18. Polley MJ, Phillips ML, Warner E, et al. CD62 and endothelial cell leukocyte adhesion molecule (ELAM-1) recognize the same carbohydrate ligand, sialyl Lewis^X. *Proc Natl Acad Sci USA* 1991;88: 624–628.

19. Albelda SM, Smith CW, Ward PA. Adhesion molecules and inflammatory injury. *FASEB J* 1994;5:2529–2537.

20. Springer TA. Traffic signals for lymphocyte recirculation and leukocyte emigration: the multistep paradigm. *Cell* 1994;76:301–314.

21. Shimizu Y, Newman W, Tanaka Y, Shaw S. Lymphocyte interactions with endothelial cells. *Immunol Today* 1992;13:106–112.

22. Paine R III, Ben-Ze'ev AB, Farmer SR, Brody JS. The pattern of cytokeratin synthesis is a marker of cytokeratin synthesis is a marker of type 2 cell differentiation in adult and maturing fetal lung alveolar cells. *Dev Biol* 1988;129:505–515.

23. Osborn L. Leukocyte adhesion to endothelium in inflammation. *Cell* 1990;62:3–6.

24. Miyake K, Medina K, Ishihara K, Kimoto M, Auerbach R, Kincade PW. A VCAM-like adhesion molecule on murine bone marrow stromal cells mediates binding of lymphocyte precursors in culture. *J Cell Biol* 1991;114:557–565.

25. Hemler ME. VLA proteins in the integrin family;structure, functions and their role on leukocytes. *Annu Rev Immunol* 1990;8:365–400.

26. Albelda SM, Muller WA, Buck CA, Newman PJ. Molecular and cellular properties of PeCAM-1 (endoCAM/CD31): a novel vascular cell–cell adhesion molecule. *J Cell Biol* 1991;114:1059–1068.

27. Albelda SM, Oliver P, Romer L, Buck CA. EndoCAM: a novel endothelial cell–cell adhesion molecule. *J Cell Biol* 1990;110:1227.

28. Muller WA, Weigl SA, Deng X, Phillips DM. PECAM-1 is required for transendothelial migration of leukocytes. *J Exp Med* 1993;178:449–450.

29. Vaporciyan AA, DeLisser HM, Yan HC, et al. Involvement of platelet–endothelial cell adhesion molecule in neutrophil recruitment *in vivo. Science* 1993;262:1580–1582.

30. Bogn S, Pak J, Garifallou M, Deng X, Muller WA. Monoclonal antibody to murine PECAM-1 (CD31) blocks acute inflammation *in vivo. J Exp Med* 1994;79:1059–1064.

31. Carlos TM, Harlan JM. Leukocyte–endothelial cell adhesion molecules. *Blood* 1994;84:2068–2101.

32. Smith CW, Rothlein R, Hughes BJ, et al. Recognition of an endothelial determinant for CD18-dependent human neutrophil adherence and transendothelial migration. *J Clin Invest* 1988;82:1746–1756.

33. Smith CW, Marlin SD, Rothlein R, Toman C, Anderson DC. Cooperative interaction of LFA-1 and Mac-1 with intercellular adheion molecule-1 in facilitating adherence and transendothelial migration of neutrophils *in vivo. J Clin Invest* 1989;83:2008–2017.

34. Anderson DC, Springer TA. Leukocyte adhesion deficiency: an inherited defect in the Mac-1, LFA-1, and p150,95 glycoprotein. *Annu Rev Med* 1987;38:175–194.

35. Lasky LA, Singer MS, Dowbenko D, et al. An endothelial ligand for L-selectin is a novel mucin-like molecule. *Cell* 1992;69:927–938.

36. Lawrence MB, Springer TA. Leukocytes roll on a selectin at physiologic flow rates: distinction from and prerequisite for adhesion through integrins. *Cell* 1991;65:859–873.

37. Von Andrian UH, Chambers JD, McEvoy LM, Bargatze RF, Arfors K-E, Butcher EC. Two-step model of leukocyte-endothelial cell interaction in inflammation: distinct roles for LECAM-1 and the leukocyte b2 integrins *in vivo. Proc Natl Acad Sci USA* 1991;88:7538–7542.

38. Hynes RO. Integrins: versatility, modulation, and signaling in cell adhesion. *Cell* 1992;69:11–20.

39. Butcher EC. Leukocyte-endothelial cell recognition: three (or more) steps to specificity and diversity. *Cell* 1991;67:1033–1036.

40. Lawrence MB, Springer TA. Leukocytes roll on a selectin at physiologic flow rates: distinction from and prerequisite for adhesion through integrins. *Cell* 1991;65:859–873.

41. Le J, Vlcek J. Tumor necrosis factor and interleukin-1: cytokines with multiple overlapping biological activities. *Lab Invest* 1987;56:234–248.

42. Larrick JW, Kunkel SL. The role of tumor necrosis factor and interleukin 1 in the immunoinflammatory response. *Pharm Res* 1988;5: 129–139.

43. Murphy PM. The molecular biology of leukocyte chemoattractant receptors. *Annu Rev Immunol* 1994;12:593–633.

44. Baggiolini M, Boulay F, Badwey JA, Curnutte J. Activation of neutrophil leukocytes: chemoattractant receptors and respiratory burst. *FASEB J* 1993;7:1004–1010.

45. Lindley IJ, Westwick J, Kunkel SL. Nomenclature announcement—the chemokines. *Immunol Today* 1993;14:24.

46. Baggiolini M, Dewald B, Walz A. Interleukin-8 and related chemokines. In: Gallin JI, Goldstein IM, Synderman R, eds. *Inflammation: basic principles and clinical correlates*, 2nd ed. New York: Raven Press, 1992;247–263.

47. Oppenheim JJ, Zachariae OC, Mukaida N, Matsushima K. Properties of the novel proinflammatory supergene "intercrine" cytokine family. *Annu Rev Immunol* 1991;9:617–648.

48. Strieter RM, Kunkel SL. Chemokines and the lung. In: Crystal R, West J, Weible E, Barnes T, eds. *Lung: scientific foundations*, 2nd ed. New York, Lippincott-Raven Publishers, 1996;1:155–186.

49. Taub DD, Oppenheim JJ. Chemokines, inflammation and immune system. *Therapeutic Immunol* 1994;1:229–246.

50. Mukaida N, Okamoto S, Ishikawa Y, Matsushima K. Molecular mechanism of interluekin-8 gene expression. *J Leuk Biol* 1994;56:554–558.

51. Clore GM, Gronenborn AM. Three-dimensional structures of α and β chemokines. *FASEB J* 1995;9:57–62.

52. Rot A. Endothelial cell binding of NAP-1/IL-8: role in neutrophil emigration. *Immunol Today* 1992;13:291–264.

53. Leonard EJ, Yoshimura T, Tanaka S, Raffeld M. Neutrophil recruitment by intradermally injected neutrophil attractant/activation protein. *J Invest Dermatol* 1991;96:690–694.

54. Shanley TP, Schmal H, Friedl HP, Jones ML, Ward PA. Role of macrophage inflammatory protein-1α (MIP-1α) in acute lung injury in rats. *J Immunol* 1995;154:4793–4802.

55. Gautam SC, Chikkala NF, Hamilton TA. Anti-inflammatory action of IL-4: negative regulation of contact sensitivity to trinitrochlorobezene. *J Immunol* 1992;148:1411–1415.

56. Hart PH, Vitti GF, Burgess DR, Whitty GA, Piccoli DS, Hamilton JA. Potential antiinflammatory effects of interleukin 4: suppression of human monocyte tumor necrosis factor alpha, interleukin 1, and prostaglandin E2. *Proc Natl Acad Sci USA* 1989;86:3803–3807.

57. de Waal Malefyt R, Abrams J, Bennett B, Figdor CG, de Vries JE. Interleukin 10 (IL-10) inhibits cytokine synthesis by human monocytes: an autoregulatory role of IL-10 produced by monocytes. *J Exp Med* 1991;174:1209–1220.

58. Cunha FQ, Moncada S, Liew FY. Interleukin-10 (IL-10) inhibits the induction of nitric oxide synthase by interferon-gamma in murine macrophages. *Biochem Biophys Res Commun* 1992;182–1155–1159.

59. Mulligan MS, Jones ML, Vaporciyan AA, Howard MC, Ward PA. Protective effects of IL-4 and IL-10 against immune complex–induced lung injury. *J Immunol* 1993;151:5666–5674.

60. Dinarello CA. Biology of interleukin 1. *FASEB J* 1988;2:108–115.

61. Hannum CH, Wilcox CJ, Arend P, et al. Interleukin-1 receptor antagonist activity of a human interleukin-1 inhibitor. *Nature* 1990;343:336–341.

62. Mulligan MS, Ward PA. Immune complex–induced lung and dermal vascular injury—differing requirements for tumor necrosis factor-α and IL-1. *J Immunol* 1992;149:331–339.

63. Seekamp A, Warren JS, Remick DG, Till GO, Ward PA. Requirements for tumor necrosis factor-α and interleukin-1 in limb ischemia/reperfusion injury and associated lung injury. *Am J Pathol* 1993;143: 453–463.

64. Curnutte JT, Babior BM. Chronic granulomatous disease. In: Harris H, Hirchhorn K, eds. *Advances in human genetics.* New York: Plenum, 1987;16:229–297.

65. Kubes P, Suzuki M, Granger DN. Nitric oxide: an endogenous modulator of leukocyte adhesion. *Proc Natl Acad Sci USA* 1991;88: 4651–4655.

66. Beckman JS, Beckman TW, Chen J, Marshall PA, Freeman BA. Apparent hydroxyl radical production by peroxynitrite: implications for endothelial injury from nitric oxide and superoxide. *Proc Natl Acad Sci USA* 1990;87:1620–1624.

67. Gazzinelli RT, Oswald IP, James SL, Sher A. IL-10 inhibits parasite killing and nitrogen oxide production by IFN-γ-activated macrophages. *J Immunol* 1992;148:1792–1796.

68. Oswald IP, Gazzinelli RT, Sher A, James SL. IL-10 synergizes with IL-4 and transforming growth factor-β to inhibit macrophage cytotoxic activity. *J Immunol* 1992;148:3578–3582.

69. Weiss SJ. Tissue destruction by neutrophils. *N Engl J Med* 1989;320: 365–376.

70. Van Wark H, Birkedal-Hansen H. The cysteine switch: A principle of regulation of metalloproteinase activity with potential applicability to the entire matrix metalloproteinase gene family. *Proc Natl Acad Sci USA* 1990;87:5578–5582.

71. Reddy VY, Zhang QY, Weiss SJ. Pericellular mobilization of the tissue-destructive cysteine proteinases, cathepsins B, L and S, by human monocyte-derived macrophages. *Proc Natl Acad Sci USA* 1995;92: 3849–3853.

72. Shapiro SD, Campbell EJ, Welgus HG, Senior RM. Elastin degradation by mononuclear phagocytes. *Ann NY Acad Sci* 1990;624:69–80.

Asthma, edited by P.J. Barnes, M.M. Grunstein,
A.R. Leff, and A.J. Woolcock.
Lippincott–Raven Publishers, Philadelphia © 1997.

■ 20 ■

Immunoglobulin E

Donata A. Vercelli

TWO-SIGNAL MODEL FOR THE INDUCTION OF IMMUNOGLOBULIN E (IGE) SYNTHESIS

During an immune response, a B lymphocyte can express different immunoglobulin (Ig) heavy chain isotypes sharing the same VDJ region. This phenomenon (isotype switching) allows a single B-cell clone to produce antibodies with the same fine specificity, but different effector functions. To switch to a particular isotype, a B cell needs to receive two signals: signal 1 is cytokine-dependent, results in the activation of transcription at a specific region of the Ig locus, and thus determines isotype specificity. Signal 2 activates the recombination machinery, resulting in DNA switch recombination.

The two signals required for switching to IgE are delivered to B cells by T cells through a complex series of interactions. Allergen-specific B cells capture the antigen through their surface Ig molecules, internalize it, and process it into peptides that are then presented on the B-cell surface in association with major histocompatibility complex (MHC) class II molecules. Recognition of the antigen/MHC class II complex by the T-cell receptor leads to two crucial events: the secretion of lymphokines, in particular interleukin-4 (IL-4), which provides the first signal for IgE induction, and the expression of CD40 ligand (CD40L). Notably, CD40L is absent on resting T

cells, and it is the expression of this molecule after activation that renders T cells fully competent to induce IgE. Engagement of CD40 on B cells by its ligand on T cells delivers the signal that triggers switch recombination to IgE. Amplification circuits involving accessory molecules then lead to high-rate IgE synthesis.

Signal 1: IL-4 and IL-13

The interaction between IL-4 and IL-4 receptors (R) delivers the first signal for switching to IgE. Evidence from different lines of inquiry consistently shows that IL-4 is essential for IgE production:

1. IL-4 was the only cytokine able to induce IgE synthesis *in vitro,* when added in recombinant form; injection of an anti–IL-4 antibody abolished IgE production in parasite-infected mice (1)
2. IL-4R exist *in vivo* not only as cell-bound molecules, but also in a soluble, circulating form. A recombinant extracellular IL-4R domain blocked switching to IgE by blocking lL-4/IL-4R interactions (2)
3. The same result was obtained using an IL-4 mutant in which a tyrosine at position 124 was replaced by aspartic acid (3). The mutation preserves the ability to bind IL-4R, but destroys the capacity to transmit a signal upon receptor binding (4). Both these experiments show that it is sufficient to block the IL-4 signal in order to block isotype switching to IgE, and IgE production

D. A. Vercelli: Molecular Immunoregulation Unit, San Raffaele Scientific Institute, 20312 Milano, Italy .

4. The most compelling evidence for the central role of IL-4 in IgE induction comes from gene-targeting experiments. Mice in which the IL-4 gene had been knocked out by homologous recombination (IL-4 KO mice) were unable to mount an antiparasite IgE response; the IgG1 response was also suppressed, although to a lesser extent, whereas the production of other isotypes was unaffected (5)

5. Genetic linkage analysis has shown that IL-4, or a nearby gene in the 5q31.1 region (IL-13, IL-5, IL-9), is responsible for the regulation of overall IgE production (6). Polymorphism(s) in the regulatory region of these gene(s) may result in a predisposition to secrete abnormally high levels of IgE-inducing cytokines in response to antigen.

More recently, it has become clear that another cytokine, IL-13, shares many of the functional properties of IL-4, including the ability to induce IgE synthesis (7). Although the sequence homology between IL-13 and IL-4 is only ≈30%, all residues that contribute to the hydrophobic core of IL-4 are conserved, or have conservative hydrophobic replacements in IL-13 (4). Furthermore, receptors for IL-4 and IL-13 share a subunit (4). Indeed, an IL-4 mutant protein, which binds IL-4R with high affinity, competitively inhibits receptor binding of both IL-4 and IL-13 and blocks induction of IgE synthesis by both cytokines (3). However, IL-4 and IL-13, as well as their receptors, are by no means identical. IL-13 does not bind to COS-3 cells transfected either with cDNAs for the 130-kDa IL-4R and/or the γ chain (8) and, unlike IL-4, has no effects on human T cells (4). The elucidation of the respective roles of IL-4 and IL-13 in physiologic conditions will require information about the structure and distribution of IL-13R, as well as a detailed analysis of the mechanisms that control the expression of these cytokines. The molecular events dependent on the delivery of signal 1 are discussed below.

Signal 2: CD40/CD40L interactions

The engagement of CD40 on B cells by CD40L expressed on T cells provides the second signal required for switching to IgE. CD40L can be replaced *in vitro* by anti-CD40 monoclonal antibodies (mAbs). Indeed, this was the first experimental system in which the B-cell activating signal for human IgE synthesis was delivered by antibody-induced engagement of a discrete B-cell surface antigen.

CD40 is a 50-kDa surface glycoprotein expressed on human B lymphocytes (9), cytokine-activated monocytes (10), follicular dendritic cells (11), epithelial cells (including thymic epithelium) (12), and by certain carcinomas and melanomas, but not by T cells (13,14). CD40 plays a key role in the survival, growth, and differentiation of B cells. Signaling through CD40 rescues B cells

from apoptosis induced by Fas (CD95) or by cross-linking of the IgM complex (15,16). Selected anti-CD40 mAbs trigger significant proliferation of highly purified resting B cells, in the absence of other co-stimuli (17).

CD40 belongs to the TNFR superfamily, which includes TNFRI and TNFRII, NGFR, CD30, CD27, Fas (CD95) (reviewed in ref. 18). Members within this family share sequence similarity through their extracellular regions that contain multiple cysteine-rich repeats. The common structural framework of the extracellular domain is reflected by the ability of the TNFR superfamily members to interact with a parallel family of TNF-related molecules, which includes the ligands for CD40, CD27, and CD30, TNF-α, and lymphotoxin. CD40L is a 261 aa type 2 membrane glycoprotein that is transiently expressed on activated, but not on resting, TH1 and TH2 cells (19). Cells transfected with CD40L induced IgE synthesis by both murine (19) and human B cells (20), in the presence of IL-4, whereas a soluble CD40-Ig fusion protein inhibited IL-4–dependent IgE synthesis in human PBMC (21). These results clearly indicated that CD40/CD40L interactions are critical in delivering the second signal required for IgE production. The central role of the CD40/CD40L pathway in IgE synthesis and in isotype switching, was confirmed by the finding that defective switching in patients with X-linked hyper-IgM (HIM) syndrome is due to mutations in CD40L that result in impaired CD40/CD40L interactions (22,23). Furthermore, no IgG, IgA, and IgE response to thymus-dependent antigens was detectable in CD40 (24,25) and CD40L (26) KO mice, and no germinal centers were recognizable in lymphoid organs. In contrast, responses to thymus-independent antigens were preserved. Finally, the inability of human newborn B cells to switch has been ascribed to the decrease observed in both CD40L expression (27) and responses to CD40 agonists (28). Thus, data from a number of *in vitro* and *in vivo* models consistently point to the crucial role of CD40/CD40L interactions in germinal center formation, B-cell activation, isotype switching, and antibody production. The molecular events that lead to isotype switching after CD40 engagement are discussed below.

The interactions between CD40 and CD40L are tightly regulated. T cells become competent to activate B cells through CD40 only after they express CD40L, and this in turn requires TCR-dependent T cell activation. The latter process seems to be anatomically constrained, i.e., CD40L is expressed only in secondary lymphoid tissues at the site of cognate T/B cell interactions. Interestingly, a subset of CD4+ memory T cells in germinal centers contains preformed CD40L that is rapidly, but transiently, expressed on the cell surface after TCR-mediated activation (29). The speed at which T cells can express CD40L on their surface may be crucial in germinal centers, because centrocytes either leave the light zone within a few hours of activation or die by apoptosis *in situ*. On the other hand, the availability of CD40L is limited drastically, because the interaction with CD40 induces rapid endocytosis of surface CD40L (30), and release of soluble CD40 by B cells downregulates CD40L mRNA (31).

γ/δ T cells and IgE regulation

CD40L has been shown to be expressed by both α/β and γ/δ activated T cells (32,33). Because CD40L expression is lower on γ/δ than on α/β T cells, γ/δ T cells are less efficient in inducing IgE synthesis, but they are competent to induce isotype switching to IgE *in vitro* in the presence of exogenous IL-4. The recent finding that mice congenitally deficient in α/β T cells produce Ig of all isotypes, with high concentrations of IgE and IgG1 (34), suggests that γ/δ T cells play a role in directing isotype switching *in vivo* as well. The potential role of γ/δ T cells in the induction of IgE responses is further emphasized by the recent observation that γ/δ T cells are able to discriminate early in infection between TH1- and TH2-inducing pathogens, and produce cytokines associated with the appropriate pattern of response. Cytokines produced by γ/δ T cells may not only aid in the direct elimination of certain pathogens, but also contribute to the cytokine milieu that influences the differentiation of CD4+ T cells into either TH1 or TH2 (35).

Interestingly, adoptive transfer of small numbers of γ/δ T cells from OVA-tolerant mice selectively suppressed TH2-dependent IgE synthesis, without affecting IgG responses. These γ/δ cells were CD8+ and produced large amounts of interferon (IFN)-γ. Similar results were obtained in rats (36). These findings confirm the potential role of γ/δ T cells in the regulation of IgE responses, pointing to potentially different roles in different models.

IgE amplification

Several pairs of accessory molecules (CD28/B7, LFA-1/ICAM-1, CD2/CD58) have been shown to participate in T/B cell interactions conducive to IgE synthesis. Interactions within these ligand/receptor pairs complement and/or upregulate the T cell–dependent activation of B cells that follows the engagement of CD40 by CD40L. A major accessory role likely is played by the CD28/B7 ligand receptor pair. CD28 KO mice have reduced basal Ig levels and decreased class switching after infection with viruses (37). The T cell molecule CD28 and its B-cell counter-receptors, B7.1 and B7.2, are part of a reciprocal amplification mechanism that amplifies T/B cell interactions mediated via CD40/CD40L. Engagement of CD40 is known to result in B7 expression on B cells (38). On the other hand, engagement of CD28 results in increased expression of CD40L on T cells (39) and, most importantly, in increased IL-4 secretion (39) and TH2 differentiation, particularly when B7.2 is involved in the co-stimulation (40,41). IL-4 in turn upregulates B7 expression

(42). Thus, CD28/B7 interactions may enhance both IL-4 secretion and CD40-mediated B cell activation and ultimately may potentiate both signal 1 and signal 2. Consistent with this view, IgE synthesis has recently been shown to be inhibited by anti-CD28 blocking mAbs (43).

A marked increase in B7 expression also is induced by cross-linking MHC class II molecules on B cells, particularly when ICAM-1 is engaged simultaneously. Thus, interactions through MHC class II and ICAM-1 complement T cell help provided via CD40/CD40L interactions (44). In contrast, the weak IgE-inducing signal provided by engagement of CD58 (LFA-3) seems to be independent of the CD40 pathway (45).

Human basophils and mast cells recently have been reported to secrete IL-4 (46,47) and to express CD40L (48). Thus, basophils and mast cells may, in principle, provide both signal 1 and signal 2 for IgE synthesis. However, these non–T cells conceivably play a role in IgE amplification, rather than in IgE induction. The optimal physiologic stimulus for secretion of IL-4 and IL-13 seems to be allergen-dependent cross-linking of receptor-bound, allergen-specific IgE (46,47). Thus, cytokine secretion would be predicated on the production of allergen-specific IgE, and this in turn requires the signals and the cells (including allergen-specific T cells) discussed above. Once IgE has been produced, it can recruit basophils and mast cells by binding to their IgE receptors, thus inducing IL-4/IL-13 secretion and CD40L expression. Only at this point may non–T cells trigger an IgE response, which would not necessarily be allergen-specific, but may be polyclonal, as well. This scenario is consistent with the observation that a significant proportion of the IgE response in hyper-IgE states is frequently polyclonal, rather than allergen-specific.

CD40L was recently found to be constitutively expressed on eosinophils from one patient with the hypereosinophilic syndrome; however, these cells were not able to induce IgE synthesis in the presence of exogenous IL-4 (49). The significance of this isolated observation remains therefore to be understood.

Final Reminder

The complexity in the interplay between T cells, B cells, and cytokines involved in IgE induction makes it difficult to establish unambiguously a chronology of the events leading to IgE synthesis. On the other hand, the molecular studies discussed below clearly point to a hierarchy in the steps to IgE induction, and in the signals that trigger such steps. The initial event in switching to IgE is the determination of isotype specificity through cytokine (IL-4)-dependent induction of germline transcription, which is followed by CD40-mediated DNA switch recombination. Our terminology of "signal 1" and "signal 2" therefore reflects a B cell–centered perspective, although high-rate IL-4 secretion (signal 1), and full B-cell activation via CD40/CD40L (signal 2) may well enhance each other and require CD28/B7 interactions.

TH1/TH2 DICHOTOMY AND POTENTIAL TH2 MARKERS

Studies with T-cell clones obtained from patients with atopic disease and parasitic infections indicate clearly that the lymphokine profile of T-cell clones specific for an antigen is determined both by the nature of the antigen and by the genetic background of the individual (reviewed in ref. 50). Most helper T-cell clones specific for parasitic antigens, isolated from patients with no history of atopic disease, had a TH2 lymphokine profile, i.e., they produced high concentrations of IL-4, low IL-2 and IFN-γ, and induced vigorous IgE synthesis. On the other hand, allergen-specific CD4+ T-cell clones established from atopic patients had a TH2 lymphokine profile and provided help for IgE synthesis, whereas helper T-cell clones from the same patients, specific for nonallergenic antigens, or CD4+ clones from nonatopic individuals, had a TH1 profile (51–53). Thus, antigens such as those expressed on parasites seem to be able to evoke a TH2/IgE response regardless of the genetic background. In contrast, the genetic background seems to be critical for the generation of a TH2/IgE response against allergens.

The factors ultimately responsible for skewing the T-helper repertoire toward TH1 or TH2 are discussed elsewhere in this book. Here, it is important to underline the existence of complex cytokine amplification loops that significantly influence both T-helper differentiation and IgE regulation. TH2-derived IL-4 markedly inhibits IFN-γ production by human T cells (54,55) and furthermore directs the differentiation of precursor T cells into TH2 cells, which will secrete more IL-4 (56,57). By contrast, IFN-γ promotes the differentiation of CD4+ T cells into TH1 cells (56). Thus, once an antigen has initially triggered a response—which will be TH1 or TH2 depending on the nature of the antigen and the genetic background of the individual—the antigen-specific T-cell repertoire will be progressively skewed, and more T cells with the same lymphokine profile will be recruited. IL-13, an IgE-inducing TH2 lymphokine, may represent an exception, in that it is not active on T cells (4), and therefore it does not contribute to TH2 skewing. The inability of IL-13 to promote TH2 differentiation may explain why TH2 responses were severely impaired in mice in which the IL-4 gene had been disrupted but the IL-13 gene was intact (5,58). The importance of the local lymphokine milieu in determining the pattern of the TH response has been confirmed recently by studies in a mouse model of virus-stimulated CD8+ T-cell responses in the lung. Bystander CD4+ TH2 responses to ovalbumin switched the virus-specific lung CD8+ cells to IL-5 production. Upon viral challenge via the airways, these cells induced a significant eosinophil infiltration (59). These results could explain the link between viral infection and acute exacerbations of asthma.

IL-12 has been shown to skew the profile of the TH response toward TH1 (60). IL-12 may provide a link between natural and specific immune responses, because some viruses and intracellular bacteria can stimulate macrophages to produce IL-12, which in turn induces IFN-γ production by both T cells and NK cells. Thus, TH cells may be presented simultaneously with processed antigen plus cytokines that induce them to differentiate toward a TH1 phenotype (61).

Further understanding of the mechanisms underlying the TH1/TH2 dichotomy may be provided by ongoing studies, aimed at identifying potential markers for TH1 and TH2 cells. It has been proposed recently that the ability of TH clones to produce TH2-type lymphokines may correlate positively or negatively with the expression of two molecules, CD30 and CD27, that belong to the TNFR superfamily. Most human TH2 clones stimulated with the relevant allergen express CD30, and concomitantly secrete IL-4 and IL-5 (62), suggesting that CD30 may be associated with the differentiation/activation pathway of human T cells producing TH2-type cytokines. Furthermore, CD30 was expressed on TH2-like T-cell clones isolated from HIV patients with hyper-IgE syndrome (63). These clones produced IL-4 and provided help for IgE synthesis, despite their CD8 phenotype (64,65). These findings suggest that CD30 may be a marker for CD8+ T cells that have switched to the production of type 2 helper cytokines.

In patients with atopy or filariasis, the proliferative response to allergens (66) and the secretion of IL-4 and IL-5 (67) have been reported to be confined to a memory T-cell population that expresses CD4 and CD45R0, but not CD27. This seems to be true for both peripheral blood T cells and T-cell clones. Because little is known about TH2 physiology, it is not clear how the expression of CD30, and/or the lack of expression of CD27, may result in a TH2 phenotype.

T CELL–INDEPENDENT IGE INDUCTION BY EPSTEIN-BARR VIRUS AND GLUCOCORTICOIDS

It recently has been shown that stimulation with IL-4 and Epstein-Barr virus (EBV) induces T cell–independent IgE synthesis in human B cells (68,69). IgE production results from *de novo* induction of isotype switching, rather than from expansion of a precommitted sIgE+ B-cell population that has switched to IgE *in vivo* (69).

The role played by EBV in IgE induction is not clear. However, a clue recently was provided by the characterization of CD40 receptor-associated factor-1 (CRAF-1), a novel component of the CD40 signaling pathway (70,71). The C-terminus of CRAF-1 interacts directly and specifically with the cytoplasmic tail of CD40; overexpression of CRAF-1 interferes with CD40 signaling. Interestingly, the C-terminus of CRAF-1 is homologous to the TNF-α receptor-associated factors 1 and 2 (TRAF1 and TRAF2), which can complex with the cytoplasmic tail of the related TNF-α receptor II (72). The TRAF-C (for COOH-terminal) domain shared by CRAF-1, TRAF1, and TRAF2 is necessary and sufficient for CD40 binding and for homodimerization. It is likely that other members of the TNFR superfamily use CRAF-related proteins in their signal transduction process. Interestingly, CRAF-1 also interacts with the cytoplasmic domain of EBV latent infection membrane protein 1 (LMP1) (73), an EBV-encoded integral membrane protein that is critical for B-lymphocyte transformation and, most importantly, is the only EBV gene that has transforming effects in nonlymphoid cells. The IgE-inducing properties of EBV may indeed result from the ability of EBV-encoded protein(s) to activate the CD40 signaling pathway, thus providing B cells with signal 2.

IgE synthesis can be induced in highly purified, sIgE-normal (74) and leukemic (75) B cells by a combination of IL-4 and glucocorticoids (hydrocortisone). The effects of hydrocortisone are specific, inasmuch as steroid sex hormones have no influence on IL-4–dependent IgE synthesis (76). The mechanisms by which hydrocortisone synergizes with IL-4 remain unknown. Paradoxically, *in vivo* prolonged topical steroid treatment inhibits IL-4 production (77). The observation that hormone-receptor interactions can provide a second signal for IgE synthesis warrants further investigation.

MOLECULAR EVENTS IN THE INDUCTION OF IGE SYNTHESIS

Isotype switching results from a DNA recombination event that juxtaposes different downstream CH genes to the expressed V(D)J gene (Fig. 1). Considerable evidence indicates that isotype switching is not a random event, but is "directed" by cytokines in conjunction with the regulation of B-cell proliferation and differentiation. Molecular analysis has shown that cytokine-dependent induction of

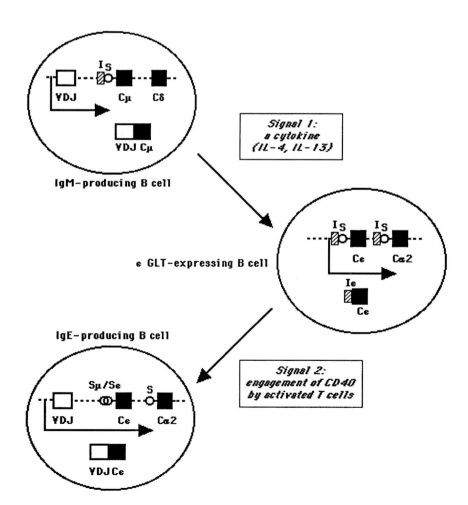

FIG. 1. Molecular events in isotype switching to IgE: the two-signal model.

isotype switching to a particular CH gene almost invariably correlates with the transcriptional activation of the same gene, in its germline configuration (reviewed in refs. 78,79). The germline transcripts (GLT) that result from this process initiate a few kilobases (kb) upstream of the switch (S) region, and proceed through one or more short exons (I exons) that are spliced to the first exon of the CH gene. GLT are unable to code for any mature protein of significant length, because the I exon contains multiple stop codons in all three reading frames. Therefore, GLT are also referred to as "sterile" transcripts. Alternatively, GLT are referred to as "truncated" transcripts, because the I exon is usually 200 to 300 base pairs (bp) shorter than the VDJ exon present in mature transcripts. Although there is no significant conservation of the sequences of GLT of different isotypes, their overall structure is conserved (79).

Expression of GLT is thought to play a key role in modulating the accessibility of a particular S region to a putative common switch recombinase, thus directing switching to the corresponding isotype. The role of GLT in the regulation of isotype switching has been recently tested by gene knock-out experiments. Deletion of the Iγ1 (80) or Iγ2b (81) exons and their promoter resulted in inhibition of class switching to the corresponding genes, indicating that transcription in the S region is necessary to direct switch recombination. However, it is apparently not sufficient: replacement of Iε with a B cell–specific promoter cassette containing the murine Eμ intronic enhancer and a VH promoter, without the Iε splice donor site, resulted in only marginal switch recombination to IgE, at about 1% of the frequency induced by IL-4 (82). In contrast, replacement of all known IL-4–inducible control elements in the Sγ1 region with the heterologous human metallothionein IIA promoter did not impair switch recombination to IgG1, provided that the Iγ1 splice donor site was included in the construct, thus allowing for the induction of artificial, but processed, GLT (83). These data indicate that a) artificial induction of structurally conserved, spliced GLT can target switch recombination, whereas transcription in the S region as such cannot, and b) spliced switch transcripts (or the process of splicing) have a functional role in switch recombination (83). The most intriguing speculation is that GLT are part of the switch recombinase, providing the specificity to target distinct S regions.

The 3' enhancer, located several kb downstream of the most 3' CH gene, has been recently identified as a novel regulatory region that controls Ig heavy chain class switching. 3' Enhancer KO mice showed a global defect in the ability to express GLT and switch to all CH genes, except one (84). Notably, the deletion affected germline transcription and class switch recombination of five CH genes spread over a 120-kb locus. Based on these data, it has been proposed that sequences within the 3' enhancer deletion may be an essential part of a locus control region

that regulates germline transcription and/or the accessibility of downstream CH genes. Further studies of this region may provide insights into the pathogenesis of human isotype deficiencies.

Regulation of ε Germline Transcription

ε Germline transcription is regulated at the transcriptional level by nuclear factors that bind to the Iε promoter and adjacent regions (Fig. 2). Nuclear factors specifically bind to relatively short (10–20 bp) DNA sequences, functionally defined as responsive elements (RE). Among the proteins that bind the εGLT promoter, some are constitutively expressed, whereas others are induced by specific cytokines. The specificity in the induction of nuclear factors provides a molecular basis for the specificity of cytokine-induced GLT expression and isotype switching.

BSAP, a transcription factor expressed in B but not T cells (85), binds to a highly conserved region upstream of the Iε transcription initiation site, and has been shown to contribute to the regulation of εGLT expression (86). An IL-4 RE more upstream has been found to bind the IL-4–inducible factor NF-IL-4 (Stat6; see below), a member of the C/EBP family, and NF-κB p50 (87). It has been proposed that these factors may have to interact physically in order to induce εGLT expression (87). The role of NF-κB in the induction of murine GLT recently has been confirmed by the finding that expression of GLT for several isotypes, including IgE, and switching to the same isotypes, is severely impaired in NF-κB p50 KO mice (88; Snapper, personal communication).

Stat6 (which is likely to be identical to NF-IL-4 and STF-IL-4) binds close to the Iε transcription initiation site and exhibits a unique pattern of rapid activation through tyrosine phosphorylation (89–92). Stat6 belongs to a newly identified family of signal transducers and activators of transcription (Stat) (93). Binding of IL-4 to its receptor leads to activation by tyrosine phosphorylation of two receptor-associated cytoplasmic tyrosine kinases, Janus kinase (JAK)-3 and, to a lesser extent, JAK-1 (94). These kinases are believed to rapidly (within minutes) phosphorylate Stat6, a latent cytoplasmic factor. The phosphorylated Stat6 would homodimerize, translocate to the nucleus, and bind to one, or possibly two, regions in the murine ε GLT promoter, contributing to the activation of transcription (91). The discovery of JAKs and Stats has finally provided an explanation for the apparent paradox that the IL-4R, as well as the receptors for a number of other cytokines, lacks kinase domains, and yet couples ligand binding to tyrosine phosphorylation (93). Stat6 is not B cell–specific, and is induced by IL-4 in monocytes, where it participates in the transcriptional regulation of the IL-4–inducible CD23b promoter. Stat6 binding sites have been identified in the promoters of a number of IL-4–respon-

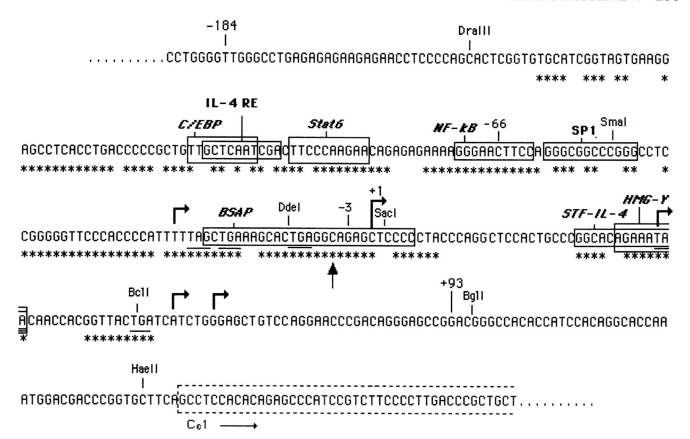

FIG. 2. Regulatory elements in the germline promoter. The binding sites for transcription factors identified in the mouse are indicated in italics. Transcription initiation site (⌐→); evolutionaly conserved sequence (***); stop condon (_). (From Ichiki T, Takahashi W, Watanabe T. Regulation of the expression of human Cε germline transcript—identification of a novel IL-4 responsive element. *J Immunol* 1993; 150:5408–5417; Köhler I, Rieber EP. Allergy-associated Iε and Fc receptor II (CD23b) genes activated via binding of an interleukin-4-induced transcription factor to a novel responsive element. *Eur J Immunol* 1993; 23:3066–3071; and Albrecht B, Peiritsch S, Woisetschläger M. A bifunctional control element in the human IgE germline promoter involved in repression and IL-4 activation. *Int Immunol* 1994; 6:1143–1151.

sive genes, such as CD23, Cγ1, and MHC class II (89, 95). The presence of homologous RE in the promoter of different genes underlies the concerted regulation of these genes by a single cytokine. Thus, the concerted increase in the expression of ε GLT, CD23, and MHC class II in B cells stimulated with IL-4 is mediated by IL-4 RE located 5' of each of these genes.

The requirements for the induction of ε GLT seem to be somewhat different in mice and humans. Two signals, IL-4 and LPS, are required for murine ε GLT expression in most murine B-cell lines, whereas IL-4 alone is sufficient in humans. The interactions between the human ε GLT promoter and transcription factors are only incompletely defined. Two contiguous IL-4 RE have been identified upstream of Iε, in a region of high human/mouse homology (95,96). The most 3' site binds NF-IL-4, which also interacts with a 9-bp binding motif in the promoter of CD23 (95). The role of both IL-4–responsive elements has been validated in reporter assays (96,97); however,

the minimal set of elements in the human ε GLT promoter required to confer full IL-4 inducibility to a heterologous promoter has not been unambiguously determined. Interestingly, the NFIL-4 binding site in the human ε GLT promoter (97) resembles the murine HMG-I(Y) site (98) because deletion or mutation results in a marked increase in basal promoter activity and in loss of IL-4 inducibility. Thus, these elements seem to have a bifunctional activity, i.e., they repress the activity of the promoter in the absence of IL-4, but they are required for IL-4–induced promoter activation.

DNA Switch Recombination

Although IL-4 (signal 1) is by itself sufficient for the initiation of transcription through the ε locus, switching and expression of mature Cε transcripts (containing VDJ spliced to Cε1-4) require signal 2 (engagement of CD40 by CD40 ligand). The molecular events that follow the delivery of the second signal for switching to IgE have been characterized only recently. The classic model, according to which switching occurs via loop-out and deletional recombination between highly repetitive S regions, has been challenged recently. Indeed, it was reported that IgE could be produced by B cells in which the immunoglobulin locus was retained in germline configuration (99,100). Thus, it became important to characterize the molecular mechanisms that underlie the expression of mature VDJ-C εmRNA in normal human B cells. This issue was investigated using polymerase chain reaction (PCR)-based approaches that allow for amplification, cloning, and sequencing of Sμ/Sε switch fragments, or of switch circles, their reciprocal products. DNA sequencing of Sμ/Sε switch fragments amplified from IgE-producing B-cell cultures proved formally that deletional switch recombination had occurred. Most of the switch fragments represented direct joining of Sμ to Sε. The recombination sites within Sμ were clustered within 900 bp at the 5'-end of the Sμ region, suggesting that there are hot spots for recombination within Sμ. In contrast, the Sε recombination sites were scattered throughout the Sε region (101–103).

Interestingly, some fragments amplified from B cells stimulated with IL-4 and hydrocortisone contained insertions at the Sμ/Sε junction that were derived from Sγ4 (103). The presence of an Sγ4-derived insertion suggested that some B cells had undergone sequential isotype switching from IgM to IgG4 to IgE. Indeed, IL-4 has been shown to induce isotype switching to IgG4 (104), as well as to IgE, and single B cells can give rise to clones that secrete IgG4 and IgE (105).

Because a B cell that first switches to IgG(4) and then to IgE may lose Sγ(4)-derived sequences during the second switch recombination, it became important to assess whether sequential and direct switching co-exist. Switch circles generated in B cells triggered to switch to IgE by IL-4 and anti-CD40 mAb were PCR-amplified. Sequencing of the circles showed the presence of μ-γ-ε switching, and of sequential events even more complex (μ-α1-γ-ε), but μ-ε circles representing direct switching events were also found, at high frequency (106). Likewise, sequence analysis of Sμ/Sε switch fragments from patients with atopic dermatitis showed a predominance of direct Sμ/Sε joining (107).

The importance of sequential switching *in vivo* was investigated by examining switching to IgE in mutant mice that lacked the Sγ1 region (80) and were therefore unable to support sequential switching via IgG1. In these mice, the frequency of switching to IgE was not affected (108). These results indicated that sequential switching merely reflects the simultaneous accessibility of two acceptor S regions for switch recombination induced by one cytokine. The apparent dominance of sequential switching observed in the generation of murine IgE-expressing cells after IL-4 stimulation is due to the

parallel activation of Sγ1 and Sε by IL-4, Sγ1 being intrinsically more accessible to recombination with Sμ (80,108). Thus, the overall low frequency of IgE switching is an autonomously determined intrinsic feature of Sε and its control elements. This may explain why, in the presence of saturating concentrations of IL-4 *in vitro,* the frequency of IgE switching reaches at most 10% of the frequency of switching to IgG1, which is also induced by IL-4.

Cytokine-dependent Modulation of IL-4–induced IgE Synthesis

Cellular studies have shown that, although IL-4 and IL-13 are the only cytokines capable of inducing IgE synthesis, IL-4/IL-13–induced IgE production can further be enhanced, or inhibited, by a number of cytokines (Table 1). However, the mechanisms responsible for the effects of these cytokines, and the event(s) that are targeted, still are mostly unclear.

TNF-α, IL-6, and IL-9 enhance IL-4–dependent IgE synthesis (109–111). IgE potentiation by TNF-α and IL-6 is detectable in both T cell—dependent and T cell—independent systems. The increase in IgE synthesis induced by TNF-α is mediated by enhanced ε GLT expression, whereas this step is not affected by IL-6 and IL-9 (110). IL-6 is not isotype-specific (112), and induces IgG secretion by selective accumulation of mRNA for the secreted form of the molecule, and possibly through differential mRNA stabilization (113). IgE secretion might be amplified by similar mechanisms; however, no direct evidence is available. Notably, engagement of CD40 triggers IL-6 and TNF-α secretion by B cells (114) and monocytes (10).

All the other cytokines listed in Table 1 inhibit IgE synthesis. Interestingly, only TGF-β has been shown to act on B cells, by targeting ε GLT expression (110). IL-8 also inhibits IgE production by purified B cells (115), but the molecular targets remain unknown. The other cytokines

TABLE 1. *Cytokines modulate molecular events in IgE induction*

	T cell-independent			T cell-dependent		
	GLT	Mature RNA	IgE	GLT	Mature RNA	IgE
TNF-α	↑	↑	↑	↑	↑	↑
IL-6	↔	↑	↑	↔	↑	↑
IL-9	↔	ND	ND	ND	ND	↑
TGF-β	↓	↓	↓	↓	↓	↓
IFN-γ	↔	↔	↔	↓	↓	↓
IFN-α	↔	↔	↔	↓	↓	↓
IL-8	ND	ND	↓	ND	ND	↓
IL-12	ND	ND	↔	↔	↓	↓
PAF-acether	ND	ND	ND	↓	↓	↓
IL-10[a]	↔	↔	↔	↓	↓	↓

[a]Monocyte-dependent.

are either inactive on germline transcription or uncharacterized so far. Interestingly, IFN-α, IFN-γ, and IL-12 inhibit IgE secretion only when tested in T cell–dependent systems (110,116,117), and IL-10 only suppresses IgE synthesis in the presence of monocytes (118). Thus, none of these cytokines acts directly on B cells.

REFERENCES

1. Finkelman FD, Katona IM, Urban JF, Snapper CM, Ohara J, Paul WE. Suppression of *in vivo* polyclonal IgE responses by monoclonal antibody to the lymphokine B-cell stimulatory factor 1. *Proc Natl Acad Sci USA* 1986;83:9675–9678.

2. Garrone P, Djossou O, Galizzi J-P, Banchereau J. A recombinant extracellular domain of the human interleukin 4 receptor inhibits the biological effects of interleukin 4 on T and B lymphocytes. *Eur J Immunol* 1991;21:1365–1369.

3. Aversa G, Punnonen J, Cocks BG, et al. An IL-4 mutant protein inhibits IL-4 or IL-13 induced human IgG4 and IgE synthesis and B cell proliferation: support for a common component shared by IL-4 and IL-13 receptors. *J Exp Med* 1993;178:2213–2216.

4. Zurawski SM, Vega F, Huyghe B, Zurawski G. Receptors for interleukin-13 and interleukin-4 are complex and share a novel component that functions in signal transduction. *EMBO J* 1993;12:2663–2670.

5. Kühn R, Rajewsky KR, Müller W. Generation and analysis of interleukin-4 deficient mice. *Science* 1991;254:707–710.

6. Marsh DG, Neely JD, Breazeale DR, et al. Linkage analysis of IL-4 and other chromosome 5q31.1 markers and total serum immunoglobulin E concentrations. *Science* 1994;264:1152–1156.

7. McKenzie ANJ, Culpepper JA, de Waal Malefyt R, et al. Interleukin-13, a T-cell-derived cytokine that regulates human monocyte and B-cell function. *Proc Natl Acad Sci USA* 1993;90:3735–3739.

8. Vita N, Lefort S, Laurent P, Caput D, Ferrara P. Characterization and comparison of the interleukin-13 receptor with the interleukin 4 receptor on several cell types. *J Biol Chem* 1995;270:3512–3517.

9. Wang CY, Fu SM, Kunkel HG. Isolation and immunological characterization of a major surface glycoprotein (gp54) preferentially expressed on certain human B cells. *J Exp Med* 1979;149:1424–1437.

10. Alderson MR, Armitage RJ, Tough TW, Strockbine L, Fanslow WC, Spriggs MK. CD40 expression by human monocytes: regulation by cytokines and activation of monocytes by the ligand for CD40. *J Exp Med* 1993;178:669–674.

11. Caux C, Massacrier C, Vanbervliet B, et al. Activation of human dendritic cells through CD40 cross-linking. *J Exp Med* 1994;180:1263–1272.

12. Galy AH, Spits H. CD40 is functionally expressed on human thymic cells. *J Immunol* 1992;149:775–782.

13. Paulie S, Ehlin-Henriksson B, Mellstedt H, Koho H, Aissa HB, Perlmann P. A p50 surface antigen restricted to human urinary bladder carcinomas and B-lymphocytes. *Cancer Immunol Immunother* 1985;20:23–30.

14. Ledbetter JA, Shu G, Gallagher M, Clark EA. Augmentation of normal and malignant B cell proliferation by a monoclonal antibody to the B cell-specific antigen Bp50 (CDw40). *J Immunol* 1987;138:788–794.

15. Liu Y-J, Joshua DE, Williams GT, Smith CA, Gordon J, MacLennan ICM. Mechanism of antigen-driven selection in germinal centres. *Nature* 1989;342:929–931.

16. Tsubata T, Wu J, Honjo T. B-cell apoptosis induced by antigen receptor crosslinking is blocked by a T-cell signal through CD40. *Nature* 1993;364:645–648.

17. Gruber MF, Bjorndahl JM, Nakamura S, Fu SM. Anti-CD45 inhibition of human B cell proliferation depends on the nature of activation signals and the state of B cell activation. *J Immunol* 1989;142:4144–4152.

18. Banchereau J, Bazan F, Blanchard D, et al. The CD40 antigen and its ligand. *Annu Rev Immunol* 1994;12:881–922.

19. Armitage RJ, Fanslow WC, Strockbine L, et al. Molecular and biological characterization of a murine ligand for CD40. *Nature* 1992;357:80–82.

20. Spriggs MK, Armitage RJ, Strockbine L, et al. Recombinant human CD40 ligand stimulates B cell proliferation and immunoglobulin E secretion. *J Exp Med* 1992;176:1543–1550.

21. Fanslow WC, Anderson DM, Grabstein KH, Clark EA, Cosman D, Armitage RJ. Soluble forms of CD40 inhibit biologic responses of human B cells. *J Immunol* 1992;149:655–660.

22. Fuleihan R, Ramesh N, Loh R, et al. Defective expression of the CD40 ligand in X-chromosome-linked immunoglobulin deficiency with normal or elevated IgM. *Proc Natl Acad Sci USA* 1993;90:2170–2173.

23. Allen RC, Armitage RJ, Conley ME, et al. CD40 ligand gene defects responsible for X-linked Hyper-IgM syndrome. *Science* 1993;259:990–993.

24. Kawabe T, Naka T, Yoshida K, et al. The immune responses in CD40-deficient mice: impaired immunoglobulin class switching and germinal center formation. *Immunity* 1994;1:167–178.

25. Castigli E, Alt FW, Davidson L, et al. CD40 deficient mice generated by RAG-2 deficient blastocyst complementation. *Proc Natl Acad Sci USA* 1994;91:12135–12139.

26. Xu J, Foy TM, Laman JD, et al. Mice deficient for the CD40 ligand. *Immunity* 1994;1:423–431.

27. Fuleihan R, Ahern D, Geha RS. Decreased expression of the ligand for CD40 in newborn lymphocytes. *Eur J Immunol* 1994;24:1925.

28. Durandy A, de Saint Basile G, Lisowska-Grospierre B, et al. Undetectable CD40 ligand expression on T cells and low B cell responses to CD40 binding agonists in human newborns. *J Immunol* 1995;154:1560–1568.

29. Casamayor-Palleja M, Khan M, MacLennan ICM. A subset of CD4-memory T cells contains preformed CD40 ligand that is rapidly but transiently expressed on their surface after activation through the T cell receptor complex. *J Exp Med* 1995;181:1293–1301.

30. Yellin MJ, Sippel K, Inghirami G, et al. CD40 molecules induce down-modulation and endocytosis of T cell surface T cell–B cell activating molecule/CD40 ligand. Potential role in regulating helper effector function. *J Immunol* 1994;152:598–608.

31. van Kooten C, Gaillard C, Galizzi J-P, et al. B cells regulate expression of CD40 ligand on activated T cells by lowering the mRNA level and through the release of soluble CD40. *Eur J Immunol* 1994;24:787–792.

32. Horner AA, Jabara H, Ramesh N, Geha RS. γ/δ T lymphocytes express CD40 ligand and induce isotype switching in B lymphocytes. *J Exp Med* 1995;181:1239–1244.

33. Gascan H, Aversa GC, Gauchat J-F, et al. Membranes of activated CD4+ T cells expressing T cell receptor (TcR) α or TcR δ induce IgE synthesis by human B cells in the presence of interleukin-4. *Eur J Immunol* 1992;22:1133–1141.

34. Wen L, Roberts SJ, Viney JL, et al. Immunoglobulin synthesis and generalized autoimmunity in mice congenitally deficient in αβ(+) cells. *Nature* 1994;369:654–658.

35. Ferrick DA, Schrenzel MD, Mulvania T, Hsieh B, Ferlin WG, Lepper H. Differential production of interferon-γ and interleukin-4 in response to TH1- and TH2-stimulating pathogens by δ T cells *in vivo*. *Nature* 1995;373:255–257.

36. McMenamin C, McKersey M, Kühnlein P, Hünig T, Holt PG. δ T cells down-regulate primary IgE responses in rats to inhaled soluble protein antigens. *J Immunol* 1995;154:4390–4394.

37. Shahinian A, Pfeffer K, Lee KP, et al. Differential T cell costimulatory requirements in CD28-deficient mice. *Science* 1993;261:609–612.

38. Ranheim EA, Kipps TJ. Activated T cells induce expression of B7/BB1 on normal or leukemic B cells through a CD40-dependent signal. *J Exp Med* 1993;177:925–935.

39. Klaus SJ, Pinchuk LM, Ochs HD, et al. Costimulation through CD28 enhances T cell-dependent B cell activation via CD40-CD40L interaction. *J Immunol* 1994;152:5643–5652.

40. King CL, Stupi RJ, Craighead N, June CH, Thyphronitis G. CD28 activation promotes TH2 subset differentiation by human CD4+ cells. *Eur J Immunol* 1995;25:587–595.

41. Freeman GJ, Boussiotis VA, Anumanthan A, et al. B7-1 and B7-2 do not deliver identical costimulatory signals, since B7-2 but not B7-1 preferentially costimulates the initial production of IL-4. *Immunity* 1995;2:523–532.

42. Vallé A, Aubry J-P, Durand I, Banchereau J. IL-4 and IL-2 upregulate the expression of antigen B7, the B cell counterstructure to T cell CD28: an amplification mechanism for T-B cell interactions. *Int Immunol* 1991;3:229–235.

43. Life P, Aubry J-P, Estoppey S, Schnuriger V, Bonnefoy J-Y. CD28

functions as an adhesion molecule and is involved in the regulation of human IgE synthesis. *Eur J Immunol* 1995;25:333–339.

44. Poudrier J, Owens T. CD54/intercellular adhesion molecule 1 and major histocompatibility complex II signaling induces B cells to express interleukin-2 receptors and complements help provided through CD40 ligation. *J Exp Med* 1994;179:1417–1427.

45. Diaz-Sanchez D, Chegini S, Zhang K, Saxon A. CD58 (LFA-3) stimulation provides a signal for human isotype switching and IgE production distinct from CD40. *J Immunol* 1994;153:10–20.

46. Schroeder JT, MacGlashan DW, Kagey-Sobotka A, White JM, Lichtenstein LM. IgE-dependent IL-4-secretion by human basophils—the relationship between cytokine production and histamine release in mixed leukocyte cultures. *J Immunol* 1994;153:1808–1817.

47. Burd PR, Thompson WC, Max EE, Mills FC. Activated mast cells produce interleukin-13. *J Exp Med* 1995;1373–1380.

48. Gauchat J-F, Henchoz S, Mazzei G, et al. Induction of human IgE synthesis in B cells by mast cells and basophils. *Nature* 1993;365:340–343.

49. Gauchat J-F, Henchoz S, Fattah D, et al. CD40 ligand is functionally expressed on human eosinophils. *Eur J Immunol* 1995;25:863–865.

50. Romagnani S. Lymphokine production by human T cells in disease states. *Annu Rev Immunol* 1994;12:227–257.

51. Parronchi P, Macchia D, Piccinni M-P, et al. Allergen- and bacterial antigen-specific T-cell clones established from atopic donors show a different profile of cytokine production. *Proc Natl Acad Sci USA* 1991;88:4538–4542.

52. Kapsenberg ML, Wierenga EA, Bos JD, Jansen HM. Functional subsets of allergen-reactive human CD4- T cells. *Immunol Today* 1991;12:392–395.

53. Del Prete GF, De Carli M, Mastromauro C, et al. Purified protein derivative of Mycobacterium tubercolosis and excretory-secretory antigen(s) of Toxocara canis expand *in vitro* human T cells with stable and opposite (type 1 T helper or type 2 T helper) profile of cytokine production. *J Clin Invest* 1991;88:346–350.

54. Peleman R, Wu J, Fargeas C, Delespesse G. Recombinant interleukin 4 suppresses the production of interferon by human mononuclear cells. *J Exp Med* 1989;170:1751–1756.

55. Vercelli D, Jabara HH, Lauener RP, Geha RS. Interleukin-4 inhibits the synthesis of interferon-γ and induces the synthesis of IgE in mixed lymphocyte cultures. *J Immunol* 1990;144:570–573.

56. Maggi E, Parronchi P, Manetti R, et al. Reciprocal regulatory effects of IFN-γ and IL-4 on the *in vitro* development of human TH1 and TH2 clones. *J Immunol* 1992;148:2142–2147.

57. Schmitz J, Thiel A, Kühn R, Rajewsky K, Müller W, Assenmacher M, Radbruch A. Induction of interleukin-4 (IL-4) expression in T helper (TH) cells is not dependent on IL-4 from non TH-cells. *J Exp Med* 1994;179:1349–1353.

58. Kopf M, Le Gros G, Bachmann M, Lamers MC, Bluethmann H, Köhler G. Disruption of the murine IL-4 gene blocks TH2 cytokine responses. *Nature* 1993;362:245–248.

59. Coyle AJ, Erard F, Bertrand C, Walti S, Pircher H, Le Gros G. Virus-specific CD8+ cells can switch to interleukin 5 production and induce airway eosinophilia. *J Exp Med* 1995;181:1229–1233.

60. Manetti R, Parronchi P, Giudizi MG, et al. Natural killer cell stimulatory factor (interleukin-12) induces T helper type 1-specific immune responses and inhibits the development of IL-4-producing TH cells. *J Exp Med* 1993;177:1199–1204.

61. Romagnani S. Induction of TH1 and TH2 responses:a key role for the "natural" immune response? *Immunol Today* 1992;13:379–381.

62. Del Prete G, De Carli M, Almerigogna F, et al. Preferential expression of CD30 by human CD4+ T cells producing TH2-type cytokines. *FASEB J* 1995;9:81–86.

63. Manetti R, Annunziato F, Biagiotti R, et al. CD30 expression by CD8- T cells producing type 2 helper cytokines. Evidence for large numbers of CD8-CD30- T cell clones in human immunodeficiency virus infection. *J Exp Med* 1994;180:2407–2411.

64. Maggi E, Giudizi MG, Biagiotti R, et al. TH2-like CD8- T cells showing B cell helper function and reduced cytolytic activity in human immunodeficiency virus type 1 infection. *J Exp Med* 1994;180:489–495.

65. Paganelli R, Scala E, Ansotegui IJ, et al. CD8+ T lymphocytes provide helper activity for IgE synthesis in human immunodeficiency virus-infected patients with hyper-IgE. *J Exp Med* 1995;181:423–428.

66. de Jong R, Brouwer M, Hooibrink B, van der Pouw-Kraan T, Miedema F, van Lier RAW. The CD27+ subset of peripheral blood memory CD4+ lymphocytes contains functionally differentiated T lymphocytes that develop by persistent antigenic stimulation *in vivo*. *Eur J Immunol* 1992;22:993–999.

67. Elson LH, Shaw S, Van Lier RAW, Nutman TB. T cell subpopulation phenotypes in filarial infections: CD27 negativity defines a population greatly enriched for TH2 cells. *Int Immunol* 1994;6:1003–1009.

68. Thyphronitis G, Tsokos GC, June CH, Levine AD, Finkelman FD. IgE secretion by Epstein-Barr virus-infected purified human B lymphocytes is stimulated by interleukin-4 and suppressed by interferon-γ. *Proc Natl Acad Sci USA* 1989;86:5580–5584.

69. Jabara HH, Schneider LC, Shapira SK, et al. Induction of germ-line and mature C transcripts in human B cells stimulated with rIL-4 and EBV. *J Immunol* 1990;145:3468–3473.

70. Hu HM, O'Rourke K, Boguski MS, Dixit VM. A novel RING finger protein interacts with the cytoplasmic domain of CD40. *J Biol Chem* 1994;269:30069–30072.

71. Cheng G, Cleary AM, Ye Z-S, Hong DI, Lederman S, Baltimore D. Involvement of CRAF1, a relative of TRAF, in CD40 signaling. *Science* 1995;267:1494–1498.

72. Rothe M, Wong SC, Henzel WJ, Goeddel DV. A novel family of putative signal transducers associated with the cytoplasmic domain of the 75 kDa tumor necrosis factor receptor. *Cell* 1994;78:681–692.

73. Mosialos G, Birkenbach M, Yalamanchili R, VanArsdale T, Ware C, Kieff E. The Epstein-Barr virus transforming protein LMP1 engages signaling proteins for the tumor necrosis factor receptor family. *Cell* 1995;80:389–399.

74. Jabara HH, Ahern DJ, Vercelli D, Geha RS. Hydrocortisone and IL-4 induce IgE isotype switching in human B cells. *J Immunol* 1991;147:1557–1560.

75. Sarfati M, Luo H, Delespesse G. IgE synthesis by chronic lymphocytic leukemia cells. *J Exp Med* 1989;170:1775–1780.

76. Wu CY, Sarfati M, Heusser C, et al. Glucocorticoids increase the synthesis of Immunoglobulin E by interleukin-4 stimulated human lymphocytes. *J Clin Invest* 1991;87:870–877.

77. Masuyama K, Jacobson MR, Rak S, et al. Topical glucocorticosteroid (fluticasone propionate) inhibits cells expressing cytokine mRNA for interleukin-4 in the nasal mucosa in allergen-induced rhinitis. *Immunology* 1994;82:192–199.

78. Vercelli D, Geha RS. Regulation of isotype switching. *Curr Opin Immuno* 1992;4:794–797.

79. Coffman RL, Lebman DA, Rothman P. The mechanism and regulation of immunoglobulin isotype switching. *Adv Immunol* 1993;54:229–269.

80. Jung S, Rajewsky K, Radbruch A. Shutdown of class switch recombination by deletion of a switch region control element. *Science* 1993;259:984–987.

81. Zhang J, Bottaro A, Li S, Stewart V, Alt FW. Targeted mutation in the Ig2b exon results in a selective Ig2b deficiency in mice. *EMBO J* 1993;12:3529–3537.

82. Bottaro A, Lansford R, Xu L, Zhang J, Rothman P, Alt FW. S region transcription per se promotes basal IgE class switch recombination but additional factors regulate the efficiency of the process. *EMBO J* 1994;13:665–674.

83. Lorenz M, Jung S, Radbruch A. Switch transcripts in immunoglobulin class switching. *Science* 1995;267:1825–1828.

84. Cogné M, Lansford R, Bottaro A, et al. A class switch control region at the 3' end of the immunoglobulin heavy chain locus. *Cell* 1994;77:737–747.

85. Adams B, Dörfler P, Aguzzi A, et al. Pax-5 encodes the transcription factor BSAP and is expressed in B lymphocytes, the developing CNS, and adult testis. *Genes Dev* 1992;6:1589–1607.

86. Liao F, Birshtein BK, Busslinger M, Rothman P. The transcription factor BSAP (NF-HB) is essential for immunoglobulin germ-line ε transcription. *J Immunol* 1994;152:2904–2911.

87. Delphin S, Stavnezer J. Characterization of an IL-4 responsive region in the immunoglobulin heavy chain germline ε promoter: regulation by NF-IL-4, a C/EBP family member, and NF-kB/p50. *J Exp Med* 1995;181:181–192.

88. Sha WC, Liou H-C, Tuomanen EI, Baltimore D. Targeted disruption of the p50 subunit of NF-κB leads to multifocal defects in immune responses. *Cell* 1995;80:321–330.

89. Kotanides H, Reich NC. Requirement of tyrosine phosphorylation for rapid activation of a DNA binding factor by IL-4. *Science* 1993;262:1265–1267.

90. Schindler C, Kashleva H, Pernis A, Pine R, Rothman P. STF-IL-4: a novel signal transducing factor. *EMBO J* 1994;13: 1350–1356.

91. Hou J, Schindler U, Henzel WJ, Ho TC, Brasseur M, McKnight SL. An interleukin-4–induced transcription factor: IL-4 Stat. *Science* 1994;265:1701–1706.

92. Quelle FW, Shimoda K, Thierfelder W, et al. Cloning of murine and human Stat6, Stat proteins that are tyrosine phosphorylated in response to IL-4 and IL-3 but are not required for mitogenesis. *Mol Cell Biol* 1995;15:3336–3343.

93. Ihle JN, Kerr IM. Jaks and Stats in signaling by the cytokine receptor superfamily. *Trends Genet* 1995;11:69-74.

94. Malabarba MG, Kirken RA, Rui H, et al. Activation of JAK3, but not JAK1, is critical to interleukin-4 stimulated proliferation and requires a membrane proximal region of IL-4 receptor α. *J Biol Chem* 1995; 270:9630–9637.

95. Köhler I, Rieber EP. Allergy-associated Iε and Fc receptor II (CD23b) genes activated via binding of an interleukin-4-induced transcription factor to a novel responsive element. *Eur J Immunol* 1993;23: 3066–3071.

96. Ichiki T, Takahashi W, Watanabe T. Regulation of the expression of human Cε germline transcript—identification of a novel IL-4 responsive element. *J Immunol* 1993;150:5408–5417.

97. Albrecht B, Peiritsch S, Woisetschläger M. A bifunctional control element in the human IgE germline promoter involved in repression and IL-4 activation. *Int Immunol* 1994;6:1143–1151.

98. Kim J, Reeves R, Rothman P, Boothby M. The non-histone chromosomal protein HMG-I(Y) contributes to repression of the immunoglobulin heavy chain germ-line ε RNA promoter. *Eur J Immunol* 1995;25:798–807.

99. MacKenzie T, Dosch HM. Clonal and molecular characteristics of the human IgE-committed B cell subset. *J Exp Med* 1989;169: 407-30.

100. Chan MA, Benedict SH, Dosch H-M, Huy MF, Stein LD. Expression of IgE from a nonrearranged ε locus in cloned B-lymphoblastoid cells that also express IgM. *J Immunol* 1990;144:3563–3568.

101. Shapira SK, Jabara HH, Thienes CP, et al. Deletional switch recombination occurs in IL-4 induced isotype switching to IgE expression by human B cells. *Proc Natl Acad Sci USA* 1991;88:7528–7532.

102. Shapira SK, Vercelli D, Jabara HH, Fu SM, Geha RS. Molecular analysis of the induction of IgE synthesis in human B cells by IL-4 and engagement of CD40 antigen. *J Exp Med* 1992;175:289–292.

103. Jabara HH, Loh R, Ramesh N, Vercelli D, Geha RS. Sequential switching from μ to ε via γ4 in human B cells stimulated with IL-4 and hydrocortisone. *J Immunol* 1993;151:4528–4533.

104. Lundgren M, Persson U, Larsson P, et al. Interleukin 4 induces synthesis of IgE and IgG4 in human B cells. *Eur J Immunol* 1989;19: 1311–1315.

105. Gascan H, Gauchat J-F, Aversa G, van Vlasselaer P, de Vries JE. Anti-CD40 monoclonal antibodies or CD4+ T cell clones and IL-4 induce IgG4 and IgE switching in purified human B cells via different signaling pathways. *J Immunol* 1991;147:8–13.

106. Zhang K, Mills FC, Saxon A. Switch circles from IL-4–directed ε class switching from human B lymphocytes—evidence for direct, sequential and multiple step sequential switch from μ to ε Ig heavy chain gene. *J Immunol* 1994;152:3427–3435.

107. van der Stoep N, Korver W, Logtenberg T. *In vivo* and *in vitro* IgE isotype switching in human B lymphocytes: evidence for a predominantly direct IgM to IgE class switch program. *Eur J Immunol* 1994;24:1307-1311.

108. Jung S, Siebenkotten G, Radbruch A. Frequency of Immunoglobulin E class switching is autonomously determined and independent of prior switching to other classes. *J Exp Med* 1994;179:2023–2026.

109. Vercelli D, Jabara HH, Arai K, Yokota T, Geha RS. Endogenous IL-6 plays an obligatory role in IL-4 induced human IgE synthesis. *Eur J Immunol* 1989;19:1419–1424.

110. Gauchat J-F, Aversa G, Gascan H, de Vries JE. Modulation of IL-4 induced germline ε RNA synthesis in human B cells by tumor necrosis factor-α, anti-CD40 monoclonal antibodies or transforming growth factor-β correlates with levels of IgE production. *Int Immunol* 1992;4: 397–406.

111. Dugas B, Renauld JC, Péne J, et al. Interleukin-9 potentiates the interleukin-4-induced immunoglobulin (IgG, IgM, and IgE) production by normal human B lymphocytes. *Eur J Immunol* 1993;1687–1692.

112. Muraguchi A, Hirano T, Tang B, et al. The essential role of B cell stimulatory factor 2 (BSF-2/IL-6) for the terminal differentiation of B cells. *J Exp Med* 1988;167:332–344.

113. Raynal M-C, Liu Z, Hirano T, Mayer L, Kishimoto T, Chen-kiang S. Interleukin 6 induces secretion of IgG1 by coordinated transcriptional activation and differential mRNA accumulation. *Proc Natl Acad Sci USA* 1989;86:8024–8028.

114. Clark EA, Shu G. Association between IL-6 and CD40 signaling. IL-6 induces phosphorylation of CD40 receptors. *J Immunol* 1990;145: 1400–1406.

115. Kimata H, Yoshida A, Ishioka C, Lindley I, Mikawa H. Interleukin-8 selectively inhibits Immunoglobulin E production induced by IL-4 in human B cells. *J Exp Med* 1992;176:1227–1231.

116. Gauchat J-F, Lebman DA, Coffman RL, Gascan H, de Vries JE. Structure and expression of germline ε transcripts in human B cells induced by interleukin 4 to switch to IgE production. *J Exp Med* 1990;172:463–473.

117. Kiniwa M, Gately M, Gubler U, Chizzonite R, Fargeas C, Delespesse G. Recombinant interleukin-12 suppresses the synthesis of immunoglobulin E by interleukin-4 stimulated human lymphocytes. *J Clin Invest* 1992;90:262–266.

118. Punnonen J, de Waal Malefyt R, van Vlasselaer P, Gauchat J-F, De Vries JE. IL-10 and viral IL-10 prevent IL-4-induced IgE synthesis by inhibiting the accessory cell function of monocytes. *J Immunol* 1993;151:1280–1289.

Asthma, edited by P.J. Barnes, M.M. Grunstein,
A.R. Leff, and A.J. Woolcock.
Lippincott–Raven Publishers, Philadelphia © 1997.

▪ 21 ▪

Animal Models

Debra J. Turner and James G. Martin

Airway Hyperresponsiveness
 Responsiveness to Challenge with Direct-Acting
  Stimuli
 Responsiveness to Challenge with Indirect-Acting
  Stimuli
 Mechanisms of Hyperresponsiveness to Directly and
  Indirectly Acting Stimuli

Induced Hyperresponsiveness
 Nonallergic Triggers
 Allergic Triggers
 Mechanisms of Allergen-Induced
  Hyperresponsiveness
Airway Inflammation

Recent definitions of asthma incorporate three characteristics of the disease, namely airway hyperresponsiveness (AHR), reversible airways obstruction, and inflammation. These defining features of asthma are presumed to account for most, if not all, of its clinical manifestations. Although presumably interrelated, the precise links among them have not been established. The effort to develop pertinent models has been prompted by the general belief that asthma is a condition unique to humans. Even if the veterinary literature contains convincing descriptions of naturally occurring airway diseases in cats and horses resembling asthma named feline asthma (1,2) and heaves (3), respectively, problems of access of investigators to animals affected by these conditions limits the practicability of their study. Useful animal models have been developed for the study of the pathogenesis and pathophysiology of both AHR and "asthmatic" airway inflammation. To date, long-term observations of airway function are lacking so that whether or not spontaneous airway narrowing occurs after induction of inflammation in hyperresponsiveness has not been investigated.

The quantification of hyperresponsiveness in human asthma is accomplished by standardized bronchial provocation tests. The most commonly used stimuli are histamine and methacholine. However, airway responses to cold air isocapnic hyperventilation and exercise have also

been used. With the exception of exercise, all these stimuli have been used to elicit airway responses in animals. It is possible to determine shifts in concentration-effect curves in animals in such a way as to quantitate the effects of various airway insults in a manner comparable with human studies.

Allergic and nonallergic stimuli have been identified for the induction of airway inflammation. Sensitization with antigens and subsequent airway challenge have permitted the identification of the typical early and late allergic responses seen in human allergic subjects, supporting the concept that allergic airway responses do not represent a diathesis unique to humans. Eosinophilic inflammation has also been evoked. Other pathologic changes reminiscent of asthma such as growth of airway smooth muscle have been identified after repeated allergen exposures. Allergen-induced hyperresponsiveness also occurs in several animal models at various times after airway challenge. Various nonallergic stimuli evoke airway narrowing, which is accompanied in some instances by airway inflammation and hyperresponsiveness, modeling potentially relevant triggers of asthma.

AIRWAY HYPERRESPONSIVENESS

There are two strategies for the study of hyperresponsiveness using animal models. One approach is to examine the mechanisms accounting for differences in responsiveness among normal animals and the second is to induce changes in responsiveness by an intervention such

---

 D. J. Turner: Department of Physiology, University of Western Australia, Nedlands, Western Australia 6907 Australia.
 J. G. Martin: Department of Medicine, Meakins-Christie Laboratories, McGill University, Montreal, Quebec H2X 2P2 Canada.

as an allergen challenge. Most studies of hyperresponsiveness are based on the assumption that differences in spontaneous or induced responsiveness are equivalent to the pathologic hyperresponsiveness of asthma. All the species studied to date show a considerable range in measures of airway responsiveness analogous to the results obtained in human surveys. The magnitude of the change in responsiveness that can be induced by airway insults is usually small, but this is not inconsistent with the situation for human studies (4).

Recently, the importance of distinguishing the maximal response that can be induced by a contractile agonist from the sensitivity to that agonist (position of the concentration-effect curve) has been stressed because these two phenomena may be determined by different factors. Shifts in both sensitivity and maximal bronchoconstrictive responses may occur independently, but usually both are strikingly abnormal in asthmatics. To date, most animal studies have used a measure of airway responsiveness that reflects the position of the concentration-effect curve without determining the maximal response of which the animal is capable. However, models of hyperresponsiveness need to address mechanisms by which both maximal responses and sensitivity are altered.

Responsiveness to Challenge with Direct-acting Stimuli

A variety of bronchoconstrictive substances has been used to quantitate airway responsiveness in various mammals. Cholinergic agonists [acetylcholine (ACh), methacholine, and carbachol] and histamine are among the most frequently employed but prostaglandin F2α, cysteinyl-leukotrienes, and serotonin have also been used. In most studies, the outcome of a challenge test with any given agonist is correlated with that of other agonists, even though each of the agonists acts through specific receptors on airway smooth muscle. Airway responsiveness is therefore not usually agonist-specific and supports the concept that differences in airway responsiveness are attributable to postreceptor phenomena.

The range of responsiveness to bronchoconstrictive agonists has been reported in cats, dogs, rats, mice, and guinea pigs. The responsiveness of a population of cats was reported to vary 23-fold (5), slightly less than the 40-fold variation found in dogs (6). The rat showed at least a 128-fold variation in its responsiveness to inhalational challenge (7). This variation is greater when challenge methodologies are employed that involve exposure of the upper airways to the contractile agonist and involve the contribution of these structures to the response (8,9). The sensitivity of small animals to the confounding effects of upper airway responses is presumably related to obligate nose breathing. Mice have also shown substantial variability in responsiveness (10–12), but differences in

methodology do not allow comparison with the rat (7,13). The variability in the responsiveness among rats and mice is much less within strains, indicating an important effect of inbreeding in reducing heterogeneity. The range of sensitivity reported for guinea pigs has varied from 22-fold to 256-fold (14,15). The lower estimates presumably were a reflection of concomitant beta-adrenergic receptor blockade, suggesting an important modulatory effect of catecholamines on airway responses in this animal. The only study to determine maximal responses in the guinea pig showed a 3.6-fold variation; sensitivity and maximal responses were not correlated (7).

There are few comparative studies in which standardized challenge and measurement techniques have been applied. A recent study showed a substantially greater maximal bronchoconstrictive response as well as a greater sensitivity to methacholine in the guinea pig compared with rat, rabbit, dog, and cat (7), suggesting that the guinea pig in its normal state is perhaps the most suitable model for AHR of a type that is comparable with the asthmatic subject. Another well characterized animal model is the Basenji-greyhound (BG) (16), which shows AHR to a variety of inhaled contractile agonists when compared with mongrel dogs.

Responsiveness to Challenge with Indirect-acting Stimuli

Certain stimuli induce bronchoconstriction indirectly through an action on cells other than airway smooth muscle. These cells in turn respond to these stimuli by release of bronchoconstrictive substances that induce the airway narrowing. As such, evaluation of the responses to these stimuli provides information concerning not only the sensitivity of the airways to bronchoconstrictors, but also the numbers and/or activation state of intermediate cells in the response. Adenosine is a good example of such a challenge agent in which airway mast cells appear to mediate the response. There is an increase in histamine in airway lavage fluid after adenosine challenge in the rat, and the effect is blocked by nedocromil sodium, presumably by an action on mast cells (17). Interestingly, adenosine responsiveness is increased in sensitized rabbits (18), whereas sensitization per se is not usually sufficient to alter airway responsiveness to other more direct forms of challenge. It also appears as if responses to neurokinin-A are at least in part mediated by effects on airway mast cells (17).

Bradykinin is another substance that appears indirectly to induce bronchoconstriction by release of tachykinin from C-fiber afferents in the airways (19). Tachykinins themselves trigger the release of cysteinyl leukotrienes from airway cells, when dry cold air is used to promote tachykinin release (20). Although it does not appear to have been tested directly, it seems likely that leukotriene release may also be involved in the airway response to bradykinin.

Propranolol is also an agent that can be used to induce bronchoconstrictive responses in the guinea pig. Few other animals show anything other than small degrees of airway narrowing after propranolol challenge. The mechanism of the response appears to involve the cholinergic nervous system. Blockade of the beta-adrenoceptor on prejunctional nerve endings in the airway wall may augment the release of ACh (21).

Mechanisms of Hyperresponsiveness to Directly and Indirectly-acting Stimuli

Mechanical Factors

The mechanisms that cause enhanced airway responsiveness *in vivo* have not been established. Mechanical limitations to the extent of smooth muscle shortening appear to be important, particularly in relationship to maximal responses. Because airway smooth muscle *in vivo* must overcome mechanical impedances to shorten, the balance of the force of contraction and the impedance to shortening should determine the airway narrowing that ultimately results (22). Various lines of evidence suggest that the elastic properties of the parenchyma (23), local airway–parenchymal interdependence (24), cartilage (25), and stiffening of the airway caused by infolding of the mucosa (26,27) are likely to be the most important impedances to shortening. However, there is little information concerning the relative or absolute magnitudes of these loads *in vivo*.

Support for mechanical determinants of airway narrowing has been obtained both from theoretical considerations (28) as well as experimental studies. The bronchodilating effect of increasing lung volume has been interpreted as the effect of the tethering of the airways by lung parenchyma (23,29). The bronchodilation is abolished in rats by elastase pretreatment, which disrupts the alveolar attachments to the airways (24). The effects of lung volume on bronchoconstriction in the guinea pig are modest compared with the rat, suggesting that part of the hyperresponsiveness of the guinea pig may be attributable to reduced airway-parenchymal interdependence in this species (30). A similar observation has been made for two rat strains differing in responsiveness. The relatively hyperresponsive Fischer strain is less sensitive to the effects of lung volume than the normoresponsive Lewis rat (31).

There is some evidence that the absolute mass of smooth muscle may be an important determinant of airway responsiveness (see also Chapter 14). Of interest in this regard is the finding that the guinea pig, which is the most hyperresponsive of the usual species studied, also has substantially more airway smooth muscle than rabbits

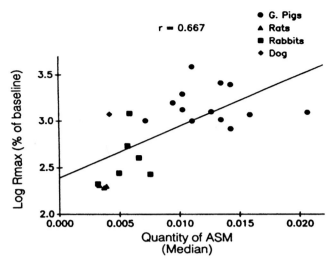

FIG. 1. Relationship of airway smooth muscle and methacholine responsiveness assessed in sedated, spontaneously breathing guinea pigs (*n*=13), rats (*n*=3), rabbits (*n*=6), and dog (*n*=1). Each animal is represented by an individual symbol. The logarithmically transformed maximal response to inhaled methacholine (log R_{max}), expressed as a percentage of the baseline value, is significantly positively correlated with the quantity of smooth muscle (*r*=0.667) for all species, suggesting that smooth muscle is a determinant of interspecies differences in maximal responses to methacholine. The quantity of smooth muscle (*ASM*) is expressed as the median value for each animal. From Martin JG, Opazo-Saez A, Du T, Tepper R, Eidelman DH. In vivo airway reactivity: predictive value of morphological estimates of airway smooth muscle. [Review]. *Can J Physiol Pharmacol* 1992;70: 597–601.

and rats (Fig. 1). Figure 1 shows the relationship of airway smooth muscle and methacholine responsiveness in guinea pigs, rats, rabbits, and dog. Maximal response is shown to be positively correlated with the quantity of smooth muscle for all species, suggesting that smooth muscle is a determinant of interspecies differences in maximal responses to methacholine. Interstrain differences in airway responsiveness in the rat are also partly explicable on the basis of differences in airway smooth muscle; however, direct proof is required before concluding that normal intra- and interspecies differences in responsiveness are linked to differences in airway smooth muscle (13).

Endogenous Factors Modulating Airway Caliber

The balance of endogenous bronchoconstrictive and bronchodilating influences has been studied as a source of variability in responsiveness. The modulatory effects of neural pathways and circulating catecholamines have been extensively evaluated. Recently, nitric oxide (NO) has been added to the list of potentially important modulating factors. NO has been reported to affect airway responsiveness in guinea pigs; inhibition of NO synthase (NOS) enhances airway responses to intravenously infused histamine (32). A comparison of the effects of NOS inhibition in two rat strains differing in airway responsiveness, the hyperresponsive Fischer strain and the normoresponsive Lewis strain, showed a resistance to NO in the Fischer rat but not the Lewis rat, accounting for part of the difference in responsiveness between the strains (33). The explanation for this observation appears to reside in the lack of response of guanylyl cyclase to NO and the formation of less cyclic guanosine monophosphate (cGMP) in the Fischer strain. There may be a link between the amount of airway smooth muscle and guanylyl cyclase activity, because cGMP is known to modulate vascular smooth muscle growth (34). The tissue of origin of NO has not been definitively established, but the epithelium is likely to be the major source (35,36).

Both the BG dog (37) and the guinea pig (38) share the common characteristic that propranolol enhances airway responsiveness. Most other species, including normal humans, do not show any modification of airway responses to inhaled contractile agonists by propranolol. This resemblance to asthmatics may be coincidental, although abnormal relaxant responses to beta-agonists have been demonstrated in the BG dog and are also a feature of asthmatic airways. In both instances, there appears to be uncoupling of the β-andrenergic receptors from adenylyl cyclase, because receptor numbers are not reduced. Prolonged treatment with corticosteroids corrects the abnormality in the BG dog (39) and also reduces AHR to methacholine (40). No impairment of β-adrenergic responses has been described in the guinea pig, making the link between resistance to β-adrenergic agonists and hyperresponsiveness uncertain.

Biochemical factors

Maturational changes in airway responsiveness have also been described. Isolated tissues from rabbit (41), cow (42), and guinea pig (43–45) show age-related changes in responsiveness to a number of agonists. These changes have also been documented *in vivo* in guinea pig (45,46) and rabbit (41). The immature rabbit has greater maximal responses to inhaled methacholine than mature animals; however, sensitivity is lower. Even though the immature animals have more airway smooth muscle, there is no relationship between the amount of muscle and maximal responses, suggesting that other mechanisms are involved. Differences in phosphoinositide metabolism have been postulated to account for the maturational differences (47). Inositol trisphosphate (IP$_3$) concentration is greater after administration of carbachol to tracheal smooth muscle from 2-week-old compared with adult rabbits. This finding is potentially important because much of the increase in intracellular calcium evoked by contractile agonists is mediated by IP$_3$. Ontogenic changes in the activities of degradative enzymes appear to be in part responsible. Changes in the sodium-potassium pump (48) and altered membrane receptor function (42,49) also have been identified and may provide additional explanations for age-related changes.

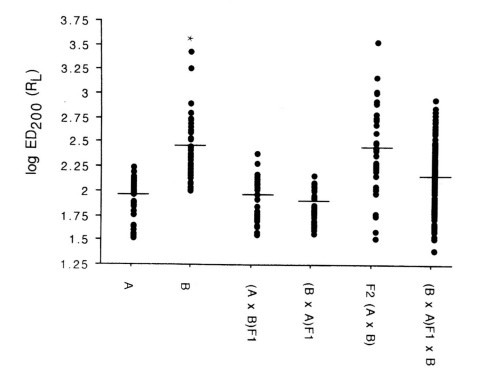

FIG. 2. Airway responsiveness to infused methacholine measured in 42 A/J mice (*A*), 40 C57BL/6J mice (*B*), 40 F$_1$(*B*×*A*), 40 F$_1$(*A*×*B*), 40 (*B*×*A*)F$_2$ intercross mice, and 321 [(*B*×*A*)F$_1$×B] backcross mice. Airway responsiveness is shown for individual animals as the log ED$_{200}$R$_L$, the effective dose required to increase R$_L$ to 200% of control values. C57BL/6J mice are significantly different from A/J mice (*p*<0.05)*. ED$_{200}$R$_L$ values for F$_1$ mice from both reciprocal crosses demonstrate airway responsiveness similar to that observed in A/J mice, suggesting that AHR is inherited as a dominant trait. (From Desanctis GT, Merchant M, Beier DR, et al. Quantitative locus analysis of airway hyperresponsiveness in A/J and C57BL/6J mice. *Nat Genet* 1995;11:150–154.)

Genetic Factors

There is evidence that suggests airway responsiveness is determined genetically. Genetic influences have been demonstrated for the Basenji-greyhound (50), rat (51), mouse (10,11), and guinea pig (52). It has been argued that responsiveness of the mouse to ACh is inherited in an autosomal recessive manner through the involvement of a single gene (10). However, a recent report (11) using linkage analysis has identified the association of several discrete regions of the genome with responsiveness. This is illustrated in Figure 2, reproduced from a study by De-Sanctis et al. (11). Figure 2 is a scatterplot of responsiveness to infused methacholine measured from individual animals in parental (A/J and C57BL/6J), F_1, F_2, and backcross mice. C57BL/6J mice were significantly different from A/J mice; however, F_1 mice from both reciprocal crosses demonstrate airway responsiveness similar to that observed in A/J mice, suggesting that AHR is inherited in a dominant trait. Likewise, various rat strains may show a different rank order of responsiveness to serotonin and carbachol (51), indicating that responsiveness may be determined by mechanisms that affect all agonists but also by mechanisms particular to specific agonists. Most studies are performed using animals that are not necessarily pathogen-free. Respiratory tract infection is therefore a potentially important confounding factor. It is possible that differences in responsiveness between animals of a given species or among inbred strains may reflect susceptibility to the effects of respiratory pathogens rather than truly genetically determined airway responses.

INDUCED HYPERRESPONSIVENESS

Nonallergic Triggers

Hyperresponsiveness to contractile agonists has been induced in a variety of animals using a range of nonallergic stimuli. The induction of airway inflammation, however, appears to be common to all these stimuli.

Ozone

Administration of ozone to the dog causes a brisk reversible neutrophilia in the epithelium and the BAL fluid and an associated increase in airway responsiveness to inhaled ACh (53,54). Rats also exhibit AHR, epithelial damage, and, usually, neutrophilia after exposure to ozone (55). The hyperresponsiveness appears to be mediated by thromboxane (54,56,57); although initial experimentation suggested that the neutrophil might be involved (58,59), more recent experimentation has raised doubts about the neutrophil as the source of thromboxane (60). This uncertainty is supported by studies in the guinea pigs, in which bronchial hyperresponsiveness to ozone exposure is dose-dependent (61,62) and occurs despite prior leukocyte depletion with cyclophosphamide (63). Several rat strains develop ozone-induced bronchial hyperresponsiveness to ACh (55,64), which has been suggested to be caused by a marked decrease in epithelial cholinesterase, resulting in increased bioavailability of the agonist. Pretreatment of dogs with antioxidants before ozone exposure abrogates the alterations in airway responsiveness despite the absence of change in neutrophil influx into the airways (65). In addition, polyethylene glycol-superoxide dismutase (an oxygen radical scavenger) has been shown to attenuate ozone-induced bronchial hyperresponsiveness in cats (66). The ozone-induced increase in hyperresponsiveness correlates with the ozone-induced increase in the capacity of BAL cells to produce oxygen radicals. The link between oxygen radicals and thromboxane production remains to be elucidated.

Sephadex

The administration of Sephadex beads to rats and guinea pigs induces blood and lung eosinophilia of a transient nature. The lung develops a granulomatous vasculitis and demonstrates perivascular and peribronchial infiltration by eosinophils. An increase in responsiveness to intravenous serotonin has been demonstrated in the rat (67,68). Excised airways and parenchymal strips are also hyperresponsive to various agonists. Corticosteroids and the immunosuppressive drug rapamycin inhibit both the inflammatory response and the hyperresponsiveness (69,70). The cells mediating the effects of Sephadex are not known; however, 5-lipoxygenase products appear to be critical in the induction of both eosinophilia and hyperresponsiveness (71). Platelet-activating factor (PAF) also appears to be involved (71).

Contractile Agonists

Several contractile agonists have been shown to enhance airway responsiveness. Among these are LTD_4 (46,72,73), bradykinin (74), and PAF (75–78). All these substances have potent effects on microvascular permeability, and it is possible that edema, either intraluminally or peribronchially, may result in excessive airway narrowing for a given degree of airway smooth muscle shortening or permit enhanced muscle shortening by uncoupling the airways from the tethering effect of the parenchyma (79). The lipid mediator PAF has been shown to induce AHR in several species including the dog (65), rabbit (76), and sheep (77), as well as humans (78). These substances are of particular interest because of the roles they appear to play in allergen-induced airways hyperresponsiveness.

Cytokines

A number of cytokines including interleukin-1 (IL-1) (80), IL-2 (81), and TNF-α (82,83) have been documented to increase airway responsiveness. IL-1, IL-2, and TNF-α have been studied in the rat and TNF-α in the sheep. More recently, antibody to IL-5 has been demonstrated to prevent the infiltration of eosinophils and the development of bronchial hyperresponsiveness in a guinea pig model of allergic asthma (84). The precise mechanism of action of these substances is not entirely clear, although they are all proinflammatory. Cyclo-oxygenase products, in particular thromboxane, mediate some of the effects of TNF-α. Endotoxin induces changes in airway responsiveness by virtue of release of TNF-α.

Viruses

Parainfluenza viral infections have been reported to cause hyperresponsiveness in the rat (85), dog (86), and guinea pig (87). Respiratory syncytial virus also is capable of inducing hyperresponsiveness in the guinea pig (88). In some cases, damage to the airway epithelium appears to be involved and to account for a selective hyperresponsiveness to tachykinins. Presumably a reduction in neutral endopeptidase activity is at least in part responsible.

Isocyanates

2,4-Toluene diisocyanate (TDI) is a causative agent in occupational asthma. Administration of TDI on the skin of TDI-sensitized guinea pigs results in immediate cutaneous reactions (89). Skin reactivity can be transferred successfully to untreated animals by injecting sera from actively sensitized animals. After 9 weeks of exposure, TDI-sensitized guinea pigs show contraction of bronchioles, hypertrophy of smooth muscle and hypersecretion of mucin, an infiltration of inflammatory cells into the peribronchial area, and an elevation of histamine-releasing activity in the lung tissues (90). Application of TDI to the nose of TDI-sensitized guinea pigs increases the histamine content, histidine decarboxylase, and histamine *N*-methyltransferase activities in the nasal mucosa and lung (91), suggesting that the turnover rate of histamine may be increased.

Trimellitic Anhydride

Trimellitic anhydride (TMA) is a small molecular weight industrial compound that can cause industrial asthma in humans. Some TMA-induced abnormalities can be reproduced in animal models such as the guinea pig (92–94), mouse (95), and rat (96). Intratracheal administration of TMA coupled to serum albumin to sensitized guinea pigs results in bronchoconstriction, microvascular leak, increased inflammatory cells in the BAL fluid, and increased eosinophil peroxidase activity in the lung tissue (92,93). The response appears to be mediated primarily by histamine release (93), and the complement system is thought to be an important source of mediators for cellular infiltration into the lung after exposure to TMA (92). Airway responsiveness to Ach also is increased in sensitized guinea pigs exposed to TMA (97). This responsiveness is significantly inhibited by pretreatment with budesonide; however, eosinophilic inflammation induced by exposure to TMA remains unaltered.

Allergic Triggers

Allergen administration to sensitized animals has been extensively studied and hyperresponsiveness to cholinergic and other agonists has been demonstrated at varying time points after the challenge. Considerable species differences are found in the patterns of allergic response. Early airway responses generally can be elicited, but not all species demonstrate late allergic bronchoconstriction. Neonatal sensitization of the rabbit (98) and dog (99) is necessary for sensitization to result in immunoglobulin E (IgE) production. Rabbits immunized with *Alternaria tenuis* extract produce significant antibody titers, which remain persistently high for 3 months when boosted every 2 weeks (100). Rabbits immunized within the first 24 hours of birth and boosted regularly have only IgE antibodies detectable, whereas rabbits immunized first at 7 days after birth produce multiple isotypes (100). The IgE titers are not greater in the neonatally immunized rabbits, suggesting that suppression of isotypes besides IgE is caused by neonatal immunization. Neonatally sensitized rabbits exhibit enhanced and persistent hyperresponsiveness to inhaled histamine compared with naive or sham-sensitized rabbits (101). Sensitization of adult guinea pigs usually results in substantial airway responses on subsequent exposure to allergen (102), but a low prevalence of late responses. The dog does not show a late response. However, this has been shown to emerge after the suppression of endogenous corticosteroid production by metyrapone by some investigators (103) but not others (104). Similarly, the pig shows a late response to *Ascaris suum* when pretreated with metyrapone (105). Rat strains vary in their propensity to develop airway narrowing after sensitization and challenge. The Sprague-Dawley (SD) rat has poor IgE responses to sensitization, and it responds to airway challenge with small early responses and very occasional late responses. By contrast, the Brown-Norway (BN) is a high IgE producer (106) and has early and late responses in high prevalence

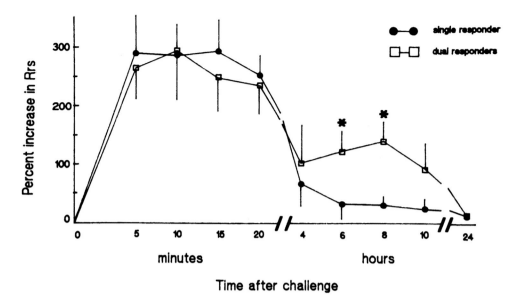

FIG. 3. Increases in respiratory system resistance (*Rrs*) during the early- and late-phase airway obstruction response after inhaled *Ascaris suum* extract in single (*closed circles*) and dual responder (*open squares*) cynomolgus monkeys. The degree of bronchoconstriction in single and dual responder monkeys was similar; however, only the dual responders had an increase in Rrs 6 to 8 hr after antigen inhalation. *Asterisk* indicates statistical significance between groups, $p<0.05$, $n=6$ per group. Data are the mean ±SEM. From Gundel RH, Wegner CD, Letts LG. Antigen-induced acute and late-phase responses in primates. *Am Rev Respir Dis* 1992;146:369–373.

(107). The BN also is distinguished by the eosinophilic infiltration of the airways that follows exposure to allergen (108). Natural sensitization to parasitic antigens has been exploited for the development of primate models; cynomolgus (109) and squirrel monkeys (110) have been explored. Figure 3 illustrates increases in respiratory system resistance during the early- and late-phase responses after inhaled *Ascaris suum* extract in cynomolgus monkeys. Some monkeys show a single response to the inhaled extract whereas others show the classic dual response. The sheep is among the best characterized animal models of allergic bronchoconstriction (111).

Allergen-induced hyperresponsiveness occurs within hours of challenge and still is present in some animals by 32 hours. The precise time course of hyperresponsiveness does not appear to have been completely mapped, but it resolves within 2 days of challenge in certain animals. Some degree of hyperresponsiveness has been reported to persist even up to a week after allergen challenge (112). Repeated antigen challenge of dogs (99), guinea pigs (113), and rats (108,114,115) also has been used to induce hyperresponsiveness. The duration of the hyperresponsiveness is often longer than the transient change after a single antigen challenge. Allergen exposures at 5-day intervals six times has been successfully used to induce hyperresponsiveness in the BN rat (114), but not either daily exposures for 14 days or six exposures at 3-day intervals (116). In addition, repeated exposure of ovalbumin (OA)-sensitized BN rats to aerosolized OA over 3 weeks induces responsiveness to Ach. This responsiveness is lost if OA exposure continues for 8 weeks (115). The timing of exposures may be of critical importance. Repeated allergen exposure at weekly intervals of neonatally sensitized rats induces a greater degree of hyperresponsiveness than comparable exposure in adult animals (R. Olivenstein, personal communication).

Mechanisms of Allergen-induced Hyperresponsiveness

Immunologic Factors

The association between atopy in human populations and increased airway responsiveness has led to an examination of these relationships in the BG dog and in high IgE-producing rat strains. Although the BG dog shows hyperresponsiveness (50), the parent Basenji dog, which is also atopic, does not have comparably increased airway responsiveness (117). Similarly, high IgE-producing rat strains do not show elevated airway responsiveness (13,51). The characteristic immune response leading to high IgE is not in itself a determinant of airway responsiveness. Presumably, exposure to aeroallergens is essential to the induction of hyperresponsiveness.

A recent report indicates the feasibility of transfer of late allergic airway responses and hyperresponsiveness to methacholine using T lymphocytes isolated from the intrathoracic lymph nodes of sensitized BN rats (118). Purification of the T cells using immunomagnetic selection has shown that CD4+ T cells but not CD8+ T cells transfer the late response (119). Figure 4 shows the time course of changes in lung resistance after ovalbumin inhalation in recipients of purified W3/25+ cells that were primed to either ovalbumin or bovine serum albumin. A significant difference was found between the two groups, illustrating that antigen-induced airway bronchoconstriction can be transferred by antigen-specific W3/25+ T cells in the BN rat. Transfer of purified spleen CD8+ T cells from ovalbumin-sensitized mice to sensitized recipients results in suppression of IgE production, a loss of immediate cutaneous reactivity, and prevention of allergen-induced increase in airway responsiveness (120). The authors propose that CD8+ T cells play an important negative regulatory role, and that interferon-gamma may be a relevant mediator of the function of CD8+ T cells in this mouse model. Primate models have also been used to illustrate the ability to transfer passively both allergic airway responses (121) and hyperresponsiveness to methacholine using unheated serum from allergic humans (122). Administration of rabbit serum containing anti-*Alternaria* IgG into rabbits that have been immunized to

produce only IgE isotypes reduces both the early and late responses (100). Transfusion of plasma containing anti-*Alternaria* IgE into nonimmunized control rabbits produces both early and late responses to aerosol challenge. This suggests that the late pulmonary response in the rabbit is IgE-dependent, is blunted in the presence of IgG, and occurs in the absence of cellular immune mechanisms resulting from the immunization procedure.

Biochemical Factors

A link between the late response and hyperresponsiveness has been suggested by studies in human allergic asthmatics, but the link between the two phenomena is now less clear. There is also a temporal relationship with the development of inflammation, but it has not been possible to identify the cell type(s) responsible for hyperresponsiveness. Pharmacologic studies using various selective antagonists have helped to implicate a number of biochemical mediators. Both PAF (78,123,124) and bradykinin (125) have been demonstrated to be important in certain species. Despite the important role for leukotriene D_4 in late allergic bronchoconstriction, a selective LTD_4 antagonist abrogates the late response in sheep without affecting hyperresponsiveness at the same time (126). A thromboxane synthetase inhibitor has re-

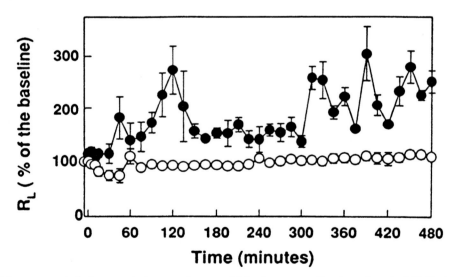

FIG. 4. Time course of changes in lung resistance (R_L) after aerosolized ovalbumin (*OVA*) challenge in the recipients of purified W3/25- cells which were primed to either OVA or bovine serum albumin (BSA). Brown Norway (BN) rats were sensitized to either OVA or BSA on Day 0. On Day 14 W3/25+ cells were isolated from the cervical lymph nodes of sensitized animals, and were transferred to naive, syngeneic BN rats. Group 1 received 20 million OVA-primed W3/25+ cells (*closed circles, n=4*), Group 2 (*control*) received 20 million BSA-primed W3/25+ cells (*open circles, n=6*). On day 16, the recipients were challenged by aerosolized OVA. A significant effect between groups was demonstrated by ANOVA (*p*<0.001), illustrating that antigen-induced airway bronchoconstriction can be transferred by antigen-specific W3/25+ T cells in the BN rat. Data are the mean ±SEM. From Watanabe A, Mishima H, Renzi PM, Xu LJ, Hamid Q, Martin JG. Transfer of allergic airway responses with antigen-primed CD4+ but not CD8+ T cells in Brown Norway rats. *J Clin Invest* 1995;96:1303–1310.

duced cholinergic hyperresponsiveness in the guinea pig at 7 hours after allergen challenge (127). Corticosteroids can prevent the development of AHR after challenge, but the multiplicity of their actions prevents any definitive information from being gleaned concerning the mechanisms of hyperresponsiveness.

The mechanism of the hyperresponsiveness induced by repeated allergen challenge has not been established, although a proliferative response of airway smooth muscle to LTD_4 released during the allergen challenge appears to be of importance in the rat (128). No such change in muscle has been demonstrated in the guinea pig despite the development of hyperresponsiveness after multiple antigen challenges; the hyperresponsiveness is inhibited by a PAF antagonist (113). Although the guinea pig does not show any morphometric evidence of increase in mass of the smooth muscle, both the guinea pig and rat have shown an increased number of smooth muscle cells entering the S phase of the growth cycle using bromodeoxyuridine incorporation (129,130). A tachykinin contribution to hyperresponsiveness is suggested by the observation that capsaicin administered to neonatal rabbits attenuates the increased responsiveness induced by allergen (131). The possibility that tachykinins and peptido-leukotrienes may be involved in each other's release warrants exploration. An interaction of this sort has been described in hyperpnea-induced bronchoconstriction in the guinea pig (20).

Biochemical alterations in sensitized canine airway smooth muscle have been identified. An increased maximal velocity of shortening without an increase in maximal isometric force has been documented (132). The change appears to be attributable to an increase in myosin adenosine triphosphatase (ATPase) activity. Because shortening of airway smooth muscle *in vivo* occurs against an auxotonic load, it is possible that an increase in maximal velocity of shortening might alter the final degree of narrowing because most of the shortening occurs in the early part of the contraction. Increased concentrations of phosphoinositides have been described in hyperresponsive guinea pigs (133), suggesting that alterations in phospholipase C or other enzymes involved in the degradation of the phosphoinositides may be important. However, the relevance of the above biochemical alterations has not been established.

AIRWAY INFLAMMATION

Airway inflammation in human asthma affects the entire airway wall and demonstrates a number of characteristic features (134–136). An increase in leukocytes, in particular eosinophils and mononuclear cells, is usually present in symptomatic asthma. The epithelium appears to be fragile and easily detachable. Subepithelial deposition of collagen, so-called thickening of the basement membrane, appears to be pathognomonic of the asthmatic condition. Thickening of the submucosa, airway smooth muscle, and adventitial tissues is present. An increase in glands, goblet cells, and bronchial vascularity also occurs. Many of these features are the result of chronic disease processes, for which there is a paucity of models.

The induction of airway inflammation, resembling asthmatic inflammation, has been most successfully achieved in allergen-driven models. Although there are no detailed studies of leukocyte kinetics, certain conclusions can be drawn from results obtained by bronchoalveolar lavage at single time points (98,108,112, 137). Sensitized animals after challenge show a rapid increase in cells retrieved from the lungs by bronchoalveolar lavage. Most of the increase in cells are neutrophils, but eosinophils and lymphocytes also increase in number with a lag time of several hours. By 24 hours after challenge, neutrophil numbers have decreased and eosinophilia is more striking. The duration of inflammation varies from species to species, lasting as long as 1 week in the sheep (112), whereas the airways of the rat (108) appear to be normal 5 days after challenge.

Chemotactic factors play a fundamental role in the process of attracting specific subsets of leukocytes from the blood to sites of inflammation. In recent years the spectrum of chemotactic factors has expanded greatly; human lung cells, including alveolar macrophages (138), airway epithelium (139), and lung endothelium in the dog (140), can produce chemotactic factors. Interleukin-8 is a recently described low-molecular-weight polypeptide with potent neutrophil chemotactic activity produced by monocytes and many other cell types. Intradermal administration of human IL-8 in rats induces a rapid and concentration-dependent neutrophil infiltration, which peaks 4 hours after IL-8 application. When injected intravenously, IL-8 induces neutrophil sequestration in the lungs, and after repeated injections causes marked septal and intra-alveolar edema and lung damage (141). Alveolar macrophages produce LTB_4, a potent neutrophil and eosinophil attractant in guinea pigs (142). Until recently, no single chemoattractant had been shown to have specific activity for eosinophils, but eotaxin now appears to be such a mediator. PAF is another humoral mediator causing eosinophil migration in animal models. PAF promotes infiltration of eosinophils into bronchoalveolar lavage in the guinea pig (143). Certain cytokines may act as eosinophil attractants; IL-5 is relatively selective in attracting eosinophils (144). Eosinophil stimulation promoter (ESP) stimulates eosinophil migration and function in the mouse (145) and has been shown to be attributable to the combined activities of granulocyte macrophage–colony stimulating factor (GM-CSF) and IL-5. *In vitro* studies suggest that locally produced chemoattractants guide leukocytes through the endothelial junctions and underlying tissue to the inflammatory site through activation of specific cell surface receptors (as reviewed in ref. 146).

Chronic allergen exposure has been used to induce some of the functional and structural changes observed in asthma. Rabbit (147), cat (148), guinea pig (102,130), and rat (115,129,149) have all been reported on to date. However, rigorous morphometric analyses are still lacking in several species. The cat shows extensive goblet cell and mucous gland hypertrophy and hyperplasia as well as epithelial erosion and eosinophilic infiltration (148). In contrast, the rat shows no morphologic alteration of the epithelium, although evidence of enhanced cell turnover has been obtained (129). There also appears to be an increase in smooth muscle mass in the cat and rat. A recent study by Bai et al. (130) showed an increase in smooth muscle DNA synthesis in ovalbumin-sensitized guinea pigs challenged twice weekly for 6 weeks compared with saline-challenged control animals. These results are consistent with the idea that airway smooth muscle proliferates as part of the chronic inflammatory response. However, despite an increase in the smooth muscle cells incorporating bromodeoxyuridine, no measurable increase was seen in smooth muscle area, suggesting increased cell turnover.

The links between airway inflammation and other manifestations of asthma, in particular hyperresponsiveness, have been extensively explored. Induced AHR, whether allergic or not, is almost invariably associated with an increase in airway leukocyte numbers. However, the precise cells responsible for the hyperresponsiveness have been difficult to pinpoint. Several strategies have been employed. Experiments involving depletion of specific leukocytes have been informative (58,150–153) but inconclusive because of uncertainty surrounding the selectivity of the drugs or antibodies used. The availability of monoclonal antibodies with selectivity for various adhesion molecules involved in leukocyte migration has helped to explore these issues further. Several studies have employed blocking antibodies to cell adhesion molecules in animal models of airway hyperreactivity (as reviewed in refs. 154,155). Figure 5 illustrates results reproduced from a study by Abraham et al. (112) investigating the protective effect of a blocking anti-alpha 4 monoclonal antibody (HP 1/2) on antigen-induced late responses in the allergic sheep. Treatment with HP1/2 blocked late-phase responses to inhaled *Ascaris suum*, indicating a role for alpha-4 integrins in the cascade of events that lead to late-phase airway responses after antigen challenge. Table 1 summarizes data obtained from primates (156,157), rats (158–160), sheep (112), guinea pigs (161), and rabbits (155). Results from these studies indicate that anti-intercellular adhesion molecule-1 (ICAM) therapy appears to be effective in blunting AHR; however, the mechanism may not be totally dependent on inhibition of inflammatory cell influx. Preliminary *in vitro* data suggest that the observed reduction in hyperresponsiveness may be due to the antibody effect on leukocyte function rather than cell recruitment (112).

CONCLUSIONS

Reversible airways narrowing, AHR, and airway inflammation encompass most of the pathophysiology of human asthma. Currently, no one animal model completely reproduces the disease process found in humans. However, the animal models discussed within this chapter have targeted one or more of these common asthmatic features, and in doing so have provided us with invaluable insight into the pathologic consequences of allergic and nonallergic inflammation in the disease process. To date, pertinent animal models have been developed for the

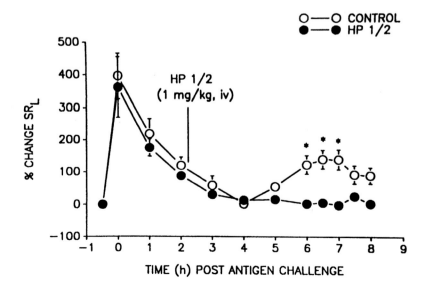

FIG. 5. Protective *in vivo* effect of a blocking anti-alpha 4 monoclonal antibody, HP 1/2, on antigen-induced late responses in the conscious, allergic sheep. In control sheep (*open circles*), *Ascaris suum* antigen challenge produced early and late increases in specific lung resistance (SR_L). Treatment with HP 1/2 (1 mg/kg iv), given 2 hrs after antigen challenge (*closed circles*) blocked late-phase airway changes (*$p<0.05$). These findings indicate a role for alpha 4-integrins in processes that lead to late-phase airway responses after antigen challenge. From Abraham WM, Sielczak MW, Ahmed A, et al. Alpha 4-integrins mediate antigen-induced late bronchial responses and prolonged airway hyperresponsiveness in sheep. *J Clin Invest* 1994;93:776–787.

TABLE 1. *Recent studies employing blocking antibodies to cell adhesion molecules in animal models of airway hyperreactivity*

Adhesion molecule	Animal model	Action	Reference
Anti-ICAM-1	Antigen-sensitized primates	Attenuates eosinophil influx into BAL and hyperreactivity	(156)
Anti-ICAM-1	Antigen-sensitized primates	No effect on BAL cell influx and late-phase response to antigen	(157)
Anti-ICAM-1	Antigen-sensitized rats	Decreases hyperresponsiveness to ACh;no change in BAL cell influx	(159)
Anti-VLA4	Antigen-sensitized guinea pigs	Prevents hyperresponsiveness post–ovalbumin challenge and the migration of eosinophils	(161)
Anti-VLA4	Allergic sheep	Blocks allergen-induced late-phase hyperresponsiveness. No reduction in BAL eosinophils or neutrophils	(112)
Anti-VLA4	Dust mite–allergic rabbit	Reduces early- and late-phase responses to house dust mite, as well as bronchial hyperresponsiveness. No reduction in BAL eosinophils	(155)
Anti-VLA4	Antigen-sensitized rat	Abrogates early and late responses to ovalbumin. No change in BAL or tissue lymphocytes and eosinophils	(158,160)
Anti-LFA-1 anti-LFA1+ anti-MAC1	Antigen-sensitized rat	Abrogates early and late responses to ovalbumin. No change in BAL or tissue lymphocytes and eosinophils	(158,160)
anti-E-selectin	Antigen-sensitized primates	Abrogates neutrophil influx into BAL and late-phase response to antigen	(157)

study of the pathogenesis and pathophysiology of both AHR and "asthmatic" airway inflammation. A model of naturally occurring airways narrowing with persistent increases in airway responsiveness is lacking. In addition, pathologic features are not fully mimicked as no current model shows the basement membrane thickening common to the human condition.

REFERENCE

1. Moses BL, Spaulding GL. Chronic bronchial disease of the cat. [Review]. *Vet Clin North Am Small Anim Pract* 1985;15:929–948.
2. Dye JA. Feline bronchopulmonary disease. [Review]. *Vet Clin North Am Small Anim Pract* 1992;22:1187–1201.
3. Thurlbeck WM, Lowell FC. Heaves in horses. *Am Rev Respir Dis* 1964;89:82–88.
4. Cockcroft DW, Killian DN, Mellon JJ, Hargreave FE. Bronchial reactivity to inhaled histamine: a method and clinical survey. *J Clin Allergy* 1977;7(3):235–243.
5. Bai TR, Macklem PT, Martin JG. Airway responses to aerosolized methacholine in the cat. *Am Rev Respir Dis* 1987;135:190–193.
6. Snapper JR, Drazen JM, Loring SH, Schneider W, Ingram RH, Jr. Distribution of pulmonary responsiveness to aerosol histamine in dogs. *J Appl Physiol Respir Environ Exerc Physiol* 1978;44:738–742.
7. Martin JG, Opazo-Saez A, Du T, Tepper R, Eidelman DH. In vivo airway reactivity: predictive value of morphological estimates of airway smooth muscle. [Review]. *Can J Physiol Pharmacol* 1992;70:597–601.
8. Bellofiore S, Di Maria GU, Martin JG. Changes in upper and lower airway resistance after inhalation of antigen in sensitized rats. *Am Rev Respir Dis* 1987;136:363–368.
9. Xu LJ, Sapienza S, Du T, Waserman S, Martin JG. Comparison of upper and lower airway responses of two sensitized rat strains to inhaled antigen. *J Appl Physiol* 1992;73:1608–1613.
10. Levitt RC, Mitzner W. Expression of airway hyperreactivity to acetylcholine as a simple autosomal recessive trait in mice. *FASEB J* 1988;2:2605–2608.
11. Desanctis GT, Merchant M, Beier DR, et al. Quantitative locus analysis of airway hyperresponsiveness in A/J and C57BL/6J mice. *Nat Genet* 1995;11:150–154.
12. Konno S, Adachi M, Matsuura T, et al. Bronchial reactivity to methacholine and serotonin in six inbred mouse strains. *Arerugi (Japan)* 1993;42:42–47.
13. Eidelman DH, DiMaria GU, Bellofiore S, Wang NS, Guttmann RD, Martin JG. Strain-related differences in airway smooth muscle and airway responsiveness in the rat. *Am Rev Respir Dis* 1991;144:792–796.
14. Douglas JS, Ridgway P, Brink C. Airway responses of the guinea pig in vivo and in vitro. *J Pharmacol Exp Ther* 1977;202:116–124.
15. Hulbert WC, McLean T, Wiggs B, Pare PD, Hogg JC. Histamine dose-response curves in guinea pigs. *J Appl Physiol* 1985;58:625–634.
16. Hirshman CA, Malley A, Downes H. Basenji-Greyhound dog model of asthma: reactivity to Ascaris suum, citric acid, and methacholine. *J Appl Physiol Respir Environ Exerc Physiol* 1980;49:953–957.
17. Pauwels R, Joos G, van der Straeten M. Effect of nedocromil sodium on bronchoconstriction induced by adenosine and tachykinins. *Drugs* 1989;37(suppl 1):87–93;discussion 127–36.
18. Ali S, Mustafa SJ, Metzger WJ. Adenosine-induced bronchoconstriction in an allergic rabbit model: antagonism by theophylline aerosol. *Agents Actions* 1992;37:165–167.
19. Lotvall JO, Tokuyama K, Barnes PJ, Chung KF. Bradykinin-induced airway microvascular leakage is potentiated by captopril and phosphoramidon. *Eur J Pharmacol* 1991;200:211–217.
20. Yang XX, Powell WS, Martin JG. Dry gas hyperpnea-induced bronchoconstriction in the guinea pig is dependent on tachykinin-induced cysteinyl-leukotriene synthesis. *J Appl Physiol* 1996;(in press).
21. Ind PW, Dixon CM, Fuller RW, Barnes PJ. Anticholinergic blockade of beta-blocker-induced bronchoconstriction. *Am Rev Respir Dis* 1989;139:1390–1394.
22. Macklem PT. Bronchial hyperresponsiveness. *Chest* 1985;87:158S–159S.
23. Sly PD, Brown KA, Bates JHT, Macklem PT, Milic-Emili J, Martin JG. The effect of lung volume on interrupter resistances in cats challenged with methacholine. *J Appl Physiol* 1988;64:360–366.
24. Bellofiore S, Eidelman DH, Macklem PT, Martin JG. Effects of elastase-induced emphysema on airway responsiveness to methacholine in rats. *J Appl Physiol* 1989;66:506–612.
25. Moreno RH, Pare PD. Intravenous papain-induced cartilage softening decreases preload of tracheal smooth muscle. *J Appl Physiol* 1989;66:1694–1698.
26. Lambert RK. Role of bronchial basement membrane in airway collapse. *J Appl Physiol* 1991;71:666–673.
27. Okazawa M, Wang L, Lambert RK, et al. Mucosal folding and airway smooth muscle shortening. *Chest* 1995;107:88S.

28. Macklem PT. Theoretical basis of airway instability. *Chest* 1995;107: 87S–88S.
29. Ding DJ, Martin JG, Macklem PT. Effects of lung volume on maximal methacholine induced bronchoconstriction in normal human subjects. *J Appl Physiol* 1987;62:1324–1330.
30. Nagase T, Ito T, Yanai M, Martin JG, Ludwig MS. Responsiveness of and interactions between airways and tissue in guinea pigs during induced constriction. *J Appl Physiol* 1993;74:2848–2854.
31. Dandurand RJ, Xu LJ, Martin JG, Eidelman DH. Airway-parenchymal interdependence and bronchial responsiveness in two highly inbred rat strains. *J Appl Physiol* 1993;74:538–544.
32. Nijkamp FP, van der Linde HJ, Folkerts G. Nitric oxide synthesis inhibitors induce airway hyperresponsiveness in the guinea pig *in vivo* and *in vitro*. Role of the epithelium. *Am Rev Respir Dis* 1993;148: 727–734.
33. Jia Y, Xu L, Heisler S, Martin JG. Airways of a hyperresponsive rat strain show decreased relaxant responses to sodium nitroprusside. *Am J Physiol* 1995;269:L85–91.
34. Jansen A, Drazen J, Osborne JA, Brown R, Loscalzo J, Stamler JS. The relaxant properties in guinea pig airways of S-nitrosothiols. *J Pharmacol Exp Ther* 1992;261:154–160.
35. Kobzik L, Bredt DS, Lowenstein CJ, et al. Nitric oxide synthase in human and rat lung: immunocytochemical and histochemical localization. *Am J Respir Cell Mol Biol* 1993;9:371–377.
36. Robbins RA, Hamel FG, Floreani AA, et al. Bovine bronchial epithelial cells metabolize L-arginine to L-citrulline: possible role of nitric oxide synthase. *Life Sci* 1993;52:709–716.
37. Hirshman CA, Downes H, Leon DA, Peters JE. Basenji-greyhound dog model of asthma: pulmonary responses after beta-adrenergic blockade. *J Appl Physiol Respir Environ Exerc Physiol* 1981;51: 1423–1427.
38. Ney UM. Propranolol-induced airway hyperreactivity in guinea-pigs. *Br J Pharmacol* 1983;79:1003–1009.
39. Tobias JD, Sauder RA, Hirshman CA. Methylprednisolone prevents propranolol-induced airway hyperreactivity in the Basenji-greyhound dog. *Anesthesiology* 1991;74:1115–1120.
40. Darowski MJ, Hannon VM, Hirshman CA. Corticosteroids decrease airway hyperresponsiveness in the Basenji-Greyhound dog model of asthma. *J Appl Physiol* 1989;66:1120–1126.
41. Tepper RS, Du T, Styhler A, Ludwig M, Martin JG. Increased maximal pulmonary response to methacholine and airway smooth muscle in immature compared with mature rabbits. *Am J Respir Crit Care Med* 1995;151:836–840.
42. Wills M, Douglas JS. Aging and cholinergic responses in bovine trachealis muscle. *Br J Pharmacol* 1988;93:918–924.
43. Duncan PG, Douglas JS. Influences of gender and maturation on responses of guinea-pig airway tissues to LTD4. *Eur J Pharmacol* 1985;112:423–427.
44. Duncan PG, Douglas JS. Age-related changes in guinea pig respiratory tissues: considerations for assessment of bronchodilators. *Eur J Pharmacol* 1985;108:39–48.
45. Douglas JS, Duncan PG, Mukhopadhyay A. The antagonism of histamine-induced tracheal and bronchial muscle contraction by diphenhydramine: effect of maturation. *Br J Pharmacol* 1984;83:697–705.
46. Arakawa H, Lotvall J, Kawikova I, Tokuyama K, Lofdahl CG, Skoogh BE. Effect of maturation on airway plasma exudation induced by eicosanoids in guinea pig. *Eur J Pharmacol* 1994;259:251–257.
47. Rosenberg SM, Berry GT, Yandrasitz JR, Grunstein MM. Maturational regulation of inositol 1,4,5-trisphosphate metabolism in rabbit airway smooth muscle. *J Clin Invest* 1991;88:2032–2038.
48. Souhrada M, Rothberg KG, Douglas JS. Membrane properties of bovine airway smooth muscle cells: effects of maturation. *Pulmon Pharmacol* 1988;1:47–52.
49. Rothberg KG, Morris PL, Douglas JS. Characterization of cholinergic muscarinic receptors in cow tracheal muscle membranes. Effect of maturation. *Biochem Pharmacol* 1987;36:1687–1695.
50. Hirshman CA, Downes H, Veith L. Airway responses in offspring of dogs with and without airway hyperreactivity. *J Appl Physiol Respir Environ Exerc Physiol* 1984;56:1272–1277.
51. Pauwels R, van der Straeten M, Weyne J, Bazin H. Genetic factors in non-specific bronchial reactivity in rats. *Eur J Respir Dis* 1985;66: 98–104.
52. Takino Y, Sugahara K, Horino I. Two lines of guinea pigs sensitive to and nonsensitive to chemical mediators and anaphylaxis. *J Allergy* 1971; 47:247–261.
53. Jones GL, O'Byrne PM, Pashley M, et al. Airway smooth muscle responsiveness from dogs with airway hyperresponsiveness after O3 inhalation. *J Appl Physiol* 1988;65:57–64.
54. Janssen LJ, O'Byrne PM, Daniel EE. Mechanism underlying ozone-induced *in vitro* hyperresponsiveness in canine bronchi. *Am J Physiol* 1991;261:L55–L62.
55. Tsukagoshi H, Haddad EB, Sun J, Barnes PJ, Chung KF. Ozone-induced airway hyperresponsiveness: role of superoxide anions, NEP, and BK receptors. *J Appl Physiol* 1995;78:1015–1022.
56. Daniel EE, O'Byrne P. Effect of inflammatory mediators on airway nerves and muscle. *Am Rev Respir Dis* 1991;143:S3–5.
57. Aizawa H, Chung KF, Leikauf GD, et al. Significance of thromboxane generation in ozone-induced airway hyperresponsiveness in dogs. *J Appl Physiol* 1985;59:1918–1923.
58. O'Byrne PM, Walters EH, Gold BD, et al. Neutrophil depletion inhibits airway hyperresponsiveness induced by ozone exposure. *Am Rev Respir Dis* 1984;130:214–219.
59. Fabbri LM, Aizawa H, Alpert SE, et al. Airway hyperresponsiveness and changes in cell counts in bronchoalveolar lavage after ozone exposure in dogs. *Am Rev Respir Dis* 1984;129:288–291.
60. Imai T, Adachi M, Horikoshi S, et al. [Relation of platelet activating factor induced airway hyperresponsiveness to thromboxane A2 and neutrophil in dogs.] *Arerugi (Japan)* 1993;42:1563–1568.
61. Nishikawa M, Ikeda H, Nishiyama H, Yamakawa H, Suzuki S, Okubo T. Combined effects of ozone and cigarette smoke on airway responsiveness and vascular permeability in guinea pigs. *Lung* 1992;170: 311–322.
62. Yeadon M, Wilkinson D, Darley-Usmar V, O'Leary VJ, Payne AN. Mechanisms contributing to ozone-induced bronchial hyperreactivity in guinea-pigs. *Pulmon Pharmacol* 1992;5:39–50.
63. Murlas C, Roum JH. Bronchial hyperreactivity occurs in steroid-treated guinea pigs depleted of leukocytes by cyclophosphamide. *J Appl Physiol* 1985;58:1630–1637.
64. Evans TW, Brokaw JJ, Chung KF, Nadel JA, McDonald DM. Ozone-induced bronchial hyperresponsiveness in the rat is not accompanied by neutrophil influx or increased vascular permeability in the trachea. *Am Rev Respir Dis* 1988;138:140–144.
65. Matsui S, Jones GL, Woolley MJ, Lane CG, Gontovnick LS, O'Byrne PM. The effect of antioxidants on ozone-induced airway hyperresponsiveness in dogs. *Am Rev Respir Dis* 1991;144:1287–1290.
66. Takahashi T, Miura M, Katsumata U, et al. Involvement of superoxide in ozone-induced airway hyperresponsiveness in anesthetized cats. *Am Rev Respir Dis* 1993;148:103–106.
67. Spicer BA, Baker R, Laycock SM, Smith H. Correlation between blood eosinophilia and airways hyper-responsiveness in rats. *Agents Actions* 1989;26:63–65.
68. Laycock SM, Smith H, Spicer BA. Airway hyper-reactivity and eosinophilia in rats treated with Sephadex particles. *Int Arch Allergy Immunol* 1987;82:347–348.
69. Piercy V, Arch JR, Baker RC, Cook RM, Hatt PA, Spicer BA. Effects of dexamethasone in a model of lung hyperresponsiveness in the rat. *Agents Actions* 1993;39:118–125.
70. Francischi JN, Conroy D, Maghni K, Sirois P. Rapamycin inhibits airway leukocyte infiltration and hyperreactivity in guinea pigs. *Agents Actions* 1993;39:C139–C141.
71. Asano M, Inamura N, Nakahara K, et al. A 5-lipoxygenase inhibitor, FR110302, suppresses airway hyperresponsiveness and lung eosinophilia induced by Sephadex particles in rats. *Agents Actions* 1992;36:215–221.
72. Kurosawa M, Yodonawa S, Tsukagoshi H, Miyachi Y. Inhibition by a novel peptide leukotriene receptor antagonist ONO-1078 of airway wall thickening and airway hyperresponsiveness to histamine induced by leukotriene C4 or leukotriene D4 in guinea-pigs. *Clin Exp Allergy* 1994;24:960–968.
73. Powell WS, Xu LJ, Martin JG. Effects of dexamethasone on leukotriene synthesis and airway responses to antigen and leukotriene D4 in rats. *Am J Respir Crit Care Med* 1995;151:1143–1150.
74. Kimura K, Inoue H, Ichinose M, et al. Bradykinin causes airway hyperresponsiveness and enhances maximal airway narrowing. Role of microvascular leakage and airway edema. *Am Rev Respir Dis* 1992; 146:1301–1305.
75. Chung KF, Aizawa H, Leikauf GD, Ueki IF, Evans TW, Nadel JA. Airway hyperresponsiveness induced by platelet-activating factor: role of thromboxane generation. *J Pharmacol Exp Ther* 1986;236:580–584.
76. Coyle AJ, Spina D, Page CP. PAF-induced bronchial hyperresponsive-

ness in the rabbit: contribution of platelets and airway smooth muscle. *Br J Pharmacol* 1990;101:31–38.

77. Christman BW, Lefferts PL, Snapper JR. Effect of platelet-activating factor on aerosol histamine responsiveness in awake sheep. *Am Rev Respir Dis* 1987;135:1267–1270.

78. Cuss FM, Dixon CMS, Barnes PJ. Effects of inhaled platelet activting factor on pulmonary function and bronchial responsiveness in man. *Lancet* 1986;July 26:189–192.

79. Yager D, Kamm RD, Drazen JM. Airway wall liquid. Sources and role as an amplifier of bronchoconstriction. [Review]. *Chest* 1995;107:105S–110S.

80. Tsukagoshi H, Sakamoto T, Xu W, Barnes PJ, Chung KF. Effect of interleukin-1 beta on airway hyperresponsiveness and inflammation in sensitized and nonsensitized Brown-Norway rats. *J Allergy Clin Immunol* 1994;93:464–469.

81. Renzi PM, Sapienza S, Du T, Wang NS, Martin JG. Lymphokine-induced airway hyperresponsiveness in the rat. *Am Rev Respir Dis* 1991;143:375–379.

82. Wheeler AP, Jesmok G, Brigham KL. Tumor necrosis factor's effects on lung mechanics, gas exchange, and airway reactivity in sheep. *J Appl Physiol* 1990;68:2542–2549.

83. Kips JC, Tavernier J, Pauwels RA. Tumor necrosis factor causes bronchial hyperresponsiveness in rats. *Am Rev Respir Dis* 1992;145:332–336.

84. Van Oosterhout AJ, Ladenius AR, Savelkoul HF, Van Ark I, Delsman KC, Nijkamp FP. Effect of anti-IL-5 and IL-5 on airway hyperreactivity and eosinophils in guinea pigs. *Am Rev Respir Dis* 1993;147:548–552.

85. Sorkness R, Clough JJ, Castleman WL, Lemanske RF, Jr. Virus-induced airway obstruction and parasympathetic hyperresponsiveness in adult rats. *Am J Respir Crit Care Med* 1995;150:28–34.

86. Lemen RJ, Quan SF, Witten ML, Sobonya RE, Ray CG, Grad R. Canine parainfluenza type 2 bronchiolitis increases histamine responsiveness in beagle puppies. *Am Rev Respir Dis* 1990;141:199–207.

87. Folkerts G, Verheyen AK, Geuens GM, Folkerts HF, Nijkamp FP. Virus-induced changes in airway responsiveness, morphology, and histamine levels in guinea pigs. *Am Rev Respir Dis* 1993;147:1569–1577.

88. Hegele RG, Hayashi S, Hogg JC, Pare PD. Mechanisms of airway narrowing and hyperresponsiveness in viral respiratory tract infections. *Am J Respir Crit Care Med* 1995;151:1659–1665.

89. Sugawara Y, Okamoto Y, Sawahata T, Tanaka K. Skin reactivity in guinea pigs sensitized with 2,4-toluene diisocyanate. *Int Arch Allergy Immunol* 1993;100:190–196.

90. Sugawara Y, Okamoto Y, Sawahata T, Tanaka K. An asthma model developed in the guinea pig by intranasal application of 2,4-toluene diisocyanate. *Int Arch Allergy Immunol* 1993;101:95–101.

91. Abe Y, Ogino S, Irifune M, et al. Histamine content, synthesis and degradation in nasal mucosa and lung of guinea-pigs treated with toluene diisocyanate (TDI). *Clin Exp Allergy* 1993;23:512–517.

92. Fraser DG, Regal JF, Arndt ML. Trimellitic anhydride-induced allergic response in the lung: role of the complement system in cellular changes. *J Pharmacol Exp Ther* 1995;273:793–801.

93. Hayes JP, Kuo HP, Rohde JA, et al. Neurogenic goblet cell secretion and bronchoconstriction in guinea pigs sensitised to trimellitic anhydride. *Eur J Pharmacol* 1995;292:127–134.

94. Arakawa H, Lotvall J, Linden A, Kawikova I, Lofdahl CG, Skoogh BE. Role of eicosanoids in airflow obstruction and airway plasma exudation induced by trimellitic anhydride-conjugate in guinea-pigs 3 and 8 weeks after sensitization. *Clin Exp Allergy* 1994;24:582–589.

95. Dearman RJ, Ramdin LS, Basketter DA, Kimber I. Inducible interleukin-4-secreting cells provoked in mice during chemical sensitization. *Immunology* 1994;81:551–557.

96. Zeiss CR, Hatoum NS, Ferguson J, et al. Localization of inhaled trimellitic anhydride to lung with a respiratory lymph node antibody secreting cell response. *J Allergy Clin Immunol* 1992;90:944–952.

97. Hayes JP, Barnes PJ, Taylor AJ, Chung KF. Effect of a topical corticosteroid on airway hyperresponsiveness and eosinophilic inflammation induced by trimellitic anhydride exposure in sensitized guinea pigs. *J Allergy Clin Immunol* 1993;92:450–456.

98. Marsh WR, Irvin CG, Murphy KR, Behrens BL, Larsen GL. Increases in airway reactivity to histamine and inflammatory cells in bronchoalveolar lavage after the late asthmatic response in an animal model. *Am Rev Respir Dis* 1985;131:875–879.

99. Becker AB, Hershkovich J, Simons FER, Simons KJ, Lilley MK, Ke-

pron WM. Development of chronic airway hyperresponsiveness in ragweed-sensitized dogs. *J Appl Physiol* 1989;66:2691–2697.

100. Shampain MP, Behrens BL, Larsen GL, Henson PM. An animal model of late pulmonary responses to Alternaria challenge. *Am Rev Respir Dis* 1982;126:493–498.

101. Minshall EM, Riccio MM, Herd CM, et al. A novel animal model for investigating persistent airway hyperresponsiveness. *J Pharmacol Toxicol Methods* 1993;30:177–188.

102. Hutson PA, Church MK, Clay TP, Miller P, Holgate ST. Early and late-phase bronchoconstriction after allergen challenge of nonanesthetized guinea pigs. I. The association of disordered airway physiology to leukocyte infiltration. *Am Rev Respir Dis* 1988;137:548–557.

103. Sasaki H, Yanai M, Shimura S, et al. Late asthmatic response to Ascaris antigen challenge in dogs treated with metyrapone. *Am Rev Respir Dis* 1987;136:1459–1465.

104. Richards IM, Griffin RL, Shields SK, Reid MS, Fidler SF. Chasing the elusive animal model of late-phase bronchoconstriction: studies in dogs, guinea pigs and rats. *Agents Actions* 1992;37:178–180.

105. Fornhem C, Lundberg JM, Alving K. Allergen-induced late-phase airways obstruction in the pig—the role of endogenous cortisol. *Eur Respir J* 1995;8:928–937.

106. Pauwels R, Bazin H, Platteau B, van der Straeten M. The influence of antigen dose on IgE production in different rat strains. *Immunology* 1979;36:151–157.

107. Eidelman DH, Bellofiore S, Martin JG. Late airway responses to antigen challenge in sensitized inbred rats. *Am Rev Respir Dis* 1988;137:1033–1037.

108. Elwood W, Lotvall JO, Barnes PJ, Fan Chung K. Characterization of allergen-induced bronchial hyperresponsiveness and airway inflammation in actively sensitized Brown-Norway rats. *J Allergy Clin Immunol* 1991;88:951–960.

109. Gundel RH, Wegner CD, Letts LG. Antigen-induced acute and late-phase responses in primates. *Am Rev Respir Dis* 1992;146:369–373.

110. Hamel R, McFarlane CS, Ford-Hutchinson AW. Late pulmonary responses induced by Ascaris allergen in conscious squirrel monkeys. *J Appl Physiol* 1986;61:2081–2087.

111. Abraham WM, Sielczak MW, Wanner A, Perruchoud AP, et al. Cellular markers of inflammation in the airways of allergic sheep with and without allergen-induced late responses. *Am Rev Respir Dis* 1988;138:1565–1571.

112. Abraham WM, Sielczak MW, Ahmed A, et al. Alpha 4-integrins mediate antigen-induced late bronchial responses and prolonged airway hyperresponsiveness in sheep. *J Clin Invest* 1994;93:776–787.

113. Ishida K, Thomson RJ, Beattie LL, Wiggs B, Schellenberg RR. Inhibition of antigen-induced airway hyperresponsiveness, but not acute hypoxia nor airway eosinophilia, by an antagonist of platelet-activating factor. *J Immunol* 1990;144:3907–3911.

114. Bellofiore S, Martin JG. Antigen challenge of sensitized rats increases airway responsiveness to methacholine. *J Appl Physiol* 1988;65:1642–1646.

115. Haczku A, Moqbel R, Elwood W, et al. Effects of prolonged repeated exposure to ovalbumin in sensitized brown Norway rats. *Am J Respir Crit Care Med* 1994;150:23–27.

116. Kips JC, Cuvelier CA, Pauwels RA. Effect of acute and chronic antigen inhalation on airway morphology and responsiveness in actively sensitized rats. *Am Rev Respir Dis* 1992;145:1306–1310.

117. Downes H, Austin DR, Parks CM, Hirshman CA. Comparison of *in vitro* drug responses in airways of atopic dogs with and without *in vivo* airway hyperresponsiveness. *Pulmon Pharmacol* 1989;2:209–216.

118. Watanabe A, Rossi P, Renzi PM, Xu LJ, Guttmann RD, Martin JG. Adoptive transfer of allergic airway responses with sensitized lymphocytes in BN rats. *Am J Respir Crit Care Med* 1995;152:64–70.

119. Watanabe A, Mishima H, Renzi PM, Xu LJ, Hamid Q, Martin JG. Transfer of allergic airway responses with antigen–primed CD4+ but not CD8+- T cells in Brown Norway rats. *J Clin Invest* 1995;96:1303–1310.

120. Renz H, Lack G, Saloga J, et al. Inhibition of IgE production and normalization of airways responsiveness by sensitized CD8 T cells in a mouse model of allergen-induced sensitization. *J Immunol* 1994;152:351–360.

121. Dykewicz MS, Patterson R, Harris KE. Induction of antigen-specific bronchial reactivity to trimellityl-human serum albumin by passive transfer of serum from humans to rhesus monkeys. *J Lab Clin Med* 1988;111:459–465.

122. Fink JN, Schlueter DP, Barboriak JJ. Passive transfer of methacholine sensitivity from man to monkey. *J Allergy Clin Immunol* 1987;79: 427–432.

123. Abraham WM, Stevenson JS, Garrido R. A possible role for PAF in allergen-induced late responses: modifications by a selective antagonist. *J Appl Physiol* 1989;66:2351–2357.

124. Soler M, Sielczak MW, Abraham WM. A PAF antagonist blocks antigen-induced airway hyperresponsiveness and inflammation in sheep. *J Appl Physiol* 1989;67:406–413.

125. Abraham WM, Burch RM, Farmer SG, Sielczak MW, Ahmed A, Cortes A. A bradykinin antagonist modifies allergen-induced mediator release and late bronchial responses in sheep. *Am Rev Respir Dis* 1991;143:787–796.

126. Soler M, Sielczak M, Abraham WM. Separation of late bronchial responses from airway hyperresponsiveness in allergic sheep. *J Appl Physiol* 1991;70:617–623.

127. Kagoshima M, Tomomatsu N, Aratani H, Terasawa M. Effect of Y-20811, a long-lasting thromboxane A2 synthetase inhibitor, on antigen-induced airway hyperresponsiveness in guinea pigs. *Int Arch Allergy Immunol* 1991;96:238–243.

128. Wang CG, Du T, Xu LJ, Martin JG. Role of leukotriene D4 in allergen-induced increases in airway smooth muscle in the rat. *Am Rev Respir Dis* 1993;148:413–417.

129. Panettieri RA, Murray RK, Bilgen G, Eszterhas AJ, Martin JG. Repeated allergen inhalations induce DNA synthesis in airway smooth muscle and epithelial cells *in vivo*. *Chest* 1995;107:S 94–S 95.

130. Bai TR, Wang ZL, Walker B, Pare PD. Chronic allergic inflammation induces replication of airway smooth muscle cells *in vivo* in guinea pigs. *Chest* 1995;107:93S

131. Riccio MM, Manzini S, Page CP. The effect of neonatal capsaicin on the development of bronchial hyperresponsiveness in allergic rabbits. *Eur J Pharmacol* 1993;232:89–97.

132. Jiang H, Rao K, Halayko AJ, Liu X, Stephens NL. Ragweed sensitization-induced increase of myosin light chain kinase content in canine airway smooth muscle. *Am J Respir Cell Mol Biol* 1992;7: 567–573.

133. Salari H, Yeung M, Howard S, Schellenberg RR. Increased contraction and inositol phosphate formation of tracheal smooth muscle from hyperresponsive guinea pigs. *J Allergy Clin Immunol* 1992;90: 918–926.

134. Saetta M, Fabbri LM, Danieli D, Picotti G, Allegra L. Pathology of bronchial asthma and animal models of asthma. [Review]. *Eur Respir J Suppl* 1989;6:477s–482s.

135. Jeffery PK. Pathology of asthma. [Review]. *Br Med Bull* 1992;48: 23–39.

136. Arm JP, Lee TH. The pathobiology of bronchial asthma. [Review]. *Adv Immunol* 1992;51:323–382.

137. Chung KF, Becker AB, Lazarus SC, Frick OL, Nadel JA, Gold WM. Antigen-induced airway hyperresponsiveness and pulmonary inflammation in allergic dogs. *J Appl Physiol* 1985;58:1347–1353.

138. Martin TR, Raugi G, Merritt TL, Henderson WR, Jr. Relative contribution of leukotriene B4 to the neutrophil chemotactic activity produced by the resident human alveolar macrophage. *J Clin Invest* 1987; 80:1114–1124.

139. Shoji S, Rickard KA, Ertl RF, Robbins RA, Linder J, Rennard SI. Bronchial epithelial cells produce lung fibroblast chemotactic factor: fibronectin. *Am J Respir Cell Mol Biol* 1989;1:13–20.

140. Farber HW, Fairman RP, Millan JE, Rounds S, Glauser FL. Pulmonary response to foreign body microemboli in dogs: release of neutrophil chemoattractant activity by vascular endothelial cells. *Am J Respir Cell Mol Biol* 1989;1:27–35.

141. Zwahlen R, Walz A, Rot A. *In vitro* and *in vivo* activity and pathophysiology of human interleukin-8 and related peptides. [Review]. *Int Rev Exp Pathol* 1993;34:27–42.

142. Sehmi R, Cromwell O, Taylor GW, Kay AB. Identification of guinea pig eosinophil chemotactic factor of anaphylaxis as leukotriene B4 and 8(S),15(S)-dihydroxy-5,9,11, 13(Z,E,Z,E)-eicosatetraenoic acid. *J Immunol* 1991;147:2276–2283.

143. Lellouch-Tubiana A, Lefort J, Simon MT, Pfister A, Vargaftig BB. Eosinophil recruitment into guinea pig lungs after PAF-acether and allergen administration. Modulation by prostacyclin, platelet depletion, and selective antagonists. *Am Rev Respir Dis* 1988;137: 948–954.

144. Sanderson CJ, Campbell HD, Young IG. Molecular and cellular biology of eosinophil differentiation factor (interleukin-5) and its effects on human and mouse B cells. [Review]. *Immunol Rev* 1988;102: 29–50.

145. Secor WE, Stewart SJ, Colley DG. Eosinophils and immune mechanisms. VI. The synergistic combination of granulocyte-macrophage colony-stimulating factor and IL-5 accounts for eosinophil-stimulation promoter activity in Schistosoma mansoni-infected mice. *J Immunol* 1990;144:1484–1489.

146. Furie MB, Randolph GJ. Chemokines and tissue injury. [Review]. *Am J Pathol* 1995;146:1287–1301.

147. Larsen GL, Wilson MC, Clark RA, Behrens BL. The inflammatory reaction in the airways in an animal model of the late asthmatic response. [Review]. *Fed Proc* 1987;46:105–112.

148. Padrid P, Snook S, Finucane T, et al. Persistent airway hyperresponsiveness and histologic alterations after chronic antigen challenge in cats. *Am J Respir Crit Care Med* 1995;151:184–193.

149. Sapienza S, Du T, Eidelman DH, Wang NS, Martin JG. Structural changes in the airways of sensitized brown Norway rats after antigen challenge. *Am Rev Respir Dis* 1991;144:423–427.

150. Murphy KR, Wilson MC, Irvin CG, et al. The requirement for polymorphonuclear leukocytes in the late asthmatic response and heightened airways reactivity in an animal model. *Am Rev Respir Dis* 1986; 134:62–68.

151. Hinson JM, Jr., Hutchison AA, Brigham KL, Meyrick BO, Snapper JR. Effects of granulocyte depletion on pulmonary responsiveness to aerosol histamine. *J Appl Physiol Respir Environ Exerc Physiol* 1984; 56:411–417.

152. Thompson JE, Scypinski LA, Gordon T, Sheppard D. Hydroxyurea inhibits airway hyperresponsiveness in guinea pigs by a granulocyte-independent mechanism. *Am Rev Respir Dis* 1986;134:1213–1218.

153. Bethel RA, Worthen GS, Henson PM, Lien DC. Effects of neutrophil depletion and repletion on PAF-induced hyperresponsiveness of canine trachea. *J Appl Physiol* 1992;73:2413–2419.

154. Pilewski JM, Albelda SM. Cell adhesion molecules in asthma: homing, activation, and airway remodeling. [Review]. *Am J Respir Cell Mol Biol* 1995;12:1–3.

155. Metzger WJ. Therapeutic approaches to asthma based on VLA-4 integrin and its counter receptors. *Springer Semin Immunopathol* 1995; 16:467–478.

156. Wegner CD, Gundel RH, Reilly P, Haynes N, Letts G, Rothlein R. Intracellular adhesion molecule-1 (ICAM-1) in the pathogenesis of asthma. *Science* 1990;247:456–459.

157. Gundel RH, Wegner CD, Torcellini CA, et al. Endothelial leukocyte adhesion molecule-1 mediates antigen-induced acute airway inflammation and late-phase airway obstruction in monkeys. *J Clin Invest* 1991;88:1407–1411.

158. Rabb HA, Olivenstein R, Issekutz TB, Renzi PM, Martin JG. The role of the leukocyte adhesion molecules VLA-4, LFA-1 and Mac-1 in allergic airway responses in the rat. *Am J Respir Crit Care Med* 1994; 149:1186–1191.

159. Sun J, Elwood W, Haczku A, Barnes PJ, Hellewell PG, Chung KF. Contribution of intercellular-adhesion molecule-1 in allergen-induced airway hyperresponsiveness and inflammation in sensitised brown-Norway rats. *Int Arch Allergy Immunol* 1994;104:291–295.

160. Nagase T, Fukuchi Y, Matsuse T, Sudo E, Matsui H, Orimo H. Antagonism of ICAM-1 attenuates airway and tissue responses to antigen in sensitized rats. *Am J Respir Crit Care Med* 1995;151: 1244–1249.

161. Pretolani M, Ruffie C, Lapa eS, JR, Joseph D, Lobb RR, Vargaftig BB. Antibody to very late activation antigen 4 prevents antigen-induced bronchial hyperreactivity and cellular infiltration in the guinea pig airways. *J Exp Med* 1994;180:795–805.

Asthma, edited by P.J. Barnes, M.M. Grunstein,
A.R. Leff, and A.J. Woolcock.
Lippincott–Raven Publishers, Philadelphia © 1997.

■ 22 ■

Animal Models for Studying Genetics of Asthma

Romain A. Pauwels, Guy F. Joos, and Johan C. Kips

Immunoglobulin E Synthesis	Plasma Protein Extravasation
Airway Responsiveness	Inflammatory Cell Activation
Airway Inflammation	

Animal models have been used for many years to study the pathogenesis of bronchial asthma, but none of the animal models reproduces all the characteristics of human bronchial asthma. Animal models are therefore generally used to investigate one or more particular characteristics of human asthma, hoping that the findings in the animal model will help to understand the human disease better. The study of genetic factors involved in asthma using animal models started several years ago and has focused on the inheritance of one or more characteristics of human asthma, such as increased airway responsiveness to various bronchoconstrictor agents, the tendency to develop an anaphylactic response upon immunization, the tendency to produce immunoglobulin E (IgE) antibodies, etc. The initial studies in animal models mainly focused on identifying the mendelian mode of inheritance of these asthmalike characteristics. It became rapidly clear that the genetic factors controlling one single characteristic of bronchial asthma in animal models are multiple and that the genetic factors involved in human asthma are almost sure to be multiple and very complex.

There is currently a renewed interest in animal models of human asthma with respect to the genetic factors involved. Indeed, it is hoped that identification of the genes that control certain asthma-linked characteristics in these animal models might help in elucidating impor-

tant pathogenetic mechanisms in human asthma and also help to identify the relevant genes that control the pathogenesis of human asthma.

This chapter reviews the studies that have investigated the influence of genetic factors in animal models of human asthma. The relevance of these findings to human asthma will serve as a *leitmotif.*

IMMUNOGLOBULIN E SYNTHESIS

The synthesis of IgE antibodies to environmental allergens is an important risk factor for the development of bronchial asthma. Studies in mice and rats have demonstrated clearly that the capacity to synthesize IgE antibodies is under the control of genetic factors (1). One set of genes, linked to the major histocompatibility genes, controls the immune response to the antigen. A second set is responsible for the preferential production of IgE versus IgG antibodies. The discovery of the immunocytomas in the rat made the development of specific immune reagents for the various immunoglobulin classes and subclasses possible, including reagents for the measurement of total and specific IgE. Studies in inbred rat strains demonstrated that these strains vary considerably with respect to the total serum IgE before active immunization. Inbred rat strains also differ significantly in their production of specific IgE antibodies after active immunization. There was a significant relationship between the total serum IgE concentration before immunization and the IgE antibody response after intraperitoneal immunization.

R. A. Pauwels, G. F. Joos, and J. C. Kips: Department of Respiratory Diseases, University Hospital Ghent, B-9000 Ghent, Belgium.

Studies in the rat also confirmed the influence of other factors on the production of IgE. These factors included age, antigen dose, parasitic infection, type of adjuvant, way of administration, and the breeding conditions (1).

Studies in other species such as guinea pig and dog have never clearly shown a genetic influence on IgE synthesis, mainly because of the lack of analytical tools. It is interesting to mention, however, the selective breeding of a guinea pig strain especially prone to anaphylaxis (2).

The studies in mice and in rats have the advantage that a high number of inbred strains are available and that breeding studies can be performed easily to confirm the genetic control mechanisms of the characteristic under study. The mapping of the mouse and rat genome should also be helpful for a further localization of the genes involved in the synthesis of IgE antibodies, especially those developing after antigen inhalation.

AIRWAY RESPONSIVENESS

Airway hyperresponsiveness (AHR) to a variety of stimuli is an important physiopathologic characteristic of asthma. It now is thought that this AHR in asthma is largely acquired through the development of chronic airway inflammation after sensitization of the individual. The role of increased baseline airway responsiveness in the pathogenesis of human asthma never has been clearly shown. There are many indications that humans differ with regard to baseline airway responsiveness to different stimuli. However, the difference in airway responsiveness among healthy individuals is usually much less than between healthy individuals and asthmatics, suggesting that most of the latter difference is indeed acquired over time. Family studies have suggested that, the baseline airway responsiveness is genetically controlled and that an increased baseline airway responsiveness is a risk factor for the development of asthma (3).

Most of the animal studies on genetic factors controlling airway responsiveness have focused on baseline airway responsiveness to a number of stimuli. Initial studies on the genetic control of baseline airway responsiveness were carried out in the rat (4,5). These were later complemented by studies in mice (6,7).

Many of the experiments that we performed in the rat were set up to understand better the mechanisms involved in the acute airway narrowing. During these experiments it became clear that inbred rat strains differ significantly with regard to their baseline airway responsiveness to a number of bronchoconstrictor stimuli. 5-Hydroxytryptamine (5-HT) is the major bronchoconstrictor mediator released from activated rat mast cells. There are significant differences between different inbred rat strains with regard to the airway responsiveness to 5-HT (4). By crossing a low-responder strain with a high-responder strain and back-crossing the F1 hybrids with the parental strains, a recessive Medalian mode of inheritance was found for high responsiveness to 5-HT.

Carbachol, a muscarinic agonist, also causes bronchoconstriction in the rat by a direct action on airway smooth muscle. Inbred rat strains differ significantly in their airway responsiveness to carbachol, but no relationship exists between airway responsiveness to 5-HT and to carbachol in the rat strains that we studied (8).

Most of the natural stimuli that cause airway narrowing in asthma do not act directly on airway smooth muscle but cause airflow limitation by indirect mechanisms such as the activation of inflammatory cells and the activation of local or central nervous reflexes (9). Examples of such indirect stimuli are adenosine and the tachykinins. In studying the acute effect of adenosine on the airway resistance in rats, significant differences in airway responsiveness were observed between various inbred rat strains (10). The BDE and the Brown Norway (BN) strain are high responders to adenosine whereas the F344 strain is a low responder to this agonist. In further studies, we explored the possibility that the differences in adenosine responsiveness between these three inbred rat strains were related to strain-related different mechanisms of adenosine-induced bronchoconstriction. In all three strains, methysergide (a 5-HT antagonist) inhibited the adenosine-induced bronchoconstriction, suggesting that mast cell activation and 5-HT release were responsible for part of the adenosine-induced bronchoconstriction (5). Similarly, atropine inhibited in all three strains the adenosine-induced bronchoconstriction. Further experiments proved that adenosine activates postganglionic nerve endings.

A comparison of the dose-response curve to N^6-2-(4-aminophenyl) ethyladenosine (APNEA), the adenosine analog that is supposed to act on the A3 receptor located on mast cells in the BDE and F344 strains, showed that the BDE strain is much more responsive to APNEA (11). These data on the difference in APNEA responsiveness between the two inbred rat strains BDE and F344 suggest that the greater responsiveness to adenosine and analogs observed in the BDE strain is due to the presence of a higher number of A3 receptors on the airway mast cells of the BDE strain compared with the F344 strain. A difference in coupling of the A3 receptor to the intracellular mechanisms involved in mast cell activation cannot be excluded.

The picture is still more complex for the airway response to the tachykinin neurokinin A (NKA). Inbred rat strains demonstrate significant differences in airway responsiveness to tachykinins such as substance P (SP) and neurokinin A (5,12,13). F344 rats are high responders to SP and NKA and BDE rats are low responders to these neuropeptides. No relationship was observed between the airway responsiveness to adenosine and to tachykinins in the different inbred rat strains that we tested. This observation suggests that the mechanisms of the indirect bronchoconstriction caused by adenosine and tachykinins differ at least at some points. The effect of NKA in F344 rats is comparable with the adenosine-induced bronchoconstriction involving simultaneous activation of mast cells and postganglionic nerve endings. The NKA-induced bronchoconstriction in BDE rats, however, is not influenced by either methysergide or atropine, suggesting that NKA acts directly on the airway smooth muscle in this strain. The bronchoconstriction induced by NKA in BN rats is partly inhibited by atropine and methysergide. Further evidence of mechanistic differences in NKA-induced bronchoconstriction between different inbred rat strains was obtained by comparing the effect of selective tachykinin receptor agonists and antagonists in F344 and BDE rats (12).

In F344 rats, SP and NKA caused a dose-dependent bronchoconstriction and a dose-dependent increase in 5-HT in bronchoalveolar lavage (BAL) fluid. The effects of SP and NKA were comparable. The specific NK_1 agonists $[Sar^9,Met(O_2)^{11}]SP$ and $Ac[Arg^6,Sar^9,Met(O_2)^{11}]SP$ (6–11) caused a dose-dependent bronchoconstriction and increase in BAL serotonin, which mimicked the effects of SP and NKA and occurred at similar molar concentrations. The NK_2 agonist $[\beta ala^8]NKA$ (4–10) caused a small increase in lung resistance but had no effect on BAL serotonin.

In BDE rats SP and NKA also caused a dose-dependent bronchoconstriction. However, in this rat strain, the effect of NKA was more pronounced than the effect of SP. Neither SP nor NKA caused an increase in BAL 5-HT. The NK_1 agonists $[Sar^9,Met(O_2)^{11}]SP$ and $Ac[Arg^6,Sar^9,Met(O_2)^{11}]SP$ (6–11) had no effect on R_L, whereas the NK_2 agonist $[\beta ala^8]NKA$ (4–10) caused a modest increase in R_L. None of the specific tachykinin receptor agonists caused an increase in BAL 5-HT.

In F344 rats, the nonpeptide NK_1 receptor antagonists, CP-96,345, 5 mg/kg BW ip, and RP 67580, 1.0 mg/kg BW i.v., significantly reduced the NKA-induced increase in R_L and BAL 5-HT. The nonpeptide NK_2 receptor antagonist SR 48968, 1 mg/kg BW i.v., had a nonsignificant effect on the increase in R_L induced by NKA and no effect on BAL 5-HT. After pretreatment with a combination of RP 67580, 1 mg/kg BW i.v., and SR 48968, 1 mg/kg BW i.v., the bronchoconstrictor effect of NKA and its effect on BAL 5-HT were abolished.

The increase in lung resistance caused by NKA in BDE rats was not affected by pretreatment with the NK_1 receptor antagonist RP 67580, 1 mg/kg BW, but was largely reduced by pretreatment with the NK_2 receptor antagonist, SR 48968, 1 mg/kg BW i.v. These experiments therefore showed that different mechanisms are involved in the bronchoconstriction induced by the intravenous administration of the tachykinins in the F344 and BDE rat strain. In the F344 rat, NKA and SP cause bronchoconstriction mainly by indirect mechanisms, involving mast cells and cholinergic nerves, an effect that de-

pends on the activation of NK_1 receptors. In the BDE rat, and to some extent also in the F344 rat, a direct bronchoconstrictor effect was observed, occurring at higher concentrations of the tachykinins and mediated by interaction with NK_2 receptors.

Levitt and Mitzner (6) reported that the AHR to acetylcholine (Ach) is inherited as an autosomal recessive trait in A/J and C3H/HeJ mice and the progeny of crosses between them. The same investigators extended their findings by studying the airway responsiveness to 5-HT in inbred strains of mice (7). The pattern of airway responsiveness to 5-HT differed significantly from that of the airway responsiveness to Ach in nine inbred mouse strains. Crosses between A/J and C3H/HeJ mice and the study of the 5-HT airway responsiveness in these crosses were consistent with the hypothesis that the airway responsiveness to 5-HT in these strains is primarily determined by an autosomal recessive gene. Linkage studies suggested that the airway responsiveness to 5-HT and to ACh are inherited independently. The mouse studies undoubtedly allow much more detailed analysis of the genetic mechanisms involved in baseline airway responsiveness, but they essentially confirm the findings in rats, namely that the baseline airway responsiveness to various agonists are controlled by genes that seem not to be linked to each other.

Levitt and Ewart (14) also studied the airway responsiveness in the mouse to the neuromuscular blocking agent atracurium. The airway response to atracurium in the mouse is inhibited by pretreatment with atropine or pancuronium. As for ACh and 5-HT, large differences in airway responsiveness to atracurium were observed in the nine inbred mouse strains studied. Although the investigators did not report on cross-breeding studies, they observed a remarkably similar strain distribution pattern for the airway response to atracurium and 5-HT in the nine strains and suggested that the same gene might influence the bronchoconstriction to both agents. Quantitative trait loci-mapping studies found only one site of linkage with atracurium hyperresponsiveness on the three mouse chromosome regions that are homologous to human chromosome 5q31-q33 region, where a major gene regulating bronchial hyperresponsiveness in humans is believed to be located (15).

AIRWAY INFLAMMATION

Plasma Protein Extravasation

Plasma protein extravasation is an important part of the acute inflammatory response. The role of plasma protein extravasation in asthma still is incompletely understood, but this mechanism possibly contributes to the acute and chronic airflow limitation in this disease. We compared the plasma protein extravasation in F344 and BDE rats challenged by the intravenous administration of SP or the tachykinin-releasing substance capsaicin (16). In both strains SP and capsaicin caused a dose-dependent plasma protein extravasation in trachea and main bronchi. In F344 rats, the maximal SP-induced plasma protein extravasation was higher than in the BDE rats. In both strains, a similar maximal capsaicin-induced plasma protein extravasation was observed, but with a shift of the dose-response curve to the left in the F344 rats. The NK$_1$ antagonist, RP67580, but not the NK$_2$ antagonist, SR48968, significantly inhibited the SP- and the capsaicin-induced plasma protein extravasation in both strains. Methysergide inhibited both the SP- and capsaicin-induced plasma protein extravasation in the F344 rats but not in the BDE rats, although 5-HT provoked a dose-dependent plasma protein extravasation in both strains. These two strains therefore also differ in the mechanisms involved in the plasma protein extravasation induced by SP or capsaicin. In both the F344 and BDE strains, the plasma protein extravasation caused by SP and capsaicin is caused by activation of the NK$_1$ receptor. However, in the F344—but not in the BDE strain—the plasma protein extravasation is at least partly mediated by mast cell activation and the release of 5-HT from these cells.

Inflammatory Cell Activation

Inbred rat strains differ significantly with regard to the capacity of their peritoneal and pleural mast cells to become sensitized with IgE and to release histamine after cross-linking of the surface-bound IgE (17). Both the sensitization and the activation of mast cells via IgE may therefore be controlled by genetic influences.

As discussed in the paragraphs on airway responsiveness, it is now generally accepted that the major part of the AHR in asthma is due to airway inflammation and the inflammation-induced airway remodeling. This is fundamentally different from the baseline airway responsiveness that has been studied in inbred and crossbred rat and mouse strains. The relationship has been investigated between airway inflammation and hyperresponsiveness in the rat model. Airway inflammation was induced by exposing the animals to an aerosol of endotoxin (18). Exposure to endotoxin induces rapidly a neutrophilic airway inflammation that persists for at least 24 hours. The exposure to endotoxin is also followed, 1 to 2 hours later, by an increase in airway responsiveness to a variety of stimuli such as 5-HT, carbachol, adenosine, NKA, and electrical field stimulation. The increase in airway responsiveness persists for a few hours and is followed by hyporesponsiveness, 9 to 12 hours after exposure. Later on, the airway responsiveness again normalizes. The increased airway responsiveness is at least partly due to the release of tu-

mor necrosis factor-α (TNF-α) in the airways, whereas the temporary decrease in airway responsiveness is caused by the production of nitric oxide (19,20). The effect of endotoxin inhalation was examined in five inbred rat strains. The aerosol exposure induced in all five strains a comparable neutrophil influx in the airways, but only four of the five strains became hyperresponsive to 5-HT, 90 minutes after the end of the endotoxin exposure. The inbred strains RA, F344, OM/N, and Wistar became hyperresponsive, whereas the airway responsiveness did not change in the BN strain. No studies have been done in the mouse looking at genetic factors that influence airway inflammation and its relationship with airway responsiveness.

Winthereik et al. (21,22) have selectively bred guinea pigs for their high or low anaphylactic responsiveness after sensitization with ovalbumin. They could demonstrate that this anaphylactic responsiveness is inherited independently of the tendency to develop blood or tissue eosinophilia, spontaneously or upon immunization. The development of eosinophilia either spontaneously or after immunization in these selectively bred guinea pig strains appears to be controlled by a few genes. However, spontaneous and antigen-induced eosinophilia probably are controlled by different genes.

CONCLUSIONS

Asthma is a clinical syndrome that results from a response of the airways to exogenous stimuli and the complex interaction between a number of cells in the airways. Family studies and linkage studies have clearly demonstrated that genetic factors are involved in this disease. Studies in animals and especially in the mouse and rat have indicated that genetic factors control the airway reaction to exogenous stimuli at many different levels (Table 1). The studies in inbred mice and rats suggest genetic control at the level of antigen recognition, synthesis of IgE, binding of IgE to mast cells, activation of mast cells, interaction between airway inflammation and airway re-

TABLE 1. *Potential genetically controlled mechanisms involved in asthma, according to animal models*

Antigen responsiveness
IgE synthesis
Mast cell sensitization
Eosinophil accumulation
Airway responsiveness to various agonists
Interaction between inflammation and airway responsiveness
Plasma protein extravasation

sponsiveness, airway responsiveness to direct and indirect stimuli, and airway plasma protein extravasation. It is therefore likely that the genetic control mechanisms in human asthma will be very complex and that multiple genes will be involved in the development of the clinical syndrome. Studies on the genetic factors involved in animal models of asthma may help to identify possible genetic control mechanisms and help to focus studies in humans. It is not yet clear if studies on genetic linkage and the identification of genes involved in animal models can help identify the genes and molecular mechanisms involved in human asthma, but it is certainly an interesting approach.

REFERENCES

1. Bazin H, Pauwels RA. IgE and IgG2a isotypes in the rat. *Prog Allergy* 1982;32:52–104.
2. Lundberg L. Guinea pigs inbred for studies of respiratory anaphylaxis. *Acta Pathol Microbiol Scand* 1979;87:55–66.
3. Townley RG, Bewtra A, Wilson AF, et al. Segregation analysis of bronchial response to methacholine inhalation challenge in families with and without asthma. *J Allergy Clin Immunol* 1986;77:101–107.
4. Pauwels RA, Van Der Straeten M, Weyne J, Bazin H. Genetic factors in non-specific bronchial reactivity in rats. *Eur J Respir Dis* 1985;66:98–104.
5. Pauwels RA, Germonpré PR, Kips JC, Joos GF. Genetic control of indirect airway responsiveness in the rat. *Clin Exp Allergy* 1995;25(suppl 2):55–60.
6. Levitt RC, Mitzner W. Expression of airway hyperreactivity to acetylcholine as a simple autosomal recessive trait in mice. *FASEB J* 1988;2:2605–2608.
7. Levitt RC, Mitzner W. Autosomal recessive inheritance of airway hyperreactivity to 5-hydroxytryptamine. *J Appl Physiol* 1989;67:1125–1132.
8. Pauwels RA, Van Der Straeten M, Weyne J, Bazin H. An animal model for the study of the relation between non-specific bronchial reactivity and immunological hypersensitivity. *Agents Actions Suppl* 1983;13:55–63.
9. Pauwels RA, Joos GF, Van Der Straeten M. Bronchial hyperresponsiveness is not bronchial hyperresponsiveness is not bronchial asthma. *Clin Allergy* 1988;18:317–321.
10. Pauwels RA, Van Der Straeten M. An animal model for adenosine-induced bronchoconstriction. *Am Rev Respir Dis* 1987;136:374–378.
11. Pauwels RA, Joos GF. Characterization of the adenosine receptors in the airways. *Arch Int Pharmacodyn Ther* 1995;329:151–160.
12. Joos GF, Kips JC, Pauwels RA. *In vivo* characterization of the tachykinin receptors involved in the direct and indirect bronchoconstrictor effect of tachykinins in two inbred rat strains. *Am J Respir Crit Care Med* 1994; 149:1160–1166.
13. Joos GF, Pauwels RA. The *in vivo* effect of tachykinins on airway mast cells of the rat. *Am Rev Respir Dis* 1993;148:922–926.
14. Levitt RC, Ewart SL. Genetic susceptibility to atracurium-induced bronchoconstriction. *Am J Respir Crit Care Med* 1995;151:1537–1542.
15. Levitt RC, Eleff SM, Zhang L-Y, Kleeberger SR, Ewart SL. Linkage homology for bronchial hyperresponsiveness between DNA markers on human chromosome 5q31-q33 and mouse chromosome 13. *Clin Exp Allergy* 1995;25(suppl 2):61–63.
16. Germonpré PR, Joos GF, Everaert E, Kips JC, Pauwels RA. Characterization of neurogenic inflammation in the airways of two highly inbred rat strains. *Am J Respir Crit Care Med* 1995;152:1796–1804.
17. Bergstrand H, Pauwels RA, Bazin H. Is there a functional heterogeneity among IgE type mast cell-sensitizing antibodies? *Allergy* 1986;41:11–25.
18. Pauwels RA, Kips JC, Peleman RA, Van Der Straeten M. The effect of endotoxin inhalation on airway responsiveness and cellular influx in rats. *Am Rev Respir Dis* 1990;141:540–545.
19. Kips JC, Tavernier J, Pauwels RA. Tumor necrosis factor causes bronchial hyperresponsiveness in rats. *Am Rev Respir Dis* 1992;145:332–336.
20. Kips JC, Lefebvre RA, Peleman RA, Joos GF, Pauwels RA. The effect of a nitric oxide synthase inhibitor on the modulation of airway responsiveness in rats. *Am J Respir Crit Care Med* 1995;151:1165–1169.
21. Winthereik MP, Sparck JV, Lundberg L, Sompolinsky D. Genetic control of eosinophilia in guinea pig strains inbred for high or low bronchial allergic reactivity. 2. A genetic study of spontaneous and immunization-induced eosinophilia. *Allergy* 1992;47:164–167.
22. Winthereik MP, Lundberg L, Sparck JV, Katzenstein T, Sompolinsky D. Genetic control of eosinophilia in guinea pig strains inbred for high or low bronchial allergic reactivity. *Allergy* 1992;47:103–109.

Asthma, edited by P.J. Barnes, M.M. Grunstein, A.R. Leff, and A.J. Woolcock.
Lippincott–Raven Publishers, Philadelphia © 1997.

▪ 23 ▪

Receptor Mechanisms

Peter J. Barnes and Michael M. Grunstein

Nearly all hormones, neurotransmitters, mediators, and growth factors produce their effects by interacting in target cells with specific protein recognition sites or receptors. Because receptors are specific, they allow a cell to recognize only selected signals from the myriad of chemicals that come into contact with the cell (1). Receptors play an important role in asthma because their function may be altered, resulting in altered cellular responsiveness. Many drugs used in the treatment of airway diseases act by stimulating (agonists) or blocking (antagonists) specific receptors (2).

There have been major advances in elucidating the function, regulation, and structure of receptors. This has been made possible by the development of radioligand

binding, in which highly potent radiolabeled agonists or antagonists are used to characterize and quantify receptors. More recently, many different receptors have been cloned, which has made it possible for the first time to deduce their amino acid structure and to determine the critical parts of the receptor protein involved in ligand binding and interaction with second messenger systems (3). Receptor cloning and production of pure receptor proteins has also made it possible to produce specific antibodies for use in immunocytochemical studies (4). Furthermore, molecular biology has made it possible to study the regulation of receptor genes (5).

RECEPTOR TYPES

Most receptors are proteins located within the cell membrane that interact with specific ligands outside the cell, leading to a conformational change that results either in activation or inhibition of a second messenger system and, subsequently, to the typical cell response. Cell surface receptors include:

P. J. Barnes: Department of Thoracic Medicine, Imperial College of Medicine at The National Heart and Lung Institute, London SW3 6LY United Kingdom.

M. M. Grunstein: Division of Pulmonary Medicine, The Children's Hospital of Philadelphia, University of Pennsylvania School of Medicine, Philadelphia, Pennsylvania 19104.

1. guanine-nucleotide binding protein (G protein)–coupled receptors (e.g., β-adrenoceptors)
2. ion channel–linked receptors (e.g., nicotinic receptors)
3. enzyme-linked receptors (e.g., platelet-derived growth factor receptors)
4. cytokine receptors (e.g., interleukin-5 receptors)

Some receptors, such as steroid and thyroid receptors, are intracellular and the ligand diffuses into the cell to bind to a cytosolic receptor, which then interacts with DNA in the cell nucleus. Molecular cloning techniques have made it possible to recognize several families of receptors that share common structures and to trace the evolutionary lineage of receptors within receptor families.

G PROTEIN–COUPLED RECEPTORS

Many different receptors interact with G proteins that act as a coupling mechanism linking receptor activation to second messenger systems. All these receptors appear to have structural similarities and are members of a large supergene family (6). More than 150 G protein–coupled receptors have now been cloned and their amino acid sequences determined (7). Each receptor is a single polypeptide chain, ranging in size from ≈400 to >1,000 amino acids.

Rhodopsin as a Model Receptor

The first and most carefully characterized receptor in this category was rhodopsin in light-sensitive rods of the retina, which is linked to a unique G protein called transducin; this has served as a useful structural model for other receptors in this group that were later cloned (8). Analysis of the amino acid sequence of rhodopsin revealed seven hydrophobic (lipophilic) stretches of 20 to 25 amino acids that are linked to hydrophilic regions of variable length. The most likely spatial arrangement of the receptor in the cell surface membrane is for the seven hydrophobic sections (each of which is in the form of an α-helix) to span the cell membrane. The intervening hydrophilic sections are exposed alternately intracellularly and extracellularly with the amino (N)-terminal exposed to the outside and the carboxy (C)-terminal within the cytoplasm (Fig. 1). The extracellular regions of rhodopsin recognize the specific ligand (retinal) and the intracellular regions interact with transducin. All other G protein–coupled receptors probably share this serpentine motif.

G Protein–Coupled Receptors Relevant to Asthma

G protein–coupled receptors relevant to airway diseases that have now been cloned and sequenced include neurotransmitter receptors such as β-adrenergic receptors ($\beta_1, \beta_2, \beta_3$), three α_1 and three α_2-adrenoceptors, m_1–m_5 muscarinic receptors, adenosine receptors (A_1, A_2, A_3), tachykinin receptors (NK_1, NK_2, NK_3), and VIP receptors ($VIP_1, VIP_2,$ PACAP). Inflammatory mediator receptors, such as platelet-activating factor (PAF), histamine (H_1, H_2), thromboxane (TP), and bradykinin B_2 receptors, which are also linked to G proteins, have also been cloned.

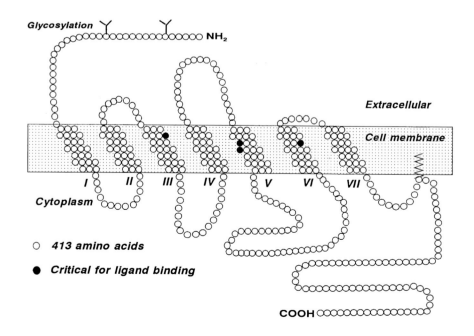

FIG. 1. Structure of the human β2-adrenergic receptor, a typical member of the G protein–coupled receptor superfamily. Each *circle* represents an amino acid; *filled circles* are amino acids critical for β-agonist binding.

Structure

All G protein–coupled receptors share the common feature of seven similar hydrophobic membrane-spanning segments. There is also some sequence homology of the intracellular loops (which interact with various species of G protein), but less similarity in the extracellular domains. For example, there is a 50% homology between rat β_2-adrenergic and muscarinic M_2-receptors (9). There is also close homology between the same receptor in different species. Thus there is 95% homology between rat and pig heart M_2-receptors (9). These similarities demonstrate that G receptor–linked receptors form part of a supergene family that may have a common evolutionary origin (10).

Members of the G protein receptor supergene family are generally 400 to 500 amino acids in length and the receptor cDNA sequence consists of 2,000 to 4,000 nucleotide bases (2–4 kb). The molecular weight of the cloned receptors predicted from the cDNA sequence is 40 to 60 kDa, which is usually less than the molecular mass of the native receptor when assessed by sodium dodecyl sulfate–polyacrylamide gel electrophoresis (SDS-PAGE). This discrepancy is due to glycosylation of the native receptor. For example, β_2-receptors contain two sites for glycosylation on asparagine (Asn/N) residues near the amino terminus, and it is estimated that N-glycosylation accounts for 25% to 30% of the molecular mass of the native receptor. The functional significance of glycosylation is not clear (11); it does not affect receptor affinity for ligand or coupling to G proteins but may be important for the trafficking of the receptor through the cell during downregulation, or for keeping the receptor correctly oriented in the lipid bilayer.

Another feature of these receptors is palmitoylation, when cysteine residues covalently bind palmitic acid via a thioester bond, thus anchoring the receptor chain to the cell membrane. This confers three-dimensional stability on the receptor; disruption of this bond in β-receptors (by mutation of Cys341) alters both binding characteristics and coupling to G proteins and may affect desensitization of the receptor (12).

Deletion mutagenesis and site-directed mutagenesis (substitution of single amino acids in the polypeptide chain) have established that the ligand binding domain is well conserved between members of the same family. In the case of β-adrenoceptors, there is good evidence for a ligand-binding cleft between the transmembrane spanning domains within the cell membrane (3,7). Critical amino acids for the interaction of endogenous adrenergic agonists (norepinephrine and epinephrine) are asparagine in the third transmembrane loop (TM3) (Asp113) and serines in the TM5 (Ser204, Ser207), which interact with the hydroxy groups on the catechol ring (Fig. 2).

The binding site for antagonists differs from those of naturally occurring ligands, and for antagonist binding to β-receptors TM7 appears to be critical. Binding of substance P to the NK_1-receptor occurs at extracellular domains of the receptor, whereas antagonist binding of the nonpeptide NK_1-antagonist, CP96,345, binds to a transmembrane domain (His197) (13).

G PROTEINS

G proteins link activation of serpentine receptors to enzymes or ion channels that then mediate the characteristic response (14). All G proteins have guanosine triphosphatase (GTPase) activity and catalyze the conversion of GTP to guanosine diphosphate (GDP). More than 20 distinct G proteins have now been characterized and most

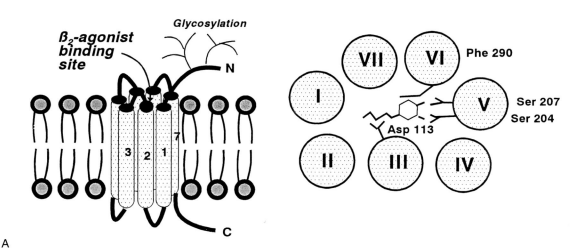

A   B

FIG. 2. Ligand-binding domain of the β_2-receptor, showing the clustering of the seven transmembrane domains to form a binding cleft (**A**) and the interaction between the catecholamine and critical amino acids in the transmembrane domains (**B**).

have been cloned (15,16). They are made up of three separate units; the α-subunit interacts with the receptor, binds GTP, and interacts with the enzyme such as adenylyl cyclase, whereas the β- and γ-subunits are very hydrophobic and are associated as a complex within the cytoplasmic surface of the cell membrane. The distinction between G proteins is largely contained within the α-subunits. These have been classified into four principle classes based on their amino acid sequences, including Gs, Gq, Gi, G_{12}, and each class contains various α-subunit members (Fig. 3). G proteins are freely diffusible within the cell membrane and the pool of G proteins may interact with several receptors. In the resting state, the G protein exists as an αβγ trimer with GDP occupying the binding site on the α-subunit. When a receptor is occupied by an agonist, a conformational change occurs and the intracellular loops of the receptor protein acquire a high affinity for αβγ, resulting in the dissociation of GDP and its replacement with GTP, which in turn causes α-GTP to dissociate from the subunits (Fig. 4). α-GTP is the active form of the G protein and diffuses to associate with effector molecules such as enzymes and ion channels. This process is terminated by hydrolysis of GTP to GDP via the intrinsic GTPase activity of the α-subunit. The resulting α-GDP dissociates from the effector molecule and reassociates with βγ, in readiness for reactivation of G protein signaling.

Several receptors, such as β-receptors and VIP receptors, stimulate adenylyl cyclase via the stimulatory G protein Gs, whereas activation of other receptors, such as muscarinic M_2-receptors, inhibits adenylyl cyclase via Gi (14). Gs may be stimulated directly by cholera toxin, whereas Gi is inhibited by pertussis toxin, so that these toxins may be useful in elucidating the involvement of a particular G protein in a particular receptor-mediated response. Other G proteins are now recognized that couple receptors that activate phosphoinosidide hydrolysis (G_0, G_q) and activate particular ion channels in the cell membrane (e.g., G_k, which is coupled to potassium channels) (17). G proteins may thus play a diverse and important role in the regulation of cell responsiveness, and there is evidence that receptors may become uncoupled from G proteins under certain conditions. For example, in fatal asthma there is evidence for a reduced responsiveness of airway smooth muscle to β-agonists (18–20), yet the number and affinity of β-receptors on airway smooth muscle is not reduced (21,22) and the response to other smooth muscle relaxants is not impaired, suggesting that the receptors have become uncoupled in severe asthma.

Although receptors affect the function of G proteins, G proteins also influence the interaction of ligands with the receptor. Thus, when coupled to an inactive G protein, the receptor exists in a state of high affinity for the agonist. Agonist binding releases G_α from contact with the recep-

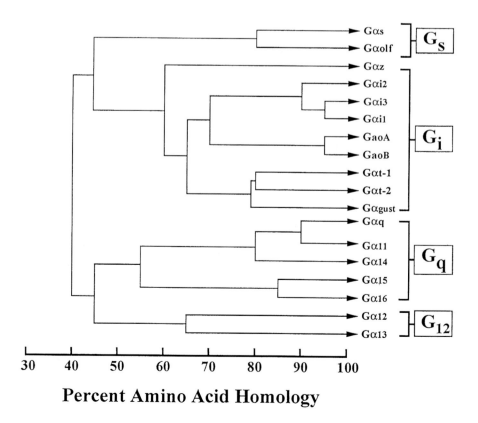

Percent Amino Acid Homology

FIG. 3. Classification of G protein α subunits and their structural homology. Members of four classes of G proteins are grouped according to their amino acid homology, with branch junctions corresponding with comparative percentage homology for the different α subunits.

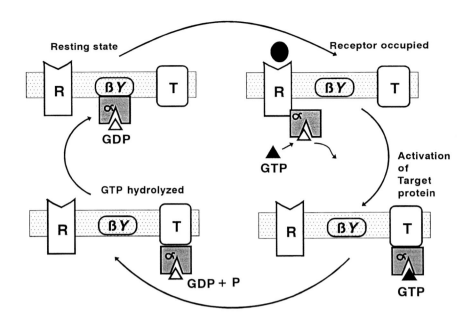

FIG. 4. G proteins. When a receptor (R) is occupied by an agonist, the α-subunit associates with the receptor, binding GTP and then activating a target protein (T) with hydrolysis of GTP to GDP. The $\beta\gamma$ units act as an anchoring mechanism for the shuttling of the α-subunit.

tor, resulting in a reduction in agonist affinity, referred to as the "guanine-nucleotide shift."

G PROTEIN–COUPLED EFFECTOR SYSTEMS

The ligand that activates a receptor is described as the first messenger and leads, via activation of a G protein, to the typical cellular response via a second messenger, such as a change in intracellular calcium ion (Ca^{2+}) concentration or cyclic adenosine monophosphate (cAMP) concentration. Although the number of surface receptors that may respond on any particular cell is large, only a limited number of signal transduction and second messenger systems have been described. These are discussed in detail in Chapter 25. Thus, the surface receptors determine cellular responsiveness and sensitivity, rather than the intracellular mechanisms that are activated by the receptor-ligand interaction. Considerable progress has been made in understanding the intracellular mechanisms involved in receptor-mediated effects, through the development of techniques such as intracellular dye indicators that reflect intracellular concentrations of ions (e.g., fura-2, which detects intracellular Ca^{2+} concentrations), by more sensitive biochemical assays, and by the development of patch clamping techniques (23).

Adenylyl Cyclase

Many receptors produce their effects by interaction with the membrane-bound enzyme adenylyl cyclase (AC) to increase or decrease production of cAMP (Fig. 5). At least eight distinct forms of AC have now been

differentiated and there is increasing evidence that these isoforms may be differentially regulated (24). Thus, PKC phosphorylates and activates certain isoforms (types 1,2,3), which may be a mechanism for receptor cross-talk, whereas it has no effect on other isoforms (4,5,6) (25). The formation of cAMP leads to the characteristic cellular response via the activation of a specific protein kinase, protein kinase A (PKA), by dissociating a regulatory (inhibitory) subunit. PKA then phosphorylates serine and threonine residues on specific proteins, such as regulatory proteins, ion channels, and enzymes within the cell, which leads to the characteristic response. For example, in airway smooth muscle cells PKA phosphorylates a certain potassium (K^+) channel that opens leading to K^+ efflux from the cell, hyperpolarization, and relaxation (26). PKA also phosphorylates and therefore inactivates myosin light chain kinase, resulting in a direct relaxant effect on the contractile machinery (27).

cAMP is hydrolyzed within cells by a family of enzymes termed phosphodiesterases (PDEs). At least seven PDE families have now been distinguished on the basis of substrate specificity and inhibition by selective inhibitors (28,29). In airway smooth muscle the PDE3 and PDE4 isoenzymes are involved in cAMP-mediated relaxation (30,31).

Phosphatidylinositol Hydrolysis

An alternative signaling system involves breakdown of a membrane phospholipid, phosphatidylinositol (PI), which results in increased intracellular Ca^{2+} concentration. Certain receptors are coupled via G_q or G_0 to the

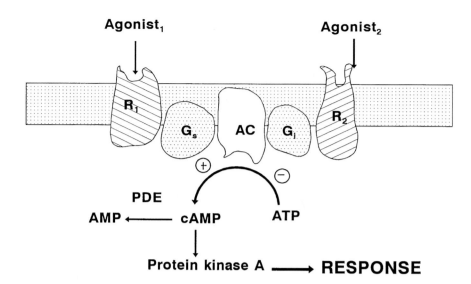

FIG. 5. AC may be activated by some receptors (R_1) via a stimulatory G protein (G_s) and inhibited by others (R_2) via an inhibitory G protein (G_i). The balance between these effects determines the level of AC activity and the intracellular concentration of cAMP.

membrane-associated enzyme phosphoinositidase or phospholipase C (PLC), which converts phosphoinositide (4,5)bisphosphate to inositol (1,4,5)trisphosphate (IP₃) and 1,2 sn-diacylglycerol (DAG) (Fig. 6). Three main groups of PLC have now been identified (PLC-β, PLC-γ, PLC-δ), each of which has subclasses (PLC-β1, PLC-β2, PLC-β3, etc.) based on amino acid structure of different cloned genes (32). These isoenzymes are differentially coupled to different receptors and are subject to differential regulation.

IP₃ binds to a specific receptor on endoplasmic/sarcoplasmic reticulum that leads to the release of Ca²⁺ from intracellular stores. Thus, PI hydrolysis links occupation of a surface receptor to intracellular Ca²⁺ release (33). Most of the mediators that contract airway smooth muscle act on receptors that activate PI hydrolysis in airway smooth muscle (34,35). IP₃ is broken down into the inactive IP₂ by an IP₃ phosphatase and subsequently to inositol, which is reincorporated into phophoinositides in the cell membrane. IP₃ may also be

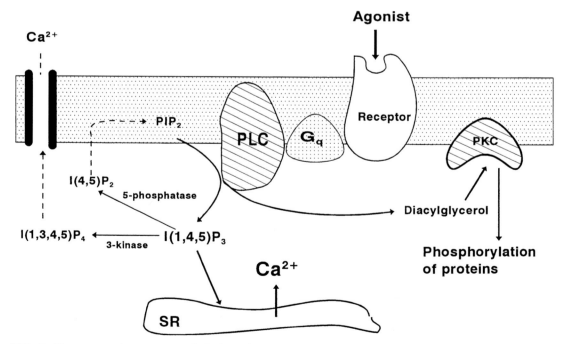

FIG. 6. Some receptors are coupled via a G protein (G_q) to phospholipase C (*PLC*), which converts membrane-bound phosphoinositide biphosphate (*PIP*) to inositol 1,4,5 triphosphate [*I(1,4,5)P₃*] and diacylglycerol. The former releases calcium ions (*Ca²⁺*) from internal stores, such as sarcoplasmic reticulum (*SR*) and the latter activates protein kinase C (*PKC*).

phosphorylated by IP₃ kinase to IP₄, which may be involved in opening receptor-operated calcium channels and the refilling of intracellular stores (33).

Using the fluorescence indicator dye fura-2, it has been possible to monitor changes in intracellular (Ca²⁺) in response to receptor-mediated activation. In addition, IP₃ has been introduced into cells in a "caged," inactive form that may then be activated by a flash of light to allow the kinetics of activation to be investigated. The use of these techniques in single cells has demonstrated that calcium release in response to agonists or IP₃ occurs in a series of oscillations, which is probably mediated via calcium-induced calcium release and the opening of calcium channels on the cell membrane (23,33). The frequency of oscillation may be important in the type of cell activation that ensues.

The formation of diacylglycerol (DAG) may activate the enzyme protein kinase C (PKC) by causing it to translocate to the cell membrane and by dramatically increasing its sensitivity to Ca²⁺. Activated PKC is then capable of phosphorylating various cell membrane–associated proteins, including some receptors, G proteins, and regulatory proteins. Several distinct isoenzymes of PKC are now recognized (36), although the role of individual isoenzymes in regulating cell function is not clear. One isoenzyme may be activated by arachidonic acid, a product of phospholipase A₂ hydrolysis. DAG is also formed by the activation of phospholipase D on phosphatidic acid, representing yet another level of complexity (37). PKC may be activated directly by tumor-promoting phorbol esters, such as phorbol myristate acetate (PMA), which have therefore been useful in examining the role of PKC. In some species PMA and other phorbol esters cause prolonged contractile responses in airway smooth muscle, but in other species bronchodilatation is observed. It has been suggested that PKC may be important for the prolonged contractile responses seen in asthmatic airways. PKC inhibitors, such as staurosporine (which is not selective) and Ro 31-8220, have been developed that are proving to be useful in elucidating the role of PKC. PKC is involved in activation of inflammatory cells and in particular the release of oxygen-derived free radicals from these cells.

Guanylyl Cyclase

It was previously believed that, whereas relaxation of smooth muscle is brought about by receptors that activate cAMP, contraction is due to the production of another cyclic nucleotide, cyclic 3',5'guanosine monophosphate (cGMP), formed by the activation of guanylyl cyclase. This is now known to be incorrect and the increase in cGMP is secondary to a rise in intracellular Ca²⁺ concentration. Indeed, cGMP causes relaxation of smooth muscle and is the major mechanism of vasodilatation in re-

sponse to nitrovasodilators (such as sodium nitroprusside) and dilators (such as acetylcholine) that release NO from endothelial cells (38). cGMP is also involved in the relaxant response of airway smooth muscle to nitrovasodilators (39) and to atrial natriuretic peptide, which is a potent bronchodilator in vitro (40,41). cGMP is broken down by PDEs, and in particular the type 5 isoenzyme (29).

Ion Channel–Coupled Signaling

G proteins may also couple receptors to ion channels. Thus, certain muscarinic receptors are coupled via G proteins (G₀) to K⁺ channels and Ca²⁺ channels. In airway smooth muscle β₂-receptors are directly coupled via Gs to the opening of a large conductance K+ (maxi-K) channel, and the same channel is inhibited by muscarinic M₂-receptors via Gᵢ (42,43).

CYTOKINE RECEPTORS

The effects of cytokines are mediated via specific surface receptors, several of which have now been cloned (44). Many of the cloned cytokine receptors have a primary structure that is quite different from the seven transmembrane spanning segments associated with G protein–linked receptors (Fig. 7). Thus, the receptor for TNF-α is a 55-kDa peptide that has a single transmembrane spanning helical segment, an extracellular domain that binds TNF-α, and an intracellular domain (45). The intracellular domain leads to activation of several kinases and ceramide, which subsequently lead to the activation of transcription factors, such as nuclear factor kappa B (NF-κB) and activator protein 1 (AP-1). The structure of the receptor is analogous to the nerve growth factor receptor. A second receptor for TNF has also been cloned, but differs markedly in sequence and may be linked to different intracellular pathways (45).

Molecular cloning has now revealed that although cytokines may be structurally diverse, their receptors may be grouped into various families that share structural homology. One family of receptors includes the receptors for interleukin-1 (IL-1) and platelet-derived growth factor; these receptors belong to the immunoglobulin superfamily, which includes T-cell antigen receptors and certain cell-surface adhesion molecules (46). Another cytokine receptor superfamily, the hematopoietin receptor superfamily, includes receptors for IL-2, IL-3, IL-4, IL-5, IL-6, IL-7, interferons, and granulocyte macrophage colony-stimulating factor (GM-CSF) (47). Prolactin, growth factor, and erythropoietin receptors are also included in this family. The receptor proteins are oriented with an extracellular N-terminal domain and a single hydrophobic transmembrane spanning segment.

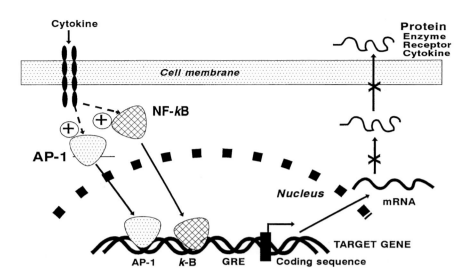

FIG. 7. Cytokine receptors are linked to the activation of transcription factors, such as activator protein 1 (*AP-1*) and nuclear factor-kappa B (*NF–κB*), which regulate expression of various inflammatory genes.

There is striking homology in the extracellular ligand binding domain with four conserved cysteine residues. There is close homology between the receptors for IL-3, IL-5, and GM-CSF, all of which stimulate growth of eosinophils. Molecular cloning has demonstrated that each of these receptors consists of an α and β chain and share a common β-chain. This explains why they have overlapping biologic activities.

The chemokines, such as IL-8, RANTES, and eotaxin, bind to receptors that are linked to G proteins and their receptors have the typical seven transmembrane spanning motifs typical of such receptors (48). Many chemokines have overlapping activities and interact with common receptors on target leukocytes. Six chemokine receptors have now been characterized and they appear to be differentially expressed on different inflammatory cells, thus explaining the differential chemotactic effects of these cytokines (49). Thus, eosinophils express the CC CK$_3$ receptor activated by RANTES, MCP-3, MCP-4, and eotaxin, thus accounting for the selective chemotactic effects of these chemokines on eosinophil migration.

The second messenger systems activated by cytokines are highly complex (50), involving many interacting pathways that allow for the possibility of signal splitting, so that the same activating signal may result in the activation of several parallel pathways, and what signal pathway predominates is determined by other signals impinging on the cell. Most cytokines activate a group of transcription factors (see Chapter 26).

ENZYME-LINKED RECEPTORS

Some receptors contain an enzyme domain within their structure, so that when the enzyme is activated by a ligand the enzyme becomes activated, leading to signal transduction through the formation of a specific substrate within the cell. The best characterized of these enzyme-linked receptors are receptor tyrosine kinases (RTK) that have protein tyrosine kinase activity.

Receptor Tyrosine Kinases

Activation of RTKs results in phosphorylation of tyrosine residues on certain target proteins that are usually associated with cell growth and chronic activation of cells (51). More than 50 different RTKs belonging to at least 14 distinct families have now been identified (52). These receptors include the growth factor receptors epithelial growth factor and platelet-derived growth factor and insulin (Fig. 8).

All RTKs share a similar general structure, consisting of a large extracellular amino-terminal portion that contains the ligand recognition domain, a single short membrane-spanning region (α-helix), and a cytoplasmic carboxy-terminal portion (≈250 amino acids) that contains the tyrosine kinase activity and autophosphorylation sites. The extracellular domain usually contains cysteine-rich regions and/or immunoglobulin-like motifs, with a large number of disulfide bonds forming a highly specific tertiary structure that is needed to establish ligand binding specificity. All RTKs (with the exception of the insulin receptor family) undergo a transition from a monomeric to a dimeric state (either homodimers or heterodimers) after binding of their specific ligands.

Another characteristic of RTKs is that they undergo internalization into two types of intracellular vesicles: pitted vesicles coated with the protein clathrin and smooth vesicles lacking clathrin. There is a spontaneous internalization, but this is rapidly accelerated when the receptor is occupied by a ligand. A proportion of the receptors is degraded, whereas a proportion is recycled to the cell surface.

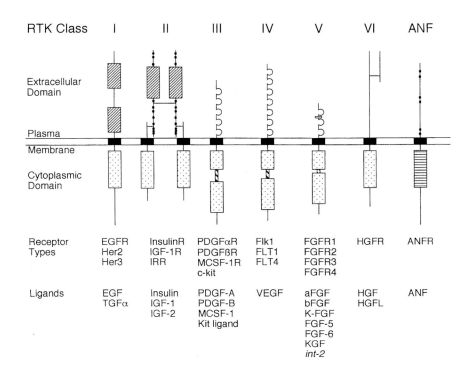

RTK Class	I	II	III	IV	V	VI	ANF
Receptor Types	EGFR Her2 Her3	InsulinR IGF-1R IRR	PDGFαR PDGFβR MCSF-1R c-kit	Flk1 FLT1 FLT4	FGFR1 FGFR2 FGFR3 FGFR4	HGFR	ANFR
Ligands	EGF TGFα	Insulin IGF-1 IGF-2	PDGF-A PDGF-B MCSF-1 Kit ligand	VEGF	aFGF bFGF K-FGF FGF-5 FGF-6 KGF int-2	HGF HGFL	ANF

FIG 8. Enzyme-linked receptors. Several classes of receptor tyrosine kinases (*RTK*) are now recognized with differing structures and signaling mechanisms. Receptors for atrial natriuretic factor (*ANF*) also belong to this receptor family.

Signal Transduction

RTKs phosphorylate intracellular molecules containing Src homology 2 and 3 (SH2 and SH3) domains. These SH2 and SH3 domains are short sequences of about 100 and 50 to 60 amino acids, respectively, that function to specify the interaction with a target protein (53). The SH2 motifs recognize phosphotyrosine residues and are responsible for interactions with autophosphorylated RTKs, the specificity of which depends on the amino acid sequences surrounding both the tyrosine autophosphorylation site on the RTK and the substrate's SH2 domain. RTK substrate proteins containing SH2 and SH3 motifs may contain enzymatic activity. The best characterized RTK enzyme substrates are cytoplasmic protein tyrosine kinases, such as Src, Syk, the p21^{ras}-GTPase-activating protein (GAP) and PLC-γ1. Alternatively, the substrate may function as adaptor proteins, composed almost entirely of SH2 and SH3 domains. Examples include Grb2 and the p85 subunit of phosphatidylinositol 3 kinase (PI3K).

Most RTKs stimulate the mitogen-activated kinase (MAPK) pathway through a complex multistep signaling cascade initiated by translocation of the adaptor protein Grb2 to the cytoplasmic membrane (53) (Fig. 9). This results in the activation of Ras proteins, which are small molecular weight GTPases that, in turn, activate Raf, which is a serine/threonine kinase that activates the MAPK pathway (54).

There is increasing evidence that RTKs may interact with several cell signaling pathways to elicit their effects, and it now seems likely that specific pathways are selected under certain conditions. For example, PDGF, which may exist in the dimeric forms AA, BB, or AB, may interact with different receptor dimers (αα,αβ,ββ), resulting in activation of different signal transduction pathways.

Receptor Serine/Threonine Kinases

Similar to RTKs, there are some receptors that are linked to serine/threonine kinase activity. The best known example is transforming growth factor-β (TGF-β), which exists in three mammalian isoforms encoded by separate genes, all of which may have complex and divergent effects on cell activity (55). Some of the effects of TGF-β are mediated via inhibition of cyclins, which regulate the cell cycle. This may account for the diverse effects of TGF-β, depending on the stage of the cycle.

Receptor Protein Tyrosine Phosphatases

Little is known about this third type of enzyme-linked receptors, which have a high level of intrinsic enzyme activity (56). Occupation by a ligand may turn this enzyme activity off, thus resulting in cell activation. These receptors appear to be important in cell differentiation and include CD45 (also known as leukocyte common antigen), which is involved in T-lymphocyte signaling.

ION CHANNEL RECEPTORS

Although several receptors are linked via G proteins to ion channels, such as Ca^{2+} and K^+ channels as discussed

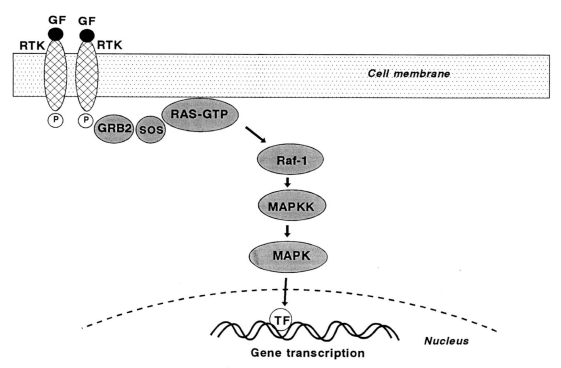

FIG. 9. Activation of receptor tyrosine kinase receptors (*RTK*) by growth factors (*GF*) results in a cascade of enzyme activation, leading to the activation of mitogen-activated protein kinases (*MAPK*) that activate transcription factors (*TF*) to regulate expression of genes involved in cell proliferation.

above, other receptors are ion channels themselves. The best characterized example is the nicotinic acetylcholine receptor, which is made up of four subunits that form a cation channel. When activated by acetylcholine, the channel opens to allow the passage of Na$^+$ ions (57). This type of receptor, which can respond rapidly because no intracellular mechanisms are involved, is known as a fast receptor and is usually involved in synaptic transmission. Nicotinic receptors are involved in ganglionic transmission in parasympathetic ganglia within the airways and are blocked by hexamethonium, which therefore blocks ganglionic transmission and cholinergic reflex bronchoconstriction. Ion channel receptors are oligomeric proteins containing about 20 transmembrane segments arranged around a central aqueous channel. Binding of the ligand and channel opening occurs very rapidly (within milliseconds). Other examples include glutamate and γ-amino acid receptors. This is in contrast to the slow receptors, such as G protein–coupled receptors, which involve a series of catalytic steps.

INTRACELLULAR RECEPTORS

Steroids interact with intracellular (cytosolic) receptors rather than surface receptors. There is a family of steroid receptors that recognize different endogenous steroids such as glucocorticoids, mineralocorticoids, an-

drogens, and estrogens. Indeed, steroid receptors belong to a supergene family that also includes thyroid hormone, retinoic acid (vitamin A), and vitamin D receptors (58). The exploration of cDNA libraries for related sequences has led to the discovery of more than 40 orphan receptors whose ligands have not been identified. Intracellular receptors share a common general structure. There is a central DNA-binding domain, characterized by the presence of two zinc fingers that are loops stabilized by four cysteine/histidine residues around a zinc ion. These zinc fingers anchor the receptor to the double helix at specific hormone response elements (HRE) in the promoter region of target genes. Ligands bind in the carboxy-terminal domain, which also contains sequences important for binding of associated chaperone proteins (e.g., heat shock proteins) and a nuclear localization signal involved in transporting the receptor from the cytoplasm into the nucleus. The amino-terminal domain is involved in transcriptional regulation (trans-activation) and in the interaction with other transcription factors (Fig. 10).

Steroid Receptors

Several steroid receptors have now been cloned and their structures have been shown to differ (59). However, there is some homology between these receptors because they all interact with nuclear DNA, where they act as

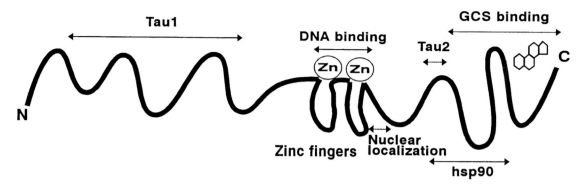

FIG. 10. Structural domains of a typical intracellular receptor, the glucocorticoid receptor. Glucocorticosteroids (*GCS*) bind to the C-terminal domain. Zinc fingers are coordinated by zinc ions (*Zn*) bound to cysteine residues.

modulators of the transcription of a specific gene (60). Only a limited number of genes appear to respond directly to steroids. Glucocorticoid receptors (GR) are normally present in the cytosol in an inactive form bound to two molecules of a 90-kDa heat shock protein (hsp90), which covers the DNA binding domain. Binding of a steroid to its receptor results in the dissociation of hsp90 and the occupied receptor then undergoes a conformational change that allows it to bind to DNA (61).

The DNA-binding domain of steroid receptors is rich in Cys residues. Formation of a complex with zinc can fold the peptide chain into a finger-shaped conformation and the zinc is coordinated by four Cys residues. GRs have two "zinc fingers" that are loops of approximately 15 residues, each of which is held in shape by four cysteine residues surrounding an atom of zinc (Fig. 10). Zinc fingers are essential for the interaction with the DNA

double helix. Steroid receptors recognize specific DNA sequences—the so-called glucocorticoid response elements (GREs) that have the consensus sequence GGTAnnnTGTTCT (62). Dimers of GR occupied by steroid bind to the GRE on the DNA double helix and either increase (+GRE) or much less commonly decrease (-GRE) the rate of transcription by influencing the promoter sequence in the target gene. Indeed, repression of target genes may be the most important aspect of steroid action in inflammatory diseases such as asthma because steroids may inhibit the transcription of many cytokines that are involved in the chronic inflammatory response. The major mechanism of gene repression is mediated via a direct interaction between the activated glucocorticoid receptor and transcription factors, such as NF-κB and AP-1 activated via inflammatory signals such as cytokines (63,64) (Fig. 11).

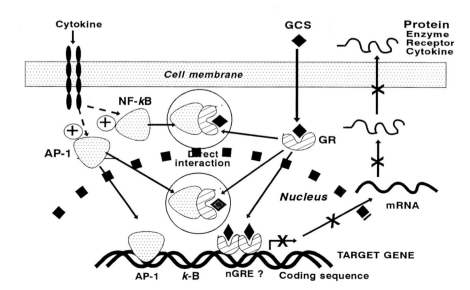

FIG. 11. Diagram of interaction between glucocorticoid receptors (*GR*) and the activated transcription factors activator protein 1 (*AP-1*) and nuclear factor-kappa B (*NF–κB*), thus blocking the chronic inflammatory response.

RECEPTOR SUBTYPES

The existence of receptor subtypes is often first indicated by differences in the potency of a series of agonists in different tissues. This could be due to differing proportions of co-existent receptor subtypes, or may indicate the existence of a novel receptor subtype. Molecular biology can resolve these possibilities because molecular techniques can clearly discriminate between different subtypes of receptor and show that they are encoded by different genes. Thus, the human β_1-receptor is clearly different from the β_2-receptor in its amino acid sequence, with a 54% homology (65), and the NK_1-receptor that is selectively activated by substance P has a 48% homology with the NK_2-receptor that is activated by the related tachykinin neurokinin A (66). A third tachykinin receptor, NK_3-receptor, which is selectively activated by neurokinin B, has also been cloned (67). Molecular biology techniques have thus confirmed the existence of receptor subtypes initially characterized by classic pharmacologic techniques, using the rank order of potency of different agonists and antagonists.

Using cross-hybridization, in which a known receptor cDNA sequence is hybridized with a genomic library, it has also been possible to detect previously unknown subtypes of a receptor. For example, an atypical β-receptor, which does not clearly fit into the β_1- or β_2-receptor subtypes, has been suspected in adipose tissue and some smooth muscle preparations. A distinct β_3 receptor has now been identified, cloned, sequenced, and expressed (68). The β_3-receptor is clearly different from either β_1- or β_2-receptors (about 50% amino acid sequence homology). β_3-Receptors appear to be important in the regulation of metabolic rate and have not been detected in lung homogenates (69). Without the techniques of molecular biology, this receptor would probably still remain undiscovered.

Molecular biology has been particularly useful in advancing our understanding of muscarinic receptors. Five distinct muscarinic receptors have been cloned from rat and human tissues (70,71). The m1-, m2-, and m3-receptors correspond to the M_1-, M_2-, and M_3-receptors identified pharmacologically, whereas m4- and m5-receptors are previously unrecognized pharmacologic subtypes that occur predominantly in the brain, and for which no selective drugs have been developed. Interestingly, m4-receptors have been demonstrated in rabbit lung using antibodies against the cloned m4-receptor (72), and their presence has been confirmed by cDNA probes for the m4-receptor (73). These m4-receptors are localized to vascular smooth muscle and alveolar walls, but have not been observed in lungs of other species, including humans (74). Other related, but as yet uncharacterized, genes could represent additional subtypes and up to nine subtypes have been predicted in rat (71). The reason for so many different subtypes of a receptor that recognize a single agonist is still not certain, but it seems likely that they are linked to different intracellular pathways and that the regulation of the intracellular portion of the amino acid sequence may be unique to each subtype. The m1-, m3-, and m5-receptors stimulate phosphoinositide (PI) hydrolysis through a pertussis toxin–insensitive G protein, whereas m2- and m4-receptors inhibit AC via G_i (75,76). It is possible that the difference in protein structure may reflect regulation at a transcriptional level from DNA through different promoters, leading to variations in tissue or developmental expression, or to differences at a post-translational level, allowing regulation by intracellular mechanisms such as phosphorylation at critical sites on intracellular loops.

RECEPTOR CROSS-TALK

Activation of one receptor may influence the function of a separate receptor via a number of interacting mechanisms. The opposing effects of receptors that increase and decrease AC activity via G_s and G_i, respectively, is well described. In airway smooth muscle where M_2-receptors inhibit AC, and β_2-receptors stimulate this enzyme, there are opposing effects (77). This may explain why it is more difficult for β-agonists to reverse contraction of airway smooth muscle induced by cholinergic agonists compared with histamine. Conversely, β-agonists may also influence the expression of M2-receptors (78). Several other interactions between receptors are recognized. Receptors that increase cAMP will oppose the effects of receptors that elevate intracellular Ca^{2+} via several mechanisms, including stimulation of Ca^{2+} sequestration and exchange (79).

PI hydrolysis leads to activation of PKC, which then phosphorylates receptors and G proteins, resulting in impaired receptor function (80) (Fig. 12). In airway smooth muscle this may be an important interaction in inflammation because inflammatory mediators will stimulate PI hydrolysis in airway smooth muscle cells and, via activation of PKC, will phosphorylate G proteins, leading to uncoupling of β_2-receptors. This may explain the reduced bronchodilator response to β-agonists *in vitro* observed in airways taken from patients with fatal asthma attacks.

An additional type of interaction may operate at the level of gene transcription. Cytokines may activate transcription factors that have an effect on a target gene and steroid receptors may interact with the same gene with an opposing effect. There may also be a direct interaction between transcription factors within the cytoplasm. For example, activated glucocorticoid receptors bind directly to the AP-1 complex, and thereby prevent its interaction with the target gene (81). In human lung, for example, cytokines such as TNF-α and phorbol esters that activate

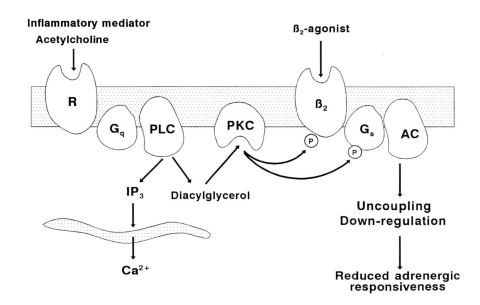

FIG. 12. Cross-talk between receptors may occur at several levels. Inflammatory mediator receptors may activate phospholipase C (*PLC*), which in turn activates protein kinase C (*PKC*). PKC may phosphorylate stimulatory G proteins (G_s) or β_2-receptors (β_2), resulting in uncoupling and downregulation, with desensitization of the response to β_2-agonists.

PKC lead to activation of AP-1 and NK-κB binding to DNA; this effect is blocked by glucocorticoids (64). Cyclic AMP may exert a profound modulatory effect on MAPK signaling pathways (82) and may activate the transcription factor CREB, which itself interacts with glucocorticoid receptors and with AP-1 (83,84).

DRUG-RECEPTOR INTERACTIONS

The binding of drug to its receptor is a dynamic process that follows the laws of mass action. At equilibrium there is a balance between the rate of association and the rate of dissociation of a drug. The concentration of drug giving half maximal activation is the EC_{50}, which describes the potency of the drug. The affinity of the drug describes the balance between association and dissociation and can be quantified as the dissociation constant K_d, which is the logarithm of the concentration of drug needed to occupy 50% of the receptors. Drugs with a low K_d therefore have a high affinity for their receptor.

Radioligand Binding

Binding between a hormone or drug and its receptor may be studied directly by radioligand binding. A radiolabeled ligand (usually a high affinity antagonist, such as [^{125}I] iodocyanopindolol for β-receptors) is incubated with a receptor preparation (either a membrane preparation from the tissue of interest or, in the case of some ligands, with intact cells). The binding interaction between ligand and receptor obeys the law of mass action. As the concentration of ligand is increased, the proportion of ligand binding to receptors increases until saturation occurs when all the receptors are occupied. Nonspecific binding to nonreceptor sites is determined by parallel incubations

with radioligand in the presence of an excess of unlabeled agonist or antagonist (e.g., 200 μM isoproterenol or 1 μM propranolol for β-receptors). Specific binding (i.e., total nonspecific binding) may be analyzed by a Scatchard plot, which will give a straight line if a single class of binding site is involved, the slope of which is related to binding affinity (1/K_d), and the intercept on the x-axis gives the maximum number of binding sites (B_{max}), a measure of receptor density (Fig. 13). Alternatively, a curvilinear Scatchard plot may signify the presence of two or more binding sites, the respective K_d and B_{max}, which may be determined by computerized curve-fitting programs (Fig. 13). Radioligand binding studies can also be used to investigate selectivity of drugs for the receptor using competition between the competitor drug and a fixed concentration of radioligand. Receptors may be characterized in this way using the rank order of potency of agonists or antagonists.

Binding studies can also be used to determine the distribution of receptor in tissues using autoradiography. The radioligand is incubated with frozen sections of the tissue of interest using optimal conditions and using an excess of nonradiolabeled competitor to define nonspecific binding, as in membrane binding studies. The distribution of specific binding is then used to indicate the tissue localization of receptors.

Agonists and Antagonists

After binding to the receptor, the response is activated via second messenger systems described above. Different agonists may elicit variable degrees of response, which is described as efficacy. A drug that produces less than a maximal response (E_{max}) is known as a partial agonist. In airway smooth muscle, isoproterenol is a full agonist and

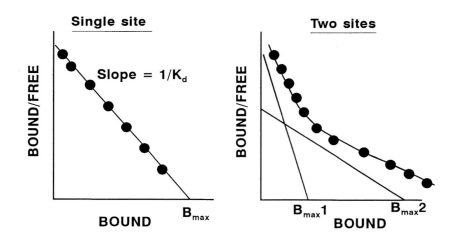

FIG. 13. Scatchard plots of receptor binding. With a single receptor population a plot of bound/free against bound ligand gives a straight line with a slope inversely related to the dissociation constant (K_d) and an intercept equal to the maximal number of binding sites (B_{max}). When two sites are involved the line is curvilinear and may be fitted to two binding sites of differing affinity and capacity ($B_{max}1, B_{max}2$).

produces a maximal response, whereas albuterol acts as a partial agonist, giving less than 50% of the maximal relaxation seen with isoproterenol.

Antagonists have zero efficacy. Antagonists block the effects of an agonist by interfering with its binding to the receptor. When antagonists interact with agonists at a common receptor, the antagonism is competitive. This can be demonstrated by a rightward shift in the log concentration-response curve (Fig. 14). For true competitive antagonism (e.g., between a β_2-antagonist and β-agonist in airway smooth muscle) the shift is parallel. The amount of shift observed with each concentration of agonist can be used to calculate the affinity of the antagonist for the particular receptor. This can be quantified in a Schild plot that gives a measure of receptor affinity (pA_2).

Sometimes a drug interferes with an agonist effect in a noncompetitive manner by inhibiting any of the steps that lead to the typical agonist effect. This results in a nonparallel shift in the agonist dose-response curve and a reduced maximal response.

Another type of antagonism relevant to lung diseases is functional antagonism, which describes an interaction between two agents that have opposite functional effects on the same cell system. Thus, agonists act as functional antagonists in airway smooth muscle because they counteract the contractile effects of any spasmogen, including histamine, leukotriene D_4, thromboxane, bradykinin, and acetylcholine.

Two drugs may interact to produce effects that are more than additive. Synergism is the term used when two drugs given together produce an effect that is greater than the additive effect of the drugs given separately. Potentiation is when one drug given alone has no effect, but increases the response to a second drug. Tolerance refers to a diminishing response to a drug that is administered repeatedly, whereas tachyphylaxis usually describes tolerance of rapid onset, so that it may be seen after only one administration of the drug. Desensitization is a term that includes rapid and long-term loss of response.

The interaction between a ligand and its receptor has several characteristics. Binding is rapid and reversible.

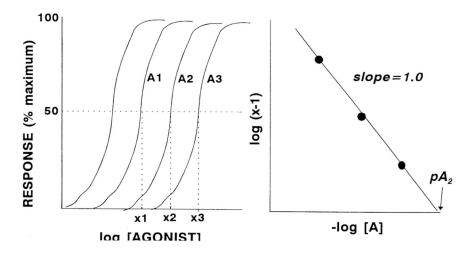

FIG. 14. Competitive binding to a receptor. Increasing concentrations of antagonist shift the dose-response curve to an agonist to the right in a parallel manner. A Schild plot plots a function of the shift with antagonist concentration against the agonist concentration. For true competitive antagonists, the slope of the line is 1 and the interaction gives the pA_2 value—a measurement of antagonist affinity for the receptor.

There is stereoselectivity with the levoisomer binding more effectively than the dextroisomer.

RECEPTOR REGULATION

Receptors are subject to many regulatory factors that may operate at several sites. Some factors influence the gene transcription of receptors, either increasing or decreasing transcription. Other factors influence the stability of mRNA and thus the amount of receptor protein formed (3). Translation of receptor protein may also be regulated. Once the receptor protein is inserted into the membrane, the receptor may be regulated by phosphorylation as a result of various kinases.

Desensitization

Desensitization occurs with most receptors when exposed to an agonist. Short-term desensitization is often termed tachyphylaxis and long-term desensitization is termed downregulation. This phenomenon has been studied in some detail with β_2-receptors and involves several molecular processes (65,85).

In the short term, desensitization involves phosphorylation that uncouples the receptor from G_s, via the action of an enzyme called β-adrenergic receptor-specific kinase (βARK) (83,86,87). The site of this phosphorylation appears to be on the Ser/Thr–rich region of the third intracellular loop and the carboxy-terminal tail, because their replacement reduces the rate of desensitization (85,88). Another protein, β-arrestin, is also involved in uncoupling the phosphorylated β-receptor from the G protein. Short-term desensitization (i.e., within minutes) after agonist exposure can also occur by the process of sequestration, involving internalization of the receptor within intracellular compartments. For β_2-receptors, the proximal portion of the C-terminal domain is important for conferring the sequestration property (89).

Longer term mechanisms include downregulation of surface receptor number, a process that may involve internalization of the receptor and its subsequent degradation. Moreover, in a cultured hamster cell line, downregulation of β_2-receptors results in a rapid decline in the steady-state level of β_2-receptor mRNA (90,91). This suggests that downregulation is achieved in part, either by inhibiting the gene transcription of receptors or by increased post-transcriptional processing of the mRNA in the cell. Using actinomycin D to inhibit transcription, it has been found that β_2-receptor mRNA stability is markedly reduced in these cells after exposure to β-agonists. Furthermore, by isolating nuclei and performing a nuclear run-on transcription assay, it is apparent that β-agonist exposure does not directly alter receptor gene transcription (91). Longer term exposure to β-agonists may also result in inhibition of β-receptor gene transcription, mediated via the effects of a cAMP-specific transcription factor (CREB) (87). Long-term exposure to β-agonists results in reduced transcription of β_2-receptors in the airways (92–94).

Steroid Modulation

Certain G protein–linked receptors are also influenced by glucocorticoids. Thus, rat pulmonary β-receptors are increased in density by pretreatment with glucocorticoids (95) and glucocorticoids increase the expression of β-receptors in rabbit fetal lung (96) and in human lung (97). Steroids also prevent the desensitization and downregulation of β-receptors on human leukocytes (98); this has also recently been demonstrated in rat lung in vivo (94). Corticosteroids increase the steady-state level of β_2-receptor mRNA in cultured hamster smooth muscle cells, thus indicating that steroids may increase β-receptor density by increasing the rate of gene transcription (91,99). The increase in mRNA occurs rapidly (within 1 hour), preceding the increase in β-receptors, and then declines to a steady-state level about twice normal. The cloned β-receptor gene contains three potential glucocorticoid responsive elements (100) and incubation of human lung with glucocorticoids results in a doubling of the rate of transcription (97) .

Glucocorticoids also regulate their own receptors. Incubation of various cells with corticosteroids may result in a downregulation of steroid receptors (101). This appears to be due to a decrease in gene transcription of the receptors, and the glucocorticoids receptor gene itself has GREs. In human lung the inhibition of receptor transcription is marked, with almost complete inhibition of transcription after incubation with a high concentration of dexamethasone (1 μM) for 24 hours (102). This may have important implications for long-term management of airway disease by high doses of inhaled steroids, because this may lead to reduced steroid responsiveness, which may be an explanation for the apparent progression of asthma in some patients.

Ontogeny

Another area in which molecular biology of receptors may be relevant is in studying the development of receptors and the factors that determine expression of particular receptor genes during development. In fetal lung there is a marked increase in the expression of β_2-receptors in the perinatal period that is critically dependent on glucocorticoids (96).

Disease

There are several pulmonary diseases in which altered expression of receptors may be relevant to understanding their pathophysiology. Molecular biology offers a new perspective in investigating these abnormalities of receptor expression by providing insights into whether the abnormality arises through altered transcription of the receptor gene, or abnormalities in post-transcriptional or post-translational processing.

There is some evidence that β-adrenoceptor function may be impaired in airway smooth muscle of patients with fatal asthma (18–20). However, binding and autoradiographic studies have not demonstrated any reduction in β-adrenoceptors in airway smooth muscle, suggesting that the reduced bronchodilator responses to β-agonists may be due to uncoupling of the receptor (102). Similarly, no differences in muscarinic receptors have been detected in asthmatic lungs using binding approaches (103).

Relatively few studies have explored whether there are any differences in the expression of mediator receptors in asthmatic airways. There is some evidence for increased expression of PAF-receptor mRNA in lungs of asthmatic patients, although whether this has functional significance is not known (104). There is also evidence for increased NK$_1$-receptor expression in the lungs of patients with asthma and chronic obstructive lung disease (105, 106).

Transcriptional Control

Receptor genes, like any other genes, may be regulated by transcription factors, which may be activated within the cell under certain conditions, leading to increased or decreased receptor gene transcription, which may in turn alter the expression of receptors at the cell surface. Little is known about the transcription factors that regulate receptors, but these may be relevant to disease such as chronic inflammation. The transcription factor AP-1, a Fos-Jun heterodimer, may be activated via PKC. AP-1 increases transcription of several genes, including some receptor genes. For example, the gene coding for the NK$_1$-receptor has an AP-1 site, which leads to increased gene transcription and a GRE that conversely results in decreased transcription (107). Chronic cell stimulation, via activation of protein kinase C, may therefore lead to an increase in NK$_1$-receptor gene expression, which could lead to increased neurogenic inflammation. An increase in NK$_1$-receptors has been reported in the colons of patients with inflammatory bowel disease (108), and an increased NK$_1$-receptor gene expression is present in asthmatic airways (105). By contrast, glucocorticoids reduce NK$_1$-specific mRNA in human lung, probably via an inhibitory effect of glucocorticoid receptors on AP-1 (105).

REFERENCES

1. Barnes PJ. Receptors and second messengers: chairman's summary. *Am Rev Respir Dis* 1990;141:S97–S98.
2. Barnes PJ. Molecular biology of lung receptors. In: Barnes PJ, Stockley RA, eds. *Molecular biology of lung disease.* Oxford: Blackwell, 1994;192–215.
3. Barnes PJ. Molecular biology of receptors. *Q J Med* 1992;301:339–353.
4. Bahouth SW, Wang H, Malbon CC. Immunological approaches for probing receptor structure and function. *Trends Pharmacol Sci* 1991; 12:338–343.
5. Barnes PJ. Molecular biology of receptors in the respiratory tract. In: Chung KF, Barnes PJ, eds. *Pharmacology of the respiratory tract: experimental and clinical research.* New York: Marcel Dekker, 1993;1–26.
6. Venter JC, Fraser CM. Structure and molecular biology of transmitter receptors. *Am Rev Respir Dis* 1990;141:S99–105.
7. Strader CD, Fong TM, Graziano MP, Tota MR. The family of G protein coupled receptors. *FASEB J* 1995;9:745–754.
8. Hargrave PA, McDowell JH. Rhodopsin and phototransduction: a model system for G protein–linked receptors. *FASEB J* 1992;6:2323–2331.
9. Gokayne J, Robinson DA, Fitzgerald MG, et al. Primary structure of rat cardiac β-adrenergic and muscarinic receptors obtained by automated DNA sequence analysis: further evidence for a multigene family. *Proc Natl Acad Sci USA* 1987;89:8296–8300.
10. Venter JC, Fraser CM, Kerlavage AR, Buck MA. Molecular biology of adrenergic and muscarinic cholinergic receptors: a perspective. *Biochem Pharmacol* 1989;38:1197–1208.
11. George ST, Ruoho AE, Malbon CC. N-glycosylatcos in expression and function of β-adrenergic receptors. *J Biochem* 1986;261:16559–16564.
12. Inglese J, Freedman NJ, Koch WJ, Lefkowitz RJ. Structure and mechanism of the G protein–coupled receptor kinases. *J Biol Chem* 1993; 268:23735–23738.
13. Fong TM, Cascieri MA, Yu H, Bonsal A, Swain C, Strader CD. Amino-aromatic interaction between histidine 197 of the neurokinin-1 receptor. *Nature* 1993;362:350–353.
14. Birnbaumer L, Brown AM. G proteins and the mechanism of action of hormones, neurotransmitters and autocrine and paracrine regulatory factors. *Am Rev Respir Dis* 1990;141:S106–114.
15. Gilman AG. G proteins: transducers of receptor-generated signals. *Annu Rev Biochem* 1987;56:615–649.
16. Bourne HR, Sanders DA, McCormick F. The GTPase superfamily: conserved structure and molecular mechanism. *Nature* 1991;349:117–127.
17. Neer EJ, Clapham DE. Roles of G protein subunits in transmembrane signaling. *Nature* 1988;133:129–134.
18. Goldie RG, Spina D, Henry PJ, Lulich KM, Paterson JW. In vitro responsiveness of human asthmatic bronchus to carbachol, histamine, β-adrenoceptor agonists and theophylline. *Br J Clin Pharmacol* 1986; 22:669–676.
19. Cerrina J, Ladurie ML, Labat C, Raffestin B, Bayol A, Brink C. Comparison of human bronchial muscle response to histamine *in vivo* with histamine and isoproterenol agonists *in vitro*. *Am Rev Respir Dis* 1986;134:57–61.
20. Bai TR. Abnormalities in airway smooth muscle in fatal asthma: a comparison between trachea and bronchus. *Am Rev Respir Dis* 1991; 143:441–443.
21. Spina D, Rigby PJ, Paterson JW, Goldie RG. Autoradiographic localization of beta-adrenoceptors in asthmatic human lung. *Am Rev Respir Dis* 1989;140:1410–1415.
22. Bai TR, Mak JCW, Barnes PJ. A comparison of beta-adrenergic receptors and *in vitro* relaxant responses to isoproterenol in asthmatic airway smooth muscle. *Am J Respir Cell Mol Biol* 1992;6:647–651.
23. Tsien RW, Tsien RY. Calcium channels, stores, and oscillations. *Annu Rev Cell Biol* 1990;6:715–760.
24. Tang WO, Gilman AG. Adenylyl cyclases. *Cell* 1992;70:869–872.
25. Jacobowitz O, Chen J, Premont RT, Iyengar R. Stimulation of specific types of G$_s$-stimulated adenylyl cyclases by phorbol ester treatment. *J Biol Chem* 1993;268:3829–3832.
26. Kume H, Takai A, Tokuno H, Tomita T. Regulation of Ca^{2+}-dependent K$^+$-channel activity in tracheal myocytes by phosphorylation. *Nature* 1989;341:152–154.
27. Gerthoffer UT. Calcium dependence of myosin phosphorylation and airway smooth muscle contraction and relaxation. *Am J Physiol* 1986; 250:C597–604.
28. Beavo JA, Reifsnyder DH. Primary sequence of cyclic nucleotide

phosphodiesterase isoenzymes and the design of selective inhibitors. *Trends Pharmacol Sci* 1990;11:150–155.

29. Nicholson CD, Challiss RAJ, Shahid M. Differential modulation of tissue function and therapeutic potential of selective inhibitors of cyclic nucleotide phosphodiesterase isoenzymes. *Trends Pharmacol Sci* 1991;12:19–27.

30. Torphy TJ, Undem RJ. Phosphodiesterase inhibitors: new opportunities for the treatment of asthma. *Thorax* 1991;46:512–523.

31. Barnes PJ. Cyclic nucletodies, phosphodiesterases and airway function. *Eur Respir J* 1995;8:457–462.

32. Cockroft S, Thomas GMH. Inositol-lipid–specific phospholipase C isoenzymes and their differential regulation by receptors. *Biochem J* 1992;288:1–14.

33. Berridge MJ, Irvine RF. Inositol phosphates and cell signaling. *Nature* 1989;341:197–205.

34. Grandordy BM, Barnes PJ. Phosphoinositide turnover in airway smooth muscle. *Am Rev Respir Dis* 1987;136:S17–S20.

35. Hall I, Chilvers ER. Inositol phosphates and airway smooth muscle. *Pulm Pharmacol* 1989;2:113–120.

36. Nishizuka Y. The molecular heterogeneity of protein kinase C and its implications for cellular regulation. *Nature* 1988;334:661–665.

37. Thompson NT, Bonser RW, Garland LG. Receptor-coupled phospholipase D and its inhibition. *Trends Pharmacol Sci* 1991;12:404–407.

38. van Oosterhoot AJM, Nijkamp FP. Effects of lymphokines on beta-adrenoceptor function of human peripheral blood mononuclear cells. *Br J Clin Pharmacol* 1990;30:150–152S.

39. Gruetter CA, Childers CC, Bosserman MK, Lemke SM, Ball JG, Valentovic MA. Comparison of relaxation induced by glycerl trinitate, isosorbide dinitrate and sodium nitroprusside in bovine airways. *Am Rev Respir Dis* 1989;139:1192–1197.

40. Ishii K, Murad F. ANP relaxes bovine tracheal smooth muscle and increase cGMP. *Am J Physiol* 1989;256:C495–500.

41. Angus RM, Mecallaum MJA, Hulks G, Thomson NC. Bronchodilator, cardiovascular and cyclic guanylyl monophosphate response to high dose infused atrial natriuretic peptide in asthma. *Am Rev Respir Dis* 1993;147:1122–1125.

42. Kume H, Graziano MP, Kotlikoff MI. Stimulatory and inhibitory regulation of calcium-activated potassium channels by guanine nucleotide binding proteins. *Proc Natl Acad Sci USA* 1992;89:11051–11055

43. Kume H, Hall IP, Washabau RJ, Takagi K, Kotlikoff MI. b-Adrenergic agonists regulate K_{Ca} channels in airway smooth muscle by cAMP-dependent and -independent mechanisms. *J Clin Invest* 1994;93:371–379.

44. Shepherd VL. Cytokine receptors in lung. *Am J Respir Cell Mol Biol* 1991;5:403–410.

45. Sprang SR. The divergent receptors for TNF. *Trends Biochem Sci* 1990;15:366–368.

46. Williams AF, Barclay AN. The immunoglobulin superfamily—domains for cell surface recognition. *Annu Rev Immunol* 1988;6:381–405.

47. Bazan JF. Structural design and molecular evolution of a cytokine receptor superfamily. *Proc Natl Acad Sci USA* 1990;87:6934–6938.

48. Holmes WE, Lee J, Kuang W, Rice GC, Wood WI. Structure and functional expression of a human interleukin-8 receptor. *Science* 1991;253:1278–1280.

49. Horuk R. Molecular properties of the chemokine receptor family. *Trends Pharmacol Sci* 1994;15:159–165.

50. Kishimoto T, Taga T, Akira S. Cytokine signal transduction. *Cell* 1994;76:253–262.

51. Michell RH. Peptide regulatory factors: post-receptor signaling pathways. *Lancet* 1989;i:765–768.

52. van der Geek P, Hunter T, Lindberg RA. Receptor protein-tyrosine kinases and their signal transduction pathways. *Annu Rev Biol* 1994;10:251–337.

53. Schlessinger J. SH2/SH3 signaling proteins. *Curr Opin Genet Dev* 1994;4:25–30.

54. Burgering BMT, Bos JL. Regulation of Ras-mediated signaling: more than one way to skin a cat. *Trends Biochem Sci* 1995;20:18–22.

55. Massague J, Attasano L, Wrana JL. The TGF-β family and its composite receptors. *Trends Cell Biol* 1994;4:172–178.

56. Walton KM, Dixon JE. Protein tyrosine phosphatases. *Annu Rev Biochem* 1993;12:101–120.

57. Galzi JL, Changeux JP. Neuronal nicotinic receptors: molecular organization and regulation. *Neuropharmacology* 1995;34:563–582.

58. Evans RM. The steroid and thyroid hormone receptor superfamily. *Science* 1988;247:889–895.

59. Thompson BC. The structure of the human glucocorticoid receptor and its gene. *J Steroid Biochem* 1987;27:105–108.

60. Beato M. Gene regulation by steroid hormones. *Cell* 1989;56:335–344.

61. Munck A, Mendel DB, Smith LI, Orti E. Glucocorticoid receptors and actions. *Am Rev Respir Dis* 1991;141:S2–S10.

62. Miesfield RL. Molecular genetics of corticosteroid action. *Am Rev Respir Dis* 1990;141:S11–S17.

63. Barnes PJ, Adcock IM. Antiinflammatory actions of steroids: molecular mechanisms. *Trends Pharmacol Sci* 1993;14:436–441.

64. Barnes PJ. Molecular mechanisms of steroid action in asthma. *J Allergy Clin Immunol* 1996;97:159–168.

65. Lefkowitz RJ, Caron MG. Adrenergic receptors. Models for the study of receptors coupled to guanine nucleotide regulatory proteins. *J Biol Chem* 1988;263:4993–4996.

66. Yokota Y, Sasai Y, Tanaka K, et al. Molecular characterization of a functional cDNA for rat substance P receptor. *J Biol Chem* 1989;264:17649–17652.

67. Shigemoto R, Yokota Y, Tsuchida K, Nakanishi S. Cloning and expression of a rat neuromedin K receptor cDNA. *J Biol Chem* 1990;265:623–628.

68. Emorine LJ, Marullo S, Briend-Sutren M, et al. Molecular characterization of the human β3-adrenergic receptor. *Science* 1989;245:1118–1121.

69. Kriff S, Lonnqvist F, Raimbault S, et al. Tissue distribution of β3–adrenergic receptor mRNA in man. *J Clin Invest* 1993;91:344–349.

70. Hulme EC, Birdsall NJM, Buckley NJ. Muscarinic receptor subtypes. *Annu Rev Pharmacol* 1990;30:633–673.

71. Bonner TI. New subtypes of muscarinic acetylcholine receptors. *Trends Pharmacol Sci* 1989;10(suppl):11–15.

72. Dorje F, Levey AI, Brann MR. Immunological detection of muscarinic receptor subtype proteins (m1–m5) in rabbit peripheral tissues. *Mol Pharmacol* 1991;40:459–462.

73. Lazareno S, Buckley NJ, Roberts FF. Characterization of muscarinic M_4 binding sites in rabbit lung, chicken heart and NG 108-15 cells. *Mol Pharmacol* 1990;38:805–815.

74. Mak JCW, Haddad E, Buckley NJ, Barnes PJ. Visualization of muscarinic m4 mRNA and M_4-receptor subtypes in rabbit lung. *Life Sci* 1993;53:1501–1508.

75. Buckley NJ, Bonner TI, Buckley CM, Brann MR. Antagonist binding properties of cloned muscarinic receptors expressed in CHO–K1 cells. *Mol Pharmacol* 1989;35:469–476.

76. Kurtenbach E, Curtis CAM, Pedder EK, Aiken A, Harris ACM, Hulme EC. Muscarinic acetylcholine receptors. *J Biol Chem* 1990;265:13702–13708.

77. Yang CM, Chow S, Sung T. Muscarinic receptor subtypes coupled to generation of different second messengers in isolated tracheal smooth muscle cells. *Br J Pharmacol* 1991;104:613–618.

78. Rousell J, Haddad E-B, Webb BLJ, Giembycz MA, Mak JCW, Barnes PJ. β-Adrenoceptor–mediated down-regulation of M_2-muscarinic receptors: role of cAMP-dependent protein kinases and protein kinase C. *Mol Pharmacol* 1996;49:629–635.

79. Rasmussen H, Kelley G, Douglas JS. Interactions between Ca^{2+} and cAMP messenger system in regulation of airway smooth muscle contraction. *Am J Physiol* 1990;258:L279–L288.

80. Grandordy BM, Mak JCW, Barnes PJ. Modulation of airway smooth muscle β-adrenoceptor function by a muscarinic agonist. *Life Sci* 1994;54:185–191.

81. Jonat C, Rahsdorf HJ, Park KK, et al. Anti tumor promotion and antiinflammation: down-modulation of AP-1 (fos/jun) activity by glucocorticoid hormone. *Cell* 1990;62:1189–1204.

82. Masquilier D, Sassone-Corsi P. Transcriptional cross talk: nuclear factors CREM and CREB bind to AP-1 sites and inhibit activation by Jun. *J Biol Chem* 1992;267:22460–22466.

83. Barnes PJ. Beta-adrenergic receptors and their regulation. *Am J Respir Crit Care Med* 1995;152:838–860.

84. Adcock IM, Stevens DA, Barnes PJ. Interactions between steroids and β2-agonists. *Eur Respir J* 1996;9:160–168.

85. Bouvier M, Collins S, O'Dowd BF, et al. Two distinct pathways for cAMP-mediated down-regulation of the β2-adrenergic receptor. *J Biol Chem* 1989;264:16786–16792.

86. Benovic JL, Strasser RH, Daniel K, Lefkowitz RJ. Beta-adrenergic receptor kinase : identification of a novel protein kinase that phospho-

rylates the agonist-occupied form of the receptor. *Proc Natl Acad Sci USA* 1986;83:2797–2801.

87. Collins S, Caron MG, Lefkowitz RJ. From ligand binding to gene expression: new insights into the regulation of G protein–coupled receptors. *Trends Pharmacol Sci* 1992;17:37–39.

88. Bouvier MW, Hausdorff A, DeBlasi A, et al. Removal of phosphorylation sites from the β-adrenergic receptor delays the onset of agonist-promoted desensitization. *Nature* 1988;333:370–373.

89. Hausdorff WP, Campbell PT, Ostrowski I. A small region of beta-adrenergic receptor is selectively involved in its rapid regulation. *Proc Natl Acad Sci USA* 1991;88:2979–2985.

90. Hadcock JR, Williams DL, Malbon CC. Physiological regulation at the level of mRNA: analysis of steady state levels of specific mRNAs by DNA-excess solution hybridization. *Am J Physiol* 1989;256:C457–C465.

91. Hadcock JR, Wang HY, Malbon CC. Agonist-induced destabilization of β-adrenergic receptor mRNA: attenuation of glucocorticoid-induced up-regulation of β-adrenergic receptors. *J Biol Chem* 1989;264:19928–19933.

92. Nishikawa M, Mak JCW, Shirasaki H, Barnes PJ. Differential down-regulation of pulmonary β_1- and β_2-adrenoceptor messenger RNA with prolonged *in vivo* infusion of isoprenaline. *Eur J Pharmacol* (Molecular Section) 1993;247:131–138.

93. Nishikawa M, Mak JCW, Shirasaki H, Harding SE, Barnes PJ. Long term exposure to norepinephrine results in down-regulation and reduced mRNA expression of pulmonary β-adrenergic receptors in guinea pigs. *Am J Respir Cell Mol Biol* 1994;10:91–99.

94. Mak JCW, Nishikawa M, Shirasaki H, Miyayasu K, Barnes PJ. Protective effects of a glucocorticoid on down-regulation of pulmonary β_2-adrenergic receptors *in vivo*. *J Clin Invest* 1995;96:99–106.

95. Mano K, Akbarzadeh A, Townley RG. Effect of hydrocortisone on beta-adrenergic receptors in lung membranes. *Life Sci* 1979;25:1925–1930.

96. Barnes PJ, Jacobs MM, Roberts JM. Glucocorticoids preferably increase fetal alveolar beta-receptors: autoradiographic evidence. *Pediatr Res* 1984;18:1191–1194.

97. Mak JCW, Nishikawa M, Barnes PJ. Glucocorticosteroids increase β_2-adrenergic receptor transcription in human lung. *Am J Physiol* 1995;12:L41–L46.

98. Davis AO, Lefkowitz RJ. Regulation of beta–adrenergic receptors by steroid hormones. *Annu Rev Physiol* 1984;46:119–130.

99. Collins S, Caron MG, Lefkowitz RJ. β-Adrenergic receptors in hamster smooth muscle cells are transcriptionally regulated by glucocorticoids. *J Biol Chem* 1988;263:9067–9070.

100. Strader CD, Sigal IS, Dixon RAF. Structural basis of β-adrenergic receptor function. *FASEB J* 1989;3:1825–1832.

101. Okret S, Dong Y, Brönnegård M, Gustafsson J–Å. Regulation of glucocorticoid receptor expression. *Biochimie* 1991;73:51–59.

102. Adcock IM, Gilbey T, Gelder CM, Chung KF, Barnes PJ. Glucocorticoid receptor localization in normal human lung and asthmatic lung. *Am J Respir Crit Care Med* 1996;154:771–782.

103. Haddad E-B, Mak JCW, Barnes PJ. Expression of β-adrenergic and muscarinic receptors in human lung. *Am J Physiol* 1996; (*in press*).

104. Shirasaki H, Nishikawa M, Adcock IM, et al. Expression of platelet activating factor receptor mRNA in human and guinea-pig lung. *Am J Respir Cell Mol Biol* 1994;10:533–537.

105. Adcock IM, Peters M, Gelder C, Shirasaki H, Brown CR, Barnes PJ. Increased tachykinin receptor gene expression in asthmatic lung and its modulation by steroids. *J Mol Endocrinol* 1993;11:1–7.

106. Bai TR, Zhou D, Weir T, et al. Substance P (NK_1)- and neurokinin A (NK_2)-receptor gene expression in inflammatory airway diseases. *Am J Physiol* 1995;269:L309–L317.

107. Ihara H, Nakanishi S. Selective inhibition of expression of the substance P receptor mRNA in pancreatic acinar AR42J cells by glucocorticoids. *J Biol Chem* 1990; 36:22,441–22,445.

108. Mantyh CR, Gates TS, Zimmerman RP, et al. Receptor binding sites for substance P but not substance K or neuromedin K are expressed in high concentrations by arterioles, venules and lymph nodes in surgical specimens obtained from patients with ulcerative colitis and Crohns disease. *Proc Natl Acad Sci* 1988; 85:3235–3259.

Asthma, edited by P.J. Barnes, M.M. Grunstein,
A.R. Leff, and A.J. Woolcock.
Lippincott–Raven Publishers, Philadelphia © 1997.

▪ 24 ▪

Molecular and Genetic Basis of β-Adrenergic Receptor Function and Regulation

Stephen B. Liggett

Classification and Structure of Adrenergic Receptors
Agonist Binding Domains of the β₂AR
G Protein-Coupling Domains of the β₂AR
Desensitization of the β₂AR via Phosphorylation
Determinants of β₂AR Sequestration

Determinants of β₂AR Downregulation
β₂AR Desensitization to Agonist in the Treatment
of Asthma
Genetic Variation of β₂AR Structure

Adrenergic receptors (AR) are cell surface proteins which are the receptors for the endogenous catecholamines. In addition, they are the targets for a large number of therapeutic agents acting as agonists or antagonists. Adrenergic receptors are members of a superfamily of receptors that accomplish signal transduction through their interaction with membrane-bou nd G proteins which, in turn, alter the activity of several different effector systems. In the lung, the adrenergic receptor that is most relevant to asthma is the β₂AR [reviewed in (1,2)]. In this chapter the molecular basis of β₂AR function will be discussed, with particular emphasis on the relationship between receptor structure and function. In addition, the relatively new findings of genetically based variation in β₂AR structure within the human population, due to polymorphisms in the gene encoding for the receptor, will be discussed as they relate to asthma.

CLASSIFICATION AND STRUCTURE OF ADRENERGIC RECEPTORS

The structure of a typical G protein–coupled receptor is shown in Figure 1. The membrane topology of these receptors is predicted to consist of seven α-helixes which putatively span the cell membrane seven times. The amino-terminus is extracellular and the carboxy-terminus is intracellular. Each transmembrane domain is connected by amino acids which make up intracellular and extracellular loops. A number of posttranslational modifications occur with many G protein–coupled receptors, including glycosylation of the amino terminus, disulfide bonding in the extracellular loops, palmitoylation of residues in the proximal portion of the cytoplasmic tail, and phosphorylation of residues in the intracellular domains. There are nine cloned human adrenergic receptors. Three adrenergic receptors are classified as βAR, three are α₁AR, and three are α₂AR. The β₁, β₂ and β₃AR subtypes have a high degree of sequence homology (~70%) in their transmembrane domains. In contrast, the homology is considerably less (~40%) between a βAR and an α₁AR or an α₂AR in these regions. All βAR couple to the same G protein (the stimulatory guanine nucleotide-binding regulatory protein, G_s), resulting in activation of adenylyl cyclase and an increase in intracellular cyclic 3'5" adenosine monophosphate (cAMP). α₁AR are coupled to G_q, activating phospholipase C and causing an increase in second messengers diacylglycerol and inositil—1, 4, 5 triphosphate. α₂AR couple to G_i which decreases the activity of adenylyl cyclase resulting in a decrease in intracellular cAMP.

β₂AR are expressed on a number of cells in the lung relevant to asthma [reviewed in (2)]. These include bronchial epithelial cells, submucosal glands, bronchial smooth muscle, vascular endothelium and smooth muscle, presynaptic cholinergic nerve terminals, and multiple immune cells including eosinophils, mast cells, neutrophils, lymphocytes, and macrophages. The most obvi-

S. B. Liggett: Department of Internal Medicine, University of Cincinnati College of Medicine, Cincinnati, Ohio 45267-0564.

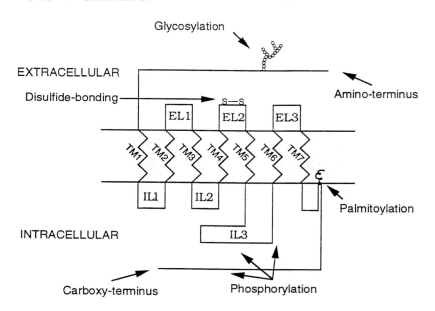

FIG. 1. General topography of a prototypical G protein–coupled receptor. Shown is the proposed orientation within the membrane, with the amino-terminus being extracellular, seven transmembrane spanning segments (TM1–TM7), three extracellular loops (ELI–EL3), three intracellular loops (IL1–IL3), and an intracellular carboxy-terminus. The four most common posttranslational modifications are shown.

ous results of administering β-adrenergic agonists in asthma is relaxation of bronchial smooth muscle via the receptors localized to these cells, with consequent increases in airway caliber and relief of airway obstruction. Other potentially therapeutic effects of β-adrenergic agonists in asthma, such as increased ciliary beat frequency and improved mucociliary clearance, decreases in acetylcholine release from cholinergic nerve fibers, alterations in vascular tone and permeability, and alterations in immune cell function are more speculative.

AGONIST BINDING DOMAINS OF THE β₂AR

The primary amino-acid sequence and proposed membrane topography of the human β₂AR is shown in Figure 2. Using site-directed mutagenesis and recombinant expression, the sites of attachment of agonists have been mapped to several key locations. It has been shown that Ser204 and Ser207 of the fifth transmembrane spanning domain interact with the metahydroxyl and parahydroxyl groups on the catecholamine ring (3) (Fig. 2). Mutant receptors where these serines were replaced with alanines have been studied using isoproterenol and isoproterenol derivatives lacking these hydroxyl groups. The data suggest that the catecholamine can be positioned and can activate β₂AR by forming hydrogen bonds with either serine, but that with endogenous catecholamines (and most synthetic β-agonists), interactions occur at both serines. This was elucidated by the use of isoproterenol derivatives lacking the parahydroxyl group, which were unable to activate the receptor that lacked Ser207, while the derivative lacking the metahydroxyl group, was unable to activate the receptor lacking Ser204. Isoproterenol itself could activate both mutant receptors. Another key inter-

action of the receptor with catecholamines occurs at the amine head group of the carboxylate group on Asp113 of the third transmembrane spanning domain (4,5). Mutant β₂AR having a serine for this aspartate are not activated by catecholamines, but can be activated by catechol esters which can form hydrogen bonds to serines. In addition to these key determinants in transmembrane spanning domains 3 and 5, recent data suggest that transmembrane spanning domain 4 also plays a role in establishing the agonist-binding pocket. A naturally occurring polymorphism at position 164, where serine is replaced by threonine, was found to alter the affinity of isoproterenol, epinephrine, and norepinephrine (6). All of these agonists have hydroxyl groups on their β-carbons. It has been hypothesized, based on computer modeling, that this hydroxyl group may interact with the serine in position 165 (which is conserved in all catecholamine receptors). When the affinities of two agonists that lack such β-hydroxyl groups (dopamine and dobutamine) were assessed, it was found that there was no difference between the Thr164 and Ile164 receptors (6). Taken together, these data suggest that the polymorphism at position 164 affects the milieu established by the serine at position 165, which interacts with the β-carbon hydroxyl groups of most agonists. It should be noted that a direct mutation of Ser165 results in a receptor that fails to properly fold in the membrane (7).

Based on the traditional theory of agonist-receptor-G protein interaction, agonist binding at the critical points in the transmembrane domains alters the conformations of the second and third intracellular loops, which then bind and activate Gs. Recent studies have suggested that the activated state of the receptor may occur spontaneously, but that this is highly unfavorable (8–10). Based on this model, agonists stabilize the activated receptor increasing the net number of activated receptors on the cell. This model (often referred to as the "two-state model") also predicts that a certain degree of basal coupling to G_s, in the absence of agonist, is present in cells. Recently, certain traditional antagonists (now referred to as inverse agonists) when bound to the receptor, shift the equilibrium to very few activated receptors, i.e., they favor the inactivated form. If basal coupling is, indeed, of a significant magnitude, then inverse agonists would cause a decrease in intracellular cAMP. Neutral antagonists favor neither state, and, thus, result in no change in cAMP levels; they block access of the receptor to agonist. The clinical relevance of such findings is not clear. On hypothetical grounds, certain βAR antagonists used for treating other conditions such as angina or hypertension, which are, in fact, inverse agonists, may decrease intracellular cAMP in bronchial smooth muscle and exacerbate asthma. However, the inverse agonist phenomenon has only been shown with overexpression of the receptor in cell lines or transgenic animals, and the applicability of the concept to normal physiologic conditions is uncertain.

G PROTEIN-COUPLING DOMAINS OF THE β₂AR

The G protein-coupling domains of the receptor appear to be localized to intracellular loop (IL)2, IL3, and, possibly, to the most proximal portion of the cytoplasmic tail (Fig. 2). Deletion and substitution mutagenesis of the two regions adjacent to the membrane in IL3 have resulted in receptors with depressed coupling to G_s (11–13). The conclusions derived from the results of deletion mutations, however, are subject to debate since the global conformation of the loop may be substantially altered with such deletions. Studies where these regions have been

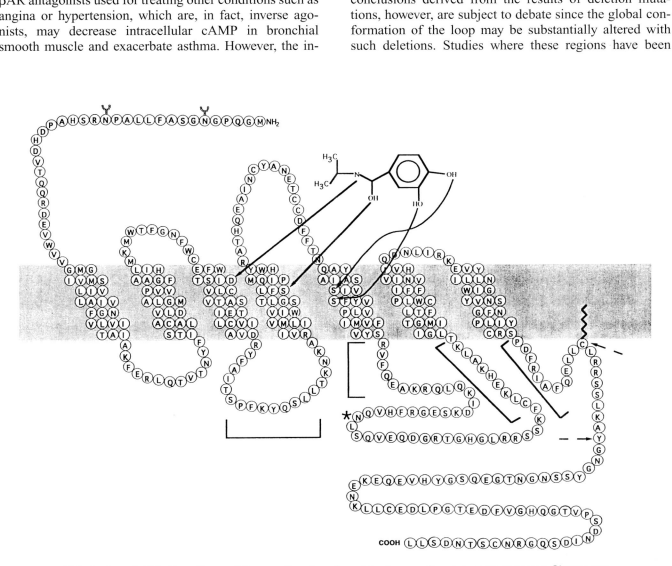

FIG. 2. Agonist-binding sites and G_s coupling domains of the human β₂-adrenergic receptor. Shown are the regions of contact between the agonist isoproterenol and specific residues in the third, fourth, and fifth transmembrane spanning segments that have been found to be critical for agonist binding. *Brackets* indicate regions that have been found to be important for G_s coupling. *Dashed arrows* indicate specific residues that are important for coupling. The *asterisk* in the third intracellular loop is where the β₂AR lacks a stretch of prolines found in the β₁AR that alters G_s coupling.

substituted with analogous regions of other G protein–coupled receptors have revealed interesting results. When expressed in *Xenopus laevis* oocytes, mutant β_2AR having substitutions of α_2AR sequence in the amino- and carboxy terminal portions of IL3 and the cytoplasmic tail, revealed depressed coupling to G_s (11). However, when expressed in mammalian cells (Chinese hamster fibroblasts), only the substitution within the carboxy-portion of IL3 had a significant effect on functional coupling (12). Subsequently, it was shown that the α_2AR can also couple to G_s, although much less efficiently than to G_i, and that at least one determinant within the α_2AR that is necessary for G_s coupling is the amino-terminal portion of IL3 (14–16). Thus, the relevance of the finding that there was no loss of G_s coupling in the β_2AR chimera, consisting of α_2AR substitution in the amino-terminus, is not clear. Other studies, using point mutations and deletions, have demonstrated that both the N- and C-terminal portions of the β_2AR are important determinants of receptor-Gs coupling, although it is not clear whether these regions perform specific functions in the binding and activation of G_s, or whether they establish a global conformation necessary for coupling (17,18).

Studies utilizing substitutions in IL2 also have indicated that this loop plays an important role in G protein coupling (11). More detailed studies within the carboxy-terminal portion of IL3 have indicated that certain residues maintain the loop in a nonfavorable conformation for coupling in the absence of agonist. With the α_1AR, substitution of Ala293 with any other amino acid results in a receptor that is activated in the absence of agonists (constituitive activation) (19). An analogous residue in the β_2AR has also been found (20). Agonist activation, then, may be thought of as relieving the constraining effect imposed by this region. Mutagenesis studies also have shown that the palmitoylated cystein of the β_2AR plays a role in G_s coupling (21). About 70% of G protein–coupled receptors are palmitoylated; however, the role of such palmitoylcysteins may be different for any given receptor. For the β_2AR, it has been shown that mutation of Cys341 to Ala results in functional uncoupling of the receptor from G_s. Subsequently, this was shown to be due to enhanced phosphorylation of the receptor which leads to the uncoupling. In contrast, we have found that mutation of the analogous cystein (residue 442) of the $\alpha_{2A}AR$ has no affect on coupling or phosphorylation, but rather disrupted the ability of the receptor to undergo agonist-promoted downregulation (22). Thus, this feature appears to impart different properties within the context of different G protein–coupled receptors. A tyrosine residue in the carboxy-terminal portion of the receptor may play a role in G_s coupling (23). Removal of tyrosine 350 of the β_2AR results in a receptor that is only partially coupled to G_s, compared to wild-type. While the aforementioned regions of the receptor appear to be key determinants of G_s coupling, the conformation of these regions can be affected by other areas of the receptor. For example, the ICL3 of β_1AR and β_2AR differ by a large proline-rich region located in the middle portion of the loop of the β_1AR (Fig. 2). The β_1AR couples less efficiently to G_s, compared to the β_2AR (24). Removal of this proline-rich region from the β_1AR increases G_s coupling, while insertion of this region into the β_2AR decreases G_s coupling (25).

DESENSITIZATION OF THE β_2AR VIA PHOSPHORYLATION

During continuous exposure to agonist, many G protein–coupled receptors display the property of desensitization (26). Desensitization is defined as a waning of the response to a stimulus, despite the continuous exposure to such stimulus. The β_2AR, indeed, displays agonist-promoted desensitization, which has been shown to be due to three different mechanisms—uncoupling due to phosphorylation, sequestration, and downregulation. The earliest event, occurring within seconds to minutes of agonist exposure, is phosphorylation of the receptor by two kinases. Early studies suggested that at least one mechanism of β_2AR phosphorylation was cAMP-dependent. Subsequently, protein kinase A (PKA) was implicated, suggesting a classic negative feedback-type of regulation. Activation of the receptor results in increases in intracellular cAMP, which induces PKA activity that both phosphorylates downstream components of the signal transduction pathway leading to the physiologic response and also phosphorylates the receptor itself, resulting in depressed coupling to G_s and a waning of the response. However, studies with mutant S49 lymphoma cells lacking G_s or PKA showed that agonist occupancy leads to receptor phosphorylation in a noncAMP-dependent manner as well. The kinase responsible for this was subsequently purified and cloned and was termed the βAR kinase or βARK (27,28).

The structural requirements of the β_2AR for PKA and βARK-mediated phosphorylation (Fig. 3) have been explored using site-directed mutagenesis and recombinant expression (29,30). A classic consensus sequence for PKA (Arg-Arg-X-Ser) is located in IL3 and the proximal portion of the cytoplasmic tail (Fig. 3). These serines have been mutated to alanine. Within its cytoplasmic tail, the human β_2AR has 11 Ser or Thr which are potential sites for βARK phosphorylation. These were mutated to Ala or Gly. When expressed in Chinese hamster fibroblasts (CHW cells), receptors lacking both PKA and βARK sites showed little short-term (<30 minutes) agonist-promoted desensitization (30). Similarly, receptors lacking either PKA or βARK sites showed attenuated desensitization as compared to wild-type (29,30). Mutated receptors underwent depressed agonist-mediated phosphorylation, confirming the concept that phosphorylation is the key mediator of the short-term desensitization process (30). Similar studies using inhibitors of PKA and βARK in cell systems have shown the importance of both kinases, as have studies us-

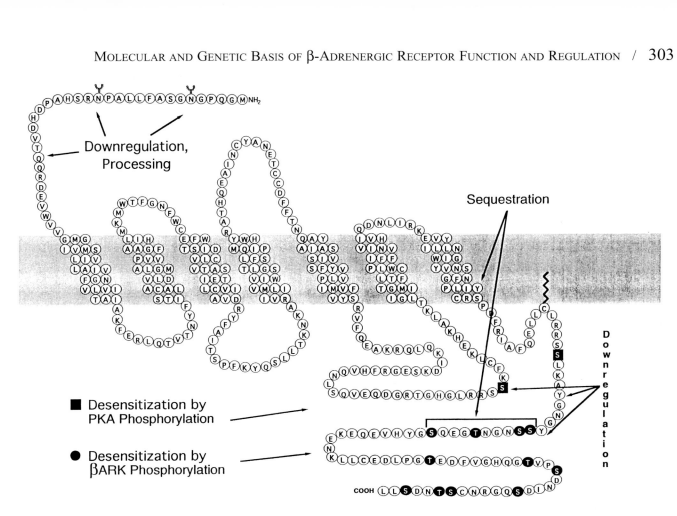

FIG. 3. Phosphorylation, sequestration and downregulation domains of the human β₂-adrenergic receptor. Each of the mechanisms contributes to agonist-promoted desensitization as described in the text.

ing purified receptor and kinases in a reconstituted phospholipid vesicle system (31,32). With the cloning of the β₃AR, it was noticed that this receptor lacks PKA sites and has few serines or threonines in the cytoplasmic tail, suggesting that this receptor might undergo little or no agonist-promoted desensitization. In recombinant expression studies, this was, indeed, found to be the case (33). In addition, a mutated β₃AR having a cytoplasmic tail substituted with the analogous region of the β₂AR did display phosphorylation and desensitization by βARK (33). These studies point further toward the cytoplasmic tail of the β₂AR as a key regulatory site and to the ubiquitous nature of βARK phosphorylation.

From studies of purified βARK, it is clear that an additional protein is required to provide for the receptor-G protein–uncoupling observed (34). In the rhodopsin/rhodopsin kinase system, such a protein had been identified and termed "arrestin." Arrestin binds to phosphorylated rhodopsin, inducing the uncoupling of rhodpsin from transducin. A similar group of proteins (termed "β-arrestins") have now been identified which subserve the same role with βARK and β₂AR (35).

While the previous studies have delineated the general area of the β₂AR that is the site for βARK-mediated

phosphorylation, the precise serines or threonines phosphorylated by this kinase in this receptor are not yet known. However, such sites have been determined in another adrenergic receptor, the α₂AAR. In this receptor, the sites for phosphorylation were known to be present in IL3 (36). The sequence EESSSS is present in this loop, and peptide-based studies using purified βARK in a reconstituted phospholipid vesicle system have shown that this was an excellent substrate for βARK (37). Removal of each serine reduced the extent of agonist-promoted phosphorylation by 25%, and when all four serines were removed, the mutated receptors exhibited no agonist-promoted phosphorylation (38). In functional studies, loss of phosphorylation correlated with the loss of desensitization. Indeed, even in receptors that were partially phosphorylated, desensitization was ablated. This suggests that in order for βarrestin to bind and induce uncoupling, a very precise conformational change induced by phosphorylation via βARK is required. With the identification of this precise sequence that is phosphorylated by βARK in this receptor, examination of the sequences of other G protein–coupled receptors indicates many potential sites where βARK may subserve similar roles. Three sites are potential candidates in the human β_2AR, and mutagenesis studies are underway to assess this.

It now is recognized that βARK is one of several G protein–coupled receptor kinases (termed "GRKs"), which phosphorylate receptors during agonist occupancy (39,40). Recently, rhodopsin kinase, which phosphorylates the light activated form of rhodopsin, has been cloned and has been designated GRK1. βARK (also called $\beta ARK1$) is designated GRK2, and $\beta ARK2$ is designated GRK3 (41). Additional kinases termed GRK4, GRK5, and GRK6 also have been cloned and partially characterized (42–44). GRKs 2, 3, 5 and 6 are all expressed in the lung. The primary structures of these kinases suggest that they may have different regulatory properties or utilize different receptors for substrates. The most extensive studies in regard to substrates have been carried out using βARK. This kinase is known to phosphorylate β_1AR, β_2AR, $\alpha_{2A}AR$, $\alpha_{2B}AR$, M2 muscarinic receptors, substance P receptors, the thrombin receptor, and the delta-opioid receptor. As such results accumulate, it appears that GRKs may subserve a broad role in G protein–coupled receptor biology, where they act to phosphorylate agonist-occupied receptors quenching signal transduction. It should be noted that some G protein–coupled receptors do not undergo phosphorylation during agonist occupancy. Neither the β_3AR nor the $\alpha_{2C}AR$ appear to undergo phosphorylation by βARK or any other kinase during agonist occupancy (45,46). Presumably, desensitization is disadvantageous for these receptors, and they have evolved to lack the structural features necessary for this rapid form of regulation.

DETERMINANTS OF β_2AR SEQUESTRATION

After more prolonged agonist exposure (maximal effect observed in ~30 minutes), cell surface β_2AR undergoes a translocation from the cell surface to a subcellular compartment. This internalization process is termed "sequestration." The mechanism of sequestration is not known; however, the process occurs only in response to agonist-occupancy, is cAMP-independent, does not require palmitoylation or phosphorylation, and is not dependent on receptor coupling to G_s [reviewed in (47)]. In some cells, sequestration effectively removes as many as 70% of cell surface receptors. If there is not much "receptor reserve," sequestration then becomes an important mechanism of desensitization. Given that it occurs after phosphorylation, but before downregulation, the process may play a role in this intermediate time period. Data also suggest that the sequestered receptor can be rapidly recycled to the cell surface. The compartment(s) where the sequestered receptors have been localized are rich in phosphatases, and evidence suggests that sequestration may also serve as a mechanism of dephosphorylation of the receptor (48). Little is known about the molecular determinants of sequestration. A sequence in the seventh trans-

membrane spanning domain, NPLIY, is similar to the NPXXY motif that has been shown to be critical for internalization of the LDL receptor. When this region was mutated in the β_2AR, agonist-promoted sequestration was abolished (49). However, several adrenergic receptors that do not sequester (β_3AR and $\alpha_{2C}AR$) also have similar sequences, suggesting that this motif may be necessary, but not sufficient for the process.

DETERMINANTS OF β_2AR DOWNREGULATION

After more prolonged exposure to agonist, a net loss of cellular receptors (regardless of the compartment) occurs. This process, termed *downregulation*, is first observed after 3 to 6 hours of agonist exposure. Downregulation of β_2AR is due to both receptor-protein degradation and to a decrease in receptor production. The latter is due to both a decrease in transcription and to a degradation of messenger ribonucleic acid (mRNA) transcripts (50,51). Destabilization of β_2AR mRNA is apparently due to the binding of a cAMP-dependent protein to a destabilization sequence in the $3'$ untranslated region of the gene (52). Interestingly, in the $5'$ untranslated region of the gene, a cAMP response element is present that has been shown to increase transcription (53). However, the effect is short-lived and may serve to dampen downregulation response during the first few hours of agonist exposure.

The molecular requirements at the level of the receptor for downregulation are not well-defined. Neither phosphorylation, palmitoylation, G protein–coupling, or sequestration are required for downregulation, and the process occurs during exposures to both high (micromolar) and low (nanomolar or less) concentrations of agonist. It is attractive to consider that downregulation during low-dose agonist exposure is caused by cAMP-dependent events primarily operating at the level of transcription or message stability, while during high doses of agonist exposure, other events such as sequestration, lead to protein degradation. This, however, is purely speculative. One study suggests that PKA-mediated phosphorylation of the receptor is required for full downregulation (54). Tyrosine residues in the cytoplasmic tail also are necessary for agonist-promoted downregulation (55). Downregulation can be conferred to the β_3AR by substitution of its cytoplasmic tail with that of the β_2AR, implying that a key determinant may lie in this region (33). Finally, as will be discussed, regions in the extracellular amino terminus appear to be important in dictating the extent of agonist-promoted downregulation of the β_2AR (56).

β_2AR DESENSITIZATION TO AGONIST IN THE TREATMENT OF ASTHMA

The processes discussed earlier, which result in β_2AR desensitization, likely have evolved to meet homeostatic needs of intact organisms. It is intriguing to consider whether desensitization might limit the therapeutic effectiveness of administered agonist. This has been studied by a number of investigators in regard to tachyphylaxis to chronic β-agonist administration in the treatment of asthma. Some studies have found tachyphylaxis to the bronchodilating effects of β-agonist during long-term administration, while other studies have not (57–64). To explore this at the cellular level, a recent study determined whether administration of standard doses of inhaled β-agonist in humans caused desensitization of lung-cell β_2AR (65). Normal subjects underwent bronchoscopy with harvesting of bronchial epithelial cells and alveolar macrophages. β_2AR expression and function were assessed *in vitro* with both cell types. Subjects then were administered inhaled metaproterenol (10mg) every 4 hours for 6 consecutive doses. After such treatment, bronchoscopy with cell harvesting from the contralateral lung was then carried out as before, and receptor expression and function determined. The results are summarized in Figure 4. β_2AR expression decreased ~65% in both bronchial epithelial cells and alveolar macrophages after the *in vivo* metaproterenol exposure. Receptor function also was depressed in both cell types. For alveolar macrophage β_2AR, a very extensive desensitization was observed. Prior to *in vivo* β-agonist treatment, stimulation by 10μM isoproterenol *in vitro* caused a ~12-fold increase in macrophage intracellular cAMP. After *in vivo* β-agonist exposure, the harvested macrophages showed virtually no response to isoproterenol (Fig. 4). In contrast, forskolin-stimulated cAMP responses were not decreased. Prostaglandin (PG)E₂ responses also decreased somewhat, but not nearly to the level found with the isoproterenol responses. In bronchial epithelial cells, *in vivo* exposure to inhaled metaproterenol induced a desensitization of the β_2AR which was not as profound, amounting to ~50% desensitization. Again, no decrements in forskolin-stimulated levels were noted, and PGE₂ responses were not depressed. Taken together, these results indicate that at the cellular level, administration of β-agonists in conventional doses causes desensitization of macrophage and epithelial β_2AR.

However, these results are not evidence for clinical tachyphylaxis to the bronchodilating effects of β-agonist. Because of the limitations of the cell types which are available by bronchoscopy, it is not possible to address whether desensitization occurs at β_2AR expressed on bronchial smooth muscle cells, which are the major sites of therapeutic action of β-agonists in the treatment of asthma. Furthermore, it should be stressed that whether physiologic refractoriness actually occurs at the level of a given organ function depends on the relationship between the second messenger (in this case, cAMP) and the biologic response. Ultimately, whether tachyphylaxis occurs depends on whether the residual level of cAMP stimulation in a given cell is sufficient to provide for the required

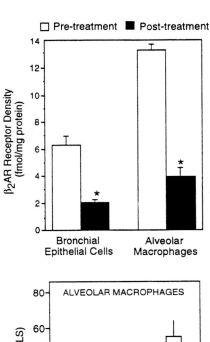

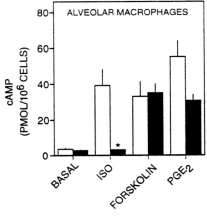

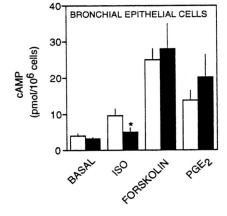

FIG. 4. Effects of *in vivo* agonist administration on human lung-cell β_2AR expression and function. Normal subjects underwent bronchoscopy with harvesting of epithelial cells and macrophages. They were then treated with 10 mg metaproterenol by inhalation every 4 hours for 6 doses, and underwent a second bronchoscopy with cell harvesting. β_2AR expression on the cells was determined by radioligand binding and function assessed *in vitro* by measuring cAMP accumulation during exposure to the indicated stimulants. Both β_2AR expression and function were significantly reduced by *in vivo* agonist administration. Shown are the mean results from 8 subjects. *,P value is 0.007 or less as compared to pretreatment.

clinical response. Finally, small degrees of tachyphylaxis, as have been reported in some of the aforementioned studies, may not necessarily be clinically relevant, such tachyphylaxis may not limit the therapeutic usefulness of a pharmacologic agent and may be evident only upon laboratory testing.

The mechanisms responsible for the lung-cell desensitization observed in these types of studies is unknown. The concentration of inhaled β-agonist in the fluid of the large airways has been estimated to be 100 μM to 1.0 mM, and in the smaller airways to be 1.0 to 10 μM (66). If such concentrations of agonist are, in fact, present at the level of the receptor, then all three of the mechanisms previously noted are possible. Given the potential for there to be little receptor reserve in these cells, the extent of receptor loss that is encountered probably accounts for some portion of depressed β2AR cellular responses that were observed. Both cell types demonstrated downregulation of receptor expression to the same extent, yet macrophage β2AR-desensitization was considerably more extensive than that observed with epithelial cell β2AR. This suggests that mechanisms other than downregulation may be important under the conditions of this study. Recently, using site-directed mutagenesis and recombinant expression, cell lines that express physiologic levels of β2AR lacking the ability to undergo downregulation, phosphorylation by PKA, and phosphorylation by βARK were developed. These were then exposed to 1 μm isoproterenol for 24 hours, and the receptor function assessed using whole-cell cAMP assays. Using this approach, it was found that both downregulation and phosphorylation by βARK were important determinants of desensitization during long-term agonist exposure (McGraw D., Liggett S., unpublished observations).

GENETIC VARIATION OF β2AR STRUCTURE

A number of studies using various human and nonhuman models have suggested that β2AR dysfunction occurs during asthma [reviewed in (1)]. Early studies utilizing circulating lymphocyte or neutrophil β2AR (acting as potential surrogates for lung receptors) showed depressed expression or function of these β2AR, and, in some cases, a correlation with the severity of asthma. On the other hand, a number of studies showed no differences between asthmatics and nonasthmatics in regard to circulating-cell β2AR expression or function. It is also clear that in some studies, altered receptor function was the result of concomitant use of β-adrenoceptor agonists in the asthmatic group. In guinea-pig ovalbumin-sensitized models of asthma, β2AR expression has shown to be depressed (67,68). In another animal model, the Basenji greyhound dog, which displays bronchial hyperreactivity, a dysfunctional β2AR has been reported (69). In viral models, β2AR responsiveness has been reported to be depressed

(70,71). Studies of autopsy-derived tissues from normal subjects and from those who had died of asthma have shown varied results, including increases and decreases in expression, and no changes or decreased function of the receptor (72–74). Taken together, the previous studies suggest a dysfunctional β2AR may have some role in the pathogenesis of asthma, or accompanies asthma in some individuals, contributing to the asthmatic phenotype. It is possible that altered β2AR function in asthmatics and/or the interindividual variation in the response to β-agonist may be caused by mutations in the gene encoding the receptor (6,56,75–79). Reishaus et al. (75) developed a screening technique for identification of variations from wild-type β2AR deoxyribonucleic acid (DNA) sequence using temperature gradient gel electrophoresis (TGGE). Blood samples were obtained from 56 normal and 51 asthmatic subjects, and genomic DNA was extracted from lymphocytes. DNA samples were then subjected to five overlapping polymerase chain reactions, and the products subjected to TGGE. All samples that were positive for a deviation from wild-type by TGGE were subsequently directly sequenced by the dideoxy method. Using the previously mentioned approach, a deviation from wild-type sequence was identified at nucleic acids 46, 79, 100, 252, 491, 523, 1053, 1098, and 1239. These correspond to the triplet codons at positions 16, 27, 34, 84, 164, 175, 351, 366, and 413 (Fig. 5). Most of these deviations were common and, henceforth, will be termed "polymorphisms." In some cases, the polymorphisms at the nucleotide level did not result in a change in the amino acid (darkened residues of Fig. 5). However, nucleotide changes at codons 16, 27, 34, and 164, resulted in a change in the encoded amino acids, and have been referred to as Arg16→Gly, Gln27→Glu, Met34→Val, and Thr164→Ile. In this initial study, no differences in the distribution of these polymorphisms between the normal and the asthmatic group were found. The Arg16→Gly polymorphism occurred in the homozygous state in approximately 50% of the subjects, and the Gln27→Glu polymorphism occurred in the homozygous state in approximately 25% of subjects. It is clear that the frequency of these variants is sufficiently high to raise the issue of what sequence is, indeed, "wild-type." For purposes of continuity, it is useful to consider the sequence as originally reported by Kobilka et al. (80) with the cloning of the human β2AR as wild-type. The Val34→Met polymorphism was found in only one subject in the heterozygous state. The Thr164→Ile polymorphism was only found in the heterozygous state, in 3% of subjects. Subsequent studies have revealed that the frequency of heterozygotes for this polymorphism appears to be in the range of 6% to 8%. In some cases, the Art16→Gly and Gln27→Glu polymorphisms occur together; however, the frequency of this form of the receptor was the same between the two groups. It was considered that some of the subjects in the normal group had subclinical asthma and, thus, were not

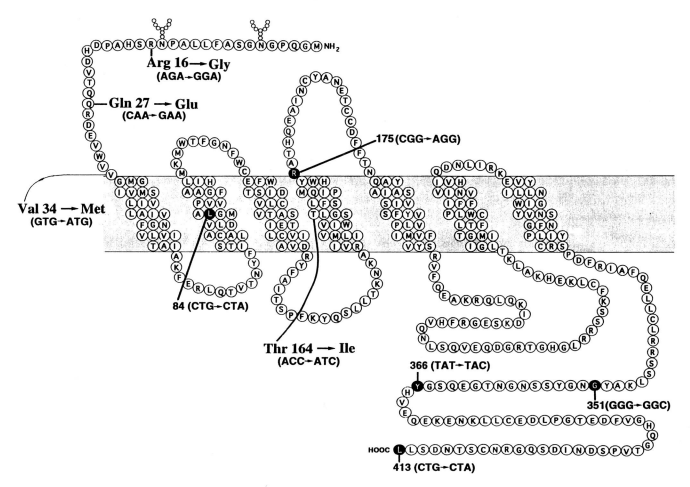

FIG. 5. Polymorphisms of the human β₂-adrenergic receptor. Shown are the 9 polymorphisms that have been identified in cohorts of normal subjects and asthmatics. The darkened residues indicate codons where the nucleic acid change did not result in a change in the encoded amino acid. Four polymorphisms did result in amino-acid changes at positions 16, 27, 34 and 164 as shown. In parentheses are the nucleic-acid sequences for the codon at the indicated polymorphic site.

truly normal. Methacholine challenge testing, therefore, was performed in 10 subjects who were homozygous for the double polymorphism at positions of 16 and 27. All had normal baseline pulmonary function, and 9 of 10 were not reactive to methacholine. This suggests that mutations in the β₂AR coding block region were not a major cause of asthma. However, a clustering of severe, chronic oral steroid-dependent asthmatics with the Arg16→Gly polymorphism was noted, and asthmatics who required immunotherapy were more likely to have this polymorphism.

While β₂AR polymorphisms may not be major causes of asthma, *they may act as disease modifiers.* One approach to study this is to mimic each polymorphism by site-specific oligonucleotide-directed mutagenesis of the β₂AR "wild-type" cDNA. These constructs can then be subcloned into mammalian expression vectors and transfected into cells such as Chinese hamster fibroblasts. [These cells do not natively express β₂AR]. These per-

manent cell lines expressing β₂AR variants then can be studied to assess their biochemical and pharmacologic properties (6,56). The Val34→Met polymorphism is indistinguishable from wild-type. The Thr164→Ile receptor displays a number of different abnormalities (6). In agonist competition studies, this receptor has lower affinity (~4-fold) for epinephrine, norepinephrine, and isoproterenol. These agonists have hydroxyl group on their β-carbons, and it has been hypothesized that these interact with Ser165 in the ligand-binding pocket of the receptor. Dopamine and dobutamine do not have β-hydroxyl groups: these agonists had equal affinities for wild-type and the Thr164→Ile variant, supporting the concept that the binding affinities of catecholamines is decreased in this mutant due to an altered interaction between the β-hydroxyl group and the receptor.

In functional studies, the Thr164→Ile receptor was found to be substantially impaired (Fig. 6). Maximal agonist-stimulated adenylyl cyclase activities of this recep-

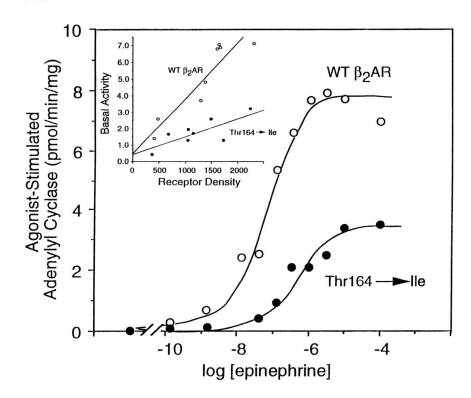

FIG. 6. Receptor phenotype of the Thr164→Ile β2-adrenergic receptor polymorphism. As compared to wild-type β2AR, this variant displayed a decreased maximal agonist stimulation of adenylyl cyclase and an increased EC_{50} (decreased potency) for stimulation by catecholamines. In addition, regardless of the level of expression, the basal level of adenylyl cyclase activity was also lower for the Thr164→Ile receptor (*inset*).

tor were only ~50% that of the wild-type β2AR. In addition, the concentration that attained 50% maximal stimulation (EC_{50}) for the response was ~3-fold higher with this mutant. Figure 6 also demonstrates that the basal (agonist-independent) adenylyl cyclase levels also were decreased with this mutant as compared to wild-type. The basis for this functional defect appears to be in an impairment of the receptor to form the high-affinity-agonist-receptor-G protein complex (6).

On further studies, which are more extensively detailed elsewhere, it was shown that the different polymorphic forms of the receptor undergo different degrees of agonist-promoted downregulation (56). The results of these studies are summarized in Figure 7A. Under these conditions, wild-type β2AR-expressed CHW cells underwent a ~26% downregulation. On the other hand, the Arg16→Gly receptor underwent an enhanced downregulation, amounting to a ~41% decrease in expression. In contrast, the Gln27→Glu receptor underwent no detectable downregulation. These differences were found to be due to alterations at the level of receptor protein degradation, rather than at the level of transcription or message stability.

Green et al. (77) have undertaken studies of receptor regulation using human bronchial smooth muscle cells in primary culture that natively express these different polymorphisms. This was done for several reasons. In these recombinant studies, β2AR expression was being driven by promoter elements in the expression vector that was utilized for the transfections. Thus, the effects of polymorphisms on downregulation when expression is under

control of the natural promoter was not known. In addition, it was not clear that events in fibroblasts accurately reflected similar events in a relevant cell type, such as smooth muscle. Finally, because the cells used in recombinant studies do not natively express βAR, they may lack cell-specific components, which may be involved in the process of receptor downregulation. The only defect that was noted was the level of agonist-promoted downregulation between the different polymorphic forms of the receptor at positions 16 and 27 (Fig. 7B). After 24 hours of agonist exposure, wild-type receptor underwent a ~77% downregulation in these bronchial smooth muscle cells. The Arg16→Gly form of the receptor displayed substantially greater downregulation which amounted to a ~96% loss of receptor expression. On the other hand, the Gln27→Glu form of the receptor displayed much less downregulation, amounting to only ~30% loss of receptor after 24 hours of agonist exposure. The results from these studies with bronchial smooth muscle cells confirmed what was found in the recombinant studies: the Arg16→Gly receptor undergoes enhanced agonist-promoted downregulation while the Gln27→Glu receptor is relatively resistant to such regulation.

Having defined the phenotypic characteristics of the different receptors, Liggett and co-workers have begun to investigate their potential role in asthma (78,79,81,83). The first study undertaken assessed whether the Arg16→Gly polymorphism was associated with nocturnal asthma (81). In this asthmatic phenotype, β2AR have been reported to undergo downregulation between 4:00 P.M. and 4:00 A.M.

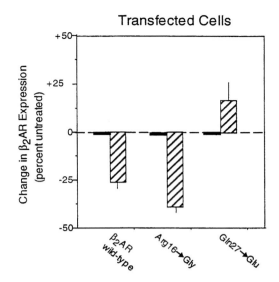

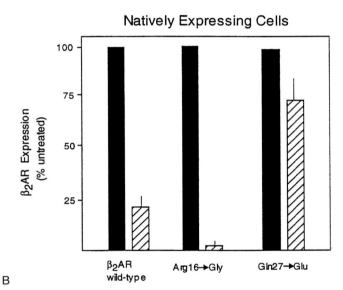

FIG. 7. Receptor phenotypes of β₂-adrenergic receptor polymorphisms at positions 16 and 27. Cells were exposed to media alone or media with 10 μM isoproterenol for 24 hours. Results using Chinese hamster fibroblasts transfected with wild-type or mutated cDNA for the β₂AR or a polymorphic receptor are shown in **A**. In **B**, human bronchial smooth muscle cells obtained at autopsy were cultured, the β₂AR genotype determined by allele specific polymerase chain reactions, and cells with the indicated genotypes exposed to agonist. Taken together, the results of both types of studies reveal that the Arg16→Gly receptor downregulates to a greater extent, and that the Gln27→Glu receptor is relatively resistant to agonist-promoted downregulation.

(82). In nonnocturnal asthmatics and normal individuals, such downregulation is not observed (82). The stimuli for downregulation presumably are endogenous catecholamines, which peak earlier in the evening. Since the

Arg16→Gly receptor undergoes extensive downregulation, we considered that this may represent the genetic basis of this asthmatic phenotype. Consecutive asthmatics who were not receiving oral corticosteroids underwent evening and morning peak expiratory flow rate (PEFR) measurements and were categorized as nocturnal if the PEFR decreased by 20% overnight for 5 consecutive nights. Nonnocturnal asthmatics were defined as those who had less than 10% PEFR overnight decrements for 5 consecutive nights. Twenty-three nocturnal asthmatics and 22 nonnocturnal asthmatics then underwent β₂AR genotyping in a blinded fashion at loci 16, 27, and 164. The results are summarized in Figure 8. The data clearly indicate an overrepresentation of Arg16→Gly allele (here referred to as Gly16) in the nocturnal group. In patients with nocturnal asthma, there were 37 Gly16 alleles as compared to 9 Arg16 alleles. In the nonnocturnal asthmatic group, there was an equal distribution of these alleles. This was significant at P = 0.007 with an odds ratio of 3.8. No differences in the allele frequencies at position 27 between the 2 groups were noted. The Ile164 polymorphism was found in the heterozygous state in only 3 subjects. The overrepresentation of Gly16 was also evident when only the homozygous states were analyzed. Of the 18 nocturnal asthmatic patients who were homozygous at this position, 16 (89%) were homozygous for Gly16. Nonnocturnal asthmatics had an equal distribution of homozygotes for Gly16 and Arg16. The odds ratio for this comparison was 7.0 for having nocturnal asthma if one was homozygous for Gly16. Similar findings were obtained when patients were categorized as homozygous for Gly16 or not homozygous for Gly16 (i.e., heterozygotes and Arg16 homozygotes).

It was also intriguing to assess the prevalence of the Gly16 polymorphism with nocturnal asthma as defined historically, rather than the more strict PEFR decrement criteria. Of the 31 asthmatics with histories of nocturnal awakening occurring at least once per week for 12 consecutive months, 74% had the homozygous Gly16 polymorphism, while among those without nocturnal histories, only 7% were homozygous for Gly16 (p<0.0001, odds ratio = 33). It also was determined that these findings with the Gly16 polymorphism were not simply a reflection of more severe asthma in the nocturnal group. Overall, the nocturnal group did have a lower-percent predicted forced expiratory volume in one second (FEV₁) as compared to the nonnocturnal group. However, the percent predicted FEV₁ for those patients who did or did not have the homozygous 16 polymorphisms, regardless of their nocturnal vs. nonnocturnal phenotype, were not statistically different. In addition, the prevalence for the Gly16 polymorphisms in these asthmatics based on whether they were defined as mild (FEV₁>70% predicted) or moderate, was assessed, and there was no overrepresentation of the polymorphism in the moderately severe group. Of 13 moderate asthmatics defined, 61% had the Gly16 polymorphism; of the 32 mild asthmatics, 50% had the polymorphism. Finally, of those

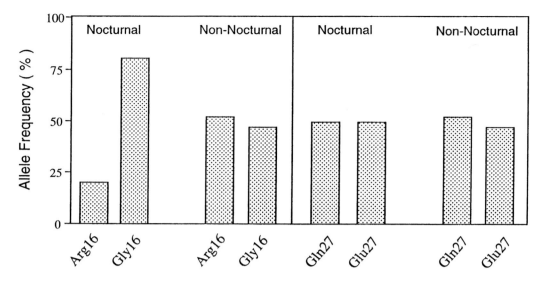

FIG. 8. Allele frequencies of β₂-adrenergic receptor polymorphisms at positions 16 and 27 in nocturnal and nonnocturnal asthmatics. The overrepresentation of the Gly16 allele in nocturnal asthma was significant at P = 0.007 (odds ratio 3.8). No differences were noted in the distribution of polymorphisms at position 27.

originally assigned to the nonnocturnal cohort by PEFR criteria, but who had the homozygous Gly16 polymorphism, 88% had positive histories of nocturnal asthma, whereas in the same group in those without homozygous Gly16, only 7% had positive nocturnal histories. These data are consistent with the Gly16 polymorphism predisposing patients with asthma to develop the nocturnal asthma.

An issue to be explored further is whether β₂AR polymorphisms may play a role in establishing bronchial hyperreactivity (83). The basis for this is the concept that β₂AR are under constant dynamic regulation by either endogenous catecholamines, or by exogenously administered β-agonists. Thus, the level of receptor expression of the Glu27 variant (relatively resistent to downregulation) would be expected to be higher than that of the "wild-type" (Gln27) receptor. As such, the Glu27 receptor might provide a protective effect against nonspecific bronchial hyperreactivity. To address this, 65 asthmatics underwent methacholine challenge testing, and in a blinded fashion were genotyped at positions 16 and 27. As was predicted from the *in vitro* phenotyping, patients with the Glu27 polymorphism had lower bronchial hyperreactivity (higher $PD_{20}s$). Patients who were homozygous for Gln27 had a geometric mean PD_{20} of 0.86 μmol. By contrast, those who were homozygous for Glu27 had geometric mean $PD_{20}s$ of 3.23 μM (p = 0.03). Heterozygotes had an intermediate value. The methacholine pD_{20} values for patients with different alleles at position 16 were not statistically different.

CONCLUSIONS

The β₂AR has been extensively studied at the molecular level. Indeed, the greatest amount of structure/func-

tion information has accumulated with this receptor as compared to any other G protein–coupled receptor. The key domains of the receptor responsible for ligand binding, and the events of G protein–coupling and agonist regulation through receptor phosphorylation, sequestration, and downregulation now are known. Thus, we are now in a position to understand the signal transduction process at a fundamental mechanistic level, how it occurs under normal physiologic conditions, how the process is modified by agonists and other agents, as well as pathologic processes, and how to modulate receptor function for therapeutic purposes. It also appears that β₂AR structure is polymorphic within the population, with some of these polymorphisms having different pharmacologic properties. Initial studies do not suggest that any polymorphism is a major cause of asthma. However, a contribution in combination with other genetic factors cannot be excluded. Studies to date do suggest that certain polymorphic forms may correlate with various asthmatic subphenotypes, the degree of severity, or the response to therapy. As such, β₂AR polymorphisms may act primarily as disease modifiers in asthma.

ACKNOWLEDGMENTS

The work reported here is funded by NIH grants HL45967, HL53436, and HL41496.

REFERENCES

1. Liggett SB. Molecular basis of G-protein coupled receptor signalling. In: Crystal R, West JB, Weibel ER, Barnes PJ, eds. *The lung: scientific foundations.* New York: Raven Press, 1995.

2. Barnes PJ. β-adrenergic receptors and their regulation. *Am J Respir Crit Care Med* 1995;152:838–860.

3. Strader CD, Candelore MR, Hill WS, Sigal IS, and Dixon RAF. Identification of two serine residues involved in agonist activation of the β-adrenergic receptor. *J Biol Chem* 1989;264:13572–13578.

4. Strader CD, Sigal IS, Candelore MR, Rands E, Hill WS, Dixon RAF. Conserved aspartic acid residues 79 and 113 of the β-adrenergic receptor have different roles in receptor function. *J Biol Chem* 1988; 263:10267–10271.

5. Strader CD, Gaffney T, Sugg EE, Candelore MR, Keys R, Patchett AA, Dixon RAF. Allele-specific activation of genetically engineered receptors. *J Biol Chem* 1995;266:5–8.

6. Green SA, Cole G, Jacinto M, Innis M, Liggett SB. A polymorphism of the human β2-adrenergic receptor within the fourth transmembrane domain alters ligand binding and functional properties of the receptor. *J Biol Chem* 1993;268:23116–23121.

7. Strader CD, Candelore MR, Hill WS, Dixon RAF, Sigal IS. A single amino acid substitution in the β-adrenergic receptor promotes partial agonist activity from antagonists. *J Biol Chem* 1989;264:16470–16477.

8. Samama P, Pei G, Costa T, Cotecchia S, Lefkowitz RJ. Negative antagonists promote an inactive conformation of the β2-adrenergic receptor. *Mol Pharmacol* 1994;45:390–394.

9. Bond RA, Leff P, Johnson TD, et al. Physiological effects of inverse agonists in transgenic mice with myocardial overexpression of the β2-adrenoceptor. *Nature* 1995;374:272–275.

10. Milano CA, Allen LF, Rockman HA, et al. Enhanced myocardial function in transgenic mice overexpressing the β2-adrenergic receptor. *Science* 1994;264:582–586.

11. O'Dowd BF, Hnatowich M, Regan JW, Leader WM, Caron MG, Lefkowitz RJ. Site-directed mutagenesis of the cytoplasmic domains of the human β2-adrenergic receptor. *J Biol Chem* 1988;263: 15985–15992.

12. Hausdorff WP, Hnatowich M, O'Dowd BF, Caron MG, Lefkowitz RJ. A mutation of the β2-adrenergic receptor impairs agonist activation of adenylyl cyclase without affecting high affinity agonist binding. *J Biol Chem* 1990;265:1388–1393.

13. Liggett SB, Caron MG, Lefkowitz RJ, Hnatowich M. Coupling of a mutated form of the human β2-adrenergic receptor to Gi and Gs. *J Biol Chem* 1991;266:4816–4821.

14. Eason MG, Kurose H, Holt BD, Raymond JR, Liggett SB. Simultaneous coupling of α2-adrenergic receptors to two G-proteins with opposing effects: Subtype-selective coupling of α2C10, α2C4 and α2C2 adrenergic receptors to Gi and Gs. *J Biol Chem* 1992;267:15795–15801.

15. Eason MG, Jacinto MT, Liggett SB. Contribution of ligand structure to activation of α2AR subtype coupling to Gs. *Mol Pharmacol* 1994;45:696–702.

16. Eason MG, Liggett SB. Identification of a Gs coupling domain in the amino-terminus of the third intracellular loop of the α2A-adrenergic receptor. Evidence for distinct structural determinnants that confer Gs and Gi coupling. *J Biol Chem* 1995;270:24753–24760.

17. Cheung AH, Huang RC, Strader CD. Involvement of specific hydrophobic, but not hydrophilic, amino acids in the third intracellular loop of the β-adrenergic receptor in the activation of Gs. *Mol Pharmacol* 1992;41:1061–1065.

18. Strader CD, Dixon RAF, Cheung AH, Candelore MR, Blake AD, Sigal IS. Mutations that uncouple the β-adrenergic receptor from Gs and increase agonist affinity. *J Biol Chem* 1987;262:16439–16443.

19. Kjelsberg MA, Cotecchia S, Ostrowski J, Caron MG, Lefkowitz RJ. Constitutive activation of the α1B-adrenergic receptor by all amino acid substitutions at a single site. *J Biol Chem* 1992;267:1430–1433.

20. Samama P, Cotecchia S, Costa T, Lefkowitz RJ. A mutation-induced activated state of the β2-adrenergic receptor. *J Biol Chem* 1993;268: 4625–4636.

21. O'Dowd BF, Hnatowich M, Caron MG, Lefkowitz RJ, Bouvier M. Palmitoylation of the human β2-adrenergic receptor. Mutation of Cys341 in the carboxyl tail leads to an uncoupled nonpalmitoylated form of the receptor. *J Biol Chem* 1989;264:7564–7569.

22. Eason MG, Jacinto MT, Theiss CT, Liggett SB. The palmitoylated cysteine of the cytoplasmic tail of α2A-adrenergic receptors confers subtype-specific agonist-promoted downregulation. *Proc Natl Acad Sci U S A* 1994;91:11178–11182.

23. Valiquette M, Bonin H, Bouvier M. Mutation of tyrosine-350 impairs the coupling of the β2-adrenergic receptor to the stimulatory guanine nucleotide binding protein without interfering with receptor down-regulation. *Biochem* 1993;32:4979–4985.

24. Green SA, Holt BD, Liggett SB. β1- and β2-adrenergic receptors display subtype-selective coupling to Gs. *Mol Pharmacol* 1992;41: 889–893.

25. Green S, Liggett SB. A proline-rich region of the third intracellular loop imparts phenotypic β1- versus β2-adrenergic receptor coupling and sequestration. *J Biol Chem* 1994;269:26215–26219.

26. Liggett SB, Lefkowitz RJ. Regulation of receptor function by phosphorylation, sequestration and downregulation. In: Sibley D, Houslay M, eds. *Regulation of cellular signal transduction pathways by desensitization and amplification.* London: John Wiley & Sons, 1993; 71–97.

27. Benovic JL, Mayor F, Staniszewski E, Lefkowitz RJ, Caron MG. Purification and characterization of β-adrenergic receptor kinase. *J Biol Chem* 1987;262:9026–9032.

28. Benovic JL, Deblasi A, Stone WC, Caron MG, Lefkowitz RJ. β-adrenergic receptor kinase: primary structure delineates a multigene family. *Science* 1989;246:235–240.

29. Liggett SB, Bouvier M, Hausdorff WP, O'Dowd B, Caron MG, Lefkowitz RJ. Altered patterns of agonist-stimulated cAMP accumulation in cells expressing mutant β2-adrenergic receptors lacking phosporylation sites. *Mol Pharmacol* 1989;36:641–646.

30. Hausdorff WP, Bouvier M, O'Dowd BF, Irons GP, Caron MG, Lefkowitz RJ. Phosphorylation sites on two domains of the β2-adrenergic receptor are involved in distinct pathways of receptor desensitization. *J Biol Chem* 1989;264:12657–12665.

31. Lohse MJ, Benovic JL, Caron MG, Lefkowitz RJ. Multiple pathways of rapid β2-adrenergic receptor desensitization. *J Biol Chem* 1990;265: 3202–3209.

32. Pitcher J, Lohse MJ, Codina J, Caron MG, Lefkowitz RJ. Desensitization of the isolated β2-adrenergic receptor by β-adrenergic receptor kinase, cAMP-dependent protein kinase, and protein kinase C occurs via distinct molecular mechanisms. *Biochem* 1992;31:3193–3197.

33. Liggett SB, Freedman NJ, Schwinn DA, Lefkowitz RJ. Structural basis for receptor subtype specific regulation revealed by a chimeric β2/β2-adrenergic receptor. *Proc Natl Acad Sci U S A* 1993;90:3665–3669.

34. Benovic JL, Kuhn J, Weyland I, Codina J, Caron JG, Lefkowitz RJ. Functional desensitization of the isolated β-adrenergic receptor by the β-adrenergic receptor kinase: potential role of an analog for the retinal protein arrestin. *Proc Natl Acad Sci U S A* 1987;84:8879–8882.

35. Lohse MJ, Benovic JL, Codina J, Caron MG, Lefkowitz RJ. β-arrestin: a protein that regulates β-adrenergic receptor function. *Science* 1990;248:1547–1550.

36. Liggett SB, Ostrowski J, Chestnut LC, Kurose H, Raymond JR, Caron MG, Lefkowitz RJ. Sites in the third intracellular loop of the α2A-adrenergic receptor confer short term agonist-promoted desensitization: evidence for a receptor kinase-mediated mechanism. *J Biol Chem* 1992;267:4740–4746.

37. Onorato JJ, Palczewski K, Regan JW, Caron MG, Lefkowitz RJ, Benovic JL. The role of acidic amino acids in peptide substrates of the β-adrenergic receptor kinase and rhodopsin kinase. *Biochem* 1991;30: 5118–5125.

38. Eason MG, Moreira SP, Liggett SB. Four consecutive serines in the third intracellular loop are the sites for βARK-mediated phosphorylation and desensitization of the α2A-adrenergic receptor. *J Biol Chem* 1995;270:4681–4688.

39. Lefkowitz RJ. G protein-coupled receptor kinases. *Cell* 1993;74:409–412.

40. Inglese J, Freedman NJ, Koch WJ, Lefkowitz RJ. Structure and mechanism of the G protein-coupled receptor kinases. *J Biol Chem* 1993;268:23735–23738.

41. Benovic JL, Onorato JJ, Arriza JL, et al. Cloning, expression, chromosolmal localization of β-adrenergic receptor kinase 2. A new member of the receptor kinase family. *J Biol Chem* 1991;266:14939–14946.

42. Ambrose C, James M, Barnes G, et al. A novel G protein-coupled receptor kinase gene cloned from 4p16.3. *Human Molecular Genetics* 1992;1:697–703.

43. Kunapuli P, Benovic JL. Cloning and expression of GRK5: a member of the G protein-coupled receptor kinase family. *Proc Natl Acad Sci, USA* 1993;90:5588–5592.

44. Benovic JL, Gomez J. Molecular cloning and expression of GRK6. A new member of the G protein-coupled receptor kinase family. *J Biol Chem* 1993;268:19521–19527.

45. Liggett SB, Freedman NJ, Schwinn DA, Lefkowitz RJ. Structural basis for receptor subtype-specific regulation revealed by a chimeric β3/β2-adrenergic receptor. *Proc Natl Acad Sci U S A* 1993;90:3665–3669.

46. Eason MG, Liggett SB. Subtype-selective desensitization of α2-adren-

ergic receptors: different mechanisms control short and long term agonist-promoted desensitization of α_2C10, α_2C4 and α_2C2. *J Biol Chem* 1992;267:25473–25479.

47. Liggett SB, Lefkowitz RJ. Adrenergic receptor-coupled adenylyl cyclase systems: regulation of receptor function by phosphorylation, sequestration and downregulation. In: Sibley D, Houslay M, eds. *Regulation of cellular signal transduction pathways by desensitization and amplification.* London: John Wiley & Sons, 1993;71–97.

48. Yu SS, Hausdorff WP, Lefkowitz RJ. β-adrenergic receptor sequestration. *J Biol Chem* 1993;268:337–341.

49. Barak LS, Tiberi M, Freedman NJ, Kwatra MM, Lefkowitz RJ, Caron MG. A highly conserved tyrosine residue in G protein-coupled receptors is required for agonist-mediated β_2-adrenergic receptor sequestration. *J Biol Chem* 1994;269:2790–2795.

50. Nishikawa M, Mak JCW, Shirasaki H, Barnes PJ. Differential downregulation of pulmonary β_1-and β_2-adrenoceptor messenger RNA with prolonged *in vivo* infusion of isoprenaline. *Eur J Pharmacol* 1993; 247:131–138.

51. Hadcock JR, Wang H, Malbon CC. Agonist-induced destabilization of β-adrenergic receptor mRNA. Attenuation of glucocorticoid induced upregulation of β-adrenergic receptors. *J Biol Chem* 1992;267: 4740–4746.

52. Huang L, Tholanikunnel BG, Vakalopoulou E, Malbon CC. The M_r35,000 β-adrenergic receptor mRNA-binding protein induced by agonists requires both an AUUUA pentamer and U-rich domains for RNA recognition. *J Biol Chem* 1993;268:26769–26775.

53. Collins S, Bouvier M, Bolanowski MA, Caron MG, Lefkowitz RJ. cAMP stimulates transcription of the β_2-adrenergic receptor gene in response to short-term agonist exposure. *Proc Natl Acad Sci U S A* 1989;86:4853–4857.

54. Bouvier M, Collins S, O'Dowd BF, et al. Two Distinct Pathways for cAMP-mediated Down-regulation of the β_2-Adrenergic Receptor. *J Biol Chem* 1989;264:16786–16792.

55. Valiquette M, Bonin H, Hnatowich M, Caron MG, Lefkowitz RJ, Bouvier M. Involvement of tyrosine residues located in the carboxyl tail of the human β_2-adrenergic receptor in agonist-induced down-regulation of the receptor. *Proc Natl Acad Sci U S A* 1990;87:5089–5093.

56. Green SA, Turki J, Innis M, Liggett SB. Amino-terminal polymorphisms of the human β_2-adrenergic receptor impart distinct agonist-promoted regulatory properties. *Biochem* 1994;33:9414–9419.

57. Cockroft DW, McPharland CP, Britto SA, Swystun VA. Regular inhaled salbutamol and airway responsiveness to allergen. *Lancet* 1993; 342:833–836.

58. Newnham DM, McDevitt DG, Lipworth BJ. Bronchodilator subsensitivity after chronic dosing with eformoterol in patients with asthma. *Am J Med* 1994;97:29–37.

59. Repsher LH, Anderson JA, Bish RK, et al. Assessment of tachyphylaxis following prolonged therapy of asthma with inhaled albuterol. *Chest* 1984;85:34–38.

60. Vathenen AS, Knox AJ, Higgins BG, Britton JR, Tattersfield AE. Rebound increase in bronchial responsiveness after treatment with inhaled terbutaline. *Lancet* 1988;1:554–558.

61. Weber RW, Smith JA, Nelson HS. Aerosolised terbutaline in asthmatics: development of subsensitivity with long term administration. *J Allergy Clin Immunol* 1982;70:417–422.

62. van Wheel E, van Herwaarden CLA. Increased bronchial hyperresponsiveness after inhaling salbutamol during 1 year is not caused by subsensitization to salbutamol. *J Allergy Clin Immunol* 1990;86: 793–800.

63. O'Connor BJ, Aikman S, Barnes PJ. Tolerance to the nonbronchodilator effects of inhaled β-2 agonists in asthma. *N Engl J Med* 1992;327: 1204–1208.

64. Larsson S, Svedmyr N, Thiringer GJ. Lack of bronchial β-adrenoceptor resistance in asthmatics during long-term treatment with terbutaline. *J Allergy Clin Immunol* 1977;59:93–100.

65. Turki J, Green SA, Newman KB, Meyers MA, Liggett SB. Human lung cell β_2-Adrenergic receptors desensitize in response to *in vivo* administered β-agonist. *Am J Physiol* 1995;269:L708–L714.

66. Kerrebijn KF. Beta agonists. In: Kaliner MA, Barnes PJ, Persson CGA, eds. *Asthma: its pathology and treatment.* New York: Marcel Dekker, Inc. 1991;526–527.

67. Barnes PJ, Dollery CT, MacDermot J. Increased pulmonary α-adrenergic and reduced β-adrenergic receptors in experimental asthma. *Nature* 1980;285:569–571.

68. Gatto C, Green TP, Johnson MG, Marchessault RP, Seybold V, Johnson DE. Localization of quantitative changes in pulmonary β-receptors in ovalbumin-sensitized guinea pigs. *Am Rev Respir Dis* 1987;136:150–154.

69. Parker CW, Smith JW. Alternations in cyclic adenosine monophosphate metabolism in human bronchial asthma. Luekocyte responsiveness to β-adrenergic agents. *J Clin Invest* 1973;52:48–59.

70. Buckner CK, Clayton DE, Ain-Shoka AA, Busse WW, Dick EC, Shult P. Parainfluenza 3 infection blocks the ability of a β- adrenergic receptor agonist to inhibit antigen-induced contraction of guinea pig isolated airway smooth muscle. *J Clin Invest* 1981;376–384.

71. Busse WW. Decreased granulocyte response to isoproterenol in asthma during upper respiratory infections. *Am Rev Respir Dis* 1977;115: 783–791.

72. Sharma R, Jeffery P. Airway β-adrenoceptor number in cystic fibrosis and asthma. *Clin Sci* 1990;78:409–417.

73. Goldie RG, Spina D, Henry PJ, Lulich KM, Paterson JW. *In vitro* responsiveness of human asthmatic bronchus to carbachol, histamine, β-adrenoceptor agonists and theophylline. *Br J Clin Pharmac* 1986;22: 669–676.

74. Spina D, Rigby PJ, Paterson JW, Goldie RG. Autoradiogrphic localization of β-adrenoceptors in asthmatic human lung. *Am Rev Respir Dis* 1989;140:1410–1415.

75. Reihsaus E, Innis M, MacIntyre N, Liggett SB. Mutations in the gene rncoding for the β_2-adrenergic receptor in normal and asthmatic subjects. *Am J Resp Cell Mol Biol* 1993;8:334–339.

76. Green SA, Turki J, Hall IP, Liggett SB. Implications of genetic variability of human β_2-adrenergic receptor structure. *Pulm Pharmacol* 1995;8:1–11.

77. Green SA, Turki J, Bejarano P, Hall IP, Liggett SB. Influence of β_2-adrenergic receptor genotypes on signal transduction in human airway smooth muscle cells. *Am J Resp Cell Mol Biol* 1995;13:25–33.

78. Liggett SB. Genetics of β_2-adrenergic receptor variants in asthma. *Clin and Exp Allergy* 1995;25:89–94.

79. Liggett SB. The genetics of β_2-adrenergic receptor polymorphisms: relevance to receptor function and asthmatic phenotypes. In: Liggett SB, Meyer DA, eds. *The genetics of asthma.* New York: Marcel Dekker, 1996;455–478.

80. Kobilka BK, Dixon RA, Frielle T, et al. cDNA for the human β_2-adrenergic receptor: a protein with multiple membrane-spanning domains and encoded by a gene whose chromosomal location is shared with that of the receptor for platelet-derived growth factor. *Proc Natl Acad Sci U S A* 1987;84:46–50.

81. Turki J, Pak J, Green S, Martin R, Liggett SB. Genetic polymorphisms of the β_2-adrenergic receptor in nocturnal and non-nocturnal asthma: evidence that Gly 16 correlates with the nocturnal phenotype. *J Clin Invest* 1995;95:1635–1641.

82. Szefler SJ, Ando R, Cicutto LC, Surs W, Hill MR, Martin RJ. Plasma histamine, epinephrine, cortisol, and leukocyte β-adrenergic receptors in nocturnal asthma. *Clin Pharmacol Ther* 1991;49:59–68.

83. Hall IP, Wheatley A, Wilding P, Liggett SB. Association of the Glu27 β_2-adrenoceptor polymorphism with lower airway reactivity in asthmatic subjects. *Lancet* 1995;345:1213–1214.

Asthma, edited by P.J. Barnes, M.M. Grunstein, A.R. Leff, and A.J. Woolcock.
Lippincott–Raven Publishers, Philadelphia © 1997.

▪ 25 ▪

Intracellular Signaling Mechanisms

The Second Messengers

David A. Bass

Vocabulary of Signal Transduction—"Second Messengers"
  Calcium
  Protein-protein Binding: The Src and Pleckstrin Homology Domains
  Guanine Nucleotide-binding Proteins
  Protein Phosphorylation and Dephosphorylation by Kinases and Phosphatases
Protein Kinase A (cAMP-activated Protein Kinase)
Protein Kinase C Family
Tyrosine Kinases and Associated Signaling Pathways
  Receptor-associated Tyrosine Kinases: Src, Syk, and Janus Kinase Families
  Ras/MAP Kinase Pathways

Phosphatases
Coordinated Regulation of Related Signaling Enzymes
Lipids as Second Messengers and Autocrine Signaling Molecules
  Phospholipase C Releases Diglyceride and IP3, Which Activate Protein Kinase C and Mobilize Intracellular Calcium
  Phospholipase D and Phosphatidic Acid
  Phospholipases A2 Yield Fatty Acids and Lysophospholipids
Lipid Kinases: The PI 3-Kinase
Sphingomyelinase Releases Ceramide

Virtually every aspect of cell behavior, from growth to death, is regulated carefully in multicellular organisms. To achieve such activities as coordinated growth, muscle contraction, etc., communication between cells is necessary. For such communication, the signaling cell expresses a molecule that may either be on the cell surface (for communication during cell-cell contact) or is released into the extracellular environment as a soluble signaling molecule. Such signaling molecules can be of any chemical type, from complex proteins to dissolved gases such as nitric oxide. The signaling molecule interacts with a specific receptor on or within the "target" cell. Such receptors show great specificity for the signaling molecules. Upon bind-

ing of the signaling molecule (often now referred to as the "agonist" or "ligand"), a change is induced in the receptor that in turn causes activation of further intracellular biochemical events, which in the end result in the appropriate functional response, such as muscle contraction. For example, catecholamine (the "first messenger") interacts with the β-adrenergic receptor, which activates adenyl cyclase to increase intracellular cyclic adenosine monophosphate (cAMP) (the "second messenger"). The signaling cascades involve many carefully regulated intracellular "messengers" of diverse types. Although signaling events appear complex, it is amazing that such a limited number of signals could be combined in ways to allow highly specific regulation of every aspect of cell function. This has prompted a fine analogy: "Signal transduction is, in some ways, reminiscent of classical symphonies. Nature, like all the great composers that it created, relies on masterful variations on themes" (1).

D.A. Bass: Section of Pulmonary and Critical Care Medicine, Bowman Gray School of Medicine of Wake Forest University, Winston-Salem, North Carolina 27157-1054.

Regarding asthma, relatively little is known about the precise disruption of signaling that occurs in this disease. Bronchial hyperreactivity almost certainly reflects abnormalities of cell signaling. However, it is unknown to what degree the problem resides in the over- or underproduction of soluble intracellular signaling molecules or if it represents abnormal reactions within cells to a "normal" amount of stimulating agonists. Abnormalities of membrane receptors are discussed in Chapters 23 and 24. This chapter provides an overview of the "language" of signaling, that is, the intracellular mechanisms or "messengers" that provide the rapid on/off biochemical regulation of cellular processes.

VOCABULARY OF SIGNAL TRANSDUCTION— "SECOND MESSENGERS"

To achieve appropriate signaling, the mechanism must be able to turn on and off within the time frame of the desired response. In most cases, the signaling molecule must be capable of activation and deactivation rapidly, but also in a precisely controlled manner. Signaling can involve one of a limited number of mechanisms: a) the rapid synthesis (and then catabolism or inactivation) of a new molecule, such as cAMP, b) the mobilization (and resequestration) of a molecule, such as Ca^{2+}, which is stored in an inaccessible intracellular compartment, such as the endoplasmic reticulum, and is abruptly mobilized in response to receptor activation, c) release of a lipid mediator by hydrolysis of a membrane glycerophospholipid or sphingolipid (and rapid metabolism or reincorporation of the mediator), and d) a rapidly reversible covalent modification, such as phosphorylation by a kinase or dephosphorylation by a phosphatase, that alters the structure and function of the target molecule. These limited scenarios are played out in many specific variations.

Calcium

Functional properties of many proteins are regulated by divalent cations, especially Ca^{2+}. Calcium is a paradigm signaling molecule, as its concentration at subcellular sites is tightly regulated and can be rapidly increased or decreased. Within the cytosol, Ca^{2+} is maintained at low concentrations, 20 to 200 nM. For signaling, this concentration can be abruptly increased either by allowing influx of Ca^{2+} from the extracellular milieu (where the concentration is about 10,000 times higher than in the cytosol) or by allowing Ca^{2+} release from intracellular storage sites. Entry from the outside is controlled by voltage-operated Ca^{2+} channels, receptor-operated channels, or second messenger–operated channels (2). In nonexcitable cells, the regulation of the second messenger–operated channel may be important,

but its regulation remains a topic of controversy. In most cells, rapid increase in cytosolic Ca^{2+} is regulated by mobilization from intracellular stores.

Within cells, calcium is stored in membrane-bound compartments, including the sarcoplasmic reticulum in striated muscle, endoplasmic reticulum in most nonexcitable cells, and small vesicles separable from the endoplasmic reticulum (termed "calciosomes") in some cells, including granulocytes (3). These intracellular compartments share several important properties. The membrane of each contains a large amount of a Ca^{2+}–adenosine triphosphatase (ATPase) capable of pumping calcium against a concentration gradient from the cytosol into the intracellular vesicle. Within the vesicle, large concentrations of calcium are retained, largely by binding to a protein, calsequestrin. Calsequestrin has a high capacity and relatively low affinity for calcium. Its presence reduces the concentration gradient of free calcium between the cytosol and the intracellular storage site, thus easing the energy gradient confronted by the calcium pump. The low affinity of calsequestrin, conversely, allows rapid release of the calcium during signaling.

Three messengers can induce release from these Ca^{2+} stores: Ca^{2+} itself, cyclic adenosine diphosphate (ADP) ribose, or inositol-1,4,5-trisphosphate (IP_3) (2). Ca^{2+}-induced Ca^{2+} release (CICR) recently has been recognized as an important aspect of Ca^{2+} regulation, and is discussed further below. Cyclic ADP ribose acts on intracellular stores bearing ryanodine receptors, which are expressed in some neurons and striated muscle; the regulation of this compartment is not well understood (2) and not a major source of increased cytosolic free calcium concentrations $[(Ca^{2+})i]$ in lung cells or inflammatory cells, where the IP_3-regulated compartment predominates. Activation of this receptor by IP_3 causes opening of a Ca^{2+} channel in the vesicle membrane, allowing a sudden rush of calcium from within the vesicle to the cytosol (Fig. 1).

Activation of PLCβ1 by G protein–coupled receptors or of PLCγ1 by tyrosine kinase associated receptors results in hydrolysis of phosphatidylinositol-4,5-bisphosphate, causing a rapid increase in IP_3 within a few seconds. This causes a similarly rapid rise in $[Ca^{2+}]i$. The release of Ca^{2+} is probably hastened by the fact that Ca^{2+} itself increases the sensitivity of IP_3 receptors to IP_3 and/or can directly stimulate enhanced Ca^{2+} release. When measuring $[Ca^{2+}]i$ as an average of many cells (as in a cuvette), the mean $[Ca^{2+}]i$ begins to decrease after about 1 minute (or less), largely due a decrease in IP_3. IP_3 can be rapidly removed from the cytosol by either of two mechanisms: a phosphatase can convert it to inositol-1,4-bisphosphate, which is inactive in calcium release, or it can be phosphorylated by an IP_3-kinase to form inositol-1,3,4,5-tetrakisphosphate [Ins-1,3,4,5-P_4],

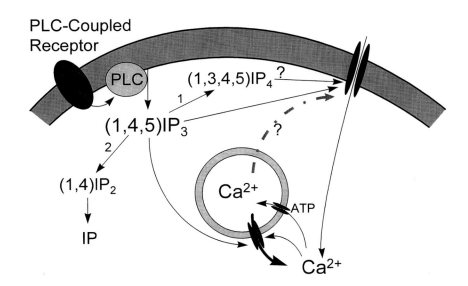

FIG. 1. Main mechanism(s) for elevation of cytosolic Ca^{2+} in lung cells and in inflammatory cells. Receptor activation is coupled to activation of phospholipase C, which cleaves membrane phosphatidylinositol-4,5-bisphosphate to release inositol-1,4,5-trisphosphate (IP_3). Initially, IP_3 releases Ca^{2+} from intracellular stores. Subsequently IP_3, probably with IP_4, may activate Ca^{2+} channels in plasma membrane, allowing influx into the cytosol. An alternative theory is that depletion of intracellular Ca^{2+} stores causes formation of a soluble messenger (*shaded gray arrow*) that activates Ca^{2+} influx.

which itself may be a messenger (see PI 3-kinase, below). The inactivation of IP_3 is rapidly followed by pumping of the free calcium out of the cell or into other intracellular storage compartments.

In many cells, there is a subsequent return to an increase in mean cytosolic calcium or a persistence of elevated Ca^{2+} that persists for a relatively prolonged period (for 10–15 min in neutrophils). This prolonged increase depends on extracellular calcium and therefore appears to involve influx of extracellular calcium through calcium channels in the plasma membrane. Ca^{2+} influx can be mediated by several mechanisms: one is by inositol phosphates themselves. Injection of 1,4,5-IP_3 (helped by some 1,3,4,5-IP_4) can induce Ca^{2+} influx, and IP_3 binding to plasma membrane has been reported (reviewed in ref. 4). Another concept is that depletion of intracellular Ca^{2+} stores causes activation of Ca^{2+} entry (5–8). The mechanism of this capacitative calcium influx is not well defined, but it may be that depletion of Ca^{2+} stores releases a small (<500 kDa) messenger and/or a small G protein that activates a Ca^{2+} current (9–14).

Signaling via $[Ca^{2+}]i$ may be manifest not only by the magnitude (peak and duration) of the mean $[Ca^{2+}]i$, but also by rapid temporal and spatial events within the cell. Studies of single cells have revealed that the elevation of $[Ca^{2+}]i$ often occurs in a series of oscillations or repeated transient spikes (15,16). For example, stimulation of neutrophils by chemotactic factors (at concentrations that stimulate motility) induce such oscillations of Ca^{2+} (16), whereas greater concentrations of such agonists (which stimulate actin polymerization and the respiratory burst) are associated with a constantly elevated $[Ca^{2+}]i$ (17,18). At low agonist concentrations, the frequency of calcium oscillations also is increased with in-

creasing concentrations of agonist, suggesting that this might be a form of digital communication to modulate subsequent cellular responses.

The increase in intracellular free calcium initially occurs at localized regions within the cell, e.g., at the site of phagocytosis (19). In many cells, the calcium transient then may spread through the cell in the form of waves, perhaps by a proposed mechanism of calcium-induced calcium release (12,15). It has also been shown that such calcium waves may spread from one cell to the next. Sanderson et al. (20) developed a preparation of ciliated pulmonary epithelium labeled with a Ca^{2+}-dependent fluorochrome, and showed that simple physical contact with one cell (or the injection into the cell of IP_3) initiated a wave of increased $[Ca^{2+}]i$ that spread between cells throughout the epithelial layer.

Many proteins directly bind calcium with affinity and specificity, which allow the calcium molecule to regulate directly that protein function. For this activity, the protein calcium binding site must have a high affinity, effective at the low concentration of calcium present even in the stimulated cell. The calcium binding site must also be highly specific and not recognize the magnesium ion present in the cytosol at about a 1,000-fold higher concentration than calcium. Other proteins interact indirectly with calcium by having a highly specific recognition of a Ca^{2+}-binding protein, calmodulin. Calmodulin is a 150–amino acid polypeptide with four high-affinity calcium binding sites. When Ca^{2+} binds to calmodulin, it causes a conformational change that allows the calmodulin to be recognized by and activate its target proteins. The most important family of calmodulin-binding proteins are the Ca^{2+}/calmodulin-dependent kinases that indirectly mediate most of the signaling by Ca^{2+} in animal cells (21).

Protein-protein Binding: The Src and Pleckstrin Homology Domains

Many signaling events involve binding of one protein to another, thus appropriately positioning the effector and its target. Such proteins contain defined regions that mediate protein-protein binding. The best characterized of these are the Src-homology 2 (SH2), Src-homology 3 (SH3), and the more recently defined pleckstrin homology (PH) domains. Each of these can fold into a compact functional module within the protein polypeptide. These modules are physically well defined (looplike) and can recognize and bind complementary motifs on target proteins.

The SH2 and SH3 domains (22) consist of about 100 and 60 amino acids, respectively. SH2 and SH3 domains mediate protein-protein binding by distinct mechanisms. The binding of the SH2 domain is to specific amino acid motifs containing a phosphotyrosine residue. Proteins with SH2 domains control biochemical pathways involving phospholipid metabolism, tyrosine phosphorylation and dephosphorylation, activation of Ras-like GTPases, gene expression, protein trafficking, and cytoskeletal architecture (23). The SH2 domains have two binding regions: one region, which is completely conserved, binds the phosphate and the tyrosine ring of the phosphotyrosine; the second binding region is more variable and provides recognition of amino acids adjacent to the phosphotyrosine. Thus, phosphorylation of the tyrosine functions as an on-off switch for SH2 binding, and binding by the adjacent residues determines which SH2 signaling protein is bound (23).

The mechanism of binding to the SH3 domain is less well defined but appears to involve binding SH3 to specific sequences of about 10 amino acids in length which are rich in proline (23,24). The proline-rich region binding SH3 usually has a characteristic helical configuration. In addition to intermediary signaling molecules, SH3 domains may be involved in activation of multiprotein enzyme complexes, such as assembly of the reduced nicotinamide adenine dinucleotide phosphate (NADPH) oxidase of neutrophils or eosinophils (25).

SH2 and SH3 domains often are present on the same protein. An interesting variation on this are "adapter" proteins, mediating the binding of two other proteins into a functional complex. An example of this is the adapter protein, Grb2, which has the structure of two SH3 motifs flanking a single SH2 domain. For example, it mediates coupling between the EGF receptor and the GDP-GTP exchange protein Sos1. Grb2 forms a complex with Sos1 through the Grb2 SH3 domains (26). With activation and autophosphorylation of the EGF receptor, the SH2 domains of GRB2 bind to the phosphotyrosine site on the receptor, which thus also recruits the Sos1 (bound to the Grb2). This brings the Sos1 to the membrane, where it is activated and in turn causes activation of Ras (27,28) (see below).

The targets of the pleckstrin homology (PH) domains are being defined; several lines of evidence suggest that they may tether signaling proteins to membranes (23,29–31).

Guanine Nucleotide-binding Proteins

Proteins regulated by binding of guanine nucleotides (GTP and GDP) fall into two groups: a) large heterotrimeric G proteins, which are coupled to a family of surface receptors (the G protein–coupled receptors discussed in Chapter 23), and b) low molecular weight G proteins (LMWG), with sizes of 18 to 26 kDa, which have intrinsic guanosine triphosphatase (GTPase) activity and act as regulatory proteins. The premier example is the Ras superfamily of monomeric GTPases, which includes several subfamilies (32,33): a) the Ras proteins, which help signaling from receptor-linked tyrosine kinases to the nucleus to stimulate cell proliferation or differentiation and other effects of activation of the Ras/MAP kinase pathway (see below), b) the Rho and Rac proteins, which are involved in relating signals to the actin cytoskeleton, to phospholipase D, and to activation of the granulocyte NADPH oxidase (34–37), c) the Rab family, which is involved in trafficking of intracellular transport vesicles and in phagocytosis (38), d) the ARF family, which is also involved in vesicular trafficking and in activation of phospholipase D (32), and e) the Ran family, which is necessary for nuclear transport through the nuclear pores (39).

Virtually all the heterotrimeric G proteins and monomeric GTPases function as switches, cycling between two conformational states, active when GTP is bound and inactive with GDP is bound. This is analogous to activation of a protein by phosphorylation; the difference is that here the phosphate group is transferred to and from the associated guanine nucleotide, rather than the protein itself. To function as messengers, the cell must control the timing and duration of these GTP-bound versus GDP-bound states. The Ras protein provides an example (Fig. 2, 40). Ras is active when bound to GTP. GTP is present in the cytosol at a 10-fold higher concentration than GDP, and Ras hydrolyzes GTP slowly. Thus, once Ras binds GTP, it would, if left alone, remain in the activated GTP-bound state. The switching between the GDP and GTP bound state is regulated and facilitated by two other proteins. Guanine nucleotide dissociation stimulators (GDS, also termed guanine nucleotide exchange factors or GEFs) promote activation of Ras by promoting the release of the bound GDP from Ras, which in turn allows the binding of GTP from its high concentration in the cytosol. Once activated, Ras-GTP can be deactivated by participation of GTPase-activating proteins (GAPs), which stimulate Ras to hydrolyze the bound GTP, thus inactivating Ras. Examples of this regulatory mechanism appear throughout the rest of the chapter.

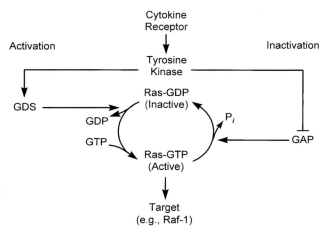

FIG. 2. Regulation of the activity of Ras. Ras is normally inactive, bound to GDP; it must bind GTP for activation. A stimulated receptor usually causes activation of a GDP dissociation stimulator (*GDS*) (also called a GDP/GTP exchange factor, or GEF) that dissociates GDP from Ras, allowing binding of GTP. The GTP-activated Ras then activates the next signaling enzyme, e.g., Raf-1. Activation of Ras is terminated by a GTPase activating protein (*GAP*) that promotes hydrolysis of Ras-GTP to Ras-GDP, thus inactivating Ras. In some cases, receptor activation also suppresses (for a time) activation of GAP.

Protein Phosphorylation and Dephosphorylation by Kinases and Phosphatases

The most common mechanism of signaling involves phosphorylation or dephosphorylation of target proteins. Addition of the strong negative charge of a phosphate group is a potent mechanism to alter protein conformation and hence function (41). Each of the second messengers being discussed, including Ca^{2+}, cAMP, diacylglycerol, arachidonic acid, and phosphatidic acid, exert their final effects most commonly by activating a protein kinase or phosphatase. About 10% of cell proteins are phosphoproteins (i.e., they are or can be phosphorylated). Recent genomic sequencing reveals that perhaps 2% to 3% of all eukaryotic genes may code for protein kinases (42). The kinases all contain a catalytic domain of about 250 amino acids, with differing adjacent structures that determine the substrate specificity and allow regulation of the enzyme. The gradually varying structures have allowed description of the evolutionary tree of the enzymes and their classification into different kinase families (43,44).

The kinases often are grouped by substrate specificity: kinases that phosphorylate tyrosine residues and kinases that phosphorylate serine or threonine residues. Phosphotyrosine has an elongated structure and has a particular role in targeted and regulated protein-protein binding. The specific phosphotyrosine and its adjacent amino acids on one protein bind a phosphotyrosine-recognition

motif (the SH2 domain) on another protein (see above). Tyrosine kinases may constitute a cytoplasmic domain of a membrane receptor, may be associated closely with receptors, or may be activated elsewhere in the cell as part of the sequential signaling cascade. Most tyrosine kinases activate other signaling molecules.

In contrast with the structural specificity of phosphotyrosines, phosphorylation of serine and threonine often can be mimicked by insertion of acidic amino acids, suggesting that these phosphopeptides act through a charge alteration in a manner to change the conformation or substrate binding sites of the target proteins (45). Serine/threonine kinases include, as examples, protein kinase A (the cAMP-activated kinase), protein kinase C (activated by Ca^{2+}, diacylglycerol and phosphatidylserine, and/or by arachidonic acid), Ca^{2+}/calmodulin-activated kinase, and the MAP kinases. One group of receptor kinases, those expressed on the TGFb receptor family, are serine-threonine kinases (46) (other receptor kinases phosphorylate protein tyrosines).

PROTEIN KINASE A (cAMP-ACTIVATED PROTEIN KINASE)

In the mid-1960s the role of cAMP was clarified, leading to a Nobel prize. Stimulation of certain cells, such as stimulation of myocytes by a catecholamine, was found to cause activation of adenyl cyclase to produce a rapid increase in intracellular cAMP.

cAMP causes activation of the cAMP-dependent protein kinase (protein kinase A, PKA). Inactive PKA exists as a complex of two subunits of the catalytic portion of the enzyme and two regulatory subunits. cAMP binds to the regulatory subunits, causing dissociation of the complex and the release of the catalytically active PKA. PKA then is capable of serine or threonine phosphorylation of certain proteins; often these phosphorylated proteins are also regulatory proteins that in turn activate the next target protein in a chain of regulatory events. For example, this pathway is of central importance in regulation of intermediary metabolism via regulation of synthesis and breakdown of glycogen, thus, controlling the level of glucose-1-phosphate for glycolysis. PKA activates phosphorylase kinase, which in turn activates glycogen phosphorylase, causing release of glucose-1-phosphate for further metabolism. Simultaneously, PKA phosphorylates and inactivates glycogen synthase, causing inhibition of glycogen synthesis synchronously with activation of glycogenolysis. Finally, PKA also phosphorylates and activates triacylglycerol lipase, promoting lipolysis. PKA also can inhibit many functions of certain cells. For example, it interacts with the Ras pathway by phosphorylation of Raf-1 at a site that prevents Raf-1 activation (47–49).

Another aspect of cAMP signaling involves induction of transcription of certain genes. Genes that are activated by cAMP contain a cAMP response element (CRE). A regulatory protein, CRE-binding protein (CREB), binds to the CRE but has little transcriptional activity until it is phosphorylated by PKA (see Chapter 26).

Phosphodiesterases (PDEs) terminate the activity of PKA by hydrolyzing the 3′-ribose phosphate bond of 3′,5′-cAMP, yielding biologically inactive 5′-AMP. PDEs have been grouped into five to seven isoenzyme classes coded by four genes with distinct proteins produced by alternative splicing, resulting in multiple subfamilies and 20 or more different PDE isoenzymes (50,51). Although increase in cAMP concentration is a positive signal for many cellular responses, a prolonged increase in cAMP concentration can be induced by PDE inhibitors, and this actually causes inhibition of many cell activities. For example, stimulation of granulocytes is associated with an abrupt and brief (15 s) increase in cAMP (52), but prolonged cAMP elevation inhibits many functions of the same cells (e.g., see ref. 53). Pharmacologic increases in cAMP inhibit contraction of smooth muscle, responses of mast cells and eosinophils, etc., and PDE inhibitors long have been used in asthma therapy. Unfortunately, the therapeutic value of PDE inhibition has been limited by effects of the agents on all PDE isoenzymes in many tissues, causing side effects at or near minimally therapeutic concentrations (54). The PDE isoenzymes are differentially expressed in various tissues, allowing the possibility of therapeutic agents with greater effect and specificity. Inhibitors of PDE IV may have particular relevance to asthma. In addition to suppression of bronchoconstriction, inhibitors of PDE IV suppress responses of eosinophils, mast cells, and basophils and may protect vascular endothelial permeability induced, for example, by H_2O_2 (reviewed in ref. 55). Effective increases in smooth muscle cAMP probably will require inhibition of both PDE III and IV, which are present in smooth muscle (56,57). Such increased specificity may improve the value of PDE inhibitors compared with less specific agents, such as theophylline.

PROTEIN KINASE C FAMILY

Protein kinase C (PKC) initially was described as a cytosolic kinase that is translocated to membrane and activated by the concerted actions of increased cytosolic Ca^{2+}, diacylglycerol, and phosphophatidylserine (58). It has been found to be important in an immense number of cell functions. PKC exists in at least 11 isoforms, which can be divided into three groups: conventional Ca^{2+}-dependent PKC (cPKC), new or non-Ca^{2+}–dependent PKC (nPKC), and atypical PKC (aPKC) (59–61) (Fig. 3). All require phosphatidylserine for activity. The co-existence of other acidic and basic phospholipids, e.g., at the enzyme-membrane interface, have positive and negative effects, respectively, on PKC activation.

In the cPKC isoforms (α, β, and γ), the amino-terminal half of the regulatory domain contains two conserved regions, C1 and C2 (Fig. 3). The C1 region has a pseudo-substrate sequence followed by two tandem repeats of a cysteine-rich zinc-finger–like motif that is responsible for binding of diacylglyerol and phorbol ester. The C2 region in the regulatory domain of cPKC isoforms is needed for calcium sensitivity. This region has been

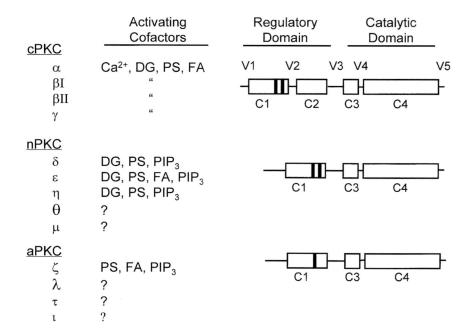

FIG. 3. Currently known isotypes of PKC, which are divided into the classical, Ca^{2+}- and lipid-dependent cPKC, the non–Ca^{2+}-dependent nPKC, and the atypical aPKC groups. The cofactors involved in activation of each are shown. In the schematic of the proteins, the constant regions are denoted by C and the variable regions by V. In the regulatory region, C1 contains the diglyceride-binding domain and C2 contains the Ca^{2+}-binding domain. In the catalytic domain, C3 contains the ATP-binding site. (Modified from Nishizuka Y. Protein kinase C and lipid signaling for sustained cellular responses. *FASEB J* 1995; 9:484–496, and Khan WA, Blobe GC, Hannun YA. Arachidonic acid and free fatty acids as second messengers and the role of protein kinase C. *Cellular Signalling* 1995;7:171–184.)

termed the calcium- and lipid-binding motif (CaLB) and is found in a number of lipid-binding proteins including cytosolic PLA_2 and $PLC\gamma$. The region interacts with phospholipids in a Ca^{2+}-dependent fashion, which facilitates translocation of PKC to membranes when there is an increase in cytosolic Ca^{2+} concentration.

Diacylglycerol activates the cPKC isoforms by causing an increase in affinity for calcium in the micromolar range. *cis*-unsaturated fatty acids, including oleic and linoleic as well as arachidonic acids, cannot directly activate the cPKC but may act in concert with activation by diglyceride, one mechanism being to increase further the affinity of the cPKC for Ca^{2+} (61). Thus, cPKC activation depends on the interplay of the relative amounts of diacylglycerol, calcium, and free fatty acids during cell stimulation.

The nPKC isoforms (δ,ϵ, η, θ, μ) lack the C2 region and do not require Ca^{2+} for activation. They vary in their relative responses to *cis*-unsaturated fatty acids and diacylglycerols. The δ-, ϵ-, and η-isoforms are activated by PIP_3, which is a product of the PI 3-kinase. In cultured cells overexpressing PI 3-kinase and individual PKC isoforms, PI 3-kinase was found to potentiate reporter gene expression in cells overexpressing the δ- and ϵ-isoforms but not the α-isoform of PKC (60).

The aPKC isoforms (ζ, λ, τ, ι) also lack the C2 region and are therefore calcium-independent (61,62). The signaling pathway leading to activation of the aPKC isoforms is unknown. Best characterized is the ζ-isoform, which depends on phosphatidylserine and is activated by *cis*-unsaturated fatty acids and by PIP_2 and PIP_3 (59). This isoform does not respond to diacylglycerol or phorbol esters. A role in signaling is supported by the observation that overexpression of these enzymes enhances transcriptional activation of *cis*-acting elements in response to certain growth factors. Chinese hamster ovary cells (which are used often for studying gene regulation by transfection) overexpressing the α or δ PKC isoforms also had prolonged activation of MAP kinases upon treatment by phorbol esters (61).

There are a number of differences in activation of PKC isoforms by diacylglycerols (DAG) and by free fatty acids (FAs) (63). Activation by FAs (especially of the nPKC and aPKC isoforms) is independent of Ca^{2+} and of phosphatidylserine. The FAs appear to act at a site separate from the DAG binding site. Some PKC inhibitors (e.g., staurosporine) are less inhibitory to the FA-mediated PKC activity. Perhaps most importantly, FA appears to activate soluble PKC isoforms preferentially over membrane-bound PKC, which is the opposite of DAG-mediated PKC activation. Finally, the Ca^{2+}-independent PKC isoforms are more potently activated by FA than are Ca^{2+}-dependent PKCs. This suggests different activation scenarios for PKC affected by DAG (dependent on Ca^{2+}, active at the cell membrane) versus FA (independent of DAG and Ca^{2+} increases, occurring in the cytosol) (discussed in ref. 63).

PKC can activate gene transcription either by its role in facilitating activation of the MAP kinase pathway or by the activation of NF-κB. NF-κB is normally held in an inactive form in the cytosol by its binding to Iκ-B. PKC phosphorylates Iκ-B and causes disruption of the Iκ-B/NF-κB complex. Such regulation of transcription is described further in Chapter 26.

TYROSINE KINASES AND ASSOCIATED SIGNALING PATHWAYS

Receptor-associated Tyrosine Kinases: Src, Syk, and Janus Kinase Families

Many receptors, especially those for many growth factors (e.g., epidermal growth factor, platelet-derived growth factor, insulin), have intrinsic tyrosine kinase domains within the cytoplasmic region (see Chapter 23). Other receptors may lack enzymatic activity but are closely associated with cytoplasmic tyrosine kinase(s). Such receptors include the T-cell receptor, mIg receptor of B cells, and several immunoglobulin receptors (see Chapter 23). These cytosolic kinases are usually grouped in the closely related Src, Syk, and the recently described Tec families and in the Janus family (typified by the Jak kinases, which are coupled to gene transcription). The Src kinases are common receptor-associated kinases and include (at least) Src, Lck, Lyn, Yes, Fgr, Fyn, Hck, Blk, and Yrk (64). The functions mediated by these are protean, e.g., molecular inactivation of the *fyn* gene causes T-cell receptor defects but also causes hippocampal defects and impaired learning (64).

The initial steps coupling Src family kinases with the Ras pathway occur at the cell membrane. Src family members have a unique terminal domain containing a myristylated glycine at position 2; the myristoyl lipid chain is responsible for membrane association. In contrast, Syk kinases (Syk and ZAP-70) are not myristylated and probably not constitutively localized by the plasma membrane. The Syk members have two N-terminal SH2 domains and a C-terminal catalytic domain but lack an SH3 domain and the C-terminal negative regulatory site tyrosine phosphorylation (reviewed in ref. 65). Thus, there are several differences in regulation of the Src and Syk kinases. The Tec kinases are active in hematopoietic cells, and apparently couple to Src kinases; their functions are currently being defined (66,67).

The Src kinases phosphorylate cytoplasmic subunits of receptors at characteristic sequences that have been referred to as tyrosine activation motifs (TAMs) (65,68–70) or "antigen recognition activation motifs" (reviewed in ref. 65). Such characteristic receptor motifs are found in the ϵ and ζ chains of the multisubunit T-cell receptor, the Ig-α and Ig-β chains of the mIg receptor, and in the β and γ chains of the heterotrimeric FcϵR1. This tyrosine phosphorylation of the receptor TAM provides sites for binding and activation of members of the Syk family of tyrosine kinases as well as binding a range of SH2 domain–containing tyrosine kinase substrates (65).

An example is provided by a Src family kinase, Lck, in lymphocyte signaling. Both CD4 and CD8 bind cytoplasmic tyrosine kinase Lck through a cysteine-containing motif shared by their cytoplasmic domains (69). Studies of the functional significance of Lck in cell receptor signaling have employed mice deficient in Lck or expressing a dominant negative Lck transgene, T-cell lines deficient in Lck kinase function, T-cell clones deficient in Lck or, conversely, overexpression of activated Lck in a T-cell hybridoma (65,71,72). Lck-mediated tyrosine phosphorylation of the receptor TAM allows recruitment of Syk family kinases, Syk or ZAP-70, via their SH2 domains. ZAP-70 is expressed exclusively in T cells and NK cells, whereas Syk is expressed in B-cell myeloid cells and monocytes (65).

Syk already has been shown to be coupled to the activation of the IgE receptor in mast cells (73–75), to activation of integrins and Fc$_\gamma$RIIIa in monocytes, to cross-linking of either high- (Fc$_\gamma$RI) or low- (Fc$_\gamma$RII) affinity receptors on myelomonocytic cells (76–78), and to lectin stimulation of neutrophils (79).

It has been suggested that simple clustering events may activate directly these kinases (80,81). Kolanus et al. (80) used chimeric transmembrane proteins bearing a CD16 extracellular domain and an extracellular domain expressing one or more of these kinases in a cytolytic T-cell line. The chimeras were then aggregated by interaction of the cells with hybridomas expressing surface IgE. They found that aggregation of the Syk chimera alone or co-aggregation of chimeras bearing the Src family kinase Fyn and the Syk family kinase ZAP-70 sufficed to initiate cytolytic effector function (80).

The Ras/MAP Kinase Pathways

A multitude of cell functions, extending from proliferation and differentiation to programmed cell death, are controlled by a signaling sequence leading to the activation of Ras and eventually to an MAP kinase. These pathways involve activation of several molecules at the cell membrane followed by sequential activation of several cytoplasmic protein kinases. This complex series is complicated further by the presence of several similar but distinct pathways with remarkable parallels in the number and type of enzymes activated at each step (82–84). Krebs (85) has suggested that a generic nomenclature be applied such that the enzyme at the level at the MAP kinase be abbreviated MAPK, the level of the MAP kinase kinase be MAPKK, the MAP kinase kinase kinase be MAP3K, etc. Unfortunately, this does not avoid the necessity for retaining the individual acronyms of the specific enzymes at each level, but it will simplify communication of where in the cascade the individual enzyme is active (Fig. 4).

At the level of the MAP kinase, the three currently known parallel pathways in humans activate the ERK kinases, Jun kinase (JNK), and p38 kinase. The targets of these pathways may overlap, e.g., both ERKs and at least one of the other two MAP kinases can activate cytosolic PLA$_2$ (86–90).

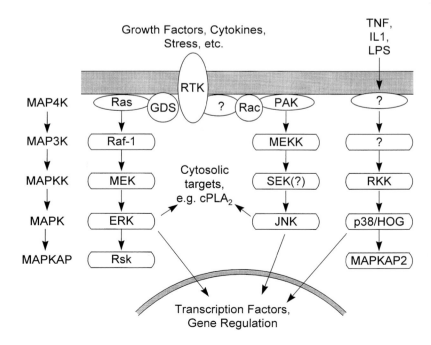

FIG. 4. The MAP kinase pathways. See text for details.

The multiple pathways of the MAP kinase family may interact in important manners. One example is the regulation of a transcriptional activator complex, AP-1, which probably causes the most significant effects of the ERK/MAP kinases on cellular proliferation. AP-1 is a dimer composed of Jun and Fos DNA binding proteins. Transcriptional regulation of expression of the c-*Fos* and c-*Jun* genes are controlled by the kinases ERK and JNK, respectively. The Fos and Jun proteins combine to form the AP-1 heterodimers. A further increase in AP-1 activity requires the activity of JNK kinases and Frk kinases, which phosphorylate Jun and Fos, respectively. Thus, the activation of this one transcription activator complex requires the activation and participation of three separate kinase pathways (91).

Conversely, blocking activation of Ras can prevent critical cell functions. For example, anergy of T cells has been found to involve a blockade at Ras. Anergy is caused when a T cell receives a signal through the T-cell receptor without a co-stimulatory signal from the B7 molecules on an antigen-presenting cell interacting with CD28 on the T cell. For reasons unknown, this causes a blockade at Ras when the T cells are subsequently stimulated (92,93). Also, such cells have reduced activation of the alternative pathway leading to activation of JNK, suggesting crosstalk between the Ras/MAP kinase pathway and the Rac/JNK pathways. Because the Ras/ERK pathway is the best defined, it is discussed in some detail.

Coupling to the Ras Pathway

The Ras pathway was characterized initially as being coupled to receptor tyrosine kinases such as receptors for PDGF, EGF, and FGF. Ligand binding to the extracellular domain of such receptors causes receptor dimerization, stimulation of receptor tyrosine kinase activity, and autophosphorylation of the receptor cytoplasmic chain (see Chapter 23). After tyrosine phosphorylation of these sites, they act as high-affinity binding sites for SH2 domains of signaling molecules (see above) and cause direct or indirect (via an adapter protein such as Grb2) binding and activation of proteins such as the GDP/GTP exchange factor Sos1, which can then activate Ras.

The Ras/MAP kinase pathway can also be linked to G protein–coupled receptors (see Chapter 23). For example, the IgE receptor is coupled to the MAP kinase pathway via the cytosolic tyrosine kinase Syk, and activation of Syk results in tyrosine phosphorylation of the GDP/GTP exchange factor Vav (75,76,94). Guanine nucleotide exchange would then cause activation of Ras. Another pathway to Ras involves activation by the G protein bg subunits causing phosphorylation (perhaps by the kinase Tsk and Btk) of Shc (33,95). Phosphory-lated Shc can then recruit Grb2/Sos1 to the membrane, where Sos1 can activate Ras.

Ras

The ras gene is conserved through evolution, from yeasts and nematodes to humans. It was discovered as an oncogene, with mutations occurring in human and animal cancers (96). Mutation of a single amino acid resulted in constitutively active Ras, leading to uncontrolled cell growth. Ras normally hydrolyzes bound GTP to GDP, and in the process switches from the active to inactive state. Oncogenic Ras has a reduced ability to hydrolyze GTP and hence remains activated, which in turn stimulates uncontrolled growth of the tissue. Oncogenic mutations of several members of the Ras pathway illustrate the importance of this series of GTPases in cell growth and differentiation. Ras is normally bound to the cell membrane through a lipid (prenyl) chain (97), and bound to GDP in the inactive form of Ras (98). As discussed above, receptor-coupled activation of a guanine nucleotide exchange factor (e.g., hSos1 or Vav) causes release of the GDP, allowing binding of cytosolic GTP to Ras. This induces a conformational change in plasma membrane–associated Ras. Cytosolic Raf-1 can then associate with Ras through interactions with the Ras effector region (98–100).

Raf-1

Raf-1 is a serine-threonine kinase that is activated in association with Ras. Ras interacts directly with a conserved 81 residue region of the N-terminal portion of Raf-1, which causes recruitment of Raf to the plasma membrane (101–104), although this itself is not sufficient to activate Raf-1. Several lines of study suggest that Ras functions to recruit inactive, cytosolic Raf-1 to the plasma membrane, where additional protein-protein and/or protein-lipid interactions may regulate the further activation of Raf-1. Activation of Raf-1 is accompanied by phosphorylation at sites distinct from its autophosphorylation sites, suggesting the involvement of an unknown kinase in Raf-1 activation. PKC has been reported to active Raf-1 (105,106), but the role of PKC phosphorylation of Raf-1 is controversial (85,107). Raf contains a zinc-containing cysteine-enriched ("zinc finger") motif similar to the C1 domain of PKC, which is involved in binding diacylglycerol to PKC (108). This could suggest involvement of such an additional second messenger in Raf activation (85). In addition, Raf-1 has a different domain that is capable of binding phosphatidic acid (109), and inhibition of phosphatidic acid release results in decreased translocation of Raf-1 kinase from the cytosol to the membrane of cells after agonist stimulation (73).

Raf-1 is also a site for regulation of the Ras/MAP kinase pathway by other signaling paths. As noted, PKC can activate Raf-1, suggesting a possible modulation by the phospholipase C ∅ diacylglycerol ∅ PKC pathway. The possible role of PA also suggests participation of the PLD pathway. Conversely, PKA, activated by cAMP, can phosphorylate Raf-1 at a site that prevents Raf-1 activation (47–49).

It has been found that the Raf protein kinase exists within cells in a complex of Raf, together with the molecular chaperone SHP-90 and P50. SHP-90 had previously been described to be regulatory for other proteins including the glucocorticoid receptor (110) and other kinases (111). The presence of Raf in a large protein complex that interacts with Raf and MEK has suggested that protein-protein interactions may present another mechanism of regulation of the Raf protein kinase (111).

Raf-1 gene expression is regulated in distinct manners in different cells. In neutrophils, Raf-1 is expressed constitutively and is unaffected by agonists such as TNF or endotoxin. By contrast, simple adherence of monocytes or mitogen stimulation of lymphocytes causes increased levels of Raf-1 (112). The effects of such increased cellular Raf-1 on cell function need further study.

The function of activated Raf-1 is very specific for phosphorylation of the MAP kinase kinase, MEK (108,113).

MAP Kinase Kinase

The next enzyme in this pathway of kinases is the MAP kinase kinase (MEK). Activation of MEK involves phosphorylation on serine residues, usually by activated Raf-1, although it can also be induced through inhibition of serine/threonine phosphatases. MEK is a dual specificity kinase with a unique ability to phosphorylate both the regulatory tyrosine and threonine residues of ERK-1 and ERK-2. Thus, this MAP kinase kinase provides the specificity and an amplification step in the MAP kinase cascade (85).

MAP Kinase

MAP kinase (for microtubule-associated kinase or mitogen-activated kinase), more specifically identified by the term ERK (for extracellular regulated kinase), was one of the first enzymes identified in this pathway, is capable of activating functional enzymes (e.g., cytosolic PLA$_2$, phospholipase Cg, and tyrosine hydroxylase), gene transcription, or other signaling kinases, and has thus received intense interest. There are three ERK kinases, ERK1 and ERK2 with molecular weights of 42 and 44 kDa, and an alternatively spliced form at 40 kDa (85). The predominant

ERK1 and ERK2 are functionally identical. For activation, they require phosphorylation of both threonine and tyrosine residues in a -TXY- motif (85,114). MEK is exclusively localized in the cytoplasm; ERK is thus phosphorylated in the cytoplasm before translocation to the nucleus (85,115).

ERK1 and ERK2 can phosphorylate many proteins at membrane, cytosolic, or nuclear localizations in the cell. ERKs are "proline-directed" protein kinases in that they phosphorylate serine or threonine residues that are near proline residues, the substrate recognition sequence being Pro-Leu-Ser/Thr-Pro (116). In the nucleus, ERKs can phosphorylate transcription factors including c-Fos, c-Myc, c-Myb, Ets2, NF-IL6, TAL-1, p53, and RNA polymerase II (85) and thus have a role in the transition in the early cell cycle from the G$_0$ to the G$_1$ phase (117). They also can amplify further the Ras/MAP kinase cascade by phosphorylating certain receptors (e.g., EGF receptor) or upstream proteins of the cascade itself, such as protein tyrosine phosphatase 2C, Sos, Raf-1, and MEK. ERK1 and ERK2 can also phosphorylate cytoskeletal elements such as MAP-1, MAP-2, MAP-4, and Tau and thereby regulate cytoskeletal rearrangements and cellular morphology (85).

RSK (ribosomal protein S6 kinase) is a protein kinase activated by the MAP kinase ERKs, which would appear to extend the MAP kinase pathway through yet another generation of activatable kinases. Its role is currently being defined.

Representative Cell Functions Regulated by the MAP Kinase Pathways

Cell Proliferation and Differentiation

Many growth hormones and mitogens cause activation of the Ras/MAP kinase pathways. Downregulation of the pathway, for example using antisense Raf-1, inhibitory Raf-1 mutants, or expression of nonactivable forms of MEK-1, reduced the proliferation of cells such as NIH-3T3 cells (118); conversely, transfection with constitutively activated Raf-1 or MEK1 increased proliferation (118). The extreme natural experiment is the development of Ras or Raf mutations, which are oncogenes, associated with established cancers (i.e., uncontrolled proliferation). However, this is not the only pathway regulating proliferation. Interleukin 4–dependent proliferation occurs without activation of the MAP kinases (119). Also, certain cytokines that activate the MAP kinase cascade can induce cellular differentiation (i.e., terminate ongoing cell proliferation) (120–124).

Interestingly, in some cells activation of MAP kinase cascades can cause more than one physiologic response. For example, in certain cells where both EGF and NGF activate the MAPK cascade, EGF treatment induces proliferation but NGF induces differentiation. How such distinct responses occur by the same cascade in a single cell is currently being defined. One controlling mechanism appears to be the strength and duration of the signals transmitted through the cascade (85).

Programmed Cell Death (Apoptosis)

Although the mechanism is not well defined, cytokines that activate the MAP kinase pathway in eosinophils or in neutrophils cause a delay of the normal apoptosis (programmed cell death) of the cell (125–127). It is a reasonable hypothesis that this delay in apoptosis of eosinophils may contribute to the pathogenesis of asthma, either by prolonged release of toxic products or by eventual cellular necrosis. With death by necrosis, the cells lyse and release their granule constituents into the extracellular milieu, allowing the induction of local tissue damage. Conversely, during apoptosis, apoptotic cells are recognized by macrophages, are phagocytized, and are cleared without the induction of local tissue damage. On the other hand, it is reasonable to speculate that a cytokine-induced delay in apoptosis of neutrophils or eosinophils might have evolutionary value, as it would allow the prolongation of the cell's availability for acting in host defense.

Priming

Exposure of cells to certain agonists may cause a change in the cell such that later exposure to a second agonist results in increased ("primed") responses. Priming may be induced by exposure to substimulatory concentrations of certain agonists (128–130), exposure to cell-permeable analogs of the normal second messengers of the cell (131–133), and by cytokines (134–137). Exposure of neutrophils to GM-CSF or of eosinophils to interleukin-5 causes priming associated with MAP kinase activation (138,139), and subsequent stimulation results in increased adherence, chemotaxis, degranulation, eicosanoid release, and oxidant (superoxide) production (136,140). Some priming events, such as the induction of the prostaglandin G/H synthase 2, require activation of transcription and de novo protein synthesis (141–143).

Other priming events do not require protein synthesis but involve activation of certain kinases. For example, optimal activation of cytosolic PLA$_2$ requires at least two events. One is phosphorylation of the enzyme, resulting in increased enzymatic activity. The other is an increase in the cytosolic Ca^{2+} concentration that mediates translocation of the enzyme to the membrane substrate. In unprimed cells, stimulation causes a brief rise in cytosolic Ca^{2+}, which ceases before optimal phosphorylation of cPLA$_2$. Cytokine priming activates the MAP kinase, causing phosphorylation of cPLA$_2$; subse-

quent stimulation causes a transient burst of elevated cytosolic Ca^{2+} that can then translocate the phosphorylated enzyme and induce optimal membrane lipid hydrolysis.

PHOSPHATASES

Phosphatases reverse the effects of kinases. As noted above, the regulation by phosphorylation is especially effective for transient events because of the coordinated regulation of kinases and phosphatases done first phosphorylate and dephosphorylate the protein. In eukaryotic cells, phosphatases may be divided into three groups: the nonspecific phosphatases, the phosphoprotein (serine/threonine) phosphatases, and the protein tyrosine phosphatases (144). Nonspecific phosphatases include enzymes such as alkaline phosphatases and acid phosphatase that typically function in degradative or catabolic pathways. The serine/threonine phosphoprotein phosphatases and protein tyrosine phosphatases in general counter the activities of kinases in maintaining the desired balance between phosphorylation and dephosphorylation of proteins.

Protein tyrosine phosphatases (PTPases) may be subcharacterized into three groups: a) receptor-like, b) intracellular, and c) dual specificity protein tyrosine phosphatases. The receptor-like PTPases include an extracellular domain of varying structure, a single-membrane spanning region, and one or two intracellular catalytic domains and may be involved in cell-cell interaction. The intracellular PTPases typically contain a single catalytic domain; the variability of the remainder of the structure is believed to have targeting or regulatory function. PTPases appear to have important roles in ontogeny, cell growth and proliferation, the cell cycle and cytoskeletal integrity; many of the specific functions of these phosphatases are currently being defined (reviewed in ref. 144).

Dual specificity phosphatases, which hydrolyze both serine/threonine and tyrosine phosphate groups, are important in the dephosphorylation of activated MAP kinase, but the roles of phosphatases are not limited to termination of signaling. CD45 protein tyrosine phosphatase is a plasma membrane protein expressed in hematopoietic cells that is, e.g., essential for coupling through the T-cell antigen receptor and mast cell Fc$_\varepsilon$R1 (145,146). PTPase 1C is linked to the c-kit receptor (147), IL-3 receptor (148), and B-cell antigen receptor (149), as well as receptors for hormones such as insulin (150). PTPase 1D is coupled to receptors for EGF and PDGF (151–153).

How phosphatases positively affect signaling can be complex and may appear counterintuitive. Crosslinking Fc$_\varepsilon$R1 on mast cells is associated with tyrosine phosphorylation of multiple proteins. Surprisingly, tyrosine phosphatase activity is also essential to induction of degranulation through the IgE receptor (154,155). It has been suggested that effective signaling through the FcεR1 requires continuous phosphorylation and dephosphorylation of the receptor, without the need for formation of new receptor aggregates (156,157).

The CD45 phosphatase has an unusual role in activation of T cells. Kinases of the Src family are capable of inhibition by phosphorylation of a C-terminal tyrosine. Phosphorylation at this site may cause an intramolecular interaction, which blocks the SH2 domain of Lck. The CD45 is capable of removing the phosphate from the negative regulatory site, thus allowing binding of Lck through its SH2 domain with the T-cell receptor (65).

Another interesting example of the complex kinase/phosphatase interplay relates to the regulation of glycogen metabolism by cAMP. Here, protein phosphatase I is capable of terminating the activity of the cAMP response element-binding (CREB) protein. But there is a phosphatase inhibitor that also is activated by PKA, and phosphorylation of this inhibitor blocks the activity of phosphatase I. Thus, PKA activates an inhibitor of phosphatase while it activates CREB protein, providing a synergistic action for CREB protein activity in transcription (158).

COORDINATED REGULATION OF RELATED SIGNALING ENZYMES

The broad substrate specificities of these multiple intracellular kinases and phosphatases prompted the concept that mechanisms must exist to restrict the actions of these enzymes to their intended substrate *in vivo*. Some enzymes are seen as having a targeting subunit that restricts the enzyme to a specific intracellular site. The targeting may be to a substrate protein itself (such as the targeting of protein phosphatase 1 to glycogen; 42) or to anchoring proteins such as microtubules in the microenvironment where the enzymatic activity is appropriate (159,160). For example, a single "scaffold" protein can anchor PKA, phosphatase 2B (calcineurin), and PKC together, close to key substrates (160).

LIPIDS AS SECOND MESSENGERS AND AUTOCRINE SIGNALING MOLECULES

Phospholipase C Releases Diglyceride and IP3, Which Activate Protein Kinase C and Mobilize Intracellular Calcium

Many extracellular molecules including hormones, peptide growth factors, neurotransmitters, chemotactic factors, and immunoglobulins elicit intracellular responses by activating inositol phospholipid-specific phospholipase C (PLC) (161–163). Activated PLC hydrolyzes phosphatidylinositol 4,5-bisphosphate (PIP2),

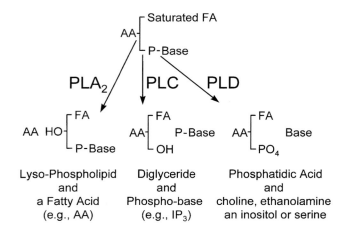

FIG. 5. Schematic of the three types of phospholipases active in signaling. PLA_2 hydrolyzes the second position of the glycerol backbone, releasing FA and lyso-phospholipid. PLC hydrolyzes the third position of the backbone, releasing a diglyceride and a phospho-base that could be phosphorylcholine, etc., but is most important when the substrate is phosphatidylinositol-bisphosphate, and the released product is IP_3. PLD hydrolyzes the phospho-ester bond, releasing a phosphatidic acid and the base (e.g., choline).

which releases diacylglycerol and inositol 1,4,5-trisphosphate (IP_3) (Fig. 5). Diacylglyercol can activate PKC, and IP_3 induces mobilization of calcium from intracellular stores. Multiple distinct PLC enzymes have been identified and 14 or more isoforms have been deduced from nucleotide sequences of their corresponding cDNAs (163). The PLCs have been divided into three types: PLC-β, PLC-γ, PLC-δ. The catalytic activity of all three depend on calcium. The PLCγ has a region homologous to that of the calcium and lipid-binding domain of PKC and cytosolic PLA_2; for these proteins, the calcium also has a role in binding the enzyme to membrane lipid.

PLC-β is activated by stimulation of receptors coupled to the Gq subfamily of trimeric G proteins. The α chain of the Gq proteins was found to activate PLC-β1 but not PLC-γ1 and PLC-δ1 (163). The interaction of Gαq causes an increase in the intrinsic activity of PLC-β. Receptors for thromboxane A_2, bradykinin, angiotensin, histamine, vasopressin ,and acetylcholine (muscarinic) were reported to be coupled to PLC by this mechanism (163). In at least some cells, it is the βγ subunit of the heterotrimeric G protein that activates PLCβ (164,165).

PLCγ1 and PLCγ2 (but not PLC-β or PLC-δ) are activated by receptor-tyrosine kinases. For example, the EGF receptor has intrinsic tyrosine kinase activity. It dimerizes on ligand binding, allowing phosphorylation crosswise of the dimerized receptor's cytoplasmic chains. The phosphotyrosine on the receptor chain then can bind the SH2 domains of the PLCγ molecule. This precedes phosphorylation of the PLC-γ1 itself by the receptor tyrosine kinase, and this tyrosine phosphorylation of PLC-γ1 is essential for activation of the enzyme. It has been hypothesized that the phosphorylation of SH2 domains on the PLC-γ1 may allow the SH3 domain on the PLC to be exposed and bind to membrane cytoskeleton, resulting in the positioning of the catalytic domains of PLC at the membrane (163).

Certain receptors, such as the T-cell receptor (TCR), activate PLC-γ1 (166), even though the receptor does not itself contain a tyrosine kinase activity. Ligation of the T-cell receptor complex activates the intracellular kinases Fyn and Lck, which in turn activate PLC-γ1 (80). Similar activation of PLC-γ1 is an early event after ligand binding by the high-affinity IgE receptor (167), IgG receptors (FcγR1 and FcγR2) (163), and the immunoglobulin receptor of B lymphocytes (168).

All PLC isoforms isolated from mammalian tissue hydrolyze phosphatidylinositol (PI), PI-4-phosphate (PIP), and PI-4,5-bisphosphate (PIP2), but not PI-3-phosphate, PI-3,4-bisphosphate, or PI-3-4,5-trisphosphate (PIP3) (61) (Fig. 6) (The PI species phosphorylated on the 3 position are discussed under PI-3 kinase).

With stimulation of cellular receptors, activation of PLC results in immediate release of diacylglycerol (DAG) from inositol phospholipids, most rapidly from PIP$_2$. This DAG molecule disappears quickly. A second wave of DAG appearance often follows that is relatively slow in onset and persists for minutes to hours (61). This sustained elevation of DAG is often observed after stimulation by long-acting signals such as growth factors and

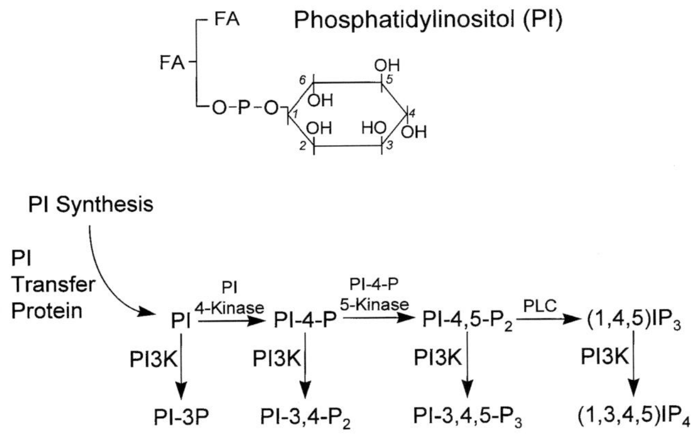

FIG. 6. Structure of phosphatidylinositol (*top*) with positions on the inositol ring numbered in italics. Metabolism of PI, showing the sites of action of PI3K (*bottom*). See text for details. (Modified from Lew DP. Receptor signalling and intracellular calcium in neutrophil activation. *Eur J Clin Invest* 1989;19:338–346; Clark JD, Lin L-L, Kriz RW, et al. A novel arachidonic acid–selective cytosolic PLA2 contains a Ca^{2+}-dependent translocation domain with homology to PKC and GAP. *Cell* 1991;65:1043–1051; and Stephens LR, Hughes KT, Irvine RF. Pathway of phosphatidylinositol(3,4,5)-trisphosphate synthesis in activated neutrophils. *Nature* 1991;351:33–39.)

cytokines. Mitogenic signals sometimes initiate only this second phase of DAG elevation (61). The fatty acid composition of this DAG matches that of phosphatidylcholine. It is controversial whether there is a PLC capable of hydrolysis of phosphatidylcholine to produce this prolonged diglyceride elevation (61,169). The alternative hypothesis is that the phosphatidylcholine is hydrolyzed by phospholipase D, releasing phosphatidic acid (the effects of which are described further below) that is converted to diglyceride by the action of a phosphomonoesterase that removes the phosphate group.

Phospholipase D and Phosphatidic Acid

It long has been known that acidic lipids (such as AA or phosphatidic acid, PA) could alter physical properties of membranes or of some proteins. These agents alter packing of phospholipid membranes allowing, e.g., enhanced hydrolysis by phospholipases. They (especially PA) facilitate fusion of membranes. They can replace Ca^{2+}-calmodulin in activation of certain proteins that have a hydrophobic pocket at the enzyme regulatory site. PA is produced when PLD hydrolyzes membrane glycerophospholipids (see Fig. 5); PA phosphohydrolase removes the phosphate, yielding a diglyceride; thus, PLD can be a source of two signaling molecules, PA and diglyceride. It was long thought that PLD occurred only in plants. In the late 1980s, the presence and importance of PLD in signaling in mammalian cells became apparent. The ability of mammalian PLD to hydrolyze phosphatidylcholine (170) provided a novel signaling pathway yielding diglycerides (as well as PA) independently of the PI-PLC pathway. It now appears that there are at least two isoforms of mammalian PLD, under separate control (171–174). One PLD isoform has been cloned (175).

Stimulation of PLD can be induced in probably all cells by many agonists, extending from mechanical strain (176) to certain cytokines (177) to receptor-mediated signaling in inflammatory cells (e.g., refs. 178–181). In turn, PA can directly activate one or more PA-dependent kinases (182,183) (involved, e.g., in activation of the granulocyte NADPH oxidase; 180,184–187). It may influence many levels of signaling pathways: a) the Ras/MAP kinase pathway by regulating translocation of Raf-1 (109), b) the PI-PLC pathway by activating the phosphatidyl-4-phosphate 5-kinase or PKCζ (188,189), c) G protein-coupled receptors, e.g., by activating PTP1C phosphatase to dephosphorylate the EGF receptor (190), and d) by activating other small G proteins such as the ARF GTPase activating protein, which would inactivate ARF and thereby inactivate PLD (191). PA may also activate small G proteins by dissociating their inhibitor; such PA-mediated activation of Rac participates in activation of the NADPH oxidase (192). PA affects many cell functions. It has a central role in vesicular transport and in secretion

(32,193), including surfactant secretion (194). It stimulates proliferation of multiple cell types (195,196). PA signaling also has been reported to be important in lung injury after hemorrhage in mice (197), by mechanisms yet to be defined.

Mechanisms activating PLD have been controversial. Dependence on the PLC-PKC pathway (198–200), e.g., showing that overexpression of PKCβ caused parallel changes in PLD activation (201), was matched by data indicating a PKC-independent path involving a G protein (e.g., ref. 202), e.g., showing that microinjection of Ras into Xenopus oocytes caused PLD activation (201). Recent data support at least two distinct forms of PLD. The PKC-dependent PLD may hydrolyze phospholipids coupled with an ether linkage in the *sn*-1 position, and the G protein-linked PLD preferentially hydrolyzes lipid with an ester *sn*-1 linkage (203). Stimulatory effects of diglycerides are controlled by *sn*-1 linkages (132,133,204,205), and such differential production of distinct diglyceride species could have specific regulatory roles in cell function.

Small G proteins regulating PLD include ARF (172,191,206,207), Rho (34,172–174,208) and possibly a 50-kDa protein (172,174). Rho could be replaced by related small G proteins Rac1 or Cdc42, but of these three, Rho appeared to be the active GTPase in the cells tested (173). In cell fractions, the Rho-dependent PLD localized in membrane, whereas ARF-dependent PLD was in both cytosol and membrane (173). The cloned human PLD1 is membrane associated, stimulated by ARF-1 and by PIP$_2$, inhibited by a *cis*-unsaturated FA (oleate), and specific for PC (175). Thus, available data indicate that PLDs occur at different physical sites in the cell, are regulated by distinct pathways, and yield products that can have different regulatory mechanisms. It is unknown if these separate PLDs have different roles in disease pathogenesis. Given their distinct regulation, and the importance of PLD products in signaling, this could become a focus of novel therapeutics.

Phospholipases A2 Yield Fatty Acids and Lysophospholipids

Fatty Acids as Second Messengers

Numerous studies have suggested that *cis*-unsaturated free fatty acids (FAs), especially arachidonic acid (AA), can act as second messengers in many cells. Such second messenger roles are difficult to delineate with certainty because the fatty acids also can take part in intermediary metabolism. For AA, the complexity is increased by potential metabolism to highly active eicosanoids, which in turn can stimulate diverse cell functions through activation of specific receptors. Such receptor-mediated paracrine and perhaps autocrine effects are reviewed in Chapters 40–42.

Direct application of exogenous AA (or other *cis*-unsaturated fatty acids) to cells causes stimulation of many cell functions. However, such exogenous AA (delivered, e.g., as a micelle) may interact with the cell in ways that are distinct from effects of AA released enzymatically within the cell (137). Other studies have used inhibition of PLA$_2$ enzymes to block putative AA-mediated pathways (e.g., refs. 209,210). PLA$_2$ inhibitors are often characterized as nonspecific, but similar inhibition of cell function by inhibitors with diverse mechanisms of action (including antisense oligonucleotides; 211) prompt further attention to FAs in signaling. Nevertheless, proof of the exact targets of AA *in vivo* remains elusive (63). One potential role is the activation of small G proteins (such as Rac) by dissociation from their endogenous inhibitors (such as Rac-GDI) (192). Other examples include inhibition of myosin light chain phosphatase causing sensitization of smooth muscle to Ca^{2+} (212) and the activation of potassium channels in myocytes (213,214).

A direct second messenger role for AA probably is best defined in its ability to activate PKC (as described above and recently reviewed in ref. 63). In particular, AA is particularly potent in activation of the Ca^{2+}-independent PKC isoenzymes and can activate them without the need for translocation to a membrane, as is necessary for activation of cPKC isoenzymes by Ca^{2+} and diacylglycerol. This suggests that AA and Ca^{2+}-DAG may regulate activation of different substrates at distinct sites within cells.

Release of Free Fatty Acids

AA typically is esterified at the *sn*-2 position of cellular phospholipids, and free AA is maintained at very low levels in resting cells. Phospholipases A$_2$ (PLA$_2$) hydrolyze the *sn*-2 position and are critically important in the release of AA (Fig. 5). PLA$_2$s may be activated by receptor-mediated stimulation of many cells, but the amount of AA released, as well as the specific eicosanoids formed, differs widely between species and between cell types. The functional status of cells may also modulate the quantities of AA and products in a manner that is probably important to disease pathogenesis. For example, receptor-mediated stimulation of human neutrophil or eosinophil granulocytes causes modest release of AA or eicosanoid products, but during inflammatory diseases, granulocytes can be "primed" to have markedly increased functional responses (215,216), including eicosanoid release (217–221).

Several distinct PLA$_2$ isoforms may mediate AA release. In most cells, stimulated AA release is Ca^{2+}-dependent, and studies have predominantly focused on the Ca^{2+}-dependent PLA$_2$s, in particular a PLA$_2$ that is cytosolic in resting cells (cPLA$_2$) and a family of secretory PLA$_2$s (sPLA$_2$). Other PLA$_2$s that might be involved in signaling include a Ca^{2+}-independent PLA$_2$, activated by ATP, reported in myocardial cells (222). Mast cells contain another PLA$_2$, which specifically hydrolyzes phosphatidylserine (223).

cPLA$_2$ is an 85-kDa protein found in soluble fractions from resting cells (224–226). It was cloned from the U937 macrophage cell line (226,227) but it is probably ubiquitous. cPLA$_2$ is specific for release of AA, whereas sPLA$_2$s do not show fatty acid specificity. Optimal cPLA$_2$ activation requires two events. cPLA$_2$ activity is increased by phosphorylation of the enzyme, induced by a member of the MAP kinase family (86,89,90). Activation also requires translocation of cPLA$_2$ to cell membranes that is induced by nanomolar concentrations of free Ca^{2+} (224–226,228,229), such as occur in cytosol of cells after membrane receptor stimulation. This Ca^{2+}-dependent membrane binding involves a region of the cPLA$_2$ homologous to the Ca^{2+}- and lipid-binding domains of PKC and GTPase-activated protein (226). Certain qualities of the cPLA$_2$, in particular phosphorylation by receptor-activated kinases and translocation by "cytosolic" concentrations of Ca^{2+}, have led to assertions that cPLA$_2$ is responsible for AA and eicosanoid release after activation of cellular receptors (225,227).

In some tissues, cPLA$_2$ activity can be enhanced (primed) by certain cytokines. For example, interferon γ induces both synthesis and phosphorylation of cPLA$_2$ in respiratory epithelial cells (230); stem cell factor induces cPLA$_2$ synthesis in mast cells (231), and IL-1 induces cPLA$_2$ synthesis in fibroblasts (232). Priming of granulocytes involves cPLA$_2$ phosphorylation (90,233,234). In asymptomatic asthmatics, cPLA$_2$ in blood eosinophils is partially phosphorylated, and becomes further phosphorylated after allergen inhalation (235). Thus, such kinase-mediated regulation of cPLA$_2$ may be of importance in the increased eicosanoid release observed in asthma.

Secretory PLA$_2$s (sPLA$_2$) are low molecular weight (~14 kDa) isoforms released by many types of mammalian cells (236–238). One sPLA$_2$ hypothesis is that the PLA$_2$, contained within granules or vesicles in cells, is mobilized to the cell exterior by exocytosis (Fig. 7). The externalized sPLA$_2$ could bind to the external membrane, perhaps via heparin sulfate proteoglycans (239) or a specific sPLA$_2$ receptor (240–243). Activity of sPLA$_2$ requires high μM to mM Ca^{2+}, which is too high to occur within cells but would be matched by extracellular Ca^{2+}. Activated sPLA$_2$ could then hydrolyze the external leaflet of the plasma membrane, and thus release AA. This scenario has been proposed, e.g., in mouse and rat mast cells (244,245), human endothelial cells (246), P388D1 macrophage cells (247), and HL-60 myelomonocytic cells (248). Others have found that sPLA$_2$ has little effect on most cells, although cell membrane hydrolysis might be enhanced after cell stimulation (137) with resultant changes in membrane phospholipid packing or symmetry (249–251) or new expression of an sPLA$_2$ receptor.

The secretory group II phospholipase A$_2$ may have a role in autocrine and paracrine signaling beyond that of hydrolysis of membrane lipids. A cellular receptor for the secretory PLA$_2$ has been defined that appears to be identical to a mannose receptor (240–243). The sPLA$_2$s bind to the receptor via carbohydrate recognition domains (252). This receptor binding can act to transduce signals into cells including activation of the MAP kinase cascade, and anti-sPLA$_2$ antibody blocks the late phase of activation of MAP kinase induced by interleukin-1 (253). Eicosanoid release, induced by such events, is independent of the enzymatic activity of the sPLA$_2$ (254), further supporting a role for receptor-mediated events as another possible function of sPLA$_2$ in allergic inflammation.

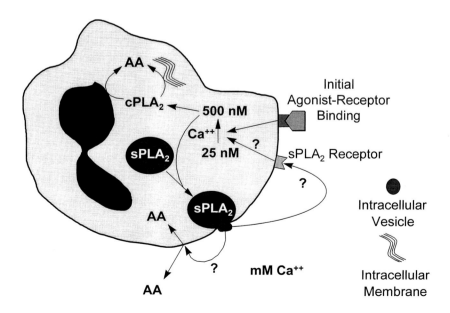

FIG. 7. A depiction of distinct, possible roles of cytosolic PLA$_2$ (cPLA$_2$) and secretory PLA$_2$ (sPLA$_2$) in cell function (here, a granulocyte). Most of the signaling pathways, including kinases, have been left out for simplicity. Receptor binding of an agonist causes an increase in cytosolic Ca^{2+} to the high nM range, which is sufficient to translocate cPLA$_2$ to nuclear or other membranes where membrane hydrolysis occurs. The cytosolic Ca^{2+} cannot activate sPLA$_2$ directly, but it is associated with exocytosis, which mobilizes sPLA$_2$ to the exterior; there it can be activated by extracellular Ca^{2+} and/or might interact in an autocrine manner via a specific sPLA$_2$ receptor.

Lysophospholipids

Lysophospholipid (such as lysophosphatidylcholine [lyso-PC]) is the other product of PLA_2. Lyso-PC may be particularly important in asthma as levels of this lipid are markedly elevated in bronchoalveolar lavage (BAL) of asthmatics after antigen challenge (255). The source of the lyso-PC within the airway lumen is currently being defined. It could be derived from airway cells or inflammatory cells, or be related to the release of secretory phospholipases A_2 into the airway lumen of asthmatics after antigen challenge, followed by hydrolysis of surfactant. Lyso-PC has multiple potential biologic activities. It can enhance cellular responses such as T-lymphocyte activation (256), cellular differentiation (257), chemotaxis (258), and increased expression of certain genes (259). In these models, lyso-PC markedly enhances responses to diacylglycerols or phorbol esters, suggesting that lyso-PC acts in synergy with diglycerides in the stimulation of PKC (61,256,260,261), although the mechanism of such synergy is unknown. At higher levels, lysolipids can be cytotoxic.

Lysophosphatidic acid is a platelet-derived phospholipid that serves as an extracellular agonist for multiple cell types via activation of a G protein–coupled receptor (262–264). This receptor is coupled to the G_i-p21 Ras pathway (265).

LIPID KINASES: THE PI 3-KINASE

In the "canonical pathway" (266) of phosphatidylinositol (PI) turnover, there is sequential phosphorylation of PI by PI 4-kinase and PI-4-P 5-kinase to yield $PI-4,5-P_2$, the preferred substrate for PLC, as discussed above. A new PI kinase was found that associates with receptor-associated protein tyrosine kinases and was subsequently found to phosphorylate the D-3 position of the inositol ring, producing PI-3-P, $PI-3,4-P_2$ or $PI-3,4,5-P_3$ (see Fig. 6) (reviewed in ref. 266). The 3-P products are being found to have important roles in signaling through diverse receptors.

Stimulation of many cells involves a rapid release of $PI-3,4-P_2$ and $PI-3,4,5-P_3$. Prevention of the PI3K response by mutation of cellular receptors or oncogenes also prevents, e.g., stimulation of mitogenesis, chemotaxis, actin assembly, and vesicle transport (reviewed in refs. 266,267). Other functions transduced via PI3K have been implicated by extensive use of PI3K inhibitors, especially wortmannin. These include stimulation of mast cell lines by $Fc_{\varepsilon}R1$ (268), of granulocytes by IgG receptors (269), or by chemotactic factor receptors (270,271) and activation of the T-cell receptor (272).

The best characterized isoform of PI3K is coupled to receptor-associated tyrosine kinases. It is a heterodimer of two peptides with masses of 85 and 110 kDa (p85 and p100, respectively). Cloning has revealed the p85 to be regulatory and contain two SH2 and one SH3 Src homology domains. The region between the two SH2 domains of p85 binds to the N-terminal region of p100. The SH2 regions of p85 are responsible for binding to tyrosine-phosphorylated domains on tyrosine kinase–associated receptors such as receptors for many growth factors. The 100-kDa subunit contains the catalytic site. How p85 achieves activation of p100 is being defined, but occupation of both p85 SH2 sites may be necessary and could involve a conformational shift in p85 that is somehow communicated to p100 (266).

It has been reported that another isoform of PI3K is coupled to the $\beta\gamma$ subunits of heterotrimeric G proteins in myeloid cells (35,273). Thus, as with PLC, specific isoforms of the enzyme may be required for interaction with G protein–coupled versus tyrosine kinase–coupled receptors.

Most intracellular targets for the products of PI3K remain unknown. One group of targets includes several isotypes of PKC. Although Ca^{2+}-activated isotypes (α,βI, βII,γ) were unaffected by $PI-3,4-P_2$ and $PI-3,4,5-P_3$, several Ca^{2+}-independent isotypes including δ,ε,η, and ζ are activated by these PI3K products, especially $PI-3,4,5-P_3$ (267,274,275). Interestingly, whereas Ca^{2+}-dependent isotypes of PKC require PS for activity, activation of the Ca^{2+}-independent PKCs by PI3K products was inhibited by PS (267). These studies showed direct effects of the PI3K products on isolated PKC isotypes *in vitro*. They have been extended to whole cells using a transgenic approach. In cultured cells overexpressing PI3K and individual PKC isotypes, PI3K was found to potentiate reporter gene expression in cells overexpressing the δ- and ε-isoforms but not the α-isoform of PKC (60). In addition to the PKC pathway, signaling from PI3K also may be coupled to Ras; however, it is uncertain if Ras directly activates a PI3K (276) or, conversely, if PI3K acts upstream of Ras (277).

PI3K also provides a potentially important site for therapeutics, as the inhibitory effects of elevated cAMP may be due to inhibition of PI3K in neutrophils (278).

SPHINGOMYELINASE RELEASES CERAMIDE

The hydrolysis of cellular sphingolipids is being recognized as a signaling path somewhat analogous to PLA_2-glycerophospholipid signaling. Sphingolipids contain a sphingoid base (such as sphingosine) at the 3 position, an amide-linked fatty acid at the 2 position, and various lipid chains in the 1 position. Sphingomyelinases (SMase) are phospholipase C–type enzymes with a specificity for sphingolipids that generate ceramide, which is thought to act as a second messenger in signaling. A membrane-associated SMase active at neutral pH has received most attention, although an endosomal acidic SMase may have distinct functions (279–281).

Most functions of the neutral SMase suggest roles in cellular differentiation, growth suppression, senescence, and/or death by apoptosis induced by agents such as TNFα, IL1β, interferon γ, NGF, glucocorticosteroids, and Fas (CD65) (282–284). Exact intracellular mechanisms are being defined. Ceramide activates specific protein kinase (ceramide-activated protein kinase; CAPK [283]) and phosphatase (ceramide-activated protein phosphatase; CAPP [282,285,286]) enzymes as well as the zeta isoform of PKC (PKCz) (287). CAPK is a 97-kDa proline-directed protein kinase that recognizes the substrate sequence Leu-Thr-Pro (283). Its activity is increased rapidly about 10-fold in cells stimulated with substances such as TNF-α or with exogenous SMase, but its natural substrates within the cell are not yet defined. CAPP belongs to the protein phosphatase 2A family (286) and is a prime candidate for intracellular actions of ceramide. The specificity of CAPP activation by various ceramide analogs paralleled their activity in inducing cellular apoptosis. Inhibition of PP2A phosphatases causes growth arrest and apoptosis, mimicking the effects of ceramide. As an example, the retinoblastoma gene product Rb is an important inhibitor of growth arrest and is activated by dephosphorylation of Rb. Ceramide analogs can induce Rb dephosphorylation. Moreover, Rb-deficient cell lines were resistant to ceramide-induced growth suppression (288). Rb mediates cell-cycle arrest but has no effect on apoptosis and the Rb-deficient deficient cells displayed normal ceramide-induced apoptosis.

Activation of PKC (e.g., by diacylglycerol) inhibited apoptosis induced by TNF or by ceramides; however, PKC activation did not affect growth arrest or the dephosphorylation of Rb. It appears that PKC and SMase have opposing effects on apoptosis induction. Thus, as suggested by Pushkareva et al. (282), the decision of cells to live or die may result from relative activity of two distinct signaling paths involving diacylglycerol and ceramide, respectively.

CONCLUSIONS

This chapter introduces the many mechanisms of signaling. Signaling pathways offer immense opportunities for improving therapeutic interventions. The baroque complexity (33) of signaling pathways renders a bit daunting the thought of intentionally manipulating them. But such manipulations are effected with therapeutic agents now available. Further knowledge of these events will allow for more effective and specific interventions in the future.

ACKNOWLEDGMENT

This work was supported in part by NIH grant HL-50395.

REFERENCES

1. Feller SM, Ren R, Hanafusa H, Baltimore D. SH2 and SH3 domains as molecular adhesives: the interactions of Crk and Abl. *Trends Biochem Sci* 1994;19:453–458.
2. Berridge MJ. The biology and medicine of calcium signaling. *Mol Cell Endocrinol* 1994;98:119–124.
3. Volpe P, Krause K-H, Hashimoto S, et al. "Calciosome," a cytoplasmic organelle: the inositol 1,4,5-trisphosphate-sensitive Ca^{2+} store of nomnuscle cells? *Proc Natl Acad Sci USA* 1988;85:1091–1095.
4. Putney JWJ, Bird GSJ. The inositol phosphate-calcium signaling system in nonexcitable cells. *Endocr Rev* 1993;14:610–631.
5. Pittet D, Lew DP, Mayr GW, Monod A, Schlegel W. Chemoattractant receptor promotion of Ca^{2+} influx across the plasma membrane of HL-60 cells. A role for cytosolic free calcium elevations and inositol 1,3,4,5-tetrakisphosphate production. *J. Biol Chem* 1989;264:7251–7261.
6. Krause K-H, Welsh MJ. Voltage-dependent and Ca^{2+}-activated ion channels in human neutrophils. *J Clin Invest* 1990;85:491–498.
7. Hoth M, Penner R. Depletion of intracellular stores activates a calcium current in mast cells. *Nature* 1992;355:353–356.
8. Zweifach A, Lewis RS. Mitogen-regulated Ca^{2+} current of T lymphocytes is activated by depletion of intracellular Ca^{2+}. *Proc Natl Acad Sci USA* 1993;90:6295–6299.
9. Demaurex N, Schlegel W, Varnai P, Mayr G, Lew DP, Krause K-H. Regulation of Ca influx in myeloid cells. Role of plasma membrane potential, inositol phosphates, cytosolic free $[Ca^{2+}]$, and filling state of intracellular Ca^{2+} stores. *J Clin Invest* 1992;90:830–839.
10. Bird GSJ, Putney JW, Jr. Inhibition of thapsigargin-induced calcium entry by microinjected guanine nucleotide analogues. Evidence for a small G-protein in capacitative calcium entry. *J Biol Chem* 1993;268:21486–21488.
11. Fasolato C, Hoth M, Penner R. A GTP-dependent step in the activation mechanism of capacitative calcium flux. *J Biol Chem* 1993;268:20737–20740.
12. Galione A, McDougall A, Busa WB, Willmott N, Gillot 1, Whitaker M. Redundant mechanisms of calcium-induced calcium release underlying calcium waves during fertilization of sea urchin eggs. *Science* 1993;261:348–352.
13. Parekh AB, Terlau H, Stuhmer W. Depletion of InSP3 stores activates a Ca^{2+} and K^+ current by means of a phosphatase and a diffusable messenger. *Nature* 1993;364:814–818.
14. Randriamampita C, Tsien RY. Emptying of intracellular Ca^{2+} stores releases a small messenger that stimulates Ca^{2+} influx. *Nature* 1993;364:809–814.
15. Berridge MJ. Calcium oscillations. *J Biol Chem* 1990;265:9583–9586.
16. Lew DP. Receptor signaling and intracellular calcium in neutrophil activation. *Eur J Clin Invest* 1989;19:338–346.
17. Omann GM, Porasik MM, Sklar LA. Oscillating actin polymerization/depolymerization responses in human polymorphonuclear leukocytes. *J Biol Chem* 1989;264:16355–16358.
18. Wymann MP, Kernen P, Deranleau DA, Baggiolini M. Respiratory burst oscillations in human neutrophils and their correlation with fluctuations in apparent cell shape. *J Biol Chem* 1989;264:15829–15834.
19. Hoffiman T, Lizzio EF, Suissa J, et al. Dual stimulation of phospholipase activity in human monocytes: role of calcium-dependent and calcium-independent pathways in arachidonic acid release and eicosanoid formation. *J Immunol* 1988;140:3912–3918.
20. Sneyd J, Wetton BT, Charles AC, Sanderson MJ. Intercellular calcium waves mediated by diffusion of inositol trisphosphate: a two-dimensional model. *Am J Physiol* 1995;268:C1537–45.
21. Schulman H. The multifunctional Ca^{2+}/calmodulin-dependent protein kinases. *Curr Opin Cell Biol* 1993;5:247–253.
22. Matsuda M, Mayer BJ, Hanafusa H. Identification of domains of the v-crk oncogene product sufficient for association with phosphotyrosine-containing proteins. Mol *Cell Biol* 1991;11:1607–1613.
23. Pawson T. Protein modules and signaling networks. *Nature* 1995;373:573–580.
24. Ren R, Mayer BJ, Cicchetti P, Baltimore D. Identification of a ten–amino acid proline-rich SH3 binding site. *Science* 1993;259:1157–1161.

25. de Mendez I, Garrett MC, Adams AG, Leto TL. Role of p67-phox SH3 domains in assembly of the NADPH oxidase system. *J Biol Chem* 1994;269:16326–16332.

26. Buday L, Downward J. Epidermal growth factor regulates p2 ras through the formation of a complex of receptor, Grb2 adapter protein, and Sos nucleotide exchange factor. *Cell* 1993;73:611–620

27. Chardin P, Camonis JH, Gale NW, et al. Human Sosl: a guanine nucleotide exchange factor for Ras that binds to GRB2. *Science* 1993; 260:1338–1343.

28. Schlessinger J. How receptor tyrosine kinases activate Ras. *TIBS* 1993;18:273–275.

29. Musacchio A, Gibson T, Rice P, Thompson J, Saraste M. The PH domain: a common piece in the structural patchwork of signaling proteins. *TIBS* 1993;18:343–348.

30. Pitcher JA, Touhara K, Payne ES, Lefkowitz RJ. Pleckstrin homology domain-mediated membrane association and activation of the β-adrenergic receptor kinase requires coordinate interaction with G βγ subunits and lipid. *J Biol Chem* 1995;270:11707–11710.

31. Harlan JE, Hajduk PJ, Yoon HS, Fesick SW. Pleckstrin homology domains bind to phosphatidylinositol-4,5-bisphosphate. *Nature (Lond)* 1994;371:168–170.

32. Moss J, Vaughan M. Structure and function of ARF proteins: activators of cholera toxin and critical components of intracellular vesicular transport processes. J *Biol Chem* 1995;270:12327–12330.

33. Macara IG, Lounsbury KM, Richards SA, McKieman C, Bar-Sagi D. The Ras superfamily of GTPases. *FASEB J* 1996;10:625–630.

34. Bowman EP, Uhlinger DJ, Lambeth JD. Neutrophil phospholipase D is activated by a membrane-associated Rho family small molecular weight GTP-binding protein. *J Biol Chem* 1993;268:21509–21512.

35. Takaishi K, Kikuchi A, Kuroda S, Kotani K, Sasaki T, Takai Y. Involvement of rho p2l and its inhibitor GDP/GTP exchange protein (rho GDI) in cell motility. *Mol Cell Biol* 1993;13:72.

36. Bokoch GM. Regulation of the human neutrophil NADPH oxidase by the Rac GTPbinding proteins. *Curr Opin Cell Biol* 1994;6:212–218.

37. Nobes CD, Hall A. Rho, Rac and Cdc42p GTPases regulate the assembly of multimolecular focal complexes associated with actin stress fibers, lamellipodia and filopodia. *Cell* 1995;81:53–62.

38. Pffeffer S. Rab GTPases: master regulators of membrane trafficking. *Curr Opin Cell Biol* 1994;6:522

39. Melchior F, Gerace L. Mechanisms of nuclear protein import. *Curr Opin Biol* 1995;7:310–318.

40. Polakis P, McCormick F. Structural requirements for the interaction of p2I ras, with GAP, exchange factors, and its biological effector target. *J Biol Chem* 1993;268:9157–9160.

41. Johnson LN, Barford D. The effects of phosphorylation of the structure and function of proteins. *Annu Rev Biophys Biomol Struct* 1993; 22:199–232.

42. Hubbard MJ, Cohen P. On target with a new mechanism for the regulation of protein phosphorylation. *TIBS* 1993;18:172–177.

43. Hanks SK, Quinn AM, Hunter T. The protein kinase family: conserved features and deduced phylogeny of the catalytic domains. *Science* 1988;241:42–52.

44. Taylor SS, Knighton DR, Zheng J, Ten Eyck LF, Sowadski JM. Structural framework for the protein kinase family. *Annu Rev Cell Biol* 1992;8:429–462.

45. Pawson T. Introduction: protein kinase. *FASEB J* 1994;8:1112–1113.

46. Wrana JL, Atlisano L, Wieser R, Ventura F, Massague J. Mechanism of activation of the TGF-P receptor. *Nature* 1994;370:341–347.

47. Wu J, Dent P, Jelinek T, Wolfman A, Weber MJ, Sturgill TW. Inhibition of the EGF-activated MAP kinase signaling pathway by adenosine 3′,5′-monophosphate. *Science* 1993;262:1065–1069.

48. Cook SJ, McCormick F. Inhibition by cAMP of Ras-dependent activation of Raf. *Science* 1993;262:1069–1072.

49. Chuang E, Barnard D, Hettich L, Zhang XF, Avruch J, Marshall MS. Critical binding and regulatory interactions between Ras and Raf occur through a small, stable N-terminal domain of Raf and specific Ras effector residues. *Mol Cell Biol* 1994;14:5318–5325.

50. Bolger GB. Molecular biology of the cyclic AMP-specific cyclic nucleotide phosphodiesterases: a diverse family of regulatory enzymes. *Cell Signal* 1994;6:851–859.

51. Manganiello VC, Murata T, Taira M, Belfrage P, Degerman E. Diversity in cyclic nucleotide phosphodiesterase isoenzyme families. *Arch Biochem Biophys* 1995;322:1–13.

52. Smolen JE, Korchak HM, Weissmann G. Increased levels of cyclic adnosine-3′,5′monophosphate in human polymorphonuclear leukocytes after surface stimulation. *J Clin Invest* 1980;65:1077–1085.

53. Fonteh AN, Winkler JD, Torphy TJ, Heravi J, Undem BJ, Chilton FH. Influence of isoproterenol and phosphodiesterase inhibitors on platelet-activating factor biosynthesis in the human neutrophil. *J Immunol* 1993;151:339–350.

54. Weinberger M, Hendeles L. Theophylline in asthma. *N Engl J Med* 1996;21:1380–1388.

55. Giembycz MA. Could isoenzyme-selective phosphodiesterase inhibitors render bronchodilator therapy redundant in the treatment of bronchial asthma?. *Biochem Pharmacol* 1992;43:2041–2051.

56. Torphy TJ, Undem BJ, Cieslinski LB, Luttmann MA, Reeves ML, Hay DW. Identification, characterization and functional role of phosphodiesterase isozymes in human airway smooth muscle. *J Pharmacol Exp Ther* 1993;265:1213–1223.

57. Underwood DC, Kotzer CJ, Bochnowicz S, et al. Comparison of phosphodiesterase III, IV and dual III/IV inhibitors on bronchospasm and pulmonary eosinophil influx in guinea pigs. *J Pharmacol Exp Ther* 1994;270:250–259.

58. Kishimoto A, Takai Y, Mori T, Kikkawa U, Nishizuka Y. Activation of calcium and phospholipid-dependent protein kinase by diacylglycerol, its possible relation to phosphatidylinositol turnover. *J Biol Chem* 1980;255:2273–2276.

59. Liscovitch M, Cantley LC. Lipid second messengers. *Cell* 1994;77:329–334.

60. Jaken S, Kiley SC. Protein kinase C: interactions and consequences. *Trends Cell Biol* 1994;4:223–227.

61. Nishizuka Y. Protein kinase C and lipid signaling for sustained cellular responses. *FASEB J* 1995;9:484–496.

62. Selbie LA, Schmitz-Peiffer C, Sheng Y, Biden TJ. Molecular cloning and characterization of PKC iota, an atypical isoform of protein kinase C derived from insulin-secreting cells. *J Biol Chem* 1993;268: 24296–24302.

63. Khan WA, Blobe GC, Hannun YA. Arachidonic acid and free fatty acids as second messengers and the role of protein kinase C. *Cell Signal* 1995;7:171–184.

64. Cooper JA, Howell B. The when and how of Src regulation. *Cell* 1993; 73:1051–1054.

65. Weiss A, Littman DR. Signal transduction by lymphocyte antigen receptors. *Cell* 1994;76:263–274.

66. Mano H, Yamashita Y, Sato K, Yazaki Y, Hirai H. Tec protein-tyrosine kinase is involved in interleukin-3 signaling pathway. *Blood* 1995;85: 343–350.

67. Mano H, Yamashita Y, Miyazato A, Miura Y, Ozawa K. Tec protein-tyrosine kinase is an effector molecule of Lyn protein-tyrosine kinase. *FASEB J* 1996;10:637–642.

68. Samelson LE, Klausner RD. Tyrosine kinases and tyrosine-based activation motifs. Current research on activation via the T cell antigen receptor. *J Biol Chem* 1992;267:24913–24916.

69. Veillette A, Abraham N, Caron L, Davidson D. The lymphocyte-specific tyrosine kinase p56-lck. *Semin Immunol* 1991;3:143–152.

70. Johnson SA, Pleiman CM, Pao L, Schneringer J, Hippen K, Cambier JC. Phosphorylated immunoreceptor signaling motifs (ITAMS) exhibit unique abilities to bind and activate Lyn and Syk tyrosine kinases. *J Immunol* 1995;155:4596–4603.

71. Karnitz L, Sutor SL, Torigoe T, et al. Effects of p56-lck deficiency on the growth and cytolytic effector function of an interleukin-2-dependent cytotoxic T-cell line. *Mol Cell Biol* 1992;12:4521–4530.

72. Straus DB, Weiss A. Genetic evidence for the involvement of the lck tyrosine kinase in signal transduction through the T cell antigen receptor. *Cell* 1992;70:585–593.

73. Benhamou M, Ryba NJP, Kihara H, Nishikata H, Siraganian RP. Protein-tyrosine kinase p72 syk in high affinity IgE receptor signaling. Identification as a component of pp72 and association with the receptor gamma chain after receptor aggregation. *J Biol Chem* 1993; 268:23318–23324.

74. Shiue L, Zoller MJ, Brugge JS. Syk is activated by phosphotyrosine-containing peptides representing the tyrosine-based activation motifs of the high affinity receptor for IgE. *JBiol Chem*.1995;270:10498–10502.

75. Hirasawa N, Scharenberg A, Yamamura H, Beaven MA, Kinet J-P. A requirement for Syk in the activation of the microtubule-associated protein kinase/phospholipase A^2 pathway by Rc-R1 is not shared by a G protein-coupled receptor. *J Biol Chem* 1995;270:10960–10967.

76. Darby C, Geahlen RL, Schreiber AD. Stimulation of macrophage Fc-γRIIIA activates the receptor-associated protein tyrosine kinase Syk and induces phosphorylation of the multiple proteins including p95Vav and p62/GAP-associated protein. *J Immunol* 1994;152:5429.

77. Lin TH, Rosales C, Mondal K, Bolen JB, Haskill S, Juliano RL. Integrin-mediated tyrosine phosphorylation and cytokine message induction in monocytic cells. A possible signaling role for the Syk tyrosine kinase. *J Biol Chem* 1995;270:16189–16197.

78. Agarwal A, Salem P, Robbins KC. Involvement of p72^{syk}, a protein-tyrosine kinase, in Fcγ receptor signaling. *J Biol Chem* 1993;268: 15900–15905.

79. Asahi M, Taniguchi T, Hashimoto E, Inazu T, Maeda H, Yamamura H. Activation of protein-tyrosine kinase p72^{syk} with concanavalin A in polymorphonuclear neutrophils. *J Biol Chem* 1993;268:23334–23338.

80. Kolanus W, Romeo C, Seed B. T cell activation by clustered tyrosine kinases. *Cell* 1993;74:171–813.

81. Wilson BS, Kapp N, Lee RJ, et al. Distinct functions of the Fc εR1 gamma and subunits in the control of FcεR1-mediated tyrosine kinase activation and signaling responses in RBL-2H3 mast cells. *J Biol Chem* 1995;270:4013–4022.

82. Davis RJ. The mitogen-activated protein kinase signal transduction pathway. *J Biol Chem* 1993;268:14553–14556.

83. Drijard B, Hibi M, Wy I-H, et al. JNK1: a protein kinase stimulated by UV light and Ha-Ras that binds and phosphorylates the c-Jun activation domain. *Cell* 1994;76:1025–1037.

84. Raingeaud J, Gupta S, Rogers JS, et al. Pro-inflammatory cytokines and environmental stress cause p38 mitogen-activated protein kinase activation by dual phosphorylation on tyrosine and threonine. *J Biol Chem* 1995;270:7420–7426.

85. Seger R, Krebs EG. The MAPK signaling cascade. *FASEB J* 1995;9: 726–735.

86. Lin LL, Wartmann M, Lin AY, Knopf JL, Seth A, Davis RJ. cPLA2 is phosphorylated and activated by MAP kinase. *Cell* 1993;72:269–278.

87. Han J, Lee J-D, Bibbs L, Ulevitch RJ. A MAP kinase targeted by endotoxin and hyperosmolarity in mammalian cells. *Science* 1994;265: 808–812.

88. Nemenoff RA, Winitz S, Qian N-X, Van Putten V, Johnson GL, Heasley LE. Phosphorylation and activation of a high molecular weight form of phospholipase A₂ by p42 microtubule-associated protein 2 kinase and protein kinase C. *J Biol Chem* 1993;268:1960–1964.

89. Kramer RM, Roberts EF, Hyslop PA, Utterback BG, Hui KY, Jakubowski JA. Differential activation of cytosolic phospholipse A₂ by thrombin and thrombin receptor antagonist peptide in human platelets. *J Biol Chem* 1995;270:14816–14823.

90. Fouda SI, Molski TFP, Ashour MS, Sha'afi RI. Effect of lipopolysaccharide on mitogen-activated protein kinases and cytosolic phospholipase A₂. *Biochem J* 1995;308:815–822.

91. Karin M. The regulation of AP-1 activity by mitogen-activated protein kinases. *J Biol Chem* 1995;270:16483–16486.

92. Li W, Whaley CD, Mondino A, Mueller DL. Blocked signal transduction to the ERK and JNK protein kinases in anergic DC⁺ T cells. *Science* 1996;271:1272–1276.

93. Fields PE, Gajewski TF, Fitch FW. Blocked Ras activation in anergic CD4+ T cells. *Science* 1996;271:1276–1278.

94. Genot EM, Parker PJ, Cantrell DA. Anaysis of the role of protein kinase C-α, -ε, and -xi in T cell activation. *J Biol Chem* 1995;270:9833–9839.

95. Van Biesen T, Hawes BE, Luttrell DK, et al. Receptor-tyrosine-kinase and G beta gamma-mediated MAP kinase activation by a common signalling pathway. *Nature* 1995;376:781–784.

96. Satoh T, Nakafuku M, Kaziro Y. Function of Ras as a molecular switch in signal transduction. *J Biol Chem* 1992;267:24149–24152.

97. Porfiri E, Evans T, Chardin P, Hancock JF. Prenylation of Ras proteins is required for efficient hSOS1-promoted guianine nucleotide exchange. J Biol Chem 1994;269:22672–22677.

98. Grand RJ, Owen D. The biochemistry of ras p21 *Biochem J* 1991;279: 609–631.

99. Pronk GJ, Bos JL. The role of p2I ras in receptor tyrosine kinase signalling. *Biochim Biophys Acta* 1994;1198:131–147.

100. Barnard D, Diaz B, Hettich L, et al. Identification of the sites of interaction between c-Raf-I and Ras-GTP. *Oncogene* 1995;10:1283–1290.

101. Vojtek AB, Hollenberg SM, Cooper JA. Mammalian Ras interacts with the serine/threonine kinase Raf. *Cell* 1993;74:205–214.

102. Hallberg B, Rayter SI, Downward J. Interaction of Ras and Raf in intact mammalian cells upon extracellular stimulation. *J Biol Chem* 1994;269:3913–3916.

103. Stokoe D, MacDonald SG, Cadwallader K, Symons S, Hancock JF. Activation of Raf as a result of recruitment to the plasma membrane. *Science* 1994;264:1463–1467.

104. Leevers SJ, Paterson HF, Marshall CJ. Requirement for Ras in Raf activation is overcome by targeting Raf to the plasma membrane. *Nature* 1994;369:411–414.

105. Kolch W, Heidecker G, Kochs G, et al. Protein kinase C alpha activates Raf-1 by direct phosphorylation. *Nature* 1993;364:249–252.

106. Carroll MP, May WS. Protein kinase C-mediated serine phosphorylation directly activates Raf-I in murine hematopoietic cells. *J Biol Chem* 1994;269:1249–1256.

107. Morrison DK, Heidecker G, Rapp UR, Copeland TD. Identification of the major phosphorylation sites of the Raf-1 kinase. *J Biol Chem* 1993;268:17309–17316.

108. Force T, Bonventre JV, Heidecker G, Rapp U, Avruch J, Kyriakis JM. Enzymatic charactersistics of the c-raf- I protein kinase. *Proc Natl Acad Sci USA* 1994;91:1270–1274.

109. Ghosh S, Strum JC, Sciorra VA, Daniel L, Bell RM. Raf-I kinase possesses distinct binding domains for phosphatidylserine and phosphatidic acid. Phosphatidic acid regulates the translocation of Raf-1 in 12-0-tetradecanooylphorbol-13-acetate-stimulated Madin-Darby canine kidney cells. *J Biol Chem* 1996;271:8472–8480.

110. Picard D, Khursheed B, Garabedian MJ, Fortin MG, Lindquist S, Yamamoto KR. Reduced levels of hsp9O compromise steroid receptor action *in vivo*. *Nature* 1990;348:166–168.

111. Wartmann M, Davis RJ. The native structure of the activated Raf protein kinase is a membane-bound multi-subunit complex. *J Biol Chem*.1994;269:6695–6701.

112. Colotta F, Polentarutti N, Mantovani A. Differential expression of Raf-1 protooncogene in resting and activated human leukocyte populations. *Exp Cell Res* 1991;194:284–288.

113. Marshall MS. Ras target proteins in eukaryotic cells. *FASEB J* 1995; 9:1311–1318.

114. Anderson NG, Maller JL, Tonks NK, Sturgill TW. Requirement for integration of signals from two distinct phosphorylation pathways for activation of MAP kinase. *Nature* 1990;343:651–653.

115. Zheng C-F, Guan K-L. Cytoplasmic localization of the mitogen-activated protein kinase activator MEK. *J Biol Chem* 1995;269:19947–19952.

116. Gonzales FA, Raden DL, Davis RJ. Identification of substrate recognition determinants for human ERKI and ERK2 protein kinases. *J Biol Chem* 1991;266:22159–22163.

117. Boulton TC, Yancopoulos GD, Gregory SJ, et al. An insulin-stimulated protein kinase similar to yeast kinases involved in cell cycle control. *Science* 1990;249:64–67.

118. Miltenberger RJ, Cortner J, Farnham PJ. An inhibitory Raf-1 mutant suppresses expression of a subset of v-raf–activated genes. *J Biol Chem* 1993;268:15674–15680.

119. Wang LM, Keegan AD, Paul WE, Heidaran MA, Gutkind JS, Pierce JH. IL-4 activates a distinct signal transduction cascade from IL-3 in factor-dependent myeloid cells. *EMBO J* 1992;11:4899–4908.

120. Yamaguchi Y, Suda T, Suda J, et al. Purified interleukin-5 supports the terminal differentiation and proliferation of murine eosinophilic precursors. *J Exp Med* 1988;167:43–56.

121. Ishizaka T, Saito H, Hatake K, Dvorak AM, Leiferman KM, Arai N, Ishizaka K. Preferential differentiation of inflammatory cells by recombinant human interleukins. *Int Arch Allergy Appl Immunol* 1989; 88:46–49.

122. Lu L, Lin Z-H, Shen R-N, Warren DJ, Leemhuis T, Broxmeyer HE. Influence of interleukins-3,-5, and -6 on the growth of eosinophil progenitors in highly enriched human bone marrow in the absence of serum. *Exp Hematol* 1990;18:1180–1186.

123. Han J, Lee JD, Tobias PS, Ulevitch RJ. Endotoxin induces rapid protein phosphorylation in 7OZ/3 cells expressing CD14. *J Biol Chem* 1993;268:25009–25014.

124. Alberola-Ila J, Forbush KA, Seger R, Krebs EG, Perlmutter RM. Selective requirement for MAP kinase activation in thymocyte differentiation. *Nature* 1995;373:620–623.

125. Her E, Frazer J, Austen KF, Owen WF, Jr. Eosinophil hematopoietins

antagonize the programmed cell death of eosinophils. Cytokine and glucocorticoid effects on eosinophils maintained by endothelial cell-conditioned medium. *J Clin Invest* 1991;88:1982–1987.

126. Stem M, Meagher L, Savill J, Haslett C. Apoptosis in human eosinophils: programmed cell death in the eosinophil leads to phagocytosis by macrophages and is modulated by IL-5. *J Immunol* 1992; 148:3543–3549.

127. Ohnishi T, Sur S, Collins DS, Fish JE, Gleich GJ, Peters SP. Eosinophil survival activity identified as interleukin-5 is assocaited with eosinophil recruitment and degranulation and lung injury twenty-four hours after segmental antigen lung challenge. *J Allergy Clin Immunol* 1993;92:607–615.

128. McCall CE, Bass DA, DeChatelet LR, Link ASJ, Mann M. *In vitro* responses of human neutrophils to N-formyl-methionyl-leucyl-phenylalanine: correlation with effects of acute infection. *J Infect Dis* 1979; 140:277–286.

129. Guthrie LA, McPhail LC, Henson PM, Johnston RB, Jr. Priming of neutrophils for enhanced release of oxygen metabolites by bacterial lipopolysaccharide. Evidence for increased activity of the superoxide-producing enzyme. *J Exp Med* 1984;160:1656–1671.

130. McPhail LC, Clayton CC, Snyderman R. The NADPH oxidase of human polymorphonuclear leukocytes. Evidence for regulation by multiple signals. *J Biol Chem* 1984;259:5768–5775.

131. Bass DA, Gerard C, Olbrantz P, Wilson J, McCall CE, McPhail LC. Priming of neutrophil respiratory burst by diacylglycerol. Independence from activation or translocation of protein kinase C. *J Biol Chem* 1987;262:6643–6649.

132. Bass DA, McPhail LC, Schmitt JD, Morris-Natschke S, McCall CE, Wykle RL. Selective priming of rate and duration of the respiratory burst of neutrophils by 1,2-diacyl and I 0-alkyl-2-acyl diglycerides. Possible relation to effects on protein kinase C. *J Biol Chem* 1988; 263:19610–19617.

133. Bauldry SA, Wykle RL, Bass DA. Phospholipase A2 activation in human neutrophils. Differential actions of diacylglycerols and alkylacylglycerols in priming cells for stimulation by N-formyl-Met-Leu-Phe. *J Biol Chem* 1988;263:16787–16795.

134. Brunner T, de Weck AL, Dahinden CA. Platelet-activating factor induces mediator release by human basophils primed with IL-3, granulocyte-macrophage colony-stimulating factor, or IL-5. *J Immunol* 1991;147:237–242.

135. Takaftiji S, Bischoff SC, de Weck AL, Dahinden CA. IL-3 and IL-5 prime normal human eosinophils to produce leukotriene C4 in response to soluble agonists. *J Immunol* 1991;147:3855–3861.

136. Fabian I, Kletter Y, Mor S, et al. Activation of human eosinophil and neutrophil functions by haematopoietic growth factors: comparisons of IL-1, IL-3, IL-5 and GM-CSF. *Br J Haematol* 1992;80:137–143.

137. Ely EW, Seeds MC, Jones DF, Chilton FH, Bass DA. Primed release of arachidonic acid and oxidants from human neutrophils: causally related or independent? *Biochim Biophys Acta Lipids Lipid Metab* 1995;1258:135–144.

138. Raines MA, Golde DW, Daeipour M, Nel AE. Granulocyte-macrophage colony-stimulating factor activates microtubule-associated protein 2 kinase in neutrophils via a tyrosine kinase-dependent pathway. *Blood* 1992;79:3350–3354.

139. Pazdrak K, Schreiber D, Forsythe P, Justement L, Alam R. The intracellular signal transduction mechanism of interleukin 5 in eosinophils: the involvement of lyn tyrosine kinase and the Ras-Raf-1-MEK-microtubule-associated protein kinase pathway. *J Exp Med* 1995;181:1827–1834.

140. Lopez AF, Sanderson CJ, Gamble JR, Campbell HD, Young IG, Vadas MA. Recombinant human interleukin-5 is a selective activator of human eosinophil function. *J Exp Med* 1988;167:219–224.

141. O'Sullivan MG, Chilton FH, Huggins EM, Jr, McCall CE. Lipopolysaccharide priming of alveolar macrophages for enhanced synthesis of prostanoids involves induction of a novel prostaglandin H synthase. *J Biol Chem* 1992;267:14547–14550.

142. Pueringer RJ, Hunninghake GW. Lipopolysaccharide stimulates de novo synthesis of PGH synthase in human alveolar macrophages. *Am J Physiol Lung Cell Mol Physiol* 1992;262:L78–L85.

143. Kawata R, Reddy ST, Wolner B, Herschman HR. Prostaglandin synthase I and prostaglandin synthase 2 both participate in activation-induced prostaglandin D2 production in mast cells. *J Immunol* 1995; 155:818–825.

144. Stone RL, Dixon JE. Protein-tyrosine phosphatases. J Biol *Chem* 1994;260:31323–31326.

145. Koretzky GA, Pincus J, Thomas ML, Weiss A. Tyrosine phosphatase CD45 is essential for coupling T cell antigen receptor to the phosphatidylinositol pathway. *Nature* 1990;346:66.

146. Berger SA, Mak TW, Paige CJ. Leukocyte common antigen (CD45) is required for immunoglobulin E-mediated degranulation of mast cells. *J Exp Med* 1994;180:471

147. Yi T, lhle JN. Association of hematopoietic cell phosphatase with c-kit after stimulation with c-kit ligand. *Mol Cell Biol* 1993;13:3350

148. Yi T, Mui ALF, Krystal G, lhle JN. Hematopoietic cell phosphatase associates with the interleukin-3 (IL-3) receptor P chain and down-regulates IL-3 induced tyrosine phosphorylation and mitogenesis. *Mol Cell Biol* 1993;13:7577

149. Pani G, Kozlowski M, Cambier JC, Mills GB, Siminovitch KA. Identification of the tyrosine phosphatase PTP IC as a B cell antigen receptor-associated protein involved in the regulation of B cell signaling (see comments). *J Exp Med* 1995;181:2077–2084.

150. Uchida T, Matozaki T, Noguchi T, et al. Insulin stimulates the phosphorylation of Tyr'18 and the catalytic activity of PTP IC, a protein tyrosine phosphatase with Src homology-2 domains. *J Biol Chem* 1994;269:12230

151. Feng GS, Hui CC, Pawson T. SH2-containing phosphotyrosine phosphatase as a target of protein-tyrosine kinases. *Science* 1993;259: 1607

152. Case RD, Piccione E, Wolf G, Benett AM, Lechleider RJ, Neel BG, Shoelson SE. SH-PTP2/Syp SH2 domain binding specificity is defined by direct interactions with platelet- derived growth factor P-receptor, epidermal growth factor receptor, and insulin receptor substrate-I-derived phosphopeptides. *J Biol Chem* 1994;269:10467

153. Li W, Nishimura R, Kashishian A, Batzer AG, Kim WJH, Cooper JA, Schlessinger J.A new function for a phosphotyrosine phosphatase: linking GRB2-Sos to a receptor tyrosine kinase. *Mol Cell Biol* 1994; 14:509

154. Benhamou M, Gutkind JS, Robbins KC, Siraganian RP. Tyrosine phosphorylation coupled to IgE receptor-mediated signal transduction and histamine release. Proc Natl *Acad Sci USA* 1990;87:5327

155. Paolini R, Jouvin MH, Kinet JP. Phosphorylation and dephosphorylatin of the highaffinity receptor for immunoglobulin E immediately after receptor engagement and disengagement. *Nature* 1991;353:885.

156. Kent UM, Mao S-Y, Wofsy C, Goldstein B, Ross S, Metzger H. Dynamics of signal transduction after aggregation of cell-surface receptors: studies on the type I receptor for IgE. *Proc Natl Acad Sci USA* 1994;91:3087–3091.

157. Swieter M, Berenstein EH, Siraganian RP. Protein tyrosine phosphatase activity associates with the high affinity IgE receptor and dephosphorylates the receptor subunits, but not Lyn or Syk. *J Immunol* 1995;155:5330–5336.

158. Cohen P. Structure and regulation of protein phosphatases. *Annu Rev Biochem* 1992;58:453–508.

159. Mochly-Rosen D. Localization of protein kinases by anchoring proteins: a theme in signal transduction. *Science* 1995;268:247–251.

160. Klauck TM, Faux MC, Labudda K, Langeberg LK, Jaken S, Scott JD. Coordination of three signaling enzymes by AKAP79, a mammalian scaffold protein. *Science* 1996;271:1589–1592.

161. Majerus PW. Inositol phosphate biochemistry. *Annu Rev Biochem* 1992;61:225–250.

162. Majerus PW. Inositol phosphate biochemistry. *Annu Rev Biochem* 1992;61:225–250.

163. Rhee SG, Choi KD. Regulation of inositol-specific phospholipase C isozymes. *J Biol Chem* 1992;267:12393–12396.

164. Camps M, Hou C, Sidiropoulos D, Stock JB, Jacobs KH, Gierschik P. Stimulation of phospholipase C by guanine-nucleotide-binding protein βγ subunits. *Eur J Biochem* 1992;206:821.

165. Blank JL, Brattain KA, Exton JH. Activation of cytosolic phosphoinositide phospholipase C by G-protein βγ subunits. *J Biol Chem* 1992;267:23069.

166. Secrist JP, Kamitz L, Abraham RT. T-cell antigen receptor ligation induces tyrosine phospholipasec-γ 1. *J Biol Chem* 1991;266:12135–12139.

167. Li W, Deanin GG, Margolis B, Schlessinger J, Oliver JM. FcεR1 -mediated tyrosine phosphorylation of multiple proteins, including phospholipase Cγ1 and the receptor βγ complex, in RBL-2H3 rat basophilic leukemia cells. *Mol Cell Biol* 1992;12:3176–3182.

168. Carter RH, Park JD, Rhee SG, Fearon DT. Tyrosine phosphorylation of phospholipase C induced by membrane immunoglobulin in B lymphocytes. Proc *Natl Acad Sci* 1991;88:2745–2749.

169. Exton JH. Phosphatidylcholine breakdown and signal transduction. *Biochim Biophys Acta* 1994;1212:26–42.

170. Daniel LW, Waite M, Wykle RL. A novel mechanism for diglyceride formation. 120-tetradecanoylphorbol-13-acetate stimulates the cyclic breakdown and resynthesis of phosphatidylcholine. *J Biol Chem* 1986 261:9128–9132.

171. Huang C, Wykle RL, Daniel LW, Cabot MC. Identification of phosphatidylcholineselective and phosphatidylinositol-selective phospholipases D in Madin-Darby canine kidney cells. *J Biol Chem* 1992; 267:16859–16865.

172. Lambeth JD, Kwak JY, Bowman EP, Perry D, Uhlinger DJ, Lopez 1. ADPribosylation factor functions synergistically with a 50-kDa cytosolic factor in cell-free activation of human neutrophil phospholipase D. *J Biol Chem* 1995;270:2431–2434.

173. Siddiqi AR, Smith JL, Ross AH, Qiu RG, Symons M, Exton JH. Regulation of phospholipase D in HL60 cells. Evidence for a cytosolic phospholipase D. *J Biol Chem* 1995;270:8466–8473.

174. Kwak JY, Lopez 1, Uhlinger DJ, Ryu SH, Lambeth JD. RhoA and a cytosolic 50kDa factor reconstitute GTP γ S-dependent phospholipase D activity in human neutrophil subcellular fractions. *J Biol Chem* 1995;270:27093–27098.

175. Hammond SM, Altshuller YM, Sung TC, et al. Human ADP-ribosylation factoractivated phosphatidylcholine-specific phospholipase D defines a new and highly conserved gene family. *J Biol Chem* 1995; 270:29640–29643.

176. Liu M, Xu J, Liu J, Kraw ME, Tanswell AK, Post M. Mechanical strain-enhanced fetal lung cell proliferation is mediated by phospholipase C and D and protein kinase C. *Am J Physiol* 1995;268:L729–38.

177. Koike T, Hirai K, Morita Y, Nozawa Y. Stem cell factor-induced signal transduction in rat mast cells. Activation of phospholipase D but not phosphoinositide-specific phospholipase C in c-kit receptor stimulation. *J Immunol* 1993;151:359–366.

178. Pai J-K, Siegel MI, Egan RW, Billah MM. Phospholipase D catalyzes phospholipid metabolism in chemotactic peptide-stimulated HL-60 granulocytes. *J Biol Chem* 1988;263:12472–12477.

179. Agwu DE, McPhail LC, Chabot MC, Daniel LW, Wykle RL, McCall CE. Cholinelinked phosphoglycerides. A source of phosphatidic acid and diglycerides in stimulated neutrophils. *J Biol Chem* 1989;264:1405–1413.

180. Agwu DE, McPhail LC, Sozzani S, Bass DA, McCall CE. Phosphatidic acid as a second messenger in human polymorphonuclear leukocytes: effects on activation of the NADPH oxidase. *J Clin Invest* 1991; 88:531–539.

181. Lin P, Wiggan GA, Gilfillan AM. Activation of phospholipase D in a rat mast (RBL 2H3) cell line. A possible unifying mechanism for IgE-dependent degranulation and arachidonic acid metabolite release. *J Immunol* 199 1;146:1609–1616.

182. Khan WA, Blobe GC, Richards AL, Hannun YA. Identification, partial purification, and characterization of a novel phospholipid-dependent and fatty acid-activated protein kinase from human platelets. *J Biol Chem* 1994;269:9729–9735.

183. McPhail LC, Qualliotine-Mann D, Waite KA. Cell-free activation of neutrophil NADPH oxidase by a phosphatidic acid-regulated protein kinase. *Proc Natl Acad Sci USA* 1995;92:7931–7935.

184. Bonser RW, Thompson NT, Randall RW, Garland LG. Phospholipase D activation is functionally linked to superoxide generation in the human neutrophil. *Biochem J* 1989;264:617–620.

185. Bauldry SA, Bass DA, Cousart SL, McCall CE. Tumor necrosis factor cc priming of phospholipase D in human neutrophils: correlation between phosphatidic acid production and superoxide generation. *J Biol Chem* 1991;266:4173–4179.

186. Kessels GCR, Roos D, Verhoeven AJ. fMet-Leu-Phe-induced activation of phospholipase D in human neutrophils. Dependence on changes in cytosolic free Ca^{2+} concentration and relation with respiratory burst activation. *J Biol Chem* 1991;266:23152–23156.

187. Bauldry SA, Elsey KL, Bass DA. Activation of NADPH oxidase and phospholipase D in penneabilized human neutrophils: correlation between oxidase activation and phosphatidic acid production. *J Biol Chem* 1992;267:25141–25152.

188. Jenkins GH, Fisette PL, Anderson RA. Type I phosphatidylinositol 4-phosphate 5kinase isoforms are specifically stimulated by phosphatidic acid. *J Biol Chem* 1994;269:11547–11554.

189. Limatola C, Schaap D, Moolenaar WH, van Blitterswijk WJ. Phosphatidic acid activation of protein kinase C–zeta overexpressed in COS cells: comparison with other protein kinase C isotypes and other acidic lipids. *Biochem J* 1994;304:1001–1008.

190. Tomic S, Greiser U, Lammers R, et al. Association of SH2 domain protein tyrosine phosphatases with the epidermal growth factor receptor in human tumor cells. Phosphatidic acid activates receptor dephosphorylation by PTPLC. *J Biol Chem* 1995;270:21277–21284.

191. Kahn RA, Yucel JK, Malhotra V. ARF signaling: a potential role for phospholipase D in membrane traffic (comment). *Cell* 1993;75:1045–1048.

192. Chuang T-H, Bohl BP, Bokoch GM. Biologically active lipids are regulators of RacxGDI complexation. *J Biol Chem* 1993;268:26206–26211.

193. Stutchfield J, Cockcroft S. Correlation between secretion and phospholipase D activation in differentiated HL60 cells. *Biochem J* 1993; 293:649–655.

194. Gobran LI, Xu ZX, Lu Z, Rooney SA. P2u purinoceptor stimulation of surfactant secretion coupled to phosphatidylcholine hydrolysis in type 11 cells. *Am J Physiol* 1994;267:L625–L633.

195. Fukami K, Takenawa T. Phosphatidic acid that accumulates in platelet-derived growth factor-stimulated Balb/c 3T3 cells is a potential mitogenic signal. *J Biol Chem* 1992;267:10988–10993.

196. Boarder MR. A role for phospholipase D in control of mitogenesis (see comments). *Trends Pharmacol Sci* 1994;15:57–62.

197. Abraham E, Bursten S, Shenkar R, et al. Phosphatidic acid signaling mediates lung cytokine expression and lung inflammatory injury after hemorrhage in mice. *J Exp Med* 1995;181:569–575.

198. Lee YH, Kim HS, Pai JK, Ryu SH, Suh PG. Activation of phospholipase D induced by platelet-derived growth factor is dependent upon the level of phospholipase C-gamma 1. *J Biol Chem* 1994;269:26842–26847.

199. Yeo EJ, Exton JH. Stimulation of phospholipase D by epidermal growth factor requires protein kinase C activation in Swiss 3T3 cells. *J Biol Chem* 1995;270:3980–3988.

200. Lopez 1, Bums DJ, Lambeth JD. Regulation of phospholipase D by protein kinase C in human neutrophils. Conventional isoforms of protein kinase C phosphorylate a phospholipase D-related component in the plasma membrane. *J Biol Chem* 1995;270:19465–19472.

201. Pachter JA, Pai JK, Mayer-Ezell R, Petrin JM, Dobek E, Bishop WR. Differential regulation of phosphoinositide and phosphatidylcholine hydrolysis by protein kinase C-β I overexpression. Effects on stimulation by α-thrombin, guanosine 5'-O-(thiotriphosphate), and calcium. *J Biol Chem* 1992;267:9826–9830.

202. Malcolm KC, Trammell SE, Exton JH. Purinergic agonist and G protein stimulation of phospholipase D in rat liver plasma membranes. Independence from phospholipase C activation. *Biochim Biophys Acta* 1995;1268:152–158.

203. Huang C, Wykle RL, Daniel LW. Phospholipase D hydrolyzes ether- and esterlinked glycerophospholipids by different pathways in MDCK cells. *Biochem Biophys Res Commun* 1995;213:950–957.

204. Daniel LW, Small GW, Schmitt JD, Marasco CJ, Ishaq K, Piantadosi C. Alkyllinked diglycerides inhibit protein kinase C activation by diacylglycerols. Alkyl–linked diglycerides inhibit protein kinase C activation by diacylglycerols. *Biochem Biophys Res Commun* 1988;151:291–297.

205. Bauldry SA, Wykle RL, Bass DA. Differential actions of diacyl- and alkylacylglycerols in priming phospholipase A2, 5-lipoxygenase and acetyltransferase activation in human neutrophils. *Biochim Biophys Acta* 1991;1084:178–184.

206. Brown HA, Gutowski S, Moomaw CR, Slaughter C, Sternwels PC. ADPribosylation factor, a small GTP-dependent regulatory protein, stimulates phospholipase D activity. *Cell* 1993;75:1137–1144.

207. Cockcroft S, Thomas GMH, Fensome A, et al. Phospholipase D: A downstream effector of ARF in granulocytes. *Science* 1994;263:523–526.

208. Singer WD, Brown HA, Bokoch GM, Stemweis PC. Resolved phospholipase D activity is modulated by cytosolic factors other than Arf. *J Biol Chem* 1995;270:14944–14950.

209. Henderson LM, Chappell JB, Jones OTG. Superoxide generation is inhibited by phospholipase A2 inhibitors. Role for phospholipase A2 in the activation of the NADPH oxidase. *Biochem J* 1989;264:249–255.

210. White SR, Strek ME, Kulp GVP, Spaethe SM, Burch RA, Neeley SP, Leff AR. Regulation of human eosinophil degranulation and activation by endogenous phospholipase A2. *J Clin Invest* 1993;91:2118–2125.

211. Locati M, Lamorte G, Luini W, et al. Inhibition of monocyte chemotaxis to C–C chemokines by antisense oligonucleotide for cytosolic phospholipase A₂. *J Biol Chem* 1996;271:6010–6016.

212. Cui Gong M, Fuglsang A, Alessi D, et al. Arachidonic acid inhibits myosin light chain phosphatase and sensitizes smooth muscle to calcium. *J Biol Chem* 1992;267:21492–21498.

213. Kim D, Clapham DE. Potassium channels in cardiac cells activated by arachidonic acid and phospholipids. *Science* 1989;244:1174–1176.

214. Ordway RW, Walsh JV Jr, Singer JJ. Arachidonic acid and other fatty acids directly activate potassium channels in smooth muscle cells. *Science* 1989;244:1176–1179.

215. McCall CE, DeChatelet LR, Cooper MR, Shannon C. Human toxic neutrophils. 111. Metabolic characteristics. *J Infect Dis* 1973;127:26–33.

216. Bass DA, Grover WH, Lewis JC, Szejda P, DeChatelet LR. Comparison of human eosinophils from normals and patients with eosinophilia. *J Clin Invest* 1980;66:1265–1273.

217. Schauer U, Eckhart A, Müller R, Gemsa D, Rieger CHL. Enhanced leukotriene C4 production by peripheral eosinophilic granulocytes from children with asthma. *Int Arch Allergy Appl Immunol* 1989;90:201–206.

218. Aizawa T, Tamura G, Ohtsu H, Takishima T. Eosinophil and neutrophil production of leukotriene C4 and B4: Comparison of cells from asthmatic subjects and healthy donors. *Ann Allergy* 1990;64:287–292.

219. Taniguchi N, Mita H, Saito H, Yui Y, Kajita T, Shida T. Increased generation of leukotriene C4 from eosinophils in asthmatic patients. *Allergy* 1985;40:571–573.

220. Roberge CJ, Laviolette M, Boulet LP, Poubelle PE. *In vitro* leukotriene (LT) C4 synthesis by blood eosinophils from atopic asthmatics: Predominance of eosinophil subpopulations with high potency for LTC4 generation. *Prostaglandins Leukotrienes Essen Fatty Acids* 1990;41:243–249.

221. Mehta D, Gupta S, Gaur SN, Gangal SV, Agrawal KP. Increased leukocyte phospholipase A2 activity and plasma lysophosphatidylcholine levels in asthma and rhinitis and their relationship to airway sensitivity to histamine. *Am Rev Respir Dis* 1990;142:157–161.

222. Hazen SL, Gross RW. Human myocardial cytosolic Ca²⁺-independent phospholipase A2 is modulated by ATP. *Biochem J* 1991;280:581–587.

223. Murakami M, Kudo I, Umeda M, et al. Detection of three distinct phospholipase A2 in cultured mast cells. *J Biochem* 1992;111: 175–181.

224. Channon JY, Leslie CC. A calcium-dependent mechanism for associating a soluble arachidonoyl-hydrolyzing phospholipase A2 with membrane in the macrophage cell line RAW 264.7. *J Biol Chem* 1990;265:5409–5413.

225. Kramer RM, Roberts EF, Manetta J, Putnam JE. The Ca2—sensitive cytosolic phospholipase A2 is a 100-kDa protein in human monoblast U93 7 cells. *J Biol Chem* 1991;266:5268–5272.

226. Clark JD, Lin L-L, Kriz RW, et al. A novel arachidonic acid-selective cytosolic PLA2 contains a Ca²⁺-dependent translocation domain with homology to PKC and GAP. *Cell* 1991;65:1043–1051.

227. Sharp JD, White DL, Chiou XG, et al. Molecular cloning and expression of human Ca²⁺-sensitive cytosolic phospholipase A₂. *J Biol Chem* 1991;266:14850–14853.

228. Diez E, Mong S. Purification of a phospholipase A2 from human monocytic leukemic U937 cells. Calcium-dependent activation and membrane association. *J Biol Chem* 1990;265:14654–14661.

229. Nalefski EA, Sultzman LA, Martin DM, Kriz RW, Towler PS, Knopf JL, Clark JD. Delineation of two functionally distinct domains of cytosolic phospholipase A2, a regulatory Ca(²⁺)-dependent lipid-binding domain and a Ca(2+)-independent catalytic domain. *J Biol Chem* 1994;269:18239–18249.

230. Wu T, Levine SJ, Lawrence MG, Logun C, Angus CW, Shelhamer JH. Interferongamma induces the synthesis and activation of cytosolic phospholipase A2. *J Clin Invest* 1994;93:571–577.

231. Fonteh AN, Samet JM, Chilton FH. Regulation of arachidonic acid, eicosanoid, and phospholipase A2 levels in murine mast cells by recombinant stem cell factor. *J Clin Invest* 1995;96:1432–1439.

232. Lin L-L, Lin AY, DeWitt DL. Interleukin-1α induces the accumulation of cytosolic phospholipase A2 and the release of prostaglandin E2 in human fibroblasts. *J Biol Chem* 1992;267:23451–23454.

233. Doerfler ME, Weiss J, Clark JD, Elsbach P. Bacterial lipopolysaccharide primes human neutrophils for enhanced release of arachidonic acid and causes phosphorylation of an 85 kD cytosolic phospholipase A2. *J Clin Invest* 1994;93:1583–1591.

234. Rodewald E, Tibes U, Maass G, Scheuer W. Induction of cytosolic phospholipase A2 in human leukocytes by lipopolysaccharide. *Eur J Biochem* 1994;223:743–749.

235. Seeds MC, Burke HL, Bowton DL, Bass DA. cPLA2 is primed in peripheral blood eosinophils of asthmatics before and after antigen challenge. *Am J Respir Crit Care Med* 1996;153:A58(abstr).

236. Kramer RM, Hession C, Johansen B, et al. Structure and properties of a human nonpancreatic phospholipase A₂. *J Biol Chem* 1989;264: 5768–5775.

237. Seilhamer JJ, Pruzanski W, Vadas P, Plant S, Miller JA, Kloss J, Johnson LK. Cloning and recombinant expression of phospholipase A2 present in rheumatoid arthritic synovial fluid. *J Biol Chem* 1989;264: 5335–5338.

238. Kudo 1, Murakami M, Hara S, Inoue K. Mammalian non-pancreatic phospholipases A2. *Biochim Biophys Acta Lipids Lipid Metab* 1993; 1170:217–231.

239. Murakami M, Kudo I, Inoue K. Molecular nature of phospholipases A2 involved in prostaglandin I2 synthesis in human umbilical vein endothelial cells. Possible participation of cytosolic and extracellular type phospholipases A₂. *J Biol Chem* 1993;268:839–844.

240. Tohkin M, Kishino J, Ishizaki J, Arita H. Pancreatic-type phospholipase A2 stimulates prostaglandin synthesis in mouse osteoblastic cells (MC3T3-EI) via a specific binding site. *J Biol Chem* 1993;268:2865–2871.

241. Ishizaki J, Kishino J, Teraoka H, Ohara 0, Arita H. Receptor-binding capability of pancreatic phospholipase A2 is separable from its enzymatic activity. *FEBS Lett* 1993;324:349–352.

242. Lambeau G, Ancian P, Barhanin J, Lazdunski M. Cloning and expression of a membrane receptor for secretary phopsholipases A2. *J Biol Chem* 1994;269:1575–1578.

243. Ancian P, Lambeau G, Lazdunski M. Multiftmctional activity of the extracellular domain of the M-type (I 80 kDa) membrane receptor for secretary phospholipases A2. *Biochemistry* 1995;34:13146–13151.

244. Murakami M, Kudo 1, Inoue K. Eicosanoid generation from antigen-primed mast cells by extracellular mammalian 14-kDa group 11 phospholipase A2. *FEBS Lett* 1991;294:247–251.

245. Fonteh AN, Bass DA, Marshall LA, Seeds MC, Samet JM, Chilton FH. Evidence that secretory phospholipase A2 plays a role in arachidonic acid release and eicosanoid biosynthesis by mast cells. *J Immunol* 1994;152:5438–5446.

246. Lin LL, Lin AY, DeWitt DL. Interleukin-1 alpha induces the accumulation of cytosolic phospholipase A2 and the release of prostaglandin E2 in human fibroblasts. *J Biol Chem* 1992;267:23451–23454.

247. Balsinde J, Barbour SE, Bianco ID, Dennis EA. Arachidonic acid mobilization in P388DI macrophages is controlled by two distinct Ca(²⁺)-dependent phospholipase A2 enzymes. *Proc Natl Acad Sci USA* 1994;91:11060–11064.

248. Hara S, Kudo 1, Inoue K. Augmentation of prostaglandin E2 production by mammalian phospholipase A2 added exogenously. *J Biochem* 1991;110:163–165.

249. Bratton DL, Kailey JM, Clay KL, Henson PM. A model for the extracellular release of PAF: the influence of plasma membrane phospholipid asymmetry. *Biochim Biophys Acta* 1991;1062:24–34.

250. Bratton DL, Dreyer E, Kailey JM, Fadok VA, Clay KL, Henson PM. The mechanism of internalization of platelet-activating factor in activated human neutrophils: enhanced transbilayer movement across the plasma membrane. *J Immunol* 1992;148:514–523.

251. Bratton DL. Release of platelet activation factor from activated neutrophils. Transglutaminase-dependent enhancement of transbilayer movement across the plasma membrane. *J Biol Chem* 1993;268: 3364–3373.

252. Nicolas JP, Lambeau G, Lazdunski M. Identification of the binding domain for secretary phospholipases A2 on their M-type 180-kDa membrane receptor. *J Biol Chem* 1995;270:28869–28873.

253. Sugiura T, Wada A, Itoh T, et al. Group II phospholipase A2 activates mitogenactivated protein kinase in cultured rat mesangial cells. *FEBS Lett* 1995;370:141–145.

254. Kishino J, Kawamoto K, Ishizaki J, Verheij HM, Ohara O, Arita H. Pancreatic-type phospholipase A2 activates prostaglandin E2 production in rat mesangial cells by receptor binding reaction. *J Biochem* 1995;17:420–424.

255. Chilton FH, Averill FJ, Hubbard WC, Fonteh AN, Triggiani M, Lui MC. Antigeninduced generation of lyso phospholipids in human airways. *J Exp Med* 1996;183:2235–2245.

256. Asaoka Y, Oka M, Yoshida K, Sasaki Y, Nishizuka Y. Role of lysophosphatidylcholine in T-lymphocyte activation: involvement of phospholipase A2 in signal transduction through protein kinase C. *Proc Natl Acad Sci USA* 1992;89:6447–6451.

257. Asaoka Y, Yoshida K, Sasaki Y, Nishizuka Y. Potential role of phospholipase A2 in HL-60 cell differentiation to macrophages induced by protein kinase C activation. *Proc Natl Acad Sci USA* 1993;90:4917–4921.

258. Quinn MT, Parthasarathy S, Steinberg D. Lysophosphatidylcholine: a chemotactic factor for human monocytes and its potential role in atherogenesis. *Proc Natl Acad Sci USA* 1988;85:2805–2809.

259. Nakano T, Raines EW, Abraham JA, Klagsbrun M, Ross R. Lysophosphatidylcholine upregulates the level of heparin-binding epidermal growth factor-like growth factor MRNA in human moncoytes. *Proc Natl Acad Sci USA* 1994;91:1069–1073.

260. Oishi K, Raynor RL, Charp PA, Kuo JF. Regulation of protein kinase C by lysophospholipids. *J Biol Chem* 1988;263:6865–6871.

261. Sasaki Y, Asaoka Y, Nishizuka Y. Potentiation of diacylglycerol-induced activation of protein kinase C by lysophospholipids: Subspecies difference. *FEBS Lett* 1993;320:47–51.

262. Jalink K, Van Corven EJ, Moolenaar WH. Lysophosphatidic acid, but not phosphatidic acid, is a potent Ca^{2+}-mobilizing stimulus for fibroblasts. Evidence for an extracellular site of action. *J Biol Chem* 1990; 265:12232–12239.

263. Ha KS, Yeo EJ, Exton JH. Lysophosphatidic acid activation of phosphatidylcholinehydrolysing phospholipase D and actin polymerization by a pertussis toxin-sensitive mechanism. *Biochem J* 1994;303:55–59.

264. Jalink K, Hordijk PL, Moolenaar WH. Growth factor-like effects of lysophosphatidic acid, a novel lipid mediator. *Biochim Biophys Acta* 1994;1198:185–196.

265. Hordijk PL, Verlaan 1, Van Corven EJ, Moolenaar WH. Protein tyrosine phosphorylation induced by lysophosphatidic acid in rat-1 fibroblasts. Evidence that phosphorylation of MAP kinase is mediated by the Glp2lras pathway. *J Biol Chem* 1994;269:645–651.

266. Kapeller R, Cantley LC. Phosphatidylinositol 3-kinase. *Bioessays* 1994;16:565–576.

267. Toker A, Meyer M, Reddy KK, et al. Activation of protein kinase C family members by the novel polyphosphoinositides Pidlns-3,4-PS2S and Ptdlns-3,4,5-p₃.. *J Biol Chem* 1994;269:32358–32367.

268. Yano H, Nakanishi S, Kimura K, et al. Inhibition of histamine secretion by Wortmannin through the blockade of phosphatidylinositol 3-kinase in RBL-2H3 cells. *J Biol Chem* 1993;268:25846–25856.

269. Ninomiya N, Hazeki K, Fukui Y, Seya T, Okada T, Hazeki O, Ui M. Involvement of phosphatidylinositol 3-kinase in Fcγ receptor signaling. *J Biol Chem* 1994;269:22732–22737.

270. Ding J, Vlahos CJ, Liu R, Brown RF, Badwey JA. Antagonists of phosphoatidylinositol 3-kinase block activation of several novel protein kinases in neutrophils. *J Biol Chem* 1995;270:11684–11691.

271. Okada T, Sakuma L, Fukui Y, Hazeki O, Ui M. Blockage of chemotactic peptideinduced stimulation of neutrophils by Wortmannin as a result of selective inhibition of phosphatidylinositol 3-kinase. *J Biol Chem* 1994;269:3563–3567.

272. Ward SG, Parry R, LeFeuvre C, Sansom DM, Westwick J, Lazarovits AI. Antibody ligation of CD7 leads to association with phosphoinositide 3-kinase and phosphatidylinositol 3,4,5-trisphosphate formation in T lymphocytes. *Eur J Immunol* 1995;25:502–507.

273. Stephens L, Smrcka A, Cooke FT, Jackson TR, Stemweis PC, Hawkins PT. A novel phosphoinositide 3 kinase activity in myeloid-derived cells is activated by G protein βγ subunits. *Cell* 1994;77:83–93.

274. Nakanishi H, Brewer KA, Exton JH. Activation of the zeta isozyme of protein kinase C by phosphatidylinositol 3,4,5-trisphosphate. *J Biol Chem* 1993;268:13–16.

275. Beffa E, Diaz-Meco MT, Dominguez 1, et al. Protein kinase C-zeta isoform is critical for mitogenic signal transduction. *Cell* 1993;74:555–563.

276. Rodriquez-Viciana P, Wame P, Dhand R, et al. Phosphatidylinositol-3-OH kinase as a direct target of Ras. *Nature* 1994;370:527.

277. Hu Q, Klippel A, Muslin AJ, Fantl WJ, Williams LT. Ras-dependent induction of cellular responses by constitutively active phosphatidylinositol-3 kinase. *Science* 1994;268:100–102.

278. Ahmed MU, Hazeki K, Hazeki 0, Katada T, Ui M. Cyclic AMP-increasing agents interfere with chemoattractant-induced respiratory burst in neutrophils as a result of the inhibition of phosphatidylinositol 3-kinase rather than receptor-operated Ca^{2+} influx. *J Biol Chem* 1995;270:23816–23822.

279. Wiegmann K, Schutze S, Machleidt T, Witte D, Kronke M. Functional dichotomy of neutral and acidic sphingomyelinases in tumor necrosis factor signaling. *Cell* 1994;78:1005–1015.

280. Cifone MG, De Maria R, Roncaioli P, et al. Apoptotic signaling through CD95 (Fas/Apo-1) activates an acidic sphingomyelinase. *J Exp Med* 1994;180:1547–1552.

281. Boucher LM, Wiegmann K, Futterer A, et al. CD28 signals through acidic sphingomyelinase [see comments]. *J Exp Med* 1995;181:2059–2068.

282. Pushkareva M, Obeid LM, Hannun YA. Ceramide: an endogenous regulator of apoptosis and grwoth suppression. *Immunol Today* 1995; 16:294–302.

283. Kolesnick R, Golde DW. The sphingomyelin pathway in tumor necrosis factor and interleukin-I signaling. *Cell* 1994;77:325–328.

284. Venable ME, Lee JY, Smyth MJ, Bielawska A, Obeid LM. Role of ceramide in cellular senescence. *J Biol Chem* 1995;270:30701–30708.

285. Dobrowsky RT, Hannun YA. Ceramide stimulates a cytosolic protein phosphatase. *J Biol Chem* 1992;267:5048–5051.

286. Hannun YA. The sphingomyelin cycle and the second messenger function of ceramide. *J Biol Chem* 1994;269:3125–3128.

287. Lozano J, Berra E, Municio MM, Diaz-Meco MT, Dominguez L, Sanz L, Moscat J. Protein kinase C zeta isoform is critical for kappa B-dependent promoter activation by sphingomyelinase. *J Biol Chem* 1994;269:19200–19202.

288. Dbaibo GS, Pushkareva MY, Jayadev S, et al. Retinoblastoma gene product as a downstream target for a ceramide-dependent pathway of growth arrest. *Proc Natl Acad Sci USA* 1995;92:1347–1351.

289. Stephens LR, Hughes KT, Irvine RF. Pathway of phosphatidylinositol(3,4,5)- trisphosphate synthesis in activated neutrophils. *Nature* 1991;351:33–39.

Asthma, edited by P.J. Barnes, M.M. Grunstein,
A.R. Leff, and A.J. Woolcock. Philadelphia © 1997.
Lippincott–Raven Publishers, Philadelphia © 1997.

▪ 26 ▪

Transcription Factors

Ian M. Adcock and Peter J. Barnes

DESCRIPTION AND DEFINITION

The production of messenger ribonucleic acid (mRNA) from deoxyribonucleic acid (DNA) (transcription) by a cell is strictly regulated. Transcriptional control results from the interaction between regulatory DNA sequences (promoters, enhancers, and silencers) and sequence-specific DNA-binding proteins or transcription factors. The binding of these proteins to these DNA sequences results in an increase or decrease in the transcription rate of the associated gene. Transcription factors therefore act as nuclear messengers that transfer information from the surface of the cell and the cytoplasm to the nucleus. Transcription factors form a tertiary structure that is compatible with the DNA sequence with which they must interact. Activation of transcription enhancers appears to require the assembly of a highly specific three-dimensional nucleoprotein complex involving extensive protein-DNA and protein-protein interactions; the transcriptional efficiency of these complexes can be altered by subtle changes in the relative positions or orientations of proteins within the complex. Understanding of these interactions has been simplified by the recognition of common structural motifs within the many different proteins that recognize DNA (1) (Table 1).

DNA binding proteins can achieve rapid target localization by initially binding to a nonspecific site on the DNA and then finding the specific site by one-dimensional diffusion along the DNA, by intersegment transfer, or both (2). The greater affinity of these proteins for specific sites provides the discrimination energy and thus determines their binding specificity.

Recognition of the cognate binding sequence requires the formation of specific contacts between the protein and the DNA and is often accompanied by conformational changes in the protein, the DNA, or both (3). Many DNA binding proteins, especially transcription regulatory proteins, induce DNA bending on specific binding (3,4). The protein-DNA complex requires 10 to 20 hydrogen bonds between the side chains of amino acids and with the DNA backbone. Most of these contacts are made by α-helical regions within the protein motifs that fit into the major groove, interacting with specific bases, especially with purines, which are larger and offer more opportunities for hydrogen bonding. Folding and docking of the entire protein controls the meaning any particular side chain has in site-specific recognition. Multiple DNA-binding domains are usually required for site-specific recognition. The same motif may be used more than once, as in binding by monomers and dimers, or when a single polypeptide contains tandem repeat motifs. Different motifs also may be used in the same complex. Several structural families of transcription factors can be recognized.

Helix-Turn-Helix

The first DNA-recognition motif identified was the helix-turn-helix (HTH) structure in which an α-helical region

---

I. M. Adcock and P J. Barnes: Department of Thoracic Medicine, Imperial College of Medicine at The National Heart and Lung Institute, London SW3 6LY United Kingdom.

TABLE 1. *Classification of transcription factors as structural families[a]*

Helix-Turn-Helix
Eukaryotic regulatory proteins
Homeodomain / POU
Antp, engrailed
Zinc Finger
Steroid receptors
Sp1, Zfy, Zif 268
Serendipity, Kruppel, Hunchback
Gal 4
Basic Protein-Leucine Zipper (bZIP)
C/EBP
Myc, Fos, Jun, CREB[b]
c-Rel, NFκB
MyoD
β-Sheet Motifs
Met J repressor
HU

[a]The large number of DNA binding proteins can be grouped together into a small number of families depending on their common structural motifs.

[b]Cyclic adenosine 3',5'-monophosphate response element binding protein

is followed by a sharp β-turn and then another α-helical region (5). The proteins bind as dimers, each monomer recognizes a half-site, and the approximate symmetry of the DNA-binding site is reflected in the symmetry of the complexes. Mutations within this region allow dramatic changes in the specificity of DNA binding (6).

Examples of these HTH transcription factors include the *Drosophila* homeotic genes, yeast mating factors, and a variety of mammalian proteins such as the *Hox* genes (7). Although an isolated homeodomain can fold correctly and bind DNA with a specificity similar to that of the intact protein, it seems likely that the precise DNA-binding specificity is modulated by other regions of the protein and by protein-protein interactions.

The high level of sequence similarity between different homeoboxes predicts that the target DNA sequences of many of these proteins will be similar or even identical, and indeed footprinting experiments have shown this to be the case (8). These observations pose the problem as to how proteins with similar DNA-binding specificities execute different regulatory roles. They are important because they illustrate the important roles that heterodimer formation can play in the regulation of gene expression.

Leucine Zipper and Basic DNA Binding Domain

The leucine zipper element is found in many transcription factors throughout the animal kingdom, such as the proto-oncogenes Myc, Fos, and Jun (9). In this structure leucine residues occur every seven amino acids in an α-helical structure over 30 to 40 residues such that the leucines occur every two turns on the same side of the helix. The leucine zipper facilitates the dimerization of the protein by interdigitation of two leucine-containing helices on different molecules. Dimerization results in the correct protein structure for DNA binding by the adjacent highly basic region that can interact directly with the acidic DNA (10).

Leucine zipper proteins can form heterodimers, and these mixed dimers have important roles in the regulation of the biologic activity of bZIP proteins. Both Fos and Jun proteins bind to sequences in DNA known as AP-1 or TRE sites, which mediate gene induction after phorbol ester (e.g., TPA) treatment (11). Although Jun can bind to DNA as a homodimer, Fos is unable to homodimerize and cannot bind to DNA without the formation of a Fos-Jun heterodimer (12). The requirement for dimer formation before DNA binding allows for regulatory control of AP-1 activity and thus gene expression. Heterodimers can limit activity: CREB, a cyclic adenosine monophosphate (cAMP) response regulator, is antagonized by formation of heterodimers with a modulator CREM (13). Heterodimers may also acquire new DNA-binding specificities (14) and thus be targeted to sites different from homodimers. In other cases, heterodimer formation may allow for different combinations of activation and/or repression domains and thus change the regulatory properties of a molecule bound at a fixed DNA site.

Zinc Fingers

Zinc fingers, of the type first described for the *Drosophila* transcription factor TFIIIA (15), are another of the major structural motifs involved in protein-protein interaction (16). The DNA binding region of these factors usually contain tandem repeats of the 30-residue zinc-finger motif, $Cys-X_{2/4}-Cys-X_{12}-His-X_{3-5}-His$. Each of these repeats contains two pairs of cysteine and histidine residues that coordinate a single atom of zinc and hold the protein in a compact globular structure (12). This results in a fingerlike structure that projects from the surface of the protein. The tips of these fingers make direct contact with the major groove of the DNA with alternate fingers binding on opposite sides of the helix (17).

The steroid receptors are an important family of regulatory proteins that include the receptors for the steroid hormones, retinoids, vitamin D, thyroid hormone, and other important compounds. These proteins contain separate regions for hormone binding, DNA binding, and transcriptional activation (18). The DNA-binding domains contain two zinc atoms that are each held in place by four cysteine residues (19). Therefore, this ≈70–amino acid region consists of two zinc fingers only, as opposed to the multiple fingers (2–37) found in genes having Cys-His fingers, and probably are not related to evolution (20). The glucocorticoid receptor binds as a dimer. The first helix of each subunit fits into the major groove, and side chains from this helix make contact with the edges of the base pairs. The second major helix provides phosphate contacts with the DNA backbone and provides the dimerization interface (21).

ROLE OF TRANSCRIPTION FACTORS IN CELL REGULATION

Cell proliferation, differentiation, and activation are largely stimulated by extracellular molecules that interact with receptors on the cell surface. Ligand-receptor interaction sets in motion intracellular signaling cascades that cause the rapid transcriptional induction of selected genes. In the final steps of these cascades, specific transcription activators are phosphorylated and bind to sites in the control regions of the required genes to stimulate their transcription. This binding of the phosphorylated activator must then be communicated to the basal transcription machinery sitting some distance from the start site of transcription. Much of this transcriptional control is governed by the action of sequence-specific DNA binding proteins (22).

Cytokines play an important role in chronic inflammation; the pattern of cytokine expression largely determines the nature and persistence of the inflammatory response. Cytokines produce their cellular effects by activation of various transcription factors such as AP-1, NF-κB, and the signal transduction and activation of transcription (STAT) family, which activate or repress target genes. Furthermore, analysis of the promoter regions of many cytokine and cytokine receptor genes reveals numerous sites for regulation of these genes by the above transcription factors. Because cytokines do not act alone but are produced and released in a coordinate network, the relative levels of these transcription factors are believed to be responsible for the prolonged inflammatory action of cytokines and their activators. During inflammation, numerous other mediators are released, such as nitric oxide (NO) and eicosanoids. Mediators, such as those mentioned above, along with various adhesion molecules and receptors, are all capable of being induced by AP-1 and NF-κB. This may, at least partially, account for the proinflammatory actions of these transcriptions factors.

AP-1 FAMILY

The AP-1 family of transcription factors are dimeric bZIP DNA-binding proteins that have become a model for understanding stimulus-invoked gene regulation (23). AP-1 proteins activate a wide assortment of genes in various cell types in response to extracellular agents that stimulate protein kinase C (PKC), such as tumor-promoting phorbol esters. This activation occurs via sequence-specific interactions between AP-1 and a DNA consensus sequence (5'-TGAC/GTCA-3')(TRE) commonly found in numerous phorbol-ester-responsive genes (24). The

AP-1 proteins bind these elements with low affinity as Jun:Jun homodimers; however, they bind with much greater affinity in association with members of the Fos family as Fos:Jun heterodimers (25).

Although AP-1 activity is widely distributed, and its constituents show a large degree of homology, the roles played by these complexes in different cells and tissue types are extremely diverse. Jun and Fos family members are known to be distinct in their tissue distribution, level of induced expression, and DNA-binding affinities as homodimers and heterodimers (26). Moreover, these proteins have been shown to form a diverse array of functionally distinct dimeric complexes with members of the related bZIP transcription factor family ATF/CREB (14). The Fos and Jun proteins preferentially form a heterodimer that is thought to be the predominant species in many cell types (27). Many other factors affect the formation, targeting, and functional specificity of AP-1 complexes through protein-specific interactions (28), and a significant role is played by the modulation of pre-existing AP-1 complexes by post-translational modifications such as phosphorylation and reduction-oxidation (29).

Because activation of AP-1–responsive genes and an increase in AP-1 activity can occur in the absence of new protein synthesis (24,30), it is believed that post-translational modification of pre-existing AP-1 regulates AP-1 activation. Because TPA directly activates PKC (31), it is likely that phosphorylation is a crucial modification for upregulation of AP-1 activity (Fig. 1).

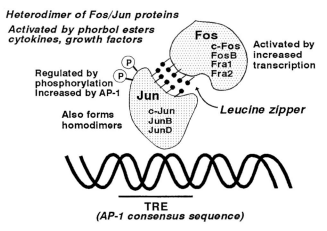

FIG. 1. AP-1 consists of Jun/Jun homodimers or, more commonly, as Fos/Jun heterodimers that dimerize through a leucine zipper motif. Upon activation by phorbol esters, cytokines, or growth factors, AP-1 binds to specific sequences within DNA (*TRE*) and modulates transcription of responsive genes. Both Fos and Jun exist as families of related proteins with altered DNA binding or transcriptional activation abilities that can modulate the final effect of AP-1 on particular genes. Jun proteins are activated by phosphorylation and are part of a positive feedback loop, as they are activated by AP-1 itself. Fos proteins, in contrast, are activated solely by regulation of gene transcription.

Jun kinases (JNK) can phosphorylate c-Jun at Ser[63] and Ser[73] and are activated by the same signals that potentiate c-Jun's activity (32). PMA functions in part by causing dephosphorylation of residues adjacent to the DNA binding domain in the carboxyl-terminal half of c-Jun (33).

AP-1 activity is also modulated by an inhibitory protein (IP-1), present both in the nucleus and cytoplasm of several cell types. IP-1 specifically blocks DNA binding of AP-1 from nuclear extracts and of *in vitro*-synthesized Fos/Jun proteins (34).

NF-KB FAMILY

The transcription factor NF-κB is important for the induction of a wide variety of cellular genes, including cytokines, cytokine receptors, inflammatory enzymes, adhesion molecules, and stress proteins (35). NF-κB is considered to be a heterodimer of proteins that belong to the Rel family of transcription factors. The members of the family in mammalian cells include the proto-oncogene c-rel, p50/p105 (NF-κB1), p65 (RelA), p52/p100 (NF-κB2), and RelB. All these proteins share an ≈300-amino acid rel homology region (RHR). A common feature of the regulation of transcription factors belonging to the Rel family is their sequestration in the cytoplasm as inactive complexes with a class of inhibitory molecules known as IκBs (36). Treatment of cells with different inducers, e.g., IL-1, TNFα, LPS, or PMA, results in the dissociation of the cytoplasmic complexes and translocation of free NF-κB to the nucleus. The dissociation of the cytoplasmic complexes is thought to be triggered by phosphorylation and subsequent degradation of the IκB protein (37) (Fig. 2).

The p50/p65 heterodimer is usually the most abundant of the trans-activating complexes, whereas p50 homodimers are also present in many cells, but these are located constitutively in the nucleus (38). The genes for each subunit have close relatives, making a family of five known vertebrate proteins (35). RHR proteins bind to DNA as either homodimers or as heterodimers of various combinations because the RHR has both dimerization and DNA-binding ability.

There are two major characterized forms of IκB proteins in mammalian cells, IκBα and IκBβ (39). IκBα regulates NF-κB through an autoregulatory feedback loop. Signals that lead to an induction of NF-κB activity results in phosphorylation and rapid loss of IκBα protein through proteolysis (40). The induced nuclear NF-κB causes the subsequent upregulation of IκBα mRNA levels because of the presence of NF-κB sites in the IκBα promoter (41). The newly synthesized IκBα mRNA is translated, and the accumulated IκBα protein helps to shut down the NF-κB response, thus ensuring that responsive genes are activated only transiently.

This model, however, failed to explain how some inducers such as LPS could cause a persistent long-term activation of NF-κB for as long as 48 hours. IκB protein is present in lung tissue in equal amounts to IκBα and interacts with equal affinity to p65 and c-Rel and does not exhibit a preference between these Rel proteins. IκBβ is not induced by NF-κB as is the case with IκBα, suggesting that IκBβ is not regulated by an autoregulatory feedback mechanism.

Inducers such as PMA and TNFα cause rapid but transient activation of NF-κB by primarily affecting IκBα complexes, whereas other inducers such as LPS and IL-1 cause persistent activation of NF-κB by affecting both

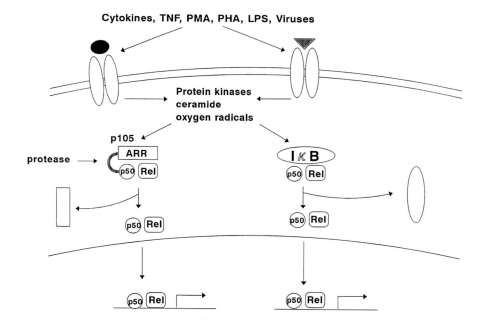

FIG. 2. Mechanism of NF-κB activation. Cytokines, lipopolysaccharides, and viruses can stimulate NF-κB DNA binding via either common or unique second-messenger systems. NF-κB is held in an inactive form by the presence of inhibitory proteins (I-κB) binding to the p50/Rel A complex or by the Rel A protein binding to the p105 precursor of p50. The presence of ankyrin repeat regions (ARR) in both p105 and IκB prevent nuclear localization and DNA binding of NF-κB. After protease digestion of p105 or phosphorylation and subsequent degradation of I-κB, activated NF-κB can translocate to the nucleus and stimulate transcription of κB-responsive genes.

IκBα and IκBβ complexes. Therefore, the overall activation of NF-κB consists of two overlapping phases, a transient phase mediated through IκBα and a persistent phase mediated through IκBα (42). Stimulation of IκB synthesis may represent a means of controlling NF-κB activation that may be exploited therapeutically (Fig. 3).

GLUCOCORTICOID RECEPTORS

Glucocorticoids are effective in controlling inflammatory and immune lung diseases and endogenous glucocorticoids are important in homeostasis. There recently have been important advances in understanding the molecular mechanisms of glucocorticoid actions. Target genes for transcription are selected by the glucocorticoid receptors (GR) through the recognition of defined palindromic sequences in the control regions of these genes (GRE, GGTACAnnnTGTTCT) (18). Recognition is brought about by discrete sequences in the zinc finger DNA binding region of the GR and by dimer formation of the GR (18). The ligands are essential for trans-activation and determine dimerization by recruiting specific regions in the ligand binding domain (43). After ligand binding, the active form of the receptor forms a homodimeric entity containing two molecules of ligand that are stabilized on DNA binding (44). In some cases an interaction of receptor monomers with DNA has been reported (45,46).

Based on cell activation studies, the unliganded receptors originally were thought to be localized in the cytoplasm and to translocate to the cell nucleus upon binding of the ligand (47). Recently it has been shown that the GR is loosely associated with the cell nucleus in the absence of hormone, and that binding of ligand leads to a tighter nuclear binding (48). GRs are expressed in almost all cell types; the density of GR varies from 2,000 to 30,000 binding sites per cell. *In situ* hybridization studies in human lung suggest a high level of GR expression in airway epithelium and endothelium of bronchial vessels (49). The affinity of GR for cortisol is approximately 30 nM, which falls within the normal range for plasma concentrations of free hormone.

The GR has several functional domains. The glucocorticoid binding domain is at the carboxy terminus of the molecule and is separated from the DNA binding domain (≈70 amino acids) by a hinge region (50). There is an N-terminal domain (τ_1) that is involved in transactivation of genes once binding to DNA has occurred. This region may also be involved in binding to other transcription factors (51). In the human GR there is another transactivating domain (τ_2) adjacent to the steroid binding domain; this region is also important for the nuclear translocation of the receptor. GR is phosphorylated (predominantly on serine residues at the N-terminal end), but the role of phosphorylation in steroid actions is not yet certain (52).

The inactive GR is bound to a protein complex (≈300 kDa) that includes two subunits of the heat shock protein hsp90, which thus act as molecular chaperones preventing the nuclear localization of unoccupied GR. There is also evidence for the presence of other associated proteins, including a 59-kDa immunophilin protein and various other inhibitory proteins (53). It appears that hsp90 is necessary for ligand binding to GR and may facilitate the proper folding of the GR into an optimal DNA binding conformation. Once the steroid molecule binds to GR, hsp90 dissociates, allowing the nuclear localization of the activated GR-steroid complex and its binding to DNA (54).

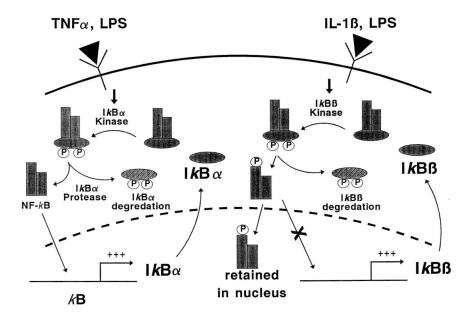

FIG. 3. Regulation of NF-κB is achieved by the presence of I-κBα and in various tissues. Some inducers, such as IL-1, elicit a transient activation of NF-κB by affecting only I-κBα complexes, whereas other inducers, such as LPS, yield a more permanent change by affecting both I-κBα and I-κBβ. NF-κB can stimulate the synthesis of new I-κBα by an autoregulatory feedback mechanism that limits the activation of signal. NF-κB released from I-κBβ complexes, in contrast, cannot induce the transcription of I-κBβ mRNA and, furthermore, the degradation of I-κB requires a modification of NF-κB, such as phosphorylation, which enables NF-κB to be retained in the nucleus for longer periods.

The number of GREs and their position relative to the transcriptional start site may be an important determinant of the magnitude of the transcriptional response to steroids. Thus, an increased number of GREs and proximity to the TATA box increase the steroid inducibility of a gene. Other transcription factors binding in the vicinity of GRE may have a powerful influence on steroid inducibility, and the relative abundance of different transcription factors may contribute to the steroid responsiveness of a particular cell type. GR-DNA interactions change Dnase1 sensitivity, indicating that there may be a change in DNA or chromatin configuration, which may expose previously masked areas, resulting in increased binding of other transcription factors and the formation of a more stable transcription initiation complex.

The mechanisms involved in gene repression are less well understood. In some instances this may be because GR binding to nGRE results in steric hindrance to the binding of transcription factors that may induce the same gene. Alternatively, GR/nGRE binding may induce bending of the DNA in a direction that prevents the distal promoter region from coming into contact with the transcription initiation complex. GR also may form complexes with activating transcription factors in the nucleus and cytoplasm and so inhibit their action, so that steroids may exert an inhibitory action on the transcription of genes (such as interleukin-2; IL-2) that do not have a nGRE within their promoter sequence. Most of the genes that are repressed by glucocorticoids do not possess a GRE sequence in their promoter region, suggesting that direct inhibition of transcription factors is the predominant mechanism for gene repression and mediates the anti-inflammatory action of steroids (55).

Although it is not yet possible to be certain of the most critical aspects of steroid action in the suppression of inflammation, it is likely that their inhibitory effects on cytokine synthesis are particularly important. Steroids inhibit the transcription of several cytokines relevant in inflammatory lung diseases, including IL-1, TNFα, granulocyte macrophage colony-stimulating factor (GM-CSF), IL-3, IL-4, IL-5, IL-6, and IL-8 (56). There may be differences in the sensitivity of different cytokines to inhibition by glucocorticoids. Thus, in alveolar macrophages and peripheral blood monocytes, GM-CSF secretion is more potently inhibited by glucocorticoids than IL-1 or IL-6 secretion (57). For some cytokines, such as IL-1β, IL-3, IL-6, and GM-CSF, increased breakdown of mRNA also has been demonstrated (58). Steroids not only may block the synthesis of cytokines, but also may block their effects in several ways: a) steroids may inhibit the synthesis of certain cytokine receptors, such as the IL-2 receptor (59), and b) steroids may block the effects of transcription factors such as AP-1 and NF-κB, which are activated by many cytokines through binding to their cognate receptors (60).

ATF/CREB FAMILY

The consensus cAMP response element, CRE, is constituted by the palindromic sequence TGACGTCA, which is similar but distinct from the AP-1 DNA binding site (61). The first nuclear protein that bound to CRE to be cloned was CREB (62). Several others have since followed and can be classified into various groups or subfamilies according to their sequences. They all belong to the bZIP family of transcription factors and can thus form protein dimers using the leucine zipper region (10). Although heterodimerization potentially is able to occur with all factors, there appears to be a limited number of allowed heterodimers in practice (63). In addition, certain members of the family of activating transcription factors (ATF-2, ATF-3, and ATF-4) can bind to other bZIP proteins such as Fos and Jun, allowing the interaction of two distinct pathways at the nuclear level (64). Another level of complexity in the CRE binding factor family is that caused by alternative splicing, which exploits their multiexonic, modular structure. Alternative splicing has been shown for CREB (65) and the modulator CREM (13). CREM splicing is of great interest because it can encode both activators and repressors of CRE-mediated transcription (Fig. 4).

CREB expression has been detected in a wide range of tissues, whereas the tissue-specific production of CREB and CREM isoforms only recently has been defined (64). Interactions of transcription factors with either DNA or proteins are affected by differences in the primary sequence, secondary and tertiary structures, and degree of phosphorylation of the individual CREB subfamily homo- or heterodimers (66). CREB and CREM play pivotal roles in basal and hormone-regulated transcription and differentiation. ATF1 is thought to be a weaker activator than either CREB or CREM, and ATF1-mediated activation is enhanced by heterodimer formation with other subfamily members via the leucine zipper (64). Activation of ATF1, CREB, and CREM proteins has been shown to occur through phosphorylation-induced allosteric changes in secondary structure.

In either of the two forms of CREB (CREB[327] and CREB[341]) that result from alternative splicing, a phosphate group in the transactivating domain is essential for a transcriptionally active protein. It is now recognized that multiple protein phosphorylation is the norm rather than the exception. Furthermore, in several instances the multiple phosphorylations do not occur randomly (67) but follow a set pattern involving "primary" and "secondary" kinase phosphorylation (68).

The adapter molecule CBP (CREB-binding protein) (69) interacts with CREB and the basal transcription factor TFIIB (70). There is a phosphorylation-induced increase in the affinity of CREB for CBP, thereby enabling CBP to couple the CRE-CREB complex and the basal transcription factor TFIIB and the remainder of the transcription initiation complex (71). Participation of TATA-

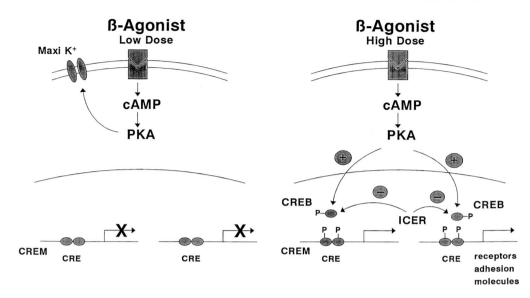

FIG. 4. Mechanisms of β-agonist activation of CREB. Short-term exposure to lower doses of β-agonist leads to a brief generation of cAMP that can activate PKA in the cytoplasm and can lead to the modification of channels and other proteins. Alternatively, the G protein-coupled receptor can interact directly with Ca^{2+}-activated K^+ channels to modulate cell responses. Long-term exposure at higher doses leads to the generation of increased amounts of cAMP, allowing the catalytic subunit of PKA to translocate to the nucleus. There it can phosphorylate CREB and other CRE-binding proteins and thus activate the transcription of immediate early genes (IEGs). The protein products of many IEGs are themselves transcription factors that can activate the transcription of late response genes, perhaps in concert with CREB. These IEGs can activate transcription from the CREM intronic P2 promoter via the CREs and ultimately lead to a rapid increase in inducible cAMP early repressor ICER protein levels. ICER represses cAMP-induced transcription, including that from its own promoter. The subsequent fall in ICER protein levels eventually leads to a release of repression and permits a new cycle of transcriptional activation.

box binding protein (TBP) and possibly some TBP-associated factors (TAFS) seems probable because of the functional characteristics of TFIIB. CBP also cooperates with upstream activators such as c-Jun, which are involved in mitogen-responsive transcription, suggesting that CBP may be involved in the transmission of several different induction signals (72).

The CREB subfamily of transcription factors has overlapping functions; the ability to substitute another transcription factor with an overlapping function may be important. This conclusion is supported by the generation of healthy mice even after homozygous deletion of CREB through recombination (73). Therefore, blocking CRE binding using antibodies or other inhibitors is not likely to prevent completely transcription of CRE controlled genes in animals or intact cells. The inhibition of transcription factors may have therapeutic applications, however, if their tissue-specific effects are better understood and if appropriate structural targets are identified.

JAK-STAT FAMILY

Cytokines and chemokines are small secreted proteins that act to modify the growth and differentiation function of cells with cognate receptors (74). Cytokines are typically expressed under tight regulation with respect to cell type and to physiologic state. The biologic effects of a given cytokine are, in turn, limited to target cells bearing the corresponding receptor. Growth factors and cytokines act through cell-surface receptors with different biochemical properties. Each type of receptor can elicit similar, as well as different, responses, suggesting that distinct classes of receptors activate common gene sets. EGF, IFNγ, and IL-6 all activate latent cytoplasmic transcription factors that recognize similar DNA-binding elements. Different ligands activate different patterns of factors with distinct DNA-binding specificities in the same and different cells. Thus, unrelated receptors may activate a common nuclear signal transduction pathway that, through differential use of latent cytoplasmic proteins, permits these receptors to regulate both common and unique sets of genes (75).

Biochemical and somatic cell genetic studies have begun to resolve the mechanisms by which cytokines selectively modify receptor-bearing target cells. A signal transduction pathway that involves Janus kinases (JAKs) and STAT proteins has been found to be regulated by a number of cytokine receptors (76). The cytoplasmic domains of cytokine receptors initiate intracellular signaling by activated members of the JAK family. These kinases are constitutively associated with the membrane-proximal portions of the cytokine receptor cytoplasmic domains and become activated upon ligand-induced receptor homo- or heterodimerization (77).

The next stage of activation of the STAT pathway seems to involve specificity of the STAT proteins rather than of the JAK proteins. The mechanism for this specificity lies with the receptor components. Dimerization of the receptors allows intermolecular phosphorylation and activation of the associated JAKs, which then phosphorylate tyrosines on the cytokine receptor components. These receptor phosphotyrosines act as docking sites that selectively bind particular STATs and other SH2-containing downstream targets, which in turn can be phosphorylated by the associated JAK. However, the associated JAKs also may activate some signaling molecules without recruitment by the receptor component (78). The selection of the specific STAT at the IFN receptor as well as specific STAT dimer formation depends on the presence of specific SH2 groups. Thus, SH2 groups in STAT proteins may play crucial roles in specificity at the receptor kinase complex and in subsequent dimerization, whereas the kinases are relatively nonspecific (79) (Fig. 5).

STAT proteins form homo- and heterodimeric complexes upon stimulation and tyrosine phosphorylation. These complexes then migrate to the nucleus, where they interact with specific DNA sequences to effect gene expression (80). To date, six members of this family have been identified (78). STAT1 and STAT2 were originally characterized in the IFNα signaling pathway as components of the IFN-stimulated gene factor 3 (ISGF3; 81). In response to IFNα, STAT1 and STAT2 become tyrosine phosphorylated and a STAT1/STAT2 complex is generated. This complex interacts with a 48-kDa protein designated ISGF3γ and binds to IFN-activated response elements (ISREs) upstream of IFNα-inducible genes (82). IFNγ induces tyrosine phosphorylation of STAT1, but not STAT2, thereby generating specific DNA-binding complexes comprising STAT1 homodimers that interact with IFNγ activation sequences (GAS; 83).

IL-4 is an immunomodulatory cytokine secreted by activated T lymphocytes, basophils, and mast cells. It plays an important role in modulating the balance of T-helper (TH) cell subsets, favoring expansion of the TH2 lineage over the TH1 subset. Imbalance of these lymphocyte subsets has been implicated in immunologic diseases including allergy, inflammation, and autoimmune disease. IL-4 may mediate its biologic effects, at least in part, by activating a tyrosine-phosphorylated DNA-binding protein, IL4-STAT (STAT6) (84).

IL-2 is a pivotal mediator of an immune response because this cytokine induces the proliferation and functional differentiation of T lymphocytes, B cells, and natural killer (NK) cells (85). IL-2 is secreted by antigen-activated T cells and mediates its effects through interaction with a specific high-affinity receptor (IL-2R) comprising three subunits α, β, and γ (85). IL-2 produces activation and tyrosine phosphorylation of DNA-binding protein complexes. One of these complexes contains a STAT1-related protein, and the second contains a novel STAT-related protein transcription factor, STAT5 (86). Although IL-2 and IFNα both stimulated JAK1 to a comparable degree, tyrosine phosphorylation of STAT1 and

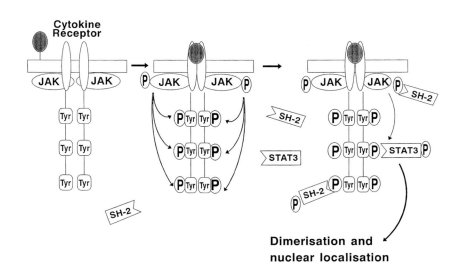

FIG. 5. Signal-transducing cytokine receptor components specify activation of particular pathways. Cytokine receptor components, which contain tyrosine-based domains, are associated with inactive JAK kinases at the membrane proximal region. Ligand binding induces receptor dimerization, resulting in tyrosine phosphorylation and activation of the JAK kinases. The phosphorylated JAK kinases then phosphorylate the tyrosine motifs on the cytosolic domain of the receptor to produce SH-2 binding sites, such as those found in STAT3 and other tertiary messengers. STAT3 binds to the receptor and itself becomes tyrosine phosphorylated by the associated JAK kinase. STAT3 subsequently dissociates, dimerizes with itself or with STAT1, and translocates to the nucleus. The sequence of the tyrosine-based motifs in the cytosolic receptor domains and not the identity of the associated JAK kinase, therefore, specifies the choice of STAT substrate.

Dimerisation and nuclear localisation

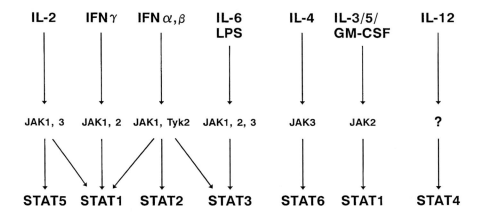

FIG. 6. Specific cytokines activate a variety of JAK kinases, which in turn leads to the activation of STAT proteins. The specificity of JAK/STAT interactions is weak and supports the hypothesis that regions within the cytokine receptor enable cytokine-specific activation of STAT proteins.

STAT3 was detected only in response to IFNα. This suggests that JAK1 activation is not the only factor determining the tyrosine phosphorylation of STATs (86) (Fig. 6).

Activation of the same JAKs by multiple cytokines raises the question of how these cytokines activate distinct intracellular signaling pathways. Selection of particular substrates, STATs, and protein tyrosine phosphatases that characterize the responses to particular cytokine families depend not on which JAK is activated but on specific SH2 motifs in the receptor components shared by these cytokines. Mutation studies have shown that these SH2 motifs are modular and confer STAT activation specifically, irrespective of the ligand (79).

NUCLEAR FACTOR OF ACTIVATED T CELLS

In activated human T lymphocytes both dexamethasone and CsA inhibited IL-2 gene transcription through interference with transcription factors AP-1 and nuclear factor of activated T cells (NF-AT) (87). NFAT, a DNA binding protein required for IL-2 gene transcription, is a potential target for glucocorticoid receptors, calcineurin, cyclosporin A, and FK506. NF-AT contains a preformed subunit (NFAT$_p$) that is present in unstimulated T cells and forms a complex with Fos and Jun proteins in the nucleus of activated T cells (88). NFAT$_p$ is a DNA binding phosphoprotein of 120 kDa and is a substrate for calcineurin *in vitro* (89). Purified NFAT$_p$ forms DNA-protein complexes with recombinant Jun homodimers or Fos-Jun heterodimers; the DNA binding domain of Fos and Jun is essential for the formation of the NFAT$_p$–AP-1–DNA complex. The interaction between the lymphoid-specific factor NFATp and the transcription factors Fos and Jun provides a novel mechanism for regulation of IL-2 gene transcription, which integrates the calcium-dependent and PKC-dependent pathways in T-cell activation. It is proposed that whereas maximum inhibition may involve interaction with both transcription factors, AP-1 is the primary target of dexamethasone (90). More recently, a synergistic interaction between dexamethasone, via the

GR, and CsA has been reported that inhibited the NF-AT DNA binding the release of IL-2 (91) (Fig. 7).

TRANSCRIPTION FACTOR INTERACTIONS

Repression by steroids, thyroid hormone, or retinoic acid affects the expression of many genes (18). One important class of target genes that are repressed by the hormones are those under positive control by certain members of the AP-1 family (Fos, Jun, and ATF) (92). As AP-1 also prevents hormone-dependent activation of GR-regulated promoters, a mutually inactive complex formed either by a direct protein-protein interaction of the receptor and AP-1 or through a third partner has been postulated (93), although the models derived from transient-transfection studies are contradictory (94–101). Cross-linking and immunoprecipitation experiments have suggested that GR interacts directly with Fos or Jun (99). However, others have not detected complexes between Fos or Jun and nuclear receptors (95,102,103), suggesting that any interaction between the proteins must be weak or indirect. Furthermore, both positive and negative regulatory interactions between Fos/Jun and nuclear hormone receptors have been described (104). Two mechanisms have been proposed to account for these observations: either GR blocks Fos/Jun DNA binding or represses their transcriptional activation (Fig. 8).

The transactivation function of the receptor is not required for the repression of AP-1 activity. The bZIP region of AP-1 is part of the target required for the repression (95). Using point mutations and by the choice of steroid ligands, it is possible to dissociate repression of AP-1 activity and the transactivation functions of the GR (105). DNA binding and activation of glucocorticoid-regulated promoters require GR dimerization, whereas AP-1 repression may be mediated by GR monomers.

These studies suggest that the exact interaction between GR and AP-1 may depend on the cell type and stimulus given and also suggests that more than one mechanism of interaction may occur at any one time

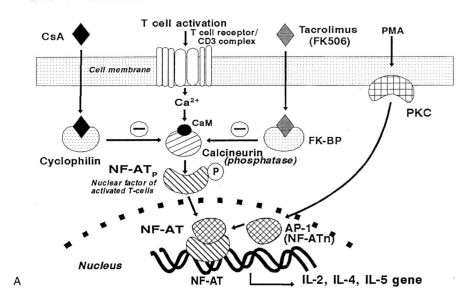

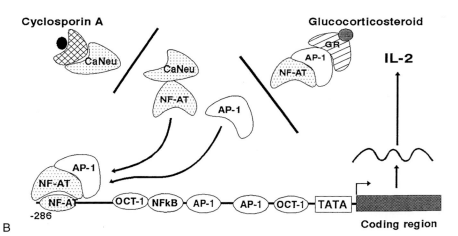

FIG. 7. Cross-linking of Tcell surface receptors causes a Ca²⁺ modulated activation of the calmodulin-dependent serine/threonine phosphatase calcineurin. Dephosphorylation of the cytosolic component of NF-AT by calcineurin allows this component to enter the nucleus, where it combines with AP-1, the nuclear component of NF-AT, to form active NF-AT, which regulates the transcription of many genes, including those for IL-2, IL-4, and IL-5. Activation of NF-AT can be inhibited by cyclosporin A and FK506 via interaction of their respective binding proteins (cyclophilin and FK-BP) with calcineurin and prevention of dephosphorylation of the cytosolic component of NF-AT (**A**). Glucocorticosteroids also can inhibit NF-AT DNA binding by interacting with AP-1 and preventing the formation of active NF-AT and reducing transcription from responsive genes such as the IL-2 gene (**B**).

(106). These results also suggest that cell specificity of GR inhibition of AP-1 activity may be due to the presence of different endogenous AP-1 family proteins in different cell types.

Yamamoto and colleagues (107) have proposed an alternative model for AP-1/GR interaction in the nucleus involving overlapping atypical GREs and TREs, termed a composite GRE. C-Jun homodimers interact with GR to cause a synergistic effect, increasing transcription of responsive genes, whereas c-Fos/c-Jun heterodimers interact with DNA-bound GR to switch off transcription. Thus, transcription rate is controlled by the level of c-Fos in the cell.

Cross-coupling between transcription factors such as that described above between Fos and Jun and the nuclear receptors for glucocorticoids and retinoic acid (94,102) are now being described for many other DNA binding proteins. Antisense c-Fos and c-Jun oligonucleotides reduce the phorbol ester response of the NF-κB-dependent

HIV1 LTR promoter, which suggests synergism between c-Fos and c-Jun at a promoter that carries no AP-1 binding site (28). Further, it has been shown that NF-κB can interact with the C/EBP family of transcription factors (108). Together, these findings illustrate an interplay of diverse transcription factor families to form novel complexes displaying enhanced biologic activity.

Glucocorticoids downregulate the expression of the IL-6, IL-8, RANTES, and other cytokine and inducible genes involved in the inflammatory response. The activation of these genes, and others, involved in the early processes of immune and inflammatory responses are regulated by NF-κB. However, activation of the IL-6 promoter by a combination of NF-IL6 and the p65 subunit of NF-κB is inhibited by the glucocorticoid receptor. Conversely, activation of the MMTV-LTR promoter by dexamethasone and the glucocorticoid receptor is inhibited by overexpression of p65. These studies suggest that direct interactions between NF-κB and the glucocorticoid

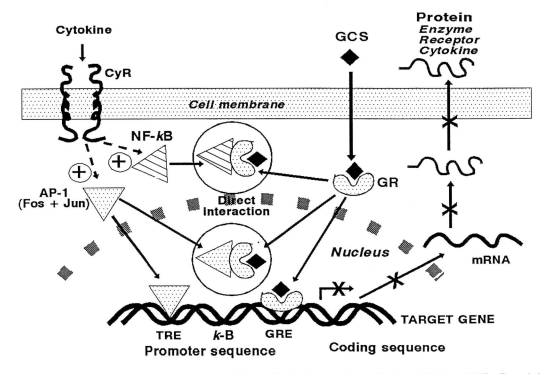

FIG. 8. Direct interaction between the cytokine activated transcription factors AP-1 and NF-κB and the GR may result in mutual repression of gene transcription. This interaction may occur either in the nucleus or the cytoplasm; in this way glucocorticoids may counteract the chronic inflammatory effects of cytokines that activate these transcription factors.

receptor may partly account for the anti-inflammatory properties of glucocorticoids (106,109,110) (see Fig. 8).

Transcription of the glycoprotein hormone α-subunit gene in placental cells is repressed by glucocorticoids, an effect that is mediated through the glucocorticoid receptor (GR). Mutation of the previously identified GR-binding sites in the α-subunit promoter fails to abolish repression, indicating that specific DNA binding to the α-subunit gene is not important for repression. Inhibition by GR is effective only when the α-subunit promoter is activated by CREB, implicating CREB as the target for GR-mediated repression. Reciprocally, overexpression of CREB interferes with GR-mediated transcriptional activation of MMTV. Despite the mutual cross-interference with activation of gene expression, GR and CREB do not appear to have a high-affinity protein:protein interaction in placental cells. GR and CREB may interact directly *in vivo,* possibly through a third protein, or may sequester a mutually required target protein (111). More recently, a direct protein:protein interaction between CREB and GR, which prevents mutual DNA binding, has been found in human and rat tissues and cells (112,113). In contrast, glucocorticoid responsiveness of the PEPCK gene involves a functional interaction between the glucocorticoid response element and the CRE through a physical association of the glucocorticoid receptor with CREB while attached to DNA (114).

TRANSCRIPTION FACTORS IN ASTHMA

Low levels of c-fos are detectable in most cells and its expression is rapidly and markedly increased by many factors that are involved in the airway inflammation associated with asthma. These factors include multiple cytokines (106), histamine (115), and various eicosanoids (116). The effect of these inflammatory mediators on c-Fos expression may account for the reported increased levels of c-Fos found in the airway epithelial of asthmatic patients (117).

NF-κB in its various forms, along with their regulators and coactivators, is intimately connected with the pathologic processes in various conditions such as toxic shock/adult respiratory distress syndrome (ARDS), graft versus host reactions, acute inflammatory conditions such as asthma, and cancer (35). NF-κB is activated by many cytokines, such as TNFα and IL-1β, and other inflammatory mediators known to be upregulated during the inflammatory state, and as such is likely to be important in the control of lung cells and tissue responses to inflammatory stress. At present there is no conclusive evidence to suggest that NF-κB activity is present in higher levels either in particular cells or in inflamed lung tissue in the inflammatory state, although increased levels of p65 subunit have been reported in asthmatic airways (Dr. V. Krishnan, personal communication). NF-κB is activated by oxidants in human epithelial cells (118); this may be relevant in the context of air pollution (119). Oxidant pollutants such as ozone increase NF-κB activation; this is associated with increased expression of chemokines resulting in neutrophil influx (120). Reactive oxygen species are also generated by inflammatory cells in asthmatic airways, such as eosinophils and macrophages, thus enhancing NF-κB expression (121). NF-κB regulates many of the genes involved in asthma, including inducible NO synthase (122), cyclo-oxygenase-2 (123), chemokines such as RANTES (124) and MIP-1α (125), adhesion molecules such as ICAM-1 (126), and VCAM (127).

Studies of transcription factor interactions may have therapeutic potential in the control of lung disease. Glucocorticoids exert their anti-inflammatory effects largely by binding to transcription factors that have been activated by inflammatory cytokines. Other drugs that regulate the activity of specific transcription factors also may be developed. The identification of enzyme targets, such as Jun kinases, also may lead to the development of new drugs that are able to control oncogenesis and inflammation. Cell-specific transcription factors may be a more attractive target, as this may lead to the development of drugs with a reduced risk of adverse effects.

REFERENCES

1. Tjian R, Maniatis T. Transcriptional activation: a complex puzzle with few easy pieces. *Cell* 1994;77:5–8.
2. Fickert R, Muller-Hill B. How Lac repressor finds lac operator *in vitro*. *J Mol Biol* 1992;226:59–68.
3. Pabo CO, Sauer RT. Transcription factors: structural families and principles of DNA recognition. *Annu Rev Biochem* 1992;61:1053–1095.
4. Travers AA. Why bend DNA?. *Cell* 1990;60:177–180.
5. Anderson WF, Ohlendorf DH, Takeda Y, Matthews BW. Structure of the cro repressor from bacteriophage lambda and its interaction with DNA. *Nature* 1981;290:754–758.
6. Koudelka GB, Harbury P, Harrison SC, Ptashne M. DNA twisting and the affinity of bacteriophage 434 operator for bacteriophage 434 repressor. *Proc Natl Acad Sci USA* 1988;85:4633–4637.
7. Scott MP, Tamkun JW, Hartzell GW. The structure and function of the homeodomain. *Biochim Biophys Acta* 1989;989:25–48.
8. Desplan C, Theis J, O'Farrell PH. The sequence specificity of homeodomain-DNA interaction. *Cell* 1988;54:1081–1090.
9. Abel T, Maniatis T. Gene regulation. Action of leucine zippers. *Nature* 1989;341:24–25.
10. Landschulz WH, Johnson PF, McKnight SL. The DNA binding domain of the rat liver nuclear protein C/EBP is bipartite. *Science* 1989;243:1681–1688.
11. Ginsberg AM, King BO, Roeder RG. Xenopus 5S gene transcription factor, TFIIIA: characterization of a cDNA clone and measurement of RNA levels throughout development. *Cell* 1984;39:479–489.
12. Pavletich NP, Pabo CO. Crystal structure of a five-finger GLI–DNA complex: new perspectives on zinc fingers. *Science* 1993;261:1701–1707.
13. Foulkes NS, Borrelli E, Sassone-Corsi P. CREM gene: use of alternative DNA-binding domains generates multiple antagonists of cAMP-induced transcription. *Cell* 1991;64:739–749.
14. Hai T, Curran T. Cross-family dimerization of transcription factors Fos/Jun and ATF/CREB alters DNA binding specificity. *Proc Natl Acad Sci USA* 1991;88:3720–3724.
15. Miller J, McLachlan AD, Klug A. Repetitive zinc-binding domains in the protein transcription factor IIIA from Xenopus oocytes. *EMBO J* 1985;4:1609–1614.
16. Berg JM. Zinc finger domains: hypotheses and current knowledge. *Annu Rev Biophys Biophys Chem* 1990;19:405–421.
17. Klug A, Rhodes D. Zinc fingers: a novel protein fold for nucleic acid recognition. *Cold Spring Harb Symp Quant Biol* 1987;52:473–482.
18. Truss M, Beato M. Steroid hormone receptors: interaction with deoxyribo-nucleic acid and transcription factors. *Endocr Rev* 1993;14:459–479.
19. Hollenberg SM, Giguere V, Segui P, Evans RM. Colocalization of DNA-binding and transcriptional activation functions in the human glucocorticoid receptor. *Cell* 1987;49:39–46.
20. Frankel AD, Pabo CO. Cellular uptake of the tat protein from human immunodeficiency virus. *Cell* 1988;55:1189–1193.
21. Luisi BF, Xu WX, Otwinowski Z, Freedman LP, Yamamoto KR, Sigler PB. Crystallographic analysis of the interaction of the glucocorticoid receptor with DNA. *Nature* 1991;352:497–505.
22. Johnson PF, McKnight SL. Eukaryotic transcriptional regulatory proteins. *Annu Rev Biochem* 1989;58:799–839.
23. Ransone LJ, Verma IM. Nuclear proto-oncogenes fos and jun. *Annu Rev Cell Biol* 1990;6:539–557.
24. Angel P, Imagawa M, Chiu R, et al. Phorbol ester-inducible genes contain a common cis element recognized by a TPA-modulated trans-acting factor. *Cell* 1987;49:729–739.
25. Nishina H, Sato H, Suzuki T, Sato M, Iba H. Isolation and characterization of fra-2, an additional member of the fos gene family. *Proc Natl Acad Sci USA* 1990;87:3619–3623.
26. Ryseck RP, Bravo R. c-JUN, JUN B, and JUN D differ in their binding affinities to AP-1 and CRE consensus sequences: effect of FOS proteins. *Oncogene* 1991;6:533–542.
27. Curran T, Van Beveren C, Verma IM. Viral and cellular fos proteins are complexed with a 39,000-dalton cellular protein. *Mol Cell Biol* 1985;5:167–172.
28. Stein B, Cogswell PC, Baldwin AS. Functional and physical associations between NF-κB and C/EBP family members: a Rel domain-bZIP interaction. *Mol Cell Biol* 1993;13:3964–3974.
29. Hunter T, Karin M. The regulation of transcription by phosphorylation. *Cell* 1992;70:375–387.
30. Angel P, Hattori K, Smeal T, Karin M. The jun proto-oncogene is positively autoregulated by its product, Jun/AP-1. *Cell* 1988;55:875–885.
31. Nishizuka Y. Studies and perspectives of protein kinase C. *Science* 1986;233:305–312.
32. Derijard B, Hibi M, Wu IH, et al. JNK1: a protein kinase stimulated by UV light and Ha-Ras that binds and phosphorylates the c-Jun activation domain. *Cell* 1994;76:1025–1037.
33. Boyle WJ, Smeal T, Defize LH, et al. Activation of protein kinase C decreases phosphorylation of c-Jun at sites that negatively regulate its DNA-binding activity. *Cell* 1991;64:573–584.
34. Auwerx J, Sassone-Corsi P. AP-1 (Fos-Jun) regulation by IP-1: effect of signal transduction pathways and cell growth. *Oncogene* 1992;7:2271–2280.
35. Sienbenlist U, Franzoso G, Brown K. Structure, regulation and function of NF-κB. *Annu Rev Cell Biol* 1994;10:405–455.
36. Beg AA, Baldwin AS. The I κ B proteins: multifunctional regulators of Rel/NF-κB transcription factors. *Genes Dev* 1993;7:2064–2070.
37. Beg AA, Finco TS, Nantermet PV, Baldwin AS. Tumor necrosis factor and interleukin-1 lead to phosphorylation and loss of IκB α: a mechanism for NF-κB activation. *Mol Cell Biol* 1993;13:3301–3310.
38. Franzoso G, Bours V, Park S, Tomita-Yamaguchi M, Kelly K, Sienbenlist U. The candidate oncoprotein Bcl-3 is an antagonist of p50/NF-κB-mediated inhibition. *Nature* 1992;359:339–342.
39. Ghosh S, Baltimore D. Activation *in vitro* of NF-κB by phosphorylation of its inhibitor I κ B. *Nature* 1990;344:678–682.
40. Brown K, Gerstberger S, Carlson L, Franzosa G, Sienbenlist U. Control of IκB-α proteolysis by site-specific, signal-induced phosphorylation. *Science* 1995;267:1485–1488.
41. de Martin R, Vanhove B, Cheng Q, Hofer E, Csizmadia V, Winkler H, Bach FH. Cytokine-inducible expression in endothelial cells of an IκB α-like gene is regulated by NFκB. *EMBO J* 1993;12:2773–2779.
42. Thompson JE, Phillips RJ, Erdjument-Bromage H, Tempst P, Ghosh S. IκB-β regulates the persistent response in a biphasic activation of NF-κB. *Cell* 1995;80:573–582.
43. Tsai SY, Carlstedt-Duke J, Weigel NL, et al. Molecular interactions of steroid hormone receptor with its enhancer element: evidence for receptor dimer formation. *Cell* 1988;55:361–369.
44. Eriksson P, Wrange O. Protein-protein contacts in the glucocorticoid

receptor homodimer influence its DNA binding properties. *J Biol Chem* 1990;265:3535–3542.

45. Chalepakis G. Schauer M, Cao X, Beato M. Efficient binding of glucocorticoid receptor to its responsive element requires a dimer and DNA flanking sequences. *DNA Cell Biol* 1990;9:355–368.

46. Hirst MA, Hinck L, Danielsen M, Ringold GM. Discrimination of DNA response elements for thyroid hormone and estrogen is dependent on dimerization of receptor DNA binding domains. *Proc Natl Acad Sci USA* 1992;89:5527–5531.

47. Jensen EV, Suzuki T, Kawashima T, Stumpf WE, Jungblut PW, DeSombre ER. A two-step mechanism for the interaction of estradiol with rat uterus. *Proc Natl Acad Sci USA* 1968;59:632–636.

48. Brink M, Humbel BM, DeKloet ER, Vandriel R. The unliganded glucocorticoid receptor is localized in the nucleus, not in the cytoplasm. *Endocrinol* 1992;130:3575–3581.

49. Adcock IM, Brönnegård M, Barnes PJ. Glucocorticoid receptor mRNA localisation and expression in human lung. *Am Rev Respir Dis* 1991;143:A628.

50. Webster NJ, Green S. Jin JR, Chambon P. The hormone binding domains of the estrogen and glucocorticoid receptors contain an inducible transcription activation function. *Cell* 1988;54:199–207.

51. Hollenberg SM, Evans RM. Multiple and cooperative transactivation domains of the human glucocorticoid receptor. *Cell* 1988;55:899–906.

52. Muller M, Renkawitz R. The glucocorticoid receptor. *Biochem Biophys Acta* 1991;1088:171–182.

53. Orti E, Bodwell JE, Munck A. Phosphorylation of steroid hormone receptors. *Endocr Rev* 1992 13:105–128.

54. Picard D, Khursheed B. Garabedian ME, Fortin MG, Lindquist S, Yamamoto KR. Reduced levels of hsp90 compromise steroid receptor action *in vivo*. *Nature* 1990;348:166–168.

55. Adcock IM, Barnes PJ. Actions of the glucocorticoid receptor on transcription factors within the cytoplasm. *Am J Respir Crit Care Med* 1995;151:A195.

56. Guyre PM, Girard MT, Morganelli PM, Manginiello PD. Glucocorticoid effects on the production and actions of immune cytokines. *J Steroid Biochem* 1988;30:89–93.

57. Linden M, Brattsand R. Effects of a corticosteroid, budesonide, on alveolar macrophages and blood monocyte secretion of cytokines: differential sensitivity of GM-CSF, IL-1 and IL-6. *Pulm Pharm* 1994;7:43–47.

58. Kern JA, Lamb RJ, Reed JL, Danielle RP, Nowell PL. Dexamethasone inhibition of interleukin-1 β production by human monocytes. Posttranscriptional mechanisms. *J Clin Invest* 1988;81:237–244.

59. Grabstein K, Dower S, Gillis S, Urdal V, Larsen A. Expression of interleukin-2, interferon-γ, and the IL-2 receptor by human peripheral blood lymphocytes. *J Immunol* 1986;136:4505–4508.

60. Barnes PJ, Adcock I. Anti-inflammatory actions of steroids: molecular mechanisms. *Trends Pharm Sci* 1993;14:436–441.

61. Borrelli E, Montmayeur JP, Foulkes NS, Sassone-Corsi P. Signal transduction and gene control: the cAMP pathway. *Crit Rev Oncog* 1992;3:321–338.

62. Montminy MR, Bilezikjian LM. Binding of a nuclear protein to the cyclic-AMP response element of the somatostatin gene. *Nature* 1987;328:175–178.

63. Hoeffler JP, Lustbader JW, Chen CY. Identification of multiple nuclear factors that interact with cyclic adenosine 3',5'-monophosphate response element-binding protein and activating transcription factor-2 by protein-protein interactions. *Mol Endocrinol* 1991;5:256–266.

64. Masquilier D, Sassone-Corsi P. Transcriptional cross-talk: nuclear factors CREM and CREB bind to AP-1 sites and inhibit activation by Jun. *J Biol Chem* 1992;267:22460–22466.

65. Yamamoto KK, Gonzalez GA, Menzel P, Rivier J, Montminy MR. Characterization of a bipartite activator domain in transcription factor CREB. *Cell* 1990;60:611–617.

66. Meyer TE, Habener JF. Cyclic adenosine 3',5'-monophosphate responsive element binding protein (CREB) and related transcription-activating deoxyribonucleic acid-binding proteins. *Endocrine Rev* 1993;14:269–290.

67. Fiol CJ, Mahrenholz AM, Wang Y, Roeske RW, Roach PJ. Formation of protein kinase recognition sites by covalent modification of the substrate. Molecular mechanism for the synergistic action of casein kinase II and glycogen synthase kinase 3. *J Biol Chem* 1987;262:14042–14048.

68. Roach PJ. Multisite and hierarchichal protein phosphorylation. *J Biol Chem* 1991;266:14139–14142.

69. Chrivia JC, Kwok RP, Lamb N, Hagiwara M, Montminy MR, Goodman RH. Phosphorylated CREB binds specifically to the nuclear protein CBP. *Nature* 1993;365:855–859.

70. Kwok RPS, Lundblad JR, Chrivia JC, Richards JP, Bachinger HP, Brennan RG, Roberts SGE, Green MR, Goodman RH. Nuclear protein CBP is a coactivator for the transcription factor CREB. *Nature* 1994;370:223–226.

71. Carey M. Transcription. Simplifying the complex. *Nature* 1994;368:402–403.

72. Arias J, Alberts AS, Brindle P, et al. Activation of cAMP and mitogen responsive genes relies on a common nuclear factor. *Nature* 1994;370:226–229.

73. Hummler E, Cole TJ, Blendy JA, et al. Targeted mutation of the CREB gene: compensation within the CREB/ATF family of transcription factors. *Proc Nat Acad Sci USA* 1994;91:5647–5651.

74. Paul WE, Seder RA. Lymphocyte responses and cytokines. *Cell* 1994;76:241–251.

75. Sadowski HB, Shuai K, Darnell JE, Gilman MZ. A common nuclear signal transduction pathway activated by growth factor and cytokine receptors. *Science* 1993;261:1739–1744.

76. Ihle JN, Witthuhn BA, Quelle FW, et al. Signaling by the cytokine receptor superfamily: JAKs and STATs. *Trends Biochem Sci* 1994;19:222–227.

77. Stahl N, Yancopoulos GD. The alphas, betas, and kinases of cytokine receptor complexes. *Cell* 1993;74:587–590.

78. Stahl N, Farruggella, TJ, Boulton TG, Zhong Z, Darnell JE, Yancopoulos GD. Choice of STATs and other substrates specified by modular tyrosine-based motifs in cytokine receptors. *Science* 1995;267:1349–1353.

79. Heim MH, Kerr IM, Stark GR, Darnell JE. Contribution of STAT SH2 groups to specific interferon signalling by the Jak-STAT pathway. *Science* 1995;267:1347–1349.

80. Shuai K. Interferon-activated signal transduction to the nucleus. *Curr Opin Cell Biol* 1994;6:253–259.

81. Fu XY, Kessler DS, Veals SA, Levy DE, Darnell JE. ISGF3, the transcriptional activator induced by interferon-α, consists of multiple interacting polypeptide chains. *Proc Natl Acad Sci USA* 1990;87:8555–8559.

82. Muller M, Laxton C, Briscoe J, et al. Complementation of a mutant cell line: central role of the 91 kDa polypeptide of ISGF3 in the interferon-alpha and -gamma signal transduction pathways. *EMBO J* 1993;12:4221–4228.

83. Schindler C, Shuai K, Prezioso VR, Darnell JE. Interferon-dependent tyrosine phosphorylation of a latent cytoplasmic transcription factor. *Science* 1992;257:809–813.

84. Hou J, Schindler U, Henzel WJ, Ho TC, Brasseur M, McKnight SL. An interleukin-4-induced transcription factor: IL-4 Stat. *Science* 1994;265:1701–1706.

85. Takeshita T, Asao H, Ohtani K, et al. Cloning of the gamma chain of the human IL-2 receptor. *Science* 1992;257:379–382.

86. Beadling C, Guschin D, Witthuhn BA, et al. Activation of JAK kinases and STAT proteins by interleukin-2 and interferon-α, but not the T cell antigen receptor, in human T lymphocytes. *EMBO J* 1994;13:5605–5615.

87. Schreiber SL, Crabtree GR. The mechanism of action of cyclosporin A and FK506. *Immunol Today* 1992;13:136–142.

88. McCaffrey PG, Jain J, Jamieson C, Sen R, Rao A. A T cell nuclear factor resembling NF-AT binds to an NF-κB site and to the conserved lymphokine promoter sequence "cytokine-1." *J Biol Chem* 1992;267:1864–1871.

89. Jain J, McCaffrey PG, Miner Z, et al. The T-cell transcription factor NFATp is a substrate for calcineurin and interacts with Fos and Jun. *Nature* 1993;365:352–355.

90. Paliogianni F, Raptis A, Ahuja SS, Najjar SM, Boumpas DT. Negative transcriptional regulation of human interleukin-2 (IL-2) gene by glucocorticoids through interference with nuclear transcription factors AP–1 and NF-AT. *J Clin Invest* 1993;91:1481–1489.

91. Wright LC, Cammisuli S, Baboulene L, Fozzard J, Adcock IM, Barnes PJ. Cyclosporin A and glucocorticoids interact synergistically in T lymphocytes: implications for asthma therapy. *Am J Respir Crit Care Med* 1995;151:A675.

92. Ponta H, Cato AC, Herrlich P. Interference of pathway specific transcription factors. *Biochim Biophys Acta* 1992;1129:255–261.

93. Pfahl M. Nuclear receptor/AP-1 interaction. *Endocr Rev* 1993;14:651–658.

94. Jonat C, Rahmsdorf HJ, Park KK, et al. Antitumor promotion and antiinflammation: down-modulation of AP-1 (Fos/Jun) activity by glucocorticoid hormone. *Cell* 1990;62:1189–1204.

95. Schule R, Rangarajan P, Kliewer S, et al. Functional antagonism between oncoprotein c-Jun and the glucocorticoid receptor. *Cell* 1990; 62:1217–1226.

96. Konig H, Ponta H, Rahmsdorf HJ, Herrlich P. Interference between pathway-specific transcription factors: glucocorticoids antagonize phorbol ester-induced AP-1 activity without altering AP-1 site occupation *in vivo*. *EMBO J* 1992;11:2241–2246.

97. Nicholson RC, Mader S, Nagpal S, Leid M, Rochette-Egly C, Chambon P. Negative regulation of the rat stromelysin gene promoter by retinoic acid is mediated by an AP1 binding site. *EMBO J* 1990;9: 4443–4454.

98. Schule R, Rangarajan P, Yang N, et al. Retinoic acid is a negative regulator of AP-1-responsive genes. *Proc Natl Acad Sci USA* 1991;88: 6092–6096.

99. Yang-Yen HF, Chambard JC, Sun YL, et al. Transcriptional interference between c-Jun and the glucocorticoid receptor: mutual inhibition of DNA binding due to direct protein-protein interaction. *Cell* 1990; 62:1205–1215.

100. Yang-Yen HF, Zhang XK, Graupner G, et al. Antagonism between retinoic acid receptors and AP-1: implications for tumor promotion and inflammation. *New Biol* 1991;3:1206–1219.

101. Kerppola TK, Luk D, Curran T. Fos is a preferential target of glucocorticoid receptor inhibition of AP-1 activity *in vitro*. *Mol Cell Biol* 1993;13:3782–3791.

102. Lucibello FC, Slater EP, Jooss KU, Beato M, Muller R. Mutual transrepression of Fos and the glucocorticoid receptor: involvement of a functional domain in Fos which is absent in FosB. *EMBO J* 1990;9: 2827–2834.

103. Shemshedini L, Knauthe R, Sassone-Corsi P, Pornon A, Gronemeyer H. Cell-specific inhibitory and stimulatory effects of Fos and Jun on transcription activation by nuclear receptors. *EMBO J* 1991;10:3839–3849.

104. Miner JN, Diamond MI, Yamamoto KR. Joints in the regulatory lattice: composite regulation by steroid receptor-AP1 complexes. *Cell Growth Differ* 1991;2:525–530.

105. Heck S, Kullmann M, Gast A, et al. A distinct modulating domain in glucocorticoid receptor monomers in the repression of activity of the transcription factor AP-1. *EMBO J* 1994;13:4087–4095.

106. Adcock IM, Shirasaki H, Gelder CM, Peters MJ, Brown CR, Barnes PJ. The effects of glucocorticoids on phorbol ester and cytokine stimulated transcription factor activation in human lung. *Life Sci* 1994;55: 1147–1153.

107. Diamond MI, Miner JN, Yoshinaga SK, Yamamoto KR. Transcription factor interactions: selectors of positive or negative regulation from a single DNA element. *Science* 1990;249:1266–1272.

108. LeClair KP, Blanar MA, Sharp PA. The p50 subunit of NF-κB associates with the NF-IL6 transcription factor. *Proc Natl Acad Sci USA* 1992;89:8145–8149.

109. Mukaida N, Morita M, Ishikawa Y, Rice N, Okamoto S, Kasahara T, Matsushima K. Novel mechanism of glucocorticoid-mediated gene repression. Nuclear factor-κB is target for glucocorticoid-mediated interleukin 8 gene. *J Biol Chem* 1994;269:13289–13295.

110. Ray A, Prefontaine KE. Physical association and functional antagonism between the p65 subunit of transcription factor NF-κB and the glucocorticoid receptor. *Proc Nat Acad Sci USA* 1994;91:752–756.

111. Stauber C, Altschmied J, Akerblom IE, Marron JL, Mellon PL. Mutual cross-interference between glucocorticoid receptor and CREB inhibits transactivation in placental cells. *New Biol* 1992;4:527–540.

112. Peters MP, Adcock IM, Brown CR, Barnes PJ. β-Adrenoceptor agonists interfere with glucocorticoid receptor DNA binding in rat lung. *Eur J Pharm (Mol Pharm)* 1995;289:275–281.

113. Adcock IM, Brown CR, Gelder CM, Shirasaki H, Peters MJ, Barnes PJ. Effects of glucocorticoids on transcription factor activation in human peripheral blood mononuclear cells. *Am J Physiol* 1995;268: C331–C338.

114. Imai E, Miner JN, Mitchell JA, Yamamoto KR, Granner DK. Glucocorticoid receptor-cAMP response element-binding protein interaction and the response of the phosphoenolpyruvate carboxykinase gene to glucocorticoids. *J Biol Chem* 1993;268:5353–5356.

115. Panettieri RA, Yadvish PA, Kelly AM, Rubinstein NA, Kotlikoff MI. Histamine stimulates proliferation of airway smooth muscle and induces c-fos expression. *Am J Physiol* 1990;259:L365–L371.

116. Mazer B, Domenico J, Sawami H, Gelfand EW. Platelet-activating factor induces an increase in intracellular calcium and expression of regulatory genes in human B lymphoblastoid cells. *J Immunol* 1991; 146:1914–1920.

117. Demoly P, Basset-Seguin N, Chanez P, et al. c-fos proto-oncogene expression in bronchial biopsies of asthmatics. *Am J Respir Cell Mol Biol* 1992;7:128–133.

118. Adcock IM, Brown CR, Kwon O, Barnes PJ. Oxidative stress induces NF-κB DNA binding and inducible NOS mRNA in human epithelial cells. *Biochem Biophys Res Commun* 1994;199:1518–1524.

119. Jany B, Betz R, Schreck R. Activation of the transcription factor NF-κB in human tracheobronchial epithelial cells by inflammatory stimuli. *Eur Respir J* 1995;8:387–391.

120. Haddad EB, Salmon M, Sun J, et al. Dexamethasone inhibits ozone-induced gene expression of macrophage inflammatory protein-2 in rat lung. *FEBS Lett* 1995;363:285–288.

121. Schreck R, Rieber P, Baeuerle PA. Reactive oxygen intermediates as apparently widely used messengers in the activation of the NF-κ B transcription factor and HIV-1. *EMBO J* 1991;10:2247–2258.

122. Xie QW, Kashiwabara Y, Nathan C. Role of transcription factor NF-κ B/Rel in induction of nitric oxide synthase. *J Biol Chem* 1994;269: 4705–4708.

123. Newton R, Adcock IM, Barnes PJ. Stimulation of COX-2 message by cytokines or phorbol ester is preceded by a massive and rapid induction of NF-κB binding activity. *Am J Respir Crit Care Med* 1995;151: A165.

124. Nelson PJ, Kim HT, Manning WC, Goralski TJ, Krensky AM. Genomic organization and transcriptional regulation of the RANTES chemokine gene. *J Immunol* 1993;151:2601–2612.

125. Grove M, Plumb M. C/EBP, NF-κB, and c-Ets family members and transcriptional regulation of the cell-specific and inducible macrophage inflammatory protein-1 α immediate-early gene. *Mol Cell Biol* 1993;13:5276–5289.

126. Ledebur HC, Parks TP. Transcriptional regulation of the intercellular adhesion molecule-1 gene by inflammatory cytokines in human endothelial cells. Essential roles of a variant NF-κ B site and p65 homodimers. *J Biol Chem* 1995;270:933–943.

127. Ahmad M, Marui N, Alexander RW, Medford RM. Cell type-specific transactivation of the VCAM-1 promoter through an NF-κB enhancer motif. *J Biol Chem* 1995;270:8976–8983.

■ 4 ■

Inflammatory Cells

Asthma, edited by P.J. Barnes, M.M. Grunstein,
A.R. Leff, and A.J. Woolcock.
Lippincott–Raven Publishers, Philadelphia © 1997.

▪ 27 ▪

Mast Cell Involvement in Asthma

Yuji Shimizu and Lawrence B. Schwartz

Growth, Differentiation, Recruitment, and Programmed Cell Death of Mast Cells
Mediators of Mast Cells
   Preformed granule-associated mediators
   Lipid mediators
   Cytokines
	Surface Markers of Mast Cells
	Activation of Mast Cells
	Mast Cells and Asthma
	   Mast cell numbers and distribution
	   Mast cell activation

Human mast cells, principal effector cells of immediate-type hypersensitivity reactions, will be reviewed as to their involvement in asthma and contrasted with human basophils. Both cell types stain metachromatically with basic dyes, store histamine in secretory granules (1), and express abundant numbers of high-affinity receptors for immunoglobulin (Ig) E on their surfaces (2,3). Distinguishing features include nuclear morphology, mediator content, cell surface molecules, response to chemical activating agents, and pathway of differentiation. Basophils complete their differentiation in bone marrow before entering the circulation as a mature cell. Basophils are not normally found in connective tissue, but migrate into tissues at sites of inflammation. Mast cell progenitors leave the bone marrow as progenitors and complete their differentiation after arriving in peripheral tissues. Mast cell concentrations are particularly high throughout the lung, bowel, dermis, nasal, and conjunctival mucosa and around blood vessels, consistent with the clinical alterations known to occur in allergic diseases at these sites.

Y. Shimizu: First Department of Internal Medicine, Gunma University School of Medicine, Maebashi, Gunma 371 Japan.

L. B. Schwartz: Department of Internal Medicine, Virginia Commonwealth University, Richmond, Virginia 23233.

GROWTH, DIFFERENTIATION, RECRUITMENT, AND PROGRAMMED CELL DEATH OF MAST CELLS (FIG. 1)

Both mast cells and basophils arise from CD34$^+$ pluripotent bone marrow cells (4). Interleukin (IL) 3 is the major growth factor for human basophils (5–7), while granulocyte-macrophage colony-stimulating factor (GM-CSF) (8), IL-5 (9), and nerve growth factor (10) also may promote basophil differentiation. IL-3, IL-5, and GM-CSF also support eosinophil differentiation. In contrast, human mast cells are deficient in receptors for IL-3, and when progenitor cells from bone marrow, cord blood, or fetal liver are exposed to human IL-3, IL-4, IL-10, or nerve growth factor, few, if any, mast cells develop (11). This is in marked contrast to rodent mast cells, which use IL-3 as a major growth factor (12–15).

Stem cell factor (SCF), the ligand for Kit (CD117) (a product of the c-*kit* protooncogene), is the major growth factor for human mast cells (11,16–18). Two alternative splice variants account for different forms of SCF, one which is primarily membrane bound and the other which is primarily soluble after being released from its site on the cell surface by proteolysis (19). However, why mast cells complete their differentiation in peripheral tissues rather than the bone marrow is not explained by avail-

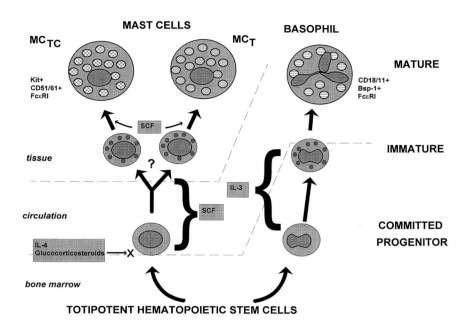

FIG. 1. Differentiation of human mast cells and basophils. *X*, inhibition; *?*, uncertainty as to the factors involved.

ability of soluble or membrane forms of SCF, because bone marrow stromal cells (20), like cells in peripheral tissues, produce both forms. One possibility is that factors produced in the bone marrow environment divert SCF-treated progenitors to non-mast-cell lineages. For example, IL-4 appears to prevent mast cell development from fetal liver, bone marrow, and peripheral blood progenitors (21,22), and may be present at higher concentrations in bone marrow than in peripheral tissue sites.

Kit, a receptor protein tyrosine kinase, is expressed on early hematopoietic progenitors and permits a synergistic response to SCF and lineage-committing growth factors such as GM-CSF for myelocytes or erythropoietin for erythrocytes. As cells mature along most hematopoietic lineages, Kit expression decreases, and is absent in the mature cells released from the bone marrow. In contrast, Kit expression on mast cells increases as the cells mature, and is abundantly and constitutively expressed on the surface of mast cells found in tissues. Thus, SCF is likely to affect mast cells throughout their life span. Indeed, membrane-bound SCF may directly influence mast cell adhesion (23), and soluble SCF is chemotactic for mast cells (24). SCF stimulates adhesion of rodent mast cells to ground substances through integrin receptors (23,25). A critical function of SCF in humans and rodents is mast cell survival; removal of mast cells from either soluble or membrane-bound SCF causes mast cells to undergo programmed cell death, called *apoptosis* (26,27). In rodent IL-3-dependent mast cells, removal of IL-3 also causes apoptosis, but this can be prevented by replacing IL-3 with SCF. The mechanisms to suppress apoptosis appear to be different for IL-3 and SCF for rodent mast cells, where IL-3 appears to act by inducing expression of the *bcl-2* protooncogene, whereas SCF does not (28).

Human mast cells have been divided into two groups based on protease composition: MC_{TC} cells contain tryptase, chymase, cathepsin G, and carboxypeptidase, whereas MC_T cells contain only tryptase (29). In normal-appearing pulmonary tissue, MC_T cells are the predominant mast cell type in the alveolar wall and in the epithelium of both the upper and the lower airway. MC_{TC} cells account for about 25% of the mast cells in bronchial subepithelium and 50% to 80% of the mast cells in nasal subepithelium. In normal skin, mast cells reside in only the dermis and are almost exclusively of the MC_{TC} type. In small bowel, MC_T cells tend to predominate in the mucosa, MC_{TC} in the submucosa. With allergic inflammation in the airway, increased numbers of mast cells, primarily of the MC_T phenotype, are found in the epithelium (30–33), whereas mast cell numbers and phenotype in subepithelial regions exhibit no apparent differences from normal tissue (34–36).

What causes mast cells to home to certain tissues and to develop as MC_T or MC_{TC} cells is unknown. Progenitors may home to tissue sites where soluble SCF is being generated. RANTES, a chemokine, also appears to chemotax human mast cells (37). Once mast cells arrive in tissues adhesion should be dictated by the adhesion molecules they express. Human mast cells express β_1 (CD29) and β_3 (CD61) integrins, but few if any of the β_2 (CD18) integrins. The predominant β_1 integrins include those with α_4 (CD49d) or α_5 (CD49e); α_v/β_3 (CD51/CD61) is the predominant β_3 integrin. These integrins recognize ground substances such as vitronectin, fibronectin, and laminin; vascular cell adhesion molecule 1 on endothelial cells; and the CD44 receptor for hyaluronan. Rodent mast cells also chemotax to IL-3 (38), laminin (39), transforming growth factor (TGF) β (40), and

C1q (41), factors that need to be evaluated with human mast cells.

Human basophils, in contrast to mast cells, do not home to tissues unless recruited into an inflamed site. Factors known to be chemotactic for human basophils include IL-3, IL-5, GM-CSF, C5a, IL-8, platelet activating factor (PAF), and various chemokines (42,43). These factors also recruit eosinophils and, in some cases, neutrophils. Thus, whereas mast cell recruitment to tissues is a component of the natural development of these cells, basophil recruitment occurs in response to inflammation.

MEDIATORS OF MAST CELLS

Activation of mast cells and basophils results in the release of mediators responsible for much of the clinical response observed during immediate-type hypersensitivity reactions. Degranulation releases preformed mediators that are stored inside secretory granules and occurs within minutes after the cells are stimulated. Metabolites of arachidonic acid are generated after cell stimulation and then are secreted over a more prolonged period. Although variable amounts of different cytokines may be present at the time of stimulation, more typical is their generation after cell stimulation, leading to their secretion over a prolonged period. These generalities are summarized in Figure 2.

Preformed Granule-Associated Mediators

Histamine, the only biogenic amine in human mast cells and basophils, is the only preformed mediator of human mast cells with direct potent vasoactive and smooth muscle spasmogenic effects. Because released histamine is metabolized rapidly, its effects are primarily local.

Several *neutral proteases* also are stored in mast cell secretory granules and released in parallel to histamine by degranulation. These enzymes account for most of the protein in secretory granules. *Tryptase* accounts for most of the trypsinlike activity first detected in human mast cells by histochemical techniques (44,45). In its enzymatically active form, tryptase is a tetramer that is uniquely stabilized by binding ionically to heparin, which resides with the protease in mast cell secretory granules (46,47). Tryptase is not inhibited by classic serine protease inhibitors present in plasma and tissues. Instead, regulation of its enzymatic activity is probably governed by this association with heparin. Although at least two genes for tryptase, α-tryptase and β-tryptase, are present on human chromosome 16, it appears that β-tryptase accounts for essentially all of the active tryptase and is the primary form stored in secretory granules. α-Tryptase appears to be inactive, is constitutively secreted from mast cells, and is the predominant immunoreactive species found in blood under conditions that do not involve mast cell activation (48).

Chymase, like tryptase, is stored fully active in mast cell secretory granules, but unlike tryptase, its activity is inhibited by classic biologic inhibitors of serine proteinases (49). Like tryptase, chymase binds tightly to heparin proteoglycan, but unlike tryptase, the stability of chymase is heparin independent (50). Chymase is encoded by a single gene on human chromosome 14 (51, 52), in a locus that also includes cathepsin G and several of the granzymes expressed in cytotoxic T cells and natural killer cells (53).

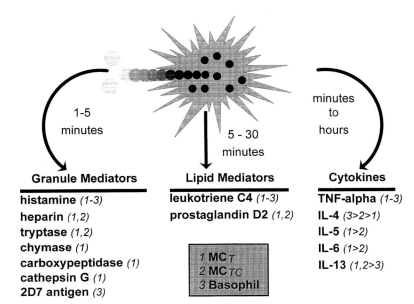

Granule Mediators	Lipid Mediators	Cytokines
histamine *(1-3)*	leukotriene C4 *(1-3)*	TNF-alpha *(1-3)*
heparin *(1,2)*	prostaglandin D2 *(1,2)*	IL-4 *(3>2>1)*
tryptase *(1,2)*		IL-5 *(1>2)*
chymase *(1)*		IL-6 *(1>2)*
carboxypeptidase *(1)*	1 MC$_T$	IL-13 *(1,2>3)*
cathepsin G *(1)*	2 MC$_{TC}$	
2D7 antigen *(3)*	3 Basophil	

FIG. 2. Mediators released by mast cells and basophils after activation by an immunoglobulin E-mediated process. Within *parentheses* next to each mediator is shown whether MC$_T$, MC$_{TC}$, or basophils are the major source.

Sensitive immunoassays have been developed to measure tryptase in blood and other body fluids. Consequently, mast cell involvement in various clinical conditions, including asthma (54,55), can be assessed. Tryptase levels provide a more precise measure of mast cell activation than available by other tests, for example, histamine or prostaglandin D_2 (PGD_2) levels, or by clinical observation alone. Similar immunoassays for chymase have not been developed, in part because chymase epitopes are obscured when the enzyme forms complexes with various inhibitors *in vivo*.

Both tryptase and chymase precursors are processed to active enzymes in a heparin-dependent manner (56–58). Conversion of β-protryptase to β-pro'tryptase involves removal of amino acids -12 through -3 of the leader peptide and is autocatalytic, heparin dependent, and optimal at acid pH, as summarized in Figure 3. This processing step is likely to occur in rodent as well as human mast cells and may best explain why mast cells of these species coexpress tryptase and heparin. Removal of the activation dipeptide (amino acids -2 and -1 from the leader peptide) from β-pro'tryptase occurs in the presence or absence of heparin, but concomitant formation of the active tetramer from the monomeric precursor occurs only in the presence of heparin (58). *In vitro*, dextran sulfate, but not monosulfated or disulfated chondroitin sulfates, may substitute for heparin. Dipeptidyl dipeptidase I also removes the activation dipeptide from prochymase, but unlike for β-pro'tryptase, this proteolytic step depends on the presence of heparin. Thus, even if tryptase is aberrantly expressed by a cell other than a mast cell, unless heparin is coexpressed, active tryptase should not be effectively produced.

Because tryptase and the other proteases present in mast cell secretory granules are so abundant, their enzymatic activities are likely to be of direct physiologic and pathophysiologic import. Bronchial hyperreactivity may be affected by chymase and tryptase. For example, dog (and apparently human) tryptase augments the contractile response of pulmonary smooth muscle to histamine (59); and human chymase enhances the cutaneous wheal response to histamine in dogs (60). Tryptase also degrades vasoactive intestinal peptide, a bronchodilator (61), and calcitonin gene-related peptide, a vasodilator (62), whereas chymase degrades both vasoactive intestinal peptide and substance P, a bronchoconstrictor (61).

Fibrogenic and fibrolytic activities of these enzymes are of interest when considering the possible associations of mast cells with airway remodeling. For example, human tryptase stimulates fibroblast proliferation (63,64), on the one hand, and activates prostromelysin (65,66), an activator of procollagenase, on the other. Human chymase directly activates procollagenase (67).

Mast cells are potent enhancers of vasopermeability through the actions of histamine, sulfidopeptide leukotrienes, and PGD_2. However, fibrinogen entering into tissue sites of mast cell activation is not typically converted into fibrin, particularly during the early phase of immediate-type hypersensitivity reactions. One possible explanation for this observation is that tryptase rapidly cleaves and inactivates fibrinogen as a substrate for thrombin (68). Additional explanations relate to the anticoagulant effects of released heparin and the antithrombotic effects of released PGD_2.

Arteriolar vasoconstriction is an activity predicted to be associated with mast cells of the MC_{TC} type because

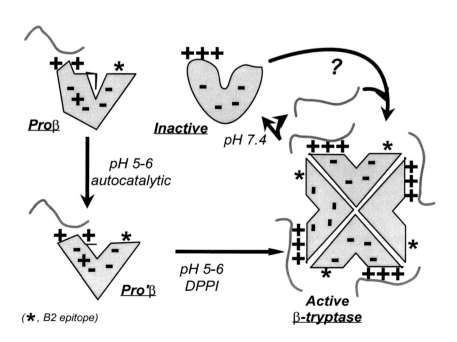

(✱, B2 epitope)

FIG. 3. Processing of β-tryptase precursor to an active tetrameric protease that binds tightly to heparin proteoglycan (*squiggly lines,* heparin). Positive and negative charges are depicted with + and −, respectively. The B2 epitope is a conformational epitope recognized by the mouse B2 monoclonal antibody. The epitope resides on tryptase precursors and active tryptase, but not on tryptase that has been inactivated by conversion of active tetramer to inactive monomer. *DPPI,* dipeptidyl peptidase I.

chymase efficiently converts angiotensin I to II (69,70). In patients taking an angiotensin-converting enzyme inhibitor, increased angiotensin I substrate may be shunted into tissues where chymase-dependent generation of angiotensin II would be anticipated. Chymase may also facilitate inflammation by activating IL-1 (71) and TGF-β (72) precursors in connective tissues.

A specific marker for basophil secretory granules has been identified by a mouse monoclonal antibody called 2D7 (73). The *2D7 antigen* is localized to secretory granules based on immunogold electron microscopy, and by a marked decrease in staining intensity of basophil cytospins prepared after the basophils had been activated with anti-FcεRI antibody compared with a buffer control. By Western blotting, the epitope was identified on two proteins of approximately 75,000 Da, which were possibly derived from a higher molecular weight protein of about 124,000 Da. The 2D7 antigen is not found in mast cells, eosinophils, neutrophils, monocytes, and lymphocytes, and is not detected in normal skin, lung, and bowel. Thus, the 2D7 antigen appears to be a specific marker of human basophils and may provide a means to measure basophil activation precisely in complex biologic fluids.

Lipid Mediators

Phospholipase A releases arachidonic acid from phospholipids when mast cells are activated, a portion of which is then oxidatively metabolized to prostaglandins, primarily PGD_2; and leukotrienes (LTs), primarily LTC_4 (74,75). Mast cells may be the major source of PGD_2 in the lung, whereas many cells, including basophils and eosinophils, produce LTC_4. Markedly elevated levels of PGD_2 and its metabolites are found in bronchoalveolar lavage fluid (BALF) obtained from atopic asthmatics at baseline, consistent with ongoing mast cell activation (76). After allergen challenge, PGD_2 and sulfidopeptide leukotriene levels markedly increase in BALF, indicating that additional activation of mast cells occurred (77–79). Mast cells dispersed both from skin (predominantly MC_{TC} cells) (80) and from lung (mostly MC_T cells) (74), when activated immunologically, produce LTC_4 and PGD_2, without a substantial difference in lipid profiles.

Atopic asthmatic patients show hyperresponsiveness to inhalation of PGD_2, which is inhibited by thromboxane receptor antagonists (81,82). However, inhibition of PGD_2 synthesis by aspirin does not normally improve the pulmonary function of atopic asthmatics. In contrast, drugs that inhibit production of sulfidopeptide leukotrienes or antagonize their interaction with receptor do produce a beneficial response in asthmatics (83), particularly in those that are aspirin sensitive (84). This observation fits with the presence of activated mast cells, eosinophils, and basophils in the asthmatic airway and the capacity of sulfidopeptide leukotrienes to contract pulmonary smooth muscle and stimulate mucus glandular secretions. Of potential relevance to therapies targeting human 5-lipoxygenase or its metabolites, mice with a targeted disruption of the 5-lipoxygenase gene develop normally, show a normal response to endotoxin, and show a markedly attenuated response to PAF (see below) (85).

PAF, another lipid mediator, is derived from phosphatidylcholine derivatives with an ether-linked alkyl group attached to the first carbon of the glycerol backbone rather than the typical ester-linked acyl group, and contains the two-carbon acetyl group attached to the second carbon of the glycerol backbone. PAF is a vasoactive proinflammatory mediator produced by many inflammatory cell types, including human eosinophils and basophils. Human mast cells produce small amounts of PAF, but whether clinically significant amounts are released from the cells is uncertain. PAF activates and recruits eosinophils and basophils (86–90). PAF does not activate human cutaneous mast cells (91). PAF-induced inflammation can be blocked by increasing its metabolism by PAF acetyl hydrolase to form inactive lyso-PAF (92). Lyso-PAF, though, can be converted back to PAF by cells with the capability of acetylating the second carbon of the glycerol backbone. Although inhaled PAF causes bronchoconstriction in humans (93), its importance in asthma remains uncertain. In the human airway, inhaled PAF does not increase airway responsiveness to methacholine in normal subjects (94) and does not increase airway inflammation in atopic subjects (95). Further, a PAF antagonist, WEB 2086, failed to diminish steroid requirements in steroid-dependent asthmatics compared with placebo (96).

Cytokines

Whereas both human mast cells and basophils when activated secrete tumor necrosis factor (TNF)-α (97–101), mast cells tend to produce IL-13 over IL-4 while basophils produce IL-4 over IL-13. Human mast cells and basophils also produce IL-5 and IL-6 to complete a T-helper type (TH)-2-like cytokine profile (102–106). In bronchial biopsy specimens from asthmatics, immunohistochemistry supports these *in vitro* observations. Preferential production of IL-4 by mast cells of the MC_{TC} type, and of IL-5 and IL-6 by those of the MC_T type, have been reported (107). The presence of cytokine mRNA and protein in tissue mast cells may signal that the mast cells are in an activated state. Percentages of cytokine-positive mast cells appear to be increased in bronchial and nasal mucosal biopsy specimens taken from active atopic asthmatic and rhinitic patients (104,108,109). IL-4 and IL-13 produced by human mast cells and basophils may affect production of IgE by influencing the development of the TH2 cell over the TH1. IL-5 may be involved in the recruitment and survival of eosinophils known to be present in sites of allergic inflammation such as the asthmatic lung. TNF-α promotes inflammation in part by facilitating recruitment of inflammatory cells. Increased levels of endothelial leukocyte adhesion molecule (ELAM) 1 on endothelial cells (98) as well as E-selectin, vascular cell adhesion molecule (VCAM) 1, and intercellular cell adhesion molecule (ICAM) 1 (110–112) are induced by TNF-α. Thus, mast cells and basophils may modulate the inflammatory phase of immediate-type hypersensitivity as well as the early humoral phase.

SURFACE MARKERS OF MAST CELLS

The most characteristic surface marker for mast cells (and basophils) is the tetrameric high-affinity receptor for IgE, FcεRI (113), which is abundantly and constitutively expressed in an active form. Other cell types capable of expressing FcεRI, such as eosinophils (114), Langerhans' cells (115,116), and monocytes (117), produce small amounts of inducible receptor or receptor that requires further activation before becoming capable of transducing signals to the cell interior. Human mast cells express neither the low-affinity receptor for IgE (CD23) nor Fcγ receptors (118) except for uterine mast cells, which are reported to express small amounts of CD64 (FcγRI) and CD32 (FcγRII) (119).

CD45, a membrane protein with tyrosine phosphatase activity, is expressed on mast cells (120), where it plays a critical role in FcεRI-mediated activation. Also noteworthy is the expression of functional CD40 ligand on human lung-derived mast cells, which stimulates B cells in the presence of IL-4 to switch from synthesis of IgM or IgG to synthesis of IgE *in vitro* (121). Mast cells do not express leukocyte markers CD1–CD8 and CD19–CD22. Mast cells do express several kinds of receptors for cytokines. As noted previously, mature and developing mast cells express Kit, the product of the c-*kit* protooncogene (CD117), and the ligand for SCF (122). Human mast cells strongly express the IL-4 receptor (21,123), but not the IL-2 (CD25) and IL-3 receptors (124), whereas human basophils strongly express both IL-3 and IL-4 receptors.

Adhesion molecules assist with cell recruitment and localization, and also may modulate cell growth, differentiation, and function. Integrins, one class of adhesion molecules, are a family of heterodimers of one α-chain and one β-chain linked noncovalently. They mediate cell-cell and/or cell-matrix adhesion in a calcium-dependent manner. β1 (CD29)/αn (CD49a–f), called very-late-activation antigen (VLA-n), β2 (CD18)/α (CD11a–c), called lymphocyte function-associated antigen (LFA), β3 (CD61)/α3 (CD51), or αIIb (CD41) and β4–7 are included in this group. The immunoglobulin superfamily of adhesion molecules includes ICAM-1 (CD54), which is a ligand for LFA-1 and leukosialin, and VCAM-1 (CD56),

which is a ligand for VLA-4 (CD29/CD49d), both being expressed on endothelial cells. The selectin adhesion molecule family includes L-, E-, and P-selectins, which are not well studied in mast cells. The phagocytic glycoprotein (Pgp)-1 homing receptor (CD44), also a receptor for hyaluronate, is expressed on both basophils and mast cells. VLA-4 and VLA-5 (CD29/CD49e) are expressed on lung and uterine mast cells. CD18/CD11n are expressed on basophils, but not on mast cells (125). During SCF-dependent differentiation of human mast cells derived from fetal liver *in vitro*, mast cells express functional CD61/CD51, an adhesion molecule for vitronectin (126). In rodents, adhesion of mast cells to extracellular matrix proteins results in enhanced FcεRI-mediated histamine release (127,128).

ACTIVATION OF MAST CELLS

Mast cells and basophils undergo regulated exocytosis when FcεRI (α, β, and γ2) molecules are dimerized by multivalent antigen, antireceptor antibody, multivalent lectins, or the p23 histamine-releasing factor with affinity for a certain subtype of IgE (129–131), as shown in Figure 4. The γ-subunit of FcεRI binds IgE. The γ-subunit is the principal signal transduction element. The β-subunit functions are somewhat uncertain. Complement anaphylatoxins activate basophils and cutaneous mast cells, but not pulmonary mast cells, consistent with the presence of C3a receptors (132). Substance P activates cutaneous mast cells, but not basophils or pulmonary mast cells. SCF also has modest direct activating capacity, but is likely to be more active in priming the mast cell response to other secretogogues (133–135). Chemokine-related histamine-releasing factors, such as monocyte chemotactic and activating factor, activate basophils, but not mast cells (136). The different agonists described above bind different cell surface molecules that in turn transduce qualitatively or quantitatively distinct signals into the interior of cells.

Immunoreceptor tyrosine activation motifs (137), 26 amino acid regions on proteins that associate with *Src*-family protein tyrosine kinases, reside on both the γ- and β-subunits of FcεRI. These two subunits are phosphorylated soon after receptor cross-linking (Fig. 4) and dephosphorylated almost immediately upon disruption of the receptor aggregates (138). *Lyn* associates with the β- and γ-chains when the cells are at rest and initiates phosphorylation of these chains after receptor aggregation (139,140). Also, a calcium-independent isoform of protein kinase C appears to associate with and phosphorylate the γ-chain. Phosphorylation of these sites increases the affinity of cytoplasmic *Syk* for these chains. *Syk* is then phosphorylated by *Lyn* and possibly by itself. *Lyn* knockout mice produce normal numbers of mast cells, but do not engage in passive cutaneous anaphylaxis, indicating

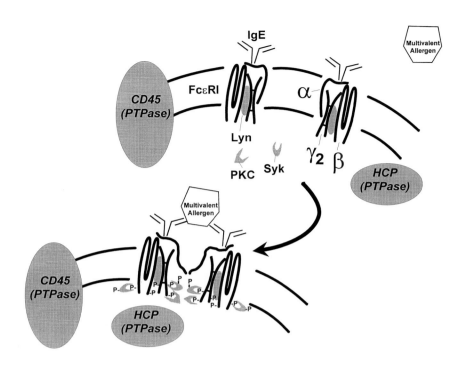

FIG. 4. Early biochemical events during immunoglobulin E-mediated activation of human mast cells. *PTPase,* protein tyrosine phosphatase; *HCP,* hematopoietic cytoplasmic phosphatase; *Lyn* and *Syk,* protein tyrosine kinases; *PKC,* protein kinase C, is a serine/threonine kinase. The FcεRI subunits are designated α, β, and γ2.

that *Lyn* plays an essential role in FcεRI-mediated signal transduction (141). These early events also are regulated by CD45, a protein tyrosine phosphatase, because mast cells from mice that are deficient in this enzyme do not exhibit IgE-dependent activation (142,143). Also, anti-CD45 antibodies inhibit FcεRI-mediated histamine release, but do not inhibit histamine release by calcium ionophore (142). The hemopoietic cytoplasmic protein tyrosine phosphatase is thought to also downregulate *Lyn*-dependent events and is phosphorylated during mast cell activation (144). Phosphorylated *Syk* then carries the activation signal to pathways involving phospholipase Cγ (PLC2), mitosis-activated protein (MAP) kinase, and phosphatidylinositol (PI)-3 kinase. Degranulation is associated with activation of small G proteins that cause actin polymerization and actin relocalization. Generation of diacylglycerol is another critical event, which results in release of calcium from the endoplasmic reticulum, which in turn stimulates calcium-dependent isoforms of protein kinase C and may directly facilitate fusion of lipid bilayers as exocytosis proceeds.

MAST CELLS AND ASTHMA

Mast Cell Numbers and Distribution

Increased numbers of mast cells are found in patients with both atopic and nonatopic asthma in BALF (145–148). This appears to reflect increased numbers of mast cells in bronchial epithelium as demonstrated by bronchial brushings (33) and biopsy specimens containing in-

tact epithelium (149,150), and also the increased epithelium denudation known to occur in asthma. Nevertheless, asthma does not appear to be a disease with generalized pulmonary mast cell hyperplasia. Most mast cells are located in subepithelial regions and in alveolar walls. No mast cell hyperplasia has been detected in these areas (151,152); consequently, the total mast cell burden in lungs of asthmatics does not appear to be substantially elevated. However, it is noteworthy that 73% of all pulmonary mast cells and most of the MC$_{TC}$ cells reside within 20 μm of bronchial/bronchiolar mucus glands (35), within striking distance of released mast cell mediators such as histamine, chymase, and LTC$_4$. Inhaled corticosteroids reduce the concentrations of mast cells, T cells, and eosinophils in epithelial and subepithelial regions, which in part may explain clinical improvement associated with their use in asthma (153).

Mast Cell Activation

Constitutive activation of mast cells appears to be a characteristic feature of the inflammation present in asthmatic lung (summarized in Table 1). In baseline samples of BALF, histamine, tryptase, PGD$_2$, and PGD$_2$ metabolite levels are elevated (76,148,154). The levels of these mediators in BALF provide the most direct measure of pulmonary mast cell activation *in vivo*. When these mediators are detected in blood, their tissue source is unclear. Supportive of ongoing mast cell activation in asthma is the observation that inhaled adenosine causes bronchospasm

TABLE 1. *Mast cell activation and asthma*

Asthmatic condition	Mast cell response
Atopic asthma	
Baseline	Degranulation
Allergen challenge	Increased degranulation
Exercise challenge (exercise response)	No increased degranulation
Aspirin challenge (aspirin sensitive)	No increased degranulation
Hypertonic saline challenge	No increased degranulation
Adenosine challenge	Increased degranulation
Atopy without asthma	
Baseline	No degranulation
Bronchial allergen challenge	
Early-phase response	Degranulation
Late-phase response	No degranulation
Rhinovirus infection	Primed response to allergen

only in asthmatics, and this response is almost totally blocked by antihistamines (155,156). Also, transmission electron microscopy of asthmatic lung tissue shows degranulating mast cells (151,153). Spontaneous release of histamine from BAL mast cells is higher in asthmatics than in control subjects, consistent with ongoing mast cell activation (157). BALF levels of histamine and tryptase in asthmatics correlate with the current severity of airway function (158). These observations suggest that ongoing mast cell activation is a component of the hyperreactive state of the airways in asthmatic patients, and that adenosine-augmented degranulation is largely responsible for the histamine-dependent clinical response to adenosine.

Response to Airway Allergen Challenge

To assess the participation of mast cells in the early phase of the pulmonary response to inhaled allergen, levels of tryptase and histamine were measured in BALF obtained 5 min after endobronchial allergen challenge (154). Four subject groups were studied: atopic and nonatopic asthmatics, and atopic and nonatopic nonasthmatics. Atopic patients elevated their tryptase levels after allergen challenge regardless of the presence of asthma, although the rise was greater in the atopic asthmatic group. No change in tryptase levels occurred after allergen challenge in the nonatopic groups, again regardless of the presence of asthma. These results showed that allergen challenge in patients with atopic asthma and, to a lesser degree, in those with atopy alone activates pulmonary mast cells. Analysis of the early and late phases of the response to endobronchial allergen challenge of sensitive atopic patients without asthma showed elevated tryptase levels only during the early phase in a dose–response fashion, elevated histamine during the early and

late phases, and elevated eosinophil cationic protein during only the late phase (159). These results are analogous to those observed in the skin after cutaneous allergen challenge and indicate that mast cell degranulation occurs only during the early phase, eosinophil activation only during the late phase, and basophil activation at least during the late phase. Viral infection may augment the mast cell response to allergen in atopic patients. Experimental rhinovirus infection in atopic rhinitis patients resulted in increased amounts of tryptase release and histamine release, and in increased eosinophil levels in BALF after bronchial allergen challenge, which also caused a late-phase decline in pulmonary function (160,161).

Aspirin-Sensitive Asthma

Two clinical subsets of immediate-type responses to aspirin have been described: one affects primarily the vasculature and causes hypotensive anaphylaxis, whereas the other affects primarily the respiratory tract and causes asthma. In aspirin-mediated anaphylaxis, mast cell activation has been documented based on elevated levels of tryptase in the blood (162,163). Mast cell activation also appeared to occur during respiratory reactions. Elevated tryptase levels in blood were only detected, however, when the clinical response extended beyond the respiratory tissues to include gastrointestinal and cutaneous signs and symptoms. This leaves open the question of whether pulmonary mast cells were involved in the response to aspirin (164). Urinary LTE4 levels in asthmatics are six times higher than in asthmatic patients who are tolerant to aspirin (165), suggesting inflammatory cells capable of generating leukotrienes are activated, but again failing to identify the tissue source. Inhibition of aspirin-induced bronchospasm by inhaling a selective sulfidopeptide leukotriene antagonist suggests that this class of lipid is generated in the airway and is largely responsible for the bronchospasm observed (166), but does not identify the cellular source of the leukotriene. Examination of nasal lavage fluid during aspirin-induced nasopulmonary reactions showed elevated levels of tryptase and sulfidopeptide leukotrienes, consistent with mast cell activation in the upper airway (167). Of interest in this study was the observation that Zileuton (Abbott Laboratories, Abbott Park, Illinois), a 5-lipoxygenase inhibitor, not only reduced signs, symptoms, and sulfidopeptide leukotriene levels, as anticipated, but also attenuated tryptase levels to an aspirin challenge. This suggests that aspirin-induced mast cell degranulation as well as production of sulfidopeptide leukotrienes is affected by 5-lipoxygenase antagonists.

Adenosine Hyperreactivity

Adenosine augments release of histamine when it is added to antigen or calcium ionophore-stimulated human mast cells, but it does not activate unstimulated mast cells. In the asthmatic airway, low levels of histamine appear to be released continuously from mast cells; inhaled adenosine augments the amounts of histamine being released and thereby results in increased bronchoconstriction (155,156,168). Because levels of PGD_2 and tryptase increase in BALF as well as those of histamine after adenosine is inhaled, mast cell activation is almost certainly enhanced (169).

Exercise-Induced Asthma

Exercise-induced asthma (EIA) is defined as an attack of bronchospasm induced by exercise and may not involve changes in airway inflammation and responsiveness (170). The relationship of mast cells to EIA is controversial. In two separate studies, histamine, tryptase, PGD_2, and LTC_4 levels were no different before and after an exercise challenge that was sufficient to cause bronchospasm (171,172). A follow-up study was performed to enable collection of BALF during the peak response to exercise. In this case, patients exercised with the bronchoscope inserted. Again, mast cell mediators did not increase with exercise (N.N. Jarjour et al., submitted). These studies suggest that mast cell activation does not occur due to an exercise challenge.

In contrast to the direct measurements of mast cell mediators in the airway, pharmacologic studies suggested mast cell activation is involved in EIA. For example, EIA is attenuated by antihistamines, inhibitors of leukotriene synthesis, β-agonists, sodium cromoglycate, and nedocromil. A unifying explanation may be that neuronal activation thresholds are lowered by mast cell mediators that are present at high levels due to constitutive mast cell activation. Neuronal activation may occur with exercise under these conditions without additional mast cell activation. Neuronal thresholds may be reset pharmacologically. In support of this hypothesis, the intrinsic tone of human bronchial smooth muscle is known to be related primarily to histamine and sulfidopeptide leukotrienes (173). In the guinea pig airway, allergen challenge potentiates excitability of sensory fibers in the airway, resulting in increased release of neuropeptides and increased parasympathetic tone (174). Therapies designed to diminish ongoing mast cell activation would be expected to decrease neuronal excitability and the airway response to exercise.

Pharmacologic Intervention

In asthma, it is unclear whether any of the drugs used by clinicians act by inhibiting mast cells activation. *In vitro*, however, treatment of human pulmonary mast cells with a β-agonist inhibits mediator release (175), preferentially decreasing LTC_4 and PGD_2 secretion over that of histamine (176). These observations suggest important potential mechanisms for the clinical efficacy of β-agonists in asthma. Cromolyn and nedocromil have limited efficacy against human mast cell activation *in vitro* and act by mechanisms *in vivo* that need further clarification (177–183). Attenuation of adenosine-induced bronchoconstriction by nedocromil may provide a partial explanation for the efficacy of this drug (184). In conclusion, development of selective pharmacologic agents that inhibit mast cell activation remains an elusive goal for the therapy of atopic asthma and other diseases in which mast cells are inappropriately activated.

ACKNOWLEDGMENTS

We thank Dr. Angela Hogan and Dr. Katherine Carias for their careful readings of the manuscript.

REFERENCES

1. Riley JF, West GB. The presence of histamine in tissue mast cells. *J Physiol* 1953;120:528–532.
2. Ishizaka K, Tomioka K, Ishizaka T. Mechanisms of passive sensitization. I. Presence of IgE and IgG molecules on human leukocytes. *J Immunol* 1970;105:1459–1467.
3. Tomioka K, Ishizaka K. Mechanisms of passive sensitization. II. Presence of receptors for IgE on monkey mast cells. *J Immunol* 1971;107:971–978.
4. Kirshenbaum AS, Kessler SW, Goff JP, Metcalfe DD. Demonstration of the origin of human mast cells from CD34+ bone marrow progenitor cells. *J Immunol* 1991;146:1410–1415.
5. Kirshenbaum AS, Goff JP, Dreskin SC, Irani AA, Schwartz LB, Metcalfe DD. IL-3-dependent growth of basophil-like cells and mastlike cells from human bone marrow. *J Immunol* 1989;142:2424–2429.
6. Valent P, Schmidt G, Besemer J, et al. Interleukin-3 is a differentiation factor for human basophils. *Blood* 1989;73:1763–1769.
7. Dvorak AM, Saito H, Estrella P, Kissell S, Arai N, Ishizaka T. Ultrastructure of eosinophils and basophils stimulated to develop in human cord blood mononuclear cell cultures containing recombinant human interleukin-5 or interleukin-3. *Lab Invest* 1989;61:116–130.
8. Tsuda T, Wong D, Dolovich J, Bienenstock J, Marshall J, Denburg JA. Synergistic effects of nerve growth factor and granulocyte-macrophage colony-stimulating factor on human basophilic cell differentiation. *Blood* 1991;77:971–979.
9. Denburg JA, Silver JE, Abrams JS. Interleukin-5 is a human basophilopoietin: induction of histamine content and basophilic differentiation of HL-60 cells and of peripheral blood basophil-eosinophil progenitors. *Blood* 1991;77:1462–1468.
10. Tsuda T, Switzer J, Bienenstock J, Denburg JA. Interactions of hemopoietic cytokines on differentiation of HL-60 cells: nerve growth factor is a basophilic lineage-specific co-factor. *Int Arch Allergy Appl Immunol* 1990;91:15–21.
11. Ishizaka T, Saito H, Furitsu T, Dvorak AM. Growth of human basophils and mast cells *in vitro*. In: Galli SJ, Austen KF, eds. *Mast cell and basophil differentiation and function in health and disease*. New York: Raven Press, 1989;39–47.
12. Nabel GJ, Galli SJ, Dvorak AM, Dvorak HF, Cantor H. Inducer T lymphocytes synthesize a factor that stimulates proliferation of cloned mast cells. *Nature* 1981;291:332–334.
13. Yung YP, Eger R, Tertian G, Moore MA. Long-term *in vitro* culture of murine mast cells. II. Purification of a mast cell growth factor and its dissociation from TCGF. *J Immunol* 1981;127:794–799.
14. Tertian G, Yung YP, Guy-Grand D, Moore MA. Long-term *in vitro* culture of murine mast cells. I. Description of a growth factor-dependent culture technique. *J Immunol* 1981;127:788–794.
15. Razin E, Cordon-Cardo C, Good RA. Growth of a pure population of

mast cells *in vitro* with conditioned medium derived from concanavalin A-stimulated splenocytes. *Proc Natl Acad Sci USA* 1981;78: 2559–2561.

16. Irani AA, Nilsson G, Miettinen U, et al. Recombinant human stem cell factor stimulates differentiation of mast cells from dispersed human fetal liver cells. *Blood* 1992;80:3009–3021.

17. Mitsui H, Furitsu T, Dvorak AM, et al. Development of human mast cells from umbilical cord blood cells by recombinant human and murine C-kit ligand. *Proc Natl Acad Sci USA* 1993;90:735–739.

18. Valent P, Spanblöchl E, Sperr WR, et al. Induction of differentiation of human mast cells from bone marrow and peripheral blood mononuclear cells by recombinant human stem cell factor/*kit*-ligand in long-term culture. *Blood* 1992;80:2237–2245.

19. Flanagan JG, Chan DC, Leder P. Transmembrane form of the kit ligand growth factor is determined by alternative splicing and is missing in the Sld mutant. *Cell* 1991;64:1025–1035.

20. Linenberger ML, Jacobsen FW, Bennett LG, Broudy VC, Martin FH, Abkowitz JL. Stem cell factor production by human marrow stromal fibroblasts. *Exp Hematol* 1995;23:1104–1114.

21. Nilsson G, Miettinen U, Ishizaka T, Ashman LK, Irani A-M, Schwartz LB. Interleukin-4 inhibits the expression of Kit and tryptase during stem cell factor-dependent development of human mast cells from fetal liver cells. *Blood* 1994;84:1519–1527.

22. Sillaber C, Sperr WR, Agis H, Spanblöchl E, Lechner K, Valent P. Inhibition of stem cell factor dependent formation of human mast cells by interleukin-3 and interleukin-4. *Int Arch Allergy Immunol* 1994; 105:264–268.

23. Kinashi T, Springer TA. Steel factor and c-*kit* regulate cell-matrix adhesion. *Blood* 1994;83:1033–1038.

24. Nilsson G, Butterfield JH, Nilsson K, Siegbahn A. Stem cell factor is a chemotactic factor for human mast cells. *J Immunol* 1994;153: 3717–3723.

25. Dastych J, Metcalfe DD. Stem cell factor induces mast cell adhesion to fibronectin. *J Immunol* 1994;152:213–219.

26. Mekori YA, Oh CK, Metcalfe DD. IL-3-dependent murine mast cells undergo apoptosis on removal of IL-3: prevention of apoptosis by c-*kit* ligand. *J Immunol* 1993;151:3775–3784.

27. Iemura A, Tsai M, Ando A, Wershil BK, Galli SJ. The c-*kit* ligand, stem cell factor, promotes mast cell survival by suppressing apoptosis. *Am J Pathol* 1994;144:321–328.

28. Yee NS, Paek I, Besmer P. Role of *kit*-ligand in proliferation and suppression of apoptosis in mast cells: basis for radiosensitivity of *white spotting* and *Steel* mutant mice. *J Exp Med* 1994;179:1777–1787.

29. Irani AA, Schwartz LB. Neutral proteases as indicators of human mast cell heterogeneity. In: Schwartz LB, ed. *Neutral proteases of mast cells*. Basel: Karger, 1990;146–162.

30. Juliusson S, Pipkorn U, Karlsson G, Enerbäck L. Mast cells and eosinophils in the allergic mucosal response to allergen challenge: changes in distribution and signs of activation in relation to symptoms. *J Allergy Clin Immunol* 1992;90:898–909.

31. Bentley AM, Jacobson MR, Cumberworth V, et al. Immunohistology of the nasal mucosa in seasonal allergic rhinitis: Increases in activated eosinophils and epithelial mast cells. *J Allergy Clin Immunol* 1992; 89:877–883.

32. Varney VA, Jacobson MR, Sudderick RM, et al. Immunohistology of the nasal mucosa following allergen-induced rhinitis. *Am Rev Respir Dis* 1992;146:170–176.

33. Gibson PG, Allen CJ, Yang JP, et al. Intraepithelial mast cells in allergic and nonallergic asthma: assessment using bronchial brushings. *Am Rev Respir Dis* 1993;148:80–86.

34. Bradley BL, Azzawi M, Jacobson M, et al. Eosinophils, T-lymphocytes, mast cells, neutrophils, and macrophages in bronchial biopsy specimens from atopic subjects with asthma: comparison with biopsy specimens from atopic subjects without asthma and normal control subjects and relationship to bronchial hyperresponsiveness. *J Allergy Clin Immunol* 1991;88:661–674.

35. Matin R, Tam EK, Nadel JA, Caughey GH. Distribution of chymase-containing mast cells in human bronchi. *J Histochem Cytochem* 1992; 40:781–786.

36. Djukanovic R, Roche WR, Holgate ST, Walls AF, Howarth PH. Quantitation of mast cells and eosinophils in the bronchial mucosa of symptomatic atopic asthmatics and healthy control subjects using immunohistochemistry: reply. *Am Rev Respir Dis* 1991;143(Suppl): 1200–1201.

37. Mattoli S, Ackerman V, Vittori E, Marini M. Mast cell chemotactic activity of RANTES. *Biochem Biophys Res Commun* 1995;209:316–321.

38. Matsuura N, Zetter BR. Stimulation of mast cell chemotaxis by interleukin 3. *J Exp Med* 1989;170:1421–1426.

39. Thompson HL, Burbelo PD, Yamada Y, Kleinman HK, Metcalfe DD. Mast cells chemotax to laminin with enhancement after IgE-mediated activation. *J Immunol* 1989;143:4188–4192.

40. Norrby K. Evidence of specificity in the action of angiogenesis antagonists. *Int J Microcirc Clin Exp* 1994;14:226–232.

41. Ghebrehiwet B, Kew RR, Gruber BL, Marchese MJ, Peerschke EIB, Reid KBM. Murine mast cells express two types of C1q receptors that are involved in the induction of chemotaxis and chemokinesis. *J Immunol* 1995;155:2614–2619.

42. Tanimoto Y, Takahashi K, Kimura I. Effects of cytokines on human basophil chemotaxis. *Clin Exp Allergy* 1992;22:1020–1025.

43. Alam R, Forsythe P, Stafford S, et al. Monocyte chemotactic protein-2, monocyte chemotactic protein-3, and fibroblast-induced cytokine: three new chemokines induce chemotaxis and activation of basophils. *J Immunol* 1994;153:3155–3159.

44. Schwartz LB, Lewis RA, Austen KF. Tryptase from human pulmonary mast cells: purification and characterization. *J Biol Chem* 1981;256:11,939–11,943.

45. Glenner GC, Cohen LA. Histochemical demonstration of species-specific trypsin-like enzyme in mast cells. *Nature* 1960;185:846–847.

46. Schwartz LB, Bradford TR. Regulation of tryptase from human lung mast cells by heparin: stabilization of the active tetramer. *J Biol Chem* 1986;261:7372–7379.

47. Craig SS, Irani A-MA, Metcalfe DD, Schwartz LB. Ultrastructural localization of heparin to human mast cells of the MC_{TC} and MC_T types by labeling with antithrombin III-gold. *Lab Invest* 1993;69:552–561.

48. Schwartz LB, Sakai K, Bradford TR, et al. The α form of human tryptase is the predominant type present in blood at baseline in normal subjects, and is elevated in those with systemic mastocytosis. *J Clin Invest* 1995;96:2702–2710.

49. Schechter NM, Sprows JL, Schoenberger OL, Lazarus GS, Cooperman BS, Rubin H. Reaction of human skin chymotrypsin-like proteinase chymase with plasma proteinase inhibitors. *J Biol Chem* 1989; 264:21,308–21,315.

50. Sayama S, Iozzo RV, Lazarus GS, Schechter NM. Human skin chymotrypsin-like proteinase chymase: subcellular localization to mast cell granules and interaction with heparin and other glycosaminoglycans. *J Biol Chem* 1987;262:6808–6815.

51. Urata H, Kinoshita A, Perez DM, et al. Cloning of the gene and cDNA for human heart chymase. *J Biol Chem* 1991;266:17,173–17,179.

52. Caughey GH, Zerweck EH, Vanderslice P. Structure, chromosomal assignment, and deduced amino acid sequence of a human gene for mast cell chymase. *J Biol Chem* 1991;266:12,956–12,963.

53. Caughey GH, Schaumberg TH, Zerweck EH, et al. The human mast cell chymase gene (CMA1): mapping to the cathepsin G/granzyme gene cluster and lineage-restricted expression. *Genomics* 1993;15: 614–620.

54. Schwartz LB. Laboratory assessment of immediate hypersensitivity and anaphylaxis: utilization of tryptase as a marker of mast cell-dependent events. In: Huston DP, ed. *Immunology and allergy clinics of North America: diagnostic laboratory immunology*. Philadelphia: WB Saunders, 1994;339–350.

55. Schwartz LB, Bradford TR, Rouse C, et al. Development of a new, more sensitive immunoassay for human tryptase: use in systemic anaphylaxis. *J Clin Immunol* 1994;14:190–204.

56. Urata H, Karnik SS, Graham RM, Husain A. Dipeptide processing activates recombinant human prochymase. *J Biol Chem* 1993;268: 24,318–24,322.

57. Murakami M, Karnik SS, Husain A. Human prochymase activation: a novel role for heparin in zymogen processing. *J Biol Chem* 1995;270: 2218–2223.

58. Sakai K, Ren S, Schwartz LB. A novel heparin-dependent processing pathway for human tryptase: autocatalysis followed by activation with dipeptidyl peptidase I. *J Clin Invest* 1995;97:988–995.

59. Sekizawa K, Caughey GH, Lazarus SC, Gold WM, Nadel JA. Mast cell tryptase causes airway smooth muscle hyperresponsiveness in dogs. *J Clin Invest* 1989;83:175–179.

60. Rubinstein I, Nadel JA, Graf PD, Caughey GH. Mast cell chymase potentiates histamine-induced wheal formation in the skin of ragweed-allergic dogs. *J Clin Invest* 1990;86:555–559.

61. Caughey GH, Leidig F, Viro NF, Nadel JA. Substance P and vasoactive intestinal peptide degradation by mast cell tryptase and chymase. *J Pharmacol Exp Ther* 1988;244:133–137.

62. Walls AF, Brain SD, Desai A, et al. Human mast cell tryptase attenuates the vasodilator activity of calcitonin gene-related peptide. *Biochem Pharmacol* 1992;43:1243–1248.

63. Ruoss SJ, Hartmann T, Caughey GH. Mast cell tryptase is a mitogen for cultured fibroblasts. *J Clin Invest* 1991;88:493–499.

64. Hartmann T, Ruoss SJ, Raymond WW, Seuwen K, Caughey GH. Human tryptase as a potent, cell-specific mitogen: role of signaling pathways in synergistic responses. *Am J Physiol* 1992;262:L528–L534.

65. Gruber BL, Schwartz LB, Ramamurthy NS, Irani AM, Marchese MJ. Activation of latent rheumatoid synovial collagenase by human mast cell tryptase. *J Immunol* 1988;140:3936–3942.

66. Gruber BL, Marchese MJ, Suzuki K, et al. Synovial procollagenase activation by human mast cell tryptase dependence upon matrix metalloproteinase 3 activation. *J Clin Invest* 1989;84:1657–1662.

67. Saarinen J, Kalkkinen N, Welgus HG, Kovanen PT. Activation of human interstitial procollagenase through direct cleavage of the Leu[83]–Thr[84] bond by mast cell chymase. *J Biol Chem* 1994;269:18,134–18,140.

68. Schwartz LB, Bradford TR, Littman BH, Wintroub BU. The fibrinogenolytic activity of purified tryptase from human lung mast cells. *J Immunol* 1985;135:2762–2767.

69. Reilly CF, Tewksbury DA, Schechter NM, Travis J. Rapid conversion of angiotensin I to angiotensin II by neutrophil and mast cell proteinases. *J Biol Chem* 1982;257:8619–8622.

70. Urata H, Kinoshita A, Misono KS, Bumpus FM, Husain A. Identification of a highly specific chymase as the major angiotensin II-forming enzyme in the human heart. *J Biol Chem* 1990;265:22,348–22,357.

71. Mizutani H, Schechter N, Lazarus G, Black RA, Kupper TS. Rapid and specific conversion of precursor interleukin 1β (IL-1β) to an active IL-1 species by human mast cell chymase. *J Exp Med* 1991;174:821–825.

72. Taipale J, Lohi J, Saarinen J, Kovanen PT, Keski-Oja J. Human mast cell chymase and leukocyte elastase release latent transforming growth factor-β1 from the extracellular matrix of cultured human epithelial and endothelial cells. *J Biol Chem* 1995;270:4689–4696.

73. Kepley CL, Craig SS, Schwartz LB. Identification and partial characterization of a unique marker for human basophils. *J Immunol* 1995;154:6548–6555.

74. Peters SP, MacGlashan DW, Schulman ES, et al. Arachidonic acid metabolism in purified human lung mast cells. *J Immunol* 1984;132:1972–1979.

75. Henderson WR Jr. The role of leukotrienes in inflammation. *Ann Intern Med* 1994;121:684–697.

76. Liu MC, Bleecker ER, Lichtenstein LM, et al. Evidence for elevated levels of histamine, prostaglandin D₂, and other bronchoconstricting prostaglandins in the airways of subjects with mild asthma. *Am Rev Respir Dis* 1990;142:126–132.

77. Liu MC, Hubbard WC, Proud D, et al. Immediate and late inflammatory responses to ragweed antigen challenge of the peripheral airways in allergic asthmatics: cellular, mediator, and permeability changes. *Am Rev Respir Dis* 1991;144:51–58.

78. Wenzel SE, Westcott JY, Smith HR, Larsen GL. Spectrum of prostanoid release after bronchoalveolar allergen challenge in atopic asthmatics and in control groups: an alteration in the ratio of bronchoconstrictive to bronchoprotective mediators. *Am Rev Respir Dis* 1989;139:450–457.

79. Wenzel SE, Larsen GL, Johnston K, Voelkel NF, Westcott JY. Elevated levels of leukotriene C4 in bronchoalveolar lavage fluid from atopic asthmatics after endobronchial allergen challenge. *Am Rev Respir Dis* 1990;142:112–119.

80. Benyon RC, Robinson C, Church MK. Differential release of histamine and eicosanoids from human skin mast cells activated by IgE-dependent and non-immunological stimuli. *Br J Pharmacol* 1989;97:898–904.

81. Featherstone RL, Robinson C, Holgate ST, Church MK. Evidence for thromboxane receptor mediated contraction of guinea-pig and human airways *in vitro* by prostaglandin (PG) D₂, 9α,11β-PGF₂ and PGF₂α. *Naunyn Schmiedebergs Arch Pharmacol* 1990;341:439–443.

82. Johnston SL, Bardin PG, Harrison J, Ritter W, Joubert JR, Holgate ST. The effects of an oral thromboxane TP receptor antagonist BAY u 3405, on prostaglandin D₂- and histamine-induced bronchoconstriction in asthma, and relationship to plasma drug concentrations. *Br J Clin Pharmacol* 1992;34:402–408.

83. Drazen JM, Evans JF, Stevens RL, Shipp MA. Inflammatory effector mechanisms in asthma. *Am J Respir Crit Care Med* 1995;152:403–407.

84. Israel E, Fischer AR, Rosenberg MA, et al. The pivotal role of 5-lipoxygenase products in the reaction of aspirin-sensitive asthmatics to aspirin. *Am Rev Respir Dis* 1993;148:1447–1451.

85. Chen X-S, Sheller JR, Johnson EN, Funk CD. Role of leukotrienes revealed by targeted disruption of the 5-lipoxygenase gene. *Nature* 1994;372:179–182.

86. Kroegel C, Yukawa T, Dent G, Chanez P, Chung KF, Barnes PJ. Platelet-activating factor induces eosinophil peroxidase release from purified human eosinophils. *Immunology* 1988;64:559–561.

87. Columbo M, Casolaro V, Warner JA, MacGlashan DW Jr, Kagey-Sobotka A, Lichtenstein LM. The mechanism of mediator release from human basophils induced by platelet-activating factor. *J Immunol* 1990;145:3855–3861.

88. Brunner T, De Weck AL, Dahinden CA. Platelet-activating factor induces mediator release by human basophils primed with IL-3, granulocyte–macrophage colony-stimulating factor, or IL-5. *J Immunol* 1991;147:237–242.

89. Kroegel C, Yukawa T, Dent G, Venge P, Chung KF, Barnes PJ. Stimulation of degranulation from human eosinophils by platelet-activating factor. *J Immunol* 1989;142:3518–3526.

90. Columbo M, Horowitz EM, Kagey-Sobotka A, Lichtenstein LM. Histamine release from human basophils induced by platelet activating factor: the role of extracellular calcium, interleukin-3, and granulocyte-macrophage colony-stimulating factor. *J Allergy Clin Immunol* 1995;95:565–573.

91. Thomas G, Church MK. Platelet activating factor does not release histamine from human dispersed cutaneous mast cells. *Clin Exp Allergy* 1990;20:377–382.

92. Tjoelker LW, Wilder C, Eberhardt C, et al. Anti-inflammatory properties of a platelet-activating factor acetylhydrolase. *Nature* 1995;374:549–553.

93. Fuller RW, Dixon CM, Dollery CT, Barnes PJ. Prostaglandin D₂ potentiates airway responsiveness to histamine and methacholine. *Am Rev Respir Dis* 1986;133:252–254.

94. Lai CKW, Jenkins JR, Polosa R, Holgate ST. Inhaled PAF fails to induce airway hyperresponsiveness to methacholine in normal human subjects. *J Appl Physiol* 1990;68:919–926.

95. Lai CKW, Djukanovic R, Wilson JW, et al. Effect of inhaled platelet-activating factor on bronchial inflammation in atopic non-asthmatic subjects. *Int Arch Allergy Appl Immunol* 1992;99:84–90.

96. Spence DPS, Johnston SL, Calverley PMA, et al. The effect of the orally active platelet-activating factor antagonist WEB 2086 in the treatment of asthma. *Am J Respir Crit Care Med* 1994;149:1142–1148.

97. Gordon JR, Galli SJ. Mast cells as a source of both preformed and immunologically inducible TNF-α/cachectin. *Nature* 1990;346:274–276.

98. Walsh LJ, Trinchieri G, Waldorf HA, Whitaker D, Murphy GF. Human dermal mast cells contain and release tumor necrosis factor α, which induces endothelial leukocyte adhesion molecule 1. *Proc Natl Acad Sci USA* 1991;88:4220–4224.

99. Gordon JR, Galli SJ. Release of both preformed and newly synthesized tumor necrosis factor-α (TNF-α)/cachectin by mouse mast cells stimulated via the FcεRI: a mechanism for the sustained action of mast cell-derived TNF-α during IgE-dependent biological responses. *J Exp Med* 1991;174:103–107.

100. Bradding P, Mediwake R, Feather IH, et al. TNF-α is localized to nasal mucosal mast cells and is released in acute allergic rhinitis. *Clin Exp Allergy* 1995;25:406–415.

101. Steffen M, Abboud M, Potter GK, Yung YP, Moore MAS. Presence of tumour necrosis factor or a related factor in human basophil/mast cells. *Immunology* 1989;66:445–450.

102. Bradding P, Feather IH, Howarth PH, et al. Interleukin-4 is localized to and released by human mast cells. *J Exp Med* 1992;176:1381–1386.

103. Okayama Y, Bradding P, Tunon-de-Lara JM, Holgate ST, Church MK. Cytokine production by human mast cells. *Chem Immunol* 1995;61:114–134.

104. Bradding P, Roberts JA, Britten KM, et al. Interleukin-4, -5, and -6 and tumor necrosis factor-α in normal and asthmatic airways: evidence for the human mast cell as a source of these cytokines. *Am J Respir Cell Mol Biol* 1994;10:471–480.

105. Okayama Y, Semper A, Holgate ST, Church MK. Multiple cytokine mRNA expression in human mast cells stimulated via FcεRI. *Int Arch Allergy Immunol* 1995;107:158–159.

106. Ying S, Durham SR, Jacobson MR, et al. T lymphocytes and mast cells express messenger RNA for interleukin-4 in the nasal mucosa in allergen-induced rhinitis. *Immunology* 1994;82:200–206.

107. Bradding P, Okayama Y, Howarth PH, Church MK, Holgate ST. Heterogeneity of human mast cells based on cytokine content. *J Immunol* 1995;155:297–307.

108. Bradding P, Feather IH, Wilson S, et al. Immunolocalization of cytokines in the nasal mucosa of normal and perennial rhinitic subjects: the mast cell as a source of IL-4, IL-5, and IL-6 in human allergic mucosal inflammation. *J Immunol* 1993;151:3853–3865.

109. Bradding P, Feather IH, Wilson S, Holgate ST, Howarth PH. Cytokine immunoreactivity in seasonal rhinitis: regulation by a topical corticosteroid. *Am J Respir Crit Care Med* 1995;151:1900–1906.

110. Osborn L, Hession C, Tizard R, et al. Direct expression cloning of vascular cell adhesion molecule 1, a cytokine-induced endothelial protein that binds to lymphocytes. *Cell* 1989;59:1203–1211.

111. Bevilacqua MP, Stengelin S, Gimbrone MA Jr, Seed B. Endothelial leukocyte adhesion molecule 1: an inducible receptor for neutrophils related to complement regulatory proteins and lectins. *Science* 1989;243:1160–1165.

112. Pober JS, Gimbrone MA Jr, Lapierre LA, et al. Overlapping patterns of activation of human endothelial cells by interleukin 1, tumor necrosis factor, and immune interferon. *J Immunol* 1986;137:1893–1896.

113. Metzger H. The high affinity receptor for IgE on mast cells. *Clin Exp Allergy* 1991;21:269–279.

114. Gounni AS, Lamkhioued B, Ochiai K, et al. High-affinity IgE receptor on eosinophils is involved in defence against parasites. *Nature* 1994;367:183–186.

115. Wang B, Rieger A, Kilgus O, et al. Epidermal Langerhans cells from normal human skin bind monomeric IgE via FcεRI. *J Exp Med* 1992;175:1353–1365.

116. Bieber T, Salle H, Wollenberg A, et al. Human epidermal Langerhans cells express the high affinity receptor for immunoglobulin E (FcεRI). *J Exp Med* 1992;175:1285–1290.

117. Maurer D, Fiebiger E, Reininger B, et al. Expression of functional high affinity immunoglobulin E receptors (FcεRI) on monocytes of atopic individuals. *J Exp Med* 1994;179:745–750.

118. Valent P, Majdic O, Maurer D, Bodger M, Muhm M, Bettelheim P. Further characterization of surface membrane structures expressed on human basophils and mast cells. *Int Arch Allergy Appl Immunol* 1990;91:198–203.

119. Guo C-B, Kagey-Sobotka A, Lichtenstein LM, Bochner BS. Immunophenotyping and functional analysis of purified human uterine mast cells. *Blood* 1992;79:708–712.

120. Reshef A, MacGlashan DW. Immunogold probe for the light-microscopic phenotyping of human mast cells and basophils. *J Immunol Methods* 1987;99:213–219.

121. Gauchat J-F, Henchoz S, Mazzei G, et al. Induction of human IgE synthesis in B cells by mast cells and basophils. *Nature* 1993;365:340–343.

122. Lerner NB, Nocka KH, Cole SR, et al. Monoclonal antibody YB5.B8 identifies the human c-kit protein product. *Blood* 1991;77:1876–1883.

123. Sillaber C, Strobl H, Bevec D, et al. IL-4 regulates c-kit proto-oncogene product expression in human mast and myeloid progenitor cells. *J Immunol* 1991;147:4224–4228.

124. Valent P, Besemer J, Sillaber C, et al. Failure to detect IL-3-binding sites on human mast cells. *J Immunol* 1990;145:3432–3437.

125. Sperr WR, Agis H, Czerwenka K, et al. Differential expression of cell surface integrins on human mast cells and human basophils. *Ann Hematol* 1992;65:10–16.

126. Shimizu Y, Irani AA, Brown EJ, Ashman LK, Schwartz LB. Human mast cells derived from fetal liver cells cultured with stem cell factor express a functional CD51/CD61 (αvβ3) integrin. *Blood* 1995;86:930–939.

127. Hamawy MM, Oliver C, Mergenhagen SE, Siraganian RP. Adherence of rat basophilic leukemia (RBL-2H3) cells to fibronectin-coated surfaces enhances secretion. *J Immunol* 1992;149:615–621.

128. Hamawy MM, Mergenhagen SE, Siraganian RP. Adhesion molecules as regulators of mast-cell and basophil function. *Immunol Today* 1994;15:62–66.

129. Ishizaka T, Ishizaka K. Triggering of histamine release from rat mast cells by divalent antibodies against IgE receptors. *J Immunol* 1978;120:800–805.

130. Ishizaka T, Conrad DH, Schulman ES, Sterk AR, Ishizaka K. Biochemical analysis of initial triggering events of IgE-mediated histamine release from human lung mast cells. *J Immunol* 1983;130:2357–2362.

131. MacDonald SM, Rafnar T, Langdon J, Lichtenstein LM. Molecular identification of an IgE-dependent histamine-releasing factor. *Science* 1995;269:688–690.

132. Füreder W, Agis H, Willheim M, et al. Differential expression of complement receptors on human basophils and mast cells: evidence for mast cell heterogeneity and CD88/C5aR expression on skin mast cells. *J Immunol* 1995;155:3152–3160.

133. Bischoff SC, Dahinden CA. c-kit Ligand: a unique potentiator of mediator release by human lung mast cells. *J Exp Med* 1992;175:237–244.

134. Wershil BK, Tsai M, Geissler EN, Zsebo KM, Galli SJ. The rat c-kit ligand, stem cell factor, induces c-kit receptor-dependent mouse mast cell activation *in vivo*: evidence that signaling through the c-kit receptor can induce expression of cellular function. *J Exp Med* 1992;175:245–255.

135. Columbo M, Horowitz EM, Botana LM, et al. The human recombinant c-kit receptor ligand, rhSCF, induces mediator release from human cutaneous mast cells and enhances IgE-dependent mediator release from both skin mast cells and peripheral blood basophils. *J Immunol* 1992;149:599–608.

136. Okayama Y, Brzezinska-Blaszczyk E, Kuna P, Kaplan AP, Church MK. Effects of PBMC-derived histamine-releasing factors on histamine release from human skin and lung mast cells. *Clin Exp Allergy* 1995;25:890–895.

137. Cambier JC, Daëron M, Fridman W, et al. New nomenclature for the Reth motif (or ARH1/TAM/ARAM/YXXL). *Immunol Today* 1995;16:110.

138. Paolini R, Jouvin M-H, Kinet J-P. Phosphorylation and dephosphorylation of the high-affinity receptor for immunoglobulin E immediately after receptor engagement and disengagement. *Nature* 1991;353:855–858.

139. Vallé A, Kinet J-P. N-acetyl-L-cysteine inhibits antigen-mediated Syk, but not Lyn tyrosine kinase activation in mast cells. *FEBS Lett* 1995;357:41–44.

140. Wilson BS, Kapp N, Lee RJ, et al. Distinct functions of the FcεR1 gamma and β subunits in the control of FcεR1-mediated tyrosine kinase activation and signaling responses in RBL-2H3 mast cells. *J Biol Chem* 1995;270:4013–4022.

141. Hibbs ML, Tarlinton DM, Armes J, et al. Multiple defects in the immune system of Lyn-deficient mice, culminating in autoimmune disease. *Cell* 1995;83:301–311.

142. Hook WA, Berenstein EH, Zinsser FU, Fischler C, Siraganian RP. Monoclonal antibodies to the leukocyte common antigen (CD45) inhibit IgE-mediated histamine release from human basophils. *J Immunol* 1991;147:2670–2676.

143. Berger SA, Mak TW, Paige CJ. Leukocyte common antigen (CD45) is required for immunoglobulin E-mediated degranulation of mast cells. *J Exp Med* 1994;180:471–476.

144. Swieter M, Berenstein EH, Swaim WD, Siraganian RP. Aggregation of IgE receptors in rat basophilic leukemia 2H3 cells induces tyrosine phosphorylation of the cytosolic protein-tyrosine phosphatase HePTP. *J Biol Chem* 1995;270:21,902–21,906.

145. Flint KC, Leung KBP, Pearce FL, Hudspith BN, Brostoff J, Johnson NM. Human mast cells recovered by bronchoalveolar lavage: their morphology, histamine release and the effects of sodium cromoglycate. *Clin Science* 1985;68:427–432.

146. Tomioka M, Ida S, Shindoh Y, Ishihara T, Takishima T. Mast cells in bronchoalveolar lumen of patients with bronchial asthma. *Am Rev Respir Dis* 1984;129:1000–1005.

147. Kirby JG, Hargreave FE, Gleich GJ, O'Byrne PM. Bronchoalveolar cell profiles of asthmatic and nonasthmatic subjects. *Am Rev Respir Dis* 1987;136:379–383.

148. Casale TB, Wood D, Richerson HB, Zehr B, Zavala D, Hunninghake GW. Direct evidence of a role for mast cells in the pathogenesis of

antigen-induced bronchoconstriction. *J Clin Invest* 1987;80:1507–1511.

149. Ollerenshaw SL, Woolcock AJ. Characteristics of the inflammation in biopsies from large airways of subjects with asthma and subjects with chronic airflow limitation. *Am Rev Respir Dis* 1992;145(4 Pt 1):922–927.

150. Laitinen LA, Laitinen A, Haahtela T. Airway mucosal inflammation even in patients with newly diagnosed asthma. *Am Rev Respir Dis* 1993;147:697–704.

151. Djukanovic R, Wilson JW, Britten KM, et al. Quantitation of mast cells and eosinophils in the bronchial mucosa of symptomatic atopic asthmatics and healthy control subjects using immunohistochemistry. *Am Rev Respir Dis* 1990;142:863–871.

152. Bradley BL, Azzawi M, Jacobson M, et al. Eosinophils, T-lymphocytes, mast cells, neutrophils, and macrophages in bronchial biopsies from atopic asthmatics: comparison with atopic non-asthma and normal controls and relationship to bronchial hyperresponsiveness. *J Allergy Clin Immunol* 1991;88:661–674.

153. Djukanovic R, Wilson JW, Britten KM, et al. Effect of an inhaled corticosteroid on airway inflammation and symptoms in asthma. *Am Rev Respir Dis* 1992;145:669–674.

154. Wenzel SE, Fowler AA III, Schwartz LB. Activation of pulmonary mast cells by bronchoalveolar allergen challenge: *in vivo* release of histamine and tryptase in atopic subjects with and without asthma. *Am Rev Respir Dis* 1988;137:1002–1008.

155. Cushley MJ, Tattersfield AE, Holgate ST. Adenosine-induced bronchoconstriction in asthma: antagonism by theophylline. *Am Rev Respir Dis* 1984;129:380–384.

156. Rafferty P, Beasley CR, Holgate ST. The contribution of histamine to bronchoconstriction produced by inhaled allergen and adenosine 5'-monophosphate in asthma. *Am Rev Respir Dis* 1987;136:369–373.

157. Jarjour NN, Calhoun WJ, Schwartz LB, Busse WW. Elevated bronchoalveolar lavage fluid histamine levels in allergic asthmatics are associated with increased airway obstruction. *Am Rev Respir Dis* 1991;144:83–87.

158. Broide DH, Gleich GJ, Cuomo AJ, et al. Evidence of ongoing mast cell and eosinophil degranulation in symptomatic asthma airway. *J Allergy Clin Immunol* 1991;88:637–648.

159. Sedgwick JB, Calhoun WJ, Gleich GJ, et al. Immediate and late airway response of allergic rhinitis patients to segmental antigen challenge: characterization of eosinophil and mast cell mediators. *Am Rev Respir Dis* 1991;144:1274–1281.

160. Calhoun WJ, Swensen CA, Dick EC, Schwartz LB, Lemanske RF Jr, Busse WW. Experimental rhinovirus 16 infection potentiates histamine release following antigen bronchoprovocation in allergic subjects. *Am Rev Respir Dis* 1991;144:1267–1273.

161. Calhoun WJ, Dick EC, Schwartz LB, Busse WW. A common cold virus, rhinovirus 16, potentiates airway inflammation after segmental antigen bronchoprovocation in allergic subjects. *J Clin Invest* 1994;94:2200–2208.

162. Schwartz LB, Metcalfe DD, Miller JS, Earl H, Sullivan T. Tryptase levels as an indicator of mast-cell activation in systemic anaphylaxis and mastocytosis. *N Engl J Med* 1987;316:1622–1626.

163. Schwartz LB, Yunginger JW, Miller JS, Bokhari R, Dull D. The time course of appearance and disappearance of human mast cell tryptase in the circulation after anaphylaxis. *J Clin Invest* 1989;83:1551–1555.

164. Bosso JV, Schwartz LB, Stevenson DD. Tryptase and histamine release during aspirin-induced respiratory reactions. *J Allergy Clin Immunol* 1991;88:830–837.

165. Christie PE, Tagari P, Ford-Hutchinson AW, et al. Urinary leukotriene E$_4$ concentrations increase after aspirin challenge in aspirin-sensitive asthmatic subjects. *Am Rev Respir Dis* 1991;143:1025–1029.

166. Christie PE, Smith CM, Lee TH. The potent and selective sulfidopeptide leukotriene antagonist, SK&F 104353, inhibits aspirin-induced asthma. *Am Rev Respir Dis* 1991;144:957–958.

167. Fischer AR, Rosenberg MA, Lilly CM, et al. Direct evidence for a role of the mast cell in the nasal response to aspirin in aspirin-sensitive asthma. *J Allergy Clin Immunol* 1994;94:1046–1056.

168. Marquardt DL, Walker LL, Wasserman SI. Adenosine receptors on mouse bone marrow-derived mast cells: functional significance and regulation by aminophylline. *J Immunol* 1984;133:932–937.

169. Polosa R, Ng WH, Crimi N, et al. Release of mast-cell-derived mediators after endobronchial adenosine challenge in asthma. *Am J Respir Crit Care Med* 1995;151:624–629.

170. Cypcar D, Lemanske RF. Asthma and exercise. *Clin Chest Med* 1994;15:351–368.

171. Broide DH, Eisman S, Ramsdell JW, Ferguson P, Schwartz LB, Wasserman SI. Airway levels of mast cell-derived mediators in exercise-induced asthma. *Am Rev Respir Dis* 1990;141:563–568.

172. Jarjour NN, Calhoun WJ, Stevens CA, Salisbury SM. Exercise-induced asthma is not associated with mast cell activation or airway inflammation. *J Allergy Clin Immunol* 1992;89:60–68.

173. Ellis JL, Undem BJ. Role of cysteinyl-leukotrienes and histamine in mediating intrinsic tone in isolated human bronchi. *Am J Respir Crit Care Med* 1994;149:118–122.

174. Undem BJ, Riccio MM, Weinreich D, Ellis JL, Myers AC. Neurophysiology of mast cell-nerve interactions in the airways. *Int Arch Allergy Immunol* 1995;107:199–201.

175. Church MK, Hiroi J. Inhibition of IgE-dependent histamine release from human dispersed lung mast cells by anti-allergic drugs and salbutamol. *Br J Pharmacol* 1987;90:421–429.

176. Undem BJ, Peachell PT, Lichtenstein LM. Isoproterenol-induced inhibition of immunoglobulin E-mediated release of histamine and arachidonic acid metabolites from the human lung mast cell. *J Pharmacol Exp Ther* 1988;247:209–217.

177. Ting S, Zweiman B, Lavker RM. Cromolyn does not modulate human allergic skin reactions *in vivo*. *J Allergy Clin Immunol* 1983;71:12–17.

178. Pearce FL, Al-Laith M, Bosman L, et al. Effects of sodium cromoglycate and nedocromil sodium on histamine secretion from mast cells from various locations. *Drugs* 1989;37(Suppl 1):37–43.

179. Enerbäck L, Bergström S. Effect of nedocromil sodium on the compound exocytosis of mast cells. *Drugs* 1989;37(Suppl 1):44–50.

180. Tainsh KR, Lau HY, Liu WL, Pearce FL. The human skin mast cell: a comparison with the human lung cell and a novel mast cell type, the uterine mast cell. *Agents Actions* 1991;33:16–19.

181. Okayama Y, Benyon RC, Rees PH, Lowman MA, Hillier K, Church MK. Inhibition profiles of sodium cromoglycate and nedocromil sodium on mediator release from mast cells of human skin, lung, tonsil, adenoid and intestine. *Clin Exp Allergy* 1992;22:401–409.

182. Pearce FL. Effect of nedocromil sodium on mediator release from mast cells. *J Allergy Clin Immunol* 1993;92(Suppl):155–158.

183. Okayama Y, Church MK. Comparison of the modulatory effect of ketotifen, sodium cromoglycate, procaterol and salbutamol in human skin, lung and tonsil mast cells. *Int Arch Allergy Appl Immunol* 1992;97:216–225.

184. Church MK, Holgate ST. Adenosine-induced bronchoconstriction and its inhibition by nedocromil sodium. *J Allergy Clin Immunol* 1993;92(Suppl):190–194.

Asthma, edited by P.J. Barnes, M.M. Grunstein, A.R. Leff, and A.J. Woolcock.
Lippincott–Raven Publishers, Philadelphia © 1997.

▪ 28 ▪

Basophils

John T. Schroeder and Lawrence M. Lichtenstein

Basophil Development	**Signal Transduction Mechanisms**
Cell Surface Markers	**Modulation of Histamine Release and Cytokine**
Inflammatory Mediators	**Secretion**
Basophil Releasability	**Basophils and Disease**
Basophil Cytokine Generation	

Chronic allergic inflammatory reactions, in particular the kind that characterize diseases such as asthma, involve the infiltration and participation of many different cell types. Although it has been evident for many years that tissue-specific mast cells have a primary role in the early stages of these reactions, in recent years much attention has focused on the events that often follow the activation of mast cells. Numerous studies now indicate that, in addition to the mast cell response, a later reaction, which includes the selective recruitment of circulating lymphocytes, eosinophils, and basophils to the site of inflammation, is a hallmark for the progression of allergic disease. In particular, the basophil seems quite suitable for fostering the development of these late responses, since this cell, like the mast cell, expresses high-affinity receptors for immunoglobulin (Ig) E antibody, which, upon cross-linking by specific antigen, results in the release of potent inflammatory mediators such as histamine and leukotrienes. This belief is further supported by the fact that basophils have been recently shown to secrete the immunoregulatory cytokine, IL-4, a protein that is known to have several important roles in allergic inflammation. It is therefore conceivable that the basophil, even though it represents the least common blood leukocyte (0.5% to 1.0% of the total population), may well help direct the immune responses of many different cells in a localized reaction site. This chapter briefly reviews some important aspects of the basophil response, with specific emphasis on more recent

findings concerning its development, the biochemical nature of its secretion of inflammatory mediators and cytokines, and its pathophysiology in allergic disease.

Much of our knowledge with respect to the biology of basophils is relatively recent, despite the fact that this cell was first described nearly 120 years ago by using basic dyes. By the 1950s, it first became apparent that basophils might represent a source of blood histamine, when it was found that this inflammatory mediator associated with fractions enriched with these granulocytes. Only after the identification of immunoglobulin (Ig)-E antibody in the early 1970s, by the Ishizakas and their colleagues (1), as the source of reaginic activity in serum, was it eventually shown that the allergic release of histamine in blood was located in basophils. This finding, and numerous others that followed, was an important first piece in assigning a function for basophils. The fact that IgE antibody bound to these cells suggested they were much like masts cells. As a result, basophils were seen as the circulating equivalent of the mast cell and, because they were readily available from blood in crude leukocyte suspensions, they soon became a surrogate with which to study mast cell function. Although this belief held for many years, the gradual accumulation of data, especially in recent years, now supports the concept that basophils are quite different then mast cells, play a greater role in the persistence of symptoms following an allergic response, and thus may contribute more to chronic inflammation. While much of this knowledge is, and continues to be, obtained from *in vitro* experiments, many studies have also shown the direct involvement of basophils at sites of experimentally induced inflammation as well as in natural disease.

J. T. Schroeder and L.M. Lichtenstein: Department of Medicine, Division of Clinical Immunology, The Johns Hopkins University School of Medicine, The Johns Hopkins Asthma and Allergy Center, Baltimore, Maryland 21224.

BASOPHIL DEVELOPMENT

Since many functional similarities exist between mature basophils and mast cells, and since, in healthy individuals, the latter are found only in tissue, an early belief developed suggesting that the basophil leukocyte might represent the circulating precursor of the tissue mast cell. This concept would imply that basophils infiltrating tissue receive some unknown signal that causes them to differentiate into mast cells. Although there is presently no evidence to disprove this hypothesis, a substantial amount of evidence suggests that these two cell types have distinct lineages. The average life span of basophils is a few days, with new cells being constantly replenished from a common pool of hematopoietic stem cells. In fact, this time course of basophil development more closely resembles that which is found for eosinophils than it does for mast cells, which are thought to have a turnover rate in tissue that is measured in months. Thus, *in vitro* cultures supplemented with supernatant derived from activated T lymphocytes showed that a common progenitor cell, colony-forming unit-eosinophil/basophil (CFU-Eo/B), is found in bone marrow, cord blood and, to a lesser extent, in peripheral blood, which can differentiate into mature basophils and eosinophils (2). Although it will become more relevant later in this chapter, it is important to note that elevated numbers of these CFU-Eo/B progenitors are found circulating in the peripheral blood during times of asthma exacerbation.

In recent years, with the help of molecular cloning techniques, a number of recombinant cytokines have been characterized that are important in the differentiation of many cell types. For basophil development, interleukin (IL)-3 or multi-CSF colony-stimulating factor (CSF) has been shown to have a profound effect in promoting the differentiation of progenitors into basophil-like cells that contain histamine, express high-affinity receptors for IgE, and resemble mature basophils both morphologically and functionally (3). However, the development of other leukocytes having a myeloid origin, including neutrophils, eosinophils, and monocytes, is also partially controlled by the actions of IL-3 and after 2 weeks in culture, a predominance of eosinophil cells are evident, with some cells taking on characteristics shared by both basophils and eosinophils. The latter differentiation is likely the result of IL-5, which appears to have an important role in the maturation of progenitors into eosinophils. Unlike the observation with respect to murine mast cells, IL-3 does not support the development of human mast cells in these cultures. It appears that the *c-kit* ligand, or stem cell factor, has a greater role in the development of mast cells from human CD34+ precursors, whereas IL-3 is important for basophil development from these same precursors (4). While, at this time, no other cytokine has been shown to have a role in basophil development, additional factors probably are needed for the generation of a stable, fully mature basophil. The cytokine, granulocyte-monocyte (GM)-CSF, which is an important granulocyte maturation cytokine, induces a disproportionate number of basophils after infusion, suggesting that it affects basophil development (5).

The KU812 cell line, derived from a patient suffering from chronic myelogenous leukemia, has been described as having a number of characteristics in common with immature basophils. Many of these cells express high-affinity receptors for IL-3 and have a tendency to differentiate more fully into basophillike cells, synthesizing and storing substantial amounts of histamine and capable of binding IgE with high affinity (6,7). Although there is some evidence that KU812 cells can differentiate into mature basophils, the conditions for this maturation have been poorly defined and the use of these cells as a substitute for investigating basophil physiology is questionable. It seems apparent that some clones, although capable of binding IgE, lack, or have a defective, β-subunit and are incapable of transmitting signals through the high-affinity receptor.

CELL SURFACE MARKERS

Basophils (and mast cells) are best known for their ability to bind IgE antibody with high affinity ($K_a > 10^{10}$) through the expression of receptors (FcεRI) found on the surface of these cells. It seems that this interaction is mediated solely through FcεRI, since the low-affinity receptor, FcεRII or CD23, as described on many other leukocytes, is not detected on basophils. Molecular cloning of the complementary deoxyribonucleic acid (cDNA) for FcεRI (8) has shown that this receptor has three subunits expressed in the membrane as $\alpha\beta\gamma_2$ with the α-subunit responsible for the binding of IgE antibody. Although FcεRI was once believed to be unique to basophils and mast cells, studies indicate that Langerhans' cells (9,10), monocytes (11), and possibly eosinophils (12) obtained from some allergic individuals also express this receptor and bind IgE antibody. However, the exact nature of the expression of FcεRI on these cells is presently unknown, since, like the KU812 cell line, the β-subunit, which is thought to have an important function in signal transduction, appears to be unexpressed. The expression of FcεRI on human basophils is highly variable among donors, ranging from 5,000 to 1,000,000 copies per cell, and is highly correlated with the serum IgE concentrations. There is some evidence that receptor expression is a function of occupancy, since studies using cell lines show that IgE-binding sites increase in the presence of IgE, indicating that the complex results in receptor stabilization (13). Since IgE binds with high affinity, almost all receptors are occupied when serum IgE levels are high. In fact, even with low IgE serum titers, occupancy remains at least 50%.

In addition to the high-affinity IgE receptor, basophils are also thought to express receptors that are capable of binding various subclasses of IgG antibody. In fact, polyclonal anti-IgG antibody has been reported to induce histamine secretion (14). However, the mechanism of release is based on the cross-linking of IgG-IgE complexes bound to the IgE receptor (15).

As a leukocyte, the basophil expresses a variety of other cell markers that function as receptors for ligands important in cell activation and adhesion. Unlike $Fc_\varepsilon RI$, many of these markers, such as HLA class I and the common leukocyte antigen, CD45, are shared with many other circulating white blood cells in addition to tissue mast cells. Basophils express a unique profile of determinants, however, that can be differentiated from most leukocytes. Many of these markers found on basophils have been detected by using dual flow cytometry. In this technique, basophils are specifically stained in leukocyte suspensions using an anti-IgE or anti-$Fc_\varepsilon RI$ antibody conjugated with a fluorescent probe (for example, fluoroscein isothiocyanate). The expression of additional markers can then be tested for by using antibodies labeled with a second fluorescent probe without concern for contaminating cells also expressing the same marker. This double-staining approach has enabled the detection of moderate levels of the adhesion molecules CD11a and b and CD18 on basophils (the CD11/CD18 complex is the α- and β-subunits that form lymphocyte function-associated antigen [LFA]-1 and membrane-attack complex [MAC]-1 adhesion molecules) in addition to very late activation antigen (VLA)-4 (CD49d/CD29) (16,17).

The selective infiltration of leukocytes into sites of allergic inflammation seems to be very much dependent on their expression of adhesion molecules that allow interaction with integrins found on vascular endothelium. In fact, recent attention has been directed at identifying the molecules expressed by many different cell types that are important in this process. As noted below, the basophil has been shown to participate in the late allergic reaction by coinfiltrating lesions along with lymphocytes and eosinophils. Therefore, these leukocytes are thought to begin migration by "rolling" along endothelium (likely a selectin-mediated process) and adhering to specific integrins. Leukocytes expressing the CD11/CD18 heterodimer are known to bind to sites having endothelial leukocyte adhesion molecules (ELAM) and intercellular adhesion molecules (ICAM). Indeed, this specific interaction seems to be an important adhesion mechanism for basophils, since cells pretreated with anti-CD18 antibody show decrease binding to cord-derived vascular endothelium (18).

With regard to activation markers (other than $Fc_\varepsilon RI$), basophils have been shown to express CD40, an antigen commonly found on B cells that has sequence homology with nerve growth factor receptor. Interestingly, recent evidence indicates that basophils also express a cell surface ligand for CD40 (CD40L), an antigen commonly found on activated T helper lymphocytes. It is important to note that the generation of IgE antibody by B cells very much depends on the costimulatory effects of IL-4 along with engagement of the CD40 antigen receptor by its ligand. As discussed below, basophils are quite efficient in secreting IL-4 protein. It has been shown, in fact, that the production of IgE *in vitro*, an event classically thought to be T cell mediated, is also possible by simply coculturing B cells with activated basophils, which, alone, can secrete IL-4 and express the CD40L (19). Whether this also occurs *in vivo* is difficult to say at this time. This finding, however, suggests that basophils have a role in the regulation of IgE synthesis.

Finally, it is important to note the recent characterization of a monoclonal antibody that appears immunologically specific for a granule-associated marker found in human basophils (20). Preliminary results show that it specifically detects a unique molecule, having a molecular weight of approximately 72 kDa, and that is released upon activation. Since this antibody does not appear to bind to mast cells or any other leukocytes, it should become a valuable tool for identifying the participation of basophils in site of allergic inflammation.

INFLAMMATORY MEDIATORS

Basophils secrete both preformed and newly synthesized mediators following activation with a wide range of stimuli. For many years, histamine and leukotriene (LT) C_4 have been studied extensively and have generally been thought to be the primary proinflammatory substances released by these cells. It has recently been shown, however, that basophils also generate and secrete high levels of IL-4, therefore making cytokines a new category to include as mediators released by these cells. It seems appropriate, however, especially in light of the immunoregulatory properties associated with IL-4, to separate cytokine production from this section and to deal with this subject below.

Histamine is synthesized from L-histidine by histidine decarboxylase and then stored in the cytoplasmic granules forming a complex with highly sulfated proteoglycans (mostly chrondroitin). It appears that both IL-3 and GM-CSF have an important role in the upregulation of this process during the latter stages of basophil maturation from progenitor cells (21). On release, histamine is a potent smooth muscle spasmogen that can also cause an increase in tissue fluid by dilating terminal arterioles and constricting postcapillary venules. It is important to note that histamine is also known to downregulate several T-cell-mediated immune responses by binding to H_2 receptors and causing elevations in intracellular cyclic adenosine monophosphate (cAMP). It seems likely that this inhibitory activity is directed at T-helper type 1 (TH1)-

like functions, particularly since basophils are increasingly thought to promote TH2-like responses through the secretion of cytokines (see below).

On activation by a variety of stimuli, basophils also synthesize and release LTC$_4$, which is generated from the metabolism of arachidonic acid. Several species of phospholipid, such as phosphatidylcholine and phosphatidylinositol, probably serve as the source of arachidonic acid. The phospholipids are cleaved directly by phospholipase A$_2$, or by the sequential action of phospholipase C and diglyceride lipase. A calcium-sensitive 5-lipoxygenase then metabolizes arachidonic acid into LTC$_4$ by glutathione transferase. The further metabolism of LTC$_4$ into LTD$_4$ and LTE$_4$ (formally referred to as slow-releasing substance of anaphylaxsis, SRS-A) does not occur in pure basophil suspensions, but apparently depends on the presence of other leukocytes. Unlike mast cells, there is little evidence for the release of prostaglandins in response to activation, suggesting that cyclooxygenase enzyme activity is not as common in basophils as is the lipoxygenase pathway.

Approximately 10 to 100 fg/basophil of LTC$_4$ is formed and released upon activation, some 100-fold less than the amount of histamine secreted by these cells (22). On a molar basis, however, LTC$_4$ is 100 to 6,000 times more potent in contracting smooth muscle. Prolonged wheal and flare reactions and mucus secretion are also stimulated, indicating that this mediator is likely a participant in the airway effects of an asthmatic attack. In other studies, leukotrienes are reported to affect the immune response of many cell types, acting as chemotactic factors in addition to promoting the production, or inhibition, of various cytokines.

BASOPHIL RELEASABILITY

The basophil is remarkably sensitive to a variety of stimuli. With respect to the cross-linking of IgE-receptor complexes with specific antigen, studies indicate that as few as 50 aggregated IgE molecules are sufficient to initiate a response (23). The formation of these aggregates seems necessary for the transmission of intracellular signals, since receptor occupancy with a single IgE molecule does not appear to generate signals resulting in secretion. As noted below, however, a receptor possessing a particular type of IgE (IgE+) might have a role in regulating the response of basophils to subsequent stimulation. In this instance, specific receptor orientations may have an important role in the generation of signals. With antigen challenge, the basophil response follows a classic bell-shaped curve over a wide range of concentrations, although the number of aggregates necessary to initiate the response appears to be far less than other antigen–antibody interactions, such as those required for the activation of B lymphocytes.

While antigen cross-linking has an important role in the basophil response, a growing list of diverse stimuli, many that are products of immune reactions, also have a profound ability to induce mediator release from these cells. It is important to note, however, that many of these same secretogogues have been shown to have little to no activity on mast cells, suggesting that the basophil is far more excitable in nature. The anaphylatoxins C5a and C3a and the bacterial peptide f-met-leu-phe (f-met peptide) were the first to show this dichotomy by inducing histamine release as univalent stimuli acting through mechanisms thought to be independent of IgE antibody (24,25). In recent years, platelet-activating factor (26,27) and the eosinophil product, major basic protein (MBP) (28), which are both known to be generated in allergic reactions, were also shown to induce histamine secretion directly from basophils. It is becoming increasingly apparent that a number of cytokines are also generated during allergic inflammatory reactions, especially in those associated with diseases such as asthma. As suspected, many of these proteins have been shown to affect the response of basophils by potentiating IgE-dependent histamine release (see below). A unique class of cytokines, the so-called histamine-releasing factors (HRFs), represent a class of proteins identified by their ability to induce histamine secretion directly from human basophils. Following their original description as soluble products found in the supernatants of mitogen- or antigen-stimulated peripheral blood mononuclear cells (PBMCs) (29), HRFs have since been recovered from cutaneous (30), bronchoalveolar (31), and nasal lavage fluids (32) during the late-phase reaction to antigen challenge. Furthermore, several different cell types are reported to generate HRF activity *in vitro*, including platelets (27,33,34), monocytes (35), B cells, and endothelial cells (36). Most of the HRFs reported thus far appear to induce histamine release independently of IgE expression and, in recent years, have been linked to a heterogeneous group of proteins, the chemokines, so named for their chemotactic activity on a number of cell types. Among the recombinant chemokines tested, monocyte chemotactic and activating factor (MCAF or MCP-1) and MCP-3 are reported to have potent activity on basophils, inducing histamine release at nanomolar concentrations (37). A second category of HRFs has been characterized based on the observation that the expression of a particular type of IgE (IgE+) is required in order for these proteins to induce histamine release from basophils. Only donors that synthesize this IgE+ have basophils responsive to the HRF. However, sensitization of nonresponsive basophils with serum containing IgE+ transfers responsiveness upon subsequent challenge with HRF. While the exact nature of IgE+ remains unknown at this time, atopic individuals appear to have increased levels of this immunoglobulin and its presence seems to correlate with disease severity (32). In fact, one study reported that children with food sensitivity and severe atopic dermatitis have PBMCs that generate an IgE-dependent HRF and have basophils that spontaneously secrete histamine. When the food was withdrawn, both activities subsided (38). Presumably, basophils migrating into reaction sites containing this HRF show enhanced releasability and, therefore, contribute to the severity of symptoms. Recently, cDNA clones have been subcloned and expressed that code for a 21-kDa protein in mice and a 23-kDa human equivalent, with the recombinant forms (rp21 and rp23, respectively) having the same IgE-dependent histamine-releasing activity as the previously described HRF found *in vivo* (39). Molecular characterization of recombinant material indicates that this HRF represents a novel cytokine, showing no homology with any known interleukin, chemokine, allergen, or antigen. Antibodies raised against recombinant protein also react with native HRF, providing strong evidence that the two are closely related and likely identical. As noted below, both rp21 and rp23 are reported to stimulate IL-4 secretion by basophils, suggesting that the IgE-dependent HRF plays a significant role in allergic inflammation by promoting mediator release as well as cytokine production.

A number of clinical investigations have confirmed many of the above *in vitro* studies, revealing striking correlations between the presence of diseases such as asthma and urticaria and the number of circulating basophils and their releasability to a number of diverse inflammatory products. There is evidence, in fact, for elevated numbers of circulating eosinophil/basophil progenitors in the blood and sputum of asthmatic patients during exacerbations of asthma, and there are decreases in these cells that correlate with resolution of symptoms following treatment with beclomethasone (40,41). Similar findings are observed for mature eosinophils and basophils, whose cell numbers correlate with airway responsiveness to antigen challenge. These increases appear to be selective for basophils and eosinophils, since there are no apparent elevations in the numbers of circulating progenitors for monocytes and neutrophils. Other studies show that the basophils isolated from asthmatics, while demonstrating releasability to a number of stimuli, also show increased spontaneous release of mediators. In the presence of deuterium oxide, this release of histamine is more pronounced, but not from subjects without asthma (42,43). There is evidence suggesting that the spontaneous release of histamine from basophils isolated from asthmatics also correlates with their baseline forced expiratory volume in one second (FEV$_1$) (44). Furthermore, chronic respiratory disease seems to correlate with enhanced IgE-dependent release of histamine from basophils. In comparing patients with either allergic rhinitis or bronchial asthma, the latter group showed significantly enhanced histamine release to specific antigen, and both of these groups had basophils having greater releasability to IgE-dependent stimulation than did cells isolated from normal

subjects. However, there is no significant correlation observed between basophil and skin mast cell sensitivity. Finally, a recent study indicates that the basophil is the only cell whose presence correlates with the hallmark of asthma, bronchial hypersensitivity, as measured by mecholyl challenge (45).

BASOPHIL CYTOKINE GENERATION

It is becoming increasingly apparent that the generation of cytokines is a common occurrence during many different immune reactions, particularly those associated with allergic inflammation (46,47). Many of these immunoregulatory proteins, in fact, are shown to have multiple functions by acting on the immune response of many different cell types. Therefore, it seems appropriate to state that cells found in allergic lesions, which secrete cytokines, have an important regulatory role in the development, progression, and outcome of the overall response. The concept that cells expressing high-affinity receptors for IgE might be capable of secreting cytokines stemmed from observations made in 1989 that IL-3-dependent murine mast cell lines generated cytokines following IgE-dependent activation (48,49). Most interesting was the observation that the cytokines generated by these mast cell lines closely resembled those made by activated TH2 lymphocytes originally described by Mosmann et al. (50) and included IL-4, IL-5, IL-6, and GM-CSF. In humans, there is now substantial evidence that basophils are, indeed, quite capable of generating IL-4 message and protein upon activation (51–54), and it is likely that these cells secrete additional cytokines important in allergic inflammation. In contrast, there is no evidence to suggest that human basophils express message or secrete protein for interferon γ (IFN-γ) and IL-2, consistent with the notion that only TH2-like cytokines are synthesized by these cells upon activation. Although one group has reported that human mast cells also secrete IL-4 (55), at this time it is difficult to say whether these cells have the same capability observed for basophils, since neither we nor any other laboratory has confirmed these findings. As noted below and elsewhere in this book, IL-4 has many regulatory roles important in the allergic response. The fact that a significant source of this cytokine may very well be derived from activated basophils underscores the significance these cells have in the pathogenesis of disease.

Unlike the release of histamine or LTC$_4$, which occurs upon degranulation or within minutes following stimulation, studies indicate that the generation of IL-4 protein by basophils occurs *de novo* upon activation, with little evidence for the storage of this protein in cytoplasmic granules. *In vitro* studies show that after IgE-dependent stimulation, IL-4 protein is first detectable only after 1 to 2 h, with levels peaking by 4 to 6 h (53,54). In these same cultures, however, histamine and LTC$_4$ are nearly completely released in just 15 to 20 min following activation. Furthermore, the addition of cycloheximide has no effect on the release of these mediators, but completely eliminates the secretion of IL-4, indicating that protein synthesis is required for the generation of this cytokine in basophils. Several other lines of evidence worth mentioning confirm the notion that IL-4 is not a preformed constituent of basophil granules. First, in the procedure referred to as sonication, by which cell membranes are broken using sound waves resulting in the release of cytoplasmic components, IL-4 protein is not detected even when using high concentrations of basophils to generate the sonicate. Secondly, there are basophil secretogogues that readily dissociate the release of histamine from the secretion of IL-4. For example, phorbol myristate acetate (PMA) is a potent degranulation stimulus for basophils, causing up to nearly 100% histamine release. Therefore, if IL-4 is stored in these granules, one would expect to measure this cytokine in the supernatants from cultures receiving this stimulus. As noted below, however, this compound does not result in IL-4 protein secretion by basophils and, in fact, actually inhibits the generation of IL-4 induced by other stimuli.

The emphasis on the ability of human basophils to generate IL-4 is demonstrated by experiments that indicate these cells are the sole source of IL-4 message and protein in mixed leukocyte cultures following IgE-dependent stimulation. In fact, this is also true during the early hours after stimulation with calcium ionophore, a stimulus known to activate many cell types. These data were obtained by using cultures in which the percentage of basophils was varied while the total cell number was kept constant. Both the presence of IL-4 protein and the expression of its messenger ribonucleic acid (mRNA) were strictly functions of the basophil purity, with no contribution by the contaminating cells (53). This finding has established the use of basophil-enriched suspensions (5% to 40%) to investigate several parameters of IgE-dependent IL-4 secretion (54). Unlike suspensions purified by using an extensive protocol of techniques that might affect their response, these preparations are easily obtained, with apparently little effect on the responsiveness of the basophils to various stimuli. In fact, with the availability of ultrasensitive enzyme-linked immunosorbent assay (ELISA) kits that detect protein levels of less than 1 pg/mL, it is now possible to measure the IL-4 protein secreted by the number of basophils found in approximately 1 mL of blood, or the same amount that is commonly used for histamine analysis. Studies using basophil-enriched suspensions have indicated that there is a correlation between the amount of IL-4 protein that is secreted and the magnitude of histamine released, with donors whose basophils show a high percentage of histamine release also secreting the highest levels of IL-4 protein (up to approximately 500 to 1,000 pg/10^6 basophils). Optimal levels of protein are secreted, however, in response to

concentrations of anti-IgE antibody (or antigen) that are 10-fold less than the amount necessary for optimal histamine release. As noted below, this observation, along with more recent findings, indicates that the intracellular mechanisms controlling histamine release and IL-4 secretion dissociate at some point after the formation of antigen-receptor complexes.

At this time, it seems that releasability to IgE-specific stimulation is the most important factor in the ability of basophils to secrete IL-4. In support of this belief are several observations made using enriched basophil suspensions. First, the IgE-independent secretogogues, f-met peptide and C5a, which are potent activators of basophil histamine release, show little to no ability to induce IL-4 secretion by basophils isolated from most donors. Secondly, there does not appear to be a difference between the amount of IL-4 protein generated by basophils obtained from allergic and nonallergic individuals when anti-IgE antibody (10 ng/mL) is used as the stimulus. As expected, however, specific antigen does trigger IL-4 protein secretion only by basophils from donors who are allergic and whose cells normally release histamine to the challenging allergen (54). Furthermore, there does appear to be evidence that basophils from allergics show slightly higher levels of spontaneous secretion of IL-4 protein. Finally, basophils from individuals releasing histamine to the IgE-dependent HRF also generate IL-4 with kinetics and protein levels essentially identical to those induced by anti-IgE antibody. In contrast, IgE-independent HRFs (for example, MCAF or MCP-1) do not appear to be potent activators of IL-4 production by basophils, inducing little to no protein secretion (56).

SIGNAL TRANSDUCTION MECHANISMS

During the past decade or so, cell biology has seen an explosion of studies focused on the mechanisms of signal transduction, or those events that occur within a cell following the binding of a ligand to its receptor. Much work has been done using rodent cell lines, including murine mast cells and the transformed rat basophilic leukemia cell, but this is of uncertain relevance to human cells. As noted earlier, both the KU812 and HMC-1 cell lines, which are characterized as human basophils and mast cells, respectively, are not working models for the study of IgE-mediated secretion mechanisms, because of their expression of nonfunctional receptors. Likewise, studies investigating the signals generated in basophils induced by the univalent stimuli (C5a and f-met peptide) have also relied heavily on other cell models (i.e., neutrophils). It is becoming increasingly possible, however, to conduct work using pure suspensions of basophils derived from blood. As a result, this section focuses primarily on the aspects of signal transduction found in human cells, with some reference made to rodent models.

Although the signals generated in different secretory cells are likely to differ from one another in specific details, there are some basic features worth generalizing. In many instances, an enzyme such as phospholipase C is converted into an active form, following the coupling of a receptor with its ligand. In basophils, this activation is believed to occur via a tyrosine kinase, resulting from receptor aggregation (for example, IgE cross-bridging), or via a guanosine triphosphate (GTP)-binding protein, which is associated with the binding of a univalent agonist (that is, C5a or f-met peptide). Both pathways result in the metabolism of phospholipid upon the activation of specific phospholipase C enzymes. With the hydrolysis of phospholipids, two important messengers are formed that relay the signal further. First, the formation of diacylglycerol is an important regulator of protein kinase C activity. Secondly, triphosphates (such as the those derived from phosphatidylinositol metabolism) seem to act on intracellular stores of calcium, causing the release of this ion into the cytosol. Increased free calcium is likely involved in the activation of calcium/calmodulin kinases that, in concert with protein kinase C, probably phosphorylate many proteins involved in secretion. It is important to note that, for the human basophil response, these signals are thought to be relatively early in the response, with little detail known of the steps beyond this point.

Although basophils generate nearly identical amounts of histamine and LTC_4 in response to either univalent or cross-linking stimuli, there are differences in the secretory mechanisms induced by these two categories of stimulation. With regard to histamine, the data clearly show that the rate of release is considerably faster with univalent stimulation. For example, release induced by f-met peptide is nearly complete by 2 min, whereas the time required for maximal release induced by an optimal concentration of anti-IgE antibody is some 5- to 10-fold greater. Both stimuli induce the metabolism of arachidonic acid, causing similar leukotriene release, with no evidence for prostaglandin generation (57). Once again, however, the rates of release are faster for f-met peptide stimulation.

As noted above, the receptor for the f-met peptide is coupled to a GTP-binding protein effector enzyme (for example, phospholipase C). The pertussis toxin (from *Bordetella pertussis*) is known to uncouple this signal transduction pathway through ADP-ribosylation of the GTP-binding proteins involved in this mechanism. As might be expected, the pertussis toxin completely inhibits basophil release induced by f-met peptide, but has no effect on the release induced by anti-IgE antibody (58). While this does not imply that IgE-mediated release functions in the absence of GTP-binding protein, it does suggest that f-met peptide uses a different protein for coupling.

There seems to be an even greater difference in the secretory mechanisms controlling the generation of cytokine in basophils compared with those important for histamine release. In fact, studies show that univalent stimuli (f-met peptide and C5a) are inconsistent activators of IL-4 secretion, compared with the signals delivered in response to cross-linking stimuli (anti-IgE antibody) (54,59). Furthermore, a body of evidence suggests that the intracellular mechanisms controlling both mediator release and cytokine secretion also differ in response to cross-linking stimuli alone. At concentrations that are suboptimal for histamine release, anti-IgE antibody (or antigen) is more potent than f-met peptide when compared with the induction of IL-4 secretion. This finding can be partially explained by evidence showing that IL-4 generation depends on elevated cytosolic calcium responses. First, studies using human basophil cultures show that calcium ionophores (for example, ionomycin and A23187) are extremely potent activators of IL-4 protein secretion. Second, studies show that the cytosolic calcium responses induced by C5a and f-met peptide are short-lived in basophils relative to those initiated by IgE-dependent stimulation. In fact, supraoptimal anti-IgE antibody also induces a briefer calcium response than does suboptimal anti-IgE (60–62). As noted earlier, basophils secrete a greater amount of IL-4 protein when challenged with suboptimal concentrations of anti-IgE antibody (or antigen). Therefore, although mediator release and cytokine secretion both require changes in cytosolic calcium, it is apparent that the latter response very much depends on stimuli that induce prolonged elevated calcium changes.

As might be expected, protein kinase (PK) C activity plays an important, yet complicated, role in the signal transduction mechanisms regulating mediator release from human basophils. In fact, several compounds that modulate PKC activity are shown to have quite opposite effects on the release induced by univalent and cross-linking stimuli. For example, the relatively specific PKC inhibitor, staurosporin, is an extremely potent inhibitor of IgE-mediated release while enhancing both the histamine and LTC_4 release that follows f-met peptide stimulation (63). With the recognition in recent years that several tyrosine kinases are involved in the early and late IgE-mediated signaling (64,65), results of experiments using staurosporin are less clear, since this compound also inhibits tyrosine kinase activity. More recently, however, several PKC inhibitors were described that inhibit specific isozymes of PKC. Two such compounds, bisindolylmaleimide II and Ro-31-8220 (both analogues of staurosporin), which are thought to inhibit PKC activity selectively, were shown to enhance anti-IgE-induced release of histamine while having modest inhibitory effect on mediator release induced by f-met peptide. In contrast, a third PKC inhibitor, Go-6976, blocks anti-IgE-mediated histamine release and is thought to inhibit the calcium-dependent PKC isozymes (α and β_1). From this analysis, along with other bits of information, including direct measurements of PKC activity, it seems that both f-met peptide and IgE-mediated release use PKC activation in both a pro- and anti-degranulatory mode.

The generation of cytokines by human basophils also appears to be modulated by PKC activity, with most of the evidence at this time clearly showing an antisecretory role (66). For example, PMA, a potent activator of PKC activity, does not induce the secretion of IL-4 protein from basophils, despite causing up to nearly 100% histamine release. This dissociation alone suggests that basophils utilize different intracellular mechanisms for the release of preformed mediators compared with those involved in cytokine secretion. More striking, however, is the observation that PMA downregulates the secretion of protein from basophils induced by calcium ionophore, this effect being completely reversed with the simultaneous addition of PKC inhibitors, either staurosporin or bisindolylmaleimide. These findings are quite surprising, since calcium influx and activation of PKC are implicated in many types of secretory function. In fact, these signals seem necessary for the expression of IL-4 mRNA and the secretion of protein by peripheral blood lymphocytes costimulated with PMA and ionophore. It is important to note that PMA also blocks IL-4 protein secretion from basophils activated with anti-IgE antibody. In this instance, however, the cytosolic calcium responses that are necessary for cytokine generation are completely ablated, unlike those that occur during stimulation with calcium ionophore. Finally, it is known that IgE-dependent mediator release uses signals involving the activation of PKC. Therefore, it seems likely that a kinase activity associated with the release of histamine may actually have a negative effect on cytokine generation. In support of this hypothesis, the secretion of IL-4 from basophils stimulated with anti-IgE antibody is actually enhanced with the addition of either bisindolylmaleimide or Ro-31-8220, suggesting that these inhibitors block a PKC isozyme having antisecretory activity for cytokine generation (J. T. Schroeder, unpublished data). It is not known at this time whether specific enzymes are necessary for cytokine secretion verses mediator release.

Studies show that elevations in cytosolic calcium highly correlate with basophil secretion. This seems particularly true for IL-4 production, but is not absolute with respect to histamine release. There is little evidence, however, that the magnitude of the response is linked to the expression density of IgE antibody found on the surface of these cells. In fact, a wide range of responses occurs in basophils isolated from different donors, with the number of IgE cross-links necessary for secretion varying some 10,000-fold. Basophils derived from some donors actually fail to release histamine in response to IgE-mediated stimuli, despite having sufficient levels of IgE antibody on their cell surface and showing normal responses when challenged with f-met peptide (61). Therefore, it seems that those stimuli capable of causing changes in cytosolic calcium in basophils are most able to induce mediator re-

lease. In fact, the duration and magnitude of this calcium response appear to be of even greater importance for the generation of IL-4 in basophils. In recent years, a considerable amount of attention has focused on the signals that occur prior to the calcium response. Many of these findings have relied on the use of rodent cell lines, such as the rat basophilic leukemia cell, to explore the nature of these signals. A monoclonal antibody directed at a cell surface protein determinant (and not FcεRI) has been shown to inhibit the release of histamine in these cells by disrupting the normal signals generated during IgE-mediated activation. As noted above, several studies have shown that tyrosine kinases are activated upon receptor aggregation and are important for both the early and late stages of degranulation. Other investigators have isolated a protein important for the movement of calcium from the extracellular space to the cytosol. Finally, as shown with f-met peptide activation, there is some evidence for the participation of a GTP-binding protein in IgE-mediated activation. All of these proteins might have a role in IgE-dependent mediator release from basophils, and variation in the expression of these proteins might explain the wide range of responses observed among different donors.

MODULATION OF HISTAMINE RELEASE AND CYTOKINE SECRETION

Basophil mediator release is also modulated by the expression of receptors that bind agents that either upregulate or downregulate the response. Increases in intracellular cAMP, or interaction with the glucocorticoid receptor, inhibit basophil histamine release. In contrast, basophils also express high-affinity receptors for a number of cytokines and chemokines that, upon binding, augment release to several secretogogues. More recent studies show that cytokine generation by basophils is also modulated through these receptors, but somewhat differently than the secretion of histamine.

In 1968, it was found that methylxanthines, which cause increases in intracellular cAMP by blocking phosphodiesterases, inhibit the release of histamine from leukocyte suspensions (67). Since many other secretion mechanisms had been shown to depend on increased levels of cAMP, this finding in basophils was novel and suggested the therapeutic use of a number of compounds for the treatment of allergic inflammation. The synthesis of cAMP occurs following the activation of adenylate cyclase. In basophils, this enzyme is coupled to receptors for prostaglandin E_2, those for β-agonists such as epinephrine, and those for histamine. The H_2 receptor for histamine appears to participate in a negative-feedback mechanism for regulating the basophil response. In fact, the IgE-dependent release of histamine is significantly increased from basophils if an H_2 antagonist is added along with stimulus (68), suggesting that histamine itself may inhibit further release. Direct measurements show that compounds that cause a sustained increase in the levels of cAMP have a greater inhibitory effect, with the formation of LTC_4 being more sensitive to inhibition than histamine release. Only IgE-dependent mechanisms appear to be inhibited by increased cAMP; mediator release induced by f-met peptide and C5a, for the most part, is unaffected (69,70). However, release induced by these secretogogues is slightly inhibited by cholera toxin, which causes very large increases in cAMP. As expected, agonists of cAMP are most effective in causing inhibition when in vitro mediator release is low, whereas relatively high concentrations are required to block additional release. In some tissues, only a small percent of total mediator release is thought to result in a large physiologic response (71), and this finding is likely the reason drugs like theophylline are more efficacious at low concentrations in vivo as compared with in vitro.

At this time, the glucocorticoids are the most potent compounds used in the management of allergic inflammation and in chronic diseases such as asthma. Although much of their effectiveness is believed to result from the inhibition of leukocyte recruitment and in the production of cytokines, glucocorticoids also block the IgE-dependent release of histamine and leukotrienes (72). Recent evidence shows that IL-4 protein secretion induced by anti-IgE antibody is also inhibited by steroids (J. T. Schroeder, unpublished data). It is important to note, however, that these compounds appear to have no effect on the mediator release induced by the univalent stimuli f-met peptide or C5a. Cortisone inhibits mediator release at concentrations in the range of 1 to 100 nM, yet, as would be expected for the steroid/receptor process, requires some 8 h to take effect, with maximal inhibition occurring after 18 h of preincubation. The sex steroids show no inhibition and, of the glucocorticoids tested, dexamethasone seems most inhibitory, with a rank ordering following their potency found in other test systems. Interestingly, a marked inhibition (about 20% to 70%) in IL-4 protein secretion is observed with as little as 1 h of pretreatment, indicating that the mechanisms controlling cytokine generation in basophils are more sensitive to glucocorticoids than are those regulating mediator release. Although steroids serve as antagonists for basophil IgE-mediated responses, both in vitro and in vivo studies show that mast cell mediator release is unaffected by these compounds. Therefore, the fact that steroids are so effective in controlling allergic inflammation may result, in part, from the ability to inhibit a multitude of basophil responses, including their recruitment (73), their secretion of histamine and IL-4 protein, and the production of cytokines by other leukocytes that upregulate the basophil response (74) (see below).

Many different cytokines, chemokines, and growth factors have been shown to modulate the IgE-mediated responses of basophils. Unlike the compounds described above, however, the coupling of receptors with these modulating factors appears, for the most part, to upregulate basophil responses. Several interleukins (including IL-1 and IL-3 and, variably, IL-5) can potentiate the antigen- or anti-IgE-driven release of histamine and/or LTC_4 from basophils (75–79). Of these, however, IL-3 is by far the most potent, with concentrations of 1 to 10 pM increasing histamine release 50% to 300% and causing increases in leukotriene release up to 100-fold (greater enhancement of leukotriene release occurs in donor basophils whose release is normally low) (76,80–82). In addition, the mediator release induced by IgE-independent stimuli is also enhanced by IL-3. For example, the release of LTC_4 is negligible with C5a stimulation, but quantities similar to those induced by f-met peptide occur with IL-3 pretreatment (81,83). There is recent evidence showing that IL-3 receptors are densely expressed on human basophils (84), perhaps accounting for its potent modulating effects. Indeed, much of the response to IL-3 occurs within 10 min of exposure, although there are clear effects that occur only with additional pretreatment. For example, in addition to maintaining basophil viability in culture, long-term pretreatment with IL-3 has the unique effect of reversing the inhibition of mediator release (and IL-4 secretion) caused by glucocorticoids (76). In contrast, the decreased response of basophils pretreated with dexamethasone is not reversed by a short exposure to IL-3. Basophils isolated from some donors release histamine in response to high concentrations of IL-3 alone (82). It appears that under these circumstances a low level of stimulation exists that the treatment with IL-3 reveals, and this may be an example of excitation by receptor occupancy without cross-linking. Indeed, IL-3-induced release is slow and bears no resemblance to activation by most other stimuli.

IL-4 secretion by basophils is similarly enhanced by pretreatment with IL-3. If pretreated for 18 h with IL-3, highly purified basophils secrete nearly 10-fold greater amounts of IL-4 upon IgE-mediated activation (53). Unlike LTC_4 release, however, IL-3 does not seem to enhance dramatically the secretion of IL-4 upon stimulation with C5a or f-met peptide (59), which, as mentioned above, are poor stimuli for cytokine release from basophils. Again, this supports the notion that IgE-mediated activation is of primary importance in the generation of IL-4 by basophils. Basophil suspensions that are prepared rapidly from whole blood also show enhancement (30% to 150%) of IL-4 secretion following a brief exposure to IL-3 (54). For reasons that are not fully understood, however, cells prepared in this manner and pretreated with IL-3 for periods longer than 15 min loose the ability to secrete IL-4 upon activation, despite retaining the ability to release histamine. It is likely that a contaminating cell fraction is responsible for downregulating IL-4 secretion in these cultures, either via cell–cell contact, by the release of a soluble inhibitor, or by some other mechanism.

There is some evidence that this inhibition is partially attributable to the presence of monocytes and possible IL-8 production (J. T. Schroeder, unpublished data), but these results are preliminary. It is not presently known what effects cytokines other than IL-3 have on the secretion of IL-4 by basophils.

The physiologic and pathophysiologic consequences of the multiple forms of basophil modulation are difficult to predict. Clearly, there are many competing influences on basophil function. If basophils are recruited to a site of allergic inflammation because mast cells have responded to antigenic challenge, then the basophils will experience high levels of prostaglandin D_2 and have their response enhanced. However, the histamine in the environment and that released by the basophil itself serves to inhibit its response. Locally generated cytokines could also significantly upregulate the basophil response while systemic glucocorticoids shut off cytokine production and further downregulate the basophil response. There have simply been too few careful studies of basophil function in tissues to appreciate the bottom line of such complex interactions. In the balance, though, the inflammatory response appears to generate more upregulators of the basophil response, and it is only through therapeutic intervention that some of these agents are brought under control.

BASOPHILS AND DISEASE

Recent studies have demonstrated the appearance of basophils in tissues following a local allergic reaction, and there is evidence that basophils increase dramatically in the airways of patients who die of severe asthma, accumulating in numbers similar to those of mast cells (85). Further, additional biopsy specimens taken from asthmatic individuals reveal a correlation between basophil number and the severity of the asthmatic symptoms (86). Although these observations strongly implicate the participation of basophils in allergic lesions, the exact nature of their role in allergic disease is not fully understood.

Studies of the clinically relevant late-phase reaction to antigen challenge best support the involvement of basophils in chronic allergic inflammation. Although the cellular infiltrates during these late reactions show a predominance of eosinophils, the early work by Okuda and Ohtsuka (87) clearly showed that basophils also migrate into the nasal mucosa. In fact, the nose of rhinitic patients provides a convenient test site for the experimental *in vivo* challenge model of the allergic late reaction. For both control and atopic patients, saline solution can be instilled into the nasal lumen and the fluid recovered after a suitable holding period of 10 s. The returned fluid contains measurable mediators of the allergic reaction and cells that have migrated into the nasal lumen by way of the nasal mucosa (88,89). The relative ease with which consistent data can be obtained with this model has meant that many therapeutic experimental maneuvers can be tested. Challenge of atopic patients with the appropriate antigen leads to the rapid appearance of mediators such as histamine, prostaglandin (PG) D_2, LTC_4, and a set of enzymes capable of generating kinins together with the usual symptoms of the allergic reaction, such as sneezing and nasal congestion. In approximately 50% of the patients, this initial response was found to subside within an hour only to return 5 to 12 h later. Both symptoms and mediators would return with the notable exception of PGD_2. This mediator would reappear only after a second antigen challenge. As discussed above, mast cells but not basophils release PGD_2 in an IgE-mediated reaction, and it was concluded that basophils contributed to the late reaction. Furthermore, a number of techniques, such as electron microscopy and flow cytometry, have confirmed that the Alcian blue-positive cells infiltrating these late reactions are not mast cells, but basophils. Also, sufficient numbers of these cells have been collected and show functional characteristics consistent with basophils, including histamine content (0.78 pg/cell) and sensitivity to both anti-IgE (0.1 mg/mL) and f-met peptide identical to peripheral blood basophils (90). If patients have been administered oral or a short course of topical steroids prior to experimental challenge, the early reaction (mast cell response) is not significantly altered, but the late phase (basophil response) is nearly stopped (73,91).

This experimental approach to studying the *in vivo* allergic reaction has been replicated in the skin and lung (92,93). For the skin studies, a blister is made and the epidermis removed and replaced with a chamber into which allergens and other substances can be instilled and fluids removed. In lung studies, a segment of the airway is isolated by wedging a bronchoscope in the lumen of a third-generation bronchus. Again, substances can be instilled and fluids removed for study. In both skin and lung studies, many of the features of the reaction observed in the nose have been replicated, including the appearance of basophils in the late reaction.

There is mounting evidence to suggest that the late reaction is characteristic of conditions in the lung tissue of asthmatic patients and thus to suggest that basophils play an important role in the pathogenesis of asthma as well as other allergic reactions. This belief may gain further support now that basophils have recently been shown to secrete large quantities of the immunoregulatory cytokine, IL-4, which, along with IL-5, have been found in late-phase reactions (47) and are implicated in the pathogenesis of allergic inflammation, including that associated with asthma. In fact, the kinetics of IL-4 secretion by basophils (protein levels peaking by 4 to 6 h following activation) are consistent with the time that these cells first appear in tissue sites during the late-phase response to antigen. Since this IL-4 release is considerably faster than the 12 to 16 h reported for the production of this cytokine by antigen-stimulated T lymphocytes (94), basophils may have a more significant role in initiating the late-phase reaction. Thus, the synthesis of IgE and IgG4 antibodies from human PBMCs, which depends on the costimulatory effects of IL-4 (95), suggests that basophil-derived cytokine may have a role in this production. The adherence and selective transmigration of eosinophils are partially controlled by the actions of IL-4 on endothelium (17,96); thus the accumulation of these cells at sites of allergic inflammation may also depend on basophil activation. Finally, a number of studies have shown that the development of TH2 and TH1 CD4+ lymphocytes is regulated by the actions of IL-4 and interferon γ on naive cells, respectively (97). Thus, basophil-derived IL-4 may upregulate the development of TH2 lymphocytes, because there is a predominance of activated cells of this phenotype at sites of allergic inflammation. Therefore, it is possible that the secretion of IL-4 (and likely other cytokines such as IL-13) from basophils might help to amplify and maintain allergic inflammatory reactions, leading to chronic conditions such as asthma.

Numerous studies have also demonstrated that basophils participate in reactions previously viewed as expressions of cellular immunity. Richerson (97a), using a guinea-pig model, first described a specific type of delayed hypersensitivity of this type, cutaneous basophil hypersensitivity, to differentiate these responses from longer delayed reactions that are predominantly lymphocytic. The Dvoraks and colleagues (98,99) have since shown that these cutaneous basophil hypersensitivity reactions also occur in humans. For example, basophils can be found in significant numbers in allergic contact dermatitis reactions. Other reactions normally associated with cellular immunity, skin allograft and tumor rejection, viral hypersensitivity, and Crohn's disease, also show an infiltrate containing a high percentage of basophils (100–102). The best described *in vivo* model of this reaction, the delayed contact skin hypersensitivity to dinitrochlorobenzene in humans, demonstrates that basophils are often the only granulocyte to infiltrate the skin during the first 3 days of the reaction (103). It is not until later that some eosinophils and neutrophils appear. In the 1970s, the Dvoraks also demonstrated that basophils secrete their granules in a piecemeal fashion in these lymphocyte-mediated reactions, a release reaction that may occur over a period of days rather than minutes (104). It has been difficult to understand the mechanism of basophil infiltration occurring in these reactions and to ascertain whether basophils play an important role. However, it has been noted that the complex rejection of schistosomes, helminthic worms, and ectoparasitic arthropods may depend on the presence of basophils. Tick rejection in guinea pigs is eliminated if the animals are first treated with a specific antibasophil antibody that leads to the specific ablation of bone marrow, peripheral blood, and infiltrating basophils (105). These data may indicate that late-phase allergic reactions result from the unfortunate expression of a response that nature has developed to combat parasitic infections. The data also indicate that basophils play a broad role in the general immune response.

CONCLUSIONS

The role of the basophil in chronic allergic inflammation has intensified in recent years with substantial evidence showing that these cells, along with eosinophils and lymphocytes, infiltrate late-phase reaction sites. These findings are supported by additional studies showing the accumulation of these cells in the airways of individuals dying from severe asthmatic reactions. The participation of basophils in allergic lesions is thought to involve the release of potent inflammatory mediators and, more recently, their secretion of proinflammatory cytokines like IL-4, which could potentially influence the functions of many different cells. The fact that basophils also demonstrate an enhanced releasability to a variety of stimuli, both related and unrelated to antigen cross-linking, further suggests that these cells are quite suitable for fostering the development allergic disease.

ACKNOWLEDGMENTS

This work was supported by grant AI07290, NIAID, NIH. J.T.S. was supported in part by a fellowship award from the American Lung Association of Maryland.

REFERENCES

1. Ishizaka T, De Bernardo R, Tomioka H, Lichtenstein LM, Ishizaka K. Identification of basophil granulocytes as a site of allergic histamine release. *J Immunol* 1972;108:1000–1008.
2. Denburg JA, Messner H, Lim B, Jamal N, Telizyn S, Bienenstock J. Clonal origin of human basophil/mast cells from circulating multipotent hemopoietic progenitors. *Exp Hematol* 1985;13:185–188.
3. Saito H, Hatake K, Dvorak AM, et al. Selective differentiation and proliferation of hematopoietic cells induced by recombinant human interleukins. *Proc Natl Acad Sci USA* 1988;85:2288–2292.
4. Kirshenbaum A, Goff J, Kessler S, Mican J, Zsebo K, Metcalfe D. Effect of IL-3 and stem cell factor on the appearance of human basophils and mast cells from CD34+ pluripotent progenitor cells. *J Immunol* 1992;148:772–777.
5. Donahue RE, Seehra J, Metzger M. IL-3 and GM-CSF act synergistically in stimulating hematopoiesis in primates. *Science* 1988;241:1820–1823.
6. Fukuda T, Kishi K, Ohnishi Y, Shibata A. Bipotential cell differentiation of KU812: evidence of a hybrid cell line that differentiates into basophils and macrophagelike cells. *Blood* 1987;70:612–619.
7. Valent P, Besemer J, Kishi K, et al. IL-3 promotes basophilic differentiation of Ku812 cells through high affinity binding sites. *J Immunol* 1990;145:1885–1889.
8. Kinet JP, Blank U, Ra C, White K, Metzger H, Kochan J. Isolation and characterization of cDNAs coding for the beta subunit of the high-affinity receptor for immunoglobulin E. *Proc Natl Acad Sci USA* 1988;85:6483–6487.
9. Wang B, Rieger A, Kilgus O, et al. Epidermal Langerhans cells from normal human skin bind monomeric IgE via FcεRI. *J Exp Med* 1992;175:1353–1365.

10. Bieber T, de la Salle H, Wollenberg A, et al. Human epidermal Langerhans cells express the high affinity receptor for immunoglobulin E (FcₑRI). *J Exp Med* 1992;175:1285–1290.

11. Maurer D, Fiebiger E, Reininger B, et al. Expression of Functional high affinity immunoglobulin E receptors (FcₑRI) on monocytes of atopic individuals. *J Exp Med* 1994;179:745–750.

12. Gounni A, Lamkhioued B, Ochiai K, et al. High-affinity IgE receptor on eosinophils is involved in defence against parasites. *Nature* 1994; 367:183–186.

13. Malveaux FJ, Conroy MC, Adkinson NF Jr, Lichtenstein LM. IgE receptors on human basophils: relationship to serum IgE concentration. *J Clin Invest* 1978;62:176–181.

14. Grant JA, Lichtenstein LM. Reversed *in vitro* anaphylaxis induced by anti-IgG: specificity of the reaction and comparison with antigen-induced histamine release. *J Immunol* 1972;109:20–25.

15. Lichtenstein LM, Kagey-Sobotka A, White JM, Hamilton RG. Anti-human IgG causes histamine release by acting on IgG-IgE complexes bound to IgE receptors. *J Immunol* 1992;148:3929–3936.

16. Bochner BS, McKelvey AA, Schleimer RP, Hildreth JE, MacGlashan DW Jr. Flow cytometric methods for the analysis of human basophil surface antigens and viability. *J Immunol Methods* 1989;125:265–271.

17. Schleimer RP, Sterbinsky SA, Kaiser J, et al. IL-4 induces adherence of human eosinophils and basophils but not neutrophils to endothelium. *J Immunol* 1992;148:1086–1092.

18. Bochner BS, MacGlashan DW Jr, Marcotte GV, Schleimer RP. IgE-dependent regulation of human basophil adherence to vascular endothelium. *J Immunol* 1989;142:3180–3186.

19. Gauchat J-F, Henchoz S, Mazzel G, et al. Induction of human IgE synthesis in B cells by mast cells and basophils. *Nature* 1993;365:340.

20. Kepley C, Craig S, Schwartz B. Identification and partial characterization of a unique marker for human basophils. *J Immunol* 1995;154:6548–6555.

21. Schneider E, Pollard H, Lepault F, Guy GD, Minkowski M, Dy M. Histamine-producing cell-stimulating activity: interleukin 3 and granulocyte–macrophage colony-stimulating factor induce *de novo* synthesis of histidine decarboxylase in hemopoietic progenitor cells. *J Immunol* 1987;139:3710–3717.

22. MacGlashan DW Jr, Peters SP, Warner J, Lichtenstein LM. Characteristics of human basophil sulfidopeptide leukotriene release: releasability defined as the ability of the basophil to respond to dimeric cross-links. *J Immunol* 1986;136:2231–2239.

23. MacGlashan DW Jr, Lichtenstein LM. Studies of antigen binding on human basophils. I. Antigen binding and functional consequences. *J Immunol* 1983;130:2330–2336.

24. Siraganian RP, Hook WA. Complement-induced histamine release from human basophils. II. Mechanism of the histamine release reaction. *J Immunol* 1976;116:639–646.

25. Siraganian RP, Hook WA. Mechanism of histamine release by formyl methionine-containing peptides. *J Immunol* 1977;119:2078–2083.

26. Okuda Y, Tsuyuguchi I, Yamatodani A. Histamine release from human leukocytes by platelet-activating factor. *Int Arch Appl Immunol* 1988; 85:341–344.

27. Columbo M, Casolaro V, Warner JA, MacGlashan DW Jr, Kagey-Sobotka A, Lichtenstein LM. The mechanism of mediator release from human basophils induced by platelet-activating factor. *J Immunol* 1990;145:3855–3861.

28. Thomas LL, Zheutlin LM, Gleich GJ. Pharmacological control of human basophil histamine release stimulated by eosinophil granule major basic protein. *Immunology* 1989;66:611–615.

29. Grant JA, Alam R, Lett-Brown MA. Histamine-releasing factors and inhibitors: historical perspectives and possible implications in human illness. *J Allergy Clin Immunol* 1991;88:683–693.

30. Warner JA, Pienkowski MM, Plaut M, Norman PS, Lichtenstein LM. Identification of histamine releasing factor(s) in the late phase of cutaneous IgE-mediated reactions. *J Immunol* 1986;136:2583–2587.

31. Liu MC, Proud D, Lichtenstein LM, et al. Human lung macrophage-derived histamine-releasing activity is due to IgE-dependent factors. *J Immunol* 1986;136:2588–2595.

32. MacDonald SM, Lichtenstein LM, Proud D, et al. Studies of IgE-dependent histamine releasing factors: heterogeneity of IgE. *J Immunol* 1987;139:506–512.

33. Brindley L, Sweet J, Goetzl E. Stimulation of histamine-release from human basophils by human platelet factor 4. *J Clin Invest* 1983;72: 1218–1223.

34. Orchard MA, Kagey SA, Proud D, Lichtenstein LM. Basophil histamine release induced by a substance from stimulated human platelets. *J Immunol* 1986;136:2240–2244.

35. Kaplan A, Haak-Frendscho M, Fauci A, Dinarello C, Halbert E. A histamine-releasing factor from activated human mononuclear cells. *J Immunol* 1985;135:2027–2032.

36. Alam R, Forsythe P, Lett-Brown M, Grant J. Cellular origin of histamine-releasing factor by peripheral blood mononuclear cells. *J Immunol* 1989;142:3951–3956.

37. Dahinden CA, Geiser T, Brunner T, et al. Monocyte chemotactic protein 3 is the most effective basophil and eosinophil-activating chemokine. *J Exp Med* 1994;179:751–756.

38. Sampson HA, Broadbent KR, Bernhisel-Broadbent J. Spontaneous release of histamine from basophils and histamine-releasing factor in patients with atopic dermatitis and food hypersensitivity. *N Engl J Med* 1989;321:228–232.

39. MacDonald S, Rafner T, Langdon J, Lichtenstein L. Molecular identification of an IgE-dependent histamine-releasing factor. *Science* 1995;269:688–690.

40. Pin I, Gibson P, Kolendowicz R, et al. Use of induced sputum cell counts to investigate airway inflammation in asthma. *Thorax* 1992;47: 25–29.

41. Gibson PG, Dolovich J, Girgis-Gabardo A, et al. The inflammatory response in asthma exacerbation: changes in circulating eosinophils, basophils, and their progenitors. *Clin Exp Allergy* 1990;20:661–668.

42. Findlay SR, Lichtenstein LM. Basophil "releasability" in patients with asthma. *Am Rev Respir Dis* 1980;122:53–59.

43. Tung R, Lichtenstein LM. *In vitro* histamine release from basophils of asthmatic and atopic individuals in D₂O. *J Immunol* 1982;128: 2067–2072.

44. Guydon L, Kagey-Sobotka A, Lichtenstein L, et al. Relationships between peripheral blood basophil releasability and lung physiology following antigen challenge in asthma. *Am J Respir Crit Care Med* 1994;149:A962(abstract).

45. Sparrow D, O'Connor G, Rosner B, Weiss S. Predictors of longitudinal change in methacholine airway responsiveness among middle-aged and older men: the normative aging study. *Am J Respir Crit Care Med* 1993;149:919.

46. Walker C, Bode E, Boer L, Hansel TT, Virchow JC Jr. Allergic and nonallergic asthmatics have distinct patterns of T-cell activation and cytokine production in peripheral blood and bronchoalveolar lavage. *Am Rev Respir Dis* 1992;146:109–115.

47. Kay AB, Ying S, Varney V, et al. Messenger RNA expression of the cytokine gene cluster, interleukin-3 (IL-3), IL-4, IL-5, and granulocyte/macrophage colony-stimulating factor, in allergen-induced late-phase cutaneous reactions in atopic subjects. *J Exp Med* 1991;173: 775–778.

48. Plaut M, Pierce JH, Watson CJ, Hanley HJ, Nordan RP, Paul WE. Mast cell lines produce lymphokines in response to cross-linkage of Fc epsilon RI or to calcium ionophores. *Nature* 1989;339:64–67.

49. Wodnar-Filipowicz A, Heusser CH, Moroni C. Production of the haemopoietic growth factors GM-CSF and interleukin-3 by mast cells in response to IgE receptor-mediated activation. *Nature* 1989;339:150.

50. Mosmann TR, Cherwinski H, Bond MW, Giedlin MA, Coffman RL. Two types of murine helper T-cell clones. I. Definition according to profiles of lymphokine activities and secreted protein. *J Immunol* 1986;136:2348–2357.

51. Brunner T, Heusser CH, Dahinden CA. Human peripheral blood basophils primed by interleukin-3 (IL-3) produce IL-4 in response to immunoglobulin E receptor stimulation. *J Exp Med* 1993;177:605–611.

52. Arock M, Merle-Beral H, Dugas B, et al. IL-4 release by human leukemic and activated normal basophils. *J Immunol* 1993;151: 1441–1447.

53. MacGlashan DW Jr, White JM, Huang SK, Ono SJ, Schroeder J, Lichtenstein LM. Secretion of interleukin-4 from human basophils: the relationship between IL-4 mRNA and protein in resting and stimulated basophils. *J Immunol* 1994;152:3006–3016.

54. Schroeder JT, MacGlashan DW Jr, Kagey-Sobotka A, White JM, Lichtenstein LM. The IgE-dependent IL-4 secretion by human basophils: the relationship between cytokine production and histamine release in mixed leukocyte cultures. *J Immunol* 1994;153:1808.

55. Bradding P, Feather IH, Howarth PH, et al. Interleukin 4 is localized to and released by human mast cells. *J Exp Med* 1992;176:1381–1386.

56. Schroeder JT, Lichtenstein LM, MacDonald SM. An IgE-dependent

recombinant histamine releasing factor induces IL-4 secretion from human basophils. *J Exp Med* 1996; 183:1265–1270.

57. Warner JA, Peters SP, Lichtenstein LM, et al. Differential release of mediators from human basophils: differences in arachidonic acid metabolism following activation by unrelated stimuli. *J Leukoc Biol* 1989;45:558–571.

58. Warner JA, Yancey KB, MacGlashan DW Jr. The effect of pertussis toxin on mediator release from human basophils. *J Immunol* 1987;139:161–165.

59. Schroeder JT, MacGlashan DW Jr, Kagey-Sobotka A, White JM, Lichtenstein LM. Cytokine generation by human basophils. *J Allergy Clin Immunol* 1994;94:1189–1195.

60. Warner JA, MacGlashan DW Jr. Protein kinase C (PKC) changes in human basophils: IgE-mediated activation is accompanied by an increase in total PKC activity. *J Immunol* 1989;142:1669–1677.

61. Nguyen KL, Gillis S, MacGlashan DW Jr. A comparative study of releasing and nonreleasing human basophils: nonreleasing basophils lack an early component of the signal transduction pathway that follows IgE cross-linking. *J Allergy Clin Immunol* 1990;85:1020–1029.

62. MacGlashan DW Jr, Guo CB. Oscillations in free cytosolic calcium during IgE-mediated stimulation distinguish human basophils from human mast cells. *J Immunol* 1991;147:2259–2269.

63. Warner JA, MacGlashan DW Jr. Signal transduction events in human basophils: a comparative study of the role of protein kinase-C in basophils activated by anti-IgE antibody and formyl-methionyl-leucyl-phenylalanine. *J Immunol* 1990;145:1897–1905.

64. Benhamou M, Stephan V, Robbins KC, Siraganian RP. High-affinity IgE receptor-mediated stimulation of rat basophilic leukemia (RBL-2H3) cells induces early and late protein–tyrosine phosphorylations. *J Biol Chem* 1992;267:7310–7314.

65. Beaven MA, Metzger H. Signal transduction by Fc receptors: the FcεRI case. *Immunol Today* 1993;14:222.

66. Schroeder JT, Lichtenstein L, Kagey-Sobotka A, MacGlashan DW Jr. Differential control of basophil histamine and IL-4 secretion with PKC activation. *J Allergy Clin Immunol* 1995;95:344.

67. Lichtenstein LM, Margolis S. Histamine release *in vitro*: inhibition by catecholamines and methylxanthines. *Science* 1968;161:902–903.

68. Tung R, Kagey SA, Plaut M, Lichtenstein LM. H₂ antihistamines augment antigen-induced histamine release from human basophils *in vitro*. *J Immunol* 1982;129:2113–2115.

69. Peachell PT, MacGlashan DW Jr, Lichtenstein LM, Schleimer RP. Regulation of human basophil and lung mast cell function by cyclic adenosine monophosphate. *J Immunol* 1988;140:571–579.

70. Warner JA, MacGlashan DW Jr, Peters SP, Kagey SA, Lichtenstein LM. The pharmacologic modulation of mediator release from human basophils. *J Allergy Clin Immunol* 1988;82:432–438.

71. Tung RS, Lichtenstein LM. Cyclic AMP agonist inhibition increases at low levels of histamine release from human basophils. *J Pharmacol Exp Ther* 1981;218:642–646.

72. Schleimer RP, Lichtenstein LM, Gillespie E. Inhibition of basophil histamine release by anti-inflammatory steroids. *Nature* 1981;292:454–455.

73. Bascom R, Wachs M, Naclerio RM, Pipkorn U, Galli SJ, Lichtenstein LM. Basophil influx occurs after nasal antigen challenge: effects of topical corticosteroid pretreatment. *J Allergy Clin Immunol* 1988;81:580–589.

74. Massey WA, Kato M, Bochner BS, et al. Inhibition of late phase reaction area, inflammatory cell appearance, and local cytokine production by topical steroid treatment in cutaneous model of allergic inflammation. 1994, *submitted*.

75. Ida S, Hooks JJ, Siraganian RP, Notkins AL. Enhancement of IgE-mediated histamine release from human basophils by viruses: role of interferon. *J Exp Med* 1977;145:892–906.

76. Schleimer RP, Derse CP, Friedman B, et al. Regulation of human basophil mediator release by cytokines. I. Interaction with antiinflammatory steroids. *J Immunol* 1989;143:1310–1317.

77. Subramanian N, Bray MA. IL-1 releases histamine from human basophils and mast cells *in vitro*. *J Immunol* 1987;138:271–275.

78. Massey WA, Randall TC, Kagey SA, et al. Recombinant human IL-1 alpha and -1 beta potentiate IgE-mediated histamine release from human basophils. *J Immunol* 1989;143:1875–1880.

79. Alam R, Welter JB, Forsythe PA, Lett-Brown MA, Grant JA. Comparative effect of recombinant IL-1, -2, -3, -4, and -6, IFN-γ, granu-locyte–macrophage-colony-stimulating factor, tumor necrosis factor-α, and histamine-releasing factor on the secretion of histamine from basophils. *J Immunol* 1989;142:3431–3435.

80. Hirai K, Morita Y, Misaki Y, et al. Modulation of human basophil histamine release by hematopoietic growth factors. *J Immunol* 1988;141:3957–3961.

81. Kurimoto Y, de Weck AL, Dahinden CA. Interleukin 3-dependent mediator release in basophils triggered by C5a. *J Exp Med* 1989;170:467–479.

82. MacDonald SM, Schleimer RP, Kagey SA, Gillis S, Lichtenstein LM. Recombinant IL-3 induces histamine release from human basophils. *J Immunol* 1989;142:3527–3532.

83. MacGlashan DW Jr, Warner JA. Stimulus-dependent leukotriene release from human basophils: a comparative study of C5a and Fmet-leu-phe. *J Leukoc Biol* 1991;49:29–40.

84. Sarmiento EU, Espiritu BR, Gleich GJ, Thomas LC. IL-3, IL-5, and granulocyte-macrophage colony-stimulating factor potentiate basophil mediator release stimulated by eosinophil granule major basic protein. *J Immunol* 1995;155:2211–2221.

85. Koshino T, Teshima S, Fukushima N, et al. Identification of basophils by immunohistochemistry in the airways of postmortem cases of fatal asthma. *Clin Exp Allergy* 1993;23:919–925.

86. Koshino T, Aria Y, Miyamoto Y, et al. Mast cell and basophil number in the airway correlate with the bronchial responsiveness of asthmatics. *Int Arch Allergy Immunol* 1995;107:378–379.

87. Okuda M, Ohtsuka H. Basophilic cells in allergic nasal secretions. *Arch Otorhinolaryngol* 1977;214:283–289.

88. Naclerio RM, Meier HL, Kagey-Sobotka A, et al. Mediator release after nasal airway challenge with allergen. *Am Rev Respir Dis* 1983;128:597–602.

89. Pipkorn U, Proud D, Lichtenstein LM, Kagey-Sobotka A, Norman PS, Naclerio RM. Inhibition of mediator release in allergic rhinitis by pretreatment with topical glucocorticoids. *N Engl J Med* 1987;316:1506–1510.

90. Guo C-B, Liu MC, Galli SJ, Bochner BS, Kagey-Sobotka A, Lichtenstein LM. Identification of IgE-bearing cells in the late phase response to antigen in the lung as basophils. *Am J Respir Cell Mol Biol* 1993;10:384–390.

91. Bascom R, Pipkorn U, Lichtenstein LM, Naclerio RM. The influx of inflammatory cells into nasal washings during the late response to antigen challenge. *Am Rev Respir Dis* 1988;138:406–412.

92. Charlesworth EN, Hood AF, Soter NA, Kagey-Sobotka A, Norman PS, Lichtenstein LM. Cutaneous late-phase response to allergen: mediator release and inflammatory cell infiltration. *J Clin Invest* 1989;83:1519–1526.

93. Liu MC, Hubbard WC, Proud D, et al. Immediate and late inflammatory responses to ragweed antigen challenge of the peripheral airways in allergic asthmatics: cellular, mediator, and permeability changes. *Am Rev Respir Dis* 1991;144:51–58.

94. Gagnon R, Akoum A, Hebert J. Lol p I-induced IL-4 and IFN-γ production by peripheral blood mononuclear cells of atopic and nonatopic subjects during and out of the pollen season. *J Allergy Clin Immunol* 1993;91:950.

95. Vercelli D, Geha RS. Regulation of IgE synthesis in humans: a tale of two signals. *J Allergy Clin Immunol* 1991;88:285–295.

96. Moser R, Fehr J. IL-4 controls the selective endothelium-driven transmigration of eosinophils from allergic individuals. *J Immunol* 1992;149:1432–1438.

97. Romagnani S. Human TH1 and TH2 subsets: doubt no more. *Immunol Today* 1991;12:256–257.

97a. Richerson HB, Dvorak HF, Leskowitz S. Cutaneous basophilic hypersensitivity: a new interpretation of the Jones-Mote reaction. *J Immunol* 1969;103:1431.

98. Dvorak HF, Dvorak AM, Simpson BA, Richerson HB, Leskowitz S, Karnovsky MJ. Cutaneous basophil hypersensitivity. II. A light and electron microscopic description. *J Exp Med* 1970;132:558.

99. Goldman MA, Simpson BA, Dvorak HF. Histamine and basophils in delayed-type hypersensitivity reactions. *J Immunol* 1973;110:1511–1517.

100. Dvorak HF. Role of basophil leukocytes in allograft reactions. *J Immunol* 1971;106:279.

101. Dvorak HF, Hirsh MS. Role of basophil leukocytes in cellular immunity to vaccinia virus infections. *J Immunol* 1971;107:1576.

102. Dvorak AM, Monahan RA. Crohn's disease: ultrastructural studies showing basophil leukocyte granule changes and lymphocyte parallel

tubular arrays in peripheral blood. *Arch Pathol Lab Med* 1982;106: 145.

103. Dvorak HF, Mihm MC Jr, Dvorak AM, et al. Morphology of delayed type hypersensitivity reactions in man. I. Quantitative description of the inflammatory response. *Lab Invest* 1974;31:111–130.

104. Dvorak AM, Mihm MC Jr, Dvorak HF. Degranulation of basophilic leukocytes in allergic contact dermatitis reactions in man. *J Immunol* 1976;116:687–694.

105. Brown SJ, Galli SJ, Gleich GJ, Askenase PW. Ablation of immunity to *Amblyomma americanum* by anti-basophil serum: co-operation between basophils and eosinophils in expression of immunity to ectoparasites (ticks) in guinea pigs. *J Immunol* 1982;129:790.380

Asthma, edited by P.J. Barnes, M.M. Grunstein, A.R. Leff, and A.J. Woolcock.
Lippincott–Raven Publishers, Philadelphia © 1997.

▪ 29 ▪

Macrophages

Galen B. Toews

Macrophages are ubiquitous cells that are distributed throughout most tissues. Macrophages play important roles in a) recognition of autologous and foreign materials, b) generation and regulation of inflammation, c) initiation of immune responses, and d) repair of injured tissues. Macrophages in the bone marrow, circulation, and tissues are often referred to as the mononuclear phagocyte system. Although these cells share a common origin and have a similar morphology, macrophages in different tissues have distinctive functional properties.

ORIGIN AND DISTRIBUTION

Macrophages originate from a common bone marrow progenitor cell for both granulocytes and monocytes/

G. B. Toews: Department of Internal Medicine, University of Michigan Medical Center, Ann Arbor, Michigan 48109-0360.

macrophages (1,2). Monocyte production is regulated by specific colony-stimulating factors that bind to progenitor cells by specific receptors. Interleukin-3 (IL-3), granulocyte macrophage colony-stimulating factor (GM-CSF), and macrophage colony-stimulating factor (M-CSF) all stimulate a sequence of differentiation steps important in monocyte development (3,5). M-CSF is the only macrophage-specific colony-stimulating factor. Monocytopoiesis is also affected by interleukin-1 (IL-1) and tumor necrosis factor (TNF)-α, which promote the release of M-CSF and GM-CSF and enhance the response of precursor cells to M-CSF and GM-CSF (6,7). The release of these cytokines during acute inflammatory responses regulate the increased cellular response found in bone marrow. Cytokines released during the inflammatory response also inhibit monocyte responses. Inhibitory cytokines include macrophage inflammatory protein 1 (MIP-1) and transforming growth factor beta (TGF-β) (8,9).

The bone marrow transit time from the first monocytic precursor to a mature monocyte is approximately 6 days (10). After differentiation in the bone marrow, monocytes enter the peripheral blood; circulating human monocytes have a half-life of approximately 3 days (11). Monocytes are also found in a marginating compartment, which may contain 60% to 70% of the total monocytes at any given time (12).

ALVEOLAR MACROPHAGES

Alveolar macrophages (AM) are derived from blood monocytes and from proliferating macrophage precursors in the interstitium of the lung. Studies of patients undergoing bone marrow or lung transplants have demonstrated that the AM population is maintained largely by movement of blood monocytes into the lung. The lifespan of AMs is months and perhaps years (13,14). Approximately 1% of the AM population in the normal lung is proliferating at any single time (15). Migration of monocytes into the lung appears to be a random phenomenon in the absence of localized inflammation. The cytokines, receptors, and ligands that modulate monocyte traffic to the normal lung have not been defined.

MACROPHAGE FUNCTIONS

Macrophages possess four critical functional attributes that allow them to accomplish a broad group of bi-ological tasks: macrophages a) recognize stimuli from the microenvironment; b) ingest particulates and debris; c) secrete large numbers of molecules, and d) migrate in response to various stimuli. Macrophages integrate these four functional capabilities to perform complex cellular functions.

RECOGNITION OF SIGNALS/INGESTION

Macrophages constantly sample their microenvironment. Macrophages ingest soluble and particulate materials by absorptive endocytosis or pinocytosis. Most endocytosed particles are taken up in clathrin-coated vesicles.

The ability of macrophages to interact with environmental agents is enhanced by surface receptors capable of binding specific ligands including immunoglobulins, cytokines, lipids, and hormones (Table 1) (16–20). Macrophages respond to these receptor ligand interactions in two ways: a) the macrophage may internalize the ligand (phagocytosis) and process and digest the ligand; and b) macrophages secrete bioactive molecules after receptor ligand interactions (Table 2). These two responses are crucial to macrophage participation in inflammatory and immune responses.

Macrophages express surface receptors that bind to the Fc fragment of immunoglobulin or to various complement proteins. These receptors that promote the uptake of antibody-coated particles are the most comprehensively studied macrophage receptors (21–23).

TABLE 1. *Molecules that bind to macrophage membranes*

Immunoglobulins	IFN-$\alpha\beta$	α_1-Antithrombin
IgG$_1$	IFN-γ	α_2-Macroglobulin-protease complexes
IgG$_2$	**Lipid mediators**	Ceruloplasmin
IgG$_3$	Leukotriene C	Coagulation factor VIIa
IgG$_4$	Leukotriene D$_4$	Fibrin
IgE	Leukotriene B$_4$	Fibrinogen products
IgA	Prostaglandin E$_2$	Fibronectin
Complement fragments	Platelet activating factor	Lactoferrin
C1q	**Adhesion molecules**	Laminin
C3b	LFA-1 (integrin αLβ_2)	Transferrin
C3bi	MAC-1 (integrin αMβ_2)	**Small molecules**
C3d	p150/95 (integrin αXβ_2)	Adenosine
C5a	ICAM-1	Bombesin
Growth factors and cytokines	GPIV (binds to thrombospondin)	Bradykinin
M-CSF	**Hormones and proteins**	Histamine (H$_1$ and H$_2$ receptors)
GM-CSF	Calcitonin	N-Formylated peptides
MCP-1	Dexamethasone	Serotonin
MIP-1α	1,25-Dihydroxyvitamin D$_3$	Substance P
MIP-1β	Epinephrine	Tuftsin
RANTES	Estrogen	Vasoactive intestinal peptide
TNF-α	Glucagon	**Pharmacologic agents**
Il-1	Glucocorticosteroids	Muscarinic and nicotinic
Il-2	Insulin	Cholinergic agonists
Il-3	Parathormone	α_1/α_2-Adrenergic agonists
Il-4	Progesterone	β_1/β_2-Adrenergic agonists
IL-6	α_1-Antiprotease-protease complexes	

TABLE 2. *Secretory products of macrophages*

Cytokines and growth factors	Growth factors	Elastase
Cytokines that promote acute inflammation and regulate lymphocytes	GM-GSF	Hyaluronidase
TNF-α	M-CSF	Lipoprotein lipase
IL-1α/β	G-CSF	Lysozyme
IL-6	Erythropoietin	Nucleases
IL-8	Factors that promote tissue repair	Phospholipase A$_2$
IL-12	Platelet-derived growth factor	Plasminogen activator
GROα/B/γ	(PDGF)	Ribonucleases
CTAPIII	Fibroblast growth factor (FGF)	Sulfatases
β Thromboglobulin	Angiogenesis factor	**Inhibitors of Enzymes**
IP-10	**Lipids**	α$_1$ Antichymotrypsin
MCP-1	PGE$_2$	α$_1$-Antiprotease
MIP-1α	PGF$_{2α}$	α$_2$-Macroglobulin
MIP-1β	Prostacylin	Inhibitors of plasminogen
Proteins involved in host defense and inflammation	Thromboxane A$_2$	Inhibitors of plasminogen activator
C$_1$	Leukotrienes B, C, D, and E	Lipomodulin
C$_4$	Mono-HETES	**Matrix proteins**
C$_2$	Di-HETES	Chondroitin sulfate proteoglycans
C$_3$	PAF	Fibronectin
C$_5$	Lysophospholipids	Gelatin-binding protein
Factor B	**Reactive oxygen intermediates**	Thrombospondin
Factor D	O$_2^-$	**Coagulation factors**
Properdin	H$_2$O$_2$	Factor X
C$_3$b inactivation	OH•	Factor IX
βIH	**Reactive nitrogen intermediates**	Factor V
Lysozyme	NO•	Thromboplastin
Interferon-γ	NO$_2$	Prothrombin
Fibronectin	NO$_3$	Thrombospondin
Lactoferrin	**Enzymes that affect conective tissues and serum proteins**	Tissue factor
Cytokines that inhibit acute inflammation and lymphocyte responses	Acid hydrolases	Factor VII/VIIA
	Acid phosphatases	Factor X activator
	Amyloid proteinase	Prothrombinase
IL-10	Amylase	**Small molecules**
TGFβ	B-Galactosidase	Purines
IL-1 receptor antagonist	B-Glucuronidase	Pyrimidines
	Cathepsins	Glutathione
	Collagenases (types I, II, III, and IV)	Thymidine
	Cytolytic proteinase	Uracil
		cAMP

Fcγ Receptors

There are three receptors that recognize the Fc domain of immunoglobulin G: FcγRI, FcγRII, and FcγRIII (24,25). The FcγRs are membrane glycoproteins that contain two to three extracellular domains with immunoglobulinlike features. FcγRI is expressed on both monocytes and macrophages. (26) Three genes for FcγRI have been identified in humans (27). Unstimulated human monocytes express 10,000 to 40,000 molecules of FcγRI on their surface; interferon-γ and complement component C5a upregulate expression of this molecule (28,29). FcγRI is a high-affinity receptor that binds both monomeric and polymeric immunoglobulin G (IgG) with high affinity. Engagement of this receptor mediates phagocytosis and superoxide and TNFα production (30). FcγRII is expressed on monocytes, macrophages, neutrophils, and eosinophils (31). Three distinct genes encoding at least six different transcripts have been identi-

fied in humans (32). AMs express approximately 260,000 FcγRII receptors; these receptors bind IgG with relatively low affinity (33). FcγRII mediates phagocytosis and superoxide and TNF-α secretion (34,35). FcγRIII is expressed by macrophages (but not monocytes), neutrophils, and eosinophils (25). FcγRIII is expressed as a transmembrane protein in macrophages and as a phosphatidyl inositol glycan-linked (GPI-linked) protein in neutrophils (36,37). Surface expression of the transmembrane form of FcγRIII depends on the co-expression of the gamma subunit of the high-affinity IgE receptor (38). The gamma subunit plays an essential role in signaling by FcγRIII. FcγRIII is remarkably homologous to FcεRI, the high-affinity IgE receptor. FcγRIII mediates phagocytosis in macrophages (34).

A low-affinity receptor for IgE (FcεRII, CD23) is present on monocytes, macrophages, and eosinophils (39). Although this 45-kDa protein is not present on resting AMs, it is expressed on the surface of AMs isolated from patients with hypersensitivity pneumonitis (40). The isoform expressed on monocytes and eosinophils (Fc$_\varepsilon$RIIb), but not the isoform expressed on B cells (Fc$_\varepsilon$RIIa), is capable of mediating phagocytosis but it is difficult to ascribe other functions to this receptor (41). Other physiologic responses observed after binding of IgE immune complexes to macrophages, such as secretion of arachidonic acid metabolites, may represent activation of receptors other than CD23. IgE immune complexes are known to bind to Fc$_\gamma$RII and Fc$_\gamma$RIII (42,43).

SECRETORY FUNCTION

Macrophages secrete more than 100 molecules (16,19,44–50). Most macrophage-secreted molecules are released after macrophage receptor ligand interactions and/or activation of macrophages. The biologic effects of these secreted molecules varies from the induction of cellular proliferation and differentiation to the induction of cell death. Several categories of macrophage secretory products are likely important in the pathogenesis of asthma (see Table 2). Macrophages secrete cytokines that promote or mediate the acute inflammatory response as well as the early proliferative response of lymphocytes. These cytokines include IL-1, TNF-α, IL-6, C-C, and C-X-C chemokines and IL-12 (51–54). Macrophages also release cytokines that inhibit inflammation. These cytokines include IL-10, TGF-β, and IL-1 receptor antagonists (55–57). Finally, macrophages release growth factors that enhance inflammatory cell proliferation, enhance inflammatory cell survival, induce growth of fibroblasts, and induce new vessel formation (47). These include GM-CSF, platelet-derived growth factor (PDGF), fibroblast growth factors (FGF), insulinlike growth factor 1 (IGF-1), and certain chemokines.

CYTOKINES THAT PROMOTE ACUTE INFLAMMATORY RESPONSES AND EARLY LYMPHOCYTE RESPONSES

Interleukin-1

Two distinct genes located on chromosome 2 encode for IL-1α and IL-1β proteins, respectively (58,59). IL-1 is rapidly synthesized by monocytes and macrophages when stimulated by microbial products or inflammatory agents (60). Endogenous agents that induce IL-1 production include C$_{5a}$ M-CSF, TNF-α, TGF-β, and IL-1 (61). Because of the lack of a leader peptide, IL-1α remains in the cytosol or membranes of cells. Surface-bound IL-1α is biologically active. In contrast to IL-1α, IL-1β is a secreted protein. The IL-1β precursor requires cleavage by an enzyme known as IL-1β-converting enzyme for optimal biologic activity (62,63).

A fundamental property of IL-1 is its ability to induce a wide variety of genes. IL-1 receptors are present on many cell types, including lymphocytes, hepatocytes, endothelial cells, fibroblasts, and neutrophils (64–66). In most instances, IL-1 induces new transcripts (chemokines), but IL-1 also stabilizes and prolongs mRNA half-life (GM-CSF). IL-1's effects on lymphocytes include augmentation of T-cell proliferation and B-cell activation in response to antigens (67). TH1 cells lack IL-1 receptors and therefore do not respond (67,68). TH2 clones produce most cytokines in response to T-cell receptor (TCR) cross-linking without IL-1, but require IL-1 to proliferate (69). Endothelial cells express new adherence molecules in response to IL-1 and change permeability characteristics (70,71). IL-1 induces fibroblast proliferation and induces fibroblast collagen and PGE$_2$ release (72,73). Neutrophils exposed to IL-1 produce increased levels of oxidants. Macrophages respond to IL-1 by increasing synthesis of IL-1, IL-6, IL-8, TNF-α, prostaglandins, procoagulants, and plasminogen activator. Antigen-presenting cells in general respond to IL-1 with a striking increase in their ability to induce T-cell proliferation (74, 75). Increased production of IL-1 has been noted in asthmatic airways (76).

Tumor Necrosis Factor-α

The gene for human tumor necrosis factor-α (TNF-α) is located on chromosome 6 within the MHC complex in humans and mice (77–80). Macrophages are believed to be the principal source of TNF-α production *in vivo* (81,82). An abridged listing of naturally occurring substances that induce TNF-α production includes lipopolysaccharide (LPS), TNF-α, IL-1, IL-2, GM-CSF, antibodies that mediate Fc receptor cross-linking, and products of complement activation (83).

TNF-α is also a potent inducer of cytokine production. Endothelial cells respond to TNF-α by expressing more ICAM-1, VCAM-1, and ELAM-1 (84). Neutrophils react to TNF-α with an increased binding to endothelial cells, respiratory burst, and degranulation (84–86). TNF-α has multiple stimulatory activities on activated T cells, including increasing the proliferative response to antigen and increasing IL-2 receptor expression and the response to IL-2 as a proliferative signal (87,88). TNF-α also induces IFN-γ production. Fibroblasts respond to TNF-α with increased PGE synthesis and collagenase release (89). TNF-α induces gene expression for numerous macrophage-produced cytokines. Cytokines induced by TNF-α include IL-1, IL-6, IL-8, IFN-γ, GM-CSF, TGF-β, PDGF, MCP-1, RANTES, and MIP-1a/b (90,91).

Increased expression of TNF-α is present in asthmatic airways (92). IgE induces increased expression of TNF-α in sensitized rat and human lungs (93,94). Allergen challenge induces TNF-α release from AMs of asthmatic patients (95). IgE triggering induces increased gene expression for TNF-α in both blood monocytes and AMs (96).

Interleukin-6

The gene for human interleukin-6 (IL-6) maps to chromosome 7 (97,98). IL-6 is produced by macrophages and many other different cell types after activation. A variety of peptide factors such as IL-1, TNF-α, IL-2, IFN-β, and PDGF induce IL-6 production in macrophages. In contrast, IL-4 and IL-13 inhibit IL-6 production in monocytes (99).

IL-6 exerts a number of important biologic effects on the immune response. An essential role has been demonstrated for IL-6 in IL-4-dependent IgE synthesis. Anti-IL-6 antibody inhibits IL-4-driven IgE production, suggesting that endogenous IL-6 plays an obligatory role in IL-4-dependent production of IgE (100). IL-6 enhances the proliferative response of thymocytes to IL-4 (101). IL-6 synergizes with GM-CSF and M-CSF in the stimulation of CFU-M, which increases both the number and size of macrophage colonies (102,103).

AMs from asthmatic patients release increased amounts of IL-6 after antigen challenge and demonstrate increased basal release when compared with nonasthmatic individuals (95). IgE stimulates secretion of IL-6 in both monocytes and AMs (96).

Macrophage Inflammatory Protein-1α

Macrophage inflammatory protein-1α (MIP-1α) is produced predominantly by leukocytes. Monocytes, macrophages, neutrophils, eosinophils, and T cells are all important cellular sources of MIP-1α (104,105). MIP-1α is expressed in activated CD4 TH1 and CD8 T-cell lines at high levels and at lower levels in CD4 TH2 cell lines (106–108). MIP-1α also can be produced by nonleukocytic cells such as pulmonary fibroblasts and epithelial cells (109). Both microbial products and cytokines induce MIP-1α production by leukocytes; LPS, IFN-γ, and IL-1 induce MIP-1α production in macrophages. Inhibitors of MIP-1α production include PGE and IL-4 (110–112).

MIP-1 is chemotactic for monocyte/macrophages, lymphocytes, basophils, and eosinophils (113–118). MIP-α stimulates phagocytic cells to produce hydrogen peroxide and release lysosomal enzymes. MIP-1α induces fibroblasts, basophils, mast cells, and macrophages to produce IL-1, IL-6, and TNF-α (119–121).

Monocyte Chemotactic Protein-1

Monocyte chemotactic protein-1 (MCP-1) is produced by almost all cells or tissues. Monocytes, en-

dothelial cells, smooth muscle cells, fibroblasts, epithelial cells, AMs, and PMN all produce MCP-1 (122–128). LPS, IL-1, TNF-α, IFN-γ, and IL-4 stimulate MCP-1 production in endothelial cells. Stimuli for MCP-1 production in fibroblasts include IL-1, TNF-α, and PDGF. IL-1 and TNF-α induce MCP-1 production by nasal, bronchial, and type II epithelial cells. MCP-1 is chemotactic for monocytes/macrophages, lymphocytes, and basophils (117,118,122,124,129). MCP-1 expression is increased in the lungs of asthmatics.

RANTES

The acronym Regulated on Activation, Normal T-Expressed and Secreted has been ascribed to RANTES, but the protein was named after a character in a science fiction film. RANTES is an 8-kDa protein produced by endothelial cells, macrophages, T cells, epithelial cells, and fibroblasts. RANTES is constitutively produced by cultured primary human bronchial epithelial cells and by human pulmonary type II epithelial cell lines (A549) after stimulation with TNF-α or IL-1β (130,131). TNF-α and IFN-γ stimulate RANTES mRNA and protein in human bronchial epithelial cell lines (BEAS-2B) (132). IFN-γ, IL-1β, and TNF-α alone cannot induce RANTES expression by endothelial cells, but the combination of TNF-α and IFN-γ induces RANTES expression (133). RANTES is chemotactic in vitro for monocytes, eosinophils, basophils, and memory CD4+ T lymphocytes (134–137). RANTES is very effective in inducing eosinophil chemotaxis and transmigration (116). In transendothelial migration assays, the effects of RANTES on eosinophils are synergistic with IL-5. RANTES also causes rapid basophil degranulation and histamine release (117,118).

Interleukin-8

Interleukin-8 (IL-8) is an 8-kDa peptide that is produced by macrophages, eosinophils, endothelial cells, epithelial cells, and fibroblasts (138). TNF-α and IL-1β are potent stimulants of IL-8 gene expression (139–144). IL-8 is a chemoattractant of neutrophils, basophils, and a small proportion (<10%) of resting CD4+ and CD8+ lymphocytes. IL-8 is capable of inducing both neutrophil and eosinophil migration through unstimulated endothelium and epithelium. Neutrophils respond much more rapidly to IL-8 than eosinophils. IL-8 is particularly chemoattractant to eosinophils primed with IL-3, IL-5, and GM-CSF. Conversely, IL-8 primes eosinophils to respond to concentrations of IL-3 and IL-5, which in themselves are only marginally chemoattractant.

IL-8 promotes the adherence of neutrophils to endothelial cells by inducing neutrophils to express β2 integrins (145). IL-8 likely plays a crucial role in the recruitment of granulocytes to the airways in patients with asthma. The local balance of cytokine synthesis within the airways likely determines the relevance of IL-8 to eosinophil airway recruitment.

Interleukin-12

Interleukin-12 (IL-12) is a 75-kDa heterodimeric cytokine consisting of disulfide-linked 35-kDa and 40-kDa subunits (146,147). The gene for P40 is located on chromosome 5 and the gene for P35 on chromosome 3 (148). Virtually all cell types examined express P35. In contrast, P40 expression has a limited range of expression. P40 is expressed in monocytes/macrophages, B cells, and to a much lesser extent T cells. The disulfide-linked heterodimer is necessary to obtain biologic activity.

Exposure of macrophages to microbial products induces IL-12 production. *Staphylococcus aureus* Cowan strain 1 (SAC) greatly increases the expression of both P40 and P70. Other inducers of IL-12 production include LPS, *Mycobacterium tuberculosis, Toxoplasma gondii,* and *Listeria monocytogenes.* Interestingly, no cytokines including IL-1α, IL-1β, IL-2, IL-4, IL-6, IFN-γ, IFN-β, TNF-α, TNF-β, or GM-CSF were found to induce IL-12 production (149).

IL-12 does not stimulate resting PBMC to proliferate but can induce proliferation of activated CD4 and CD8 lymphocytes (146,147,150). IL-12 thus appears to function *in vivo,* to focus and amplify the immune response by selectively inducing outgrowth of those T cells that have been preactivated by appropriate antigens.

IL-12 is crucially involved in the development of a TH1-type immune response. Exposure of resting or activated lymphocytes to IL-12 results in a dose-dependent induction of IFN-γ (150–152). The accessory cell required for this response does not appear to be a monocyte or a B cell, but rather a dendritic cell (151). *In vitro* models have demonstrated that antigen combined with recombinant murine IL-12 but not a number of other cytokines preferentially induced the development of TH1 cells from naive T cells (153). The effects of IL-12 on TH1/TH2 development also have been observed in human cells. CD4 T-cell lines produced from atopic individuals exposed *in vitro* to *Dermatophagoides pteronysinus* group I antigen generally exhibited a TH2-like phenotype producing IL-4 but little or no IFN-γ. Cell lines from atopic individuals exposed to this antigen generated in the presence of human IL-12 exhibited a TH0- or TH1-like cytokine profile (154).

IL-12 is also a potent inhibitor of IL-4–induced IgE synthesis from peripheral blood mononuclear cells (155). IL-12 inhibits IgE synthesis at both the transcriptional and translational levels. IL-12 is believed to mediate this effect through both an IFN-dependent and independent mechanism. Similar effects of IL-12 have been demon-

strated *in vivo* (156). Treatment of mice with IL-12 inhibited serum levels of IgE synthesis by more than 98%.

CYTOKINES THAT INHIBIT INFLAMMATION

Interleukin-10

Interleukin-10 (IL-10) is a nondisulfide-linked homodimer. Macrophages produce substantial amounts of IL-10 after activation. IL-10 is also produced by mouse TH2 and TH0 subsets of CD4 T-cell clones but not by TH1 or CD8 T-cell clones. T cells produce IL-10 only after stimulation with antigen or polyclonal activators (157). IL-10 inhibits the synthesis of several cytokines that are normally secreted by monocytes/macrophages. These cytokines include IL-1, GM-CSF, TNF-α, IL-6, IL-8, IL-10, and IL-12 (158,159). IL-10 is secreted relatively late compared with other cytokines, which may explain why macrophages are able to secrete substantial amounts of various cytokines before IL-10 inhibition occurs. IL-10 also inhibits the induction of NO synthesis. The synthesis of cytokines by TH1 clones or during TH1-like responses is inhibited by IL-10. The expression of IL-10 during *in vivo* responses usually correlates with TH2-like responses (157,160).

IL-10 enhances the proliferation of mast cells lines in synergy with IL-3 or IL-4. The synergy indicates that IL-10 acts on the mast cell by an independent mechanism (161). IL-10 also activates transcription of genes for mast cell-derived proteases. Expression of MHC class II antigens but not CD23 (Fc$_\varepsilon$ receptor) is induced on resting B cells by IL-10. IL-10 increases the survival of small resting B cells in culture and causes strong proliferation of human B cells that have been activated by anti-CD40 antibodies or cross-linking of the antigen receptor. The stimulatory effects of IL-10 are additive with those of IL-4 (162,163).

Transforming Growth Factor-β

Three transforming growth factor-β (TGF-β) isoforms, TGF-β1, -β2, and -β3, are present in mammalian species. TGF-β is produced by T and B cells, platelets, and activated macrophages. Monocytes have the necessary proteases required for TGF-β activation. The active form of TGF-β is a hydrophobic, disulfide-linked dimer of the C terminal segment of the pre-pro-TGF-β. Differentiation of monocytes into macrophages is accompanied by a decrease in TGF-β receptor levels.

TGF-β exerts a large variety of biologic functions in most cells. TGF-β–induced effects can be grouped in several categories. First, TGF-β is a potent regulator of cell growth. TGF-β stimulates proliferation or acts as a potent antiproliferative factor depending on the cell type and the cell line. Second, in cells of nonhematopoietic origin,

TGF-β modifies the cellular interaction with the extracellular matrix. TGF-β induces the synthesis and secretion of many proteins of the extracellular matrix. TGF-β also increases expression of many integrins. Third, TGF-β regulates the synthesis and activity of secreted proteases and protease inhibitors. Finally, TGF-β is a potent chemoattractant for several cell types, especially monocytes and fibroblasts. These latter activities may be important at sites of wound healing and/or repair (164).

It seems likely that, in vivo, TGF-β plays an important role as a negative regulator of various cytokine-induced effects. TGF-β knockout mice develop a multifocal mixed inflammatory disease with rapid and massive infiltration of lymphocytes and neutrophils in many tissues and subsequent death. TGF-β1 deficiency results in the increased production of several cytokine mediators of inflammation such as IFN-γ, TNF-α, and MIP-1α. TGF-β likely is an important component of the maintenance of a proper balance between different cytokine-induced effects (165).

Interleukin-1Ra

Interleukin-1Ra (IL-1Ra) peptide is produced in two different forms from the same gene by using a different transcriptional start site and differential splicing of mRNA (166–168). IL-1Ra is produced by many cell types, including monocytes and epithelial cells. Differential production of IL-1 compared with IL-1Ra can be observed in human monocytes. Cytokines exhibit differential regulation of production of IL-1Ra and IL-1. TGF-β, IL-4, IFN-α, and GM-CSF are examples of cytokines that primarily increase IL-1Ra production (169). IL-1Ra binds to IL-1RI with near equal affinity as IL-1α or IL-1β but does not transmit a signal (170). The most likely explanation for the lack of biologic activity of IL-1Ra is that the receptor binding sites for IL-1α, IL-1β, and IL-Ra are nearly the same, but that IL-Ra lacks the critical component of the three-dimensional structure required for triggering the receptor.

GROWTH FACTORS

GM-CSF

GM-CSF is one of at least 20 glycoprotein growth factors that modulate the growth and differentiation of hematopoietic cells. The gene for GM-CSF is located in close proximity to the gene for IL-3 (171). A number of cells can synthesize GM-CSF, including macrophages, T lymphocytes, endothelial cells, fibroblasts, alveolar epithelial cells, and bronchial epithelial cells (172). Stimuli known to induce GM-CSF secretion in macrophages include LPS, phagocytosis, and adherence. IL-1, TNF-α, and LPS induce expression of GM-CSF in cultured endothelial cells. Although increased transcription of the GM-CSF gene is evident after inductive stimulation of most producer cell types, quantitatively the more important mechanism of gene regulation may be post-transcriptional stabilization of the mRNA (173).

GM-CSF regulates survival, differentiation, proliferation, and the functional activities in granulocyte/macrophage populations (174). Viability of mature cells can be maintained in vitro by as little as 1/100th the concentration of GM-CSF required to stimulate cellular proliferation, implying the priority of survival (175). Given the short half-life of granulocytes, prolonging the survival of these myeloid effector cells (granulocytes, eosinophils, and basophils) may be very important in the facilitation of host inflammatory response (176–178). The mechanisms by which GM-CSF prolongs survival in hemopoietic cells are not clear, but likely involve protection against apoptotic cell death.

GM-CSF is sufficient to induce distinct granulocyte, macrophage, and dendritic cell pathways of development from a common progenitor. GM-CSF activates mature hemopoietic cells, enhances the capacity of eosinophils to release mediators, and induces histamine release from basophils.

Increased expression of GM-CSF in epithelial cells, T lymphocytes, and eosinophils has been noted after endobronchial challenge with allergen (179,180). Increased circulating concentrations of GM-CSF have been detected in patients with acute severe asthma (181); peripheral blood monocytes secrete increased amounts of GM-CSF (182). Histochemical analysis of airway biopsies have demonstrated that sevenfold more GM-CSF staining cells were present in the bronchial submucosa of asthmatic patients when compared with nonasthmatic individuals (183). Two thirds of the cells staining for GM-CSF were macrophages; three quarters of macrophages stained positively for GM-CSF. Epithelial cells also stained strongly for GM-CSF (184). In situ hybridization of BAL cells obtained 24 hours after airborne allergen challenge of allergic asthmatics revealed GM-CSF mRNA localized predominantly to T lymphocytes and AMs (179). Taken together, these data strongly suggest involvement of GM-CSF in the pathogenesis of bronchial asthma. GM-CSF likely regulates survival, differentiation, activation, and chemotaxis of macrophages, eosinophils, and basophils.

ROLE OF MACROPHAGES IN INITIATION OF IMMUNE RESPONSES

Activated T lymphocytes clearly play a central role in the pathogenesis of asthma. The activation of T lymphocytes is antigen-specific, depending on the recognition of the appropriate antigenic epitope by the T-cell receptor/CD3 complex (185). The T-cell receptor recognizes partially digested peptides (11–30 amino acids long) only when these peptides are associated with cell surface

MHC glycoproteins on another cell (186). Activation of T lymphocytes to produce cytokines requires a second distinct signal (187). This second signal depends on the interaction of B7 molecules, expressed on antigen-presenting cells and their interaction with CD28 molecules expressed on the majority of naive and memory T cells. Thus, the activation of lymphocytes is a complex biologic function that requires the participation of an antigen-presenting cell (APC). Most cell types cannot perform all these functions; "professional" antigen-presenting cells (macrophages, dendritic cells, and B cells) are required.

Antigen Processing and Presentation

At least two distinct antigen-processing pathways exist. The pathway used depends on whether the antigen is an endogenously synthesized protein, such as a viral antigen produced in an infected cell, or an exogenous protein that has been internalized by the cell. Endogenous antigens are presented in association with class I MHC molecules (HLA-A,B,C in humans), whereas exogenous antigens are usually presented in association with class II MHC molecules (HLA-DP,DQ,DR in humans) (188, 189). This discussion is limited to the processing and presenting of exogenous proteins.

Antigen processing involves five distinct steps: a) recognition and uptake of the protein antigen by the APC; b) sequestration of the antigen in intracellular vesicles of low pH; c) processing of native proteins that includes both unfolding of the protein and partial of proteolysis with generation of immunogenic peptides; d) the binding of peptides to class II MHC molecules in a distinct free lysosomal vesicle termed the MIIC; and e) transport to and display of the MHC/peptide complex on the surface of APC (190). This process occurs rapidly; immunogenic

determinants can be expressed on the surface of antigen-presenting cells in association with MHC 30 to 60 minutes after internalization (191).

Antigen Presentation

A central event in T-lymphocyte activation is the interaction between the antigenic epitope presented in association with the MHC molecule and the T-cell receptor/CD3 complex. However, three additional molecular interactions are crucial to the interaction between an antigen-presenting cell and the T lymphocyte: a) adhesion molecules that promote the physical interaction between APC and T cells; b) membrane-bound growth/differentiation molecules that promote T-cell activation (co-stimulatory molecules); and c) soluble cytokines such as TNF-α and IL-1 (192, 193) (Fig. 1).

In humans, monocytes and macrophages express a basal level of class II MHC proteins, but the level of MHC expression increases markedly after exposure to IFN-γ (194). Prostaglandin-E, TNF-α, IL-10, and corticosteroids all downregulate MHC class II expression.

The engagement of the T-cell receptor by the MHC/peptide complex of the APC provides specificity for T-cell activation. Other receptor ligand interactions occur that both promote cell-to-cell contact as well as provide important transmembrane signaling (195,196). ICAM-1 molecules on the APC interact with LFA-1 molecules on T cells; LFA-3 interacts with CD2. CD4 interacts with class II MHC molecules. Engagement of the T-cell receptor changes the affinity of the LFA molecule without increasing the number of molecules on the cell surface. Similar mechanisms appear to operate for CD4 and CD2. ICAM-1 is also upregulated during this interaction, probably in response to IL-1 and IFN-γ.

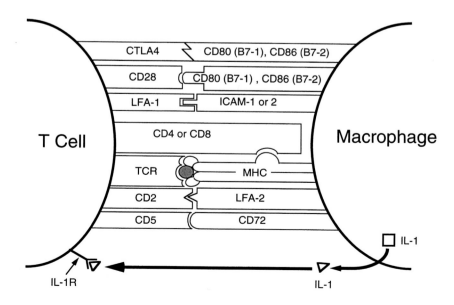

FIG. 1. Antigen presentation. The activation of T cells by antigen-presenting cells involves a) engagement of the MHC-peptide complex and the T cell receptor; b) receptor-ligand interactions that promote cell-cell contact and provide transmembrane signaling; c) obligate costimulatory receptor ligand interactions that activate T lymphocytes to produce cytokines; and d) soluble cytokine receptor interactions. These interactions take place within an immunologic synapse formed by close cell contact between antigen-presenting cells and T cells.

Co-stimulatory molecules that regulate T-cell growth and differentiation are required to activate T lymphocytes to produce cytokines (187). TH1 cell clones encountering nominal antigen/MHC complexes in the absence of appropriate co-stimulation fail to proliferate and fail to produce lymphokines, most prominently IL-2. These T cells can be rescued from this "anergic" state by the addition of exogenous IL-2. A major co-stimulatory pathway for T-cell activation involves the CD28 molecule expressed on most naive and memory T cells. CD28 antagonists alter T-cell activation, inhibit proliferation of T-cell clones, and induce anergy.

The natural ligand for CD28-mediated co-stimulation is B7. Two B7 ligands have been identified. B7-1 expression is limited normally to "professional" APC, such as dendritic cells, macrophages, thymic epithelial cells, activated B and T lymphocytes, and monocytes treated with IFN-γ. It is upregulated on APC after activation by endotoxin and cytokines or ligation of class II MHC or CD40. B7-1 can co-stimulate both antigen- and mitogen-driven T-cell proliferation and IL-2 production in a CD28-dependent manner. B7-2 is a second CD28 ligand. B7-2 is constitutively expressed on dendritic cells and macrophages and is rapidly upregulated on B cells after activation by cross-linking of the Ig receptor or cytokines. B7-2 has sequence similarity to B7-1 and binds CD28 (197).

Soluble cytokines are released during antigen presentation. IL-1 was originally believed to be a major co-stimulatory molecule, but its role in T-cell activation is more limited than initially proposed. The expression of IL-1 by macrophages is profoundly increased during antigen presentation. CD4-macrophage contact induces IL-1 mRNA. The expression and secretion of IL-1 importantly affect the local microenvironment in which T-cell activation takes place (198). The interaction between macrophages and T cells is reciprocal and symbiotic. Both cells have obligate requirements for each other for their full functional capacity; the interaction results in the activation of both cells. CD4+ lymphocytes cannot recognize antigen unless an APC processes and exhibits the peptide/class II MHC complex to the TcR/CD3 complex. Cytokines secreted by activated CD4+ T cells are required by macrophages to express their full spectrum of functions. Clearly, specific immunity and innate immunity are tightly interrelated.

Role of Alveolar Macrophages in Antigen Presentation

AMs are ineffective in presenting antigen to T cells. AMs are less effective than monocytes in inducing proliferation of blood T lymphocytes to soluble "recall" antigens and in activating T lymphocytes necessary for antibody production (199–201). AMs effectively stimulate the proliferation of T-lymphocyte lines and clones in response to soluble antigens (201,202). Thus, whereas AMs can restimulate recently activated T cells effectively, they are ineffective in stimulating the proliferation of naive T cells or resting memory cells.

AMs fail to effectively activate CD4+ T cells because of defective expression of B7 co-stimulatory cell-surface molecules. Antigen presentation by AMs can be restored by the addition of a CD28 stimulant (anti-CD28 mAb), indicating that co-stimulation by AMs via the C28 pathway is defective. AMs activated with IFN-γ fail to express B7-1 or B7-2 antigens. The mechanism by which AMs paradoxically limit their expression of B7-1 and B7-2 is not clear. Some heterogeneity exists in B7-1 and B7-2 expression. The limited expression of B7-1 and B7-2 may permit AMs to induce proliferation in already activated T cells and T-cell clones (203). The capacity of AMs to bind with T lymphocytes is also less than that of monocytes (202).

ROLE OF ALVEOLAR MACROPHAGES IN DOWNREGULATING IMMUNE RESPONSES IN THE LUNG

The findings discussed above suggest that AMs have a role distinct from other types of APC. Although the lung is frequently exposed to antigens, immune responses must be restricted or downregulated within the pulmonary parenchyma because inflammatory reactions inevitably result in significant damage to gas exchange surface. Resident pulmonary AMs actively suppress T-cell proliferation induced by antigen or polyclonal stimuli (199,200). A variety of mediators that inhibit lymphocyte proliferation are produced by AMs, including prostaglandin-E$_2$, superoxide anion, and vitamin D metabolites (204,205). Compelling evidence for the presence of active alveolar macrophage suppression *in vivo* exists; rats and mice selectively depleted of AMs by the intratracheal administration of a liposome-encapsulated macrophage cytotoxic drug displayed gross hyperresponsiveness to pulmonary antigen administration. Large numbers of activated T cells and plasma cells were found in the lung parenchyma after either intratracheal or aerosol delivery of antigens (206–208). Although the potential value of such a steady-state downregulatory control mechanism within the lung is self-evident, this suppressive activity should be reversible to allow local T-cell activation in the face of a microbial antigen. Alveolar macrophage suppressive activity can be reversed via GM-CSF (209). TNF-α amplifies the effects of GM-CSF. Thus, nonspecific inflammatory stimuli (LPS) could lessen the downregulatory tone of AMs by inducing GM-CSF production by macrophages and/or alveolar and airway epithelial cells.

Initiation of Antigen-specific Immune Responses to Pulmonary Antigens

Dendritic cells are responsible for activating naive T cells for proliferation and clonal expansion (see Chapter 33). Unprimed, naive T cells respond to virtually one type of antigen-presenting cell, the dendritic cell (210). However, phenotypic changes within the local macrophage population also may be an important factor in regulation of immune responses within the lung. The immunomodulatory function of macrophages change markedly during maturation from the monocyte to a mature alveolar macrophage. Monocytes are permissive or stimulatory to T-cell activation, whereas AMs actively suppress and fail to express B7 molecules. Thus, inflammatory stimuli that recruit fresh monocytes to the lung might theoretically dilute the resident alveolar macrophage population with recruited monocytes and convert a normally immunosuppressive tissue milieu into one that is supportive of T-cell activation (211, 212).

Evidence exists that changes occur within the local inductive milieu of the lung in patients with asthma. Alveolar macrophage suppression is reduced after exposure to allergens (213–215). Further, monocyte accumulation is a hallmark of postchallenge bronchial biopsies from asthmatics. Similar changes in the inductive microenvironment of the lung have been noted in other inflammatory diseases.

Induction of TH2 T Cells in Response to Allergen

Current models of the pathophysiology of asthma suggest that TH2 lymphocytes play a pivotal role in the bronchial inflammation characteristic of this disease (216). Production of IgE is controlled by TH2 T cells and TH2 cytokines control and modulate the functional state of effector cells, such as eosinophils, basophils, and mast cells (217). Several factors that guide T cells toward a TH2 phenotype occur during the process of antigen presentation (Fig. 2). The type of APC that presents the antigen may be crucial. Macrophages tend to favor the induction of Th1 cells and B cells favor TH2 cells (218,219). Under certain circumstances, DC preferentially activate TH2 cells (220). Hapten-specific T-cell clones derived by repeated stimulation of T cells using DC all expressed a TH2 phenotype. The mechanisms by which DC favor the expression of TH2 cells remains unclear, but may be related to the ability of LC to secrete IL-1, a co-stimulator for TH2 cells, but not TH1 cells and to the absence of IFN-γ production by LC that would inhibit the development of TH2 cells.

The first signal that naive T cells receive occurs when the TCR binds transiently to its ligand, an allergen-derived peptide bound tightly in the specialized groove of a

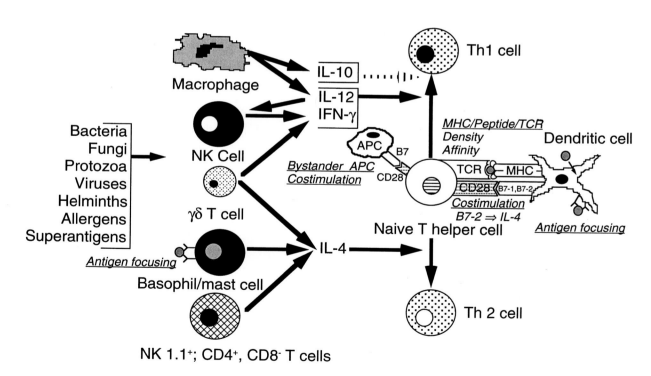

FIG. 2. Role of innate immunity in the generation of specific immune responses. The tissue microenvironment is a crucial regulator of specific immune response generation. The presence of IgE on antigen-presenting cells may focus the uptake and processing of allergens. Specific antigens deliver differentiation signals likely based on their density and affinity. Co-stimulatory signals delivered either by APC that are presenting the antigen or by bystander APC influence T-helper cell differentiation. Soluble cytokines produced by cells of the innate immune system are the major regulators of T cell differentiation (*solid arrows* indicate stimulation, *broken line arrow* indicates inhibition).

class II MHC molecule on the surface of an APC. Antigens deliver signals via the TCR that favor differentiation into TH2 T cells. Changes in ligand structure can bias the T-cell response via quantitative variation in ligand density. Peptides/MHC class II complexes that interact strongly with the TCR favor TH1 responses, whereas weak interactions result in the priming of TH2 responses. The overall binding affinity can be varied by modifying the peptide, which results in different signals (221,222). The mechanisms by which signals delivered via the TCR control differentiation and/or how these signals differ is uncertain. Two possibilities exist: a) differential TCR aggregation results in differential intracellular signals that favor distinct cytokine gene expression, or b) differential MHC/TCR interactions favor differential co-receptor expression.

Co-stimulatory molecules may direct the polarization of T cells into TH1 or TH2 cells. B7-2 is constitutively expressed on dendritic cells and macrophages, whereas B7-1 is not. These two B7 molecules bind with different kinetics to distinct regions of the CTLA-4 molecule and most likely to CD28 molecules. The outcome of B7-1 and B7-2 co-stimulation is different. B7-2 co-stimulates the production of IL-4 as well as IL-2 and IFN-γ. Thus, after B7-2 co-stimulation an initial source of IL-4 is available. B7-2 provides only a moderate signal for TH2 cell differentiation; additional signals are almost surely required to achieve high levels of IL-4 production to result in full differentiation into TH2 cells (223,224). B7-CD28 co-stimulatory signals can be delivered by bystander APC *in vitro* with the same efficiency as by the APC engaging the TcR. T cells, accordingly, might be activated *in vivo* with MHC-TCR engagement being provided by one APC whereas co-stimulation is delivered by a second APC type (225).

Soluble factors are clearly crucial in the development of TH1 responses. IL-12 secreted by macrophages drives the T-cell response toward a TH1 phenotype. IL-12 acts both directly on T cells or indirectly by the rapid induction of IFN-γ secretion by natural killer cells. IFN-γ production favors a TH1, rather than TH2, phenotype (224,225). IL-1 also favors the differentiation into a TH1 response. Activated macrophages and DC produce IL-1, but B cells do not (218). PGE-2 favors TH2 cytokine secretion profiles in murine and human CD4 T cells probably because of its inhibition of IL-2 and IFN-γ and its upregulation of IL-4 and IL-5 (226–228). IL-10 also suppresses TH1 responses and synergizes with functions mediated by IL-4. IL-10 enhances MHC class II expression on resting B cells and increases their viability (163).

Finally, the presence of IgE likely promotes antigen focusing and facilitates antigen presentation to naive T cells. IgE might thus aid in the perpetuation of a TH2 response. Dendritic cells express both FcεRI and FcεRII. These two receptors capture allergen bound to allergen-specific IgE and could focus the immune response through facilitated antigen presentation (229).

The tissue microenvironment in which the immune response is generated is clearly crucial in determining the type and intensity of an immune response. Cytokines secreted in the tissue where antigen resides are also crucial in the maintenance and/or regulation of the immune response. An understanding of these crucial signals might allow modulation of undesirable TH2 responses.

ROLE OF MACROPHAGES IN THE EFFECTOR PHASE OF IMMUNE RESPONSES

Development of an Inflammatory Response

Resident cells within the lung communicate with circulating leukocytes during the development of an inflammatory response. Both soluble mediators (cytokines and chemoattractants) and adhesion molecules are involved in this communication. This interaction is complex because soluble mediators regulate the expression of adhesion molecules and cell-cell adhesion results in the elaboration of soluble mediators.

Leukocyte recruitment to tissues requires a cascade of at least three sequential adhesion molecule events (230): a) constitutively expressed leukocyte adhesion molecules bind transiently and reversibly to ligands on endothelial cells (231); L-selectin expressed constitutively on leukocytes is important in this interaction; b) both the leukocyte and the endothelial cell are activated; Macrophage products such as IL-1 and TNF-α induce E-selectin expression on endothelial cells (232); L-selectin, P-selectin, and E-selectin are responsible for rolling of the circulating leukocyte along the surface of the endothelial cell (233); and c) firm adhesion depends on activation-induced molecules on both the leukocyte and the endothelial cell. Inflammatory cells roll and skid along the endothelial surface until a high concentration of diffusing cytokines and chemokines that activate both endothelial and inflammatory cells cause firm adhesion. The source of the cytokines and chemokines is likely intravascular monocytes, perivascular lymphocytes, and AMs. Macrophages produce early response cytokines such as IL-1, TNF-α, and IL-6. All these cytokines are released on exposure to inhaled allergens via FcεRII receptors. These cytokines upregulate VLA-4, LFA-1, and MAC-1 on leukocytes and elevate the expression of endothelial cell ICAM-1. Finally, they induce the expression of IL-8 by endothelial cells. In concert, these events allow the leukocyte to be anchored firmly at the endothelial surface, which allows for diapedesis between endothelial cells and the eventual migration through the extracellular matrix and into the air spaces (234).

Both animal studies and studies of patients with asthma have addressed leukocyte endothelial interactions in airway inflammation. Microvascular expression of E-selectin is increased in animal models involving antigen-induced acute airway inflammation and late-phase obstruction. ICAM-1 expression is increased in chronic airway inflammation (235–237). Bronchial biopsy specimens of normal humans demonstrate constitutive bronchial microvascular expression of ICAM-1 and to a lesser extent E-selection (238). Biopsies in atopic patients with mild asthma do not reveal significant differences in the expression of ICAM-1 and E-selectin when compared with nonasthmatic individuals. A role for E-selectin in allergic airway inflammation is supported from studies using segmental antigen challenge. Increased levels of soluble E-selectin are noted in BAL fluid after antigen challenge, suggesting cytokine-induced microvascular expression of E-selectin (239).

In the presence of a chemokine gradient, leukocytes move between endothelial cells, traverse the basement membrane, move through the extracellular matrix and epithelium, and eventually reach the airway. Macrophages are almost surely important sources of cell-specific chemoattractants. RANTES and MIP-1α are chemotactic for macrophages, eosinophils, and basophils. MCP-1 is chemotactic for macrophages and basophils. IL-8 is chemotactic for neutrophils, basophils, and, to a lesser extent, eosinophils. Additionally, macrophage-released early cytokines can induce epithelial cells and fibroblasts to release chemoattractants and growth factors (GM-CSF, IL-8, MCP-1, MIP-1α, RANTES). The sequential coordinated induction of parenchymal cells is likely crucial to the formation of a chemotactic gradient that allows movement of inflammatory cells from the endothelial surface to the surface of the epithelium.

Finally, ICAM-1 expression may be important in leukocyte-epithelial interactions. Both monkey and human epithelium constitutively express ICAM-1 (237,238,240). Conflicting results exist regarding the effect of cytokines on bronchial epithelial cells. In one study, TNF-α and IL-1β increased ICAM-1 expression (240), whereas in a second study, IFN-γ but not TNF-α or IL-1β induced ICAM-1 expression (241). In a monkey model of airway inflammation, ICAM-1 expression increased after chronic allergen challenge (237). No human data have demonstrated differences in epithelial ICAM-1 expression between nonasthmatic individuals and asthmatics.

Production of Leukotrienes

Leukotrienes are perhaps the best studied macrophage-produced mediators involved in the pathogenesis of asthma. Leukotriene synthesis is dependent on 5-lipoxygenase, which is found only in cells of myeloid lineage (241). Although synthesis of LTA4 is thus limited to these cells, the export of LTA4 to other cells allows a wider distribution of leukotriene-producing cell types. Most cells produce appreciable quantities of either LTB4 or LTC4 but not both, with the exception of human monocytes. Monocytes release both LTB4 and LTC4 after being ex-

posed to nonimmunologic stimuli or immunologic stimuli (IgG, IgE with cell-surface FC receptors) (242). AMs appear to produce a substantial excess of LTB4 to LTC4 after stimulation by calcium ionophore, IgE, or IgG (243,244).

LTB4 is a potent chemotactic factor for polymorphonuclear neutrophils (PMN) and a weaker chemotactic factor for eosinophils. LTB4 accounts for the majority of neutrophil chemotactic activity elaborated by AM immediately upon stimulation (244,245). LTB4 also promotes adherence of inflammatory cells to the endothelium and stimulates these cells to release reactive oxygen intermediates and proteases. Cysteinyl leukotrienes (LTC4, D4, and E4) evoke marked and prolonged contraction of smooth muscles in airways and vessels. They also increase microvascular permeability and stimulate airway mucus production. Leukotrienes also play a permissive role in inflammation by promoting the synthesis by macrophages of TNF-α, IL-8, IL-6, and AM-derived fibroblast growth factor (246). Finally, leukotrienes have direct effects on fibroblasts; they stimulate fibroblast proliferation, chemotaxis, and collagen synthesis (247).

Although intrapulmonary administration of lipid mediators promotes airway inflammation, mucus hypersecretion, and bronchoconstriction, the role of macrophage-derived leukotrienes remains unknown. Arguing against a role for AMs in leukotriene overproduction is the fact that cysteinyl leukotrienes are only minor products of AMs under usual *in vitro* circumstances. Alternatively, AMs are located on the airway surface, express plasma membrane IgE receptors, and secrete substantially more LTC4 than do PMN. Leukotriene synthesis by AM is inhibited by *in vivo* pretreatment with glucocorticoids.

ROLE OF MACROPHAGE-DERIVED GROWTH FACTORS IN FIBROGENESIS

Fibrotic changes occur in airways in response to chronic inflammation. The role of various macrophage-derived peptide growth factors in asthma has not been extensively investigated. Macrophages secrete platelet-derived growth factor (PDGF) after activation (248). PDGF induces fibroblast proliferation and collagen secretion (249). The wound-healing effects of PDGF are macrophage-dependent in most models. Macrophages also produce a TGF-β molecule with important influences in the turnover of matrix proteins and on the proliferation of fibroblasts (250).

Angiogenesis is a central biologic event encountered during chronic inflammation and during fibrogenesis. The factors that regulate angiogenesis in asthma are unknown. CXC chemokines may play an important role in angiogenesis in this disease. CXC chemokines such as IL-8 or ENA-78 that contain the sequence Glu-Leu-Arg (ELR motif) are potent angiogenic factors. In contrast,

CXC chemokines that lack the ELR motif (platelet factor 4, IFN-γ inducible protein 10) behave as potent angiostatic regulators of neovascularization. These non-ELR–containing chemokines inhibit not only the angiogenic activity of ELR-CXC chemokines, but also the structurally unrelated macrophage-derived angiogenic factor, bFGF (251). The magnitude of expression and relative concentrations of angiogenic or angiostatic CXC chemokines may thus be an important regulatory event in the angiogenesis noted during asthma.

CONCLUSIONS

Macrophages can be involved at numerous steps in the pathogenesis of asthma. Numerous questions remain, however, about their *in vivo* role in this disease process. It will be important to determine which macrophage secretory products have important *in vivo* effects and which are figments of *in vitro* assays. Because the *in vivo* milieu is complex, it will be important to determine how products work in concert and in conflict. The answers to these questions will require the judicious use of animal models and patients with asthma for detection, reconstitution, and deletion.

REFERENCES

1. Ersle VAJ, Lichtman MA. Structure and function of the marrow. In Williams WJ, Beutler E, Ersle VAJ, Lichtman MA, eds. *Hematology.* New York: McGraw-Hill, 1990;37–47.
2. Lambertsen RH, Weiss L. A model of intramedullary hematopoietic micro-environments based on stereologic study of the distribution of endocloned marrow colonies. *Blood* 1984;63:287–297.
3. Sieff CA. Hematopoietic growth factors. *J Clin Invest* 1987;79:1549–1557.
4. Metcalf D. Haemopoietic growth factors 1. *Lancet* 1989;1:825–827.
5. Metcalf D. The molecular control of normal and leukemic granulocyte and macrophages. *Proc R Soc Land [Biol]* 1987;230:389–423.
6. Bagby GC, Dinarello CA, Wallace P, Wagner C, Hefeneider S, McCall E. Interleukin-1 stimulates granulocyte-macrophage colony stimulating activity release by vascular endothelial cells. *J Clin Invest* 1986;78:1316.
7. Munker R, Gasson J, Ogawa M, Koeffler HF. Recombinant human tumor necrosis factor induces production of granulocyte-monocyte colony stimulating factor. *Nature* 1986;323:79.
8. Crocker PC, Milon G. Macrophages in the control of hematopoiesis. In Lewis CE, D Magee JO. eds. *The macrophage.* Oxford: Oxford University Press, 1992;115.
9. Broxmeyer HE, Sherry B, Lu L et al. Enhancing and suppressing effects of recombinant murine macrophage inflammatory proteins on colony formation in vitro by bone marrow myeloid progenitor cells. *Blood* 1990;76:1110–1116.
10. Whitelaw DM. The intravascular life span of monocytes. *Blood* 1966;28:445–464.
11. Whitelaw DM. Observations on human monocyte kinetics after pulse labeling. *Cell Tissue Kinet* 1972;5:311–317.
12. Meuret G, Hoffmann G. Monocyte kinetic studies in normal and disease states. *Br J Haematol* 1973;24:275–285.
13. Thomas ED, Rambergh RE, Sale GE, Sparkes RS, Golde DW. Direct evidence for bone marrow origin of the alveolar macrophage in man. *Science* 1976;192:1016–1018.
14. Winston DJ, Territo MC, Ho WG, Miller MJ, Gale RP, Golde DW. Alveolar macrophage dysfunction in human bone marrow transplant recipients. *Am J Med* 1982;73:859–866.
15. Bitterman PB, Saltzman LE, Adelberg S, Ferrans VJ, Crystal RG. Alveolar macrophage replication: one mechanism for the expansion of the mononuclear phagocyte population in the chronically inflamed lung. *J Clin Invest* 1984;74:460–469.
16. Adams, DO, Hamilton TA. The cell biology of macrophage activation. *Annu Rev Immunol* 1984;2:283–318.
17. Springer TA. Adhesion receptors of the immune system. *Nature* 1990; 346:425–434.
18. Gordon S, Perry UH, Rabinowitz S, Chung LP, Rosen H. Plasma membrane receptors of the mononuclear phagocyte system. *J Cell Sci* 1988;9(suppl):1–26.
19. Adams DO, Hamilton TA. Macrophages as destructive cells. In Gallin JI, Goldstein IM, and Snyderman R, eds. In: *Host defenses in inflammation: basic principles and clinical correlates*, 2nd ed. New York: Raven Press, 1992;637–662.
20. Uquccioni M, D'Apuzzo M, Loetscher M, Dewald B, Baggiolini M. Actions of the chemotactic cytokines MCP-1, MCP-2 RANTES MIP-1α, MIP-1β on human monocytes. *Eur J Immunol* 1995;25:64–68.
21. Ravetch JV, Kinet J. Fc receptors. *Annu Rev Immunol* 1991;9:457–492.
22. Brown EJ. Complement receptors and phagocytosis. *Curr Opin Immunol* 1991;3:76–82.
23. Rosen H, Law SKA. The leukocyte cell surface receptor(s) for the iC3b product of complement. *Curr Top Microbiol Immunol* 1989;99–122.
24. Mellman I. Relationships between structure and function in the Fc receptor family. *Curr Opin Immunol* 1988;1:16–25.
25. Funger MW, Shen L, Graziano RF, Guyre PM. Cytotoxicity mediated by human Fc receptors for IgG. *Immunol Today* 1989;111:97–99.
26. Peltz G, Frederick K. Anderson CL, Peterlin BM. Characterization of the human monocyte high affinity Fc receptor (huFcRI). *Mol Immunol* 1988;25:243–250.
27. Ernst LK, van de Winkel GJ, Chiu I-M, Anderson CL. Three genes for the human high affinity Fc receptor for IgG (Fcγ8RI) encode four distinct transcription products. *J Biol Chem* 1992;267:15692–15700.
28. Perussia B, Dayton ET, Lazarus R, Fanning V, Trinchieri G. Immune interferon induces the receptor for monomeric IgGI on human monocytic and myeloid cells. *J Exp Med* 1983;158:1092–1113.
29. Kurlander RJ, Batker J. The binding of human immunoglobulin G1 monomer and small, covalently cross-linked polymers of immunoglobulin G1 to human peripheral blood monocytes and polymorphonuclear leukocytes. *J Clin Invest* 1982;69:1–8.
30. Anderson CL, Shen L, Eicher DM, Wewers MD, Gill JK. Phagocytosis mediated by three distinct Fc receptor classes on human leukocytes. *J Exp Med* 1990;171:1333–1345.
31. Unkless JC, Scigliano E, Freedman VH. Structure and function of human and murine receptors for IgG. *Annu Rev Immunol* 1988;6:251–281.
32. Brooks DG, Qui WQ, Luster Ad, Ravetch JV. Structure and expression of human IgG FcRI(CD32). Functional heterogeneity is encoded by the alternatively spliced products of multiple genes. *J Exp Med* 1989;170:1369–1385.
33. Rossman MD, Chen E, Chien P, Rotten M, Cprek A, Schreiber AD. Fc receptor recognition of IgG ligand by human monocytes and macrophages. *Am J Respir Cell Mol Biol* 1989;1:211–220.
34. Anderson CL, Guyre PM, Whitin JC, Ryan DH, Looney RJ, Fanger MW. Soluble circulating Fc receptors on human mononuclear phagocytes. Antibody characterization and induction of superoxide production in a monocyte cell line. *J Biol Chem* 1986;261:12856–12864.
35. Debets JMH, van de Winkel JGJ, Ceuppens JL, Dieteren IEM, Buurman WA. Cross-linking of both FcγRI and FcγRII induces secretion of tumor necrosis factor by human monocytes, requiring high affinity Fc-FcgR interactions. *J Immunol* 1990;144:1304–1310.
36. Selvaraj P, Rosse WF, Silber R, Springer TA. The major Fc receptor in blood has a phosphatidylinositol anchor and is deficient in paroxysmal nocturnal haemoglobinuira. *Nature* 1988;333:565–567.
37. Huizinga TWJ, van der Schoot CE, Jost C, et al. The PI-linked receptor FcRIII is released on stimulation of neutrophils. *Nature* 1988;333:667–669.
38. Hibbs ML, Selvaraj P, Carpen O, Springer TA, Kuster H, Jouvin ME, et al. Mechanisms for regulating expression of membrane isoforms of FcγRIII(CD16). *Science* 1989;246:1608–1611.
39. Conrad DH. The low affinity receptor for IgE. *Annu Rev Immunol* 1990;8:623–633.

40. Pforte A, Breyer G, Prinz JC, et al. Expression of the Fc–receptor for IgE (Fc$_\varepsilon$RII, CD23) on AMs in extrinsic allergic alveolitis. *J Exp Med* 1990;171:1163–1169.

41. Yokota A, Yukawa K, Yamamoto A, et al. Two forms of the low-affinity Fc receptor for IgE differentially mediate endocytosis and phagocytosis: identification of the critical cytoplasmic domains. *Proc Natl Acad Sci USA* 1992;89:5030–5034.

42. Rouzer CA, Scott WA, Hamill AL, Liu F, Katz DH, Cohn ZA. Secretion of leukotriene C and other arachidonic and metabolites by macrophages challenged with immunoglobulin E immune complexes. *J Exp Med* 1982;156:1077–1086.

43. Takizawa F, Adamczewski M, Kinet J. Identification of the low affinity receptor for immunoglobulin E on mouse mast cells and as Fc$_\gamma$RII and Fc$_\gamma$RIII. *J Exp Med* 1992;176:469–476.

44. Gordon S. Biology of the macrophage. *J Cell Sci (Suppl)* 1986;4:267–286.

45. Nathan CF. Secretory products of macrophages. *J. Clin Invest* 1987;79:319–326.

46. Helin EH. Macrophage procoagulant factors-mediators of inflammatory and neoplastic tissue lesions. *Med Biol* 1986;64:167–176.

47. Rappolee DA, Werb Z. Macrophage derived growth factors. *Curr Topics in Micro and Immunol* 1992;181:87–140.

48. Unanue ER. Macrophages, antigen presenting cells and the phenomena of antigen handling and presentation Paul WE, Ed. In: *Fundamental Immunology.* 3rd ed. New York, Raven Press Ltd., 1993;111–144.

49. Takemura R, Werb Z. Secretory products of macrophages and their physiological function. *Am J Physiol* 1984;246:C1–C9.

50. Auger MJ, Ross JA. The biology of the macrophage. In: Lewis CE, McGee JO'D. ed. *The macrophage.* Oxford, Oxford University Press, 1992;1.

51. Wolpe SD, Cerami A. Macrophage inflammatory proteins 1 and 2: members of a novel superfamily of cytokines. *FASEB J* 1989;3:2565–2573.

52. Oppenheim JJ, Zachariae COC, Mukaida N, Matsushima K. Properties of the novel proinflammatory supergene intecrine cytokine family. *Annu Rev Immunol* 1991;9:617–648.

53. Wolf SF, Temple PA, Kobayashi M, Young D, Diug M, et al. Cloning of cDNA for natural killer cell stimulatory factor. *J Immunol* 1991;146:3074–3081.

54. Brunda MJ. Interleukin-12. *J Leuk Biol* 1994;55:280–288.

55. de Vries JE. Interleukin-10 (IL-10) inhibits cytokine synthesis by human monocytes: an autoregulatory role of IL-10 produced by monocytes. *J Exp Med* 1991;174:1209–1220.

56. Assoian AK, Fleurdelys BE, Stevenson HC, et al. Expression and secretion of type-β transforming growth factor by activated human macrophages. *Proc Natl Acad Sci USA* 1987;84:6020–6024.

57. Arend WP, Welgus HG, Thompson RC, Eisenberg SP. Biological properties of recombinant human monocyte-derived interleukin-1 receptor antagonist. *J Clin Invest* 1990;85:1694–1697.

58. LoMedico PT, Gubler U, Hellmann CP, et al. Cloning and expression of murine interleukin-1 cDNA in *Escherichia coli. Nature* 1984;312:458–462.

59. Auron PE, Webb AC, Rosenwasser LJ, Mucci SF, Rich A. Wolff SM, et al. Nucleotide sequence of human monocyte interleukin-1 precursor cDNA. *Proc Natl Acad Sci USA* 1984;81:7907–7911.

60. Gary I, Gershon RK, Waksman BH. Potentiation of the T lymphocyte response to mitogens. I. The responding cell. *J Exp Med* 1972;136:128–138.

61. Dinarello CA, Cannon JG, Wolff SM, et al. Tumor necrosis factor (cachectin) is an endogenous pyrogen and induces production of interleukin 1. *J Exp Med* 1986;163:1433–1450.

62. Kostura MJ, Tocci MJ, Limjuco G, et al. Identification of a monocyte specific pre-interleukin 1 β convertase activity. *Proc Natl Acad Sci USA* 1989;86:5227–5231.

63. Thornberry NA, Bull HG, Calaycay JR, et al. A novel heterodimeric cysteine protease is required for interleukin-1 β processing in monocytes. *Nature* 1992;356:768–774.

64. Dower SK, Kronheim SR, March CJ, Conlon PJ, Hopp TP, Gillis S, et al. Detection and characterization of high-affinity plasma membrane receptors for human interleukin 1. *J Exp Med* 1985;162:501–515.

65. Sims JE, March CJ, Cosman D, et al. Expression cloning of the IL-1 receptor, a member of the immunoglobulin superfamily. *Science* 1988;241:585–589.

66. McMahan CJ, Slack JL, Mosley B, et al. A novel IL-1 receptor, cloned from B cells by mammalian expression is expressed in many cell types. *EMBO J* 1991;10:2821–2832.

67. Stein PH, Singer A. Similar co-stimulation requirements of CD4+ and CD8+ primary T helper cells: role of IL–1 and IL-6 in inducing IL-2 secretion and subsequent proliferation. *Int Immunol* 1992;4:327–335.

68. Luqman M, Greenbaum L, Lu D, Bottomly K. Differential effect of interleukin 1 on naive and memory CD4- T cells. *Eur J Immunol* 1992;22:95–100.

69. Greenbaum LA, Horowitz JB, Woods A. Pasqualini T, Reich E-P, Bottomly K. Autocrine growth of CD4- T cells. Differential effects of IL-1 on helper and inflammatory T cells. *J Immunol* 1988;140:1555–1560.

70. Pober JS, Bevilacqua MP, Mendrick DL, Lapierre LA, Fiers W Jr, Gimbrone MA. Two distinct monokines, interleukin 1 and tumor necrosis factor, each independently induce biosynthesis and transient expression of the same antigen on the surface of cultured human vascular endothelial cells. *J Immunol* 1986;135:1680–1687.

71. Goldblum SE, Yoneda K, Cohen DA, McClain CJ. Provocation of pulmonary vascular endothelial injury in rabbits b human recombinant interleukin-1 β. *Infect Immun* 1988;56:2255–2263.

72. Schmidt JA, Mizel SB, Cohen D, Green I. Interleukin 1, a potential regulator of fibroblast proliferation. *J Immunol* 1982;128:2177–2182.

73. Dayer J-M, de Rochemonteix B, Burrus B, Demczuk S, Dinarello CA. Human recombinant interleukin 1 stimulates collagenase and prostaglandin E$_2$ production by human synovial cells. *J Clin Invest* 1986;77:645–648.

74. Wewers MD, Rennard SI, Hance AJ, Bitterman PB, Crystal RG. Normal human AMs obtained by bronchoalveolar lavage have a limited capacity to release interleukin-1. *J Clin Invest* 1984;74:2208–2218.

75. Koide SL, Inaba K, Steinman RM. Interleukin 1 enhances T-dependent immune responses by amplifying the function of dendritic cells. *J Exp Med* 1987;165:515–530.

76. Mattoli S, Mattoso VL, Soloperto M, Allegra L, Fasoli A. Cellular and biochemical characteristics of bronchoalveolar lavage fluid in symptomatic nonallergic asthma. *J Allergy Clin Immunol* 1991;84:794–802.

77. Pennica D, Nedwin GE, Hayflick JS, et al. Human tumor necrosis factor: precursor structure, expression and homology to lymphotoxin. *Nature* 1984;312:724–729.

78. Nedwin GE, Naylor SL, Sakaguchi AY, et al. Human lymphotoxin and tumor necrosis factor genes: structure, homology and chromosomal localization. *Nucleic Acids Res* 1985;13:6361–6373.

79. Nedospasov SA, Hirt AB, Shakob AN, Dobrynin VN, Kawashima E, Accola RS, et al. The genes for tumor necrosis factor and lymphotoxin are tandemly arranged on chromosome 17 of the mouse. *Nucleic Acids Res* 1986;14:7713–7725.

80. Gardner SM, Mock BA, Hilgers J, Huppi KE, Roeder WD. Mouse lymphotoxin and tumor necrosis factor: structural analysis of the cloned genes, physical linkage and chromosomal position. *J Immunol* 1987;139:476–483.

81. Carswell EA, Old LJ, Kassel RL, Green S, Fiore N, Williamson B. An endotoxin-induced serum factor that causes necrosis of tumors. *Proc Natl Acad Sci USA* 1975;72:3666–3670.

82. Fisch H, Gifford GE. In vitro production of rabbit macrophage tumor cell cytotoxin. *Int J Cancer* 1983;32:105–112.

83. Beutler B, Cerami A. The biology of cachectin/TNF-α primary mediator of the host response. *Annu Rev Immunol* 1989;7:625–655.

84. Gamble JR, Harlan JM, Klebanoff SJ, Vadas MA. Stimulation of the adherence of neutrophils to umbilical vein endothelium by human recombinant tumor necrosis factor. *Proc Natl Acad Sci USA* 1985;82:8667–8671.

85. Tsujumoto M, Yokota S, Vilcek J, Weissman G. Tumor necrosis factor provokes superoxide anion generation from neutrophils. *Biochem Biophys Res Commun* 1986;137:1094–1100.

86. Klebanoff SJ, Vadas MA, Harlan JM, Sparks LJ, Gamble JR, Agosti JM. Stimulation of neutrophils by tumor necrosis factor. *J Immunol* 1986;36:4220–4225.

87. Scheurich P, Thoma B, Ucer U, Pfizenmaier K. Immunoregulatory activity of recombinant human tumor necrosis factor (TNF-α): induction of TNF receptors on human T cells and TNF-α-mediated enhancement of T cell responses. *J Immunol* 1987;138:1786–1790.

88. Yokota S, Geppert TD, Lipsky PE. Enhancement of antigen-and mitogen-induced human T lymphocyte proliferation by tumor necrosis factor-α. *J Immunol* 1988;140:531–536.

89. Dayer J-M, Beutler B, Cerami A. Cachectin/tumor necrosis factor stimulates collagenase and prostaglandin E₂ production by human synovial cells and dermal fibroblasts. *J Exp Med* 1985;162:2163–2168.

90. Balkwill FR. Cytokines in Cancer Therapy. Oxford: Oxford University Press, 1989.

91. Neta R, Sayers T, Oppenheim JJ. Relationship of TNF to interleukins. In: Vilcek J, Aggarwal B. eds. *TNF: structure, function and mechanisms of action.* New York: Marcel-Dekker. 1992:499.

92. Broide DH, Lotz M, Cuomo AJ. Cytokines in symptomatic asthma. *J Allergy Clin Immunol* 191;89:958–967.

93. Ohno I, Ohkawara Y, Yamauchi K, Tanno Y, Takishima T. Production of tumor necrosis factor with IgE receptor triggering from sensitized lung tissue. *Am J Respir Cell Mol Biol* 1990;3:285–289.

94. Ohkawara Y. Yamauchi K, Tanno Y, Tamura G, Ohtani H, Ohkuda K, et al. Identification of TNF producing cells in sensitized human lung after IgE receptor triggering. *Am Rev Respir Dis* 1991;143:A201.

95. Gosset P, Tsicopoulos A, Wallaert B, Vannimenus C, Joseph M, Tonnel AB, et al. Tumor necrosis factor-α and interleukin–6 production by human mononuclear phagocytes from allergic asthmatics after IgE-dependent stimulation. *Am Rev Respir Dis* 1992;146:768–774.

96. Gosset P, Tsicopoulos A, Wallaert B, Vannimenus C, Joseph M, Tonnel AB, et al. Tumor necrosis factor a and interleukin–6 production by human mononuclear phagocytes from allergic asthmatics after IgE-dependent stimulation. *Am Rev Respir Dis* 1992;146:768–774.

97. Hirano T, Yasukawa K, Harada H, et al. Complementary NA for a novel human interleukin (BSF-2) that induces B lymphocytes to produce immunoglobulin. *Nature* 1986;324:73–76.

98. Sehgal PB, Zilbertstein A, Ruggieri RM, et al. Human chromosome 7 carries the beta 2 interferon gene. *Proc Natl Acad Sci USA* 1986;83:5219-5222.

99. Van Snick J. Interleukin 6: an overview. *Annu Rev Immunol* 1990;8:253–278.

100. Vercelli D, Jabara HH, Arai K, Yokota T, Geha RS. Endogenous interleukin-6 plays an obligatory role in interleukin-4-dependent human IgE synthesis. *Eur J Immunol* 1989;19:1419–1424.

101. Hodgkin PD, Bond MW, O Garra A, Frank G, Lee F, Coffman RL, et al. Identification of IL-6 as a T cell-derived factor that enhances the proliferative response of thymocytes to IL-4 and phorbol myristate acetate. *J Immunol* 1988;141:1529–1535.

102. Bot FJ, Van Eijk L, Broeders L, Aarden LA, Lowenber B. IL-6 synergizes with M-CSF in the formation of macrophage colonies from purified human marrow progeniter cells. *Blood* 1989;73:435–437.

103. Caracciolo D, Clark SC, Rovera G. Human interleukin-6 supports granulocytic differentiation of hematopoietic progenitor cells and acts synergistically with GM-CSF. *Blood* 1989;73:666–670.

104. VanOtteren GM, Standiford TJ, Kunkel SL, Danforth JM, Burdick MD, Abruzzo LV, et al. Expression and regulation of MIP-1α by murine alveolar and peritoneal macrophages. *Am J Respir Cell Mol Biol* 1994;10:9–15.

105. Standiford TJ, Kunkel SL, Liebler JM, Burdick MD, Gilbert AR, Strieter RM. Gene expression of MIP-1α from human blood monocytes and AMs is inhibited by interleukin-4. *Am J Respir Cell Mol Biol* 1993;9:192–198.

106. Brown KS, Zurawski T, Mosmann, Zuraski G. A family of small inducible proteins secreted by leukocytes are members of a new superfamily that includes leukocyte and fibroblast-derived inflammatory agents, growth factors and indicators of various activation processes. *J Immunol* 1989;142:679–687.

107. Cherwinski HM, Schumacher JH, Brown KD, Mosmann TR. Two types of mouse helper T cell clone. III. Further differences in lymphokine synthesis between TH1 and TH2 clones revealed by RNA hybridization, functionally monospecific bioassays and monoclonal antibodies. *J Exp Med* 1987;166:1229–1239.

108. Fong TAT, Mosmann TR. Alloreactive murine CD8- T cell clones secrete the TH1 pattern of cytokines. *J Immunol* 1990;144:1744–1752.

109. Burdick MD, Kunkel SL, Lincoln PM, Wilke CA, Strieter RM. Specific ELISAs for the detection of human macrophage inflammatory protein-1a and b. *Immunol Invest* 1993;22:441–449.

110. Standiford TJ, Kunkel SL, Liebler JM, Burdick MD, Gilbert AR, Strieter RM. Gene expression of MIP-1α from human blood monocytes and AMs is inhibited by interleukin-4. *Am J Respir Cell Mol Biol* 1993;9:192–198.

111. Danforth JM, Strieter RM, Kunkel SL, Arenberg DA, VanOtteren GM, Standiford TJ. Macrophage inflammatory protein-1 α expression *in vivo* and *in vitro*: the role of lipoteichoic acid. *Clin Immunol Immunopathol* 1995;74:77–83.

112. Martin CA, Dorf ME. Differential regulation of interleukin-6, macrophage inflammatory protein-1, and JE/MCP-1 cytokine expression in macrophage cell lines. *Cell Immunol* 1991;135:245–258.

113. VanOtteren GM, Standiford TJ, Kunkel SL, Danforth JM, Burdick MD, Abruzzo LV, et al. Expression and regulation of MIP-1α by murine alveolar and peritoneal macrophages. *Am J Respir Cell Mol Biol* 1994;10:9–15.

114. Schall TJ, Bacon K, Camp RD, Kaspazri JW, Goeddel DV. Human MIP-a and MIP-1b chemokines attract distinct populations of lymphocytes. *J Exp Med* 1993;177:1821–1826.

115. Taub D, Conlon K, Lloyd A, Oppenheim J, Kelvin D. Preferential migration of activated CD4- and CD8- T cells in response to MIP-1α. *Science* 1993;260:355–358.

116. Rot A, Krieger M, Brunner T, Bischoff SC, Schall TJ, Dahinden CA. RANTES and macrophage inflammatory protein 1 α induce the migration and activation of normal human eosinophil granulocytes. *J Exp Med* 1992;176:1489–1495.

117. Leonard EJ, Skeel A, Yoshimura T, Noer K, Kutvirt S, Van Epps D. Leukocyte specificity and binding of human neutrophil attractant/activation protein-1. *J Immunol* 1990;144:1323–1330.

118. Bischoff SC, Krieger M, Brunner T, et al. RANTES and related chemokines activate human basophil granulocytes through different G-protein-coupled receptors. *Eur J Immunol* 1993;23:761–767.

119. Oppenheim JJ, Zachariae COC. Properties of the novel proinflammatory supergene intercrine cytokine family. *Annu Rev Immunol* 1991;9:617–648.

120. Alam R, Forsythe PA, Stafford S, Lett BM, Grant JA. Macrophage inflammatory protein-1a activates basophils and mast cells. *J Exp Med* 1992;176:781–786.

121. Fahey T, Tracey KJ, Tekamp OP, Cousens LS, Jones WG, Shires GT, et al. Macrophage inflammatory protein-1 modulates macrophage function. *J Immunol* 1992;148:2764–2769.

122. Yoshimura T, Yuhki N, Moore SK, Appella E, Lerman MI, Leonard EJ. Human MCP-1. Full-length cDNA cloning, expression in mitogen-stimulated blood mononuclear leukocytes, and sequence similarity to mouse competence gene JE. *Febs Lett* 1989;244:487–493.

123. Rollins BJ, Yoshimura T, Leonard EJ, Pober JS. Cytokine-activated human endothelial cells synthesize and secrete a monocyte chemoattractant, MCP-1/JE. *Am J Pathol* 1990;136:1229–1233.

124. Valente AJ, Graves DT, Vialle VC, Delgado R, Schwartz CJ. Purification of a monocyte chemotactic factor secreted by nonhuman primate vascular cells in culture. *Biochemistry* 1988;27:4162–4168.

125. Rolfe MW, Kunkel SL, Standiford TJ, Orringer MB, Phan SH, Evanoff HL. Expression and regulation of human pulmonary fibroblast–derived monocyte chemotactic peptide-1. *Am J Physiol* 1992;L536–L545.

126. Paine R III, Rolfe MW, Standiford TJ, Burdick MD, Rollins BJ, Strieter RM. MCP-1 expression by rat type II alveolar epithelial cells in primary culture. *J Immunol* 1993;150:4561–4570.

127. Brieland JK, Jones ML, Clarke SJ, Baker JB, Warren JS, Fantone JC. Effect of acute inflammatory lung injury on the expression of monocyte chemoattractant protein-1 (MCP-1) in rat pulmonary AMs. *Am J Respir Cell Mol Biol* 1992;7:134–139.

128. Christensen PJ, Rolfe MW, Standiford TJ, Burdick MD, Toews GB, Strieter RM. Characterization of the production of monocyte chemoattractant protein-1 and IL-8 in an allogeneic immune response. *J Immunol* 1993;151:1205–1213.

129. Carr MW, Roth SJ, Luther E, Rose SS, Springer TA. Monocyte chemoattractant protein-1 acts as a T-lymphocyte chemoattractant. *Proc Natl Acad Sci USA* 1994;91:3652–3656.

130. Abdelaziz MM, Devalia JL, Khair OA, Calderon M, Sapsford RJ, Davies RJ. The effect of conditioned medium from cultured human bronchial epithelial cells on eosinophil and neutrophil chemotaxis and adherence in vitro. *Am J Respir Cell Mol Biol* 1995;13:728–737.

131. Kwon OJ, Jose PH, Robbins RA, Schall TJ, Williams TJ, Barnes PJ. Glucocorticoid inhibition of RANTES expression in human lung epithelial cells. *Am J Respir Cell Mol Biol* 1995;12:488–496.

132. Stellato, C, Beck LA, Gorgone GA, Proud D, Schall TJ, Ono SJ, et al. Expression of the chemokine RANTES by a human bronchial epithelial cell line. Modulation by cytokines and glucocorticoids. *J Immunol* 1995;155:410–418.

133. Marfaing-Koka A, Devergne O, Gorgone G, Portier A, Schall TJ, Galanaud P, et al. Regulation of the production of the RANTES chemokine by endothelial cells. Synergistic induction by IFN-γ plus TNF-α and inhibition by IL-4 and IL-13. *J Immunol* 1995;154:1870–1878.

134. Schall TJ, Bacon K, Toy KJ, Goeddel DV. Selective attraction of monocytes and T lymphocytes of the memory phenotype by cytokine RANTES. *Nature* 1990;347:669–671.

135. Taub DD, Lloyd AR, Wang JM, Oppenheim JJ, Kelvin DJ. The effects of human recombinant MIP-1α, MIP-1β and RANTES on the chemotaxis and adhesion of T cell subsets. *Adv Exp Med Biol* 1993;351:139–146.

136. Meurer R, Van RG, Feeney W, Cunningham P, Hora DJ, Springer MS, et al. Formation of eosinophilic and monocytic intradermal inflammatory sites in the dog by injection of human RANTES but not human monocyte chemoattractant protein 1, human macrophage inflammatory protein 1α, or human interleukin 8. *J Exp Med* 1993;178:1913–1921.

137. Alam R, Stafford S, Forsythe P, Harrison R, Faubion D, Lett BM, et al. RANTES is a chemotactic and activating factor for human eosinophils. *J Immunol* 1993;3442–3448.

138. Baggiolini M, Walz A, Kunkel SL. NeutrophIL-αctivating peptide-1/interleukin 8, a novel cytokine that activates neutrophils. *J Clin Invest* 1989;94:1045–1049.

139. Strieter RM, Kunkel SL, Showell HJ, et al. Endothelial cell gene expression of a neutrophil chemotactic factor by TNF-α, LPS, and IL-1β. *Science* 1989;243:1467–1469.

140. Standiford TJ, Kunkel SL, Basha MA, Chensue SW, Lynch JP III, Toews GB, et al. Interleukin-8 gene expression by a pulmonary peithelial cell line: a model for cytokine networks in the lung. *J Clin Invest* 1990;86:1945–1953.

141. Kwon OJ, Collins PD, Au B, Adcock M, Yacoub M, Chung KF, et al. Glucocorticoid inhibition of TNFα-induced IL-8 gene expression in human primary cultured epithelial cells. *Immunology* 1994;81:379–394.

142. Smart SJ, Casale TB. Interleukin-8-induced transcellular neutrophil migration is facilitated by endothelial and pulmonary epithelial cells. *Am J Respir Cell Mol Biol* 1993;9:489–495.

143. Erger RA, Casale TB. Interleukin-8 (IL-8) is a potent mediator of eosinophil chemotaxis through endothelium and epithelium. *Am J Physiol* 1995;268:L117–L122.

144. Oppenheim JJ, Zachariae COC, Mukaida W, Matsushima K. Properties of the novel proinflammatory supergene intercrine cytokine family. *Annu Rev Immunol* 1991;9:617–648.

145. Huber AR, Kunkel SL, Todd RF III, Weiss SJ. Regulation of transendothelial neutrophil migration by endogenous interleukin-8. *Science* 1991;254:99–102.

146. Stern AS, Podlaski FJ, Hulmes JD, Pan YE, Quinn PM, Wolitzky AG, et al. Purification to homogeneity and partial characterization of cytotoxic lymphocyte maturation factor from human B-lymphoblastoid cells. *Proc Natl Acad Sci USA* 1990;87:6808–6812.

147. Kobayashi M, Fitz L, Ryan M, Hewick RM, Clark SC, Chan S, et al. Identification and purification of natural killer cell stimulatory factor (NKSF), a cytokine with multiple biological effects on human lymphocytes. *J Exp Med* 1989;170:827–845.

148. Sieburth D, Jabs EW, Warrington JA, Li X, Lasota J, LaForgia S, et al. Assignment of genes encoding a unique cytokine (IL-12) composed of two unrelated subunits to chromosomes 3 and 5. *Genomics* 1992;14:59–62.

149. D Andrea A, Rengaraju M, Valiante NM, Chehimi J, Kubin M, Aste M, et al. Production of natural killer cell stimulatory factor (interleukin-12) by peripheral blood mononuclear cells. *J Exp Med* 1992;176:1387–1398.

150. Perussia B, Chan SH, D Andrea A, Tsuji K, Santoli D, Pospisil M. Natural killer (NK) cell stimulatory factor or IL-12 has differential effects on proliferation of TCR-αβ⁺, TCR-γδ⁺ T lymphocytes and NK cells. *J Immunol* 1992;149:3495–3502.

151. Chan SH, Perussia B, Gupta JW, Kobayashi M, Pospisil M, Young HA, et al. Induction of interferon-γ production by natural killer cell stimulatory factor: characterization of the responding cells and synergy with other inducers. *J Exp Med* 1991;173:869–879.

152. Naume B, Johnsen A-C, Espevik T, Sundan A. Gene expression and secretion of cytokines and cytokine receptors from highly purified CD56⁻ natural killer cells stimulated with interleukin-2, interleukin-7 and interleukin-12. *Eur J Immunol* 1993;23:1831–1838.

153. Hsieh C-S, Macatonia SE, Tripp CS, Wolf SF, O Garra A, Murphy KM. Development of Th1 CD4- T cells through IL-12 produced by Listeria-induced macrophages. *Science* 1993;260:547–549.

154. Manetti R, Parronchi P, Giudizi MG, Piccinni M-P, Maggi E, Trinchieri G, et al. Natural killer cell stimulatory factor (interleukin 12 [IL-12]) induces T helper type 1 (TH1)-specific immune response and inhibits the development of IL-4-producing Th cells. *J Exp Med* 1993;177:1199–1204.

155. Kiniwa M, Gately M, Gubler U, Chizzonite R, Fargeas C, Delespesse G. Recombinant interleukin-12 suppresses the synthesis of IgE by interleukin-4 stimulated human lymphocytes. *J Clin Invest* 1992;90:262–266.

156. Morris SC, Madden KB, Adamovicz JJ, Gause WC. Hubbard B, Gately M, et al. Effects of interleukin-12 on *in vivo* cytokine gene expression and Ig isotype selection. *J Immunol* 1994;152:1047–1056.

157. Fiorentino DF, Bond MW, Mosmann TR. Two types of mouse T helper cell. IV. Th2 clones secrete a factor that inhibits cytokine production by Th1 clones. *J Exp Med* 1989;170:2081–2095.

158. deWaal Malefyt R, Abrams J, Bennett B, Figdor CG, de Vries JE. Interleukin-10 (IL-10) inhibits cytokine synthesis by human monocytes: an autoregulatory role of IL-10 produced by monocytes. *J Exp Med* 1991;174:1209–1220.

159. Fiorentino DF, Zlotnik A, Mosmann TR, Howard M, O Garra A. IL-10 inhibits cytokine production by activated macrophages. *J Immunol* 1991;147:3815–3822.

160. LeGros G, Ben-Sasson SZ, Seder R, Finkelman FD, Paul WE. Generation of interleukin 4 (IL-4)-producing cells *in vivo* and *in vitro*: IL-2 and IL-4 are required for in vitro generation of IL-4-producing cells *J Exp Med* 1990;172:921–929.

161. Thompson-Snipes L, Dhar v, Bond MW, Mosmann TR, Moore KW, Rennick DM. Interleukin 10: a novel stimulatory factor for mast cells and their progenitors. *J Exp Med* 1991;173:507–510.

162. Go NF, Castle BE, Barrett R, Kastelein R, Dang W, Mosmann TR, et al. Interleukin-10, a novel B cell stimulatory factor: unresponsiveness of X chromosome-linked immunodeficiency B cells. *J of Exp Med* 1990;172:1625–1631.

163. Rousset F, Garcia E, Defrance T, Peronne C, Vezzio N, Hsu DH, et al. Interleukin-10 is a potent growth and differentiation factor for activated human B lymphocytes. *Proc Natl Acad Sci USA* 1992;89:1890–1893.

164. Roberts AB, Sporn MB. In: *Peptide growth factors and their receptors*. Sporn MB, Roberts AB eds. Springer-Verlag, Heidelberg 1990;421–472.

165. Shull MM, Ormsby I, Kier AB, Pawlowski S, Diebold RJ, Yin M, et al. Targeted disruption of the mouse transforming growth factor-β 1 gene results in multifocal inflammatory disease *Nature* 1992;359:693–699.

166. Eisenberg SP, Evans RJ, Arend WPL, Verderber E, Brewer MT, Hannum CH, et al. Primary structure and functional expression from complementary DNA of a human interleukin-1 receptor antagonist. *Nature* 1990;343:341–346.

167. Carter DB, Deibel MR, Dunn CJ, et al. Purification, cloning expression and biological characterization of an interleukin-1 receptor antagonist protein. *Nature* 1990;344:633–638.

168. Hannum CH, Wilcox CJ, Arend WP, et al. Interleukin-1 receptor antagonist activity of a human interleukin-1 inhibitor. *Nature* 1990;343:336.

169. Vannier E, Dinarello CA. Histamine enhances interleukin (IL-1)-induced IL-1 gene expression and protein synthesis via H2 receptors in peripheral blood mononuclear cells. Comparison with IL-1 receptor antagonist. *J Clin Invest* 1993;92:281–287.

170. Eisenberg SP, Evans RJ, Arend WP, Verderber E, Brewer MT, Hannum, et al. Primary structure and functional expression from complementary DNA of a human interleukin-1 receptor antagonist. *Nature* 1990;343:341–346.

171. Yang YC, Kovacic S, Kriz R, Wolf S, Clark SC, Wellems TE, et al. The human genes for GM-CSF and IL-3 are closely linked in tandem on chromosome 5. *Blood* 1988;71:958–961.

172. Metcalf D. *The colony-stimulating factors*. Elsevier, Amsterdam 1984.

173. Thorens B, Mermod JJ, Vassalli P. Phagocytosis and inflammatory

stimuli induce GM-CSF mRNA in macrophages through posttranscriptional regulation. *Cell* 1987;48:671–679.

174. Metcalf D. *The Molecular Control of Blood Cells.* Harvard University Press, Cambridge, MA 1988.

175. Burgess AW, Nicola NA, Johnson GR, Nice EC. Colony-forming cell proliferation: a rapid and sensitive assay system for murine granulocyte and macrophage colony-stimulating factors. *Blood* 1982;60: 1219–1223.

176. Colotta F, Re F, Polentarutti N, Sozzani S, Mantovani A. Modulation of granulocyte survival and programmed cell death by cytokines and bacterial products. *Blood* 1992;80:2012–2020.

177. Begley CG, Lopez AF, Nicola NA, Warren DJ, Vadas MA, Sanderson CJ, et al. Purified colony-stimulating factors enhance the survival of human neutrophils and eosinophils *in vitro*: a rapid and sensitive microassay for colony-stimulating factors. *Blood* 1986;68:162–166.

178. Yamaguchi M, Hirai K, Morita Y, Takaishi T. Ohta K, Suzuki S, et al. Hemopoietic growth factors regulate the survival of human basophils *in vitro*. *Int Arch Allergy Immunol* 1992;97:322–329.

179. Broide DH, Firestein GS. Endobronchial allergen challenge in asthma: demonstration of cellular source of granulocyte-macrophage colony-stimulating factor by *in situ* hybridization. *J Clin Invest* 1991; 88:1048–1053.

180. Broide DH, Lotz M, Cuomo AJ. Cytokines in symptomatic asthma. *J Allergy Clin Immunol* 1991;89:958–967.

181. Brown PA, Crompton GK, Greening AP. Proinflammatory cytokines in acute asthma. *Lancet* 1991;338:590–593.

182. Nakamura Y, Ozaki T, Kamgi T, Kawaji K, Banno K, Miki S, et al. Increased granulocyte-macrophage colony-stimulating factor production by mononuclear cells from peripheral blood of patients with bronchial asthma. *Am Rev Respir Dis* 1993;147:87–91.

183. Poston RN, Chanez P, Lacoste JY, Litchfield T, Lee TH, Bousquet J. Immunohistochemical characterization of the cellular infiltration in asthmatic bronchi. *Am Rev Respir Dis* 1992;145:918–921.

184. Sousa AR, Poston RN, Lane St, Nakhosteen JA, Lee TH. GM–CSF expression in bronchial epithelium of asthmatic airways: decrease by inhaled corticosteroids. *Am Rev Respir Dis* 1993;147:1557–1561.

185. Clevers H, Alarcon B, Wileman T, Terhorst C. The T cell receptor/CD3 complex: a dynamic protein ensemble. *Annu Rev Immunol* 1988; 6:629–662.

186. Sette A, Buus S, Colon S, Smith JA, Miles C, Grey HM. Structural characteristics of an antigen required for its interaction with Ia and recognition by T cells. *Nature* 1987;328:395–399.

187. Allison JP. Interactions in T cell activation. *Curr Opin Immunol* 1994; 6:414–419.

188. Germain RN. The ins and outs of antigen processing and presentation. *Nature* 1986;322:687–689.

189. Braciale T, Braciale U. Antigen presentation: structural themes and functional variations. *Immunology Today* 1991;12:124–129.

190. Brodsky FM, Guagliardi L. The cell biology of antigen processing and presentation. *Annu Rev Immunol* 1991;9:707–744.

191. Lanzavecchia A. Receptor-mediated antigen uptake and its effect on antigen presentation to Class II-restricted T lymphocytes. *Annu Rev Immunol* 1990;8:773–793.

192. van Seventer GA, Shimizu Y, Shaw S. Roles of multiple accessory molecules in T-cell activation. *Curr Opin Immunol* 1991;3:294–303.

193. Liu Y, Linsley PS. Costimulation of T-cell growth. *Curr Opin Immunol* 1992;4:265–270.

194. Sztein MB, Steeg PS, Johnson HM, Oppenheim J. Regulation of human peripheral blood monocyte DR antigen expression by lymphokines and recombinant interferons. *J Clin Invest* 1984;73:556–565.

195. Dustin ML, Springer TA. Adhesion receptor in the immune system. *Nature* 1989;341:619–624.

196. van Seventer GA, Shimizu Y, Horgan KJ, Shaw S. The LFA-1 ligand ICAM-1 provide an important costimulatory signal for T cell receptor mediated activation of resting T cells. *J Immunol* 1990;144:4579–4586.

197. Thompson CB. Distinct roles for the costimulatory ligands B7-1 and B7-2 in T helper cell differentiation. *Cell* 1995;81:979–982.

198. Weaver CT, Unanue ER. The costimulatory function of antigen-presenting cells. *Immunol Today* 1990;11:49–53.

199. Mayernik DG, Ul-Haq A, Rinehart JJ. Differentiation-associated alternation in human monocyte-macrophage accessory cell function. *J Immunol* 1983;130:2156–2160.

200. Toews GB, Vial WC, Dunn MM, et al. The accessory cell function of human AMs in specific T cell proliferation. *J Immunol* 1984;132: 181–186.

201. Lipscomb MF, Lyons CR, Nunez G, et al. Human AMs: HLA–DR-positive macrophages that are poor stimulators of a primary mixed leukocyte reaction. *J Immunol* 1986;136:497–504.

202. Lyons CR, Ball EJ, Toews GB, Weissler JC, Stastiny P, Lipscomb MF. Inability of human AMs to stimulate resting T cells correlates with decreased antigen-specific T cell-macrophage binding. *J Immunol* 1986;137:1173–1180.

203. Chelen CJ, Fang Y, Freeman GJ, Secrist H, Marshall JD, Hwang PT, et al. Human AMs present antigen ineffectively due to defective expression of B7 costimulatory cell surface molecules *J Clin Invest* 1995;95:1415–1421.

204. Liu MC, Proud D, Schleimer RP, Plaut M. Human lung macrophages enhance and inhibit lymphocyte proliferation. *J Immunol* 1984;132; 2895–2903.

205. Rich EA, Tweardy DJ, Fujiwara W, Ellner JJ. Spectrum of immunoregulatory functions and properties of human AMs. *Am Rev Respir Dis* 1987;136:258–265.

206. Thepen T, Van Rooijen N, Kraal G. Alveolar macrophage elimination in vivo is associated with an increase in pulmonary immune responses in mice. *J Exp Med* 1989;170:494–509.

207. Thepen T, McMenamin C, Oliver J, Kraal G, Holt PG. Regulation of immune responses to inhaled antigen by AMs (AM): differential effects of AM elimination in vivo on the induction of tolerance versus immunity. *Eur J Immunol* 1991;21:2845–2850.

208. Thepen T, McMenamin C, Girn B, Kraal G, Holt PG. Regulation of IgE production in presensitized animals: in vivo elimination of AMs selectively increases IgE responses to inhaled allergen. *Clin Exp Allergy* 1992;22:1107–1114.

209. Bilyk N, Holt PG. Inhibition of the immunosuppressive activity of resident pulmonary AMs by granulocyte macrophage colony-stimulating factors. *J Exp Med* 1993;177:1773–1777.

210. Steinman RM. The dendritic cell system and its role in immunogenicity. *Ann Rev Immunol* 1991;9:271–296.

211. Venet A, Hance AJ, Saltini C, Robinson BWS, Crystal RG. Enhanced alveolar macrophage-mediated antigen-induced T lymphocyte proliferation in sarcoidosis. *J Clin Invest* 1985;75:293–301.

212. Rich EA, Tweardy DJ, Fujiwara W, Ellner JJ. Spectrum of immunoregulatory functions and properties of human AMs. *Am Rev Respir Dis* 1987;136:258–265.

213. Aubus P, Cosso B, Godard P, Miche FB, Clot J. Decreased suppressor cell activity of AMs in bronchial asthma. *Am Rev Respir Dis* 1984; 130:875–878.

214. Spiteri MA, Knight RA, Jeremy JY, Barnes PJ, Chung KF. Alveolar macrophage-induced suppression of T-cell hyperresponsiveness in asthma is reversed following allergen exposure in vitro. *Eur Respir J* 1994;7:1431–1438.

215. Fischer HG, Frosch S, Reske K, Reske-Kunz AB. Granulocyte-macrophage colony-stimulating factor activates macrophages derived from bone marrow cultures to synthesis of Mhc class II molecules and to augment antigen presentation function. *J Immunol* 1988;141:3882–3888.

216. Robinson DS, Hamid Q, Ying S, Tsigopoulos A, Barkans T, Bentley AM, et al. Predominant TH2-type bronchoalveolar lavage T-lymphocyte population in atopic asthma. *N Engl J Med* 1992;326:298–304.

217. Mossman TR, Coffman RL. TH1 and TH2 cells: different patterns of lymphokine secretion lead to different functional properties. *Annu Rev Immunol* 1989;7:145–173.

218. Schmitz J, Assenmacher M, Radbruch A.. Regulation of T helper cytokine expression: functional dichotomy of antigen presenting cells. *Eur J Immunol* 1993;23:191–199.

219. Gajewski TF, Pinnas M, Wong T, Fitch FW. Murine TH1 and TH2 clones proliferate optimally in response to distinct antigen-presenting cell populations. *J Immunol* 1991;146:1750–1758.

220. Hauser C, Snapper CM, O Hara J, Paul WE, Katz SL. T–helper cells grown with hapten-modified cultured Langerhans cells produce interleukin-4 and stimulate IgE production by B-cells. *Eur J Immunol* 1989;19:245–251.

221. Racioppi L. Ronchese F, Matis LA, Germain R. Peptide-major histocompatibility complex class II complexes with mixed agonist/antagonist properties provide evidence for ligand-related differences in T

cell receptor-dependent intracellular signaling. *J Exp Med* 1993;177: 1047–1060.

222. Pfeiffer C, Stein J, Southwood S, Ketelaar H, Sette A, Bottomly K. Altered peptide ligands can control CD4 T lymphocyte differentiation in vivo. *J Exp Med* 1995;181:1569–1574.

223. Freeman GJ, Boussiotis VA, Anumanthan A, Bernstein GM, Ke XY, Rennert PD, et al. B7-1 and B7-2 do not deliver identical costimulatory signals, since B7-2 but not B7-1 preferentially costimulates the initial production of IL-4. *Immunity* 1995;2:523–532.

224. Bluestone JA. New perspective of CD28-B7-mediated T cell costimulation. *Immunity* 1995;2:555–559.

225. Ding L. Shevach EM. Activation of CD4+ T cells by delivery of the B7 costimulatory signal on bystander antigen-presenting cells (trans-costimulation). *Eur J Immunol* 1994;24:859–866.

226. Seder RA, Gazzinelli R, Sher A, Paul WE. IL-12 acts directly on CD4- T cells to enhance priming for IFN-γ production and diminishes IL-4 inhibition of such priming. *Proc Natl Acad Sci USA* 1993;90: 10188–10192.

227. Nabors GS, Afonso LCC, Farrell JP, Scott P. Switch from type 2 to type 1 T helper cell response and cure of established Leishmania major infection in mice is induced by combined therapy with IL-12 and Pentostam. *Proc Natl Acad Sci USA* 1995;92:3142–3146.

228. Hilkens CM, Vermeulen H, Van Neerven RJ, Snijdewint FG, Wierenga EA, Kapsenberg ML. Differential modulation of T helper type 1 (TH1) and T helper type 2 (TH2) cytokine secretion by prostaglandin E2 critically depends on interleukin-2. *Eur J Immunol* 1995;25:59–63.

229. Van der Heijden FL, Van Neerven RJI, Van Katwijk M, Bos JD, Kapsenberg ML. Serum-IgE-facilitated allergen presentation in atopic disease. *J Immunol* 1993;150:3643–3650.

230. Butcher EC. Leukocyte-endothelial cell recognition: Three (or more) steps to specificity and diversity. *Cell* 1991;67:1033–1036.

231. Lawrence MB, Springer TA. Leukocytes roll on a selectin at physiologic flow rates: distinction from and prerequisite for adhesion through integrins. *Cell* 1991;65:859–873.

232. Carlos TM, Harlan JH. Leukocyte-endothelial adhesion molecules. *Blood* 1994;84:2068–2101.

233. Picker LJ, Wrnock RA, Burns AR, Doerschuk CM, Berg EL, Butcher EC. The neutrophil selectin LECAM-1 presents carbohydrate ligands to the vascular selectins ELAM-1 and GMP-140. *Cell* 1991;66:921–933.

234. Springer TA. Adhesion receptors of the immune system. *Nature* 1990; 346:425–434.

235. Gundel RH, Wegner CD, Torcellini CA, Clarke CC, Haynes N. Rothlein R, et al. Endothelial leukocyte adhesion molecule-1 mediates antigen-induced acute airway inflammation and late-phase airway obstruction in monkeys. *J Clin Invest* 1991;88:1407–1411.

236. Gundel RH, Wegner CD, Torcellini CA, Letts LG. The role in intercellular adhesion molecule-1 in chronic airway inflammation. *Clin Exp Allergy* 1992;22:569–575.

237. Wegner CD, Gundel RH, Reilly P, Haynes N, Letts LG, Rothlein R. Intercellular adhesion molecule-1 (ICAM-1) in the pathogenesis of asthma. *Science* 1990;247:456–459.

238. Montefort S, Roche WR, Howarth PH, Djukanovic R, Gratziou C, Carroll M, et al. Intercellular adhesion molecule-1 (ICAM-1) and endothelial leucocyte adhesion molecule-1 (ELAM-1) expression in the bronchial mucosa of normal and asthmatic subjects. *Eur Respir J* 1992;5:815–823.

239. Georas SN, Liu MC, Newman W, Beall LD, Stealey BA, Bochner BS. Altered adhesion molecule expression and endothelial cell activation accompany the recruitment of human granulocytes to the lung after segmental antigen challenge. *Am J Respir Cell Mol Biol* 1992;7:261–269.

240. Tosi MF, Stark JM, Smith CW, Hamedani A, Gruenert DC, Infeld MD. Induction of ICAM-1 expression on human airway epithelial cells by inflammatory cytokines: effects on neutrophil-epithelial cell adhesion. *Am J Respir Cell Mol Biol* 1992;7:214–221.

241. Reid GK, Kargman S, Vickers PJ, Mancini JA, Leveille C, Ethier D, et al. Correlation between expression of 5-lipoxygenase-activating protein. 5-lipoxygenase and cellular leukotriene synthesis. *J Biol Chem* 1990;265:10980–10988.

242. Ferreri NR, Howalnd WC, Spiegelberg HL. Release of leukotrienes C_4 and B_4 and prostaglandin E_2 from human monocytes stimulated with aggregated IgG, IgA, and IgE. *J Immunol* 1986;136:4188–4193.

243. Fels AO, Pawlowski NA, Cramer EB, King TK, Cohn ZA, Scott WA. Human AMs produce leukotriene B4. *Proc Natl Acad Sci USA* 1982; 79:7866–7870.

244. Martin TR, Raugi G, Merritt TL, Henderson WR Jr. Relative contribution of leukotriene B_4 to the neutrophil chemotactic activity produced by the resident human alveolar macrophage. *J Clin Invest* 1987; 80:1114–1124.

245. Martin T, Pistorese B, Chi E, Goodman R, Matthay M. Effect of leukotriene B_4 in the human lung: recruitment of neutrophils into the alveolar spaces without a change in protein permeability. *J Clin Invest* 1989;84:1609–1019.

246. Phan S, McGarry B, Loeffler K, Kunkel S. Regulation of macrophage-derived fibroblast growth factor release by arachidonate metabolites. *J Leuk Biol* 1987;42:106–113.

247. Phan S, McGarry B, Loeffler K, Kunkel S. Binding of leukotriene C_4 to rat lung fibroblasts and stimulation of collagen synthesis in vitro. *Biochemistry* 1988;27:2846–2853.

248. Haynes AR, Shaw RJ. Dexamethasone-induced increased in platelet-derived growth factor (B) mRNA in human AMs and myelomonocytic HL60 macrophage-like cells. *Am J Respir Cell Mol Biol* 1992;7:198–206.

249. Rose R, Raines EW, Bowen-Pope DF. The biology of platelet-derived growth factor. *Cell* 1986;46:155–169.

250. Moses HL, Yang EL, Pietenpol JA. TGFb stimulation and inhibition of cell proliferation: new mechanistic insights. *Cell* 1990;63:245–247.

251. Strieter RM, Polverini PJ, Kunkel SL, Arenberg DA, Burdick MD, Kasper J, et al. The functional role of the ELR motif in CXC chemokine mediated angiogenesis. *J Biol Chem* 1995;270:27348–27357.

Asthma, edited by P.J. Barnes, M.M. Grunstein,
A.R. Leff, and A.J. Woolcock.
Lippincott–Raven Publishers, Philadelphia © 1997.

▪ 30 ▪

Eosinophils

Mary E. Strek and Alan R. Leff

Airway inflammation currently is thought to be the common pathophysiologic abnormality that results in the syndrome of asthma. The eosinophil is the inflammatory cell that uniquely characterizes the airway inflammation found in asthma. Experimental evidence suggests that eosinophils cause airway smooth muscle contraction, airway hyperresponsiveness, and inflammatory cell chemotaxis, similar to that noted in asthmatic patients. In this chapter, the immunobiology of eosinophils, including their morphology, intracellular protein constituents, and inflammatory products that are synthesized *de novo*, are discussed. In addition, the wealth of new information about eosinophil adhesion receptors, and factors that control their migration and activation, are covered in detail. These topics are considered in the context of airway hyperresponsiveness and asthma. The role of current asthma therapy in treating eosinophilic airway inflammation in patients with asthma also is discussed. Understanding the immunobiology of the eosinophil is an important key to understanding and treating the pathophysiologic abnormalities found in asthma.

M. E. Strek and A. R. Leff: Department of Medicine, Section of Pulmonary and Critical Care Medicine, University of Chicago, Chicago, Illinois 60637.

MORPHOLOGY AND CONSTITUENTS

Eosinophils are granulocytes with unique cytoplasmic granules that stain with eosin—hence their name. They are primarily tissue cells that are found in abundance in organs with a large epithelial interface and migrate preferentially to tissues exposed to the external environment, in particular the gastrointestinal and respiratory tracts. They secrete both unique preformed intracellular proteins and newly synthesized inflammatory mediators. They are produced in the bone marrow under the influence of cytokines that act as hemopoietins for eosinophils.

Morphology

Eosinophils are the same size as neutrophils but have bilobed nuclei and characteristic cytoplasmic granules (Fig. 1). Eosinophil granules include primary granules, specific secondary granules, smaller granules, and microgranules (1–3). These granules are present in the mature eosinophil and have different functions based on the proteins they contain (Table 1). Primary granules are round, homogeneously electron dense, lack a crystalloid core, and are noted early in eosinophil maturation (1,2,4). Some primary granules may become smaller cytoplasmic bodies that contain lysophospholipase that crystallizes to form Charcot-Leyden crystals (see below) (3,5). Secondary or

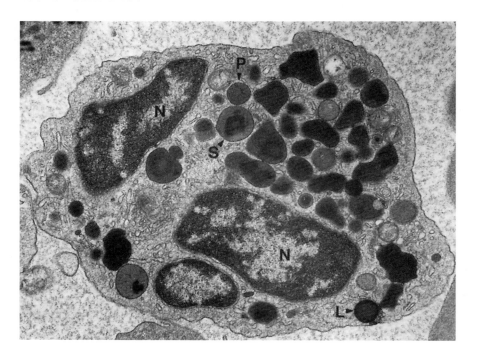

FIG. 1. Mature human eosinophil (magnification ×7,530). A mature human eosinophil has a lobulated nucleus (*N*) and cytoplasmic structures that include specific granules (*S*), with their distinctive electron-dense crystalloid core that contains major basic protein; lesser numbers of primary granules (*P*); and non-membrane-bound lipid bodies (*L*), cytoplasmic inclusions that become more numerous in cells engaged in inflammatory responses. (Courtesy of Dr. Ann M. Dvorak, Department of Pathology, Beth Israel Hospital, Harvard Medical School. From Weller PF. The immunobiology of eosinophils. *N Engl J Med* 1991;324: 1110–1118, with permission.)

specific eosinophil granules stain yellow-pink with eosin and other acid aniline dyes and allow characterization of eosinophils by light microscopy. Secondary granules have an electron-dense, crystalloid core contained in a less-electron-dense matrix. These distinct elliptical granules contain unique eosinophil proteins (see below) and lysosomal hydrolases (1). Secondary eosinophil granules typically contain one to two crystalline cores per granule (2). Small granules contain the latent inactive form of arylsulfatase and acid phosphatase in addition to other enzymes (2,6). They develop from the Golgi apparatus of the late eosinophil and increase in number as the cell matures (6). Eosinophils also contain tubulovesicular structures that previously were identified as microgranules (1). These membrane-bound C-shaped or circular-shaped cytoplasmic structures are usually empty but may play a role in cell

extrusion (3). Lipid bodies are spherical cytoplasmic structures that sometimes are mistaken for granules. They are uniformly dense non-membrane-bound osmophilic structures whose function has not been characterized fully (3,7). Lipid bodies have been shown to store and metabolize arachidonic acid (7,8). Circulating eosinophils contain more lipid bodies than neutrophils and increase in number when these cells participate in inflammatory reactions (7,9). In addition, organelles such as the rough endoplasmic reticulum, free ribosomes, a small Golgi apparatus, and mitochondria are found in eosinophils (3).

Preformed Intracellular Constituents

The eosinophil contains numerous preformed proteins, some of which have enzymatic activity. The cationic pro-

TABLE 1. *Distinct cytoplasmic structures of the human eosinophil leukocyte*

Spherical cytoplasmic structure	Appearance during differentiation	Constituents/function
Primary granule	Immature eosinophil leukocyte (promyelocyte)	Lysophosphatase
Secondary granule ("specific granule")	Mature eosinophil leukocyte	Basic proteins (MBP, ECP, EDN), hydrolases (collagenase, β-glucuronidase), eosinophil peroxidase
Small granule	Mature eosinophil leukocyte	Arylsulfatase B, acid phosphatase
Microgranules (vesiculotubular structures)	Mature eosinophil leukocyte	Transport system
Lipid bodies	Mature activated eosinophil leukocyte	Storage of unsaturated fatty acids

MBP, major basic protein; ECP, eosinophil cationic protein; EDN, eosinophil-derived neurotoxin.
From Kroegel C, Virchow JC, Luttmann W, Walker C, Warner JA. Pulmonary immune cells in health and disease: the eosinophil leukocyte (Part 1). *Eur Respir J* 1994;7:519–543, with permission.

teins of eosinophils are found in the specific or secondary granules. Major basic protein (MBP) makes up the crystalloid core of the secondary granule. The matrix of the secondary granule contains eosinophil cationic protein (ECP), eosinophil-derived neurotoxin (EDN), and eosinophil peroxidase (EPO) (10). These proteins are cloned and extensively studied (Table 2). Another protein unique to eosinophils is the lysophospholipase protein that forms Charcot-Leyden crystals that is found in the primary granule. Proteins that function as enzymes include EPO, collagenase, β-glucuronidase—all found in the secondary granule—and arylsulfatase B and acid phosphatase, which are constituents of the small granule (1,3).

Major Basic Protein

MBP accounts for the majority of the granular protein found in eosinophils (2,11). The mature protein has a molecular weight of 14,000 Da and consists of a single polypeptide chain of 117 amino acids rich in arginine (12,13). Its name reflects that it is a basic protein with an isoelectric point (pI) that is too high to measure but is calculated at 10.9 (12). Human MBP is localized mainly to

the core of the eosinophil secondary granule and is not found in other eosinophil organelles, plasma cells, mast cells, lymphocytes, or neutrophils (10). The 3.3-kilobase (kb) MBP gene consists of five introns and has been localized to chromosome 11 (12,14). Analysis of the approximately 900-nucleotide complementary deoxyribonucleic acid (cDNA) for human MBP messenger ribonucleic acid (mRNA) suggests that MBP is translated as a preproprotein with an acidic pro portion (12). It is thought that pro-MBP is translated as a relatively neutral (calculated pI is 6.2) precursor to protect the eosinophil from the toxic effects of mature MBP prior to its sequestration in the granule core (12). MBP does not have enzymatic function. It can neutralize the effect of heparin on blood clotting (2) and is bactericidal (15). While MBP is toxic to helminthic parasites, tumor cells, and other mammalian cells and may play a critical role in host defense against parasitic infections, current interest in MBP stems from recent evidence of its toxicity toward airway epithelial cells and localization to the airways of asthmatic patients (12,16). It has been shown to damage guinea-pig tracheal epithelium (17), to cause lysis of human type II pneumocytes *in vitro* (18), and to reduce ciliary beat frequency and activity on

TABLE 2. *Some properties of human eosinophil granule proteins and their cDNAs and genes*

Protein	Site	Molecular weight $\times 10^{\cdot3}$	pI[a]	Activities	cDNA	Gene	Chromosome
						Molecular biology	
MBP	Core	14	10.9	(1) Potent helminthotoxin and cytotoxin, (2) causes histamine release from basophils and rat mast cells, (3) neutralizes heparin, (4) bactericidal, and (5) causes bronchial constriction and hyperreactivity	~900 NT (prepro-MBP)	3.3 kb, 5 introns	11
ECP	Matrix	21	10.8	(1) Potent helminthotoxin, (2) potent neurotoxin, (3) inhibits cultures of peripheral blood lymphocytes, (4) causes histamine release from rat mast cells, (5) weak RNase activity, and (6) bactericidal	~725 NT (pre-ECP)	~1.2 kb, 1 intron in UTR	14
EDN	Matrix	18–19	8.9	(1) Potent neurotoxin, (2) inhibits cultures of peripheral blood lymphocytes, (3) potent RNase activity, and (4) weak helminthotoxin	~725 NT (pre-EDN)	~1.2 kb, 1 intron in UTR	14
EPO	Matrix	71–77	10.8	In the presence of H_2O_2 + halide: (1) kills microorganisms and tumor cells, (2) causes histamine release from rat mast cells, (3) inactivates leukotrienes, (4) can kill *Brugia* microfilariae and damage respiratory epithelium even in absence of H_2O_2, and (5) may contribute to bronchial hyperreactivity	~2,500 NT (2,106-NT ORF)	12 kb, 11 introns	17 (preliminary observation)

ECP, eosinophil cationic protein; EDN, eosinophil-derived neurotoxin; kb, kilobases; MBP, major basic protein; NT, nucleotides; ORF, open reading frame; UTR, untranslated region.

[a]Calculated from amino acid sequences deduced from the cDNAs.

From Hamann KJ, Barker RL, Ten RM, Gleich GJ. The molecular biology of eosinophil granule proteins. *Int Arch Allergy Appl Immunol* 1991;94:202–209, with permission.

the epithelial surface of rabbit tracheal explants (19). MBP stimulates prostaglandin E_2 production and chloride secretion by canine tracheal epithelium (20) and prostaglandin secretion by guinea-pig tracheal epithelial cells (21). In addition, MBP causes histamine release from peripheral blood basophils, human mononuclear cells, and rat peritoneal mast cells (2).

Eosinophil Cationic Protein

ECP has a molecular weight of 18,000 to 21,000 Da and a calculated pI of 10.8, and is located in the eosinophil matrix (10,12). Like MBP, it is a basic protein rich in arginine, but structurally it has significant homology with both EDN and pancreatic ribonuclease (11,22). The gene that encodes for ECP is about 1.2 kb and is located on chromosome 14 (12). ECP is toxic to helminthic parasites and host cells, and has bactericidal activity (1,15). Like EDN, ECP is a potent neurotoxin and has ribonuclease activity (see below) (22,23). ECP damages guinea-pig tracheal epithelium *in vitro* (24). Lymphocyte proliferation in culture is inhibited by ECP (2).

Eosinophil-Derived Neurotoxin

EDN received its name for its ability to cause cerebrocerebellar dysfunction after intracerebral injection into rabbits, the so-called Gordon phenomenon (23,25). It is an approximately 18,600-Da protein found in the matrix of the eosinophil granule and is less basic than either MBP or ECP with a calculated pI of 8.9 (10,12). As just discussed, it has some sequence homology with ECP and human liver and urinary ribonucleases (26,27). The EDN gene is located on human chromosome 14 in the same region as the gene for ECP and other human ribonucleases (12). Whereas EDN and ECP are equally neurotoxic (23), EDN has much greater ribonuclease activity but less cytotoxicity against helminthic parasites (2,22).

Eosinophil Peroxidase

Eosinophils contain a unique peroxidase, EPO, that is located in the eosinophil granule matrix (2). EPO has a molecular weight of 71,000 to 77,000 Da and consists of two polypeptides subunits of about 15,000 and 55,000 Da each (12,28). The protein is rich in arginine, leucine, and aspartic acid (2). It too is a basic protein with a calculated pI of 10.8 (12). The human gene for EPO consists of 11 introns spanning 12 kb and has tentatively been mapped to chromosome 17 (12,29). EPO is toxic to parasites and mammalian cells (24,30). Like myeloperoxidase, EPO in conjunction with hydrogen peroxide can oxidize halide ions to form reactive hypohalous acids that are toxic to helminthic and protozoan parasites, bacteria, tumor cells, and host cells (24,31–34). In these reactions, EPO prefer-

entially utilizes bromide over chloride (35,36). EPO, in conjunction with hydrogen peroxide and various halides, injures human type II pneumocytes in culture (37) and increases lung microvascular permeability in isolated rat lung (38). In addition, EPO causes rat mast cell secretion of histamine (39) and binds to mast cell granules, potentiating the bactericidal activity of EPO (31).

Charcot-Leyden Crystal Protein (Lysophospholipase)

Eosinophils also contain a hydrophobic protein that crystallizes *in vivo* and *in vitro* to form Charcot-Leyden crystals (1). This 17,000-Da protein has lysophospholipase activity and is immunochemically identical to eosinophil lysophospholipase (40). It is found in primary granules and is associated with eosinophil cell membranes (5). These hexagonal bipyramidal crystals are found in the sputum of patients with asthma (41).

Eosinophil-Associated Enzymes

In addition to the eosinophil protein EPO, eosinophils contain other enzymes. Eosinophil collagenase is a metalloprotein that hydrolyses collagen types I and III, the two main connective tissue components of human lung parenchyma (2). A number of other enzymes, including β-glucuronidase, arylsulfatase B, acetylcholinesterase, acid glycerophosphatase, adenosine triphosphatase, catalase, histaminase, and phospholipases, have been reported in the eosinophil (2).

Newly Synthesized Products

Eosinophils actively synthesize and secrete mediators with biological activity when stimulated. Lipid mediators such as platelet-activating factor (PAF) and eicosanoids, oxygen radicals, neuropeptides, and even cytokines and proteins are manufactured by eosinophils.

Lipid Mediators

Experimental evidence suggests that lipid bodies in eosinophils concentrate arachidonic acid and convert it to phospholipids and thus may be the site for processing arachidonic acid (2). Eosinophil lipoxygenation of arachidonic acid produces leukotrienes. The sulfidopeptide leukotrienes, leukotriene (LT) C_4 and its derivatives LTD_4 and LTE_4 cause airway smooth muscle contraction, mucus secretion, and vascular leak—all of which are noted in patients with asthma. Eosinophils preferentially synthesize LTC_4 (42,43). In addition, eosinophils can produce LTB_4 and prostanoids such as prostaglandin (PG) E, PGF_1, PGD_2, $PGF_{2\alpha}$, and thromboxane A_2 (44–47). Eosinophils also produce products of the 15-lipoxygenase pathway (48). These mediators are produced when the eosinophil is activated. Eosinophils generate PAF by acetylating lysophospholipids. Dose- and time-dependent increases in the activity of the enzyme that catalyzes PAF occur in response to stimulation with eosinophil chemotactic factor of anaphylaxis, formyl-methionyl-leucyl-phenylalanine (fMLP), or ionophore A23187 (49).

Oxygen Radicals

After stimulation, eosinophils generate a respiratory burst greater than would occur with an equal number of neutrophils and produce toxic oxygen radicals such as superoxide (O_2^-), hydrogen peroxide (H_2O_2), and OH^- (50–55). Both reduced nicotinamide adenine dinucleotide (NADPH) oxidase and cytochrome b559 are found in eosinophils and are thought to be responsible for catalyzing the production of these toxic radicals (52,56). In addition, both NADPH-oxidase activity and cytochrome b559 concentrations are greater in eosinophils than neutrophils.

Neuropeptides

Eosinophils may modulate regional inflammation by releasing neuropeptides. Mouse eosinophils synthesize vasoactive intestinal peptide (57) and substance P (58,59). Eosinophils may cause the release of substance P in vitro after H_1 receptor activation with histamine (3). Substance P can cause eosinophil degranulation (60).

Proteins and Cytokines

Recent evidence suggests that eosinophils carry the genetic information necessary for synthesizing proteins, including various cytokines, through which they may modulate inflammatory responses (3). Eosinophils express genes for granulocyte-macrophage colony-stimulating factor (GM-CSF), interleukin (IL)-3, and transforming growth factor (TGF)-β_1 and TGF-α as determined by studies utilizing in situ hybridization (61–64). Immunohistochemical staining of human eosinophils with monoclonal antibodies reveals that these cytokines are present; thus, translation of cytokine mRNA must be occurring (62). In addition, IL-3 and GM-CSF have been detected in ionomycin-activated eosinophil supernatants (61).

SURFACE RECEPTORS AND LIGANDS

Eosinophils are classified histologically as granulocytes and share common surface ligands and markers with many other hematopoietic cells. This belies what are fundamental differences in function of these cells. Unlike neutrophils, eosinophils are not phagocytic, and their granular contents are entirely different. Unlike lymphocytes and macrophages, eosinophils possess no capacity to process or present antigen during immune sensitization. Surface receptors and ligands on eosinophils that are often common to both neutrophils and lymphocytes direct selective chemotaxis of eosinophils to the conducting airways of patients with asthma, and the strong predominance of eosinophils over neutrophils and lymphocytes in the airways of human asthmatics suggests unique mechanisms for both chemotaxis and activation of these cells, which are minority constituents of the circulating leukocytes (65). Figure 2 summarizes some of the known surface ligands on the human eosinophil.

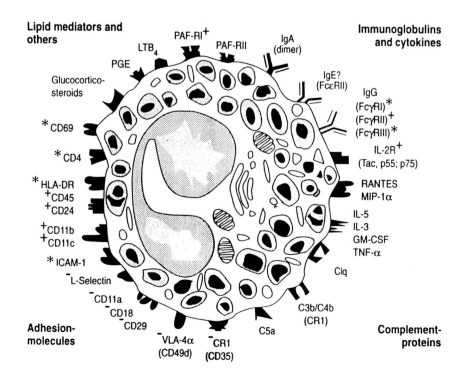

FIG. 2. Schematic representation of surface antigens identified on eosinophils. Some of the antigens are upregulated (+), downregulated (-), or induced (*) following recruitment from the circulation into tissue. The existence of an IgE receptor on eosinophils is still a matter of ongoing debate (?). CD, cluster differentiation; CR, complement receptor; FcγR, IgG receptor; GM-CSF, granulocyte–macrophage colony-stimulating factor; HLA-DR, human leukocyte antigen DR; ICAM-1, intercellular adhesion molecule 1; Ig, immunoglobulin; IL, interleukin; LTB₄, leukotriene B₄; MIP, macrophage inflammatory protein; PAF, platelet-activating factor; PAF-RI, high-affinity PAF receptor; PAF-RII, low-affinity PAF receptor; PGE, prostaglandin E; RANTES, regulated upon activation in normal T cells expressed and secreted; TNF, tumor necrosis factor; VLA, very late activation antigen. (From Kroegel C, Virchow JC, Luttmann W, Walker C, Warner JA. Pulmonary immune cells in health and disease: the eosinophil leukocyte (Part 1). Eur Respir J 1994;7: 519–543, with permission.)

Hematopoiesis

Eosinophils derive from bone marrow stem cells common to other leukocytes. Factors regulating the differential production of eosinophils have only recently been elucidated. The cytokines GM-CSF, IL-3, and IL-5 are important in promoting eosinophilopoiesis from stem cells (3,66,67). These responses can be modeled from hematopoiesis generated from human umbilical cord precursor cells (68). These highly undifferentiated cells (Fig. 3) develop into eosinophils that are functionally indistinguishable from human peripheral blood eosinophils under the influence of these cytokines. IL-5 is critically important in hematopoiesis, which is functionally complete in culture within 3 weeks; in the absence of IL-5, cell death occurs within 2 weeks. Precursor cells that develop into eosinophils are those that contain the CD34 receptor (69) (Fig. 3). Other umbilical cord stem cells that lack CD34 neither differentiate nor multiply to become eosinophils.

Development of stem cells into eosinophils also may result from interactions with matrix elements, which previously were regarded to be only structural components of the bone marrow. Hyaluronic acid causes increased proliferation and differentiation of precursor cells into eosinophils through the CD44 receptor (68). Augmented production is inhibited specifically by monoclonal antibody (mAb) directed against CD44 or through introduction of hyaluronidase into the culture medium (Fig. 4). Recent preliminary reports also suggest that heparan sulfate augments substantially the proliferation of stem cells into eosinophils through the CD31 receptor (69). This mucopolysaccharide, which exists in abundance in the environment of the bone marrow, may act by augmenting cytokine presentation (for example, IL-3 and IL-5) during the proliferation process.

Eosinophils circulate in the bloodstream after approximately 5 days of differentiation and maturation in the bone marrow with a half-life that is estimated to be 13 to 18 h (3) and then marginate along blood vessel walls or most often infiltrate tissues.

Receptors Causing Eosinophil Recruitment

The migration of eosinophils from the peripheral blood through the endothelial surface to the airway lumen is a complex process of ligation, diapedesis, and site-directed chemotaxis. Numerous specific chemotaxins have been identified, including those regulated upon activation in normal T cells expressed and secreted (RANTES) (70,71), eotaxin (72), macrophage inflammatory protein 1α (73), and IL-2 (74), and have been implicated. Eosinophils share numerous common surface ligands with the more numerous neutrophils in the circulation. These include the β_2-integrins, for example, macrophage adhesion receptor (Mac)-1 and lymphocyte function-associated antigen 1, which bind selectively to the endothelial surface ligand, intercellular adhesion molecule (ICAM) 1 (75). Recent investigations have shown that eosinophil adhesion to epithelial cells also occurs by ligation with ICAM-1 (76). Like lymphocytes, but unlike neutrophils, eosinophils also contain β_1-integrin surface ligands, which are capable of rapid binding to endothelial surface ligands (that is, vascular cell adhesion molecule [VCAM]-1) and, less rapidly, to the matrix protein, fibronectin (77). It now appears that the only β_1-integrin expressed phenotypically on the eosinophil is very late activation antigen (VLA)-4, and this expression is constitutive (77). The phenotypic expression of both VCAM-1 and ICAM-1 is upregulated by IL-1, and so the mechanism by which VLA-4 contributes to the selective migration of eosinophils (versus neutrophils) dur-

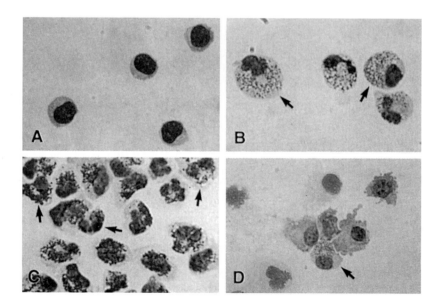

FIG. 3. Photomicrographs of **(A)** isolated (day 0) CD34$^+$ progenitor cells and cells grown in IL-3- and IL-5-stimulated cultures of **(B)** CD34$^+$ cells at day 21, **(C)** CD34$^+$ cells at day 35, and **(D)** CD34$^-$ cells at day 21. **A:** Cells are mononuclear, undifferentiated, and show no specific granulation. **B:** Bilobed nuclei and eosinophilic granulation are clearly demonstrated. Some cells (*arrows*) show less mature morphology at day 21. **C:** Differentiation to fully mature morphology (*arrows*) is complete by day 35. **D:** By contrast, there are significantly fewer eosinophils (*arrow*) differentiated from CD34$^-$ cells (compare with B). Original magnifications: A, B, C, ×600; D, ×400. *IL,* interleukin. (From Hamann KJ, Dowling TL, Neeley SP, Grant JA, Leff AR. Hyaluronic acid enhances cell proliferation during eosinopoiesis through the CD44 surface antigen. *J Immunol* 1995;154:4073–4080, with permission.)

ing asthmatic inflammation is not explained by the expression of this adhesion molecule on the eosinophil.

The process of eosinophil migration from the circulation to the lumen of conducting airways still is poorly understood. Evidence suggests that this process likely is T-helper type 2 (TH2) cell initiated (78,79). However, the actual trigger for this process is not known, and precise differences in immunologic function accounting for the pathogenesis of asthmatic airway inflammation have not been elucidated. Hence, eosinophil recruitment and corresponding airway inflammation waxes and wanes through pathogenetic triggers that still are not understood.

By whatever mechanism recruitment is triggered, the process of cellular migration is effected initially by a conversion of laminar eosinophil flow through the capillaries of the conducting airways to a rolling of these eosinophils across the endothelial surface (Fig. 5). This is modeled as a gearing of the L-selectin on the eosinophil surface to the P-selectin and E-selectin on the endothelium. This rolling causes a slowing of eosinophil flow that is terminated by strong fixation of eosinophils to the endothelial surface by ligation with β_2- and, likely, β_1-integrins on the eosinophil to endothelial ICAM-1 and VCAM-1, respec-

tively (75). Significant surface adhesion does not occur *in vitro* unless cultured endothelial cells are treated with IL-1, which upregulates both endothelial adhesion molecules (75). It is presumed that the same requirement for upregulation of endothelial ligands occurs *in vivo*, since pretreatment with anti-ICAM-1 mAb prevents eosinophil migration in *Ascaris suum*-challenged primates; this inhibition of cell migration is also accompanied by decreased airway responsiveness (80,81) (Fig. 6). However, trials to ameliorate human asthma with IL-1 antagonist have not been successful.

The process that follows fixed adhesion to the endothelial surface has been modeled largely on the behavior of neutrophils and is less well defined. Diapedesis of eosinophils through the endothelium requires cellular retraction of the endothelial junction and extreme deformation of the eosinophil (75), and the mechanism of these processes is not well understood. Once the eosinophil reaches the cellular matrix, it can bind to matrix proteins, including fibronectin, through VLA-4 (82). This is a slow process, requiring at least 60 min *in vitro*; within 120 min, eosinophils also appear to become unbound, presumably to allow for continued migration toward the lu-

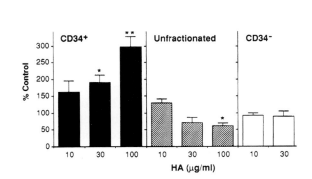
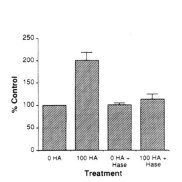
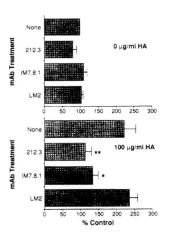

FIG. 4. Left: Effect of hyaluronic acid (*HA*) on proliferative responses of subpopulations of cord blood mononuclear cells in the presence of interleukin (IL) 3 and IL-5 as measured by total cell counts on day 21. CD34+ cell proliferation was enhanced in a dose-related fashion (*black bars*). CD34− cells were not significantly affected by HA concentration (*white bars*). Proliferation of unfractionated cells was inhibited in a dose-related fashion by HA (*hatched bars*). Values represent means ± SE of at least three separate experiments. *$p < 0.05$; **$p < 0.01$ vs. control (0 μg/mL HA) proliferation. **Middle:** Effect of hyaluronidase (*Hase*) pretreatment of control (*0 HA*) and 100-μg/mL HA-coated (*100 HA*) wells on eosinophil CD34+ progenitor cell proliferation. Proliferation in Hase-treated wells did not differ significantly from that in untreated, uncoated (0 HA) wells. Values represent mean percent of control ± SE on day 21 of four separate experiments. Similar results were obtained in three separate experiments using *Streptomyces* hyaluronidase. **Right:** Effect on antibody blockade of CD44 on CD34+ precursor cells with two anti-CD44 monoclonal antibodies (mAbs), 212.3 and IM7.8.1, and anti-CD11b mAb, LM2. **Top:** Results after pretreatment of CD34+ cells with mAbs and culture in the absence of HA. **Bottom:** Results after mAb pretreatment and culture in wells coated with 100 μg/mL HA. Values represent mean percent of control ± SE on day 21 of at least three separate experiments. *$p < 0.05$; **$p = 0.02$ vs. control (no mAb) proliferation in 100-μg/mL wells. (From Hamann KJ, Dowling TL, Neeley SP, Grant JA, Leff AR. Hyaluronic acid enhances cell proliferation during eosinopoiesis through the CD44 surface antigen. *J Immunol* 1995;154:4073–4080, with permission.)

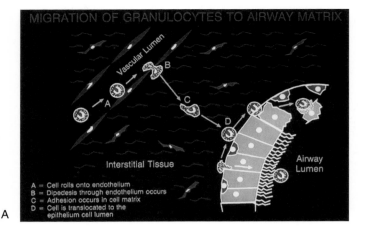

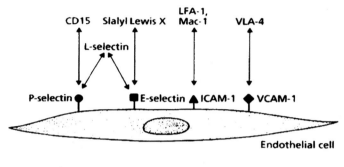

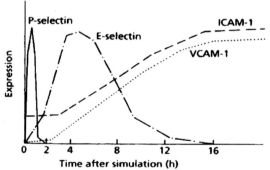

FIG. 5. Transmigration of the eosinophil into the conducting airway. **A:** Migration of granulocytes to airway matrix. Cell "rolling" is caused by interaction of P-selectin and E-selectin on the capillary endothelium to L-selectin on the eosinophil surface. Firm fixation to the endothelial surface is mediated by ICAM-1 (via β₂-integrin on the eosinophil surface) and VCAM-1 through β₁-integrin on the eosinophil. Diapedesis and migration then occur as described in text. (Drawing courtesy of Dr. K. J. Hamann, University of Chicago.) **B:** Temporal expression of adhesion molecules on the endothelial surface during early stages of migration. Note that P-selectin and E-selection, which cause initial stages of cell rolling, are first expressed. L-selectin then is shed from the eosinophil (see the text), an action of IL-5 (113). Later expression of VCAM-1 and ICAM-1 correspond to the stage of firm fixation. *ICAM-1,* intercellular adhesion molecule 1; *VCAM-1,* vascular cell adhesion molecule 1; *IL,* interleukin. (Schema from Gundel RH, et al., Leukocyte–endothelial adhesion. In: Busse WW, Holgate ST, eds. *Asthma and rhinitis.* Boston: Blackwell Scientific, 1995;752–763.)

men. Further specific ligands facilitating this process have not been identified.

CELL-CELL INTERACTIONS

Relationship Between Adhesive Ligation and Priming of Eosinophil Secretion

Although the factors that trigger eosinophil secretion are not known, there is a definite relationship between eosinophil adhesion and priming of stimulated eosinophil secretion. To date, this has been modeled largely *in vitro* using pharmacologic activators of eosinophil secretion (for example, PAF, fMLP, phorbol ester, and calcium ionophore) (44,47,50,83,84). Incubation of eosinophils for 60 min with fibronectin causes substantial augmentation of secretion of EPO (82) and LTC₄ (85) and persists beyond 120 min after eosinophils are no longer adherent. This translates directly to augmented contraction of human bronchial explants *in vitro* by a mechanism that is blocked completely by either mAb directed against VLA-4 or by 5-lipoxygenase inhibition (85). Thus, adhesion in the cellular matrix and physiologically relevant augmentation of eosinophil secretion of bronchoactive substances are intrinsically linked.

Preliminary reports also have suggested that ligation of eosinophils to the endothelium through either VLA-4 or β₂-integrin also may prime stimulated eosinophil secretion (86). However, the relative importance of each of these ligation reactions awaits confirmation. IL-5 also is capable of priming substantially eosinophil secretion. *In vitro* stimulation of eosinophils isolated from the peripheral blood of atopic subjects results in substantially augmented secretion of eosinophil granular protein (as indexed by EPO activity) as compared with nonatopic subjects (unpublished observation). This corresponds to the observation that comparable numbers of eosinophils derived from umbilical cord blood precursor cells, which are cultured in the continuous presence of IL-5 (87), cause substantially greater contraction of airway smooth muscle after activation than do cells isolated from the peripheral blood of nonatopic individuals, where circulating IL-5 concentrations are presumed to be minimal (83).

Immunologic Activation

Like mast cells, eosinophil secretion can be activated by a variety of immunoglobulin-mediated reactions. However, the pathophysiologic significance of these reactions remains to be defined. In these interactions, the eosinophil differs substantially from the neutrophil. Because eosinophils do not express the CD16 receptor, which is present on the neutrophil, they can be separated from neutrophils by negative immunoselection (88). The CD16 receptor is an immunoglobulin (Ig) G receptor of the FcᵧRIII class. Eosinophils do not express the FcᵧRI

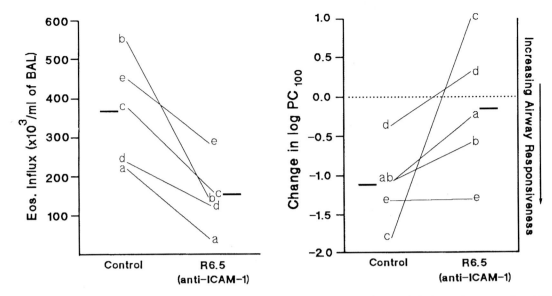

FIG. 6. Effects of monoclonal antibody R6.5 to ICAM-1 (1.76 mg · kg^{-1} · day^{-1}, i.v.) on airway eosinophilia (assessed by bronchoalveolar lavage, *BAL*) and increase in airway responsiveness (inhaled methacholine *PC$_{100}$*) induced by three alternate-day antigen inhalations by monkeys. Studies with R6.5 treatment are compared with mean of bracketing control studies with each animal. *Bars,* mean of five monkeys individually identified by letters *a* to *e*. R6.5 treatment significantly attenuated eosinophil influx when tested versus bracketing control values by two-way analysis of variance ($p = 0.0133$) and, correspondingly, significantly inhibited decrease in log PC$_{100}$ vs. pre-R6.5 control ($p = 0.0002$). *ICAM-1,* intercellular adhesion molecule 1. (From Leff AR, Hamann KJ, Wegner CD. Inflammation and cell–cell interactions in airway hyperresponsiveness. *Am J Physiol* 1991;260:L189–L206, with permission.)

(CD64) receptor but do share the Fc$_\gamma$RII (Cdw32) receptor on their membrane surface (89,90).

Prior investigations have indicated that eosinophil secretion can be stimulated by secretory IgA in substantial quantities; however, the pathophysiologic significance of this observation remains to be elucidated. The role of IgE-mediated reactions in causing eosinophil secretion is a subject of significant debate. Moqbel and co-workers (91) reported significant IgE binding to eosinophils that was augmented substantially by PAF and LTB$_4$. However, specific IgE receptors were not identified. Capron and co-workers (92,93) have identified a specific CD23 receptor on the eosinophil of the FC$_\epsilon$RII class. As these receptors are not identified consistently by mAb directed against this receptor, it has been suggested that a specific subclass of this receptor (FC$_\epsilon$RIIb) may be unique to the eosinophil (92). The concept is tantalizing, since IL-4, which stimulates IgE production from lymphocytic B cells also may upregulate this receptor (94). At present, the role of immunoglobulins in the direct regulation of eosinophil secretion in asthma remains unknown.

β-Adrenergic Regulation of Eosinophil Secretion

Yukawa and co-workers (95) first suggested from studies in guinea pigs that eosinophil secretion, like mast cell secretion, could be regulated by the β-adrenoceptor through the adenylyl cyclase/cyclic adenosine monophosphate system. Subsequent studies of human eosinophils indicated that the β$_2$-adrenoceptor caused potent downregulation of stimulated secretion of EPO and LTC$_4$ from isolated human eosinophils. This inhibition was 50% of maximal stimulated degranulation after 10^{-8} M albuterol but was not further facilitated at greater concentrations of β-adrenoceptor stimulation (96). The β-adrenoceptor of the eosinophil possesses other peculiar properties that suggest that it is either a unique receptor subtype (for example, β$_4$) or uniquely coupled to its inhibitory G protein. Treatment of isolated eosinophils with salmeterol, an extremely potent β$_2$-adrenoceptor agonist in airway smooth muscle, causes no change in intracellular cyclic adenosine monophosphate (cAMP), whereas albuterol causes a near threefold increase in cAMP (97) (Fig. 7). In like manner, pretreatment of eosinophils with salmeterol prior to administration of albuterol blocks completely the inhibitory effect of albuterol on stimulated secretion of EPO (Fig. 8).

ROLE OF EOSINOPHILS IN ASTHMA

Pathologic Evidence for Eosinophil Inflammation

The definition of asthma now includes airway inflammation (98,99). The airway inflammation found in asthma

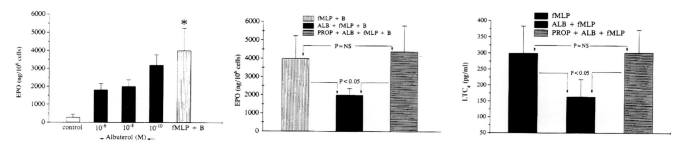

FIG. 7. Effect of β₂-adrenoceptor stimulation on eosinophil secretion caused by formyl-met-leu-phe (*fMLP*) and cytochalasin B (*B*). **Left:** Secretion of eosinophil peroxidase (*EPO*) is blocked by 10⁻⁸ M albuterol and not substantially changed with increased concentration of agonist. **Middle:** Inhibition of fMLP + B-stimulated eosinophil secretion of EPO by albuterol is blocked comparably by propranolol (*PROP*) indicating β-adrenoceptor specificity. **Right:** Leukotriene C₄ secretion, which also is inhibited comparably by albuterol, also is blocked with PROP. (From Munoz NM, Vita AJ, Neeley SP, et al. Beta adrenergic modulation of formyl–methionine–leucine–phenylalanine-stimulated secretion of eosinophil peroxidase and leukotriene C₄. *J Pharmacol Exp Ther* 1994;268:139–143, with permission.)

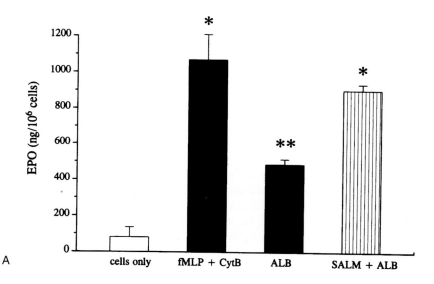

A

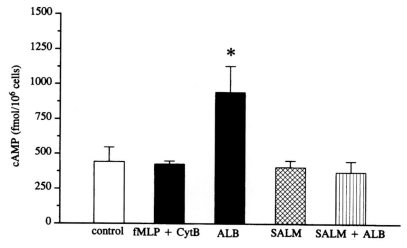

B

FIG. 8. A: Effect of SALM on EPO secretion by ALB-treated eosinophils. Eosinophils first were treated with 10⁻⁸ M SALM for 5 min before 10⁻⁸ M ALB (5 min) and fMLP + CytB (30 min) activation. *p < 0.001 vs. untreated cells; **p < 0.01 vs. fMLP + CytB (n = 4 for each group). **B:** Effect of ALB and SALM on intracellular concentration of cAMP in eosinophils. SALM blocked paradoxically the stimulatory effect on eosinophil cAMP caused by ALB. *p < 0.05 vs. individual group (n = 4 for each group). *SALM,* salmeterol; *EPO,* eosinophil peroxidase; *ALB,* albuterol; *fMLP + CytB,* formyl-met-leu-phe + cytochalasin B. (From Munoz NM, Rabe KF, Vita AJ, et al. Paradoxical blockade of beta adrenergically mediated inhibition of stimulated eosinophil secretion by salmeterol. *J Pharmacol Exp Ther* 1995;273: 850–854, with permission.)

is unique, being mediated in large part by the eosinophil rather than the neutrophil as is typical in other disease states. The pathology of asthma is characterized by eosinophil infiltration into bronchial walls and airway lumen, and airway epithelial denudation and destruction. Autopsy specimens from patients who have died of asthma reveal extensive eosinophilia lining the bronchi (100) with release of MBP from the eosinophil protein (101). Immunofluorescence studies of lung tissue from patients who have died in status asthmaticus reveal MBP in mucus plugs, in areas of necrosis below the basement membrane, and on damaged respiratory epithelial surfaces (101). As reviewed above, there is extensive evidence that the eosinophil MBP and ECP damage guinea-pig and human airway epithelium (16,17,24). Pathologically, edema may be present in the asthmatic airway, and some have proposed that this edema contributes to airway narrowing in asthma (102,103). Two studies of isolated perfused rat lungs demonstrated that activated eosinophils can cause significant lung edema (104,105) associated with epithelial injury (104) and increased peak airway pressures (105).

Eosinophils are found in the peripheral blood of patients with asthma (106,107). Sputum from asthmatic patients contains large numbers of eosinophils that have been shown to be activated and express ICAM-1 and human leukocyte antigen DR (108). There is evidence that IL-5 and GM-CSF are present in the sputum of asthmatic patients during attacks and contribute to eosinophil viability (109). The concentration of MBP in the sputum is increased in patients with asthma (41,110). ECP can be measured in the sputum of patients with asthma (111). Bronchoalveolar lavage (BAL) fluid from asthmatic patients contains increased numbers of eosinophils (112,113). Endobronchial biopsy has revealed the presence of eosinophilic airway inflammation even in mildly asymptomatic asthmatic patients (114).

Relationship to Airway Hyperresponsiveness and Clinical Severity

As discussed above, there is considerable evidence that eosinophilia of blood, sputum, BAL fluid, and airways is found in asthmatic patients. While such pathologic observations suggest that eosinophils are important in the pathophysiology of asthma, there is emerging physiologic evidence to confirm this hypothesis. Airway hyperresponsiveness, a cardinal feature of asthma clinically, is associated with increased numbers of eosinophils and their secretory products in the airway. MBP augments cholinergic contraction of canine tracheal smooth muscle (115). In ovalbumin-sensitized guinea pigs, a significant correlation between the concentrations of MBP or EPO and methacholine hyperresponsiveness was noted (116). A significant correlation between eosinophil count and MBP concentration in BAL fluid to methacholine responsiveness has been noted in patients with mild asthma

(112). Airway responsiveness to inhaled bradykinin correlated negatively with eosinophil count in BAL fluid, epithelium, lamina propria, and submucosa in asthmatic patients in a recent study by Roisman et al. (117). Serum ECP concentration and bronchial hyperresponsiveness to allergen challenge have been correlated in patients with asthma (118). Pretreatment with a monoclonal antibody to ICAM-1 decreased airway eosinophilia and hyperresponsiveness to methacholine in a primate model of asthma (80). In isolated guinea-pig tracheal smooth muscle, pretreatment with a 5-lipoxygenase inhibitor blocked hyperresponsiveness to histamine caused by activated eosinophil supernatant (119).

There is now increasing evidence that eosinophils and their inflammatory products cause direct airway smooth muscle contraction. MBP causes significant airway smooth muscle contraction in guinea-pig tracheal smooth muscle (120) and in primates (81). Both activated human eosinophils (83) and activated human umbilical cord blood-derived eosinophils (87) cause tracheal smooth muscle contraction *in situ* in guinea pigs. In addition, evidence exists that human eosinophils cause human airway smooth muscle contraction. Zymosan-activated human eosinophils caused contraction of isolated human bronchial rings that was decreased by about 70% with 5-lipoxygenase inhibition or LTD_4 receptor antagonism (121). Activation of isolated human peripheral blood eosinophils with PAF caused a 31% decrease in airway caliber and a 37% increase in wall thickness in explanted human bronchi *in vitro* (122). Pretreatment with a 5-lipoxygenase inhibitor caused significant inhibition of airway narrowing in human bronchial explants *in vitro* (Fig. 9).

An association between clinical asthma severity and blood, sputum, and BAL fluid eosinophil number and release of inflammatory products has been found in patients with asthma. In a recent study of 43 patients with chronic asthma, a significant increase in the number of peripheral blood eosinophils was noted as compared with eosinophil counts in 10 normal subjects (107). Peripheral blood eosinophilia correlated with the clinical severity of asthma and pulmonary function as assessed by forced expiratory volume in 1 second (FEV_1) (107). In addition, eosinophil number and ECP level were increased in BAL fluid in the asthmatic patients; this again correlated with clinical asthma severity (Fig. 10). Sputum ECP levels were correlated with airflow obstruction as assessed by FEV_1 in 14 asthmatic patients (111). A significant increase in BAL fluid eosinophil count and MBP concentration was noted in asthmatic patients who were symptomatic and required daily β_2-adrenergic agonist use (112). Broide et al. (123) found that patients with symptomatic asthma had significantly lower FEV_1 and significantly increased concentrations of EDN, MBP, and percent eosinophils in BAL fluid when compared with asymptomatic asthmatic patients. Eosinophils from patients with asthma are hypodense when compared with eosinophils

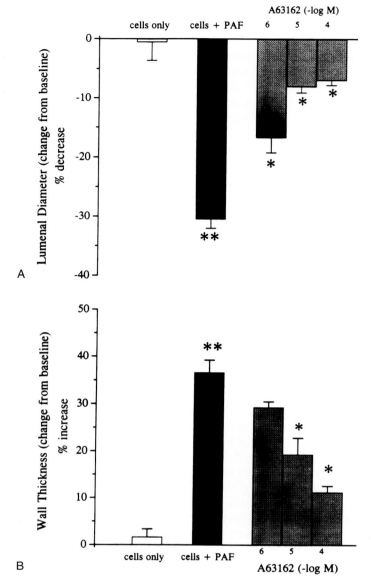

FIG. 9. Effect of A63162, a 5-lipoxygenase inhibitor, on airway narrowing and wall thickness. Increasing concentrations of A63162 inhibited decrease in luminal diameter **(A)** and airway wall thickness **(B)** in a concentration-dependent manner. $**p < 0.001$; $*p < 0.05$ vs. untreated eosinophils (cells only). PAF, platelet-activating factor. (Adapted from Rabe KF, Munoz NM, Vita AJ, Morton BE, Magnussen H, Leff AR. Contraction of human bronchial smooth muscle caused by activated human eosinophils. *Am J Physiol* 1994;267:L326–L334, with permission.)

from normal volunteers (124). Frick et al. (125) found that antigen bronchoprovocation increased the number of circulating hypodense eosinophils in patients with both an immediate and late-phase asthmatic reaction. The percent of hypodense eosinophils in the peripheral blood also was correlated with airflow obstruction. The authors concluded that because hypodense eosinophils may be

more active than normodense eosinophils, these cells may contribute to the late-phase asthma response and asthma severity.

There is evidence that eosinophils may be important contributors to aspirin-induced and nocturnal asthma. Immunohistochemical staining of bronchial tissue from asthmatic patients reveals increased numbers of activated eosinophils as a percentage of all cells containing 5-lipoxygenase in patients that are aspirin-sensitive as compared with non-aspirin-sensitive controls (126). The authors speculate that the increased numbers of eosinophils may be the source of enhanced leukotriene production that characterizes aspirin-sensitive asthma. Circulating eosinophils are present in greater numbers in asthmatic patients with more frequent episodes of nocturnal asthma and correlate with average percent decrease in FEV_1 (127). Peripheral blood eosinophilia is greatest at 4:00 a.m. as compared with eosinophil counts at 4:00 p.m. in patients with nocturnal asthma (128). A greater percentage of the eosinophils collected at 4:00 a.m. were of low density, indicating increased activity of eosinophils in the early morning in patients with nocturnal asthma.

Effect of Therapy on Eosinophils

Many of the drugs used to treat asthma affect eosinophil function (129) (Table 3). These medications include anti-inflammatory therapy, such as corticosteroids and chromones, and bronchodilators having possible anti-inflammatory action, such as β_2-adrenergic agonists and methylxanthines. Improved understanding of the pathogenesis of asthma has led to the development of pathway antagonists such as 5-lipoxygenase inhibitors and LTD_4 receptor antagonists that block a specific inflammatory pathway generated by the eosinophil.

Corticosteroids

Corticosteroids remain the most effective anti-inflammatory therapy available for the treatment of asthma. Their precise mechanism of action in asthma has yet to be delineated, but they act to suppress upregulation of eosinophil migration and secretion (129). Corticosteroids inhibit the synthesis of cytokines that control eosinophil production, survival, chemotaxis, and function (130). In a recent study by Robinson et al. (131), 2 weeks of treatment with oral prednisolone caused a reduction in the number of BAL cells per 1,000 expressing mRNA for IL-4 and IL-5. In addition, a decrease in BAL fluid eosinophils was accompanied by a decrease in airway methacholine responsiveness (131). Oral glucocorticoid therapy caused a reduction in the percentages of CD4 T lymphocytes expressing mRNA for IL-3, IL-5, and GM-CSF, and decreased secretion of eosinophil survival-prolonging activity in a study of asthmatic patients, and was

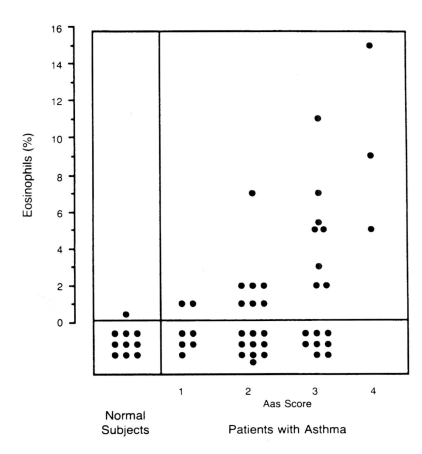

FIG. 10. Percentage of eosinophils in broncho-alveolar lavage (*BAL*) fluid from normal subjects and from patients with asthma. The percentage of eosinophils in BAL fluid correlated with the clinical severity of asthma as assessed by a clinical scoring system (*Aas*). (From Bousquet J, Chanez P, Lacoste JY, et al. Eosinophilic inflammation in asthma. *N Engl J Med* 1990;323:1033–1039, with permission.)

associated with improved lung function (132). Corticosteroids decrease eosinophilia of sputum (133) and peripheral blood (134) possibly by inhibiting release from the bone marrow (135), reducing eosinophil survival (132,136), and decreasing eosinophil tissue infiltration by inhibiting eosinophil chemotaxis (137) and adherence (138). Oral prednisone and inhaled budesonide decrease ECP concentrations in BAL fluid (139,140), serum, and sputum (129). In 14 patients hospitalized for asthma, treatment with glucocorticoids caused a decrease in blood eosinophils and a decrease in serum and sputum concentration of MBP (110). In a 6-week study of inhaled beclomethasone therapy in atopic asthmatic patients, a significant reduction in mucosal eosinophils was associated with decreased asthma symptoms, improved airflow, and decreased hyperresponsiveness to methacholine (141). Prolonged therapy with inhaled beclomethasone caused a decrease in total and activated eosinophils in endobronchial biopsy specimens of 25 mildly asthmatic patients (142). Corticosteroid therapy also decreases the number of peripheral blood eosinophils of low density (143). Corticosteroids inhibit eosinophil activation by preventing the expression of Fc receptors, degranulation, formation of leukotrienes, and release of EPO (129,144,145).

Chromones

Both disodium cromoglycate (DSCG) and nedocromil sodium have demonstrated inhibitory effects on numerous inflammatory cells, including eosinophils. Nedocromil sodium prevents eosinophil chemotaxis (146) and surface antigen expression (147). In a study of human peripheral blood eosinophils by Sedgwick et al. (148), nedocromil sodium inhibited eosinophil secretion of LTC_4 and decreased the percentage of eosinophils becoming hypodense. Incubation of human nasal epithelial cells with nedocromil sodium prevented the attenuation of ciliary beat frequency caused by activated human eosinophils (149). Nedocromil sodium prevents eosinophil recruitment and secretion of granule proteins (150,151). DSCG reduces the number of eosinophils in bronchial mucus and BAL fluid in patients with asthma and inhibits *in vitro* activation of eosinophils (129,152). It prevents tissue eosinophilia during the late reaction to allergen in IgE-sensitized rabbits and to PAF in guinea pigs (153,154).

β-Adrenergic Receptor Agonists

In addition to their potent ability to relax airway smooth muscle, $β_2$-adrenergic agonists may act to sup-

TABLE 3. *Effect of various drugs on cellular functions of the eosinophil leukocyte*

Eosinophil function	Anti-eosinophil drug
Tissue infiltration	Corticosteroids
	Ketotifen
	DSCG
	PDE type IV inhibitors
	Cetirizine
	PAF receptor antagonists
	Anti-IL-5 receptor antagonists
Chemotaxis	Corticosteroids
	Nedocromil
	PDE type IV inhibitors?
	Cetirizine
	PAF receptor antagonists
Surface receptor expression	Corticosteroids
	Nedocromil
	Cetirizine
Adhesion	Corticosteroids
	Cetirizine
Hypodensity	Corticosteroids
	Nedocromil
	Azelastine
Survival	Corticosteroids
Granular protein secretion	Corticosteroids
	Nedocromil
	DSCG
	Ketotifen
	β_2-Agonists
Oxygen radical production	Corticosteroids
	DSCG
	β_2-Agonists
Lipid mediator release	Corticosteroids
	Nedocromil
Cytotoxicity	Corticosteroids
	Nedocromil
	Cetirizine

DSCG, disodium cromoglycate; PDE, phosphodiesterase; PAF, platelet-activating factor; IL-5, interleukin 5.

From Kroegel C, Warner JA, Virchow JC, Matthys H. Pulmonary immune cells in health and disease: the eosinophil leucocyte (Part II). *Eur Respir J* 1994;7:743–760, with permission.

press asthmatic airway inflammation. Human eosinophils express β_2-adrenoceptors at a relatively low density (155). β_2-Adrenergic agonists inhibit EPO release and LTC_4 secretion from activated human eosinophils *in vitro* (96). Immunoglobulin-induced degranulation of human eosinophils is weakly inhibited in the presence of a phosphodiesterase inhibitor (155). Inhalation of low concentrations of β_2-adrenergic agonists by sensitized guinea pigs blocked BAL fluid eosinophilia in response to allergen challenge (156). Treatment with β_2-adrenergic agonists and theophylline decreases serum ECP concentrations in asthmatic patients (129).

Methylxanthines

Methylxanthines, such as theophylline, act as bronchodilators by an as yet undetermined mechanism that may include inhibition of phosphodiesterase. Although claims for anti-inflammatory effects of theophylline have been made, there is little evidence at present to substantiate this. In a study by Auffermann et al. (157), treatment with the phosphodiesterase inhibitor zardaverine decreased the number of eosinophils harvested from the peritoneum of sensitized guinea pigs after challenge with human serum. Eosinophil migration was slightly reduced in eosinophils isolated from these animals. The clinical efficacy of phosphodiesterase inhibitors in preventing inflammation in asthma has not been demonstrated.

Antihistamines

Antihistamines are not currently used as conventional asthma therapy; however, new evidence suggests that they may have anti-inflammatory properties that may be of benefit to patients with asthma. Cetirizine, a selective histamine$_1$ receptor antagonist, significantly decreased fMLP-augmented adhesion of human eosinophils to cultured human umbilical vein endothelial cells (158). In a study of inflammatory cell recruitment to the skin of pollen-sensitive patients, cetirizine significantly decreased eosinophil recruitment 24 h after pollen challenge (159). In addition, cetirizine decreases eosinophil receptor complement expression and cytotoxicity caused by PAF (160) and blocks ICAM-1 expression *in vitro* in response to IL-5 (161). Clinically, cetirizine has been shown to block decreased FEV_1 and increased airway resistance during the late allergic response to allergen in atopic asthmatic patients (162). Azelastine, a new antihistamine, significantly inhibits activated human peripheral blood eosinophil generation of O_2^- in a dose-dependent manner (163). Clinically, azelastine has recently been reported to reduce the need for inhaled corticosteroids in patients with chronic asthma (164).

Leukotriene Synthesis Inhibitors and Receptor Antagonists

Leukotriene synthesis inhibitors and receptor antagonists are a new class of compounds targeted at a specific pathway found in the eosinophil and other inflammatory cells noted in asthmatic airway inflammation. There is now significant evidence of their clinical efficacy in the treatment of asthma and emerging evidence of their anti-inflammatory properties. In a recent study, zileuton, a 5-lipoxygenase inhibitor, decreased eosinophil number in BAL fluid sampled 24 h after segmental antigen challenge in atopic patients (165). Wenzel et al. (166) noted significant reductions in 4 a.m. BAL fluid and blood eosinophil percentages in patients receiving zileuton associated with decreases in LTB_4 concentrations and improvement in FEV_1.

Other Agents

Other agents that may have anti-inflammatory effects on eosinophil function are listed in Table 3 and discussed extensively in a review by Kroegel et al. (129). None, at present, have been clearly proven to be of benefit in patients with asthma.

CONCLUSIONS

Eosinophils are granulocytes that differ substantially in function from other circulating granulocytes with which they share common surface ligands. For most people of the world, these cells function as an important line of defense against parasitic diseases, particularly helminthic infestations. In another, pathologic role, eosinophils appear to be important components of the inflammatory response characterizing human asthma. Eosinophils develop in the bone marrow and are transported to the peripheral circulation for short periods (Fig. 11). This presents the first opportunity to intervene therapeutically in the action of these cells that are rather unique to the inflammatory process of asthma, for eosinophilopoiesis is critically dependent on certain cytokines (for example, IL-5) and matrix proteins during development. To date, no therapy has been directed against selective eosinophilopoiesis.

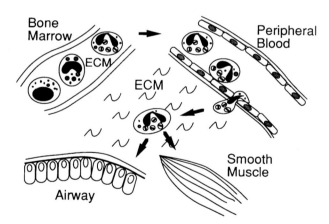

FIG. 11. Eosinophils in airway disease. Eosinophilopoiesis begins in the bone marrow, where specific cytokines and matrix components are essential to cell ontogeny and differentiation. This process requires about 5 days, after which cells are released for a short time into the peripheral blood. During this time, endothelial adhesion and diapedesis into conducting airways occur. No therapies currently have been directed that intervene in either of these two events. After migration into the airway interstices, release of products secreted by eosinophils causes both direct and indirect activation of airway smooth muscle contractility and loss of epithelial integrity. At present, therapies are directed against preventing the effect of asthmatic inflammation occurring in the conducting airways after cell genesis and migration have occurred.

The mechanism by which these minority constituents of circulating granulocytes are honed selectively to conducting airways in human asthma remains unknown. In the late asthmatic response, eosinophils are, however, often the majority granulocytic constituent. A fuller understanding of the mechanisms by which these cells adhere and migrate thus presents a second potential line of defense against asthmatic inflammation caused by eosinophils. Although specific therapies have not yet been developed that prevent molecular adhesion and eosinophil migration, this currently is an area of active research and product development.

Current therapies are directed largely against the effects of asthmatic inflammation after airways are infiltrated with eosinophils (Fig. 11). Eosinophil secretion of leukotrienes is blocked either by inhibition of the 5-lipoxygenase pathway or by receptor antagonism at the end organ itself—that is, the LTC_4/LTD_4 receptor on airway and vascular smooth muscle—thus decreasing airway constriction and edema. Although the correlative evidence for a critical relationship between eosinophilic infiltration and human asthma is strong, determination of the extent to which eosinophils are causative in the bronchoconstriction of human asthma awaits development of therapies that eliminate selectively all components of eosinophilic inflammation in human airways.

ACKNOWLEDGMENT

The author thanks Ted Slusarczyk and Nancy Trojan for their dedicated assistance in typing the manuscript.

REFERENCES

1. Weller PF. The immunobiology of eosinophils. *N Engl J Med* 1991; 324:1110–1118.
2. Gleich GJ, Adolphson CR. The eosinophilic leukocyte: structure and function. *Adv Immunol* 1986;39:177–253.
3. Kroegel C, Virchow JC, Luttmann W, Walker C, Warner JA. Pulmonary immune cells in health and disease: the eosinophil leukocyte (Part 1). *Eur Respir J* 1994;7:519–543.
4. Bainton DF, Farquhar MG. Segregation and packaging of granule enzymes in eosinophilic leukocytes. *J Cell Biol* 1970;45:54–73.
5. Dvorak AM, Letourneau L, Login GR, Weller PF, Ackerman SJ. Ultrastructural localization of the Charcot-Leyden crystal protein (lysophospholipase) to a distinct crystalloid-free granule population in mature human eosinophils. *Blood* 1988;72:150–158.
6. Parmley RT, Spicer SS. Cytochemical and ultrastructural identification of a small type granule in human late eosinophils. *Lab Invest* 1974;30:557–567.
7. Weller PF, Dvorak AM. Arachidonic acid incorporation by cytoplasmic lipid bodies of human eosinophils. *Blood* 1985;65:1269–1274.
8. Weller PF, Monahan-Earley RA, Dvorak HF, Dvorak AM. Cytoplasmic lipid bodies of human eosinophils. *Am J Pathol* 1991;138: 141–148.
9. Weller PF, Ackerman SJ, Nicholson-Weller A, Dvorak AM. Cytoplasmic lipid bodies of human neutrophilic leukocytes. *Am J Pathol* 1989; 135:947–959.
10. Peters MS, Rodriguez M, Gleich GJ. Localization of human eosinophil granule major basic protein, eosinophil cationic protein, and eosinophil-derived neurotoxin by immunoelectron microscopy. *Lab Invest* 1986;54:656–662.

11. Ackerman SJ, Loegering DA, Venge P, et al. Distinctive cationic proteins of the human eosinophil granule: major basic protein, eosinophil cationic protein, and eosinophil-derived neurotoxin. *J Immunol* 1983; 131:2977–2982.

12. Hamann KJ, Barker RL, Ten RM, Gleich GJ. The molecular biology of eosinophil granule proteins. *Int Arch Allergy Appl Immunol* 1991; 94:202–209.

13. Wasmoen TL, Bell MP, Loegering DA, Gleich GJ, Prendergast FG, McKean DJ. Biochemical and amino acid sequence analysis of human eosinophil granule major basic protein. *J Biol Chem* 1988;263:12, 559–12,563.

14. Barker RL, Loegering DA, Arakawa KC, Pease LR, Gleich GJ. Cloning and sequence analysis of the human gene encoding eosinophil major basic protein. *Gene* 1990;86:285–289.

15. Lehrer RI, Szklarek D, Barton A, Ganz T, Hamann KJ, Gleich GJ. Antibacterial properties of eosinophil major basic protein and eosinophil cationic protein. *J Immunol* 1989;142:4428–4434.

16. Hamann KJ, Gundel RH, Gleich GJ, White SR. Interactions between respiratory epithelium and eosinophil granule proteins in asthma. In: Farmer SG, Hay DWP, eds. *The airway epithelium.* New York: Marcel Dekker, 1991;255–300.

17. Frigas E, Loegering DA, Gleich GJ. Cytotoxic effects of the guinea pig eosinophil major basic protein on tracheal epithelium. *Lab Invest* 1980;42:35–43.

18. Ayars GH, Altman LC, Gleich GJ, Loegering DA, Baker CB. Eosinophil- and eosinophil granule-mediated pneumocyte injury. *J Allergy Clin Immunol* 1985;76:595–604.

19. Hastie AT, Loegering DA, Gleich GJ, Kueppers F. The effect of purified human eosinophil major basic protein on mammalian ciliary activity. *Am Rev Respir Dis* 1987;135:848–853.

20. Jacoby DB, Ueki IF, Widdicombe JH, Loegering DA, Gleich GJ, Nadel JA. Effect of human eosinophil major basic protein on ion transport in dog tracheal epithelium. *Am Rev Respir Dis* 1988;137:13–16.

21. White SR, Sigrist KS, Spaethe SM. Prostaglandin secretion by guinea pig tracheal epithelial cells caused by eosinophil major basic protein. *Am J Physiol* 1993;265:L234–L242.

22. Barker RL, Loegering DA, Ten RM, Hamann KJ, Pease LR, Gleich GJ. Eosinophil cationic protein cDNA: comparison with other toxic proteins and ribonucleases. *J Immunol* 1989;143:952–955.

23. Gleich GJ, Loegering DA, Bell MP, Checkel JL, Ackerman SJ, McKean DJ. Biochemical and functional similarities between human eosinophil-derived neurotoxin and eosinophil cationic protein: homology with ribonuclease. *Proc Natl Acad Sci USA* 1986;83:3146–3150.

24. Motojima S, Frigas E, Loegering DA, Gleich GJ. Toxicity of eosinophil cationic proteins for guinea pig tracheal epithelium *in vitro.* *Am Rev Respir Dis* 1989;139:801–805.

25. Durack DT, Suml SM, Klebanoff SJ. Neurotoxicity of human eosinophils. *Proc Natl Acad Sci USA* 1979;76:1443–1447.

26. Rosenberg HF, Tenen DG, Ackerman SJ. Molecular cloning of the human eosinophil-derived neurotoxin: a member of the ribonuclease gene family. *Proc Natl Acad Sci USA* 1989;86:4460–4464.

27. Hamann KJ, Barker RL, Loegering DA, Pease LR, Gleich GJ. Sequence of human eosinophil-derived neurotoxin cDNA: identity of deduced amino acid sequence with human nonsecretory ribonucleases. *Gene* 1989;83:161–167.

28. Olsen RL, Little C. Purification and some properties of myeloperoxidase and eosinophil peroxidase from human blood. *Biochem J* 1983; 209:781–787.

29. Sakamaki K, Tomonaga M, Tsukui K, Nagata S. Molecular cloning and characterization of a chromosomal gene for human eosinophil peroxidase. *J Biol Chem* 1989;264:16,828–16,836.

30. Hamann KJ, Gleich GJ, Checkel JL, Loegering DA, McCall JW, Barker RL. *In vitro* killing of microfilariae of *Brugia pahangi* and *Brugia malayi* by eosinophil granule proteins. *J Immunol* 1990;144: 3166–3173.

31. Henderson WR, Jong EC, Klebanoff SJ. Binding of eosinophil peroxidase to mast cell granules with retention of peroxidatic activity. *J Immunol* 1980;124:1383–1388.

32. Jong EC, Mahmoud AAF, Klebanoff SJ. Peroxidase-mediated toxicity to schistosomula of *Schistosoma mansoni.* *J Immunol* 1981;126: 468–471.

33. Nogueira NM, Klebanoff SJ, Cohn ZA. *T. cruzi:* sensitization to macrophage killing by eosinophil peroxidase. *J Immunol* 1982;128: 1705–1708.

34. Jong EC, Klebanoff SJ. Eosinophil-mediated mammalian tumor cell cytotoxicity: role of the peroxidase system. *J Immunol* 1980;124: 1949–1953.

35. Weiss SJ, Test ST, Eckmann CM, Roos D, Regiani S. Brominating oxidants generated by human eosinophils. *Science* 1986;234:200–203.

36. Mayeno AN, Curran AJ, Roberts RL, Foote CS. Eosinophils preferentially use bromide to generate halogenating agents. *J Biol Chem* 1989;264:5660–5668.

37. Agosti JM, Altman LC, Ayars GH, Loegering DA, Gleich GJ, Klebanoff SJ. The injurious effect of eosinophil peroxidase, hydrogen peroxide, and halides on pneumocytes *in vitro.* *J Allergy Clin Immunol* 1987;79:496–504.

38. Yoshikawa S, Kayes SG, Parker JC. Eosinophils increase lung microvascular permeability via the peroxidase-hydrogen peroxide-halide system. *Am Rev Respir Dis* 1993;147:914–920.

39. Henderson WR, Chi EY, Klebanoff SJ. Eosinophil peroxidase-induced mast cell secretion. *J Exp Med* 1980;152:265–279.

40. Weller PF, Bach DS, Austen KF. Biochemical characterization of human eosinophil Charcot–Leyden crystal protein (lysophospholipase). *J Biol Chem* 1984;259:15,100–15,105.

41. Dor PJ, Ackerman SJ, Gleich GJ. Charcot-Leyden crystal protein and eosinophil granule major basic protein in sputum of patients with respiratory diseases. *Am Rev Respir Dis* 1984;130:1072–1077.

42. Owen WF, Soberman RJ, Yoshimoto T, Sheffer AL, Lewis RA, Austen KF. Synthesis and release of leukotriene C4 by human eosinophils. *J Immunol* 1987;138:532–538.

43. Shaw RJ, Cromwell O, Kay AB. Preferential generation of leukotriene C4 by human eosinophils. *Clin Exp Immunol* 1984;56:716–722.

44. Kroegel C, Matthys H. Platelet-activating factor-induced human eosinophil activation: generation and release of cyclo-oxygenase metabolites in human blood eosinophils from asthmatics. *Immunol* 1993;78:279–285.

45. Giembycz MA, Kroegel C, Barnes PJ. Platelet-activating factor stimulates cyclo-oxygenase activity in guinea pig eosinophils. *J Immunol* 1990;144:3489–3497.

46. Morley J, Bray MA, Jones RW, Nugteren DH, van Dorp DA. Prostaglandin and thromboxane production by human and guinea-pig macrophages and leucocytes. *Prostaglandins* 1979;17:729–746.

47. Kroegel C, Hubbard WH, Lichtenstein LM. Spectrum of prostanoid generation by human blood eosinophils stimulated with platelet-activating factor and calcimycin. *Eur Respir J* 1990;3:347s.

48. Sigal E, Grunberger D, Cashman JR, Craik CS, Caughey GH, Nadel JA. Arachidonate 15-lipoxygenase from human eosinophil-enriched leukocytes: partial purification and properties. *Biochem Biophys Res Commun* 1988;150:376–383.

49. Lee T-C, Lenihan DJ, Malone B, Roddy LL, Wasserman SI. Increased biosynthesis of platelet-activating factor in activated human eosinophils. *J Biol Chem* 1984;259:5526–5530.

50. Kroegel C, Yukawa T, Dent G, Venge P, Chung KF, Barnes PJ. Stimulation of degranulation from human eosinophils by platelet-activating factor. *J Immunol* 1989;142:3518–3526.

51. Learn DB, Brestel EP. A comparison of superoxide production by human eosinophils and neutrophils. *Agents Actions* 1982;12:485–488.

52. Dechatelet LR, Shirley PS, McPhail LC, Huntley CC, Muss HB, Bass DA. Oxidative metabolism of the human eosinophil. *Blood* 1977; 50:525–535.

53. Klebanoff SJ, Durack DT, Rosen H, Clark RA. Functional studies on human peritoneal eosinophils. *Infect Immun* 1977;17:167–173.

54. Weiss SJ, Test ST, Eckmann CM, Roos D, Regiani S. Brominating oxidants generated by human eosinophils. *Science* 1986;234:200–203.

55. Kanofsky JR, Hoogland H, Wever R, Weiss SJ. Singlet oxygen production by human eosinophils. *J Biol Chem* 1988;263:9692–9696.

56. Segal AW, Garcia R, Goldstone AH, Cross AR, Jones OTG. Cytochrome b-245 of neutrophils is also present in human monocytes, macrophages and eosinophils. *Biochem J* 1981;196:363–367.

57. Weinstock JV, Blum AM. Detection of vasoactive intestinal peptide and localization of its mRNA within granulomas of murine schistosomiasis. *Cell Immunol* 1990;125:291–300.

58. Weinstock JV, Blum AM. Tachykinin production in granulomas of murine *Schistosomiasis mansoni.* *J Immunol* 1989;142:3256–3261.

59. Weinstock JV, Blum A, Walder J, Walder R. Eosinophils from granulomas in murine *Schistosomiasis mansoni* produce substance P. *J Immunol* 1988;141:961–966.

60. Kroegel C, Giembycz MA, Barnes PJ. Characterization of eosinophil

cell activation by peptides: differential effects of substance P, melittin and FMET-Leu-Phe. *J Immunol* 1990;145:2581–2587.

61. Kita H, Ohnishi T, Okubo Y, Weiler D, Abrams JS, Gleich GJ. Granulocyte-macrophage colony-stimulating factor and interleukin 3 release from human peripheral blood eosinophils and neutrophils. *J Exp Med* 1991;174:745–748.

62. Moqbel R, Hamid Q, Ying S, et al. Expression of mRNA and immunoreactivity for the granulocyte/macrophage colony-stimulating factor in activated human eosinophils. *J Exp Med* 1991;174:749–752.

63. Wong D, Weller PF, Galli SJ, et al. Human eosinophils express transforming growth factor-α. *J Exp Med* 1990;172:673–681.

64. Ohno I, Lea RG, Flanders KC, et al. Eosinophils in chronically inflamed human upper airway tissues express transforming growth factor-β₁ gene (TGF-β₁). *J Clin Invest* 1992;89:1662–1668.

65. Leff AR. Will there be a cure for asthma? *Chest* (Suppl) 1996, (*in press*).

66. Silberstein DS, Austen KF, Owen WF. Hemopoietins for eosinophils: glycoprotein hormones that regulate the development of inflammation in eosinophilia-associated disease. *Hematol Oncol Clin North Am* 1989;3:511–533.

67. Clutterbuck EJ, Hirst EMA, Sanderson CJ. Human interleukin-5 (IL-5) regulates the production of eosinophils in human bone marrow cultures: comparison and interaction with IL-1, IL-3, IL-6, and GM-CSF. *Blood* 1989;73:1504–1512.

68. Hamann KJ, Dowling TL, Neeley SP, Grant JA, Leff AR. Hyaluronic acid enhances cell proliferation during eosinopoiesis through the CD44 surface antigen. *J Immunol* 1995;154:4073–4080.

69. Tyler TL, Grant JA, Dowling TL, Leff AR, Hamann KJ. Proliferation of developing umbilical cord blood-derived eosinophils is enhanced by heparan sulfate. *Am J Respir Crit Care Med* 1995;151:A218(abstr).

70. Kameyoshi Y, Dörschner A, Mallet AI, Christophers E, Schröder JM. Cytokine RANTES released by thrombin-stimulated platelets is a potent attractant for human eosinophils. *J Exp Med* 1992;176:587–592.

71. Schal TJ. Biology of the RANTES/SIS cytokine family. *Cytokine* 1991;3:165–183.

72. Chung KF. Chemokines. In: Leff AR, ed. *Pulmonary pharmacology & therapeutics* New York: McGraw-Hill, 1996;285–296.

73. Rot A, Krieger M, Brunner T, Bischoff SC, Schall TJ, Dahinden CA. RANTES and macrophage inflammatory protein-1α induce the migration and activation of normal human eosinophil granulocytes. *J Exp Med* 1992;176:1489–1495.

74. Rand TH, Silberstein DS, Kornfeld H, Weller PF. Human eosinophils express functional interleukin-2 receptors. *J Clin Invest* 1991;88:825–832.

75. Leff AR, Hamann KJ, Wegner CD. Inflammation and cell-cell interactions in airway hyperresponsiveness. *Am J Physiol* 1991;260:L189–L206.

76. Godding V, Stark JM, Sedgwick JB, Busse WW. Adhesion of activated eosinophils to respiratory epithelial cells is enhanced by tumor necrosis factor-α and interleukin-1β. *Am J Respir Cell Mol Biol* 1995;13:555–562.

77. Neeley SP, Hamann KJ, White SR, Baranowski SL, Burch RA, Leff AR. Selective regulation of expression of surface adhesion molecules Mac-1, L-selectin, and VLA-4 on human eosinophils and neutrophils. *Am J Respir Cell Mol Biol* 1993;8:633–639.

78. Padrid PA, Mitchell RW, Cozzi PJ, et al. Cyclosporine treatment *in vivo* inhibits the development of airway hyperresponsiveness and histologic alterations after chronic antigen challenge in cats. *Am Rev Respir Dis* 1994;149:A771(abstr).

79. Alexander AG, Barnes NC, Kay AB. Trial of cyclosporin in corticosteroid-dependent chronic severe asthma. *Lancet* 1992;339:324–328.

80. Wegner CD, Gundel RH, Reilly P, Haynes N, Letts LG, Rothlein R. Intercellular adhesion molecule-1 (ICAM-1) in the pathogenesis of asthma. *Science* 1990;247:456–459.

81. Gundel RH, Letts LG, Gleich GJ. Human eosinophil major basic protein induces airway constriction and airway hyperresponsiveness in primates. *J Clin Invest* 1991;87:1470–1473.

82. Neeley SP, Hamann KJ, Dowling TL, McAllister KT, White SR, Leff AR. Augmentation of stimulated eosinophil degranulation by VLA-4 (CD49d)-mediated adhesion to fibronectin. *Am J Respir Cell Mol Biol* 1994;11:206–213.

83. Strek ME, White SR, Hsiue TR, Kulp GVP, Williams FS, Leff AR. Effect of mode of activation of human eosinophils on tracheal smooth muscle contraction in guinea pigs. *Am J Physiol* 1993;264:L475–L481.

84. Sedgwick JB, Vrtis RF, Gourley MF, Busse WW. Stimulus-dependent differences in superoxide anion generation by normal human eosinophils and neutrophils. *J Allergy Clin Immunol* 1988;81:876–883.

85. Munoz NM, Rabe KF, Neeley SP, et al. Eosinophil VLA-4 binding to fibronectin causes augmented narrowing of human bronchial explants through 5-lipoxygenase activation. *Am J Physiol* 1996;270:L587–L594.

86. Munoz NM, Herrnreiter A, Rabe KF, et al. Induction by interleukin (IL)-1 augments eosinophil secretion and luminal narrowing of explanted human airways. *Am J Respir Crit Care Med* 1995;151:A369(abstr).

87. Hamann KJ, Strek ME, Baranowski SL, et al. Effects of activated eosinophils cultured from human umbilical cord blood on guinea pig trachealis. *Am J Physiol* 1993;L301–L307.

88. Hansel TT, De Vries IJM, Iff T, et al. An improved immunomagnetic procedure for the isolation of highly purified human blood eosinophils. *J Immunol Methods* 1991;145:105–110.

89. Kroegel C, Liu MC, Lichtenstein LM, Bochner BS. Antigen-induced eosinophil activation and recruitment in the lower airways. *J Allergy Clin Immunol* 1991;87:303.

90. Tosi MF, Berger M. Functional differences between the 40 kDa and 50 to 70 kDa IgG Fc receptors on human neutrophils revealed by elastase treatment and antireceptor antibodies. *J Immunol* 1988;141:2097–2103.

91. Moqbel R, Walsh GM, Nagakura T, et al. The effect of platelet-activating factor on IgE binding to, and IgE-dependent biological properties of human eosinophils. *Immunology* 1990;70:251–257.

92. Capron M, Truong M-J, Aldebert D, et al. Eosinophil IgE receptor and CD23. *Immunol Res* 1992;11:252–259.

93. Capron M, Prin L. The IgE receptor of eosinophils. *Springer Semin Immunopathol* 1990;12:327–348.

94. Munoz NM, Zhu X, Rabe KF, et al. Passive sensitization of purified human peripheral blood eosinophils: effect on CD23/FεRII expression and eosinophil degranulation. *Am J Respir Crit Care Med* 1995;151:A238(abstract).

95. Yukawa T, Ukena D, Kroegel C, et al. Beta₂-adrenergic receptors on eosinophils. *Am Rev Respir Dis* 1990;141:1446–1452.

96. Munoz NM, Vita AJ, Neeley SP, et al. Beta adrenergic modulation of formyl-methionine-leucine-phenylalanine-stimulated secretion of eosinophil peroxidase and leukotriene C₄. *J Pharmacol Exp Ther* 1994;268:139–143.

97. Munoz NM, Rabe KF, Vita AJ, et al. Paradoxical blockade of beta adrenergically mediated inhibition of stimulated eosinophil secretion by salmeterol. *J Pharmacol Exp Ther* 1995;273:850–854.

98. Barnes PJ. A new approach to the treatment of asthma. *N Engl J Med* 1989;321:1517–1527.

99. Gleich GJ. The eosinophil and bronchial asthma: current understanding. *J Allergy Clin Immunol* 1990;85:422–436.

100. Dunnill MS. The pathology of asthma. In: Porter R, Birch J, eds. *The identification of asthma*. Edinburgh: Churchill-Livingstone, 1971;35–46.

101. Filley WV, Holley KE, Kephart GM, Gleich GJ. Identification by immunofluorescence of eosinophil granule major basic protein in lung tissues of patients with bronchial asthma. *Lancet* 1982;2:11–16.

102. Djukanovic R, Roche WR, Wilson JW, et al. Mucosal inflammation in asthma. *Am Rev Respir Dis* 1990;142:434–457.

103. Moreno RH, Hogg JC, Paré PD. Mechanics of airway narrowing. *Am Rev Respir Dis* 1986;133:1171–1180.

104. Rowen JL, Hyde DM, McDonald RJ. Eosinophils cause acute edematous injury in isolated perfused rat lungs. *Am Rev Respir Dis* 1990;142:215–220.

105. Fujimoto K, Parker JC, Kayes SG. Activated eosinophils increase vascular permeability and resistance in isolated perfused rat lungs. *Am Rev Respir Dis* 1990;142:1414–1421.

106. Horn BR, Robin ED, Theodore J, Van Kessel A. Total eosinophil counts in the management of bronchial asthma. *N Engl J Med* 1975;292:1152–1155.

107. Bousquet J, Chanez P, Lacoste JY, et al. Eosinophilic inflammation in asthma. *N Engl J Med* 1990;323:1033–1039.

108. Hansel TT, Braunstein JB, Walker C, et al. Sputum eosinophils from asthmatics express ICAM-1 and HLA-DR. *Clin Exp Immunol* 1991;86:271–277.

109. Adachi T, Motojima S, Hirata A, Fukuda T, Makino S. Eosinophil vi-

ability-enhancing activity in sputum from patients with bronchial asthma. *Am J Respir Crit Care Med* 1995;151:618–623.

110. Frigas E, Loegering DA, Solley GO, Farrow GM, Gleich GJ. Elevated levels of the eosinophil granule major basic protein in the sputum of patients with bronchial asthma. *Mayo Clin Proc* 1981;56:345–353.

111. Virchow JC, Hölscher U, Virchow C. Sputum ECP levels correlate with parameters of airflow obstruction. *Am Rev Respir Dis* 1992;146:604–606.

112. Wardlaw AJ, Dunnette S, Gleich GJ, Collins JV, Kay AB. Eosinophils and mast cells in bronchoalveolar lavage in subjects with mild asthma. *Am Rev Respir Dis* 1988;137:62–69.

113. Smith DL, Deshazo RD. Bronchoalveolar lavage in asthma. *Am Rev Respir Dis* 1993;148:523–532.

114. Beasley R, Roche WR, Roberts JA, Holgate ST. Cellular events in the bronchi in mild asthma and after bronchial provocation. *Am Rev Respir Dis* 1989;139:806–817.

115. Brofman JD, White SR, Blake JS, Munoz NM, Gleich GJ, Leff AR. Epithelial augmentation of trachealis contraction caused by major basic protein of eosinophils. *J Appl Physiol* 1989;66:1867–1873.

116. Pretolani M, Ruffié C, Joseph D, et al. Role of eosinophil activation in the bronchial reactivity of allergic guinea pigs. *Am J Respir Crit Care Med* 1994;149:1167–1174.

117. Roisman GL, Lacronique JG, Desmazes-Dufeu N, Carré C, Le Cae A, Dusser DJ. Airway responsiveness to bradykinin is related to eosinophilic inflammation in asthma. *Am J Respir Crit Care Med* 1996;153:381–390.

118. Dahl R, Venge P, Olsson I. Variations of blood eosinophils and eosinophil cationic protein in serum in patients with bronchial asthma. *Allergy* 1978;33:211–215.

119. Aizawa T, Sekizawa K, Aikawa T, et al. Eosinophil supernatant causes hyperresponsiveness of airway smooth muscle in guinea pig trachea. *Am Rev Respir Dis* 1990;142:133–137.

120. White SR, Ohno S, Munoz NM, et al. Epithelium-dependent contraction of airway smooth muscle caused by eosinophil MBP. *Am J Physiol* 1990;259:L294–L303.

121. Jongejan RC, De Jongste JC, Raatgeep RC, Bonta IL, Kerrebijn KF. Effects of zymosan-activated human granulocytes on isolated human airways. *Am Rev Respir Dis* 1991;143:553–560.

122. Rabe KF, Munoz NM, Vita AJ, Morton BE, Magnussen H, Leff AR. Contraction of human bronchial smooth muscle caused by activated human eosinophils. *Am J Physiol* 1994;267:L326–L334.

123. Broide DH, Gleich GJ, Cuomo AJ, et al. Evidence of ongoing mast cell and eosinophil degranulation in symptomatic asthma airway. *J Allergy Clin Immunol* 1991;88:637–648.

124. Fukuda T, Dunnette SL, Reed CE, Ackerman SJ, Peters MS, Gleich GJ. Increased numbers of hypodense eosinophils in the blood of patients with bronchial asthma. *Am Rev Respir Dis* 1985;132:981–985.

125. Frick WE, Sedgwick JB, Busse WW. The appearance of hypodense eosinophils in antigen-dependent late phase asthma. *Am Rev Respir Dis* 1989;139:1401–1406.

126. Nasser SMS, Pfister R, Christie PE, et al. Inflammatory cell populations in bronchial biopsies from aspirin-sensitive asthmatic subjects. *Am J Respir Crit Care Med* 1996;153:90–96.

127. Bates ME, Clayton M, Calhoun W, et al. Relationship of plasma epinephrine and circulating eosinophils to nocturnal asthma. *Am J Respir Crit Care Med* 1994;149:667–672.

128. Calhoun WJ, Bates ME, Schrader L, Sedgwick JB, Busse WW. Characteristics of peripheral blood eosinophils in patients with nocturnal asthma. *Am Rev Respir Dis* 1992;145:577–581.

129. Kroegel C, Warner JA, Virchow JC, Matthys H. Pulmonary immune cells in health and disease: the eosinophil leucocyte (Part II). *Eur Respir J* 1994;7:743–760.

130. Barnes PJ, Pedersen S. Efficacy and safety of inhaled corticosteroids in asthma. *Am Rev Respir Dis* 1993;148:S1–S26.

131. Robinson D, Hamid Q, Ying S, et al. Prednisolone treatment in asthma is associated with modulation of bronchoalveolar lavage cell interleukin-4, interleukin-5, and interferon-γ cytokine gene expression. *Am Rev Respir Dis* 1993;148:401–406.

132. Corrigan CJ, Hamid Q, North J, et al. Peripheral blood CD4 but not CD8 T-lymphocytes in patients with exacerbation of asthma transcribe and translate messenger RNA encoding cytokines which prolong eosinophil survival in the context of a TH2-type pattern: effect of glucocorticoid therapy. *Am J Respir Cell Mol Biol* 1995;12:567–578.

133. Brown HM. Treatment of chronic asthma with prednisolone: significance of eosinophils in the sputum. *Lancet* 1958:2:1245–1247.

134. Baigelman W, Chodosh S, Pizzuto D, Cupples LA. Sputum and blood eosinophils during corticosteroid treatment of acute exacerbations of asthma. *Am J Med* 1983;75:929–936.

135. Slovick FT, Abboud CN, Brennan JK, Lichtman MA. Modulation of in vitro eosinophil progenitors by hydrocortisone: role of accessory cells and interleukins. *Blood* 1985;66:1072–1079.

136. Wallen N, Kita H, Weiler D, Gleich GJ. Glucocorticoids inhibit cytokine-mediated eosinophil survival. *J Immunol* 1991;147:3490–3495.

137. Clark RAF, Gallin JI, Fauci AS. Effects of in vivo prednisone on in vitro eosinophil and neutrophil adherence and chemotaxis. *Blood* 1979;53:633–641.

138. Altman LC, Hill JS, Hairfield WM, Mullarkey MF. Effects of corticosteroids on eosinophil chemotaxis and adherence. *J Clin Invest* 1981;67:28–36.

139. Dworski R, Fitzgerald GA, Oates JA, Sheller JR. Effect of oral prednisone on airway inflammatory mediators in atopic asthma. *Am J Respir Crit Care Med* 1994;149:953–959.

140. Ädelroth E, Rosenhall L, Johansson SA, Linden M, Venge P. Inflammatory cells and eosinophilic activity in asthmatics investigated by bronchoalveolar lavage. *Am Rev Respir Dis* 1990;142:91–99.

141. Djukanovic R, Wilson JW, Britten KM, et al. Effect of an inhaled corticosteroid on airway inflammation and symptoms in asthma. *Am Rev Respir Dis* 1992;145:669–674.

142. Trigg CJ, Manolitsas ND, Wang J, et al. Placebo-controlled immunopathologic study of four months of inhaled corticosteroids in asthma. *Am J Respir Crit Care Med* 1994;150:17–22.

143. Evans PM, O'Conner BJ, Fuller RW, Barnes PJ, Chung KF. Effect of inhaled corticosteroids on peripheral blood eosinophil counts and density profiles in asthma. *J Allergy Clin Immunol* 1993;91:643–650.

144. Oliver RC, Glauert AM, Thorne KJI. Mechanism of Fc-mediated interaction of eosinophils with immobilized immune complexes. I. Effects of inhibitors and activators of eosinophil function. *J Cell Sci* 1982;56:337–356.

145. Yukawa T, Dent G, Kroegel C, Evans P, Barnes PJ, Chung KF. Inhibition of guinea-pig and human eosinophil function by corticosteroids in vitro. *Thorax* 1989;44:883p.

146. Bruijnzeel PLB, Warringa RAJ, Kok PTM, Hamelink ML, Kreukniet J. Inhibitory effects of nedocromil sodium on the in vitro induced migration and leukotriene formation of human granulocytes. *Drugs* 1989;37(Suppl 1):9–18.

147. Moqbel R, Walsh GM, Kay AB. Inhibition of human granulocyte activation by nedocromil sodium. *Eur J Respir Dis* 1986;69:227–229.

148. Sedgwick JB, Bjornsdottir U, Geiger KM, Busse WW. Inhibition of eosinophil density change and leukotriene C_4 generation by nedocromil sodium. *J Allergy Clin Immunol* 1992;90:202–209.

149. Davies RJ, Sapsford RJ, McCloskey DT, Devalia JL. Influence of nedocromil sodium (N) on eosinophil-induced changes in human nasal epithelial cell (HNE) activity, in vitro. *J Allergy Clin Immunol* 1991;87:282.

150. Twentyman OP, Sams VR, Holgate ST. Albuterol and nedocromil sodium affect airway and leukocyte responses to allergen. *Am Rev Respir Dis* 1993;147:1425–1430.

151. Spry CJF, Kumaraswami V, Tai PC. The effect of nedocromil sodium on secretion from human eosinophils. *Eur J Respir Dis* 1986;69:241–243.

152. Moqbel R, Walsh GM, MacDonald AJ, Kay B. Effect of disodium cromoglycate on activation of human eosinophils and neutrophils following reversed (anti-IgE) anaphylaxis. *Clin Allergy* 1986;16:73–83.

153. Sanjar S, Colditz I, Aoki S, Boubekeur K, Morley J. Pharmacological modulation of eosinophil accumulation in guinea-pig airways. In: Morley J, Colditz I, eds. *Perspectives in asthma: eosinophils and asthma.* London: Academic,1989;202–212.

154. Larson GL. The rabbit model of the late asthmatic response. *Chest* 1985;87:1845–1885.

155. Barnes PJ. Beta-adrenergic receptors and their regulation. *Am J Respir Crit Care Med* 1995;152:838–860.

156. Fügner A. Formation of oedema and accumulation of eosinophils in the guinea-pig lung: inhibition by inhaled beta-stimulants. *Int Arch Allergy Appl Immunol* 1989;88:225–227.

157. Auffermann K, Virchow JC Jr, Norgauer J, et al. Effects of the selective type III/IV PDE-inhibitor, zardaverine, on peritoneal guinea pig

eosinophils *in vivo*: inhibition of eosinophil recruitment *in vivo* correlates with decreased actin polymerisation. *Am Rev Respir Dis* 1993; 147:A818(abstract).

158. Kyan-Aung U, Hallsworth M, Haskard D, De Vos C, Lee TH. The effects of cetirizine on the adhesion of human eosinophils and neutrophils to cultured human umbilical vein endothelial cells. *J Allergy Clin Immunol* 1992;90:270–272.

159. Michel L, De Vos C, Rihoux JP, Burtin C, Benveniste J, Dubertret L. Inhibitory effect of oral cetirizine on *in vivo* antigen-induced histamine and PAF-acether release and eosinophil recruitment in human skin. *J Allergy Clin Immunol* 1988;82:101–109.

160. Walsh GM, Moqbel R, Hartnell A, Kay AB. Effects of cetirizine on human eosinophil and neutrophil activation *in vitro*. *Int Arch Allergy Appl Immunol* 1991;95:158–162.

161. Walsh GM, Wardlaw AJ, Hartnell A, Sanderson CJ, Kay AB. IL-5 enhances *in vitro* eosinophil, but not neutrophil, adhesion in a CD11/18-dependent manner. *Immunology* 1990;20:8.

162. Wasserfallen JB, Leuenberger P, Pècoud A. Effect of cetirizine, a new H$_1$ antihistamine, on the early and late allergic reactions in a bronchial provocation test with allergen. *J Allergy Clin Immunol* 1993;91: 1189–1197.

163. Busse WW, Randley B, Sedgwick J. The effect of azelastine on neutrophil and eosinophil generation of superoxide. *J Allergy Clin Immunol* 1989;83:400–405.

164. Busse WW, Middleton E, Storms W, et al. Corticosteroid-sparing effect of azelastine in the management of bronchial asthma. *Am J Respir Crit Care Med* 1996;153:122–127.

165. Tolino M, Kane G, Pollice M, et al. Sulfidopeptide leukotrienes in IgE-mediated early and late airway reactions in humans. *Am Rev Respir* 1994;149:A531(abstract).

166. Wenzel SE, Trudeau JB, Kaminsky DA, Cohn J, Martin RJ, Westcott JY. Effect of 5-lipoxygenase inhibition on bronchoconstriction and airway inflammation in nocturnal asthma. *Am J Respir Crit Care Med* 1995;152:897–905.

Asthma, edited by P.J. Barnes, M.M. Grunstein, A.R. Leff, and A.J. Woolcock.
Lippincott–Raven Publishers, Philadelphia © 1997.

▪ 31 ▪

Neutrophils and Asthma

Leonardo Fabbri, Gaetano Caramori, Marco Piattella, and Piero Maestrelli

Neutrophils are considered as major effector cells in acute inflammatory processes and their role in the defense of the host against infections is well documented (1–3). In the absence of an inflammatory process, the neutrophils are confined to the intravascular compartment, where they comprise the majority of circulating leukocytes.

These cells measure about 10 to 15 mm in diameter, the nucleus is condensed and lobulated, and the lobes are joined by thin filaments of chromatin, although the filaments may not be easily visible if the lobes are partially superimposed.

Neutrophil cytoplasm is filled with granules. The smaller peroxidase-negative specific granules are more numerous secondary granules (4–8). Some small, irregularly shaped azurophils granules (primary granules), hav-

ing been reduced in number by cell divisions after the promyelocyte stage, are also present. These granules are membrane-bound lysosomes that contain many enzymes and other molecules (5–8). Tertiary granules also have been described in human neutrophil (9). These granules readily release gelatinase when stimulated by low levels of formyl methionyl-leucyl-phenylanine (FMLP) and phorbol myristic acetate (PMA) (10). They appear during the late myelocyte, metamyelocyte, and segmented neutrophils stages.

ORIGIN, DIFFERENTIATION, AND APOPTOSIS OF NEUTROPHILS

Neutrophils have an estimated lifespan of 6 to 8 hours in peripheral blood (6,11). Like other leukocytes, neutrophils originate from a common stem cell in the bone marrow. The totipotent stem cells are the progenitors for all blood cells, including lymphocytes, and can be recognized by their ability to form blast colonies *in vitro* (6,7).

The totipotent stem cells are the progenitors of the colony-forming unit's (CFU) multipotential cell for gran-

L. Fabbri, G. Caramori and M. Piattella: Institute of Respiratory Diseases, University of Ferrara, 44100 Ferrara, Italy.

P. Maestrelli: Institute of Occupational Diseases, University of Padua, 35127 Padua, Italy.

ulocytes, erythrocytes, monocytes, and megakaryocytes (CFU-GEMoMe), which is characterized by a limited ability of self-renewal.

The CFU-GEMoMe differentiates to the CFU-granulocyte/monocyte (CFU-GM) and then to the CFU-granulocyte cell (CFU-G), the progenitor of neutrophils (6,7). CFU-4 progenitors differentiate into different precursors.

Myeloblasts are undifferentiated cells with a large oval nucleus, large nucleoli, and cytoplasm lacking granule. Subsequently there are two stages, the promyelocyte and the myelocyte, each of which produces a distinct type of secretory granule, i.e., the azurophyl granules, which are produced only during the promyelocyte stage, and the specific granules that are produced only during the myelocyte stage. The metamyelocyte and band forms are nonproliferative stages that develop into the mature polymorphonuclear granulocyte characterized by a multilobulated nucleus (11–13).

A series of growth factors for bone marrow hematopoietic stem cells have been identified (14). Some of them, e.g., interleukin-1 (IL-1), interleukin-4 (IL-4), interleukin-6 (IL-6), and interleukin-8 (IL-8), act preferentially on early progenitor cells and, unlike true growth factors, they stimulate cell differentiation and act synergistically with other molecules (14). A second group acts as true growth factor (14,15). It includes interleukin-3 (IL-3) and granulocyte macrophage colony-stimulating factor (GM-CSF) and granulocyte colony-stimulating factor (G-CSF), which regulates the differentiation of more committed stem cells toward mature granulocytes (14,16).

At the time of leaving the bone marrow, neutrophils are completely differentiated and equipped with the complete spectrum of surface receptors and intracytoplasmic granules with their secretory products (7,14,17). Neutrophil granulocytes contain many inflammatory mediators with the capacity to injure tissues and amplify the inflammatory response (Table 1) (5,6,18). These inflammatory mediators have been implicated in the pathogenesis of many inflammatory diseases, including bronchial asthma.

TABLE 1. *Inflammatory mediators produced by neutrophils*

Proteolytic enzymes	Serine elastase, cathepsin G, proteinase 3, collagenase, gelatinase
Microbicidal proteins	Lactoferrin, defensins, bacterial permeability-increasing protein CAP37/asurocidin, lysozyme
Nitric oxide	Myeloperoxidase
Lipid mediators	LTB4, PAF, TXA2
Oxygen radicals	Superoxide anion, hydrogen peroxide, radical hydroxyl
Cytokines	IL-1β, IL-6, IL-8, TNF-α, TGF-β1

LTB4, leukotriene B4; PAF, platelet activating factor; TAX2, thromboxane 2; IL, interleukin; TNF-α, tumor necrosis factor-α; TGF-β1, transforming growth factor-β1

Neutrophils undergo apoptosis, a physiologic or programmed form of cell death distinct from accidental cell death or necrosis, which is responsible for deletion of unwanted cells in different processes as immunologic tolerance, embryologic tissues remodeling, neoplasia, inflammation, and normal tissue turnover (19). Clearance of neutrophils from inflamed tissue is a prerequisite for inflammatory resolution (20). Macrophage phagocyte impact apoptotic neutrophil (19,21,22). Fibroblasts are able, *in vitro,* to recognize and ingest apoptotic neutrophils with participation of the fibroblast vitronectin receptor (CD51) and the involvement of a mannose/fucose-specific lectine (23). The cellular changes in apoptosis are numerous, such as condensation of the nucleus and condensation and vacuolation of the cytoplasm, but it is still not clear which of them is directly associated with cell death and which is of the greatest physiologic importance (19).

MEMBRANE RECEPTORS AND SURFACE MARKERS OF NEUTROPHILS

Numerous membrane receptors have been identified on the surface of neutrophils that modulate the neutrophil functions, including adherence, migration, degranulation, and phagocytosis (6,8).

Two receptors for the complement-activating fragment (Fc) portion of immunoglobulin G (IgG) (CD16[FcγRII] and Cdw32 [FcγRIIIb]) and one receptor for the crystallizable fragment (Fc) of IgA (FcaR) have been characterized on neutrophils (24,25). These immunoglobulins have been implicated in the recruitment and activation of neutrophils in inflammatory processes (26).

Neutrophils also can interact with IgE through its binding to the Mac-2/e-binding protein (Mac-2/e-BP) of the S-lectin family present on their surface (27). This interaction appears to account for the activation of the neutrophil respiratory burst by IgE immune complexes (27).

Bacteria-derived polypeptides interact with neutrophils via a specific FLMP receptor (FPR); several molecules, including GM-CSF, can upregulate the cell-surface expression of these receptors (28).

Endotoxin (lypopolysaccharide, LPS) derived from gram-negative bacteria also interacts with the neutrophil surface via the binding of several ligands, including CD14 (LPS-binding protein) and the bacterial permeability–increasing protein (BIP) (29,30).

Most of the neutrophil chemoattractants also act by binding to specific membrane receptors. IL-8 shares two classes of receptors with two other activators of neutrophils, neutrophil-activating protein-2 (NAP-2) and gro/melanoma growth-stimulatory activity (gro/MGSA) (31). There are also, on neutrophils, specific receptors for colony-stimulating factors (G-CSF, GM-CSF) (6).

The arachidonic acid metabolites leukotriene B4 (LTB4) and platelet-activating factor (PAF) bind to specific receptors present on neutrophils (32,33). Several receptors (CR1, CR3, CR4 decay accelerating factor [DAF], membrane co-factor protein [MCP]) for the complement component C3 have been reported in neutrophils (34); C5a receptors also are present on neutrophils and mediate adherence, chemotaxis, degranulation, and oxygen radical release induced by C5a (35).

Moreover, neutrophils express on their cell membrane receptors for adenosine (A$_2$) (36) tumor necrosis factor-alpha (TNF-α) and atrial natriuretic peptide (ANP), although as single agents the TNF-α and ANP have minimal effect on neutrophils, and they can potentiate activation of neutrophil induced by other factors (37,38).

ADHERENCE AND MIGRATION OF NEUTROPHILS

At a local site of tissue damage or infection, adherence of the neutrophils to the endothelial cells of the blood microvasculature and their subsequent emigration into the tissue can be seen within minutes (5,6). Leukocyte adhesion to human endothelial cells and other substrata appears to be mediated principally by three glycoprotein receptors Mac-1 (CD11b/CD18), leukocyte function antigen 1 (LAF-1, [CD11a/CD18]), and p150,95 (CD11c/CD18), which are found exclusively on white blood cells and hemopoietic precursors. These receptors belong to the larger category of adhesion molecules called integrins, are heterodimers, and have a b-chain CD18 in common (39–41).

Antibodies against the membrane glycoprotein complex decrease chemotaxis and neutrophil adhesion to endothelial cell *in vitro* and markedly decrease neutrophil accumulation at sites of inflammation *in vivo* (41,42). Compared with neutrophils, the role of the endothelial cells in the regulation of migratory processes is likely to be equally important (40). Thus, binding properties for neutrophils have now been demonstrated for a series of endothelial cell surface molecules including P-selectin and intercellular adhesion molecule 1 and 2 (ICAM-1 and ICAM-2), members of the Ig supergene family (41–44). ICAM-1 is expressed on unstimulated endothelial cells and represents the corresponding binding site for both LFA-1 and Mac-1 of the neutrophils, whereas ICAM-2 binds only LFA-1 (42). Binding of ICAM-1 to β_2-integrins is involved in adherence and appears to play a major role in transendothelial migration of neutrophils (41,43,44).

Several mechanisms can increase neutrophils' adherence to endothelial cells; β_2-integrins and ICAM-1 expression on the cell surface can be upregulated, providing an increased number of anchorage sites. This upregulation can be induced by cytokines such as TNF-α, IL-1 for endothelial cells, and GM-CSF, PAF, and bacteria-derived formyl peptides for neutrophils (41,42,45).

Moreover, other factors can modulate the interaction between endothelial cells and neutrophils such as configuration modulation involving cytoskeletal changes and protein kinase C (PKC) activation (46), increased local concentration of divalent cations (Mn^{2+}, Mg^{2+}), autocrine secretion of binding factors by neutrophils such as integrin modulating factor (47,48), and synthesis and expression of PAF on endothelial cells surface (33,45). Most of the mediators involved in the adherence process are also implicated in the regulation of neutrophil migration (6).

SECRETORY AND PHAGOCYTIC FUNCTION

Several stimuli, including bacterial peptides (FMLP), LPS, complement fragments (C5a), GM-CSF, IL-6, IL-8, TNF-α, LTB$_4$, and PAF, can activate neutrophils (6,8). They release a series of secretory products able to react with pathogens and host tissues (5,6,18). These neutrophil-derived products are mostly stored in lysosomal granules; they migrate to the cell membrane and the fusion with the membrane initiates the exocytosis, followed by the release of the granule content into the extracellular medium (6). In addition to these intracellular products, neutrophils can undergo a respiratory burst and release substantial amounts of reactive oxygen metabolites including superoxide anion (O_2^-) and hydrogen peroxide (H_2O_2). These molecules, through the catalytic effect of myeloperoxidase and halide, appear to be of major importance in bacterial killing (49). Neutrophils play an important role as inflammatory cells in the defense of the organism against infections both through secretory and phagocytic functions (1–3). The presence of inhibitory mechanisms of neutrophil activation is equally important because they can prevent an inadequate and prolonged activation of neutrophils, which could lead to tissue damage. Such inhibitors of neutrophil functions have been identified as secretory products derived from endothelial cells such as prostacyclin (PGI$_2$), adenosine, and nitric oxide (NO), from macrophages such as prostaglandin E$_2$ (PGE$_2$) and alveolar macrophage–derived neutrophil inhibitor, and from platelets (lipoxin A$_4$, LXA$_4$) (5,6,50).

The principal role of neutrophils in inflammatory and immune responses has long been thought to be the phagocytosis and killing of bacteria via the generation of reactive oxygen intermediates and the release of lytic enzymes stored in granules. Neutrophil granules contain more than 20 enzymes (6); lysozyme, present in both azurophil and specific granules, can induce the hydrolysis of glycosidic linkages in bacterial cell wall (51). Lactoferrin, a protein stored in neutrophil-specific granules, is also considered to have a bactericidal and fungicide activity (52); other enzymes including cathepsin G, defensins, and bacterial permeability-increasing protein have a well defined role in antibacterial defenses (3,53,54). Different proteinases are considered to have the greatest potential for tissue destruction at inflammatory sites: neutrophil elastase (55), neutral serine protease (56) (active on elastin fibers and type I, II, III, and IV collagens), and collagenase (preferentially active on type I as compared with type III collagen) (57), and gelatinase, a metalloprotein with specific activity on type V collagen, a major constituent of the basement membrane (58).

These proteinases, however, are rapidly and irreversibly degraded by antiproteinases such as α_1-antiproteinase (α_1-PI) and α_2-macroglobulin (α_2-MG), which are present in plasma and interstitial fluid. Gelatinase and other plasma proteins such as albumin, transferrin, IgG, tetranectin, alkaline phosphatase, cytochrome b558, and CR1 are internalized in intracytoplasmatic vesicles (59). The exocytosis of these vesicles is induced by concentrations of chemotactic factors lower than those required for degranulation of azurophil and specific granules (59). Lipid mediators, which cause the influx of inflammatory cells, such as LTB$_4$, PAF, and thromboxane A$_2$ (TXA$_2$), are released from neutrophils at sites of inflammation (60).

Recent *in vitro* studies have raised the possibility that neutrophils might be a significant source of cytokines in inflammatory lesions because neutrophils can release IL-1β, IL-6 IL-8, tumor necrosis factor-α (TNF-α), and transforming growth factor β1 (TGF-β1) (6,61–64). Animal studies have suggested that cytokine production by neutrophils might significantly affect processes such as modulation of the immune or antitumor responses (65).

Neutrophils are terminally differentiated, short-lived cells incapable of proliferation or self-renewal; however, increasing evidence indicates that neutrophil survival can be greatly extended after exposure to microenvironmental signals involved in infection and immunity (66). Neutrophils should be considered not only as active and central elements of the inflammatory response, but also as cells that, through cytokine and other mediators, may significantly influence the direction and evolution of immune processes (67) (Table 1).

ROLE OF NEUTROPHILS IN ACUTE AND CHRONIC AIRWAYS INFLAMMATION

Infections

Neutrophils are considered as a major cellular component in the defense of lung against respiratory infections (1–3,68–75). The success of the neutrophil granulocytes in the defense against micro-organisms depends not only on its ultimate action, killing of the ingested microorganism, but also on the ability of neutrophil to perform the necessary related activities, i.e., to recognize and to move toward the intruding bacteria and fungi and to seize and internalize them (1,3). An understanding of the microbicidal mechanism of neutrophils is based on the recognition that morphologic and biochemical changes that take place in the neutrophil are intimately connected and not simply epiphenomena triggered by phagocytosis (1,3).

It is well recognized that patients with marked neutropenia or severe defects in neutrophil function often present with respiratory problems and other types of life-threatening bacterial and fungal infections (1,3,76,77). However, in these patients infections do not always occur, suggesting that other host defense mechanisms are involved and could compensate for the decrease in neutrophil number and/or function. The adherence properties of neutrophils influence their transendothelial migration and indirectly their antibacterial role at the site of infection. Both gram-positive and gram-negative infections are observed in patients with neutropenia, although the latter are more frequent (78). Some organisms such as virulent staphylococci may survive and multiply within neutrophils and actually may kill them, overcoming the defense mechanism (79). In certain streptococcal and other infections, bacterial exotoxins (e.g., streptolysin) are released and damage the phagosomal membrane (80). Also, vitamin A and certain drugs, when incorporated into phagosomal membranes, rend them fragile and readily susceptible to rupture, thereby leading to inflammation (81). Hydrocortisone has been shown to inhibit neutrophil oxidase activity and reduce bacterial killing (82).

Smoking

Smoking can cause a decrease in lung function, but only a minority of smokers develop severe chronic obstructive pulmonary disease (83). In cigarette smokers, there is an increase of both venous peripheral blood and bronchoalveolar lavage (BAL) neutrophils in comparison with nonsmoking controls (84). Recent studies have shown a close correlation between the venous peripheral blood neutrophil count and serum lactoferrin protein contained in granules of neutrophils, which may protect the respiratory epithelium from oxygen radical damage by acting as an iron scavenger (85). The magnitude of the increase in serum lactoferrin in smokers compared with lifetime nonsmokers was larger than the increase in neutrophil counts; this is probably the result of the combination of an increase in the number of these cells and an enhanced secretory activity of the granulocytes in smokers compared with lifetime nonsmokers and an expression of activation of the cells (85). Nicotine is chemotactic for neutrophils and enhances neutrophil responsiveness to chemotactic peptides but does not affect degranulation or superoxide production (86). However, the relevance of active smoking on neutrophil function *in vivo* remains speculative (87).

Pulmonary Emphysema and Chronic Bronchitis

The prevalent hypothesis in the pathogenesis of pulmonary emphysema is an abnormal balance between proteases and antiproteases in the lung (88,89). This theory proposes that increased numbers of neutrophils and/or alveolar macrophages, activated by cigarette smoke or other inflammatory stimuli, release large amounts of proteases and oxidants responsible for tissue destruction, with the contribution of smoking-related oxidation and inactivation of α_1-antitrypsin, the major antiproteases of the lung (89). However, recent studies correlated the degree of pulmonary emphysema to overall alveolar wall cellularity and suggest that so long as the inflammatory reaction is predominantly of neutrophils, there is no destruction of the lung (90) and that alveolar macrophages and T lymphocytes might be more important in the pathogenesis of emphysema in smokers (90).

Increased numbers of neutrophils have been found in BAL fluid in patients with chronic bronchitis (91) and in sputum of patients with severe airflow limitation (92). By contrast, the dominant cell in the sputum of patients with stable chronic bronchitis is the macrophage, with few neutrophils, eosinophils, or metachromatic cells (93). Mild exacerbations of chronic bronchitis are associated with marked sputum eosinophilia and with a milder increase in the number of neutrophils (94), whereas severe exacerbations of chronic bronchitis are associated with marked sputum neutrophilia (95).

Whether the increase of the number of neutrophils and/or eosinophils in BAL and sputum of patients with chronic obstructive pulmonary disease (COPD) represents a cause or a consequence of the disease is unknown. However, through the release of many mediators (see Table 1), neutrophils could contribute to inflammation, bronchial damage, and mucus hypersecretion, three characteristics of chronic bronchitis.

NEUTROPHILS AND ASTHMA

Asthma is considered a chronic inflammatory disease of the airways that undergoes recurrent exacerbations of symptoms and airflow limitation. The exacerbations of asthma are associated with a change of the characteristics of airway inflammation, which become transiently acute.

It has long been recognized that fatal asthma is associated with marked inflammatory changes (96). A mild but significant increase of inflammatory cells has been consistently reported in BAL, tracheobronchial biopsies, and sputum of asthmatic individuals examined between attacks (97,98). Taking into account these findings, the most recent consensus documents on asthma define this disease as a chronic inflammatory disorder of the airways (99).

Although the relative role of each inflammatory cell for the pathogenesis of asthma remains unclear, the consensus underlines that eosinophils, mast cells, and T lymphocytes may be particularly relevant, and that a particular type of airway inflammation, including an increase and activation of these three cells, may be responsible for the airway hyperresponsiveness to a variety of stimuli, which is the physiologic hallmark of the disease (99).

As suggested by this definition of asthma, which underlines the particular role of lymphocytes, eosinophils, and mast cells, neutrophils seem to have no role in the chronic inflammation of the airways and with the airway hyperresponsiveness associated with stable asthma.

LONG-LASTING AND TRANSIENT AIRWAY HYPERRESPONSIVENESS

Airway hyperresponsiveness is an exaggerated bronchoconstrictive response to physical, chemical, or pharmacologic stimuli (100). It is a common and important feature of bronchial asthma. There is some evidence that asthma airway hyperresponsiveness is associated with the presence of airway inflammation (97,98,101,102), but the relative role of each inflammatory cell remains unclear. In stable mild asthmatics, airway hyperresponsiveness significantly correlates with bronchoalveolar eosinophils, methachromatic cells, or epithelial cells (98), but not with neutrophils.

Similar to the variable nature of the disease, the degree of airway hyperresponsiveness also is variable, being often, but not invariably (103), further increased when asthma is active or exacerbated, and decreased, sometimes to normal levels, when asthma is in remission (100, 104). The involvement of neutrophils in the transient increase of airway responsiveness has been first suggested by studies in animals.

ANIMAL STUDIES

In dogs, the transient increase of airway responsiveness induced by allergen inhalation (105), ozone (106), PAF (107), and LTB_4 (108) is associated with neutrophilia in BAL and/or biopsies. The transient increase of airway responsiveness and the associated neutrophilia in BAL and in biopsies induced by exposure to ozone are all prevented by depletion of circulating neutrophils induced with the cytotoxic agent hydroxyurea (109). However, pretreatment of dogs with an antibody against neutrophil adhesion molecules does not prevent ozone-induced hyperresponsiveness, even if it totally prevents the bronchoalveolar neutrophilia induced by ozone (110). Similarly, the prevention of ozone-induced airway hyperresponsiveness by indomethacin (111), and by antioxidant agents (112), is not associated with prevention of ozone-induced neutrophilia. These data, taken together, suggest that, in dogs, airway neutrophilia and airway hyperresponsiveness may represent separate effects of ozone.

Bronchoalveolar neutrophilia and eosinophilia occur during late asthmatic reactions and hyperresponsiveness induced by extracts of *Ascaris suum* in sheep spontaneously allergic to *A. suum* (113,114). A transient bronchoalveolar neutrophilia and airway hyperresponsiveness occur in nonsensitized sheep after inhalation of aerosolized endotoxins (115), and granulocyte depletion decreases the degree of airway responsiveness present in these animals (116).

In rabbits actively sensitized to *Alternaria,* an increased number of neutrophils in the airway mucosa is present during the late asthmatic reactions and during the transient increase of airway responsiveness induced by inhalation of *Alternaria* extracts (117). These effects of the inhalation challenge with *Alternaria* are prevented by neutrophil depletion and are reconstituted by neutrophil repletion of the animals with concentrated (i.e., 97%) neutrophils (118). Also in rabbits, the number of neutrophils transiently increases in the airway mucosa during the transient increase of airway responsiveness induced by aerosolized C5A desArg, a complement fragment with marked neutrophil chemotactic activity; this effect is prevented by neutrophil depletion (119). All these studies, taken together, suggest a significant pathogenetic role of neutrophils for late asthmatic reactions and for the transient increase of airway responsiveness induced by allergen challenge or complement fragments in rabbits.

In monkeys with a natural-occurring hypersensitivity to *A. suum,* a single *Ascaris* inhalation of *Ascaris* extract induces acute airway obstruction associated with a marked but transient bronchoalveolar neutrophililia, associated with a mild but prolonged bronchoalveolar eosinophilia (120). Interestingly, pretreatment with a monoclonal antibody against neutrophil adhesion molecules specifically prevents bronchoalcveolar neutrophilia and airway obstruction induced by allergen, suggesting a significant role of neutrophils for the development of asthmatic reactions in this animal model. However, in the same model, both the transient and the sustained increase of airway responsiveness and the bronchoalveolar eosinophilia induced by inhalation of *Ascaris* extract are both prevented by a monoclonal antibody against ICAM-1, the adhesion molecule for eosinophils, suggesting a major role of eosinophils rather than neutrophils for the transient and sustained increase of airway responsiveness induced by the allergen challenge (121–123).

In a similar animal model, recent studies have shown that a neutralizing monoclonal antibody to interleukin-5 (IL-5) has a long-lasting preventing effect on both increased responsiveness and airway eosinophilia and neutrophilia induced by *Ascaris* challenge (124).

IN VITRO EVIDENCE FOR THE INVOLVEMENT OF NEUTROPHILS IN THE PATHOGENESIS OF ASTHMA

In vitro studies have produced conflicting results. Products generated by activation with calcium ionophore of human neutrophils and eosinophils increase the responsiveness of human bronchial tissue to histamine and electrical field stimulation, suggesting that both cells may have an active role in regulating airway responsiveness *in vivo* (125). However, it is not known whether other more physiologic inflammatory cell activators such as cytokines and bacterial factors can induce from neutrophils the release of mediators that increase airway smooth muscle responsiveness. For example, neutrophil activation by GM-CSF and FMLP does not result in the release of products that increase bronchial responsiveness *in vitro* (126).

Interestingly, the antiasthma drug nedocromil sodium inhibits the airway hyperresponsiveness induced *in vitro* by ionophore-activated human neutrophils (126), possibly by preventing the release of mediators such as arachidonic acid metabolites, which are active on airway smooth muscle (126,127).

Because inflammatory cells are thought to play an active role in the pathogenesis of asthma, the inhibitory effect of nedocromil sodium on the mobilization, activation, and mediator release from neutrophils has been investigated *in vitro,* the results suggesting that nedocromil sodium may interfere with a receptor-mediated intracellular signal transduction process (128).

Other *in vitro* studies have shown that neutrophils obtained from asthmatics exhibit a heightened respiratory burst compared with normal control, such as enhanced secretion of superoxide that may contribute to the airway inflammation characteristic of asthma (129). Whether such an increase in secretion of superoxide may modify airway responsiveness remains to be established.

EVIDENCE AGAINST THE INVOLVEMENT OF NEUTROPHILS IN AIRWAY HYPERRESPONSIVENESS AND ASTHMA

Indeed, neutrophils are neither increased nor activated in biopsies (97,99,130–133), sputum (93,134–136), or BAL (95,98,101,102,137–139) of asthmatics examined in stable conditions, and their number and state of activation does not correlate, except in a few studies (101,102), with the degree of airway hyperresponsiveness (95,97–99,101, 102,130–139).

Both human and animal studies suggest that the long-lasting hyperresponsiveness present between asthmatic exacerbations is associated with mild airway inflammation, but neutrophils are not increased in the bronchial mucosa and in BAL of these patients. Indeed, the bronchial biopsies (97) and BAL fluid (98) from asthmatic patients examined between asthmatic exacerbations show a slight increase of inflammatory cells, particularly eosinophils, mast cells, and lymphocytes, but not neutrophils. Although several studies have shown a correlation between the number of eosinophils, mast cells, and/or epithelial cells in BAL and the degree of airway responsiveness (reviewed in ref. 98), only one study has reported a significant correlation between the degree of bronchial hyperresponsiveness (PD$_{20}$ FEV$_1$) and the number of neutrophils (101).

Apart from the specific role of the single inflammatory cells, the observation that airway responsiveness remains increased in most asthmatic patients even after long-term treatment with inhaled glucocorticoids (140–142), or after cessation of exposure to occupational sensitizing agent (143,144), at a time when either all inflammatory cells have returned to normal or close to normal (140,144,145) or the subepithelial fibrosis has disappeared (143,146), suggests that the long-lasting airway hyperresponsiveness inherited or experimentally induced in animals is not associated with airway inflammation.

Although some of the human and animal studies reviewed in this chapter would suggest that neutrophils may be involved in the development of asthma exacerbations, no studies, not even the leukocyte depletion studies performed so far, rule out the possibility that asthma exacerbations are merely associated and not causally related to the increase of inflammatory cells, particularly neutrophils, in airway tissues.

Also, in guinea pigs the airway hyperresponsiveness induced by inhalation of ozone develops before the increase of neutrophils infiltration of the airway mucosa, i.e., in the exudative noncellular phase of the inflammatory reaction (147) (similar results have been obtained with smoke [148]), and is not prevented by administration of steroids or leukocyte depletion (147), suggesting that leukocytes may not be required for airway hyperresponsiveness to develop. Also, in guinea pig, neutrophil depletion induced with cyclophosphamide, in contrast to neutrophil depletion induced by hydroxyurea, does not prevent the increase of airway responsiveness induced by toluene diisocyanate (TDI) (149), suggesting that the effect observed in other studies might be related to a nonspecific effect of hydroxyurea and might not be mediated by neutrophil depletion.

Finally, a recent study has shown that *ex vivo*–activated human eosinophils, but not similarly activated human neutrophils, increase the muscarinic airway responsiveness of guinea pigs, confirming that neutrophils may not be involved in the regulation of airway smooth muscle responsiveness in this animal species (150).

EXPERIMENTAL HYPERRESPONSIVENESS IN HUMANS

Neutrophils have been shown to be involved in the acute inflammatory reaction of the airways occurring af-

ter bronchoprovocation with allergens or sensitizing agents (151–155), during spontaneous asthma attacks (156,157), nocturnal asthma (158,159), and even in the dramatic bronchopulmonary inflammation associated with asthma death (160,161).

The importance of neutrophils for asthma exacerbations has been examined in experimentally induced airway hyperresponsiveness in nonasthmatic and asthmatic individuals. Exposure to ozone (162–166), nitrogen dioxide (165,166), and inhalation of inflammatory mediators such as PAF (167) increases the airway responsiveness of normal individuals and causes transient airway neutrophilia.

Interestingly, asthmatics exposed to ozone develop a significant BALF neutrophilia and increased levels of the cytokines IL-8 and IL-6, even at a level of ozone exposure that does not reduce pulmonary function (164). Similarly, aerosolized TNF-α causes a transient increase of airway responsiveness associated with sustained sputum neutrophilia and not eosinophilia in normal individuals (168), further suggesting the potential involvement of neutrophils in asthma exacerbations.

An association does not prove a cause-effect relationship. Indeed, in dogs, although there is ample evidence that the transient airway hyperresponsiveness induced by ozone is associated with neutrophilia both in the airway mucosa and in BAL, complete prevention of the neutrophilia with an antiadhesion molecule antibody (110) does not prevent airway hyperresponsiveness, suggesting the lack of a cause-effect relationship between neutrophilia and hyperresponsiveness.

In conclusion, although there is no evidence that neutrophils play a significant role in the maintenance of long-lasting airway hyperresponsiveness, there is some evidence that neutrophils are involved in the transient increase of airway responsiveness induced by different inflammatory stimuli both in animal and humans. Whether the increase of neutrophils is associated only with late asthmatic reactions and/or the transient increase of airway responsiveness, or neutrophils are in fact involved in the development of late asthmatic reactions and/or the transient increase of airway responsiveness, remains to be determined.

EVIDENCE FOR THE INVOLVEMENT OF NEUTROPHILS IN THE PATHOGENESIS OF HUMAN ASTHMA

As previously mentioned, the evidence that neutrophils play a role in asthma is controversial. Neutrophils appear to be normal resident cells of the larger airway. We now examine the evidence for and against the role of neutrophils in the pathogenesis of asthma of different severity or cause, and thus in patients with stable asthma, in asthmatics after experimental challenge with allergens, occupational sensitizers, or atmospheric pollutants, in spontaneous and experimental exacerbations of asthma, and in fatal asthma.

STABLE ASTHMA

Similar numbers of neutrophils have been found in bronchial biopsies, BAL, and sputum of stable asthmatic patients and healthy control subjects (95,97–99,101,102, 130–139). Only one study has reported that individuals with occupational asthma have a significant increase of neutrophils in bronchial biopsies, but not in BAL, even after removal from the causal agent (169). In addition, only one study (101) has reported a significant correlation between the number of bronchoalveolar neutrophils and the degree of airway hyperresponsiveness in stable asthmatics.

The fact that the number of neutrophils found in BAL and in bronchial biopsies in stable asthmatic patients and healthy control subjects is not different does not exclude the possibility that neutrophils may have a different degree of activation. For example, in steroid-resistant asthmatics there is an increased production of LTB_4 by neutrophils in response to cytokines produced by peripheral blood mononuclear cells (170).

ASTHMA EXACERBATIONS INDUCED BY BRONCHOPROVOCATION

In humans, bronchoalveolar neutrophilia is present before the onset and during the first few hours of late asthmatic reactions induced by allergens (152,153), TDI (154), and plicatic acid (171), and a striking increase of neutrophils has been described recently in bronchial biopsies obtained after a local allergen challenge (155). Although the percentage increase is similar, the increase of the number of airway neutrophils is much larger than the increase of the number of airway eosinophils. The increase of neutrophils usually precedes, but sometimes parallels or follows, the increase of eosinophils, metachromatic cells, or lymphocytes (152–155,172).

Some recent studies question the mechanism of allergen-induced bronchoalveolar neutrophilia, suggesting that it might be due either to a nonspecific effect of the maneuvers involved in local bronchoprovocation (172, 173) or to endotoxin contamination of the allergen extracts (174). However, previous studies have shown bronchoalveolar neutrophilia during late reactions to allergens (151,152) or isocyanates (154) even in sites not previously lavaged, suggesting that indeed neutrophilia may be specific, and that the nonspecific increase observed after saline is linked to the specific maneuver of lavaging twice the same segment at short intervals. The specificity of airway neutrophilia occurring during the first few hours after allergen challenge is also suggested by the biopsy studies, where it is present only in allergen-challenged airways (155).

The serum heat stable neutrophil chemotactic activity (HS-NCA) is increased during early and late asthmatic reactions induced by allergens (175–177), toluene diisocyanate (178), and adenosine (179). Interestingly, during asthmatic reactions induced by inhalation of toluene diisocyanate the percentage increase in plasma neutrophil chemotactic activity correlates with the percentage decline of FEV_1 of the early asthmatic reaction (178).

Bronchoalveolar or airway neutrophilia or circulating neutrophil activation induced by bronchoprovocation is inhibited by some antiasthma drugs such as steroids (180,181) and cromones (182,183), but not by others (theophylline [184,185], formoterol, salmeterol), suggesting that some agent (e.g., steroids) may prevent the asthmatic reactions by preventing the inflammatory cascade, whereas others (e.g., theophylline or long-acting $β_2$-agonists) may prevent the asthmatic reaction by preventing bronchoconstriction and/or airway edema, without having any effect on the inflammatory cascade (186).

LY293111, a leukotriene B_4-receptor antagonist, given before allergen challenge to asthmatic persons reduces the numbers of BAL neutrophils in BAL but has no effect on early and late asthmatic responses, suggesting that neutrophils might in fact parallel the asthmatic reactions, but may not be involved in their development (187).

SPONTANEOUS ASTHMA EXACERBATIONS

Neutrophilia is associated with eosinophilia in sputum (156) and BAL fluid (157,188) during spontaneous asthma exacerbations, particularly if severe (156). By contrast, mild asthma exacerbations occurring during tapering of inhaled steroid treatment is associated with sputum eosinophilia but not with neutrophilia (134), suggesting that time course and triggers of exacerbations may be critical for the type of cellular response.

In exercise-induced asthma, many studies have shown an increased serum NCA (189–191), even if there is no clear-cut evidence of acute airway inflammation of the airways after exercise-induced asthma (192).

The chain of events leading to the acute airway inflammation associated with exacerbations of asthma can be hypothesized as follows: inflammatory stimuli activate immunocompetent and other resident cells of the airways that, once activated, release mediators that mobilize inflammatory cells from the circulation. The recruited inflammatory cells may then release inflammatory mediators that may cause directly or indirectly, via the nervous system, smooth muscle contraction, bronchial vasodilation, increase in microvascular leakage, epithelial damage, mucus hypersecretion, and efferent endings nerve stimulation (193,194). The precise mechanisms by which various inflammatory cells, and particularly neutrophils, are recruited to the lung during asthma exacerbations are unknown. It is believed that specific chemotactic factors and adhesion molecules are responsible for the recruitment of various inflammatory cells to the lung, particularly cells such as granulocytes, which are normally found in large numbers in the circulation (6). Leading candidates for chemotaxis of neutrophils include LTB$_4$, C5a, and IL-8 (6,195).

Recent studies have shown that neutrophils recruited to the lung of asthmatics by local allergen challenge display a marked inhibition of their chemotactic response to LTB$_4$, probably caused by a neutrophil desensitization produced by LTB$_4$, suggesting that LTB$_4$ might be responsible for their recruitment to the lung (196).

ACUTE SEVERE ASTHMA

Although mild controlled exacerbations of asthma are associated with sputum eosinophilia (134), severe asthma exacerbations are associated with a predominant sputum neutrophilia (156). Interestingly, the high IL-8 levels and free neutrophil elastase activity observed in the sputum of patients with severe exacerbations suggest that IL-8 may mediate airway neutrophilia and neutrophil elastase mucin glycoprotein hypersecretion that occurs in acute severe asthma (156). Interestingly, the arterial blood concentrations of the neutrophil chemotaxin LTB$_4$ correlate with the severity of asthma exacerbations and are sensitive to steroids, further suggesting the importance of neutrophils for severe asthma exacerbations (197).

Previous studies have shown that acute severe asthma is associated with an increase of serum neutrophil chemotactic activity (198) and with peripheral blood mononuclear cells that spontaneously elaborate an NCA distinct from IL-8 (199).

NOCTURNAL ASTHMA

The involvement of neutrophils in nocturnal asthma is still controversial. One study showed a significant increase of bronchoalveolar neutrophils and eosinophils at night in persons with nocturnal asthma, but other studies showed either no increase of inflammatory cells (200) or an increase of bronchoalveolar eosinophils and lymphocytes, but not of neutrophils (159).

SUDDEN-ONSET FATAL ASTHMA

Asthma has been considered in the past a relatively mild disease, and not a life-threatening disease. In fact, asthma mortality remains a relatively rare event. Overall, asthma mortality at 5 to 34 years of age is approximately four deaths per million persons per year in the United States. Even among the highest risk subgroups, the mor-

tality rates are around 10 per million per year (201). Even though the absolute number of deaths from asthma remains low, the rate of death from asthma has increased steadily in the United States (202). Pathologically, asthma is characterized by increased numbers of activated T lymphocytes, eosinophils, and mast cells in the airway mucosa and by thickening of the reticular basement membrane (203).

Two scenarios may lead to death from asthma, one associated with slow progression of the disease, and one characterized by sudden death (202). Asthma death associated with a slow progression of the disease is characterized by a dramatic increase of eosinophils in the submucosa (204), whereas sudden onset fatal asthma is characterized by fewer eosinophils and more neutrophils in the airway submucosa (160), and less mucus in the airways lumen (160,203). These observations raise the possibility that the mechanism of airway inflammation as well as of airway narrowing in sudden-onset fatal asthma may be different from that in slow-onset fatal asthma (160,161), and again that time course of the asthma exacerbation and possibly the nature of the trigger may be critical for the type of cellular response.

CONCLUSIONS

Airway inflammation appears to be central to the pathogenesis of most clinical manifestations of asthma. Indeed, chronic airway inflammation is present in stable asthmatics, and exacerbations of asthma are associated with exacerbation of the inflammation of the airways.

Neutrophils are not increased in the airway mucosa of stable asthmatics, suggesting that they may not be involved in the chronic airway inflammation associated with stable asthma. By contrast, there is substantial evi-

TABLE 2. *Role of neutrophils in the pathophysiology of human asthma*

Stable asthma	
Nonoccupational stable asthma	0
Nocturnal asthma	+/−
Occupational asthma	+
Steroid-resistant Asthma	+/−
RADS	−
Experimental asthmatic exacerbations	
Allergen challenge	+
Occupational sensitizers	+
Atmospheric pollutants	++
Spontaneous asthma exacerbations	
Mild-moderate spontaneous asthma exacerbations	+/−
Exercise-induced asthma	+/−
Acute severe asthma	++
Sudden-onset fatal asthma	++

0, Apparently no role of neutrophils; +/−, controversial role of neutrophils; +, significant role of neutrophils; ++ definite involvement of neutrophils.

dence, particularly in humans, that neutrophils may be involved in exacerbations of asthma, and particularly in the early stages of sudden and severe asthma exacerbations (Table 2). Also, the predominant involvement of neutrophils in some type of asthma exacerbations (i.e., induced by occupational sensitizers, or severe asthma exacerbations) with respect to others (e.g., allergens) suggests that different triggers of asthma may induce airway inflammation through different mechanisms.

ACKNOWLEDGMENTS

Supported by National Council of Research (Project FATMA 95.00820.PF41), MURST (fondi 60% e 40%), Consortium Ferrara Ricerche, and European Community (Project Concerted Action on Severe Asthma as part of the Project Biomed 2).

REFERENCES

1. Klempner MS, Malech HL. Phagocytes: normal and abnormal neutrophil host defenses. In: Gorbach SL, Bartlett JG, Blacklow NR, eds. *Infectious diseases*. Philadelphia: WB Saunders, 1992;43–62.
2. Phair JP, et al. Phagocytosis and algicidal activity of human polymorphonuclear neutrophils against *Prototheca wickerhamii*. *J Infect Dis* 1981;144:72–76.
3. Lehrer RI, Ganz T, Selsted ME, Babior BM, Curnutte JT. Neutrophils and host defense. *Ann Intern Med* 1988;109:127–142.
4. Scott RE, Horn RG. Ultrastructural aspects of neutrophil granulocyte development in humans. *Lab Invest* 1970;23:202–215.
5. Sibille Y, Reynolds HY. Macrophages and polymorphonuclear neutrophils in lung, defense and injury. *Am Rev Respir Dis* 1990;141:471–501.
6. Sibille Y, Marchandise F-X. Pulmonary immune cells in health and disease: polymorphonuclear neutrophils. *Eur Respir J* 1993;6:1529–1543.
7. Bainton DF. Development biology of neutrophils and eosinophils. In: Gallin JI, Goldstein IM, Snyderman R, eds. *Inflammation: basic principles and clinical correlates*. New York: Raven Press, 1992;303–325.
8. Abramson SL, Malech HL, Gallin JI. Major components. Neutrophils. In: Crystal RG, West JB, eds. *The lung: scientific foundation*. New York: Raven Press, 1991;553–574.
9. Payne DN, Ackerman GA. Ultrastructural autoradiographic study of the uptake and intracellular localization of ^{35}S-sulfate by developing human neutrophils. *Blood* 1977;50:841–856.
10. Dewald B, Bretz U, Baggiolini M. Release of gelatinase from a novel secretory compartment of human neutrophils. *J Clin Invest* 1982;70:518–525.
11. Bainton DF, Ullyot JL, Farquhar MG. The development of neutrophilic polymorphonuclear leukocytes in human bone marrow: origin and content of azurophil and specific granules. *J Exp Med* 1971;134:907–934.
12. Boll I, Kuhn A. Granulocytopoies in human bone marrow cultures studies by means of kinematography. *Blood* 1965;26:449–453.
13. Quesenberry P, Levitt L. Hematopoietic stem cells. *N Engl J Med* 1979;301:755,819,868.
14. Ogawa M. Hematopoiesis. *J Allergy Clin Immunol* 1994;94:645–650.
15. Vancheri C, Ohtoshi T, Cox G, et.al. Neutrophilic differentiation induced by human upper airway fibroblast-derived granulocyte/macrophage colony-stimulating factor (GM-CSF). *Am J Respir Cell Mol Biol* 1991;4:11–17.
16. Boogaerts M, Cavalli F, Cortès-Funes H, Gatell JM, Khayat D, Levy Y, Link H. Granulocyte growth factors: achieving a consensus. *Ann Oncol* 1995;6:237–44.
17. Yoshimura K, Crystal RG. Transcriptional and posttranscriptional modulation of human neutrophil elastase gene expression. *Blood* 1992;79:2733–2740.
18. Weiss SJ. Tissue destruction by neutrophils. *N Engl J Med* 1989;320:365–376.
19. Cohen JJ. Apoptosis. *Immunol Today* 1993;14:126–133.
20. Weissman G. Inflammation: historical perspectives. In: Gallin JI, Goldstein IM, Snyderman R, eds. *Inflammation: basic principles and clinical correlates*, 2nd ed. New York: Raven Press, 1992;5–13.
21. Savill J, Fadok V, Henson P, Haslett C. Phagocyte recognition of cells undergoing apoptosis. *Immunol Today* 1993;14:131–136.
22. Newman SL, Henson JE, Henson PM. Phagocytosis of senescent neutrophils by human monocyte-derived macrophages and rabbit inflammatory macrophages. *J Exp Med* 1982;156:430–442.
23. Hall SE, Savill JS, Henson PM, Haslett C. Apoptotic neutrophils are phagocytosed by fibroblasts with partecipation of the fibroblast vitronectin receptor and involvement of a mannose/fucose-specific lectine. *J Immunol* 1994;153:3218–3227.
24. Unkeless JC. Function and heterogeneity of human Fc receptors for immunoglobulin G. *J Clin Invest* 1989;83:355–361.
25. Albrechtsen M, Yeaman GR, Kerr MA. Characterization of the IgA receptor from human polymorphonuclear neutrophils. *Immunology* 1988;64:201–205.
26. Reynolds HY. Mechanisms of inflammation in the lungs. *Am Rev Med* 1987;38:295–331.
27. Truoug MJ, Gruart V, Kusnierz JP, et al. Human neutrophils express immunoglobulin E (IgE)-binding proteins (Mac-2/eBP) on the S-type lectine family: role in IgE-dependent activation. *J Exp Med* 1993;177:243–248.
28. Becker EL. The formylpeptide receptor of the neutrophil. *Am J Pathol* 1987;38:295–331.
29. Worthen GS, Avdi N, Vukajlovich S, Tobias PS. Neutrophil adherence induced by lipopolysaccharide *in vitro*. Role of plasma component interaction with lipopolysaccharide. *J Clin Invest* 1992;90:2526–2535.
30. Weersink AJL, van Kessel KPM, van den Tol ME, et al. Human granulocytes express a 55 Kda lipopolysaccharide-binding protein on the cell surface that is identical to the bactericidal/permeability-increasing protein. *J Immunol* 1993;150:253–263.
31. Moser B, Schumacher C, von Tscharner V, Clarck-Lewis I, Baggiolini M. Neutrophil-activating peptide 2 and gro-melanoma growth-stimulatory activity interact with neutrophil activating peptide 1/interleukin-8 receptors on human neutrophils. *J Biol Chem* 1991;266:10666–10671.
32. Martin TR, Pistorese BP, Chi EY, Goodman RB, Matthay MA. Effects of leukotriene B4 in the human lung. Recruitment of neutrophils into the alveolar spaces without a change in protein permeability. *J Clin Invest* 1989;84:1609–1619.
33. Dent G, Ukena D, Chanez P, Sybrecht G, Barnes P. Characterization of PAF receptors on human neutrophils using the specific antagonist, WEB 2086: correlation between receptor binding and function. *FEBS Lett* 1989;244:365–368.
34. Holers VM, Kinoshita T, Molina H. The evolution of mouse and human complement C3-binding proteins: divergence of form but conservation of function. *Immunol Today* 1992;13:231–236.
35. Chenoweth DE, Hugli TE. Demonstration of specific C5a receptors on intact human polymorphonuclear leukocytes. *Proc Nat Acad Sci U S A* 1978;75:3943–3954.
36. Rose FR, Hirschhorn R, Weissmann G, Cronstein BN. Adenosine promotes neutrophil chemotaxis. *J Exp Med* 1988;167:1186–1194.
37. Wiedermann CJ, Niedermuhlbichler M, Braunsteiner H. Priming of polymorphonuclear neutrophils by atrial natriuretic peptide *in vitro*. *J Clin Invest* 1992;89:1580–1586.
38. Shalaby MR Jr, Palladino MA, Hirabayash SE, et al. Receptor binding and activation of polymorphonuclear neutrophils by tumor-necrosis-alpha. *J Leukocyte Biol* 1987;41:196–203.
39. Zimmerman GA, Prescott SM, McIntyre TM. Endothelial cell interactions with granulocytes: tethering and signaling molecules. *Immunol Today* 1992;13:93–99.
40. Tedder TF, Steeber DA, Chen A, Engel P. The selectins: vascular adhesion molecules. *FASEB J* 1995;9:866–873.
41. Adams DH, Shaw S. Leucocyte-endothelial interactions and regulation of leucocyte migration. *Lancet* 1994;343:831–835.
42. Carlos TM, Harlen JM. Leukocyte-Endothelial adhesion molecules. *Blood* 1994;84:2068–2101.
43. Nakajima S, Look DC, Roswit WT, Bragdon MJ, Holtzman MJ. Selective differences in vascular endothelial vs. airway epithelial. T- cell adhesion mechanism. *Am J Physiol* 1994;263:2422–2432.

44. Albelda SM. Endothelial and epithelial cell adhesion molecules. *Am J Respir Cell Mol Biol* 1991;4:195–203.

45. Kuijpers TW, Hakkert BC, Hoogerwerf M, Leeuwenberg JFM, Roos D. Role of endothelial leukocyte adhesion molecule-1 and platelet-activating factor in neutrophil adherence to IL-1 prestimulated endothelial cells. Endothelial leukocyte adhesion molecule-1-mediate CD18 activation. *J Immunol* 1991;147:1369–1376.

46. Pardi R, Inverardi L, Bender JR. Regulatory mechanisms in leukocyte adhesion: flexible receptors for sophisticated travelers. *Immunol Today* 1992;13:224–230.

47. Altieri DC. Occupancy of CD11b/CD18 (Mac-1) divalent ion binding site(s) induces leukocyte adhesion *J Immunol* 1991;147:1891–1898.

48. Elices MJ, Urry LA, Hemler ME. Receptor functions for the integrin VLA-3: fibronectin, collagen and laminin binding are differentially influenced by Arg-Gly-Asp peptide and by divalent cations. *J Cell Biol* 1991;112:169–181.

49. Fantone JC, Ward PA. Role of oxygen-derived free radicals and metabolites in leukocyte dependent inflammatory reactions. *Am J Pathol* 1982;107:397–418.

50. Clancy RM, Leszczynska-Piziak J, Abramson SB. Nitric oxide an endothelial cell relaxation factors, inhibits neutrophil superoxide anion production via a direct action on the NADPH oxidase. *J Clin Invest* 1992;90:1116–1121.

51. Konstan MW, Chen PW, Sherman JM, Thomassen MJ, Wood RE, Boat TF. Human lung lysozyme: sources and properties. *Am Rev Respir Dis* 1981;123:120–124.

52. Brok JH. Iron-binding proteins. *Acta Paediatr Scand* 1989;361 (suppl):31–43.

53. Spitznagel JK. Bactericidal mechanism of the granulocyte. *Pro Clin Biol Res* 1976;13:103–108.

54. Spitznagel JK. Antibiotic proteins of human neutrophils. *J Clin Invest* 1990;86:1381–1384.

55. Smedly CA, Tonnesen MG, Sendhaus RA, et al. Neutrophil mediated injury to endothelial cells. Enhancement by endotoxin and essential role of neutrophil elastase. *J Clin Invest* 1986;77:1233–1243.

56. Kao RC, Wehner NG, Skubitz KM, Gray BH, Hoidal JR. Proteinase 3. A distinct human polymorphonuclear leukocyte proteinase that produces emphysema in hamsters. *J Clin Invest* 1988;82:1963–1973.

57. Macartney HW, Tschesche H. Latent and active human polymorphonuclear leukocyte collagenases. Isolation, purification and characterization. *Eur J Biochem* 1983;130:71–78.

58. Hibbs MS, Bainton DF. Human neutrophil gelatinase is a component of specific granules. *J Clin Invest* 1989;84:1395–1402.

59. Borregaard N, Kjeldsen L, Rygaard K, et al. Stimulus dependent secretion of plasma proteins from human neutrophils. *J Clin Invest* 1992;90:86–96.

60. Valone FH, Boggs JM, Goetzel EJ. Lipid mediators of hypersensitivity and inflammation. In: Middleton E Jr, Reed CE, Ellis EF, Adkinson NF Jr, Yunginger JW, Busse WW, eds. *Allergy: principles and practice.* St. Louis: CV Mosby, 1993;84:501–510.

61. Haziot A, Tsuber BZ, Goyert SM. Neutrophil CD14: biochemical properties and role in the secretion of tumor necrosis factor-α in response to lipopolysaccharide *J Immunol* 1993;150:5556–5565.

62. Malyak M, Smith ME, Abel AA, Azend WP. Peripheral blood neutrophil production of interleukin-1 receptor antagonist and interleukin-1 beta *J Clin Immunol* 1994;14:20–30.

63. Cassatella MA, Bazzoni F, Ceska M, Ferro I, Baggiolini M, Berton G. IL-8 production by human polymorphonuclear leukocytes. The chemoattractant formyl-methionyl-leucyl-phenylalanine induces the gene expression and release of IL-8 through a Pertussis toxin–sensitive pathway *J Immunol* 1992;148:3216–3220.

64. Fava RA, Olsen NJ, Postlebyaite AE, et al. Tranforming growth factor-β1 (TGF-β1) induced neutrophil recruitment to synovial tissues: implications for TGF-β-driven synovial inflammation and hyperplasia *J Exp Med* 1991;173:1121–1132.

65. Kudo C, Yamashita T, Terashita M, Sendo F. Modulation of *in vivo* immune response by selective depletion of neutrophils using a monoclonal antibody RP-3. *J Immunol* 1993;150:3739–3746.

66. Colotta FR, Polentarutti N, Sozzani S, Mantovani A. Modulation of granulocyte survival and programmed cell death by cytokines and bacterial products. *Blood* 1992;80:2012–2020.

67. Cassatella MA. The production of cytokines by polymorphonuclear neutrophils. *Immunol Today* 1995;16:21–25.

68. Diamont RD, et al. Damage to hyphal forms of fungi by human leukocytes *in vitro*. *Am J Pathol* 1978;91:313–323.

69. Gerson SL, et al. Prolonged granulocytopenia: the major risk factor for invasive pulmonary aspergillosis in patients with acute leukemia. *Ann Intern Med* 1984;100:345–351.

70. Lehrer RI, Jan RG. Interaction of Aspergillus fumigatus spores with human leukocytes and serum. *Infect Immun* 1970;1:345–350.

71. Levitz SM, Diamond RD. Mechanisms of resistance of Aspergillus fumigatus conidia to killing by neutrophils *in vitro*. *J Infect Dis* 1985;152:33–42.

72. Levitz SM, Farrell TP. Human neutrophil degranulation stimulated by Aspergillus fumigatus. *J Leukocyte Biol* 1990;47:170–175.

73. Schaffner A, Douglas H, Braude A. Selective protection against conidia by polymorphonuclear and against mycelia by polymorphonuclear phagocytes in resistance to Aspergillus. *J Clin Invest* 1982;69:617–631.

74. Diamond Rd, Root RK, Bennett JE. Factors influencing killing of Cryptococcus neoformans by human leukocytes *in vitro*. *J Infect Dis* 1972;125:367–376.

75. Schaffner A, et al. *In vitro* susceptibility of fungi to killing by neutrophil granulocytes discriminates between primary pathogenicity and opportunism. *J Clin Invest* 1986;78:511–524.

76. Gallin JI. Disorders of phagocytic cells. In: Gallin JI, Goldstein IM, Snyderman R, eds. *Inflammation: basic principles and clinical correlates.* New York: Raven Press, 1992;859–874.

77. Borregaard N. Bactericidal mechanisms of the human neutrophil. *Scand J Haematol* 1984;32:225–230.

78. Russin SJ, Fillipo BH, Adler A. Neutropenia in adults. What is its clinical significance? *Postgrad Med* 1990;88:209–219.

79. Rogers DE, Tompsett R. The survival of staphylococci within human leukocytes. *J Exp Med* 1952;95:209–214.

80. Zucker-Franklin D. Electron microscope study of the degranulation of polymorphonuclear leukocytes following treatment with streptolysin. *Am J Pathol* 1965;47:419–423.

81. Weissman G. Effect on lysosomes of drugs useful in connective tissue disease. In: Campbell PN, ed. *Interaction of drugs and subcellular components in animal cells.* London: J&A Churchill, 1968;150–169.

82. Mandell GL, Rubin W, Hooks EW. The effect of an NADH oxidase inhibitor (Hydrocortisone) on polymorphonuclear leukocyte bactericidal activity. *J Clin Invest* 1970;49:1381–1388.

83. Fletcher C, Peto R. the natural history of chronic airflow obstruction. *Br Med J* 1977;1:1645–1648.

84. Hunninghake GW, Crystal RG. Cigarette smoking and lung destruction: accumulation of neutrophils in the lungs of cigarette smokers. *Am Rev Respir Dis* 1983;128:833–838.

85. Jensen EJ, Pedersen B, Schimidt E, Venge P, Dahl R. Serum eosinophilic cationic protein and lactoferrin related to smoking history and lung function. *Eur Respir J* 1994;7:927–933.

86. Totti N III, McCusker KT, Campbell EJ, Griffin GL, Senior RM. Nicotine is chemotactic for neutrophils and enhances neutrophil responsiveness to chemotactic peptides. *Science* 1984;223:169–171.

87. MacNee W, Wiggs B, Belzerg AS, Hogg JC. The effect of cigarette smoking on neutrophil kinetics in human lungs. *N Engl J Med* 1989;321:924–928.

88. Janoff A. Elastases and emphysema: current assessment of the protease-antiprotease hypothesis. *Am Rev Respir Dis* 1985;132:417–433.

89. Wewers MD, Gadek JE. The protease theory of emphysema. *Ann Intern Med* 1987;107:761–763.

90. Finkelstein R, Fraser RS, Ghezzo H, Cosio MG. Alveolar inflammation and its relation to emphysema in smokers. *Am J Respir Crit Care Med* 1995;152:1666–1672.

91. Thompson AB, Daughton D, Robbins RA, et al. Intraluminal airway inflammation in chronic bronchitis. Characterization and correlation with clinical parameters. *Am Rev Respir Dis* 1989;140:1527–1537.

92. Keating VM, Collins PD, Scott DM, Barnes PJ. Differences in Interleukin-8 and tumor necrosis factor-α in induced sputum from patients with chronic obstructive pulmonary disease or asthma. *Am J Respir Crit Care Med* 1996;153: 530–4.

93. Gibson PG, Girgis-Gabardo A, Morris MM, et al. Cellular characteristics of sputum from patients with asthma and chronic bronchitis. *Thorax* 1989;44:693–699.

94. Saetta M, Di Stefano A, Maestrelli P, et al. Airway eosinophilia in chronic bronchitis during exacerbations. *Am J Crit Care Respir Med* 1994;150:1646–1652.

95. Piattella M, Maestrelli P, Saetta M, et al. Sputum eosinophilia during mild vs. sputum neutrophilia during severe exacerbations of COPD. *Am J Respir Crit Care Med* 1997 (submitted).

96. Holloway L, Beasley R, Roche WR. The pathology of fatal asthma. In: Busse WW, Holgate ST, eds. *Asthma and rhinitis*. London: Blackwell Scientific Publications, 1995;109–117.

97. Djukanovic R. Bronchial biopsies. In: Busse WW, Holgate ST, eds. *Asthma and rhinitis*. London: Blackwell Scientific Publications, 1995;118–129.

98. Calhoun WJ, Liu MC. Broncholaveolar lavage and bronchial biopsies. In: Busse WW, Holgate ST,eds. *Asthma and rhinitis*. London: Blackwell Scientific Publications, 1995;1130–144.

99. Sheffer AL, ed. *Global initiative for asthma*. NHLBI/WHO Workshop report. National Institutes of Health, National Heart, Lung and Blood Institute. Publication No. 95–3659. January 1995.

100. Sterk PJ, Fabbri LM, Quanjer PhH, et al. Airway responsiveness: standardized challenge testing with pharmacological, physical and sensitizing stimuli in adults. Report Working party, Standardization of Lung Function Tests, European Community for Steel and Coal, Official Statement of the European respiratory Society. *Eur Respir J* 1993;6(suppl 16):53–83.

101. Kelly C, Ward C, Stenton CS, Bird G, Hendrick DJ, Walters EH. Number and activity of inflammatory cells in the bronchoalveolar lavage fluid in asthma and their relation to airway hyperresponsiveness. *Thorax* 1988;43:684–692.

102. Kelly C, Stenton SC, Ward C, et al. Lymphocyte subsets in bronchoalveolar lavage fluid obtained from stable asthmatics and their correlation with bronchial responsiveness. *Clin Exp Allergy* 1989;19: 169–175.

103. Josephs LK, Gregg I, Holgate ST. Does nonspecific bronchial responsiveness indicate the severity of asthma?. *Eur Respir J* 1990;3: 220–227.

104. Mapp CE, Dal Vecchio L, Boschetto P, De Marzo N, Fabbri LM. Toluene diisocyanate-induced asthma without airway hyperresponsiveness. *Eur J Respir Dis* 1986;68:89–95.

105. Chung KF, Becker AB, Lazarus SC, et al. Antigen induced airway hyperresponsiveness and pulmonary inflammation in allergic dogs. *J Appl Physiol* 1985;58:1347–1353.

106. Fabbri LM, Aizawa H, Alpert SE, et al. Airway hyperresponsiveness abd changes in cell counts in bronchoalveolar lavage after exposure to ozone in dogs. *Am Rev Respir Dis* 1984;129:288–291.

107. Bethel RA, Curtis SP, Lien DC, et al. Trachealis muscle hyperresponsivennes induced by platelet activating factor (PAF) in the dog. *Am Rev Respir Dis* 1987;135(suppl):A159.

108. O'Byrne PM, Leikauf GD, Aizawa H, et al. Leukotriene B4 induces airway hyperresponsiveness in dogs. *J Appl Physiol* 1985;59:1941–1946.

109. O'Byrne PM, Walters EH, Gold BD, et al. Neutrophil depletion inhibits airway hyperresponsiveness iniduced by ozone exposure. *Am Rev Respir Dis* 1984;130:214–219.

110. Li ZY, Daniel EE, Lane CG, Arnaout MA, O'Byrne PM. Effect of an anti-Mo1 Mab on ozone-induced airway inflammation and airway hyperresponsiveness in dogs. *Am J Physiol* 1992;263:L723–L726.

111. O'Byrne PM, Walters EH, Aizawa H, Fabbri LM, Holtzman MJ, Nadel JA. Indomethacin inhibits the airway hyperresponsiveness but not the neutrophil influx induced by ozone in dogs. *Am Rev Respir Dis* 1984;130:220–224.

112. Matsui S, Jones GL, Woolley MJ, Lane CG, Gontovnick LS, O'Byrne PM. The effect of antioxidants on ozone-induced airway hyperresponsiveness in dogs. *Am Rev Respir Dis* 1991;144:1287–1290.

113. Wanner A, Mezey RJ, Reihart ME, Eyre P. Antigen-induced bronchospasmin conscious sheep. *J Appl Physiol* 1979;47:917–922.

114. Abraham WMN, Stevenson JS, Sielkzak MS. Preliminary report on the effect of nedocromil sodium on antigen-indiuced early and late reactions in allergic sheep. *Eur J Respir Dis* 1986;69:(suppl 147):192–195.

115. Hutchinson AA, Hinson JM,Brigham KL, Snapper JR. Effect of endotoxin on airway responsiveness to aerosol histamine in sheep. *J Appl Physiol* 1983;54:1463–1468.

116. Hinson JM, Hutchinson AA, Brigham KL, Meyrick BO, Snapper JR. Effect of granulocyte depletion on pulmonary responsiveness to aerosol histamine. *J Appl Physiol* 1984;56:411–417.

117. Marsh WR, Irvin CG, Murphy KR, Behrens BL, Larsen GL. Increases in airway reactivity to histamin and inflammatory cells in

118. Murphy KR, Wilson MC, Irvin CG, et al. The requirement for polymorphonuclear leukocytes in the late asthmatic respons an hightened airways reactivity in an animal model. *Am Rev Respir Dis* 1986;134: 62–68.

119. Irvin CG, Henson PM, Berend N. Airway hyperreactivity and inflammation produced by aerosolization of human C5a desArg. *Am Rev Respir Dis* 1986;134:777–783.

120. Wegner CD, Rothlein R, Gundel RH. Adhesion molecules in the pathogenesis of asthma. *Agents Actions* 1990;34:529–534.

121. Gundel RH, Gerritsen ME, Wegner CD. Antigen-coated sepharose beads induce airway eosinophilia and airway hyperresponsiveness in cynomolgus monkeys. *Am Rev Respir Dis* 1989;140:629–633.

122. Gundel RH, Gerritsen ME, Gleich GJ, Wegner CD. Repeated antigen inhalation results in a prolonged airway eosinophilia and airway hyperresponsiveness in primates. *J Appl Physiol* 1990;68:779–786.

123. Gundel RH, Gerritsen ME, Wegner CD. Polymyxin B-induced bronchial neutrophilia does not alter airway responsiveness to methacholine in cynomolgus monkeys. *Clin Exp Allergy* 1992;22:357–363.

124. Mauser PJ, Pitman AM, Fernandez X, et al. Effects of an antibody to interleukin-5 in a monkey model of asthma. *Am J Respir Crit Care Med* 1995;152:467–472.

125. Hallahan AR, Armour CL, Black JL. Products of neutrophils and eosinophils increase the responsiveness of human isolated bronchial tissue. *Eur Resp J* 1990;3:554–558.

126. Hughes JM, McKay KO, Johnson PR, Tragoulias S, Black JL, Armour CL. Neutrophil-induced human bronchial hyperresponsiveness *in vitro*: pharmacological modulation. *Clin Exp Allergy* 1993;23:251–256.

127. Radeau T, Chavis C, Godard PH, Michel FB, Crastes de Paulet A, Damon M. Arachidonate 5-lipoxygenase metabolism in human neutrophils from patients with asthma: *in vitro* effect of nedocromil sodium. *Int Arch Allergy Appl Immunol* 1992;97:209–215.

128. Bruijnzeel PLB, Warringa RAJ, Kok PTM, Hamelink ML, Kreukniet H, Koenderman L. Effects of nedocromil sodium on *in vitro* induced migration, activation, and mediator release from human granulocytes. *J Allergy Clin Immunol* 1993;92:159–164.

129. Joseph BZ, Routes JM, Borish L. Activities of superoxide dismutases and NADPH oxidase in neutrophils obtained from asthmatic and normal donors. *Inflammation* 1993;17:361–370.

130. Bousquet J, Chanez P, Lacoste JY. Eosinophilic inflammation in asthma. *N Engl J Med* 1990;323:1033–1039.

131. Djukanovic R, Roche WR, Wilson JW, et al. Mucosal inflammation in asthma. *Am Rev Respir Dis* 1990;142:357–434.

132. Saetta M, Di Stefano A, Maestrelli P, et al. Airway mucosal inflammation in occupational asthma induced by toluene diisocyanate. *Am Rev Respir Dis* 1992;145:160–168.

133. Roisman GL, Peiffer C, Lacronique JG, Le Cae A, Dusser DJ. Perception of bronchial obstruction in asthmatic patients: relationship with bronchial eosinophilic inflammation and epithelial damage and effect of corticosteroid treatment. *J Clin Invest* 1995;96:12–21.

134. Gibson PG, Wong BJO, Hepperle MJE, et al. A research method to induce and examine a mild exacerbation of asthma by withdrawal of inhaled corticosteroids. *Clin Exp Allergy* 1992;22:525–532.

135. Pin I, Gibson PG, Kolendowicz R, et al. Use of induced sputum cell counts to investigate airway inflammation in asthma. *Thorax* 1992;47: 25–29.

136. Fahy JV, Liu J, Wong H, Boushey HA. Analysis of cellular and biochemical constituents in induced sputum after allergen challenge: a method for studying allergic airway inflammation. *J Allergy Clin Immunol* 1994;93:1031–1039.

137. Kirby GJ, Hargreave FE, Gleich GJ, O Byrne PM. Bronchoalveolar cell profiles of asthmatic and nonasthmatic subjects. *Am Rev Respir Dis* 1987;136:379–383.

138. Fabbri LM, De Rose, Godard P, Boschetto P, Rossi GA. Guidelines and recommendations for the clinical use of bronchoalveolar lavage in asthma. *Eur Respir Rev* 1992;2:116–123.

139. Fabbri LM, Ciaccia A. Investigative bronchoscopy in asthma and other airway diseases. *Eur Respir J* 1992;5:8–11.

140. Lundgren R, Soderberg M, Horstedt P, Stenling R. Morphological studies of bronchial mucosa biopsies from asthmatics before and after ten years of treatment with inhaled steroids. *Eur Respir J* 1988;1: 883–889.

141. Juniper EF, Kline PA, vanzieleghem MA, Ramsdale EH, O Byrne PM, Hargreave FE. Effect of long term treatment with an inhaled corticosteroid (budesonide) on airway hyperresponsiveness and clinical asthma in non-teroid-dependent asthmatics. *Am Rev Respir Dis* 1990; 142:832–836.

142. Haahtela T, Jarvinen M, Kava T, et al. Comparison of a β_2-agonist, terbutaline, with an inhaled corticosteroid, budesonide, in newly detected asthma. *N Engl J Med* 1991;325:388–392.

143. Saetta M, Maestrelli P, Di Stefano A, et al. Effect of cessation of exposure to toluene diisocyanate (TDI) on bronchial mucosa of subjects with TDI-induced asthma. *Am Rev Respir Dis* 1992;145:169–174.

144. Saetta M, Maestrelli P, Mapp CE, et al. Airway remodeling in isocyanate induced asthma. *Am J Respir Crit Care Med* 1995;151:489–494.

145. Laitinen LA, Laitinen A, Heino M, Haahtel T. Eosinophilic airway inflammation during exacerbation of asthma and its treatment with inhaled corticosteroid. *Am Rev Respir Dis* 1991;143:423–427.

146. Trigg CJ, Manolitsas ND, Wang J, et al. Placebo-controlled immunopathologic study of four months of inhaled corticosteroids in asthma. *Am J Respir Crit Care Med* 1994;150:17–22.

147. Murlas C, Roum JH. Bronchial hyperreactivity occurs in steroid-treated guinea pigs depleted of leukocytes by cyclophosphamide. *J Appl Physiol* 1985;58:1630–1637.

148. Hulbert WC, Walker DC, Jackson A, Hogg JC. Airway permeability to horseradish peroxidase in guinea pigs: the repair phase after injury by cigarette smoke. *Am Rev Respir Dis* 1981;123:320–325.

149. Thomson JE, Scypinsky LA, Grodon T, Sheppard D. Hydroxyurea inhibits airway hyperresponsiveness in guinea pigs by a granulocyte-independent mechanism. *Am Rev Respir Dis* 1986;134:1213–1218.

150. Munoz NM, Hamann KJ, Vita A, et al. Activation of tracheal smooth muscle responsiveness by FMLP-treated HL-60 cells and neutrophils. *Am J Physiol* 1993;264:L222–L226.

151. Metzger WJ, Mosely P, Nugent K, Richerson HB, Hunninghake GW. Local antigen challenge in bronchoalveolar lavage in asthmatic patients. *Chest* 1985;87:155–156.

152. Metzger WJ, Richerson HB, Worden K, Monick M, Hunninghake GW. Bronchoalveolar lavage of allergic asthmatic patients following allergen bronchoprovocation. *Chest* 1986;89:483–481.

153. Diaz P, Gonzales C, Galleguillos FR, et al. Leucocyte and mediators in bronchjolaveolar lavage during allergen-induced late–phase asthmatic reactions. *Am Rev Respir Dis* 1989;139:1383–1389.

154. Fabbri LM, Boschetto P, Zocca E, et al. Bronchoalveolar neutrophilia during late asthmatic reactions induced by toluene diisocyanate. *Am Rev Respir Dis* 1987;136:36–42.

155. Montefort S, Gratziou C, Goulding D, et al. Bronchial biopsy evidence for leukocyte infiltration and upregulation of leukocyte-endothelial cell adhesion molecules 6 hours after local allergen challenge of sensitized asthmatic subjects. *J Clin Invest* 1994;93:1411–1421.

156. Fahy JV, Kim KW, Liu J, Boushey HA. Prominent neutrophilic inflammation in sputum from subjects with asthma exacerbation. *J Allergy Clin Immunol* 1995;95:843–852.

157. Sur S, Gleich GJ, Swanson MC, Bartemes KR, Broide DH. Eosinophilic inflammation is associated with elevation of interleukin-5 in the airways of patients with spontaneous symptomatic asthma. *J Allergy Clin Immunol* 1995;96:661–668.

158. Martin RJ, Cicutto LC, Smith HR, Ballard RD, Szefler SJ. Airway inflammation in nocturnal asthma. *Am Rev Respir Dis* 1991;143:351–357.

159. Mackay TW, Wallace WAH, Howie SEM, et al. Role of inflammation in nocturnal asthma. *Thorax* 1994;49:257–262.

160. Sur S, Crotty TB, Kephart GM, et al. Sudden-onset fatal asthma. *Am Rev Respir Dis* 1993;148:713–719.

161. Carroll N, James A. Neutrophils and eosinophils in fatal asthma. *Eur Respir J* 1994;7(suppl 18):19S (abstr 0168).

162. Holtzman MJ, Cunningham JH, Sheller JR, Irsigler GB, Nadel JA, Boushey HA. Effect of ozone on bronchial reactivity in atopic and nonatopic subjects. *Am Rev Respir Dis* 1979;120:1059–1067.

163. Seltzer J, Bigby BG, Stulbarg M, et al. Ozone-induced changes in bronchial reactivity to metacholine and airway inflammation in humans. *J Appl Physiol* 1986;60:1321–1326.

164. Basha MA, Gross KB, Gwizdala CJ, Haidar AH Popovich J. Bronchoalveolar lavage neutrophilia in asthmatic and healthy volunteers after controlled exposure to ozone and filtered purified air. *Chest* 1994;106:1757–1765.

165. Bascom R, Bromberg PA, Costa DL, et al. Health effects of outdoor air pollution: part II. *Am J Respir Crit Care Med* 1996;153:477–498.

166. Chitano P, Hosselet JJ, Fabbri LM. Effects of oxidant pollutants on the respiratory system: insights from experimental research. *Eur Respir J* 1995;8:1357–1371.

167. Louis R, Bury T, Corhay J-L, Radermecker MF. Acute bronchial and hematologic effects following inhalation of a single dose of PAF: comparison between asthmatics and normal subjects. *Chest* 1994; 106:1094–1099.

168. Thomas PS, Yates DH, Barnes PJ. Tumor necrosis factor-α increases airway responsiveness and sputum neutrophilia in normal human subjects. *Am J Respir Crit Care Med* 1995;152: 76–80.

169. Boulet LP, Boulet M, Laviolette M, et al. Airway inflammation after removal from the causal agent in occupational asthma due to high and low molecular weight agents. *Eur Respir J* 1994;7:1567–1575.

170. Wilkinson JRW, Crea AEG, Clark TJH, et al. Identification and characterization of monocyte-derived neutrophil activating peptide in corticosteroid resistant bronchial asthma. *J Clin Invest* 1989;4:1930–1941.

171. Lam S, LeRiche J, Phillips D, Chan-Yeung M. Cellular and protein changes in bronchoalveolar lavage fluid after late asthmatic reactions in patients with red cedar asthma. *J Allergy Clin Immunol* 1987;80: 44–50.

172. Gratzious C, Carroll M, Montefort S, Teran L, Howarth PH, Holgate ST. Inflammatory and T cell profile of asthmatic airways 6 hours after local allergen challenge. *Am J Respir Crit Care Med* 1996;53: 515–520.

173. Teran LM, Carroll M, Frew AJ, et al. Leucocyte recruitment following local endobronchial allergen challenge in asthma: its relationship to procedure and to airway interleukin-8 release. *Am J Respir Crit Care Med* 1996, submitted.

174. Hunt LW, Gleich GJ, Ohnishi T, et al. Endotoxin contamination causes neutrophilia following pulmonary allergen challenge. *Am J Respir Crit Care Med* 1994;149:1471–1475.

175. Nagy L, Lee TH, Kay AB. Neutrophil chemotactic activity in antigen-induced late asthmatic reactions. *N Engl J Med* 1982;306:497–501.

176. Hakansson L, Rak S, Dahl R, Venge P. The formation of eosinophil and neutrophil chemotactic activity during a pollen season and after allergen challenge. *J Allergy Clin Immunol* 1989;83:933–939.

177. Metzger WJ, Richerson HB, Wasserman SI. Generation and partial characterization of eosinophil chemotactic activity and neutrophil chemotactic activity during early and late phase asthmatic response. *J Allergy Clin Immunol* 1986;78:282–290.

178. Sastre J, Banks DE, Lopex M, Barkman HW, Salvaggio JE. Neutrophil chemotactic activity in toluene diisocyanate induced asthma. *J Allergy Clin Immunol* 1990;85:567–572.

179. Driver AG, Kukoly CA, Metzger WJ, Mustafa SJ. Bronchial challenge with adenosine causes the release of serum neutrophil chemotactic factor in asthma. *Am Rev Respir Dis* 1991;143:1002–1007.

180. Boschetto P, Fabbri LM, Zocca E, et al. Prednisone inhibits late asthmatic reactions and airway inflammation induced by toluene diisocyanate in sensitized subjects. *J Allergy Clin Immunol* 1987;80:261–267.

181. Gin W, Kay AB. The effect of corticosteroids on monocyte and neutrophil activation in bronchial asthma. *J Allergy Clin Immunol* 1985; 76:675–682.

182. Kay AB, Walsh GM, Moqbel R, et al. Disodium cromoglycate inhibits activation of human inflammatory cells *in vivo*. *J Allergy Clin Immunol* 1987;80:1–9.

183. Mirone C, Fontana A, Mosca S, et al. Effects of nedocromil sodium on bronchospasm and HS-NCA release induced by allergen inhalation in asthmatic patients. *Clin Exp Allergy* 1994;24:281–287.

184. Venge P, Dahl R, Karlstrom R, Pedessen B, Peterson CGB. Eosinophil and neutrophil activity in asthma in a one year double-blind trial with theophylline and two doses of inhaled budesonide. *J Allergy Clin Immunol* 1993;89:141–144.

185. Condino-Neto A, Vilela MM, Cambiucci EC, et al. Theophylline therapy inhibits neutrophil and mononuclear cell chemotaxis from chronic asthmatic children. *Br J Clin Pharmacol* 1991;32:557–561.

186. Bradding P. Anti-inflammatory effects of long-acting β-agonists in asthma. *Clin Exp Allergy* 1995;25:912–914.

187. Evans DJ, Coulby LJ, Spaethe SM, et al. The inflammatory response to allergen challenge in atopic asthmatic is modulated by the leukotriene receptor B4 antagonist LY293111. Abstract presented at the conference: *Asthma 95: theory to treatment*. Chicago, July 15–17 1995.

188. Noppen M, Vincken W, Dewaele M, Demanet C. Increase in bronchoalveolar lavage fluid neutrophils following acute asthma. *Eur Respir J* 1994;7(suppl 18):458S (abstr P2035).
189. Lee TH, Nagy L, Nagakura T, Wallport MJ, Kay AB. Identification and partial characterization of an exercise-induced neutrophil chemotactic factor in bronchial asthma. *J Clin Invest* 1982;69:889–899.
190. Lee TH, Nagakura T, Papageorgiou N, Iikura J, Kay AB. Exercise-induced late asthmatic reactions. *N Engl J Med* 1983;308:1502–1505.
191. Venge P, Henriksen J, Dahl R, Hakansson L. Exercise-induced asthma and the generation of neutrophil chemotactic activity. *J Allergy Clin Immunol* 1990;85:498–504.
192. Crimi E, Balbo A, Milanese M, Miadonna A, Rossi G, Brusasco V. Airway inflammation and occurrence of delayed bronchoconstriction in exercise-induced asthma. *Am Rev Respir Dis* 1992;146:507–512.
193. O'Byrne PM. Pathogenesis. In: O Byrne P, Thomson NC, eds. *Manual of asthma management*. Cambridge: University Press, 1995;36–49.
194. Barnes PJ, Holgate ST, Laitinen LA, Pauwels R. Asthma mechanisms, determinants of severity and treatment: the role of nedocromil sodium. *Clin Exp Allergy* 1995;25:771–787.
195. Horuk R. The interleukin-8-receptor family: from chemokines to malaria. *Immunol Today* 1994;15:169–174.
196. Koh YY, Dupuis R, Pollice M, Albertine KH, Fish JE, Peters SP. Neutrophils recruited to the lungs of humans by segmental antigen challenge display a reduced chemotactic response to leukotriene B4. *Am J Respir Cell Mol Biol* 1993;8:493–499.
197. Shindo K, Fukumura M, Miyakawa K. Leukotriene B$_4$ levels in the arterial blood of asthmatic patients and the effect of prednisolone. *Eur Respir J* 1995;8:605–610.
198. Buchanan DR, Cromwell O, Kay AB. Neutrophil chemotactic activity in acute severe asthma ("status asthmaticus"). *Am Rev Respir Dis* 1987;136:1397–1402.
199. Corrigan CJ, Collard P, Nagy L, Kay AB. Cultured peripheral blood mononuclear cells derived from patients with acute severe asthma ("status asthmaticus") spontaneously elaborate a neutrophil chemotactic activity distinct from interleukin-8. *Am Rev Respir Dis* 1991;143:538–544.
200. Oosterhoff Y, Hoogsteden HC, Rutgers B, Kauffman HF, Postma DS. Lymphocyte and macrophage activation in bronchoalveolar lavage fluid in nocturnal asthma. *Am J Respir Crit Care Med* 1995;151:75–81.
201. Strunk RC. Death due to asthma. *Am Rev Respir Dis* 1993;148:550–552.
202. Arrighi HM. US asthma mortality: 1941 to 1989. *Ann Allergy Asthma Immunol* 1995;74:321–326.
203. Reid LM. The presence or absence of bronchial mucus in fatal asthma. *J Allergy Clin Immunol* 1987;80:415–416.
204. Saetta M, Di Stefano A, Maestrelli P, Mapp CE, Ciaccia A, Fabbri LM. Pathology of the airway mucosa: similarities and discrepancies between asthma and chronic bronchitis. *Allergy Clin Immunol News* 1993;5:102–104,114.

Asthma, edited by P.J. Barnes, M.M. Grunstein, A.R. Leff, and A.J. Woolcock.
Lippincott–Raven Publishers, Philadelphia © 1997.

▪ 32 ▪

T Lymphocytes in Asthma Pathogenesis

Chris J. Corrigan, and A. Barry Kay

T lymphocytes play a fundamental role in the initiation and regulation of inflammatory responses. Through their specific antigen receptors, they can recognize invading foreign antigens and initiate appropriate immune responses, which may be characterized predominantly by "cell-mediated" reactions, in which effector immune cells play a major role, or "humoral" reactions, in which antibody responses are more prominent. Although immature B lymphocytes express surface immunoglobulin (Ig) M with low binding affinity for foreign antigens, these cells are largely dependent on T lymphocytes for their subsequent activation and proliferation, and for antibody affinity maturation. There is now abundant evidence that T lymphocytes orchestrate both the initiation and the propagation of immune responses largely through the secretion of cytokines, and that the particular combinations of cytokines secreted during the course of these inflammatory responses are responsible for the type of inflammatory reaction that ensues, including whether the reaction is predominantly cellular or humoral in nature. This chapter describes the fundamental properties of T lymphocytes and the factors that govern their secretion of cytokines in asthma, and how these cytokines influence immunoglobulin synthesis, particularly that of IgE, by B lymphocytes. Finally, it will be shown how the secretion of various patterns of cytokines can influence the course and nature of the ensuing inflammatory response.

Asthma is a disease characterized clinically by reversible obstruction of the airways, or bronchi, and bronchial nonspecific hyperresponsiveness (BHR), which refers to the tendency of the bronchi in asthmatics to constrict in response to a wide range of pharmacologic, immunologic, and irritant stimuli. It is now widely accepted that chronic inflammation of the bronchial mucosal lining plays a fundamental role in the genesis of these clinical manifestations.

The most striking feature of the histopathology of asthma is the intense infiltration of the bronchial mucosa with eosinophils, macrophages, and lymphocytes (1–3). In fact, the disease has many histopathologic features of a chronic, cell-mediated immune response. It will be seen later in this chapter how cytokine and chemokine products of activated T lymphocytes can bring about selective eosinophil accumulation and activation at mucosal surfaces. The eosinophil appears to be a key cell in producing injury to the bronchial mucosa (4). This in turn is be-

C. J. Corrigan: Department of Medicine, Charing Cross and Westminster Medical School, University of London, London W6 8RF United Kingdom.
A. B Kay: Department of Allergy and Clinical Immunology, Imperial College of Medicine at the National Heart and Lung Institute, London SW3 6LY United Kingdom.

lieved to result in bronchial obstruction and irritability, although the precise mechanisms by which this occurs are not clear.

ATOPIC DIATHESIS AND ASTHMA

Asthma is often, although not invariably, associated with atopy, particularly in children. Atopy refers to the genetic predisposition of certain individuals to synthesize, inappropriately, IgE specific for protein components of inhaled aeroallergens such as grass pollen. Cells with high- and low-affinity IgE Fc receptors bind to allergen-specific IgE, thus sensitizing them. Further allergen exposure then brings about the release of inflammatory agents from these sensitized cells. One principal feature of this process is its immediacy, which has resulted in the term "immediate hypersensitivity." IgE-mediated mechanisms are assumed to play a fundamental role in the pathogenesis of allergic diseases such as rhinitis and conjunctivitis because many of the symptoms of these diseases occur immediately in relation to aeroallergen exposure, and they can be alleviated at least partly by antagonists of mediators released by sensitized IgE Fc receptor-bearing cells such as antihistamines. Furthermore, with few exceptions, these diseases are seen only in sensitized, atopic individuals, although not all atopic individuals develop them. Similarly, some atopic asthmatics sensitized to environmental aeroallergens experience an exacerbation of their disease on exposure to these allergens. Such patients have traditionally been referred to as "extrinsic" asthmatics, reflecting the clear relationship of their disease to external environmental factors (although unlike rhinitics these patients do not respond to antihistamines). Nonatopic asthmatics, who are not apparently sensitized to a wide range of environmental allergens (although it is impossible to make such a list exhaustive), and in whom IgE-mediated mechanisms do not obviously operate, have been labeled "intrinsic." Following Rackemann's initial description of intrinsic asthma (5,6), it is now generally accepted that this term be used to describe a group of asthmatics who are skin-prick-test–negative in response to extracts of common aeroallergens and have serum total IgE concentrations within the normal range. As a group, these patients tend to develop symptoms for the first time in adulthood (although some child asthmatics are nonatopic), and their disease is often relatively difficult to control. There is a higher incidence of nasal polyposis and aspirin sensitivity (the so-called aspirin triad) in patients with intrinsic asthma (7). Some patients develop asthma after exposure to specific proteins or small molecular weight chemicals at work (see Chapter 85); these "occupational" asthmatics form a third clinical category. An IgE response specific for the sensitizing agent can sometimes, but not always, be demonstrated in these patients.

The relative roles of IgE-mediated mechanisms and chronic inflammation of mucosal surfaces brought about by interactions of activated T lymphocytes with eosinophils in asthma and allergic diseases therefore remain unclear. Perhaps "rhinitis without asthma" and "intrinsic asthma" represent the two ends of a continuous spectrum of the relative prominence of these processes. It will be argued later in this chapter that activated T lymphocytes may drive asthmatic inflammation independently of IgE-mediated mechanisms, although the nature of the antigen(s) involved in this activation process remains a subject for speculation. The concept that there are indeed fundamental pathogenetic differences between "extrinsic" and "intrinsic" asthma also has been challenged by an epidemiologic study showing that, irrespective of atopic status as defined by skin-prick tests, the prevalence of self-reported asthma in individuals related closely to their serum concentrations of IgE corrected for age and sex (8). On the other hand, a second epidemiologic study (9) showed that, whereas serum total IgE concentrations were strongly correlated in pairs of asthmatic siblings concordant for BHR, suggesting that these traits are co-inherited, BHR was not correlated with serum total IgE concentrations. Analysis of pairs of siblings showed linkage of BHR with several genetic markers on chromosome 5q, near a locus previously shown to be linked to a locus regulating total serum IgE concentrations (9). At least one distinct locus linked to regulation of total serum IgE concentrations has been identified on chromosome 11q13 (10). One candidate gene at this locus is that encoding the β-subunit of the high-affinity IgE receptor: a common allelic variant of this gene (Ile-Leu substitution at amino acid 181) has been demonstrated in unrelated nuclear families with extrinsic asthmatic probands (11). These data raise the possibility that IgE-mediated mechanisms may play at least some role in the pathogenesis of asthma in all patients, although distinct genes regulating susceptibility to BHR, as distinct from inappropriate IgE synthesis, are beginning to be identified. Whatever the case, it is clear that IgE-mediated mechanisms are not sufficient for the development of asthma because not all atopic individuals develop the disease. It is possible to speculate that, as has been proposed for many other diseases, asthma develops after environmental influences on individuals with an inherited predisposition (see Chapters 11 and 12). Some of these genetic influences may become clearer in the near future.

In summary, although IgE-mediated mechanisms may clearly be important in allergen-induced short-term exacerbations of asthma in atopic individuals, their role in the pathogenesis of chronic disease, in both atopic and nonatopic individuals alike, is less certain. Despite these observations, many studies on the "pathogenesis" of asthma address changes in cell numbers and activation after experimental allergen challenge of atopic asthmatics.

T LYMPHOCYTE ANTIGEN RECOGNITION

T lymphocytes recognize antigens through specific cell surface receptors composed of a pair of polypeptide chains (either α/β or γ/δ). Unlike antibodies, which recognize the shape of antigens, T-lymphocyte receptors specifically recognize the sequence of small peptide fragments ("epitopes") derived from the intact antigen. These fragments are presented to T lymphocytes after partial hydrolysis, or "denaturation" of the antigen by antigen-presenting cells (APC). Antigenic epitopes cannot be recognized in isolation, but must be "presented" to T lymphocytes bound to major histocompatibility complex (MHC) molecules on the surface of APC (MHC class I molecules in the case of CD8 T lymphocytes and class II molecules in the case of CD4 T lymphocytes). As with immunoglobulins, the presence of multiple germ-line gene segments encoding "hypervariable" regions in those parts of the T-lymphocyte receptor proteins that contact both the epitope and its associated MHC molecules accounts for variable specificity of epitope binding. Again, analogously with immunoglobulins, the T-lymphocyte receptor gene rearrangements that take place during maturation of individual T lymphocytes from their precursors is fixed during ontogeny, so that each mature T lymphocyte can recognize only a limited range of epitopes. The potential variability of these gene rearrangements is more than enough, however, to ensure that T lymphocytes recognizing any particular epitope will be generated during maturation of T cells in the thymus.

Epitopes derived from both "self" and "nonself" proteins can associate with MHC molecules. Indeed, "self" peptides are processed as efficiently as those derived from foreign proteins (12), and so mechanisms must exist whereby the potential ability of T lymphocytes to recognize and respond to "self" epitopes is eliminated. Experimental data from several systems (13–16) provide strong evidence that most self-reactive T lymphocytes are removed either by clonal deletion (cell death) or the induction of clonal "anergy," probably by encounter with their specific epitopes under conditions incompatible with cell activation during their development in the thymus. Most cells leaving the thymus possess receptors that are capable of recognizing "nonself" or "foreign" antigenic peptides in association with self-MHC molecules, but not "self" peptides associated with self-MHC molecules (Fig. 1).

In addition to presentation of specific antigenic peptides on appropriate MHC molecules, additional signals are required for T lymphocyte activation. One important signal is interleukin (IL)-1 secreted by the APC (17). In addition, cell contact between the APC and the antigen-specific T lymphocytes is required (Fig. 2). This conclusion is supported by the observation that antigen-pulsed APC fixed with agents such as ECDI fails to stimulate antigen-specific T lymphocytes, even in the presence of IL-1, and furthermore induce a state of nonresponsiveness (18). If the APCs are activated before fixation, tolerance is not induced, suggesting that one or more cell surface molecules, whose expression is increased during activation, are responsible for this "contact signal."

There is now considerable evidence implicating the homologous glycoproteins CD28 and CTLA-4, expressed on the surface of T lymphocytes, as co-stimulator molecules responsible for this requirement for contact with APC during T lymphocyte activation (Fig. 2). Cellular signals induced by engagement of these molecules synergize with signals arising from the engaged T lymphocyte antigen receptor to induce T lymphocyte proliferation (19). Both CD28 and CTLA-4 interact with the same ligands on APC, namely CD80 (previously known as B7) and CD86 (previously known as B70 or B7-2) (20–22). These molecules are highly homologous and are expressed on most activated APC including B lymphocytes and also, interestingly, on activated T lymphocytes and natural killer (NK) cells. Currently available evidence suggests that successful T lymphocyte activation involves upregulation of both CD28/CTLA-4 and CD80/CD86. Evidence that CD28 is a co-stimulatory molecule for T

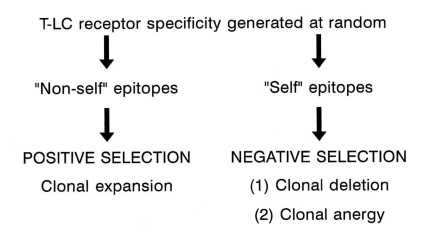

FIG. 1. Clonal selection in the thymus. T-lymphocyte (T-LC) epitope specificity is generated at random during thymic development. "Nonself" reactive cells are positively selected for expansion in the periphery. "Self" reactive cells are negatively selected by deletion (death) or induction of anergy.

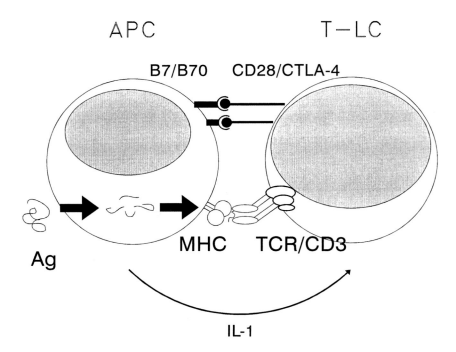

FIG. 2. Role of accessory molecules in T-lymphocyte activation/anergy. Antigen *(Ag)* processed by antigen-presenting cells *(APC)* is presented as small peptides to T cells on major histocompatibility *(MHC)* molecules. Additional cytokine signals such as interleukin-1 *(IL-1)* are important for T-cell activation. In addition, engagement of the T-cell ligands CD28/CTLA-4 and their counter-receptors B7/B70 on APC are also essential. If these signals are not provided then the T cell is rendered nonresponsive or "anergic" to the particular epitope. This may represent at least one mechanism for physiologic anergy.

lymphocytes has been provided by the finding that nonstimulatory anti-CD28 antibody Fab fragments completely inhibit the provision of co-stimulation to T lymphocytes by activated B lymphocytes (19). CD28 cross-linking in the presence of phorbol ester results in IL-2 production by T lymphocytes that is resistant to inhibition by cyclosporin A (23), suggesting that CD28 signals by a biochemical pathway distinct from that used by the T lymphocyte antigen receptor.

The CD28 ligands CD80 and CD86 are heavily glycosylated membrane glycoproteins. Both molecules are expressed on activated APC, although the time courses of their expression differ. In addition, CD80 is constitutively expressed on dendritic cells, whereas CD86 is constitutively expressed on monocytes. Expression of CD80 on B lymphocytes was induced by cross-linking of their surface immunoglobulin or MHC class II molecules (24,25), as may occur during presentation of antigen to T lymphocytes. Anti-CD80 antibodies or a fusion protein comprised of the extracellular domain of CTLA-4 fused to the human IgG₁ Fc region (CTLA-4-Ig) blocked the proliferation of T lymphocytes in response to antigen presented by a variety of CD80-expressing accessory cells (26). A similar series of effects was observed with anti-CD86 antibodies (22).

T LYMPHOCYTES, B LYMPHOCYTES, AND IGE SYNTHESIS

Primary antibody responses are mounted by antibodies of the IgM class. Because these antibodies generally ex-

press germ-line–determined variable region genes that have not been modified by somatic mutation, they bind antigen only with low affinity. Antibodies of the IgG, IgA, and IgE classes are made later than IgM during a primary immune response, but account for most of the antibody made during a memory response. Although isotype switching and affinity maturation are independent processes, they usually occur simultaneously (27), so that the increased affinity of bivalent antibodies of isotypes other than IgM is rapidly enhanced. IgG antibody is the predominant isotype in plasma and lymph, whereas IgA antibody predominates at mucosal surfaces and in secretions from these surfaces. Little is known about the precise site of antibody synthesis in secondary immune responses; this might be of considerable relevance to the pathogenesis of "extrinsic" asthma, where local allergen-specific IgE synthesis might enhance IgE-mediated inflammatory mechanisms, and in "intrinsic" asthma, where local IgE synthesis might enable such mechanisms to participate in bronchial mucosal inflammation even though elevated IgE concentrations are undetectable in the peripheral blood. The regulation of IgE synthesis in humans is covered in some detail in Chapter 20 of this volume. It is relevant here, however, to emphasize briefly the important role that T lymphocyte–derived cytokines play in this process.

The antigen-binding specificity of an immunoglobulin molecule is determined by the amino-termini of its heavy and light chains, which are highly variable in structure. By contrast, the carboxy-terminus of the heavy chain has a constant sequence that determines the effector functions of the immunoglobulin molecule, such as binding to

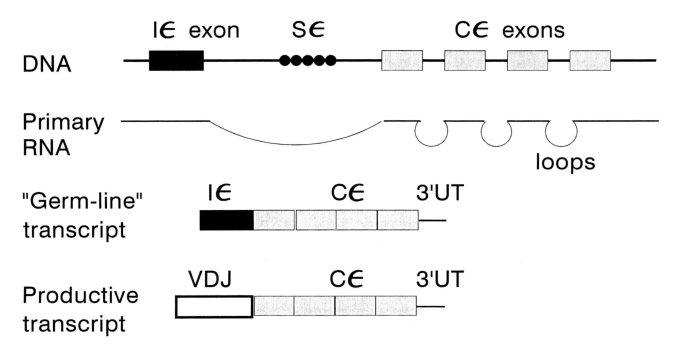

FIG. 3. Switching to IgE synthesis in B lymphocytes. During switching, Cε exons encoding the constant region of the IgE heavy chain are juxtaposed to the variable *(VDJ)* region genes by looping out of intervening DNA sequences at the adjacent switch recombinase site *(Sε)*. During the switching process, the Cε exons are brought near to the Iε exon, the transcription of which product results after RNA processing in a "germ-line" transcript. Later, the Cε exons are juxtaposed to the VDJ regions, the transcription of which product results in a productive IgE heavy chain transcript.

particular Fc receptors. The variable region of immunoglobulin is encoded by multiple germ-line elements that are assembled into complete V(D)J variable regions during B lymphocyte differentiation by a common enzymatic activity termed "recombinase." These variable region genes are then juxtaposed to germ-line constant region (C_H) genes that determine the isotype, and thus the functional properties of, the immunoglobulin. During an immune response, a B lymphocyte can express different heavy-chain isotypes sharing the same V(D)J region. This phenomenon, known as class switching, allows a single B-lymphocyte clone to secrete antibodies of the same antigen specificity in association with different C_H region genes. Intervening sequences, including previously expressed C_H region genes, are deleted. Class switching involves characteristic repetitive sequences (S regions), composed of short tandem repeats, located upstream of the Cμ gene and corresponding regions located immediately upstream of each C_H gene except Cδ. In B lymphocytes predisposed to undergo class switching to a particular isotype such as ε, the C_H locus to which switching is directed is transcribed before switching into a "germline" transcript (Fig. 3). These transcripts initiate approximately 2 kb upstream of the S region involved in switch recombination and are processed to a messenger ribonucleic acid (mRNA) in which an exon (designated I exon)

located 100 to 500 bp upstream of the relevant C_H exon, and the C_H exon itself are spliced directly together. The resulting "germ-line" transcripts do not appear to be capable of encoding for protein products, because the I exon contains stop codons in all three reading frames. The I exon is 200 to 300 bp shorter than the V(D)J region present in mature transcripts, so that "germ-line" transcripts are also correspondingly shorter (Fig. 3). The precise significance of "germ-line" transcripts remains to be defined, but they appear in the course of switching in B lymphocytes and are a useful marker of switching when studying the effects of cytokines on this process.

Role of Cytokines in Regulating IgE Synthesis

Cytokines play an important role in the control of switching of antibody isotypes in humans away from IgM during the evolution of the immune response, and also in regulating the amounts of antibody that are secreted through their growth-regulating effects on B lymphocytes. In the case of IgE, cytokines that play a role in this process may be classified as follows:

1. cytokines that specifically induce IgE switching in B lymphocytes. These cytokines have in common the ability to induce the transcription of "germ-line" C_H

transcripts. IL-4 induces switching to IgE synthesis in human B lymphocytes, which is preceded by the synthesis of "germ-line" Cε transcripts (28). Until recently, it was thought that no other cytokine could substitute for IL-4 in this process; it is now clear, however, that IL-13 can also cause Cε "germ-line" transcript expression and IgE switching in human B lymphocytes (29). There is some evidence that IL-13 competes with IL-4 for binding to its receptor (30). The gene encoding IL-13 is located in chromosome 5q31 in the same region as the genes encoding IL-3, IL-4, IL-5, and granulocyte-macrophage colony-stimulating factor (GM-CSF) (31). In addition to IgE, IL-4 also stimulates switching of human B lymphocytes to synthesis of IgG4, although IgG4 is detectable earlier, consistent with the interpretation that the switch from IgM to IgE typically involves an initial switch to an IgG4 and then a second switch to IgE (32).

2. cytokines that influence IgE production by B lymphocytes through effects other than the induction of switching. Some of these cytokines are generally facilitatory or inhibitory to B lymphocyte activation and clonal expansion. Thus, interferon (IFN)-α, IFN-γ, transforming growth factor (TGF)-β, IL-8, and IL-12 inhibit IL-4–induced IgE synthesis whereas IL-2, IL-5, IL-6, and tumor necrosis factor (TNF)-α enhance it (33–39). Endogenous IL-6 is crucially involved in IL-4–dependent IgE induction *in vitro,* because anti–IL-6 antibodies strongly inhibit IgE synthesis (39).

A Second B Lymphocyte–activating Signal is Required for IgE Synthesis

IL-4 and IL-13 are necessary, but not sufficient, for the induction of IgE synthesis by B lymphocytes. A variety of second IgE-inducing signals have been described that are necessary for IgE secretion and that synergize with IL-4/13 in this process. Allergen-specific CD4 T lymphocytes are activated when processed fragments of allergen are presented to their T-cell receptor/CD3 complex by APC on MHC class II molecules. B lymphocytes process and present antigen in this way. After presentation, the activated, allergen-specific T lymphocytes secrete cytokines, including IL-4 and IL-13. In addition to these "cognate" interactions between allergen-specific T lymphocytes and B lymphocytes, additional signals are provided to B lymphocytes through T-lymphocyte contact that, along with IL-4/13, are essential for subsequent secretion of allergen-specific IgE. At least two signals are important in this respect:

1. CD40/CD40 ligand interaction. CD40 is a surface glycoprotein expressed on immature and mature B lymphocytes as well as thymic epithelial cells and dendritic cells (40). The importance of this interaction was first inferred when it was discovered that anti-CD40 monoclonal antibodies could replace contact with activated T lymphocytes in induction of IgE synthesis (32,41). These experiments conversely suggested the presence of a ligand for CD40 (CD40L) on T lymphocytes. Recently, CD40L has been cloned from complementary deoxyribonucleic acid (cDNA) libraries constructed from activated T lymphocytes (42). In contrast to activated CD4 T lymphocytes, resting cells do not express CD40L. Interestingly, human mast cells have also been shown to express CD40L, which was functional in the sense that mast cells could induce IgE synthesis by human B lymphocytes in the presence of IL-4 (43).

2. CD21/CD23 interaction. CD23 is the low-affinity receptor for IgE present on many cells including B lymphocytes, monocytes, and a subset of T lymphocytes, whereas CD21, identified as the Epstein-Barr virus (EBV) and C3 desArg receptor on B lymphocytes, is also found on some T lymphocytes as well as follicular dendritic cells. It was shown recently (44) that triggering of CD21 either with anti-CD21 antibody or recombinant soluble CD23 increased IL-4–induced IgE production by B lymphocytes.

Interactions between these ligand pairs may explain why noncognate interactions between T lymphocytes and B lymphocytes may result in IgE synthesis in the presence of exogenous IL-4 (45).

In summary, it is clear that many T lymphocyte–derived cytokines play an indispensable role in the initiation and propagation of IgE synthesis by B lymphocytes. The need for both cytokines and cellular contact mediated by specific receptor/ligand interactions in this process bears many similarities to the requirements for T lymphocyte activation by APC. Conversely, APCs themselves may influence cytokine synthesis by allergen-specific T lymphocytes, for example by their differential capacity to present soluble antigen to Th1- and Th2-like T cells.

T LYMPHOCYTES, CYTOKINES, AND EOSINOPHIL RECRUITMENT

The proinflammatory properties of eosinophils and a summary of the evidence implicating them in the pathogenesis of asthma is found in Chapters 30 and 45 of this volume. It is relevant here, however, to consider the role of T lymphocyte–derived cytokines in the genesis of the marked and specific infiltration of eosinophils into the asthmatic bronchial mucosa, which is the hallmark of this disease.

Eosinophils are nondividing granular cells that arise principally in the bone marrow. Eosinophil differentiation, like that of all leukocytes, is influenced by cytokines. Of the cytokines secreted by activated T lymphocytes, IL-3, IL-5, and GM-CSF promote maturation, activation, and prolonged survival of the eosinophil (46–48). IL-5 is unique in that, unlike IL-3 and GM-CSF, it acts specifically on eosinophils in terms of activation, hyperadhesion, and terminal differentiation of the eosinophil precursor (49,50). IL-5 may be the most important cytokine for eosinophil differentiation because it is released principally by T lymphocytes, and eosinophilia associated with parasitic infections is T lymphocyte–dependent (51). This hypothesis is supported further by the observation that transgenic mice constitutively expressing the gene for IL-5 show a marked, specific expansion of blood and tissue eosinophils (52).

One fundamental problem with asthma pathogenesis is the mechanism by which eosinophils preferentially accumulate in the inflamed mucosa. Established eosinophil chemoattractants such as platelet activating factor (PAF), although highly potent (53), are nonspecific because they also attract neutrophils. Local expression of eosinophil-specific cytokines such as IL-5 may partly account for this phenomenon by selectively enhancing eosinophil differentiation and survival, although these cytokines exhibit only weak eosinophil chemotactic activity *in vitro*. Chemoattractants may also play a role. Cytokines such as IL-5, IL-3, and GM-CSF have been shown to prime eosinophils for an enhanced chemotactic response to other chemoattractants including chemokines such as IL-8 (54, 55). The T lymphocyte–derived cytokines, lymphocyte chemoattractant factor (LCF), and IL-2 are also relatively potent eosinophil chemoattractants (56,57). The LCF protein exerts its activity by binding to CD4 molecules, so that in addition to affecting lymphocytes it also specifically acts on eosinophils as compared with other granulocytes, because only eosinophil granulocytes express CD4 (56). An exciting recent observation has been that the chemokines RANTES, monocyte chemotactic protein-3 (MCP-3), and, to a lesser extent, macrophage inflammatory protein-1α (MIP-1α) are powerful and selective chemoattractants for eosinophils and basophils *in vitro* (58). Furthermore, RANTES was shown to be expressed in the bronchial epithelium of mild asthmatics (59) and to induce transepithelial migration of eosinophils *in vitro* (60). A full assessment of the possible origins of these proteins, which are likely to be secreted by other cells including T lymphocytes, and their role in promoting eosinophil recruitment to the bronchial mucosa of asthmatic patients, is now urgently required.

Another revealing field of study has been the role of adhesion molecules in selective eosinophil migration. Three major families of adhesion molecules have been defined as being involved in leukocyte migration: (a) the immunoglobulin superfamily, including intercellular adhesion molecule 1 (ICAM-1), vascular cell adhesion molecule 1 (VCAM-1), and platelet endothelial cell adhesion molecule (PECAM), (b) the integrins, including leukocyte functional antigen (LFA)-1, Mac-1, and VLA-4, and (c) the selectins, including E-selectin, P-selectin, and L-selectin (see also Chapter 38). Leukocyte migration is initiated by an interaction between receptors on the cell surface with their ligands on the surface of vascular endothelial cells. Selectins mediate the initial weak tethering of leukocytes to the endothelial wall. Eosinophils can bind to endothelium using all three selectins, with no apparent differences between these cells and neutrophils. Both eosinophils and neutrophils exhibit surface shedding of L-selectin on activation, which may facilitate endothelial transmigration (61). Integrins such as LFA-1 and Mac-1, also on the leukocyte surface, mediate firm adhesion and transmigration by binding to immunoglobulinlike molecules such as ICAM-1 and VCAM-1 on the endothelium (62,63). Eosinophils appear to be unique, however, in that IL-3 and IL-5 upregulate eosinophil, but not neutrophil, adhesion to unstimulated endothelial cells (51). Furthermore, eosinophils, but not neutrophils, express the β1-integrin VLA-4, which is a ligand for VCAM-1 on the surface of stimulated endothelial cells (64). The expression of VCAM-1 on endothelial cells is increased by exposure to IL-4 and IL-13, which enhanced VLA-4/VCAM-1–dependent adherence of eosinophils, but not neutrophils, to endothelium (65). Bronchial mucosal endothelial cells do not express VCAM-1, at least in mild atopic asthmatics, but this molecule does appear after allergen bronchial challenge (66). Eosinophils may also use VLA-4 for binding to tissue fibronectin (67), which prolongs their survival *in vitro,* possibly by inducing autocrine secretion of IL-3 (68). Such mechanisms offer further possible explanations for the selective recruitment and activation of eosinophils observed in asthmatic inflammation. The important role of T lymphocyte–derived cytokines in this process is self-evident.

FUNCTIONAL HETEROGENEITY OF T LYMPHOCYTES

In recent years it has become clear that the nature of the immune response initiated by CD4 T lymphocytes is at least partly dependent on the "selection" or preferential activation of particular subsets of CD4 T lymphocytes that secrete defined patterns of cytokines (Table 1). These patterns of cytokine release result in the initiation and propagation of distinct immune effector mechanisms. Initial studies of mouse CD4 T-lymphocyte clones revealed that these could be divided into two basic functional subsets termed TH1 and TH2. TH1 T lymphocytes were characterized by the predominant secretion of IL-2, IFN-γ, and TNF-β, whereas TH2 cells characteristically predominantly secreted IL-4, IL-5, IL-6, and IL-10. Other cytokines, such as TNF-α, IL-3, and GM-CSF, were produced by both TH1 and TH2 cell subsets (69,70). These differing patterns of cytokine secretion by CD4 T lymphocytes result in distinct effector functions (71). Broadly speak-

TABLE 1. *Functional properties of subsets of human T lymphocytes*

	TH0	TH1	TH2
Cytokine secretion			
IL-2	+++	+++	–
IFN-γ	+++	+++	–
TNF-β	+	+++	–
TNF-α	++	+++	–
IL-3	+	+	++
IL-10	+	±	++
GM-CSF	++	+	++
IL-4	+	+	+++
IL-5	+	+	+++
IL-6	+	+	++
IL-13	+	+	+++
IL-9		+	++
Cytolytic activity	++	+++	±
Help for IgE synthesis	±	–	+++
Help for IgG/A/M synthesis			
Low T/B cell ratios	++	++	++
High T/B cell ratios	±	+++	

IL, interleukin; TNF, tumor necrosis factor; GM-CSF, granulocyte-macrophage colony-stimulating factor; Ik, immunoglobulin.

ing, TH1 cells participate in delayed-type hypersensitivity reactions (72), but also provide help for B lymphocyte immunoglobulin synthesis under certain circumstances. TH2 cells, on the other hand, by their pattern of secretion of B lymphocyte co-stimulatory cytokines, enhance the synthesis of all immunoglobulins, including IgE, in immune responses. In the center of this spectrum, T-lymphocyte clones secreting cytokines characteristic of both TH1 and TH2 cells, termed TH0 cells, were also described (73). It is still not clear whether these TH0 cells represent distinct functional subsets or precursor cells in the process of differentiating into TH1 or TH2 cells.

Initial studies on mitogen-stimulated or alloreactive human T-lymphocyte clones raised from the peripheral blood of normal donors suggested that only a few CD4 T-lymphocyte clones showed clear-cut TH1 or TH2 phenotypes, whereas most resembled TH0 cells (74). A different picture emerged, however, when human T-lymphocyte clones specific for particular antigens were raised, particularly when these antigens were implicated in prototype immunologic mechanisms such as delayed type hypersensitivity to mycobacterial antigens or nickel, on the one hand, and IgE-mediated responses to helminth allergens on the other. For example, study of a large series of T-lymphocyte clones raised from the peripheral blood of healthy individuals specific for purified protein derivative (PPD) of *Mycobacterium tuberculosis* or the excretory/secretory antigens of *Toxocara canis* (TES) revealed that most of the PPD-specific clones showed a TH1-like cytokine profile, with excess secretion of IL-2 and IFN-γ, whereas the TES-specific clones showed a TH2-like profile, with excess IL-4 and IL-5 secretion (75). Similarly, many T-lymphocyte clones specific for intracellular organisms such as *Borrelia burgdorferi* showed a Th1-like pattern of cytokine secretion (76). In patients with atopic dermatitis, T-lymphocyte clones specific for house dust mite (*Dermatophagoides pteronyssinus*) allergen raised from the peripheral blood secreted IL-4 and not IFN-γ, whereas all clones specific for *Candida albicans* or tetanus toxoid raised from the same donors secreted an excess of IFN-γ and relatively little IL-4 (77). CD8 T lymphocytes also appear to exhibit functional hetero-

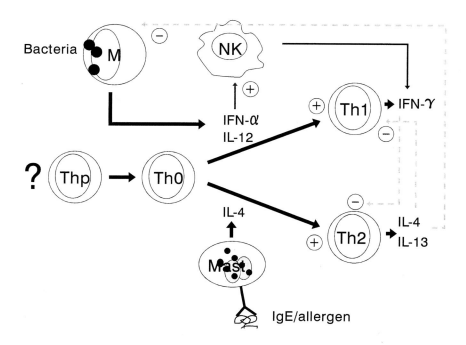

FIG. 4. Factors thought to influence development of TH1- and TH2-like T lymphocytes. Although it is suggested in this figure that both TH1- and TH2-like T cells arise from precursor *(Thp)* and Th0-like cells, this is by no means certain. Intracellular infection of monocytes *(M)* by organisms such as bacteria and viruses results in secretion of IFN-α and IL-12, which promote TH1-like development of T cells and activate NK cells *(NK)* to secrete IFN-γ, which is inhibitory to TH2-like cell development. It is not known precisely what favors TH2-like T cell development *in vivo*, although local IL-4 released, for example, from allergen-triggered mast cells *(Mast)* may play a role. Once established, TH2-like T cells inhibit TH1-like development through the synthesis of IL-4 and IL-13, which also inhibit the activation of monocytes.

geneity in terms of their cytokine secretion profile. For example, CD8 T-lymphocyte clones specific for *M. leprae* antigens showed patterns of cytokine secretion consistent with both TH1- and TH2-like phenotypes (78).

There is some evidence for mutual cross-inhibition of proliferation and cytokine secretion by TH1 and TH2 T lymphocytes, which is mediated by particular cytokines (Fig. 4). For example, exogenous IL-4 favors the growth and proliferation of TH2 T lymphocytes, whereas TH2 clones are exquisitely sensitive to inhibition by IFN-γ. IL-2 is a growth factor for both TH1 and TH2 cells. Whereas in mice, IL-10 significantly inhibits the proliferation and cytokine secretion of TH1 cells (79), human IL-10 significantly inhibits proliferation of and cytokine secretion by both TH1- and TH2-like clones raised in response to specific antigen or lectin, and is itself a product of both TH1- and TH2-like clones (80).

Human TH1 and TH2 cells also differ in the nature of their help for immunoglobulin synthesis by autologous B lymphocytes and in their cytolytic potential. In the presence of specific antigen, TH2-like clones were able to induce the synthesis of IgM, IgG, IgA, and IgE by autologous B lymphocytes (81). Under the same conditions, TH1-like clones induced synthesis of IgM, IgG, and IgA, but not IgE, with a peak response at a T cell/B cell ratio of 1:1. At higher T cell/B cell ratios, immunoglobulin synthesis was reduced, possibly reflecting the cytolytic activity of the TH1-like clones against autologous B lymphocytes at higher T cell/B cell ratios. This inhibition of immunoglobulin synthesis by TH1-like cells may represent an important mechanism whereby the production of antibodies other than IgE in immune responses is self-regulated. In contrast, the failure of such an intrinsic regulatory mechanism in the case of Th2 cells may explain, at least partly, why IgE antibody responses may persist despite the cessation of antigen exposure.

Mechanisms of Differentiation of Human TH1- and TH2-like CD4 T Lymphocytes

The experimental data discussed above suggest that TH1 and TH2 CD4 T-lymphocyte clones exist in humans, and that one factor determining their profiles of cytokine secretion is their antigen specificity. The observation, however, that T-lymphocyte clones specific for any given antigen, such as tetanus toxoid, can exhibit TH1, TH2, and TH0 phenotypes (77) suggests that the cytokine secretion profile of individual T lymphocytes is not irrevocably "set" in a TH1- or TH2-like pattern by the criterion of antigen specificity alone. Indeed, it is hard to envisage how this could occur, because T-lymphocyte antigen specificity is acquired at random during differentiation in the thymus, and therefore predetermination of a particular cytokine secretion profile according to antigen specificity would have to invoke some mechanism whereby

such a profile is "imprinted" on a T lymphocyte before it has encountered its specific antigen, which is not impossible but seems unlikely.

To address this problem, it has been suggested that, at least in mice, TH1 and TH2 cells may represent memory cells that have matured into different functional phenotypes in the face of repeated stimulation by specific antigen. This hypothesis invokes the putative existence of antigen-naive precursor T lymphocytes (Thp) that secrete principally IL-2 and develop into early memory TH0 effector cells after first encounter with specific antigen (Fig. 4) (82). These cells then terminally differentiate into TH1 or TH2 cells after repetitive antigen stimulation.

The concept that TH0, TH1, and TH2 effector cells differentiate from a common pool of precursor cells raises the question of which factors influence the differentiation of a T lymphocyte to the TH1- or TH2-like phenotype. There is some evidence that exogenous cytokines may play a role in this differentiation process. For example, early addition of IL-4 to uncloned peripheral blood mononuclear cells stimulated with PPD shifted the subsequent differentiation of PPD-specific T lymphocytes from a TH1-like toward a TH0- or TH2-like phenotype. Conversely, in similar cultures, early addition of both IFN-γ and anti–IL-4 antibody induced many allergen- or TES-specific T-lymphocyte clones to differentiate into TH0- and TH1-like, instead of TH2-like clones (83). These data suggest that the presence or absence of exogenous IL-4 or IFN-γ at the time of antigen stimulation of resting T lymphocytes may influence their subsequent development into TH1- or TH2-like clones, regardless of any pre-existing functional bias. In addition, the cytokines IFN-α and IL-12 (both activators of NK cells that induce IFN-γ synthesis) were also found to promote the differentiation of allergen- or TES-specific T-lymphocyte clones toward a TH0- or TH1-like phenotype instead of the usual TH2-like phenotype, whereas neutralization of endogenous IL-12 by specific antibody promoted the differentiation of PPD-specific T lymphocytes toward a TH0- or TH2-like phenotype instead of the typical TH1-like phenotype (84). These observations have led to the hypothesis (84) that infection of cells such as macrophages with viruses and intracellular bacteria may favor a TH1-like response through local release of IFN-α and IL-12 that might in turn activate NK cells, resulting in local release of IFN-γ (Fig. 4). It is less clear what could favor the differentiation of Th2-like effector T lymphocytes from precursors *in vivo*, although it is possible to speculate that allergens or helminth-derived antigens, in contrast with intracellular parasites, might invoke relatively little IL-12 release from monocytes and therefore low local concentrations of IFN-γ. This, coupled with the presence of local IL-4 released from IgE-sensitized mast cells in patients with atopic disease or helminthic infections, might favor the local differentiation of TH2-like effector T lymphocytes. In addition, IL-13, like IL-4, inhibits secretion of IFN-α and IL-12 by monocytes (85). The local emergence of TH2-like T lymphocytes, themselves a rich source of IL-4 and IL-13 (32), might therefore be expected to encourage the further development of TH2-like T lymphocytes and discourage the development of Th1-like cells.

The nature of the APCs that activate antigen-naive T lymphocytes may also play a role in their subsequent development toward a TH1- or TH2-like phenotype. This possibility has been strengthened by recent preliminary evidence, yet to be confirmed by scientific consensus, suggesting that TH1 and TH2 T-lymphocyte responses display differential dependence on co-stimulation by CD80 (B7-1) and CD86 (B7-2) (86). For example, repetitive co-stimulation of naive T lymphocytes with CD86-expressing APC favored IL-4 secretion, whereas repetitive co-stimulation with CD80-expressing APC resulted in high IL-2, but low IL-4 secretion (87). In the murine model of experimental allergic encephalomyelitis, an autoimmune disease induced by immunization with axonal proteolipid and mediated by TH1-type T lymphocytes, simultaneous treatment with anti-CD80 antibodies resulted in the evolution of TH2-type effector T lymphocytes and disease amelioration, whereas treatment with anti-CD86 antibodies produced TH1-type T lymphocytes and disease exacerbation (88). It is possible to speculate that, at sites where the dominant APC are dendritic cells, which constitutively express CD80, TH1-like responses might be favored. On the other hand, soluble antigen present at low concentrations in the periphery, such as at a mucosal surface, might be preferentially taken up and presented by resting, CD80-negative B lymphocyte expressing antigen-specific surface immunoglobulin. Such cells are a poor stimulus for TH1-like T lymphocyte activation (89) but favor TH2-like development, at least in murine systems (90,91). IL-4 and IL-10 secreted by activated TH2-like T lymphocytes might then inhibit macrophage co-stimulation. This, coupled with the lack of secretion of IFN-γ, which is required for the induction of CD80 expression on resting macrophages, might further downregulate TH1-like responses in the presence of low concentrations of antigen.

The spectrum of APC available to present allergens to T lymphocytes may also depend on the atopic status of the individual. APCs such as B lymphocytes and monocytes may internalize and process allergens captured by their binding to surface-bound, allergen-specific IgE. This IgE may bind to low- and high-affinity IgE Fc receptors (FC$_\varepsilon$RI and FC$_\varepsilon$RII, CD23) on monocytes and to CD23 on B lymphocytes. It was shown recently that allergen-specific IgE bound to monocyte Fc$_\varepsilon$RI receptors (92), and monomeric IgE bound to surface CD23 on EBV-transformed B lymphocytes (93), may be used to capture and process allergens. In the latter study, exposure of specific IgE-pulsed B lymphocytes to allergen concentrations of <10^{-12} M was sufficient to induce an immune response in specific T lymphocytes, whereas monomeric, specific IgG antibodies were not able similarly to bind to IgG Fc$_\gamma$RII receptors (CD32) on B lymphocytes and activate T lymphocytes in this manner. These observations suggest that allergen-specific IgE responses, once established in atopic individuals, may profoundly influence the spectrum of APC that maintains these responses. This, coupled with the possible differential expression of co-stimulatory molecules on different APC, might play a major role in maintaining distinct cytokine secretion profiles of allergen-specific T lymphocytes in atopic and nonatopic individuals.

Roles of TH1 and TH2 T Lymphocytes in Immune Responses

The existence of CD4 and CD8 T lymphocytes that secrete defined combinations of cytokines in response to various antigenic stimuli, and a consideration of the properties of these cytokines, allow the view that particular patterns of cytokine release during inflammatory responses play an important role in determining the type of immune effector mechanism that a foreign antigen may elicit. Thus, TH1-like cells, through their predominant secretion of IL-2 and IFN-γ, might be expected to promote the development of cytotoxic T lymphocytes, enhance the bactericidal activity of macrophages, and stimulate the activity of NK and lymphokine-activated killer (LAK) cells. These effector mechanisms would be particularly effective for the elimination of viruses and other intracellular pathogens. On the other hand, the secretion of cytokines such as IL-4, IL-6, and IL-10 by TH2-like T lymphocytes would be expected to inhibit local activation of macrophages and dendritic cells but would favor the synthesis and release of specific antibody, including IgE, by activated B lymphocytes. Such humoral responses have a well defined role in the elimination of invading extracellular micro-organisms such as bacteria and their secreted products.

In addition to their possible role in eliminating certain infections, there is also some evidence that secretion of TH2 cytokines may be detrimental to the host. In several infectious diseases of humans, a TH1-like pattern of cytokine secretion is associated with resistance to infection, whereas a TH2-like pattern may be associated with progressive, uncontrolled infection. A good example of how TH2-like cytokines might impair host responses to infection is provided by leprosy, which presents as a clinical and immunologic spectrum of disease where, on the one hand, patients with tuberculoid leprosy exemplify the resistant response restricting growth of the pathogen, and on the other hand patients with lepromatous leprosy suffer from uncontrolled proliferation of the *M. leprae* organism despite demonstrating a marked humoral response to the pathogen. These clinical patterns of disease are associated with distinct cytokine patterns in skin lesions of patients with leprosy (94), with elevated concentrations of mRNA including IL-2 and IFN-γ in tuberculoid lesions, and elevated concentrations of mRNA encoding IL-4, IL-5, and IL-10 in lepromatous lesions. Spontaneous "conversion" of the disease from the lepromatous to the tuberculoid form was associated with an alteration of the corresponding cytokine pattern observed in skin lesions. These differences in cytokine profiles were confirmed in both CD4 and CD8 T lymphocytes at the clonal level (78). In addition to providing further evidence for the existence of TH1 and TH2 CD4 and CD8 T lymphocytes, these studies also implicate TH2 cytokines in suppressing cell-mediated immunity to such an extent that infection is allowed to proceed unabated.

Some of the most convincing evidence for a role for TH1- and TH2-like cytokines in orchestrating distinct inflammatory responses *in vivo* has, however, come from studies of allergic inflammation and asthma, as described in detail below.

EVIDENCE FOR MUCOSAL INFLAMMATION IN ASTHMA

Most recent studies on the histopathology of asthma have compared mild asthmatic and normal volunteers, using the techniques of BAL and bronchial biopsy. Elevated numbers of eosinophils, both in the bronchial mucosa and in BAL fluid, were constant features of mild asthma (95–97). Similarly, increased numbers of activated lymphocytes, identified either as irregular, atypical lymphocytes by transmission electron microscopy (98) or as CD25+ cells as shown by immunocytochemistry, were also invariably seen. Most of the CD25-expressing cells in these biopsies were shown to be T lymphocytes (99). The numbers of activated, "memory" T lymphocytes were also increased in the BAL fluid of mild atopic asthmatics as compared with controls (100). There is evidence that activation of T lymphocytes and subsequent eosinophil recruitment and secretion may contribute both to epithelial damage and to BHR (101–103). In contrast, these studies demonstrated no significant changes in the numbers of mast cells and their subtypes or neutrophils in the bronchial mucosa (98,103–108). Cell numbers do not, however, necessarily correlate with function: It was shown, for example, that spontaneous release of mediators from mast cells is elevated in asthmatic patients (96).

The present clinical classification of asthma discussed above (intrinsic, extrinsic, and occupational) implies possible variability in its pathogenesis. Are such distinctions apparent in histopathologic terms? Preliminary studies addressing this question would suggest that they are not: An autopsy study of the bronchial mucosa of a patient who had died with severe occupational asthma showed histologic changes similar to those seen in fatal nonoccu-

pational asthma (106), whereas immunocytochemical studies (107,108) comparing bronchial biopsies from extrinsic, intrinsic, and occupational asthmatics showed marked similarities in terms of their inflammatory cell infiltrate. Examination of BAL fluid obtained from a group of intrinsic asthmatics (109) showed increased numbers of activated T lymphocytes, eosinophils, and neutrophils as compared with normal controls. These observations suggest that the bronchial response in patients with asthma has similar characteristics regardless of the nature of identifiable provoking agents, and lend support to the hypothesis that the pathogenesis of asthma is independent of co-existing atopy. On the other hand, the recent demonstration that elevated numbers, compared with nonatopic controls, of cells expressing high-affinity (FcεRI) IgE receptors were present in the bronchial mucosa of both atopic and nonatopic asthmatics (110) suggests that IgE-mediated mechanisms may also play a role in "intrinsic" asthma.

CD4 T LYMPHOCYTES AND ASTHMA PATHOGENESIS

CD4 T Lymphocytes and Eosinophils

CD4 T lymphocytes are clearly an important source of the cytokines IL-5, IL-3, and GM-CSF, and may be an important source of chemokines such as RANTES, MIP-1α, and MCP-3. The possible roles of these agents in enhancing eosinophil survival, maturation, activation, and local accumulation have been discussed above. These observations emphasize the fact that cytokines and other products of activated CD4 T lymphocytes can bring about selective accumulation and activation of eosinophils in tissues, and that this need not involve immunologic processes dependent on the presence of antibodies, including IgE.

Cytokine Secretion by Cells Other than T Lymphocytes

In addition to T lymphocytes, it is clear that many other cells that are normally present in the bronchial mucosa, or that migrate into it in association with asthmatic inflammation, are potential sources of cytokines and chemokines. For example, eosinophils also have the capacity to elaborate cytokines and chemokines including TGF-α, TGF-β, TNF-α, MIP-1α, IL-1, IL-3, IL-4, IL-5, IL-6, IL-8, and GM-CSF (111–119). The secretion of such mediators by eosinophils may enable them to participate in the propagation of asthmatic inflammation, for example by autocrine prolongation of their own survival. It is also clear that mast cells and basophils can store a number of cytokines, including IL-4, IL-5, IL-6, and TNF-α (120–122), probably in their intracytoplasmic granules. In a study comparing bronchial biopsies from mild atopic asthmatics and nonatopic normal controls (120), serial thin glycol methacrylate sections were used to define the cellular provenance of IL-4, IL-5, IL-6, and TNF-α using immunocytochemistry with monoclonal antibodies directed against these cytokines and cellular phenotypic markers. Both the asthmatic and normal bronchial mucosae contained numerous cells staining positively for all four cytokines, with most identified as mast cells owing to their tryptase content. The total number of mucosal mast cells was similar in the asthmatics and the controls, as has been observed in other studies (98,103–108). The number of mast cells staining positively with antibodies against IL-4 and TNF-α were elevated in the asthmatics as compared with the controls, whereas the number of cells staining with IL-5 and IL-6 antibodies was similar in both groups. This study suggests that mast cells have a potential role in the initiation and propagation of asthmatic mucosal inflammation, at least in atopic individuals. In particular, mast cell–derived IL-4 and IL-5 may play a role in eosinophil recruitment, whereas IL-4 may direct T-lymphocyte maturation toward a Th2-like phenotype during the initiation of mucosal inflammation. Interestingly, the authors were unable to demonstrate cytokine staining of T lymphocytes in this study (120), whereas T lymphocytes were shown to be the predominant source of IL-4 and IL-5 mRNA in BAL T lymphocytes from atopic asthmatics and the nasal mucosa of patients with atopic rhinitis (123,124), with a smaller but significant contribution from mast cells and eosinophils. Aside from an idiosyncrasy of the staining technique in these heavily fixed sections, these observations suggest the possibilities that secretion and storage of cytokine proteins in leukocytes may not be synchronous with transcription of their mRNA, and that T lymphocytes may secrete cytokines rapidly, without storage, after synthesis such that intracytoplasmic cytokines are not detectable by immunocytochemistry. The resolution of these important questions, and the relative contributions to local cytokine release, must await further studies. Nevertheless, T lymphocytes are unique among inflammatory cells because they can recognize and respond to processed antigens directly, and almost certainly play a pivotal role in initiating and sustaining immunologically driven chronic asthma, particularly perhaps in situations where the IgE response is absent or minimal.

T Lymphocytes and Asthmatic Inflammation

Immunocytochemical studies of bronchial biopsies taken from patients with asthma (95,98,104,107,108) have shown that activated (CD25+) T lymphocytes can be detected in the bronchial mucosa, and that their numbers can be correlated both with the numbers of local activated eosinophils and with disease severity. Activated (CD25+, HLA-DR+) CD4, but not CD8 T, lymphocytes were also detected in the peripheral blood of patients with severe asthma (125–127), and their numbers were reduced after glucocorticoid therapy to a degree that correlated with the degree of clinical improvement. Similarly, activated CD4 and CD8 T lymphocytes were observed in the peripheral blood of child asthmatics (128), and the numbers of activated CD4 cells correlated with both disease severity and the number of peripheral blood eosinophils. In one of these studies (127), elevated serum concentrations of IL-5 were also detected in a proportion of the asthmatics, but not in nonasthmatic controls, and again concentrations were reduced in association with glucocorticoid therapy. Elevated serum concentrations of IL-5 were also seen in a proportion of patients with severe, glucocorticoid-dependent asthma (129). As shown (130) by semiquantitative polymerase chain amplification of reverse transcribed cytokine-specific mRNA, peripheral blood T lymphocytes from both atopic and nonatopic severe asthmatics contained elevated quantities (relative to β-actin) of mRNA encoding IL-5 as compared with controls, although elevated quantities of IL-4 mRNA in these cells were seen in all atopic individuals as compared with nonatopic controls regardless of their asthmatic status. The quantities of IL-5 mRNA were reduced in association with oral glucocorticoid therapy of the asthmatics and clinical improvement. Peripheral blood T lymphocytes from asthmatics clinically resistant to glucocorticoid therapy were shown to express activation markers *in vivo* (131) and to be refractory to the inhibitory effects of glucocorticoids *in vitro* (132,133). These studies suggest that glucocorticoids exert their antiasthma effect at least partly by inhibiting the release of cytokines from activated T lymphocytes.

Some (134), but not all (96), studies have demonstrated increased numbers of lymphocytes in the BAL fluid of patients with mild asthma, and preferential activation of memory CD4 T lymphocytes in the BAL fluid of mild atopic asthmatics was observed to correlate with asthma symptoms and BHR (100). In another study of intrinsic and extrinsic asthmatics (135), it was shown that whereas both CD4 and CD8 T lymphocytes in BAL fluid expressed activation markers, only the numbers of activated CD4 cells correlated with the numbers of BAL eosinophils and disease severity.

Measurement of cytokines *in vivo* is problematic because of their low concentrations, rapid metabolism, and unquantifiable degree of dilution. Furthermore, "physiologic" concentrations of cytokines have in general not been defined, so it is often unknown whether a specific assay, such as ELISA, is sufficiently sensitive. This problem is illustrated by a recent study of BAL fluid from mild asthmatics (136), in whom cytokines were detectable only after considerable concentration of the BAL fluid. Clearly, such a procedure might result in variable loss of specific proteins. On the other hand, challenge of sensitized atopic asthmatics with allergen or diluent control in separate bronchial segments was associated with increased numbers of eosinophils, neutrophils, and activated (CD25+) T lymphocytes in the allergen, but not the diluent-challenged segments, along with elevated quantities of various cytokines including IL-1, IL-2, IL-5, TNF-α, IL-6, IL-8, and GM-CSF in the concentrated lavage fluid (137). The fact that the extrapolated concentrations of IL-5 in the concentrated lavage fluid could be correlated with the numbers of infiltrating eosinophils suggests that concentration may preserve, at least semiquantitatively and in the case of at least some cytokines, relative cytokine concentrations.

One alternative to the direct measurement of cytokines is the detection of their mRNA using the technique of *in situ* hybridization with cytokine-specific cRNA probes or riboprobes. Although this is not a strictly quantitative technique, and with the proviso that mRNA synthesis does not necessarily equate with secretion of the corresponding protein, it does have the advantage that it can localize the secretion of cytokines within cells and tissues. Using this technique, it was demonstrated that IL-5 mRNA was elaborated by cells in bronchial biopsies from a majority of mild asthmatics but not normal controls (138). The amount of mRNA correlated broadly with the numbers of activated T lymphocytes and eosinophils in biopsies from the same individuals. In another study (139), it was shown that significantly elevated percentages of BAL cells expressed mRNA encoding IL-2, IL-3, IL-4, IL-5, and GM-CSF but not IFN-γ in mild atopic asthmatics as compared with nonatopic normal controls. Separation of CD2+ T lymphocytes from the remainder of the BAL cells showed that most (>90%) of the cells expressing IL-5 and IL-4 mRNA were T lymphocytes. Over a broad range of asthma severity, the percentages of BAL fluid cells from atopic asthmatics expressing mRNA encoding IL-5, IL-4, IL-3, and GM-CSF, but not IL-2 and IFN-γ, could be correlated with the severity of asthma symptoms and BHR (140). Elevated percentages of peripheral blood CD4, but not CD8 T lymphocytes, from patients with exacerbation of asthma expressed mRNA encoding IL-3, IL-4, IL-5, and GM-CSF but not IL-2 and IFN-γ as compared with controls (141). Elevated spontaneous secretion of IL-3, IL-5, and GM-CSF was also demonstrable in these patients using an eosinophil survival-prolonging assay. Again, the percentages of CD4 T lymphocytes expressing mRNA encoding IL-3, IL-5, and GM-CSF, as well as spontaneous secretion of these cytokines by the CD4 T lymphocytes, were reduced in association with glucocorticoid therapy and clinical improvement. In a double-blind, parallel group study, therapy of mild atopic asthmatics with oral prednisolone, but not placebo, resulted in clinical improvement associated with a reduction in the percentages of BAL fluid cells expressing IL-5 and IL-4 and an increase of those expressing IFN-γ (142). Conversely, artificial exacerba-

tion of asthma by allergen bronchial challenge of sensitized atopic asthmatics was associated with increased numbers of activated T lymphocytes and eosinophils and increased expression of mRNA encoding IL-5 and GM-CSF in the bronchial mucosa (143).

Taken together, these studies provide overwhelming evidence in support of the general hypothesis that, in asthma, activated CD4 T lymphocytes secrete cytokines that are relevant to the accumulation and activation of eosinophils in the bronchial mucosa, and that glucocorticoids exert their antiasthma effect at least partly by reducing the synthesis of cytokines by these cells. They also suggest that the properties of CD4 T lymphocytes in the peripheral blood of asthmatics closely resemble those of T lymphocytes in the bronchial mucosa and BAL fluid, owing perhaps to a "spill-over" effect of these cells from the mucosa into the peripheral blood. Thus, there seems considerable scope for examining the properties of asthmatic T lymphocytes at the level of the peripheral blood, obviating the problem of performing fiberoptic bronchoscopy in patients with severe disease.

Are Asthmatic CD4 T Lymphocytes "TH2-like"?

Some of the most convincing evidence for a role for TH1 and TH2 cytokines in orchestrating distinct inflammatory responses *in vivo* has come from the studies of cytokine mRNA expression in asthma, as described above. In other studies employing *in situ* hybridization, the cutaneous inflammatory responses to challenge with allergen in atopic individuals and tuberculin in nonatopic individuals were compared (144,145). Both types of response (delayed-type hypersensitivity late-phase allergic and [DTH]) were associated with an influx of activated CD4 T lymphocytes, but whereas mRNA molecules encoding IL-2 and IFN-γ were abundant within the tuberculin reactions, little mRNA encoding of these cytokines was observed in the late-phase allergic reactions. Conversely, mRNA encoding IL-4 and IL-5 was abundant in the late-phase allergic but not the tuberculin reactions. Furthermore, the relative numbers and types of granulocytes infiltrating these reactions reflected these different patterns of cytokine release (146). Similar differences were observed in the mRNA profiles of BAL T lymphocytes from patients with atopic asthma and pulmonary tuberculosis (147). These observations provide direct evidence in support of the hypothesis that activated T lymphocytes, through their patterns of cytokine secretion, regulate the types of granulocyte that participate in inflammatory reactions. Furthermore, they demonstrate that TH1 and TH2 CD4 T lymphocyte responses can be detected in humans under physiologic conditions, and that the antigen specificity of the T lymphocytes might be one factor that determines that that type of response is initiated. Taken together, they provide a considerable body of evidence for the existence of TH1 and TH2 patterns of cytokine secretion *in vivo* in human asthma, although it cannot be ascertained from such studies whether or not these cytokines originate from the same cells. In support of clonal TH2-like differentiation in allergic diseases, it was shown that, after mitogen stimulation, most T lymphocytes derived from the conjunctival infiltrates of patients with vernal conjunctivitis developed into TH2 clones (148). Similarly, high proportions of TH2 clones were obtained from the skin lesions of patients with atopic dermatitis (149,150). A proportion of these skin-derived T-lymphocyte clones were specific for house dust mite or grass pollen allergens. On the other hand, a recent study (151) suggested that co-expression of IL-4 and IL-5 by cloned T lymphocytes *in vitro* may reflect an artifactual effect of T-lymphocyte activation, and that T lymphocytes isolated *ex vivo* rarely co-express IL-4 and IL-5. Furthermore, whereas studies on T-lymphocyte clones provide information about patterns of cytokine synthesis, they do not allow comparison of the amount of secretion of cytokines in asthmatic T lymphocyte populations. In this regard, it was shown recently that CD4 T-lymphocyte lines propagated from BAL fluid of atopic asthmatics using an anti-CD3 antibody stimulus secreted elevated quantities, on a per cell basis, of the eosinophil-active cytokines IL-5 and GM-CSF as compared with lines derived from atopic nonasthmatics and nonatopic controls (152). These data may reflect an increased frequency of T lymphocytes secreting IL-5 at the clonal level in the asthmatic bronchial mucosa, or elevated IL-5 secretion by individual T lymphocytes without clonal differentiation, or both.

THE "CAUSE" OF ASTHMA AND ALLERGIC DISEASE

The studies described above have provided considerable insight into the role of TH2-like T lymphocytes in the pathogenesis of the chronic eosinophil-rich mucosal infiltration seen in asthma, and in the regulation of IgE synthesis. They do not, however, explain why some individuals develop allergen-specific IgE antibodies, atopic disease, and/or asthma while others do not.

The phenomenon of atopy defined in its broadest sense as the inappropriate synthesis of allergen-specific IgE and without reference to the development of disease, shows a strong heritable tendency. How precisely allelic variability in candidate genes such as that encoding the β-subunit of the high-affinity IgE receptor might predispose to the development of atopy is not clear, although dysregulation of the expression of IgE receptors on inflammatory effector cells or dysregulation of the expression of cytokines such as IL-4 that enhance IgE synthesis

(possibilities for which there is as yet little good evidence) may play a role.

It is clear from many of the studies discussed above that both atopic and nonatopic adults have T lymphocytes in the peripheral blood that recognize epitopes derived from inhalant allergens. In atopic individuals, however, these T lymphocytes are more likely to be TH2-like, whereas in nonatopics they are more likely to be TH1-like. There is increasing interest in the so-called window of susceptibility to atopy in infancy and early childhood, during which persistent IgE responses to both inhaled and dietary allergens may or may not be initiated. One view expounded by Holt (153) is that exposure of mucosal surfaces to potential allergens, whether inhaled or consumed, results in active immunologic recognition comprising cross-competing TH1-like and TH2-like allergen-specific T-lymphocyte clones. During repeated rounds of normal environmental restimulation, either a TH1-like or a TH-2 like response eventually becomes dominant, resulting in a reservoir of memory T lymphocytes that directs the nature of the response to these allergens throughout later life. In support of this theory, it has been shown that most children develop transient serum IgE antibody responses against common food allergens during the first year of life, the magnitude and duration of which reflect the incidence of atopy in their parents (154). A similar pattern is seen with inhalant allergens (155), although the IgE responses commence later and persist longer. It is possible that, in those children who go on to develop atopic disease, this transient TH2-like response persists rather than being "overwhelmed" by TH1-like responses. In addition to genetic predisposition, environmental factors that are known to influence the risk of sensitization to allergens (156) may play a role in "tipping the balance" of the TH1/TH2-like responses.

Both atopic and nonatopic individuals may develop asthma, and here even less is known about the key factors that influence this process. The heritability of asthma is more complex than that of atopy, and no single pattern of inheritance has emerged. Perhaps the clearest evidence that asthma may be initiated in previously disease-free individuals by exposure to novel, inhaled antigens comes from occupational asthma. Interestingly, in these individuals there is again a "window of susceptibility" to asthma and allergic disease in the sense that most individuals who are going to develop this disease as a consequence of occupational exposure do so within about 3 years of the initiation of this exposure. The influences of environmental factors, such as cigarette smoking, and genetic predisposition to atopy are also apparent. Sensitizing antigen-specific IgE and TH2-like T-lymphocyte responses can be detected with varying prominence, according to the nature of the sensitizing agent. Nevertheless, of those individuals who develop these responses *de novo*, not all develop asthma. Clearly, further critical factors, be they environmental, immunologic, physiologic, or heritable, need to be taken into account before the true "cause" of asthma can be defined.

NEW THERAPEUTIC STRATEGIES IN ASTHMA

New therapeutic strategies for asthma therapy are considered in other chapters of this volume, but it is relevant here briefly to consider those strategies based on our knowledge of the role of T lymphocytes in asthma pathogenesis. Data from many of the studies discussed above are consistent with the hypothesis that glucocorticoids ameliorate asthma at least partly by inhibiting the local synthesis of TH2-like cytokines in the inflamed mucosa. This raises the possibility that other drugs that inhibit activated CD4 T lymphocytes or their cytokine products may also be useful for the therapy of asthma. Although glucocorticoids form the mainstay of antiasthma therapy for most patients, the rising mortality and morbidity from this disease attest to the possibility that not all asthmatics respond well to this therapy. It was recently shown that cyclosporin A, a T-lymphocyte inhibitory drug that also has inhibitory effects on granulocytes such as eosinophils and basophils, was effective in improving disease severity in a proportion of chronic, severe, glucocorticoid-dependent asthmatics (157), and also reduced the frequency of disease exacerbations requiring elevated oral glucocorticoid therapy. There are also preliminary suggestions that cyclosporin A therapy improves BHR in severe, glucocorticoid-dependent asthmatics (158). This may be partly related to its activity in suppressing the secretion by activated T lymphocytes of eosinophil-active cytokines such as IL-5 (159). Intravenous immunoglobulin therapy may also exert an antiasthma effect at least partly through T-lymphocyte inhibition (see Chapter 115). Other possible novel approaches to drug therapy include cytokine antagonists, adhesion molecule antagonists, and therapy with antibodies that temporarily ablate CD4 T lymphocytes or asthma-relevant cytokines.

CONCLUSION

There now exists considerable support for the hypothesis that asthma represents a specialized form of cell-mediated immunity, in which cytokines and possibly other mediators secreted by activated T lymphocytes bring about the specific accumulation and activation of eosinophils in the bronchial mucosa (Fig. 5). These cytokines are secreted in the context of a TH2-type pattern and putatively reflect a locally directed T-lymphocyte response against mucosal antigens, including aeroallergens. The relative roles of T lymphocyte–dependent and IgE-mediated mechanisms in the pathogenesis of asthma in various clinical settings remain to be defined, although there is some evidence that IgE-mediated mechanisms may play a role even in so-called intrinsic asthma. These observations suggest that T–lymphocyte inhibition is likely to

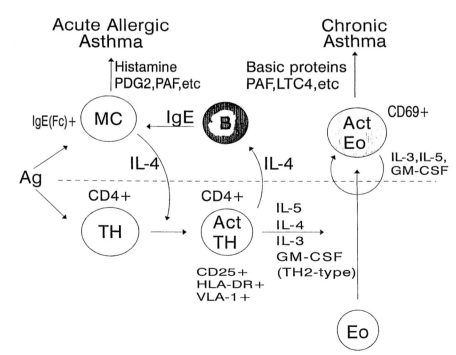

FIG. 5. Inflammatory mechanisms in asthma and allergic inflammation. Activation of TH2-like CD4+ T cells *(TH)* by specific antigen *(Ag)* results in the secretion of cytokines, particularly IL-5, IL-4, IL-3, and GM-CSF that influence eosinophil survival, differentiation, activation, and adherence *(Eo, Act Eo)*, and are implicated in orchestrating the specific eosinophil infiltration that characterizes mucosal inflammation in allergic disease and asthma. In parallel, allergens may trigger inflammatory processes through the cross-linking of surface IgE on mast cells *(MC)*, resulting in the release of mediators such as histamine and leukotrienes. The relative importance of these processes in asthmatic and allergic inflammation in different clinical settings remains to be determined. The two systems are interdependent in the sense that IL-4 derived from TH2-like TH cells is essential for IgE switching by B lymphocytes *(B)*, and thus mast cell sensitization, whereas IL-4 release from IgE-triggered mast cells may further promote TH2-like T-lymphocyte development.

continue to form part of the fundamental basis for the future therapy of asthma. Finally, further documentation of the cytokines involved in asthma of varying clinical associations might allow a pathophysiologic classification of the disease.

REFERENCES

1. Houston JC, De Navasquez S, Trounce JR. A clinical and pathological study of fatal cases of status asthmaticus. *Thorax* 1953;8:207–213.
2. Dunnill MS. The pathology of asthma with special reference to changes in the bronchial mucosa. *J Clin Pathol* 1960;13:27–33.
3. Dunnill MS, Massarella GR, Anderson JA. A comparison of the quantitative anatomy of the bronchi in normal subjects, in status asthmaticus, in chronic bronchitis and in emphysema. *Thorax* 1969;24:176–179.
4. Filley WV, Holley KE, Kephart GM, Gleich GJ. Identification by immunofluorescence of eosinophil granule major basic protein in lung tissues of patients with bronchial asthma. *Lancet* 1982;ii:11–16.
5. Rackemann FM. A working classification of asthma. *Am J Med* 1947;3:601–606.
6. Rackemann FM. Intrinsic asthma. *J Allergy* 1940;11:147–162.
7. Settipane GA, Chafee FH. Nasal polyps in asthma and rhinitis. *J Allergy Clin Immunol* 1977;59:17–21.
8. Burrows B, Martinez FD, Halonen M, Barbee RA, Cline MG. Association of asthma with serum IgE levels and skin-test reactivity to allergens. *N Engl J Med* 1989;320:271–277.
9. Postma DS, Bleeker ER, Amelung PJ, Holroyd KJ, Xu J, Panhuysen CIM, Meyers DA, Levitt RC. Genetic susceptibility to asthma—bronchial hyperresponsiveness coinherited with a major gene for atopy. *N Engl J Med* 1995;333:894–900.
10. Sandford AJ, Shirakawa T, Moffatt MF, et al. Localisation of atopy and b subunit of high-affinity IgE receptor (FcₑRI) on chromosome 11q. *Lancet* 1993; 341:332–334.
11. Shirakawa T, Li A, Dubowitz M, et al. Association between atopy and variants of the b subunit of the high-affinity immunoglobulin E receptor. *Nature Genet* 1994;7:125–130.
12. Adorini L, Muller S, Cardinaux F, Lehmann PV, Falcioni F, Nagy ZA. *In vivo* competition between self peptides and foreign antigens in T cell activation. *Nature* 1988;334:623–625.
13. MacDonald HR, Pedrazzini T, Schneider R, Louis JA, Zinkernagel RM. Intrathymic elimination of Mlsa-reactive (V(β6)+) cells during neonatal tolerance induction to Mlsa-encoded antigens. *J Exp Med* 1988; 167;2005–2010.
14. Kisielow P, Bluthmann H, Staerz UD, Steinmetz M, Von Boehmer H. Tolerance in T cell receptor transgenic mice involves deletion of nonmature CD4+ and CD8+ T-lymphocytes. *Nature* 1988;333:742–746.
15. Kappler JW, Staerz U, White J, Marrack PC. Self tolerance eliminates T cells specific for Mls-modified products of the major histocompatibility complex. *Nature* 1988;332:35–40.
16. McDuffie M, Roehm N, Born W, Marrack P, Kappler JW. T cell receptor/MHC interactions in the thymus and the shaping of the T cell repertoire. *Transpl Proc* 1987;19(S7):111–116.
17. Durum SK, Schmidt JA, Oppenheim JJ. Interleukin 1: an immunological perspective. *Annu Rev Immunol* 1985;3:263–282.
18. Mueller DL, Jenkins MK, Schwartz RH. Clonal expansion versus functional clonal inactivation: a costimulatory signalling pathway determines the outcome of T cell receptor occupancy. *Annu Rev Immunol* 1989;7:445–463.
19. Harding FA, McArthur JG, Gross JA, Raulet DH, Allison HP. CD28-mediated signalling co-stimulates murine T cells and prevents induction of anergy in T cell clones. *Nature* 1992;356:607–609.
20. Linsley PS, Brady W, Urnes M, Grosmaire LS, Damle NK, Ledbetter JA. CTLA-4 is a second receptor for the B-cell activation antigen B7. *J Exp Med* 1991;174:561–569.
21. Engel P, Gribben JG, Freeman GJ, et al. The B7-2 (B70) cosimulatory molecule expressed by monocytes and activated B lymphocytes is the CD86 differentiation antigen. *Blood* 1994;84:1402–1407.
22. Lanier LL, O'Fallon S, Somoza C, et al. CD80 (B7) and CD86 (B70) provide similar costimulatory signals for T cell proliferation, cytokine production and generation of CTL. *J Immunol* 1995;154:97–105.
23. June CH, Ledbetter JA, Linsley PS, Thompson CB. Role of the CD28 receptor in T cell activation. *Immunol Today* 1990;11:211–216.
24. Nabavi N, Freeman GJ, Gault A, Godfrey D, Nadler LM, Glimcher LH. Signalling through the MHC class II cytoplasmic domain is required for antigen presentation and induces B7 expression. *Nature* 1992;360:266–268.
25. Schwartz RH. Co-stimulation of T lymphocytes: the role of CD28, CTLA-4 and B7/BB1 in IL-2 production and immunotherapy. *Cell* 1992;71:1065–1068.
26. Jenkins MK, Taylor PS, Norton SD, Urdhal KB. CD28 delivers a co-stimulatory signal involved in antigen-specific IL-2 production by human T cells. *J Immunol* 1991;147:2461–2466.
27. Fish S, Zenowich E, Fleming M, Manser T. Molecular analysis of original antigenic sin. I. Clonal selection, somatic mutation and isotype switching during a memory B cell response. *J Exp Med* 1989; 170:1191–1209.
28. Gauchat J-F, Lebman DA, Coffman RL, Gascan H, De Vries JE. Structure and expression of germline ε transcripts in human B cells induced by IL-4 to switch to IgE production. *J Exp Med* 1990;172:463–473.
29. Punnonen J, Aversa G, Cocks BG, et al. Interleukin-13 induces interleukin-4-independent IgG4 and IgE synthesis and CD23 expression by human B-cells. *Proc Natl Acad Sci USA* 1993;90:3730–3734.
30. Zurawski SM, Vega F, Huyghe G, Zurawski G. Receptors for interleukin-13 and interleukin-4 are complex and share a novel component that functions in signal transduction. *EMBO J* 1993;12:2663–2670.
31. Zurawski G, De Vries JE. Interleukin-13, an interleukin-4-like cytokine that acts on monocytes and B-cells, but not on T cells. *Immunol Today* 1994;15:19–26.
32. Gascan H, Gauchat J-F, Aversa G, Van Vlasselaer P, De Vries JE. Anti-CD40 monoclonal antibodies or CD4- T cell clones induce IgG4 and IgE switching in purified human B cells via different signalling pathways. *J Immunol* 1991;147:8–13.
33. Pene J, Rousset F, Briere F et al. IgE regulation by normal human lymphocytes is induced by interleukin-4 and suppressed by interferons γ and α and prostaglandin E₂. *Proc Natl Acad Sci USA* 1988;85:6880–6884.
34. Pene J, Rousset F, Briere F, et al. Interleukin-5 enhances interleukin-4-induced IgE production by normal human B-cells. The role of soluble CD23 antigen. *Eur J Immunol* 1988;18:929–935.
35. Gauchat J-F, Aversa GG, Gascan H, De Vries JE. Modulation of IL-4 induced germline e mRNA synthesis in human B-cells by tumor necrosis factor-α, anti-CD40 monoclonal antibodies or transforming growth factor-β correlates with levels of IgE production. *Int Immunol* 1992;4:397–406.
36. Kimata H, Yoshida A, Ishioka C, Lindley L, Mikawa H. Interleukin-8 selectively inhibits immunoglobulin E production induced by IL-4 in human B-cells. *J Exp Med* 1992;176:1227–1231.
37. Kinawa M, Gately M, Gabler V, Chizzonite R, Fargeas C, Delespesse G. Recombinant interleukin-12 suppresses the synthesis of IgE by interleukin-4-stimulated human lymphocytes. *J Clin Invest* 1992;90;262–269.
38. Miyajima H, Hirano T, Hirose S, Karasuyama H, Okumara K, Ovary Z. Suppression by IL-2 of IgE production by B cells stimulated by IL-4. *J Immunol* 1991;146:457–462.
39. Vercelli D, Jabara HH, Arai K-I, Yokota T, Geha RS. Endogenous IL-6 plays an obligatory role in IL-4-induced human IgE synthesis. *Eur J Immunol* 1989;19:1419–1424.
40. Clark EA, Leadbetter JA. How B- and T cells talk to each other. *Nature* 1994;367:425–428.
41. Jabara HH, Fu SM, Geha RS, Vercelli D. CD40 and IgE: synergism between anti-CD40 monoclonal antibody and IL-4 in the induction of IgE synthesis by highly purified human B cells. *J Exp Med* 1990;172:1861–1864.
42. Hollenbaugh D, Grosmaire LS, Kullas CD, et al. The human T cell antigen gp39, a member of the TNF gene family, is a ligand for the CD40 receptor: expression of a soluble form of gp39 with B cell co-stimulatory activity. *EMBO J* 1992;11:4313–4321.
43. Gauchat J-F, Henchoz S, Mazzei G, et al. Induction of human IgE synthesis by mast cells and basophils. *Nature* 1993;365:340–343.
44. Aubry J-P, Pochon S, Graber P, Jansen KU, Bonnefoy J-Y. CD21 is a ligand for CD23 and regulates IgE production. *Nature* 1992;358:505–507.
45. Parronchi P, Tiri A, Macchia D, et al. Noncognate contact-dependent

B-cell activation can promote IL-4-dependent *in vitro* human IgE synthesis. *J Immunol* 1990;144:2102–2106.

46. Rothenberg ME, Owen WF, Silberstein DS, et al. Human eosinophils have prolonged survival, enhanced functional properties and become hypodense when exposed to human interleukin-3. *J Clin Invest* 1988; 81:1986–1992.

47. Lopez AF, Williamson DJ, Gamble JR, et al. Recombinant human granulocyte-macrophage colony stimulating factor stimulates *in vitro* mature human eosinophil and neutrophil function, surface receptor expression and survival. *J Clin Invest* 1986;78:1220–1228.

48. Rothenberg ME, Petersen J, Stevens RL, et al. IL-5 dependent conversion of normodense human eosinophils to the hypodense phenotype uses 3T3 fibroblasts for enhanced viability, accelerated hypodensity and sustained antibody-dependent cytotoxicity. *J Immunol* 1989;143:2311–2316.

49. Lopez AF, Sanderson CJ, Gamble JR, Campbell HD, Young IG, Vadas MA. Recombinant human interleukin-5 is a selective activator of eosinophil function. *J Exp Med* 1988;167:219–224.

50. Walsh GM, Hartnell A, Wardlaw AJ, Kurihara K, Sanderson CJ, Kay AB. IL-5 enhances the *in vitro* adhesion of human eosinophils, but not neutrophils, in a leucocyte integrin (CD11/CD18)-dependent manner. *Immunology* 1990;71:258–265.

51. Basten A, Beeson PB. Mechanism of eosinophilia. II: role of the lymphocyte. *J Exp Med* 1970;131:1288–1305.

52. Dent LA, Strath M, Mellor AL, Sanderson CJ. Eosinophilia in transgenic mice expressing interleukin-5. *J Exp Med* 1990;172:1425–1431.

53. Wardlaw AJ, Moqbel R, Cromwell O, Kay AB. Platelet activating factor: a potent chemotactic and chemokinetic factor for human eosinophils. *J Clin Invest* 1986;78:1701–1706.

54. Sehmi R, Wardlaw AJ, Cromwell O Kurihara K, Waltmann P, Kay AB. IL-5 selectively enhances the chemotactic response of eosinophils obtained from normal but not eosinophilic subjects. *Blood* 1992;79: 2952–2959.

55. Warringa RA, Koenderman L, Kok PT, Kreukniet J, Bruijnzeel PL. Modulation and induction of eosinophil chemotaxis by granulocyte/ macrophage colony stimulating factor and IL-3. *Blood* 1991;77: 2694–2700.

56. Rand TH, Cruikshank WW, Center DM, Weller PF. CD4-mediated stimulation of human eosinophils: lymphocyte chemoattractant factor and other CD4-binding ligands elicit eosinophil migration. *J Exp Med* 1991;173:1521–1528.

57. Rand TH, Silberstein DS, Kornfeld H, Weller PF. Human eosinophils express functional IL-2 receptors. *J Clin Invest* 1991;88:825–832.

58. Baggiolini M, Dahinden CA. CC chemokines in allergic inflammation. *Immunol Today* 1994;15:127–133.

59. Davies RJ, Wang JH, Trigg CJ, Devalia JL. Expression of granulocyte-macrophage colony-stimulating factor, interleukin-8 and RANTES in the bronchial epithelium of mild asthmatics is down-regulated by inhaled beclomethasone dipropionate. *Int Arch Allergy Immunol* 1995;107:428–429.

60. Ebisawa M, Yamada T, Bickel C, Klunk D, Schleimer RP. Eosinophil transendothelial migration induced by cytokines. III. Effect of the chemokine RANTES. *J Immunol* 1994;153:2153–2160.

61. Smith JB, Kunjummen RD, Kishimoto TK, Anderson, DC. Expression and regulation of L-selectin on eosinophils from human adults and neonates. *Pediatr Res* 1992;32:465–471.

62. Kyan-Aung U, Haskard DO, Poston RN, Thornhill MH, Lee TH. Endothelial leukocyte adhesion molecule 1 and intercellular adhesion molecule 1 mediate adhesion of eosinophils to endothelial cells *in vitro* and are expressed by endothelium in allergic cutaneous inflammation *in vivo*. *J Immunol* 1991;146:521–528.

63. Bochner BS, Luscinskas FW, Gimbrone MAJ, et al. Adhesion of human basophils, eosinophils and neutrophils to IL-1 activated human vascular endothlial cells: contributions of endothelial cell adhesion molecules. *J Exp Med* 1993;173:1553–1557.

64. Walsh GM, Hartnell A, Mermod J-J, Kay AB, Wardlaw AJ. Human eosinophil, but not neutrophil adherence to IL-1 stimulated HUVEC is a4b1 (VLA-4) dependent. *J Immunol* 1991;146:3419–3423.

65. Schleimer RP, Sterbinsky SA, Kaiser J, et al. IL-4 induces adherence of human eosinophils and basophils but not neutrophils to endothelium: association with expression of VCAM-1. *J Immunol* 1992;148: 1086–1092.

66. Bentley AM, Durham SR, Robinson DS, et al. Expression of the endothelial and leucocyte adhesion molecules ICAM-1, E-selectin and VCAM-1 in the bronchial mucosa in steady state and allergen-induced asthma. *J Allergy Clin Immunol* 1993;92:857–868.

67. Elices MJ, Osborn L, Takada Y, et al. VCAM-1 on activated endothelium interacts with the leucocyte integrin VLA-4 at a site distinct from the VLA-4/fibronectin binding site. *Cell* 1990;60:577–584.

68. Anwar ARE, Moqbel R, Walsh GM, Kay AB, Wardlaw AJ. Adhesion to fibronectin prolongs eosinophil survival. *J Exp Med* 1993;177: 819–824.

69. Mosmann TR, Cherwinski H, Bond MW, Gedlin MA, Coffman RL. Two types of murine helper T cell clones. I. Definition according to profiles of lymphokine activities and secreted proteins. *J Immunol* 1986;136:2348–2357.

70. Mosmann TR, Moore KW. The role of IL-10 in cross-regulation of TH1 and TH2 responses. *Immunoparasitol Today* 1991;12:49–53.

71. Mosmann TR, Coffman RL. TH1 and TH2 cells: different patterns of lymphokine secretion lead to different functional properties. *Annu Rev Immunol* 1989;7:145–173.

72. Cher DJ, Mosmann TR. Two types of murine helper T cell clone. II: delayed-type hypersensitivity is mediated by TH1 clones. *J Immunol* 1987;138:3688–3694.

73. Firestein GS, Roeder WD, Laxer JA, et al. A new murine CD4– T cell subset with an unrestricted cytokine profile. *J Immunol* 1989;143: 518–525.

74. Paliard X, De Waal Malefyt R, Yssel H, et al. Simultaneous production of IL-2, IL-4 and interferon-gamma by activated human CD4+ and CD8+ T cell clones. *J Immunol* 1988;141:849–855.

75. Del Prete GF, De Carli M, Mastromauro C, et al. Purified protein derivative of Mycobacterium tuberculosis and excretory-secretory antigen(s) of Toxocara canis expand *in vitro* human T cells with stable and opposite (type 1 T helper or type 2 T helper) profile of cytokine production. *J Clin Invest* 1991;88:346–350.

76. Yssel H, Shanafelt MC, Soderberg C, Schneider PV, Anzola J, Peitz G. *Borrelia burgdorferi* activates a T helper type 1-like T cell subset in lyme arthritis. *J Exp Med* 1991;174:593–601.

77. Parronchi P, Macchia D, Piccinni MP, et al. Allergen and bacterial antigen-specific T cell clones established from atopic donors show a different profile of cytokine production. *Proc Natl Acad Sci USA* 1991; 88:4538–4542.

78. Salgame P, Abrams JS, Clayberger C, et al. Differing cytokine profiles of functional subsets of human CD4 and CD8 T cell clones. *Science* 1991;254:279–282.

79. Fiorentino DF, Bond MW, Mossmann TR. Two types of mouse T helper cells. IV. TH2 clones secrete a factor that inhibits cytokine production by TH1 clones. *J Exp Med* 1989;170:2081–2095.

80. Del Prete GF, De Carli M, Almerigogna F, Giudizi MG, Biagiotti R, Romagnani S. Human IL-10 is produced by both type 1 helper (TH1) and type 2 helper (TH2) T cell clones and inhibits their antigen–specific proliferation and cytokine production. *J Immunol* 1993;150: 353–360.

81. Del Prete GF, De Carli M, Ricci M, Romagnani S. Helper activity for immunoglobulin synthesis of TH1 and TH2 human T cell clones. The help of TH1 clones is limited by their cytolytic capacity. *J Exp Med* 1991;174:809–813.

82. Swain SL, Weinberg AD, English M. CD4+ T cell subsets: lymphokine secretion of memory cells and effector cells which develop from precursors *in vitro*. *J Immunol* 1990;144:1788–1798.

83. Maggi E, Parronchi P, Manetti R, et al. Reciprocal regulatory role of IFN-γ and IL-4 on the *in vitro* development of human TH1 and TH2 clones. *J Immunol* 1992;148:2142–2147.

84. Romagnani S. Induction of TH1 and TH2 response: a key role for the "natural" immune response? *Immunol Today* 1992;13:379–381.

85. De Waal-Malefyt R, Figdor CG, Huijbens R, et al. Effects of IL-13 on phenotype, cytokine production and cytotoxic function of human monocytes. *J Immunol* 1993;191:6370–6381.

86. Thompson CB. Distinct roles for the costimulatory ligands B7-1 and B7-2 in T helper cell differentiation? *Cell* 1995;81:979–982.

87. Freeman GJ, Boussiotis VA, Anumanthan A, et al. B7-1 and B7-2 do not deliver identical co-stmulatory signals, since B7-2 but not B7-1 preferentially co-stimulates the initial production of IL-4. *Immunity* 1995;2:523–532.

88. Kuchroo VK, Das MP, Brown JA, et al. B7-1 and B7-2 co-stimulatory molecules activate differentially the TH1/TH2 developmental pathways: application to autoimmune disease therapy. *Cell* 1995;80: 707–718.

89. Gilbert KM, Weigle WO. B cell presentation of a tolerogenic signal to TH clones. *Cell Immunol* 1992;139:58–71.

90. Gajewski TF, Pinnas M, Wong T, Fitch FW. Murine TH1 and TH2 clones proliferate optimally in response to distinct antigen-presenting cell populations. *J Immunol* 1991;146:1750–1758.

91. Williams ME, Shea CM, Lichtman AH, Abbas AK. Antigen receptor-mediated anergy in resting lymphocytes and T cell clones. *J Immunol* 1992;149:1921–1926.

92. Maurer D, Ebner C, Reininger B, et al. The high affinity IgE receptor (FcεRI) mediates IgE-dependent allergen presentation. *J Immunol* 1995;154:6285–6290.

93. Van der Heijden FL, van Neerven RJ, Kapsenberg ML. Relationship between facilitated allergen presentation and the presence of allergen-specific IgE in the serum of atopic patients. *Clin Exp Immunol* 1995; 99:289–293.

94. Yamamura M, Wagn X-H, Ohmen JD, et al. Cytokine patterns of immunologically mediated tissue damage. *J Immunol* 1992;149: 1470–1475.

95. Azzawi M, Bradley B, Jeffery PK, et al. Identification of activated T lymphocytes and eosinophils in bronchial biopsies in stable atopic asthma. *Am Rev Respir Dis* 1990;142:1410–1413.

96. Wardlaw AJ, Dunnette S, Gleich GJ, Collins JV, Kay AB. Eosinophils and mast cells in bronchoalveolar lavage in mild asthma: relationship to bronchial hyperreactivity. *Am Rev Respir Dis* 1988;137:62–69.

97. Kirby JG, Hargreave FE, Gleich GJ, O'Byrne PM. Bronchoalveolar cell profiles of asthmatic and nonasthmatic subjects. *Am Rev Respir Dis* 1987;136:379–383.

98. Jeffery PK, Wardlaw AJ, Nelson FC, Collins JV, Kay AB. Bronchial biopsies in asthma: an ultrastructural, quantitative study and correlation with hyperreactivity. *Am Rev Respir Dis* 1989;140:1745–1753.

99. Hamid Q, Barkans J, Robinson DS, Durham SR, Kay AB. Co-expression of CD25 and CD3 in atopic allergy and asthma. *Immunology* 1992;75:659–663.

100. Robinson DS, Bentley AM, Hartnell A, Kay AB, Durham SR. Activated memory T helper cells in broncoalveolar lavage from atopic asthmatics. Relationship to asthma symptoms, lung function and bronchial responsiveness. *Thorax* 1993;48:26–32.

101. Salvato G. Some histological changes in chronic bronchitis and asthma. *Thorax* 1968;23:168–172.

102. Laitinen LA, Heino M, Laitinen A, Kava T, Haahtela T. Damage of airway epithelium and bronchial reactivity in patients with asthma. *Am Rev Respir Dis* 1985;131:599–606.

103. Beasley R, Roche W, Roberts JA, Holgate ST. Cellular events in the bronchi in mild asthma and after bronchial provocation. *Am Rev Respir Dis* 1989;139:806–817.

104. Bradley BL, Azzawi M, Assoufi B, et al. Eosinophils, T-lymphocytes, mast cells, neutrophils and macrophages in bronchial biopsies from atopic asthmatics: comparison with atopic nonasthma and normal controls and relationship to bronchial hyperresponsiveness. *J Allergy Clin Immunol* 1991;88:661–674.

105. Jeffery PK, Godfrey RW, Adelroth E, Nelson F, Rogers A, Johansson S-A. Effects of treatment on airway inflammation and thickening of reticular collagen in asthma: a quantitative light and electron microscopic study. *Am Rev Respir Dis* 1992;145:890–899.

106. Fabbri LM, Danielli D, Crescioli S, et al. Fatal asthma in a subject sensitized to toluene diisocyanate. *Am Rev Respir Dis* 1988;137: 1494–1498.

107. Bentley AM, Maestrelli P, Saetta M, et al. Activated T-lymphocytes and eosinophils in the bronchial mucosa in isocyanate-induced asthma. *J Allergy Clin Immunol* 1992;89:821–829.

108. Bentley AM, Menz G, Storz C, et al. Identification of T-lymphocytes, macrophages and activated eosinophils in the bronchial mucosa in intrinsic asthma: relationship to symptoms and bronchial responsiveness. *Am Rev Respir Dis* 1992;146:500–506.

109. Mattoli S, Mattoso VL, Soloperto M, Allegra L, Fasoli A. Cellular and biochemical characteristics of bronchoalveolar lavage fluid in symptomatic nonallergic asthma. *J Allergy Clin Immunol* 1991;87:794–802.

110. Humbert M, Grant JA, Taborda-Barata L, et al. High affinity IgE receptor (FcεRI)-bearing cells in bronchial biopsies from atopic and non-topic asthma. *Am Rev Respir Crit Care Med* 1996;153:1931–1937.

111. Wong DT, Weller PF, Galli SJ, et al. Human eosinophils express transforming growth factor alpha. *J Exp Med* 1990;172:673–681.

112. Weller PF, Rand TH, Barrett T, Elovic A, Wong DTW, Finberg RW. Accessory cell function of human eosinophils: HLA-DR dependent, MHC-restricted antigen presentation and interleukin-1α formation. *J Immunol* 1993;150:2554–2562.

113. Moqbel R, Hamid Q, Ying S, et al. Expression of mRNA and immunoreactivity for the granulocyte/macrophage colony stimulating factor (GM-CSF) in activated human eosinophils. *J Exp Med* 1991; 174:749–752.

114. Kita H, Ohnishi T, Okubo Y, Weiler D, Abrams JS, Gleich GJ. GM-CSF and interleukin-3 release from human peripheral blood eosinophils and neutrophils. *J Exp Med* 1991;174:743–748

115. Broide DH, Paine MM, Firestein GS. Eosinophils express interleukin-5 and granulocyte-macrophage colony-stimulating factor mRNA at sites of allergic inflammation in asthmatics. *J Clin Invest* 1992;90: 1414–1424.

116. Hamid Q, Barkans J, Abrams JS, Meng Q, Ying S, Kay AB, Moqbel R. Human eosinophils synthesize and secrete interleukin-6 in vitro. *Blood* 1992;80:1496–1501.

117. Braun RK, Franchini M, Erard F, et al. Human peripheral blood eosinophils produce and release interleukin-8 on stimulation with calcium ionophore. *Eur J Immunol* 1993;23:956–960.

118. Costa JJ, Matossian K, Resnick MB, et al. Human eosinophils can express the cytokines tumour necrosis factor-α and macrophage inflammatory protein-1 α. *J Clin Invest* 1993;91:2673–2684.

119. Moqbel R, Ying S, Barkans J, et al. Identification of messenger RNA for IL-4 in human eosinophils with granule localisation of the translated product. *J Immunol* 1995;155:4939–4947.

120. Bradding P, Roberts JA, Britten KM, et al. Interleukin-4, -5, -6 and tumor necrosis factor-α in normal and asthmatic airways: evidence for the human mast cell as a source of these cytokines. *Am J Respir Cell Mol Biol* 1994;10:471–480.

121. Ohkawara Y, Yamauchi K, Tanno Y, et al. Human lung mast cells and pulmonary macrophages produce tumor necrosis factor-α in sensitized lung tissue after IgE receptor triggering. *Am J Resp Cell Mol Biol* 1992;7:385–392.

122. Arock M, Merle-Beral H, Dugas B, et al. IL-4 release by human leukemic and activated normal basophils. *J Immunol* 1993;151:1441–1447.

123. Ying S, Durham SR, Barkans J, et al. T cells are the principal source of interleukin-5 mRNA in allergen-induced rhinitis. *Am J Respir Cell Mol Biol* 1993;9:356–360.

124. Ying S, Durham SR, Corrigan CJ, Hamid Q, Kay AB. Phenotype of cells expressing mRNA for TH2-type (interleukin-4 and interleukin-5) and TH1-type (interleukin-2 and interferon-γ) cytokines in bronchoalveolar lavage and bronchial biopsies from atopic asthmatics and normal control subjects. *Am J Respir Cell Mol Biol* 1995;12: 477–487.

125. Corrigan CJ, Hartnell A, Kay AB. T-lymphocyte activation in acute severe asthma. *Lancet* 1988;i:1129–1131.

126. Corrigan CJ, Kay AB. CD4 T-lymphocyte activation in acute severe asthma. Relationship to disease severity and atopic status. *Am Rev Respir Dis* 1990;141:970–977.

127. Corrigan CJ, Haczku A, Gemou-Engesaeth V, et al. CD4 T-lymphocyte activation in asthma is accompanied by increased concentrations of interleukin-5: effect of glucocorticoid therapy. *Am Rev Respir Dis* 1993;147:540–547.

128. Gemou-Engesaeth V, Kay AB, Bush A, Corrigan CJ. Activated peripheral blood CD4 and CD8 T-lymphocytes in childhood asthma: correlation with eosinophilia and disease severity. *Pediatr Allergy Immunol* 1994;5:170–177.

129. Alexander AG, Barkans J, Moqbel R, Barnes NC, Kay AB, Corrigan CJ. Serum interleukin-5 concentrations in atopic and nonatopic patients with glucocorticoid-dependent chronic severe asthma. *Thorax* 1994;49:1231–1233.

130. Doi S, Gemou-Engesaeth V, Kay AB, Corrigan CJ. Polymerase chain reaction quantification of cytokine messenger RNA expression in peripheral blood mononuclear cells of patients with severe asthma: effect of glucocorticoid therapy. *Clin Exp Allergy* 1994;24:854–687.

131. Corrigan CJ, Brown PH, Barnes NC, Tsai JJ, Kay AB. Glucocorticoid resistance in chronic asthma: peripheral blood T-lymphocyte activation and a comparison of the T-lymphocyte inhibitory effects of glucocorticoids and cyclosporin A. *Am Rev Respir Dis* 1991;144:1026–1032.

132. Corrigan CJ, Brown PH, Barnes NC, Tsai JJ, Kay AB. Glucocorticoid resistance in chronic asthma: glucocorticoid pharmacokinetics, glu-

cocorticoid receptor characteristics and inhibition of peripheral blood T cell proliferation by glucocorticoids *in vitro. Am Rev Respir Dis* 1991;144:1016–1025.

133. Haczku A, Alexander A, Brown P, Kay AB, Corrigan CJ. The effect of dexamethasone, cyclosporin A and rapamycin on T-lymphocyte proliferation *in vitro*: comparison of cells from corticosteroid sensitive and corticosteroid resistant chronic asthmatics. *J Allergy Clin Immunol* 1994;93:510–519.

134. Graham DR, Luksza AR, Evans CC. Bronchoalveolar lavage in asthma. *Thorax* 1985;40:717.

135. Walker C, Kaegi MK, Braun MD, Blaser K. Activated T cells and eosinophils in bronchoalveolar lavages from subjects with asthma correlated with disease severity. *J Allergy Clin Immunol* 1991;88: 935–942.

136. Broide DH, Lotz M, Cuomo AJ, Cobum DA, Federman EC, Wasserman SI. Cytokines in symptomatic asthma airways. *J Allergy Clin Immunol* 1992;89:958–967.

137. Virchow J-C, Walker C, Hafner D, et al. T cells and cytokines in bronchoalveolar lavage fluid after segmental allergen provocation in atopic asthma. *Am J Respir Crit Care Med* 1995;151:960–968.

138. Hamid Q, Azzawi M, Ying S, et al. Expression of mRNA for interleukin-5 in mucosal bronchial biopsies from asthma. *J Clin Invest* 1991;87:1541–1546.

139. Robinson DS, Hamid Q, Ying S, et al. Evidence for a predominant "TH2-type" bronchoalveolar lavage T-lymphocyte population in atopic asthma. *N Engl J Med* 1992;326:298–304.

140. Robinson DS, Ying S, Bentley AM, et al. Relationships among numbers of bronchoalveolar lavage cells expressing messenger ribonucleic acid for cytokines, asthma symptoms, and airway methacholine responsiveness in atopic asthma. *J Allergy Clin Immunol* 1993;92: 397–403.

141. Corrigan CJ, Hamid Q, North J, et al. Peripheral blood CD4, but not CD8 T-lymphocytes in patients with exacerbation of asthma transcribe and translate messenger RNA encoding cytokines which prolong eosinophil survival in the context of a TH2-type pattern: effect of glucocorticoid therapy. *Am J Respir Cell Mol Biol* 1995;12: 567–578.

142. Robinson DS, Hamid Q, Ying S, et al. Prednisolone treatment in asthma is associated with modulation of bronchoalveolar lavage cell interleukin-4, interleukin-5 and interferon-γ cytokine gene expression. *Am Rev Respir Dis* 1993;148:402–406.

143. Bentley AM, Meng Q, Robinson DS, Hamid Q, Kay AB, Durham SR. Increases in activated T-lymphocytes, eosinophils and cytokine messenger RNA for IL-5 and GM-CSF in bronchial biopsies after allergen inhalation challenge in atopic asthmatics. *Am J Respir Cell Mol Biol* 1993;8:35–42.

144. Kay AB, Ying S, Varney V, et al. Messenger RNA expression of the cytokine gene cluster IL-3, IL-4, IL-5 and GM-CSF in allergen-induced late phase cutaneous reactions in atopic subjects. *J Exp Med* 1991;173:775–778.

145. Tsicopoulos A, Hamid Q, Varney V, et al. Preferential messenger RNA expression of TH1-type cells (IFN-γ+, IL-2+) in classical delayed-type (tuberculin) hypersensitivity reactions in human skin. *J Immunol* 1992;148:2058–2061.

146. Gaga M, Frew AJ, Varney VA, Kay AB. Eosinophil activation and T-lymphocyte infiltration in allergen-induced late phase skin reactions and classical delayed-type hypersensitivity. *J Immunol* 1991;147: 816–822.

147. Robinson DS, Ying S, Taylor IK, et al. Evidence for a TH1-like bronchoalveolar T cell subset and predominance of IFN-gamma gene activation in pulmonary tuberculosis. *Am J Respir Crit Care Med* 1994; 149:989–993.

148. Maggi E, Biswas P, Del Prete G, et al. Accumulation of TH2-like helper T cells in the conjunctiva of patients with vernal conjunctivitis. *J Immunol* 1991;146:1169–1174.

149. Van der Heijden FL, Wierenga EA, Bos JD, Kapsenberg ML. High frequency of IL-4 producing CD4+ allergen-specific T lymphocytes in atopic dermatitis leisonal skin. *J Invest Dermatol* 1991;97:389–394.

150. Ramb-Lindhauer C, Feldmann A, Rotte M, Neumann C. Characterization of grass pollen reactive T cell lines derived from lesional atopic skin. *Arch Dermatol Res* 1991;283:71–76.

151. Jung T, Schauer U, Rieger C, Interleukin-4 and interleukin-5 are rarely co-expressed by human T cells. *Eur J Immunol* 1995;25: 2413–2416.

152. Till SJ, Li B, Durham S, et al. Secretion of the eosinophil-active cytokines IL-5, GM-CSF and IL-3 by bronchoalveolar lavage CD4- and CD8- T cell lines in atopic asthmatics and atopic and nonatopic controls. *Eur J Immunol* 1995;25:2727–2731.

153. Holt PG. A potential vaccine strategy for asthma and allied atopic diseases during early childhood. *Lancet* 1994;344:456–458.

154. Hattevig G, Kjellman B, Bjorksten B. Clinical symptoms and IgE responses to common proteins and inhalants in the first 7 years of life. *Clin Allergy* 1987;17:571–578.

155. Hattevig G, Kjellman B, Bjorksten B. Appearance of IgE antibodies to ingested and inhaled allergens during the first 12 years of life in atopic and nonatopic children. *Pediatr Allergy Immunol* 1993;4: 182–186.

156. Holt PG, McMenamin C, Nelson D. Primary sensitization to inhalant allergens during infancy. *Pediatr Allergy Immunol* 1990;1:3–13.

157. Alexander AG, Barnes NC, Kay AB. Trial of cyclosporin A in corticosteroid-dependent chronic severe asthma. *Lancet* 1992;339: 324–328.

158. Fukuda T, Asakawa J, Motojima S, Makino S. Cyclosporine A reduces T lymphocyte activity and improves airway hyperresponsiveness in corticosteroid-dependent chronic severe asthma. *Ann Allergy Asthma Immunol* 1995;75:65–69.

159. Mori A, Suko M, Nishizaki Y, et al. IL-5 production by CD4- T cells of asthmatic patients is suppressed by glucocorticoids and the immunosuppressants FK506 and cyclosporin A. *Int Immunol* 1995;7: 449–457.

Asthma, edited by P.J. Barnes, M.M. Grunstein, A.R. Leff, and A.J. Woolcock.
Lippincott–Raven Publishers, Philadelphia © 1997.

▪ 33 ▪

Dendritic Cell Populations in the Lung and Airway Wall

Patrick G. Holt

THE ROLE OF THE DENDRITIC CELL SYSTEM IN IMMUNOBIOLOGY

The dendritic cell (DC) system comprises two distinct lineages of bone marrow-derived cells, characterized by highly pleiomorphic morphology and constitutive surface expression of a variety of function-associated molecules that facilitate their stable interaction with lymphocytes (1). The first of these is a sessile population of long-lived cells found in the germinal centers of lymph nodes, known as follicular dendritic cells, which are specialized for the presentation of antigen to B cells. These cells are not discussed further in this review.

The second DC population was first described within the paracortical (T cell) regions of lymph nodes and were originally named interdigitating cells (IDCs). They represent the end stage in the life cycle of a bone marrow-derived cell population that migrates initially into peripheral tissues and that finally "home" to the paracortical regions of draining lymph nodes after a variable period of residence in their host tissues (1). Recent evidence sug-

gests that the immediate precursors of the tissue DCs are monocytelike cells in peripheral circulation, some of which may be pluripotential, with the capacity to differentiate into macrophages or DCs, depending upon the microenvironment (and cytokine milieu) into which they migrate from the blood (2,3).

The archetypal example of the peripheral tissue DC population is the Langerhans cells (LCs) of the epidermis. Their prime function is to acquire samples of incoming foreign antigens and subsequently present them to T cells in the adjacent lymph nodes. They are specialized for presentation of these antigens to *naive* T cells and, in this regard, are in the order of 1,000 times more potent (on a cell-for-cell basis) than any other type of antigen-presenting cell (APC) yet described: that is, they represent the major cellular source of processed immunogen for the induction of primary immune responses (1). They are also considerably more efficient than other APC types in reactivation of T-memory cells.

These DCs exhibit a number of hallmark properties that distinguish them from other recognized APCs such as macrophages. These include poor adherence to substrata *in vitro*, a generally low capacity for phagocytosis (although they appear able to take up some particles including certain microorganisms) (4,5), and constitutive expression of both

P. G. Holt: Department of Cell Biology, TVW Telethon Institute for Child Health Research, Subiaco, Western Australia 6008 Australia.

class II major histocompatibility complex (MHC) and T-cell costimulator molecules (1,4). They appear to sample antigens from their surrounding tissue microenvironment by receptor-mediated endocytosis and pinocytosis, processes that they carry out with greater efficiency than conventional phagocytes or B cells, and to "store" them in intracellular vesicles that have a relatively high pH (around 5.4) relative to equivalent vesicles in phagocytes (6), which may account for the longer survival of internalized antigen in immunogenic form in DCs compared with macrophages. In addition, they have the capacity to form very stable "clusters" with T cells, during which they display processed antigen complexed to MHC class I and class II, together with costimulator molecules, to the clustered CD8+ and CD4+ lymphocytes. Unlike other potential APC types, their expression of the principal T-cell costimulators B7.1 and B7.2 is constitutive and at a high level (7); these latter properties are believed to underlie collectively their unique potency in priming naive T cells.

While the existence of an equivalent DC population in the lung has been recognized for several years, it is only very recently that accurate information has become available on the large size and widespread distribution of these cells throughout the respiratory tree. This information, together with data on their high turnover rate and rapid responses to inflammation (reviewed below), suggest potentially important roles in both the induction and expression of immunoinflammatory diseases in the respiratory tract.

IMMUNOMORPHOLOGIC CHARACTERISTICS OF RESPIRATORY TRACT DENDRITIC CELLS

In frozen sections of respiratory tract tissues, DCs can be identified on the basis of their characteristic pleiomorphic morphology, expression of high levels of class II MHC, and lack of expression of markers defining mature tissue macrophages (8–13) (see also below). They exhibit heterogeneous expression of function-associated molecules including β_1/β_2 integrins, lymphocyte function-associated antigens, and intracellular adhesion molecules (12, 14–16), Fc receptors (15,17), and the T-200 and S-100 antigens (18). Heterogeneous expression of CD1a and CD1c is also observed in different tissue microenvironments within the respiratory tract (19), and Birbeck granule expression is infrequent and variable (18), possibly reflecting differing levels of stimulation at different sites (20).

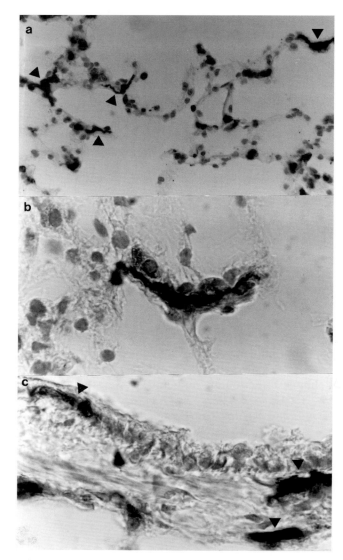

FIG. 1. Dendritic cell (DC) distribution in peripheral lung tissue. Frozen sections of rat lung immunostained for immune-associated antigen (Ia) with monoclonal antibodies 0 × 6. **a:** Low magnification: note the highly pleiomorphic Ia+ DCs (*arrowheads*) in the alveolar wall. **b:** High magnification: typical DCs at the alveolar septal junction. **c:** Ia+ DCs (*arrowheads*) within the epithelium of a peripheral airway and in underlying connective tissue. (From Holt PG, Oliver J, McMenamin C, Schon-Hegrad MA. Studies on the surface phenotype and functions of dendritic cells in parenchymal lung tissue of the rat. *Immunology* 1992;75:582–587, with permission.)

DISTRIBUTION OF DENDRITIC CELLS THROUGHOUT THE LUNG AND AIRWAYS

In the peripheral lung, DCs are widely distributed throughout the pleura (8) and in parenchymal tissue (8,9, 13,14,18). In particular, they are found in the connective tissue between the vessels and the small airways, and in the alveolar septa, most frequently at interseptal junctions (Fig. 1). The accurate localization of these DCs is facilitated by preinflation of lung tissue prior to fixation and staining.

Studies on the distribution of DCs in immunostained airway tissues, in particular the airway epithelium, have been complicated by the potential colocalization of other

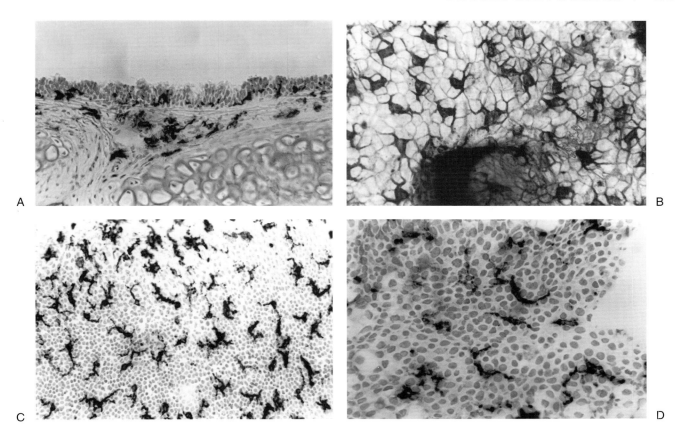

FIG. 2. Dendritic cell (DC) network in the airway epithelium. Frozen sections of airway and epidermis. **A:** Longitudinal section of rat trachea; note immune-associated antigen (Ia+) DCs above and below the epithelial basement membrane. **B:** Ia+ epidermal Langerhans' cell network (*dark area,* hair follicle). **C:** Rat tracheal tissue used in A, sectioned through the epithelium in a plane parallel to the underlying basement membrane. **D:** Human bronchial epithelium sectioned and stained as per C.

cell types expressing surface markers (such as class II MHC) that are used to identify DCs. As shown in Figure 2A, a conventional vertical or longitudinal plane of section through the large airways reveals an apparently heterogeneous population of class II MHC-bearing cells within the epithelium, which could readily be classified as a mixture of monocytes and/or B cells and/or DCs. However, we reasoned that the airway epithelium may instead contain predominantly class II MHC-positive DCs distributed as a network, analogous to the LC population discernible in the skin via immunostaining of epidermal sheets (Fig. 2B), and in order to test this hypothesis we have devised a procedure to section isolated airway segments in a tangential plane, parallel to the underlying basement membrane (11). Immunostaining of such sections revealed a tightly meshed network of intraepithelial DCs in the airways of rats (Fig. 2C) and humans (Fig. 2D), and in both species these cells account for virtually all class II MHC immunostaining, at least in the steady state.

Employing this technique, the distribution of these cells in the epithelium of the conducting airways at different levels of the respiratory tree has been studied in detail in the rat model. As shown in Figure 3, the intraepithelial density of DCs is inversely related to airway diameter, particularly in young animals, varying from 500 to 700/mm^2 epithelium in the trachea down to less than 100/mm^2 by the fifth airway generation; this gradation is less obvious in older rats, possibly reflecting differences in the net inflammatory "experience" of the tissues in the different age groups (further discussion below). Comparable studies have yet to be reported for humans; our observations suggest that DC density in the epithelium of the small bronchioles in humans (as per an earlier study [10]) is of a similar order to that of rat trachea.

In addition to these DC populations, large numbers are found in the nasal mucosa, particularly in the epithelium lining the nasal turbinates (for example, see Nelson et al. [21]). A further (considerably smaller) population has been described on the alveolar surface (22–24); these DCs are accessible by bronchoalveolar lavage (BAL), but are difficult to study because they usually comprise less than 0.5% of the BAL population.

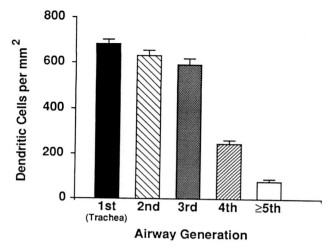

FIG. 3. Dendritic cell (DC) density in the conducting airways of rats. Data shown are DCs/mm² airway epithelium. (From Schon-Hegrad MA, Oliver J, McMenamin PG, Holt PG. Studies on the density, distribution, and surface phenotype of intraepithelial class II major histocompatibility complex antigen (Ia)-bearing dendritic cells (DC) in the conducting airways. *J Exp Med* 1991;173:1345–1356, with permission.)

TABLE 1. *Estimated turnover times for dendritic cells in various tissues*

Tissue	Species	Turnover time
Lymphoid		
Spleen	Mouse	10 days
Mesenteric lymph node[a]	Rat	3 days
Peripheral lymph	Rat	3–10 days
Spleen	Rat	2–4 weeks
Thymus	Rat	4 weeks
Nonlymphoid		
Heart	Rat	2–4 weeks
Kidney	Rat	2–4 weeks
Skin	Mouse, rat	2–7 weeks
Skin	Human, guinea pig	>9 weeks
Airway epithelium	Rat	2 days

[a]Derived from gut wall.

PRIMARY FUNCTION OF LUNG AND AIRWAY DENDRITIC CELLS

Our group has obtained formal proof of the capacity of both peripheral lung (13) and airway epithelial DCs (9) to "sample" inhaled antigens in the rat model. The crucial experiments involved exposure of disease-free animals to low levels of soluble protein antigen in an aerosol, followed by isolation and purification of DCs from the lung and airway wall, and demonstration of their capacity to present antigen-specific activation signals to T cells following their introduction into cocultures. As discussed in detail below, however, their capacity to express such APC activity efficiently is not constitutive and is subject to very tight regulation.

ORIGIN AND TURNOVER OF RESPIRATORY TRACT DENDRITIC CELLS

Recent studies from our laboratory have employed a radiation chimera model to study the population dynamics of rat airway and lung DCs (25). This system employs congenic PVG rats that are genetically identical apart from a minor allotypic variant in CD45, which is distinguishable via the use of monoclonal antibodies against respective CD45s. Bone marrow can be transplanted from one congenic partner to the other without elicitation of graft-versus-host reactions, and transplanted leukocytes can be "tracked" in tissues of the recipients employing the monoclonal antibodies described above.

Our experiments employing this model involved sublethal X-irradiation of rats in order to interrupt the supply of "precursors" required to maintain the lung DC populations that are continuously being depleted as a result of emigration of mature DCs to regional lymph nodes. In some cases, the thorax was lead shielded to control for potential radiation damage to epithelial tissues in the lung.

By sampling animals at varying time points after irradiation, it was possible to determine the rate of decline of airway epithelial DCs due to normal emigration to regional lymph nodes and thus obtain an estimate of population half-life, which was on the order of 1.5 to 2 days (25). In parallel experiments, other X-irradiated animals received congenic bone marrow; after an initial lag for establishment of the marrow graft, the airway DC populations were rapidly replenished by congenic precursors, with similar rapid kinetics. It was noteworthy that the lung DC population in the same animals displayed a significantly longer half-life (≥6 days), and epidermal LCs turned over even more slowly (25).

The only other nonlymphoid peripheral tissue DC population that displays a comparably rapid turnover is that from the gastrointestinal tract (Table 1; data derived from the study by Fossum [26]), reflecting the unique requirements for efficient antigen "surveillance" at the two main mucosal surfaces of the body that are in most direct contact with the outside environment.

RESPONSE OF LUNG DENDRITIC CELL POPULATIONS TO IMMUNOINFLAMMATORY CHALLENGE

Animal Models

The initial indication that these cell populations may be responsive to inhaled stimuli came from the studies detailed above, which mapped their distribution throughout the respiratory tree of healthy young rats. The decline in the intraepithelial density of DCs through successive airway generations reflected the known pattern of differential deposition of inhaled particles on airway surfaces, suggesting that the "drive" for maintenance of local population density was provided by direct stimulation of the airway mucosa by inhaled irritants (12).

Further support for this possibility came from observations on the effects of chronic exposure of animals to dusty bedding, notably to pine shavings (12). These animals displayed focal areas of class II MHC expression on airway epithelial cells with a concomitant eosinophil infiltrate, together with an increase (on the order of 50%) in the density of airway DCs. The DCs in these chronically inflamed airway tissues displayed a number of hallmark characteristics of activation, including increased branching of processes, upregulation of surface class II MHC, and expression of integrins such as the common β-chain of CD11a/CD18 (12).

However, even more extensive changes were observed in these cell populations during acute inflammation. Our initial studies relating to this question involved challenge of normal animals with aerosolized bacterial lipopolysaccharide (LPS); these demonstrated a transient increase in airway epithelial DC density during the first 24 h following challenge, reminiscent of the time course followed by infiltrating neutrophils (12). In more detailed follow-up experiments (27), heat-killed whole bacteria were used, employing the organism *Moraxella catarrhalis*, which has been implicated as a potential causative agent in inflammatory diseases, including otitis media. As shown in Figure 4A, exposure to aerosols containing this organism elicits a classic acute cellular inflammatory response detectable in BAL, involving a rapid early neutrophil influx, followed much later by a mononuclear cell component. No significant infiltrate of DCs was observed in the BAL.

However, immunostaining of the airway epithelium of the same animals (Fig. 4B) indicated the presence of a hitherto undetected "early" DC response, involving the rapid influx of monocytelike DC precursors within the first 2 h following challenge; these immature DCs do not progress into the airway lumen, but instead remain tightly adherent to the epithelium, presumably via cell–cell interaction molecules such as E-cadherin. These recruited DCs progressively increased in size and attained characteristic dendritiform morphology over the ensuing 8 h (27). Between 2 and 24 h after challenge, the intraepithelial density of DCs in the airway epithelium was maintained at a level equivalent to 200% to 300% above steady-state density, prior to declining to starting (normal) levels by the 72-h time point (Fig. 4).

Analysis of DC density in regional lymph nodes indicated that the "inflammatory" DCs migrate to these areas during the latter stages of the response (Table 2 [27]), presumably carrying samples of the antigens encountered in the inflammatory milieu of the epithelium. We view this as a highly efficient "front-line defense" mechanism, permitting rapid signalling of the T-cell system as to the

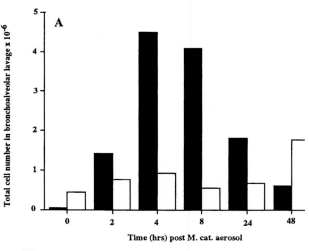

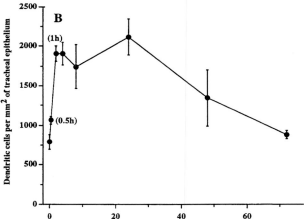

FIG. 4. Recruitment of dendritic cells (DCs) into the airway epithelium during acute inflammation: cellular inflammatory response in the lung and airways after inhalation of whole bacteria. Adult PVG rats were exposed to aerosolized *Moraxella catarrhalis*. At various times after aerosol exposure, bronchoalveolar lavage was performed. Cytospin preparations of the cells obtained were stained with Leishman's stain and differential counts performed. Tracheas were removed at each time point and frozen sections prepared and immunostained. **A:** Recovery of neutrophils *(solid bars)* and macrophages *(open bars)* from bronchoalveolar lavage fluids. Cytospin preparations stained with 0×6 contained few or no immune-associated antigen (Ia+) cells. **B:** Fluctuations in the density of Ia+ DCs in the tracheal epithelium during the inflammatory response. The data shown are derived from three to five rats per time point. (From Sallusto F, Lanzavecchia A. Efficient presentation of soluble antigen by cultured human dendritic cells is maintained by GM-CSF plus IL-4 and downregulated by TNF-α. *J Exp Med* 1994;179:1109–1118, with permission.)

TABLE 2. *Dendritic cell "traffic" from the airway and lung wall to respective draining lymph nodes during acute inflammation*

Lymph node	Mean number of dendritic cells per lymph node $\times 10^{-5}$			
	Control	*Moraxella catarrhalis* aerosol	Difference	Percent increase
Superficial cervical	20.7	24.3	3.6	17
Internal jugular	0.88	2.67	1.79	203
Parathymic	0.40	1.53	1.13	282
Posterior mediastinal	1.39	2.54	1.15	83

Data shown are mean number of dendritic cells (DCs) per lymph node from groups of three PVG rats, which were exposed to an aerosolized bacterial preparation as in Figure 4. After 48 h, the superficial cervical, internal jugular, and parathymic lymph nodes draining the upper respiratory tract and conducting airways, and the posterior mediastinal nodes draining the peripheral lung, were removed, a single-cell suspension was prepared, and macrophages were depleted by adherence to nylon wool. DCs were enumerated by flow-cytometric analysis. Parallel analysis of lymph nodes performed at the 24-h time point revealed a similar order of increase in DC numbers; however, the changes were more consistent at 48 h. (From McWilliam AS, Nelson D, Thomas JA, Holt PG. Rapid dendritic cell recruitment is a hallmark of the acute inflammatory response at mucosal surfaces. *J Exp Med* 1994;179:1331–1336, with permission.)

presence of incoming pathogenic antigens; it appears to operate also in the gastrointestinal tract (GIT) (28), in which lipopolysaccharide challenge has been observed to purge resident DCs rapidly (also observed during the early stage of the lung response [27]), but we have been unable to demonstrate a similar mechanism in the skin.

Recent studies in our lab suggest a similar DC component in the acute airway mucosal response to virus infection, or following inhalation of an antigen to which animals have been presensitized, suggesting that this represents a virtually universal first line of defense in this tissue microenvironment. We are investigating the possible role of this mechanism in "bystander" immune responses, in particular in the context of primary allergic sensitization to inhaled allergens encountered during airway inflammation.

It has also been demonstrated that local challenge via the intratracheal administration of bacillus Calmette–Guerin recruits significant numbers of DCs into the airway lumen (24).

Human Data

A number of observations indicate that human lung and airway DC populations are capable of upregulation in response to local stimulation. For example, it is clear that chronic inflammation in response to tobacco smoke exposure increases the number of DCs in both the airway mucosa (13) and peripheral lung, including on the alveolar surface (24). Additionally, the surface phenotype of the recruited DCs exhibit a variety of changes suggestive of activation.

Secondly, nasal mucosal DCs in rhinitics increase in number and surface expression of function-associated molecules during the spring (29), presumably in response to repeated exposure to pollens to which the patients were allergic. It has been suggested that atopic asthmatics may exhibit similar changes (30); however, supporting evidence is as yet scanty, and this important issue requires further detailed investigation. Progress in this area has been disappointingly slow because of the considerable difficulties associated with quantifying DCs in small bronchoscopic biopsy samples.

A recent study has clearly demonstrated hyperplasia of parenchymal DCs associated with certain lung tumors (31); this was in turn associated with local production of granulocyte-macrophage colony-stimulating factor (GM-CSF), underscoring the importance of this cytokine in regulation of DC turnover and maturation in the lung (further discussion below).

REGULATION OF DENDRITIC CELL FUNCTIONS

Previous studies on epidermal LCs have established that, while present in the skin, these cells are specialized for the uptake and processing of antigen, but are relatively poor as "presenters" of the processed antigen to T cells; under the influence of GM-CSF, particularly in combination with tumor necrosis factor-α and/or interleukin-1 (32,33) or interleukin-4 (34), the LCs functionally mature into the most potent APCs known. The LCs have thus been described as "sentinel" cells, their main role being to internalize, process, and store foreign antigens encountered in the skin, but to delay the presentation of resultant immunogenic signals to T cells until they are exposed to a milieu rich in GM-CSF and associated cytokines, which normally only occurs *in vivo* after their migration to the paracortical regions of draining lymph nodes (1).

Such a "partitioning" of the DC functions would effectively limit the frequency of T-cell activation events at the periphery, thus minimizing potential tissue damage resulting from local release of T-cell cytokines. Such a mechanism would have obvious advantages at delicate tissue sites such as the airway epithelium, which is essentially in constant contact with a wide range of environmental antigens. Recent studies from our lab indicate that, at least in the rat model, this mechanism does indeed operate for both airway and lung wall DCs (19,35), which require overnight exposure to GM-CSF-containing medium in order to "mature" their APC functions. We have additionally established that the capacity of the DCs to respond to GM-CSF activation signals is under active negative control via inhibitors produced by lung macrophages (19,35). The latter include nitric oxide and tumor necrosis factor-α (particularly in combination). Direct evidence that this mechanism operates *in vivo* has been provided by experiments demonstrating that selective *in situ* depletion of alveolar macrophages leads to rapid upregulation of the APC activity of lung wall DCs, which is associated with the development of hyperresponsiveness

of alvelolar macrophage-depleted animals to inhaled antigens to which they had been previously primed (36); interestingly, T-helper type-2 (TH-2) dependent antibody production was the most prominent aspect of the altered responder status of these animals (36).

SENSITIVITY OF LUNG AND AIRWAY DENDRITIC CELLS TO STEROIDS

Studies in the rat model have examined the sensitivity of these DC populations to both topical and systemic steroids. As shown in Figure 5, exposure of normal animals to steroids rapidly depletes resident DCs, and cessation of steroid treatment results in an equally rapid "rebound" (Fig. 6). Moreover, both systemic and topical

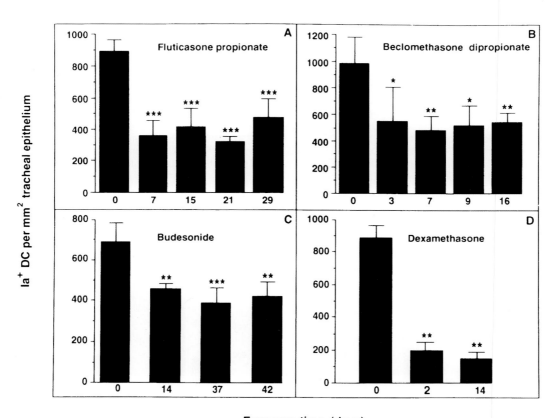

Exposure time (days)

FIG. 5A–D. Effects of repeated exposure to topical or system steroids upon airway epithelial dendritic cells (DCs). Data shown are from individual experiments and are representative of a larger series, and indicate mean number of DCs/mm^2 epithelium ± SD (n = 3–6 animals per group for each time point; minimum of 200 DCs counted per sample). Control rats exposed to aerosols containing carrying buffer alone (that is, without added steroid) were tested at each time point, and DC densities in these animals were not significantly different from untouched control animals (results not shown). The estimated dosages delivered per animal per day to the large airways (as milligrams per kilogram body weight) of adult animals in these experiments were fluticasone propionate, 0.012 mg; budesonide, 0.014 mg; and beclomethasone dipropionate, 0.11 mg. Dexamethasone was administered intraperitoneally at a dose of 10 mg/kg per day. Exposed < control animals by t test: *$p < 0.05$, **$p < 0.01$, ***$p < 0.001$. (From Nelson D, McWilliam AS, Haining S, Holt PG. Downmodulation of airway intraepithelial dendritic cell populations following local and system exposure to steroids. *Am J Respir Crit Care Med* 1995;151:475–481, with permission.)

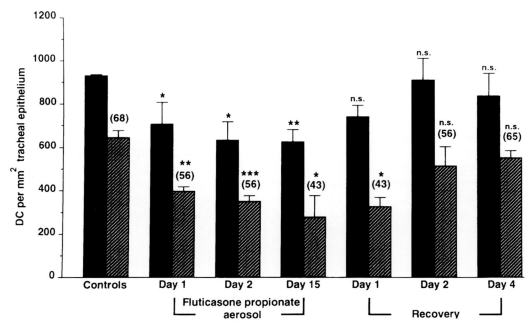

FIG. 6. Kinetics of fluticasone propionate aerosol-mediated changes in airway dendritic cell (DC) density. Data shown are mean ± SD derived from fewer than three animals per time point. *Black bars* indicate total numbers of DCs (as determined by 0 × 62 staining). *Hatched bars* indicate 0 × 6+ per immune-associated antigen (Ia+) DCs (*data in parentheses* are percent overall DC population that was Ia+). Exposed < control animals: *$p < 0.05$, **$p < 0.01$, ***$p < 0.001$; *NS,* not significantly different from control animals. (From Nelson D, McWilliam AS, Haining S, Holt PG. Downmodulation of airway intraepithelial dendritic cell populations following local and system exposure to steroids. *Am J Respir Crit Care Med* 1995;151:475–481, with permission.)

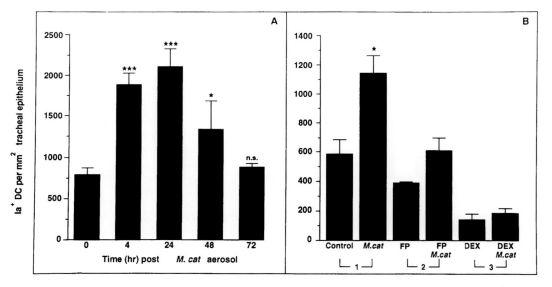

FIG. 7. Steroids downmodulate the dendritic cell (DC) component of the acute inflammatory response in the airways. **A:** Rats in groups of three to six were exposed for 30 min to aerosolized *Moraxella catarrhalis*, and airway intraepithelial DC density determined up to 72 h thereafter. **B:** Paired groups of rats (n = 3–6 rats per group) were exposed to aerosolized *M. catarrhalis* as above and airway epithelial DC density compared at the peak (24 h) of the acute inflammatory response: *pair 1,* untouched control rats; *pair 2,* rats exposed daily for 14 days to aerosolized fluticasone propionate *(FP); pair 3,* rats injected daily with dexamethasone. *Moraxella catarrhalis* exposed > control rats: *$p < 0.05$, **$p < 0.01$, ***$p < 0.001$; *NS,* not significant. The DC response in fluticasone-propionate-treated and dexamethasone-treated rats was less than that of control rats ($p < 0.01$). (From Nelson D, McWilliam AS, Haining S, Holt PG. Downmodulation of airway intraepithelial dendritic cell populations following local and system exposure to steroids. *Am J Respir Crit Care Med* 1995;151:475–481, with permission.)

steroid treatment prevents the recruitment of DCs during acute inflammation (Fig. 7). The site of action of steroids in this system appears to be at the level of inhibition of the influx of bloodborne DC precursors (Fig. 8), possibly via abrogation of local generation of chemokines and/or prevention of expression of cell trafficking-associated integrins on local vascular endothelial cells.

More recent studies (37) have examined the effects of *in vitro* exposure of lung DCs to dexamethasone, during culture in GM-CSF-containing medium. Levels of dexamethasone as high as 10^{-6} M are completely ineffective in prevention of GM-CSF-mediated upregulation of the APC functions of DCs. These steroid levels are considerably higher than those achievable *in vivo*, which casts doubt on their potential efficacy as therapeutic agents in this context.

It is of interest to note that local production of high levels of GM-CSF within the airway epithelium is a hallmark of atopic asthma (38); it has not been formally established that this actually leads to local DC "activation," but this must be considered at least a likely possibility,

and, if so, anti-inflammatory drugs other than steroids would appear to be required to modulate the process.

DENDRITIC CELLS AND PRIMARY ALLERGIC SENSITIZATION TO AIRBORNE ENVIRONMENTAL ANTIGENS

As noted above, DCs are specialized for the presentation of immunogenic signals to naive T cells and are considerably more potent in this regard than any other APC type that has been identified. Importantly, they are the only cell type normally resident at the interface of the airway epithelium and the outside environment, which expresses constitutive APC function, and it is hence axiomatic that they must play an important role in "priming" the immune system for responses to inhaled allergens.

It is now evident from the human seroepidemiologic literature (which I have reviewed [39]) that initial antibody responses to these allergens are most commonly initiated during the early postnatal period, and these findings are borne out by recent evidence of inhalant allergen-specific T-cell reactivity in infants (40).

No formal data are yet available on the status of respiratory tract DC populations in humans in the perinatal period, but recent studies on the ontogeny of these populations in rodents provide potentially important pointers for future work with corresponding human tissues. In rats, seeding of DC precursors into airway tissue commences during late fetal life, such that, by birth, the airway DC network is approximately one-third the density of that in adults (21). However, the neonatal DCs express only very low levels of class II MHC, the principal surface molecule involved in presentation of processed peptide to T cells (Fig. 9). During the early postnatal period, the density of airway DCs increases (Fig. 9A), and mean levels of class II MHC expression by individual DCs also progressively increase (Fig. 9B), until the network approximates the typical adult pattern by shortly after weaning (21). This maturation process proceeds most rapidly in the epithelium lining the nasal turbinates, suggesting that it is driven by inflammatory stimuli in inspired air (21). The APC activity of DCs isolated from neonatal lung and airway tissues is additionally relatively refractory to GM-CSF stimulation, and moreover their capacity for recruitment during acute inflammation is markedly attenuated relative to adults, suggesting overall low functional capacity (41).

During this period of early life, the T-cell system commences its "education" for subsequent responses to all manner of airborne antigens, including allergens. It is clear that this education process requires the development of appropriate nonpathogenic T-cell immunity to allergens, culminating in the nonatopic adult, in the expression of apparently stable TH1-like allergen-specific immunity (39). This involves a complex cognate immu-

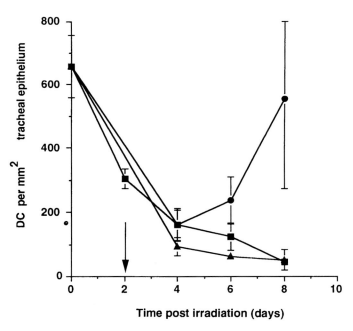

FIG. 8. Kinetics of epithelial dendritic cell (DC) repopulation following irradiation and fluticasone-propionate treatment. Rats in groups of three to six were exposed to lethal irradiation and immune-associated antigen (Ia+) epithelial DCs were quantitated following either no treatment *(solid squares)*, injection with donor bone marrow *(solid circles)*, or injection of bone marrow plus exposure to a daily aerosol of fluticasone-propionate *(solid triangles)*. Steroid treatment was started 2 days after irradiation *(arrow)*. Data are mean ± SD. (From Nelson D, McWilliam AS, Haining S, Holt PG. Downmodulation of airway intraepithelial dendritic cell populations following local and system exposure to steroids. *Am J Respir Crit Care Med* 1995;151:475–481, with permission.)

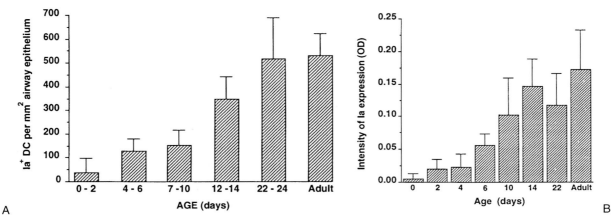

FIG. 9. Postnatal development of the airway epithelial dendritic cell (DC) network in rats. **A:** Postnatal development of the airway intraepithelial DC network. Data shown are mean ± SD derived from five to seven rats in each age group; at least 200 cells were counted for each rat. **B:** Immune-associated antigen (Ia) expression on individual airway epithelial DCs in rats. Frozen sections of tracheal epithelium were immunoperoxidase stained with monoclonal antibodies 0 × 6 and the intensity of staining determined on randomly selected DCs; data shown are mean ± SD derived from three litters in each age group and from seven adult rats. (From Nelson DJ, McMenamin C, McWilliam AS, Brenan M, Holt PG. Development of the airway intraepithelial dendritic cell network in the rat from class II MHC (Ia) negative precursors: differential regulation of Ia expression at different levels of the respiratory tract. *J Exp Med* 1994;179:203–212, with permission.)

nologic process of antigen-driven T-cell "selection," in which APCs must by definition play a central role (39). It is conceivable that the kinetics of postnatal maturation of the functional capacity of these respiratory tract DC populations may be a key rate-limiting factor in this process and hence a determinant of allergen-responder phenotype in adulthood.

Studies are in progress in our laboratory to map the normal ontogeny of these populations in humans, as a necessary prelude to more detailed investigations in atopic infants.

REFERENCES

1. Steinman RM. The dendritic cell system and its role in immunogenicity. *Annu Rev Immunol* 1991;9:271–296.
2. Inaba K, Inaba M, Deguchi M, et al. Granulocytes, macrophages, and dendritic cells arise from a common major histocompatibility complex class II-negative progenitor in mouse bone marrow. *Immunology* 1993; 90:3038–3042.
3. Inaba K, Steinman RM, Pack MW, et al. Identification of proliferating dendritic cell precursors in mouse blood. *J Exp Med* 1992;175:1157–1167.
4. Sousa CR, Stahl PD, Austyn JM. Phagocytosis of antigens by Langerhans cells *in vitro*. *J Exp Med* 1993;178:509–519.
5. Inaba K, Inaba M, Naito M, Steinman RM. Dendritic cell progenitors phagocytose particulates, including bacillus Calmette–Guerin organisms, and sensitize mice to mycobacterial antigens *in vivo*. *J Exp Med* 1993;178:479–488.
6. Stossel H, Koch F, Kampgen E, et al. Disappearance of certain acidic organelles (endosomes and Langerhans cell granules) accompanies loss of antigen processing capacity upon culture of epidermal Langerhans cells. *J Exp Med* 1990;172:1471–1482.
7. Larsen CP, Ritchie SC, Pearson TC, Linsley PS, Lowry RP. Functional expression of the costimulatory molecule, B7/BB1, on murine dendritic cell populations. *J Exp Med* 1992;176:1215.
8. Holt PG, Schon-Hegrad MA. Localization of T cells, macrophages and dendritic cells in rat respiratory tract tissue: implications for immune function studies. *Immunology* 1987;62:349–356.
9. Holt PG, Schon-Hegrad MA, Oliver J. MHC class II antigen-bearing dendritic cells in pulmonary tissues of the rat: regulation of antigen presentation activity by endogenous macrophage populations. *J Exp Med* 1988;167:262–274.
10. Holt PG, Schon HM, Phillips MJ, McMenamin PG. Ia-positive dendritic cells form a tightly meshed network within the human airway epithelium. *Clin Exp Allergy* 1989;19:597–601.
11. Holt PG, Schon-Hegrad MA, Oliver J, Holt BJ, McMenamin PG. A contiguous network of dendritic antigen-presenting cells within the respiratory epithelium. *Int Arch Allergy Appl Immunol* 1990;91:155–159.
12. Schon-Hegrad MA, Oliver J, McMenamin PG, Holt PG. Studies on the density, distribution, and surface phenotype of intraepithelial class II major histocompatibility complex antigen (Ia)-bearing dendritic cells (DC) in the conducting airways. *J Exp Med* 1991;173:1345–1356.
13. Holt PG, Oliver J, McMenamin C, Schon-Hegrad MA. Studies on the surface phenotype and functions of dendritic cells in parenchymal lung tissue of the rat. *Immunology* 1992;75:582–587.
14. Kradin RL, McCarthy KM, Xia WJ, Lazarus D, Schneeberger EE. Accessory cells of the lung. I. Interferon-γ increases Ia+ dendritic cells in the lung without augmenting their accessory activities [see comments]. *Am J Respir Cell Mol Biol* 1991;4:210–218.
15. Gong JL, McCarthy KM, Telford J, Tamatani T, Miyasaka M, Schneeberger EE. Intraepithelial airway dendritic cells: a distinct subset of pulmonary dendritic cells obtained by microdissection. *J Exp Med* 1992;175:797–807.
16. Nicod LP, El Habre F. Adhesion molecules on human lung dendritic cells and their role for T-cell activation. *Am J Respir Cell Mol Biol* 1992;7:207–213.
17. Pollard AM, Lipscomb MF. Characterization of murine lung dendritic cells: similarities to Langerhans cells and thymic dendritic cells. *J Exp Med* 1990;172:159–167.
18. Sertl K, Takemura T, Tschachler E, Ferrans VJ, Kaliner MA, Shevach EM. Dendritic cells with antigen-presenting capability reside in airway epithelium, lung parenchyma, and visceral pleura. *J Exp Med* 1986; 163:436–451.
19. Soler P, Moreau A, Basset F, Hance AJ. Cigarette smoking-induced changes in the number and differentiated state of pulmonary dendritic cells/Langerhans cells. *Am Rev Respir Dis* 1989;139:1112–1117.

20. Hanau D, Fabre M, Lepoittevin JP, Stampf JL, Grosshans E, Benezra C. Formation of Langerhans granules seems linked to membrane AT-Pase activity of epidermal Langerhans cells. *C R Acad Sci III* 1985; 301:167–172.

21. Nelson DJ, McMenamin C, McWilliam AS, Brenan M, Holt PG. Development of the airway intraepithelial dendritic cell network in the rat from class II MHC (Ia) negative precursors: differential regulation of Ia expression at different levels of the respiratory tract. *J Exp Med* 1994;179:203–212.

22. van Haarst JMW, Hoogsteden HC, de Wit HJ, Verhoeven GT, Havenith CEG, Drexhage HA. Dendritic cells and their precursors isolated from human bronchoalveolar lavage: immunocytologic and functional properties. *Am J Respir Cell Mol Biol* 1994;11:344–350.

23. Havenith CE, Breedijk AJ, Hoefsmit EC. Effect of bacillus Calmette–Guerin inoculation on numbers of dendritic cells in bronchoalveolar lavages of rats. *Immunobiology* 1992;184:336–347.

24. Casolaro MA, Bernaudin JF, Saltini C, Ferrans VJ, Crystal RG. Accumulation of Langerhans' cells on the epithelial surface of the lower respiratory tract in normal subjects in association with cigarette smoking. *Am Rev Respir Dis* 1988;137:406–411.

25. Holt PG, Haining S, Nelson DJ, Sedgwick JD. Origin and steady-state turnover of class II MHC-bearing dendritic cells in the epithelium of the conducting airways. *J Immunol* 1994;153:256–261.

26. Fossum S. The life history of dendritic leukocytes. In: Iversen OH, ed. *The cell kinetics of the inflammatory reaction.* Berlin: Springer-Verlag, 1989;101–124.

27. McWilliam AS, Nelson D, Thomas JA, Holt PG. Rapid dendritic cell recruitment is a hallmark of the acute inflammatory response at mucosal surfaces. *J Exp Med* 1994;179:1331–1336.

28. MacPherson GG, Fossum S, Harrison B. Properties of lymph-borne (veiled) dendritic cells in culture. II. Expression of the IL-2 receptor: role of GM-CSF. *Immunology* 1989;68:108–113.

29. Fokkens WJ, Vroom TM, Rijntjes E, Mulder PG. Fluctuation of the number of CD1(T6)-positive dendritic cells, presumably Langerhans cells, in the nasal mucosa of patients with an isolated grass-pollen allergy before, during, and after the grass-pollen season. *J Allergy Clin Immunol* 1989;84:39–43.

30. Bellini A, Vittori E, Marini M, Ackerman V, Mattoli S. Intraepithelial dendritic cells and selective activation of TH2-like lymphocytes in patients with atopic asthma. *Chest* 1993;103:997–1005.

31. Tazi A, Bouchonnet F, Grandsaigne M, Boumsell L, Hance AJ, Soler P. Evidence that GM-CSF regulates the distribution and differentiated state of dendritic cells/Langerhans cells in human lung and lung cancers. *J Clin Invest* 1993;91:566–576.

32. Koch F, Heufler C, Kampgen E, Schneeweiss D, Bock G, Schuler G. Tumor necrosis factor alpha maintains the viability of murine epidermal Langerhans cells in culture, but in contrast to granulocyte-macrophage colony-stimulating factor, without inducing their functional maturation. *J Exp Med* 1990;171:159–171.

33. Heufler C, Koch F, Schuler G. Granulocyte-macrophage colony-stimulating factor and interleukin-1 mediate the maturation of murine epidermal Langerhans cells into potent immunostimulatory dendritic cells. *J Exp Med* 1988;167:700–705.

34. Sallusto F, Lanzavecchia A. Efficient presentation of soluble antigen by cultured human dendritic cells is maintained by GM-CSF plus IL-4 and downregulated by TNF-α. *J Exp Med* 1994;179:1109–1118.

35. Holt PG, Oliver J, Bilyk N, et al. Downregulation of the antigen presenting cell function(s) of pulmonary dendritic cells *in vivo* by resident alveolar macrophages. *J Exp Med* 1993;177:397–407.

36. Nelson D, McWilliam AS, Haining S, Holt PG. Downmodulation of airway intraepithelial dentritic cell populations following local and system exposure to steroids. *Am J Respir Crit Care Med* 1995;151: 475–481.

37. Holt PG, Thomas J, Nelson DS, McWilliam A. Steroids modulate dendritic cell recruitment into the airway mucosa, but do not affect GM-CSF-mediated upregulation of antigen presentation function(s). (*Submitted*).

38. Poston RN, Chanez P, Lacoste JY, Litchfield T, Lee TH, Bousquet J. Immunohistochemical characterisation of the cellular infiltration in asthmatic bronchi. *Am Rev Respir Dis* 1992;145:918–921.

39. Holt PG. Immunoprophylaxis of atopy: light at the end of the tunnel? *Immunol Today* 1994;15:484–489.

40. Holt PG, O'Keefe PO, Holt BJ, et al. T-cell "priming" against environmental allergens in human neonates: sequential deletion of good antigen specificities during infancy with concomitant expansion of responses to ubiquitous inhalant allergens. *Pediatr Allergy Immunol* 1995;6:1–5.

41. Nelson DJ, Thomas JA, Holt PG. Defective regional immunity in the respiratory tract of neonates is attributable to hyporesponsiveness of local dendritic cells to activation signals. *J Immunol* 1995;155:3517–3524.

Asthma, edited by P.J. Barnes, M.M. Grunstein, A.R. Leff, and A.J. Woolcock.
Lippincott–Raven Publishers, Philadelphia © 1997.

▪ 34 ▪

Platelets

Clive P. Page

Platelet-Derived Mediators
Platelet Membrane Proteins
Platelet Activation
Platelets and Allergic Asthma

Experimental evidence for platelet activation in
   allergic responses
Clinical evidence
Therapeutic Perspectives

The platelet has been traditionally associated with disorders of the cardiovascular system, a well-recognized cell type actively involved in the maintenance of hemostasis and the initiation of repair after tissue injury. However, increasing evidence now suggests an important role for platelets in allergic inflammation and asthma (1–3).

Platelets possess many of the features of classic inflammatory cells such as polymorphonuclear leukocytes (PMNs). They are capable of undergoing chemotaxis (4, 5), have been shown to phagocytose foreign particles (6); contain and release various adhesive proteins; activate complement; interact with parasites, viruses, and bacteria; alter vascular tone; and enhance vascular permeability (7,8). Furthermore, platelets synthesize, store, take up, and release a variety of inflammatory mediators (3).

PLATELET-DERIVED MEDIATORS

Platelets are a rich source of a wide range of biologically active substances that, when released from the cell following activation, are capable of inducing or augmenting inflammatory responses. Platelet-dense granules contain ADP and ATP, 5-hydroxytryptamine (5-HT or serotonin), and Ca^{2+}, and the more numerous α-granules store mediators synthesized by the megakaryocyte or taken up from the circulation. α-Granules also contain a variety of proteins, some platelet specific, which include adhesive

proteins, the antiheparinoid platelet factor 4 (PF4), platelet-derived growth factor (PDGF), β-thromboglobulin (β-TG), and transforming growth factor-β (TGF-β).

5-HT, stored in large amounts in human platelets, may contribute to the inflammatory response via its vasoconstrictor properties and ability to increase vascular permeability. Human platelets synthesize, take up, and release histamine (9–11), a potent inflammatory mediator capable of inducing bronchoconstriction, vasodilatation, edema caused by leakage of plasma proteins from post-capillary venules, stimulation of bronchoconstrictor reflexes, and mucus secretion. In addition, human platelets activated with thrombin, collagen, and platelet activating factor (PAF) have been shown to liberate a substance that stimulated the release of histamine from mast cells and basophils, platelet-derived histamine-releasing factor (PDHRF) (12,13). PDHRF has also been shown to be chemotactic toward eosinophils and to induce early- and late-onset airway obstruction and airway hyperresponsiveness in experimental animals (14). Adenosine, which can be formed from the nucleotides stored and released by platelets, may play a role in bronchoconstriction (15), and receptors for adenosine have been shown to be upregulated in allergic rabbits compared with normal rabbits (16).

Platelets contain cationic proteins that can increase vascular permeability (17) in addition to a cationic protein that cleaves the fifth component of complement to form a factor that is chemotactic for leukocytes (18). The platelet-specific protein PF4 possesses many properties that suggest a key role in allergy and inflammation. It has been shown to increase the expression of Fc-immunoglobulin (Ig) G and Fc-IgE receptors (19) and to stimulate

C. P. Page: Sackler Institute of Pulmonary Pharmacology, King's College, University of London, London SW3 6LX United Kingdom.

the release of histamine from basophils (20). PF4 is not only chemotactic for PMNs, monocytes, and fibroblasts (21), but also for eosinophils (19). The ability of PF4 to activate eosinophils is of particular interest as it has been suggested that these cells contribute to the tissue damage observed in asthma that may be associated with airway hyperresponsiveness (22). Furthermore, PF4 has been shown to increase airway responsiveness in rats (23).

PDGF may act as a mediator of inflammation and repair by affecting vascular tone (24), exerting chemotactic effects toward monocytes and neutrophils, and by activating monocytes (25) and neutrophils (26). Smooth muscle cells and fibroblasts are strongly attracted to PDGF, suggesting that these cells may migrate to injured sites where subsequent mitogenic stimulation contributes to repair processes (26). Similarly, TGF-β has been shown to be chemotactic for neutrophils and fibroblasts (26). Bronchial smooth muscle hypertrophy and hyperplasia are characteristic of the asthmatic lung at autopsy (27,28), and it is possible that continuous platelet activation, recruitment, and extravascular diapedesis into the airways with consequent release of mitogens, could contribute to this feature of asthma. The role of platelet activation in the induction of myofibroblast proliferation and bronchial smooth muscle thickening remains to be elucidated, although PDGF (29) and TGF-β (30) have both been reported to act as mitogens for airway smooth muscle cells in culture.

Platelet activation also leads to the generation of the cytokine RANTES (31) which is chemoattractant for eosinophils (31) and monocytes and T lymphocytes (32). Following platelet stimulation and activation, products of the metabolism of membrane arachidonic acid (AA) are synthesized via the enzymes cyclooxygenase and lipoxygenase, many of which may contribute to the allergic response. Thromboxane A$_2$ (TXA$_2$) and prostaglandin F$_{2\alpha}$ (PGF$_{2\alpha}$) are potent vasoconstrictors and bronchial smooth muscle spasmogens, whereas PGE$_2$ is a vasodilator and inducer/modulator of pain and fever. It has been suggested that PGF$_{2\alpha}$ may cause heightened reflex bronchoconstriction by sensitizing nerve endings in the airway and platelet-derived 12-HETE has been shown to exert chemotactic activity toward eosinophils (33).

Platelets and PMNs have been shown to cooperate in processing AA or AA-derived intermediate metabolites into novel biologically active substances (34). In the presence of activated platelets, leukocytes can produce increased amounts of leukotrienes due to the ability of platelet 12-HPETE to stimulate leukocyte 5-lipoxygenase (35). Neutrophils can utilize AA from stimulated platelets for the synthesis of 5-HETE and leukotriene B$_4$ (LTB$_4$) (36,37), a mediator with a broad proinflammatory profile (38,39).

Human PMNs stimulated *in vitro* by several specific agonists are able to activate coincubated platelets, inducing aggregation, cytoplasmic Ca^{2+} increase and TXA$_2$

production (40). The major platelet activator released by PMNs in this system appears to be cathepsin G, a neutral serine protease released from azurophilic granules of activated PMNs (41). TXB$_2$ production, however, is the result of transcellular metabolism of AA between activated PMNs and cathepsin G-stimulated platelets, where platelets use PMN-derived unmetabolized AA to synthesize TXB$_2$ (42). Cathepsin G released from activated PMNs induces expression of P-selectin on platelet membranes that modulates cell–cell contact and transcellular metabolism of AA (43).

Both neutrophils and platelets can liberate PAF from membrane phospholipids in modest amounts in response to activation stimuli (44,45). The presence, however, of a small number of platelets in a suspension of neutrophils results in the generation of significantly increased amounts of PAF, far in excess of that predicted from the individual cell types (46). PAF is an extremely potent inflammatory agent and has been implicated as a mediator of inflammation and asthma (47).

PLATELET MEMBRANE PROTEINS

Platelet surface glycoproteins play a primary role in the adhesion of platelets to exposed subendothelial matrix proteins, interaction with ligands such as collagen and thrombin, and exposure of fibrinogen receptors to facilitate aggregation (48). Several glycoproteins of the integrin superfamily of adhesion receptors are present on the plasma membrane (49). Platelets (and endothelial cells) express an adhesion protein of the selectin family (P-selectin, GMP-140, PADGEM, and CD62) following degranulation that permits the interaction of platelets with leukocytes (8,49). It is of interest that recently platelets have been observed to undergo rolling analogous to that seen with neutrophils, that is, dependent on P-selectin (50).

The transmembrane-4 superfamily (TM4SF) of membrane proteins, to date, comprises 15 members that are variously expressed on leukocytes and a variety of other mammalian tissues (51). The precise biochemical function of the TM4SF is not yet clear, but a role in the regulation of cell development, proliferation, activation, and motility is suggested from the available data (51). Expression of CD9 antigen has been described on platelets, and functional data suggest a role in signal transduction and cell adhesion. CD63 is expressed on activated platelets and on lysosomal and dense granule membranes in resting platelets. A role of this molecule in cell adhesion of platelets and endothelial cells has been suggested, and recent experiments provide evidence that there is differential expression of the platelet adhesion molecules CD62P and CD63 in patients with aspirin-sensitive asthma (51).

Platelets possess a glycoprotein receptor for the third component of complement (C3b), which resembles that located on mononuclear cells (52), and Fc receptors for both IgG and IgE antibodies (53,54). Human platelets can bind IgE *in vitro*, and cross-linking of surface-bound IgE with anti-IgE or the specific antigens induces platelet activation and secretion. A specific receptor for the Fc fragment of IgE, the Fc epsilon-receptor type II (Fc$_\epsilon$RII), has been demonstrated on the platelet membrane, which is of low affinity (10^{-7} M) compared with that found on mast cell or basophil surfaces (Fc$_\epsilon$RI) (10^{-9} M) (54), but of comparable affinity to the IgE receptor located on other inflammatory cell types such as alveolar macrophages and eosinophils (55). Only a small number (20–30%) of platelets from normal individuals bind IgE, but more than 50% of the platelets from patients with aspirin-induced asthma, allergic patients, and patients with parasitic diseases bind IgE (54–56).

The physiologic relevance of the platelet IgE receptor may be associated with a mechanism for aiding the removal of parasitic infections, as the passive transfer of platelets bearing IgE receptors toward schistosomes to naive rats can protect these animals from parasitic challenge (56). The platelet IgE receptor appears not to be associated in any way with the formation of aggregates, but with the ability of platelets to mount a reaginic antibody-dependent cytotoxic response against helminth parasites, such as *Schistosoma mansoni*, through oxidative killing (57,58).

PLATELET ACTIVATION

A distinction may exist between the mechanism of platelet activation resulting in the generation of free radicals and that resulting in degranulation (58). Platelets that release free radicals do not aggregate, and platelet aggregation itself will inhibit any subsequent free-radical release (58). This type of activation can be elicited by a range of stimuli thought to be involved in the inflammatory response, including C-reactive protein (57), substance P (59), the complement-derived peptides C3b and C5b–C9, the eosinophil-specific major basic protein (60), and the cytokines, interferon-γ (61) and tumor necrosis factor-α (62). Antiallergic compounds such as disodium cromoglycate (63) and nedocromil sodium (64) inhibit IgE-dependent release of free radicals from platelets, yet these drugs are ineffective against classic platelet aggregation (65). Furthermore, the therapeutic efficacy of certain antiparasite drugs such as diethylcarbamazine may to some extent be related to their ability to generate free radicals from platelets (66).

It has been shown that a suppressive lymphokine released by activated mononuclear cells can inhibit the production of cytotoxic free radicals by IgE-coated platelets (67). This lymphokine has been termed *platelet activity suppressive lymphokine*, a heat-stable molecule of molecular weight 15,000 to 20,000 and a product of a T-lymphocyte subpopulation bearing the CD8+ antigen (67). Furthermore, CD4+/CD8– lymphocytes have been observed to release factors, including interferon-γ, which can induce cytotoxic activity in normal platelets (61).

PLATELETS AND ALLERGIC ASTHMA

Asthma is characterized clinically by hyperresponsiveness of airway smooth muscle to various spasmogens, resulting in the widespread narrowing of the airways. In recent years, it has been recognized that asthma is a chronic inflammatory disease associated pathologically by eosinophil infiltration and damaged airway epithelium (68). These underlying inflammatory events are considered important in the development of the enhanced airway responsiveness observed in asthmatic individuals. Airway inflammation is complex, triggered by inflammatory stimuli interacting with primary effector cells resident in the airway, of which numerous cell types have been implicated. Release of inflammatory mediators from these cells may recruit and activate other effector cells, thus augmenting the inflammatory process. Evidence now exists in support of a role of platelets in the pathogenesis of asthma, acting as inflammatory cells.

Experimental Evidence for Platelet Activation in Allergic Responses

Platelets have been observed to undergo diapedesis into the extravascular tissue of the lungs of guinea pigs following challenge with antigen or PAF (69). The extravasated platelets have been observed in close proximity to bronchial smooth muscle and to infiltrating eosinophils, suggesting a possible link between the two cell types. Treatment of experimental guinea pigs with other platelet agonists such as ADP, although inducing platelet aggregation in the pulmonary vasculature, does not elicit extravascular diapedesis of platelets and eosinophils (69). Platelets have also been detected in bronchoalveolar lavage (BAL) fluid obtained from rabbits undergoing late-onset airway obstruction following antigen challenge (70), and markers of platelet activation, such as PF4, have been shown to be elevated in plasma following antigen challenge of allergic rabbits (71).

In several animal species, the intravenous injection of selected platelet agonists induces thrombocytopenia associated with bronchospasm (72), a phenomenon that also occurs in sensitized animals challenged with specific antigen (73,74). Similarly, the intravenous administration of PAF or allergen into guinea pigs induces bronchospasm associated with the accumulation of platelets in the lung (75), with the bronchospasm being platelet-dependent since platelet depletion abolishes the response (76). Under these circumstances platelet aggregates have been located histologically (73,77) and by the use of radiolabeled platelets (75) within the lung vasculature. Furthermore, several classes of drugs, including the anti-asthma drugs ketotifen and theophylline, inhibit the platelet-release reaction *in vitro* and platelet-dependent bronchospasm *in vivo* (78,79), but do not affect platelet accumulation within the lung (78), suggesting that the bronchospasm is unlikely to be due to the mere presence of aggregates in lung vasculature. These observations indicate that platelet-derived mediators contribute to the bronchospasm as well as, or instead of, physical obstruction of lung vasculature by platelet aggregates. The dissociation of platelet release and aggregation *in vivo* led to the hypothesis that platelet activation plays a central role in the pathogenesis of asthma (80). Furthermore, the pharmacologic inhibition of the platelet-release reaction (79,81) or TXA_2 production (81) can abrogate the bronchospasm, suggesting the response is related to the release of bronchoactive agents from platelets rather than the retention of platelet aggregates per se. It is of interest therefore that PAF only contracted isolated human bronchus when platelets were present (82).

The late-onset response to antigen challenge in allergic rabbits can be abrogated by prior treatment with a selective antiplatelet antiserum (83). This phenomenon may be attributable to an interaction between platelets and eosinophils, as the antigen-induced pulmonary eosinophil infiltration is also inhibited in thrombocytopenic animals (83). In guinea pigs and rabbits, PAF-induced airway hyperresponsiveness is platelet dependent since it can be abrogated by rendering animals selectively thrombocytopenic by the intravenous administration of a specific lytic antiplatelet antiserum (84,85). Activation of platelets by PAF differs from activation by other agonists, since ADP, collagen, thrombin, or the TXA_2 mimetic U46619, in amounts sufficient to cause comparable pul-

monary platelet retention *in vivo*, did not induce airway hyperresponsiveness (86–88). Therefore, as with the bronchoconstrictor response, the pulmonary retention of platelets is not central for the induction of airway hyperresponsiveness.

PAF injected into thrombocytopenic guinea pigs does not induce an acute bronchoconstrictor response or enhanced airway responsiveness. In platelet-depleted guinea pigs, however, the supernatant obtained from normal guinea-pig platelet-rich plasma (PRP) incubated with PAF induced airway hyperresponsiveness (87). A factor released from platelets has been reported to induce airway hyperresponsiveness (platelet-derived hyperreactivity factor [PDHF] [87]). The generation of PDHF was inhibited by prior incubation of PRP with the stable prostacyclin mimetic iloprost. The secretion or formation of this mediator of hyperresponsiveness appears to be PAF specific, as neither platelet disruption nor activation of platelets with ADP induced its production. The chemical nature of this material remains as yet unidentified. Ketotifen and prednisolone have been shown to inhibit the airway hyperresponsiveness induced by PAF-stimulated platelet supernatants, whereas cromoglycate and aminophylline were without effect (89). Similarly, when ketotifen or prednisolone were incubated with PRP prior to the addition of PAF, the injection of supernatants into thrombocytopenic guinea pigs resulted in reduced airway hyperresponsiveness (89). In addition, a human PDHRF has been shown to induce airway hyperresponsiveness as well as selective pulmonary eosinophil infiltration in allergic rabbits (14,90).

Eosinophils and their products such as major basic protein have been implicated in the pathogenesis of asthma (22). It is of interest therefore that platelet depletion has been shown to reduce PAF and antigen-induced

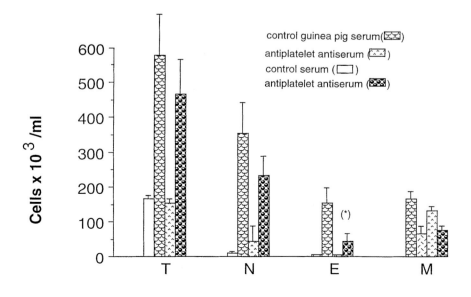

FIG. 1. The effect of administration of control guinea-pig serum or antiplatelet antiserum on allergen-induced total leukocytes *(T)*, neutrophils *(N)*, eosinophils *(E)*, and mononuclear cells *(M)* 24 h after allergen challenge. Cell numbers prior to allergen challenge in animals receiving control serum or antiplatelet antiserum are shown for comparison. Results are shown as the mean ± SEM of seven rabbits and are expressed as the number of cells × 103/ml. The *asterisk* indicates *p* < 0.03, determined by a Mann–Whitney sum-rank test. (From Coyle AJ, Page CP, Atkinson L, Flanagan R, Metzger WJ. The requirement for platelets in allergen-induced late asthmatic airway obstruction. *Am Rev Respir Dis* 1990;142:587–593, with permission.)

eosinophil infiltration into the lungs of experimental animals (83,84,91) (Fig. 1), suggesting a central role for platelets in this response. The mechanism by which platelets attract eosinophils into the lung may be via the release of PF4 (19) or RANTES (31), which are both platelet-derived eosinophil chemoattractants (Fig. 2). Both platelet depletion and treatment with the PAF antagonist BN 52021 have been shown to inhibit antigen-induced late-onset airway obstruction, airway hyperresponsiveness, and eosinophil infiltration in experimental animals (91–95). These findings suggest that antigen-induced release of PAF may play a role in the platelet activation necessary to initiate the eosinophil infiltration into the airways which, in turn, contributes to airway hyperresponsiveness.

Thrombin activation, suggested by the presence of fibrinopeptide A, has been described in early- and late-phase allergic responses (70) and may therefore contribute to

the activation of platelets during allergen-induced responses. Further evidence in favor of the platelet as an important effector cell in the lung has been provided by *in vitro* studies where platelets potentiate mucous glycoprotein release from tracheal submucosal glands induced by PAF (96).

Clinical Evidence

A number of clinical studies have demonstrated platelet activation in asthma, although this disease is not normally associated with thrombosis. Platelets from asthmatics have been shown to behave abnormally *in vitro*, lacking the second wave of aggregation (97–100) or defective release of platelet 5-HT, PF4 (97), and platelet nucleotides (100) following stimulation with platelet agonists. These *in vitro* abnormalities are suggestive of overstimulation *in vivo* (101).

In asthmatic patients, the uptake of 5-HT by platelets has been shown to be reduced, possibly due to exposure of the cells to an increased concentration of this amine (102). Increased plasma levels of 5-HT have been reported in asthmatics (103), as well as elevated resting levels of platelet cytoplasmic Ca^{2+} and inositol-triphosphate production (104), findings suggestive of *in vivo* platelet stimulation.

Thrombocytopenia was first reported to accompany asthmatic attacks in 1955 (105) and has been subsequently been confirmed by others (106,107). Platelet activation *in vivo* during provoked or spontaneous asthmatic attacks has also been shown by the detection of circulating platelet aggregates (108,109) and activated platelets in the circulation (110). A number of studies have demonstrated elevated plasma levels of PF4 and β-TG associated with bronchoconstriction induced by antigen or exercise (108,109,111–114). Release of these platelet-derived markers was not observed following comparable bronchoconstriction induced by methacholine, suggesting that platelet activation occurs as a consequence of the allergic reaction rather than of the bronchoconstriction.

Evidence of platelet activation has also been reported during exacerbations of nocturnal asthma (115,116) (Fig. 3). In another study, increased levels of PF4 and β-TG have been demonstrated in BAL fluid after antigen challenge in asthmatic patients (117), although no evidence of platelet activation was observed in another study (107). Platelet markers were significantly elevated during the late inflammatory response to antigen and were significantly correlated with elevations in albumin, eosinophil granule proteins, and inflammatory prostanoids (PGE_2 and $PGF_{2\alpha}$). A study investigating the possible involvement of platelets under three different conditions (chronic asthma, following allergen challenge with house dust mite, and during *status asthmaticus*) suggested that platelet activation is sometimes provoked in asthma, but

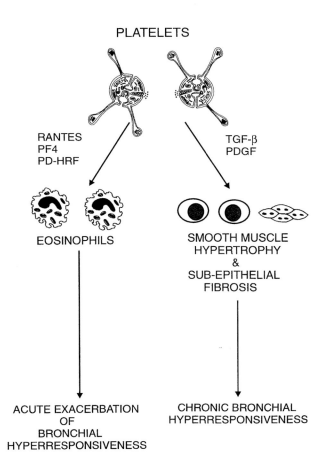

PLATELETS

RANTES
PF4
PD-HRF

TGF-β
PDGF

EOSINOPHILS

SMOOTH MUSCLE
HYPERTROPHY
&
SUB-EPITHELIAL
FIBROSIS

ACUTE EXACERBATION
OF
BRONCHIAL
HYPERRESPONSIVENESS

CHRONIC BRONCHIAL
HYPERRESPONSIVENESS

FIG. 2. Schematic representation of the relationship between platelet activation and the induction of acute exacerbations of bronchial hyperresponsiveness via recruitment of eosinophils, as well as the possible contribution of platelet-derived growth factors to structural changes in the airways and chronic bronchial hyperresponsiveness. *PD-HRF,* platelet-derived histamine-releasing factor; *PF4,* platelet factor 4; *TGF-β,* transforming growth factor-β.

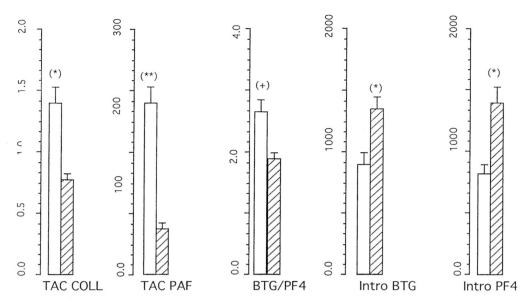

FIG. 3. The individual and overall mean difference in the threshold aggregation concentration of collagen *(TAC COLL)* required to activate platelets from normal subjects (slashed columns) and asthmatic patients (empty columns) is depicted, as well as the ratio of plasma β-thromboglobulin to platelet factor 4 *(B-TG/PF4)*, intraplatelet β-TG *(Intro BTG)*, or intraplatelet PF4 *(Intro PF4)* in normal subjects or asthmatic patients. The results are expressed as the mean ± SEM. $p < 0.01$; **$p < 0.03$, *$p < 0.04$, + < 0.07. (From Gresele P, Dottorini M, Selli ML, et al. Altered platelet function associated with the bronchial hyperresponsiveness accompanying nocturnal asthma. *J Allergy Clin Immunol* 1993;91:894–902, with permission.)

plasma levels of α-derived proteins did not reflect the intensity or severity of asthma (118). The authors of this study suggested that PAF is the likely mediator responsible for the platelet activation (118). Both urinary and plasma TXB_2 (stable metabolite of TXA_2) have been shown to be elevated following allergen challenge in allergic asthmatics (119,120).

Evidence of platelet activation has not been consistently observed (121–125). In other studies, pulmonary platelet sequestration was not found to follow antigen challenge in asthmatic volunteers (125,126). However, numerous other clinical observations support the proposed role of platelets in asthma. In lung tissue removed at autopsy from patients dying of *status asthmaticus*, abnormal megakaryocytes have been observed in abundance (127,128), suggestive of a potential abnormality in this system. Platelet survival time in atopic asthmatics is severely shortened (129), a finding suggestive of continuous cell activation (130). Shortened platelet regeneration time, an index of *in vivo* platelet activation associated with accelerated platelet consumption (that is, increased platelet turnover) (109), has been reported in asthmatics undergoing acute asthma attacks (109), and increased bleeding time has been observed in a group of atopic asthmatics (131). In addition, altered responsiveness of platelets from allergic patients has been observed by numerous investigators (reviewed by Gresele et al.

[109]), the incidence of which was greatest in patients presenting with high serum IgE titers (56). Furthermore, platelet size (132), platelet count, and platelet mass (131) have been found to be increased in asthmatics.

Accumulated platelets have been observed in lung microvasculature of patients undergoing bronchial provocation with allergen (68) and have also been detected by electron microscopy in BAL fluid obtained from asthmatics undergoing late-onset airway obstruction following antigen provocation (70). In addition, platelets have been observed undergoing diapedesis in sections biopsied from asthmatics (133), and platelets have been observed at sites of denuded epithelium in bronchial biopsy specimens from symptomatic asthmatics along with fibrinous material (134). Furthermore, platelets from asthmatic patients have been shown to migrate *in vitro* in response to antigen, possibly by interaction with platelet-bound antigen-specific IgE (5).

THERAPEUTIC PERSPECTIVES

The PAF antagonist BN 52063 has been shown to inhibit the platelet activation accompanying exercise-induced bronchoconstriction in asthmatic patients (135) (Fig. 4). These results suggest that the release of PAF may be central to the platelet activation accompanying exer-

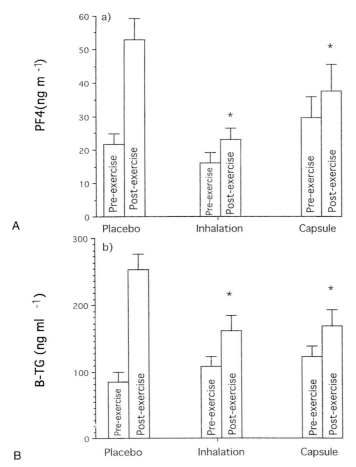

FIG. 4. Effects of the platelet-activating factor antagonist BN52063 on the plasma concentrations of platelet factor 4 *(PF4)* (**A**) and β-thromboglobulin *(B-TG)* (**B**) before and 5 min after the exercise challenge. (From Wilkens JH, Wilkens H, Uffman J, Bovers J, Fabel H, Froelich JC. Effects of a PAF antagonist (BN52063) on bronchoconstriction and platelet activation during exercise induced asthma. *Br J Clin Pharmacol* 1990;29:85–91, with permission.)

oratory, thrombocytopenia was evident 24 h following antigen challenge. However, after 6 weeks of treatment with low-dose theophylline, this thrombocytopenia induced by allergen was almost abolished (107). Therefore, part of the therapeutic efficacy of these drugs may reside in their ability to restore normal platelet behavior.

There is overwhelming evidence that platelets are involved and play an active role in primary defense mechanisms such as antibody-dependent cytotoxicity of parasites. Inappropriate activation of this system in allergic asthmatic patients may contribute to the eosinophil infiltration and subsequent damage to the host tissue, contributing to the heightened airway responsiveness characteristic of bronchial asthma. The recent awareness that platelets are capable of behaving like, and interacting with, other inflammatory cells opens up whole new areas of potential ways to influence the allergic inflammatory response and suggests that we should indeed consider platelets as playing a role in the pathogenesis of bronchial asthma.

REFERENCES

1. Capron A, Joseph M, Ameisen J-C, Capron M, Pancre V, Auriault C. Platelets as effectors in immune and hypersensitivity reactions. *Int Arch Allergy Appl Immunol* 1987;82:307–312.
2. Gresele P. The platelet in asthma. In: Page CP, ed. *The platelet in health and disease.* Oxford: Blackwell Scientific, 1991;132–157.
3. Herd CM, Page CP. Do platelets have a role as inflammatory cells? In: Joseph M, ed. *The immunopharmacology of platelets.* New York: Academic, 1995;1–20.
4. Lowenhaupt RW. Human platelet chemotaxis can be induced by low molecular substance(s) derived from the interaction of plasma and collagen. In: Jamieson GA, Scipio AR, eds. *Interaction of platelets and tumour cells.* New York: Alan R Liss, 1982;269–280.
5. Zhang X, Selli ML, Baglioni S, et al. Platelets from asthmatic patients migrate *in vitro* in response to allergen stimulation. *Thromb Haemost* 1993;69:1356.
6. Mustard SJ, Ali S, Metzger WJ. The reaction of the blood to injury. In: Movart HZ, ed. *Inflammation, immunity and hypersensitivity.* New York: Harper and Row, 1991;61.
7. Weksler BB. Platelets. In: Gallin JI, Goldstein IM, Snyderman R, eds. *Inflammation: basic principles and clinical correlates.* New York: Raven, 1983.
8. McGregor JL. The role of human platelet membrane receptors in inflammation. In: Joseph M, ed. *The immunopharmacology of platelets.* New York: Academic, 1995;67–82.
9. Saxena SP, Brandes LJ, Becker AB, Simons KJ, La Bella FS, Gerrard JM. Histamine is an intracellular messenger mediating platelet aggregation. *Science* 1989;243:1596–1599.
10. Mannaioni PF, Pistelli A, Di Bello MG, Gambassi F, Masini E. H1-receptor dependent increase in platelet aggregation is mediated by intracellular calcium. *Agents Actions* 1992;35:C401–C405.
11. Mannaioni PF, Di Bello MG, Raspanti S, Pistelli A, Masini E. Histamine release by human platelets. *Agents Actions* 1993;38:C203–C205.
12. Knauer KA, Kagey-Sobotka A, Adkinson NE, Lichtenstein LM. Platelet augmentation of IgE-dependent histamine release from human basophils and mast cells. *Int Arch Allergy Appl Immunol* 1984;74:29–35.
13. Orchard MA, Kagey-Sobotka A, Proud D, Lichtenstein LM. Basophil histamine release induced by a substance from stimulated human platelets. *J Immunol* 1986;136:2240–2244.
14. Fisher RH, Henriksen RA, Wirfel-Svet KL, Atkinson LB, Metzger WJ. Bronchial challenge with platelet-derived histamine releasing factor (PD-HRF) induces prolonged changes in dynamic compliance

cise-induced bronchoconstriction as has been suggested in nocturnal attacks of asthma (116). Although early studies with the PAF antagonists UK74,505 (136), WEB 2086 (137), and MK-287 (138) have shown no effect on the early or late response to inhaled allergen in mild atopic asthmatics or on the subsequent airway hyperresponsiveness, recent studies with Y24180 (139) and SR27417 (140) have shown activity in asthmatics, raising the possibility that PAF may play a role in allergic asthma.

It is also of interest that treatment of atopic asthmatic individuals with antiasthma drugs such as glucocorticoids and ketotifen has been shown to correct abnormal platelet survival (141). Furthermore, in asthmatic patients, the antiasthma drug nedocromil sodium has been shown to inhibit platelet activation induced by PAF *ex vivo* (64). In a recent study of mild asthmatics in our lab-

(Cdyn) and hyperreactivity in the allergic asthmatic rabbit model. *J Allergy Clin Immunol* 1990;85:261.

15. Holgate ST, Church MK, Polosa R. Adenosine: a positive modulator of airway inflammation in asthma. *Ann NY Acad Sci* 1991;629:227–236.

16. Mustafa SJ, Ali S, Metzger WJ. Adenosine induced bronchoconstriction in allergic rabbits: evidence for receptor involvement. *Jpn J Pharmacol* 1991;52:113.

17. Sasaki M, Paul W, Douglas GJ, Page CP. Cutaneous responses to poly-L-lysine in the rabbit. *Br J Pharmacol* 1991;104:444P.

18. Weksler B, Coupal CE. Platelet dependent generation of chemotactic activity in serum. *J Exp Med* 1973;137:1419–1430.

19. Chihara J, Fukuda K, Yasuba H, et al. Platelet factor 4 enhances eosinophil IgG and IgE Fc receptors and has eosinophil chemotactic activity. *Am Rev Respir Dis* 1988;137:A421(abstr).

20. Brindley LL, Sweet JM, Goetzl EJ. Stimulation of histamine release from human basophils by human platelet factor 4. *J Clin Invest* 1983;72:1218–1223.

21. Deuel TF, Senior RM, Chang D, Griffin GL, Heinrickson RL, Kaiser ET. Platelet factor 4 is chemotactic for neutrophils and monocytes. *Proc Natl Acad Sci USA* 1981;78:4584–4587.

22. Frigas E, Gleich GJ. The eosinophil and the pathophysiology of asthma. *J Allergy Clin Immunol* 1986;77:527–537.

23. Coyle AJ, Ackerman SJ, Irvin CG. Cationic proteins induce airway hyperresponsiveness dependent on charge interactions. *Am Rev Respir Dis* 1993;147:896–900.

24. Berk BC, Alexander RW, Brock TA, Gimbrone MA, Webb RC. Vasoconstriction: a new activity for platelet-derived growth factor. *Science* 1986;232:87–90.

25. Tzeng DY, Deuel TF, Huang JS, Boehner RL. Platelet-derived growth factor promotes human peripheral monocyte activation. *Blood* 1985;66:179–183.

26. Duel TF, Huang JS. Platelet-derived growth factor: structure, function, roles in normal and transformed cells. *J Clin Invest* 1984;74:669–676.

27. Ebina M, Yaegashi H, Chiba R, Takahashi T, Motomiya M, Tanemura M. Hyperreactive site in the airway tree of asthmatic patients revealed by thickening of bronchial muscles. *Am Rev Respir Dis* 1990;141:1327–1332.

28. Carroll N, Elliot J, Morton A, James J. The structure of large and small airways in nonfatal and fatal asthma. *Am Rev Respir Dis* 1993;147:405–410.

29. Hirst SJ, Barnes PJ, Twort CHC. Quantifying proliferation of cultured human and rabbit airway smooth muscle cells in response to serum and platelet-derived growth factor. *Am J Respir Cell Mol Biol* 1992;7:574–581.

30. Kilfeather SA, Okona-Mensha KB, Tagoe S, Costello J, Page CP. Stimulation of airway smooth muscle cell mitogenesis by TGF-beta, inhibition by heparin and smooth muscle explant conditioned media. *Eur Respir J* 1995;8:547S.

31. Kameyoshi Y, Dorschner A, Mallet AI, Christophers E, Schroder JM. Cytokine RANTES released by thrombin-stimulated platelets is a potent attractant for human eosinophils. *J Exp Med* 1992;176:587–592.

32. Schall TJ, Bacon K, Toy KJ, Goeddel DV. Selective attraction of monocytes and T lymphocytes of the memory phenotype by cytokine RANTES. *Nature* 1990;347:669–671.

33. Goetzl EJ, Woods JM, Gorman RR. Stimulation of human eosinophil and neutrophil polymorphonuclear leukocyte chemotaxis and random migration by 12-L-hydroxy-5,8,10,14-eicosatetraenoic acid. *J Clin Invest* 1977;59:179–183.

34. Marcus AJ, Safier LB, Ullman HL, et al. Platelet neutrophil interactions. *J Biol Chem* 1988;263:2223–2229.

35. Maclouf J, Fruteau de Laclos B, Borgeat P. Stimulation of leukotriene biosynthesis in human blood leukocytes by platelet derived 12-hydroperoxy-icosatetraenoic acid. *Proc Natl Acad Sci USA* 1982;79:6042–6046.

36. Marcus AJ, Broekman MJ, Safier LB, et al. Formation of leukotrienes and other hydroxy acids during platelet-neutrophil interactions *in vitro*. *Biochem Biophys Res Commun* 1982;109:130–137.

37. Maclouf JA, Murphy RC. Transcellular metabolism of neutrophil-derived leukotriene A_4 by human platelets: a potential source of leukotriene C_4. *J Biol Chem* 1988;263:174–181.

38. Seeds EAM, Kilfeather S, Okiji S, Shoupe TS, Gale DG, Page CP. Role of lipoxygenase metabolites in PAF and antigen induced bronchial hyperresponsiveness and eosinophil infiltration. *Eur J Pharmacol* 1995;293:369–376.

39. Ford-Hutchinson AW. Leukotriene B_4 in inflammation. *CRC Crit Rev Immunol* 1990;10:1–12.

40. Chignard M, Selak MA, Smith JB. Direct evidence for the existence of a neurophil-derived platelet activator (neurophilin). *Proc Natl Acad Sci USA* 1986;83:8609–8613.

41. Evangelista V, Piccardoni P, de Gaetano G, Cerletti C. Difibrotide inhibits platelet activation by cathepsin G released from stimulated polymorphonuclear leukocytes. *Thromb Haemost* 1992;67:660–664.

42. Maugeri N, Evangelista V, Piccardoni P, et al. Transcellular metabolism of arachidonic acid: increased platelet thromboxane generation in the presence of activated polymorphonuclear leukocytes. *Blood* 1992;80:447–451.

43. Maugeri N, Evangelista V, Celardo A, et al. Polymorphonuclear leukocyte–platelet interaction: role of P-selection in thromboxane B_2 and leukotriene C_4 cooperative synthesis. *Thromb Haemost* 1994;72:450–456.

44. Chignard M, le Couedic JP, Vargaftig BB, Benveniste J. Platelet activating factor (PAF-acether) from platelets: effects of aggregating agents. *Br J Haemotol* 1980;46:455–464.

45. Bratton D, Henson PM. Cellular origins of PAF. In: Barnes PJ, Page CP, Henson PM, eds. *Platelet activating factor and human disease.* Oxford: Blackwell Scientific, 1989;23–57.

46. Coeffier E, Chignard M, Delautier D, Benveniste J. Cooperation between platelets and neutrophils for PAF-acether formation. *Fed Proc* 1984;43:781.

47. Heuer HO. Current status of PAF antagonists. *Clin Exp Allergy* 1992;22:980–983.

48. Tuffin DP. The platelet surface membrane, ultrastructure, receptor binding and function. In: Page CP, ed. *The platelet in health and disease.* Oxford: Blackwell Scientific, 1991;10–60,

49. Parentier S, Kaplan C, Catimel B, McGregor JL. New families of adhesion molecules play a vital role in platelet functions. *Immunol Today* 1990;11:225–227.

50. Frenette PS, Johnson RC, Hynes RO, Wagner DD. Platelets roll on stimulated endothelium *in vivo*: an interaction mediated by endothelial P-selectin. *Proc Natl Acad Sci USA* 1995;92:7450–7454.

51. Taylor ML, Misso NLA, Stewart GA, Thomson PJ. Differential expression of platelet activation markers in aspirin-sensitive asthmatics and normal subjects. *Clin Exp Allergy* 1996;26:202–215.

52. Yu GH, Holers VM, Seya T, Ballard L, Atkinson JP. Identification of a third component of complement-binding glycoprotein of human platelets. *J Clin Invest* 1986;78:494–501.

53. Rosenfeld SJ, Looney RJ, Leddy JP, Phipps DC, Abraham GN, Anderson CL. Human platelet Fc receptor for immunological G. *J Clin Invest* 1985;76:2317–2322.

54. Joseph M, Capron A, Ameisen J-C, et al. The receptor for IgE on blood platelets. *Eur J Immunol* 1986;16:306–312.

55. Capron M, Jouault T, Prin L, et al. Functional study of a monoclonal antibody to IgE Fc receptor (FceR2) of eosinophils, platelets and macrophages. J Exp Med 1986;164:72–89.

56. Joseph M, Auriault C, Capron A, Vorng H, Viens P. A new function for platelets: IgE-dependent killing of schistosomes. *Nature* 1983;303:810–812.

57. Bout D, Joseph M, Pontet M, Vorng H, Deslee D, Capron A. Rat resistance to schistomasiasis: platelet-mediated cytotoxicity induced by C-reactive protein. *Science* 1986;231:153–156.

58. Joseph M. The generation of free radicals by blood platelets. In: Joseph M, ed. *The Immunopharmacology of platelets.* New York: Academic, 1995;209–225.

59. Damonneville M, Monte D, Auriault C, et al. The neuropeptide substance P stimulates the effector functions of platelets. *Clin Exp Immunol* 1990;81:346–351.

60. Rohrbach MS, Wheatley CL, Slifman NR, Gleich GJ. Activation of platelets by eosinophil granule proteins. *J Exp Med* 1990;172:1271–1274.

61. Pancre V, Joseph M, Capron A, et al. Recombinant human interferon induced increased IgE receptor expression on human platelets. *Eur J Immunol* 1988;18:829–832.

62. Damonneville M, Wietzerbin J, Pancre M, Joseph M, Capron A, Auriault C. Recombinant tumor necrosis factors mediate platelet cytotoxicity to *Schistosoma mansoni* larvae. *J Immunol* 1988;140:3962–3965.

63. Tsicopoulos A, Lassalle P, Joseph M, Tonnel T, Dessaint JP, Capron A. Effect of disodium cromoglycate on inflammatory cells bearing the Fc epsilon receptor type II (Fc$_\varepsilon$RII). *Int J Immunopharmacol* 1988;10: 227–236.

64. Roth M, Soler M, Lefkowitz H, et al. Inhibition of receptor-mediated platelet activation by nedocromil sodium. *J Allergy Clin Immunol* 1993;91:1217–1225.

65. Lewis AJ, Dervinis A, Chang J. The effects of antiallergic and bronchodilator drugs on platelet activating factor (PAF-acether) induced bronchospasm and platelet aggregation. *Agents Actions* 1984;15:636–642.

66. Cesbron JY, Capron A, Vargaftig BB, et al. Platelets mediate the action of diethylcarbamazine on microfilariae. *Nature* 1987;325:533–536.

67. Pancre V, Auriautl C, Joseph M, Cesbon JY, Kusnierz JP, Capron A. A suppressive lymphokine on platelet cytotoxic functions. *J Immunol* 1986;137:585–591.

68. Beasley R, Roche WR, Roberts JA, Holgate ST. Cellular events in the bronchi in mild asthma and after bronchial provocation. *Am Rev Respir Dis* 1989;139:806–817.

69. Lellouch-Tubiana A, Lefort J, Pirotzky E, Vargaftig BB, Pfister A. Ultrastructural evidence for extravascular platelet recruitment in the lung upon intravenous injection of platelet activating factor (PAF-acether) to guinea-pigs. *Br J Exp Pathol* 1985;66:345–355.

70. Metzger WJ, Sjoerdsma K, Richerson HB, et al. Platelets in bronchoalveolar lavage from asthmatic patients and allergic rabbits with allergen-induced late phase responses. *Agents Actions* 1987;21:151–159.

71. McManus LM, Morley CA, Levine SP, Pinckard RN. Platelet activating factor (PAF) induced release of platelet factor 4 (PF4) *in vitro* during IgE anaphylaxis in the rabbit. *J Immunol* 1979;123:2835–2841.

72. Vargaftig BB, Lefort J. Differential effects of prostacyclin and prostaglandin E$_1$ on bronchoconstriction and thrombocytopaenia during collagen and arachidonate infusions and anaphylactic shock in the guinea pig. *Prostaglandins* 1979;18:519–528.

73. Pinckard RN, Halonen M, Palmer JD, Butler C, Shaw JO, Henson PM. Intravascular aggregation and pulmonary sequestration of platelets during IgE induced systemic anaphylaxis in the rabbit: abrogation of lethal anaphylactic shock by platelet depletion. *J Immunol* 1977;119:2185–2193.

74. Halonen M, Palmer JD, Lohman C, McManus LM, Pinckard RN. Differential effects of platelet depletion on the physiologic alterations of IgE anaphylaxis and acetyl glyceryl ether phosphorycholine infusion in the rabbit. *Am Rev Respir Dis* 1981;124:416–421.

75. Page CP, Paul W, Morley J. Platelets and bronchospasm. *Int Arch Allergy Appl Immunol* 1984;74:347–350.

76. Vargaftig BB, Lefort J, Chignard M, Benveniste J. Platelet activating factor induces a platelet-dependent bronchoconstriction unrelated to the formation of prostaglandin derivatives. *Eur J Pharmacol* 1980;65: 185–192.

77. Dewar A, Archer CB, Paul W, Page CP, MacDonald DM, Morley J. Cutaneous and pulmonary histopathological responses to platelet activating factor (PAF-acether) in the guinea pig. *J Pathol* 1984;144: 25–34.

78. Page CP, Tomiak RHH, Sanjar S, Morley J. Suppression of PAF-acether responses: an anti-inflammatory effect of anti-asthma drugs. *Agents Actions* 1985;16:33–35.

79. Chignard M, Wal F, Lefort J, Vargaftig BB. Inhibition by sulphinpyrazone of the platelet-dependent bronchoconstriction due to platelet activating factor (PAF-acether) in the guinea pig. *Eur J Pharmacol* 1982;78:71–79.

80. Morley J, Sanjar S, Page CP. The platelet in asthma. *Lancet* 1984;2: 1142–1144.

81. Vargaftig BB, Lefort J, Wal F, Chignard M, Medeiros M. Nonsteroidal antiinflammatory drugs if combined with antihistamine and antiserotonin agents interfere with the bronchial and platelet effects of platelet activating factor (PAF-acether). *Eur J Pharmacol* 1982;82: 121–130.

82. Schellenberg RR, Walker B, Snyder F. Platelet-dependent contraction of human bronchus by platelet activating factor. *J Allergy Clin Immunol* 1983;71:145.

83. Coyle AJ, Page CP, Atkinson L, Flanagan R, Metzger WJ. The requirement for platelets in allergen-induced late asthmatic airway obstruction. *Am Rev Respir Dis* 1990;142:587–593.

84. Coyle AJ, Spina D, Page CP. PAF-induced bronchial hyperresponsiveness in the rabbit: contribution of platelets and airway smooth muscle. *Br J Pharmacol* 1990;101:31–38.

85. Mazzoni L, Morley J, Page CP, Sanjar S. Induction of airway hyperreactivity by platelet activating factor in the guinea-pig. *J Physiol* 1985;365:107P.

86. Robertson DN, Page CP. Effect of platelet agonists on airway reactivity and intrathoracic platelet accumulation. *Br J Pharmacol* 1987;82: 105–111.

87. Sanjar S, Smith D, Kristersson A. Incubation of platelets with PAF produces a factor which causes airway hyperreactivity in guinea-pigs. *Br J Pharmacol* 1989;96:75P.

88. Smith D, Sanjar S, Morley J. Platelet activation and PAF-induced airway hyperreactivity in the anaesthetised guinea-pig. *Br J Pharmacol* 1989;96:74P.

89. Morley J, Chapman ID, Sanjar S, Schaeublin E. Actions of ketotifen on PAF-induced airway hyperreactivity in the anesthetised guinea-pig. *Br J Pharmacol* 1989;96:76P.

90. Metzger WJ, Henriksen RA, Atkinson LB, Wirfel-Svet KL, Fisher RH. Bronchial challenge with platelet derived histamine releasing factor (PD-HRF) induces a pulmonary eosinophilic infiltrate. *J Allergy Clin Immunol* 1990;85:262A.

91. Lellouch-Tubiana A, Lefort J, Simon M-T, Pfister A, Vargaftig BB. Eosinophil recruitment into guinea pig lungs after PAF-acether and allergen administration. *Am Rev Respir Dis* 1988;137:948–954.

92. Coyle AJ, Urwin SC, Page CP, Touvay C, Villain B, Braquet P. The effect of the selective PAF antagonist BN 52021 on PAF and antigen-induced bronchial hyperreactivity and eosinophil accumulation. *Eur J Pharmacol* 1988;148:51–58.

93. Coyle AJ, Page CP, Atkinson L, Sjoerdsma K, Touvay C, Metzger WJ. Modification of allergen-induced airway obstruction and airway hyperresponsiveness in an allergic rabbit model by the selective PAF antagonist BN 52021. *J Allergy Clin Immunol* 1989;84:960–967.

94. Smith HR, Henson PM, Clay KL, Larsen GL. Effect of the PAF antagonist L-659,989 on the late asthmatic response and increased airway reactivity in the rabbit. *Am Rev Respir Dis* 1988;137:A283.

95. Seeds EAM, Coyle AJ, Page CP. The effect of the selective PAF antagonist WEB 2170 on PAF and antigen induced airway hyperresponsiveness and eosinophil infiltration. *J Lipid Mediators* 1991;4:111–122.

96. Sasaki T, Shimura S, Ikeda K, Sasaki H, Takishima T. Platelet-activating factor increase platelet-dependent glycoconjugate secretion from tracheal submucosal gland. *Am J Physiol* 1989;257:L373–L378.

97. Maccia CA, Gallagher JS, Ataman G, Gluek HI, Brooks SM, Bernstein IL. Platelet thrombopathy in asthmatic patients with elevated immunoglobulin E. *J Allergy Clin Immunol* 1977;59:101–108.

98. Fishel CW, Zwemer RJ. Aggregation of platelets from *Bordetella pertussis*-injected mice and atopically sensitive human individuals. *Fed Proc* 1970;29:640.

99. Soliner A, Bernstein IL, Glueck HI. The effect of epinephrine on platelet aggregation in normal and atopic subjects. *J Allergy Clin Immunol* 1973;51:29–34.

100. D'Souza L, Glueck HI. Measurement of nucleotide pools in platelets using high pressure liquid chromatography. *Thromb Haemost* 1977; 38:990–1001.

101. Harker LA, Malpass TW, Branson HE, Hessel EA, Slichter SJ. Mechanism of abnormal bleeding in patients undergoing cardiopulmonary bypass: acquired transient platelet dysfunction associated with selective alpha granule release. *Blood* 1980;56:824–834.

102. Malmgren R, Grubbstrom J, Olsson P, Theorell H, Tornling G, Unge G. Defective serotonin (5-HT) transport mechanism in platelets from patients with endogenous and allergic asthma. *Allergy* 1982;37: 29–39.

103. Bakulin MP, Joffe EJ. Content of biologically active substances, histamine and serotonin in patients with bronchial asthma. *Teraputicheskii Arkh* 1979;51:45–49.

104. Block LH, Imhof E, Emmons LR, Roth M, Perruchoud AP. PAF-dependent phosphatidylinositol turnover in platelets: differences between asthmatics and normal individuals. *Respiration* 1990;57:373–378.

105. Storck H, Hoigne R, Koller F. Thrombocytes in allergic reactions. *Int Arch Allergy* 1955;6:372–384.

106. Maestrelli P, Boschetto P, Zocca E, et al. Venous blood platelets decrease during allergen-induced asthmatic reactions. *Clin Exp Allergy* 1990;20:367–372.

107. Jaffar Z, Sullivan P, Restrick L, Costello J, Page CP. Modification of platelet activation in allergic asthmatics by regular low dose theophylline therapy. *Eur Respir J* 1996; (*in press*).

108. Gresele P, Todisco T, Merante F, Nenci GG. Platelet activation and allergic asthma [Letter]. *N Engl J Med* 1982;306:549.

109. Gresele P, Ribaldi E, Grasselli S, Todisco T, Nenci GG. Evidence for platelet activation in asthma. *Agents Actions Suppl* 1987;21:119–128.

110. Traietti P, Marmaggi S, Dardes N, Moscatelli B, Bologna E, Vulterini S. Circulating platelet activation in respiratory diseases: differences between arterial and venous blood in cold and asthmatic patients. *Respiration* 1984;46:62–63.

111. Knauer KA, Lichtenstein LM, Adkinson NF Jr, Fish JE. Platelet activation during antigen-induced airway reactions in asthmatic subjects. *N Engl J Med* 1981;304:1404–1406.

112. Toga H, Ohya N, Kitagawa S. Clinical studies on plasma platelet factor 4 in patients with bronchial asthma. *Jpn J Allergy* 1984;33:474–479.

113. Gresele P, Grasselli S, Todisco T, Nenci GG. Platelets and asthma [Letter]. *Lancet* 1985;1:347.

114. Johnson CE, Belfield PW, Davis S, Cooke NJ, Spencer A, Davies JA. Platelet activation during exercise-induced asthma: effect of prophylaxis with salbutamol. *Thorax* 1986;42:290–294.

115. Morrison JFJ, Pearson SB, Dean HG, Craig IR, Bramley PN. Platelet activation in nocturnal asthma. *Thorax* 1991;146:197–200.

116. Gresele P, Dottorini M, Selli ML, et al. Altered platelet function associated with the bronchial hyperresponsiveness accompanying nocturnal asthma. *J Allergy Clin Immunol* 1993;91:894–902.

117. Averill FJ, Hubbard WC, Proud D, Gleich GJ, Liu MC. Platelet activation in the lung after antigen challenge in a model of allergic asthma. *Am Rev Respir Dis* 1992;145:571–576.

118. Jian S, Gua-Xing W, Jia-Yonhg M. Platelet function in acute asthma. *Chest* 1992;102:1535.

119. Lupinetti MD, Sheller JR, Catella F, Fitzgerald GA. Thromboxane biosynthesis in allergen-induced bronchospasm: evidence for platelet activation during exercise induced asthma. *Am Rev Respir Dis* 1989;140:932–935.

120. Yamamoto H, Nagata M, Tabe K, et al. The evidence of platelet activation in bronchial asthma. *J Allergy Clin Immunol* 1993;91:79–87.

121. Greer IA, Winter JH, Gaffiney D, et al. Platelets in asthma [Letter]. *Lancet* 1984;2:1479.

122. Durham SR, Dawes J, Kay AB. Platelets in asthma. *Lancet* 1985;2:36–36.

123. Greer IA, Winter JH, Gaffiney D, et al. Platelet activation in allergic asthma [Letter]. *Thromb Haemost* 1985;53:438.

124. Shephard EG, Malan L, Macfarlane CM, Mouton W, Joubert JR. Lung function and plasma levels of thromboxane B$_2$, 6-ketoprostaglanding F$_{1\alpha}$ and β-thromboglobulin in antigen-induced asthma before and after indomethacin pretreatment. *Br J Clin Pharmacol* 1985;19:459–470.

125. Hemmendinger S, Pauli G, Tenabene A, et al. Platelet function: aggregation by PAF or sequestration in lung is not modified during immediate or late allergen-induced bronchospasm in man. *J Allergy Clin Immunol* 1989;83:990–996.

126. Ind PW, Peters AM, Malik F, Lavender JP, Dollery CT. Pulmonary platelet kinetics in asthma. *Thorax* 1985;40:412–417.

127. Martin JF, Levine RF. Evidence in favour of the lungs as the site of platelet production. In: Page CP, ed. *The platelet in health and disease.* Oxford: Blackwell Scientific, 1991;1–9.

128. Martin JF, Slater DN, Trowbridge EA. Platelet production in the lungs. *Agents Actions Suppl* 1987;37–57.

129. Taytard A, Guenard H, Vuilemin L, et al. Platelet kinetics in stable atopic asthmatic patients. *Am Rev Respir Dis* 1986;134:983–985.

130. Harker LA. Platelet survival time: its measurement and use. *Prog Hemost Thromb* 1978;4:321–347.

131. Szczeklik A, Milner PC, Birch J, Watkins J, Martin JF. Prolonged bleeding time, reduced platelet aggregation, altered PAF-acether sensitivity and increased platelet mass are a trait of asthma and hay fever. *Thromb Haemost* 1986;56:283–287.

132. Audera C, Rocklin R, Vaillancourt R, Jakubowski JA, Deykin D. Altered arachidonic acid metabolism and platelet size in atopic subjects. *Clin Immunol Immunopathol* 1988;46:571–576.

133. Page CP. Platelets. In: Holgate ST, Church MK, eds. *Allergy illustrated.* London: Gower Medical, 1993.

134. Jeffery PK, Wardlaw AJ, Nelson FC, Collins JV, Kay AB. Bronchial biopsies in asthma: an ultrastructural, quantitative study and correlation with hyperreactivity. *Am Rev Respir Dis* 1989;140:1745–1753.

135. Wilkens JH, Wilkens H, Uffman J, Bovers J, Fabel H, Froelich JC. Effects of a PAF antagonist (BN52063) on bronchoconstriction and platelet activation during exercise induced asthma. *Br J Clin Pharmacol* 1990;29:85–91.

136. Kuitert LM, Hui KP, Uthayarkumar S, et al. Effect of the platelet-activating factor antagonist UK-74,505 on the early and late response to allergen. *Am Rev Respir Dis* 1993;147:82–86.

137. O'Byrne PM. Effect of platelet activating factor antagonist WEB 2086, on allergen-induced asthmatic responses. *Thorax* 1993;48:594–598.

138. Bel EH, De Smet M, Rossing TH, Timmers MC, Dijkman JH, Sterk PJ. The effects of a specific oral PAF-antagonist, MK-287, on antigen-induced early and late asthmatic reactions in man. *Am Rev Respir Dis* 1991;143:A811(abstract).

139. Hozawa S, Haruta Y, Ishioka S, Yamakido M. Effects of a PAF antagonist, Y-24180, on bronchial hyperresponsiveness in patients with asthma. *Am J Respir Crit Care Med* 1995;152:1198–1202.

140. O'Connor BJ, Evans DJ, Coulby LJ, Cluzel M. Treatment with a PAF receptor antagonist, SR 27417A, inhibits the late asthmatic response. *J Allergy Clin Immunol* 1997; (*in press*).

141. Taytard A, Vuillemin L, Guenarg H, Rio P, Vergeret J, Ducassou D. Platelet kinetics in stable asthma patients: effect of ketotifen. *Am Rev Respir Dis* 1987;135:388A(abstr).

Asthma, edited by P.J. Barnes, M.M. Grunstein,
A.R. Leff, and A.J. Woolcock.
Lippincott–Raven Publishers, Philadelphia © 1997.

▪ 35 ▪

Interstitial and Bronchial Fibroblasts

Patricia J. Sime, Guy M. Tremblay, Zhou Xing,
Bengt O. Sarnstrand, and Jack Gauldie

Fibroblasts and the Extracellular Matrix
  Fibroblast-Derived Structural Components of the
    Extracellular Matrix
  Effector Functions of the Extracellular Matrix
Fibroblasts as Targets of Inflammatory and Fibrotic
  Mediators
  Fibroblast Cytokine Release
  Fibroblast Proliferation
  Fibroblast Extracellular Matrix Synthesis
  Fibroblast Phenotypic Modulation

Fibroblasts as Effector Cells in Asthma
  Prostaglandins
  Chemokines (MIP-1α, MCP-1, and IL-8)
  Interleukin 6
  Colony-Stimulating Factors
  Transforming Growth Factor-β
  Matrix Metalloproteinases and Inhibitors
  Fibroblast-Epithelial Interactions
  Modulation of Effector Functions by Corticosteroids

Asthma is a disease characterized pathologically by bronchial epithelial injury and chronic inflammation with prominent tissue eosinophilia, and more recently it has been recognized that there is discernible tissue remodeling with bronchial fibrosis (1,2). Although many studies have examined the contribution of inflammatory cells in this disease, much less attention has been focused on the role of tissue structural cells such as the fibroblast. Evidence is now accumulating that these cells too, may be critical in inducing and perpetuating the pathophysiologic changes that characterize asthma. Fibroblasts are structural cells and, once activated by cytokines and other mediators produced during the inflammatory response, can proliferate and synthesize extracellular matrix (ECM) proteins (3). As such, it is likely that it is the fibroblast which is responsible for the subepithelial bronchial wall fibrosis seen in asthmatics, even those with mild disease of short duration (4). Aside from its struc-

tural role, the fibroblast has many other important effector functions. Much data now indicate that fibroblasts, particularly those activated by cytokines such as interleukin (IL)-1 and tumor necrosis factor (TNF)-α, are capable of synthesizing and releasing many of the same cytokines as inflammatory cells (5–7). This is important because the large number of fibroblasts in the lung represent a potentially very extensive reservoir of cytokines and, unlike many of the inflammatory cells, the resident fibroblasts are long-lived. They are therefore capable of producing inflammatory mediators over a prolonged period, which may contribute to the chronic nature of inflammation in asthma. Recent data also suggest that the fibroblast may be phenotypically altered after exposure to such a chronically inflamed milieu, and this altered phenotype may derive either from the intrinsic heterogeneity within the fibroblast population or develop by induction or selection following exposure to signals generated during prolonged inflammation. In this chapter, we discuss our understanding of the potential role of the fibroblast in the pathogenesis of asthma. Since there have only been a few studies of fibroblast cell biology in asthma, we also review relevant data from studies of fibroblasts *in vitro* and *in vivo* from other pulmonary inflammatory and fibrotic conditions.

  P. J. Sime, Z. Xing, and J. Gauldie: Department of Pathology, McMaster University, Hamilton, Ontario L8N 3Z5 Canada.
  G. M. Tremblay: Centre de Recherche, Université Laval, Laval Hospital, Sainte-Foy, Quebec G1V 4G5 Canada.
  B. O. Sarnstrand: Department of Pharmacology, Astra Draco AB, S-221 00 Lund, Sweden.

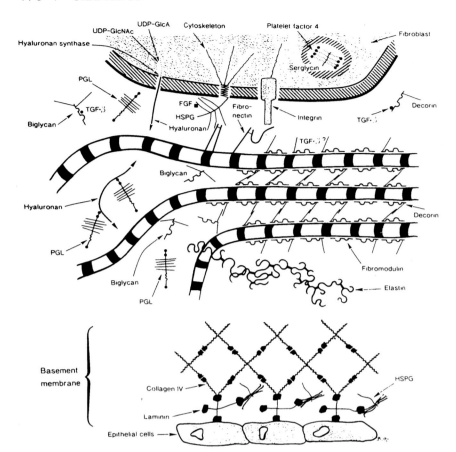

FIG. 1. Scheme showing the organization of the extracellular matrix. (Diagram courtesy of G. Westergren Thorsson.)

FIBROBLASTS AND THE EXTRACELLULAR MATRIX

Fibroblasts are the cells of the lung that contribute the major portion of the proteins and complex carbohydrates that comprise the ECM. The ECM not only provides mechanical support for the pulmonary tissues, but is a source of signals for cell migration, localization, differentiation, and activation (8,9). Deposition of a number of these ECM proteins increases in the bronchus of some asthmatic patients. In addition to important effects on the mechanical properties of the lung, ECM abnormalities may also directly affect accumulation and activation of cells with important effector functions in asthma such as eosinophils, T lymphocytes, and mast cells (10,11). Figure 1 illustrates organization of the ECM components.

Fibroblast-Derived Structural Components of the Extracellular Matrix

Collagens

Twelve different types of collagens have been identified in lung (12). Interstitial fibrillar collagens such as types I and III comprise the major portion, with smaller contributions from types V and VI. In contrast to these fibrillar subtypes, type IV collagen has a large sheetlike structure and forms the basic framework of the basement membrane (13). Abnormalities in collagen deposition have been shown to occur in the bronchus of asthmatic subjects. Histologic and electron-microscopic studies of lung tissue from biopsies of asthmatic patients demonstrate an apparent thickening of the bronchial basement membrane (4,14,15). However, this is not due to true thickening of the basement membrane proper (lamina lucida and lamina densa), but rather to deposition of interstitial collagen III, collagen V and, to a lesser extent, collagen I plus fibronectin, proteoglycans, and tenasin in the lamina reticularis (Fig. 2) beneath the true basement membrane. In this region, there is also an accumulation of a population of fibroblastlike cells (myofibroblasts) with characteristics of both smooth muscle cells and fibroblasts. These cells have abundant ribosomes indicative of active protein metabolism, thin filaments with focal densities, and after immunohistochemical staining may demonstrate the smooth muscle-associated isotype of the contractile protein actin (α-smooth muscle actin). Although such cells are also present in normal subjects, they are increased in asthma, and their number correlates

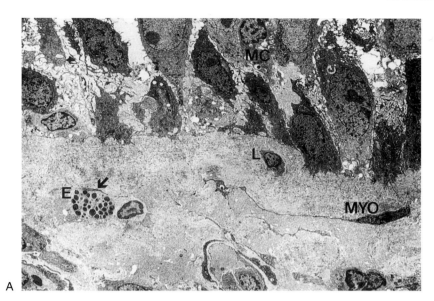

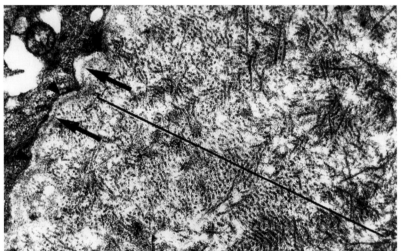

FIG. 2. A: Ultrastructure of the bronchial mucosa in allergic asthma. There is separation of the epithelial cells, thickening of the lamina reticularis of the basement membrane, and an infiltrate of inflammatory cells. A partially degranulated mast cell *(MC)* is present in the epithelium. The nucleus and elongated cytoplasm of a subepithelial myofibroblast *(MYO)* are shown. An eosinophil leukocyte *(E)* is seen in close contact with a strand of myofibroblast cytoplasm *(arrow)*. A lymphocyte *(L)* is migrating through the collagen of the lamina reticularis. Electron microscopy, original magnification, ×500. **B:** High magnification of the ultrastructure of the bronchial basement membrane and subepithelial myofibroblast in allergic asthma. Basement membrane showing lamina lucida *(arrowheads)*, lamina densa *(arrows)*, and lamina reticularis *(bar)*. (From Roche WR. Fibroblasts and extracellular matrix in bronchial asthma. In: Busse WW, Holgate ST, eds. *Asthma and rhinitis.* Boston: Blackwell Scientific, 1995;554–562.)

well with the depth of subepithelial collagen deposited (15). It has been postulated that these cells are responsible for the abnormal accumulation of interstitial collagens described above. The origin of these cells is not yet established, but it is likely that they are derived after phenotypic modulation of the resident fibroblast population. This is discussed in the following section.

It is interesting that this accumulation of collagen can be seen in all types of asthma (intrinsic, extrinsic, and occupational), and the depth of the extent of the collagen deposition does not seem to be related to disease duration or severity. In addition, these changes may not always be permanent. For example, in isocyanate-induced asthma, avoidance of isocyanate results in a decrease in subepithelial collagens, myofibroblasts, and inflammatory cells, and is accompanied by clinical improvement (16). While fibroblasts synthesize collagens and other ECM components, they are also a source of the matrix metallopro-

teinases (collagenases, stromolysins, and gelatinases) that degrade them, and abnormalities in these degradative pathways may also be involved in abnormal collagen deposition (17). This aspect of fibroblast cell biology and ECM turnover has not yet been investigated in the context of asthma.

Proteoglycans and Hyaluronan

The proteoglycans are a class of macromolecules with a core protein linked to unusual carbohydrates: glycosaminoglycans (GAGs). The GAG chains consist of repeating disaccharide units arranged linearly. The carbohydrate backbones of the GAGs comprise hexosamine and either hexuronic acid or galactose arranged in an alternating sequence, with sulfate substitutions in various positions. The sulfates give the GAGs a negative charge.

The alterations in the disaccharide unit result in different types of GAG chains, such as heparan sulfate, heparin, or chondroitin sulfate (CS) and dermatan sulfate (DS). This diversity in GAG chains and the different core proteins produces a family of proteoglycans that is appropriately large, considering the many different functions and locations of proteoglycans (18–20).

Some of the proteoglycans are intracellular, such as serglycine, whereas others are either cell surface associated or extracellular. The cell surface proteoglycans, such as the syndican family, seem to be important in forming links between the cell cytoskeleton and the ECM, and so are important in controlling the shape and organization of cells. The extracellular proteoglycans range greatly in size from large molecules such as aggrecan and versican, with core proteins of 200 kDa, to small proteoglycans such as decorin, biglycan, and fibromodulin, with core proteins of only 40 kDa. The high-molecular-weight proteoglycans form very large aggregates with hyaluronan (HA), with up to 100 proteoglycans bound per molecule of HA. These aggregates have high-charge density, which leads to high osmotic swelling pressures. This swelling is counteracted by collagen and elastin, and enables the tissue to support compressive loads (21). HA is a long polymer consisting of repeating disaccharide units of glucosamine–glucuronic acid and has no protein core. It is thought to play an important role in tissues into which cells are migrating, such as during inflammation and repair, as it provides a highly hydrated matrix, maintaining water within the collagen network and so providing a looser matrix for cell mobility.

Bousquet et al. (22) have found an increase in HA in the bronchoalveolar lavage (BAL) fluid of asthmatics and moreover have shown that there was a significant correlation between hyaluronic acid levels and the severity of asthma. The family of small extracellular proteoglycans includes decorin, biglycan, and fibromodulin. Decorin and biglycan carry one or two CS/DS chains, respectively, whereas fibromodulin bears keratan-sulfate chains. Decorin and fibromodulin are likely to be important in organizing the ECM, as both bind collagen and can result in delayed and thinner fiber formation (23). Decorin is found associated with collagen fibrils, whereas biglycan accumulates at the cell surface and in the pericellular environment. Decorin, biglycan, and fibromodulin can all bind to the potentially fibrogenic cytokine transforming growth factor (TGF)-β by their core proteins, but only decorin neutralizes its biological activity (9,24).

Abnormal expression of these proteoglycans occurs in fibrotic conditions in the lung and other organs such as the liver and skin (25,26). In the bleomycin-induced pulmonary fibrotic model in rats, Westergren-Thorsson et al. (27) showed that decorin messenger ribonucleic acid (mRNA) was downregulated while biglycan and collagen gene expression were increased. Decreased decorin expression may lead to increased available and bioactive TGF-β that could then act on fibroblasts to increase expression of collagen genes and biglycan. Indeed, it has been shown that delivering decorin to the kidney either as recombinant protein or using gene-transfer techniques can protect the kidney from fibrosis in a model of renal glomerulonephritis (28,29). Recent data in vitro from our own laboratory have demonstrated that fibroblast clones isolated from normal human neonatal and fibrotic pulmonary tissues produce different amounts of proteoglycans and HA. In particular, fibroblast clones isolated

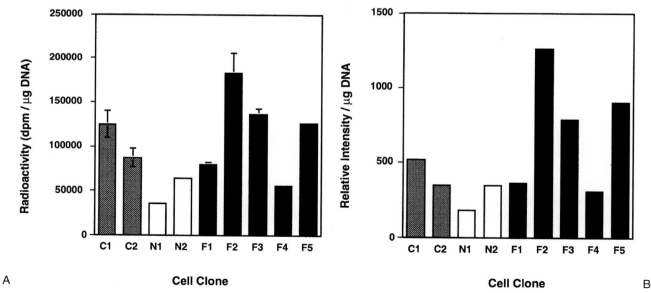

FIG. 3. A: Production of total proteoglycans by fibroblast clones from control (C), neonatal (N), and fibrotic (F) lung tissue. **B:** Production of small proteoglycans by fibroblast clones from control (C), neonatal (N), and fibrotic (F) lung tissue.

from patients with idiopathic pulmonary fibrosis (IPF) secrete more proteoglycans, particularly those of the small proteoglycan family (Fig. 3). In addition, there appeared to be an inverse correlation between production of these small proteoglycans and the proliferation rates of the clones (30). This suggests that at least some fibrotic clones are phenotypically altered in terms of proteoglycan and HA production, and these clones might have important roles in the pathogenesis of fibrosis. It would be interesting to examine the proteoglycan expression from the airways of asthmatics to determine whether such abnormalities in proteoglycan expression also exist in this inflammatory and remodeling disease.

Glycoproteins

Fibroblasts synthesize a number of different glycoproteins such as fibronectin and tenasin. Fibronectin is a large glycoprotein of 220 kDa that contains specific domains for binding to cell surface receptors or integrins, as well as to other ECM molecules, for example, collagen and heparan sulfate. The cell-binding amino acid sequence in fibronectin is RGD (Arg-Gly-Asp), which it shares with many other matrix molecules (31). Through this and other specific binding sites on the fibronectin molecule, it promotes cell adhesion and migration, differentiation, phagocytosis, and cell growth. Fibronectin is produced by fibroblasts and macrophages and is chemotactic for fibroblasts themselves. Fibronectin is localized in the interstitium and on the surface of collagen, and has been detected in the alveolar lining fluid, where it increases during inflammation (32). Tenacin expression is also increased in fibrotic tissues and has been detected close to the basement membrane (14).

Elastin

Elastin is an essential and abundant component of the lung ECM, is important in maintaining the elastic properties of the lung, and is produced predominantly by fibroblasts. Abnormalities of elastic fibers occur in the asthmatic bronchi. Superficial fibers are fragmented, and fibers in the deeper layers are often patchy, disordered, and thickened (14).

Effector Functions of the Extracellular Matrix

As well as its structural role, the ECM is likely to be influential by providing signals for the localization, differentiation, and activation of T lymphocytes, eosinophils, mast cells, and even fibroblasts themselves, which are all important in the inflammation and repair that characterize asthma (8). These signals either result from the interaction of the ECM with specific cell surface receptors or by the action of ECM-bound reservoirs of cytokines such as TGF-β, granulocyte-macrophage colony-stimulating factor (GM-CSF), and basic fibroblast-derived growth factor (bFGF) (33–35).

Cell surface receptor ECM interactions are exemplified by lymphocytes that express CD44 (a membrane glycoprotein), the ligand for which is the glycosaminoglycan HA (36). Interestingly, it has been shown that while many normal cells express CD44, they do not bind HA, unless ligand activation has occurred that requires an additional signal (37). This CD44-HA interaction may be important in T-lymphocyte homing specifically to sites of inflammation. Similarly, eosinophil survival and activation are also influenced by ECM components such as fibronectin, which prolongs eosinophil survival by stimulating auto-

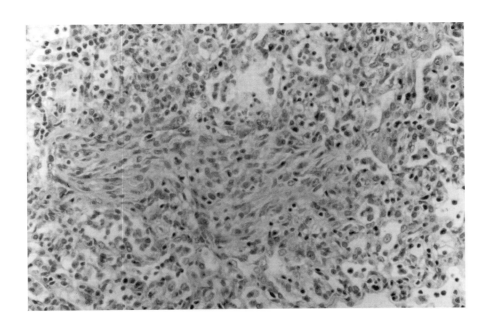

FIG. 4. Hematoxylin-eosin stain of rat lung 7 days after intratracheal injection of a recombinant adenovirus expressing the core protein of biglycan. Note the fibroblastic changes.

crine production of GM-CSF (38), and mast cell and laminin interactions may be relevant to recruitment of these cells in allergic disorders (39).

There are a number of examples of cytokines that associate with ECM components. These include the binding of bFGF, GM-CSF, and IL-3 to the heparan-sulfate moiety of proteoglycans, and the binding of TGF-β to the core protein of the proteoglycan decorin (discussed above) (34,40). It has been suggested that the binding of such molecules to proteoglycans provides a tissue reservoir for these products, which could be released immediately during inflammation. Release of these cytokines from the proteoglycans could be mediated, for example, by displacement by mast cell-derived heparin or alternatively by proteolytic cleavage of the proteoglycan (41,42). In some cases, binding of cytokines to the proteoglycans—for example, bFGF (whose biological activity is maintained when bound to proteoglycans)—may also protect them from degradation (43). This may therefore result in the long-term biological function of this and other such biologically active cytokines in the tissue.

There are undoubtedly many other unrecognized effector functions of the ECM. For example, work from our lab suggests that overexpression of the proteoglycan biglycan, but not the closely related proteoglycan decorin, in rat lung has novel effects. Using adenovirus-mediated gene transfer of the complementary deoxyribonucleic acid (cDNA) for biglycan to the rat respiratory tract, we have shown that there is a transient but pronounced fibroblastic response with increased collagen deposition in the lung parenchyma and pleura (44) (Fig. 4). This response is maximal between days 7 and 14 after gene transfer, and has begun to resolve by 3 weeks after the transient overexpression. These data suggest that biglycan may have previously unrecognized but interesting effects on fibroblast cell biology that require further investigation.

FIBROBLASTS AS TARGETS OF INFLAMMATORY AND FIBROTIC MEDIATORS

Fibroblasts are targets for a wide variety of inflammatory mediators potentially produced during inflammatory and fibrotic processes in asthma, eliciting profound effects on fibroblast biology and influencing many aspects of fibroblast behavior such as secondary cytokine release, cell proliferation, and ECM turnover. Only a few studies have examined the effects of these mediators in asthma. However, using data from studies of fibroblasts *in vitro*, and from studies *in vivo* of patients and animals with remodeling and fibrotic diseases, we can suggest a potential role for similar factors in the pathogenesis of asthma.

Fibroblast Cytokine Release

Fibroblasts are generally regarded as rather inert or quiescent cells. Much evidence, however, now indicates that fibroblasts become activated following exposure to the "early wave" of inflammatory cytokines such as IL-1α, IL-1β, and TNF-α. They are then capable of synthesizing and secreting a wide range of mediators such as the cytokines IL-1, IL-8, IL-6, monocyte chemoattractant protein (MCP) 1, macrophage inflammatory protein (MIP) 1α, platelet-derived growth factor (PDGF), bFGF, CSFs, and TGF-β (45–48), as well as lipid mediators such prostaglandin (PG) E$_2$ (49). Production of these mediators by the large number of fibroblasts resident in the lung is important in amplifying the inflammatory and immune responses. IL-1 and TNF-α are both produced by activated monocyte/macrophages (50) as well as the activated structural cells themselves (51). Recently, it has also been shown that eosinophils can produce both IL-1 and TNF-α, and that resident mast cells may be an important source of TNF-α (52). Certainly, increased IL-1 and TNF-α expression has been detected in asthmatic patients (53). An interesting phenomenon relevant to the stimulation of cytokines from fibroblasts is the process of autoinduction, whereby a cell stimulated by a cytokine such as IL-1, PDGF, or TGF-β can induce further production of the same cytokine from the target cell. This autocrine progression may help explain the chronicity of the inflammatory process in tissues (6).

In vitro, fibroblasts can also be activated directly by viral infection to produce cytokines such as IL-8, IL-6, and MCP-1 (45,54). This may have important implications because a significant number of asthmatic exacerbations are preceded by viral infections (55).

Fibroblast Proliferation

Fibroblast proliferation can be stimulated by a variety of mediators that are likely to be present in the inflamed asthmatic bronchus, including cytokines, products of activated eosinophils and mast cells, and even components of the ECM.

The cytokines IL-1, bFGF, PDGF, and TGF-β have all been shown to be mitogenic for fibroblasts *in vitro*. IL-1, PDGF, and TGF-β are all produced by activated macrophages and structural cells. IL-1 effects are mediated through binding to the specific IL-1 receptor. Most of these receptors on the surface of the fibroblasts are localized to binding sites of ECM, suggesting that interactions between IL-1 and ECM components could affect fibroblast functions (56). PDGF is both chemoattractant and mitogenic for fibroblasts. It is the prototype of the competence factors, inducing proliferation of fibroblasts and other mesenchymal cells by initiating their transition from quiescent nonreplicating cells into the G$_1$ phase of the cell cycle (57). PDGF is also important in autocrine loops as a mediator of the mitogenic effects of weakly mitogenic cytokines such as IL-1, TNF-α, and TGF-β (58, 59). TGF-β (through induction of PDGF) is also capable *in vitro* of inducing fibroblasts from both normal and remodeling lung to proliferate (60). Increased TGF-β immunoreactivity has been detected in the bronchial epithelium of asthmatic patients (61).

Resident mast cells, as well as being a source of cytokines, contain an impressive array of vasoactive mediators and enzymes. Some of these mast cell products have also been shown to be mitogenic for fibroblasts *in vitro*. Histamine, heparin, and tryptase, for example, can all induce fibroblast proliferation (62,63) and are found in the BAL after antigen bronchoprovocation of allergic asthmatics, or in lavage fluid of patients with chronic asthma. In addition, the possible interactions of mast cells and fibroblasts are highlighted by the finding of mast cell hyperplasia *in vivo* during repairing and fibrotic processes of the lung and other tissues (63–65).

Like the mast cell, the eosinophil too is capable of producing a variety of mediators with potential mitogenic effects on fibroblasts. In addition to cytokines, these include eosinophilic cationic protein and major basic protein, both of which stimulate fibroblast proliferation *in vitro* (66). These products are found in the BAL and biopsy specimens from asthmatics, and the level of eosinophilic cationic protein correlates with asthma severity (67).

Several other potentially mitogenic stimuli are likely to exist in the inflamed asthmatic bronchus. These include collagen fragments, fibronectin, and endothelin (ET)-1 (68–70). ET-1 is a peptide produced by epithelial and endothelial cells that has a number of actions relevant to asthma, including bronchoconstriction, vasoconstriction, and stimulation of fibroblast proliferation (71,72). Springall et al. (70) have shown by immunohistochemistry that ET-1 is localized to the epithelium of 70% of asthmatics compared with only 10% of controls, and ET-1 concentrations are increased in the BAL and serum of patients with exacerbations of asthma and indeed in other fibrotic diseases such as IPF (73). It is conceivable therefore that ET-1 produced by epithelial cells could play a role in fibroblast proliferation.

Fibroblast Extracellular Matrix Synthesis

The major contribution of the fibroblast to the synthesis of the ECM has been outlined in the preceding sections. Production of these proteins, proteoglycans, and glycoproteins can be stimulated by a variety of cytokines. TGF-β is the archetypal profibrotic cytokine. *In vitro*, it stimulates production of many ECM components, including collagens (74), fibronectin (75) and the fibronectin receptor, CS and DS (76), HA (27), and various integrins. Conversely, TGF-β decreases the synthesis of matrix-degrading enzymes such as collagenases and increases the synthesis of protease inhibitors (60), the net result being increased deposition of ECM. Support for its fibrogenic role *in vivo* comes from both animal and human studies. Many authors have demonstrated increased TGF-β in animals developing fibrosis (77). Hoyt and Lazo (78), for

example, demonstrated increased TGF-β in the bleomycin model of experimental pulmonary fibrosis, with maximal expression preceding the increase in gene expression for collagens, fibronectin, and laminin. TGF-β has also been localized in studies of human pulmonary disorders such as IPF. Limper et al. (79) demonstrated TGF-β mRNA in areas of macrophage accumulation, and TGF-β protein in alveolar buds populated by fibroblasts, whereas Khalil et al. (80) demonstrated TGF-β production in the bronchiolar epithelium, and Broekelmann et al. (81) found TGF-β mRNA and protein in tissue sites where active ECM deposition was occurring. It is thus not difficult to conceive that TGF-β derived from either subepithelial fibroblasts, bronchial epithelium, or macrophages could be important in the subepithelial collagen deposition found in asthma. IL-1, like TGF-β, has been shown to increase collagen, fibronectin, and proteoglycan synthesis (6), and recently it has been demonstrated that IL-4 is capable of inducing some subsets of murine lung fibroblasts to produce collagen (82).

Fibroblast Phenotypic Modulation

There is now a significant amount of evidence that there is heterogeneity among fibroblasts from different tissues and even within any one tissue. In addition, it appears there are important differences between pulmonary fibroblast lines isolated from chronically inflamed and repairing tissues, and fibroblasts isolated from normal tissues (83–86). These differences include increases in proliferation rates (87–89), alterations of matrix gene (30) and integrin expression, and abnormal cytokine production (51). The mechanism of production of such phenotypic differences is uncertain at present. Data from *in vitro* studies, though, would certainly suggest that some of the cytokines and other mediators just discussed might be responsible. In a series of studies in which normal pulmonary fibroblasts are exposed to inflammatory mediators such as IL-1 and PGE₂ for a protracted period, fibroblast lines emerge that exhibit a phenotype different from the parent (89). These data suggest that altered phenotypes present in diseased tissue may evolve by persistent pressure from chronic or repeated episodes of inflammation and exposure to inflammatory mediators (90–92). *In vivo* support for similar changes of fibroblast phenotype in inflamed tissue derives from studies of acute lung injury where fibroblasts with enhanced proliferative activities can be isolated (87,88). The nature of fibroblast heterogeneity within the airway and the potential for contribution to chronic disease have been summarized by Phipps in a major review (93). Of particular relevance to asthma is the development of cells with a phenotype of the contractile cell of granulation tissue: the myofibroblast. These cells have ultrastructural features of both smooth muscle cells and fibroblasts, and have contractile elements that are identified in many cases as α-smooth muscle actin (α-SMA) (94,95). They are present in a variety of inflamed and repairing tissues, including in asthma, where they are found in increased numbers below the bronchial epithelium (11,96–98). It has been speculated that these cells may be important in producing the excess collagens that accumulate in the lamina reticularis (11) (see Fig. 2). The derivation of these cells is unclear. However, it is interesting to speculate that exposure to inflammatory mediators such as TGF-β, GM-CSF, interferon-γ, or mast cell-derived products such as heparin, released by adjacent inflammatory and stromal cells, may induce α-SMA and result in the tissue appearance of myofibroblasts (98–101). Data *in vitro* certainly support this hypothesis, since all of these mediators have been shown to induce α-SMA. In fibroblasts, we and others have shown that TGF-β is particularly effective in inducing the phenotype *in vitro*. Figure 5 shows the dose-dependent upregulation of α-SMA in asthmatic bronchial fibroblast. Interestingly, it was not possible to block this α-SMA induction by coincubation of these fibroblasts with steroid and TGF-β. In contrast, however, the α-SMA expression in myofibroblasts isolated from a chronically inflamed respiratory tissue (a nasal polyp) was downregulated by steroid. These data suggest that the steroid effects were

mediated in this case by interruption of an autocrine loop (102). These findings are particularly relevant to asthma, since topical steroids are widely used in the treatment of asthma. Both TGF-β and GM-CSF are also capable of inducing this phenotype *in vivo*, as evidenced by a set of experiments where these cytokines were infused subcutaneously in rats, resulting in production of granulation tissue rich in α-SMA-expressing myofibroblasts (101, 103). Using adenovirus-mediated gene-transfer techniques, we have also been able to show that overexpression of GM-CSF in the respiratory tract of rats results in pulmonary granulation tissue formation and myofibroblast development (104). Although such cytokine- or mediator-induced phenotypic change may explain the increase in myofibroblast in asthma, it is of course also possible that they may arise from other precursors, such as perivascular pericyte, in the lung (105). Further studies are required to investigate the genesis and contribution of the myofibroblast to the tissue remodeling and/or altered physiology of the airways in asthma.

FIBROBLASTS AS EFFECTOR CELLS IN ASTHMA

In addition to an important role in the synthesis of ECM proteins, recent studies demonstrate that the pulmonary fibroblast is an important effector cell secreting a broad spectrum of mediators, including prostaglan-

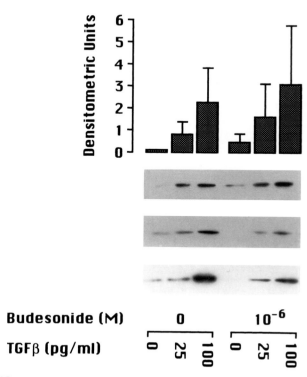

FIG. 5. Effect of transforming growth factor-β (TGF-β) on α-smooth muscle actin (α-SMA) expression in asthmatic bronchial fibroblasts. Shown are the Western blots from three different cell lines and the mean ± SEM intensity of the bands expressed in arbitrary densitometric units for each treatment. The dose-dependent upregulation of α-SMA by TGF-β was not prevented by budesonide at 10^{-6} M.

TABLE 1. *Cytokine production by fibroblasts*

Cytokines	Possible effects in asthma	Inhibited by steroids
IL-8	Chemotaxins of inflammatory cells	+
MIP-1	Chemotaxins of inflammatory cells	+
MCP-1	Chemotaxins of inflammatory cells	+
RANTES	Chemotaxins of inflammatory cells	+
IL-6	Immune regulation	+
IL-1	Inflammation	+
CSFs		
GM-	Eosinophil viability	+
G	Neutrophil viability	+
M-	Monocyte viability	−
TGF-β	Myofibroblast differentiation Collagen synthesis	+
bFGF	Fibroblast proliferation	?
PDGF	Proliferation and chemotaxis of structural cells	?
SCF	Mast cell proliferation	?
HGF	Epithelial cell growth and differentiation	+

bFGF, basic fibroblast growth factor; CSFs, colony-stimulating factors; G, granulocyte; GM, granulocyte–macrophage; HGF, hepatocyte growth factor; IL, interleukin; M, macrophage; MCP, monocyte chemoattractant protein; MIP, macrophage inflammatory protein; PDGF, platelet-derived growth factor; SCF, stem cell factor; TGF, transforming growth factor.

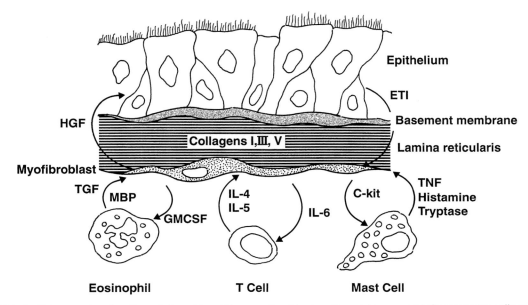

FIG. 6. Scheme showing the relationship of the myofibroblast, collagen layer, and inflammatory cells with cytokine interactions. *GM-CSF,* granulocyte-macrophage colony-stimulating factor; *MBP,* major basic protein; *IL-4, IL-5,* and *IL-6,* interleukins; *c-kit,* stem cell factor; *TNF,* tumor necrosis factor; *ET-1,* endothelin 1. (Adapted from Roche WR. Fibroblasts and extracellular matrix in bronchial asthma. In: Busse WW, Holgate ST, eds. *Asthma and rhinitis.* Boston: Blackwell Scientific, 1995;554–562, with permission).

dins, immune and inflammatory regulating cytokines, and growth factors (Table 1). These mediators have effects on mast cells, eosinophils, T cells, and even structural cells themselves through autocrine and paracrine mechanisms. Figure 6 illustrates some of these cellular interactions. The result of these effector functions is to amplify inflammatory and immune responses, and probably also to prolong them, since fibroblasts, unlike many of the inflammatory cells, have a long half-life in the tissue.

Prostaglandins

Pulmonary fibroblasts release prostaglandins such as PGE_2 after stimulation by IL-1 and TNF-α (106). The PGE_2 induces smooth muscle cell constriction, inhibits fibroblast proliferation (potentially providing a feedback mechanism for IL-1- or TNF-α-induced mitogenesis), and modulates immune functions (107). T-cell proliferation as well as IL-2 and interferon-γ production are inhibited by PGE_2 (108). However, this T-cell suppression is rather selective, since only T-helper type 1 (TH1) cytokines (IL-2 and interferon-γ) are inhibited, with no effect on the expression of TH2 cytokines IL-4 and IL-5 (109). Hence, as suggested by Phipps et al. (110), PGE_2 should be considered as a regulator rather than a suppressor of immunity, with a net effect of favoring the TH2 phenotype. This has important implications in asthma. In particular, PGE_2 has recently been used as a therapy to pro-

tect against exercise-induced bronchoconstriction (111). However, in the light of the data above, longer-term use of these inhibitors should perhaps be cautioned because they could result in an unfavorable phenotypic switch of pulmonary lymphocytes.

Chemokines (MIP-1α, MCP-1, and IL-8)

The chemokines are a family of low-molecular-weight proteins that are potent chemoattractants for leukocytes, are frequently found in inflamed lung tissue (112), and may play a role in the accumulation of inflammatory cells within airway tissue in asthma. There are two different types of chemokines—C-X-C and C-C—depending on the presence or absence of an amino acid between the first two cysteines in a highly conserved motif. IL-8 is a member of the C-X-C family, and MCP-1 and MIP-1α are members of the C-C family. The C-X-C family primarily recruits neutrophils, and the C-C family is relatively specific for the accumulation of monocytes and lymphocytes. They are produced in the lung by immune cells as well as fibroblasts, particularly after stimulation by "early wave" cytokines such as IL-1 and TNF-α (113).

IL-8 is a potent chemokine for neutrophils and is known to activate the respiratory burst and superoxide radical generation in these cells (114). In addition, there is enhanced expression of the cell surface β_2-integrin, CD11b/CD18. While neutrophil presence is not a prominent feature of asthma, the release of such a factor during episodes of fibroblast activation may exacerbate tissue damage and/or remodeling.

More relevant to asthma is the release by cytokine-activated fibroblasts of MCP-1 and MIP-1α. In particular, MIP-1α is a potent inducer of both migration and activation of eosinophils (115) and may play a role in pulmonary granuloma formation as it does in hepatic granuloma associated with eosinophil presence (116,117). A further chemokine, MCP-1, is chemotactic for mononuclear cells, and in addition can result in their activation (118). The chemokine is elevated in lung tissue of patients with a variety of pulmonary and other fibrotic disorders (119). Recently, increased MCP-1 has been detected in the bronchial tissue of asthmatic patients (120).

Most notable is the recent demonstration in a mouse model of antigen-induced airway hyperresponsiveness, known to be associated with eosinophil accumulation (121), that MIP-1α is involved in mediating the eosinophil recruitment to the lung (122). The presence of MIP-1α and association with eosinophil accumulation in this animal model and the presence of MCP-1 in asthmatic tissue suggest that tissue cell-derived chemokines, possibly from the altered myofibroblast, can contribute to the localization of eosinophils to the bronchial tissue and to the pathophysiology of asthma.

Interleukin 6

IL-6 is a potent multifunctional cytokine produced by most nucleated cells, including IL-1- and TNF-α-stimulated pulmonary fibroblasts (45,123). This cytokine is the principal mediator of the acute-phase response associated with pulmonary inflammation and has a role in promoting B-cell differentiation and T-cell proliferation and activation. These effects on lymphocyte activation and differentiation are likely to be important in regulating T-cell effector functions in asthma.

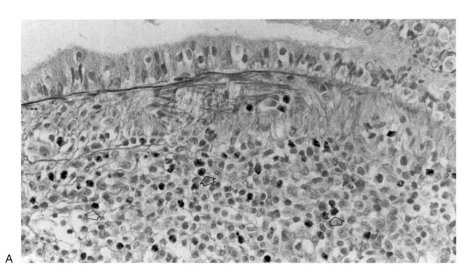

A

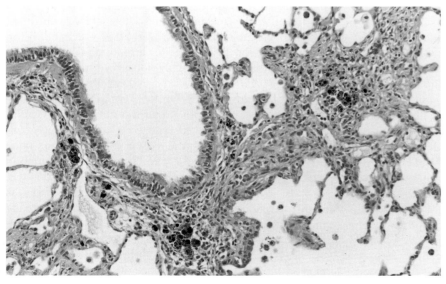

B

FIG. 7. A: Rat lung 12 days after intratracheal injection of an adenovirus expressing murine granulocyte-macrophage colony-stimulating factor *(Ad5m GM-CSF)*. There is a prominent peribronchial eosinophilia *(arrows)*. **B:** Rat lung 36 days after intratracheal injection of Ad5mGM-CSF adenovirus. There is peribronchial and interstitial fibrosis.

Colony-Stimulating Factors

Colony-stimulating factors (CSFs) are acidic glycoproteins produced by activated fibroblasts, T cells, and monocyte/macrophages that influence the differentiation, activation, and survival of granulocytes. There are three members of the family that are defined by the type of colony they induce through stem-cell differentiation. Macrophage development is governed by macrophage (M) CSF, granulocyte development by granulocyte (G) CSF, and mixed granulocyte and monocyte development by granulocyte-macrophage (GM) CSF (3). While these factors stimulate bone marrow progenitor differentiation, they may also regulate similar differentiation locally within the tissue and could contribute to local inflammatory cell accumulation. *In vitro* studies demonstrate that CSFs prolong survival of leukocytes by delaying apoptosis, and this process may further contribute to tissue accumulation of an activated population of inflammatory cells (124). GM-CSF has been detected in the BAL, lung tissue, and serum of asthmatics (52,125). *In vitro*, GM-CSF has been shown to activate eosinophil functions including differentiation, chemotaxis, chemotaxis priming, survival, transendothelial migration, expression of CD11b, CD4, and HLA-DR, and mediator release (126). Recent data from our lab confirm that GM-CSF has effects on eosinophils *in vivo*. Using adenoviral-mediated gene-transfer techniques, we have shown that transient overexpression of GM-CSF in rat lung leads to a sustained but self-limiting accumulation of eosinophils and macrophages (Fig. 7A). This was associated with pulmonary tissue damage and irreversible fibrotic reactions at a later stage (Fig. 7B). The finding of fibrotic changes and tissue remodeling was unexpected, and the details of the underlying mechanism are still under investigation. However, coordinate signals from both eosinophils and macrophages might be involved. It is worth noting that both eosinophils and macrophages are sources of TGF-β (127) and, indeed, TGF-β levels are elevated in the BAL of these GM-CSF-exposed animals. These studies have interesting implications for the potential role of GM-CSF in bronchial eosinophilic inflammation and airway remodeling in asthma.

Transforming Growth Factor-β

As discussed in the preceding sections, it is clear that TGF-β has many important effects on fibroblast function, particularly on matrix protein metabolism. Several cellular sources of TGF-β have been identified *in vitro* (60). These include eosinophils, macrophages, and epithelial cells, as well as activated fibroblasts themselves. This fibroblast-derived TGF-β can be induced by cytokines such as IL-1 and TNF-α, or by TGF-β itself acting in an autocrine or paracrine fashion. Data *in vivo* support these varied cellular sources of TGF-β. For example, Zhang et al. (127) identified eosinophils as an important source of lung TGF-β in the bleomycin model of fibrosis, Limper et al. (79) found TGF-β in alveolar buds populated by fibroblasts, and Khalil et al. (80) demonstrated macrophage and epithelial sources of TGF-β in the rodent bleomycin model.

While the effects of TGF-β *in vitro* have been well investigated, it has only been with the recent advent of technology such as transgenic animal models that its *in vivo* functions are now being unraveled. TGF-β "knockout" animals, for example, develop a fatal and widespread (including pulmonary) inflammation, indicating an important anti-inflammatory role for this molecule (128). TGF-β-overexpressing permanent transgenic models in contrast are not viable, and die *in utero*. Using a transient transgenic model in rats, we have been able to investigate the effects of overexpression of TGF-β in rat lung using recombinant adenoviruses expressing the cDNA for TGF-β₁. TGF-β is produced physiologically as an inactive precursor or latent form that is rendered active by dissociation of the latency-associated peptide (which constitutes the amino terminal of the prepro TGF-β molecule) (60). *In vitro*, this activation can be achieved by extremes of pH, heat, chaotropic agents, or enzymes such as plasmin and cathepsin D (129). Its *in vivo* activation has not yet been elucidated. We have shown that overexpression of the full-length "latent" molecule by itself does not produce fibrosis, whereas overexpression of TGF-β cDNA that has a mutation (interfering with latency-associated peptide function) rendering it spontaneously biologically active results in extensive fibrotic changes in the interstitium and pleura (77). Overexpression and activation of TGF-β in the asthmatic bronchus may therefore be important in bronchial wall fibrosis.

Matrix Metalloproteinases and Inhibitors

Whereas fibroblasts are the major source of collagen in the lung, they are also an important source of metalloproteinases such as collagenase, stromelysin, and gelatinase. These enzymes degrade collagens and other ECM products, and so contribute to tissue remodeling (130). In turn, the action of these metalloproteinases is inhibited by tissue inhibitors of metalloproteinases that are also produced by fibroblasts particularly following stimulation by cytokines such as IL-6 and oncostatin M (131,132). The fibroblast is therefore not only a producer of the ECM, but also has effector functions in its remodeling. These aspects of fibroblast biology have not yet been studied in asthma.

Fibroblast-Epithelial Interactions

During the process of mammalian lung development, there are a series of coordinated and well-regulated interactions between the mesenchyme and epithelium (3). Similar interactions between mesenchymally derived cells such as the fibroblast and epithelium are also likely to be important in mature adult lung, particularly during the course of injury and repair. Epithelial injury is one of the hallmarks of asthma, and the fibroblast is a source of a variety of different growth factors and cytokines that are likely to have effects on epithelial growth, differentiation, and activation (Fig. 6). TGF-α, epidermal growth factor, hepatocyte growth factor, and FGF can all stimulate epithelial cell proliferation and differentiation *in vitro*, with TGF-α and epidermal growth factor also promoting epithelial migration (133), and it is likely that these factors will prove to be important in repair of damaged epithelial in asthma.

Modulation of Effector Functions by Corticosteroids

Topical corticosteroids are a widely used and effective therapy for asthma of all types. While there is no doubt that they improve the bronchial inflammation that is characteristic of the disease, their effects on collagen metabolism and fibroblast/myofibroblast accumulation are much less clear. For example, Trigg et al. (134) found reduced deposition of type III collagen in the lamina reticularis on biopsies of asthmatic patients treated with inhaled steroid for 4 months, whereas other investigators have found no effect on collagen deposition (135,136) and even an increase in fibroblast numbers (137).

Steroids can potentially modulate fibroblast effector functions in several ways. Firstly, steroids could directly affect collagen and other ECM component synthesis. Leitman et al. (138) have shown *in vitro* that steroid can stimulate collagen secretion in pulmonary vascular smooth muscle cells, and this may be true for other structural cells including fibroblasts. In contrast, Ekblom et al. (139) have shown downregulation of tenasin and laminin in bone marrow stromal fibroblasts after exposure to corticosteroids, and similar downregulation of these ECM components was also recently demonstrated by Laitinen et al. (140) in a study examining biopsy specimens from patients treated with inhaled budesonide for 4 to 6 weeks. Secondly, steroids can inhibit cytokine and growth factor functions, either by directly inhibiting their production (Table 1) or by altering their bioactivity by modulating cytokine-binding proteoglycans such as heparan sulfate and decorin. Finally, there is evidence that inhaled steroids can inhibit the development of abnormal phenotypes such as the myofibroblast. In a study of nasal polyp-derived cell lines, topical steroid effectively inhibited α-SMA expression that is a hallmark of myofibroblast development (102). It is evident therefore that steroids can affect a variety of fibroblast functions, and further studies are required to evaluate the impact of these effects in terms of the fibroblast and bronchial wall remodeling.

CONCLUSIONS

The role of the pulmonary fibroblast in the pathophysiology of asthma has not been well studied. However, it is increasingly recognized that, in addition to eosinophilic inflammation, asthma is also a disease of bronchial wall remodeling, and it is likely that the fibroblast and phenotypic modulations thereof, such as the myofibroblast, are involved in this remodeling. In addition, the fibroblast may also contribute to the amplification and chronicity of inflammation by virtue of its ability to produce a wide range of inflammatory cytokines and growth factors with effects on adjacent inflammatory and structural cells.

Much of the data presented above are based on *in vitro* observations, and over the next few years further studies will be required to understand fully the contributions of the fibroblast in asthma, perhaps offering new insights into therapy of this common and chronic disease.

REFERENCES

1. Jeffrey PK, Wardlaw AJ, Nelson FC, Collins JV, Kay AB. Bronchial biopsies in asthma: an ultrastructural, quantitative study and correlation with hyperreactivity. *Am Rev Respir Dis* 1989;140:1745–1753.
2. Jeffery PK. Comparative morphology of the airways in asthma and chronic obstructive pulmonary disease. *Am J Respir Crit Care Med* 1994;150:S6–S13.
3. Kirpalani H, Gauldie J. Differentiation and effector function of pulmonary fibroblasts. In: Busse WW, Holgate ST, eds. *Asthma and rhinitis.* Boston: Blackwell Scientific, 1995;539–553.
4. Roche WR, Beasley R, Williams JH, Holgate ST. Subepithelial fibrosis in the bronchi of asthmatics. *Lancet* 1989;2:520–524.
5. Sheppard MN, Harrison NK. Lung injury, inflammatory mediators, and fibroblast activation in fibrosing alveolitis. *Thorax* 1992;47:1064–1074.
6. Tremblay GM, Sarnstrand B, Jordana M, Gauldie J. Fibroblasts as effector cells in fibrosis. In: Phan SH, Thrall RS, eds. *Pulmonary fibrosis.* New York: Marcel Dekker, 1994;541–577.
7. Strieter RM, Phan SH, Showell HJ, et al. Monokine-induced neutrophilic chemotactic factor gene expression in human fibroblasts. *J Biol Chem* 1989;264:10,621–10,626.
8. Damsky CH, Werb Z. Signal transduction by integrin receptors for extracellular matrix: cooperative processing of extracellular information. *Curr Opin Cell Biol* 1992;4:772–781.
9. Yamaguchi Y, Mann DM, Ruoslahti E. Negative regulation of transforming growth factor-β by the proteoglycan decorin. *Nature* 1990; 346:281–284.
10. Boulet L-P, Belanger M, Carrier G. Airway responsiveness and bronchial-wall thickness in asthma with or without fixed airflow obstruction. *Am J Crit Care Med* 1995;152:865–871.
11. Roche WR. Fibroblasts and extracellular matrix in bronchial asthma. In: Busse WW, Holgate ST, eds. *Asthma and rhinitis.* Boston: Blackwell Scientific, 1995;554–562.
12. Adams SL. Collagen gene expression. *Am J Respir Cell Mol Biol* 1989;1:161–168.
13. Yurchenco PD. Assembly of basement membrane. *Ann NY Acad Sci* 1990;580:55–63.
14. Bousquet J, Vignola AM, Chanez P, Campbell AM, Bonsignore G, Michel F-B. Airways remodelling in asthma: no doubt, no more? *Int Arch Allergy Immunol* 1995;107:211–214.
15. Brewster CE, Howarth PH, Djukanovic R, Wilson J, Holgate ST, Roche WR. Myofibroblasts and subepithelial fibrosis in bronchial asthma. *Am J Respir Cell Mol Biol* 1990;3:507–511.
16. Saetta M, Maestrelli P, Turato G, et al. Airway wall remodelling after cessation of exposure to isocyanates in sensitized asthmatic subjects. *Am J Respir Crit Care Med* 1995;151:489–494.

17. Emonard H, Grimaud JA. Matrix metalloproteinases: a review. *Cell Mol Biol* 1990;36:131–153.

18. Hardingham TE, Fosang AG. Proteoglycans: many forms and many functions. *FASEB J* 1992;6:861–870.

19. Kjellen L, Lindahl U. Proteoglycans: structures and interactions. *Annu Rev Biochem* 1991;60:443–475.

20. Ruoslahti E. Structure and biology of proteoglycans. *Annu Rev Cell Biol* 1988;4:229–255.

21. Heinegard D, Oldberg A. Structure and biology of cartilage and bone matrix noncollagenous macromolecules. *FASEB J* 1989;3:2042–2051

22. Bousquet J, Chanez P, Lacoste JY, et al. Indirect evidence of bronchial inflammation assessed by titration of inflammatory mediators in BAL fluid of patients with asthma. *J Allergy Clin Immunol* 1991;88:649–660.

23. Fleischmajer R, Fisher LW, MacDonald ED, Jacobs L, Perlish JS, Termine JD. Decorin interacts with fibrillar collagen of embryonic and adult human skin. *J Struct Biol* 1991;106:82–90.

24. Hildebrand A, Romaris M, Rasmussen LM, et al. Interaction of the small interstitial proteoglycans biglycan, decorin, and fibromodulin with transforming growth factor-β. *Biochem J* 1994;302:527–543.

25. Krull NB, Zimmermann T, Gressner AM. Spatial and temporal patterns of gene expression for the proteoglycans biglycan and decorin and for the transforming growth factor-β₁ revealed by *in situ* hybridization during experimentally induced liver fibrosis in the rat. *Hepatology* 1993;18:581–589.

26. Bernstein EF, Fisher LW, Li K, Le Baron RG, Tan EML, Uitto J. Differential expression of the versican and decorin genes in photoaged and sun-protected skin. *Lab Invest* 1995;72:662–669.

27. Westergren-Thorsson G, Sarnstrand B, Fransson LA, Malmstrom A. TGF-β enhances the production of hyaluronan in human lung but not in skin fibroblasts. *Exp Cell Res* 1990;186:192–195.

28. Border WA, Noble NA, Yamamoto T, et al. Natural inhibitor of transforming growth factor-β protects against scarring in experimental kidney disease. *Nature* 1992;360:361–364.

29. Isaka Y, Brees DK, Ikegaya K, et al. Gene therapy by skeletal muscle expression of decorin prevents fibrotic disease in rat kidney. *Nature Med* 1996;2:418–423.

30. Sarnstrand B, Westergren-Thorsson G, Sime PJ, Jordana M, Gauldie J, Malmstrom A. Fibroblast clones differ in proliferation rates and proteoglycan production. (Submitted).

31. Yamada KM. Adhesive recognition sequences. *J Biol Chem* 1991;266:12,809–12,812.

32. Aota S, Nagai T, Olden K, Akiyama SK, Yamada KM. Fibronectin and integrins in cell adhesion and migration. *Biochem Soc Trans* 1991;19:830–835.

33. Folkman J, Klagsbrun M, Sasse J, Wadziniski M, Ingber D, Vodavsky I. A heparin-binding angiogenic protein-basic fibroblast growth factor is stored within basement membrane. *Am J Pathol* 1988;130:393–400.

34. Roberts R, Gallagher J, Spooncer E, Allen TD, Bloomfield F, Dexter TM. Heparan sulphate bound growth factors: a mechanism for stromal cell mediated haemopoiesis. *Nature* 1988;332:376–378.

35. Ruoslahti E, Yamaguchi Y. Proteoglycans as modulators of growth factor activities. *Cell* 1991;64:867–869.

36. Aruffo A, Stamenkovic I, Melnick M, Underhill CB, Seed B. CD44 is the principal cell surface receptor for hyaluronate. *Cell* 1990;61:1303–1313.

37. David G. Integral membrane heparan sulfate proteoglycans. *FASEB J* 1993;7:1023–1030.

38. Anwar ARF, Moqbel R, Walsh GM, Kay AB, Wardlaw AJ. Adhesion to fibronectin prolongs eosinophil survival. *J Exp Med* 1993;177:839–843.

39. Thompson HL, Burbelo PD, Yamada Y, Kleinman HK, Metcalfe DD. Mast cells chemotax to laminin with enhancement after IgE-mediated activation. *J Immunol* 1989;143:4188–4192.

40. Burgess WH, Maciag T. The heparin binding (fibroblast) growth family of proteins. *Annu Rev Biochem* 1989;58:575–606.

41. Thompson RW, Whalen GF, Saunders KB, Hores T, D'Amore PA. Heparin-mediated release of fibroblast growth factor-like activity into the circulation of rabbits. *Growth Factors* 1990;3:221–229.

42. Saksela O, Rifkin DB. Release of basic fibroblast growth factor–heparan sulphate complexes from endothelial cells by plasminogen activator mediated proteolytic activity. *J Cell Physiol* 1989;138:221–226.

43. Damon DH, Lobb RR, De Amour PA, Wagner JA. Heparin potentiates the action of acidic fibroblast growth factor by prolonging its biological half life. *J Cell Physiol* 1989;138:221–226.

44. Sime PJ, Sarnstrand B, Graham FL, Weindel K, Fisher LW, Gauldie J. Recombinant human adenovirus 5 vectors expressing the core proteins of the proteoglycans decorin and biglycan. *Am J Respir Crit Care Med* 1996;153:A112(abstr).

45. Cox C, Gauldie J, Jordana M. Bronchial epithelial cell derived cytokines (G-CSF and GM-CSF) promote the survival of peripheral blood monocytes *in vitro. Am J Respir Cell Mol Biol* 1992;7:507–513.

46. Elias JA, Trinchieri G, Beck J, et al. A synergistic interaction between IL-6 and IL-1 mediates the thymocyte-stimulating activity produced by recombinant IL-1 stimulated fibroblasts. *J Immunol* 1989;142:509–514.

47. Strieter RM, Wiggins R, Phan SH, et al. Monocyte chemotactic protein gene expression by cytokine treated human fibroblasts and endothelial cells. *Biochem Biophys Res Commun* 1989;162:694–700.

48. Gauldie J, Sarnstrand B, Sime PJ, Tremblay G, Torry D, Jordana M. Tissue remodelling and fibroblast heterogeneity in asthma and other chronic airways inflammatory diseases. In: Schleimer R, Busse W, O'Byrne P, eds. *Topical glucocorticoids in asthma: mechanisms and clinical actions.* New York: Marcel Dekker, 1997;151–166.

49. Lin LL, Lin AY, De Witt DL. Interleukin-1α induces the accumulation of cytosolic phospholipase A₂ and the release of prostaglandin E₂ in human fibroblasts. *J Biol Chem* 1992;267:23,451–23,454.

50. Kelley J. Cytokines of the lung. *Am Rev Respir Dis* 1990;141:765–788.

51. Gauldie J, Torry D, Cox G, Xing Z, Ohno I, Jordana M. Effector functions of tissue structural cells in inflammation. In: Holgate ST, Austen KF, Lichtenstein LM, Kay AB, eds. *Asthma: physiology, immunopharmacology and treatment. Fourth international symposium.* London: Academic, 1993;211–225.

52. Barnes PJ. Cytokines as mediators of chronic asthma. *Am J Respir Crit Care Med* 1994;150:S42–S49.

53. Broide DH, Lotz M, Cuomo AJ, et al. Cytokines in symptomatic asthma airways. *J Allergy Clin Immunol* 1992;89:958–967.

54. Van Damme J, Decock B, Bertini R, et al. Production and identification of natural monocyte chemotactic protein from virally infected murine fibroblasts. *Eur J Biochem* 1991;199:223–229.

55. Bardin PG, Johnston SL, Pattemore PK. Viruses as precipitants of asthma symptoms. II. Physiology and mechanisms. *Clin Exp Allergy* 1992;22:809–822.

56. Quarnstrom EE, MacFarlane SA, Page RC, Dower SK. Interleukin 1β induces rapid phosphorylation and redistribution of talin: a possible mechanism for modulation of fibroblast focal adhesion. *Proc Natl Acad Sci USA* 1991;88:1232–1236.

57. Larsson O, Latham C, Zicket P, et al. Cell cycle regulation of human diploid fibroblasts: possible mechanisms of platelet-derived growth factor. *J Cell Physiol* 1989;139:477–483.

58. Raines EW, Dower SK, Ross R. IL1 mitogenic activity for fibroblasts and smooth muscle cells is due to PDGF-AA. *Science* 1989;243:393–396.

59. Paulsson Y, Austgulen R, Hofsli E, et al. Tumor necrosis factor-induced expression of platelet derived growth factor-α-chain messenger RNA in fibroblasts. *Exp Cell Res* 1989;180:490–496.

60. Kelley J. Transforming growth factor-β. In: Kelley J, ed. *Cytokines of the lung.* New York: Marcel Dekker, 1992;101–132.

61. Sousa AR, Poston RN, Lane SJ, Nakhosteen JA, Lee TH. Detection of GM-CSF in asthmatic bronchial epithelium and decrease by inhaled corticosteroids. *Am Rev Respir Dis* 1993;147:1557–1561.

62. Wasserman SI. Mast cells and airway inflammation in asthma. *Am J Respir Crit Care Med* 1994;150(Suppl):S39–S41.

63. Hebeds PA, Collins MA, Tharp MD. Mast cell and myofibroblast in wound healing. *Dermatol Clin* 1993;11:685–696.

64. Jordana M. Mast cells and fibrosis: who's on first? *Am J Respir Cell Mol Biol* 1993;8:7–8.

65. Claman HN. Mast cells, T cells and abnormal fibrosis. *Immunol Today* 1985;6:192–195.

66. Bousquet J, Chanez P, Vignola AM, Lacoste J-Y, Michel FB. Eosinophil inflammation in asthma. *Am J Respir Crit Care Med* 1994;150(Suppl):S33–S38.

67. Van Vyve T, Chanez P, Lacoste J, Bousquet J, Michel F, Godard P. Comparison between bronchial and alveolar samples of bronchoalveolar lavage fluid in asthma. *Chest* 1992;102:356–361.

68. Katayama K, Seyer JM, Raghow R, Kang AH. Regulation of extracellular matrix production by chemically synthesized subfragments of type I collagen carboxy propeptide. *Biochemistry* 1991;30:7097–7104.

69. Katayama K, Armendariz-Borunda J, Raghow R, Kang AH, Seyer JM. A pentapeptide from type I procollagen promotes extracellular matrix production. *J Biol Chem* 1993;268:9941–9944.

70. Springall DR, Howarth PH, Counihan H, Djukanovic RD, Holgate ST, Polak JM. Endothelin immunoreactivity of airway epithelium in asthmatic patients. *Lancet* 1991;337:697–701.

71. Lagente V, Chabrier PE, Mencia Huerta JM, Braquet P. Pharmacological modulation of the bronchopulmonary action of the vasoactive peptide, endothelin, administered by aerosol in the guinea pig. *Biochem Biophys Res Commun* 1989;158:625–632.

72. Takuwa N, Takuwa Y, Yanagisawa M, Yamashita K, Masaki T. A novel vasoactive peptide endothelin stimulates mitogenesis through inositol lipid turnover in Swiss 3T3 fibroblasts. *J Biol Chem* 1989;264:7856–7861.

73. Sofia M, Mormile M, Faraone S, et al. Increased endothelin-like immunoreactive material on bronchoalveolar lavage fluid from patients with bronchial asthma and patients with interstitial lung disease. *Respiration* 1993;60:89–95.

74. Fine A, Goldstein RH. The effect of transforming growth factor-β on cell proliferation and collagen formation by lung fibroblasts. *J Biol Chem* 1987;262:3897–3902.

75. Dean DC, Newby RF, Bourgeois S. Regulation of fibronectin biosynthesis by dexamethasone, transforming growth factor-β, and cAMP in human cell lines. *J Cell Biol* 1988;263:3039–3045.

76. Bassols A, Massague J. Transforming growth factor-β regulates the expression and structure of extracellular matrix chondroitin/dermatan sulfate proteoglycans. *J Biol Chem* 1988;263:3039–3045.

77. Sime PJ, Xing Z, Graham FL, Gauldie J. Adenoviral mediated transfer of transforming growth factor-β₁ cDNA to the respiratory tracts of rats, alone, and in combination with acute neutrophilic lung inflammation. *Am J Respir Crit Care Med* 1996;153:A793(abstr).

78. Hoyt DG, Lazo JS. Alterations in pulmonary mRNA encoding procollagens, fibronectin and transforming growth factor-β precede bleomycin-induced pulmonary fibrosis in mice. *J Pharmacol Exp Ther* 1988;246:765–771.

79. Limper AH, Broekelmann TJ, Colby TV, Malizia G, McDonald JA. Analysis of local mRNA expression for extracellular matrix proteins and growth factors by *in situ* hybridisation in fibroproliferative lung disorders. *Chest* 1991;99(Suppl):55S–56S.

80. Khalil N, O'Connor RN, Unruh HW, et al. Increased production and immunohistochemical localization of transforming growth factor-β in idiopathic pulmonary fibrosis. *Am J Respir Cell Mol Biol* 1991;5:155–162.

81. Broekelmann TJ, Limper AH, Colby TV, et al. Transforming growth factor-β₁ is present at sites of extracellular matrix gene expression in human pulmonary fibrosis. *Proc Natl Acad Sci USA* 1991;88:6642–6646.

82. Sempowski GD, Beckmann MP, Derdak S, Phipps RP. Subsets of murine lung fibroblasts express membrane bound and soluble IL4 receptors. *J Immunol* 1994;152:3606–3614.

83. Raghu G, Chen Y, Rusch V, Rabinovitch PS. Differential proliferation of fibroblasts cultured from normal and fibrotic human lungs. *Am Rev Respir Dis* 1988;138:703–708.

84. Breen E, Falco VM, Absher M, Cutroneo KR. Subpopulations of rat lung fibroblasts with different amounts of type I and III collagen mRNAs. *J Biol Chem* 1990;265:6286–6290.

85. Maxwell DB, Grotendorst CA, Grotendorst GR, Le Roy EC. Fibroblast heterogeneity in scleroderma:C1q studies. *J Rheumatol* 1987;14:756–759.

86. Jordana M, Schulman J, McSharry C. Heterogeneous proliferation characteristics of human adult lung fibroblast lines and clonally derived fibroblasts from control and fibrotic tissue. *Am Rev Respir Dis* 1988;137:579–584.

87. Chen B, Polunovsky V, White J, et al. Mesenchymal cells isolated after acute lung injury manifest an enhanced proliferative phenotype. *J Clin Invest* 1992;90:1778–1785.

88. Dubaybo BA, Rubei GL, Fligiel SEG. Dynamic changes in the functional characteristics of the interstitial fibroblast during lung repair. *Exp Lung Res* 1992;18:461–477.

89. Jordana M, Kirpalani H, Gauldie J. Heterogeneity of human lung fibroblast proliferation in relation to disease expression. In: Phipps RP, ed. *Pulmonary fibroblast heterogeneity.* Boca Raton, FL: CRC, 1992; 229–249.

90. Worrall JG, Whiteside TL, Prince RK, Buckingham RB, Stachura I, Rodnan GP. Persistence of scleroderma-like phenotype in normal fibroblasts after prolonged exposure to soluble mediators from mononuclear cells. *Arthritis Rheum* 1986;29:54–64.

91. Botstein GR, Sherer GK, Le Roy EC. Fibroblast selection in scleroderma: an alternative model of fibrosis. *Arthritis Rheum* 1982;25:189–195.

92. Korn JH, Torres D, Downie E. Clonal heterogeneity in the fibroblast response to mononuclear cell derived mediators. *Arthritis Rheum* 1984;27:174–179.

93. Phipps RP, ed. *Pulmonary fibroblast heterogeneity.* Boca Raton, FL: CRC, 1992.

94. Foo ITH, Naylor IL, Timmons MJ, Trejdosiewicz LK. Intracellular actin as a marker for myofibroblasts *in vitro*. *Lab Invest* 1992;67:727–733.

95. Oda D, Gown AM, Vande Berg JS, Stern R. The fibroblast-like nature of myofibroblasts. *Exp Mol Pathol* 1988;49:316–329.

96. Adler KB, Low RB, Leslie KO, Mitchell J, Evans JN. Contractile cells in normal and fibrotic lung. *Lab Invest* 1989;60:473–485.

97. Schmitt-Graff A, Chakroun G, Gabbiani G. Modulation of perisinusoidal cell cytoskeletal features during experimental hepatic fibrosis. *Virchows Arch [A]* 1993;422:99–107.

98. Schmitt-Graff A, Desmouliere A, Gabbiani G. Heterogeneity of myofibroblast phenotypic features: an example of fibroblastic cell plasticity. *Virchows Arch* 1994;425:3–24.

99. Desmouliere A, Rubbia-Brandt L, Grau G, Gabbiani G. Heparin induces α-smooth muscle actin expression in cultured fibroblasts and in granulation tissue myofibroblasts. *Lab Invest* 1992;67:716–726.

100. Desmouliere A, Rubbia-Brandt L, Abdiu A, Walz T, Macieira-Coelho A, Gabbiani G. α-Smooth muscle actin is expressed in a population of cultured and cloned fibroblasts and is modulated by γ interferon. *Exp Cell Res* 1992;201:64–73.

101. Desmouliere A, Rubbia-Brandt L, Grau G, Gabbiani G. Transforming growth factor-β₁ induces α-smooth muscle actin expression in granulation tissue myofibroblasts and in quiescent and growing cultured fibroblasts. *J Cell Biol* 1993;122:103–111.

102. Tremblay GM, Nonaka M, Sarnstrand B, Dolovich J, Gauldie J, Jordana M. Myofibroblasts in nasal polyposis: regulation by topical steroids. *Canadian Respiratory Journal* 1996 (*in press*).

103. Rubbia-Brandt L, Sappino AP, Gabbiani G. Locally applied GM-CSF induces the accumulation of α-smooth muscle actin containing myofibroblasts. *Virchows Arch [B]* 1991;60:73–82.

104. Xing Z, Ohkawara Y, Braciak T, et al. Disparate functional consequences of transient overexpression of GM-CSF and IL-5 in the lung. *Am J Respir Crit Care Med* 1996;153:A793(abstr).

105. Sappino AP, Schurch W, Gabbiani G. Differentiation repertoire of fibroblastic cells: expression of cytoskeletal proteins as marker of phenotypic modulations. *Lab Invest* 1990;63:144–161.

106. Dayer JM, Beutler B, Cerami A. Cachectin/tumor necrosis factor stimulates collagenases and prostaglandin E production by human synovial cells and dermal fibroblasts. *J Exp Med* 1985;162:2163–2166.

107. Jordana M, Sarnstrand B, Sime PJ, Ramis I. Immune-inflammatory functions of fibroblasts. *Eur Respir J* 1994;7:2212–2222.

108. Snijdewint FGM, Kalinski P, Wierenga EA, Bos JD, Kapsenberg ML. Prostaglandin E₂ differentially modulates cytokine secretion profiles of human T-helper lymphocytes. *J Immunol* 1993;150:5321–5329.

109. Betz M, Fox BS. Prostaglandin E₂ inhibits production of TH1 lymphokines but not of TH2 lymphokines. *J Immunol* 1991;146:108–113.

110. Phipps RP, Stein SH, Roper RL. A new view of prostaglandin E regulation of the immune response. *Immunol Today* 1991;12:349–352.

111. Melillo E, Woolley KL, Manning PJ, Watson RM, O'Byrne PM. Effect of inhaled PGE₂ on exercise-induced bronchoconstriction in asthmatic subjects. *Am J Respir Crit Care Med* 1994;149:1138–1141.

112. Streiter RM, Koch AE, Antony VB, Fink RB Jr, Standiford TJ, Kunkel SL. The immunopathology of chemotactic cytokines: the role of interleukin-8 and monocyte chemoattractant protein-1. *J Lab Clin Med* 1994;123:183–197.

113. Sime PJ, Gauldie J. Mechanisms of scarring in the adult respiratory distress syndrome. In: Haslett C, Evans T eds. *ARDS: acute respiratory distress in adults.* London: Chapman and Hall, 1996;215–231.

114. Baggiolini M, Walz A, Kunkel SL. Neutrophil-activating peptide-1/interleukin 8, a novel cytokine that activates neutrophils. *J Clin Invest* 1989;84:1045–1049.
115. Rot A, Krieger M, Brunner T, Bischoff SC, Schall TJ, Dahinden CA. RANTES and macrophage inflammatory protein 1α induce the migration and activation of normal human eosinophil granulocytes. *J Exp Med* 1992;176:1489–1495.
116. Lukacs NW, Kunkel SL, Strieter RM, Warmington K, Chensue SW. The role of macrophage inflammatory protein 1 alpha in *Schistosoma mansoni* egg-induced granulomatous inflammation. *J Exp Med* 1993;177:1551–1559.
117. Chensue, SW, Warmington KS, Lukacs NW, et al. Monocyte chemotactic protein expression during schistosome egg granuloma formation: sequence of production, localization, contribution, and regulation. *Am J Pathol* 1995;146:130–138.
118. Schall TJ. Biology of RANTES/sis cytokine family. *Cytokine* 1991;3:165–183.
119. Standiford TJ, Rolfe MR, Kunkel SL, et al. Altered production and regulation of monocyte chemoattractant protein-1 from pulmonary fibroblasts isolated from patients with idiopathic pulmonary fibrosis. *Chest* 1993;103:121S.
120. Sousa AR, Lame SJ, Nakhostee JA, Yoshimura T, Lee TH, Poston RN. Increased expression of the monocyte chemoattractant protein-1 in bronchial tissue from asthmatic subjects. *Am J Respir Cell Mol Biol* 1994;10:142–147.
121. Lukacs NW, Strieter RM, Chensue SW, Kunkel SL. Interleukin-4 dependent pulmonary eosinophil infiltration in a murine model of asthma. *Am J Respir Cell Mol Biol* 1994;10:526–532.
122. Lukacs NW, Strieter RM, Shaklee CL, Chensue SW, Kunkel SL. Macrophage inflammatory protein-1α influences eosinophil recruitment in antigen-specific airway inflammation. *Eur J Immunol* 1995;25:245–251.
123. Gauldie J, Richards C, Harnish D, Lansdorp P, Baumann H. Interferon-β2/B-cell stimulatory factor type 2 shares identity with monocyte-derived hepatocyte-stimulating factor and regulates the major acute phase protein response in liver cells. *Proc Natl Acad Sci USA* 1987;84:7251–7255.
124. Vancheri C, Gauldie J, Bienenstock J, et al. Human lung fibroblast-derived granulocyte-macrophage colony stimulating factor (GM-CSF) mediates eosinophil survival *in vitro*. *Am J Respir Cell Mol Biol* 1989;1:289–295.
125. Brown PH, Crompton GK, Greening AP. Proinflammatory cytokines in acute asthma. *Lancet* 1991;338:590–593.
126. Xing Z, Ohkawara Y, Jordana M, Graham FL, Gauldie J. Transfer of granulocyte–macrophage colony-stimulating factor gene to rat lung induces eosinophilia, monocytosis and fibrotic reactions. *J Clin Invest* 1996;97:1102–1110.
127. Zhang K, Flanders KC, Phan SH. Cellular localisation of transforming growth factor-β expression in bleomycin-induced pulmonary fibrosis. *Am J Pathol* 1995;147:352–361.
128. Shull MM, Ormsby I, Kier AB, et al. Targeted disruption of the mouse transforming growth factor-β1 gene results in multifocal inflammatory disease. *Nature* 1992;359:693–699.
129. Lyons RM, Keski-Oja J, Moses HL. Proteolytic activation of latent transforming growth factor-β from fibroblast-conditioned medium. *J Cell Biol* 1988;106:1659–1665.
130. Woessner JF Jr. Matrix metalloproteinases and their inhibitors in connective tissue remodelling. *FASEB J* 1991;5:2145–2154.
131. Murphy G, Reynolds JJ, Werb Z. Biosynthesis of tissue inhibitor of metalloproteinases by human fibroblasts in culture. *J Biol Chem* 1985;260:3079–3083.
132. Raghu G, Kinsella M. Cytokine effects on extracellular matrix. In: Kelley J, ed. *Cytokines of the lung.* New York: Marcel Dekker, 1993;491–543.
133. Madtes DK. Transforming growth factor-α and epidermal growth factor. In: Kelley J, ed. *Cytokines of the lung.* New York: Marcel Dekker, 1992;139–181.
134. Trigg CJ, Manolitsas ND, Wang J, et al. Placebo-controlled immunopathologic study of four months of inhaled corticosteroids in asthma. *Am J Respir Crit Care Med* 1994;150:17–22.
135. Jeffrey PK, Godfrey RW, Adelroth E, Nelson F, Rogers A, Johansson SA. Effects of treatment on airway inflammation and thickening of basement membrane reticular collagen in asthma: a quantitative light and electron microscopic study. *Am Rev Respir Dis* 1992;145:890–899.
136. Altraja A, Laitinen A, Kämpe M, et al. Inhaled budesonide has no effect on the distribution of collagen types III and VII in bronchial epithelial basement membrane in allergic asthmatics. *Am J Respir Crit Care Med* 1994;149:A632(abstr).
137. Laitinen LA, Laitinen A, Haahtela T. A comparative study of the effects of an inhaled corticosteroid, budesonide, and a B2-agonist, terbutaline, on airway inflammation in newly diagnosed asthma: a randomized, double-blind, parallel-group controlled trial. *J Allergy Clin Immunol* 1992;90:32–42.
138. Leitman DC, Benson SC, Johnson LK. Glucocorticoids stimulate collagen and noncollagen protein synthesis in cultured vascular smooth muscle cells. *J Cell Biol* 1984;98:541–549.
139. Ekblom M, Fassler R, Tomasini-Johansson B, Nilsson K, Ekblom P. Downregulation of tenascin expression by glucocorticoids in bone marrow stromal cells and in fibroblasts. *J Cell Biol* 1993;123:1037–1045.
140. Laitinen A, Altraja A, Linden M, et al. Treatment with inhaled budesonide and tenascin expression in bronchial mucosa of allergic asthmatics. *Am J Respir Crit Care Med* 1994;149:A942(abstr).

Asthma, edited by P.J. Barnes, M.M. Grunstein, A.R. Leff, and A.J. Woolcock.
Lippincott–Raven Publishers, Philadelphia © 1997.

▪ 36 ▪

Epithelial Cells as Inflammatory Cells

Albert J. Polito and David Proud

Lipid Mediators	**Reactive Oxygen Species/Nitric Oxide**
Peptide Mediators	**Expression of Adhesion Molecules**
Catabolic Enzymes/Inhibitors	**Immunoregulation**
Cytokine Release	**Repair and Remodeling**

The traditional depiction of the airway epithelium assigns it the role of acting as a physical barrier to a variety of potentially harmful inhaled agents. Research within the last decade, however, has revealed that the epithelium has a much broader functional scope. It is metabolically active and, as such, can play a central part in modulating airway inflammation. Epithelial cells exert their influence over the inflammatory response by acting as both *target* cells and *effector* cells (1,2). Exogenous and endogenous stimuli *target* the epithelial cell, resulting in a variety of responses ranging from altered modulation of airway secretions, mucociliary apparatus, and ion transport to cell death; the concept of the epithelial cell as a target is addressed in detail in Chapter 62. Conversely, in an *effector* capacity, the epithelial cell can respond to such stimuli by generating inflammatory mediators, including arachidonic acid metabolites, peptide products, cytokines, and reactive oxygen species; it expresses adhesion molecules for interaction with leukocytes, potentially acts as an antigen presenting cell, and mediates repair in the injured airway. It is this active role in the inflammatory response that is addressed in this chapter.

LIPID MEDIATORS

Airway epithelial cells of all species examined to date have demonstrated the ability to convert arachidonic acid

to a variety of biologically active products that can modulate airway inflammation. Three distinct lipoxygenase pathways have been observed in mammalian respiratory epithelia, 5-, 12-, and 15-lipoxygenase, and the dominant pathway varies among species (3). For example, 5-lipoxygenase activity is present in canine and ovine epithelial cells (4–6), whereas rabbit and bovine tracheal epithelial cells display primarily 12-lipoxygenase activity (7,8). In contrast, human airway epithelial cells have a highly active 15-lipoxygenase pathway (9). This enzyme converts arachidonic acid not only to 15-hydroxyeicosatetraenoic acid (15-HETE) but also to a range of hydroperoxy, epoxyhydroxy, keto, and dihydroxy acids (6,9).

It has been reported that 15-lipoxygenase activity is increased in asthmatic bronchial epithelium (10), a finding that is supported by immunohistochemical staining techniques (11). These studies have demonstrated minimal levels of 15-lipoxygenase antigen in the bronchial epithelium of normal subjects (it being confined to the nose and trachea) but markedly elevated levels in the bronchi of asthmatics and chronic bronchitics. Moreover, the major metabolite of this pathway, 15-HETE, is found in bronchoalveolar lavage (BAL) fluid from chronic stable asthmatics and increases after antigen provocation (12). In this latter instance, however, it is difficult to ascribe a cellular origin to the 15-HETE, since eosinophils also contain high levels of 15-lipoxygenase (13).

Thus, inflammation in the airways may induce 15-lipoxygenase in epithelial cells. The metabolites of this enzyme have been shown to have potentially important effects on airway function and biology. For example, 15-HETE causes the release of leukotriene (LT) C_4 from mast cells through activation of the 5-lipoxygenase path-

A. J. Polito: Department of Medicine, The Johns Hopkins University School of Medicine, Baltimore, Maryland 21205.

D. Proud: Department of Medicine, The Johns Hopkins University School of Medicine, The Johns Hopkins Asthma and Allergy Center, Baltimore, Maryland 21224.

way (14). It also enhances mucus glycoprotein production by cultured human airways (15) and augments the acute response to antigen challenge in asthmatics (16). Another important metabolite, 8S,15S-diHETE, has been shown to induce chemotaxis of neutrophils both *in vitro* (17) and *in vivo* (18). The recruited neutrophils can then utilize 15-HETE in a pathway catalyzed by 5-lipoxygenase to generate lipoxin A (19), a trihydroxy acid with a variety of physiologic actions. Lipoxin A activates protein kinase C (20), inhibits the cytotoxic activity of human natural killer cells (21), causes the generation of superoxide radicals by neutrophils (19,22), and contracts guinea-pig lung strips (19,23) and human bronchi (24). The 15-lipoxygenase pathway in airway epithelial cells,

therefore, has the capacity to induce a cascade of inflammatory responses on the molecular and cellular levels.

While the lipoxygenase pathway often predominates, airway epithelial cells from a variety of animal species also metabolize arachidonic acid via the cyclooxygenase pathway (5,6,8,25). Both freshly isolated and cultured human epithelial cells synthesize nearly equivalent amounts of prostaglandin (PG) E_2 and $PGF_{2\alpha}$ (6,26) (Fig. 1). PGE_2 mediates relaxation of airway smooth muscle (3) and regulates mucus glycoprotein secretion (27). Inhalation of this mediator has been reported to block the early and late bronchoconstrictor responses to inhaled allergen and to abolish allergen-induced increases in bronchial reactivity (28), as well as to attenuate exercise-in-

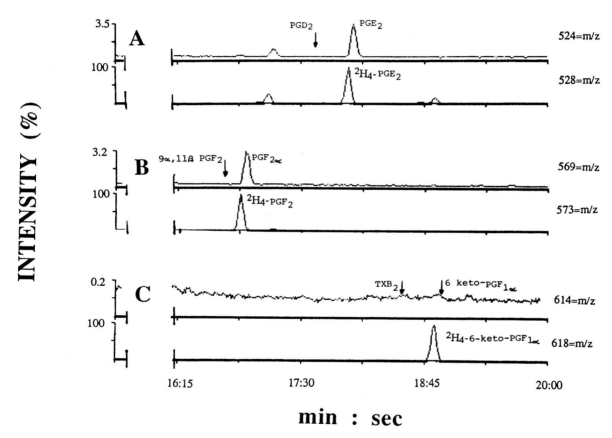

FIG. 1. Capillary gas chromatography-negative-ion mass spectrometry of prostanoids synthesized by human tracheal epithelial cells *(HTE)*. Fragment ions at m/z 524 [**A:** characteristic of prostaglandin (PG) D_2 and PGE_2), m/z 528 (**A:** derived from $^2H_4$-$PGE_2$$2H_4$ be defined?), m/z 569 (**B:** common ion generated from 9α,11β-PGF_2 and $PGF_{2\alpha}$), m/z 573 (**B:** fragment ion of $^2H_4$-PGF_2), m/z 614 [**C:** fragment ion common to thromboxane (TX) B_2 and 6-keto-$PGF_{1\alpha}$], and m/z 618 (**C:** fragment ion from $^2H_4$-6-keto-$PGF_{1\alpha}$) were monitored simultaneously. Signal intensity is normalized in each panel to that derived from the $^2H_4$ analogues employed as internal standards. Retention times in minutes and seconds are indicated along the *abscissa. Arrows* indicate the position at which PGD_2, 9α,11β-PGF_2, TXB_2, and 6-keto-$PGF_{1\alpha}$ would elute if they were present. This particular mass chromatograph reveals that PGE_2 and $PGF_{2\alpha}$ were the only prostanoids biosynthesized by HTE preincubated with serum-containing medium and stimulated with bradykinin (10^{-6} M). Similar profiles were obtained (n = 4), however, regardless of preincubation conditions and the presence or absence of stimuli (bradykinin or calcium ionophore A23187). (From Churchill L, Chilton FH, Resau JH, Bascom R, Hubbard WC, Proud D. Cyclooxygenase metabolism of endogenous arachidonic acid by cultured human tracheal epithelial cells. *Am Rev Respir Dis* 1989;140:449–459, with permission.)

duced bronchoconstriction (29). Among its *in vitro* effects are the inhibition of mast cell degranulation (30) and LTB$_4$ production by alveolar macrophages (31). PGE$_2$ has been shown to increase cough sensitivity and may play a role in the cough associated with angiotensin-converting enzyme inhibitor therapy (32). In a counter-regulatory role, PGF$_{2\alpha}$ acts as a potent bronchoconstrictor (3). Epithelial prostanoid production can be enhanced in response to a variety of inflammatory mediators, including bradykinin, platelet-activating factor (PAF), and histamine (26,33).

The predominant arachidonic acid products produced by epithelial cells may vary depending on the available substrate concentration (3), since maximal epithelial cyclooxygenase activity occurs at lower concentrations of arachidonic acid than for the lipoxygenases (6,8).

The epithelium is also capable of producing low levels of another lipid mediator: PAF. In some cell types, synthesis of PAF is directly linked to the release of arachidonic acid from the membrane phospholipid 1-*O*-alkyl-phosphatidylcholine (34,35). PAF has been reported to have important inflammatory effects in the lung, including increased vascular permeability, airway hyperreactivity, and recruitment of neutrophils and eosinophils (36). Studies of baseline PAF generation by airway epithelial cells have shown complete lack of synthesis in guinea-pig tracheal tissue (33) and low-level production in human cells, with most of the PAF remaining associated with the cell (37). Synthesis of PAF by primary bronchial epithelial cells significantly increases, however, in response to calcium ionophore A23187 (37) or ozone (38). A cultured human lung epithelial cell line (ATC-CCL-185) has also been shown to produce PAF when stimulated with phorbol myristate acetate (PMA) (39).

PEPTIDE MEDIATORS

Lipids are not the only class of mediator to be synthesized by the epithelium. Research has begun to focus on peptide products, most notably the endothelin family. Endothelins are potent constrictors of both vascular and airway smooth muscles (40). Three closely related peptides, designated endothelins 1, 2, and 3, have been described (41). BAL fluids from asthmatic patients have been reported to contain elevated levels of endothelin 1 and endothelin 3 (42,43); indeed, levels of endothelin paralleled the severity of symptoms, leading some investigators to suggest that endothelin plays a central role in the regulation of airway smooth muscle tone (44). Canine, porcine, and human tracheobronchial epithelial cells secrete these peptides (45,46), and there is evidence for increased epithelial expression of endothelin in asthma (47,48). Moreover, treatment of asthmatic bronchial epithelial cell cultures with hydrocortisone significantly decreases release of endothelin (48). An increase in synthesis of endothelin

occurs in response to a variety of proinflammatory stimuli, including thrombin (49), bacterial endotoxin (50,51), tumor necrosis factor (TNF) (50), interleukin (IL)-1, IL-2, IL-6, IL-8, and transforming growth factor (TGF)-β (52). By contrast, interferon (IFN)-γ and platelet-derived growth factor have been reported to decrease endothelin release (53). In addition to modulating bronchoconstriction, endothelin may contribute to the pathogenesis of asthma by inducing the release of both cyclooxygenase and lipoxygenase pathway products from the epithelium (54,55), as well as by stimulating smooth muscle proliferation (56) and promoting subepithelial fibrosis (57,58).

There is increasing evidence that a number of other peptide mediators are also synthesized by epithelial cells, but these have been less well investigated than endothelin. Vasopressin and substance P have been demonstrated in cultured and intact rabbit tracheal epithelium (59). In response to thrombin, vasopressin, but not substance P, is released from these cells (49). Calcitonin gene-related peptide, another neuropeptide that is colocalized with substance P in sensory nerves (60,61), has known bronchoconstrictor (62) and vasodilatory (63) functions and has been localized to serous cells in rat tracheal epithelium (64).

CATABOLIC ENZYMES/INHIBITORS

While most of this chapter focuses on epithelial production of proinflammatory mediators, it must be remembered that inflammation can also be enhanced if protective functions of the epithelium are lost. Several early studies in this regard focused on a putative epithelium-derived relaxing factor analogous to endothelium-derived relaxing factor (65). The initial suggestion of such a mediator came from the finding that removal of epithelium from canine bronchial rings markedly potentiates the bronchoconstrictor effects of histamine, 5-hydroxytryptamine, and acetylcholine (66,67). These results have been replicated in many different *in vitro* systems (68–70), but the identity of the proposed factor remains elusive (see chapter 63). It has been suggested that PGE$_2$, which is known to be produced by epithelial cells and acts as a smooth muscle relaxant, may contribute to epithelial-derived relaxation. The finding that indomethacin, a cyclooxygenase inhibitor, reverses the epithelium-dependent attenuation of contractile responses lends credence to this hypothesis (68), but some investigators have demonstrated contradictory results (71).

The protective role of the epithelium need not be confined, however, to the possible production of a mediator. Epithelial cells can also reduce effects of mediators on airway smooth muscle, glands, nerves, and vessels by actively degrading them. The best studied example of this is the ability of the epithelium to degrade peptide mediators via the actions of cell surface peptidases, such as neutral metalloendopeptidase 24.11 (NEP; also called EC 3.4.24.11, CD10, common acute lymphoblastic leukemia antigen or CALLA, and enkephalinase). Substrates for NEP include tachykinins, such as substance P and neurokinin A (72), bradykinin, and enkephalins. In animal models, NEP has been shown to modulate the effects of several of these peptides on mucus secretion, cough, and bronchoconstriction. Selective inhibitors of NEP (most notably phosphoramidon and thiorphan) potentiate tachykinin- and bradykinin-induced bronchoconstriction in rodents in a similar manner to epithelial removal (73–76). This holds true for both endogenously released and exogenously applied tachykinins. Exposure to inhaled irritants such as cigarette smoke (77) and toluene 2,4-diisocyanate (TDI) (78), an industrial chemical implicated in occupational asthma, decreases airway tissue NEP activity and increases bronchomotor response to substance P; administration of NEP inhibitors causes no further potentiatory effect. Similar observations have been made in animal models of viral respiratory infections (79,80), although, in such models, viral infection increased bronchoconstrictor, but not secretory, responses to substance P (81).

These data suggest that the shedding of epithelium in environmentally, or virally, induced asthmatic exacerbations could promote inflammation and induce hyperreactivity through the loss of a catabolic protective barrier. This idea remains controversial, however, because studies in humans have shown that, while inhibitors of NEP cause a modest increase in airway reactivity to neurokinin A, the magnitude of this shift is not significantly different between normal and asthmatic subjects, and the NEP inhibitor has no effect on baseline lung function, or bronchial responsiveness to methacholine, in asthmatic patients (82,83). Another area of controversy concerns the potential effects of glucocorticoids on the expression of NEP. Although initial studies showed that glucocorticoids upregulate NEP in an immortalized human bronchial epithelial cell line (84), more recent work has demonstrated no alteration in NEP expression upon exposure to glucocorticoids (85).

In addition to NEP, epithelial cells express cell surface aminopeptidase M (also referred to as EC 3.4.11.2, CD13, and aminopeptidase N) but not carboxypeptidase M or angiotensin-converting enzyme (85). Aminopeptidase M is expressed both by a human bronchial epithelial cell line (85) and by rat type II alveolar epithelial cells (86), and expression of the human enzyme is not modified by glucocorticoid exposure (85). Aminopeptidase M converts lysylbradykinin to bradykinin and could modify airway inflammation by degrading enkephalins (85), which have been shown to modulate the release of acetylcholine and neuropeptides from airway nerves.

The epithelium also has the ability to degrade PAF. Guinea-pig tracheal epithelial cell cultures degrade 50% of exogenously added PAF within 15 min via the deacetylation-reacylation pathway (33). Thus, the epithelium can either promote or depress inflammation through its ability to both synthesize and degrade PAF.

Another protease, cathepsin B, is stored as an inactive proenzyme in the lysosomes of epithelial cells (87). It is secreted and converted, via the actions of neutrophil elastase, to the active form that is usually found in airway secretions. Cathepsin B hydrolyzes extracellular matrix proteins (88) and may mediate the airway damage seen in emphysema, chronic bronchitis, and bronchiectasis, since it is found in increased levels in BAL fluids and sputum of patients with these diseases (89–91).

Airway epithelial cells not only express catabolic enzymes but also produce protease inhibitors. These include cystatin C, the major inhibitor of cathepsin B (87), as well as secretory leukocyte protease inhibitor (SLPI) and elastase-specific inhibitor (ESI or elafin) (92), which regulate the destructive activity of leukocyte elastase in the airway.

It is clear, therefore, that the contribution of the epithelium to the regulation of airway inflammation during asthma can be quite complex. Initial activation of the epithelium may produce a range of inflammatory mediators and cytokines (see below) but, at the same time, the epithelium can regulate the activity of several mediators. Subsequent loss of the epithelium results in a reduction of mediator generation but also in an imbalance in this regulatory function.

CYTOKINE RELEASE

Cytokines play a central role in the pathogenesis of lung inflammation (93). While their production has classically been ascribed to lymphocytes and macrophages, it is now known that numerous cell types within the airways synthesize a broad variety of cytokines. Epithelial cells can be an active contributor to the cytokine network in the lung, and several relevant stimuli can result in the generation of epithelial cytokines that can act to modulate the inflammatory response (1). Although there is general agreement regarding the ability of epithelial cells to synthesize several cytokines, including IL-6, IL-8, IL-11, granulocyte-macrophage colony-stimulating factor (GM-CSF), G-CSF, and the chemokine RANTES (regulated on activation, normal T cell expressed and secreted), there is still some dispute about the full spectrum of cytokines that can be produced by epithelial cells.

GM-CSF, one of the most extensively studied epithelial cytokines, could contribute to the inflammation that is characteristic of asthma via its abilities to prolong eosinophil survival and to activate neutrophils, eosinophils, and macrophages to display enhanced cytotoxic activity, generation of mediators, and phagocytosis (94–97). The first suggestion of GM-CSF production by epithelium was the demonstration that supernatants from human nasal epithelial cell cultures demonstrated hematopoietic activity, promoting the formation of granulocyte-macrophage and metachromatic cell colonies from progenitor cells (98). Moreover, cells obtained from atopic individuals displayed a higher level of activity than those from nonatopics. GM-CSF has since been shown to be constitutively synthesized and released by airway epithelial cells *in vitro* (99,100). The levels of GM-CSF produced are clearly of biological relevance, since conditioned media from human bronchial epithelial cells markedly prolong survival of eosinophils in culture and this effect is abrogated by antibodies to GM-CSF (101). The constitutive production of GM-CSF by human epithelial cells *in vitro* is inhibited by exposure to glucocorticoids (99). Increased *in vitro* production of GM-CSF is seen upon exposure to several stimuli, including histamine (99), IL-1 (99,102) (Fig. 2), and common respiratory viruses (103, 104). In rats, surfactant protein A has also been shown to upregulate secretion of GM-CSF (105). There is some controversy, however, regarding responsiveness to lipopolysaccharide, which has been reported to increase GM-CSF release from rat tracheal epithelial cells (106) but has no effect on human cells (99).

Levels of GM-CSF are significantly elevated in the BAL fluids of patients with asthma, as compared with normal subjects (107). This difference also holds true for bronchial biopsy specimens from asthmatic patients, where increased GM-CSF gene expression is detected and increased protein production has been observed by direct immunohistochemical staining of the epithelium

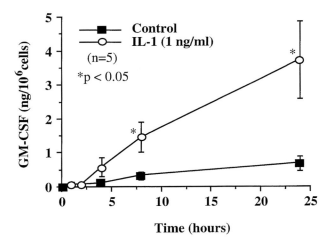

FIG. 2. Kinetics of granulocyte-macrophage colony-stimulating factor (GM-CSF) release from human tracheal epithelial cells *(HTE)*. Conditioned media was collected from HTE cultured in serum-supplemented medium with or without interleukin 1 (1 ng/mL) for the time periods indicated and was assayed for GM-CSF activity. *Values* represent the mean ± standard error. (From Churchill L, Friedman B, Schleimer RP, Proud D. Production of granulocyte–macrophage colony-stimulating factor by cultured human tracheal epithelial cells. *Immunology* 1992;75:189–195, with the permission of Blackwell Science Ltd.)

(108–110). In addition, a correlation between GM-CSF expression and the degree of eosinophil infiltration of the bronchial epithelium has been reported (111). Glucocorticoids have been shown to downregulate expression of GM-CSF in bronchial epithelial cells from asthmatics, both when cells are exposed to glucocorticoids *in vitro* (108,109) and after inhalation therapy *in vivo* (110–112). The mechanisms by which epithelial expression of GM-CSF is increased during asthma are unknown, but stimulation by IL-1 may play some role in this regard, since IL-1 levels are increased in the airways of asthmatic patients (107). Marini et al. (113) observed that nedocromil sodium, an inhaled anti-inflammatory agent useful in the treatment of asthma, reduces the IL-1-induced increase in epithelial-derived GM-CSF by more than 40%, but it has no effect on constitutive production of this cytokine; these data, however, have not been reproduced and remain controversial.

There have been reports that epithelial cells produce other CSFs capable of supporting the development of granulocytic or monocytic cell populations. These include G-CSF (114,115) and CSF-1 (116). M-CSF may also be produced, but this needs further clarification (117,118).

Epithelial cells also generate other cytokines that have been postulated to contribute to the asthmatic disease process. IL-8 gene expression has been established in several transformed human bronchial epithelial cell lines (114,116,119,120) as well as in primary cell cultures (100). An increase in IL-8 synthesis is seen in bronchial epithelial cells of asthmatic patients (108,109,111). This intriguing observation may be clinically relevant because IL-8 functions as a chemoattractant for neutrophils (121) and some T lymphocytes (122,123) and has the potential to be chemotactic for eosinophils that have been preexposed to GM-CSF or IL-3 (124). Each of these cell types has been implicated in the pathophysiology of asthma. IL-6, a factor involved in T-cell activation and proliferation (125), is also produced by bronchial epithelial cells (100,114,116,126) and, in a comparable way to IL-8, its expression is increased in bronchial biopsy specimens of asthmatic patients (108,109). BAL collections from symptomatic asthmatics show increased levels of IL-6 (107), as do supernatants from TDI-stimulated bronchial epithelial cells (127). The secretion of IL-6 is reported to be vectorial in nature, with release from epithelial monolayers exposed to histamine being primarily in the apical direction (128). The release of IL-6 in asthma actually might represent a normal healing response in the dysfunctional airway and be an attempt by the host to normalize airway physiology. This is supported by the finding that transgenic mice that overexpress IL-6 in airway epithelial cells demonstrate hyporesponsiveness to methacholine, despite the development of a chronic peribronchial lymphocytic infiltrate (129). IL-1β and TNF-α enhance epithelial cell production of IL-6 and IL-8 (100, 119), whereas inhaled glucocorticoid therapy attenuates expression of these cytokines *in vivo* (109,111). In contrast, glucocorticoid exposure of cultured cells has minimal effects on IL-8 and IL-6 production (114). Nedocromil sodium has been reported to inhibit IL-1-induced production of IL-8 by primary human bronchial epithelial cells in a manner analogous to its effect on GM-CSF production (130).

In addition to producing GM-CSF, IL-6, and IL-8, epithelial cells also produce IL-11, a cytokine with IL-6-like properties (131). At baseline, IL-11 secretion is low, but an increase is seen upon stimulation with IL-1 or TGF-β. Retinoic acid differentially regulates these stimuli, with inhibition of IL-1-stimulated IL-11 release and synergistic augmentation of TGF-β-stimulated release (131). IL-11 may play a significant role in airway diseases, such as asthma. Increased levels of IL-11 have been detected in the nasal secretions of children with upper respiratory symptoms, and administration of IL-11 to mice induces pronounced airways hyperresponsiveness (132).

Another chemokine that has become the focus of recent attention is RANTES. It has been established that, whereas unstimulated human lung epithelial cells produce little or no RANTES, production of this chemokine is increased in response to a variety of stimuli, including IL-1, TNF-α, and IFN-γ (133,134). The combination of TNF-α and IFN-γ is synergistic in inducing RANTES expression (133). Induction of RANTES expression is probably due to transcriptional activation, since mRNA levels for RANTES are markedly upregulated and, once induced, the mRNA is quite stable (133,134). Pretreatment with glucocorticoids inhibits cytokine induction of both mRNA and protein for RANTES (133,134). The production of RANTES by stimulated epithelial cells could contribute to the recruitment of eosinophils to the airways of asthmatics, since RANTES is chemotactic for eosinophils, memory T lymphocytes, and monocytes (135,136), and intradermal injection of RANTES into dogs (137) or humans (138) causes a profound eosinophilic infiltrate. Elevated levels of this chemokine are, in fact, found in BAL fluids of allergic asthmatics, compared with normal subjects (139), and RANTES and IL-5 have been identified as the major chemoattractant stimuli for eosinophils in asthmatic lungs (140).

In addition to RANTES and IL-8, epithelial cells produce other members of both the C-C and C-X-C chemokine families that may contribute to airway inflammation. Monocyte chemoattractant protein (MCP)-1, a member of the C-C chemokine family that is chemotactic for monocytes, basophils (141), and memory T lymphocytes (142), is produced by epithelial cells *in vitro* (143). Increased epithelial expression of MCP-1 has been observed by immunohistochemistry in biopsy specimens of patients with atopic asthma (144), and increased levels of this chemokine are also seen in BAL fluids of allergic asthmatics, compared with normal subjects (139). Increased levels of MCP-1 are also seen in the bronchial epithelium of pa-

tients with idiopathic pulmonary fibrosis (145). Eotaxin is another C-C chemokine that was first identified in the bronchoalveolar lavage fluid of allergen-challenged guinea-pigs (146). Both guinea-pig (147) and human (148,149) genes have now been cloned, and it has been shown that eotaxin is produced by human epithelial cells stimulated with TNF-α and IFN-γ (148,149). Increased production of eotaxin is also observed in epithelium from nasal polyps (148). This chemokine has attracted considerable interest because it is a selective chemoattractant for eosinophils (148,149). The C-X-C chemokines, GROα and GROγ, which are chemotactic for neutrophils, have also been reported to be produced by cultured epithelial cells (143).

Epithelial cells make one additional chemoattractant cytokine that does not belong to either the C-C or C-X-C chemokine families, namely, IL-16 (150,151). Levels of this cytokine, which is a selective chemoattractant for CD4-+ cells, such as lymphocytes and eosinophils, are increased in BAL fluids from antigen-challenged asthmatics (152), raising the possibility that IL-16 may contribute to the increased numbers of CD4-+ cells seen in the airway mucosa of asthmatics.

The search for additional cytokines elaborated by the airway epithelium is an active area of investigation from which conflicting data have arisen. For example, recent studies have reported the production of TGF-β₁ and TGF-β₂ from cultured epithelial cells (153,154), and immunohistochemical localization studies have also shown the presence of TGF-β protein in human bronchial epithelial cells (155,156). A study in murine lung, however, while also detecting the presence of TGF-β₁, TGF-β₂, and TGF-β₃ proteins in epithelial cells, found mRNA transcripts for each of these isoforms in smooth muscle and connective tissue cells adjacent to the epithelium, but not in epithelial cells themselves (157). This raises the possibility that this cytokine is not synthesized in the epithelium, but that product from adjacent cells is internalized when TGF-β acts on the epithelium. Further studies are necessary to clarify this. Similarly, several studies have identified the presence of mRNA for IL-1 in epithelial cells but, to date, protein product has been detected primarily upon cell lysis (158) or upon exposure to cytotoxic stimuli, such as TDI (127). IL-10, also known as cytokine synthesis inhibitory factor, is present in epithelial cells obtained by bronchial brushings of normal, healthy subjects and is downregulated in patients with cystic fibrosis (159). To date, this cytokine is not detectable in immortalized epithelial cell lines (D. Proud, unpublished data). Production of other cytokines, such as TNF-α (160) and macrophage inflammatory protein 2 (161), by airway epithelial cells is still somewhat controversial and confirmation by additional research is needed.

Although it is apparent that proinflammatory cytokines, such as IL-1 and TNF-α, are among the most potent stimuli for epithelial cytokine production, other stimuli may be of equal or greater importance in triggering epithelial cytokine generation during asthma. For example, viral infections of the airway, long considered an important trigger of asthma exacerbations, induce production of proinflammatory cytokines by epithelial cells. Infection of epithelial cells by rhinoviruses, the most common upper respiratory viruses experienced by humans, stimulates secretion of IL-8 (Fig. 3), IL-6, and GM-CSF within 24 h of infection but has no adverse effects on cell viability. Induction of IL-8 protein levels parallels rhinovirus replication during the first 24 h (104). IL-8 production also increases upon infection of epithelial cells with influenza virus (162). Respiratory syncytial virus (RSV), the most common cause of lower respiratory tract infection in infants, causes a sequential generation of cytokines. IL-8 gene expression occurs soon after infection (during the "eclipse" phase) with release of the cytokine within the first 24 h, whereas IL-6 and GM-CSF are not detected until 96 h after RSV infection (during the replicative phase) (103). IL-11 (131) and soluble TNF receptor type I (163) are also released from RSV-infected epithelium.

Bacterial infections also mediate cytokine production by airway epithelium. Pertussis is characterized by destruction of ciliated epithelial cells lining the large airways, and a muramyl peptide known as tracheal cytotoxin has been implicated as the causative agent in this cytopathology (164). Recent work in a hamster model has shown that the toxic effects of tracheal cytotoxin may be mediated by IL-1α produced by tracheal epithelial cells (165). Bacterial alterations of epithelial cytokine production may have important implications for other diseases in addition to asthma. For example, cystic fibrosis (CF) is characterized by colonization of the airways with *Staphylococcus aureus* and *Pseudomonas aeruginosa*, and by a chronic recruitment of neutrophils to the lung, resulting in a progressive, destructive bronchitis. *Pseudomonas* infections are known to stimulate IL-8 expression in airway epithelial cells (166,167), providing a possible explanation for the neutrophil influx seen in the lungs of patients with CF. Other recent investigations of CF have shown that IL-6 and IL-8 are secreted under baseline conditions by an immortalized CF respiratory epithelial cell line (168), and their secretion is increased by exposure to IL-1β and neutrophil elastase (168,169). As mentioned above, epithelial cells regulate elastase-mediated inflammation and destruction through the production of inhibitors, including SLPI and elastase-specific inhibitor. IL-1β and TNF-α induce significant expression of these antiproteases (92). In a study of 20 individuals with CF, therapy with aerosolized recombinant SLPI resulted in a significant reduction in IL-8 in BAL fluid, and there was a clear association between BAL active neutrophil elastase and IL-8 levels (170). IL-8 produced by epithelial cells has also been implicated in the pathogenesis of asbestos-associated lung diseases (171).

REACTIVE OXYGEN SPECIES/NITRIC OXIDE

Although reactive oxygen species are important mediators of inflammation and tissue injury, it is only recently that the role of these mediators in airway diseases, such as asthma, has become a focus of significant research. It has been suggested that airway inflammation is associated with the generation of reactive oxygen species that ultimately contribute to the pathologic changes seen in asthma (for example, epithelial shedding and hypersecretion of mucus) (172,173). In support of this is the demonstration that catalase is partially protective against the cytotoxic effects of PAF-activated eosinophils on tracheal epithelial cells (174). Macrophages, eosinophils, and neutrophils are classically invoked as major sources of reactive oxygen species (175,176), but it is now known that epithelial cells also generate these products. Hydrogen peroxide is released by guinea-pig tracheal and bovine bronchial epithelial cells in response to PAF or the protein kinase C activator, PMA (172,177,178). Inactivation of protein kinase C abolishes the PAF- and PMA-induced release in the guinea-pig model (172,177). In addition, cigarette smoke promotes production of hydrogen peroxide and superoxide anion at the apical surface of rat tracheal explants (179). The amount of hydrogen peroxide released by epithelial cells is approximately 100-fold less

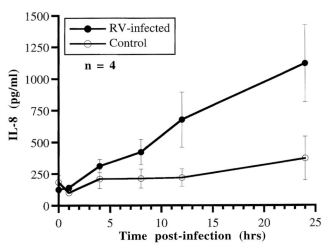

FIG. 3. Time course of interleukin 8 production after infection of the BEAS-2B respiratory epithelial cell line with rhinovirus 14. Data are expressed as the mean ± standard error; $p < 0.05$, compared with control values. Control data are those from uninfected cells at the same time points. (From Subauste MC, Jacoby DB, Richards SM, Proud D. Infection of a human respiratory epithelial cell line with rhinovirus: induction of cytokine release and modulation of susceptibility to infection by cytokine exposure. *J Clin Invest* 1995;96:549–557, by copyright permission of the American Society for Clinical Investigation.)

than that generated by macrophages (180), but the total amount derived from the entire respiratory epithelium may be a significant contributor to inflammatory states. Indeed, an autocrine effect of epithelial production of hydrogen peroxide must also be considered, since hydrogen peroxide has been shown to upregulate epithelial production of IL-8 (181).

Nitric oxide (NO) is an important signaling molecule that initially came to prominence when it was identified as being responsible for the vasodilatory effects of what had previously been called endothelium-derived relaxing factor. In the last few years, attention has begun to focus on the potential role of NO in airway diseases. Production of NO occurs via the actions of the enzyme NO synthase, which exists in at least three isoforms, sometimes referred to as the constitutive form (cNOS), the neuronal form (nNOS) and the inducible form (iNOS). It has recently been shown that both cNOS and iNOS can be produced from cultured respiratory epithelial cells (182,183) and that lipopolysaccharide, IL-1β, and zymosan-activated serum each enhance NO production by epithelial cells. It has also been reported that IFN-γ and TNF-α may cause an increase in NO formation (182), but conflicting data exist in this regard (184). Immunohistochemical staining of transbronchial biopsy specimens from asthmatic patients has convincingly demonstrated increased iNOS activity compared with nonasthmatic controls (185), and levels of NO in exhaled air are also increased in asthmatic patients (186,187). It remains unclear, however, whether increased production of NO in asthma is primarily beneficial or if it exacerbates the inflammatory state. Thus, while inhaled NO has bronchodilatory effects, leading to the suggestion that it may be a contributor to the putative epithelium-derived relaxing factor discussed previously (188,189), it has been hypothesized that NO derived from airway epithelial cells may serve to amplify and perpetuate asthmatic inflammation (190). NO is a potent vasodilator in the bronchial circulation and could exacerbate plasma leakage by increasing blood flow to affected postcapillary venules. Moreover, NO has been reported to have suppressive effects on the T-helper type 1 subtype of lymphocytes (191), leading to possible proliferation of T-helper type 2 cells and increased production of IL-4 (which is responsible for local production of immunoglobulin E) and IL-5 (which promotes eosinophil recruitment). In addition, NO is capable of interacting with superoxide anion to produce highly toxic peroxynitrite radicals that could contribute to tissue damage in asthma.

Epithelial cells not only produce reactive oxygen species, but they also have mechanisms to degrade them. Cultured epithelial cells are known to contain manganese superoxide dismutase (SOD), copper/zinc SOD, catalase, and the glutathione redox cycle (192). Expression of manganese SOD can be induced by exposure to TNF-α (192). Antioxidant gene expression can also be induced in epithelial cells in response to hyperoxia (193) or influenza virus (194). In contrast to endothelial cells, where the major mechanism for scavenging hydrogen peroxide is the glutathione oxidation-reduction cycle, airway epithelial cells use a catalase-dependent pathway in addition to the glutathione redox cycle (192,195). Moreover, epithelial cell scavenging ability is polar, with faster consumption of hydrogen peroxide at the apical surface (196).

EXPRESSION OF ADHESION MOLECULES

Adhesion molecules play a central role in mediating interactions between leukocytes and cellular barriers. Although leukocyte–endothelial interactions have been extensively characterized (197), it is only in recent years that investigators have begun to focus on the mechanisms by which leukocytes interact with, and migrate through, the respiratory epithelium. The spectrum of adhesion molecules expressed by epithelial cells is by no means fully defined. Epithelial cells apparently do not express E-selectin or vascular cell adhesion molecule-1, but do show marked expression of intercellular adhesion molecule (ICAM)-1. The first demonstration of the potential importance of epithelial ICAM-1 in this cell recruitment was provided using a nonhuman primate model of asthma, in which ICAM-1 expression was increased on both endothelium and airway epithelium in response to antigen inhalation (198). More recently, it has been shown not only that ICAM-1 expression is enhanced on epithelial cells of asthmatic patients compared to normals or to patients with chronic bronchitis, but that ICAM-1 expression correlates with disease severity (199). In addition to being the receptor for the majority of rhinovirus serotypes (200,201), ICAM-1 is the counterligand for the β2-integrins (CD11/CD18) that are expressed on the surface of leukocytes (202). The interaction of ICAM-1 with β2-integrins results in strong adhesion. Mediators and cytokines that play a role in inflammation in the lung, including histamine, IL-1β, TNF-α, and IFN-γ, have all been shown to augment ICAM-1 expression in both primary human airway epithelial cells and immortalized epithelial cell lines (203–206). The effects of viral infection are variable. Although parainfluenza virus infection also results in upregulation of ICAM-1 and increased neutrophil adhesion to epithelium (207), infection with rhinovirus does not alter ICAM-1 expression or leukocyte adhesion (104). Interestingly, several studies have shown that antibodies against ICAM-1 only partially inhibit leukocyte adhesion to epithelial cells under a variety of experimental conditions, suggesting an as yet unidentified, ICAM-1-independent pathway for leukocyte binding to epithelial cells (203,204, 207,208). Further support for this concept comes from studies with mice in which the genes for both P-selectin and ICAM-1 were mutated, yet neutrophil emigration into the alveolar spaces of these mice during acute *Streptococcus pneumoniae* infection was normal (209).

Despite the evidence that additional epithelial surface ligands may play a role in leukocyte adhesion to, and migration through, the respiratory epithelium, the phenotype of adhesion molecules on epithelial cells has not been fully characterized. In addition to E-cadherin, which plays a role in adhesive interactions between epithelial cells, it is known that several β_1-integrins, predominantly $\alpha_2\beta_1$, $\alpha_3\beta_1$, and $\alpha_6\beta_1$, are expressed on epithelial cells (210,211). These β_1-integrins are presumably primarily involved in anchorage to structural proteins of the basement membrane, such as collagen, fibronectin, and laminin. Other adhesion molecules that are known to be expressed on human bronchial epithelial cells include leukocyte function-associated antigen 3 (CD58) and CD44, the receptor for hyaluronic acid, but their role in modulating leukocyte adhesion to epithelial cells remains uninvestigated (206).

IMMUNOREGULATION

Airway epithelial cells express class II major histocompatibility (MHC) antigens at all levels of the bronchial tree (212). Normal airway epithelium has relatively low levels of human leukocyte antigen (HLA)-DR on the cell membrane, but expression is increased upon exposure to IFN-γ (213,214). TNF-α may also have a role in potentiating the effects of IFN-γ (214). Bronchial epithelial cells of patients with asthma show significantly increased expression of HLA-DR in comparison with cells from normal subjects (199,215), and similar results are seen in nasal epithelial cells of patients with nasal polyps (216).

As the function of class II HLA antigens is to regulate the immune response by modulating the interaction between T-helper cells and foreign antigenic determinants, this raises the possibility that epithelial cells may act as antigen-presenting cells in their associations with lymphocytes. Support for a role of epithelial cells as immune accessory cells is provided by the demonstration of their ability to stimulate proliferation of CD4 and CD8 T cells in mixed lymphocyte cultures (217). Moreover, it has been shown that IFN-γ-treated epithelial cells are capable of presenting antigens to autologous T lymphocytes in an HLA-DR-restricted manner (218). Although less efficient as antigen-presenting cells than macrophages, it is attractive to suggest that epithelial cells may play a role in antigen presentation in respiratory viral infections. It has also been postulated that increased MHC expression on epithelial cells in transplanted lungs mediates rejection and consequent obliterative bronchiolitis (219).

REPAIR AND REMODELING

Inflammatory injury to the airway often results in sloughing of epithelial cells and a partially denuded basement membrane. Repair of any such defect depends on epithelial cell-fibroblast interactions and on the production of extracellular matrix proteins. Bronchial epithelial cells produce at least two matrix glycoproteins: fibronectin and tenascin (220,221). Fibronectin acts not only as a matrix component but as a substrate for cell adhesion during tissue repair and fibrosis. Moreover, fibronectin has been reported to be a chemoattractant stimulus for fibroblasts (220). Tenascin shows structural homology to fibronectin and is expressed in tissues during wound healing and inflammation (221). It has also been reported that immunoreactive tenascin is increased in airway tissues of patients with asthma, and that the amount of tenascin detected correlates with disease severity (222). Epithelial production of fibronectin and tenascin can be modified upon exposure to several cytokines, including TGF-β (223), IFN-γ, and TNF-α (221).

Not only do epithelial cells influence fibroblast migration (220,224), but they affect DNA synthesis (225) and matrix production from fibroblasts (226). Many epithelial-derived mediators and cytokines, including IL-1, IL-6, and PGE$_2$, directly alter extracellular matrix production (227).

Epithelial cells themselves also migrate chemotactically to the fibronectin produced by fibroblasts or by other epithelial cells (228). This is important because the basal cells of the epithelium are relatively resistant to insult, and the epithelial damage that is characteristic of asthma is characterized by a split at the junction between basal cells and columnar cells (229). Thus, epithelial repair may involve cells at the margin of a damaged area being recruited into the field of injury by products produced by the remaining basal cells within the area (230).

CONCLUSIONS

Our understanding of the airway epithelium has evolved from a static viewpoint invoking its function as simply a physical barrier to a much more active description of its central role in the inflammatory process. Epithelial cells generate a wide variety of lipid mediators, peptide products, and cytokines that act to modulate airway tone, regulate secretions, and attract circulating leukocytes to the airway. Inflammation is both promoted and inhibited by the actions of the epithelium. Alterations in the release of specific epithelial cell products and in the expression of surface markers have been extensively described in clinical entities such as asthma and are likely to play a significant role in the pathogenesis of the disease state. These derangements may serve as future targets for therapeutic intervention.

REFERENCES

1. Proud D. The epithelial cell as a target and effector cell in airway inflammation. In: Holgate ST, Austen KF, Lichtenstein LM, Kay AB,

eds. *Asthma: physiology, immunopharmacology, and treatment (fourth international symposium)*. London: Academic, 1993;199–209.

2. Adler KB, Fischer BM, Wright DT, Cohn LA, Becker S. Interactions between respiratory epithelial cells and cytokines: relationships to lung inflammation. *Ann NY Acad Sci* 1994;725:128–145.

3. Holtzman MJ. Arachidonic acid metabolism in airway epithelial cells. *Annu Rev Physiol* 1992;54:303–329.

4. Holtzman MJ, Aizawa H, Nadel JA, Goetzl EJ. Selective generation of leukotriene B₄ by tracheal epithelial cells from dogs. *Biochem Biophys Res Commun* 1983;114:1071–1076.

5. Eling TE, Danilowicz RM, Henke DC, Sivarajah K, Yankaskas JR, Boucher RC. Arachidonic acid metabolism by canine tracheal epithelial cells: product formation and relationship to chloride secretion. *J Biol Chem* 1986;261:12,841–12,849.

6. Holtzman MJ, Hansbrough JR, Rosen GD, Turk J. Uptake, release and novel species-dependent oxygenation of arachidonic acid in human and animal airway epithelial cells. *Biochim Biophys Acta* 1988;963: 401–413.

7. Alpert SE, Kramer CM, Brashler JR, Bach MK. Generation of lipoxygenase metabolites of arachidonic acid by monolayer cultures of tracheal epithelial cells and intact tracheal segments from rabbits. *Exp Lung Res* 1990;16:211–233.

8. Hansbrough JR, Atlas AB, Turk J, Holtzman MJ. Arachidonate 12-lipoxygenase and cyclooxygenase: PGE isomerase are predominant pathways for oxygenation in bovine tracheal epithelial cells. *Am J Respir Cell Mol Biol* 1989;1:237–244.

9. Hunter JA, Finkbeiner WE, Nadel JA, Goetzl EJ, Holtzman MJ. Predominant generation of 15-lipoxygenase metabolites of arachidonic acid by epithelial cells from human trachea. *Proc Natl Acad Sci USA* 1985;82:4633–4637.

10. Kumlin M, Hamberg M, Granström E, et al. 15(S)-Hydroxyeicosatetraenoic acid is the major arachidonic acid metabolite in human bronchi: association with airway epithelium. *Arch Biochem Biophys* 1990;282:254–262.

11. Shannon VR, Chanez P, Bousquet J, Holtzman MJ. Histochemical evidence for induction of arachidonate 15-lipoxygenase in airway disease. *Am Rev Respir Dis* 1993;147:1024–1028.

12. Murray JJ, Tonnel AB, Brash AR, et al. Release of prostaglandin D₂ into human airways during acute antigen challenge. *N Engl J Med* 1986;315:800–804.

13. Holtzman MJ, Pentland A, Baenziger NL, Hansbrough JR. Heterogeneity of cellular expression of arachidonate 15-lipoxygenase: implications for biological activity. *Biochim Biophys Acta* 1989;1003: 204–208.

14. Goetzl E, Phillips MJ, Gold WM. Stimulus specificity of the generation of leukotrienes by dog mastocytoma cells. *J Exp Med* 1983;158: 731–737.

15. Marom Z, Shelhamer JH, Sun F, Kaliner M. Human airway monohydroxyeicosatetraenoic acid generation and mucus release. *J Clin Invest* 1983;72:122–127.

16. Lai CKW, Polosa R, Holgate ST. Effect of 15-(s)-hydroxyeicosatetraenoic acid on allergen-induced asthmatic responses. *Am Rev Respir Dis* 1990;141:1423–1427.

17. Shak S, Perez HD, Goldstein IM. A novel dioxygenation product of arachidonic acid possesses potent chemotactic activity for human polymorphonuclear leukocytes. *J Biol Chem* 1983;258:14,948–14,953.

18. Kirsch CM, Sigal E, Djokic TD, Graf PD, Nadel JA. An *in vivo* chemotaxis assay in the dog trachea: evidence for chemotactic activity of 8,15-diHETE. *J Appl Physiol* 1988;64:1792–1795.

19. Serhan CN, Nicolaou KC, Webber SE, et al. Lipoxin A: stereochemistry and biosynthesis. *J Biol Chem* 1986;261:16,340–16,345.

20. Hansson A, Serhan CN, Haeggström J, Ingelman-Sundberg M, Samuelsson B. Activation of protein kinase C by lipoxin A and other eicosanoids: intracellular action of oxygenation products of arachidonic acid. *Biochem Biophys Res Commun* 1986;134:1215–1222.

21. Ramstedt U, Ng J, Wigzell H, Serhan CN, Samuelsson B. Action of novel eicosanoids lipoxin A and B on human natural killer cell cytotoxicity: effects on intracellular cAMP and target cell binding. *J Immunol* 1985;135:3434–3438.

22. Sigal E, Nadel JA. The airway epithelium and arachidonic acid 15-lipoxygenase. *Am Rev Respir Dis* 1991;143:S71–S74.

23. Dahlén S-E, Raud J, Serhan CN, Björk J, Samuelsson B. Biological activities of lipoxin A include lung strip contraction and dilation of arterioles *in vivo*. *Acta Physiol Scand* 1987;130:643–647.

24. Dahlén S-E, Franzén L, Raud J, et al. Actions of lipoxin A₄ and related compounds in smooth muscle preparations and on the microcirculation *in vivo*. In: Wong PYK, Serhan CN, eds. *Lipoxins: biosynthesis, chemistry, and biological activities*. New York: Plenum, 1988;107–130.

25. Duniec ZM, Eling TE, Jetten AM, Gray TE, Nettesheim P. Arachidonic acid metabolism in normal and transformed rat tracheal epithelial cells and its possible role in the regulation of cell proliferation. *Exp Lung Res* 1989;15:391–408.

26. Churchill L, Chilton FH, Resau JH, Bascom R, Hubbard WC, Proud D. Cyclooxygenase metabolism of endogenous arachidonic acid by cultured human tracheal epithelial cells. *Am Rev Respir Dis* 1989;140: 449–459.

27. Marom Z, Shelhamer JH, Kaliner M. Effects of arachidonic acid, monohydroxyeicosatetraenoic acid and prostaglandins on the release of mucus glycoproteins from human airways *in vitro*. *J Clin Invest* 1981;67:1695–1702.

28. Pavord ID, Wong CS, Williams J, Tattersfield AE. Effect of inhaled prostaglandin E₂ on allergen-induced asthma. *Am Rev Respir Dis* 1993;148:87–90.

29. Melillo E, Wooley KL, Manning PJ, Watson RM, O'Byrne PM. Effect of inhaled PGE₂ on exercise-induced bronchoconstriction in asthmatic subjects. *Am J Respir Crit Care Med* 1994;149:1138–1141.

30. Peters SP, Schulman ES, Schleimer RP, MacGlashan DW Jr, Newball HH, Lichtenstein LM. Dispersed human lung mast cells: pharmacologic aspects and comparison with human lung tissue fragments. *Am Rev Respir Dis* 1982;126:1034–1039.

31. Christman BW, Christman JW. Prostaglandin E₂ decreases leukotriene B₄ production by A23187-stimulated rat alveolar macrophages: analysis by gas chromatography/mass spectrometry. *Am Rev Respir Dis* 1990;141:A393.

32. Choudry NB, Fuller RW, Pride NB. Sensitivity of the human cough reflex: effect of inflammatory mediators prostaglandin E₂, bradykinin, and histamine. *Am Rev Respir Dis* 1989;140:137–141.

33. Churchill L, Chilton FH, Proud D. Interaction of platelet-activating factor with cultured guinea pig tracheal epithelial cells. *Biochem J* 1991;276:593–598.

34. Albert DH, Snyder F. Release of arachidonic acid from 1-alkyl-2-acyl-*sn*-glycero-3-phosphocholine, a precursor of platelet-activating factor, in rat alveolar macrophages. *Biochim Biophys Acta* 1984;796: 92–101.

35. Lee TC. Biosynthesis of platelet activating factor: substrate specificity of 1-alkyl-2-lyso-*sn*-glycero-3-phosphocholine:acetyl CoA acetyltransferase in rat spleen microsomes. *J Biol Chem* 1985;260: 10,952–10,955.

36. McManus LM, Deavers SI. Platelet activating factor in pulmonary pathobiology. *Clin Chest Med* 1989;10:107–118.

37. Holtzman MJ, Ferdman B, Bohrer A, Turk J. Synthesis of the 1-*O*-hexadecyl molecular species of platelet-activating factor by airway epithelial and vascular endothelial cells. *Biochem Biophys Res Commun* 1991;177:357–364.

38. Samet JM, Noah TL, Devlin RB, et al. Effect of ozone on platelet-activating factor production in phorbol-differentiated HL60 cells, a human bronchial epithelial cell line (BEAS S6), and primary human bronchial epithelial cells. *Am J Respir Cell Mol Biol* 1992;7:514–522.

39. Salari H, Wong A. Generation of platelet activating factor (PAF) by a human lung epithelial cell line. *Eur J Pharmacol* 1990;175:253–259.

40. Uchida Y, Ninomiya H, Saotome M, et al. Endothelin, a novel vasoconstrictor peptide, as potent bronchoconstrictor. *Eur J Pharmacol* 1988;154:227–228.

41. Sakurai T, Yanagisawa M, Masaki T. Molecular characterization of endothelin receptors. *Trends Pharmacol Sci* 1992;13:103–108.

42. Mattoli S, Soloperto M, Marini M, Fasoli A. Levels of endothelin in the bronchoalveolar lavage fluid of patients with symptomatic asthma and reversible airflow obstruction. *J Allergy Clin Immunol* 1991;88: 376–384.

43. Marini M, Fasoli A, Mattoli S. Release of endothelin in the airways of patients with symptomatic asthma and reversible airflow obstruction. *Am Rev Respir Dis* 1991;143:A158.

44. Nomura A, Uchida Y, Kameyama M, Saotome M, Oki K, Hasegawa S. Endothelin and bronchial asthma. *Lancet* 1989;1:747–748.

45. Black PN, Ghatei MA, Takahashi K, et al. Formation of endothelin by cultured airway epithelial cells. *FEBS Lett* 1989;255:129–132.

46. Mattoli S, Mezzetti M, Riva G, Allegra L, Fasoli A. Specific binding of endothelin on human bronchial smooth muscle cells in culture and

secretion of endothelin-like material from bronchial epithelial cells. *Am J Respir Cell Mol Biol* 1990;3:145–151.

47. Springall DR, Howarth PH, Counihan H, Djukanovic R, Holgate ST, Polak JM. Endothelin immunoreactivity of airway epithelium in asthmatic patients. *Lancet* 1991;337:697–701.

48. Vittori E, Marini M, Fasoli A, De Franchis R, Mattoli S. Increased expression of endothelin in bronchial epithelial cells of asthmatic patients and effect of corticosteroids. *Am Rev Respir Dis* 1992;146:1320–1325.

49. Rennick RE, Milner P, Burnstock G. Thrombin stimulates release of endothelin and vasopressin, but not substance P, from isolated rabbit tracheal epithelial cells. *Eur J Pharmacol* 1993;230:367–370.

50. Nakano J, Takizawa H, Ohtoshi T, et al. Endotoxin and pro-inflammatory cytokines stimulate endothelin-1 expression and release by airway epithelial cells. *Clin Exp Allergy* 1994;24:330–336.

51. Ninomiya H, Uchida Y, Ishii Y, et al. Endotoxin stimulates endothelin release from cultured epithelial cells of guinea-pig trachea. *Eur J Pharmacol* 1991;203:299–302.

52. Endo T, Uchida Y, Matsumoto H, et al. Regulation of endothelin-1 synthesis in cultured guinea pig airway epithelial cells by various cytokines. *Biochem Biophys Res Commun* 1992;186:1594–1599.

53. Markewitz BA, Kohan DE, Michael JR. Endothelin-1 synthesis, receptors, and signal transduction in alveolar epithelium: evidence for an autocrine role. *Am J Physiol* 1995;268:L192–L200.

54. Wu T, Rieves RD, Larivee P, Logun C, Lawrence MG, Shelhamer JH. Production of eicosanoids in response to endothelin-1 and identification of specific endothelin-1 binding sites in airway epithelial cells. *Am J Respir Cell Mol Biol* 1993;8:282–290.

55. Nagase T, Fukuchi Y, Jo C, et al. Endothelin-1 stimulates arachidonate 15-lipoxygenase activity and oxygen radical formation in the rat distal lung. *Biochem Biophys Res Commun* 1990;168:485–489.

56. Nakaki T, Nakayama M, Yamamoto S, Kato R. Endothelin-mediated stimulation of DNA synthesis in vascular smooth muscle cells. *Biochem Biophys Res Commun* 1989;158:880–883.

57. Takuwa N, Takuwa Y, Yanagisawa M, Yamashita K, Masaki T. A novel vasoactive peptide endothelin stimulates mitogenesis through inositol lipid turnover in Swiss 3T3 fibroblasts. *J Biol Chem* 1989;264:7856–7861.

58. Roche WR, Williams JH, Beasley R, Holgate ST. Subepithelial fibrosis in the bronchi of asthmatics. *Lancet* 1989;1:520–524.

59. Rennick RE, Loesch A, Burnstock G. Endothelin, vasopressin, and substance P like immunoreactivity in cultured and intact epithelium from rabbit trachea. *Thorax* 1992;47:1044–1049.

60. Lundberg JM, Franco-Cereceda A, Hua X, Hökfelt T, Fischer JA. Coexistence of substance P and calcitonin gene-related peptide-like immunoreactivities in sensory nerves in relation to cardiovascular and bronchoconstrictor effects of capsaicin. *Eur J Pharmacol* 1985;108:315–319.

61. Martling CR, Saria A, Fischer JA, Hökfelt T, Lundberg JM. Calcitonin gene-related peptide and the lung: neuronal coexistence with substance P, release by capsaicin and vasodilatory effect. *Regul Pept* 1988;20:125–139.

62. Palmer JBD, Cuss FMC, Mulderry PK, et al. Calcitonin gene-related peptide is localised to human airway nerves and potently constricts human airway smooth muscle. *Br J Pharmacol* 1987;91:95–101.

63. McCormack DG, Salonen RO, Barnes PJ. Effect of sensory neuropeptides on canine bronchial and pulmonary vessels *in vitro*. *Life Sci* 1989;45:2405–2412.

64. Baluk P, Nadel JA, McDonald DM. Calcitonin gene-related peptide in secretory granules of serous cells in the rat tracheal epithelium. *Am J Respir Cell Mol Biol* 1993;8:446–453.

65. Mehta JL. Endothelium, coronary vasodilation, and organic nitrates. *Am Heart J* 1995;129:382–391.

66. Flavahan NA, Aarhus LL, Rimele TJ, Vanhoutte PM. Respiratory epithelium inhibits bronchial smooth muscle tone. *J Appl Physiol* 1985;58:834–838.

67. Flavahan NA, Vanhoutte PM. The respiratory epithelium releases a smooth muscle relaxing factor. *Chest* 1985;87:189S–190S.

68. Butler GB, Adler KB, Evans JN, Morgan DW, Szarek JL. Modulation of rabbit airway smooth muscle responsiveness by respiratory epithelium: involvement of an inhibitory metabolite of arachidonic acid. *Am Rev Respir Dis* 1987;135:1099–1104.

69. Vanhoutte PM. Epithelium-derived relaxing factor(s) and bronchial reactivity. *Am Rev Respir Dis* 1988;138:S24–S30.

70. Burgaud JL, Javellaud J, Oudart N. Do perfused small caliber airways of guinea-pig release an epithelium-dependent relaxing factor? *Pulm Pharmacol* 1993;6:217–224.

71. Tamaoki J, Yamawaki I, Takeyama K, Chiyotani A, Yamauchi F, Konno K. Interleukin-1β inhibits airway smooth muscle contraction via epithelium-dependent mechanism. *Am J Respir Crit Care Med* 1994;149:134–137.

72. Nadel JA, Borson DB. Modulation of neurogenic inflammation by neutral endopeptidase. *Am Rev Respir Dis* 1991;143(Suppl):S33–S36.

73. Sekizawa K, Tamaoki J, Graf PD, Basbaum CB, Borson DB, Nadel JA. Enkephalinase inhibitor potentiates mammalian tachykinin-induced contraction in ferret trachea. *J Pharmacol Exp Ther* 1987;243:1211–1217.

74. Dusser DJ, Nadel JA, Sekizawa K, Graf PD, Borson DB. Neutral endopeptidase and angiotensin converting enzyme inhibitors potentiate kinin-induced contraction of ferret trachea. *J Pharmacol Exp Ther* 1988;244:531–536.

75. Frossard N, Rhoden KJ, Barnes PJ. Influence of epithelium on guinea pig airway responses to tachykinins: role of endopeptidase and cyclooxygenase. *J Pharmacol Exp Ther* 1989;248:292–298.

76. Kohrogi H, Graf PD, Sekizawa K, Borson DB, Nadel JA. Neutral endopeptidase inhibitors potentiate substance P- and capsaicin-induced cough in awake guinea pigs. *J Clin Invest* 1988;82:2063–2068.

77. Dusser DJ, Djokic TD, Borson DB, Nadel JA. Cigarette smoke induces bronchoconstrictor hyperresponsiveness to substance P and inactivates airway neutral endopeptidase in the guinea pig: possible role of free radicals. *J Clin Invest* 1989;84:900–906.

78. Sheppard D, Thompson JE, Scypinski L, Dusser D, Nadel JA, Borson DB. Toluene diisocyanate increases airway responsiveness to substance P and decreases airway neutral endopeptidase. *J Clin Invest* 1988;81:1111–1115.

79. Jacoby DB, Tamaoki J, Borson DB, Nadel JA. Influenza infection causes airway hyperresponsiveness by decreasing enkephalinase. *J Appl Physiol* 1988;64:2653–2658.

80. Dusser DJ, Jacoby DB, Djokic TD, Rubinstein I, Borson DB, Nadel JA. Virus induces airway hyperresponsiveness to tachykinins: role of neutral endopeptidase. *J Appl Physiol* 1989;67:1504–1511.

81. Murray TC, Jacoby DB. Viral infection increases contractile but not secretory responses to substance P in ferret trachea. *J Appl Physiol* 1992;72:608–611.

82. Cheung D, Bel EH, Den Hartigh J, Dijkman JH, Sterk PJ. The effect of an inhaled neutral endopeptidase inhibitor, thiorphan, on airway responses to neurokinin A in normal humans *in vivo*. *Am Rev Respir Dis* 1992;145:1275–1280.

83. Cheung D, Timmers MC, Bel EH, et al. An inhaled neutral endopeptidase inhibitor, thiorphan, enhances airway narrowing to neurokinin A in asthmatic subjects *in vivo*. *Am Rev Respir Dis* 1992;145:A682 (abstract).

84. Borson DB, Gruenert DC. Glucocorticoids induce neutral endopeptidase in transformed human tracheal epithelial cells. *Am J Physiol* 1991;260:L83–L89.

85. Proud D, Subauste MC, Ward PE. Glucocorticoids do not alter peptidase expression on a human bronchial epithelial cell line. *Am J Respir Cell Mol Biol* 1994;11:57–65.

86. Funkhouser JD, Tangada SD, Jones M, OS-J, Peterson RDA. p146 type II alveolar epithelial cell antigen is identical to aminopeptidase N. *Am J Physiol* 1991;260:L274–L279.

87. Burnett D, Abrahamson M, Devalia JL, Sapsford RJ, Davies RJ, Buttle DJ. Synthesis and secretion of procathepsin B and cystatin C by human bronchial epithelial cells *in vitro*: modulation of cathepsin B activity by neutrophil elastase. *Arch Biochem Biophys* 1995;317:305–310.

88. Burleigh MCA, Barrett AJ, Lazarus GL. Cathepsin B1: a lysozomal enzyme that degrades native collagen. *Biochem J* 1974;137:387–398.

89. Orlowski M, Orlowski J, Lesser M, Kilburn KH. Proteolytic enzymes in bronchopulmonary lavage fluids: cathepsin B-like activity and prolyl endopeptidase. *J Lab Clin Med* 1981;97:467–476.

90. Burnett D, Crocker J, Stockley RA. Cathepsin B-like cysteine proteinase activity in sputum and immunohistologic identification of cathepsin B in alveolar macrophages. *Am Rev Respir Dis* 1983;128:915–919.

91. Burnett D, Stockley RA. Cathepsin B-like cysteine proteinase activity in sputum and bronchoalveolar lavage samples: relationship to in-

flammatory cells and effects of corticosteroids and antibiotic treatment. *Clin Sci* 1985;68:469–474.

92. Sallenave J-M, Shulmann J, Crossley J, Jordana M, Gauldie J. Regulation of secretory leukocyte proteinase inhibitor (SLPI) and elastase-specific inhibitor (ESI/elafin) in human airway epithelial cells by cytokines and neutrophilic enzymes. *Am J Respir Cell Mol Biol* 1994; 11:733–741.

93. Kelley J. Cytokines of the lung. *Am Rev Respir Dis* 1990;141:765–788.

94. Lopez AF, Williamson DJ, Gamble JR, et al. Recombinant human granulocyte-macrophage colony-stimulating factor stimulates *in vitro* mature human neutrophil and eosinophil function, surface receptor expression, and survival. *J Clin Invest* 1986;78:1220–1228.

95. Heidenreich S, Gong J-H, Schmidt A, Nain M, Gemsa D. Macrophage activation by granulocyte/macrophage colony stimulating factor: priming for enhanced release of tumor necrosis factor-α and prostaglandin E₂. *J Immunol* 1989;143:1198–1205.

96. Burke LA, Hallsworth MP, Litchfield TM, Davidson R, Lee TH. Identification of the major activity derived from cultured human peripheral blood mononuclear cells, which enhances eosinophil viability, as granulocyte macrophage colony-stimulating factor (GM-CSF). *J Allergy Clin Immunol* 1991;88:226–235.

97. Ruef C, Coleman DL. Granulocyte–macrophage colony-stimulating factor: pleiotropic cytokine with potential clinical usefulness. *Rev Infect Dis* 1990;12:41–62.

98. Otsuka H, Dolovich J, Richardson M, Bienenstock J, Denburg JA. Metachromatic cell progenitors and specific growth and differentiation factors in human nasal mucosa and polyps. *Am Rev Respir Dis* 1987;136:710–717.

99. Churchill L, Friedman B, Schleimer RP, Proud D. Production of granulocyte-macrophage colony-stimulating factor by cultured human tracheal epithelial cells. *Immunology* 1992;75:189–195.

100. Cromwell O, Hamid Q, Corrigan CJ, et al. Expression and generation of interleukin-8, IL-6 and granulocyte-macrophage colony-stimulating factor by bronchial epithelial cells and enhancement by IL-1β and tumour necrosis factor-α. *Immunology* 1992;77:330–337.

101. Cox G, Ohtoshi T, Vancheri C, et al. Promotion of eosinophil survival by human bronchial epithelial cells and its modulation by steroids. *Am J Respir Cell Mol Biol* 1991;4:525–531.

102. Marini M, Soloperto M, Mezzetti M, Fasoli A, Mattoli S. Interleukin-1 binds to specific receptors on human bronchial epithelial cells and upregulates granulocyte-macrophage colony-stimulating factor synthesis and release. *Am J Respir Cell Mol Biol* 1991;4:519–524.

103. Noah TL, Becker S. Respiratory syncytial virus-induced cytokine production by a human bronchial epithelial cell line. *Am J Physiol* 1993;265:L472–L478.

104. Subauste MC, Jacoby DB, Richards SM, Proud D. Infection of a human respiratory epithelial cell line with rhinovirus: induction of cytokine release and modulation of susceptibility to infection by cytokine exposure. *J Clin Invest* 1995;96:549–557.

105. Blau H, Riklis S, Kravtsov V, Kalina M. Secretion of cytokines by rat alveolar epithelial cells: possible regulatory role for SP-A. *Am J Physiol* 1994;266:L148–L155.

106. Smith SM, Lee DKP, Lacy J, Coleman DL. Rat tracheal epithelial cells produce granulocyte-macrophage colony-stimulating factor. *Am J Respir Cell Mol Biol* 1990;2:59–68.

107. Mattoli S, Mattoso VL, Soloperto M, Allegra L, Fasoli A. Cellular and biochemical characteristics of bronchoalveolar lavage fluid in symptomatic nonallergic asthma. *J Allergy Clin Immunol* 1991;87:794–802.

108. Mattoli S, Marini M, Fasoli A. Expression of the potent inflammatory cytokines, GM-CSF, IL6, and IL8, in bronchial epithelial cells of asthmatic patients. *Chest* 1992;101:27S–29S.

109. Marini M, Vittori E, Hollemborg J, Mattoli S. Expression of the potent inflammatory cytokines, granulocyte–macrophage colony-stimulating factor and interleukin-6 and interleukin-8, in bronchial epithelial cells of patients with asthma. *J Allergy Clin Immunol* 1992;89:1001–1009.

110. Sousa AR, Poston RN, Lane SJ, Nakhosteen JA, Lee TH. Detection of GM-CSF in asthmatic bronchial epithelium and decrease by inhaled corticosteroids. *Am Rev Respir Dis* 1993;147:1557–1561.

111. Wang JH, Trigg CJ, Devalia JL, Jordan S, Davies RJ. Effect of inhaled beclomethasone dipropionate on expression of proinflammatory cytokines and activated eosinophils in the bronchial epithelium of patients with mild asthma. *J Allergy Clin Immunol* 1994;94:1025–1034.

112. Trigg CJ, Manolitsas ND, Wang J, et al. Placebo-controlled immuno-

113. Marini M, Soloperto M, Zheng Y, Mezzetti M, Mattoli S. Protective effect of nedocromil sodium on the IL1-induced release of GM-CSF from cultured human bronchial epithelial cells. *Pulm Pharmacol* 1992;5:61–65.

114. Levine SJ, Larivée P, Logun C, Angus CW, Shelhamer JH. Corticosteroids differentially regulate secretion of IL-6, IL-8, and G-CSF by a human bronchial epithelial cell line. *Am J Physiol* 1993;265:L360–L368.

115. Cox G, Gauldie J, Jordana M. Bronchial epithelial cell-derived cytokines (G-CSF and GM-CSF) promote the survival of peripheral blood neutrophils *in vitro*. *Am J Respir Cell Mol Biol* 1992;7:507–513.

116. Bédard M, McClure CD, Schiller NL, Francoeur C, Cantin A, Denis M. Release of interleukin-8, interleukin-6, and colony-stimulating factors by upper airway epithelial cells: implications for cystic fibrosis. *Am J Respir Cell Mol Biol* 1993;9:455–462.

117. Ohtoshi T, Vancheri C, Cox G, et al. Monocyte-macrophage differentiation induced by human upper airway epithelial cells. *Am J Respir Cell Mol Biol* 1991;4:255–263.

118. Xing Z, Ohtoshi T, Ralph P, Gauldie J, Jordana M. Human upper airway structural cell-derived cytokines support human peripheral blood monocyte survival: a potential mechanism for monocyte/macrophage accumulation in the tissue. *Am J Respir Cell Mol Biol* 1992;6:212–218.

119. Standiford TJ, Kunkel SL, Basha MA, et al. Interleukin-8 gene expression by a pulmonary epithelial cell line: a model for cytokine networks in the lung. *J Clin Invest* 1990;86:1945–1953.

120. Nakamura H, Yoshimura K, Jaffe HA, Crystal RG. Interleukin-8 gene expression in human bronchial epithelial cells. *J Biol Chem* 1991; 266:19,611–19,617.

121. Leonard EJ, Yoshimura T. Neutrophil attractant/activation protein-1 (NAP-1 [interleukin-8]). *Am J Respir Cell Mol Biol* 1990;2:479–486.

122. Larsen CG, Anderson AO, Appella E, Oppenheim JJ, Matsushima K. The neutrophil activating protein (NAP-1) is also chemotactic for T lymphocytes. *Science* 1989;243:1464–1466.

123. Taub DD, Anver M, Oppenheim JJ, Longo DL, Murphy WJ. T lymphocyte recruitment by interleukin-8 (IL-8): IL-8-induced degranulation of neutrophils releases potent chemoattractants for T lymphocytes both *in vitro* and *in vivo*. *J Clin Invest* 1996;97:1931–1941.

124. Warringa RAJ, Koenderman L, Kok PTM, Kreukniet J, Bruijnzeel PLB. Modulation and induction of eosinophil chemotaxis by granulocyte-macrophage colony-stimulating factor and interleukin-3. *Blood* 1991;77:2694–2700.

125. Kishimoto T. The biology of interleukin-6. *Blood* 1989;74:1–10.

126. Takizawa H, Ohtoshi T, Ohta K, et al. Interleukin 6/B cell stimulatory factor-II is expressed and released by normal and transformed human bronchial epithelial cells. *Biochem Biophys Res Commun* 1992;187: 596–602.

127. Mattoli S, Miante S, Calabrò F, Mezzetti M, Fasoli A, Allegra L. Bronchial epithelial cells exposed to isocyanates potentiate activation and proliferation of T-cells. *Am J Physiol* 1990;259:L320–L327.

128. Noah TL, Paradiso AM, Madden MC, McKinnon KP, Devlin RB. The response of a human bronchial epithelial cell line to histamine: intracellular calcium changes and extracellular release of inflammatory mediators. *Am J Respir Cell Mol Biol* 1991;5:484–492.

129. Di Cosmo BF, Geba GP, Picarella D, et al. Airway epithelial cell expression of interleukin-6 in transgenic mice: uncoupling of airway inflammation and bronchial hyperreactivity. *J Clin Invest* 1994;94: 2028–2035.

130. Vittori E, Sciacca F, Colotta F, Mantovani A, Mattoli S. Protective effect of nedocromil sodium on the interleukin-1-induced production of interleukin-8 in human bronchial epithelial cells. *J Allergy Clin Immunol* 1992;90:76–84.

131. Elias JA, Zheng T, Einarsson O, et al. Epithelial interleukin-11: regulation by cytokines, respiratory syncytial virus, and retinoic acid. *J Biol Chem* 1994;269:22,261–22,268.

132. Einarsson O, Geba GP, Zhu Z, Landry M, Elias JA. Interleukin-11: stimulation *in vivo* and *in vitro* by respiratory viruses and induction airways hyperresponsiveness. *J Clin Invest* 1996;97:915–924.

133. Stellato C, Beck LA, Gorgone GA, et al. Expression of the chemokine RANTES by a human bronchial epithelial cell line: modulation by cytokines and glucocorticoids. *J Immunol* 1995;155:410–418.

134. Kwon OJ, Jose PJ, Robbins RA, Schall TJ, Williams TJ, Barnes PJ.

Glucocorticoid inhibition of RANTES expression in human lung epithelial cells. *Am J Respir Cell Mol Biol* 1995;12:488–496.

135. Rot A, Krieger M, Brunner T, Bischoff SC, Schall TJ, Dahinden CA. RANTES and macrophage inflammatory protein 1α induce the migration and activation of normal human eosinophil granulocytes. *J Exp Med* 1992;176:1489–1495.

136. Schall TJ, Bacon K, Toy KJ, Goeddel DV. Selective attraction of monocytes and T lymphocytes of the memory phenotype by cytokine RANTES. *Nature* 1990;347:669–671.

137. Meurer R, van Riper G, Feeney W, et al. Formation of eosinophilic and monocytic intradermal inflammatory sites in the dog by injection of human RANTES but not human monocyte chemoattractant 1, human macrophage inflammatory protein 1α, or human interleukin 8. *J Exp Med* 1993;178:1913–1921.

138. Beck L, Bickel C, Sterbinsky S, et al. Injection of human subjects with RANTES causes dermal infiltration of eosinophils (EOS) and mononuclear cells (MNC). *FASEB J* 1995;9:A804(abstr).

139. Alam R, York J, Boyars M, et al. Increased MCP-1, RANTES, and MIP-1α in bronchoalveolar lavage fluid of allergic asthmatic patients. *Am J Respir Crit Care Med* 1996;153:1398–1404.

140. Venge J, Lampinen M, Hakansson L, Rak S, Venge P. Identification of IL-5 and RANTES as the major eosinophilic chemoattractants in the human lung. *J Allergy Clin Immunol* 1996;97:1110–1115.

141. Leonard EJ, Skeel A, Yoshimura T. Biological aspects of monocyte chemoattractant protein-1 (MCP-1). In: Westwick J, ed. *Chemotactic cytokines.* New York: Plenum, 1991;57–64.

142. Carr MW, Roth SJ, Luther E, Rose SS, Springer TA. Monocyte chemoattractant protein-1 acts as a T-lymphocyte chemoattractant. *Proc Natl Acad Sci USA* 1994;91:3652–3656.

143. Becker S, Quay J, Koren HS, Haskill JS. Constitutive and stimulated MCP-1, GROα, β, and γ expression in human airway epithelium and bronchoalveolar macrophages. *Am J Physiol* 1994;266:L278–L286.

144. Sousa AR, Lane SJ, Nakhosteen JA, Yoshimura T, Lee TH, Poston RN. Increased expression of the monocyte chemoattractant protein-1 in bronchial tissue from asthmatic subjects. *Am J Respir Cell Mol Biol* 1994;10:142–147.

145. Antoniades HN, Neville-Golden J, Galanopoulos T, Kradin RL, Valente AL, Graves DT. Expression of monocyte chemoattractant protein 1 mRNA in human idiopathic pulmonary fibrosis. *Proc Natl Acad Sci USA* 1992;89:5371–5375.

146. Jose PJ, Griffiths-Johnson DA, Collins PD, et al. Eotaxin: a potent eosinophil chemoattractant cytokine detected in a guinea pig model of allergic airway inflammation. *J Exp Med* 1994;179:881–887.

147. Jose PJ, Adcock IM, Griffiths-Johnson DA, et al. Eotaxin: cloning of an eosinophil chemoattractant cytokine and increased mRNA expression in allergen challenged guinea-pig lungs. *Biochem Biophys Res Commun* 1994;205:788–794.

148. Ponath PD, Qin S, Ringler DJ, et al. Cloning of the human eosinophil chemoattractant, eotaxin: expression, receptor binding, and functional properties suggest a mechanism for the selective recruitment of eosinophils. *J Clin Invest* 1996;97:604–612.

149. Garcia-Zepeda EA, Rothenberg ME, Ownbey RT, Celestin J, Leder P, Luster AD. Human eotaxin is a specific chemoattractant for eosinophil cells and provides a new mechanism to explain tissue eosinophilia. *Nature Med* 1996;2:449–456.

150. Bellini A, Yoshimura H, Vitori E, Marini M, Mattoli S. Bronchial epithelial cells of patients with asthma release chemoattractant factors for T lymphocytes. *J Allergy Clin Immunol* 1993;92:412–424.

151. Laberge S, Ernst P, Ghaffar O, et al. Bronchial epithelial cells are the major source of interleukin-16 (IL-16) in asthma. *Am J Respir Crit Care Med* 1996;153:A880(abstract).

152. Cruikshank WW, Long AR, Tarpy RE, et al. Early identification of interleukin-16 (lymphocyte chemoattractant factor) and macrophage inflammatory protein 1α (MIP1α) in bronchoalveolar lavage fluid on antigen-challenged asthmatics. *Am J Respir Cell Mol Biol* 1995;13:738–747.

153. Cazals V, Mouhieddine B, Maitre B, et al. Insulinlike growth factors, their binding proteins, and transforming growth factor-β₁ in oxidant-arrested lung alveolar epithelial cells. *J Biol Chem* 1994;269:14,111–14,117.

154. Sacco O, Romberger D, Rizzino A, Beckmann JD, Rennard SI, Spurzem JR. Spontaneous production of transforming growth factor-β₂ by primary cultures of bronchial epithelial cells: effects on cell behavior *in vitro. J Clin Invest* 1992;90:1379–1385.

155. Magnan A, Frachon I, Rain B, et al. Transforming growth factor-β in normal human lung: preferential location in bronchial epithelial cells. *Thorax* 1994;49:789–792.

156. Khalil N, O'Connor RN, Unruh HW, et al. Increased production and immunohistochemical localization of transforming growth factor-β in idiopathic pulmonary fibrosis. *Am J Respir Cell Mol Biol* 1991;5:155–162.

157. Pelton RW, Johnson MD, Perkett EA, Gold LI, Moses HL. Expression of transforming growth factor-β₁, -β₂, and -β₃ mRNA and protein in murine lung. *Am J Respir Cell Mol Biol* 1991;5:522–530.

158. Kenney JS, Baker C, Welch MR, Altman LC. Synthesis of interleukin-1α, interleukin-6, and interleukin-8 by cultured human nasal epithelial cells. *J Allergy Clin Immunol* 1994;93:1060–1067.

159. Bonfield TL, Konstan MW, Burfeind P, Panuska JR, Hilliard JB, Berger M. Normal bronchial epithelial cells constitutively produce the anti-inflammatory cytokine interleukin-10, which is downregulated in cystic fibrosis. *Am J Respir Cell Mol Biol* 1995;13:257–261.

160. Devalia JL, Campbell AM, Sapsford RJ, et al. Effect of nitrogen dioxide on synthesis of inflammatory cytokines expressed by human bronchial epithelial cells *in vitro. Am J Respir Cell Mol Biol* 1993;9:271–278.

161. Driscoll KE, Hassenbein DG, Carter J, et al. Macrophage inflammatory proteins 1 and 2: expression by rat alveolar macrophages, fibroblasts, and epithelial cells and in rat lung after mineral dust exposure. *Am J Respir Cell Mol Biol* 1993;8:311–318.

162. Choi AMK, Jacoby DB. Influenza virus A infection induces interleukin-1 gene expression in human airway epithelial cells. *FEBS Lett* 1992;309:327–329.

163. Arnold R, Humbert B, Werchau H, Gallati H, König W. Interleukin-8, interleukin-6, and soluble tumour necrosis factor receptor type I release from a human pulmonary epithelial cell line (A549) exposed to respiratory syncytial virus. *Immunology* 1994;82:126–133.

164. Goldman WE, Klapper DG, Baseman JB. Detection, isolation, and analysis of a released *Bordetella pertussis* product toxic to cultured tracheal cells. *Infect Immun* 1982;36:782–794.

165. Heiss LN, Moser SA, Unanue ER, Goldman WE. Interleukin-1 is linked to the respiratory epithelial cytopathology of pertussis. *Infect Immun* 1993;61:3123–3128.

166. Massion PP, Inoue H, Richman-Eisenstat J, et al. Novel *Pseudomonas* product stimulates interleukin-8 production in airway epithelial cells *in vitro. J Clin Invest* 1994;93:26–32.

167. Inoue H, Massion PP, Ueki IF, et al. *Pseudomonas* stimulates interleukin-8 mRNA expression selectively in airway epithelium, in gland ducts, and in recruited neutrophils. *Am J Respir Cell Mol Biol* 1994;11:651–663.

168. Ruef C, Jefferson DM, Schlegel-Haueter SE, Suter S. Regulation of cytokine secretion by cystic fibrosis airway epithelial cells. *Eur Respir J* 1993;6:1429–1436.

169. Nakamura H, Yoshimura K, McElvaney NG, Crystal RG. Neutrophil elastase in respiratory epithelial lining fluid of individuals with cystic fibrosis induces interleukin-8 gene expression in a human bronchial epithelial cell line. *J Clin Invest* 1992;89:1478–1484.

170. McElvaney NG, Nakamura H, Birrer P, et al. Modulation of airway inflammation in cystic fibrosis: *in vivo* suppression of interleukin-8 levels on the respiratory epithelial surface by aerosolization of recombinant secretory leukoprotease inhibitor. *J Clin Invest* 1992;90:1296–1301.

171. Rosenthal GJ, Germolec DR, Blazka ME, et al. Asbestos stimulates IL-8 production from human lung epithelial cells. *J Immunol* 1994;153:3237–3244.

172. Kinnula VL, Adler KB, Ackley NJ, Crapo JD. Release of reactive oxygen species by guinea pig tracheal epithelial cells *in vitro. Am J Physiol* 1992;262:L708–L712.

173. Adler KB, Holden-Stauffer WJ, Repine JE. Oxygen metabolites stimulate release of high-molecular-weight glycoconjugates by cell and organ cultures of rodent respiratory epithelium via an arachidonic acid-dependent mechanism. *J Clin Invest* 1990;85:75–85.

174. Yukawa T, Read RC, Kroegel C, et al. The effects of activated eosinophils and neutrophils on guinea pig airway epithelium *in vitro. Am J Respir Cell Mol Biol* 1990;2:341–353.

175. DeChatelet LR, Shirley PS, McPhail LC, Huntley CC, Muss HB, Bass DA. Oxidative metabolism of the human eosinophil. *Blood* 1977;50:525–535.

176. Rossi F. The O₂-forming NADPH oxidase of the phagocytes: nature,

mechanisms of activation and function. *Biochim Biophys Acta* 1986; 853:65–89.

177. Adler KB, Kinnula VL, Akley N, Lee J, Cohn LA, Crapo JD. Inflammatory mediators and the generation and release of reactive oxygen species by airway epithelium *in vitro*. *Chest* 1992;101(Suppl):53S–54S.

178. Lopez A, Shoji S, Fujita J, Robbins R, Rennard S. Bronchoepithelial cells can release hydrogen peroxide in response to inflammatory stimuli. *Am Rev Respir Dis* 1988;137:A81(abstract).

179. Hobson J, Wright J, Churg A. Histochemical evidence for generation of active oxygen species on the apical surface of cigarette-smoke-exposed tracheal explants. *Am J Pathol* 1991;139:573–580.

180. Kinnula VL, Everitt JI, Whorton AR, Crapo JD. Hydrogen peroxide production by alveolar type II cells, alveolar macrophages, and endothelial cells. *Am J Physiol* 1991;261:L84–L91.

181. DeForge LE, Preston AM, Takeuchi E, Kenney J, Boxer LA, Remick DG. Regulation of interleukin 8 gene expression by oxidant stress. *J Biol Chem* 1993;268:25,568–25,576.

182. Asano K, Chee CBE, Gaston B, et al. Constitutive and inducible nitric oxide synthase gene expression, regulation, and activity in human lung epithelial cells. *Proc Natl Acad Sci USA* 1994;91:10,089–10,093.

183. Shaul PW, North AJ, Wu LC, et al. Endothelial nitric oxide synthase is expressed in cultured human bronchiolar epithelium. *J Clin Invest* 1994;94:2231–2236.

184. Gutierrez HH, Pitt BR, Schwarz M, et al. Pulmonary alveolar epithelial inducible NO synthase gene expression: regulation by inflammatory mediators. *Am J Physiol* 1995;268:L501–L508.

185. Hamid Q, Springall DR, Riveros-Moreno V, et al. Induction of nitric oxide synthase in asthma. *Lancet* 1993;342:1510–1513.

186. Kharitonov SA, Yates D, Robbins RA, Logan-Sinclair R, Shinebourne E, Barnes PJ. Increased nitric oxide in exhaled air of asthmatic patients. *Lancet* 1994;343:133–135.

187. Massaro AF, Gaston B, Kita D, Fanta C, Stamler JS, Drazen JM. Expired nitric oxide levels during treatment of acute asthma. *Am J Respir Crit Care Med* 1995;152:800–803.

188. Dupuy PM, Shore SA, Drazen JM, Frostell C, Hill WA, Zapol WM. Bronchodilator action of inhaled nitric oxide in guinea pigs. *J Clin Invest* 1992;90:421–428.

189. Hogman M, Frostell CG, Hedenstrom H, Hedenstierna G. Inhalation of nitric oxide modulates adult human bronchial tone. *Am Rev Respir Dis* 1993;148:1474–1478.

190. Barnes PJ, Liew FY. Nitric oxide and asthmatic inflammation. *Immunol Today* 1995;16:128–130.

191. Taylor-Robinson AW, Liew FY, Severin A. Regulation of the immune response by nitric oxide differentially produced by T helper type 1 and T helper type 2 cells. *Eur J Immunol* 1994;24:980–984.

192. Kinnula VL, Yankaskas JR, Chang L, et al. Primary and immortalized (BEAS 2B) human bronchial epithelial cells have significant antioxidant capacity *in vitro*. *Am J Respir Cell Mol Biol* 1994;11:568–576.

193. Freeman BA, Mason RJ, Williams MC, Crapo JD. Antioxidant enzyme activity in alveolar type II cells after exposure of rats to hyperoxia. *Exp Lung Res* 1986;10:203–222.

194. Jacoby DB, Choi AMK. Influenza virus induces expression of antioxidant genes in human epithelial cells. *Free Radic Biol Med* 1994;16: 821–824.

195. Kinnula VL, Chang L, Everitt JI, Crapo JD. Oxidants and antioxidants in alveolar epithelial type II cells: *in situ*, freshly isolated, and cultured cells. *Am J Physiol* 1992;262:L69–L77.

196. Cohn LA, Kinnula VL, Adler KB. Antioxidant properties of guinea pig tracheal epithelial cells *in vitro*. *Am J Physiol* 1994;266:L397–L404.

197. Adams DH, Shaw S. Leucocyte-endothelial interactions and regulation of leucocyte migration. *Lancet* 1994;343:831–836.

198. Wegner CD, Gundel RH, Reilly P, Haynes N, Letts LG, Rothlein R. Intercellular adhesion molecule-1 (ICAM-1) in the pathogenesis of asthma. *Science* 1990;247:456–459.

199. Vignola AM, Campbell AM, Chanez P, et al. HLA-DR and ICAM-1 expression on bronchial epithelial cells in asthma and chronic bronchitis. *Am Rev Respir Dis* 1993;148:689–694.

200. Greve JM, Davis G, Meyer AM, et al. The major human rhinovirus receptor is ICAM-1. *Cell* 1989;56:839–847.

201. Staunton DE, Merluzzi VJ, Rothlein R, Barton R, Marlin SD, Springer TA. A cell adhesion molecule, ICAM-1, is the major surface receptor for rhinoviruses. *Cell* 1989;56:849–853.

202. Kishimoto TK, Larson RS, Corbi AL, Dustin ML, Staunton DE, Springer TA. The leukocyte integrins. *Adv Immunol* 1989;46:149–182.

203. Tosi MF, Stark JM, Smith CW, Hamedani A, Gruenert DC, Infeld MD. Induction of ICAM-1 expression on human airway epithelial cells by inflammatory cytokines: effects on neutrophil–epithelial cell adhesion. *Am J Respir Cell Mol Biol* 1992;7:214–221.

204. Look DC, Rapp SR, Keller BT, Holtzman MJ. Selective induction of intercellular adhesion molecule-1 by interferon-γ in human airway epithelial cells. *Am J Physiol* 1992;263:L79–L87.

205. Vignola AM, Campbell AM, Chanez P, et al. Activation by histamine of bronchial epithelial cells from normal subjects. *Am J Respir Cell Mol Biol* 1993;9:411–417.

206. Bloemen PGM, van den Tweel MC, Henricks PAJ, et al. Expression and modulation of adhesion molecules on human bronchial epithelial cells. *Am J Respir Cell Mol Biol* 1993;9:586–593.

207. Tosi MF, Stark JM, Hamedani A, Smith CW, Gruenert DC, Huang YT. Intercellular adhesion molecule-1 (ICAM-1)-dependent and ICAM-1-independent adhesive interactions between polymorphonuclear leukocytes and human airway epithelial cells infected with parainfluenza virus type 2. *J Immunol* 1992;149:3345–3349.

208. Tosi MF, Hamedani A, Brosovich J, Alpert SE. ICAM-1-independent, CD18-dependent adhesion between neutrophils and human airway epithelial cells exposed *in vitro* to ozone. *J Immunol* 1994;152:1935–1942.

209. Bullard DC, Qin L, Lorenzo I, et al. P-selectin/ICAM-1 double mutant mice: acute emigration of neutrophils into the peritoneum is completely absent but is normal into pulmonary alveoli. *J Clin Invest* 1995;95:1782–1788.

210. Albelda SM. Endothelial and epithelial cell adhesion molecules. *Am J Respir Cell Mol Biol* 1991;4:195–203.

211. Manolitsas ND, Trigg CJ, McAulay AE, et al. The expression of intercellular adhesion molecule-1 and the β₁-integrins in asthma. *Eur Respir J* 1994;7:1439–1444.

212. Glanville AR, Tazelaar HD, Theodore J, et al. The distribution of MHC class I and II antigens on bronchial epithelium. *Am Rev Respir Dis* 1989;139:330–334.

213. Rossi GA, Sacco O, Balbi B, et al. Human ciliated bronchial epithelial cells: expression of the HLA-DR antigens and of the HLA-DR alpha gene, modulation of the HLA-DR antigens by gamma-interferon and antigen-presenting function in the mixed leukocyte reaction. *Am J Respir Cell Mol Biol* 1990;3:431–439.

214. Spurzem JR, Sacco O, Rossi GA, Beckmann JD, Rennard SI. Regulation of major histocompatibility complex class II gene expression on bovine bronchial epithelial cells. *J Lab Clin Med* 1992;120:94–102.

215. Vignola AM, Chanez P, Campbell AM, et al. Quantification and localization of HLA-DR and intercellular adhesion molecule-1 (ICAM-1) molecules on bronchial epithelial cells of asthmatics using confocal microscopy. *Clin Exp Immunol* 1994;96:104–109.

216. Stoop AE, Hameleers DMH, van Run PEM, Biewenga J, van der Baan S. Lymphocytes and nonlymphoid cells in the nasal mucosa of patients with nasal polyps and of healthy subjects. *J Allergy Clin Immunol* 1989;84:734–741.

217. Kalb TH, Chuang MT, Marom Z, Mayer L. Evidence for accessory cell function by class II MHC antigen-expressing airway epithelial cells. *Am J Respir Cell Mol Biol* 1991;4:320–329.

218. Mezzetti M, Soloperto M, Fasoli A, Mattoli S. Human bronchial epithelial cells modulate CD3 and mitogen-induced DNA synthesis in T cells but function poorly as antigen-presenting cells compared to pulmonary macrophages. *J Allergy Clin Immunol* 1991;87:930–938.

219. Burke CM, Glanville AR, Theodore J, Robin ED. Lung immunogenicity, rejection, and obliterative bronchiolitis. *Chest* 1987;92:547–549.

220. Shoji S, Rickard KA, Ertl RF, Robbins RA, Linder J, Rennard SI. Bronchial epithelial cells produce lung fibroblast chemotactic factor: fibronectin. *Am J Respir Cell Mol Biol* 1989;1:13–20.

221. Härkönen E, Virtanen I, Linnala A, Laitinen LL, Kinnula VK. Modulation of fibronectin and tenascin production by human bronchial epithelial cells by inflammatory cytokines *in vitro*. *Am J Respir Cell Mol Biol* 1995;13:109–115.

222. Laitinen A, Altraja A, Linden M, et al. Treatment with inhaled budes-

onide and tenascin expression in bronchial mucosa of allergic asthmatics. *Am J Respir Crit Care Med* 1994;149:A942.

223. Romberger DJ, Beckmann JD, Claassen L, Ertl RF, Rennard SI. Modulation of fibronectin production of bovine bronchial epithelial cells by transforming growth factor-beta. *Am J Respir Cell Mol Biol* 1992; 7:149–155.

224. Infeld MD, Brennan JA, Davis PB. Human tracheobronchial epithelial cells direct migration of lung fibroblasts in three-dimensional collagen gels. *Am J Physiol* 1992;262:L535–L541.

225. Nakamura Y, Tate L, Ertl R, et al. Bovine bronchial epithelial cells stimulate fibroblast DNA synthesis. *Am Rev Respir Dis* 1993;147:A278(abstr).

226. Kawamoto M, Nakamura Y, Tate L, Ertl RF, Romberger DJ, Rennard SI. Modulation of fibroblast type I collagen and fibronectin produc-

tion by bronchial epithelial cells. *Am Rev Respir Dis* 1992;145:A842 (abstr).

227. McGowan SE. Extracellular matrix and the regulation of lung development and repair. *FASEB J* 1992;6:2895–2904.

228. Shoji S, Ertl RF, Linder J, Romberger DJ, Rennard SI. Bronchial epithelial cells produce chemotactic activity for bronchial epithelial cells: possible role for fibronectin in airway repair. *Am Rev Respir Dis* 1990;141:218–225.

229. Montefort S, Herbert CA, Robinson C, Holgate ST. The bronchial epithelium as a target for inflammatory attack in asthma. *Clin Exp Allergy* 1992;22:511–520.

230. Rennard SI, Beckmann JD, Robbins RA. Biology of airway epithelial cells. In: Crystal RG, West JB, Barnes PJ, Cherniak NS, Weibel ER, eds. *The lung: scientific foundations.* New York: Raven, 1991;157–167.

Asthma, edited by P.J. Barnes, M.M. Grunstein,
A.R. Leff, and A.J. Woolcock.
Lippincott–Raven Publishers, Philadelphia © 1997.

▪ 37 ▪

The Role of Endothelial Cells in Asthma

Philippe Gosset, Pascale Jeannin, Philippe Lassalle,
Michel Joseph, and André-Bernard Tonnel

**Production of Mediators Involved in Allergic
  Reaction by the Endothelial Cell**
  Mediators Modulating the Vascular Tone
  Production of Proinflammatory Mediators by the
  Endothelial Cell
**Mechanisms of Leukocyte Recruitment in Allergic
  Reaction**
  Leukocyte-Endothelial Cell Adhesion Molecule
  Cascade
  Specificity and Selectivity of Adhesion Processes
  with Each of the Cells Involved in Allergic
  Inflammation
**Endothelial Cells in Asthma: Experimental and
  Clinical Approaches**

Experimental Models of Asthma
Adhesion Molecule Expression on the
  Microvasculature in Allergic Diseases
**The Vascular Endothelium as a Target Organ of
  Allergic Inflammation**
  Interaction between Macrophages and Endothelial
  Cells
  Interaction between Mast Cells and Endothelial
  Cells
  Interaction between Eosinophils and Endothelial
  Cells
  Interaction between T Lymphocytes and Endothelial
  Cells
Future Developments

The role of endothelial cells (ECs) in the allergic reaction has long been limited to the regulation of vasomotricity in gaseous and liquid exchanges or in hemostasis. Mast cell-derived mediators were known to induce activation of ECs leading to vasodilatation, and plasma exudation with protein leakage (1,2). The resulting edema was considered as increasing plasma proteins in airways, with a dual role: protective by chelating ferric ions, unavailable for the production of damaging free radicals (3), and negative by increasing mucus viscosity (4). However, allergic reaction induces also inflammation characterized by the accumulation of leukocytes at the site of the reaction. Evaluation of the inflammatory processes involved in bronchial asthma has resulted from pathologic observations obtained from bronchial biopsies (5) as well as from bronchoalveolar

lavage findings in asthmatics (6) or postmortem histologic analysis (7). All of these studies showed that the bronchial inflammation is mainly characterized by a cell infiltration where mast cells, T lymphocytes, activated eosinophils, and monocytes are present (8,9).

The recruitment of leukocytes into area of inflammation requires interactions with endothelium leading to the binding of leukocytes to the endothelium followed by their transmigration into tissues. Only in the last decade, the molecular mechanisms underlying leukocyte migration have been elucidated with the identification of cell adhesion molecules and mediators (with chemoattractant and/or activating properties). Paradoxically, each particular adhesion molecule participates in multiple leukocyte-EC interactions that are quite independently regulated *in vivo*. The role of ECs in this process is not limited to the expression of cell adhesion molecules and includes also the production of a large panel of mediators involved in the regulation of vascular tone and inflammation. The expression of cell adhesion molecules as well as the synthesis of potent mediators is modulated by compounds produced by leukocytes and mast cells, as related by nu-

  P. Gosset, P. Jeannin, P. Lassalle: INSERM U416, Institut Pasteur, F-59019 Lille, France.
  M. Joseph: Department of Immuno-Allergology, INSERM U416, Institut Pasteur, F-59019 Lille, France.
  A-B. Tonnel: Department of Respiratory Medicine, Calmette Hospital; and INSERM U416, Institut Pasteur, F-59019 Lille, France.

merous papers. In contrast, a limited number of studies evaluated the cooperation between ECs and the cells involved in the physiopathology of asthma (such as mast cells, lymphocytes, macrophages, and eosinophils) in order to define the respective role of these effector cells in the activation of endothelium observed in asthma. To explain the constitution of the cell infiltration inside the bronchial mucosa from asthmatic patients and its relative specificity, all of these different and often concomitant events involved in the development of allergic inflammation are successively described:

- The EC produces potent vasoactive and proinflammatory mediators.
- Leukocytes and ECs express adhesion molecules and secrete activating and chemoattractant factors that control leukocyte recruitment.
- The role of some of these adhesion molecules and mediators has been evaluated in allergic reaction.
- Specific interactions between effector cells and ECs have been demonstrated in allergy.

PRODUCTION OF MEDIATORS INVOLVED IN ALLERGIC REACTION BY THE ENDOTHELIAL CELL

Mediators produced by ECs might be classified into two groups depending on their properties: modulation of vascular tone and proinflammatory effect.

Mediators Modulating the Vascular Tone

Upon stimulation, the EC is capable of intrinsic modulation of the vascular tone by the production of vasoactive products. Prorelaxant factors like prostacyclin and endothelial-derived relaxing factor, at least in part composed of nitric oxide, are released upon various stimuli (hypoxia, acetylcholine, bradykinin, and thrombin but also mediators present in allergic inflammation like histamine and serotonin). The effects of these relaxant factors that determine a local vasodilation with an accumulation of fluid and plasma proteins are counterbalanced by procontractile factors like endothelin 1, which elicits potent and prolonged vasoconstrictive properties.

Production of Proinflammatory Mediators by the Endothelial Cell

Besides vasoactive components, the EC has the capacity to generate mediators directly implicated in the allergic reaction, including phospholipid mediators like platelet-activating factor (PAF), cytokines, and chemokines. Lastly, endothelium has been proved to control inflammation by its ability to express EC surface molecules that support the adhesion of blood leukocytes and their further emigration toward the sites of the allergen conflict (10).

These various factors confer on the EC a crucial role in the development of the allergic inflammatory reaction.

Some acute endothelial modifications occur within the first 15 min following stimulation. Among proinflammatory mediators, a local generation of PAF has been evidenced (11) as a consequence of hydrogen peroxide production. PAF, which is produced by the vascular endothelium, was shown to exert a potent chemotactic activity on eosinophils and then to participate in their further emigration through human umbilical cord vein EC (HUVEC) preparations. This eosinophil transendothelial migration was blocked in the presence of the PAF-receptor antagonist WEB 2086 that did not affect neutrophil migration (12), demonstrating a specific role for PAF in this process and suggesting its involvement in allergic reaction. ECs can also generate the peptide leukotriene (LT) C_4 and LTD_4, from LTA_4 provided by neutrophils (13). These components interfere in the allergic reaction by the induction of bronchoconstriction and vasodilatation.

ECs can also produce various cytokines and chemokines. In response to injury or inflammatory stimuli, ECs demonstrate long-term complex responses that require a *de novo* messenger ribonucleic acid (mRNA) expression and protein synthesis (14). Following exposure to lipopolysaccharide (LPS), interleukin (IL)-1α/β, or tumor necrosis factor (TNF)-α, ECs regulate hematopoiesis through the release of colony-stimulating factors (CSFs), not only granulocyte-macrophage (GM)-CSF but also G-CSF and M-CSF. If ECs do not constitutively secrete IL-1, IL-1 itself, LPS, and TNF-α may activate ECs to release IL-1 and to express membrane-associated IL-1. IL-6, which regulates immune reaction and acute-phase protein synthesis, is also produced by ECs activated by the same stimuli as for IL-1 synthesis. In addition, IL-6 production by ECs is triggered by several mediators, including histamine (15).

Among chemokines, several molecules have been identified as secreted by ECs, like IL-8, monocyte chemotactic protein 1 (MCP-1), and RANTES (regulated on activation in normal T cell expressed and secreted). IL-8, first characterized as a product of LPS-activated monocytes, is effectively secreted by a number of cell types, including ECs; moreover, it is also associated with the membrane. Initially considered as chemoattractant for neutrophils, it also exerts chemotactic activities toward T lymphocytes (16) and eosinophils (17,18) and, in this way, is directly implicated in allergic inflammation. MCP-1, a very potent chemotactic factor for monocytes, is also produced by ECs activated by LPS and proinflammatory cytokines. Similarly RANTES, initially identified as a chemoattractant for monocytes and memory T lymphocytes, is recognized to be *in vitro* a chemoattractant and activating factor for human eosinophils (19) with a more efficient migratory response after eosinophil priming with IL-5 (20). Moreover, intradermal injection of human RANTES in dogs demonstrated a local eosinophil infiltration, pointing to a potential role in allergic diseases (21). A number of potential sources of RANTES have been identified, including ECs. A recent study (22) observed that the production of RANTES by ECs was potentiated by a combination of TNF-α and interferon (IFN)-γ, whereas both cytokines alone are ineffective. In addition, IL-4 and IL-13 inhibited the effects of TNF-α and IFN-γ on RANTES secretion. Another activity shared by IL-8, MCP-1 and, at a lower level, RANTES was the triggering of histamine release by basophils. Thus, the vascular endothelium appears as a direct participant in the secretion of a large series of chemokines.

MECHANISMS OF LEUKOCYTE RECRUITMENT IN ALLERGIC REACTION

Leukocyte-Endothelial Cell Adhesion Molecule Cascade

Leukocyte recruitment requires selective leukocyte-EC recognition that can display specificity in relation to the stimulus, the stage of inflammatory response, and the localization. Some typical examples are illustrated by the preferential attachment of eosinophils to venules in allergic reaction, the specific recruitment of neutrophils early in acute inflammation, and the interaction of lymphocyte subsets with high endothelium venules in organized lymphoid tissues. Under the effect of chemotactic or activating factors, adhesion of leukocytes is increased (23) and, at the same time, ECs upon stimulation become more adhesive for leukocytes (24,25). Cell adhesion molecules mediate direct leukocyte-EC interactions (reviewed by Carlos and Harlan [26]). Chemically, they are glycoproteins present on all surfaces involved in cell-cell contact and have multiple functions, including (a) the promotion of the cell-cell or cell-tissue matrix adhesion, (b) the activation of cells, and (c) the promotion of cell migration.

Cell Adhesion Molecules

On the basis of their chemical structural similarities, four major groups of adhesion molecules have been described.

The *selectins* are considered as playing a crucial role in the initial binding of leukocytes to endothelium. This family comprises three proteins designated by the prefix E (endothelial), P (platelet), and L (lymphocyte). E- and P-selectins are expressed by ECs, and L-selectin is expressed only by leukocytes. Structural similarities are the presence of an NH_2 terminal C-type lectinlike binding domain, an epidermal growth factor-like region, and a variable number of consensus repeats of sequences present in complement-regulatory proteins. Upon cell stimulation, P- and E-selectins are rapidly and transiently expressed on the cell surface. *E-selectin* is an induced adhesion structure; after

exposure to endotoxin, IL-1, or TNF-α, cultured ECs synthesize and express E-selectin with a major expression between 4 and 6 h (27). Initially reported to support neutrophil adhesion, E-selectin has been shown to participate in the adhesion of most circulating leukocytes (monocytes, eosinophils, basophils, and some subsets of T lymphocytes). E- as well as P-selectin recognize fucosylated and sialylated saccharides present on neutrophils, monocytes, and activated lymphocytes. The cutaneous lymphocyte-associated antigen (CLA) that exhibits a sialylated Lewis x antigen different from sLe^x allows the binding of a subset of skin-homing lymphocyte to E-selectin (28). *P-selectin* (granule membrane protein [GMP]-140) is found on ECs and platelets (29). In both cell types, it is synthesized and stored in granules: in α-granules for platelets and in Weibel-Palade bodies for ECs. With appropriate activation (that is, by thrombin, C5a, or histamine), P-selectin is mobilized to the external plasma membrane in 15 min, and its level of expression returns to baseline in 30 min. Treatment with LPS and TNF-α induces the expression and protein synthesis of P-selectin mRNA between 2 and 4 h after treatment (30,31). A mucinlike protein designated P-selectin glycoprotein ligand 1 has been identified as a P-selectin ligand and cloned (32). Interestingly, mediators that stimulate P-selectin expression are also responsible for endothelial retraction with a subsequent increase in vascular permeability. *L-selectin* is found only on leukocytes. It is constitutively expressed and is shed by proteolytic cleavage upon activation of leukocytes. L-selectin is involved in leukocyte adherence to nonlymphoid microvasculature where an sLe^x antigen serves as a ligand (33). CD34, a sialomucin, has been described as a protein ligand of L-selectin and is present on the surface of hematopoietic precursors and endothelium (34).

Among the adhesion molecules belonging to the *immunoglobulin supergene family*, intercellular adhesion molecules (ICAMs)-1 and -2, vascular cell adhesion molecule (VCAM)-1 and, more accessorily, platelet EC adhesion molecule (PECAM)-1 (or CD31) are present at the surface of the vascular endothelium. ICAM-1 (CD54) is constitutively expressed at a low level on unstimulated ECs; its expression is largely enhanced after stimulation by IL-1 and TNF-α (35), with a different pattern compared with E-selectin. Overexpression of ICAM-1 increases progressively and peaks at a maximum value at 24 h. ICAM-1 and ICAM-2 also present on ECs interact with most leukocytes through binding with β2-integrins represented by the complex CD11/CD18.

The third cytokine-inducible endothelial adhesion molecule is *VCAM-1*, primarily described as INCAM-110. Like ICAM-1, the expression of VCAM-1 is upregulated in the presence of IL-1 and TNF-α (36–39) with maximal activity reached between 6 and 12 h. Of particular interest is the capacity of IL-4 and IL-13, two cytokines directly implicated in allergy, to enhance VCAM-1 expression on ECs. This effect of IL-4 on VCAM-1 expression

TABLE 1. *Adhesion molecules present on endothelial cells (ECs) and their counterligands*

	Expressed on			
	ECs	Other cells	Induced by	Counter-ligand
Selectins				
E-selectin (ELAM-1)	+		IL-1, TNF-α	Sialyl-Lewis x/a
P-selectin (GMP-140)	+	*Platelets*	Thrombin, histamine	Sialyl-Lewis x/L-selectin
Immunoglobulin supergene family				
ICAM-1	+	*Epithelial cells* (eosinophils, macrophages)	TNF, IL-1, IFN-γ	LFA-1/MAC-1
ICAM-2	+	—	Constitutive	LFA-1
VCAM-1	+	(Lymphocytes)	TNF, IL-1, IL-4	VLA-4
PECAM-1	+	Platelets (neutrophils, subsets of T cells)	Constitutive	PECAM-1

ELAM, endothelial leukocyte adhesion molecule; ICAM, intercellular adhesion molecule; IL, interleukin; LFA, leukocyte function-associated antigen; MAC, macrophage; PECAM, platelet EC adhesion molecule; TNF, tumor necrosis factor; VCAM, vascular cell adhesion molecule; VLA, very late antigen.

differentiates this adhesion molecule from ICAM-1 and E-selectin that are insensitive to IL-4. The counterligand for VCAM-1 is the $\alpha_4\beta_1$-integrin also called very late antigen (VLA) 4 (or CD29/CD49d), present on lymphocytes and monocytes but not neutrophils. VCAM-1 is also involved in eosinophil and basophil adhesion to activated endothelium.

PECAM-1 (or CD31), which belongs to the same immunoglobulin supergene family, is also found on ECs, platelets, and some leukocytes, but its role is not as well defined; it binds to glycosaminoglycans or to PECAM-1 itself by an homotypic adhesion process. Its expression is not increased by treatment with TNF, IL-1, or combination with IFN-γ (40). CD31 has been localized only at intercellular junctions where it could participate in the control of vascular permeability (41). However, the treatment of leukocytes or ECs with either soluble CD31 or blocking anti-CD31 monoclonal antibody (mAb) prevented monocyte or neutrophil (42) but not lymphocyte transmigration, confirming the involvement of CD31 in leukocyte-EC interaction (43).

Mucosal addressin cell adhesion molecule (MadCAM) 1, the last integrin described that shares also homologies with the sialomucins, was initially identified on high endothelial venules in mucosal lymph nodes (44). Its counterreceptors include $\alpha_4\beta_7$-integrin and L-selectin for a subset of MadCAM-1 expressing the specific carbohydrate (45,46).

Integrins are noncovalent heterodimers composed of an α-subunit and a β-subunit. Eight groups of integrins exist as determined by β-chain diversity: each β-subunit may be associated with from one to eight different α-chains. Integrins, which are transmembrane cell surface proteins, bind to cytoskeleton and communicate extracellular signals. Most of them are involved in the link between the intracellular cytoskeleton and the extracellular matrix: some β_1-integrins are expressed on ECs (VLA-2

and VLA-5). As a consequence, integrins are essential in epithelium attachment to the basement membrane. In addition, some integrins of the β_1, β_2, and β_7 groups are the counterreceptors for some members of the immunoglobulin (Ig)-like family (Table 1).

Adhesive Interactions during Leukocyte Emigration

Elegant studies by intravital microscopy have identified a sequence of adhesive interactions involved in leukocyte emigration from the bloodstream. As reported in Table 2, five steps can be distinguished: rolling, activation, stable binding, transendothelial migration, and subendothelial migration. After initial contact due in a large part to a random event, some of the leukocytes are observed to roll along the vessel wall adjacent to the site of inflammation. Rolling greatly slows the transit of neutrophils through inflamed venules; this may allow time for the leukocytes to produce activating and chemoattractant factors in the local environment or surface. Evidence from both *in vitro* and *in vivo* studies indicates that selectins are involved in the leukocyte rolling; L-selectin seems to play a key role in this process (47) by its interaction with the vascular E- and P-selectins (48,49).

After exposure to proinflammatory mediators, a portion of the rolling leukocytes is observed to flatten and spread on the ECs and then to adhere firmly, whereas a *de novo* expression of endothelial adhesion proteins occurs. EC activation by cytokines such as TNF-α also induces the production of PAF and chemokines. Activation of leukocytes (for example, by chemoattractant factors such as IL-8, IL-5, C5a, and formyl-methionyl-leucyl-phenylalanine [fMLP]) triggers increased avidity of integrins caused by a conformational change in heterodimers, resulting in a greater affinity for ligands. This increased avidity of integrins associated with the enhanced expres-

TABLE 2. *Adhesive interactions during leukocyte emigration*

	Rolling	Activation	Stable binding	Transendothelial migration	Subendothelial migration
Leukocyte	sLe^x, CLA, and other glycoproteins L-selectin	Cytokines, chemokines, and chemoattractant receptors	Integrins	PECAM-1, integrins	Integrins
Endothelium	P-selectin L-selectin ligand E-selectin CD34 MadCAM-1	Chemokines PAF PECAM-1 E-selectin	ICAM-1, ICAM-2 VCAM-1, MadCAM-1	PECAM-1 ICAM-1 VCAM-1	
Tissue	Histamine Thrombin Oxidants Leukotrienes Cytokines (IL-1, TNF-α)	Cytokines (GM-CSF, IL-5) Chemoattractants Chemokines (IL-8, MCP-1)	Cytokines (TNF-α, IL-1, IFN-γ, IL-4)	Chemokines Chemoattractants	Extracellular matrix components Chemokines Chemoat-

CLA, cutaneous lymphocyte-associated antigen; GM-CSF, granulocyte-macrophage colony-stimulating factor; ICAM, intercellular adhesion molecule; IFN, interferon; IL, interleukin; MadCAM, mucosal addressin cell adhesion molecule; MCP, monocyte chemotactic protein; PAF, platelet-activating factor; PECAM, platelet endothelial cell adhesion molecule; sLe^x, sialylated Lewis x antigen; TNF, tumor necrosis factor; VCAM, vascular cell adhesion molecule.

sion of ICAM-1, ICAM-2, and VCAM-1 (mainly regulated by cytokines) allows the development of a stable binding for activated leukocytes.

Some of the adherent leukocytes crawl on the surface of ECs, seeming to probe for an opening, and then emigrate between ECs: this is the transendothelial migration. TNF-α and other related cytokines also induce structural changes of the EC by a rearrangement of actin and the loss of tight junctions that probably facilitate transmigration. This step also depends on the interactions between integrins and Ig-like molecules. The crawling over the EC surface requires reversible adhesion, namely, the modulation of integrin receptor avidity and the opening of intercellular junctions (50). For this, the presence of activating factors and a gradient of chemotactic factors is also required. CD11/CD18 integrins and ICAM-1 are important determinants of neutrophil transmigration across confluent cultures of ECs. *In vitro* studies of monocyte and eosinophil transmigration have shown that both E-selectin and VCAM-1 are involved. PECAM-1 seems to be directly implicated in neutrophil and monocyte diapedesis across ECs but not in their adherence to ECs. Indeed, leukocytes blocked during transmigration by anti-PECAM-1 antibodies remain bound to the EC surface over the intercellular junction (42). Adherence to ECs is a prerequisite for the transmigration. However, it seems that only half of the leukocytes adhering to the apical surface of ECs transmigrate under optimal conditions (51).

Once in subendothelial tissue, the extravasated leukocytes continue to migrate toward the inflammatory site. The interactions between extracellular matrix compo-

nents and their specific receptor of the integrin family, as well as the presence of a gradient of chemotactic factors, are involved in this step.

Specificity and Selectivity of Adhesion Processes with Each of the Cells Involved in Allergic Inflammation

The possible mechanism to account for the selective recruitment of leukocyte subtypes is a model combining strategies to achieve diversity and specificity. There are three key components in this model: primary adhesion receptors (selectins), then activating factors, and finally activation-dependent adhesion receptors (integrins). The diversity and the specificity seem not to be the consequence of adhesion molecule expression, given the limited number of selectin-carbohydrate or integrin-Ig-like interactions and the redundancy of their expression *in vivo*. In contrast, a plethora of potent activating factors, including cytokines, peptides, and lipid mediators, are implicated in the inflammatory reaction. A combination of selectin, carbohydrate ligand, integrin, and the Ig-like ligand provides sufficient diversity to allow selective recruitment of leukocytes. In allergic inflammation, continuous exchanges do exist between soluble mediators generated by peripheral blood leukocytes or cells present into bronchial mucosa and the endothelial surface. All of these factors constantly mediate, modulate, and alter the expression of adhesion molecules. Therefore, during the development of the allergic reaction, mediators of allergy, cytokines, chemokines, and cell adhesion molecules expressed on ECs and on leukocytes (like integrins and L-selectin) interfere bidirectionally to induce, regulate, and eventually reverse the cellular influx. Moreover, processes that regulate cell trafficking differ according to the cell type implicated: eosinophils, T lymphocytes, and basophils are responding to different leukocyte-EC adhesion pathways, which may explain the apparent selectivity of migration.

Lymphocytes

Although activated T lymphocytes represent a major component of cell infiltrates seen in allergic asthma, little is known about the control of lymphocyte migration in the airway mucosa. The selectin and CD18 integrin pathways as well as other pathways not used by neutrophils are involved in their migration. As an example, the $\alpha_4\beta_1$-integrin (VLA-4) and $\alpha_4\beta_7$-integrin, which preferentially bind to the EC counterligands VCAM-1 and MadCAM-1, have been implicated in lymphocyte migration through the endothelial barrier.

Moreover, evidence exists for a selectivity of lymphocyte traffic. This is supported by the fact that naive and memory T lymphocytes have different recirculation pathways: memory lymphocytes are programmed so as to be predisposed to return to the tissue where they were first exposed to the allergen (for example, skin or respiratory mucosa) (52). In the skin, T lymphocytes localized at the site of the allergen conflict were shown to express a carbohydrate termed CLA, which represents a homing structure that primarily interacts during the rolling step with E-selectin (28). In the second phase of transmigration, CLA engagement is required for using the VLA-4/VCAM-1 pathway (53). Thus, CLA-dependent transendothelial T-cell migration appears as a complex system in which mutual interactions between CLA and E-selectin as well as VLA-4/VCAM-1 are successively involved for T-lymphocyte homing.

Lymphocyte chemoattractants are also implicated in lymphoaccumulation at inflammatory sites. A number of chemokines, among which are some produced by ECs, are found to be chemoattractive for lymphocyte subpopulations: monocyte chemotactic protein 1 is a major lymphocyte chemoattractant; macrophage-inflammatory protein (MIP) 1β enhances the binding of naive T cells to VCAM-1 (54); RANTES selectively attracts the memory T lymphocytes (55). Lymphocyte chemoattractant factor is also a potent chemotactic factor for CD4+ lymphocytes and is produced by lymphocytes activated by various stimuli, including histamine. Moreover, an increased concentration of lymphocyte chemoattractant factor was found in bronchoalveolar fluid from allergen-challenged asthmatic patients.

In allergic asthma, the exact traffic signals for lymphocyte emigration are presently unknown. Specific bronchial homing molecules that might explain the influx of activated T lymphocytes in target tissues remain to be discovered. Conditions of lymphocyte recirculation in asthmatics are also incompletely understood. Some indirect data, though, indicate that T lymphocytes in bronchial asthma can circulate and migrate toward other parts of the mucosal associated lymphoid tissue (MALT). In a prospective study, we evaluated the histologic abnormalities of the minor salivary glands (MSGs) in a series of 58 asthmatics (29 with allergic asthma and 20 with nonallergic asthma) compared with 15 healthy subjects and 15 patients with chronic obstructive pulmonary disease (56). Results are summarized in Table 3: 43 (74%) of 58 asthmatic patients had MSG abnormalities with a large T-lymphocyte infiltration, with partly degranulated mast cells and basement membrane thickening. Abnormalities were more often observed in nonallergic (97%) than in allergic asthmatics (52%, $p < 0.01$). They were practically absent in the two control groups (6%, $p < 0.001$ versus asthmatics). Thus, these intriguing observations showed that, except for eosinophil infiltration which was absent in MSGs, the glandular tissue of MSGs in bronchial asthma expressed an airwaylike inflammation that might be due to the homing of T lymphocytes in another part of the MALT system. Interestingly, endothelium changes

TABLE 3. *Abnormalities in minor salivary glands from patients with bronchial asthma, chronic obstructive pulmonary disease (COPD), or from healthy subjects*

	Patients with allergic asthma (n = 29)	Patients with nonallergic asthma (n = 29)	Patients with COPD (n = 15)	Healthy subjects (n = 15)
Mean Chisholm's score[a]	0.45 ± 0.14	1.5 ± 0.18	0.07 ± 0.07	0.07 ± 0.07
Lymphocyte infiltration	9 (31%)	24 (83%)	1 (6.5%)	1 (6.5%)
Eosinophils	1 (3.5%)	1 (3.5%)	0	0
Mast cells	13 (45%)	27 (93%)	3 (20%)	4 (27%)
Basement membrane thickening	11 (38%)	26 (90%)	1 (6.5%)	0
Vascular wall edema	1 (3.5%)	14 (48%)	0	0
ICAM-1 expression (on vascular sections)	0/6	10/16 (62.5%)	0/4	0/4

ICAM, intercellular adhesion molecule.
[a]The Chisholm's score quantifies the number of focal inflammatory cell aggregates containing ≥50 lymphocytes or plasma cells in each 4 mm^2 of salivary gland.

with turgescent ECs, vascular wall edema, and narrowing of capillary and venule lumens were detectable in 15 patients (26%). Morphologic alterations of vessels, the vascular expression of ICAM-1 observed mainly in nonallergic asthmatics, support the hypothesis that ECs were activated and suggest that at least an ICAM-1-dependent pathway may be involved in the T-lymphocyte sequestration into the MSG tissue of asthmatics.

Eosinophils

The prominent role of eosinophils in allergy and its marked accumulation at the sites of allergic inflammation (57) have been widely described. Many structures expressed on the surface of eosinophils, particularly after eosinophil activation, are susceptible to interaction with counterligands on ECs and on extracellular matrix components (Table 4) (58,59).

Like other leukocytes, eosinophils express the β_2-integrins (leukocyte function-associated antigen 1, macrophage 1, and glycoprotein 150-95), which can bind, among others, ICAM-1. When eosinophils are exposed to a range of chemotactic or activating stimuli, expression of CD11b rapidly increases (60,61); an upregulation of CD11b levels is also induced by IL-5, GM-CSF, and PAF addition (62), with additive or synergistic effects when various combinations are used. In parallel, it has been reported (63) that eosinophils from sputum, nasal polyps, and bronchoalveolar lavage fluid (BAL) from asthmatics demonstrated a marked increase of CD11b (macrophage 1) compared with blood eosinophils.

Other adhesion receptors present on eosinophils, however, appear to be more specific: they are represented by the group of α_4-integrins. One part of the specificity may be explained by the presence of a counterreceptor for VCAM-1: the VLA-4 present on eosinophils but not on neutrophils (64–66). More recent studies showed that $\alpha_4\beta_7$, a ligand of VCAM-1 and MadCAM-1, was detected on eosinophils. Experimental studies with mAb to α_4-in-

tegrins managed to block eosinophil infiltration in allergy lung models (67). Moreover, α_4-integrin antagonists have been synthesized and thus inhibited binding to components of the extracellular matrix, more precisely at the site of the α_4-recognition motif.

L-selectin acts differently; it is likely to be involved in leukocyte rolling on the vessel wall, a process that precedes firm adhesion and extravasation. L-selectin, unlike the P- and E-selectins, is constitutively expressed at the surface of most leukocytes, and eosinophils from peripheral blood currently express L-selectin. After cellular activation during extravasation, however, L-selectin is shed, as shown by eosinophils that migrate into the alveolar spaces after allergen challenge. This downregulation of L-selectin enables eosinophils to detach themselves from the endothelial surface, this de-adhesion consecutive to the shedding of L-selectin favoring the subsequent migration (68).

The issue of eosinophil migration is now still more complicated. Indeed, cytokines active on eosinophil trafficking were originally considered to be derived predominantly from lymphocytes and mast cells: they are now known to be elaborated by many other cell types, including the eosinophil itself. Eosinophils synthesize and store in their granules several important inflammatory and regulating cytokines including IL-1, IL-3, IL-5, IL-6, IL-8, GM-CSF, transforming growth factor (TGF)-α, TGF-β, TNF-α, and MIP-1α (69–73). Moqbel et al. (72) have presented new evidence that human eosinophils could synthesize IL-4 and RANTES in airway tissue and/or in late-phase reaction lesions. Thus, eosinophils certainly contribute to the modification of their own environment and facilitate, by an autocrine cytokine release, their emigration through the vascular endothelium.

Basophils

The mechanisms by which circulating human basophils migrate toward the site of allergic reaction are not well defined. Several studies have specified that basophils have been involved in the late-phase reaction for allergic asthmatics (74). Similarly, after nasal allergen challenge, the analysis of mediators locally released showed two peaks of histamine release in lavage fluids. The first is related to a local mast cell degranulation, and the second, which is not accompanied by a rise of prostaglandin D_2 and tryptase, is considered to be basophil dependent (75). These data suggest, therefore, that circulating basophils were actively recruited during the late phase, implying the existence of specific adherence and migration process across the vascular barrier. Bochner and colleagues (76, 77) showed effectively that human basophils can adhere to cultured HUVECs by a mechanism that is somewhat similar to the interaction between ECs and eosinophils. Indeed, the interactions between VCAM-1 and VLA-4, and perhaps also between $\alpha_4\beta_7$-integrin and MadCAM-1, seem to be implicated in the specificity of the influx.

TABLE 4. *Eosinophil adherence to human endothelial cells*

Adhesion molecules expressed on	
Eosinophils	Endothelial cells
β_2-Integrins	
CD11a/CD18 (LFA-1)	ICAM-1 and ICAM-2
CD11b/CD18 (MAC-1)	ICAM-1
α_4-Integrins	
VLA-4	VCAM-1
$\alpha_4\beta_7$	MadCAM
L-selectin	Sialoglycoproteins

ICAM, intercellular adhesion molecule; LFA, leukocyte function-associated antigen; MAC, macrophage; MadCAM, mucosal addressin cell adhesion molecule; VCAM, vascular cell adhesion molecule; VLA, very late antigen.

ENDOTHELIAL CELLS IN ASTHMA: EXPERIMENTAL AND CLINICAL APPROACHES

Histopathologic studies performed on patient biopsy specimens, and therapeutic effects of antibodies directed against some of the adhesion structures present on ECs, have led to a better, although incomplete and sometimes controversial, understanding of the role of ECs in allergic diseases.

Experimental Models of Asthma

Several animal models have been used—guinea pigs, sheep, and primates—in the perspective of evaluating endothelial and/or epithelial adhesion molecules in the experimental situations comparable to acute or chronic asthma.

In primate models of asthma, acute or chronic airway responses can be reproduced consecutive to allergen inhalation (78). A single inhalation of *Ascaris suum* in cynomolgus monkeys induced a rapid and short neutrophil infiltration, followed by a long-term eosinophil infiltration (6 h to 6–7 days) and only a weak increase in bronchial hyperresponsiveness (BHR). In contrast, repeated antigen exposures produced a massive and pure eosinophil infiltration concomitantly with a severe increase of airway responsiveness thought to be related to eosinophil cationic proteins.

In the model of repeated antigen inhalations, an enhanced expression of adhesion molecules was detected in bronchial biopsy specimens (ICAM-1 on epithelium and endothelium of airways, but E-selectin only on airway microvessels). When monkeys received anti-ICAM-1 mAb, both eosinophil infiltration and BHR were corrected (79). In the case of a single *Ascaris* antigen inhalation in sensitized animals, bronchial challenge resulted in an immediate bronchoconstriction followed in some of them by a late-phase response characterized by an acute neutrophilic infiltration, correlated with the intensity of the bronchospastic response (80). To determine the respective role of ICAM-1 and E-selectin in both situations, neutralizing antibodies for each adhesion molecule were injected intravenously prior to *Ascaris* challenge: anti-ICAM-1 antibodies did not affect the neutrophil infiltration in airways, whereas anti-E-selectin antibodies clearly inhibited the late-phase bronchoconstriction as well as the number of neutrophils and myeloperoxidase activity present in BAL fluids. In this model of experimental acute asthma, E-selectin appears therefore to play a crucial role in the allergen-induced late bronchoconstriction response, whereas, in the model of multiple antigen inhalations, ICAM-1 is predominantly implicated in BHR and eosinophil infiltration. In addition, when allergen exposure is chronically repeated with a persistent inflammation and airway responsiveness, daily intravenous administration of anti-ICAM-1 and E-selectin antibodies given *a posteriori* fails to reverse both phenomena, suggesting that an anti-adhesion-molecule treatment is unable to reverse an established persistent airway inflammation (81). In a rat model, treatment of sensitized rats with anti-CD18 or anti-ICAM-1 mAb reduced the eosinophil infiltrate and the hyperreactivity induced by allergen challenge.

More recent studies have explored an alternative adhesion pathway represented by the VCAM-1/VLA-4 couple. In guinea pigs, the eosinophil accumulation obtained by passive cutaneous anaphylaxis is inhibited by an anti-VLA-4 antibody (82). In ovalbumin-sensitized guinea pigs, anti-VLA-4 mAb also blocks the eosinophil influx into alveolar spaces as well the BHR obtained in response to carbachol (83). Similar results were obtained in rats and sheep challenged with allergen: treatment with an anti-VLA-4 mAb restricted the accumulation of lymphocytes and eosinophils in BAL 24 h after aerosol ovalbumin challenge (84); in sheep, mAb to VLA-4 also prevented the late-phase bronchospastic response and BHR but without effect on eosinophil attraction (85). In fact, multiple experimental models are presently being tested that are directed against EC adhesion molecules but also against integrins (from the group of α_4-integrins such as VLA-4 or $\alpha_4\beta_7$, or those belonging to the CD11-CD18 complex). Although these data look very promising, the variability in results suggests that the experimental model and the treatment protocol make their interpretation difficult.

Adhesion Molecule Expression on the Microvasculature in Allergic Diseases

After the initial demonstration in 1990 that the intravenous administration of antibodies against ICAM-1 and E-selectin could prevent the development of BHR and cell infiltration in sensitized monkeys (79,80), many studies were initiated in patients developing allergic reactions at different sites: in the skin, the nose, and the bronchial mucosa. Adhesion molecule expression was evaluated at baseline and after allergen challenge.

Analysis of mechanisms for accumulation of inflammatory cells at the site of a cutaneous late-phase allergic reaction enabled the crucial role of adhesion molecules to be demonstrated for the first time in human beings (86). In that report, expression of endothelial leukocyte adhesion molecule 1, presently named E-selectin, was quantified in sequential skin biopsy specimens from patients with respiratory allergy between 20 min and 24 h after intradermal allergen challenge. In all seven atopics tested, allergen injection determined the appearance of E-selectin on ECs simultaneously to the influx of inflammatory cells: E-selectin expression was detected 3 to 4 h after allergen administration, increased in intensity at 6 h, and declined after 24 h, reproducing the well-known kinetics of E-selectin expression. Cytokines involved in the process were identified as IL-1 and TNF-α, as proved by the inhibition of the expression of E-selectin by allergen when skin biopsy specimens were incubated with a combination of anti-TNF-α and anti-IL-1 antibodies. Many cell types are potentially presumed to secrete IL-1 and TNF-α. Klein et al. (87) and Walsh et al. (88) have reported the presence of preformed TNF-α in mast cells of human skin fragments and its release upon allergen challenge. Both suggested that upregulation of E-selectin on ECs by antigen addition could be related to TNF-α release from IgE-triggered mast cells.

In perennial allergic rhinitis, immunostaining of nasal biopsy specimens showed that the number of ECs expressing ICAM-1 and VCAM-1 were significantly elevated (89). Another study (90) compared data obtained with nasal biopsies performed at baseline and 24 h after nasal challenge: ICAM-1 appeared as the predominantly expressed molecule in ECs of the nasal mucosa but was considered as constitutive. More interestingly, an enhanced percentage of vessels expressing VCAM-1 was observed after allergen challenge, whereas no change was found for ICAM-1 and E-selectin. The low expression of E-selectin may be explained by the timing of the study: biopsies were performed at 24 h after challenge, that is, at a period when E-selectin, which is known to be induced early (between 4 and 6 h), had already declined.

Results obtained by asthma studies confirm this modulation of cell adhesion molecules on the microvasculature. When allergic asthmatic patients were studied at baseline, Gosset et al. (91) found that ICAM-1 and, to a lesser degree, E-selectin and VCAM-1 were overexpressed at the surface of the vascular endothelium (Fig. 1). An increased expression of ICAM-1 on the bronchial epithelium was also detectable. Our results differ from those reported by Bentley et al. (92) and Montefort et al. (93), who observed no difference between normal donors and asthmatics. This apparent discrepancy might be explained by the fact that most of our patients were symptomatic at the time of bronchoscopy and the asthma symptom (Aas) score was higher. In contrast, in the nonallergic asthma group, adhesion molecule expression in bronchial biopsy specimens was not significantly different from that in the control population: as patients in this subgroup demonstrated a higher degree of severity, a probable role for corticosteroids, used more widely in treating intrinsic asthma, is therefore suspected. *In vitro* treatment of ECs with glucocorticoids is known to inhibit ICAM-1 expression.

There is also evidence that EC activation occurs within the human airways after local allergen challenge. By using an endobronchial allergen instillation (94), morphologic and histochemical modifications consecutive to allergen challenge can be compared in the same patient. Specimens from biopsies performed 6 h after challenge were compared with specimens recovered at the same time from saline-instilled bronchial segments. Parallel with a submucosal infiltration by neutrophils, eosinophils, mast cells, and CD3+ lymphocytes, a marked increase in ICAM-1 and E-selectin—but not VCAM-1—was detectable on the microvasculature. The mechanisms sustaining the dissociation of VCAM-1 and ICAM-1 expressions are not understood, since ICAM-1 and VCAM-1 have theoretically similar patterns of upregulation. Nevertheless, it seems possible to postulate that, following allergen exposure, cell emigration through the vascular endothelium proceeds in two successive steps: (a) an early upregulation of E-selectin and ICAM-1, which is responsible for the eosinophil and T-cell response at 6 h, followed by (b) the enhancement of VCAM-1 persistence for 24 h, which may account for more selective eosinophil and basophil attraction through interaction with VLA-4. Another important issue is represented by the relationships between an enhanced expression of adhesion molecules and the level of airflow limitation. In asthmatic patients monitored with a peak-flow meter (95), the BAL procedure and bronchial biopsies were performed as soon as peak expiratory flow values were below 80% of the control values. Under these conditions, they clearly demonstrated a marked upregulation of ICAM-1, VCAM-1, and E-selectin in vascular ECs concomitantly with local eosinophil accumulation. Interestingly, immunoelectron microscopy enabled a specific immunoreactivity to be detected for the three structures, especially for VCAM-1, in the perinuclear space and on the luminal surface of

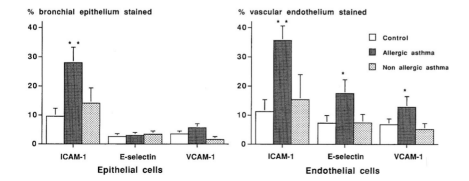

FIG. 1. Adhesion molecule expression quantified on sections of bronchial biopsies from allergic and nonallergic asthmatics. Comparison of endothelial and epithelial staining (*p<0.05 and **p<0.01 compared with controls).

ECs, suggesting an active *in vivo* synthesis by the bronchial microvasculature. Nevertheless, this upregulation of adhesion molecules in submucosal tissues of bronchi is not specific for allergic or nonallergic asthma. In patients with chronic obstructive bronchitis (96), a quantitative analysis by immunohistochemical techniques demonstrated an enhanced expression of E-selectin on bronchial vessels and of ICAM-1 on basal epithelial cells. The increased number of vessels positive for E-selectin was correlated with the level of airway obstruction and with the number of neutrophils present in the submucosa of bronchitics.

Another approach to the study of the role of adhesion molecules in asthma is represented by the evaluation of soluble forms of adhesion molecules. Not surprisingly, during inflammation, serum levels of circulating ICAM-1, VCAM-1, and E-selectin, as well as the leukocyte L-selectin, have been measured to follow the inflammatory process, including its severity or reversal under treatment (97,98). In acute asthma, circulating soluble ICAM-1 and soluble E-selectin, but not VCAM-1, were enhanced, which probably reflected the intense inflammatory reaction in airways. Enhancement of a soluble form of E-selectin was also detected in BAL fluids after local endobronchial allergen challenge (99). In patients with stable asthma, however, no difference in circulating forms of adhesion molecules could be demonstrated when compared with nonatopic asthmatics and with healthy subjects (100).

There was also no correlation between the concentrations of the three circulating adhesion molecules or between serum levels and the degree of disease severity. In dual asthmatic responders, a significant increase in serum levels of the soluble form of ICAM-1 was associated with the upregulation of ICAM-1 on peripheral blood T lymphocytes and the secondary decrease of ICAM-1 expression on CD8+ and CD4+ T cells at the time when the late bronchospastic reaction developed (101).

THE VASCULAR ENDOTHELIUM AS A TARGET ORGAN OF ALLERGIC INFLAMMATION

During the induction of the inflammatory reaction, different effector cells, including recruited leukocytes, release the first activation signals that trigger the cascade of events leading to an increased leukocyte recruitment. The EC is one target of these mediators. In allergic reaction,

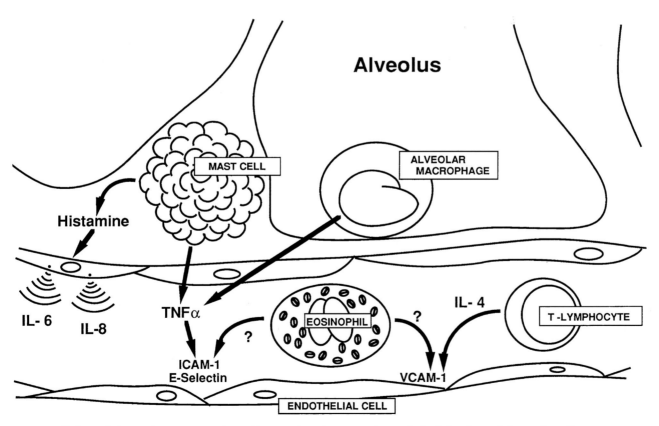

FIG. 2. Schematic representation of interactions between the endothelial cells and the main cell types involved in allergic inflammation.

exposure to allergen induces the rapid activation of mast cells and alveolar macrophages followed, during the late-phase reaction, by the activation of other cell types, including eosinophils and lymphocytes, which secrete various mediators in the lung tissue (Fig. 2). Although activation of ECs in allergic reaction has been largely postulated to occur through the expression of adhesion molecules, the mechanisms implicated in this stimulation are not well defined. Some *in vitro* models of EC monolayers have provided precious information about the behavior of the endothelium in the presence of leukocyte products. These observations have been fruitful for the understanding of the physiopathology of vascular endothelium in inflammatory reactions and are summarized next.

Interaction between Macrophages and Endothelial Cells

In asthmatics, alveolar macrophages stimulated *in vitro* with anti-human IgE antibody or with IgE-specific allergens produce large amounts of TNF-α and IL-6, with an amplification in the case of costimulation with IFN-γ. An increased release of TNF-α and IL-6 by alveolar macrophages has been observed in patients who develop a late asthmatic response (102). After bronchial allergen challenge, a bronchoalveolar lavage performed 18 h after allergen exposure enabled alveolar macrophages to be recovered that produced large amounts of TNF-α and IL-6 (a 10- to 12-fold increase when compared with patients studied at baseline or exhibiting only an immediate bronchospastic response). The direct addition of AM supernatants on EC cultures mediated an enhanced expression of ICAM-1 and E-selectin that was completely abolished in the presence of anti-TNF-α antibodies. Our results suggest therefore that macrophages—by their capacity to induce expression of cell adhesion molecules in their local environment—might participate in the induction of the local inflammation reaction observed in bronchial asthma (103).

Interaction between Mast Cells and Endothelial Cells

Among mast cell mediators, histamine interacts directly with ECs: Histamine is known to induce such early changes in endothelium as increased permeability, a transient expression of P-selectin and the secretion, and/or the surface expression of early mediators (for example, prostaglandin I_2, PAF, and LTB_4) (104). However, later effects of histamine on ECs, in particular on cytokine production, have not been estimated. We have evaluated the action of histamine on IL-8 and IL-6 production by HUVECs (105,106). IL-8 secretion by histamine-stimulated HUVECs was concentration dependent, with the largest

amount of IL-8 obtained with histamine concentration of 10^{-3} M. After a 24-h incubation, however, lower concentrations of histamine (10^{-6} M) also induced a significant increase in IL-8 production (Fig. 3). IL-8 neosynthesis was assessed by Northern blot analysis: when ECs were cultured for 4 h in the presence of histamine, there was an increase of 1.8-kilobase mRNA expression compared with basal expression in resting cells. Moreover, histamine and TNF-α (a mediator present in mast cell granules and released concomitantly with histamine) had synergistic effects on IL-8 production. TNF-α used alone at 50 units/mL induced a low but significant IL-8 production by ECs, largely enhanced in the case of coincubation with histamine. Histamine-induced cytokine production by ECs probably reflects a mechanism involved in inflammatory reaction. Although it was difficult to define histamine concentrations exactly in the target organs, concentrations of histamine (from 10^{-6} to 10^{-4} M) were compatible with those measured in tissues after mast cell degranulation. Furthermore, since histamine-induced IL-8 production by ECs was detected from 4 to 24 h after stimulation, it might participate in the late-phase reaction: *in vitro* IL-8 exerted a chemotactic activity for neutrophils, eosinophils, and basophils. IL-8 has also been demonstrated to modulate basophil histamine release. This point is of importance in allergic rhinitis, where different observations suggest that basophils are implicated as effector cells in the late-phase reaction (107).

The same results were obtained for IL-6. After incubation with increasing concentrations of histamine, IL-6 was also secreted by ECs within the same time span and at similar concentrations as for IL-8 (108).

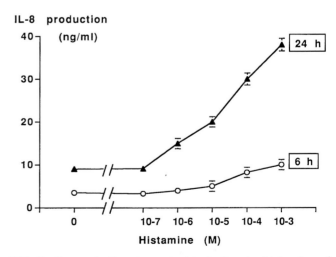

FIG. 3. Concentration-dependent induction by histamine of interleukin (IL)-8 production from HUVEC monolayers. IL-8 measured by an immunoassay in supernatants at the end of a 6-h or a 24-h incubation with the indicated concentrations of histamine.

Interaction between Eosinophils and Endothelial Cells

It has long been known that proteins from eosinophil granules can activate other cells associated with allergic inflammation. Micromolar concentrations of major basic protein (MBP) and eosinophil peroxidase affect functional activities of basophils and neutrophils. MBP stimulates histamine release from human basophils and rat mast cells (108); it also activates neutrophils by enhancing the expression of CR3 and glycoprotein 150-95 (109). All of these experiments indicate that MBP and various eosinophil products can activate other participants of the inflammatory reaction.

To test whether eosinophils and their degranulation products are susceptible to interfere with vascular endothelium, we evaluated the effects of eosinophil supernatants on the cell adhesion molecule expression of HUVEC preparations. Eosinophils from patients with circulating hypereosinophilia (hypereosinophilic syndrome, chronic eosinophilic pneumonia, allergic asthma, and various atopic diseases, including atopic dermatitis), purified by adsorption of CD16 (FcγRIII)-positive cells on magnetic beads, were stimulated through IgE or IgG activation. Supernatants were transferred to HUVEC monolayers, and the subsequent expression of ICAM-1, E-selectin, and VCAM-1 appreciated by enzyme-linked immunosorbent assay after 6 and 24 h. With 1-h supernatants, a clear-cut enhancement of ICAM-1 and E-selectin was obtained

in the case of IgE-dependent stimulation. VCAM-1 expression compared with unstimulated eosinophils did not significantly vary. In contrast, with eosinophil supernatants collected after 18 h, the expression of all three cell adhesion molecules was largely enhanced (200%), with similar levels in all conditions (Fig. 4).

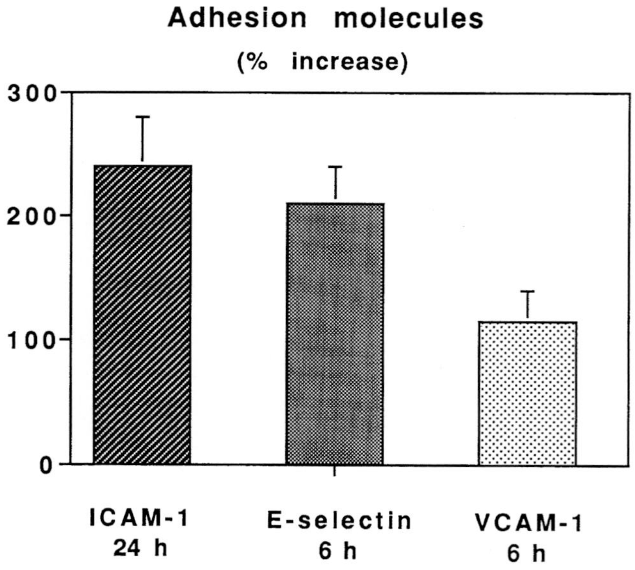

The addition of eosinophil supernatants on ECs appears therefore able to enhance CAM expression greatly, the role of contaminant cells having been excluded by the high degree of purity of the eosinophil preparation. The problem is presently to identify the factor(s) present in eosinophil supernatants that is (are) responsible for the over-expression of CAM. Several potential candidates need to be considered: arachidonic acid metabolites and PAF-acether are not involved; the role of basic proteins or of cytokines produced after eosinophil activation, or the association of both, is presently under investigation. Whatever its (their) exact nature, eosinophils recovered from patients with hypereosinophilia appear to be able to activate the vascular endothelium directly and to create a kind of autoamplification loop of the inflammatory process.

Interaction between T Lymphocytes and Endothelial Cells

As for the other cells and cytokines just discussed, lymphokines also upregulate adhesion molecule expression on ECs, but to a lesser extent. IFN-γ modulates ICAM-1 and HLA class II expression, favoring mainly the adherence of neutrophils and T lymphocytes. IL-4, a lymphokine with a broad range of immune functions, upregulates VCAM-1 expression specifically, allowing preferential eosinophil, basophil, and T-lymphocyte adhesion to endothelium (110–112).

The inflammatory response in allergic diseases is characterized by infiltrates of activated T lymphocytes (8). In bronchial asthma, activated T cells secrete IL-3, IL-4, IL-5, or GM-CSF (9). Therefore, the T lymphocyte, by the production of IL-4 and IL-5, could be one of the most potent cells able to create the specificity of the infiltrate associated with allergic reaction. In this context, we have recently explored the activation of ECs by T-cell-derived lymphokines produced by peripheral blood T cells from mite-sensitive asthmatics in the presence of the related allergen presented by paraformaldehyde-fixed antigen-presenting cells (113). T-lymphocyte supernatants from these patients induced an increase of VCAM-1 (Fig. 5) and ICAM-1 expression, but not of E-selectin. IL-6 synthesis by ECs was also significantly enhanced. The induction of VCAM-1 expression was inhibited by adding neutralizing antibodies against IL-4, whereas IL-6 expression and ICAM-1 expression were inhibited by anti-IFN-γ antibodies. An enhanced production of both lymphokines was in fact detected in the supernatants of allergen-stimulated T cells from allergic patients, com-

Adhesion molecules
(% increase)

FIG. 4. Adhesion molecule expression induced on human umbilical cord vein cell monolayers by supernatants of purified eosinophils from patients with hypereosinophilic diseases of various etiologies. Enhancement of adhesion molecule expression was evaluated after 6 h for E-selectin and vascular cell adhesion molecule-1, and after 24 h for intercellular adhesion molecule-1.

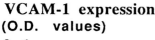

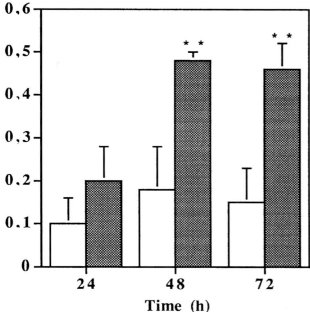

FIG. 5. Vascular cell adhesion molecule-1 expression induced on human umbilical cord vein cell monolayers after addition of supernatants of T lymphocytes from mite-sensitive asthmatics; T lymphocytes were incubated in the presence of *Dermatophagoides pteronyssinus* allergen *(dark bars)* or in the presence of an unrelated allergen *(light bars)* (**p<0.001 compared with unrelated allergen). Supernatants of activated T-lymphocytes were collected after 24, 48, and 72 h.

pared with unstimulated cells from asthmatics or allergen-stimulated cells from healthy controls. These data showed that both allergen-specific T-helper type 1 (TH1) and TH2 T cells were present in the circulation of allergic patients, a situation certainly different from that observed in lung tissue where a predominant TH2 T-cell infiltrate has been evidenced.

FUTURE DEVELOPMENTS

In allergic asthma, an exciting field of research is represented by the evaluation of the mechanisms modulating the functions of ECs. Indeed, among the numerous mediators produced by the cells involved in the development of allergic reaction, it is very difficult to define those really implicated in this process. Some *in vitro* studies have approached these mechanisms, but nothing has been done *in vivo*.

The definition and the molecular cloning of integrins, members of the Ig-like superfamily, and selectins have already enabled the construction of a model for adhesive interactions involved in leukocyte emigration. However, the modulation of adhesion molecule expression by che-

moattractant and activating factors needs to be studied further, particularly *in vivo*. Additional studies with animal models are required to dissect the contribution of individual adhesion molecules in the development of inflammatory reaction, but such studies could also help in the understanding of the relationships between the different adhesion pathways. Although numerous reports describe the effects of specific antibodies against adhesion molecules, these studies need to be improved. Several methods of administration must still be evaluated; the question of the best route of administration—systemic or inhaled—is still being debated and changes according to the chosen target: circulating blood leukocytes, ECs, or airway epithelial cells. Another exciting area is the definition of the functions of the soluble form of adhesion molecules that are released in biological fluid following inflammatory reaction.

We recently described the isolation and molecular characterization of a novel human endothelial cell molecule designated EC-specific molecule (ESM) 1 (114), which displays several unique features of interest that can confer on it a putatively important role in local inflammation. Sequence analysis confirmed the unique identity of ESM-1, which contains a hydrophobic NH_2-terminal amino acid sequence of 19 residues consistent with a signal sequence. There is no transmembrane region, suggesting that ESM-1 is a secretory molecule. The ESM-1 cDNA sequence predicts a mature ESM-1 polypeptide of 165 amino acids corresponding to a molecular weight of 20 kDa. An important finding is that ESM-1 mRNA is regulated by the cytokines. TNF-α induced accumulation of ESM-1 mRNA detectable early at the second hour and peaking at the 18th hour of TNF incubation. In addition, IL-1β was also shown to increase ESM-1 gene expression in a very similar pattern as did TNF-α. Also interesting is the particular action of IFN-γ on ESM-1 mRNA expression. Unexpectedly, our results clearly indicate that IFN-γ, which was without any effect when used alone, has inhibitory effects on TNF-α-induced ESM-1 gene expression. This suggests that ESM-1 may exhibit unusual functions during the inflammatory reaction depending on cytokines. A second finding is that this molecule is highly restricted to the EC, and that the ESM-1 is synthesized, distributed, and restricted to the lung vascular ECs. This would suggest that ESM-1 may participate in specialized endothelial functions, particularly in the lung vascular spaces. These data indicate a link between ESM-1 and inflammation, and provide new insights in areas of vascular cell biology and human lung pathology, particularly in asthma.

CONCLUSIONS

Considering the general economy of vascular endothelium in allergic inflammation, and more particularly in asthma, this structure appears to be both a target and an effector organ in the physiopathology of the disease, which means that the balance between adhesion molecule expression and secreted mediators has to be regulated not only at the vascular endothelium level but also at the level of migrating leukocytes. Therefore, among all functions served by the microvasculature during the allergic conflict, complex and persistent interactions between ECs and neighboring tissues permanently modify the reactivity of circulating and migrating cells. Among them, cells of the immune system induce, through a large panel of mediators, cytokines and chemokines, a constant adaptation of EC behavior, evidenced by the modulation of adhesion molecule expression. The dysregulation of such a critical equilibrium leads easily to the overexpression of inflammatory components, which is detrimental to patients. An extensive understanding of this complex network should enable more accurate therapy to be developed and provide new insights for the prophylaxis of allergic diseases.

REFERENCES

1. Persson CGA. Role of plasma exudation in asthmatic airways. *Lancet* 1986;2:1126–1129.
2. Persson CGA. Tracheobronchial microcirculation in asthma. In: Kaliner MA, Barnes PJ, Persson CGA, eds. *Asthma: its pathology and treatment.* New York: Marcel Dekker, 1991;209–229.
3. Lamm WJE, Selfe S, Albert RK. Pharmacologic and pulmonary physiologic effects of leukotrienes binding to albumin. *Am Rev Respir Dis* 1988;137:398(abstr).
4. Forstner JF, Jabbal I, Findlay BP, Forstner GG. Interaction of mucins with calcium, H^+ ion and albumin. *Mod Probl Paediatry* 1977;19: 54–65.
5. Jeffery PK, Wardlaw A, Nelson FC, Collins JV, Kay AB. Bronchial biopsies in asthma: an ultrastructural quantification study and correlation with hyperreactivity. *Am Rev Respir Dis* 1989;140:1745–1753.
6. Bousquet J, Chanez P, Lacoste JY, et al. Eosinophilic inflammation in asthma. *N Engl J Med* 1990;323:1033–1039.
7. Saetta M, Distefano A, Rosina C, Thiene G, Fabbri LM. Quantitative structural analysis of peripheral airways and arteries in sudden fatal asthma. *Am Rev Respir Dis* 1991;143:138–143.
8. Corrigan CJ, Kay AB. T cells and eosinophils in the pathogenesis of asthma. *Immunol Today* 1992;13:501–506.
9. Robinson DS, Hamid Q, Ying S, et al. Predominant TH2-like bronchoalveolar T-lymphocyte population in atopic asthma. *N Engl J Med* 1992;326:298–304.
10. Albelda SM. Endothelial and epithelial cell adhesion molecules. *Am J Respir Cell Mol Biol* 1991;4:195–203.
11. Lewis MS, Whatley RE, Cain P, McIntyre TM, Prescott SM, Zimmerman GA. Hydrogen peroxide stimulates the synthesis of platelet activating factor by endothelium and induces endothelial cell dependent adhesion. *J Clin Invest* 1988;82:2045–2055.
12. Casale TB, Erger RA, Little MM. Platelet-activating factor-induced human eosinophil transendothelial migration: evidence for a dynamic role of the endothelium. *Am J Respir Cell Mol Biol* 1993;8:77–82.
13. Feinmark SJ, Cannon PJ. Endothelial cell leukotriene C_4 synthesis results from intercellular transfer of LTA_4 synthesized by polymorphonuclear leukocytes. *J Biol Chem* 1986;261:16,466–16,472.
14. Gerritsen ME, Bloor CM. Endothelial cell gene expression in response to injury. *FASEB J* 1993;7:523–532.
15. Delneste Y, Lassalle P, Jeannin P, Joseph M, Tonnel AB, Gosset P. Histamine induces IL-6 production by human endothelial cells. *Clin Exp Immunol* 1994;98:344–349.
16. Larsen CG, Anderson AO, Appella E, Oppenheim JJ, Matsushima K. The neutrophil-activating peptide (NAP-1) is also chemotactic for T-lymphocytes. *Science* 1989;243:1464–1466.
17. Collins PD, Weg WB, Gaccioli LH, Watson ML, Moqbel R, Williams TJ. Eosinophil accumulation induced by human interleukin 8 in guinea pig *in vivo. Immunology* 1993;79:312–318.
18. Erger RA, Casale TB. Interleukin-8 is a potent mediator of eosinophil chemotaxis through endothelium and epithelium. *Am J Physiol* 1995; 268:L117–L122.
19. Alam R, Stafford P, Forsythe P, et al. RANTES is a chemotactic and activating factor for human eosinophils. *J Immunol* 1993;150:3442–3447.
20. Schweizer RC, Walmers BAC, Raaijmakers JA, Zanen P, Lammers JWJ, Koenderman L. RANTES and Interleukin 8 induced responses in normal human eosinophils: effects of priming with interleukin 5. *Blood* 1994;83:3697–3704.
21. Meurer R, Van Riper G, Feeney W, et al. Formation of eosinophilic and monocytic intradermal inflammatory sites in the dog by injection of human RANTES but not human MCP-1, human MIP-1α or human IL-8. *J Exp Med* 1993;178:1913–1921.
22. Marfaing-Koka A, Devergne O, Gorgone G, et al. Regulation of the production of the RANTES chemokine by endothelial cells: synergistic induction by IFN-gamma plus TNF-alpha and inhibition by IL-4 and IL-13. *J Immunol* 1995;154:1870–1878.
23. Worthen GS, Lien DC, Tonnesen MG, Hensen PM. Interaction of leukocytes with the pulmonary endothelium. In: Ryan US, ed. *Pulmonary endothelium in health and disease.* New York: Marcel Dekker, 1987;123–160.
24. Bevilacqua MP, Pober JS, Wheeler ME, Cotran RS, Gimbrone MJ. Interleukin-1 acts on cultured human vascular endothelium to increase the adhesion of polymorphonuclear leukocytes, monocytes and related leukocyte cell lines. *J Clin Invest* 1985;76:2003–2011.
25. Gamble JR, Harlan JM, Klebanoff SJ, Vadas MA. Stimulation of the adherence of neutrophils to umbilical vein endothelium by human recombinant tumor necrosis factor. *Proc Natl Acad Sci USA* 1985;82: 8667–8671.
26. Carlos TM, Harlan JM. Leukocyte-endothelial adhesion molecules. *Blood* 1994;84:2068–2101.
27. Bevilacqua MP, Pober JS, Mendrick DL, Cotran RS, Gimbrone MA. Identification of an inducible endothelial-leukocyte adhesion molecule. *Proc Natl Acad Sci USA* 1987;84:9238–9243.
28. Berg EL, Yoshino T, Rott LS, et al. The cutaneous lymphocyte antigen is a skin lymphocyte homing receptor for the vascular lectin endothelial cell–leukocyte adhesion molecule-1. *J Exp Med* 1991;174:1461–1466.
29. McEver RP, Beckstead JH, Moore KL, Marshall-Carlson L, Bainton DF. GMP-140, a platelet α granule membrane protein, is also synthesized by vascular endothelial cells and is localized in Weibel–Palade bodies. *J Clin Invest* 1989;84:92–99.
30. Sanders WE, Wilson RW, Ballantyne CM, Beaudet AL. Molecular cloning and analysis of *in vivo* expression of murine P-selectin. *Blood* 1992;80:795–802.
31. Weller A, Isenmann S, Vestweber D. Cloning of the mouse endothelial selectins: expression of both E- and P-selectin is inducible by tumor necrosis factor. *J Biol Chem* 1992;267:15,176–15,182.
32. Sako D, Chang XJ, Barone KM, et al. Expression cloning of a functional glycoprotein ligand for P-selectin. *Cell* 1993;75:1179–1185.
33. Berg EL, Magnani J, Warnock RA, Robinson MK, Butcher EC. Comparison of L-selectin and E-selectin ligand specificities: the L-selectin can bind the E-selectin ligands sialyl Le^x and sialyl Le^a. *Biochem Biophys Res Commun* 1992;184:1048–1054.
34. Dowbenko D, Andalibi A, Young PE, Lusis AJ, Lasky LA. Structure and chromosomal localization of the murine gene encoding glycan-1: a mucin-like endothelial ligand for L-selectin. *J Biol Chem* 1993;268: 4525–4532.
35. Pober JSM, Gimbrone MA Jr, Lapierre LA, et al. Overlapping patterns of activation of human endothelial cells by interleukin 1, tumor necrosis, and immune interferon. *J Immunol* 1986;137:1893–1896.
36. Briscoe DM, Cotran RS, Pober JS. Effects of tumor necrosis factor, lipopolysaccharide, and IL-4 on the expression of vascular cell adhesion molecule-1 *in vivo. J Immunol* 1992;149:2954–2960.
37. Ebisawa M, Bochner BS, Georas SN, Schleimer RP. Eosinophil transendothelial migration induced by cytokines. I. Role of endothelial and eosinophil adhesion molecules in IL-1β-induced transendothelial migration. *J Immunol* 1992;149:4021–4025.

38. Osborn L, Hession C, Tizard R, et al. Direct expression cloning of vascular cell adhesion molecule-1 (VCAM-1), a cytokine-induced endothelial protein that binds to lymphocytes. *Cell* 1989;59:1203–1211.

39. Petzelbauer P, Bender JR, Wilson J, Pober JS. Heterogeneity of dermal microvascular endothelial cell antigen expression and cytokine responsiveness *in situ* and in cell culture. *J Immunol* 1993;151:5062–5072.

40. Simmons DL, Walker C, Power C, Pigott R. Molecular cloning of CD31, a purative intercellular adhesion molecule closely related to carcinoembryonic antigen. *J Exp Med* 1990;171:2147–2154.

41. Newman PJ, Albelda SM. Cellular and molecular aspects of PECAM-1. *Nouv Rev Fr Hematol* 1992;34:S7–S11.

42. Muller WA, Weigl SA, Deng X, Phillips DM. PECAM-1 is required for transendothelial migration of leukocytes. *J Exp Med* 1993;178:449–454.

43. Bird IN, Spragg JH, Ager A, Mathews N. Studies of lymphocyte transendothelial migration: analysis of migrated cell phenotypes with regard to CD31 (PECAM-1), CD45RA and CD45RO. *Immunology* 1993;80:553–559.

44. Nakache M, Berg EL, Streeter PR, Butcher EC. The mucosal vascular addressin is a tissue-specific endothelial cell adhesion molecule for circulating lymphocytes. *Nature* 1989;337:179–181.

45. Berlin C, Berg EL, Brislin MJ, et al. α4β7 Integrin mediates lymphocyte binding to the mucosal vascular addressin MAdCAM-1. *Cell* 1993;74:185–189.

46. Berg EL, McEvroy LM, Berlin C, Bargatze RF, Butcher EC. L-selectin-mediated lymphocyte rolling on MAdCAM-1. *Nature* 1993;366:695–699.

47. Ley K, Gaehtgens P, Fennie C, Singer MS, Lasky MS, Rosen SD. Lectin-like cell adhesion molecule 1 mediates leukocyte rolling in mesenteric venules *in vivo*. *Blood* 1991;77:2553–2560.

48. Lawrence MB, Springer TA. Leukocytes roll on a selectin at physiologic flow rates: distinction from and prerequisite for adhesion through integrins. *Cell* 1991;65:859–864.

49. Lawrence MB, Springer TA. Neutrophils roll on E-selectin. *J Immunol* 1993;151:6338–6344.

50. Stossel TP. On the crawling of animal cells. *Science* 1993;260:1086–1087.

51. Smith CW. Transendothelial migration. In: Harlan JM, Liu DY, eds. *Adhesion: its role in inflammatory diseases*. New York: Freeman, 1992;83.

52. Mackay CR, Marston WL, Dudler L, Spertini O, Tedder TF, Hein WR. Tissue specific migration pathways by phenotypically distinct subpopulations of memory T-cells. *Eur J Immunol* 1992;22:887–895.

53. Santamaria-Babi LF, Moser R, Perez-Soler MT, Picker LJ, Blaser K, Hauser C. Migration of skin-homing T cells across cytokine-activated human endothelial cell layers involves interaction of the cutaneous lymphocyte-associated antigen (CLA), the very late antigen-4 (VLA-4), and the lymphocyte function-associated antigen-1 (LFA-1). *J Immunol* 1995;154:1543–1550.

54. Tanaka Y, Adams DH, Hubscher S, Hirano H, Siebenlist U, Shaw S. T cell adhesion induced by proteoglycan immobilized MIP-1β. *Nature* 1993;361:79–82.

55. Schall TJ, Bacon K, Toy KJ, Goeddel DV. Selective attraction of monocytes and T-lymphocytes of the memory phenotype by cytokine RANTES. *Nature* 1990;347:669–671.

56. Wallaert B, Janin A, Lassalle P, et al. Airway-like inflammation of the salivary gland in bronchial asthma. *Am J Respir Crit Care Med* 1994;150:802–809.

57. Resnick MB, Weller PF. Mechanisms of eosinophil recruitment. *Am J Respir Cell Mol Biol* 1993;8:345–355.

58. Moser R, Fehr J, Bruijnzeel PLB. IL-4 controls the selective endothelium-driven transmigration of eosinophils from allergic individuals. *J Immunol* 1992;149:1432–1438.

59. Moser R, Fehr J, Olgiati L, Bruijnzeel PL. Migration of primed human eosinophils across cytokine-activated endothelial cell monolayers. *Blood* 1992;79:2937–2945.

60. Hartnell A, Moqbel R, Walsh GM, Bradley B, Kay AB. Fc gamma and CD11/CD18 receptor expression on normal density and low density eosinophils. *Immunology* 1990;69:264–270.

61. Walker C, Rihs S, Braun RK, Betz S, Bruijnzeel PL. Increased expression of CD11b and functional changes in eosinophils after migration across endothelial cell monolayers. *J Immunol* 1993;150:4061–4071.

62. Warringa RAJ, Koenderman L, Kok PTM, Kreukniet J, Bruijnzeel PLB. Modulation and induction of eosinophil chemotaxis by granulocyte macrophage colony stimulating factor and IL-3. *Blood* 1991;77:2694–2700.

63. Hansel TT, Braunstein JB, Walker C, et al. Sputum eosinophils from asthmatics express ICAM-1 and HLA-DR. *Clin Exp Immunol* 1991;86:271–277.

64. Bochner BS, Luscinskas FW, Gimbrone MA Jr, et al. Adhesion of human basophils, eosinophils, and neutrophils to interleukin 1-activated human vascular endothelial cells: contributions of endothelial cell adhesion molecules. *J Exp Med* 1991;173:1553–1557.

65. Dobrina A, Menegazzi R, Carlos TM, et al. Mechanisms of eosinophil adherence to cultured vascular endothelial cells: eosinophils bind to the cytokine-induced endothelial ligand VCAM-1 via the very late activation antigen-4 integrin receptor. *J Clin Invest* 1991;88:20–26.

66. Walsh GM, Mermod JJ, Hartnell A, Kay AB, Wardlaw AJ. Human eosinophil, but not neutrophil, adherence to IL-1-stimulated human umbilical vascular endothelial cells is α4β1 (very late antigen-4) dependent. *J Immunol* 1991;146:3419–3423.

67. Lobb RR, Hember ME. The pathophysiologic role of α4 integrins *in vivo*. *J Clin Invest* 1994;94:1722–1728.

68. Mengelers HJJ, Maikoe T, Hooibrink B, et al. Down modulation of L-selectin expression on eosinophils recovered from bronchoalveolar lavage fluid after allergen provocation. *Clin Exp Allergy* 1993;23:196–204.

69. Braun RK, Franchini M, Erard F, et al. Human peripheral blood eosinophils produce and release interleukin-8 on stimulation with calcium ionophore. *Eur J Immunol* 1993;23:956–960.

70. Desreumaux P, Janin A, Colombel JF, et al. Interleukin-5 messenger RNA expression by eosinophils in the intestinal mucosa of patients with coeliac disease. *J Exp Med* 1992;175:293–296.

71. Hamid Q, Barkans J, Meng Q, et al. Human eosinophils synthesize and secrete interleukin-6 in vitro. *Blood* 1992;80:1496–1501.

72. Moqbel R, Hamid Q, Ying S. Expression of mRNA and immunoreactivity for the granulocyte-macrophage colony-stimulating factor (GM-CSF) in activated human eosinophils. *J Exp Med* 1991;174:749–752.

73. Wong DT, Weller PF, Galli SJ, et al. Human eosinophils express transforming growth factor α. *J Exp Med* 1990;172:673–681.

74. Guo CB, Liu MC, Galli SJ, Bochner BS, Kagey-Sobotka A, Lichtenstein LM. Identification of IgE-bearing cells in the late-phase response to antigen in the lung as basophils. *Am J Respir Cell Mol Biol* 1994;10:384–390.

75. Naclerio RM, Baroody FM, Kagey-Sobotka A, Lichtenstein LM. Basophils and eosinophils in allergic rhinitis. *J Allergy Clin Immunol* 1994;94:1303–1309.

76. Bochner BS, Peachell PT, Brown KE, Schleimer RP. Adherence of human basophils to cultured umbilical vein endothelial cells. *J Clin Invest* 1988;81:1355–1364.

77. Bochner BS, Schleimer RP. The role of adhesion molecules in human eosinophil and basophil recruitment. *J Allergy Clin Immunol* 1994;94:427–438.

78. Wegner CD, Torcellini CA, Clarke CC, Letto LG, Gundel RH. Effects of single and multiple inhalations of antigen on airway responsiveness in monkeys. *J Allergy Clin Immunol* 1991;87:835–841.

79. Wegner CD, Gundel RH, Reilly P, Haynes N, Letts LG, Rothlein R. Intercellular adhesion molecule-1 (ICAM-1) in the pathogenesis of asthma. *Science* 1990;247:456–459.

80. Gundel RH, Wegner CD, Torcellini CA, et al. Endothelial leukocyte adhesion molecule-1 mediates antigen-induced acute airway inflammation and late-phase airway obstruction in monkeys. *J Clin Invest* 1991;88:1407–1411.

81. Gundel RH, Wegner CD, Torcellini CA, Letts LG. The role of intercellular adhesion molecule-1 in chronic airway inflammation. *Clin Exp Allergy* 1992;22:569–575.

82. Weg WB, Williams TJ, Lobb RR, Nourshargh S. A monoclonal antibody recognizing very late activation antigen-4 inhibits eosinophil activation *in vivo*. *J Exp Med* 1993;177:561–566.

83. Pretolani M, Ruffi C, Lapa e Silva JR, Joseph D, Lobb RR, Vargaftig BB. Antibody to very late activation antigen 4 prevents antigen induced bronchial hyperreactivity and cellular infiltration in the guinea pig airways. *J Exp Med* 1994;180:795–805.

84. Richards IM, Kolbasa KP, Hatfield CA, et al. Role of VLA-4 in the antigen accumulaton of eosinophil and lymphocyte in the lungs and

airway lumen of sensitized Brown Norway rats. *Am J Respir Cell Mol Biol.* 1996;15:172–183.

85. Abraham WM, Sielczak MW, Ahmed A, et al. Alpha-4 integrins mediate antigen-induced late bronchial responses and prolonged airway hyperresponsiveness in sheep. *J Clin Invest* 1994;93:776–787.

86. Leung DYM, Pober JS, Cotran RS. Expression of endothelial-leukocyte adhesion molecule-1 in elicited late phase allergic reactions. *J Clin Invest* 1991;87:1805–1809.

87. Klein LM, Lavker RM, Mates WL, Murphy GF. Degranulation of human mast cells induces an endothelial antigen central to leukocyte adhesion. *Proc Natl Acad Sci USA* 1989;86:8972–8976.

88. Walsh LJ, Trinchieri G, Waldorf HA, Whitaker D, Murphy GF. Human dermal mast cells contain and release tumor necrosis factor α, which induces endothelial leukocyte adhesion molecule-1. *Proc Natl Acad Sci USA* 1991;88:4220–4224.

89. Montefort S, Feather IH, Wilson SJ, et al. The expression of leukocyte–endothelial adhesion molecules is increased in perennial allergic rhinitis. *Am J Respir Cell Mol Biol* 1992;7:393–398.

90. Lee BJ, Naclerio RM, Bochner BS, Taylor RM, Lim MC, Baroody F. Nasal challenge with allergen up regulates the local expression of vascular endothelial adhesion molecules. *J Allergy Clin Immunol* 1994;94:1006–1016.

91. Gosset P, Tillie Leblond I, Janin A, et al. Expression of E-selectin, ICAM-1 and VCAM-1 on bronchial biopsies from allergic and non-allergic asthmatic patients. *Int Arch Allergy Immunol* 1995;106:69–77.

92. Bentley AM, Durham SR, Robinson DS, et al. Expression of endothelial and leukocyte adhesion molecules (ICAM-1, E-selectin and VCAM-1) in the bronchial mucosa in steady state and allergen induced asthma. *J Allergy Clin Immunol* 1993;92:857–868.

93. Montefort S, Roche WR, Howarth PH, et al. Intercellular adhesion molecule-1 (ICAM-1) and endothelial leukocyte adhesion molecule-1 (ELAM-1) expression in the bronchial mucosa of normal and asthmatic subjects. *Eur Respir J* 1992;5:815–823.

94. Montefort S, Gratziou C, Goulding D, et al. Bronchial biopsy evidence for leukocyte infiltration and upregulation of leukocyte–endothelial cell adhesion molecules 6 hs after local allergen challenge of sensitized asthmatic airways. *J Clin Invest* 1994;93:1411–1421.

95. Ohkawara Y, Yamauchi K, Maruyama N, et al. *In situ* expression of the cell adhesion molecules in bronchial tissues from asthmatics with air flow limitation: *in vivo* evidence of VCAM-1/VLA-4 interaction in selective eosinophil infiltration. *Am J Respir Cell Mol Biol* 1995;12:4–12.

96. Di Stefano A, Maestrelli P, Roggeri A, et al. Upregulation of adhesion molecules in the bronchial mucosa of subjects with chronic obstructive bronchitis. *Am J Respir Crit Care Med* 1994;149:803–810.

97. Gearing AJH, Hemingway I, Pigott R, Hughes J, Rees AJ, Cashman SJ. Soluble forms of vascular adhesion molecules, E selectin, ICAM-1 and VCAM-1: pathological significance. *Ann NY Acad Sci* 1992; 667:324–331.

98. Seth R, Raymond FD, Makgoba MW. Circulating ICAM-1 isoforms: diagnostic prospects for inflammatory and immune disorders. *Lancet* 1991;338:83–84.

99. Georas SN, Liu MC, Newman W, Beall LD, Stealey BA, Bochner BS. Altered adhesion molecule expression and endothelial cell activation accompanies the recruitment of human granulocytes to the lung after segmental antigen challenge. *Am J Respir Cell Mol Biol* 1992;7:261–269.

100. Montefort S, Lai CK, Kapahi P, et al. Circulating adhesion molecules in asthma. *Am J Respir Crit Care Med* 1994;149:1149–1152.

101. De Rose V, Rolla G, Bucca C, et al. Intercellular adhesion molecule-1 is upregulated on peripheral blood T lymphocyte subsets in dual asthmatic responders. *J Clin Invest* 1994;94:1840–1845.

102. Gosset P, Tsicopoulos A, Wallaert B, Joseph M, Tonnel AB, Capron A. Increased secretion of tumor necrosis factor and interleukin 6 by alveolar macrophages during late asthmatic reaction after bronchial allergen challenge. *J Allergy Clin Immunol* 1991;88:561–571.

103. Lassalle P, Gosset P, Delneste Y, et al. Modulation of adhesion molecule expression on endothelial cells during the late asthmatic reaction: role of macrophage-derived tumour necrosis factor-alpha. *Clin Exp Immunol* 1993;94:105–110.

104. Falus A, Meretey K. Histamine: an early messenger in inflammatory and immune reaction. *Immunol Today* 1992;13:154–158.

105. Jeannin P, Delneste Y, Gosset P, et al. Histamine induces Interleukin-8 secretion by endothelial cells. *Blood* 1994;84:2229–2233.

106. Delneste Y, Lassalle P, Jeannin P, Joseph M, Tonnel AB, Gosset P. Histamine induces IL-6 production by endothelial cells. *Clin Exp Immunol* 1994;98:344–349.

107. Naclerio RM. The role of histamine in allergic rhinitis. *J Allergy Clin Immunol* 1990;86:628–635.

108. O'Donnell MA, Ackerman SJ, Gleich GJ, Thomas LL. Activation of basophil and mast cell histamine release by eosinophil granule proteins. *J Exp Med* 1983;157:1981–1988.

109. Moy JN, Thomas LL, Wisler LC. Eosinophil major basic protein enhances the expression of neutrophil CR3 and p150-95. *J Allergy Clin Immunol* 1993;92:598–604.

110. Masinovski B, Urdal D, Gallatin WM. IL-4 acts synergistically with IL-1β to promote lymphocyte adhesion to microvascular endothelium by induction of vascular cell adhesion molecule-1. *J Immunol* 1990; 145:2886–2893.

111. Schleimer RP, Sterbinsky SA, Kaiser J, et al. IL-4 induces adherence of human eosinophils and basophils but not neutrophils to endothelium: association with expression of VCAM-1. *J Immunol* 1992;148: 1086–1092.

112. Thornhill MH, Kyan-Aung U, Haskard DO. IL-4 increases human endothelial cell adhesiveness for T cells but not for neutrophils. *J Immunol* 1990;144:3060–3065.

113. Delneste Y, Jeannin P, Gosset P, et al. Allergen stimulated T lymphocytes from allergic patients induce vascular cell adhesion molecule-1 (VCAM-1) expression and IL-6 production by endothelial cells. *Clin Exp Immunol* 1995;101:164–171.

114. Lassalle P, Molet S, Janin A, et al. ESM-1 is a novel human endothelial cell-specific molecule expressed in lung and regulated by cytokines. *J Biol Chem* 1996;271:20,458–20,464.

Asthma, edited by P.J. Barnes, M.M. Grunstein,
A.R. Leff, and A.J. Woolcock.
Lippincott–Raven Publishers, Philadelphia © 1997.

▪ 38 ▪

Cell Adhesion Molecules

Joseph M. Pilewski and Steven M. Albelda

Families of Cell Adhesion Molecules
Adhesion Molecules in Normal Lung Structure
  Cell-Matrix Adhesion
  Cell-Cell Adhesion
Adhesion Molecules in Airway Inflammation
  Leukocyte-Endothelial Cell Adhesion Cascade
  Leukocyte Adhesion Deficiencies
  Adhesion Molecules in Airway Inflammation and
    Asthma

Adhesive Steps Involved in Airway Inflammation
Role of Endothelial Cell Adhesion Molecules in
  Leukocyte Homing
Adhesion Molecules in Leukocyte Activation
Adhesion Molecules in Airway Remodeling
Leukocyte-Epithelial Adhesion
Future Directions

The adhesion of cells to one another and to the extracellular matrix is crucial to embryonic development, maintenance of tissue architecture, the inflammatory response, tumor metastasis, and wound healing. Over the last decade, much progress has been made toward determining the specific cell surface receptors that mediate these adhesive interactions. More recently, investigators have begun to address the role of adhesion molecules in bronchial epithelial homeostasis and airway inflammation. This chapter summarizes our current understanding of the cell adhesion molecule (CAM) families and then discusses their role in lung structure and the inflammatory response observed in asthma. For a more detailed discussion of cell adhesion molecules, the reader is referred to a number of recent reviews (1–18).

FAMILIES OF CELL ADHESION MOLECULES

The known CAMs can be grouped into distinct families based on their molecular structure: integrins, cadherins, members of the immunoglobulin supergene family,

selectins, vascular addressins, and surface carbohydrates. Table 1 includes some of the adhesion molecules significant for lung structure, and Table 2 lists those determined to be important in the inflammatory response.

Integrins. The integrins are a family of transmembrane glycoproteins that function in both cell-cell and cell-substratum adhesion (2,4,6), signal transduction (4, 19), and internalization of adenoviruses (20,21). Structurally they are highly disulfide-linked, noncovalently associated heterodimers consisting of α- and β-subunits. Originally thought to consist of three subfamilies with a common β-subunit capable of associating with a specific group of α-(alpha)-subunits, it is now clear that certain α-subunits can associate with more than one β-subunit. These molecules are ubiquitous, with at least one heterodimer present on all nucleated cells *in vivo.*

Cadherins. The cadherins are a family of adhesion molecules characterized by calcium-dependent cell-cell adhesion (8). Structurally they are single polypeptide chains with a short cytoplasmic domain that interacts indirectly with the cytoskeleton. Three cytoplasmic proteins—α-, β-, and γ-catenin—bind noncovalently to the cytoplasmic domain of cadherins and are required for cadherin function in cell-cell adhesion (22–24). Unlike integrins, cadherins bind to one another on adjacent cells and appear to function only in cell-cell adhesion.

Immunoglobulin supergene family. This family of adhesion molecules is characterized structurally by repeated immunoglobulinlike domains in the extracellular portion

J. M. Pilewski: Department of Medicine, University of Pittsburgh Medical Center, Pittsburgh, Pennsylvania 15261.
S. M. Albelda: Department of Medicine, Pulmonary and Critical Care Division, University of Pennsylvania Medical Center, Philadelphia, Pennsylvania 19104.

TABLE 1. *Structural cell adhesion molecules*

Family	Molecule or subunit	Ligand(s)
Integrin	$\alpha_1\beta_1$ (VLA-1)	Collagen, laminin
	$\alpha_2\beta_1$ (VLA-2)	Collagen, laminin
	$\alpha_3\beta_1$ (VLA-3)	Collagen, laminin, fibronectin
	$\alpha_4\beta_1$ (VLA-4)	Fibronectin, VCAM-1
	$\alpha_5\beta_1$ (VLA-5)	Fibronectin
	$\alpha_6\beta_1$ (VLA-6)	Laminin
	$\alpha_7\beta_1$	Laminin
	$\alpha_8\beta_1$	?
	$\alpha_9\beta_1$	Tenascin
	$\alpha_v\beta_1$	Vitronectin, fibronectin
	$\alpha_v\beta_3$	Vitronectin, fibrinogen, von Willebrand factor, fibronectin, thrombospondin
	$\alpha_6\beta_4$	Laminin
	$\alpha_v\beta_5$	Vitronectin
	$\alpha_v\beta_6$	Fibronectin
	$\alpha_4\beta_7$	Fibronectin, VCAM-1
Cadherin	Epithelial (E)-cadherin (uvomorulin)	E-cadherin, $\alpha_E\beta_7$
	Placental (P)-cadherin	P-cadherin
	Vascular (V)-cadherin	?
Immunoglobulin supergene	PECAM-1	PECAM-1, glycosaminoglycans
Others	CD44	Hyaluronic acid, vascular addressins
	Syndecan	Collagens, fibronectin

PECAM, platelet endothelial cell adhesion molecule; VCAM, vascular cell adhesion molecule; VLA, very late antigen.

of the molecule (9). Members of this family function as cell-cell adhesion molecules and are especially important in leukocyte-endothelial cell interactions.

Selectins. The selectins are a group of transmembrane glycoproteins characterized by an N-terminal lectin domain, an epidermal growth factor domain, and a series of complement-regulatory domains (11–15). These adhesion molecules function in cell-cell interactions and appear crucial for the initial binding of leukocytes to endothelial cells in inflammatory responses.

Vascular addressins. This family consists of several recently discovered glycoproteins on endothelial cells responsible for the direction or "homing" of lymphocytes to organ-specific lymph nodes or extranodal tissue (18). The role of these molecules in pulmonary function and disease remains an area for investigation, as the members of this family may provide the mechanism for organ-specific cell movement.

Carbohydrate and other ligands. Specific carbohydrate moieties have been identified that serve as ligands for the selectins (12,25). Strictly speaking, the carbohydrates are not a distinct adhesion molecule family, but

their unique structure and importance in leukocyte-endothelial adhesion merit separation from other CAMs. The Lewis x antigen and sialylated Lewis x are the best characterized of the carbohydrate ligands. More recent work has identified the receptors for P-selectin and E-selectin. The glycoprotein receptor for P-selectin has been cloned (26), and a glycoprotein receptor with homology to a fibroblast growth factor receptor has been identified as a myeloid cell ligand for E-selectin (27).

ADHESION MOLECULES IN NORMAL LUNG STRUCTURE

In order for the pulmonary epithelium and endothelium to form and maintain functional permeability barriers, there must be firm adhesion to the extracellular matrix and tight contact between adjacent cells. Molecules in the integrin family are the most important for cell-matrix adhesion, with some contribution from other proteins and proteoglycans. For cell-cell adhesion, the cadherins and integrins interact with cytoplasmic proteins to form the structures that characterize epithelial and endothelial junctions.

Cell-Matrix Adhesion

Maintenance of tissue integrity requires the adhesion of cells to a variety of matrix proteins, including laminin, various types of collagen, elastin, fibronectin, glycosaminoglycans, and hyaluronic acid. For simplicity, it is useful to consider the integrins involved in cell-matrix adhesion by their ligand specificities (28). One group binds primarily to components of the basement membrane (collagen and laminin), whereas the second group binds primarily to proteins found during inflammation, wound repair, and development (fibronectin, fibrinogen, vitronectin, and thrombospondin).

Using monoclonal antibodies specific for individual integrin subunits, the distribution of β_1-integrin (very late antigen or VLA), β_3-integrin (cytoadhesin), and β_4-integrin in normal lung tissue has been determined (29–31) (Table 3). The bronchial epithelium (large and small airways), bronchial smooth muscle, and the submucosal endothelium predominantly express integrin subunits that serve as collagen and/or laminin receptors (α_2, α_3, and α_6). The α_6- and β_4-subunits localize to the subbasal portion of epithelial cells, suggesting that the α_6/β_4-heterodimer is part of the hemidesmosomes that are responsible for adhesion of endothelial and basal epithelial cells to the basement membrane (32). There is limited expression of fibronectin/fibrinogen-binding subunits (α_4, α_5, β_3, and β_6) on bronchial epithelial and microvascular endothelial cells. The α_3- and α_v-subunits are the only fibronectin-binding integrins present normally on these cells

TABLE 2. *Adhesion molecules involved in inflammation*

Family	Molecule	Distribution	Counterreceptor(s)
Integrin	$\alpha_L\beta_2$ (CD11a/CD18, LFA-1)	All leukocytes	ICAM-1, ICAM-2
	$\alpha_M\beta_2$ (CD11b/CD18, MAC-1, CR3)	Neutrophils, monocytes, some lymphocytes	ICAM-1, fibrinogen, C3bi
	$\alpha_X\beta_2$ (CD11c/CD18, gp150-95)	Granulocytes, monocytes	Fibrinogen, C3bi(?)
	$\alpha_4\beta_1$ (VLA-4)	Eosinophils, lymphocytes, monocytes	VCAM-1
	$\alpha_E\beta_7$	Lymphocytes	E-cadherin
	$\alpha_{IIb}\beta_3$	Platelets	Fibrinogen, fibronectin, von Willebrand factor, vitronectin, thrombospondin
Immunoglobulin supergene	CD2 (LFA-2)	All T lymphocytes	LFA-3
	LFA-3	Widespread	CD2
	ICAM-1	Endothelial and epithelial cells, eosinophils (induced), other cells	$\alpha_L\beta_2$ (LFA-1), $\alpha_M\beta_2$ (MAC-1)
	ICAM-2	Endothelial and other cells	$\alpha_L\beta_2$ (LFA-1)
	VCAM-1	Endothelial cells (induced)	$\alpha_4\beta_1$ (VLA-4)
	PECAM-1	Endothelial cells, platelets, some leukocytes	PECAM-1, glycosaminoglycans
Selectin	E-selectin (ELAM-1, LECAM-1)	Endothelial cells (induced)	sLe^x, sLe^a, ESL-1, L-selectin?
	P-selectin (GMP-140, PADGEM)	Endothelial cells (induced), platelets	P-selectin glycoprotein ligand, sLe^x, L-selectin?
	L-selectin	Lymphocytes, neutrophils, eosinophils	E- and P-selectin?, MECA-79 antigen
Carbohydrate	sLe^x (CD15)	Neutrophils, monocytes, platelets	E- and P-selectin

ESL, E-selectin ligand; GMP, granule-associated membrane protein; ICAM, intercellular adhesion molecule; LECAM, lectin-like cell adhesion molecule; LFA, lymphocyte function-associated antigen; MAC, membrane-attack complex; PADGEM, platelet activation-dependent granule-external membrane protein; PECAM, platelet endothelial cell adhesion molecule; sLe, sialyl Lewis; VCAM, vascular cell adhesion molecule; VLA, very late antigen.

in vivo, and it appears that β_5 is a major β-subunit expressed with α_v on bronchial epithelium (33, and unpublished observations).

Recent evidence indicates that the expression of epithelial CAMs is altered in epithelial injury and repair. In human skin, there is increased expression of the α_5- and α_v-integrins and a redistribution of α_6 on the migrating epithelial cells (34). Similar changes in epithelial integrin expression have been described in airway epithelium (35,36), suggesting that changes in integrin expression facilitate epithelial repair. Expression of $\alpha_v\beta_6$ on the epithelium of airway from smokers undergoing lung resection is additional indirect evidence that integrins function in epithelial repair (37). A similar programmed expression is likely to occur during the reepithelialization that occurs after injury in the asthmatic airway epithelium.

The role of non-integrin cell-matrix adhesion molecules in the lung remains to be defined. The hyaluronic acid receptor CD44 is found on smooth muscle and on bronchial and alveolar epithelium but not on endothelium (18). It is likely that elastin-binding proteins (5) and proteoglycans, such as heparan sulfate (38) and syndecan (39,40), are also important in the adhesion of epithelial and endothelial cells to their basement membranes.

TABLE 3. *Distribution of integrin cell adhesion receptors in lung tissue*

Tissue	Integrin subunit								
	Collagen/laminin receptors					Fibronectin/fibrinogen receptors			
	α_1	α_2	α_3	α_6	β_4	α_4	α_5	α_v	β_3
Bronchial epithelium	□	●	●	●	●	○	○	●	○
Large vessel endothelium	●	●	●	●	●	○	●	●	●
Microvessel endothelium	●	□	●	●	●	○	○	○	○
Bronchial smooth muscle	●	●	●	○	○	○	○	●	□
Vascular smooth muscle	●	□	●	○	○	○	○	●	□

●, readily detectable staining; □, trace staining; ○, no detectable staining.
From Damjanovich L, Albelda SM, Mette SA, Buck CA. Distribution of integrin cell adhesion receptors in normal and malignant lung tissue. *Am J Respir Cell Mol Biol* 1992;6:197–206.

Cell-Cell Adhesion

The adhesion of cells to one another can be considered in terms of homotypic (to a cell of the same type) or heterotypic (to a different cell type) interactions. Heterotypic adhesion is most relevant for inflammation (see below) and tumor metastasis. Homotypic adhesion in bronchial epithelium is maintained primarily by desmosomes (macula adherens) and intermediate junctions (zonula adherens). Tight junctions (zonula occludens) and gap junctions (nexus) also contribute to epithelial cell-cell adhesion. These structures consist of CAMs interacting indirectly with cytoplasmic junctional proteins (reviewed in references 41–43), such as cingulin, the desmoplakins, and the connexins (22–24).

Members of the cadherin family are the best characterized of the adhesion molecules participating in homotypic adhesion in the lung. Epithelial cadherin (E-cadherin, uvomorulin) and placental cadherin (P-cadherin) have been localized to epithelial cell-cell junctions and are constituents of intermediate junctions (41). Both E- and P-cadherin have been identified at epithelial contacts in bronchial epithelium, but only E-cadherin has been detected in alveolar lining cells (44). The physiologic importance of the cadherins *in vivo* remains unclear. *In vitro* experiments using kidney epithelial cells have demonstrated that antibodies to E-cadherin cause an increase in epithelial permeability by interfering with cell-cell junctions (45). Moreover, several investigators have found loss of E-cadherin expression in the invasive phase of epithelial malignancies (46,47). These data suggest that E-cadherin is important for maintenance of epithelial integrity.

Other adhesion molecules potentially contributing to homotypic adhesion include certain β_1-integrins and at least one member of the immunoglobulin supergene family. The α_2-subunit of the β_1-integrins has been localized to cell-cell borders in bronchial epithelium *in situ*, whereas the α_2-, α_3-, and α_5-subunits have been detected at cell-cell borders in some cultured cells (48,49). Antibodies against these subunits have been shown to disrupt cell-cell contacts, providing further evidence for their importance in homotypic adhesion. Lastly, platelet endothelial cell adhesion molecule (PECAM) 1, a member of the immunoglobulin supergene family, appears to function as an endothelial cell-cell adhesion molecule *in vitro* (50). The physiologic importance of PECAM-1 and the cell-cell binding integrins in pathologic states is not yet known.

ADHESION MOLECULES IN AIRWAY INFLAMMATION

The development of an inflammatory response requires that the resident cells of a given tissue communicate with circulating effector cells. This communication can occur through the production of soluble mediators (cytokines and chemoattractants) and/or through cell-cell adhesion. *In vivo*, there are complex interactions between soluble mediators and adhesion molecules: the soluble mediators can alter the expression of adhesion molecules, and cell adhesion can result in the elaboration of soluble mediators.

A major goal of adhesion molecule research has been elucidating the adhesive mechanisms that regulate the inflammatory response. Leukocytes flowing in a vessel lumen must first adhere to an endothelial cell, then migrate between adjacent endothelial cells, and finally move through the extracellular matrix to perform effector functions in a given tissue. An evolving paradigm to explain the molecular mechanisms involved in this process has been termed the *leukocyte-endothelial cell adhesion cascade* (51–53): cytokines, cell adhesion molecules, and chemoattractants are expressed in a programmed and interactive manner to create a specific inflammatory response. The relevance of this paradigm to pulmonary health and disease remains an area of intensive investigation. For the purpose of this chapter, we present the existing paradigm and some of the data addressing its role in airway disease.

Leukocyte-Endothelial Cell Adhesion Cascade

The process whereby leukocytes are recruited from vascular lumen to tissue appears to require a cascade of at least four sequential adhesion molecule events (52). In the first step, constitutively expressed leukocyte adhesion molecules bind transiently and reversibly to specific ligands on endothelial cells. This results in a slowing or rolling of the circulating leukocyte along the surface of the endothelial cell in postcapillary venules (54). In the second step, the leukocyte or endothelial cell becomes activated, that is, the adhesion molecule repertoire changes in response to either a soluble mediator or the initial adhesion event. This activation event may involve expression of new so-called inducible adhesion molecules (55), increased expression of constitutive adhesion molecules, or an increase in adhesion molecule avidity (through soluble factors such as integrin-modulating factor [56], through phosphorylation events [19,57], or through cation-induced changes in integrin conformation [58]). In the third step, there is firm adhesion between activation-dependent molecules on the leukocyte or endothelial cell. In the final step, the leukocyte, anchored at the endothelial surface, migrates between endothelial cells and moves into the extracellular matrix.

In simplest terms, the leukocyte-endothelial interaction can be considered as a series of ligand-receptor pairs (Table 4), but the paradigm of a leukocyte-endothelial cascade requires that these adhesive steps be considered

TABLE 4. *Ligand-receptor pairs involved in leukocyte-endothelial adhesion*

	Leukocyte ligand	Endothelial receptor(s)
Rolling adhesion	L-selectin	P-selectin, E-selectin, carbohydrates
	Lewis x	P-selectin
	Sialyl Lewis x	P-selectin, E-selectin, MECA-79 antigen
Firm adhesion	$\alpha_L\beta_2$ (CD11a/CD18)	ICAM-1, ICAM-2
	$\alpha_M\beta_2$ (CD11b/CD18)	ICAM-1
	$\alpha_4\beta_1$ (VLA-4)	VCAM-1

ICAM, intercellular adhesion molecule; VCAM, vascular cell adhesion molecule; VLA, very late antigen.

within the richer context of soluble mediators (16,52,59). The leukocyte-endothelial interaction is often initiated by chemotactic factors or cytokines, which stimulate adhesion through activation of either leukocytes or endothelial cells. In the resting state, the endothelium expresses few adhesion molecules and is relatively nonadhesive. Leukocytes, however, express L-selectin constitutively and have other carbohydrate ligands bound to undetermined glycoproteins. The β_2 (CD18)-integrins are present at the cell surface but are in a low-avidity state. The inflammatory response begins with rolling of leukocytes on postcapillary venular endothelium and appears to be mediated by selectins. L-selectin on leukocytes interacts with P-selectin, E-selectin, or other carbohydrate ligands on endothelial cells (60). This is followed by shedding of L-selectin, an increase in the avidity of other leukocyte adhesion molecules (such as the β_2-integrins), and new expression or upregulation of adhesion molecules on the endothelial surface (E-selectin, vascular cell adhesion molecule [VCAM]-1, or intercellular adhesion molecule [ICAM]-1). These secondary activation events may be mediated by cytokines (such as tumor necrosis factor), chemoattractants (such as interleukin 8), or adhesion molecule interactions (such as binding of E-selectin causing increased β_2-integrin avidity [61]). The resulting activation provides for firm adhesion between integrins such as $\alpha_M\beta_2$ on neutrophils and ICAM-1 on endothelial cells or $\alpha_4\beta_1$ on eosinophils and VCAM-1 on endothelial cells. This firm adhesion then allows for diapedesis between endothelial cells, a process that may also require expression of PECAM-1, down a chemoattractant gradient.

Leukocyte Adhesion Deficiencies

The importance of adhesion molecules in inflammatory responses *in vivo* is best demonstrated by two rare congenital diseases. In the first, termed leukocyte adhesion deficiency (62), there is an autosomal recessively inherited defect in the β_2-subunit of leukocyte integrins. The result is absence of functional $\alpha_L\beta_2$ and $\alpha_M\beta_2$ on all leukocytes, resulting in failure of neutrophils to adhere to endothelial cells. Neutrophils accumulate intravascularly but are unable to exit the vessel lumen. This manifests clinically as recurrent severe bacterial infections, with inability to mount a pyogenic inflammatory response despite increased numbers of circulating neutrophils. These patients also have abnormalities in T-cell function, but lymphocyte migration is not affected. This rare disorder demonstrates the critical role of β_2-integrins in the firm adhesion phase of neutrophilic inflammatory responses.

The second recently described adhesion deficiency results from absence of the sialyl Lewis x ligand of E-selectin (63). Neutrophils from these patients have functional β_2-integrins and L-selectin but complete absence of the sialyl Lewis x antigen. This results in an inability of neutrophils to bind to E-selectin on activated endothelial cells *in vitro* and absence of normal adhesion under flow conditions. Like the individuals with abnormalities in β_2-integrins, these patients have recurrent episodes of bacterial infection, including pneumonia, without the formation of pus. This second congenital disorder indicates that E-selectin-mediated adhesion of neutrophils is crucial for pyogenic responses *in vivo*. Considered together, the leukocyte adhesion deficiencies support the paradigm of a leukocyte-endothelial cascade, since deficiencies in either the initial selectin-mediated adhesion or later integrin-mediated firm adhesion result in abnormal neutrophil responses to bacterial infection.

Adhesion Molecules in Airway Inflammation and Asthma

The specific role of adhesion molecules in airway inflammation is an area of increasing investigation. Studies have relied on *in vitro* systems, animal models, including transgenic or "knockout mice" (64,65), and the use of monoclonal antibodies against a particular adhesion molecule to demonstrate its function in a given experimental model.

For normal host defense against inhaled pathogens, leukocytes must migrate from the circulating pool to the airway lumen. In asthma, accumulation of leukocytes, specifically eosinophils and lymphocytes, appears excessive and detrimental to normal airway function. Several important questions remain unanswered: What is the initiating stimulus for leukocyte accumulation? What are the mechanisms of selective leukocyte infiltration, especially eosinophil recruitment in the asthmatic airway? How are bronchial microvascular and epithelial cells different from those in other tissues such as the skin? Can knowledge of the adhesion molecules or soluble mediators involved in these processes be applied therapeutically?

In recent years, great progress has been made toward elucidating the cellular and molecular mechanisms responsible for the development of inflammation. Numerous investigators have begun to dissect the relative contributions of CAMs, cytokines, and other soluble mediators in specific inflammatory diseases, such as asthma. Much of this effort has focused on the role of CAMs with the hope that a better understanding of adhesion pathways will lead to useful anti-inflammatory therapies. Recent data suggest multiple roles for CAMs in asthma, not only in directing leukocyte homing, but in immune activation and the regulation of interstitial cell-cell interactions.

Adhesive Steps Involved in Airway Inflammation

The adhesive mechanisms involved in airway inflammation can be considered as sequential steps (see Fig. 1). In the initial step (a), an inflammatory stimulus results in the production of cytokines and/or chemoattractants (66). The nature of this stimulus in asthma is still unknown in many cases, but likely involves viral infection or an im-

mune response to an inhaled antigen. Notably, the epithelium is itself capable of mediator production and may function as an effector cell and not simply as a passive target cell. For example, bronchial epithelial cells express HLA-DR class II molecules (67) and may contribute to antigen presentation.

Following the initial stimulus, the cytokines and chemoattractants activate bronchial microvascular endothelial cells and/or circulating leukocytes, thereby initiating a leukocyte-endothelial adhesion cascade (b). Once arrested in the microcirculation, leukocytes then diapedese between endothelial cells and migrate through extracellular matrix (c) along a chemoattractant gradient. At this stage, there may be interactions with airway smooth muscle cells and other interstitial cells. In a final step, some leukocytes traverse the basement membrane and pseudostratified columnar epithelium to gain access to the airway lumen (d). This step of epithelial transmigration is thought to include leukocyte-epithelial cell adhesion and

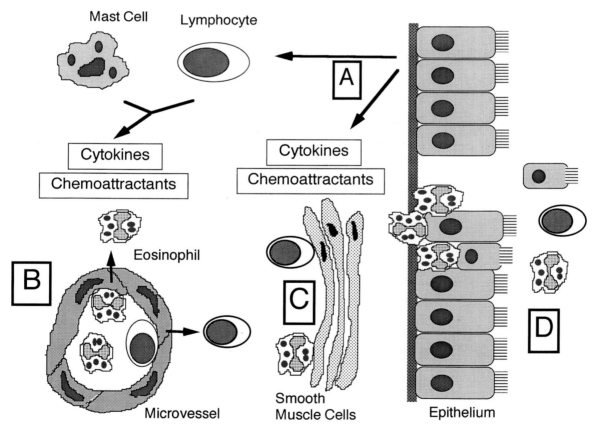

FIG. 1. Proposed steps in the development of airway inflammation. After an inflammatory stimulus, epithelial cells, lymphocytes, and mast cells release cytokines and chemoattractants **(A)**. This results in activation of the leukocyte-endothelial adhesion cascade and leukocyte adhesion to the endothelium **(B)** (see the text). In the presence of a chemoattractant gradient, leukocytes migrate between endothelial cells and through the extracellular matrix **(C)**, where they may interact with interstitial cells such as airway smooth muscle cells. Leukocytes then traverse the basement membrane and epithelium to reach the airway **(D)**. In asthma, epithelial desquamation may occur as activated leukocytes release toxic mediators while adhering to and migrating through the epithelium.

de-adhesion or, in some instances, direct leukocyte interaction with epithelial cells that eventuates in cytotoxicity (68) (reviewed in references 41 and 69). Completion of these steps allows for normal host defense or, as depicted in the figure, results in epithelial desquamation of the asthmatic airway.

Role of Endothelial Cell Adhesion Molecules in Leukocyte Homing

In the simplest paradigm, adhesion molecules play a crucial role in the leukocyte-endothelial step (Fig. 1B) and thereby direct circulating cells into the asthmatic airway. A plausible schema is that, in allergic asthma, antigen exposure leads to activation of mast cells and T-helper type-2 lymphocytes that release a number of soluble mediators, including tumor necrosis factor α, interleukins 3, 4, and 5, granulocyte-monocyte colony-stimulating factor, or specific eosinophil or lymphocyte chemoattractants. These mediators, in turn, induce airway endothelial cells to increase expression of E-selectin, ICAM-1, and VCAM-1. The combination of upregulation of the appropriate CAMs along with the proper chemoattractants subsequently mediates the migration of leukocytes, particularly eosinophils, into the airway.

In this pathway, endothelial adhesion molecules could function in the selective recruitment of eosinophils into the bronchial mucosa (reviewed in reference 70). *In vitro* studies using umbilical vein endothelial cells suggest that VCAM-1 on activated endothelial cells binds $\alpha_4\beta_1$ (VLA-4) on eosinophils (71), leading to the hypothesis that eosinophils could be selectively recruited from the vasculature via this mechanism.

What *in vivo* data support this hypothesis? In humans, the evidence comes from studies of CAM expression in asthmatic or allergic airway tissue. In patients with perennial allergic rhinitis, nasal biopsies have demonstrated increased expression of VCAM-1 and ICAM-1 on endothelial cells, but expression did not correlate with the number of eosinophils in biopsy specimens or with the severity of disease (72). Using a primate model of antigen-induced airway eosinophilia and hyperresponsiveness, Wegner et al. (73) demonstrated enhanced ICAM-1 expression on bronchial microvessels and epithelium after chronic antigen challenge. Subsequent human studies using bronchial biopsy with or without segmental antigen challenge have provided further evidence that ICAM-1 and E-selectin are upregulated in the bronchial microvasculature in allergic asthma. Investigators found increased soluble E-selectin in bronchoalveolar lavage fluid 18 h after antigen challenge (74), and increased serum levels of soluble E-selectin and ICAM-1 in patients with acute asthma compared with stable asthmatics and normal subjects (75,76). Using immunohistochemical analysis of bronchial biopsy specimens 6 h after segmental allergen challenge, Montefort et al. (77) demonstrated an increase in neutrophils, eosinophils, mast cells, and T lymphocytes that was associated with increased expression of E-selectin and ICAM-1 on bronchial microvessels. Of note, however, was a lack of endothelial VCAM-1 expression 6 h after allergen challenge. In contrast to upregulation of E-selectin and ICAM-1 in this study, an earlier study comparing symptomatic asthmatics and normal subjects failed to demonstrate differences in E-selectin and ICAM-1 expression (78), but this may have been due to the small numbers of patients or to the semiquantitative method used to assess CAM expression.

In more recent studies, however, Ohkawara et al. (79) and Gosset et al. (80) presented evidence that the endothelial expression of VCAM-1, as well as E-selectin and ICAM-1, is increased in asthmatics. Using immunohistochemistry, Ohkawara et al. found that when bronchial microvessels were examined in a heterogeneous population of asthmatics during periods of airflow limitation, there was increased endothelial expression of these CAMs compared with control subjects. Immunoelectron microscopy was used to demonstrate E-selectin, ICAM-1, and VCAM-1 in both the luminal membrane and the intracellular organelles, suggesting *de novo* synthesis. The authors showed increased numbers of lymphocyte function-associated antigen (LFA) 1, membrane-attack complex (MAC) 1, and VLA-4-expressing leukocytes in the submucosa; however, they did not attempt to correlate this with endothelial CAM expression. These findings are similar to those reported by Gosset et al. (80), who found increased expression of ICAM-1 (on both epithelium and endothelium) and of E-selectin and VCAM-1 (on endothelium alone) in allergic, but not nonallergic, asthmatics.

In addition to E-selectin, ICAM-1, and VCAM-1, a recent study suggests that P-selectin may be important for eosinophil homing to sites of allergic inflammation. Immunohistochemistry of nasal polyps revealed increased expression of ICAM-1 and both E- and P-selectin on endothelium, with weak or absent expression of VCAM-1 (81). More importantly, eosinophil adhesion to frozen sections was almost completely inhibited by antibodies to P-selectin or to the P-selectin ligand on leukocytes. Antibodies to MAC-1 partially inhibited adhesion, while antibodies to E-selectin, ICAM-1, VCAM-1, VLA-1, and LFA-1 had no effect. This study suggests that P-selectin may be required for eosinophil adhesion to airway endothelium. To date, there are no available data in animal models of airway eosinophilia to confirm this interesting finding.

Data from a number of studies thus provide evidence that airway inflammation in various populations of asthmatics is associated with upregulation of E-selectin and ICAM-1. However, it appears that VCAM-1 expression may be increased in only a subset of patients or only transiently during periods of increased inflammation.

Although these human studies provide important associations, it is difficult to make any mechanistic conclusions. To this end, several studies have employed blocking antibodies to endothelial or leukocyte CAMs in animal models of airway hyperreactivity or eosinophil recruitment (see Table 5 for a summary). In their primate models of chronic antigen challenge, Wegner et al. (73) found that administration of an anti-ICAM-1 antibody attenuated both eosinophil influx and the induction of chronic airway hyperresponsiveness. In companion studies, an antibody against E-selectin abrogated the neutrophil influx and late-phase response observed with acute antigen challenge, but the anti-ICAM-1 antibody had no effect (82,83). These data suggested that E-selectin was necessary for neutrophil influx, and ICAM-1 for eosinophil influx in these models of acute and chronic antigen challenge and that inhibition of cell homing may block airway hyperreactivity.

In contrast to the primate studies, studies employing a guinea-pig model of antigen-induced eosinophil infiltration revealed that blockade of the VCAM-1/VLA-4 pathway with antibodies against either VCAM-1 or VLA-4, but not blockade of the ICAM-1/LFA-1 pathway, significantly reduced eosinophil accumulation 24 h after antigen inhalation (84). In addition, blockade of VCAM-1/VLA-4 reduced T-cell infiltration to a greater degree than did blockade of ICAM-1/LFA-1. The authors speculate that binding of LFA-1 to its constitutively expressed alternate ligand, ICAM-2, may in part explain the minor effects of ICAM-1/LFA-1-blocking antibodies. However,

differences in the species (primate versus rodent) or antigen-sensitization model (chronic versus acute) could explain the disparate findings in these two studies.

Additional studies targeting the leukocyte CAMs suggest that both CD18 and VLA-4 mediate eosinophil migration into the lung. In a guinea-pig model in which airway and lung eosinophilia are induced by intravenous delivery of Sephadex particles, administration of anti-CD18 *or* anti-VLA-4 antibodies resulted in a 50% decrement in eosinophil accumulation. Administration of *both* antibodies, however, completely inhibited eosinophil influx (85). These data, in contrast to the findings reported by Nakajima et al. (84) in ovalbumin-sensitized guinea pigs, suggest that eosinophils may use *either* CD18 or VLA-4 for endothelial adherence and transmigration in the lung, and that, for some stimuli, multiple adhesion pathways may need to be blocked to inhibit eosinophil migration to the airways *in vivo*. The conflicting results among several different animal species, or different models in the same species, highlight the problem with extrapolating from any animal model of eosinophil or lymphocyte accumulation to the pathologic eosinophil accumulation observed in the asthmatic airway.

Other, more recent, studies have suggested that the paradigm of CAMs as simple adhesive gatekeepers regulating leukocyte accumulation is too simplistic. In an allergic sheep model of airway hyperresponsiveness, Abraham et al. (86) demonstrated that intravenous or aerosol administration of an anti-VLA-4 antibody blocked allergen-induced late-phase hyperresponsiveness *without* sig-

TABLE 5. *Summary of in vivo studies using anti-CAM-blocking antibodies*

Author	Targeted CAM	Species	Model	Physiologic endpoint
Wegner et al. (73)	ICAM-1	Primate	Chronic allergen challenge	Reduced eosinophil influx and hyper-responsiveness
Gundel et al. (82)	E-selectin	Primate	Acute allergen challenge	Reduced neutrophil influx
Abraham et al. (86)	VLA-4	Sheep	Allergen challenge	Reduced airway hyperresponsiveness without reduced leukocyte influx
Rabb et al. (87)	VLA-4 or LFA-1/MAC-1	Rat	Ovalbumin sensitization	Reduced hyperresponsiveness without consistent changes in BAL/lung leukocytes
Laberge et al. (88)	LFA-1 or VLA-4	Rat	Ovalbumin sensitization	Reduced response to ovalbumin with either antibody; reduced eosinophils in lavage/lung with LFA-1 but not VLA-4 antibodies
Das et al. (85)	CD18/VLA-4	Guinea pig	i.v. Sephadex particles	Reduced eosinophil recruitment by combination of blocking antibodies
Milne et al. (104)	CD18	Guinea pig	Allergen sensitization	Reduced hyperresponsiveness and BAL eosinophilia with one antibody; reduced eosinophilia without reduced hyperresponsiveness with second antibody
Nakajima et al. (84)	VLA-4/VCAM-1, LFA-1/ICAM-1	Mice	Allergen sensitization	No reduction in airway eosinophilia after systemic administration
Nakao et al. (105)	ICAM-1/LFA-1	Mice	Allergen sensitization	Reduction in eosinophilia by T-cell tolerance (induced by administering antibodies plus antigen prior to sensitization)

BAL, bronchoalveolar lavage; CAM, cell adhesion molecule; ICAM, intercellular adhesion molecule; LFA, lymphocyte function-associated antigen; MAC, membrane-attack complex; VCAM, vascular cell adhesion molecule; VLA, very late antigen.

nificantly reducing the numbers or percentages of neutrophil and eosinophils in bronchoalveolar lavage fluid. Similarly, in the ovalbumin-sensitized brown Norway rat, administration of an anti-VLA-4 or both anti-LFA-1 and anti-MAC-1 antibodies abrogated the early and late-phase (less than 8 h) responses after ovalbumin challenge *without* reducing eosinophil or lymphocyte numbers in BAL or tissue 8 h after challenge (87,88). Another study in Norway rats demonstrated a reduction in hyperresponsiveness *without* a reduction in airway inflammation after administration of an anti-ICAM-1 antibody (89). These data (which should be considered within the context of the experimental limitations of any animal model of asthma) indicate that although anti-CAM therapy appears to be effective in blunting airway hyperresponsiveness, the mechanism may not be totally dependent on inhibition of inflammatory cell influx.

Adhesion Molecules in Leukocyte Activation

What might these other mechanisms be? One well-established function of CAMs is as accessory molecules in leukocyte activation (reviewed in reference 10). Inhibition of leukocyte β_1- or β_2-integrin function can inhibit T-helper and B-lymphocyte responses to antigen and antigen-independent-induced activation stimuli. In addition, binding of T cells to VCAM-1-expressing endothelial cells contributes to the induction of matrix metalloproteinases (90), which may be a necessary prerequisite to T-cell migration through matrix. *In vitro* experiments have also demonstrated that anti-VLA-4 antibody can reduce platelet-activating factor-induced eosinophil peroxidase release (86). These data suggest that eosinophil activation is, in part, mediated by VLA-4 and that the observed reduction in hyperresponsiveness may have been due to the antibody effect on leukocyte function rather than recruitment. Finally, the importance of CAMs in leukocyte activation is supported by the observation that pretreatment of mice with anti-ICAM-1 and anti-LFA-1 antibodies effectively induces tolerance to subsequent antigen challenge in mice (91). Thus, a number of studies indicate that blockade of adhesion molecules might blunt the responses of airway leukocytes, or preclude effective antigen presentation, independent of the recruitment of circulating cells.

Adhesion Molecules in Airway Remodeling

Recent evidence also suggests that CAMs mediate a number of inflammatory cell-interstitial cell interactions (depicted in Fig. 1C) and may thereby contribute to the inflammatory response in the airway. Lazaar et al. (92) have recently demonstrated that activated T lymphocytes, via LFA-1 and VLA-4, adhere to cytokine-inducible ICAM-1 and VCAM-1 on cultured human airway smooth muscle cells. Moreover, an integrin-independent component of lymphocyte-smooth muscle adhesion appeared to be mediated by CD44 and hyaluronate. Functionally, adhesion of stimulated T lymphocytes induced deoxyribonucleic acid (DNA) synthesis in smooth muscle, suggesting that CAM-mediated T-lymphocyte adhesion to smooth muscle may induce smooth muscle growth and thereby contribute to the airway remodeling that occurs in asthmatics. Other interactions of lymphocytes with interstitial cells may also be mediated by CAMs.

Leukocyte-Epithelial Adhesion

Leukocyte-epithelial cell interactions may also be regulated by adhesion molecules, especially ICAM-1 (Fig. 1D). Biopsies of human and monkey bronchial epithelium have shown constitutive ICAM-1 expression (73,77,93). In the monkey model (73), ICAM-1 expression appears to increase after chronic allergen challenge. Upregulation of ICAM-1 on epithelial cells, as noted by Wegner et al. (73), may be important in mediating the binding of activated eosinophils with subsequent release of toxic mediators and epithelial damage. Indeed, immunostaining of epithelial cells from bronchial brushing suggests that there is increased expression of ICAM-1, and of HLA-DR, in asthmatic airway compared with normal subjects (94). Moreover, the distribution of ICAM-1 and HLA-DR appeared altered in asthmatics insofar as both molecules were localized to the apical membrane in asthmatics but not controls (95). The discrepancies in ICAM-1 expression between these studies and those of Montefort et al. (78) suggest that further studies will be necessary. The pathophysiologic importance of epithelial ICAM-1 expression *in vivo* remains unclear, but intriguing possibilities are that the apical upregulation of ICAM-1 and HLA-DR increases the retention of leukocytes in the airway lumen or facilitate antigen presentation.

In vitro studies have implicated ICAM-1 in the adhesion of neutrophils to primary tracheal epithelial cells, but the evidence suggests that there are other epithelial ligands for leukocytes. After infection with parainfluenza virus and adenovirus, epithelial cells were found to have increased ICAM-1 expression and neutrophil adhesion (96,97). Antibodies against ICAM-1 only partially blocked adhesion, suggesting that there are additional adhesion mechanisms for leukocyte binding to epithelial cells (94). Indeed, recent data suggest that the cadherins may be involved in leukocyte-epithelial adhesion. Specifically, in intestinal epithelia, Brenner and colleagues showed that intraepithelial lymphocytes bind to epithelial cells via both LFA-1 and $\alpha_E\beta_7$ (98), and interestingly that the epithelial ligand is E-cadherin (99). Additional studies in airway epithelium are necessary to determine whether similar mechanisms are involved in the localization of lymphocytes in respiratory epithelium.

Other studies have addressed the effects of histamine and cytokines on adhesion molecule expression by epithelial cells. Incubation of normal human bronchial epithelial cells with histamine has been shown to result in increased ICAM-1 (and HLA-DR) expression, suggesting that mast cells may upregulate adhesion molecules on epithelial cells (100). In one study, tumor necrosis factor and interleukin 1β increased ICAM-1 expression and neutrophil adherence (93) while, in another, interferon-γ (but not tumor necrosis factor or interleukin 1β) induced ICAM-1 expression on bronchial epithelial cells (101). Interferon-γ was shown to induce ICAM-1 expression on tracheal epithelial cells but not umbilical vein endothelial cells, suggesting that the cellular regulation of ICAM-1 expression differs between endothelial and epithelial cells (101). Moreover, the adhesion of peripheral blood lymphocytes to cytokine-stimulated epithelial monolayers could be completely abrogated by anti-CD18 and anti-ICAM antibodies, whereas lymphocyte adhesion to endothelial monolayers required blockade of both the LFA-1/ICAM-1 and VLA-4/VCAM-1 interactions (102).

CONCLUSIONS

The accumulated data thus suggest that CAMs potentially mediate cell migration, leukocyte activation, and interstitial cell-cell interactions in inflammatory airway diseases such as asthma. Identification of these complex, and perhaps interrelated, functions leads to an increasingly sophisticated paradigm and underscores the need for additional studies to define further the *in vivo* function of the known CAMs in the airway. In addition, the possibility of unidentified, or lung-specific, CAMs needs to be explored further.

FUTURE DIRECTIONS

Research over the last decade has identified some of the important cell adhesion molecules on pulmonary epithelial and endothelial cells, but many questions remain to be answered. In terms of lung structure, the integrins, cadherins, and other molecules are important for epithelial integrity. One area for future work is the expression and regulation of these molecules in epithelial repair after inhalational or infectious damage. Development of new therapeutic modalities will, however, require knowledge of the complex regulatory interplay between leukocyte-endothelial and leukocyte-epithelial molecules, cytokines, and chemoattractants *in vivo*. For example, detailed understanding of the CAMs involved in leukocyte activation may lead to new classes of drugs for asthma, such as cyclic arginine-glycine-aspartic acid (RGD) peptides. In addition, future studies will need to determine the impact of specific cytokines on both expression and function, and define the genetic regulation of CAM expression (103). This in turn will facilitate rational therapeutic approaches to CAM function in the asthmatic airway.

ACKNOWLEDGMENTS

The authors acknowledge support from the American Cancer Society, the Polly Annenberg Levee Charitable Trust, and the National Institutes of Health (H2 RO1 HL 49591 to S.M.A.). J.M.P. is supported by an American Lung Association Research Grant and the Cystic Fibrosis Foundation. S.M.A. is an Established Investigator of the American Heart Association.

REFERENCES

1. Albelda SM, Smith CW, Ward PA. Adhesion molecules and inflammatory injury. *FASEB J* 1994;8:504–512.
2. Albelda SM, Buck CA. Integrins and other cell adhesion molecules. *FASEB J* 1990;4:2868–2880.
3. Carlos TM, Harlan J. Leukocyte-endothelial adhesion molecules. *Blood* 1994;84:2061–2101.
4. Hynes RO. Integrins: versatility, modulation, and signaling in cell adhesion. *Cell* 1992;69:11–25.
5. McDonald JA. Receptors for extracellular matrix components. *Am J Physiol* 1989;257:L331–L337.
6. Hemler ME. VLA proteins in the integrin family: structures, functions and their role on leukocytes. *Annu Rev Immunol* 1990;8:365–400.
7. Ruoslahti E, Pierschbacher MD. New perspectives in cell adhesion: RGD and integrins. *Science* 1987;238:491–497.
8. Takeichi M. Cadherin cell adhesion receptors as a morphogenetic regulator. *Science* 1991;251:1451–1455.
9. Williams AF, Barclay AN. The immunoglobulin supergene family-domains for cell surface recognition. *Annu Rev Immunol* 1988;6:381–405.
10. Springer TA. Adhesion receptors of the immune system. *Nature* 1990;46:425–434.
11. Bevilacqua MP, Nelson RM. Selectins. *J Clin Invest* 1993;91:379–387.
12. Springer TA, Lasky LA. Sticky sugars for selectins. *Nature* 1991;349:196–197.
13. Lasky LA. Selectins: interpreters of cell-specific carbohydrate information during inflammation. *Science* 1992;258:964–969.
14. Rosen SD. The LEC-CAMs: an emerging family of cell-cell adhesion receptors based upon carbohydrate recognition. *Am J Respir Cell Mol Biol* 1990;3:397–402.
15. Brandley BK, Swiedler SJ, Robbins PW. Carbohydrate ligands of the LEC cell adhesion molecules. *Cell* 1990;63:861–863.
16. Adams DH, Shaw S. Leucocyte-endothelial interactions and the regulation of leucocyte migration. *Lancet* 1994;343:831–836.
17. Butcher EC. Cellular and molecular mechanisms that direct leukocyte traffic. *Am J Pathol* 1990;136:3–11.
18. Picker LJ, Nakache M, Butcher EC. Monoclonal antibodies to human lymphocyte homing receptors define a novel class of adhesion molecules on diverse cell types. *J Cell Biol* 1989;109:927–937.
19. Clark EA, Brugge JS. Integrins and signal transduction pathways: the road taken. *Science* 1995;268:233–239.
20. Wickham TJ, Mathias P, Cheresh DJ, Nemerow GR. Integrins $\alpha_v\beta_3$ and $\alpha_v\beta_5$ promote adenovirus internalization but not virus attachment. *Cell* 1993;73:309–319.
21. Mathias P, Wickham T, Moore M, Nemerow G. Multiple adenovirus serotypes use α_v integrins for infection. *J Virol* 1994;68:6811–6814.
22. Ozawa M, Baribault H, Kemler R. The cytoplasmic domain of the cell adhesion molecule uvomorulin associates with three independent proteins structurally related in different species. *EMBO J* 1989;8:1711–1717.
23. Ozawa M, Kemler R. Molecular organization of the uvomorulin-catenin complex. *J Cell Biol* 1992;116:989–996.

24. Nathke IS, Hinck L, Swedlow JR, Papkoff J, Nelson WJ. Defining interactions and distributions of cadherin and catenin complexes in polarized epithelial cells. *J Cell Biol* 1994;125:1341–1352.
25. Berg EL, Robinson MK, Mansson O, Butcher EC, Magnani JL. A carbohydrate domain common to both sialyl Lea and sialyl Lex is recognized by the endothelial cell adhesion molecule ELAM-1. *J Biol Chem* 1991;266:14,869–14,872.
26. Sako D, Chang X-J, Barone KM, et al. Expression cloning of a functional glycoprotein ligand for P-selectin. *Cell* 1993;75:1179–1186.
27. Steegmaier M, Levinovitz A, Isenmann S, et al. The E-selectin-ligand ESL-1 is a variant of a receptor for fibroblast growth factor. *Nature* 1995;373:615–620.
28. Albelda SM. Endothelial and epithelial cell adhesion molecules. *Am J Respir Cell Mol Biol* 1991;4:195–203.
29. Damjanovich L, Albelda SM, Mette SA, Buck CA. Distribution of integrin cell adhesion receptors in normal and malignant lung tissue. *Am J Respir Cell Mol Biol* 1992;6:197–206.
30. Mette SA, Pilewski J, Buck CA, Albelda SM. The distribution of integrin cell adhesion receptors on normal bronchial epithelial cells and lung cancer cells *in vitro* and *in vivo*. *Am J Respir Cell Mol Biol* 1993; 8:562–572.
31. Sapsford RJ, Devalia JL, McAulay AE, d'Ardenne AJ, Davies RJ. Expression of $\alpha_{1-6}1-\beta_6$? integrin cell surface receptors in normal human bronchial biopsies and cultured bronchial epithelial cells. *J Allergy Clin Immunol* 1991;87:A303.
32. Sonnenberg A, Calafat J, Jannsen H, et al. Integrin α_6/β_4 complex is located in hemidesmosomes, suggesting a major role in epidermal cell-basement membrane adhesion. *J Cell Biol* 1991;113:907–917.
33. Pasqualini R, Bodorova J, Ye S, Hemler ME. A study of the structure, function and distribution of β_5 integrins using novel anti-β_5 monoclonal antibodies. *J Cell Science* 1993;105:101–111.
34. Juhasz I, Murphy GF, Yan H-C, Herlyn M, Albelda SM. Regulation of extracellular matrix proteins and integrin cell substratum adhesion receptors on epithelium during cutaneous human wound healing *in vivo*. *Am J Pathol* 1993;143:1458–1469.
35. Horiba K, Fukuda Y. Synchronous appearance of fibronectin, integrin $\alpha_5\beta_1$, vinculin and actin in epithelial cells and fibroblasts during rat tracheal wound healing. *Virchows Arch* 1994;425:425–434.
36. Pilewski JM, Chilkitowsky J, Albelda SM. Epithelial expression of ICAM-1 and integrin cell adhesion receptors during airway epithelial repair *in vivo*. *Am J Respir Crit Care Med* 1995;151:A301(abstract).
37. Weinacker A, Ferrando R, Elliott M, Hogg J, Balmes J, Sheppard D. Distribution of integrins $\alpha_v\beta_6$ and $\alpha_9\beta_1$ and their known ligands, fibronectin and tenascin, in human airways. *Am J Respir Cell Mol Biol* 1995;12:547–557.
38. Ruoslahti E. Proteoglycans in cell regulation. *J Biol Chem* 1989;264: 13,369–13,372.
39. Saunders S, Jalkanen M, O'Farrell S, Bernfield M. Molecular cloning of syndecan, an integral membrane proteoglycan. *J Cell Biol* 1989; 108:1547–1556.
40. Elenius K, Salmivirta M, Inki P, Mali M, Jalkanen M. Binding of human syndecan to extracellular matrix proteins. *J Biol Chem* 1990;265: 17,837–17,843.
41. Montefort S, Herbert CA, Robinson C, Holgate ST. The bronchial epithelium as a target for inflammatory attack in asthma. *Clin Exp Allergy* 1992;22:511–520.
42. Cowin P, Franke WW, Grund C, Kapprell H, Kartenbeck J. The desmosome-intermediate filament complex. In: Edelman GM, Thiery J-P, eds. *The cell in contact: adhesions and junctions as morphogenetic determinants.* New York: John Wiley and Sons 1985;427–460.
43. Stevenson BR, Paul DL. The molecular constituents of intercellular junctions. *Curr Opin Cell Biol* 1989;1:884–891.
44. Shimoyama Y, Hirohashi S, Hirano S, et al. Cadherin cell-adhesion molecules in human epithelial tissues and carcinomas. *Cancer Res* 1989;49:2128–2133.
45. Behrens J, Birchmeir W, Goodman SL, Imhof BA. Dissociation of Madin-Darby canine kidney epithelial cells by the monoclonal antibody anti-Arc-1: mechanistic aspects and identification of the antigen as a component related to uvomorulin. *J Cell Biol* 1985;101:1307–1315.
46. Albelda SM. Role of integrins and other cell adhesion molecules in tumor progression and metastasis. *Lab Invest* 1993;68:4–17.
47. Vleminckx K, Vakaet L, Mareel M, Fiers W, Van Roy F. Genetic manipulation of E-cadherin expression by epithelial tumor cells reveals an invasive suppressor role. *Cell* 1991;66:107–119.
48. Carter WG, Wayner EA, Bouchard TS, Kaur P. The role of integrins

49. $\alpha_2\beta_1$ and $\alpha_3\beta_1$ in cell-cell and cell-substrate adhesion of human epidermal cells. *J Cell Biol* 1990;110:1387–1404.
49. Lampugnani MG, Resnati M, Dejana E, Marchisio PC. The role of integrins in the maintenance of endothelial monolayer integrity. *J Cell Biol* 1991;112:479–490.
50. Newman PJ, Albelda SM. Cellular and molecular aspects of PECAM-1. *Nouv Rev Fr Hematol* 1992;34:S7–S11.
51. Pober JS, Cotran RS. The role of endothelial cells in inflammation. *Transplantation* 1990;50:537–544.
52. Butcher EC. Leukocyte-endothelial cell recognition: three (or more) steps to specificity and diversity. *Cell* 1991;67:1033–1036.
53. Pober JS, Cotran RS. What can be learned from the expression of endothelial adhesion molecules in tissues? *Lab Invest* 1991;64:301–305.
54. Lawrence MB, Springer TA. Leukocytes roll on a selectin at physiologic flow rates: distinction from and prerequisite for adhesion through integrins. *Cell* 1991;65:859–873.
55. Bevilaqua MP, Stengalin S, Gimbrone MA, Seed B. Endothelial leukocyte adhesion molecule 1: an inducible receptor for neutrophils related to complement regulatory proteins and lectins. *Science* 1989; 243:1160–1165.
56. Hermanowski-Vosatka A, Van Strijp JAG, Swiggard WJ, Wright SD. Integrin modulating factor 1: a lipid that alters the function of leukocyte integrins. *Cell* 1992;68:341–352.
57. Hibbs ML, Stacker JS, Wallace SA, Springer TA. The cytoplasmic domain of the integrin lymphocyte function-associated antigen-1 beta subunit: sites required for binding to intercellular adhesion molecule 1 and the phorbol ester-stimulated phosphorylation sites. *J Exp Med* 1991;174:1227–1238.
58. Elices MJ, Urry LA, Hemler ME. Receptor functions for the integrin VLA-3: fibronectin, collagen, and laminin binding are differentially influenced by ARG-GLY-ASP peptide and by divalent cations. *J Cell Biol* 1991;112:169–181.
59. Osborn L. Leukocyte adhesion to endothelium in inflammation. *Cell* 1990;62:3–6.
60. Picker LJ, Warnock RA, Burns AR, Doerschuk CM, Berg EL, Butcher EC. The neutrophil selectin LECAM-1 presents carbohydrate ligands to the vascular selectins ELAM-1 and GMP-140. *Cell* 1991; 66:921–933.
61. Lo SK, Lee S, Ramos RA, et al. Endothelial-leukocyte adhesion molecule 1 stimulates the adhesive activity of leukocyte integrin CR3 (CD11b/CD18, MAC-1) on human neutrophils. *J Exp Med* 1991;173: 1493–1500.
62. Anderson DC, Springer TA. Leukocyte adhesion deficiency: an inherited defect in the MAC-1, LFA-1, and p150,95 glycoproteins. *Annu Rev Med* 1987;38:175–194.
63. Etzioni A, Frydman M, Pollack S, et al. Recurrent severe infections caused by a novel leukocyte adhesion deficiency. *N Engl J Med* 1992; 327:1789–1792.
64. Mayadas TN, Johnson RC, Rayburn H, Hynes RO, Wagner DD. Leukocyte rolling and extravasation are severely compromised in P selectin-deficient mice. *Cell* 1993;74:541–554.
65. Arbones ML, Ord DC, Ley K, et al. Lymphocyte homing and leukocyte rolling and migration are impaired in L-selectin-deficient mice. *Immunity* 1994;1:247–260.
66. Schleimer RP, Benenati SV, Friedman B, Bochner BS. Do cytokines play a role in leukocyte recruitment and activation in the lungs? *Am Rev Respir Dis* 1991;143:1169–1174.
67. Rossi GA, Sacco O, Balbi B, et al. Human ciliated bronchial epithelial cells: expression of the HLA-DR antigens by gamma-interferon and antigen-presenting function in the mixed leukocyte reaction. *Am J Respir Cell Mol Biol* 1990;3:431–439.
68. Robbins RA, Koyama S, Spurzem JR, et al. Modulation of neutrophil and mononuclear cell adherence to bronchial epithelial cells. *Am J Respir Cell Mol Biol* 1992;7:19–29.
69. Leff AR, Hamann KJ, Wegner CD. Inflammation and cell-cell interactions in airway hyperresponsiveness. *Am J Physiol* 1991;260:L189–L206.
70. Hansel TT, Walker C. The migration of eosinophils into the sputum of asthmatics: the role of adhesion molecules. *Clin Exp Allergy* 1992;22: 345–356.
71. Dobrina A, Menegazzi R, Carlos TM, et al. Mechanisms of eosinophil adherence to cultured vascular endothelial cells: eosinophils bind to the cytokine-induced endothelial ligand vascular cell adhesion molecule 1 via the very late activation antigen-4 integrin receptor. *J Clin Invest* 1991;88:20–26.

72. Montefort S, Feather IH, Wilson SJ, et al. The expression of leukocyte-endothelial adhesion molecules is increased in perennial allergic rhinitis. *Am J Respir Cell Mol Biol* 1992;7:393–398.

73. Wegner CD, Gundel RH, Reilly P, Haynes N, Letts LG, Rothlein R. Intercellular adhesion molecule 1 (ICAM-1) in the pathogenesis of asthma. *Science* 1990;247:456–459.

74. Georas SN, Liu MC, Newman W, Beall LD, Stealey BA, Bochner BS. Altered adhesion molecule expression and endothelial cell activation accompany the recruitment of human granulocytes to the lung after segmental antigen challenge. *Am J Respir Cell Mol Biol* 1992;7:261–269.

75. Montefort S, Lai CKW, Kapahi P, et al. Circulating adhesion molecules in asthma. *Am J Respir Crit Care Med* 1994;149:1149–1152.

76. Kobayashi T, Hashimoto S, Imai K, et al. Elevation of serum soluble intercellular adhesion molecule 1 (sICAM-1) and sE-selectin levels in bronchial asthma. *Clin Exp Immunol* 1994;96:110–115.

77. Montefort S, Gratziou C, Goulding D, et al. Bronchial biopsy evidence for leukocyte infiltration and upregulation of leukocyte–endothelial cell adhesion molecules 6 hours after local antigen challenge of sensitized asthmatic airways. *J Clin Invest* 1994;93:1411–1421.

78. Montefort S, Roche WR, Howarth PH, et al. Intercellular adhesion molecule 1 (ICAM-1) and endothelial leukocyte adhesion molecule 1 (ELAM-1) expression in the bronchial mucosa of normal and asthmatic subjects. *Eur Respir J* 1992;5:815–823.

79. Ohkawara Y, Yamauchi K, Maruyama N, et al. *In situ* expression of the cell adhesion molecules in bronchial tissues from asthmatics with airflow limitation: *in vivo* evidence of VCAM-1/VLA-4 interaction in selective eosinophil infiltration. *Am J Respir Cell Mol Biol* 1994;12:4–12.

80. Gosset P, Tillie-Lebiond I, Janin A, et al. Expression of E-selectin, ICAM-1 and VCAM-1 on bronchial biopsies from allergic and non-allergic patients. *Int Arch Allergy Immunol* 1995;106:69–77.

81. Symon FA, Walsh GM, Watson SR, Wardlaw AJ. Eosinophil adhesion to nasal polyp endothelium is P-selectin-dependent. *J Exp Med* 1994;180:371–376.

82. Gundel RH, Wegner CD, Torcellini CA, et al. Endothelial leukocyte adhesion molecule 1 mediates antigen-induced acute airway inflammation and late-phase airway obstruction in monkeys. *J Clin Invest* 1991;88:1407–1411.

83. Gundel RH, Wegner CD, Torcellini CA, Letts LG. The role of intercellular adhesion molecule 1 in chronic airway inflammation. *Clin Exp Allergy* 1992;22:569–575.

84. Nakajima H, Sano H, Nishimura T, Yoshida S, Iwamoto I. Role of VCAM-1/VLA-4 and ICAM-1/LFA-1 interactions in antigen-induced eosinophil and T cell recruitment into the tissue. *J Exp Med* 1994;179:1145–1154.

85. Das AM, Williams TJ, Lobb R, Nourshargh S. Lung eosinophilia is dependent on IL-5 and the adhesion molecules CD18 and VLA-4, in a guinea pig model. *Immunology* 1995;84:41–46.

86. Abraham WM, Sielczak MW, Ahmed A, et al. α-4-Integrins mediate antigen-induced late bronchial responses and prolonged airway hyperresponsiveness in sheep. *J Clin Invest* 1994;93:776–787.

87. Rabb HA, Olivenstein R, Issekutz TB, et al. The role of the leukocyte adhesion molecules VLA-4, LFA-1, and MAC-1 in allergic airway responses in the rat. *Am J Respir Crit Care Med* 1994;149:1186–1191.

88. Laberge S, Rabb H, Issekutz TB, Martin JG. Role of VLA-4 and LFA-1 in airway hyperresponsiveness and lung inflammation following allergen challenge in the rat. *Am J Respir Crit Care Med* 1995;151:822–829.

89. Sun J, Elwood W, Haczku A, Barnes PJ, Hellewell PG, Chung KF. Contribution of intercellular adhesion molecule 1 in allergen-induced airway hyperresponsiveness and inflammation in sensitized brown-Norway rats. *Int Arch Allergy Immunol* 1994;104:291–295.

90. Romanic AM, Madri JA. The induction of 72-kd gelatinase in T cells upon adhesion to endothelial cells is VCAM-1 dependent. *J Cell Biol* 1994;125:1165–1178.

91. Nakai A, Nakajima H, Tomioka H, Nishimura T, Iwamoto I. Induction of T cell tolerance by pretreatment with anti-ICAM-1 and anti-lymphocyte function-associated antigen-1 antibodies prevents antigen-induced eosinophil recruitment into the mouse airways. *J Immunol* 1994;153:5819–5825.

92. Lazaar AL, Albelda SM, Pilewski JM, Brennan B, Pure E, Panettieri RA. T lymphocytes adhere to airway smooth muscle cells via integrins and CD44 and induce smooth muscle cell DNA synthesis. *J Exp Med* 1994;180:807–816.

93. Tosi MF, Stark JM, Smith CW, Hamedani A, Gruenert DC, Infeld MD. Induction of ICAM-1 expression on human airway epithelial cells by inflammatory cytokines: effects on neutrophil–epithelial cell adhesion. *Am J Respir Cell Mol Biol* 1992;7:214–221.

94. Vignola AM, Campbell AM, Chanez P, et al. HLA-DR and ICAM-1 expression on bronchial epithelial cells in asthma and chronic bronchitis. *Am Rev Respir Dis* 1993;148:689–694.

95. Vignola AM, Chanez P, Campbell AM, et al. Quantification and localization of HLA-DR and intercellular adhesion molecule 1 (ICAM-1) molecules on bronchial epithelial cells of asthmatics using confocal microscopy. *Clin Exp Immunol* 1994;96:104–109.

96. Tosi MF, Stark JM, Hamedani A, Smith CW, Gruenert DC, Huang YT. ICAM-1-dependent and ICAM-1-independent adhesive interactions between PMN leukocytes and human airway epithelial cells infected with parainfluenza virus type 2. *J Immunol* 1992;149:3345–3349.

97. Pilewski JM, Sott DJ, Wilson JM, Albelda SM. Expression of ICAM-1 on bronchial epithelium after recombinant adenovirus infection. *Am J Respir Cell Mol Biol* 1995;12:142–148.

98. Cepek KL, Parker CM, Madara JL, Brenner MB. Integrin $\alpha_E\beta_7$ mediates adhesion of T lymphocytes to epithelial cells. *J Immunol* 1993;150:3459–3470.

99. Cepek KL, Shaw SK, Parker CM, et al. Adhesion between epithelial cells and T lymphocytes mediated by E-cadherin and the $\alpha_E\beta_7$ integrin. *Nature* 1994;372:190–193.

100. Vignola AM, Campbell AM, Chanez P, et al. Activation by histamine of bronchial epithelial cells from nonasthmatic subjects. *Am J Respir Cell Mol Biol* 1993;9:411–417.

101. Look DC, Rapp SR, Keller BT, Holtzman MJ. Selective induction of intercellular adhesion molecule 1 by interferon-γ in human airway epithelial cells. *Am J Physiol* 1992;263:L79–L87.

102. Nakajima S, Look DC, Roswit WT, Bragdon MJ, Holtzman MJ. Selective differences in vascular endothelial versus airway epithelial T cell adhesion mechanisms. *Am J Physiol* 1994;267:L422–432.

103. Holtzman MJ, Look DC. Cell adhesion molecules as targets for unraveling the genetic regulation of airway inflammation. *Am J Respir Cell Mol Biol* 1992;7:246–247.

104. Milne AA, Piper PJ. Role of VLA-4 integrin in leukocyte recruitment and bronchial hyperresponsiveness in the guinea pig. *Eur J Pharm* 1995;282:243–249.

105. Nakao A, Nakajima H, Tomioka H, Nishimura T, Iwamoto I. Induction of T-cell tolerance by pretreatment with anti-ICAM-1 and antilymphocyte function-associated antigen-1 antibodies prevents antigen-induced eosinophil recruitment into the mouse airways. *J Immunol* 1994;1953:5819–5825.

▪ 5 ▪

Inflammatory Mediators

Asthma, edited by P.J. Barnes, M.M. Grunstein,
A. R. Leff, and A. Woolcock.
Lippincott–Raven Publishers, Philadelphia © 1997.

■ 39 ■

Histamine

Mary Beth Hogan and Paul A. Greenberger

Histamine: Synthesis and Degradation
Histamine: Airway Pathophysiology
   Control of Histamine Release
   Intracellular Control of Histamine Release

   Extracellular Control of Histamine Release
Histamine as a Mediator of Immunologic Function
Antihistamines: A Role in Treating Asthma?

The first observation of the vasoactive properties of histamine occurred in the early 1900s. This cellular mediator has been studied extensively since then. Histamine, however, is more than a vasoactive mediator. It is a ubiquitous mediator of cellular function that affects the immune system. It is well-known that histamine is stored in mast cells and basophils. Subsequent stimulation of these cells residing in the human airway results in the release of histamine and other mediators, which cause bronchoconstriction. However, histamine also is synthesized by other cells including lymphocytes, macrophages, and platelets (1–2). In this review of the role of histamine in causing the asthmatic response, particular attention is given to how the inflammatory cascade of histamine production is released. In addition, the role of histamine as a secondary messenger in the inflammatory cascade of asthma will be discussed.

HISTAMINE: SYNTHESIS AND DEGRADATION

Histamine is a product of the enzyme, histidine decarboxylase, acting upon the amino acid histidine (1). Inducers of the inflammatory cascade can influence the activity of this enzyme. For instance, lipopolysaccharide, concanavalin A, and interleukin-1 have stimulated histi-

dine decarboxylase in macrophages and T lymphocytes to make histamine (3). Oh and Nakano (4) investigated the *in vitro* macrophage and lymphocyte histidine decarboxylase response to glucocorticoids. They showed that histamine synthesis is inhibited by this anti-inflammatory agent. This is particularly interesting since inhaled glucocorticosteroids are the current mainstay of asthma management.

Once histamine is made, it can be excreted by the kidneys in an unmodified form. However, only 1% of the histamine produced is detectable in this unchanged form in the urine. The most important enzymes degrading histamine are histamine N-methyltransferase and diamine oxidase (5). N- methyltransferase converts histamine to methyl histamine. This enzyme is the major enzyme-metabolizing histamine in the human nasal mucosa (5). It would be reasonable to expect the enzyme to be found in lung tissue. Nakazawa et al. (6) used a guinea pig model to investigate the results of viral infections on histamine metabolism. In this model, histamine N-methyltransferase activity was decreased after viral infection by 86% in the guinea pig bronchi. The authors of this study concluded that bronchial hyperresponsiveness secondary to viral infections may be the result of decreased enzymatic catabolism of histamine. In fact, Jarjour et al. (7) have found a correlation between increased bronchoalveolar lavage (BAL) fluid histamine concentrations in human subjects and increased bronchoconstriction. Increased BAL histamine concentrations were associated with hyperresponsiveness as measured by methacholine challenge (8).

These *in vitro* and *in vivo* studies suggest that pulmonary inflammation induced by infections and other triggers, may increase histamine concentrations by af-

M. B. Hogan: Department of Pediatrics, West Virginia University School of Medicine, Morgantown, West Virginia 26506-9214.

P. A. Greenberger: Department of Medicine, Division of Allergy / Immunology, Northwestern University Medical School, Chicago, Illinois 60611-3008.

fecting both the synthesis and degradation of histamine. These increased histamine concentrations may be contributing to bronchoconstriction and asthmatic symptoms. Anti-inflammatory therapy may intervene in this upregulation of histamine production. Further study of histamine metabolism should clarify the role the inflammatory cascade plays in increasing local bronchial histamine concentrations during exacerbations of asthma.

HISTAMINE: AIRWAY PATHOPHYSIOLOGY

Histamine has multiple actions throughout many human tissues. Our understanding of the effect of histamine on various tissues has progressed since the discovery of the histamine receptor. There are three distinct histamine receptors (9). Specific agonists and antagonists of these receptors have been used to study the response histamine induces as a mediator (9). Broadly, H_1-receptors mediate vasodilation, bronchoconstriction, and stimulate bronchial irritant receptors. H_2-receptors modulate bronchial mucus secretion, gastric acidity, and various immune functions. H_3-receptors play a role as an inhibitory feedback mechanism to limit further histamine release by mast cells. Multiple sub-types of histamine receptors may be located in the same organ.

Studies of histamine infused intravenously have identified many of its vasoactive properties. Patients given intravenous histamine have developed bronchoconstriction, accelerated heart rate, reduced diastolic pressure, flushing, increased cutaneous temperature, and headache (10). Both H_1-and H_2-receptors control pulmonary blood flow through the pulmonary arteries (11). However, Braude et al. (12) found that pulmonary vascular permeability is mediated by the H_2-receptor.

Histamine receptors also are found in the peripheral nervous system. Specifically, H_3-receptors are present on cholinergic nerve fibers in the lung (13). H_3-receptors present on neural fibers may act as the feedback mechanism that inhibits acetylcholine release and, thereby, limits reflex bronchoconstriction. Ichinose et al. (14) examined the relationship of H_3-receptors and neurogenically induced bronchoconstriction in the guinea pig. In this model, H_3-receptor activation downregulated nonadrenergic, noncholinergic induced bronchoconstriction. The role of the nervous system and its influence on bronchial hyperreactivity is just beginning to be understood.

Mast cells tend to congregate near nerve endings. The presence of histamine receptors on neural tissue also could imply that a neural-immunologic communication pathway exists. This interaction between the nervous system and the immunologic system has been investigated in several *in vivo* models. Dixon et al. (15) discovered that upper respiratory infections due to *Bordetella bronchisep-*

tica in the canine model caused an increased lung irritant response to histamine challenge. Undem et al. (16) delivered a pulmonary challenge of aerosolized ovalbumin to previously sensitized guinea pigs. The increase in pulmonary resistance after antigen challenge was abolished by vagotomy. In addition, a depolarization of sympathetic, parasympathetic, and sensory neuron action potentials occurred simultaneously with the antigen-induced release of histamine by most cells. This finding of neuronal excitability secondary to histamine also was found in a study by Empey et al. (17). In this study, patients with viral infections had a greater response to bronchial challenge of histamine compared to uninfected normal subjects. This response was inhibited by atropine, indicating that histamine interacted with the cholinergic neural pathway to cause the increase in bronchoconstriction.

In the asthmatic patient, histamine induces bronchospasm. H_1-receptors mediate antigen-induced concentration of bronchial smooth muscle in the canine model of asthma (18). The presence of histamine receptors on smooth muscle fibers also has been demonstrated in *ex vivo* studies of human bronchi (19). Human studies also have been performed that demonstrated the predominance of the H_1-receptor mediating bronchoconstriction (20).

Another major histaminic effect on pulmonary physiology is the stimulation of mucus secretion. Shelhamer et al. (21) reported increased mucus glycoprotein release upon addition of histamine to resected human lung tissue. The release of mucus was inhibited by cimetidine and enhanced by an H_2-agonist. H_1-receptor activity was not associated with mucus production.

Airway obstruction is enhanced by mucosal edema, and this is influenced by histamine as well. Prolonged neural stimulation can lead to mast cell release of histamine and increased vascular permeability (22). In the canine model, pulmonary alveolar membrane permeability is enhanced by histamine (23) acting through H_1-receptors (24). These receptors cause a sodium and chloride influx toward the tracheal lumen, creating a fluid shift. This increased vascular permeability may contribute to the epithelial damage seen in the asthmatic airway (25). In the guinea pig, H_3-receptors appear to act as a feedback mechanism to moderate, nonadrenergic noncholinergic-induced plasma leakage (26). The mechanism of airway obstruction caused by mucus plugging and mucosal edema clearly is an area deserving more research.

Histamine obviously has multiple physiologic effects upon pulmonary tissue. BAL fluid from asthmatic patients has higher concentrations of histamine than BAL fluid from normal subjects. This finding suggests that histamine contributes to resting bronchomotor tone. In addition, mucus secretion, smooth muscle contractility, neural excitability, and vascular permeability all are affected by histamine.

Control of Histamine Release

Mast cells and basophils are the primary histamine storage cells in humans. Mast cells are located in the alveolar walls and the bronchi of the lung (25,27). As early as 1953, Riley et al. (28) associated histamine storage function with the tissue mast cell. Intracellular histaminic effects are controlled by storing histamine bound to heparin (29). A direct *in vivo* link between allergen-induced immediate hypersensitivity reactions and mast cell degranulation has been verified (30).

Histamine release from basophils and mast cells also occurs by other mechanisms. Cytotoxic phenomenon can cause cellular release of stored histamine. The mediators of the inflammatory cascade also can initiate non-cytotoxic histamine release without the requirement for antigen. Non-cytotoxic mediators capable of acting as a secretagogue in humans include bradykinin, substance P, adenosine, c-kit ligand, major basic protein, C3a, and C5a (31–34).

Exogenous substances also have been noted to cause histamine release from mast cells, e.g., compound 48/80 (35). Other histamine- releasing substances have frequent medical uses including radiocontrast media, d-tubocurarine, neuromuscular blocking agents, thiopental, morphine, ketamine, and dextran (36–39). The reactions to these medical agents may be severe enough to cause bronchospasm or life-threatening anaphylactic reactions.

Intracellular Control of Histamine Release

There are several proposed mechanisms by which basophils and mast cells release store histamine. Histamine release is initiated by antigen binding to its specific IgE antibody occupying the FcεRI receptor of the basophil. Initially, this binding is associated with two or more IgE receptors cross-linking. Seagrave et al.(40) found that the FcεRI receptors must move into closer proximity to each other for cross-linking and activation to occur. Antigen-induced activation results in tyrosine kinases becoming coupled to the IgE receptor. The kinases are also rapidly uncoupled from the receptor to stop ongoing tyrosine phosphorylation when the receptor is deactivated (41). The tyrosine kinases phosphorylate antigen recognition activation motif sequences on the β and μ chains of the IgE receptor (42). Once phosphorylated, these motifs synergistically activate phopholipase C (42). Phospholipase C hydrolyses phosphatidyl inositol to inositol 1,4,5 triphosphate, causing the release of intracellular calcium stores. The resulting calcium flux causes the exocytosis of stored histamine.

There are two phenotypes of basophils. These phenotypes are "releasers" (as previously described) and "non-

releasers." Basophils, which readily release histamine and other mediators, play an important role in allergen-induced asthma. The differences in the intracellular control mechanism for "non-releaser" basophils appear to occur after IgE receptor aggregation and activation (43). These "non-releaser" basophils may have a separate mechanism initiated by IgE receptor activation which inhibits the intracellular calcium flux and histamine release (43). Further study of these "non-releasing" basophils may yield information that would help generate new therapeutic options for the future treatment of asthmatic patients. This is particularly true if this control mechanism is found to apply to mast cell physiology also.

Other non-cytolytic mechanisms of histamine release occur in basophils. Baxter et al. (44) noted that basophil surface polysaccharides interact with substances such as dextran and concanavalin A to induce histamine release. Antigen and anti-IgE antibody-induced histamine release also was dependent on the presence of phosphatidylserine (44). It is likely that polysaccharide-induced conformational changes in either the IgE antibody or its receptor are involved in initiating receptor activation.

Immunologic mediators, such as C5a generated by the inflammatory cascade, induce histamine release through its specific receptor on basophils (45). Other mediators like bradykinin cause mast cell histamine release by activating GTP-binding regulatory proteins (G proteins) (46). Subsequent GTPase activity then activates the inositol triphosphate pathway to cause histamine exocytosis (46). It is not surprising with the presence of multiple histamine-releasing pathways in basophils and mast cells, that multiple, unrelated mediators are capable of releasing histamine.

Extracellular Control of Histamine Release

It appears that at least some basophils have an intracellular means for controlling histamine release. In addition, a complex external histamine control pathway with an inhibitory feedback mechanism exists to regulate histamine release. Cytokines are noted for acting as messengers in the inflammatory process and can interact with basophils to influence histamine release. Histamine-releasing factors (HRF) have been defined as products of activated cells that cause histamine release from basophils or mast cells. These activated cells producing HRF include T and B lymphocytes, macrophages, neutrophils, and platelets (47–49).

HRF cytokines are heterogeneous in their ability to induce histamine release. For instance, interleukin-3 (Il-3), interleukin-5 (Il-5), c-kit ligand, granulocyte-macrophage colony-stimulating factor (GM-CSF), and insulinlike growth factor prime basophils for subsequent histamine release induced by C3a, platelet activating factor, and neutrophil activating peptide (33, 50–53). IL-5 and other priming cytokines will not cause histamine release even in basophils from atopic subjects (52). However, the basophils from some atopic individuals release histamine when challenged with IL-3 (54) or GMCSF (55).

Some members of the chemokine family of cytokines are particularly adept at causing basophil histamine release. Macrophage inflammatory protein-1α, RANTES, connective tissue activating peptide III, and neutrophil activating peptide-II are all histamine releasing members of this family (51,56). One of the most potent histamine releasing factors in this family is monocyte chemotactic and activating factor (MCAF) (57). It is significant that even "normal" basophils respond to MCAF. However, basophils from atopic subjects will release more histamine than "normal" basophils when challenged with MCAF. This seems to indicate that MCAF may be a major HRF *in vivo*.

In this discussion of histamine releasing factors, two subgroups of cytokines are noted. The first group includes cytokines that can cause histamine release in any basophil (MCAF). The second group initiates basophil histamine release only in specific "responder" allergic donors (IL-3). MacDonald et al. (58) stripped the IgE antibody from these allergic donor "responder" basophils and challenged them with an HRF. These basophils with empty FcεRI receptors lost the ability to release histamine to HRF. This HRF-responding IgE antibody was termed "IgE+," and the non-responding IgE antibody was termed "IgE+." The implication for asthmatic patients who have generated IgE+ antibody is that the presence of antigen is no longer needed to trigger histamine release. HRF and IgE+ antibody together short circuit the basophil. Potentially, this enables an "endless loop" of HRF-induced histamine and mediator release to cause inflammation. The resultant inflammation increases HRF production and so on.

Histamine releasing factor is not unique to allergic individuals. Comparisons of allergic rhinitis patients with normal patients demonstrated HRF in both sets of nasal washings (59). However, normal basophils did not release histamine when challenged with HRF. The atopic basophils lost their ability to respond to HRF when the IgE antibody was removed.

Direct bronchial challenge of HRF in asthmatic patients induces bronchospasm (60). Production of HRF by mononuclear cells from asthmatic patients correlated with the degree of bronchial hyperreactivity in these patients (61). Another *in vivo* study found an IgE-independent HRF in BAL fluid after diisocyanate challenge in asthmatics sensitized to this substance (62). These studies suggest that HRF production may be an important factor in generating inflammation in the airways of asthmatic patients.

Other investigators have assessed the clinical relevance of HRF by measuring HRF concentrations in patients undergoing treatment for allergic diseases. Sim et al. (63) noted that HRF concentrations in the nasal mucosa of allergic rhinitis patients decreased after a six-day trial of topical beclomethasone dipropionate. In another study, a correlation was noted between improving symptom scores and declining HRF concentrations in BAL fluid from asthmatic patients receiving allergen-specific immunotherapy (64). Patients receiving placebo immunotherapy had a seasonal increase in both HRF and symptoms.

Alam et al. (65) hypothesized that a counterregulatory feedback mechanism to HRF-induced histamine release should exist. They reported that histamine causes the production of histamine release inhibitory factors (HRIF) from T cells, B cells, and monocytes (66). By a process of elimination, they found that interleukin-8 (IL-8), a chemokine, inhibited HRF-induced histamine release from basophils (66). These HRIFs were specific to HRF-induced histamine release. Interleukin-8 abolished histamine release in those donors whose basophils did release histamine to CTAP II and IL-3 (66). HRIF does not inhibit histamine release caused by anti-IgE antibody, or C5a. Further investigation of HRIF action as a histamine release inhibitory pathway *in vivo* is warranted.

The previous discussion of HRF and HRIF started with the premise that basophils from atopic patients were most notable for histamine release. This model also may apply to non-allergic asthma. Infections appear to play an important role in generating bronchoconstriction in some patients with non-allergic asthma. Kuna et al. (67) found that *Moroxella catarrhalis*, *Haemophilus influenza*, and *Streptococcus viridans* cause mononuclear cells obtained from non-allergic asthmatics to produce HRF. Although a specific HRF was not identified, MCAF would be a likely candidate for the active HRF in these non-atopic asthmatics.

Bacterial agents can directly cause histamine release (68). In this study, the time required for bacteria-induced histamine release was the same as for antigen-induced basophil activation. This release was caused by either endotoxin or by lectin polysaccharide binding on the basophil or IgE receptor (68). Lastly, the link between viral infections and the onset of asthma has not been ignored. Clementsen et al. (69) reported that influenza A virus can potentiate histamine release from basophils. In non-allergic asthma, viral agents may act as basophil-priming agents with other inflammatory mediators, subsequently inducing the histamine release.

IgE is not the only antibody capable of activating basophils and mast cells. Monoclonal antibodies to IgG induce *in vitro* histamine release (70). In addition, antigen-specific histamine release occurs in an IgE knock out mouse model. Anaphylaxis, not mediated by complement, was induced after antigen challenge in these sensitized IgE-deficient mice (71). The authors suggested that an antibody other than IgE was responsible for the antigen-specific anaphylaxis.

Hapten modified basophils stripped of IgE antibody have been shown to interact with hapten-specific IgG antibody resulting in basophil activation (72). Toluene diisocyanate or plicatic acid-induced asthma is associated with the development of IgG antibodies (but not IgE antibody) to these low molecular weight compounds (73–74). *In vivo* models of these occupationally induced diseases have demonstrated a possible IgG antibody-mediated mechanism for the subsequent development of asthma (73–74). These data suggest that, in some forms of asthma, an antibody-specific immunologic sensitization and subsequent histamine release may be possible without the development of antigen-specific IgE antibody.

HISTAMINE AS A MEDIATOR OF IMMUNOLOGIC FUNCTION

The effect the immunologic response has on the production of histamine is varied. However, histamine itself has multiple effects on the inflammatory cascade. Histamine acts as a secondary messenger in the immune response. This mediator can provide an upregulatory signal to the immune system of atopic-type individuals. For instance, histamine stimulates prostaglandin $F_{2\alpha}$ synthesis in human umbilical vein endothelial cells and lung tissue (75). The resultant increase in prostaglandins could contribute to the degree or duration of bronchospasm experienced by asthmatic patients. Histamine can act as a chemotactic agent for eosinophils (76). In addition, interleukin-6 (IL-6) production in B cells is increased in response to histamine (77). The increased IL-6 production then results in increased antibody production. This upregulation of the immune response is mediated by cells with H_1-receptors (78).

Histamine more consistently provides a dampening effect on the immune response. Downregulatory messages are conveyed by cells carrying the H_2-receptor (78). Allergen-induced histamine release through the basophil H_2-receptor was inhibited by increasing extracellular histamine concentrations (79). However, these data may not apply to mast cells (80). Other granulocytes also are downregulated by histamine. Histamine may decrease the number of Fc receptors and complement receptors on neutrophils (81).

Downregulation of other inflammatory cells can be induced by histamine. HLA DR expression on macrophages is diminished by histamine (82). Monocyte production of complement and factor B also was decreased (83). One could hypothesize that less local production of complement ensures less C3a and C5a availability for initiating

further basophil histamine release. Production of other inflammatory cytokines such as interleukin-2, interferon δ and tumor necrosis factor α also was attenuated (84). T cell help of B cell differentiation and immunoglobulin production also is diminished by histamine (83,85).

Histamine activates T suppressor cells to decrease the expression of delayed hypersensitivity reactions and suppress mixed lymphocyte reactions (83,86). In humans, this dampening of the delayed hypersensitivity reaction occurred only if histamine was present early in the development of the reaction (86). Beer et al. (87) noted that atopic individuals had no histamine activation of their T suppressor cells. This finding correlated with a decreased number of H_2-receptors present on the T suppressor cells when compared to normal controls. One mechanism responsible for the ongoing inflammation seen in asthma may be this inability of T suppressor cells to become activated after histamine release.

The central role of histamine as a secondary messenger in modulating the immune response is remarkable. Basophils, neutrophils, macrophages, and lymphocytes all receive important immunomodulatory messages from histamine. More investigations are needed to clarify how feedback pathways used by histamine are altered in patients with asthma.

ANTIHISTAMINES: A ROLE IN TREATING ASTHMA?

Histamine has a prominent role in the pathophysiology and immunologic control of asthma. It would be reasonable to assume that antihistamine therapy could inhibit the asthmatic response. However, histamine is one of many inflammatory mediators released during an antigen response, and histamine antagonists do not serve as useful anti-asthma medications.

Bronchomotor tone may be influenced by histamine. Bronchodilation was documented in one study in which chlorpheniramine was delivered intravenously to achieve high concentrations of the drug in the bronchi (88). In another study, high local concentrations of antihistamine were achieved by aerosolizing clemastine (89). Clemastine increased the FEV_1 by 21% in the study subjects, while the comparison bronchodilator salbutamol increased the FEV_1 by 29%. However, bronchial hyperreactivity is not altered by H_1-antagonists (90). Terfenadine did not provide a significant protective effect against cold air-induced bronchospasm (91). These contradictory studies leave unanswered the question of whether antihistamines could ever be clinically useful for treating all patients with hyperreactive airways.

Several studies of antihistamines exist that demonstrate a protective effect in allergen-induced asthma.

Most of these studies used second generation H_1-antagonists. In one trial, objective measures of pulmonary functions did not differ between the placebo and the oral cetirizine group (92). However, the cetirizine group recorded significantly better symptom scores for their asthma. Bruttmann et al. (93) showed a modest improvement in FEV_1 and symptoms in the group treated with oral cetirizine, compared to the control group. Other studies using loratidine and cetirizine did not demonstrate a protective effect on the antigen-induced early asthmatic response (94–95).

Studies investigating the antihistaminic effect on the late phase asthmatic reactions also have reported conflicting results. Cetirizine did not significantly influence the development of the late phase reaction (96). However, another study using azelastine did demonstrate an inhibitory effect on the development of a late phase asthma response (97).

The studies using a second generation H_1-antagonist indicate that these antihistamines may affect the inflammatory cascade of asthma. An *in vitro* study by Busse (98) noted azelastine had the capability of decreasing neutrophil and eosinophil superoxide production. Other inflammatory functions inhibited by a second generation antihistamine include basophil histamine and leukotriene C_4 release (99). The chemotaxis of lymphocytes and monocytes was inhibited by cetirizine (100). In an *in vivo* study by Rédier et al. (96), subjects receiving cetirizine demonstrated lower total eosinophil counts in the lung 24 hours after allergen challenge when compared to placebo subjects.

None of these studies investigated the mechanism of how these effects were achieved. For example, these effects may be mediated through an H_2-receptor feedback mechanism or may be a direct effect of the H_1-antagonist. These studies showing an anti-inflammatory effect of the second generation antihistamines are exciting for two reasons. First, there is the possibility of these drugs having a dual effect. Second, future studies investigating how these medications are exerting their anti-inflammatory effect may lead to promising pharmacotherapeutic modalities.

Studies showing an anti-inflammatory action and efficacy of antihistamines in modulating asthma are contradicted by studies showing no anti-asthma effect of H_1-and H_2-receptor antagonists. This contradiction is emphasized further by the fact that antihistamines have not found a place in the mainstream of asthma therapy. It could be that sufficient concentrations of antihistamines have not been achieved to cause an anti-asthma effect (88). Other reasons for these contradictory findings include the hypothesis that the only patients responsive to antihistamine therapy are those asthmatics without long- standing inflammation (101). Others have found that allergic rhinitis itself may contribute to hyperreactive airways in mild asthmatics. Welsh et al.

(102) treated allergic rhinitis patients for 1 month with only topical nasal steroids and found a concomitant decrease in bronchial hyperreactivity. This subpopulation may be reflected in a study by Grant et al. (92) where there was no change in pulmonary function tests, but a reduction in chest symptoms.

CONCLUSIONS

Histamine is an important inflammatory mediator of asthma. Histamine synthesis, storage, and degradation are tightly controlled, and homeostasis, thus is maintained. The intracellular and extracellular controls for histamine release are complex. Disregulation of histamine metabolism is found in asthmatic patients, but the clinical consequences, if any, remain unclear.

Histamine release from basophils and mast cells is influenced by other inflammatory mediators such as C5a and bradykinin. Histamine releasing factors (HRF) can either prime basophils (IL-5) for histamine release or directly cause exocytosis of histamine (MCAF). In atopic patients the presence of IgE+ suggests that histamine release can be induced by multiple cytokines without the participation of an antigen. An inhibitory pathway to HRF-induced histamine release has been identified. The major HRIF appears to be IL-8. Treatment of asthma with allergen immunotherapy or glucocorticosteroids decreases the amount of HRF available to induce histamine release. This indicates that an imbalance of these controls of histamine release may be clinically relevant.

Antihistamine therapy directed at modifying the physiologic results of histamine release have not been a prominent part of current asthma therapy due to doubtful efficacy. The second generation antihistamines may play a more prominent future role in the treatment of asthma if they live up to their promise as anti-inflammatory agents. Future research into the role that histamine plays in the inflammatory cascade should be very fruitful.

ACKNOWLEDGMENTS

Supported by the Ernest S. Bazley Grant to Northwestern Memorial Hospital and Northwestern University Medical School.

REFERENCES

1. Oh C, Suzuki S, Nakashima I, Yamashita K, Nakano K. Histamine synthesis by non-mast cells through mitogen- dependent induction of histidine decarboxylase. *Immunology* 1988;65:143–148.
2. Saxena SP, Brandes LJ, Becker AB, Simons KJ, LaBella FS, Gerrard JM. Histamine is an intracellular messenger mediating platelet aggregation. *Science* 1989;243:1596–1599.
3. Aoi R, Nakashima I, Kitamura Y, Asai H, Nakano K. Histamine synthesis by mouse T lymphocytes through induced histidine decarboxylase. *Immunology* 1989;66:219–223.
4. Oh C, Nakano K. Inhibition by glucocorticoids of mitogen- dependent

histamine biosynthesis caused by histidine decarboxylase in cultured mouse spleen cells and peritoneal adherent cells. *Immunology* 1988;65: 433–436.

5. Okayama M, Yamauchi K, Sekizawa K, et al. Localization of histamine N-methyltransferase messenger RNA in human nasal mucosa. *J Allergy Clin Immunol* 1995;95:96–102.

6. Nakazawa H, Sekizawa K, Morikawa M, et al. Viral respiratory infection causes airway hyperresponsiveness and decreases histamine N-methyltransferase activity in guinea pigs. *Am J Respir Crit Care Med* 1994;149:1180–1185.

7. Jarjour NN, Calhoun WJ, Schwartz LB, Busse WW. Elevated bronchoalveolar lavage fluid histamine levels in allergic asthmatics are associated with increased airway obstruction. *Am Rev Respir Dis* 1991; 144:83–87.

8. Casale TB, Wood D, Richerson HB, et al. Elevated bronchoalveolar lavage fluid histamine levels in allergic asthmatics are associated with methacholine bronchial hyperresponsiveness. *J Clin Invest* 1987;79: 1197–1203.

9. Arrang JM, Garbarg M, Lancelot JC, et al. The third histamine receptor. *Int Arch Allergy Appl Immunol* 1989;88:79–81.

10. Kaliner M, Sigler R, Summers R, Shelhamer JH. Effects of infused histamine: analysis of the effects of H_1 and H_2 histamine receptor antagonists on cardiovascular and pulmonary responses. *J Allergy Clin Immunol* 1981;68:365–371.

11. Boe J, Boe MA, Simonsson BG. A dual action of histamine on isolated human pulmonary arteries. *Respiration* 1980;40:117–122.

12. Braude S, Royston D, Coe C, Barnes PJ. Histamine increases lung permeability by an H_2-receptor mechanism. *Lancet* 1984;2:372–374.

13. Ichinose M, Barnes PJ. Inhibitory histamine H_3-receptors on cholinergic nerves in human airways. *Eur J Pharmacol* 1989;163:383–386.

14. Ichinose M, Barnes PJ. Histamine 3-receptors modulate nonadrenergic noncholinergic bronchoconstriction in guinea pig *in vivo. Eur J Pharmacol* 1989;174:49–55.

15. Dixon M, Jackson DM, Richards IM. The effect of a respiratory tract infection on histamine-induced changes in lung mechanics and irritant receptor discharge in dogs. *Am Rev Respir Dis* 1979;120:843–848.

16. Undem BJ, Myers AC, Weinreich D. Antigen-induced modulation of autonomic and sensory neurons *in vitro. Int Arch Allergy Appl Immunol* 1991;94:319–324.

17. Empey DW Laitinen LA, Jacobs L. Mechanisms of bronchial hyperreactivity in normal subjects after upper respiratory tract infection. *Am Rev Respir Dis* 1976;133:131–134.

18. Antonissen LA, Mitchell RW, Kroeger EA, Kepron W, Stephens NL, Bergen J. Histamine pharmacology in airway smooth muscle from a canine model of asthma. *J Pharmacol Exp Ther* 1980;213:150–155.

19. Kneussl MP, Richardson JB. Alpha-adrenergic receptors in human and canine tracheal and bronchial smooth muscle. *J Appl Physiol* 1978;45:307–311.

20. Eiser NM, Mills J, Snashall PD, Guz A. The role of histamine receptors in asthma. *Clin Sci* 1981;60:363–370.

21. Shelhamer JH, Marom Z, Kaliner M. Immunologic and neuropharmacologic stimulation of mucous glycoprotein release from human airways *in vitro. J Clin Invest* 1980;66:1400–1408.

22. Kowalski ML, Kaliner MA. Neurogenic inflammation, vascular permeability and mast cells. *J Immunol* 1988;140:3905–3911.

23. Propst K, Millen JE, Glauser FL. The effects of endogenous and exogenous histamine on pulmonary alveolar membrane permeability. *Am Rev Respir Dis* 1978;117:1063–1068.

24. Marin MG, Davis B, Nadel JA. Effect of histamine on electrical and ion transport properties of tracheal epithelium. *J Appl Physiol* 1977; 42:735–738.

25. Kaliner M. Asthma and mast cell activation. *J Allergy Clin Immunol* 1989;83:510–520.

26. Ichinose M, Belvisi MG, Barnes PJ. Histamine H_3-receptors inhibit neurogenic microvascular leakage in airways. *J Appl Physiol* 1990;68: 21–25.

27. Fox B, Bull TB, Guz A. Mast cells in the human alveolar wall: an electronmicroscopic study. *J Clin Pathol* 1981;34:1333–1342.

28. Riley JF, West GB. The presence of histamine in tissue mast cells. *J Physiol* 1953;120:528–537.

29. Metcalfe DD, Lewis RA, Silbert JE, Rosenberg RD, Wasserman SI, Austen KF. Isolation and characterization of heparin from human lung. *J Clin Invest* 1979;64:1537–1543.

30. Gomez E, Corrado OJ, Baldwin DL, Swanston AR, Davies RJ. Direct *in vivo* evidence for mast cell degranulation during allergen-induced reactions in man. *J Allergy Clin Immunol* 1986;78:637–645.

31. Polosa R, Djukanovic R, Rajakalasingam K, Palerino F, Holgate ST. Skin responses to bradykinin, kallidin and (des Arg⁹)-bradykinin in non-atopic and atopic volunteers. *J Allergy Clin Immunol* 1993;92: 683–689.

32. Thomas LL, Haskell MD, Sarmiento EU, Bilimoria Y. Distinguishing features of basophil and neutrophil activation by major basic protein. *J Allergy Clin Immunol* 1994;94:1171–1176.

33. Bischoff SC, Dahinden CA. c-*kit* ligand: a unique potentiator of mediator release by human lung mast cells. *J Exp Med* 1992;175:237–244.

34. Björck T, Gustafsson LE, Dahlén S-E. Isolated bronchi from asthmatics are hyperresponsive to adenosine, which apparently acts indirectly by liberation of leukotrienes and histamine. *Am Rev Respir Dis* 1992; 145:1087–1091.

35. Marks R, Greaves MW. Vascular reactions to histamine and compound 48/80 in human skin: suppression by a histamine H_2-receptor blocking agent. *Br J Clin Pharmacol* 1977;4:367–369.

36. Fisher M. Intradermal testing after anaphylactoid reactions to anaesthetic drugs: practical aspects of performance and interpretation. *Anaesth Intensive Care* 1984;12:115–120.

37. Mathieu A, Goudsouzian N, Snider MT. Reaction to ketamine: anaphylactoid or anaphylactic? *Br J Anaesth* 1975;47:624–627.

38. Watkins J, Clarke RSJ. Report of a symposium: Adverse responses to intravenous agents. *Br J Anaesth* 1978;50:1159–1164.

39. Cogen FC, Norman ME, Dunsky E, Hirschfield J, Zweiman B. Histamine release and complement changes following injection of contrast media in humans. *J Allergy Clin Immunol* 1979;64:299–303.

40. Seagrave J, Pfeiffer JR, Wofsy C Oliver JM. Relationship of IgE receptor topography to secretion in RBL2H3 mast cells. *J Cell Physiol* 1991;148:139–151.

41. Paolini R, Nunerof R, Kinet J-P. Phosphorylation / dephosphorylation of high affinity IgE receptors: a mechanism for coupling / uncoupling of a Ig signal complex. *Proc Natl Acad Sci U S A* 1992;89:10733–10737.

42. Jounvin M-H, Adamczewski M, Numerof R, Letourneur O, Valié A, Kinet J-P. Differential control of the tyrosine kinases Lyn and Syk by the two signaling chains of the high affinity immunoglobulin E receptor. *J Biol Chem* 1994;269:5918–5925.

43. Knol EF, Mul FPJ, Kuijpers TW, Verhoeven AJ, Roos D. Intracellular events in anti-IgE nonreleasing human basophils. *J Allergy Clin Immunol* 1992;90:92–103.

44. Baxter JH, Adamik R. Differences in requirements and actions of various histamine-releasing agents. *Clin Pharmacol Ther* 1978;27:497–503.

45. Grant JA, Settle L, Whorton EB, Dupree E. Complement- mediated release of histamine from human basophils. II Biochemical characterization of the reaction. *J Immunol* 1976;117:450–456.

46. Bueb J-L, Mousli M, Bronner C, Rouot BB, Landry Y. Activation of G_i-like proteins, a receptor-independent effect of kinins in mast cells. *Mol Pharmacol* 1990;38:816–822.

47. Alam R, Forsythe PA, Lett-Brown MA, Grant JA. Cellular origin of histamine-releasing factor produced by peripheral blood mononuclear cells. *J Immunol* 1989;142:3951–3956.

48. White MV, Kaliner MA. Neutrophils and mast cells. I. Human neutrophils derived histamine releasing activity. *J Immunol* 1987;139: 1624–1630.

49. Orchard MA, Kagey-Sobotka A, Proud M, Lichtenstein LM. Basophil histamine release induced by a substance from stimulated human platlets. *J Immunol* 1986;136:2240–2244.

50. Columbo M, Horowitz EM, Kagey-Sobotka A, Lichtenstein LM. Histamine release from human basophils induced by platelet activating factor: the role of extracellular calcium, Interleukin-3, and granulocyte-macrophage colony-stimulating factor. *J Allergy Clin Immunol* 1995;95:565–573.

51. Kuna P, Reddigari SR, Schall TJ, Rucinski D, Sadick M, Kaplan AP. Characterization of the human basophil response to cytokine, growth factors, and histamine releasing factors of the intercrine/chemokine family. *J Immunol* 1993;150:1932–1943.

52. Bischoff SC, Brunner T, De Weck AL, Dahinden CA. Interleukin 5 modifies histamine release and leukotriene generation by human basophils in response to diverse agonists. *J Exp Med* 1990;172:1577–1582.

53. Dahinden CA, Kurimoto Y, De Weck AL, Lindley I, Dewald B, Baggiolini M. The neutrophil-activating peptide NAF/NAP-1 induces histamine and leukotriene release by interleukin 3- primed basophils. *J Exp Med* 1989;170:1787–1792.

54. Sugiyama H, Eda R, Hopp RJ, Bewtra AK, Townley RG. Importance of interleukin-3 on histamine release from human basophils. *Ann Allergy* 1993;71:391–395.

55. Haak-Frendscho M, Arai N, Arai K, Baeza ML, Finn A, Kaplan AP. Human recombinant granulocyte-macrophage colony- stimulating factor and interleukin-3 cause basophil histamine release. *J Clin Invest* 1988;82:17–20.

56. Alam R, Forsythe PA, Stafford S, Lett-Brown MA, Grant JA. Macrophage inflammatory protein-1α activates basophils and mast cells. *J Exp Med* 1992;176:781–786.

57. Alam R, Lett-Brown MA, Forsythe PA, et al. Monocyte chemotactic and activating factor is a potent histamine- releasing factor for basophils. *J Clin Invest* 1992;89:723–728.

58. MacDonald SM, Lichtenstein LM, Proud D, et al. Studies of IgE-dependent histamine releasing factors: Heterogeneity of IgE. *J Immunol* 1987;139:506–512.

59. Sim TC, Alam R, Forsythe PA, Welter JB, Lett-Brown MA, Grant JA. Measurement of histamine-releasing factor activity in individual nasal washings: Relationship with atopy, basophil response, and membrane-bound IgE. *J Allergy Clin Immunol* 1992;89:1157–1165.

60. Alam R, Rozniecki J. A mononuclear cell-derived histamine releasing factor in asthmatic patients. II. Activity *in vivo. Allergy* 1985;40:124–129.

61. Alam R, Kuna P, Rozniecki J, Kuzminska B. The magnitude of the spontaneous production of histamine-releasing factor (HRF) by lymphocytes *in vitro* correlates with the state of bronchial hyperreactivity in patients with asthma. *J Allergy Clin Immunol* 1987;79:103–108.

62. Herd ZL, Bernstein DI. Antigen-specific stimulation of histamine releasing factors in diisocyanate-induced occupational asthma. *Am J Respir Crit Care Med* 1994;150:988–994.

63. Sim TC, Hilsmeier KA, Alam R, Allen RK, Lett-Brown MA, Grant JA. Effect of topical corticosteroids on the recovery of histamine releasing factors in nasal washings of patients with allergic rhinitis. *Am Rev Respir Dis* 1992;145:1316–1320.

64. Kuna P, Alam R, Kuzminska B, Rozniecki J. The effect of preseasonal immunotherapy on the production of histamine- releasing factor (HRF) by mononuclear cells from patients with seasonal asthma: results of a double-blind, placebo- controlled, randomized study. *J Allergy Clin Immunol* 1989;83:816–824.

65. Alam R, Forsythe PA, Lett-Brown MA Grant JA. Study of the cellular origin of histamine release inhibitory factor using highly purified subsets of mononuclear cells. *J Immunol* 1989;143:2280–2284.

66. Kuna P, Reddigari SR, Kornfeld D, Kaplan AP. Il-8 inhibits histamine release from human basophils induced by histamine- releasing factors, connective tissue activating peptide III, and Il-3. *J Immunol* 1991;147:1920–1924.

67. Kuna P, Roznieck J, Kuzminska B. Effect of autogenic bacterial antigens on the production of histamine releasing factor by mononuclear cells from intrinsic asthmatic patients. *Allergy* 1988;43:511–518.

68. Clementsen P, Norn S, Kristense KS, Bach-Mortensen C, Koch C, Permin H. Bacteria and endotoxin enhance basophil histamine release and potentiation is abolished by carbohydrates. *Allergy* 1990;45:402–408.

69. Clementsen P, Pedersen M, Permin H Espersen F, Norn S. Influenza A virus potentiates bacteria-induced histamine release. *Allergy* 1990;45:464–470.

70. Fagan DL, Slaughter CA, Capra JD, Sullivan TJ. Monoclonal antibodies to immunoglobulin G_4 induce histamine release from human basophils *in vitro. J Allergy Clin Immunol* 1982;70:399–404.

71. Oettgen HC, Martin TR, Wynshaw-Boris A, Deng C, Drazen JM, Leder P. Active anaphylaxis in IgE-deficient mice. *Nature* 1994;370:367–370.

72. Akiyama K, Pruzansky JJ, Patterson R. Hapten-modified basophils: A model of human immediate hypersensitivity that can be elicited by IgG antibody. *J Immunol* 1984;133:3286–3290.

73. Hogan MB, Harris KE, Patterson R. Toluene diisocyanate- induced reverse passive cutaneous anaphylaxis caused by IgG antibody. *J Allergy Clin Immunol* 1995;95:913–915.

74. Salari H, Howard S, Chan H, Dryden P, Chan-Yeung M. Involvement of immunologic mechanisms in a guinea pig model of Western red cedar asthma. *J Allergy Clin Immunol* 1994;93:877–884.

75. Platshon LF, Kaliner M. The effects of the immunologic release of histamine upon human lung cyclic nucleotide levels and prostaglandin generation. *J Clin Invest* 1978;62:1113–1121.

76. Turnbull LW, Kay AB. Histamine and imidazole acetic acid as chemotactic agents for human eosinophil leucocytes. *Immunology* 1976;31:797–802.

77. Falus A. Interleukin-6 biosynthesis is increased by histamine in human B-cell and glioblastoma cell lines. *Immunology* 1993;78:193–196.

78. Falus A, Merétey K. Histamine: an early messenger in inflammatory and immune reactions. *Immunol Today* 1992;13:154–156.

79. Bergstrand H, Hegardt B, Löwhagen O, Strannegord Ö, Svedmyr N. Effects of long-term treatment with low dose cimetidine on allergen-induced airway responses and selected immunological parameters in atopic asthmatics. *Allergy* 1985;40:187–197.

80. Kaliner M. Human lung tissue and anaphylaxis: the effects of histamine on the immunologic release of mediators. *Am Rev Respir Dis* 1978;118:1015–1022.

81. Hsieh K-H. The effects of histamine, antihistamines, isoproterenol and theophylline on the Fc and complement receptor functions of polymorphonuclear leukocytes of asthmatic children. *Ann Allergy* 1981;47:38–42.

82. Kawano Y, Noma T. Cell action mechanism of tranilast- effect on the expression of HLA-class II antigen. *Int J Immunopharmacol* 1993:15:487–500.

83. Beer DJ, Matloof SM. Rocklin RE. The influence of histamine on immune and inflammatory responses. *Adv Immunol* 1984:35:209–267.

84. Vannier E, Miller LC, Dinarello CA. Histamine suppresses gene expression and synthesis of tumor necrosis factor α via histamine H_2 receptors. *J Exp Med* 1991;174:281–284.

85. Birch RE, Polmar SH. Pharmacological modification of immunoregulatory T lymphocytes. I. Effect of adenosine, H_1 and H_2 histamine agonists upon T lymphocyte regulation of B lymphocyte differentiation *in vitro. Clin Exp Immunol* 1982;48:218–230.

86. Askenase PW, Schwartz A, Siegel JN, Gershon RK. Role of histamine in the regulation of cell-mediated immunity. *Int Arch Allergy Appl Immunol* 1981;66(suppl 1):225–233.

87. Beer DJ, Osband ME, McCaffrey RP, Soter NA, Rocklin RE. Abnormal histamine-induced suppressor-cell function in atopic subjects. *N Engl J Med* 1982;306:454–458.

88. Popa VT. Bronchodilating activity of an H_1 blocker, chlorpheniramine. *J Allergy Clin Immunol* 1977;59:54–63.

89. Nogrady SG, Hartley JPR, Handslip PDJ, Hurst NP. Bronchodilatation after inhalation of the antihistamine clemastine. *Thorax* 1978;33:479–482.

90. Ruffin RE, Latimer KM. Lack of effect of 4 weeks of oral H_1 antagonist on bronchial responsiveness. *Eur Respir J* 1991;4:575–579.

91. Bewtra AK, Hopp RJ, Nair NM, Townley RG. Effect of terfenadine on cold air-induced bronchospasm. *Ann Allergy* 1989;62:299–301.

92. Grant JA, Nicodemus CF, Findlay SR, et al. Cetirizine in patients with seasonal rhinitis and concomitant asthma: prospective, randomized, placebo-controlled trial. *J Allergy Clin Immunol* 1995;95:923–932.

93. Bruttmann G, Pedrali P, Arendt C, Rihoux JP. Protective effect of cetirizine in patients suffering from pollen asthma. *Ann Allergy* 1990;64:224–228.

94. Town GI, Holgate ST. Comparison of the effect of loratadine on the airway and skin responses to histamine, methacholine and allergen in subjects with asthma. *J Allergy Clin Immunol* 1990;86:886–893.

95. Kopferschmitt-Kubler MC, Couchot A, Pauli G. Evaluation of the effect of oral cetirizine on antigen-induced immediate asthmatic response. *Ann Allergy* 1990;65:501–503.

96. Rédier H, Chanez P, De Vos C, et al. Inhibitory effect of cetirizine on the bronchial eosinophil recruitment induced by allergen inhalation challenge in allergic patients with asthma. *J Allergy Clin Immunol* 1992;90:215–224.

97. Rafferty P, Ng WH, Phillips G, et al. The inhibitory actions of azelastine hydrochloride on the early and late bronchoconstrictor responses to inhaled allergen in atopic asthma. *J Allergy Clin Immunol* 1989;84:649–657.

98. Busse W, Randlev B, Segwick J. The effect of azelastine on neutrophil and eosinophil generation of superoxide. *J Allergy Clin Immunol* 1989;83:400–405.

99. Nabe M, Agrawal DK, Sarmiento EU, Townley RG. Inhibitory effect of terfenadine on mediator release from human blood basophils and eosinophils. *Clinical Exp Allergy* 1989;19:515–520.

100. Jinquan T, Reimert CM, Deleuran B, Zachariae C, Simonson C, Thestrup-Peders K. Cetirizine inhibits the *in vitro* and *ex vivo* chemotactic response of T lymphocytes and monocytes. *J Allergy Clin Immunol* 1995;95:979–986.

101. Hoshino K, Kawasaki A, Mizushima Y, Yano S. Effect of antiallergic agents and bronchial hypersensitivity in short-term bronchial asthma. *Chest* 1991;100:57–62.

102. Welsh PW, Stricker WE, Chu CP, et al. Efficacy of beclomethasone nasal solution, flunisolide, and cromolyn in relieving symptoms of ragweed allergy. *Mayo Clin Proc* 1987;62:125–134.

Asthma, edited by P.J. Barnes, M.M. Grunstein, A.R. Leff, and A.J. Woolcock.
Lippincott–Raven Publishers, Philadelphia © 1997.

■ *40* ■

Leukotrienes

Andrew R. Fischer and Jeffrey M. Drazen

Biochemistry of Leukotriene Formation and Action	**Recovery of Leukotrienes from Biological Fluids**
Biology of the Leukotrienes Relevant to Asthma	**Anti-leukotriene Drugs in Asthma**
Cells with the Capacity to Produce the Leukotrienes	Studies in Induced Asthma
Biological Effects of the Leukotrienes	Effects on Airway Tone
Chemotaxis	Effects on Airway Reactivity
Bronchoconstriction	Effects of Chronic Administration of Drugs Active on the 5-Lipoxygenase Pathway in Asthma

Leukotrienes (LTs) is the name given to the family of bioactive polyunsaturated eicosatetraenoic acids that contain a triene structure, that is, three conjugated double bonds (1–4). As detailed below, the LTs are derived from oxidative metabolism of arachidonic acid, a fatty acid that is a common constituent of biological membranes. There are two major classes of LTs: cysteinyl (Cys) LTs, so termed because they contain the amino acid cysteine attached to the fatty-acid backbone, and LTB_4, which is a dihydroxy LT and contains no cysteine. There is now abundant evidence to suggest that the LTs are effector mediators with an important role in the biology of asthma. In this chapter, the biochemistry of LT formation first is reviewed, and then four lines of evidence are considered (Table 1) that indicate the importance of LTs in asthma.

BIOCHEMISTRY OF LEUKOTRIENE FORMATION AND ACTION

The biosynthesis of the Cys-LTs has been reviewed in detail (5–9); in this chapter, an overview of these pathways is provided so that the reader can understand how the various entities in this family are related one to another. An appreciation of the biosynthetic pathways for

the LTs is useful to gain a full understanding of the mechanism of action of the various pharmaceutical agents that are used to treat asthma by interfering with the synthesis or action of the LTs.

Arachidonic acid is the fatty acid from which the LTs are derived. Prior to cell activation, arachidonic acid is found esterified in the *sn*2 position of about 80% of membrane phospholipids (10,11). When target cells are activated, arachidonic acid is cleaved from these membranes by phospholipases (Fig. 1) (12–14). Although the exact form of phospholipase responsible for cleaving arachidonic acid from membrane phospholipids is not known with certainty, it seems likely that both secretory (about 14 kDa) and cytosolic (about 100 kDa) phospholipase A_2 are involved (15–23). Once arachidonic acid is cleaved from cell membranes, a complex consisting of the 5-lipoxygenase-activating protein (FLAP) and the enzyme 5-lipoxygenase (5-LO) catalyzes the addition of molecular oxygen to the fifth carbon of arachidonic acid (19,24–32). This process results in the formation of 5-hydroperoxyeicosatetraenoic acid (5-HPETE). Our current understanding of this process is that it occurs at the perinuclear membrane, with 5-LO translocating from both nuclear and cytoplasmic pools (33). The 5-HPETE produced by 5-LO then serves as a substrate for 5-LO a second time; on this occasion, 5-LO catalyzes the formation of the epoxide LTA_4.

LTA_4 is a *branch point* in the 5-LO pathway. LTA_4 can serve as a substrate for the enzyme termed LTC_4 synthase, which catalyzes the conjugation of glutathione (a tripeptide consisting of cysteine, glycine, and glutamic

A. R. Fischer and J. M. Drazen: Division of Pulmonary and Critical Care Medicine, Department of Medicine, Brigham and Women's Hospital and Harvard Medical School, Boston, Massachusetts 02115.

TABLE 1. *Lines of evidence implicating leukotrienes (LTs) in asthma*

Cells with the capacity to produce LTs are thought to be of importance in asthmatic airway biology.
LTs transduce chemotaxis and airway obstruction, two cardinal features of asthma, via specific receptors.
LTs can be recovered from the urine of patients with spontaneous or induced asthma at average levels higher than found in normal subjects.
Agents capable of inhibiting LT action or formation have a salutary therapeutic effect in patients with asthma.

acid residues) to LTA_4 at its sixth carbon, thereby forming LTC_4 (34,35). It is interesting that this reaction also occurs at the perinuclear membrane (36). LTC_4 is transported from the cell cytosol to the extracellular microenvironment (37), where the removal of the glutamic acid residue from the glutathione moiety of LTC_4, catalyzed by γ-glutamyl transpeptidase, yields LTD_4 (2,38). LTD_4 serves as a substrate for a number of dipeptidases that catalyze the removal of the glycine moiety, thus yielding LTE_4 (3,4); LTs C_4, D_4, and E_4 are known collectively as the Cys-LTs because they each contain cysteine; together these compounds constitute the material formerly known as slow-reacting substance of anaphylaxis (SRS-A). These molecules have the capacity to initiate signal transduction at the Cys-LT_1 receptor. LTE_4 can be excreted unchanged in the urine (about 5% to 15% of exogenously administered LTE_4 can be recovered intact from the

urine) or *n*-acetylated, or the ω backbone of the LT is subject to carboxylation and β elimination (39–41). These last two modifications (that is, *n*-acetylation or ω modification) of the LT structure are associated with a loss of LT bioactivity.

LTA_4 also can serve as a substrate for LTA_4 epoxide hydrolase, which catalyzes the addition of molecular oxygen and subsequent hydration of LTA_4 to form the specific dihydroxy LT (5[S],12[R]-dihydroxy-6,14-*cis*-8,10-*trans*-eicosatetraenoic acid) known as LTB_4 (42–46). LTB_4 can initiate signal transduction through the B-leukotriene (BLT) receptor, which results in neutrophil and eosinophil chemotaxis. In the absence of either activated enzyme system, that is, LTC_4 synthase or LTA_4 epoxide hydrolase, LTA_4 undergoes spontaneous degradation to 6-trans-LTB_4, a molecule with markedly attenuated bioactivity.

BIOLOGY OF THE LEUKOTRIENES RELEVANT TO ASTHMA

Cells with the Capacity to Produce the Leukotrienes

Among the cells in the lung with the enzymatic capacity to produce the LTs are neutrophilic and eosinophilic polymorphonuclear leukocytes (47), mast cells (4,48), alveolar macrophages (49,50), airway epithelial cells (51, 52), and pulmonary vascular endothelial cells (48,53–55). Of these cells, only eosinophils (56,57), alveolar macro-

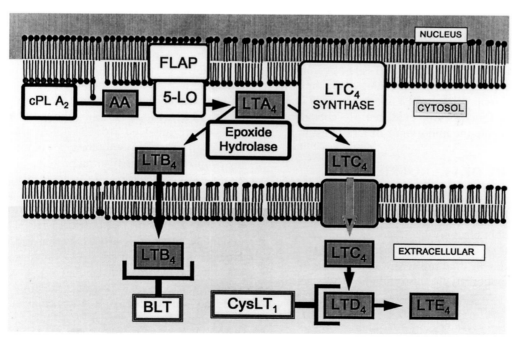

FIG. 1. Schematic diagram of the 5-lipoxygenase pathway; see the text for details. *BLT,* leukotriene B_4 receptor; *cPLA$_2$,* cytosolic phospholipase A_2; *Cys-LT$_1$,* cysteinyl leukotriene receptor; *FLAP,* 5-lipoxygenase-activating protein; *LTC$_4$,* leukotriene C_4; *5-LO,* 5-lipoxygenase.

phages (50), and mast cells (4) possess the combination of the FLAP, 5-LO, and LTC$_4$ synthase; this combination is needed for a given cell to produce the Cys-LTs from arachidonic acid. In this regard, it is of importance to note that eosinophils and mast cells have been implicated as important cell types in the biology of asthma (58–61). Indeed, it is interesting to speculate that one of the properties that makes these cells important in the biology of asthma is their capacity to elaborate the Cys-LTs.

Biological Effects of the Leukotrienes

The biological actions of the LTs arise from their capacity to transduce a variety of effects through stimulation at specific receptors. Two major classes of receptors, BLT receptors (receptors for LTB$_4$) and Cys-LT receptors (for the Cys-LTs), have been functionally characterized; as of this time (Winter 1996) neither the BLT nor the Cys-LT receptor has been molecularly cloned (62). Much of what is known about the biological effects of the LTs derives from physiological studies of the actions of the LTs or their antagonists. Among the actions of the LTs, those related to chemotaxis and bronchoconstriction are the most relevant to asthma.

Chemotaxis

LTB$_4$ is the natural ligand for the BLT; 20-OH-LTB$_4$ and 12-R-HETE can also activate the receptor but do so with potencies that are $\frac{1}{10}$ to $\frac{1}{500}$ of that of the native ligand. The BLT is a 60kDa plasma membrane protein that can exist in either a high- or a low-affinity state; the affinity appears to be regulated by the binding of GTP to a 40kDa G protein (63–65). When activated, the BLT receptor transduces chemotaxis and cellular activation (66,67). There appear to be no functional subtypes of this receptor (63,68). A number of chemically distinct, specific, and selective antagonists at the BLT with IC$_{50}$ values from 1 nM to 10 μM have been identified (69–78). Trials of the clinical utility of BLT antagonists in the treatment of asthma are in their early stages.

Bronchoconstriction

One of the reasons for the interest in the role of LTs as mediators of asthma is their capacity to effect prolonged airway constriction when administered at very low doses. Although bronchoconstriction is prominent among the biological actions of the LTs, these mediators have numerous other effects that are not considered in this chapter. The reader is referred to a number of authoritative reviews on the general pharmacology of the LTs (79–81). Inhalation of aerosols generated from solutions of LTC$_4$ or LTD$_4$ causes airway obstruction, which is mani-

fest as a decrease in specific airway conductance (SG$_{aw}$), decreases in the forced expiratory volume in 1 s (FEV$_1$), or decrements in flow rates at various points in the vital capacity. In normal subjects, nebulizer concentrations between 5 and 20 μM are required to reduce the maximal expiratory flow rate (measured near midvital capacity) by about 30%, whereas, in patients with asthma, nebulizer concentrations on the order of 0.5 to 1 μM are required to achieve the same decrement in flows (82–89). These concentrations are 3,000 to 10,000 times less than the concentrations of histamine or methacholine required to achieve the same bronchoconstrictor response; thus, the Cys-LTs are among the most potent bronchoconstrictor substances known. It is interesting that LTE$_4$ is about 100-fold less potent than LTC$_4$ or LTD$_4$ as a bronchoconstrictor agonist in both normal subjects and patients with asthma (89). This loss of bioactivity is consistent with the hypothesis that the bioconversion of LTD$_4$ to LTE$_4$ is a downregulatory event. In addition to the marked potency of the Cys-LTs as bronchoconstrictors, their duration of effect on the airways is 10 to 30 times greater than that of inhaled histamine or methacholine.

The Cys-LTs exert their effects through signal transduction at the Cys-LT$_1$ receptor, which was previously known as the LTD$_4$ receptor or the LTR$_d$ (90). This receptor is a 45-kDa membrane protein found in a variety of cell types, including airway smooth muscle (91–94). Receptor-ligand interaction initiates signal transduction via the stimulation of phosphoinositide turnover (95–98). In isolated human airway smooth muscle, LTC$_4$ and LTD$_4$ are equipotent as contractile agonists at the Cys-LT$_1$ receptor, whereas LTE$_4$ is diminished in potency as a ligand at this receptor (99–103), which agrees with the findings of intact subjects. More than a dozen chemically distinct, specific, and selective antagonists of the Cys-LT$_1$ receptor have been identified; these antagonists have pA$_2$ values between 7 and 10 in isolated airway smooth muscle contractile assays when LTD$_4$ is used as the contractile agonist (104–112). Some of these antagonists have been tested in human subjects *in vivo* and shown to decrease the sensitivity of subjects to inhaled LTD$_4$. The weaker antagonists shift the LTD$_4$ dose-response curve about fivefold, whereas the more potent antagonists shift this dose-response curve by more than 200-fold. Furthermore, a number of these antagonists have been used in clinical trials designed to ascertain whether antagonism at the Cys-LT$_1$ receptor is associated with an improvement in asthma control; these studies are considered in detail later in the chapter.

RECOVERY OF LEUKOTRIENES FROM BIOLOGICAL FLUIDS

Quantitative recovery of Cys-LTs from blood or plasma has been technically difficult and, more importantly, fraught with artifact (113); as a result, many investigators have capitalized on the observation that 5% to 15% of exogenously administered LTC_4 or LTE_4 appears unchanged in the urine (39,114–118) and have used the urinary excretion of LTE_4 as an index of the production of the Cys-LTs. Normal subjects have measurable amounts of LTE_4 in their urine (119–124), but the source(s) and biological significance of this LTE_4 excretion have not been established. It is known that the excretion rate of LTE_4 does not vary systematically over the course of a day (123).

In patients with allergen-induced asthma, allergen bronchoprovocation has been associated with the enhanced recovery of urinary LTE_4 during the early-phase but not the late-phase response (119,125–130); the greater the magnitude of the decrease in FEV_1 after allergen challenge, the greater is the amount of LTE_4 recovered in the urine (127). By contrast, the recovery of LTE_4 in the urine after exercise-induced asthma has been documented by some investigators (131,132), whereas others have been unable to recover LTE_4 in the urine after this asthmatic stimulus (125,133).

Patients with aspirin-induced asthma, in the absence of known aspirin exposure, excrete three to four times more LTE_4 in their urine than nonaspirin-sensitive asthmatic patients. After aspirin challenge (128,134–137), urinary LTE_4 levels increase over three- to fivefold in aspirin-sensitive asthmatic patients, whereas they do not increase in nonaspirin-sensitive asthmatic patients.

Asano and co-workers (123) examined urinary LTE_4 excretion in eight patients with mild chronic stable asthma (average FEV_1, 72% of predicted) whose only treatment was the intermittent use of inhaled β-agonists. A total of 16 consecutive 6h urine samples were obtained during a 4-day observation period on a metabolic ward. Although the mean urinary LTE_4 in the asthmatic group was significantly greater than that in normal subjects, there was substantial variability among these patients with otherwise identical asthma. Some of the asthmatic patients had persistently elevated concentrations of urinary LTE_4, while others had levels consistently within the normal range. This supports the hypothesis that, among patients with clinically similar asthma, there are some whose asthma is due predominantly to LT excess and others in whom LT excess is not of pathophysiological importance.

There is some evidence of excess LT excretion in patients with spontaneous asthmatic episodes. Taylor and co-workers (119,125) recovered increased amounts of LTE_4 from the urine of some patients with acute severe asthma presenting for emergency treatment, but normal amounts from many other patients with asthma of equal severity. Drazen and co-workers (122) demonstrated that, among individuals presenting to an emergency service for treatment of asthma, those with acutely reversible airway narrowing had increased urinary LTE_4 concentration. This observation suggests that acute spontaneous bronchospasm is associated with LT excess.

ANTILEUKOTRIENE DRUGS IN ASTHMA

The most important evidence supporting a role for LTs in asthma derives from studies of selective inhibitors of LT synthesis, for example, 5-LO and FLAP inhibitors, as well as studies using antagonists of the action of Cys-LTs at the Cys-LT_1. The effects of anti-LT drugs have been studied in laboratory-induced asthma, spontaneous asthmatic bronchoconstriction, and chronic stable asthma.

Studies in Induced Asthma

Allergen Challenge Studies

An asthmatic reaction may be induced in the clinical laboratory by having a patient with asthma inhale an aerosol generated from solutions containing gradually increasing concentrations of allergens to which the subject is sensitive. In such challenges, airway narrowing may occur in two *phases*. *Early-phase* bronchospasm occurs within minutes, lasts up to 3 h after allergen inhalation, and is associated with increased LT production (138). In a variable proportion of individuals, a second period of airway obstruction, the *late phase*, occurs 4 to 24 h after the allergen inhalation. In contrast to the early phase, enhanced recovery of LTs from biological fluids during the late-phase response has not been demonstrated.

The first studies conducted with LT receptor antagonists did not indicate a major role for LTs in allergen-induced asthma (139,140). As more potent receptor antagonists became available, however, a greater therapeutic response was achieved. One of the first clinical trials to demonstrate that anti-LT drugs had substantive efficacy in the allergen challenge model used the LT receptor antagonist LY 171883 (141). The investigators reported significant inhibition of the early-phase response to allergen-induced bronchoconstriction after treatment with the active Cys-LT_1 receptor antagonist. The mean maximal antigen-induced decrease in flow rate at 40% of vital capacity (V_{p40}), was 54.7% after placebo, compared with 35.8% after treatment with LY 171883 ($p < 0.05$) (Fig. 2). As similar trials were performed with more potent receptor antagonists, a greater therapeutic effect was observed. For example, the LT receptor antagonist MK-571 inhibited the early-phase decrease in FEV_1 by 62% and attenuated the late-phase response by nearly 50% (142). In other studies, the LT receptor antagonist zafirlukast (also known as ICI 204,219 or Accolate) inhibited the early-phase response to inhaled allergen by 80% and decreased the late-phase response by 45% (Fig. 3) (143). In another study, the amount of allergen required to achieve a given degree of airway narrowing in the early phase was measured in patients pretreated with either placebo or zafirlukast. There was a shift in the allergen dose-response curve such that more allergen was required to induce a

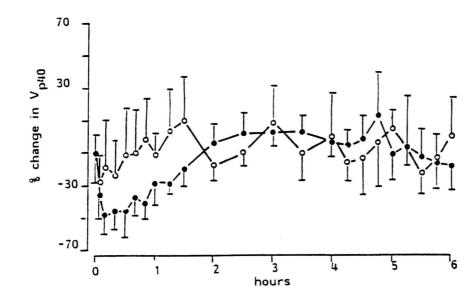

FIG. 2. The mean ± SEM percentage change in flow rate at 40% of vital capacity (V_{p40}) following antigen inhalation after placebo *(solid circles)* and LY 171883 (400 mg orally) *(open circles)*. (From Fuller RW, Black PN, Dollery CT. Effect of the oral leukotriene D_4 antagonist LY171883 on inhaled and intradermal challenge with antigen and leukotriene D_4 in atopic subjects. *J Allergy Clin Immunol* 1989;83:939–944, with permission.)

given degree of airway narrowing after zafirlukast treatment than after placebo treatment in eight subjects; there was no change in three subjects, and less allergen was required in one (144).

Despite the generally positive effects on allergen-induced asthmatic reactions reported with Cys-LT_1 receptor antagonists, only two reports have been published on 5-LO inhibitors; in both studies, only minimal effects on

early- or late-phase antigen-induced bronchospasm were observed (126,145). By contrast, two inhibitors of FLAP action, MK-886 and MK-0591, each produced significant inhibition of the early-phase response (146,147). The reasons for these discrepancies in efficacy in allergen-induced asthma are not known.

Cold-Air-Induced and Exercise-Induced Asthma

Cold air and exercise elicit airway narrowing by unknown but likely similar mechanisms. Various anti-LT drugs have been studied in models of asthma based on cold-air responses. The first study reported the effect of 2 weeks of treatment with the LT receptor antagonist LY 171883. In a double-blind, placebo-controlled crossover trial, 19 asthmatics underwent cold-air challenge after 2 weeks of treatment with LY 171883 or placebo (148). Treatment with LY 171883 produced a 24% increase in the amount of respiratory heat loss needed to produce a 20% decrease in FEV_1 ($p < 0.05$). In another study, the effects of treatment with a 5-LO inhibitor, zileuton, were assessed in patients with cold-air-induced bronchospasm by a double-blind, placebo-controlled crossover trial (149). Pretreatment with zileuton 3 h before cold-air challenge increased the amount of respiratory heat loss needed to produce a 10% decrease in FEV_1 by 47% ($p < 0.002$).

At least three LT receptor antagonists have been tested in exercise-induced asthma. Intravenous administration of MK-571 at 20 min before exercise challenge produced a significant shift in the airway response to exercise; the FEV_1 decreased 25% after placebo treatment and 9% after MK-571 treatment ($p < 0.001$) (150). SKF 104353, ad-

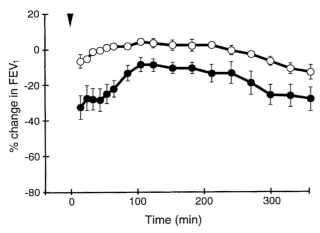

FIG. 3. The mean ± SEM percentage change in forced expiratory volume in 1 s (FEV_1) following allergen inhalation after zafirlukast *(open circles)* and placebo *(solid circles)*. The *downward arrowhead* represents the point of allergen inhalation. *Error bars* for most time points are within the confines of the symbol. (From Taylor IK, O'Shaughnessy KM, Fuller RW, Dollery CT. Effect of cysteinyl-leukotriene receptor antagonist ICI 204.219 on allergen-induced bronchoconstriction and airway hyperreactivity in atopic subjects. *Lancet* 1991;337:690–694, with permission.)

ministered by inhalation, was compared with both placebo and cromolyn sodium for its ability to inhibit exercise-induced asthma; both agents produced equivalent protection against exercise-induced bronchospasm that was significantly greater than that of placebo (151). Treatment with 20 mg p.o. zafirlukast blunted the response to exercise challenge in seven of the eight subjects; the mean maximal percentage fall was 36% after placebo and 21% after zafirlukast ($p<0.01$) (152). Treatment with zafirlukast, 400 μg by inhalation, provided significantly greater protection against exercise-induced bronchospasm than did placebo. The mean maximal decreases in FEV_1 after exercise challenge were 30% and 15% after treatment with zafirlukast and placebo, respectively ($p<0.05$) (153).

Aspirin-Induced Asthma

Approximately 5% to 10% of patients with asthma will experience bronchospasm and extrapulmonary symptoms after ingestion of aspirin or nonsteroidal anti-inflammatory drugs (NSAIDs) that inhibit type I cyclooxygenase. These asthmatics with aspirin-induced asthma (AIA) are a biochemically distinct subset of individuals who have been shown to overexcrete Cys-LTs chronically (128,135, 136,154). It is also important to note that within the first few hours after AIA patients ingest aspirin, LT production increases severalfold. The increase in urinary LTs occurs with a simultaneous development of pulmonary symptoms (128), including airway obstruction and extrapulmonary symptoms such as facial flushing, angioedema, and gastrointestinal symptoms. The mechanism of AIA has not been established; however, the fact that reactions occur with multiple agents that are structurally dissimilar makes allergy to acetylsalic acid (ASA)

or NSAIDs unlikely. The aspirin reaction is associated with mast cell activation, which, in turn, seems to be dependent on products of the 5-LO pathway (155).

The reactions to aspirin ingestion in individuals with AIA can be dramatically inhibited by administration of either antagonists of the action of LTD_4 at the Cys-LT_1 receptor or inhibitors of the action of 5-LO. Christie et al. (134) reported that aerosol administration of the LT receptor antagonist SKF 104353 at 30 min before oral aspirin challenge significantly ($p<0.02$) blunted the aspirin-induced decrease in FEV_1 in five of six patients with AIA. Israel et al. (136) treated eight patients with AIA with zileuton (600 mg four times a day) or placebo for 1 week before ASA challenge. Treatment with zileuton blocked the adverse upper and lower airway effects as well as the extrapulmonary symptoms induced by ASA ingestion in all eight patients (Fig. 4). Curiously, blockade of the clinical response to ASA challenge by zileuton treatment was not accompanied by blockade of LT production as determined by measurement of urinary LTE_4. The concentration of urinary LTE_4 after 1 week of zileuton administration decreased by 69% compared with placebo, from a mean of 469 pg LTE_4/mg urinary creatinine after 1 week of placebo to a mean of 147 pg LTE_4/mg urinary creatinine after 1 week of zileuton treatment ($p<0.02$). After ASA challenge, during the zileuton treatment arm, there was an increase in urinary LTE_4 excretion from a baseline of 147 pg/mg creatinine to 1120 pg/mg compared with an increase from a baseline urinary LTE_4 concentration of 469 pg LTE_4/mg creatinine to 3539 pg LTE_4/mg creatinine during the placebo treatment arm. Since the fractional increase in urinary LTE_4 after ASA challenge was equivalent in both groups, these data suggest that a critical absolute concentration of LT production may be needed to induce a measurable clinical response. Furthermore, these data indicate that one does

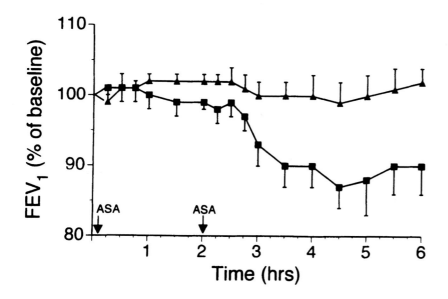

FIG. 4. The mean ± SEM percentage change in forced expiratory volume in 1 s *(FEV₁)* after aspirin challenge following 1 week of zileuton (600 mg q.i.d.) *(triangles)* and placebo *(squares)*. The *downward arrows* represent the time points of aspirin ingestion. (From Israel E, Fischer AR, Rosenberg MA, et al. The pivotal role of 5-lipoxygenase products in the reaction of aspirin-sensitive asthmatics to aspirin. *Am Rev Respir Dis* 1993;148:1447–1451, with permission.)

not have to block LT production completely to obtain a clinically relevant effect. Another 5-LO inhibitor, ZD2138, also proved efficacious in blunting the decrease in airway tone associated with ASA challenge (156). Nasser et al. (156) used a crossover design to compare the effects of a single oral dose of 350 mg of ZD2138 or placebo given 4 h before a dose of ASA previously shown to produce at least a 20% decrease in FEV_1. ZD2138 treatment blunted the adverse effects of ASA in five of seven patients. As noted above with zileuton, the enhanced excretion of urinary LTE_4 after ASA ingestion was blunted but not ablated. Taken together, these data establish a pivotal role for the LTs as effector molecules in AIA.

Effects on Airway Tone

Hui and Barnes (157) were the first to report acute bronchodilation after administration of zafirlukast, an LT receptor antagonist. They gave 10 asthmatics each 40 mg of drug (or placebo) orally, measured FEV_1 every 30 min for 4 h, and then administered a β-agonist. Compared with placebo, active treatment increased the FEV_1 modestly but significantly; there was an average increase of 8 ± 2% above baseline, which was maximal 3.5 h after drug ingestion. Zafirlukast augmented the bronchodilation achieved after salbutamol administration, which suggests that the Cys-LT_1 receptor antagonist and the β-adrenergic agonist each act at a defined site or via distinct mechanisms.

Gaddy et al. (158) have reported the salutary effects of the LT receptor antagonist MK-571 in a group of 12 male asthmatics whose baseline FEV_1 was 50% to 80% of predicted. The investigators administered MK-571 (or placebo) as an intravenous bolus followed by a continuous infusion. After 6 h of infusion, they administered albuterol to determine the maximal effect on airway tone and to observe any possible interactions between these two agents. The FEV_1 increased from a baseline of 2.79 L to 3.36 L by 20 min after the start of the infusion during MK-571 treatment; this effect was significantly greater than the increase from 2.80 L to 2.84 L, which occurred after the start of the placebo infusion. The improvement in FEV_1 was sustained for the 6-h duration of the infusion; the mean percentage increase from baseline ranged from 15% to 22%. They noted additional bronchodilation after inhalation of an albuterol aerosol, but there was no reported interaction between these two drugs. Thus, their findings are consistent with the previously described findings of Hui and Barnes.

Effects on Airway Reactivity

The airways of asthmatics are hyperresponsive to provocative stimuli. Airway reactivity may be quantified by assessing the response to bronchoprovocative challenge

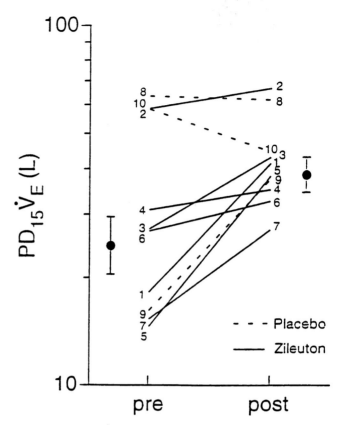

FIG. 5. The $PD_{15}\dot{V}_E$ for 10 subjects before zileuton treatment *(pre)* and after 13 weeks of zileuton treatment and a period of drug washout (range, 1 to 10 days) *(post)*. The geometric means $PD_{15}\dot{V}_E$ pretreatment and posttreatment are also shown. (From Fischer AR, McFadden CA, Franz R, et al. Effects of chronic 5-lipoxygenase inhibition on airway hyperresponsiveness in asthmatic subjects. *Am J Respir Crit Care Med* 1995;152:1203–1207, with permission.)

with pharmacologic or physical means, for example, methacholine or exercise. Such challenges are performed in stepwise fashion, thereby enabling construction of a dose-response curve. Agents that decrease airway reactivity will shift the dose-response curve to the right, that is, it will require a greater stimulus to achieve the same degree of bronchoconstriction. It has recently been demonstrated that 13 weeks of treatment with a 5-LO inhibitor, zileuton, decreased airway reactivity in a group of mild–moderate asthmatics (159). In a double-blind, placebo-controlled, parallel study, subjects were treated with 400 or 600 mg of zileuton four times a day for 13 weeks. Ten subjects underwent cold, dry-air hyperventilation challenge before randomization and after completion of 13 weeks of randomized treatment. Among the seven subjects randomized to zileuton, the minute ventilation of cold, dry air needed to induce a 15% decrease in FEV_1 ($PD_{15}\dot{V}_E$) increased by 58%, from a geometric mean baseline of 24.5 L/min to 38.8 L/min after treatment ($p = 0.01$) (Fig. 5).

Effects of Chronic Administration of Drugs Active on the 5-Lipoxygenase Pathway in Asthma

At present, only three reports of the effect on chronic asthma by treatment with agents active against LTs have been published (160–162) in the archival literature. The first study to report that chronic treatment with an anti-LT drug was beneficial to patients with asthma was conducted by Cloud et al. (161). In this study, 138 patients were enrolled at nine centers; each subject was randomized to receive either 600 mg of the LT receptor antagonist LY 171883 or placebo for 6 weeks. There were modest but significant improvements in symptoms and airway tone in the active treatment group compared with the placebo group.

Israel et al. (163) reported the effect of 4 weeks of treatment with zileuton in 139 adults with mild–moderate asthma. Subjects were nonsmokers with a baseline FEV_1 of 40% to 75% of predicted, which improved by $\geq 15\%$ after inhalation of 180 μg of albuterol. Inhaled β-agonists were the sole asthma therapy permitted before study entry. A 10-day placebo lead-in period preceded randomization to zileuton 600 mg q.i.d., zileuton 800 mg b.i.d. (alternating with placebo), or placebo. During the placebo lead-in period, subjects needed to have moderately symptomatic asthma, defined by frequency of albuterol use and symptom scores, in order to qualify for randomization to one of the treatment arms. After treatment with zileuton, the FEV_1 significantly increased in the two zileuton treatment groups compared with each group's FEV_1 after placebo lead-in. The FEV_1 of the group that received 600 mg q.i.d. improved by 13.4% (0.32 L) ($p = 0.02$), and the group that received 800 mg b.i.d. improved by 10.9% (0.24 L) ($p = 0.09$) compared with placebo lead-in. Zileuton treatment also produced other beneficial effects such as a decrease in β-agonist usage and decreased peak flow variability; this latter effect was significant only in the 600-mg q.i.d. group. The adverse effects reported with zileuton treatment were urticaria (one patient in the 800-mg b.i.d. group) and transient alterations in hepatic function, all of which resolved after discontinuation of the drug. Gastrointestinal disturbances were also reported: six patients taking zileuton reported dyspepsia, whereas none of the placebo patients reported this symptom.

Spector et al. (162) reported the results of the Accolate Asthma Trialists Group, which performed a multicenter, double-blind, placebo-controlled, dose-ranging study of the LT receptor antagonist zafirlukast. They studied asthmatics with a baseline FEV_1 of 40% to 75% of predicted who had previously been treated with only inhaled β-agonists and/or theophylline. After a single-blind placebo lead-in period during which subjects were required to report mild–moderate symptoms in order to be eligible for randomization, the subjects were randomized to receive 6 weeks of treatment with placebo or 10, 20, or 40 mg of zafirlukast per day. Study medication was administered in equal morning and evening doses. The primary efficacy variables were symptom scores, changes in pulmonary function (peak expiratory flow rate and FEV_1), and number of occasions of rescue albuterol use. There was a mean 11% improvement in FEV_1 among all zafirlukast recipients, with the greatest improvement in the group receiving the highest dose, 40 mg/day. There was no difference in the improvement in FEV_1 between the groups of patients receiving 10 mg or 20 mg of zafirlukast per day. There was a mean of 2.6 fewer nocturnal awakenings per week among the group receiving 40 mg of zafirlukast per day than among the placebo group, a decrease of 46% ($p < 0.001$). Similarly, the 40-mg dose of zafirlukast reduced "first morning" asthma symptoms by 28% and reduced the daytime asthma score by 27%. There was a mean decrease in albuterol use from baseline in the 40-mg/day group compared with the placebo group of 1 puff/day ($p < 0.02$). There were no significant differences in adverse events reported between the placebo and zafirlukast recipients.

CONCLUSIONS

The Cys-LTs are potent chemical mediators produced by a variety of inflammatory cells with relevance to asthma, for example, eosinophils and mast cells. These mediators can induce asthma symptoms when given exogenously and can be recovered from the urine of patients with induced or spontaneous asthmatic reactions. Most importantly, three different classes of novel pharmacologic agents—namely, agents capable of inhibiting 5-LO, inhibiting 5-LO-activating protein, or antagonizing the action of the Cys-LTs at the Cys-LT$_1$ receptor—have demonstrated reasonable safety and efficacy profiles in clinical trials for the treatment of asthma. Taken together, these data indicate that the Cys-LTs have a significant effector role in asthma biology.

REFERENCES

1. Murphy RC, Hammarstrom S, Samuelsson B. Leukotriene C: a slow-reacting substance from murine mastocytoma cells. *Proc Natl Acad Sci USA* 1979;76:4275–4279.
2. Lewis RA, Austen KF, Drazen JM, Clark DA, Marfat A, Corey EJ. Slow reacting substances of anaphylaxis: identification of leukotrienes C-1 and D from human and rat sources. *Proc Natl Acad Sci USA* 1980;77:3710–3714.
3. Parker CW, Huber MM, Hoffman MK, Falkenhein SF. Characterization of the two major species of slow reacting substance from rat basophilic leukemia cells as glutathionyl thioethers of eicosatetraenoic acids oxygenated at the 5 position: evidence that peroxy groups are present and important for spasmogenic activity. *Prostaglandins* 1979;18:673–686.
4. Lewis RA, Drazen JM, Austen KF, Clark DA, Corey EJ. Identification of the C(6)-S-conjugate of leukotriene A with cysteine as a naturally occurring slow reacting substance of anaphylaxis (SRS-A): importance of the 11-*cis*-geometry for biological activity. *Biochem Biophys Res Commun* 1980;96:271–277.

5. Samuelsson B. Leukotrienes: mediators of immediate hypersensitivity reactions and inflammation. *Science* 1983;220:568–575.

6. Samuelsson B, Dahlen SE, Lindgren JA, Rouzer CA, Serhan CN. Leukotrienes and lipoxins: structures, biosynthesis, and biological effects. *Science* 1987;237:1171–1176.

7. Lewis RA, Austen KF, Soberman RJ. Leukotrienes and other products of the 5-lipoxygenase pathway: biochemistry and relation to pathobiology in human diseases. *N Engl J Med* 1990;323:645–655.

8. Henderson WR. The role of leukotrienes in inflammation. *Ann Intern Med* 1994;121:684–697.

9. Murphy RC. Lipid mediators, leukotrienes and mass spectrometry. *J Mass Spectrometry* 1995;30:5–16.

10. Dennis EA. Modification of the arachidonic acid cascade through phospholipase A_2 dependent mechanisms. *Adv Prostaglandin Thromboxane Leukotriene Res* 1990;20:217–223.

11. Davidson FF, Dennis EA. Biological relevance of lipocortins and related proteins as inhibitors of phospholipase A_2. *Biochem Pharmacol* 1989;38:3645–3651.

12. Waite M. Phospholipases: enzymes that share a substrate class. *Adv Exp Med Biol* 1990;279:1–22.

13. Kaiser E, Chiba P, Zaky K. Phospholipases in biology and medicine. *Clin Biochem* 1990;23:349–370.

14. Ferguson JE, Hanley MR. The role of phospholipases and phospholipid-derived signals in cell activation. *Curr Opin Cell Biol* 1991;3:206–212.

15. Kramer RM, Hession C, Johansen B, et al. Structure and properties of a human nonpancreatic phospholipase A_2. *J Biol Chem* 1989;264:5768–5775.

16. Kramer RM, Roberts EF, Manetta J, Putnam JE. The $Ca^{2}(+)$-sensitive cytosolic phospholipase A_2 is a 100-kDa protein in human monoblast U937 cells. *J Biol Chem* 1991;266:5268–5272.

17. Kramer RM, Johansen B, Hession C, Pepinsky RB. Structure and properties of a secretable phospholipase A_2 from human platelets. *Adv Exp Med Biol* 1990;275:35–53.

18. Sharp JD, White DL, Chiou XG, et al. Molecular cloning and expression of human $Ca^{2}(+)$-sensitive cytosolic phospholipase A_2. *J Biol Chem* 1991;266:14,850–14,853.

19. Peters-Golden M, McNish RW. Redistribution of 5-lipoxygenase and cytosolic phospholipase A_2 to the nuclear fraction upon macrophage activation. *Biochem Biophys Res Commun* 1993;196:147–153.

20. Clark JD, Milona N, Knopf JL. Purification of a 110-kilodalton cytosolic phospholipase A_2 from the human monocytic cell line U937. *Proc Natl Acad Sci USA* 1990;87:7708–7712.

21. Murakami M, Kudo I, Inoue K. Molecular nature of phospholipases A_2 involved in prostaglandin I_2 synthesis in human umbilical vein endothelial cells: possible participation of cytosolic and extracellular type II phospholipases A_2. *J Biol Chem* 1993;268:839–844.

22. Balsinde J, Barbour SE, Bianco ID, Dennis EA. Arachidonic acid mobilization in P388D1 macrophages is controlled by two distinct $Ca(2+)$-dependent phospholipase A_2 enzymes. *Proc Natl Acad Sci USA* 1994;91:11,060–11,064.

23. White SR, Strek ME, Kulp GVP, et al. Regulation of human eosinophil degranulation and activation by endogenous phospholipase-A_2. *J Clin Invest* 1993;91:2118–2125.

24. Matsumoto T, Funk CD, Radmark O, Hoog JO, Jornvall H, Samuelsson B. Molecular cloning and amino acid sequence of human 5-lipoxygenase. *Proc Natl Acad Sci USA* 1988;85:26–30 [Erratum, *Proc Natl Acad Sci USA* 1988;85:3406].

25. Rouzer CA, Rands E, Kargman S, Jones RE, Register RB, Dixon RA. Characterization of cloned human leukocyte 5-lipoxygenase expressed in mammalian cells. *J Biol Chem* 1988;263:10,135–10,140.

26. Balcarek JM, Theisen TW, Cook MN, et al. Isolation and characterization of a cDNA clone encoding rat 5-lipoxygenase. *J Biol Chem* 1988;263:13,937–13,941.

27. Dixon RA, Diehl RE, Opas E, et al. Requirement of a 5-lipoxygenase-activating protein for leukotriene synthesis. *Nature* 1990;343:282–284.

28. Miller DK, Gillard JW, Vickers PJ, et al. Identification and isolation of a membrane protein necessary for leukotriene production. *Nature* 1990;343:278–281.

29. Reid GK, Kargman S, Vickers PJ, et al. Correlation between expression of 5-lipoxygenase-activating protein, 5-lipoxygenase, and cellular leukotriene synthesis. *J Biol Chem* 1990;265:19,818–19,823.

30. Woods JW, Evans JF, Ethier D, et al. 5-Lipoxygenase and 5-lipoxygenase activating protein are localized in the nuclear envelope of activated human leukocytes. *J Exp Med* 1993;178:1935–1946.

31. Mancini JA, Abramovitz M, Cox ME, et al. 5-Lipoxygenase-activating protein is an arachidonate binding protein. *FEBS Lett* 1993;318:277–281.

32. Charleson S, Evans JF, Leger S, et al. Structural requirements for the binding of fatty acids to 5-lipoxygenase-activating protein. *Eur J Pharmacol* 1994;267:275–280.

33. Brock TG, McNish RW, Petersgolden M. Translocation and leukotriene synthetic capacity of nuclear 5-lipoxygenase in rat basophilic leukemia cells and alveolar macrophages. *J Biol Chem* 1995;270:21,652–21,658.

34. Lam BK, Penrose JF, Freeman GJ, Austen KF. Expression cloning of a cDNA for human leukotriene C_4 synthase, an integral membrane protein conjugating reduced glutathione to leukotriene A_4. *Proc Natl Acad Sci USA* 1994;91:7663–7667.

35. Welsch DJ, Creely DP, Hauser SD, Mathis KJ, Krivi GG, Isakson PC. Molecular cloning end expression of human leukotriene-C_4 synthase. *Adv Prostaglandin Thromboxane Leukot Res* 1995;23:167–169.

36. Penrose JF, Spector J, Lam BK, et al. Purification of human lung leukotriene C_4 synthase and preparation of a polyclonal antibody. *Am J Respir Crit Care Med* 1995;152:283–289.

37. Lam BK, Owen WF Jr, Austen KF, Soberman RJ. The identification of a distinct export step following the biosynthesis of leukotriene C_4 by human eosinophils. *J Biol Chem* 1989;264:12,885–12,889.

38. Orning L, Hammarstrom S, Samuelsson B. Leukotriene D: a slow reacting substance from rat basophilic leukemia cells. *Proc Natl Acad Sci USA* 1980;77:2014–2017.

39. Sala A, Voelkel N, Maclouf J, Murphy RC. Leukotriene E_4 elimination and metabolism in normal human subjects. *J Biol Chem* 1990;265:21,771–21,778.

40. Stene DO, Murphy RC. Metabolism of leukotriene E_4 in isolated rat hepatocytes: identification of beta-oxidation products of sulfidopeptide leukotrienes. *J Biol Chem* 1988;263:2773–2778.

41. Maclouf J, Antoine C, Decaterina R, et al. Entry rate and metabolism of leukotriene C-4 into vascular compartment in healthy subjects. *Am J Physiol* 1992;263:H244–H249.

42. Lewis RA, Goetzl EJ, Drazen JM, Soter NA, Austen KF, Corey EJ. Functional characterization of synthetic leukotriene B and its stereochemical isomers. *J Exp Med* 1981;154:1243–1248.

43. Medina JF, Radmark O, Funk CD, Haeggstrom JZ. Molecular cloning and expression of mouse leukotriene-A_4 hydrolase cDNA. *Biochem Biophys Res Commun* 1991;176:1516–1524.

44. Wetterholm A, Medina JF, Radmark O, et al. Recombinant mouse leukotriene-A_4 hydrolase: a zinc metalloenzyme with dual enzymatic activities. *Biochim Biophys Acta* 1991;1080:96–102.

45. Bigby TD, Lee DM, Minami M, Ohishi N, Shimizu T, Baker JR. Characterization of human airway epithelial cell leukotriene A_4 hydrolase. *Am J Respir Cell Mol Biol* 1994;11:615–624.

46. Mancini JA, Evans JF. Cloning and characterization of the human leukotriene A_4 hydrolase gene. *Eur J Biochem* 1995;231:65–71.

47. Weller PF, Lee CW, Foster DW, Corey EJ, Austen KF, Lewis RA. Generation and metabolism of 5-lipoxygenase pathway leukotrienes by human eosinophils: predominant production of leukotriene C_4. *Proc Natl Acad Sci USA* 1983;80:7626–7630.

48. Murakami M, Austen KF, Bingham CO, Friend DS, Penrose JF, Arm JP. Interleukin-3 regulates development of the 5-lipoxygenase/leukotriene C_4 synthase pathway in mouse mast cells. *J Biol Chem* 1995;270:22,653–22,656.

49. Rankin JA, Hitchcock M, Merrill W, Bach MK, Brashler JR, Askenase PW. IgE-dependent release of leukotriene C_4 from alveolar macrophages. *Nature* 1982;297:329–331.

50. Schonfeld W, Schluter B, Hilger R, Konig W. Leukotriene generation and metabolism in isolated human lung macrophages. *Immunology* 1988;65:529–536.

51. Holtzman MJ. Arachidonic acid metabolism in airway epithelial cells. *Annu Rev Physiol* 1992;54:303–329.

52. Eling TE, Danilowicz RM, Henke DC, Sivarajah K, Yankaskas JR, Boucher RC. Arachidonic acid metabolism by canine tracheal epithelial cells: product formation and relationship to chloride secretion. *J Biol Chem* 1986;261:12,841–12,849.

53. Feinmark SJ, Cannon PJ. Endothelial cell leukotriene C_4 synthesis results from intercellular transfer of leukotriene A_4 synthesized by polymorphonuclear leukocytes. *J Biol Chem* 1986;261:16,466–16,472.

54. Jackson RM, Chandler DB, Fulmer JD. Production of arachidonic acid metabolites by endothelial cells in hyperoxia. *J Appl Physiol* 1986;61:584–591.

55. Piper PJ, Galton SA. Generation of leukotriene B$_4$ and leukotriene E$_4$ from porcine pulmonary artery. *Prostaglandins* 1984;28:905–914.

56. Owen WF Jr, Soberman RJ, Yoshimoto T, Sheffer AL, Lewis RA, Austen KF. Synthesis and release of leukotriene C$_4$ by human eosinophils. *J Immunol* 1987;138:532–538.

57. Bruynzeel PL, Kok PT, Vietor RJ, Verhagen J. On the optimal conditions of LTC$_4$ formation by human eosinophils *in vitro*. *Prostaglandins Leukotriene Med* 1985;20:11–22.

58. Broide DH, Gleich GJ, Cuomo AJ, et al. Evidence of ongoing mast cell and eosinophil degranulation in symptomatic asthma airway. *J Allergy Clin Immunol* 1991;88:637–648.

59. Sedgwick JB, Calhoun WJ, Gleich GJ, et al. Immediate and late airway response of allergic rhinitis patients to segmental antigen challenge: characterization of eosinophil and mast cell mediators. *Am Rev Respir Dis* 1991;144:1274–1281.

60. Broide DH, Eisman S, Ramsdell JW, Ferguson P, Schwartz LB, Wasserman SI. Airway levels of mast cell-derived mediators in exercise-induced asthma. *Am Rev Respir Dis* 1990;141:563–568.

61. Bradley BL, Azzawi M, Jacobson M, et al. Eosinophils, T-lymphocytes, mast cells, neutrophils, and macrophages in bronchial biopsy specimens from atopic subjects with asthma: comparison with biopsy specimens from atopic subjects without asthma and normal control subjects and relationship to bronchial hyperresponsiveness. *J Allergy Clin Immunol* 1991;88:661–674.

62. Coleman RA, Eglen RM, Jones RL, et al. Prostanoid and leukotriene receptors: a progress report from the IUPHAR working parties on classification and nomenclature. *Prostaglandins Relat Compounds* 1995;23:285.

63. Goldman DW, Gifford LA, Young RN, Marotti T, Cheung MK, Goetzl EJ. Affinity labeling of the membrane protein-binding component of human polymorphonuclear leukocyte receptors for leukotriene B$_4$. *J Immunol* 1991;146:2671–2677.

64. Miki I, Watanabe T, Nakamura M, et al. Solubilization and characterization of leukotriene B$_4$ receptor-GTP binding protein complex from porcine spleen. *Biochem Biophys Res Commun* 1990;166:342–348.

65. Kreisle RA, Parker CW, Griffin GL, Senior RM, Stenson WF. Studies of leukotriene B$_4$-specific binding and function in rat polymorphonuclear leukocytes: absence of a chemotactic response. *J Immunol* 1985;134:3356–3363.

66. Ford-Hutchinson AW. Leukotriene B$_4$ in inflammation. *Crit Rev Immunol* 1990;10:1–12.

67. Rola-Pleszczynski M, Thivierge M, Gagnon N, Lacasse C, Stankova J. Differential regulation of cytokine and cytokine receptor genes by PAF, LTB$_4$ and PGE$_2$. *J Lipid Mediat* 1993;6:175–181.

68. Slipetz DM, Scoggan KA, Nicholson DW, Metters KM. Photoaffinity labelling and radiation inactivation of the leukotriene B$_4$ receptor in human myeloid cells. *Eur J Pharmacol* 1993;244:161–173.

69. Jackson WT, Boyd RJ, Froelich LL, Mallett BE, Gapinski DM. Specific inhibition of leukotriene-B(4)-induced neutrophil activation by LY223982. *J Pharmacol Exp Ther* 1992;263:1009–1014.

70. Silbaugh SA, Stengel PW, Cockerham SL, et al. Pulmonary actions of LY255283, a leukotriene B$_4$ receptor antagonist. *Eur J Pharmacol* 1992;223:57–64.

71. Kishikawa K, Tateishi N, Maruyama T, Seo R, Toda M, Miyamoto T. ONO-4057, a novel, orally active leukotriene B$_4$ antagonist: effects on LTB$_4$-induced neutrophil functions. *Prostaglandins* 1992;44:261–275.

72. Ohmi N, Tani C, Yamada K, Fukui M. Pharmacological profile of a novel, orally active leukotriene B4 antagonist, SM-15178. *Inflammation* 1994;18:129–140.

73. Labaudiniere R, Dereu N, Cavy F, Guillet MC, Marquis O, Terlain B. Omega-([4,6-diphenyl-2-pyridyl]oxy)alkanoic acid derivatives: a new family of potent and orally active LTB$_4$ antagonists. *J Med Chem* 1992;35:4315–4324.

74. Huang FC, Chan WK, Warus JD, et al. 4-(2-[Methyl{2-phenethyl}amino]-2-oxoethyl)-8-(phenylmethoxy)-2-naphthalenecarboxylic acid: a high affinity, competitive, orally active leukotriene B$_4$ receptor antagonist. *J Med Chem* 1992;35:4253–4255.

75. Harper RW, Jackson WT, Froelich LL, Boyd RJ, Aldridge TE, Herron DK. Leukotriene B-4 [LTB(4)] receptor antagonists: a series of (hydroxyphenyl) pyrazoles. *J Med Chem* 1994;37:2411–2420.

76. Sarau HM, Foley JJ, Schmidt DB, et al. SB 209247, a high affinity LTB$_4$ receptor antagonist demonstrating potent antiinflammatory activity. *Prostaglandins Relat Compounds* 1995;23:277.

77. Kishikawa K, Nakao S, Matsumoto S, Kondo K, Hamanaka N. Estimation of antagonistic activity of ONO-4057 against leukotriene B$_4$ in humans. *Prostaglandins Relat Compounds* 1995;23:281.

78. Showell HJ, Pettipher ER, Cheng JB, et al. The *in vitro* and *in vivo* pharmacologic activity of the potent and selective leukotriene B$_4$ receptor antagonist CP-105696. *J Pharmacol Exp Ther* 1995;273:176–184.

79. Dahlen SE. Pulmonary effects of leukotrienes. *Acta Physiol Scand Suppl* 1983;512:1–51.

80. Piper PJ. Formation and actions of leukotrienes. *Physiol Rev* 1984;64:744–761.

81. Drazen JM, Austen KF. Leukotrienes and airway responses. *Am Rev Respir Dis* 1987;136:985–998.

82. Weiss JW, Drazen JM, Coles N, et al. Bronchoconstrictor effects of leukotriene C in humans. *Science* 1982;216:196–198.

83. Griffin M, Weiss JW, Leitch AG, et al. Effects of leukotriene D on the airways in asthma. *N Engl J Med* 1983;308:436–439.

84. Adelroth E, Morris MM, Hargreave FE, O'Byrne PM. Airway responsiveness to leukotrienes C$_4$ and D$_4$ and to methacholine in patients with asthma and normal controls. *N Engl J Med* 1986;315:480–484.

85. Barnes NC, Piper PJ, Costello JF. Comparative effects of inhaled leukotriene C$_4$, leukotriene D$_4$, and histamine in normal human subjects. *Thorax* 1984;39:500–504.

86. Smith LJ, Greenberger PA, Patterson R, Krell RD, Bernstein PR. The effect of inhaled leukotriene D$_4$ in humans. *Am Rev Respir Dis* 1985;131:368–372.

87. Greenberger PA, Smith LJ, Patterson R, et al. Comparison of cutaneous and bronchial reactivity to leukotriene D$_4$ in humans. *J Lab Clin Med* 1986;108:70–75.

88. Kern R, Smith LJ, Patterson R, Krell RD, Bernstein PR. Characterization of the airway response to inhaled leukotriene D$_4$ in normal subjects. *Am Rev Respir Dis* 1986;133:1127–1132.

89. Davidson AB, Lee TH, Scanlon PD, et al. Bronchoconstrictor effects of leukotriene E$_4$ in normal and asthmatic subjects. *Am Rev Respir Dis* 1987;135:333–337.

90. Wetmore LA, Gerard NP, Herron DK, et al. Leukotriene receptor on U-937 cells: discriminatory responses to leukotrienes C$_4$ and D$_4$. *Am J Physiol* 1991;261:L164–L171.

91. Mong S, Wu HL, Scott MO, et al. Molecular heterogeneity of leukotriene receptors: correlation of smooth muscle contraction and radioligand binding in guinea-pig lung. *J Pharmacol Exp Ther* 1985;234:316–325.

92. Lewis MA, Mong S, Vessella RL, Crooke ST. Identification and characterization of leukotriene D$_4$ receptors in adult and fetal human lung. *Biochem Pharmacol* 1985;34:4311–4317.

93. Mong S, Chi-Rosso G, Hay DW, Crooke ST. Subcellular localization of leukotriene D$_4$ receptors in sheep tracheal smooth muscle. *Mol Pharmacol* 1988;34:590–596.

94. Mong S, Wu HL, Stadel JM, Clark MA, Crooke ST. Solubilization of [^{3}H]leukotriene D$_4$ receptor complex from guinea pig lung membranes. *Mol Pharmacol* 1986;29:235–243.

95. Mong S, Wu HL, Miller J, Hall RF, Gleason JG, Crooke ST. SKF 104353, a high affinity antagonist for human and guinea pig lung leukotriene D$_4$ receptor, blocked phosphatidylinositol metabolism and thromboxane synthesis induced by leukotriene D$_4$. *Mol Pharmacol* 1987;32:223–229.

96. Mong S, Hoffman K, Wu HL, Crooke ST. Leukotriene-induced hydrolysis of inositol lipids in guinea pig lung: mechanism of signal transduction for leukotriene-D$_4$ receptors. *Mol Pharmacol* 1987;31:35–41.

97. Crooke ST, Sarau H, Saussy D, Winkler J, Foley J. Signal transduction processes for the LTD$_4$ receptor. *Adv Prostaglandin Thromboxane Leukotriene Res* 1990;20:127–137.

98. Crooke ST, Mattern M, Sarau HM, et al. The signal transduction system of the leukotriene D$_4$ receptor. *Trends Pharmacol Sci* 1989;10:103–107.

99. Hay DW, Muccitelli RM, Tucker SS, et al. Pharmacologic profile of SK andF 104353: a novel, potent and selective peptidoleukotriene receptor antagonist in guinea pig and human airways. *J Pharmacol Exp Ther* 1987;243:474–481.

100. Buckner CK, Krell RD, Laravuso RB, Coursin DB, Bernstein PR, Will JA. Pharmacological evidence that human intralobar airways do not contain different receptors that mediate contractions to leukotriene C_4 and leukotriene D_4. *J Pharmacol Exp Ther* 1986;237: 558–562.

101. Muccitelli RM, Tucker SS, Hay DW, Torphy TJ, Wasserman MA. Is the guinea pig trachea a good *in vitro* model of human large and central airways? Comparison on leukotriene-, methacholine-, histamine- and antigen-induced contractions. *J Pharmacol Exp Ther* 1987;243: 467–473.

102. Jones TR, Davis C, Daniel EE. Pharmacological study of the contractile activity of leukotriene C_4 and D_4 on isolated human airway smooth muscle. *Can J Physiol Pharmacol* 1982;60:638–643.

103. Davis C, Kannan MS, Jones TR, Daniel EE. Control of human airway smooth muscle: *in vitro* studies. *J Appl Physiol* 1982;53:1080–1087.

104. Weichman BM, Wasserman MA, Gleason JG. SK&F 88046: a unique pharmacologic antagonist of bronchoconstriction induced by leukotriene D_4, thromboxane and prostaglandins F_2 alpha and D_2 *in vitro*. *J Pharmacol Exp Ther* 1984;228:128–132.

105. Fleisch JH, Rinkema LE, Haisch KD, et al. LY171883, 1 < 2-hydroxy-3-propyl-4- < 4-(1H-tetrazol-5-yl)butoxy > phenyl > ethanone, an orally active leukotriene D_4 antagonist. *J Pharmacol Exp Ther* 1985; 233:148–157.

106. Snyder DW, Giles RE, Keith RA, Yee YK, Krell RD. *In vitro* pharmacology of ICI 198,615: a novel, potent and selective peptide leukotriene antagonist. *J Pharmacol Exp Ther* 1987;243:548–556.

107. Jones TR, Zamboni R, Belley M, et al. Pharmacology of L-660,711 (MK-571): a novel potent and selective leukotriene D_4 receptor antagonist. *Can J Physiol Pharmacol* 1989;67:17–28.

108. Jones TR, Young R, Champion E, et al. L-649,923, sodium (beta S*, gamma R*)-4-(3-[4-acetyl-3-hydroxy-2-propylphenoxy]-propylthio)-gamma-hydroxy-beta-methylbenzenebutanoate, a selective, orally active leukotriene receptor antagonist. *Can J Physiol Pharmacol* 1986; 64:1068–1075.

109. Torphy TJ, Newton JF, Wasserman MA, et al. The bronchopulmonary pharmacology of SK&F 104353 in anesthetized guinea pigs: demonstration of potent and selective antagonism of responses to peptidoleukotrienes. *J Pharmacol Exp Ther* 1989;249:430–437.

110. Dillard RD, Hahn RA, McCullough D, et al. (Phenylmethoxy)phenyl derivatives of omega-oxozolylalkanoic and omega-tetrazolylalkanoic acids and related tetrazoles: synthesis and evaluation as leukotriene-D_4 receptor antagonists. *J Med Chem* 1991;34:2768–2778.

111. O'Donnell M, Crowley HJ, Yaremko B, O'Neill N, Welton AF. Pharmacologic actions of RO 24-5913, a novel antagonist of leukotriene-D(4). *J Pharmacol Exp Ther* 1991;259:751–759.

112. Jacobs RT, Bernstein PR, Cronk LA, et al. Synthesis, structure–activity relationships, and pharmacological evaluation of a series of fluorinated 3-benzyl-5-indolecarboxamides: identification of 4-[[5-[(2R)-2-methyl-4,4,4-trifluorobutyl)carbamoyl]-1-methyl indol-3-yl]methyl]-3-methoxy-N-[(2-methylphenyl)sulfonyl]benzamide, a potent, orally active antagonist of leukotrienes D_4 and E_4. *J Med Chem* 1994;37: 1282–1297.

113. Heavey DJ, Soberman RJ, Lewis RA, Spur B, Austen KF. Critical considerations in the development of an assay for sulfidopeptide leukotrienes in plasma. *Prostaglandins* 1987;33:693–708.

114. Orning L, Norin E, Gustafsson B, Hammarstrom S. *In vivo* metabolism of leukotriene C_4 in germ-free and conventional rats: fecal excretion of N-acetylleukotriene E_4. *J Biol Chem* 1986;261:766–771.

115. Orning L, Kaijser L, Hammarstrom S. *In vivo* metabolism of leukotriene C_4 in man: urinary excretion of leukotriene E_4. *Biochem Biophys Res Commun* 1985;130:214–220.

116. Hammarstrom S, Orning L, Keppler A. Metabolism of cysteinyl leukotrienes to novel polar metabolites in the rat and endogenous formation of leukotriene D_4 during systemic anaphylaxis in the guinea pig. *Ann NY Acad Sci* 1988;524:43–67.

117. Orning L. Omega-hydroxylation of N-acetylleukotriene E_4 by rat liver microsomes. *Biochem Biophys Res Commun* 1987;143:337–344.

118. Maltby NH, Taylor GW, Ritter JM, Moore K, Fuller RW, Dollery CT. Leukotriene C_4 elimination and metabolism in man. *J Allergy Clin Immunol* 1990;85:3–9.

119. Taylor GW, Taylor I, Black P, et al. Urinary leukotriene E_4 after antigen challenge and in acute asthma and allergic rhinitis. *Lancet* 1989; 1:584–588.

120. Westcott JY, Johnston K, Batt RA, Wenzel SE, Voelkel NF. Measurement of peptidoleukotrienes in biological fluids. *J Appl Physiol* 1990; 68:2640–2648.

121. Westcott JY, Voelkel NF, Jones K, Wenzel SE. Inactivation of leukotriene C_4 in the airways and subsequent urinary leukotriene E_4 excretion in normal and asthmatic subjects. *Am Rev Respir Dis* 1993;148: 1244–1251.

122. Drazen JM, O'Brien J, Sparrow D, et al. Recovery of leukotriene-E_4 from the urine of patients with airway obstruction. *Am Rev Respir Dis* 1992;146:104–108.

123. Asano K, Lilly CM, O'Donnell WJ, et al. Diurnal variation of urinary leukotriene E_4 and histamine excretion rates in normal and mild-to-moderate asthmatic subjects. *J Allergy Clin Immunol* 1995; 96:643–651.

124. Kumlin M, Stensvad F, Larsson L, Dahlen B, Dahlen SE. Validation and application of a new simple strategy for measurements of urinary leukotriene E_4 in humans. *Clin Exp Allergy* 1995;25:467–479.

125. Taylor IK, Wellings R, Taylor GW, Fuller RW. Urinary leukotriene-E_4 excretion in exercise-induced asthma. *J Appl Physiol* 1992;73: 743–748.

126. Hui KP, Taylor IK, Taylor GW, et al. Effect of a 5-lipoxygenase inhibitor on leukotriene generation and airway responses after allergen challenge in asthmatic patients. *Thorax* 1991;46:184–189.

127. Sladek K, Dworski R, Fitzgerald GA, et al. Allergen-stimulated release of thromboxane A_2 and leukotriene E_4 in humans: effect of indomethacin. *Am Rev Respir Dis* 1990;141:1441–1445.

128. Knapp HR, Sladek K, Fitzgerald GA. Increased excretion of leukotriene-E_4 during aspirin-induced asthma. *J Lab Clin Med* 1992;119: 48–51.

129. Westcott JY, Smith HR, Wenzel SE, et al. Urinary leukotriene-E_4 in patients with asthma: effect of airways reactivity and sodium cromoglycate. *Am Rev Respir Dis* 1991;143:1322–1328.

130. Manning PJ, Rokach J, Malo JL, et al. Urinary leukotriene E_4 levels during early and late asthmatic responses. *J Allergy Clin Immunol* 1990;86:211–220.

131. Kikawa Y, Miyanomae T, Inoue Y, et al. Urinary leukotriene E_4 after exercise challenge in children with asthma. *J Allergy Clin Immunol* 1992;89:1111–1119.

132. Kikawa Y, Hosoi S, Inoue Y, et al. Exercise-induced urinary excretion of leukotriene-E_4 in children with atopic asthma. *Pediatr Res* 1991; 29:455–459.

133. Smith CM, Christie PE, Hawksworth RJ, Thien F, Lee TH. Urinary leukotriene-E_4 levels after allergen and exercise challenge in bronchial asthma. *Am Rev Respir Dis* 1991;144:1411–1413.

134. Christie PE, Tagari P, Ford-Hutchinson AW, et al. Urinary leukotriene-E_4 concentrations increase after aspirin challenge in aspirin-sensitive asthmatic subjects. *Am Rev Respir Dis* 1991;143:1025–1029.

135. Kumlin M, Dahlen B, Bjorck T, Zetterstrom O, Granstrom E, Dahlen SE. Urinary excretion of leukotriene-E_4 and 11-dehydro-thromboxane-B_2 in response to bronchial provocations with allergen, aspirin, leukotriene-D_4, and histamine in asthmatics. *Am Rev Respir Dis* 1992; 146:96–103.

136. Israel E, Fischer AR, Rosenberg MA, et al. The pivotal role of 5-lipoxygenase products in the reaction of aspirin-sensitive asthmatics to aspirin. *Am Rev Respir Dis* 1993;148:1447–1451.

137. Nasser SMS, Patel M, Bell GS, Lee TH. The effect of aspirin desensitization on urinary leukotriene E_4 concentrations in aspirin-sensitive asthma. *Am J Respir Crit Care Med* 1995;151:1326–1330.

138. Wenzel SE, Larsen GL, Johnston K, Voelkel NF, Westcott JY. Elevated levels of leukotriene C_4 in bronchoalveolar lavage fluid from atopic asthmatics after endobronchial allergen challenge. *Am Rev Respir Dis* 1990;142:112–119.

139. Britton JR, Hanley SP, Tattersfield AE. The effect of an oral leukotriene D_4 antagonist L-649,923 on the response to inhaled antigen in asthma. *J Allergy Clin Immunol* 1987;79:811–816.

140. Bel EH, Timmers MC, Dijkman JH, Stahl EG, Sterk PJ. The effect of an inhaled leukotriene antagonist, L-648,051, on early and late asthmatic reactions and subsequent increase in airway responsiveness in man. *J Allergy Clin Immunol* 1990;85:1067–1075.

141. Fuller RW, Black PN, Dollery CT. Effect of the oral leukotriene D_4 antagonist LY171883 on inhaled and intradermal challenge with antigen and leukotriene D_4 in atopic subjects. *J Allergy Clin Immunol* 1989; 83:939–944.

142. Rasmussen JB, Eriksson LO, Margolskee DJ, Tagari P, Williams VC, Andersson KE. Leukotriene-D_4 receptor blockade inhibits the imme-

diate and late bronchoconstrictor responses to inhaled antigen in patients with asthma. *J Allergy Clin Immunol* 1992;90:193–201.

143. Taylor IK, O'Shaughnessy KM, Fuller RW, Dollery CT. Effect of cysteinyl-leukotriene receptor antagonist ICI 204.219 on allergen-induced bronchoconstriction and airway hyperreactivity in atopic subjects. *Lancet* 1991;337:690–694.

144. Findlay SR, Barden JM, Easley CB, Glass M. Effect of the oral leukotriene antagonist, ICI 204,219, on antigen-induced bronchoconstriction in subjects with asthma. *J Allergy Clin Immunol* 1992;89:1040–1045.

145. Nasser SM, Bell GS, Hawksworth RJ, et al. Effect of the 5-lipoxygenase inhibitor ZD2138 on allergen-induced early and late asthmatic responses. *Thorax* 1994;49:743–748.

146. Friedman BS, Bel EH, Buntinx A, et al. Oral leukotriene inhibitor (MK-886) blocks allergen-induced airway responses. *Am Rev Respir Dis* 1993;147:839–844.

147. Diamant Z, Timmers MC, Vanderveen H, et al. The effect of MK-0591, a novel 5-lipoxygenase activating protein inhibitor, on leukotriene biosynthesis and allergen-induced airway responses in asthmatic subjects *in vivo*. *J Allergy Clin Immunol* 1995;95:42–51.

148. Israel E, Juniper EF, Callaghan JT, et al. Effect of a leukotriene antagonist, LY171883, on cold air-induced bronchoconstriction in asthmatics. *Am Rev Respir Dis* 1989;140:1348–1353.

149. Israel E, Dermarkarian R, Rosenberg M, et al. The effects of a 5-lipoxygenase inhibitor on asthma induced by cold, dry air. *N Engl J Med* 1990;323:1740–1744.

150. Manning PJ, Watson RM, Margolskee DJ, Williams VC, Schwartz JI, O'Byrne PM. Inhibition of exercise-induced bronchoconstriction by MK-571, a potent leukotriene D_4-receptor antagonist. *N Engl J Med* 1990;323:1736–1739.

151. Robuschi M, Riva E, Fuccella LM, et al. Prevention of exercise-induced bronchoconstriction by a new leukotriene antagonist (SK&F 104353). *Am Rev Respir Dis* 1992;145:1285–1288.

152. Finnerty JP, Wood-Baker R, Thomson H, Holgate ST. Role of leukotrienes in exercise-induced asthma: inhibitory effect of ICI 204219, a potent LTD_4 receptor antagonist. *Am Rev Respir Dis* 1992;145:746–749.

153. Makker HK, Lau LC, Thomson HW, Binks SM, Holgate ST. The protective effect of inhaled leukotriene-D(4) receptor antagonist ICI-204,219 against exercise-induced asthma. *Am Rev Respir Dis* 1993;147:1413–1418.

154. Sladek K, Dworski R, Soja J, et al. Eicosanoids in bronchoalveolar lavage fluid of aspirin-intolerant patients with asthma after aspirin challenge. *Am J Respir Crit Care Med* 1994;149:940–946.

155. Fischer AR, Rosenberg MA, Lilly CM, et al. Direct evidence for a role of the mast cell in the nasal response to aspirin in aspirin-sensitive asthma. *J Allergy Clin Immunol* 1994;94:1046–1056.

156. Nasser SM, Bell GS, Foster S, et al. Effect of the 5-lipoxygenase inhibitor ZD2138 on aspirin-induced asthma. *Thorax* 1994;49:749–756.

157. Hui KP, Barnes NC. Lung function improvement in asthma with a cysteinyl-leukotriene receptor antagonist. *Lancet* 1991;337:1062–1063.

158. Gaddy JN, Margolskee DJ, Bush RK, Williams VC, Busse WW. Bronchodilation with a potent and selective leukotriene D_4 (LTD_4) antagonist (MK-571) in patients with asthma. *Am Rev Respir Dis* 1992;146:358–363.

159. Fischer AR, McFadden CA, Frantz R, et al. Effect of chronic 5-lipoxygenase inhibition on airway hyperresponsiveness in asthmatic subjects. *Am J Respir Crit Care Med* 1995;152:1203–1207.

160. Alving K, Sundstrom C, Matran R, Panula P, Hokfelt T, Lundberg JM. Association between histamine-containing mast cells and sensory nerves in the skin and airways of control and capsaicin-treated pigs. *Cell Tissue Res* 1991;264:529–538.

161. Cloud ML, Enas GC, Kemp J, et al. A specific LTD_4/LTE_4-receptor antagonist improves pulmonary function in patients with mild, chronic asthma. *Am Rev Respir Dis* 1989;140:1336–1339.

162. Spector SL, Smith LJ, Glass M, et al. Effects of 6 weeks of therapy with oral doses of ICI 204,219, a leukotriene D_4 receptor antagonist, in subjects with bronchial asthma. *Am J Respir Crit Care Med* 1994;150:618–623.

163. Israel E, Rubin P, Kemp JP, et al. The effect of inhibition of 5-lipoxygenase by zileuton in mild to moderate asthma. *Ann Intern Med* 1993;119:1059–1066.

Asthma, edited by P.J. Barnes, M.M. Grunstein,
A.R. Leff, and A.J. Woolcock.
Lippincott–Raven Publishers, Philadelphia © 1997.

▪ 41 ▪

Cyclooxygenase Products

Paul M. O'Byrne

Arachidonic Acid Metabolism
Role of Cyclooxygenase Products in Asthma

Stimulatory Prostaglandins and Thromboxane
Inhibitory Prostaglandins

Events occurring in the airways as a result of acute and chronic airway inflammation are important in the pathogenesis of asthma (1). This has been known for more than 100 years in patients with severe fatal asthma (2). In these patients, a large number of inflammatory cells along with epithelial desquamation, mucosal edema, and excess secretions are present in the airways (3). It now is recognized that airway inflammation is also important in milder asthma. For example, studies have demonstrated increases in airway eosinophils and mast cells in patients with very mild, stable asthma (4–7). The severity of airway hyperresponsiveness correlates with the numbers of these inflammatory cells in the airways (4). The mechanisms by which airway inflammation causes airway hyperresponsiveness and airway narrowing in asthma still are largely unknown. It is likely, however, that mediators released from effector cells in the airways cause the influx of inflammatory cells and subsequent activation of these cells. Further release of mediators from activated cells causes the bronchoconstriction, airway hyperresponsiveness and other manifestations of inflammation such as airway edema and excess airway secretions.

The investigation of the potential role of a mediator in the pathogenesis of asthma has, to date, depended on three pieces of evidence. Firstly, the inhaled mediator mimics a component of the asthmatic response. Secondly, the mediator (or its metabolite) can be measured in a biological fluid following induction of an asthmatic response. Thirdly, a selective mediator receptor antagonist or synthetase inhibitor inhibits some component of an asthmatic response. These studies tend to be performed

initially in animal models and eventually in asthmatic subjects. While several mediators have been proposed as playing a role in the pathogenesis of asthma, problems have existed that prevent convincing evidence from being obtained. These problems include a) the difficulties in measuring the mediator or its metabolite at its site of action in the airways; b) the lack of potent, specific mediator antagonists; and c) the absence of an animal model of asthma. Several animal models of airway hyperresponsiveness exist (9–11), and studies using these models have led to interesting and potentially important insights into the pathogenesis of airway hyperresponsiveness. However, definitive studies only can be performed in human subjects, which imposes major limitations to potential experimental interventions.

This review examines the evidence that one group of mediators, cyclooxygenase products of arachidonic acid metabolism, are released in human airways and are involved in the pathogenesis of asthmatic responses. In addition, evidence is considered that suggests that some metabolites from this group of mediators provide a protective function in asthmatic airways.

ARACHIDONIC ACID METABOLISM

The release of arachidonic acid from cell membrane phospholipids through the action of a family of phospholipases can result in the production of a wide variety of mediators that may be relevant in the pathogenesis of asthma (Fig. 1). These lipid mediators have traditionally been considered in two classes: mediators formed from the action of the enzyme cyclooxygenase on arachidonic acid, which are prostaglandins (PGs) or thromboxane (Tx); and mediators synthesized from the action of the

---

P. M. O'Byrne: Department of Medicine, Health Sciences Centre, McMaster University, Hamilton, Ontario L8N 3Z5 Canada.

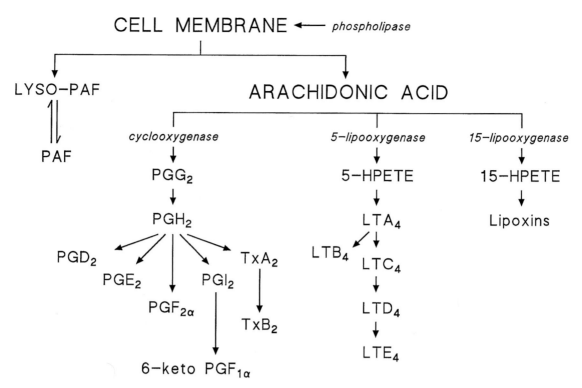

FIG. 1. The spectrum of eicosanoids produced as a consequence of arachidonic acid metabolism.

enzyme 5-lipoxygenase on arachidonic acid, which are the leukotrienes (LT). More recently, however, other products have been identified which result from the activity of different enzymes, e.g., 12- and 15-lipoxygenase. Lastly, platelet activating factor (PAF) has been recognized to be a mediator derived from arachidonic acid metabolism.

The oxidative metabolism of arachidonic acid by cyclooxygenase produces the cyclic endoperoxides PGG_2 and PGH_2. The subsequent action of prostaglandin isomerases produces either PGD_2 or PGE_2, reductive cleavage produces PGF_{2a}, while one of two terminal synthetases on the endoperoxide produces PGI_2 and TxA_2. Cyclooxygenase appears to be present in most cells; however, the cyclooxygenase metabolite(s) released from a particular cell are quite specific (for example TxA_2 from platelets, and PGI_2 from endothelial cells). This suggests that terminal synthetases are cell-specific.

The effect of 5-lipoxygenase on arachidonic acid is to produce 5-hydroperoxyeicosatetraenoic acid (5-HPETE), which is converted by dehydrase to LTA_4. This intermediate metabolite can be acted upon by epoxide hydrolase resulting in LTB_4, or by glutathione-s-transferase resulting in LTC_4, which is further metabolized to LTD_4 and LTE_4. It now is recognized that the biological activity of previously called slow reacting substance of anaphylaxis (SRS-A) is made up by the sulfidopeptide leukotrienes LTC_4, LTD_4 and LTE_4 (8). (see Chapter 40.)

PAF is derived from the activity of phospholipase A_2 on membrane phospholipids, which cleaves arachidonic acid from a glycerol backbone to form an inactive precursor, lyso-PAF. Subsequent incorporation of an acetyl group by acetyltransferase results in the active PAF. The half-life of PAF is very short, being less than 1 minute; interestingly, PAF is inactivated by removal of the acetyl group to produce the inactive precursor, lyso-PAF.

ROLE OF CYCLOOXYGENASE PRODUCTS IN ASTHMA

All of the cyclooxygenase products of arachidonic acid metabolism have been synthesized and, with the exception of thromboxane, are readily available for study. Thromboxane has an exceedingly short half-life (about 30 seconds), and studies with thromboxane have been limited to a few, very limited, experimental preparations, none of them in the airways. Fortunately, several stable thromboxane mimetics have been synthesized. These are endoperoxides, which activate the thromboxane receptor and mimic the biological actions of thromboxane.

The prostaglandins are most easily considered in two classes to evaluate their possible role in asthma. These are stimulatory prostaglandins, such as PGD_2 and PGF_{2a}, which are potent bronchoconstrictors, and inhibitory prostaglandins, such as PGE_2, which can reduce bronchoconstrictor responses and can attenuate the release of acetylcholine from airway nerves.

Prostaglandins have a variety of effects on airway function in asthma. Evidence has been obtained in both animal models of airway hyperresponsiveness and in human subjects with asthma that cyclooxygenase metabolites are involved in causing bronchoconstriction and also airway hyperresponsiveness after inhalation of allergens. There is, however, little convincing evidence that cyclooxygenase metabolites are important in causing the ongoing, persisting airway hyperresponsiveness that is characteristic of asthma. This is because several studies have not demonstrated any effect of cyclooxygenase inhibitors on stable airway hyperresponsiveness in asthmatic subjects.

The initial studies examining the role of cyclooxygenase metabolites in the pathogenesis of transient airway hyperresponsiveness after an inflammatory stimulus in animal models of airway hyperresponsiveness were carried out in dogs with airway hyperresponsiveness after inhaled ozone (9,10). The cyclooxygenase inhibitor indomethacin did not alter baseline airway responsiveness to inhaled acetylcholine, but did prevent the development of airway hyperresponsiveness after inhaled ozone (11). Despite the absence of airway hyperresponsiveness, the magnitude of the inflammatory response, as measured by the numbers of neutrophils in the airway epithelium, was not altered by indomethacin. This suggested that a cyclooxygenase product was not responsible for the chemotaxis of acute inflammatory cells into the airways after inhaled ozone; however, a cyclooxygenase product was released during the inflammatory response which caused airway hyperresponsiveness. Subsequently, a reputed combined cyclooxygenase and lipooxygenase inhibitor, BW775c, also was demonstrated to prevent the development of airway hyperresponsiveness after inhaled ozone in dogs (12). Inhibition of cyclooxygenase by indomethacin also prevents the development of airway hyperresponsiveness in other species; for example, after C_{5a} des arg in rabbits (13), and after inhaled allergen in sheep (14). The importance of cyclooxygenase products in these responses may be species-dependent. For example, BW775c, but not indomethacin, prevents airway hyperresponsiveness after inhaled ozone in guinea pigs (15), suggesting that a lipooxygenase rather than a cyclooxygenase product was causing airway hyperresponsiveness in this species.

In human subjects, cyclooxygenase products have been implicated in the pathogenesis of allergen-induced early asthmatic (16) as well as late asthmatic responses (17). This has been done by pretreating subjects with several different cyclooxygenase inhibitors. For example, Joubert et al. (18) reported that pretreatment with indomethacin inhibited the late response in 10 of 11 subjects without affecting substantially the early response. A subsequent study, however, did not confirm these observations. Pre-

treatment with indomethacin (100 mg/day) did not influence either the early or late asthmatic responses (19). These results suggested that cyclooxygenase products were not important mediators in causing these asthmatic responses. However, in this study, indomethacin significantly inhibited the development of allergen-induced airway hyperresponsiveness (19), which suggests that a cyclooxygenase product is involved in the pathogenesis of this response. The most likely candidates are the stimulatory prostaglandins PGD_2, PGF_{2a} or TxA_2.

STIMULATORY PROSTAGLANDINS AND THROMBOXANE

PGD_2 is known to be released from stimulated dispersed human lung cells *in vitro* (20) and from the airways of allergic human subjects that have been stimulated by allergen (21). PGD_2 is a bronchoconstrictor of human airways (22), and is more potent when inhaled by human subjects than PGF_{2a}. PGD_2 causes bronchoconstriction, in part, directly through stimulation of specific contractile receptors. There appears to be a single contractile receptor for all bronchoconstrictor prostaglandins and thromboxane; this is called the TP_1-receptor (23,24). Contraction also occurs indirectly through presynaptically stimulating release of acetylcholine from airway parasympathetic nerves (25,26). Subthreshold contractile concentrations of PGD_2 have been demonstrated to increase airway responsiveness to inhaled histamine and methacholine in asthmatic subjects (27). Thus, PGD_2 released in human airways after allergen inhalation has the potential to both cause acute bronchoconstriction and increase airway hyperresponsiveness to other constrictor mediators. However, specific receptor antagonists for PGD_2 or inhibitors of its production are not available to allow a precise evaluation of the importance of this cyclooxygenase metabolite in causing asthmatic responses.

PGF_{2a} also has the potential for being important in causing bronchoconstriction and airway hyperresponsiveness after inhaled allergen in human subjects. This is because it is released from human lungs, it is a potent bronchoconstrictor in asthmatic airways (28), and inhaled subthreshold constrictor concentrations can increase airway responsiveness in dogs (29) and human subjects (30,31). As with PGD_2, there are no selective PGF_{2a} receptor antagonists available, which would allow identification of the importance of these metabolites in causing these responses. Indeed, because all contractile prostaglandins may act through a single TP_1-receptor (23), differentiation of the relative importance of the contractile prostaglandins in causing asthmatic responses may prove to be extremely difficult.

Both PGD_2 and PGF_{2a} cause bronchoconstriction in human subjects through a direct effect on airway receptors and indirectly through cholinergic-mediated bronchoconstriction (26). It is not known, however, whether the cholinergic component occurs through a cholinergic reflex or through a direct presynaptic effect causing the release of acetylcholine.

TxA$_2$ is a potent constrictor of smooth muscle. TxA$_2$ originally was described as being released from platelets (32) but is now known to be released from other cells, including macrophages and neutrophils (33). As the biological half-life of TxA$_2$ is very short, implicating TxA$_2$ in disease processes has depended on measurement of its more stable metabolite thromboxane B$_2$ (TxB$_2$) in biological fluids; on the use of the stable endoperoxides U44069 or U46619, which mimic most of the biological effects of TxA$_2$ and have been used as TxA$_2$ analogs; and on the use of inhibitors of TxA$_2$ synthesis and antagonists of the TxA$_2$ receptor. Using these techniques, TxA$_2$ has been implicated in the pathogenesis of airway hyperresponsiveness in dogs (34–36) and primates (37); of the late cutaneous response to intradermal allergen (38) in humans; of the immediate response to inhaled allergen in dogs (39); of the late asthmatic response after inhaled allergen in humans (40); and of airway hyperresponsiveness in asthmatic subjects (41).

The mechanism by which TxA$_2$ causes airway hyperresponsiveness is not yet known, but possible mechanisms include presynaptic modulation of acetylcholine release or an effect on airway smooth muscle. TxA$_2$ was demonstrated to modulate acetylcholine release in airways initially by Munoz et al. (42) using the TxA$_2$ mimetic U46619, which increased the responses to field stimulation in trachealis muscle. No increase in the responses to exogenous acetylcholine by U46619 was demonstrated, suggesting that the augmentation was occurring presynaptically, through increased acetylcholine release in response to field stimulation. Further support for this hypothesis was provided by Tamaoki et al. (43), who demonstrated that aggregated platelets in an organ bath released TxA$_2$. The TxA$_2$ transiently increased the responses to field stimulation and this effect was prevented by a TxA$_2$ receptor antagonist. Once again, the responses to an exogenous cholinergic agonist was not altered by the released TxA$_2$.

Inhaled U46619 has been delivered to asthmatic airways and shown to be 178-times more potent on a molar basis than inhaled methacholine (44) (Fig. 2). Inhaled U46619 also causes very transient (< 1h) airway hyperresponsiveness (44). U46619 also causes bronchoconstriction in asthmatic airways, in part, by stimulating acetylcholine release by presynaptic stimulation of cholinergic nerves (45).

Attempts to measure the stable metabolite TxB$_2$ in human subjects during asthmatic episodes or following allergen challenge have lead to conflicting results. Both Shephard et al. (40) and Manning et al. (46) have demonstrated increased concentration of TxB$_2$ in plasma following allergen challenge. However, plasma TxB$_2$ mea-

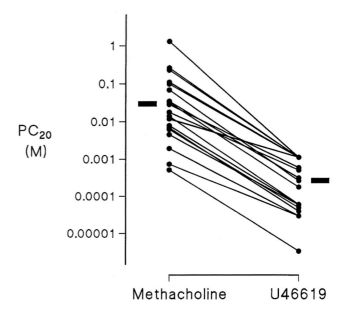

FIG. 2. The relative potency of inhaled methacholine and the inhaled thromboxane mimetic, U46619, in subjects with mild stable asthma. Airway responsiveness to each agonist is expressed as the molar provocative concentration causing a 20% fall (PC$_{20}$) in the forced expired volume in 1 second (FEV$_1$). U46619 is a mean 178 times more potent as a constrictor agonist of asthmatic airways than is methacholine. (From Saroea HG, Inman M, O'Byrne PM. U46619-induced bronchoconstriction in asthmatic subjects is mediated by acetylcholine release. *Am J Respir Crit Care Med* 1995;151: 321–324, with permission.)

surements must be viewed cautiously because of the possibility of local platelet generation of TxB$_2$. Hence, measurements should be confirmed by assaying the 2,3-dinor metabolite of TxB$_2$, which cannot come from platelet activation alone.

The TxA$_2$ synthetase inhibitor, OKY 046, administered orally, reduces acetylcholine airway hyperresponsiveness in stable asthmatic subjects (although these studies were uncontrolled), while a lipooxygenase inhibitor had no effect in these subjects (41). Thus, TxA$_2$ may be an important mediator in the pathogenesis of airway hyperresponsiveness either in stable asthma or after inhaled allergens. Subsequent studies, however, have examined the effect of the thromboxane synthetase inhibitor, CGS 13080, on airway responses after allergen challenge. CGS 13080 slightly, but significantly, inhibited the magnitude of the early, but not the late, responses after inhaled allergen (46) (Fig. 3). In addition, there was no effect on airway hyperresponsiveness to inhaled histamine measured at 24 h post allergen (46). These studies taken together suggest that thromboxane may be released following allergen challenge and is partly responsible for the early asthmatic response. However, in contrast to dogs, thromboxane is not important in causing airway hyperresponsiveness following allergen inhalation.

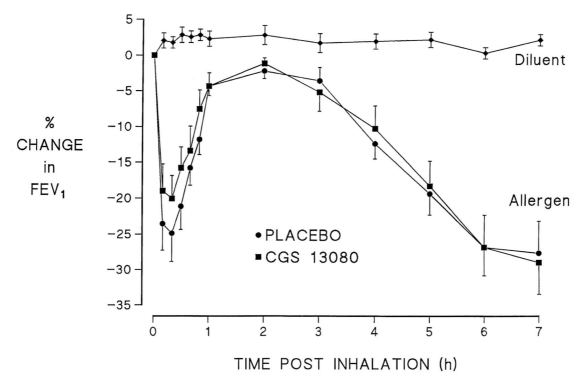

FIG. 3. The mean decrease in the forced expired volume in 1 second (FEV$_1$) after inhaled diluent (*solid circles*) and during the early and late asthmatic response after inhaled allergen after pretreatment with placebo, or with the thromboxane synthetase inhibitor CGS 13080 (*closed squares*). CGS 13080 had a small, but statistically significant (p=0.0009) effect on attenuating the magnitude of the early, but not the late, asthmatic response. (From Manning PJ, Stevens WH, Cockcroft DW, O'Byrne PM. The role of thromboxane in allergen-induced asthmatic responses. *Eur Resp J* 1991;4:667–672, with permission.)

INHIBITORY PROSTAGLANDINS

The differentiation of the prostaglandins into stimulatory and inhibitory classes is somewhat inappropriate; both PGE$_2$ and PGF$_{2a}$ can have different effects on the airways depending on the time after inhalation at which the response is measured (47,48). However, the main action of PGE$_2$ and PGI$_2$ on airway function is to relax airway smooth muscle and to antagonize the contractile responses of other bronchoconstrictor agonists. In addition PGE$_2$ is extremely effective in inhibiting the release of acetylcholine from airway cholinergic nerves (49). This effect is thought to occur through stimulation of presynaptic receptors. Inhibitory prostaglandins also are important in causing tachyphylaxis (a decreased response to repeated stimulation) to the bronchoconstrictor responses to repeated stimulation with histamine. This effect was described initially in dogs (50–54) but also has been shown to occur in guinea pigs (55) and primates (56).

The evidence that inhibitory prostaglandins play a role in modulating the contractile responses of agonists such as histamine and acetylcholine in asthmatic subjects comes from studies that have demonstrated that tachy-phylaxis occurs following repeated challenges with exercise or inhaled histamine (57,58). Both exercise refractoriness (59,60) and histamine tachyphylaxis (58) are prevented by pretreatment with indomethacin; this suggests that tachyphylaxis occurs through release of inhibitory prostaglandins in the airways. Pretreatment of asthmatic subjects with oral PGE$_1$ in doses that do not cause bronchodilation also reduces airway responsiveness to both histamine and methacholine (61). Histamine tachyphylaxis in asthmatic subjects is blocked by pretreatment with the H$_2$-receptor antagonist, cimetidine, in asthmatics (62); this suggested that H$_2$-receptor stimulation causes histamine tachyphylaxis. Stimulation of H$_2$-receptors in the lung *in vitro* previously has been shown to be associated with PGE$_2$ release in guinea-pigs (20), and PGE$_2$ release from canine trachealis by histamine is antagonized by cimetidine (63).

Contraction of asthmatic airways by histamine also reduces airway responsiveness to acetylcholine (64) and exercise (65). This lack of specificity suggests that either receptor downregulation or an alteration of the contractile properties of airway smooth muscle is occurring. Indeed, PGE causes heterologous receptor desensitization in some isolated cell systems, and airway smooth muscle has specific PGE receptors (23) mediating inhibitory effects such as relaxation. However, there is no current evidence from either *in vivo* or *in vitro* preparations to support this speculation.

These studies suggest that histamine released in asthmatic airways following exercise causes exercise-induced bronchoconstriction, but also provides partial protection against subsequent exercise-induced bronchoconstriction through PGE2 released by stimulation of histamine H_2-receptors. However, several recent studies have suggested that this notion is incorrect. First, the marked attenuation of exercise-induced bronchoconstriction by pretreatment with LTD_4-receptor antagonists (66,67) indicates that LTD_4, rather than histamine, is the main mediator of exercise-induced bronchoconstriction. Second, exercise refractoriness is not prevented by pretreatment with the H_2-receptor antagonists, cimetidine or ranitidine, which effectively prevent histamine tachyphylaxis (68). Therefore, histamine-stimulated release of inhibitory prostaglandins does not appear to be the cause of exercise refractoriness. These studies raise the possibility that exercise refractoriness is caused by leukotriene-stimulated inhibitory prostaglandin release (Fig. 4). This possibility recently has been tested in a study in asthmatic subjects who develop exercise-induced bronchoconstriction and refractoriness (69). The study demonstrated that there is an interdependence between the cyclooxygenase and lipooxygenase pathways of arachidonate metabolism in causing exercise bronchoconstriction and refractoriness in asthmatic subjects. This concept is supported by the fact that 1) exercise refractoriness and LTD_4 tachyphylaxis exist in the same subjects and the magnitude of the protection afforded by exercise correlates with that afforded by LTD_4; 2) cross refractoriness exists between exercise and LTD_4; and 3) all of these effects are attenuated by cyclooxygenase inhibition, suggesting that the release of inhibitory prostaglandins is the common mechanism affording protection after each of these stimuli. Pretreatment with inhaled PGE_2 also has been demonstrated to attenuate markedly both exercise (70) and allergen-induced bronchoconstriction (71). Thus, it appears that the mechanism of exercise-induced bronchoconstriction and refractoriness is caused by cysteinyl leukotriene release causing bronchoconstriction and leukotriene-induced PGE_2 release causing exercise refractoriness. Interestingly, bronchoconstriction after exercise is not necessary for PGE_2 release and the development of refractoriness in asthmatics (72), suggesting that the leukotriene-mediated effects in asthmatics are not dependent upon each other.

CONCLUSIONS

Despite more than 30 years of research on the release, metabolism, and clinical relevance of prostaglandins and thromboxane in lung disease, no definitive role has been identified for these mediators in the pathogenesis of persisting asthma. However, it is likely that PGD_2 and TxA_2 are involved in causing acute bronchoconstriction after stimuli such as inhaled allergen in asthmatic patients. There also is evidence that indicates that inhibitory prostaglandins can be released by asthmatic airways, reducing bronchoconstrictor responses to stimuli such as exercise, leukotrienes, and histamine. However, it is unlikely that prostaglandins are involved directly in the influx and maturation of the effector inflammatory cells or in the airway hyperresponsiveness of asthma.

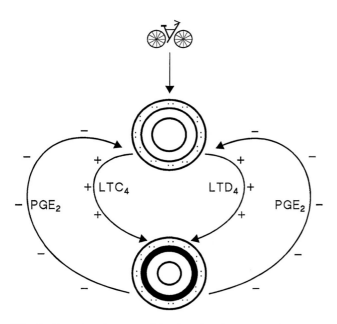

FIG. 4. Hypothesis to explain the development of exercise refractoriness in asthmatic subjects. Exercise, by cooling and drying the airways, causes release of the cysteinyl leukotrienes (LT) C4 and D4 and histamine, which are responsible for exercise-induced bronchoconstriction. The leukotrienes also cause the release of inhibitory prostaglandins, likely PGE2, which partially protect the airways against futher bronchoconstriction caused by the leukotrienes and histamine.

REFERENCES

1. O'Byrne PM, Kirby JG, Hargreave FE. Airway inflammation and hyperresponsiveness. *Am Rev Respir Dis* 1987;136:S35–S37.
2. Osler W. In: *The principals and practice of medicine.* New York: Appleton and Co., 1892;497.
3. Dunnill MS, Massarell GR, Anderson JA. A comparison of the quantitative anatomy of the bronchi in normal subjects, in status asthmaticus, in chronic bronchitis and in emphysema. *Thorax* 1969; 24:176–179.
4. Kirby JG, Hargreave FE, Gleich GJ, O'Byrne PM. Bronchoalveolar cell profiles of asthmatic and nonasthmatic subjects. *Am Rev Respir Dis* 1987;136:379–383.
5. Beasley R, Roche WR, Roberts JA, Holgate ST. Cellular events in the

bronchi in mild asthma and after bronchial provocation. *Am Rev Respir Dis* 1989;139:806–817.

6. Djukanovic R, Roche WR, Wilson JW, et al. State of the Art: mucosal Inflammation in Asthma. *Am Rev Respir Dis* 1990;142:434–457.

7. Jeffery PK, Wardlaw AJ, Nelson FC, Collins JV, Kay AB. Bronchial biopsies in asthma. An ultrastructural, quantitative study and correlation with hyperreactivity. *Am Rev Respir Dis* 1989;140:1745–1753.

8. Lewis RA, Austen KF. The biologically active leukotrienes. Biosynthesis, metabolism, receptors, functions and pharmachology. *J Clin Invest* 1984;73:889–897.

9. Lee L-Y, Bleeker ER, Nadel JA. Effect of ozone on bronchomotor response to inhaled histamine in dogs. *J Appl Physiol* 1977;43:626–631.

10. Holtzman MJ, Fabbri LM, O'Byrne PM, Gold BD, Aizawa H, Walters EH, Alpert SE, Nadel JA. Importance of airway inflammation for hyperresponsiveness induced by ozone. *Am Rev Respir Dis* 1983;127:686–690.

11. O'Byrne PM, Walters EH, Aizawa H, Fabbri LM, Holtzman MJ, Nadel JA. Indomethacin inhibits the airway hyperresponsiveness but not the neutrophil influx induced by ozone in dogs. *Am Rev Respir Dis* 1984;130:220–224.

12. Fabbri LM, Aizawa H, O'Byrne PM, et al. An anti-inflammatory drug (BW755c) inhibits airway responsiveness induced by ozone in dogs. *J Allergy Clin Immunol* 1985;76:162–166.

13. Berend N, Armour CL, Black JL. Indomethacin inhibits C5a des arg-induced airway hyperresponsiveness in the rabbit. *Am Rev Respir Dis* 1985;131:24A.

14. Lanes S, Stevenson JS, Codias E, et al. Indomethacin and FPL 55321 inhibit antigen-induced airway hyperresponsiveness in sheep. *J Appl Physiol* 1986; 61:864–872.

15. Lee HK, Murlas C. Ozone-induced bronchial hyperreactivity in guinea pigs is abolished by BW 755C or FPL 55712 but not by indomethacin. *Am Rev Respir Dis* 1985;132:1005–1009.

16. Fish JE, Ankin MG, Adkinson NF, Peterman VI. Indomethacin modification of immediate-type immunologic airway responses in allergic asthmatic and non-asthmatic subjects. *Am Rev Respir Dis* 1981; 123:609–614.

17. Fairfax AJ. Inhibition of the late asthmatic response to house dust mite by non-steroidal anti-inflammatory drugs. *Prostaglandins Leukotrienes and Medicine* 1982;8:239–248.

18. Joubert JR, Shephard E, Mouton W, Van Zyk L, Viljoen I. Non-steroid anti-inflammatory drugs in asthma: dangerous or useful therapy? *Allergy* 1985;40:202–207.

19. Kirby JG, Hargreave FE, Cockcroft DW, O'Byrne PM. The effect of indomethacin on allergen-induced asthmatic responses. *J Appl Physiol* 1989;66:578–583.

20. Yen SS, Mathe AA, Dugan JJ. Release of prostaglandins from healthy and sensitized guinea-pig lung and trachea by histamine. *Prostaglandins* 1976;11:227–239.

21. Murray JJ, Tonnel AB, Brash AR, et al. Release of prostaglandin D₂ into human airways during acute antigen challenge. *N Engl J Med* 1986;315:800–804.

22. Hardy CC, Robinson C, Tattersfield AE, Holgate ST. The bronchoconstrictor effect of inhaled prostaglandin D₂ in normal and asthmatic men. *N Engl J Med* 1984; 311:209–213.

23. Gardiner PJ. Eicosanoids and airway smooth muscle. *Pharm Ther* 1989;44:1–62.

24. Johnston SL, Freezer NJ, Ritter W, O Toole S, Howarth PH. Prostaglandin D₂-induced bronchoconstriction is mediated only in part by the tromboxane prostanoid receptor. *Eur Respir J* 1995;8:411–415.

25. Tamaoki J, Sekizawa K, Graf PD, Nadel JA. Cholinergic neuromodulation by prostaglandin D₂ in canine airway smooth muscle. *J Appl Physiol* 1987;63:1396–1400.

26. Beasley R, Varley J, Robinson C, Holgate ST. Cholinergic-mediated bronchoconstriction induced by prostaglandin D₂, its initial metabolite 9ₐ,11ᵦ-PGF₂ₐ, and PGF₂ₐ in asthma. *Am Rev Respir Dis* 1987; 136:1140–1144.

27. Fuller RW, Dixon CMS, Dollery CT, Barnes PJ. Prostaglandin D₂ potentiates airway responsiveness to histamine and methacholine. *Am Rev Respir Dis* 1986;133:252–254.

28. Thomson NC, Roberts R, Bandouvakis J, Newball H, Hargreave FE. Comparison of bronchial responses to prostaglandin F2a and methacholine. *J Allergy Clin Immunol* 1981;68:392–398.

29. O'Byrne PM, Aizawa H, Bethel RA, Chung KF, Nadel JA, Holtzman MJ. Prostaglandin F2a increases airway responsiveness of pulmonary airways in dogs. *Prostaglandins* 1984; 28:537–543.

30. Walters EH, Parrish RW, Bevan C, Smith AP. Induction of bronchial hypersensitivity: evidence for a role for prostaglandins. *Thorax* 1981;36:571–574.

31. Fish JE, Jameson A, Albright A, Norman PS. Modulation of bronchomotor effects of chemical mediators by PGF2a. *Amer Rev Respir Dis* 1984;129:A2.

32. Hamberg M, Svensson J, Samuelsson B. Thromboxanes: a new group of biologically active compounds derived from prostaglandin endoperoxides. *Proc Natl Acad Sci U S A* 1975;72:2994–2998.

33. Higgs GA, Moncada S, Salmon JA, Seager K. The source of thromboxane and prostaglandins in experimental inflammation. *Br J Pharmacol* 1983;79:863–868.

34. Aizawa H, Chung KF, Leikauf GD, et al. Significance of thromboxane generation in ozone-induced airway hyperresponsiveness in dogs. *J Appl Physiol* 1985;59:1918–1923.

35. Chung KF, Aizawa H, Becker AB, Frick O, Gold WM, Nadel JA. Inhibition of antigen-induced airway hyperresponsiveness by a thromboxane synthetase inhibitor (OKY 046) in allergic dogs. *Am Rev Respir Dis* 1986;134:258–261.

36. O'Byrne PM, Leikauf GD, Aizawa H, et al. Leukotriene B4 induced airway hyperresponsiveness in dogs. *J Appl Physiol* 1985;59:1941–1946.

37. McFarlane CS, Ford-Hutchinson AW, Letts LG. Inhibition of thromboxane (TxA₂)- induced airway hyperresponsiveness to aerosolized acetylcholine by the selective TxA₂ antagonist L655,240 in the conscious primate. *Am Rev Respir Dis* 1985;137:100A.

38. Dorsch WD, Ring J, Melzer H. A selective inhibitor of thromboxane biosynthesis enhances immediate and inhibits late cutaneous allergic reactions in man. *J Allergy Clin Immunol* 1983;72:168–174.

39. Kleeberger SR, Kolbe J, Adkinson NF Jr, Peters SP, Spannhake EW. Thromboxane contributes to the immediate antigenic response of canine peripheral airways. *J Appl Physiol* 1987;62:1589–1595.

40. Shephard EG, Malan L, Macfarlane CM, Mouton W, Joubert JR. Lung function and plasma levels of thromboxane B₂, 6-ketoprostaglandin F₁ₐ and B-thromboglobulin in antigen-induced asthma before and after indomethacin pretreatment. *Br J Clin Pharmacol* 1985;19:459–470.

41. Fujimura M, Sasaki F, Nakatsumi Y, et al. Effects of a thromboxane synthetase inhibitor (OKY-046) and a lipoxygenase inhibitor (AA-861) on bronchial responsiveness to acetylcholine in asthmatic subjects. *Thorax* 1986; 41:955–959.

42. Munoz NM, Shioya T, Murphy TM, et al. Potentiation of vagal contractile response by thromboxane mimetic U-46619. *J Appl Physiol* 1986;61:1173–1179.

43. Tamaoki J, Sekizawa K, Osborne ML, Ueki IF, Graf PD, Nadel JA. Platelet aggregation increases cholinergic neurotransmission in canine airway. *J Appl Physiol* 1987;62:2246–2251.

44. Jones GL, Saroea G, Watson RL, O'Byrne PM. The effect of an inhaled thromboxane mimetic (U46619) on airway function in human subjects. *Am Rev Respir Dis* 1992;145:1270–1275.

45. Saroea HG, Inman M, O'Byrne PM. U46619-induced bronchoconstriction in asthmatic subjects is mediated by acetylcholine release. *Am J Respir Crit Care Med* 1995;151:321–324.

46. Manning PJ, Stevens WH, Cockcroft DW, O'Byrne PM. The role of thromboxane in allergen-induced asthmatic responses. *Eur Resp J* 1991; 4:667–672.

47. Walters EH, Parrish RW, Bevan C, Parrish RW, Smith BH, Smith AP. Time-dependent effect of prostaglandin E₂ inhalation on airway responses to bronchoconstrictor agents in normal subjects. *Thorax* 1982; 37:438–442.

48. Fish JE, Newball HH, Norman PS, Peterman VI. Novel effects of PGF₂ₐ on airway function in asthmatic subjects. *J Appl Physiol* 1983;54:105–112.

49. Walters EH, O'Byrne PM, Fabbri LM, Graf PD, Holtzman MJ, Nadel JA. Control of neurotransmission by prostaglandins in canine trachealis smooth muscle. *J Appl Physiol* 1984;57:129–134.

50. Anderson WH, Krzanowski JJ, Polson JB, Szentivanyi A. Characteristics of histamine tachyphylaxis in canine tracheal smooth muscle. *Naunyn Schmiedebergs Arch Pharmacol* 1977;308:117–125.

51. Anderson WH, Krzanowski JJ, Polson JB, Szentivanyi A. Increased synthesis of prostaglandin-like material during histamine tachyphylaxis in canine tracheal smooth muscle. *Biochemical Pharmacol* 1979;28:2223–2226.

52. Anderson WH, Krzanowski JJ, Polson JB, Szentivanyi A. Prostaglan-

dins as mediators of tachyphlaxis to histamine in canine tracheal smooth mucle. In Samuelsson B, Ramwell PW, Paoletti R, eds. *Advances in prostaglandin and thromboxane research.* New York: Raven Press, 1980;7:995–1001.

53. Brink C, Duncan PG, Douglas JS. Histamine tachyphylaxis in canine isolated airways; role of endogenous prostaglandins. *J Pharm Pharmacol* 1982;34:199–201.
54. Shore S, Martin JG. Tachyphylaxis to inhaled aerosolized histamine in anesthetized dogs. *J Appl Physiol* 1985;59:1355–1363.
55. Dorsh W, Frey L. Allergen tachyphylaxis of guinea pigs *in vivo*: a prostaglandin E mediated phenomenon. *Naunyn-Schmeideberg Arch Pharmacol* 1981;317:351–356.
56. Krzanowski JJ, Anderson WH, Polsen JB, Szentivanyi A. Prostaglandin mediated histamine tachyphylaxis in subhuman primate tracheal smooth muscle. *Arch Int Pharmacodyn* 1980;247:155–162.
57. Edmunds AT, Tooley M, Godfrey S. The refractory period after exercise-induced asthma: its duration and relation to the severity of exercise. *Am Rev Resp Dis* 1978;117:247–254.
58. Manning PJ, Jones GL, O'Byrne PM. Tachyphylaxis to inhaled histamine in asthmatic subjects. *J Appl Physiol* 1987;63:1572–1577.
59. O'Byrne PM, Jones GL. The effect of indomethacin on exercise-induced bronchoconstriction and refractoriness after exercise. *Am Rev Respir Dis* 1986;134:69–72.
60. Margolskee DJ, Bigby BG, Boushey HA. Indomethacin blocks airway tolerence to repetitive exercise but not to eucapnic hyperpnea in asthmatic subjects. *Am Rev Respir Dis* 1988;137:842–846.
61. Manning PJ, Lane CG, O'Byrne PM. The effect of oral prostaglandin E$_1$ on airway responsiveness in asthmatic subjects. *Pulm Pharmacol* 1989;2:121–124.
62. Jackson PA, Manning PJ, O'Byrne PM. A new role for histamine H$_2$-receptors in asthmatic airways. *Am Rev Respir Dis* 1988;138:784–788.
63. Manning PM, Jones GL, Lane CG, O'Byrne PM. Histamine-induced prostaglandin E$_2$ release from canine tracheal smooth muscle is inhibited by H$_2$-receptor blockade. *Am Rev Respir Dis* 1988;137:373A.
64. Manning PJ, O'Byrne PM. Histamine bronchoconstriction reduces airway responsiveness in asthmatic subjects. *Am Rev Respir Dis* 1988;137:1323–1325.
65. Hamilec CM, Manning PJ, O'Byrne PM. Exercise refractoriness post histamine bronchoconstriction in asthmatic subjects. *Am Rev Respir Dis* 1988;138:794–798.
66. Manning PJ, Watson RM, Margolskee DJ, Williams V, Schartz JI, O'Byrne PM. Inhibition of exercise-induced bronchoconstriction by MK-571, a potent leukotriene D$_4$ receptor antagonist. *N Engl J Med* 1990;323:1736–1739.
67. Finnerty JP, Wood-Baker R, Thomson H, Holgate ST. Role of leukotrienes in exercsie- induced asthma. *Am Rev Respir Dis* 1992; 145:746–749.
68. Manning PJ, Watson RL, O'Byrne PM. The effect of H$_2$-receptor antagonists on exercise- induced refractoriness in asthma. *J Allergy Clin Immunol* 1992;88:125–126.
69. Manning PJ, Watson RW, O'Byrne PM. Exercise-induced refractoriness in asthmatic subjects involves leukotriene and prostaglandin interdependent mechanisms. *Am Rev Respir Dis* 1993; 148:950–954.
70. Melillo E, Woolley KL, Manning PJ, Watson RM, O'Byrne PM. Effect of inhaled PGE$_2$ on exercise-induced bronchoconstriction in asthmatic subjects. *Am J Respir Crit Care Med* 1994;149:1138–1141.
71. Pavord ID, Wong C, Williams J, Tattersfield AE. Effect of inhaled prostaglandin E$_2$ on allergen-induced asthma. *Am Rev Respir Dis* 1993;148:87–90.
72. Wilson BA, Bar-Or O, O' Byrne PM. The effects of indomethacin on refractoriness following exercise both with and without a bronchoconstrictor response. *Eur Respir J* 1994;7:2174–2178.

Asthma, edited by P.J. Barnes, M.M. Grunstein, A.R. Leff, and A.J. Woolcock.
Lippincott–Raven Publishers, Philadelphia © 1997.

▪ 42 ▪

Platelet-Activating Factor and Its Implications

Paula L. Watson and James R. Snapper

Formation and Degradation	**Inflammatory Cells and PAF**
PAF Receptors	**Microvascular Permeability**
Antagonists	**Airway Epithelium**
Asthma	**PAF Antagonists in Asthma**
Airway Obstruction and Hyperreactivity	

Platelet-activating factor (PAF) is a potent phospholipid mediator that has been implicated in a variety of inflammatory processes including asthma and the acute respiratory distress syndrome (ARDS). PAF was first identified as a product of sensitized rabbit basophils that induced histamine release from platelets (1). This finding has led to much interest and investigation of PAF in allergic rhinitis and asthma. PAF has been shown to reproduce many characteristic features of asthma such as bronchoconstriction, increased airway responsiveness, injury to bronchial epithelium, microvascular leakage, and eosinophil migration and activation.

This chapter reviews the current knowledge of PAF synthesis and degradation, receptors and antagonists, as well as the data for and against PAF's involvement of PAF in asthma.

FORMATION AND DEGRADATION

Platelet activating factor refers to a group of closely related glycerophospholipids, which contain an alkyl group at the *sn*-1 position, a acyl group at the *sn*-2 position, and a phosphocholine polar head group (Fig. 1). The structure of the classic PAF species, 1-O-alkyl-2-acetyl-*sn*-glyc-

ero-3-phosphocholine was first identified in the late 1970s and is often referred to as alkyl-PAF (2,3). The 1-O-hexadecyl (PAF_{16}) and 1-O-octadecyl (PAF_{18}) are the most common biologic forms of the mediator. Different PAF species have varying affinities for receptors and activities. The isoform tested is rarely specified in studies of PAF effects. While both PAF_{16} and PAF_{18} are active, several pharmacologic differences exist and, thus, they should not be viewed as identical (4).

Besides the basophil, PAF is formed by neutrophils, monocytes, macrophages, and eosinophils in response to activation with the calcium ionophore A23187, zymosan, and IgE (5). Early data from rat peritoneal cell populations suggested that PAF was also produced by mast cells (6). However, when these mast cells were stimulated in isolation, they failed to produce PAF, indicating that it was more than likely produced from other cells in the mixed population (7). PAF is produced by endothelial cells following stimulation with thrombin, histamine, interleukin-1, and tumor necrosis factor (8). Platelets and lymphocytes synthesize only small amounts of PAF.

PAF is often produced along with many closely related species. One such species, acyl-PAF or 1-acyl-2-alkyl-*sn*-glycero-3-phosphocholine, may be produced in greater amounts than alkyl-PAF in certain cells such as endothelial cells, basophils, and mast cells (9–11). Acyl-PAF has been demonstrated to be proinflammatory, but is less potent than alkyl-PAF (12–14). Alkyl-PAF, though produced at smaller amounts, may still be the more active species due to its greater potency. Relatively inactive species

P. L. Watson: Lung Associates, Sarasota, Florida 34239.

J. R. Snapper: Department of Medicine, Center for Lung Research, Vanderbilt University School of Medicine, Nashville, Tennessee 37232-2650.

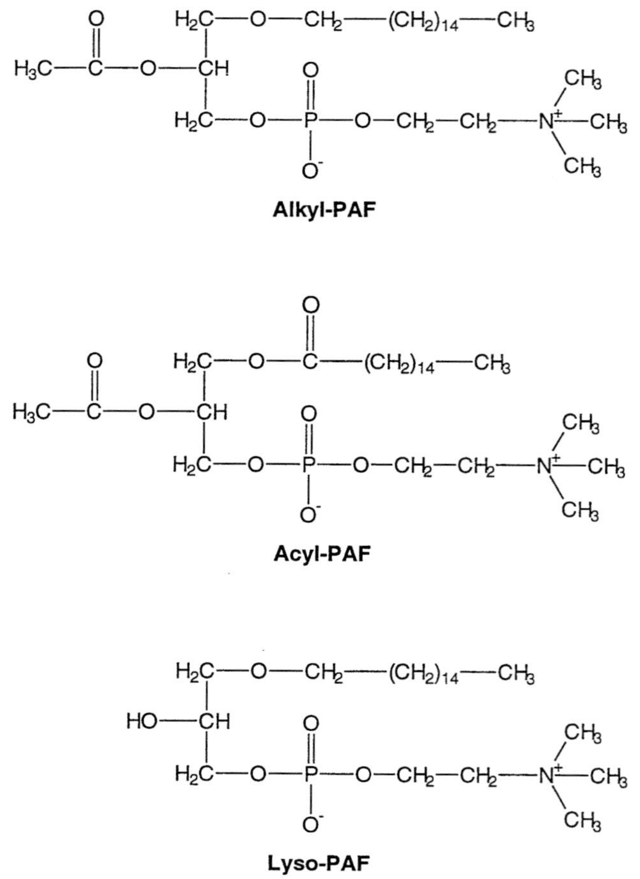

FIG. 1. Molecular structures of representative PAF species.

such as acyl-PAF may bind to PAF receptors and function as endogenously produced, competitive receptor antagonists, thus modifying the pathologic effects of "classic" PAF.

The effects of bacterial lipopolysaccharide (LPS) on PAF production by neutrophils has also been investigated. LPS does not cause neutrophils to produce PAF. However, it does have a priming effect increasing PAF production in response to stimulation with N-formyl-L-methionyl-L-leucyl-L-phenylalanine (FMLP)(15). LPS does stimulate the production of PAF by alveolar macrophages (16).

Evidence indicates that PAF is not a preformed mediator since cell damage or disruption does not lead to the release of significant amounts of the mediator. PAF is formed upon stimulation by two major enzymatic pathways (Fig. 2). The "remodeling pathway" involves a two-step process. Initially, 2-acyl groups are removed from the membrane-bound phospholipid, 1-alkyl-2-acyl-*sn*-glycero-3-phosphocholine, by phospholipase A$_2$-dependent hydrolysis, leading to the formation of 1-alkyl-2-lyso-*sn*-glycero-3-phosphocholine or lyso-PAF. This

formation of lyso-PAF is prevented by phospholipase A$_2$ inhibitors. Lyso-PAF is then converted to PAF by the addition of an acetyl group at the *sn*-2 position in a reaction catalyzed by an acetyl CoA-requiring lyso-PAF acetyltransferase. This enzyme appears to be the rate limiting step in the formation of PAF by this pathway (17). The acetyltransferase enzyme is activated by calcium ions and protein kinase phosphorylation.

The initial hydrolysis reaction of the remodeling pathway results in the liberation of a fatty acid, the most commonly produced being arachidonic acid. PAF synthesis may, thus, be accompanied by the release of free arachidonic acid which can then be used as a substrate for the production of eicosanoids. These eicosanoids may then function as secondary mediators and contribute to inflammatory effects of PAF. The simultaneous release of arachidonic acid does not fully explain the formation of eicosanoids associated with PAF since exogenous PAF has also been shown to stimulate eicosanoid production (18).

The *de novo* pathway actually consists of several mechanisms through which PAF is directly produced. The most common reaction is catalyzed by cholinephosphotransferase during which phosphorylcholine is transferred from ether-linked phospholipids. The *de novo* pathway appears to be important in the maintenance of physiologic concentrations of PAF in blood and certain tissues. This hypothesis is supported by studies of the renal medulla where PAF is produced almost exclusively by the *de novo* pathway (19). When cholinephosphotransferase is inhibited, PAF production is decreased in this tissue (20). Unlike the remodeling pathway, this pathway is not stimulated by inflammatory agents. Whereas calcium stimulates the enzymes of the remodeling pathway, it inhibits the *de novo* pathway.

While much remains to be learned regarding these two pathways, it is hypothesized that the "remodeling" pathway primarily is responsible for PAF production in inflammatory cells. Macrophages, neutrophils, and platelets have all been demonstrated to release the intermediate, lyso-PAF (21–23), whereas in cells in which PAF may function as a physiologic hormone and where it is produced on a more continuous basis, the *de novo* pathway predominates.

The inactivation of PAF is catalyzed by phosphatide-2-acetylhydrolase, which is found both intra- and extra-cellularly. This enzyme rapidly cleaves the acetate group at the *sn*-2 position to produce the lyso-PAF. Further catalysis by acyltransferase reforms the membrane phospholipid.

PAF RECEPTORS

PAF produces its effects by binding to stereospecific membrane-bound receptors belonging to the family of

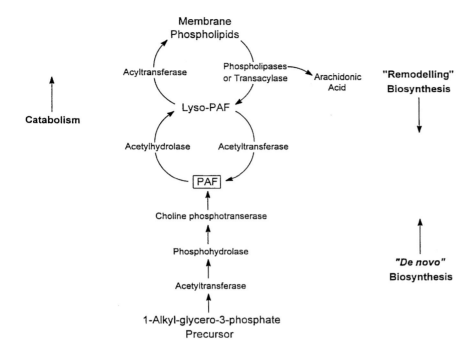

FIG. 2. Biosynthesis and catabolism of PAF.

guanine-nucleotide-binding, (G)-protein-coupled, receptors (24). PAF receptors are found in lung and heart, as well as in many inflammatory cells (e.g., eosinophils, neutrophils, and platelets), and smooth muscle (25). They have been cloned from the lung, heart, and neutrophils (26–28). Multiple conformational states for the PAF receptor have been demonstrated and the affinity of the receptors for PAF vary among these states (29). The state in which the receptors exist is influenced by the presence of certain ions such as K^+, Mg^{2+}, Ca^{2+}, and Na^+. Not only does the affinity for PAF vary with these different states, but also the cellular response secondary to the binding of the mediator. Kroegel et al. demonstrated that PAF-induced eosinophil degranulation was dependent on the presence of extracellular Ca^{2+}, and PAF-stimulated superoxide production was dependent on extracellular Mg^{2+} (30). Despite these differences, there appears to be only one major class of high affinity PAF receptors.

Both extracellular and intracellular PAF receptors have been demonstrated (31,32). Intracellular receptors

may provide a mechanism through which PAF can function as an intracellular messenger (33–35). As a result, PAF may influence the production of secondary mediators such as prostacyclin or other arachidonic metabolites (34).

Significant tachyphylaxis to PAF occurs (1,36). Possible mechanisms of this tachyphylaxis include a decrease in the number of receptor sites available, a decrease in binding affinity, an inhibition of receptor-response coupling, and an increase in acetylhydrolase activity (37–40).

ANTAGONISTS

The discovery and synthesis of multiple PAF antagonists have greatly aided in the investigation of the physiologic and pathophysiologic role. The major classes of PAF antagonists are listed in Table 1. PAF antagonists are generally competitive in nature, although irreversible antagonists exist. For instance, L-662,025, a tetrahydrofu-

TABLE 1. *PAF Receptor Antagonists*

Type	Examples
Naturally Occurring	
Ginkgolides	BN 52020, BN 52021, BN 52022, BN 52063
Lignans	Kadsurenone, fargesin, veraguensin
Semi-Synthetic or Synthetic Phospholipid analogues	CV-3988, CV-6209, E5880, SDZ 63-675, SRI 63-441
Lignan analogues	L-652,731, L-659,989
Benzodiazepine derivatives	alprazolam, WEB 2086, WEB 2170, BN 50739
Calcium channel blockers	verapamil, diltiazem
Imidazolyl derivatives	PCA-4248, UK-74,505, SDZ 64-412, BB-882
Pyridyl derivatives	RP 59227, RP 66681, SM-10661, ABT-299

ran analogue, and futoxide, isolated from the *Piper futodiadsurae* plant, are both irreversible in action (41,42).

Chinese herbal medicine includes a number of naturally occurring substances used in the treatment of asthma, allergic rhinitis, and nasal congestion, many of which have been shown over the recent years to possess PAF antagonist activity. Kadsurenone, isolated from the stem of *Piper futokadsurae*, was the first natural product found to be a potent inhibitor of PAF. *Haifenteng*, a product of the same plant, has long been used in Chinese herbal medicine for the relief of asthma. The flower buds of *Magnolia biondii*, which were used to treat allergic activity, were also shown to contain substances with significant anti-PAF activity (43). Perhaps, the most investigated of the naturally occurring antagonists are the ginkgolides. These compounds are a family of terpenoids isolated from the *Gingko biloba* tree. Of these compounds, ginkolide B (BN 52021) is the most potent PAF antagonist.

The first PAF antagonists were chemically related in structure to PAF. The first such antagonist, CV-3988, was developed by Terashita et al. in 1983 (44). This compound was then modulated to produce a more potent antagonist, CV-6209, which was 100-fold more potent than CV-3988 in inhibiting [^{3}H]PAF binding to human platelet membranes (45). Since, the list of these antagonists developed has grown rapidly. Because of their similarity to PAF, many of these antagonists also possess partial agonist activity. This has limited their usefulness, both clinically and experimentally.

Several benzodiazepines were discovered to have PAF-antagonist activity. The compounds were modified to produce agents that continued to have antagonist activity but were no longer sedating. WEB 2086 was the prototype of this class. The calcium blocking agents, diltiazem and verapamil, also have PAF-antagonist activity. A more complete discussion of PAF antagonists is included in published reviews (46,47).

ASTHMA

The measurement of PAF in body fluids is difficult because of its rapid metabolism and the lack of a simple, sensitive and specific assay. Despite this, several studies suggest an increase in PAF levels in asthmatics, alluding to a role in the pathophysiology of the disease. The bronchoalveolar lavage (BAL) fluid from asthmatics has been shown to contain PAF. By contrast, no PAF was found in the BAL fluid from normal controls or subjects with emphysema (48,49). PAF concentrations in the blood have also been demonstrated to increase in asthmatics during exacerbations of their disease, and following inhaled antigen challenge (50–52). After successful immunotherapy, PAF concentrations decrease toward normal (50). Miwa et al. (40) found reduced PAF acetylhydrolase activity in

sera from asthmatic children, which may result in increased PAF half-life and activity. Lung tissue from asthmatics contains increased concentrations of PAF receptor mRNA (53). The resulting increase in PAF receptor numbers may cause augmentation of PAF effects in these patients.

AIRWAY OBSTRUCTION AND HYPERREACTIVITY

In vivo, PAF inhalation causes a rapid onset of bronchoconstriction occurring within 2 to 3 minutes of treatment, followed by a period of bronchial hyperresponsiveness to other spasmogens such as methacholine (54). In one human study, this hyperreactivity was maximal at 3 days and persisted for up to 4 weeks (55). Airway hyperreactivity to PAF is variable and does not correlate well with the response to methacholine. PAF-induced bronchoconstriction has been demonstrated in both normal and asthmatic subjects. However, this effect is not consistent, since not even all asthmatics will experience a significant decrease in FEV$_1$ (56).

PAF induces airway smooth muscle contraction *in vitro* (57,58). This contraction is minimal in purified smooth muscle cells and appears to be the result of secondary mediator release from neighboring cells. Both serotonin and the eicosanoids have been implicated in this process (59–64). Schellenberg et al. (54) found that PAF-induced contraction of human bronchial tissue *in vitro* is dependent on the presence of platelets. It is not known if other inflammatory cells, such as neutrophils or eosinophils, may also mediate this effect.

The ability of PAF to recruit and activate inflammatory cells (as discussed following) may be the etiology of PAF-induced bronchoconstriction and hyperreactivity. Several other indirect effects may be important as well. As mentioned previously, arachidonic acid (AA) may be released during the formation of PAF. Leukotriene and cyclooxygenase products subsequently formed may exert important effects. Increased microvascular permeability and damage to the epithelium, also effects of PAF, may be important as well, and will be discussed later.

In humans, PAF-induced bronchoconstriction is not significantly decreased by treatment with the antihistamine, ketotifen, nor is it reduced by indomethacin, implying that cyclooxygenase products also are not involved (65,66). However, leukotriene-receptor antagonists have been shown to attenuate the effects of inhaled PAF (67). Bronchoconstriction induced by inhaled PAF can also be attenuated by nedocromil and, not surprisingly, by PAF antagonists (68–70).

PAF has also been implicated in the down-regulation of β-adrenergic receptors (71). Subsequent studies have failed to confirm this. PAF has not been found to alter the affinity or density of either β-adrenergic receptors, or muscarinic receptors, or H_1-histamine receptors, *in vitro* (72–74). Furthermore, the β-adrenergic agonist, albuterol, has limited effects on the reversal of PAF-induced airway obstruction (75).

Rapid tachyphylaxis is caused by PAF. Despite this, chronic inhalation and infusion both lead to smooth muscle hypertrophy and chronic epithelial damage, effects which are commonly seen in asthma (76). If, as suggested, the concentrations of PAF are greator in asthmatics, this chronic effect may represent an important pathophysiologic role for PAF, which may be even more important than the acute effects.

INFLAMMATORY CELLS AND PAF

An association between eosinophils and asthma first was described in 1908 by Ellis (77). Eosinophilic infiltration of the airways has since been recognized as a characteristic finding in patients dying of status asthmaticus (78,79). Their presence and activation in the airways of asthmatics can cause the release of various inflammatory mediators that may be important in the pathophysiology of asthma.

PAF is a potent chemotactic factor for eosinophils both *in vitro* and *in vivo* (80–82). It is, in fact, more potent than eosinophil chemotactic factor itself. PAF inhalation in guinea pigs and baboons caused a rapid increase in the eosinophils collected in bronchoalveolar lavage fluid (BAL) (83,84). Eosinophils possess PAF receptors and also produce large amounts of PAF themselves, allowing PAF to serve an autocrine function (64). *In vitro*, purified hypodense eosinophils from eosinophilic patients release PAF following IgE-mediated activation (85).

PAF also serves as an "eosinophil-activating factor." Exposure to PAF causes eosinophils to become hypodense, a change that is associated with the activation of these cells (86,87). *In vitro*, PAF leads to an increase in superoxide (O_2^-) production in human eosinophils and stimulates the formation and release of arachidonic acid products such as leukotriene C_4 (LTC_4) (88,89). In guinea pig eosinophils, PAF produces a dose-dependent increase in cyclooxygenase activity, resulting in an increase in the release of thromboxane B_2 (TXB_2) and prostaglandin E_2 (PGE_2) from these cells (90). PAF also induces the degranulation of eosinophils, releasing preformed mediators such as eosinophil peroxidase (EPO), eosinophil cationic protein (ECP), β-glucuronidase, and arylsulfatase B into the surrounding tissue (61,90,91).

The neutrophil is also a source of PAF production. PAF is a chemotactic factor to recruit other neutrophils; PAF also stimulates neutrophil activation, leading to the release of superoxide as well as granule enzymes such as β-glucuronidase and lysozyme (92,93). *In vivo*, inhalation of PAF causes activation of neutrophils and increased adherence to the endothelium (94). The antihistamine keto-

tifen has been shown to attenuate *ex vivo* PAF production by stimulated human neutrophils (95).

The lymphocyte has been increasingly implicated in the pathogenesis of asthma, especially the late phase response (96,97). An increase in CD_4+ T lymphocytes has been shown in BAL fluid from atopic asthmatics, and increased numbers of lymphocytes are found in bronchial biopsies from asthmatics (96,98–101). PAF recently has been shown to cause significant chemotaxis of lymphocytes which was attenuated by the PAF antagonist WEB 2086 (102).

In mononuclear cells, PAF regulates cytokine production and enhances alveolar macrophage production of tumor necrosis factor (103,104). This modulation of cytokines may also occur in other cell types such as the eosinophil, but this is yet unknown.

MICROVASCULAR PERMEABILITY

PAF has marked effects on the pulmonary vasculature, causing vasoconstriction and increased microvasculature permeability. This increase in permeability leads to the formation of intraluminal, mucosal, and submucosal edema resulting in a thickening of the bronchial wall. Since edema fluid is essentially incompressible, its presence will magnify the bronchoconstrictive effects of other agents, such as methacholine or allergens.

PAF is the most potent known mediator stimulating microvascular leakage. It enhances leakage of plasma tracer from airway microvasculature, as well as increases endothelial permeability to macromolecules (105–107). This effect of PAF does not appear to depend on platelets or arachidonic acid metabolites (108,109).

Structural changes in endothelial cells have been demonstrated following exposure to PAF (110). Endothelial cells are also a source of PAF production. In contrast to the inflammatory cells, the majority of PAF produced by the endothelial cell remains associated with these cells. The close association of PAF to the cell surface may function to promote the adherence and subsequent activation of eosinophils, neutrophils, and lymphocytes. The release of mediators from these recruited inflammatory cells causes further endothelial damage.

PAF antagonists have been shown to block the effect of exogenous PAF. In contrast, WEB 2086 failed to decrease the microvascular leakage following the administration of ovalbumin to sensitized guinea pigs (111). This may indicate that the microvascular leak associated with allergic phenomenon does not occur secondary to PAF release, but may involve the release of secondary mediators (112,113). Bradykinin, another mediator implicated in inflammatory states, is also a potent stimulate of microvascular leakage. This action of bradykinin is inhibited by treatment with PAF antagonists, which suggests a role for PAF in this process.

AIRWAY EPITHELIUM

Epithelial injury is a common and important finding in asthma. PAF introduced into the airways leads to a profound shedding of the epithelial cells (114–117). As with many other effects attributed to PAF, this cellular damage appears to occur secondary to the recruitment of inflammatory cells, their activation, and the subsequent release of damaging mediators (114,118). The loss of the epithelial barrier theoretically allows antigens and other airway irritants to come into direct contact with airway smooth muscle cells, stimulating bronchoconstriction.

The destruction of the epithelial barrier also results in the exposure of vagal afferent C fibers. These nerve endings contain tachykinins, which also may contribute to the findings seen with PAF exposure. For example, substance P, a tachykinin, stimulates smooth muscle contraction, epithelial ion transport, and submucosal gland secretion (119–121). PAF also causes a significant decrease in ciliary action, diminishing mucociliary transport and preventing the clearance of the increased airway secretions produced (117,122).

PAF exposure also causes an increase in mucin secretion which possibly occurs by a leukotriene mediated mechanism (123). An increase in the transepithelial secretion of chloride in canine airways has also been demonstrated (121). PAF causes a significant decrease in ciliary action, diminishing mucociliary transport, and preventing the clearance of the increased airway secretions produced (117,122).

PAF ANTAGONISTS IN ASTHMA

Several PAF antagonists have been shown to decrease antigen-induced bronchoconstriction in animal studies. Gingkolide antagonists such as BN 52021 and BN 52063 reduce bronchoconstriction and airway hyperresponsiveness in sensitized guinea pigs and rabbits (124–126). The heterocyclic antagonists SDZ 64-412 and SM-10661 and the phospholipid analogue CV-6209 block antigen-induced airway hyperreactivity in guinea pigs (127,128). The benzodiazepine derivative WEB 2086 reduces antigen-induced late, but not early, bronchoconstriction (129,130).

In human studies, 3 days of therapy with BN 52063 was shown to reduce early bronchoconstriction after antigen challenge. BN 52021 also appeared to decrease allergen-induced bronchospasm. but in only 3 of 7 subjects tested (131). In a double-blind crossover study involving 13 patients with stable asthma, Y-24180 significantly decreased the airway reactivity to methacholine when compared to placebo (132).

BN 52063 did not reduce bronchospasm induced by isocapnic hyperventilation of cold, dry air or by exercise (133). Oral UK 74,505 failed to reduce either the early or late phase allergen-induced bronchoconstriction, or the hyperresponsiveness to histamine in 8 asthmatics, despite a demonstrated reduction in platelet aggregation (134). In a crossover study, 8 atopic asthmatics treated with WEB 2086 for 1 week showed no reduction in bronchospasm or histamine responsiveness after antigen inhalation (135). In another group of atopic asthmatics on stable doses of inhaled corticosteroids, the addition of WEB 2086 did not improve the patient's ability to tolerate decreased corticosteroid doses (136). Modipafant, UK-80,067, in 120 adult asthmatics failed to improve FEV_1 or decrease use of rescue bronchodilators or airway responsiveness (137).

CONCLUSIONS

Much remains to be learned regarding the involvement of PAF with asthma. PAF is produced in asthma and allergic reactions. Unquestionably, PAF can reproduce the major characteristics of asthma such as bronchoconstriction, inflammatory infiltration of the airways, epithelial injury, microvascular leakage, and mucous secretion. While this evidence would suggest an involvement in the pathogenesis of asthma, the use of PAF antagonists has failed to consistently to produce a significant response in asthmatic subjects. The development and clinical study of more potent and pure antagonists such as ABT-299 will be helpful in further defining PAF's role in disease. Perhaps, as for inhaled corticosteroids, clinical studies employing protracted treatment with antagonists may be needed to demonstrate an effect. However, as the amount of negative data accumulates, it appears unlikely that PAF will be found to have a significant role in the pathogenesis of asthma.

ACKNOWLEDGMENTS

Supported by grants no. HL 46971 and HL 07123 from the National Institutes of Health, National Heart Lung and Blood Institute; and by the Foundation for Fellows in Asthma Research (FFAR) and the Allen & Hanburys Respiratory Institute.

REFERENCES

1. Benveniste J, PM Henson PM, CG Cochrane CG. Leukocyte- dependent histamine release form rabbit platelets. *J Exp Med* 1972; 136: 1356–1377.
2. Demopoulos CA, Pinckard RN, Hanahan DJ. Platelet-activating factor. Evidence for 1-O-alkyl-2-acetyl-sn-glyceryl-3- phosphorylcholine as the active component (a new class of lipid chemical mediators). *J Biol Chem* 1979;254:9355–9358.
3. Blank ML, Synder F, Byers LW, et al. Antihypertensive activity of an alkyl ether analog of phosphatidylcholine. *Biochem Biophys Res Commun* 1979;90:1194–1200.
4. Krell RD, McCarthy M. Pharmacologic analysis of platelet activating factor16-and 18-induced bronchoconstriction in the guinea pig. *Ann N Y Acad Sci* 1991;629:176–192.

5. Braquet P, Touqui L, Shen T, Vargaftig B. Perspectives in platelet-activating factor research. *Pharmacol Rev* 1987;39:97–145.

6. Camussi G, Mencia-Huerta J, Benveniste J. Release of platelet-activating factor and histamine I. Effect of immune complexes, complement and neutrophils on human and rabbit mastocytes and basophils. *Immunology* 1977;33:523–534.

7. Mencia-Huerta J, Benveniste J. Platelet-activating factor and macrophages I. Evidence for the release from rat and mouse peritoneal macrophages and not from mastocytes. *Eur J Immunol* 1979;9:409–415.

8. Prescott S, Zimmerman G, McIntyre T. Human endothelial cells in culture produce platelet-activating factor (1-alkyl-2- acetyl-sn-glycero-3-phosphocholine) when stimulated with thrombin. *Proc Natl Acad Sci U S A* 1984;81:3534–3538.

9. Triggiani M, Hubbard WC, Chilton FH. Synthesis of 1-acyl-2- acetyl-sn-glycero-3-phosphocholine by an enriched preparation of the human lung mast cell. *J Immunol* 1990;144:4773–4780.

10. Triggiani M, Schleimer RP, Warner JA, Chilton FH. Differential synthesis of 1-acyl-2-acetyl-sn-glyero-3- phosphocholine and platelet-activating factor by human inflammatory cells. *J Immunol* 1991;147:660–666.

11. Clay KL, Johnson C, Worthen GS. Biosynthesis of platelet activating facctor and 1-O-acyl analogues by endothelial cells. *Biochem Biophys Acta* 1991;1094:43–50.

12. Triggiani M, Goldman DW, Chilton FH. Biological effects of 1-acyl-2-acetyl-sn-glycero-3-phosphocholine in the human neutrophil. *Biochem Biophys Acta* 1991;1084:41–47.

13. Pinckard RN, Showell HJ, Castillo R, et al. Differential responsiveness of human neutrophils to the autocrine actions of 1-O-alkyl-homologs and 1-acyl analogs of platelet- activating factor. *J Immunol* 1992;148:3528–3535.

14. Columbo M, Horowitz EM, Patella V, et al. A comparative study of the effects of 1-acyl-2-acetyl-sn-glycero-3- phosphocholine and platelet activating factor on histamine and leukotriene C4 release from human leukocytes. *J Allergy Clin Immunol* 1993;92:325–333.

15. Worthen GS, Seccombe JF, Clay KL, et al. The priming of neutrophils by lipopolysaccharide for production of intracellular platelet-activating factor. Potential role in mediation of enhance superoxide secretion. *J Immunol* 1988;140:3553–3559.

16. Rylander R, Beijer L. Inhalation of endotoxin stimulates alveolar macrophage production of platelet-activation factor. *Am Rev Respir Dis* 1987;135:83–86.

17. Lee T, Lenihan D, Malone B, Roddy L, Wasserman S. Increased biosynthesis of platelet activating factor in activated human eosinophils. *J Biol Chem* 1984;259:5526–5530.

18. Lin AH, Morton DR, Gorman RR. Acetyl glyceryl ether phosphorylcholine stimulates leukotriene B4 synthesis in human polymorphonuclear leukocytes. *J Clin Invest* 1982;70:1058–1065.

19. Woodard D, Lee T, Snyder F. The final step in the de novo biosynthesis of platelet activating factor. Properties of a unique CDP-choline:1-alkyl-2-acetyl-sn-glycerol cholinephosphotransferase in microsomes from the renal inner medulla of rats. *J Biol Chem* 1987; 262:2520–2527.

20. Lee T, Malone B, Woodard D, Snyder F. Renal necrosis and the involvement of a single enzyme of the *de novo* pathway for the biosynthesis of platelet-activating factor in rat kidney inner medulla. *Biochem Biophys Res Commun* 1989;163:1002–1005.

21. Mencia-Heurta J, Ninio E, Roubin R, Benveniste J. Is platelet-activating factor (PAF-acether) synthesis by murine peritoneal cells (PC) a two-step process? *Agents and Actions* 1981;11:556–558.

22. Jouvin-Marche E, Cerrina J, Coeffier E, Duroux P, Venveniste J. Effect of the Ca2- antagonist nefedipine on the release of platelet-activating factor (PAF-acether), slow-reacting substance and -glucuronidase from human neutrophils. *Eur J Pharmacol* 1983;89:19–26.

23. Benveniste J, Chignard M, Le Couedic J, Vargaftig B. Biosynthesis of platelet-activating factor (PAF-ACETHER). II. Involvement of phospholipase A2 in the formation of PAF-ACETHER and lyso-PAF-ACETHER from rabbit platelets. *Thromb Res* 1982;25:375–385.

24. Hwang SB, Lee CS, Cheah MJ, Shen TY. Specific receptor sites for 1-O-alkyl-2-O-acetyl-sn-glycero-3-phosphocholine (platelet activating factor) on rabbit platelet and guinea pig smooth muscle membranes. *Biochemistry* 1983;22:4756–4763.

25. Hwang SB, Lam MH, Shen TY. Specific binding sites for platelet activating factor in human lung tissues. *Biochem Biophys Res Commun* 1985;128:972–979.

26. Honda Z, Nakamura M, Miki I, et al. Cloning by functional expression of platelet-activating factor receptor from guinea-pig lung. *Nature* 1991;349:342–346.

27. Nakamura M, Honda Z, Izumi T, et al. Molecular cloning and expression of platelet-activating factor receptor from human leukocytes. *J Biol Chem* 1991;266:20400–20405.

28. Sugimoto T, Tsuchimochi H, McGregor CG, et al. Molecular cloning and characterization of the platelet-activating factor receptor gene expressed in the human heart. *Biochem Biophys Res Commun* 1992;189:617–624.

29. Hwang SB, Lam MH. L-659,989: a useful probe in the detection of multiple conformational states of PAF receptors. *Lipids* 1991;26:1148–1153.

30. Kroegel C, Yukawa T, Westwick J, Barnes PJ. Evidence for two platelet activating factor receptors on eosinophils: dissociation between PAF-induced intracellular calcium mobilization degranulation and superoxides anion generation in eosinophils. *Biochem Biophys Res Commun* 1989;162:511–521.

31. Marcheselli VL, Rossowska MJ, Domingo MT, et al. Distinct platelet-activating factor binding sites in synaptic endings and in intracellular membranes of rat cerebral cortex. *J Biol Chem* 1990;265:9140–9145.

32. Hwang SB. Function and regulation of extracellular and intracellular receptors of platelet activating factor. *Ann N Y Acad Sci* 1991;629:217–226.

33. Stewart AG, Phillips WA. Intracellular platelet-activating factor regulates eicosanoid generation in guinea-pig resident peritoneal macrophages. *Br J Pharmacol* 1989;98:141–148.

34. Stewart AG, Dubbin PN, Harris T, Dusting GJ. Evidence for an intracellular action of platelet-activating factor in bovine cultured aortic endothelial cells. *Br J Pharmacol* 1989;96:503–505.

35. Tool AT, Verhoeven AJ, Roos D, Koenderman L. Platelet-activating factor (PAF) acts as an intercellular messenger in the changes of cytosolic free Ca 2- in human meutrophils induced by opsonized particles. *FEBS Lett* 1989;259:209–212.

36. O'Flaherty JT, Lees CJ, Miller CH, et al. Selective desensitization of neutrophils: further studies with 1-O-alkyl-sn-glycero-3-phosphocholine analogues. *J Immunol* 1981;127:731–737.

37. Kloprogge E, Akkerman JW. Binding kinetics of PAF-acether (1-O-alkyl-2-acetyl-sn-glycero-3-phosphocholine) to intact human platelets. *Biochem J* 1984;223:901–909.

38. Chesney CM, Pifer DD, Huch KM. Desensitization of human platelets by platelet activating factor. *Biochem Biophys Res Commun* 1985;127:24–30.

39. Homma H, Hanahan DJ. Attenuation of platelet activating factor (PAF)-induced stimulation of rabbit platelet GTPase by phorbol ester, dibutyryl cAMP, and desensitization: concomitant effects on PAF receptor binding characteristics. *Arch Biochem Biophys* 1988;262:32–39.

40. Miwa M, Miyake T, Yamanaka T, et al. Characterization of serum platelet-activating factor (PAF) acetylhydrolase. Correlation between deficiency of serum PAF acetylhydrolase and respiratory symptoms in asthmatic children. *J Clin Invest* 1988;82:1983–1991.

41. Hussaini, I, Shen T. A specific, photolavile and irreversible antagonist (L-662,025) of the PAF-receptor. *Biochem Biophys Res Commun* 1989;161:23–30.

42. Shen T, Hussaini I, Hwang S, Chang M. Recent development of platelet-activating factor antagonists. *Adv Prostaglandin Thromboxane Leukot Res* 1989;19:359–362.

43. Pan J, Hensens O, Zink D, Chang M, Hwang S. Lignans with platelet-activating factor antagonist activity from Magnoliz biondii. *Phytochem Photobiol* 1987;26:1377–1379.

44. Terashita Z, Tsushima S, Yoshioka Y, Nomura H, Inada Y, Nishikawa K. CV-3988-A specific antagonist of platelet- activating factor (PAF). *Life Sci* 1983;32:1975–1982.

45. Terashita Z, Imura Y, Takatani M, Tsushima S, Nishikawa K. CV-6209-A highly potent platelet-activating factor (PAF) antagonist in *in vitro* and *in vivo*. *J Pharmacol Exp Ther* 1987;242:263–268.

46. Hwang SB. Platelet-activating factor: Receptors and receptor antagonists. In: Cunningham FM, ed. *Lipid mediators*. London: Academic Press, 1994;297–360.

47. Koltai M, Guinot P, Hosford D, Braquet PG. Platelet-activating factor

antagonists: scientific background and possible clinical applications. *Adv Pharmacol* 1994;28:81–167.

48. Stenton SC, Court EN, Kingston WP, et al. Platelet- activating factor in bronchoalveolar lavage fluid from asthmatic subjects. *Eur Respir J* 1990;3:408–413.

49. Horii T, Okazaki H, Kino M, Kobayashi Y, Satouchi K, Saito K. Platelet-activating factor detected in bronchoalveolar lavage fluids from an asthmatic patient. *Lipids* 1991;26:(12)1292–1296.

50. Hsieh KH, Ng CK. Increased plasma platelet-activating factor in children with acute asthmatic attacks and decreased *in vivo* and *in vitro* production of platelet-activating factor after immunotherapy. *J Aller Clin Immunol* 1993;91:650–657.

51. Kurosawa M, Yamashita T, Kurimoto F. Increased levels of blood platelet-activating factor in bronchial asthmatic patients with active symptoms. *Allergy* 1994;49:60–63.

52. Chan-Yeung M, Lam S, Chan H, et al. The release of platelet- activating factor into plasma during allergen-induced bronchoconstriction. *J Aller Clin Immunol* 1991;87:667–673.

53. Shirasaki H, Nishikawa M, Adcock IM, et al. Expression of platelet-activating factor receptor mRNA in human and guinea pig lung. *Am J Respir Cell Mol Biol* 1994;10:533–537.

54. Schellenberg R, Walker B, Snyder F. Platelet-dependent contraction of human bronchi by platelet-activating factor. *J Aller Clin Immunol* 1983;71:145A.

55. Cuss F, Dixon C, Barnes P. Effects of inhaled platelet activating factor on pulmonary function and bronchial responsiveness in man. *Lancet* 1986;ii:189–192.

56. Louis R, Bury T, Corhay J, Radermecker MF. Acute bronchial and hematologic effects following inhalation of a single dose of PAF. Comparison between asthmatics and normal subjects. *Chest* 1994; 106:1094–1099.

57. Popovich KJ, Sheldon G, Mack M, et al. Role of platelets in contraction of canine tracheal muscle elicited by PAF *in vitro. J Appl Physiol* 1988;65:914–920.

58. Kaye MG, Smith LJ. Effects of inhaled leukotriene D₄ and platelet-activating factor on airway reactivity in normal subjects. *Am Rev Respir Dis* 1990;141:993–997.

59. Murphy TM, Munoz NM, Moss J, et al. PAF-induced contraction of canine trachea mediated by 5-hydroxytryptamine *in vivo. J Appl Physiol* 1989;66:638–643.

60. Underwood DC, Kadowitz PJ. Analysis of bronchoconstrictor responses to platelet-activating factor in the cat. *J Appl Physiol* 1989;67: 377–382.

61. Spencer DA, Evans JM, Green SE, et al. Participation of the cysteinyl leukotrienes in the acute bronchoconstrictor response to inhaled platelet activating factor in man. *Thorax* 1991;46:441–445.

62. Taylor IK, Ward PS, Taylor GW, et al. Inhaled PAF stimulates leukotriene and thromboxane A₂ production in humans. *J Appl Physiol* 1991;71:1396–1402.

63. Kidney JC, Ridge SM, Chung KF, Barnes PJ. Attenuation of platelet-activating factor induced bronchoconstriction by the leukotriene D₄ receptor antagonist ICI 204,219. *Am Rev Respir Dis* 1993;147:215–217.

64. Vargaftig B, Lefort J, Chignard M, Benveniste J. Platelet-activating factor induces a platelet-dependent bronchoconstriction unrelated to the formation of prostaglandin derivatives. *Eur J Pharmacol* 1980;65: 185–192.

65. Chung K, Minette P, McCusker M, Barnes P. Ketotifen inhibits the cutaneous but not the airway responses to platelet- activating factor in man. *J Allergy Clin Immunol* 1988;81:1192–1197.

66. Smith L, Rubin A, Patterson R. Mechanism of platelet activating factor-induced bronchoconstriction in humans. *Am Rev Respir Dis* 1990; 141:993–997.

67. Spencer D, Evans J, Green S, Piper P, Costello J. Bronchospasm induced by inhaled platelet-activating factor is released by a selective cysteinyl-leukotriene antagonist in normal man. *Am Rev Respir Dis* 1990;141:218.

68. Hayes JP, Chang KF, Barnes PJ. Attenuation of platelet- activating factor induced bronchoconstriction by nedocromil sodium. *Eur Respir J* 1992;5:1193–1196.

69. Roberts NM, McCusker M, Chung KF, Barnes PJ. Effect of a PAF antagonist, BN52063, on PAF-induced bronchoconstriction in normal subjects. *Br J Clin Pharmacol* 1988;26:65–72.

70. Adamus WS, Heuer HO, Meade CJ, Schilling JC. Inhibitory effects of the new PAF acether antagonist WEB-2086 on pharmacologic changes induced by PAF inhalation in human beings. *Clin Pharmacol Ther* 1990;47:456–462.

71. Agrawal D, Townley R. Effect of platelet-activating factor on beta-adrenoceptors in human lung. *Biochem Biophys Res Comm* 1987; 143:1–6.

72. Robertson DN, Coyle AJ, Rhoden KJ, et al. The effect of platelet-activating factor on histamine and muscarinic receptor vunction in guinea pig airways. *Am Rev Respir Dis* 1988;137:1317–1322.

73. Barnes PJ, Grandordy BM, Page CP, et al. The effect of platelet activating factor on pulmonary -adrenoceptors. *Br J Pharmacol* 1987;90: 709–715.

74. Agrawal DK, Bergren DR, Byorth PJ, Townley RG. Platelet- activating factor induces nonspecific desensitization to bronchodilators in guinea pigs. *J Pharmacol Exp Ther* 1991;259:1–7.

75. Chung KF, Dent G, Barnes PJ. Effects of salbutamol on bronchoconstriction, bronchial hyperresponsiveness, and leucocyte responses induced by platelet activating factor in man. *Thorax* 1989; 44:102–107.

76. Metzger W, Ogden-Ogle C, Atkinson L, Mustafa J, Park K. Chronic PAF inhalation induces inflammatory changes in allergic rabbits. *Clin Soc Clin Res* 1989;37:926A.

77. Ellis A. The pathological anatomy of bronchial asthma. *Am J Med Sci* 1908;136:407–429.

78. Huber H, Koessler K. The pathology of bronchial asthma. *Arch Intern Med* 1922;30:689–760.

79. Dunnill M. The pathology of asthma, with special reference to changes in the bronchial mucosa. *J Clin Pathol* 1960;31:27–33.

80. Wardlaw AJ, Moqbel R, Cromwell O, Kay AB. Platelet- activating factor. A potent chemotactic and chemokinetic factor for human eosinophils. *J Clin Invest* 1986;78:1701–1706.

81. Little M, Casale T. Comparison of platelet-activating factor-induced chemotaxis of normodense and hypodense eosinophils. *J Allergy Clin Immunol* 1991;88:187–192.

82. Sanjar S, Aoki S, Boubekeur K, et al. Eosinophil accumulation in pulmonary airways of guinea-pigs induced by exposure to an aerosol of platelet-activating factor: effect of anti-asthma drugs. *Br J Pharmacol* 1990;99:267–272.

83. Arnoux B, Denjean A, Page C, Nolibe N, Morley J, Benveniste J. Accumulation of platelets and eosinophils in baboon lung after PAF-acether challenge: inhibition by ketotifen. *Am Rev Respir Dis* 1988; 137:855–860.

84. Coyle A, Unwin S, Page C, Touvay C, Villain B, Braquet P. The effect of the selective antagonist BN 52021 on PAF and antigen-induced bronchial hyperreactivity and eosinophil accumulation. *Eur J Pharmacol* 1988;148:51–58.

85. Capron M, Benveniste J, Braquet P, Capron A. Role of PAF-acether in IgE-dependent activation of eosinophils. In Braquet P, ed. *New trends in lipid mediators research: the role of platelet-activating factor in immune disorders.* Basel: Karger, 1988;10–17.

86. Shult P, Lega M, Jadid S, et al. The presence of hypodense eosinophils and diminished chemiluminescence response in asthma. *J Allergy Clin Immunol* 1988;81:429–437.

87. Fukuda T, Dunnette S, Reed C, Ackerman S, Peters M, Gleich G. Increased numbers of hypodense eosinophils in the blood of patients with bronchial asthma. *Am Rev Respir Dis* 1985;132:981–985.

88. Zoratti EM, Sedgwick JB, Vrtis RR, Busse WW. The effect of platelet-activating factor on the generation of superoxide anion in human eosinophils and neutrophils. *J Aller Clin Immunol* 1991;88:749–758.

89. Bruynzeel P, Kok P, Hamelink M, Kijne A, Verhagen J. Platletlet-activating factor induces leukotriene C₄ synthesis by purified human eosinophils. *Prostaglandins* 1987;34:205–214.

90. Kroegel C, Yukawa T, Dent G, Cahnez P, Chung K, Barnes P. Platelet activating factor induces eosinophil perioxidase releases from purified human eosionphils. *Immunology* 1988;64:559–562.

91. Kroegel C, Yukawa T, Dent G, Chanez P, Chung K, Barnes P. Stimulation of degranulation from human eosinophils by platelet activating factor. *J Immunol* 1989;142:3518–3526.

92. Lellouch-Tubiana A, Lefort J, Simon M, Pfister A, Vargaftig B. Eosinophil recruitment into guinea pig lungs after PAF-aceter and allergen administration. *Am Rev Respir Dis* 1988;137:948–954.

93. O'Flaherty J. Neutrophil degranulation: evidence pertaining to its medsiation by the combined effects of leukotriene B₄, platelet-activating factor, and 5-HETE. *J Cell Physiol* 1985;122:229–239.

94. Wardlaw A, Chung K, Mogbel R, et al. Effects of inhaled PAF in humans on circulating and bronchoalveolar lavage fluid neutrophils. *Am Rev Respir Dis* 1990;141:386–392.

95. Nakamura T, Kuriyama M, Ishihara K, Matsumura Y, Miyamoto T. Platelet-activating factor (PAF) in allergic diseases: inhibitory effects of anti-allergic drugs, Ketotifen and three kampo medicines on PAF production. *Lipids* 1991;26:1297–1300.

96. Kay A. Lymphocytes in asthma. *Respir Med* 1991;85:87–90.

97. Rochester C, Rankin J. Is asthma T-cell mediated? *Am Rev Respir Med* 1991;144:1005–1007.

98. Gerblich A, Salik H, Schuyler M. Dynamic T-cell changes in peripheral blood and bronchoalveolar lavage afrter antigen bronchoprovocation in asthmatics. *Am Rev Respir Dis* 1987;91:533–537.

99. Metzger W, Zavala D, Richerson H, Moseley P, Iwamota P, Monick M, et al. Local allergen challenge and bronchoalveolar lavage of allergic asthmatic lungs: description of the model and lacal airway inflammation. *Am Rev Respir Dis* 1987;135:433–440.

100. Jeffery P, Wardlaw A, Nelson F, Collins J, Kay A. Bronchial biopsies in asthma: an ultrastructural, quantitative study and correlation with hyperreactivity. *Am Rev Respir Dis* 1989;140:1745–1753.

101. Azzawi M, Bradley B, Jeffery P, Frew A, Wardlaw A, Knowles G, et al. Identification of activated T lymphocytes and eosiophils in brochial biopsies in stable atopic asthma. *Am Rev Respir Dis* 1990; 142:1407–1413.

102. McFadden R, Bishop M, Caveney A, Fraher L. Effect of platelet activation factor (PAF) on the migration of human lymphocytes. *Thorax* 1995;50:265–269.

103. Rola-Pleszczynski M, Stankova J. Modulation of cytokine gene expression by LTB4 and PAF: transcriptional and posttranscriptional regulation. In Bailey J, ed. *Prostaglandins, leukotrienes, lipoxins, and PAF*. New York: Plenum Press, 1991;329–334.

104. Dubois C, Bissonnette E, Rola-Pleszczynski M. Platelet- activating factor (PAF) enhances tumor necrosis factor production by alveolar macrophages. Prevention by PAF receptor antagonists and lipoxygenase inhibitors. *J Immunol* 1989;143:964–970.

105. Evans TW, Chung KF, Rogers DF, Barnes PJ. Effect of platelet-activating factor on airway vascular permeability: possible mechanisms. *J Appl Physiol* 1987;63:479–484.

106. O'Donnell SR, Erjefalt I, Persson CG. Early and late tracheobronchial plasma exudation by platelet-activating factor administered to the airway mucosal surface in guinea pigs: effects of WEB 2086 and enprofylline. *J Pharmacol Exp Ther* 1990;254:65–70.

107. Handley DA, Arbeeny CM, Lee ML, et al. Effect of platelet activating factor on endothelial permeability to plasma macromolecules. *Immunopharmacol* 1984;8:137–142.

108. Evans T, Chung K, Rogers D, Barnes P. Effects of platelet-activating factor on airway vascular permeability: possible mechanisms. *J Appl Physiol* 1987;63:479–484.

109. O'Donnell S, Barnett C. Microvascular leakage to platelet activating factor in guinea-pig trachea and bronchi. *Eur J Pharmacol* 1987;138: 385–396.

110. Grigorian GY, Ryan US. Platelet-activating factor effects on bovine pulmonary artery endothelial cells. *Circ Res* 1987;61:389–395.

111. Evans TW, Dent G, Rogers DF, et al. Effect of a PAF antagonist, WEB 2086, on airway microvascular leakage in the guinea-pig and platelet aggregation in man. *Br J Pharmacol* 1988;94:164–168.

112. Sirois MG, Plante GE, Braquet P, Sirois P. Role of eicosanoids in PAF-induced increases of the vascular permeability in rat airways. *Br J Pharmacol* 1990;101:896–900.

113. Tokuyama K, Lotvall JO, Morikawa A, et al. Role of thromboxane A2 in airway microvascular leakage induced by inhaled platelet-activating factor. *J Appl Physiol* 1991;71:1729–1734.

114. Camussi G, Pawlowski I, Tetta C, et al. Acute lung inflammation induced in the rabbit by lacal instillation of 1-O-octadecyl-2-acetyl-sn-glyceryl-3-phosphorylcholine or of native platelet-activating factor. *Am J Pathol* 1983;112:78.

115. Lellouch-Tubiana A, Lefort J, Simon MT, et al. Eosinophil recruitment into guinea pig lungs after PAF-acether and allergen administration. Modulation by prostacyclin, platelet depletion, and selective antagonists. *Am Rev Respir Dis* 1988;137:948.

116. Takizawa H, Ishii A, Suzuki S, et al. Bronchoconstriction induced by platelet-activating factor in the guinea pig and its inhibition by CV-3988, a PAF antagonist: serial changes in findings of lung histology and bronchoalveolar lavage cell population. *Int Arch Allergy Appl Immunol* 1988;86:375.

117. Hisamatsu K, Ganbo T, Nakazawa T, Murakami Y. Platelet activating factor induced respiratory mucosal damage. *Lipids* 1991; 26:1287–1291.

118. Wardlaw AJ, Chung KF, Moqbel R, et al. Effects of inhaled PAF in humans on circulating and bronchoalveolar lavage fluid neutrophils. Relationship to bronchoconstriction and change in airway responsiveness. *Am Rev Respir Dis* 1988;137:948–392.

119. Tanaka D, Grunstein M. Mechanisms of substance P-induced contractionof rabbit airway smooth muscle. *J Appl Physiol* 1984; 57: 1551–1557.

120. Al-Bazzaz F, Kelsey J, Kaage W. Substance P stimulation of chloride secretion by canine tracheal mucosa. *Am Rev Respir Dis* 1985; 131: 86–89.

121. Tamaoki J, Sakai N, Isono K, et al. Effects of platelet-activating factor on bioelectric properties of cultured tracheal and bronchial epithelia. *J Allergy Clin Immunol* 1991;87:1042.

122. Nieminen MM, Moilanen EK, Nyholm JE, et al. Platelet- activating factor impairs mucociliary transport and increases plasma leukotriene B4 in man. *Eur Respir J* 1991;4:551–560.

123. Goswami SK, Ohashi M, Stathas P, Marom ZM. Platelet- activating factor stimulates secretion of respiratory glycoconjugate from human airways in culture. *J Aller Clin Immunol* 1989;84:726.

124. Lagente V, Touvay C, Randon J, et al. Interference of the PAF-acether antagonist BN 52021 with passive anaphylaxis in the guinea-pig. *Prostaglandins* 1987;33:265–274.

125. Touvay C, Etienne A, Braquet P. Inhibition of antigen-induced lung anaphylaxis in the gunea-pig by BN 52021 a new specific paf-acether receptor antagonist isolated from Ginkgo biloba. *Agents Actions* 1986;17:371–372.

126. Coyle AJ, Page CP, Atkinson L, et al. Modification of allergen-induced airway obstruction and airway hyperresponsiveness in an allergic rabbit model by the selective platelet-activating factor antagonist, BN 52021. *J Allergy Clin Immunol* 1989;84:960–967.

127. Ishida K, Thomson RJ, Beattie LL, et al. Inhibition of antigen-induced airway hyperresponsiveness, but not acute hypoxia nor airway eosinophilia, by an antagonist of platelet-activating factor. *J Immunol* 1990;144:3907–3911.

128. Morooka S, Uchida M, Imanishi N. Platelet-activating factor (PAF) plays an important role in the immediate asthmatic response in guinea-pig by augmenting the response to histamine. *Br J Pharmacol* 1992;105:756–762.

129. Abraham WM, Stevenson JS, Garrido R. A possible role for PAF in allergen-induced late responses: modification by a selective antagonist. *J Appl Physiol* 1989;66:2351–2357.

130. Soler M, Sielczak MW, Abraham WM. A PAF antagonist blocks antigen-induced airway hyperresponsiveness and inflammation in sheep. *J Appl Physiol* 1989;67:406–413.

131. Hsieh KH. Effects of PAF antagonist, BN52021, on the PAF-, methacholine-, and allergen-induced bronchocnstriction in asthmatic children. *Chest* 1991;99:877–882.

132. Hozawa S, Haruta Y, Shinichi, I, Yamakido M. Effects of a PAF antagonist, Y-24180, on bronchial hyperresponsiveness in patients with asthma. *Am J Respir Crit Care Med* 1995;152:1198–1202.

133. Wilkens JH, Wilkens H, Uffmann J, et al. Effects of a PAF-antagonist (BN 52063) on bronchoconstriction and platelet activation during exercise induced asthma. *Br J Clin Pharmacol* 1990;29:85–91.

134. Kuitert LM, Hui KP, Uthayarkumar S, et al. Effect of the platelet-activating factor antagonist UK-74,505 on the early and late response to allergen. *Am Rev Respir Dis* 1993;147:82–86.

135. Freitag A, Watson RM, Matsos G, et al. Effect of a platelet activating factor antagonist, WEB 2086, on allergen induced asthmatic responses. *Thorax* 1993;48:594–598.

136. Spence DP, Johnston SL, Calverley PM, et al. The effect of the orally active platelet-activating factor antagonist WEB 2086 in the treatment of asthma. *Am J Respir Crit Care Med* 1994;149:1142–1148.

137. Kuitert L, Angus R, Barnes N, Barnes P, Bone M, Chung K, et al. Effect of a novel potent platelet-activating factor antagonist, modipafant, in clinical asthma. *Am J Respir Crit Care Med* 1995; 151: 1331–1335.

Asthma, edited by P.J. Barnes, M.M. Grunstein, A.R. Leff, and A.J. Woolcock.
Lippincott–Raven Publishers, Philadelphia © 1997.

▪ 43 ▪

Bradykinin

Peter J. Barnes

Formation	Neural Effects
Metabolism	Vascular Actions
Receptors	Effects on Secretions
Effects on Airways	**Bradykinin Antagonists**
Airway Smooth Muscle	**Role in Asthma?**

Many mediators have been implicated in the pathophysiology of asthma, but the role of individual mediators will only become apparent with the use of potent and selective antagonists or synthesis inhibitors, which are now becoming available for many mediators, including bradykinin (1). Bradykinin has long been considered a mediator involved in asthma, since the first demonstration of bronchoconstriction after inhaled bradykinin in asthmatic patients (2). The development of potent and long-lasting bradykinin receptor antagonists has focused attention on the role of bradykinin in the pathophysiology of asthma and the potential of bradykinin antagonists in asthma therapy (3–6).

FORMATION

Kinins are vasoactive peptides formed during the inflammatory response from the α_2-globulins high and low molecular weight kininogens by the action of kininogenases (Fig. 1). Kininogenases include plasma kallikrein and tissue kallikrein. HMW and LMW kininogens are derived from the same gene (containing 11 exons and 10 introns) as a consequence of alternative splicing (7). Both kininogens are synthesized in the liver. HMW kininogen is present only is plasma, whereas LMW kininogen also occurs in tissues. Two kinins are

formed in humans—the nonapeptide bradykinin (Arg-Pro-Pro-Gly-Phe-Ser-Pro-Phe-Arg), which is generated from HMW kininogen, and the decapeptide lysyl-bradykinin (kallidin), which is generated from LMW kininogen. Kallidin is rapidly converted to bradykinin by the enzyme aminopeptidase-N (8). There is evidence for kinin activity in BAL fluid of asthmatic patients and it is likely that bradykinin is formed from plasma exuded from the inflamed airways, by the action of plasma and tissue kallikreins (9,10). The concentration of kallikrein and kinins in bronchoalveolar lavage fluid increases after allergen challenge (10). HMW kininogen is the preferred substrate for plasma kallikrein, which is generated from the inactive prekallikrein by contact with certain negatively charged surfaces, including basement membrane components and proteoglycans, such as heparin released from mast cells. Tissue kallikreins are produced in glandular secretions and release kinins from both HMW and LMW kininogens. Tissue kallikrein has been localized immunocytochemically to serous cells in the submucosal glands of human airways (11). α1-Antiprotease is an effective inhibitor of kallikrein in the circulation, but in tissues kallikrein may remain activated for prolonged periods.

Other proteases which may be produced by inflammatory cells may also generate kinins from kininogens. Mast cell tryptase is a weak kininogenase *in vitro* under conditions of low pH. It is unlikely that this occurs to any significant extent *in vivo* (12). There is also some evidence that neutrophils and platelets may release proteases with kininogen activity (13).

P. J. Barnes: Department of Thoracic Medicine, Imperial College of Medicine at The National Heart and Lung Institute, London SW3 6LY United Kingdom.

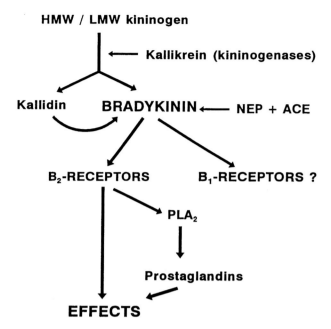

FIG. 1. The generation of bradykinin.

METABOLISM

Bradykinin is subject to rapid enzymatic degradation and has a plasma half-life of less than 30 seconds. Bradykinin is metabolized by several peptidases (collectively known as kininases) which may be present in the asthmatic airways (Fig. 2). Angiotensin converting enzyme (ACE, kininase 2) may be important for degrading bradykinin in the circulation, since it is localized to endothelial cells, but may also be present in the airway tissue (14). ACE inhibitors potentiate both the bronchoconstrictor and microvascular leakage produced by bradykinin, suggesting that this may be the mechanism of ACE inhibitor-induced cough (15,16).

The enzyme neutral endopeptidase 24.11 (NEP) appears to be the most important enzyme in degradation of bradykinin in the airways. Phosphoramidon, which inhibits NEP, enhances the bronchoconstrictor effect of bradykinin both *in vitro* and *in vivo* (15–17). Since NEP is expressed on airway epithelium, the shedding of airway epithelium in asthma may result in the enhanced airway responses to bradykinin seen in asthmatic patients.

A third enzyme, carboxypeptidase-N (kininase 1), may be important in degrading bradykinin in the circulation, but an inhibitor of this enzyme DL-2-mercaptomethyl-3-guanidinoethyl thiopropionic acid (MGPTA) does not have any effect on the bronchoconstrictor response to bradykinin *in vivo* (15). Carboxypeptidase-N converts bradykinin to [desArg^9]-bradykinin which is selective for B$_1$-receptors (18). Aminopeptidase M, which converts lysyl-bradykinin to bradykinin, is widely distributed, so that kallidin is rapidly converted to bradykinin. This enzyme is expressed in airway epithelial cells (19).

RECEPTORS

Bradykinin exerts several effects on the airways which are mediated via specific surface receptors. At least two subtypes of bradykinin receptor are recognized based on the rank order of potency of kinin agonists (18):

B$_1$: des-Arg^{10}-lysylBK > des-Arg^9-BK = lysylBK >> BK

B$_2$: BK = lysylBK >> des-Arg^{10}-lysylBK > des-Arg^9-BK

B$_1$-receptors are selectively activated by lyslybradykinin (kallidin) and des-Arg^9-bradykinin, but have only been described under certain experimental conditions, and these observations have usually been confined to rabbits (20). However, recent studies have suggested that B$_1$-receptors are expressed in chronic inflammation induced by interleukin(IL)-1β and IL-6 in rats, and may play an important role in hyperalgesia (21). The effects of bradykinin on airways are mediated via B$_2$-receptors, and there is no evidence for functional B$_1$-receptors in the airways. A B$_3$-receptor has also been proposed in airway smooth muscle of sheep, but there are doubts about its existence, since it has been defined with weak antagonists (22,23).

The B$_2$-receptor in animals and humans and a human B$_1$-receptor have now been cloned (24–26). Both have the

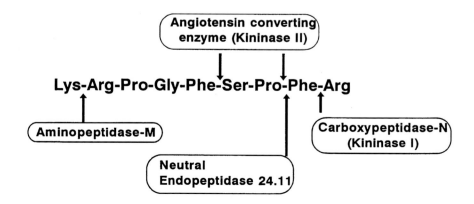

FIG. 2. The metabolism of bradykinin.

typical seven transmembrane spanning segment structure common to all G-protein coupled receptors (24). Interestingly, des-Arg^{10}-lysylbradykinin is much more potent than des-Arg^9-bradykinin at the human B$_1$-receptor, suggesting that potential B$_1$-receptor responses in human tissues may be missed if des-Arg^9-bradykinin is used as the only selective probe (26). Pharmacological studies suggest that there may be subtypes of the B$_2$-receptor which may be more clearly defined using molecular probes (27,28). Using low stringency probes, there is no evidence in human cDNA libraries for additional types of bradykinin receptor.

The distribution of B$_2$-receptors has been mapped out in human and guinea pig lung by autoradiography using [^{3}H]bradykinin (29). There is a high density of binding sites in bronchial and pulmonary vessels, particularly on endothelial cells. Epithelial cells, airway smooth muscle (particularly in peripheral airways), submucosal glands, and nerves are also labeled, indicating that bradykinin may have diverse effects on airway function. A particularly high density of labeling is observed in the lamina propria immediately beneath the epithelium; it is not clear what cellular structures are labeled, but a very similar pattern of labeling has been observed in other epithelialized structures (30). The subepithelial binding sites may be to nerves and superficial blood vessels.

EFFECTS ON AIRWAYS

Bradykinin has many effects on airway functions, some of which are mediated via direct activation of B$_2$-receptors on target cells. Others are mediated indirectly via the release of other mediators or neurotransmitters (Table 1, Fig. 3).

TABLE 1. *Effects of Bradykinin on Airways Mediated Via B2-Receptors*

Bronchoconstriction	Direct effect
	Cholinergic reflex effect
	Release of neuropeptides (NKA)
	Release of prostanoids
Neural effects	Activation of sensory nerves (C-fibers)
	Release of neuropeptides
	Activation of cholinergic reflex
Plasma exudation	Direct effect (post-capillary venules)
	Release of neuropeptides (SP)
	Release of platelet activating factor
Vasodilatation	Direct effect on arterioles
	Release of nitric oxide from endothelial cells
	Release of neuropeptides (CGRP)
Secretions	Increased ion transport from epithelial cells
	Release of prostanoids from epithelial cells
	Release of nitric oxide from epithelial cells
	Increased mucociliary clearance
	Increased mucus secretion (submucosal glands)

Airway Smooth Muscle

Inhaled bradykinin is a potent bronchoconstrictor in asthmatic patients, but has little or no effect, even in high concentrations, in normal individuals, suggesting an increased responsiveness of airway smooth muscle to bradykinin as observed with other spasmogens (31–33). *In vitro* bradykinin is only a weak constrictor of proximal human airways, proposing that its potent bronchoconstrictor effect in asthmatic patients is mediated indirectly.

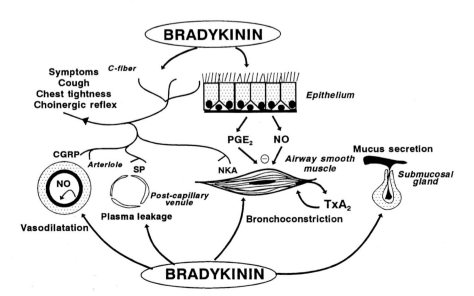

FIG. 3. The effects of bradykinin on the airways.

However, bradykinin is more potent in constricting peripheral human airways (34,35). This is partly via a direct stimulation of B_2-receptors on airway smooth muscle, and partly via the release of thromboxane. Bradykinin contracts airway smooth muscle *in vitro*, but in guinea pig airways *in vitro* bradykinin has weak and variable effects which are influenced by the presence of airway epithelium and by the activity of local degrading enzymes (36). Bradykinin causes relaxation of intact guinea pig airways *in vitro*, but constricts airways if epithelium is removed mechanically (17,37). Bradykinin releases the bronchodilator prostaglandin E_2 from epithelial cells and epithelial removal, therefore, reduces the functional antagonism, resulting in a bronchoconstrictor effect of bradykinin (37). Furthermore, NEP is strongly expressed on airway epithelial cells and, thus, epithelial removal may reduce bradykinin metabolism (38). A combination of indomethacin (to inhibit PGE_2 formation) and phosphoramidon (which inhibits NEP) mimics the effect of epithelial removal (17). Epithelial shedding, commonly observed in asthmatic airways, could be a factor contributing to the increased bronchoconstrictor effect of bradykinin in asthma. The bronchoconstrictor effect of bradykinin in ferrets *in vitro* and in guinea pig *in vivo* is enhanced by the inhibition of both NEP by phosphoramidon and of angiotensin converting enzyme by captopril (14,15). In small human bronchi *in vitro* bradykinin may cause relaxation when airway epithelium is intact, but consistently causes constriction after epithelial removal and phosphoramidon had a similar effect (35).

Intravenous bradykinin causes intense bronchoconstriction in guinea pigs, which is markedly inhibited by indomethacin, suggesting that a bronchoconstrictor cyclo-oxygenase product (probably thromboxane) largely mediates this effect (39). The bronchoconstrictor response to bradykinin instilled directly into the airways is not reduced by indomethacin, however, implying a different mechanism of bronchoconstriction after airway delivery of the mediator (39). In airway inflammation it is likely that bradykinin would be formed at the airway surface from plasma kininogens exuded into the airway lumen from leaky superficial blood vessels. In human subjects inhibition of cyclo-oxygenase by aspirin or flurbiprofen similarly has no effect on the bronchoconstrictor effect of inhaled bradykinin (32,40). Similarly, antihistamines have no effect on bradykinin-induced bronchoconstriction, suggesting that mast cell mediator release is not involved (40).

The bronchoconstrictor effect of bradykinin in guinea pigs is also modulated by nitric oxide (NO), since pretreatment with aerosolized NO synthase inhibitors significantly potentiates the bronchoconstrictor effect of bradykinin, whether administered intravenously or via inhalation (41). The source of NO is unclear, but may be from airway epithelium, which expresses constitutive and inducible forms of NO synthase (42,43).

The bronchoconstrictor response to both intravenous and inhaled bradykinin in guinea pigs is mediated via a B_2-receptor, since the B_2-receptor antagonists NPC 349 and icatibant inhibit the bronchoconstrictor response, whereas a B_1-selective antagonist is ineffective (44–46). In human airways the bronchoconstrictor effect of bradykinin is also mediated via a B_2-receptor, since icatibant blocks the bronchoconstrictor response to bradykinin *in vitro* and the B_1-selective agonist [desArg^9]-bradykinin has no effect on airway function in asthmatic patients (33–35).

Neural Effects

Perhaps the most important property of bradykinin is its ability to activate C-fiber nociceptive sensory nerve endings (47). Bradykinin is the mediator of inflammatory pain, and in the airways, this may be manifest as cough and tightness of the chest, commonly observed after inhalation of bradykinin in patients with asthma (32,48). Bradykinin stimulates bronchial C-fibers in dogs (49). In guinea pigs, the bronchoconstrictor response to instilled bradykinin is reduced by atropine and by capsaicin pretreatment which depletes neuropeptides from sensory nerves, indicating that both a cholinergic reflex and release of neuropeptides from sensory nerves are involved (39). Indeed, a combination of atropine and capsaicin pretreatment largely abolishes the bronchoconstrictor response to instilled bradykinin, but has little effect on the bronchoconstrictor response to intravenous bradykinin (largely inhibited by indomethacin) (39). Bradykinin also releases tachykinins from perfused guinea pig lung and rat trachea, and enhances the bronchoconstrictor response to electrical field stimulation (mediated by release of endogenous tachykinins) in guinea pig bronchi *in vitro*; it enhances the non-adrenergic non-cholinergic bronchoconstrictor response to vagus nerve stimulation *in vivo* as well (50–53). Tachykinin antagonists have an inhibitory effect on the bronchoconstrictor and plasma exudation response to bradykinin in guinea pigs, suggesting that release of tachykinins from sensory nerves is an important component of both responses (54). The effect of bradykinin on airway sensory nerves is blocked by icatibant, indicating that B_2-receptors are involved in the release of neuropeptides from sensory nerves (52). Although studies in human subjects are more limited, a non-selective tachykinin antagonist (FK-224) has been shown to reduce the bronchoconstrictor response to inhaled bradykinin in asthmatic patients, suggesting that bradykinin releases tachykinins in asthmatic airways (55).

Single fiber recordings from sensory nerves of guinea pig airways indicate that bradykinin is a potent activator of C-fibers, and that this is a direct action since it is not blocked by cyclo-oxygenase inhibition, but is blocked by icatibant (56). Bradykinin has no direct effect on the release of neurotransmitters from airway cholinergic nerves (52).

In asthmatic patients, the bronchoconstrictor response to bradykinin is also reduced by anticholinergic pretreatment, indicating that a cholinergic reflex is involved (32). Pre-treatment with cromolyn sodium and nedocromil sodium is very effective in inhibiting the airway response to bradykinin. This may indicate the involvement of C-fiber activation in asthmatic airways, since both drugs have been found to inhibit C-fibers in animals (57–59). This suggests that bradykinin may be an important mediator of cough and chest discomfort in asthma. Bradykinin induces cough in normal and asthmatic subjects and has been implicated in ACE inhibitor-induced cough, seen in approximately 10% of patients on chronic therapy (60, 61). ACE inhibitor cough is reduced by cyclo-oxygenase inhibitors, suggesting that prostaglandins (such as PGE_2 or $PGF_{2\alpha}$) may be involved (62). Endogenous bradykinin may stimulate the release of these prostaglandins in the larynx and trachea leading to cough, although it is not clear why only a proportion of patients are affected. ACE inhibitors do not worsen asthma, presumably because other enzymes, such as NEP, are more important in degrading bradykinin in airways. Indeed, a potent ACE inhibitor has been shown to have no effect on the bronchoconstrictor response to inhaled bradykinin in asthmatic patients, indicating that ACE is not of critical importance in degrading bradykinin in the lumen of human airways .

Vascular Actions

Bradykinin is a potent inducer of airway microvascular leak and causes a prolonged leakage at all airway levels. This is partly mediated via the release of platelet-activating factor (PAF), since a PAF antagonist markedly inhibits the prolonged leak (64). The immediate leakage response to bradykinin is partly mediated via the release of neuropeptides (probably substance P) from airway sensory nerves. The effect of bradykinin plasma exudation is partly reduced by pretreatments with the non-peptide NK_1-receptor antagonist, CP 96,345 (54). The effect of bradykinin on leakage is mediated via B_2-receptors which are localized to endothelial cells on post-capillary venules since B_2-antagonists inhibit the leakage response (45,46). The microvascular leakage induced by bradykinin is enhanced by inhibition of both NEP and ACE (65).

Bradykinin is a potent vasodilator of bronchial vessels and causes an increase in airway blood flow (66–68). This is consistent with the high density of bradykinin receptors on bronchial vessels, and suggests that a major effect of bradykinin in asthma may be hyperemia of the airways (29).

Effects on Secretions

Bradykinin stimulates airway mucus secretion from canine and feline airways in vitro, presumably indicating a direct effect of bradykinin on submucosal glands (69,70). This is consistent with the demonstration of B_2-receptors on these glands by autoradiographic mapping (29). Bradykinin also stimulates the release of mucus glycoproteins from human nasal mucosa in vitro (70).

Bradykinin stimulates ion transport in airway epithelial cells, which is mediated via the release of prostaglandins (71). The effects of bradykinin on epithelial cells are mediated via B_2-receptors (72). In animals, bradykinin also stimulates mucociliary clearance and ciliary beating via the release of prostaglandins (73,74). Inhaled bradykinin increased mucociliary clearance in normal humans, presumably reflecting the stimulatory effect of bradykinin on airway secretions (75).

BRADYKININ ANTAGONISTS

Several peptide antagonists to bradykinin (B_2-antagonists) have now been developed. The early antagonists were relatively weak and were rapidly degraded in tissues (76,77). One such antagonist D-Arg-[Hyp³,Thi⁵,⁸, D-Phe⁷]bradykinin (NPC 349) reduces the bronchoconstrictor and microvascular leakage response to bradykinin, but its effect is transient (44,45). In view of its short duration of action, it is surprising that the same antagonist appears to block allergen-induced airway hyperresponsiveness in sheep which follows many hours after allergen exposure (78,79). A related antagonist [D-Arg⁰,Hyp³,D-Phe⁷]bradykinin (NPC567) is unable to inhibit the effect of bradykinin on nasal secretions, even when given at the same time as bradykinin, presumably because of rapid local metabolism (80). Icatibant (HOE 140, D-Arg[Hyp³,Thi⁶,D-Tic⁷,Oic⁸]bradykinin is a selective B_2-receptor antagonist, which is not only potent, but has a long duration of action in animals in vivo since it is resistant to enzymatic degradation (3,4). This antagonist is potent at inhibiting the bronchoconstrictor and microvascular leakage response to bradykinin and the effect of bradykinin on airway sensory nerves (46,52,81). Clinical studies with icatibant are limited, but there is some evidence that nasal application reduces the nasal blockage induced by allergen in patients with allergic rhinitis (82). Other potent bradykinin antagonists have also been developed, such as D-Arg[Hyp³,Thi⁵,D-Tic⁷,Tic⁸]bradykinin (NPC16731), but these peptide antagonists have poor oral bioavailability and are expensive to manufacture (5). Recently, non-peptide antagonists have been identified (5). WIN 64338 is a non-peptide B_2-receptor antagonist that has been shown to block the bronchoconstrictor action of bradykinin in airway smooth muscle in vitro (83). Although this compound is not very potent, it may lead to the development of more potent non-peptide drugs in the future.

ROLE IN ASTHMA?

While the role of bradykinin in asthma is still not clear, the development of potent and stable B_2-receptor antagonists offers the possibility of clarifying its role in airway disease in the near future (84). Bradykinin is generated in asthmatic airways by the action of various kininogenases generated in the inflammatory response on HMW kininogen present in the exuded plasma and on LMW kininogens secreted in the airways. Bradykinin has been detected in bronchoalveolar lavage fluid (BAL) of asthmatic patients (10). The degradation of bradykinin may be impaired in the airways if NEP is down-regulated in asthmatic airways or epithelial shedding occurs (38). In experimental animals, exposure to interleukin-1β by aerosol markedly increases the bronchoconstrictor response to bradykinin; this may be due to reduced expression of NEP in the airways (85,86).

Bradykinin has many effects on the airway which are relevant to asthma. Perhaps the most important property of bradykinin is its ability to activate nociceptive nerve fibers in the airway, since these may mediate the cough and chest tightness, symptoms inherently characteristic of asthma. This effect of bradykinin may be enhanced by hyperesthesia of sensory nerves in the airways which have been sensitized by inflammatory mediators. Inhalation of bradykinin in asthmatic patients rather closely mimics an asthma attack; in addition to wheezing, patients observe chest tightness, coughing, and, sometimes, itching under the chin, common sensory manifestations during an asthma exacerbation. Bradykinin is also a potent bronchoconstrictor in asthmatic patients and after allergen challenge, there is a disproportionate increase in responsiveness to bradykinin compared to methacholine which may not be maximal until several days after allergen challenge and may persist for several days (88). This may be a reflection of airway sensory nerve hyperesthesia. In patients with perennial rhinitis, there is a marked increase in response to topically applied bradykinin, with evidence of enhanced reflex effects (89).

The contribution of bradykinin to asthma will only be determined with the use of potent and specific bradykinin antagonists which are now in clinical development. Since many mediators may contribute to the pathophysiology of asthma it is difficult to predict how useful bradykinin antagonists will be; they may be of particular value in controlling asthma symptoms, but it is unlikely that they will be as effective as β-agonists or steroids. Such agents may be predicted to be effective in symptom control, but it is not clear whether they will also have any anti-inflammatory effect in animal studies.

REFERENCES

1. Barnes PJ, Chung KF, Page CP. Inflammatory mediators and asthma. *Pharmacol Rev* 1988;40:49–84.
2. Herxheimer H, Streseman E. The effect of bradykinin aerosol in guinea-pigs and in man. *J Physiol* 1961;158:38P.
3. Hock FJ, Wirth K, Albus U, et al. HOE 140 a new potent and long acting bradykinin-antagonist: in vitro studies. *Br J Pharmacol* 1991;102:769–773.
4. Wirth K, Hock FJ, Albus U, et al. HOE 140, a new potent and long acting bradykinin antagonist: in vivo studies. *Br J Pharmacol* 1991;102:774–777.
5. Farmer SG, Burch RM, Kyle DJ, Martin JA, Meeker SN, Togo J. D-Arg[Hyp³-Thi⁵-D-Tic⁷-Tic⁸]-bradykinin, a potent antagonist of smooth muscle BK_2 receptors and BK_3 receptors. *Br J Pharmacol* 1991;102:785–787.
6. Barnes PJ. Bradykinin and asthma. *Thorax* 1992;47:979–983.
7. Nakanishi S. Substance P precursor and kininogen: their structures, gene organizations, and regulation. *Physiol Rev* 1987;67:1117–1142.
8. Proud D, Kaplan AP. Kinin formation: mechanisms and role in inflammatory disorders. *Annu Rev Immunol* 1988;6:49–83.
9. Christiansen SC, Proud D, Cochrane CG. Detection of tissue kallikrein in the bronchoalveolar lavage fluid of asthmatic patients. *J Clin Invest* 1987;79:188–197.
10. Christiansen SC, Proud D, Sarnoff RB, Juergens U, Cochrane CG, Zuran BL. Elevation of tissue kallikrein and kinin in the airways of asthmatic subjects after endobronchial allergen challenge. *Am Rev Respir Dis* 1992;145:900–905.
11. Proud D, Vio CP. Localization of immunoreactive tissue kallikrein in human trachea. *Am J Respir Cell Mol Biol* 1993;816:16–19.
12. Proud D, Siekierski ES, Bailey GS. Identification of human lung mast cell kininogenase as tryptase and relevance of tryptase kininogenase activity. *Biochem Pharmacol* 1988;37:1473–1480.
13. Proud D. Kinins as mediators of lung disease. In: Crystal RG, West JB, Barnes PJ, Cherniak NS, Wiebel ER, eds. *The lung scientific foundations*. New York: Raven Press, 1995.
14. Dusser DJ, Nadel JA, Sekizawa K, Graf PD, Borson DB. Neutral endopeptidase and angiotensin converting enzyme inhibitors potentiate kinin-induced contraction of ferret trachea. *J Pharmacol Exp Ther* 1988;244:531–536.
15. Ichinose M, Barnes PJ. The effect of peptidase inhibitors on bradykinin-induced bronchoconstriction in guinea-pigs in vivo. *Br J Pharmacol* 1990;101:77–80.
16. Lötvall JO, Tokuyama K, Barnes PJ, Chung KF. Bradykinin-induced airway microvascular leakage is potentiated by captopril and phosphoramidon. *Eur J Pharmacol* 1991;200:211–218.
17. Frossard N, Stretton CD, Barnes PJ. Modulation of bradykinin responses in airway smooth muscle by epithelial enzymes. *Agents Actions* 1990;31:204–209.
18. Regoli D, Barabé J. Pharmacology of bradykinin and related kinins. *Pharm Rev* 1980;32:1–46.
19. Proud D, Subauste MC, Ward RE. Glucocorticoids do not alter peptidase expression on a human bronchial epithelial cell line. *Am J Respir Cell Mol Biol* 1994;11:57–65.
20. Regoli D, Drapeau G, Rovgro P, et al. Conversions of kinins and their antagonists into bX1X-receptor activators and blockers in isolated vessels. *Eur J Pharmacol* 1986;127:219–224.
21. Davies AJ, Perkins MN. The involvement of bradykinin B_1 and B_2 receptor mechanisms in cytokine-induced mechanical hyperalgesia in rat. *Br J Pharmacol* 1994;113:63–68.
22. Farmer SG, Burch RM, Meeker SA, Wilkins DE. Evidence for a pulmonary B_3-bradykinin receptor. *Mol Pharmacol* 1989;36:1–8.
23. Farmer SG, Ensor JE, Burch RM. Evidence that cultured airway smooth muscle cells contain bradykinin B_2 and B_3 receptors. *Am J Respir Cell Mol Biol* 1991;4:273–277.
24. McEachern AE, Shelton GR, Bhakta S, et al. Expression cloning of a rat B_2-badykinin receptor. *Proc Natl Acad Sci U S A* 1991;88:7724–7728.
25. Hess JF, Borkowski JA, Young GS, Strader CD, Ransom RW. Cloning and pharmacological characterization of a human bradykinin (BK-2) receptor. *Biochem Biophys Res Commun* 1992;184:260–268.
26. Mencke JG, Borkowski JA, Bierilo KK, et al. Expression and cloning of a human B_1 bradykinin receptor. *J Biol Chem* 1995;269:21583–21586.

27. Braas KM, Manning DC, Perry DC, Snyder SH. Bradykinin analogues: differential agonist and antagonist activities suggesting multiple receptors. *Br J Pharmacol* 1988;94:3–5.

28. Hall JM. Bradykinin receptors: pharmacological properties and biological roles. *Pharmacol Ther* 1992;56:131–190.

29. Mak JCW, Barnes PJ. Autoradiographic visualization of bradykinin receptors in human and guinea pig lung. *Eur J Pharmacol* 1991;194:37–44.

30. Manning DC, Snyder SH. Bradykinin receptors localized by quantitative autoradiography in kidney, ureter and bladder. *Am J Physiol* 1989; 256:FSu9–18.

31. Simonsson BG, Skoogh BE, Bergh NP, Anderson R, Svedmyr N. *In vivo* and *in vitro* effect of bradykinin on bronchial motor tone in normal subjects and in patients with airway obstruction. *Respiration* 1973;30:378–388.

32. Fuller RW, Dixon CMS, Cuss FMC, Barnes PJ. Bradykinin-induced bronchoconstriction in man: mode of action. *Am Rev Respir Dis* 1987; 135:176–180.

33. Polosa R, Holgate ST. Comparative airway responses to inhaled bradykinin, kallidin and [desArg⁹]-bradykinin in normal and asthmatic airways. *Am Rev Respir Dis* 1990;142:1367–1371.

34. Molimard M, Martin CA, Naline E, Hirsch A, Advenier C. Contractile effects of bradykinin on the isolated human bronchus. *Am J Resp Crit Care Med* 1994;149:123–127.

35. Hulsmann AR, Raatgep HR, Saxena PR, Kerrebijn KF, de Jongste JC. Bradykinin-induced contraction of human peripheral airways mediated by both bradykinin B₂ and thromboxane receptors. *Am J Respir Crit Care Med* 1994;150:1012–1018.

36. Bhoola KD, Bewley J, Crothers DM, Cingi MI, Figeroa CD. Kinin receptors on epithelial cells and smooth muscle of trachea. *Adv Exp Med Biol* 1990;247A:1–6.

37. Bramley AM, Samhoun MN, Piper PJ. The role of epithelium in modulating the responses of guinea-pig trachea induced by bradykinin *in vitro*. *Br J Pharmacol* 1990;99:762–766.

38. Nadel JA. Neutral endopeptidase modulates neurogenic inflammation. *Eur Respir J* 1991;4:745–754.

39. Ichinose M, Belvisi MG, Barnes PJ. Bradykinin-induced bronchoconstriction in guinea-pig *in vivo*: role of neural mechanisms. *J Pharmacol Exp Ther* 1990;253:1207–1212.

40. Polosa R, Phillips GD, Lai CKW, Holgate ST. Contribution of histamine and prostanoids to bronchoconstriction provoked by inhaled bradykinin in atopic asthma. *Allergy* 1990;45:174–182.

41. Ricciardolo FLM, Nadel JA, Yoishihara S, Geppetti P. Evidence for reduction of bradykinin-induced bronchoconstriction in guinea pigs by release of nitric oxide. *Br J Pharmacol* 1994;113:1147–1152.

42. Robbins RA, Barnes PJ, Springall DR, et al. Expression of inducible nitric oxide synthase in human bronchial epithelial cells. *Biochem Biophys Res Commun* 1994;203:209–218.

43. Asano K, Chee CBE, Gaston B, et al. Constitutive and inducible nitric oxide synthase gene expression, regulation and activity in human lung epithelial cells. *Proc Natl Acad Sci U S A* 1994;91:10089–10093.

44. Jin LS, Seeds E, Page CP, Schachter M. Inhibition of bradykinin-induced bronchoconstriction in the guinea pig by synthetic B₂ receptor antagonist. *Br J Pharmacol* 1988;97:598–602.

45. Ichinose M, Barnes PJ. Bradykinin-induced airway microvascular leakage and bronchoconstriction are mediated via a bradykinin B₂-receptor. *Am Rev Respir Dis* 1990;142:1104–1107.

46. Sakamoto T, Elwood W, Barnes PJ, Chung KF. Effect of HOE 140, a new bradykinin antagonist, on bradykinin and platelet-activating factor-induced bronchoconstriction and airway microvascular leakage in guinea pig. *Eur J Pharmacol* 1992;213:376–373.

47. Geppetti P. Sensory neuropeptide release by bradykinin: mechanisms and pathophysiological implications. *Regul Pept* 1993;47:1–23.

48. Steranka LR, Manning DL, de Haas C, et al. Bradykinin as a pain mediator: receptors are localized to sensory neurons and antagonists have analgesic effects. *Proc Natl Acad Sci U S A* 1988;85:3245–3249.

49. Kaufman MP, Coleridge HM, Coleridge JCG, Baker DG. Bradykinin stimulates afferent vagal C-fibres in intrapulmonary airways of dogs. *J Appl Physiol* 1980;48:511–517.

50. Saria A, Martling CR, Yan Z, Theodorsson-Norheim E, Gamse R, Lundberg JM. Release of multiple tachykinins from capsaicin-sensitive nerves in the lung by bradykinin, histamine, dimethylphenylpiperainium, and vagal nerve stimulation. *Am Rev Respir Dis* 1988;137:1330–1335.

51. Ray NJ, Jones AJ, Keen P. Morphine, but not sodium cromoglycate, modulates the release of substance P from capsaicin-sensitive neurones in the rat trachea *in vitro*. *Br J Pharmacol* 1991;102:797–800.

52. Miura M, Belvisi MG, Barnes PJ. Effect of bradykinin in airway neural responses *in vitro*. *J Appl Physiol* 1992;73:1537–1541.

53. Miura M, Belvisi MG, Barnes PJ. Modulation of nonadrenergic noncholinergic neural bronchoconstriction by bradykinin in anesthetized guinea pigs *in vivo*. *J Pharmacol Exp Ther* 1994;268:482–486.

54. Sakamoto T, Barnes PJ, Chung KF. Effect of CP-96,345, a non-peptide NK₁-receptor antagonist against substance P-, bradykinin-, and allergen-induced airway microvascular leak and bronchoconstriction in the guinea pig. *Eur J Pharmacol* 1993;231:31–38.

55. Ichinose M, Nakajima N, Takahashi T, Yamauchi H, Inoue H, Takishima T. Protection against bradykinin-induced bronchoconstriction in asthmatic patients by a neurokinin receptor antagonist. *Lancet* 1992;340:1248–1251.

56. Fox AJ, Barnes PJ, Urban L, Dray A. An *in vitro* study of the properties of single vagal afferents innervating guinea-pig airways. *J Physiol* 1993;469:21–35.

57. Dixon CMS, Barnes PJ. Bradykinin induced bronchoconstriction: inhibition by nedocromil sodium and sodium cromoglycate. *Br J Clin Pharmacol* 1989;270:8310–8360.

58. Dixon N, Jackson DM, Richards IM. The effect of sodium cromoglycate on lung irritant receptors and left ventricular receptors in anasthetized dogs. *Br J Pharmacol* 1979;67:569–574.

59. Jackson DM, Norris AA, Eady RP. Nedocromil sodium and sensory nerves in the dog lung. *Pulm Pharmacol* 1989;2:179–184.

60. Choudry NB, Fuller RW, Pride NB. Sensitivity of the human cough reflex: effect of inflammatory mediators prostaglandin E₂, bradykinin and histamine. *Am Rev Respir Dis* 1989;140:137–141.

61. Fuller RW. Cough associated with angiotensin converting enzyme inhibitors. *J Hum Hypertens* 1989;3:159–161.

62. McEwan JR, Choudry NB, Fuller RW. The effect of sulindac on the abnormal cough reflex associated with dry cough. *J Pharmacol Exp Ther* 1990;255:161–164.

63. Dixon CMS, Fuller RW, Barnes PJ. The effect of an angiotensin converting enzyme inhibitor, ramipril, on bronchial responses to inhaled histamine and bradykinin in asthmatic subjects. *Br J Clin Pharmacol* 1987;23:91–93.

64. Rogers DF, Dijk S, Barnes PJ. Bradykinin-induced plasma exudation in guinea pig airways: involvement of platelet activating factor. *Br J Pharmacol* 1990;101:739–745.

65. Lötvall JO, Tokuyama K, Löfdahl C, Ullman A, Barnes PJ, Chung KF. Peptidase modulation of noncholinergic vagal bronchoconstriction and airway microvascular leakage. *J Appl Physiol* 1991;70:2730–2735.

66. Laitinen LA, Laitinen A, Widdicombe JG. Effects of inflammatory and other mediators on airway vascular beds. *Am Rev Respir Dis* 1987;135:567–570.

67. Parsons GH, Nichol GM, Barnes PJ, Chung KF. Peptide mediator effects on bronchial blood velocity and lung resistance in conscious sheep. *J Appl Physiol* 1992;72:1118–1122.

68. Corfield DR, Webber SE, Hanafi Z, Widdicombe JG. The actions of bradykinin and lys-bradykinin on tracheal blood flow and smooth muscle in anaesthetized sheep. *Pulm Pharmacol* 1991;4:85–90.

69. Baker AP, Hillegass LM, Holden DA, Smith WJ. Effect of kalliden, substance P and other basic polypeptides on the production of respiratory macromolecules. *Am Rev Respir Dis* 1977;115:811–817.

70. Baraniuk JN, Lundgren JD, Goff J, et al. Bradykinin receptor distribution in human nasal mucosa, and analysis of *in vitro* secretory responses *in vitro* and *in vivo*. *Am Rev Respir Dis* 1990;141:706–714.

71. Leikhauf GD, Ueki IF, Nadel JA, Widdicombe JH. Bradykinin stimulates chloride secretion and prostaglandin E₂ release by canine tracheal epithelium. *Am J Physiol* 1985;248:F48–55.

72. Proud D, Reynolds CJ, Broomfield J, Goldman DW, Bathon JM. Bradykinin effects on guinea-pig tracheal epithelial cells are mediated through B2 kinin receptors and can be inhibited by the selective antagonist HOE 140. *J Pharmacol Exp Ther* 1993;264:1124–1131.

73. Tamaoki J, Kobayashi K, Sakai N, Chitoyani A, Kanemura T, Takizawa T. Effect of bradykinin on airway ciliary motility and its modulation by neutral endopeptidase. *Am Rev Respir Dis* 1989;140:430–435.

74. Wong LB, Miller IF, Yeates DB. Regulatory pathways for the stimulation of canine tracheal ciliary beat frequency by bradykinin. *J Physiol* 1990;422:421–431.

75. Polosa R, Hasani A, Pavia D, et al. Acute effect of inhaled bradykinin on tracheobronchial clearance in normal humans. *Thorax* 1992;47: 952–956.
76. Vavrek RJ, Stewart JM. Competitive antagonists of bradykinin. *Peptides* 1985;6:161–164.
77. Burch RM, Farmer SG, Steranka LR. Bradykinin receptor antagonists. *Med Res Rev* 1990;10:237–269.
78. Soler M, Sielczak MW, Abraham WM. A bradykinin antagonist blocks antigen-induced airway hyperresponsiveness and inflammation in sheep. *Pulm Pharmacol* 1990;3:9–15.
79. Abraham WM, Burch RM, Farmer SG, Sielczak MW, Ahmed A, Cortes A. A bradykinin antagonist modifies allergen-induced mediator release and late bronchial responses in sheep. *Am Rev Respir Dis* 1991; 143:782–796.
80. Pongracic JA, Naclerio RM, Reynolds CJ, Proud D. A competitive kinin receptor antagonist, [DArg , Hyp^3, DPhe^7]-bradykinin, does not affect the response to nasal provocation with bradykin. *Br J Clin Pharmacol* 1991;31:287–294.
81. Wirth KJ, Gehring D, Schölkens BA. Effect of HOE 140 on bradykinin-induced bronchoconstriction in anesthetized guinea pigs. *Am Rev Respir Dis* 1993;148:702–706.
82. Austin CE, Foreman JC, Scadding SK. Reduction by Hoe 140, the B2 kinin receptor antagonist, of antigen-induced nasal blockage. *Br J Pharmacol* 1994;111:969–971.
83. Scherrer D, Daeffler L, Trifilieff A, Gies J. Effects of WIN 64338, a non peptide bradykinin B$_2$-receptor antagonist, on guinea-pig trachea. *Br J Pharmacol* 1995;115:1127–1128.
84. Abraham WM. The potential role of bradykinin antagonists in the treatment of asthma. *Agents Actions Suppl* 1992;38:439–449.
85. Tsukagoshi H, Robbins RA, Barnes PJ, Chung KF. Role of nitric oxide and superoxide anions in interleukin 1(β-induced airway hyperresponsiveness to bradykinin. *Am J Resp Crit Care Med* 1994;150:1019–1025.
86. Tsukagoshi H, Sun J, Kwon O, Barnes PJ, Chung KF. Role of neutral endopeptidase in bronchial hyperresponsiveness to bradykinin induced by IL-1(. *J Appl Physiol* 1995;78:921–927.
87. David TJ, Wybrew M, Hennessen U. Prodromal itching in childhood asthma. *Lancet* 1984;ii:154–155.
88. Berman AR, Togias AG, Skloot G, Proud D. Allergen-induced hyperresponsiveness to bradykinin is more pronounced than to methacholine. *J Appl Physiol* 1995; 78:1844–1852.
89. Baraniuk JN, Silver PB, Kaliner MA, Barnes PJ. Perennial rhinitis subjects have altered vascular, glandular and neural responses to bradykinin nasal provocation. *Int Arch Allergy Immunol* 1994;103:202–208.

Asthma, edited by P.J. Barnes, M.M. Grunstein, A.R. Leff, and A.J. Woolcock.
Lippincott–Raven Publishers, Philadelphia © 1997.

▪ 44 ▪

Adenosine

Diana L. Marquardt

Cell and Tissue Sources of Adenosine	**Bronchoconstriction Induced by Adenosine**
Production and Metabolism of Adenosine	**Pharmacologic Modulation of Adenosine-Induced**
Subtypes of Cell Surface Adenosine Receptors	**Bronchoconstriction**
Adenosine Effects on Mast Cell Mediator	**Animal Models of Asthma and Adenosine**
Release	**Hyperresponsiveness**
Regulation of Adenosine Receptor Expression	**Effects of Adenosine on Isolated Bronchial Tissue**

The description of the release of adenosine from hypoxic lung tissue by Mentzer and colleagues (1) provided some of the first evidence that adenosine may play a regulatory role in pulmonary homeostasis or in the pathogenesis of pulmonary disease. Extensive studies of adenosine and its actions at adenosine receptors in the ensuing 20 years have led to a number of conclusions regarding the importance of adenosine as a mediator and modulator of mast cell function and bronchoconstriction.

CELL AND TISSUE SOURCES OF ADENOSINE

Adenosine is released by a number of hypoxic tissues, including lung, and circulating adenosine concentrations in the high nanomolar to low micromolar range have been reported (2–4). Concentrations of adenosine in the venous blood of atopic asthmatic patients before and after allergen bronchoprovocation reveal that basal plasma adenosine concentrations less than 10 nanograms per milliliter prior to challenge, increase nearly 3 times baseline within minutes of allergen exposure (5). Mast cells stimulated by immunoglobulin E (IgE) receptor crosslinking or by other secretagogues, release adenosine into the extracellular space within 1 to 5 minutes of activation (6). Adenosine is released in both early- and late-phase asthmatic responses after allergen bronchoprovocation, but only the late release of adenosine has been observed with methacholine challenge (7). Thus, the physiologic presence of adenosine locally near resident mast cells, or systemically in the peripheral circulation, has been demonstrated. These data suggest that adenosine is generated during human asthma and may serve as a mediator of the bronchoconstrictive response.

PRODUCTION AND METABOLISM OF ADENOSINE

Adenosine is a naturally occurring purine nucleoside that may be produced by the hydrolysis of adenosine 5′-monophosphate (AMP) by 5′-nucleotidase or by the catabolism of s-adenosylhomocysteine. Both of these metabolic pathways are intracellular (8). When intracellular adenosine concentrations increase under conditions of hypoxia or cellular activation, adenosine may be released from the cell or tissue affected. This extracellular adenosine may be deaminated to inosine by adenosine deaminase, taken up by cells by diffusion or active transport utilizing a specific nucleoside transporter, phosphorylated to AMP by the action of adenosine kinase, or bound to adenosine receptors present on a variety of cells and tissues (9,10).

SUBTYPES OF CELL SURFACE ADENOSINE RECEPTORS

Most of the physiologic effects of adenosine are thought to take place by the action of adenosine at cell surface receptors, although high concentrations of adeno-

D. L. Marquardt: Department of Medicine, University of California at San Diego, La Jolla, California 92093-0635.

sine have been postulated to interact with an intracellular "p-site" that requires an intact purine base for activation (11,12). Adenosine receptors initially were classified on the basis of their linkage to an activation or inhibition of adenylate cyclase (13). The occupancy of A_1-adenosine receptors by an agonist induced a decrease in cyclic AMP (cAMP) levels, whereas A_2-adenosine receptor subtype occupancy by an agonist induced an increase in cAMP. This classification of adenosine receptors has become more complex over the past few years, with the molecular cloning of at least four adenosine receptor subtypes, A_1, A_{2a}, A_{2b}, and A_3 (14–20). Each of these receptor subtypes is expressed in lung and may participate in the inflammatory processes underlying asthma (Table 1).

The A_1-adenosine receptor subtype, originally defined by its negative coupling to adenylate cyclase activity through G_i proteins, can act through other effectors including phospholipase A_2, phospholipase C, guanylate cyclase, potassium ion channels, and calcium ion channels (21–25). It is expressed predominantly in brain, heart, and lung, among other tissues (26). This adenosine receptor mediates a variety of physiologic phenomena, including the inhibition of lipolysis, negative cardiac intropy, and an inhibition of renin secretion (27–29). It has been reported to be important in ischemia-reperfusion injury of the lung, and has been identified in human airway epithelial cells (30,31). As discussed in more detail following, its role in pulmonary physiology is controversial and under intense study.

The A_2-adenosine receptor has been subclassified into A_{2a}- and A_{2b}- subtypes based on distinct rank orders of potency of receptor agonists and antagonists and substantial differences in the nucleotide sequences of the two complementary deoxyribonucleic acids (cDNA). A_{2a}-receptors are expressed strongly in brain, lung, liver, neutrophils, and mast cells (32). They mediate an activation of adenylate cyclase and an increase in cAMP by G_s protein linkages. It has been postulated that this is the exclusive A_{2a}-receptor signal transduction pathway. A_{2b}-receptors are expressed in colon, brain, mast cells, and lung, and are coupled to a number of effector systems by one or more G protein subtypes (32). The details of A_{2b}-receptor function and signaling mechanisms remain uncertain, although A_{2b}-receptor occupancy by an agonist has been associated with an increase in cAMP concentration, an increase in phospholipase C activity, and with the rapid induction of a calcium transient (33).

The A_3-adenosine receptor was initially described in the rat as one present primarily in testis and linked to an inhibition of adenylate cyclase (34). However, human A_3-receptor transcripts are present in lung, liver, heart, and brain (35). A_3-receptor subtypes have been reported to couple to phospholipases, ion channels, and other effectors via multiple G protein subtypes (36). They mediate a variety of processes including activation of the cellular antioxidant defense system (37). This type of action has engendered the classification of adenosine as a cytoprotective agent in the setting of post-ischemic injury. The ongoing controversies regarding the role of A_3-receptors in the potentiation of mast cell degranulation and the induction of bronchoconstriction are described later in this chapter.

ADENOSINE EFFECTS ON MAST CELL MEDIATOR RELEASE

The observation that exogenous adenosine induces the release of histamine from uterine horns was followed by the report that adenosine augments the stimulated release of histamine from rat serosal mast cells (38,39). Adenosine alone fails to activate mast cell degranulation but is an effective potentiating signal for almost any mast cell secretagogue, including anti-IgE, compound 48/80, and calcium ionophores (40). A number of subsequent studies confirmed the ability of adenosine to enhance mediator release from mast cells of both "connective tissue" and "mucosal" phenotypes in rodents and humans (41–45). Adenosine potentiates mediator release from human lung mast cells, and this effect is partially antagonized by theophylline (46). Agents that inhibit the intracellular uptake of adenosine, such as dipyridamole, fail to reverse this effect, suggesting an extracellular site of action. Most studies of the effect of adenosine on human basophils indicate that it inhibits the stimulated release of histamine and other basophil-derived mediators, clearly contrasting with the effect of adenosine on mast cells (47,48). As noted previously, adenosine has been measured in stimulated mast cell supernatants within seconds after antigen

TABLE 1. *Evidence for adenosine receptor participation in asthma*

Subtype		Tissue Expression		Pulmonary Effect
	Lung	Mast Cell	Selected Others	
A_1	Yes	No	Airway Epithelium, Brain, Heart	Ciliary activity; cytoprotection(?)
A_{2a}	Yes	Yes	Brain, Liver, Neutrophil	cAMP[a]
A_{2b}	Yes	Yes	Fibroblasts, Brain, Colon	Mast Cell Degranulation(?)
A_3	Yes	Yes	Liver, Brain, Heart, Kidney	Modulation of Mast Cell Secretion(?)

[a]cAMP, adenosine 3′5′cyclic-monophosphate

challenge, postulating that adenosine may be a pro-inflammatory stimulus in mast cell-dependent reactions such as immediate hypersensitivity and asthma.

The nature of the adenosine receptor signal transduction pathways in the mast cell is controversial. Adenosine induces an increase in intracellular cAMP concentrations, a rapid calcium transient, and an activation of phospholipase C (49–51). The activation of adenylate cyclase is rapid but does not appear to be necessary for mast cell mediator release to occur, in that the inhibition of cAMP-dependent protein kinase, protein kinase A, does not change the ability of adenosine to enhance histamine release (52). It appears that calcium fluxes and phospholipid metabolism are more critical to the adenosine effect on mast cells. The adenosine receptor and G protein subtypes that couple to these effector systems are in the process of being defined. Many of the effects of adenosine on mast cells are at least partially pertussis toxin-dependent (53,54). Therefore, a pertussis toxin-dependent G protein such as G_i or G_o may be important in coupling of the adenosine receptor subtype responsible for the facilitation of mast cell mediator release to its second messenger effector systems.

A_3-adenosine receptors are present on rat basophilic leukemia (RBL) cells, a model of mucosal mast cells (55). However, the contention that this receptor subtype is the one responsible for the facilitation of mast cell degranulation was based partially on the inability to identify other adenosine receptor subtypes on the cells using Northern blotting. Using molecular biologic techniques, A_{2a}- and A_{2b}-receptor subtypes have been demonstrated to be present on mouse bone marrow-derived mast cells and RBL cells (18). As discussed earlier, both A_{2b}- and A_3-receptors have been shown to be coupled to a number of second messengers, whereas A_{2a}-receptors may couple exclusively to adenylate cyclase. Therefore, either A_{2b}- or A_3-receptor subtypes, or a combination of the two, is likely to be responsible for the potentiation of mast cell mediator release by adenosine.

REGULATION OF ADENOSINE RECEPTOR EXPRESSION

A number of agents have been reported to alter adenosine receptor expression. Chronic exposure to adenosine receptor agonists such as N-ethylcarboxamidoadenosine or adenosine itself in the presence of an inhibitor of adenosine deaminase, results in a down regulation of adenosine receptor numbers and a functional adenosine hyporesponsiveness (56). This is consistent with patterns of downregulation and desensitization observed in many studies of cell surface receptors (57). In airway specimens from ovalbumin-sensitized guinea pigs, the contractile response to a second adenosine exposure is consistently reduced or absent, indicative of tachyphylaxis

and consistent with a mechanism that involves mediator release (58). Chronic exposure to adenosine receptor antagonists, including aminophylline, results in a functional adenosine hyperresponsiveness in the mast cell and an increase in adenosine receptor numbers (41,59). It has been proposed that chronic theophylline therapy may augment the regulation of adenosine receptor numbers, with a resultant hypersensitivity to adenosine exposure. If this were true, the administration of theophylline should not be abruptly discontinued, and a tapering of the dose would provide less potential for a rebound hyperresponsiveness to adenosine receptor agonists.

Another agent that has been reported to alter adenosine receptor expression is the corticosteroid, dexamethasone (60). In RBL cells, dexamethasone increases the expression of the A_3-adenosine receptor subtype and in mouse bone marrow-derived mast cells, dexamethasone exposure induces an increase in A_{2a}-, but not A_{2b}-receptor transcripts, indicating some differential effects of corticosteroids on adenosine receptor expression (18,61). Mast cells *in vitro* do not develop a functional hyperresponsiveness to adenosine after dexamethasone administration, suggesting that the apparently unaffected A_{2b}-receptor subtype may be important in the potentiation of mast cell mediator release by adenosine (62).

BRONCHOCONSTRICTION INDUCED BY ADENOSINE

Inhaled adenosine induces a bronchoconstrictor response in asthmatic subjects, but not in normal subjects (63). This ability to induce bronchoconstriction is generally unrelated to atopic status and appears to be a marker for the asthmatic diathesis, as is methacholine sensitivity and enhanced bronchial reactivity to other chemical triggers (64). However, individuals with other forms of airway inflammation, such as that induced by smoking or ozone exposure, are not hyperresponsive to AMP, although they may be hyperreactive to methacholine. When administered as an inhaled aerosol to patients with asthma, adenosine induces bronchoconstriction as assessed by a decrease in specific airway conductance that reaches a peak in 1 to 3 minutes and gradually returns to baseline over the next hour. The adenosine monophosphates and diphosphates also cause bronchoconstriction upon inhalation, since these can rapidly be metabolized to adenosine under physiologic conditions (63). Adenosine 5′-monophosphate is more water soluble than adenosine, and has been used as a standard in a number of bronchoprovocation studies (65). The related nucleoside, guanosine, and the deaminated product of adenosine, inosine, fail to induce bronchospasm upon inhalation by asthmatics and nonasthmatics. The basis for this effect of inhaled adenosine is not completely understood. Several theories have been developed to suggest mechanisms whereby adenosine may induce bronchoconstriction, including stimulation of mast cell mediator release, a direct effect on neuronal pathways, and modulation of the function of other inflammatory cells. In humans, both AMP (as a source of adenosine) and histamine can induce rapid bronchoconstriction in asthmatics. Adenosine is approximately one-third as potent as histamine and one-sixth as potent as methacholine in inducing this airway contractility (66). However, the bronchoconstrictor activity of adenosine does not always parallel that of methacholine (67). Even maximally soluble doses of inhaled AMP fail to induce bronchoconstriction in the vast majority of normal individuals, whereas high doses of methacholine induce nonspecific bronchial reactivity in normal subjects (68). Three hours after allergen challenge of asthmatic patients, both methacholine- and adenosine-induced bronchial contractilities are enhanced (69). The heightened bronchial reactivity to methacholine persists for at least 24 hours, whereas 24 hours after allergen challenge, airway responses to adenosine have returned to baseline. It has been postulated that the lack of adenosine hyperresponsiveness at 24 hours after allergen challenge may be due to adenosine receptor desensitization, but no direct demonstration of this phenomenon has been reported.

PHARMACOLOGIC MODULATION OF ADENOSINE-INDUCED BRONCHOCONSTRICTION

A number of anti-asthmatic pharmacologic agents have been studied in an effort to decipher the basis of the adenosine effect on asthmatic airways (Table 2). Pretreatment with oral antihistamines a few hours before inhalation challenge completely inhibits the bronchoconstrictor response to histamine and markedly inhibits the bronchoconstrictor response to AMP, suggesting a role for mast cells and basophils in the adenosine-induced airway response (70). In similar studies, the response to inhaled allergen was only inhibited 50% by antihistamine pretreatment. These *in vivo* data correlate well with the *in vitro*

data that indicate that adenosine preferentially potentiates the release of mast cell granule-associated mediators, such as histamine, more than newly generated mediators such as leukotrienes or cytokines (71,72). However, the bronchoconstrictor effect of inhaled adenosine is more rapid than that of inhaled allergen, postulating that a more direct effect of adenosine on the airways smooth muscle is an alternative mechanistic explanation (73).

Oral theophylline and inhaled theophylline are also effective in antagonizing adenosine-induced bronchoconstriction in asthmatics (74). Other related methylxanthines, including 8-phenyltheophylline, 3-isobutyl-1-methylxanthine, and caffeine, are more potent in inhibiting adenosine-induced bronchoconstriction than that induced by histamine or methacholine (75). These observations would be most consistent with an action of adenosine on cell surface adenosine receptors, since theophylline is a non-specific antagonist at both A_1- and A_2-receptors. However, theophylline also exhibits a number of pharmacologic properties that may contribute to its anti-asthmatic activity (76–78). Disodium cromoglycate, an anti-asthmatic drug purported to stabilize mast cells, also inhibits adenosine-induced bronchoconstriction, but is not effective in alleviating histamine-induced bronchoconstriction in humans. Again, this suggests a possible role for the mast cell in this adenosine response (79). By contrast, cromolyn inhibits bronchospasm induced by some nonspecific stimulants not necessarily thought to act through mast cell mechanisms, including cold air and sulfur dioxide (80).

Pretreatment of asthmatic subjects with the cyclooxygenase inhibitor, indomethacin, shifts the dose-response curves of inhaled adenosine to the right, proposing that the effects of adenosine include inducing the release of arachidonic acid metabolites from resident cells (81). Another potent cyclooxygenase inhibitor, lysine acetylsalicylate, delivered by inhalation 15 minutes prior to AMP, methacholine, or histamine bronchoprovocation, attenuates the fall in FEV_1 induced by AMP but not by the other stimuli (82). One would speculate that a product of cyclooxygenase activity stimulated by adenosine inhalation is important in the bronchoconstrictor response.

Finally, in animal models, atropine has been demonstrated to blunt bronchoconstriction provoked by adenosine. Analyses of this effect have demonstrated that, whereas the majority of the adenosine effect is mediated by histamine, additional bronchoprotection can be noted with ipratropium bromide, an anticholinergic agent, when administered with antihistamines prior to adenosine challenge.

Taken together, the data from utilizing pharmacologic agents to modulate the ability of adenosine to induce bronchial reactivity in asthmatics, underscore the differences between adenosine and other chemical triggers of bronchospasm; they support a central role for the mast cell in this phenomenon.

TABLE 2. *Effects of drugs on adenosine-induced bronchoconstriction*

Agent	Effect	Mechanism
Terfenadine	80-90% Inhibition	H_1 Histamine Receptor Antagonism
Indomethacin	Partial Inhibition	Cyclooxygenase Inhibition
Cromolyn Sodium	Partial Inhibition	Mast Cell Stabilization(?)
Atropine	Partial Inhibition	Cholinergic Receptor Antagonism
Theophylline	Complete Inhibition	Adenosine Receptor Antagonism

ANIMAL MODELS OF ASTHMA AND ADENOSINE HYPERRESPONSIVENESS

A number of animal models of asthma have been developed to assess the ability of adenosine to induce bronchospasm under selected conditions. In an allergic rabbit model of airway sensitivity to ragweed pollen, rabbits immunized intraperitoneally with ragweed allergen extract developed allergen-specific IgE antibody, early- and late-phase asthmatic responses to aeroallergen, and bronchial hyperresponsiveness (83). In the allergic rabbits, aerosolized adenosine induced a dose-dependent bronchoconstriction *in vivo* and a contraction of bronchial airway rings *in vitro*. It has been postulated that sensitization alone may destabilize inflammatory cells for enhanced mediator release with adenosine stimulation (84). Unsensitized rabbits exhibited no effects from inhaled adenosine, and the bronchial smooth muscle tissue from normal rabbits did not contract when stimulated with the doses of adenosine studied. The smooth muscle in the peripheral airway was more responsive to adenosine than that in the central airway. Interestingly, radioligand binding studies revealed a single class of adenosine binding sites in the lung tissue from the allergic rabbits, but no demonstrable specific binding of the radiolabeled adenosine receptor antagonist, 8-cyclopentyl-1,3-dipropylxanthine, to lung tissue from unsensitized rabbits (83). These effects of adenosine in this rabbit model were postulated to be medicated by A_1-adenosine receptors because of the rank order of potency of the antagonists effective in abrogating the adenosine response.

In a rat model of experimental asthma, adenosine-induced bronchoconstriction was evident only in sensitized rats that exhibited eosinophilic airway inflammation (85). The rank order of potency of adenosine receptor agonists in inducing bronchoconstriction was not consistent with an single adenosine receptor subtype. However, A_{2a}-receptor specific agonists alone were ineffective in inducing bronchoconstriction upon inhalation under these experimental conditions, and A_{2a}-receptor specific antagonists had no significant inhibitory activity on the adenosine-induced bronchoconstriction. The authors concluded that the effects of adenosine on rat airways were secondary to binding to A_1-, A_{2b}-, and/or A_3-receptor subtypes. Similarly, guinea pigs sensitized to ovalbumin antigen developed pulmonary hyperresponsiveness to adenosine (86). Adenosine also enhanced the bronchocontractile response to histamine, but not to methacholine in guinea pigs (87).

EFFECTS OF ADENOSINE ON ISOLATED BRONCHIAL TISSUE

Studies of human airway smooth muscle further support the contention that mast cells play a central role in adenosine-induced bronchoconstriction. Surgical specimens of lung tissue obtained from asthmatics and non-asthmatic subjects revealed that bronchi from asthmatics were more sensitive to the contractile effects of adenosine (88). However, there was no difference in sensitivity to histamine or leukotriene C_4 between the two groups. Interestingly, the combination of leukotriene and histamine antagonism of the bronchial segments blocked the contractile effects of adenosine, suggesting that adenosine may act indirectly by liberating these mediators from resident cells (89). Although the airway responses to adenosine appear to be similar in human asthma and experimental asthma induced in several different animal models, there are a number of conflicting reports regarding the effects of adenosine on isolated airway smooth muscle. In the human, the contractile effect of adenosine on isolated normal airways is minimal. In airway preparations or lung tissue from asthmatic individuals, a hyperresponsiveness to adenosine has been observed that was inhibitable by theophylline. In tracheal rings from guinea pigs and other species, adenosine may induce relaxation, especially after maximal precontraction (90). One caveat in the interpretation of these data is that peripheral airways are more responsive to adenosine and more representative of the asthmatic condition than trachea or large bronchi. Secondly, because there are substantial differences between normal airways and inflamed or asthmatic airways, studies of adenosine responses in normal lung tissue may not reflect the pathophysiological state of asthma.

In spite of some of the controversies, adenosine appears to be a remarkable exception to the general notion that there is no direct correlation between *in vivo* and *in vitro* sensitivity to bronchoconstrictors (91). Standard *in vitro* challenges of airway smooth muscle with histamine, methacholine, or leukotriene C_4 do not differentiate asthmatics from normals, but adenosine can (92). As a bridge between *in vivo* and *in vitro* studies of pulmonary responses to adenosine, asthmatic subjects have been challenged with the local airway instillation of AMP or saline, followed by bronchoalveolar lavage of the challenged and unchallenged lung segments. These studies have provided additional evidence of mast cell involvement in adenosine-induced airway hyperresponsiveness. Endobronchial stimulation with AMP resulted in a prompt reduction in airway caliber and a significant rise in histamine, tryptase, and prostaglandin D_2 levels in the lavage fluid (93). No changes from baseline were observed in the saline-challenged segment. The release of these mediators, which are predominantly mast cell-derived, underscores the importance of this cell in the asthmatic response to adenosine.

CONCLUSIONS

Adenosine is a potent bronchoconstricting agent that is released by activated mast cells and hypoxic lung tissue. The concentration of adenosine is increased in the local milieu and in the peripheral circulation after allergen-induced bronchospasm. Since adenosine is a strong potentiator of mast cell mediator release, it has been postulated that adenosine acts on the mast cell to enhance the release of proinflammatory mediators and increase the asthmatic response. Adenosine also serves as a marker for the asthmatic diathesis, in that only asthmatic subjects develop bronchoconstriction after inhalation of adenosine. The cellular, molecular, and genetic bases for this adenosine hyperresponsiveness in asthma are under intensive investigation.

REFERENCES

1. Mentzer RM, Rubio R, Berne RM. Release of adenosine by hypoxic canine lung tissue and its possible role in pulmonary circulation. *Am J Physiol* 1975;229:1625–1632.
2. Rubio R, Berne RM. Relationships of adenosine concentration, lactate levels and oxygen supply in rat brain. *Am J Physiol* 1975;228:1896–1904.
3. Schrader J, Gerlach E. Compartmentation of cardiac adenine nucleotides and formation of adenosine. *Pfluger's Arch* 1976;367:129–133.
4. Mills GC, Schmalstieg FC, Trimmer KB, Goldman AS, Goldblum RM. Purine metabolism in adenosine deaminase deficiency. *Proc Natl Acad Sci U S A* 1976;73:2867–2871.
5. Mann JS, Holgate ST, Renwick AG, Cushley MJ. Airway effects of purine nucleosides and nucleotides and release with bronchial provocation in asthma. *J Appl Physiol* 1986;61:1667–1676.
6. Marquardt DL, Gruber HE, Wasserman SI. Adenosine release from stimulated mast cells. *Proc Natl Acad Sci U S A* 1984;81:6192–6196.
7. Ali S, Mustafa SJ, Driver AG, Metzger WJ. Release of adenosine in bronchoalveolar lavage fluid following allergen bronchial provocation in allergic rabbits. *Am Rev Respir Dis* 1991;143:A417.
8. Church MK, Featherstone RL, Cushley JM, Mann JS, Holgate ST. Relationships between adenosine, cyclic nucleotides, and xanthines in asthma. *J Allergy Clin Immunol* 1986;78:670–675.
9. Fleit H, Conklin M, Stebbins RD, Silber R. Function of 5′-nucleotidase in the uptake of adenosine from AMP by human lymphocytes. *J Biol Chem* 1975;250:8889–8896.
10. Collis MG, Hourani SMO. Adenosine receptor subtypes. *Trends Pharmacol Sci* 1993;14:360–366.
11. Stiles GL. Adenosine receptors: structure, function and regulation. *Trends Pharmacol Sci* 1986;7:486–490.
12. Stiles GL. Adenosine receptors. *J Biol Chem* 1992;10:6451–6454.
13. Jacobson KA, van Galen PJM, Williams M. Adenosine receptors: pharmacology, structure-activity relationships, and therapeutic potential. *J Med Chem* 1992;35:407–422.
14. Mahan LC, McVittie LD, Smyk-Randall EM, et al. Cloning and expression of an A$_1$ adenosine receptor from rat brain. *Mol Pharmacol* 1991;40:1–8.
15. Libert F, Parmentier M, Lefort A, et al. Selective amplification and cloning of four new members of the G protein-coupled receptor family. *Science* 1989;24:570–573.
16. Stehle JH, Rivkees SA, Lee JJ, Weaver DR, Deeds JD, Reppert SM. Molecular cloning and expression of the cDNA for a novel A$_2$-adenosine receptor subtype. *Mol Endocrinol* 1992;6:384–391.
17. Zhou Q, Li C, Olah ME, Johnson RA, Stiles GL, Civelli O. Molecular cloning and characterization of the A$_3$ adenosine receptor. *Proc Natl Acad Sci U S A* 1992;89:7432–7438.
18. Marquardt DL, Walker LL, Heinemann S. Cloning of two adenosine receptor subtypes from mouse bone marrow-derived mast cells. *J Immunol* 1994;152:4508–4515.
19. Fink JS, Weaver DR, Rivkees SA, Peterfreund RA, Pollack AE, Adlers EM, Reppert SM. Molecular cloning of the rat A$_2$ adenosine receptor: selective co-expression with D$_2$ dopamine receptors in rat striatum. *Brain Res Mol Brain Res* 1992:14:186–192.
20. Rivkees SA, Reppert SM. RFL9 encodes an A$_{2b}$-adenosine receptor. *Mol Endocrinol* 1992;61598–1602.
21. Van Calker D, Muller M, Hamprecht B. Adenosine regulates via two different types of receptors. The accumulation of cyclic AMP in cultured brain cells. *J Neurochem* 1979;33:999–1005.
22. Akbar M, Okajima F, Tomura H, Shimegi S, Kondo Y. A single species of A$_1$ adenosine receptor expressed in chinese hamster ovary cells not only inhibits cAMP accumulation but also stimulates phospholipase C and arachidonate release. *Mol Pharmacol* 1994;45:1036–1042.
23. Kurtz A. Adenosine stimulates guanylate cyclase activity in vascular smooth muscle cells. *J Biol Chem* 1987;262:6296–6300.
24. Belardinelli L, Linden J, Berne RM. The cardiac effects of adenosine. *Prog Cardiovasc Dis* 1989;32:73–97.
25. Iredale PA, Alexander SP, Hill SJ. Coupling of a transfected human brain A$_1$ adenosine receptor in CHO-K1 cells to calcium mobilisation via a pertussis toxin-sensitive mechanism. *Br J Pharmacol* 1994;111:1252–1256.
26. Ren H, Stiles GL. Posttranscriptional mRNA processing as a mechanism for regulation of human A$_1$ adenosine receptor expression. *Proc Natl Acad Sci U S A* 1994;91:4864–4866.
27. Schwabe U, Ebert R, Erbler HC. Adenosine release from fat cells: effect on cyclic AMP levels and hormone actions. *Adv Cyclic Nuc Res* 1975;5:569–575.
28. Barrett RJ, Droppleman DA, Wright KF. Discrimination of A$_1$ versus A$_2$ receptor subtype selectivity of adenosine receptor agonists *in vivo*. *J Pharmacol Exp Ther* 1994;268;1166–1173.
29. Weaver DR, Reppert SM. Adenosine receptor gene expression in rat kidney. *Am J Physiol* 1992;263:F991–995.
30. Neely CF, Keith IM. A$_1$ adenosine receptor antagonists block ischemia-reperfusion injury of the lung. *Am J Physiol* 1995;268:L1036–1046.
31. McCoy DE, Schwiebert EM, Karlson KH, Speilman WS, Stanton BA. Identification and function of A$_1$ adenosine receptors in normal and cystic fibrosis human airway epithelial cells. *Am J Physiol* 1995;268:C1520–1527.
32. Yakel JL, Warren RA, Reppert SM, North RA. Functional expression of adenosine A$_{2b}$ receptor in Xenopus oocytes. *Mol Pharmacol* 1993;43:277–281.
33. Strohmeier GR, Reppert SM, Lencer WI, Madara JL. The A$_{2b}$ adenosine receptor mediates cAMP responses to adenosine receptor agonists in human intestinal epithelia. *J Biol Chem* 1995;270:2387–2394.
34. Meyerhof W, Muller-Brechlin R, Richter D. Molecular cloning of a novel putative G-protein coupled receptor expressed during rat spermiogenesis. *FEBS Lett* 1991;284:155–158.
35. Linden J, Taylor He, Robeva AS, et al. Molecular cloning and functional expression of a sheep A$_3$ adenosine receptor with widespread tissue distribution. *Mol Pharmacol* 1993;44:524–530.
36. Palmer TM, Gettys TW, Stiles GL. Differential interaction with and regulation of multiple G-proteins by the rat A$_3$ adenosine receptor. *J Biol Chem* 1995;270:16895–16902.
37. Maggirwar SB, Dhanraj DN, Somani SM, Ramkumar V. Adenosine acts as an endogenous activator of the cellular antioxidant defense system. *Biochem Biophys Res Commun* 1994;201:508–515.
38. Okazaki T, Namae A. Enhancement of anaphylaxis of isolated smooth muscle by adenosine phosphates and inhibition of anaphylactic mechanisms by adenosine 3′,5′-cyclic monophosphate. *Experientia* 1972;28:426–431.
39. Marquardt DL, Parker CW, Sullivan TJ. Potentiation of mast cell mediator release by adenosine. *J Immunol* 1978;120:871–878.
40. Marquardt DL, Walker LL, Wasserman SI. Adenosine receptors on mouse bone marrow-derived mast cells: functional significance and regulation by aminophylline. *J Immunol* 1984;133:932–937.
41. Church MK, Hughes PF, Vardey CJ. studies on the receptor mediating cyclic AMP-independent enhancement by adenosine of IgE-dependent mediator release from rat mast cells. *Br J Pharmacol* 1986;87:233–237.
42. Abbracchio MP, Paolettti AM, Luini A, Cattabeni F, De Matteis MA. Adenosine receptors in rat basophilic leukaemia cells: transductional mechanism and effects on 5-hydroxytryptamine release. *Br J Pharmacol* 1992;227:317–322.
43. Peters SP, Schulman RP, Schleimer RP, MacGlashan DW, Newball HH, Lichtenstein LM. Dispersed human lung mast cells. Pharmacologic aspects and comparison with human lung tissue fragments. *Am Rev Respir Dis* 1982;126:1034–1039.
44. Auchampach JA, Caughey GH, Linden J. Molecular cloning and pharmacological characterization of the canine A$_3$ adenosine receptor from Br mastocytoma cells. *FASEB J* 1995;A122.
45. Feoktistov I, Biaggioni I. Adenosine A$_{2b}$ receptors evoke interleukin-8

secretion in human mast cells. An enprofylline-sensitive mechanism with implications for asthma. *J Clin Invest* 1995;96:1979–1986.

46. Peachell PT, Columbo M, Kagey-Sobotka A, Lichtenstein LM, Marone G. Adenosine potentiates mediator release from human lung mast cells. *Am Rev Respir Dis* 1988;138:1143–1151.

47. Marone G, Cirillo R, Genovese A, Marino O, Quattrin S. Human basophil/mast cell releasability. VII. Heterogeneity of the effect of adenosine on mediator secretion. *Life Sci* 1989;45:1745–1754.

48. Marone G, Findlay SR, Lichtenstein LM. Adenosine receptor on human basophils: modulation of histamine release. *J Immunol* 1979;123:1473–1477.

49. Marquardt DL. Adenosine and mast cell secretion. In: Londos C, Cooper D, eds. *Adenosine receptors*. New York: Alan R. Liss, Inc., 1988;87–95.

50. Lohse MJ, Klotz K-N, Salzer MJ, Schwabe U. Adenosine regulates the Ca^{2+} sensitivity of mast cell mediator release. *Proc Natl Acad Sci U S A* 1988;85:8875–8879.

51. Ali H, Cunha-Melo JR, Saul WF, Beaven MA. The activation of phospholipase C via adenosine receptors provide synergistic signals for secretion in antigen stimulated RBL-2H3 cells: evidence for a novel adenosine receptor. *J Biol Chem* 1990;265:745–751.

52. Marquardt DL, Walker LL. Inhibition of protein kinase A fails to alter mast cell adenosine responsiveness. *Agents Actions* 1994;43:7–12.

53. Marquardt DL, Walker LL. Alteration of mast cell responsiveness to adenosine by pertussis toxin. *Biochem Pharmacol* 1988;37:4019–4025.

54. Gilfillan AM, Wiggan GA, Welton AF. Pertussis toxin pretreatment reveals differential effects of adenosine analogs on IgE-dependent histamine and peptidoleukotriene release from RBL-2H3 cells. *Biochim Biophys Acta* 1990;1052:467–474.

55. Ramkumar V, Stiles GL, Beaven MA, Ali H. The A_3 adenosine receptor is the unique adenosine receptor which facilitates release of allergic mediators in mast cells. *J Biol Chem* 1993;268:16887–16890.

56. Marquardt DL, Walker LL. Inhibition of mast cell adenosine responsiveness by chronic exposure to adenosine receptor agonists. *Biochem Pharmacol* 1987;36:4297–4302.

57. Chern Y, Chiou JY, Lai HL, Tsai MH. Regulation of adenylyl cyclase type VI activity during desensitization of the A_{2a} adenosine receptor-mediated cyclic AMP response: role for protein phosphatase 2A. *Mol Pharmacol* 1995;48:1–8.

58. Thorne JR, Broadley KJ. Adenosine-induced bronchoconstriction of isolated lung and trachea from sensitized guinea pigs. *Br J Pharmacol* 1992;106:978–985.

59. Marquardt DL, Wasserman SI. [³H] Adenosine binding to rat mast cells—pharmacologic and functional characterization. *Agents Actions* 1985;16:453–461.

60. Collado-Escobar D, Cunha-Melo JR, Beaven MA. Treatment with dexamethasone down-regulates IgE-receptor-mediated signals and up-regulates adenosine-receptor-mediated signals in a rat mast cell (RBL-2H3) line. *J Immunol* 1990;144:244–250.

61. Ramkumar V, Wilson M, Dhanraj DN, Gettys TW, Ali H. Dexamethasaone up-regulates A_3 adenosine receptors in rat basophilic leukemia (RBL-2H3) cells. *J Immunol* 1995;154:5436–5443.

62. Marquardt DL, Wasserman SI. Modulation of rat serosal mast cell biochemistry by *in vivo* dexamethasone administration. *J Immunol* 1983;131:934–939.

63. Cushley MJ, Tattersfield AE, Holgate ST. Inhaled adenosine and guanosine on airway resistance in normal and asthmatic subjects. *Br J Clin Pharmacol* 1983;15:161–167.

64. Cushley MJ, Tattersfield AE, Holgate ST. Adenosine-induced bronchoconstriction in asthma. *Am Rev Respir Dis* 1984;129:380–384.

65. Mann JS, Holgate ST, Renwick AG, Cushley MJ. Airway effects of purine nucleosides and nucleotides and release with bronchial provocation in asthma. *J Appl Physiol* 1986;61:1667–1676.

66. Church MK, Featherstone RL, Cushley JM, Mann JS, Holgate ST. Relationships between adenosine, cyclic nucleotides, and xanthines in asthma. *J Allergy Clin Immunol* 1986;78:670–675.

67. Juniper EF, Frith PA, Dunnett C, Cockcroft DW, Hargreave FE. Reproducibility and comparison of responses to inhaled histamine and methacholine. *Thorax* 1978;33:705–711.

68. Cushley MJ, Holgate ST. Adenosine-induced bronchoconstriction in asthma: specificity and relationship to airway reactivity. *Thorax* 1983;705–710.

69. Aalbers R, Kauffman HF, Koeter GH, Postma DS, De Vries K, De Monchy JGR. Dissimilarity in methacholine and adenosine 5′-monophosphate responsiveness 3 and 24 h after allergen challenge. *Am Rev Respir Dis* 1991;144:352–357.

70. Rafferty P, Beasley CR, Holgate ST. The contribution of histamine to bronchoconstriction produced by inhaled allergen and adenosine 5′-monophosphate in asthma. *Am Rev Respir Dis* 1987;136:369–373.

71. Marquardt DL, Gruber HE, Wasserman SI. Aminophylline exposure alters mouse bone marrow-derived mast cell adenosine responsiveness. *J Allergy Clin Immunol* 1986;78:462–469.

72. Marquardt DL, Alongi JL, Walker LL. The phosphatidylinositol 3-kinase inhibitor, wortmannin, blocks mast cell exocytosis but not IL-6 production. *J Immunol* 1996;156:1942–1945.

73. Dahlen S-E, Hansson G, Hedqvist P, Bjorck T, Granstrom E, Dahlen B. Allergen challenge of lung tissue from asthmatics elicits bronchial contraction that correlates with the release of leukotrienes C_4, D_4, and E_4. *Proc Natl Acad Sci U S A* 1983;80:1712–1716.

74. Cushley MJ, Tattersfield AE, Holgate ST. Adenosine-induced bronchoconstriction in asthma: antagonism by inhaled theophylline. *Am Rev Respir Dis* 1984;129:380–385.

75. Mann JS, Holgate ST. Specific antagonism of adenosine-induced bronchoconstriction in asthma by oral theophylline. *Br J Clin Pharmacol* 1985;19:685–689.

76. Aubirer M, De Troyer A, Sampson M, Macklem PT, Roussos C. Aminophylline improves diaphragmatic contractility. *N Engl J Med* 1981;305:249–253.

77. Higbee MD, Kumar M, Galant SP. Stimulation of endogenous catecholamine release by theophylline: a proposed mechanism of action for theophylline effects. *J Allergy Clin Immunol* 1982;70:377–383.

78. Hendeles L, Weinberger M. Theophylline: a "state of the art" review. *Pharmacotherapy* 1983;3:2–11.

79. Cushley MJ, Church MK, Pao GJ-K, Holgate ST. Adenosine-induced bronchoconstriction is not caused by enhance immunological release of mast cell mediators. *Br J Clin Pharmacol* 1982;14:607–611.

80. Church MK, Warner JO. Sodium cromoglycate and related drugs. *Clin Exp Allergy* 1985;15:311–317.

81. Crimi N, Palermo F, Polosa R, Oliveri R, Maccarrone C, Palermo B, Mistretta A. Effect of indomethacin on adenosine-induced bronchoconstriction. *J Allergy Clin Immunol* 1989;83:921–925.

82. Crimi N, Polosa R, Magii S, et al. Inhaled lysine acetylsalicylate (L-ASA) attenuates the bronchoconstrictor response to adenosine 5′-monophosphate (AMP) in asthmatic subjects. *Eur Respir J* 1995;8:905–912.

83. Metzger WJ. Late phase asthma in allergic rabbit model. In: Dorsch W, ed. *CRC handbook*. Boca Raton: CRC Press, 1990;347–362.

84. Rafferty P, Beasley R, Southgate P, Holgate ST. The role of histamine in allergen and adenosine-induced bronchoconstriction. *Int Archs Allergy Appl Immunol* 1987:82:292–294.

85. Pauwels RA, Joos GF. Characterization of the adenosine receptors in the airways. *Arch Int Pharmacodyn Ther* 1995;329:151–160.

86. Thorne JR, Broadley KJ. Adenosine-induced bronchoconstriction in conscious hyperresponsive and sensitized guinea pigs. *Am J Respir Crit Care Med* 1994;149:392–399.

87. Breschi MC, Nieri P, Lazzeri N, Martinotti E. Adenosine enhances the bronchocontractile response to histamine in anaesthetized and curarized guinea pigs through a mechanism partly blocked by hexamethonium. *Pharmacology* 1994;49:42–51.

88. Finney MJB, Karlsson J-A, Persson CGA. Effects of bronchoconstrictors and bronchodilators on a novel human small airway preparation. *Br J Pharmacol* 1985;85:29–36.

89. Bjorck T, Gustafsson LE, Dahlen S-E. Isolated bronchi from asthmatics are hyperresponsive to adenosine, which apparently acts indirectly by liberation of leukotrienes and histamine. *Am Rev Respir Dis* 1992;145:1087–1091.

90. Advenier C, Deriflier P, Matran R, Naline E. Influence of epithelium on the responsiveness of guinea pig isolated trachea to adenosine. *Br J Pharmacol* 1988;93:295–302.

91. Vincenc KS, Black JL, Yan K, Armour CA, Donnelly PD, Woolcock AJ. Comparison of *in vivo* and *in vitro* responses to histamine in human airways. *Am Rev Respir Dis* 1983;128:875–879.

92. Roberts JA, Raeburn D, Rodger IW, Thomson NC. Comparison on *in vivo* airway responsiveness and *in vitro* smooth muscle sensitivity to methacholine in man. *Thorax* 1984;39:837–843.

93. Polosa R, Ng WH, Crimi N, et al. Release of mast-cell-derived mediators after endobronchial adenosine challenge in asthma. *Am J Respir Crit Care Med* 1995:151:624–629.

Asthma, edited by P.J. Barnes, M.M. Grunstein, A.R. Leff, and A.J. Woolcock.
Lippincott–Raven Publishers, Philadelphia © 1997.

▪ 45 ▪

Eosinophil Basic Proteins

Masayuki Kaneko, Hirohito Kita, and Gerald J. Gleich

Eosinophil Basic Proteins
  Major Basic Protein (MBP)
  Eosinophil Cationic Protein (ECP)
  Eosinophil-Derived Neurotoxin (EDN)

Eosinophil Peroxidase (EPO)
**Association of Eosinophil Basic Proteins with
  Hypersensitivity Diseases**

Eosinophil granule proteins are toxic for multicellular parasites and mammalian cells. When the toxic effects are directed toward parasites, they could function as a protective mechanism for the host. However, in some cases the toxic effects may be directed toward the host cells, causing organ damage in hypersensitivity diseases including bronchial asthma. Present evidence suggests that the eosinophil is an effector cell for hypersensitivity diseases and that the basic proteins of the eosinophil granule cause organ dysfunction. This evidence supports the hypothesis that the eosinophil importantly contributes to the pathophysiology of a variety of diseases, including bronchial asthma and atopic dermatitis (1–4). This chapter describes the biochemical properties and functions of eosinophil basic proteins in relation to hypersensitivity diseases. The properties of these basic proteins are summarized in Table 1 (5).

EOSINOPHIL BASIC PROTEINS

Major Basic Protein (MBP)

Biochemical Properties

In early studies, MBP was isolated from acid-solubilized eosinophil granules from guinea pigs (6,7). The molecular mass of this protein is about 11×10^3 Da, and it readily aggregates through formation of disulfide-linked chains. Amino acid analyses revealed that MBP is rich in arginine, tryptophan, and cysteine. Subsequently, human and rat MBP have been purified from eosinophil granules (8–10). Purified MBP from human and guinea pig eosinophils has similar biochemical properties. Both readily form disulfide bonds, are rich in arginine, and show relatively high isoelectric points (human MBP: 10.9) (8). As recently reported, human MBP contains five unpaired cysteines per molecule (11).

The amino acid sequence of MBP has been determined by protein sequencing and has been predicted from cDNA nucleotide sequence (9,12,13). Human MBP is a single polypeptide consisting of 117 amino acids with a mass of 14×10^3 Da. Interestingly, human MBP has weak homology to the lectin domain of the low affinity IgE receptor, $Fc_\varepsilon RII$ (14,15).

Cloning the MBP cDNA revealed that MBP is produced as a pre-pro-molecule with a 15 amino acid leader sequence and a 90 amino acid pro-sequence followed by the 117 amino acid sequence for granule MBP (12,13). The pro-portion of MBP is strikingly enriched in acidic amino acids, mainly glutamic acid, and the predicted isoelectric point of this portion is 3.9. Because the pro-form is as acidic as MBP itself is basic, the resulting molecule, proMBP, with 207 amino acids, has roughly equal numbers of basic and acidic amino acids with an isoelectric point of 6.2. As predicted, the recombinant pro-portion blocked the effect of MBP in two different *in vitro* systems: basophil histamine release and neutrophil activation (16). This also suggests that a major role of the proportion is to protect the cell from the injurious effects of MBP during the transport of proMBP from the Golgi apparatus to the eosinophil granule, where proMBP is converted to MBP. Recent studies have succeeded in se-

M. Kaneko: Basic Research Laboratories, Toray Industries, Inc., Kamakura, Kanagawa 248 Japan.
H. Kita and G. J. Gleich: Department of Immunology, Mayo Clinic and Mayo Foundation, Rochester, Minnesota 55905.

Table 1. *Some properties of human eosinophil granule proteins and their encoding cDNA and genes*

Protein	Site	Mr (×10⁻³)	Isoelectric point[a]	Cell content (mg/10⁶ cells)	Activities	Molecular biology[b] cDNA	Gene
MBP	Core	14	10.9	9	Potent helminthotoxin and cytotoxin; bactericidal; inhibits C3b; releases histamine from basophils and rat mast cells; strong platelet agonist; activates neutrophils and alveolar macrophages; promotes bronchospasm; increases bronchial reactivity to methacholine; blocks muscarinic M2 receptors; induces degranulation and IL-8 production from human eosinophils	~900 nt (pre-pro-MBP)	3.3kb 5 introns 6 exons
ECP	Matrix	18–21	10.8	5	Potent helminthotoxin and cytotoxin; bactericidal; potent neurotoxin; releases histamine from rat mast cells; weak RNase activity	~725 nt (pre-ECP)	~1.2 kb 1 intron in UTR
EDN	Matrix	18–19	8.9	3	Potent neurotoxin; potent RNase activity; weak helminthotoxin	~725 nt (pre-EDN)	~1.2 kb 1 intron in UTR
EPO	Matrix	66	10.8	12	In the presence of $H_2O_2+I^-$ or Br^- it kills microorganisms and tumor cells; causes histamine release from rat mast cells; inactivates leukotrienes; kills *Brugia* microfilariae and damages respiratory epithelium. In the absence of H_2O_2 it damages respiratory epithelium; causes bronchospasm; kills helminths	~2500 nt (2106 nt ORF)	12kb 11 introns

[a]Calculated from amino acid sequences deduced from the cDNAs

[b]nt = nucleotides; kb = kilobases; ORF = open reading frame; UTR = untranslated region; see text for references concerning the molecular biology of these proteins and their genes.

Modified from Gleich GJ, Kita H, Adolphson CR. The eosinophils. In: Frank MM, Austen KF, Claman HN, Unanue ER, eds. *Samter's immunologic diseases.* Boston: Little Brown, 1995;205–245, with permission.

quencing and cloning the cDNA of guinea pig MBP (MBP1 and MBP2) (17,18). As observed in human MBP, both of the guinea pig MBP molecules have a pre-pro-form and the pro-portion is rich in acidic amino acids. These observations indicate that the mechanisms for synthesis and processing of MBP in guinea pig eosinophils are similar to those in human eosinophils.

A genomic MBP clone has been identified and its nucleotide sequence determined (19). The 3.3 kb gene consists of six exons and five introns; one of the introns contains an Alu family repeat. The sequences of the exons are identical to the previously reported MBP cDNA sequences. The gene for MBP is immediately preceded by a putative promoter containing typical TATA and CCAATT boxes. Analysis of the genomic DNA from four individuals of different racial groups showed identical restriction maps, suggesting that the MBP gene exhibits limited polymorphism (13,19).

Localization

By isolation of granules and by immunoelectron microscopy, human and guinea pig eosinophils have MBP localized to the crystalline cores of their specific granules. The core appears to contain only MBP (20–22). Human eosinophils do not contain MBP in organelles other than granules, and no MBP can be detected in plasma cells, lymphocytes, or neutrophils (20,21).

Human basophils also are stained with antibody to MBP by immunofluorescence; MBP can be detected in basophil extracts at approximately 140 ng/10⁶ cells (23). One report detected 2400 ng/10⁶ cells of MBP in human basophils (24). There are two possible explanations for the existence of MBP in basophils. One is that basophils can synthesize MBP by themselves. The other is that basophils tend to internalize MBP in their granules, similar to the ability of guinea pig basophils to internalize eosinophil peroxidase (EPO) (25,26). Further studies are needed to clarify the significance of MBP in basophils.

Mast cells from nasal polyps, ileal tissue, and cutaneous mastocytosis specimens, but not normal skin, show the presence of MBP by immunofluorescence (27). When mast cells from normal skin were cultured in the presence of MBP, the mast cells showed positive staining for MBP in 3 minutes. These results suggest that mast cells in several tissues can internalize MBP by endocytosis. The MBP in mast cells could bind to heparin in their granules because of the biochemical properties of each molecule. Neutralization of the toxic protein by internalization might be one of the mast cell's functions (28,29).

Immunoreactive MBP is increased in the sera of all pregnant women, often peaking just before labor and falling rapidly after parturition (30). Serial blood samples from pregnant women show a striking rise of MBP 2 to 3 weeks before parturition, suggesting that MBP might be involved in the onset of term and preterm labor (31,32). A test of this hypothesis showed that MBP rises before labor in 80% of pregnant women, but this rise does not predict the onset of labor (33). MBP has been shown to localize to placental X cells and placental site giant cells by immunofluorescence; MBP mRNA also has been shown to be expressed in placental X cells (34–36). Analyses of the placenta-derived MBP isolated either from placental septal cyst fluid or from extracts of placental septa indicated that the pregnancy-associated MBP (pMBP) is indistinguishable from the eosinophil granule MBP (gMBP) (37). Recent studies indicate that proMBP is bound to PAPP-A and suggest that proMBP is present in the placenta and is the predominant form of MBP in the blood of pregnant women (38). Analyses of proteins accumulating in the uteri of rats after estradiol treatment (which causes a striking eosinophil infiltration) revealed a protein of 17kDa that had 28 amino-terminal residues with a strong homology to human MBP (39). Antibodies to this rat molecule reacted with rat eosinophils and cross-reacted with human MBP. Immunohistochemical staining of the rat uterus showed that this same protein was associated with eosinophils that infiltrate after estrogen treatment; MBP then spreads throughout the stroma and the deep glandular epithelium. Further investigation of the distribution of MBP in the rat uterus by immunohistochemistry revealed deposition of MBP in the cervix and the uterus, especially during proestrus and estrus (40). At present, the function of MBP during parturition is obscure.

MBP was also found in the HL-60 cell line and in alveolar macrophages of patients with asthma (41,42). Eosinophil granules were found by electron microscopy in macrophages of patients with eosinophilic pneumonia (43).

Functions of MBP

Toxicity to Parasites

Eosinophils kill schistosomula of *Schistosoma mansoni* in the presence of antibodies to the parasite obtained from patients with this infectious disease (44,45). In addition to eosinophils themselves, MBP binds and disrupts the membrane of *S. mansoni*, resulting in killing of the parasites (46). Subsequent experiments on the interactions of *S. mansoni* schistosomula with eosinophils showed that the strong, stable binding of eosinophils to the parasite target is most likely due to the release of cationic granule proteins which bind the cell to the organism (45).

MBP also damages other parasites, including newborn larvae of *Trichinella spiralis* and microfilariae of *Brugia pahangi* and *B. malayi* (47–49). MBP can kill a protozoan parasite, the bloodstream form (trypomastigote stage) of *Trypanosoma cruzi*, and the etiologic agent of Chaga's disease in humans (50,51). In addition, amastigote forms of *T. cruzi*, the intracellular form of the organism, were ingested by eosinophils and damaged (52,53). Purified MBP in the absence of eosinophils caused lysis of amastigotes, and its toxicity was inhibited by specific antibody to MBP (52).

Effects on Bacteria

Initial studies of the effect of guinea pig MBP on bacterial growth, including *Staphylococcus epidermidis*, *Proteus vulgaris*, *Staphylococcus aureus*, *Streptococcus pyogenes*, and two strains of *Escherichia coli*, failed to show striking effects except for a 50% reduction of the growth of *E. coli* 182 (7). More recently, human MBP showed marked activity against *S. aureus* 502A and *E. coli* ML-35 (54). MBP was active against *E. coli* in mediums containing 140 mM NaCl or 1 mM Ca^{2+}, but the presence of 1 mM Mg^{2+} abolished its activity. Thus, MBP causes outer- and inner-membrane permeabilization.

Toxicity to Mammalian Cells

MBP shows cytotoxicity to murine and human tumor cells and to other mammalian cells (46,55). It has been reported that the concentrations of MBP in the body fluids of patients with eosinophilia may approach the toxic range, suggesting MBP contributes to hypersensitivity diseases (55–57). Eosinophil accumulation and dysfunction or desquamation of bronchial epithelial cells are characteristic features observed in patients with asthma (58). Therefore, several investigators focused their interests on the cytotoxic effects of MBP on respiratory epithelial cells. MBP itself induced ciliostasis and exfoliation of respiratory epithelial cells (55,56,59,60), an effect that mimics the pathology of asthma. In addition, activated eosinophils, or MBP itself, damage adherent human amnion cells, as assessed by ^{51}Cr release; however, neither eosinophils nor MBP induced exfoliation of the cells (61).

Complement Activation

Initial studies of the antigenicity of MBP by quantitative complement fixation showed that concentrations of guinea pig or rat MBP higher than 50 μg/ml cause nonspecific complement activation (62). These results are in keeping with prior observations that complement activation can occur with polycationic proteins (63). Analyses of the ability of MBP to regulate generation of classic and alternative-amplification pathway C3 convertases, showed that MBP inhibits the generation of EAC1,4b,2a and EAC4b,3b,Bb,P, and that the MBP effect is greater on the classic pathway convertase than on the alternative-amplification pathway convertase. The mechanism of inhibition of convertase activity is likely through an action on C3b and through inhibition of factor B consumption (64). These results suggest that MBP (and the other eosinophil proteins; see later) act predominantly on C3b to regulate the alternative pathway activity; MBP had no effect on the later events in complement activation after the formation of C3b convertase (65).

Activation of Inflammatory Cells

Among the eosinophil basic granule proteins, only MBP induces histamine release from human basophils by a calcium-, temperature- and energy-dependent mechanism (66). This histamine release was inhibited by calmodulin antagonists, by theophylline and pertussis toxin, and partially blocked by a phospholipase A2 inhibitor (67). The effect of pertussis toxin suggests involvement of a regulatory G protein. In addition to human basophils, rat peritoneal mast cells are stimulated and release histamine in response to MBP, as well as ECP and EPO (68). This secretion was observed in both the absence and the presence of extracellular calcium (68). In contrast to these previous studies, one report showed that MBP and EPO inhibited histamine release induced by substance P from human skin mast cells (69). These results suggest that mast cells in various organs differ in their responses to MBP; a recent report shows that cardiac mast cells release histamine on incubation with MBP and ECP (70).

In addition to basophils and mast cells, MBP can stimulate neutrophils, platelets, and macrophages, as well as eosinophils. Incubation of neutrophils in the presence of MBP caused increase of chemiluminescence, superoxide anion production, lysozyme release, and CR3 expression (71,72). Stimulation of platelets by MBP or EPO induced release of 5-hydroxytryptamine, α-granule, and lysosome components (73). This secretion was not affected by the presence of indomethacin; 1 μM of prostaglandin E1 inhibited this secretion. MBP and EPO can be classified as strong platelet agonists with distinctive mechanisms of activation. MBP also stimulates lung macrophages, causing superoxide anion generation (74). Furthermore, a recent study indicates that eosinophil degranulation can be induced by MBP or EPO, and that eosinophil production of IL-8 is also induced by MBP. These effects on eosinophils were not attributed to cytotoxic effects of MBP or EPO (75). These results suggest the presence of specific receptors for MBP on these cells. Because of the abundance of neutrophils or platelets in comparison with basophils or mast cells, they should be useful for analyses of the putative MBP receptor. In contrast to these stimulative effects described previously, MBP inhibited superoxide anion production from guinea pig alveolar macrophages stimulated with PMA (74). This effect of MBP was not due to cytotoxicity and was concentration-dependent. Thus, MBP may also act as an inhibitory factor for cell activation in some conditions.

Effect on Coagulation

Early studies of MBP revealed that it neutralizes heparin by forming a precipitate and increases the clotting time of whole blood (7). Eosinophil supernatants and MBP, EPO, and ECP all inhibited Hageman factor activation by ellagic acid and sulfatide-induced activation (76). In these experiments, it seems likely that the inhibition of Hageman factor activation is related to neutralization of the negatively charged Hageman factor activators, such as ellagic acid, by the markedly cationic eosinophil granule proteins (76). MBP also binds to the anionic endothelial protein thrombomodulin and impairs its anticoagulant activities (77).

Mechanisms of Toxicity

The mechanisms by which MBP exerts its toxicity have been tested using liposomes as targets (78). MBP readily interacted with acidic lipids, causing disorder of the bilayer lipid membrane and fusion and lysis of liposomes. These results indicate that MBP associates with acidic lipids and that it disrupts, aggregates, fuses, and lyses lysosomes composed of acid lipids. This mechanism of action might account for the wide range of MBP activity as a cytostimulant and as a toxin.

Eosinophil Cationic Protein (ECP)

Biochemical Properties

ECP, with an isoelectric point of approximately 10.8, consists of a single polypeptide chain and displays striking heterogeneity, as revealed by liquid chromatography and gel electrophoresis (79,80). ECP and MBP differ in their compositions, pI, reactivity with antibodies, and abundance within the eosinophil granule (24,81). Fractionation of eosinophil granule proteins on heparin-Sepharose shows two major peaks of ECP antigenic activity, referred to as ECP1 and ECP2 (79). On gel electrophoresis, ECP1 consists of a major band with a mass of 18,300 Da and a minor band with a mass of 21,400 Da; ECP2 shows three bands: a doublet at 16,000 Da and another band at 16,900 Da. Despite this electrophoretic heterogeneity, the partial N-terminal amino acid sequences of ECP1 and ECP2 are identical, and their electrophoretic heterogeneity may be the result of posttranslational modification (79). The partial N-terminal amino acid sequence of ECP reveals marked homology to that of EDN (see following) and of pancreatic ribonuclease (RNase) (79).

The nucleotide sequence of ECP cDNA codes for a preprotein of 160 amino acids and a protein of 133 amino acids with a mass of 15,600 Da (82,83). The ECP-deduced amino acid sequence reveals 66% identity to EDN and 31% identity to human pancreatic RNase; the essential cysteine and catalytic region lysine and histidine residues are conserved. ECP is a member of the RNase gene superfamily, the other members of which include EDN, pancreatic ribonuclease, and human angiogenin. However, the RNase activity of ECP is approximately 50 to 100 times less than that of EDN, perhaps due to the lack of a positively charged residue at human pancreatic RNase position 122 (84). Comparison of the RNase activity of ECP with that of pancreatic RNase revealed that ECP possesses 70- to 200-fold less activity (85). ECP preferentially hydrolyzed synthetic polynucleotides composed of poly-U, rather than poly-C; ECP did not hydrolyze defined low molecular weight substrates, such as dinucleotide phosphates and uridine and cytidine $2',3'$-cyclic phosphates. These results link ECP ribonucleolytic activity to the "nonsecretory" liver type enzymes, rather than to the secretory pancreatic RNases.

The ECP gene has been cloned and localized to the q24-q31 region of human chromosome 14. This gene possesses a single intron of 230 bases in the 5′ untranslated region, and the structure of the ECP gene (RNS3) is remarkably similar to that of the EDN gene (RNS2) (86,87).

Monoclonal antibodies to ECP revealed differences between the stored and secreted forms of the molecule (88). Monoclonal antibody EG1 was specific for ECP and recognized both the stored and secreted forms of ECP, whereas antibody EG2 recognized only the secreted or extracted form of ECP; monoclonal antibody EG2 also reacted with EDN. EG2 did not react with resting eosinophils, but it did react with eosinophils after phagocytosis and after activation with eosinophil cytotoxicity-enhancing factor. Also, monoclonal antibody EG2 reacted with eosinophils from patients with the hypereosinophilic syndrome. Thus, EG2 appears to detect activated eosinophils, and it has been used to identify these cells in tissues and blood during disease (89,90); although a recent report claimed that EG2 does not provide reliable immunohistochemical discrimination between resting and activated eosinophils (91). Analyses of the specificity of EG2 suggest that it recognizes a polypeptide epitope that is masked in the higher molecular weight glycosylated chain, because EG2 recognizes only the low glycosylated form of ECP and the deglycosylated EDN; EG1 recognizes the more heavily glycosylated form of ECP (92).

Localization

As discussed above, MBP can be localized in the eosinophil granule crystalloid. Because the crystalloid is presumably one substance, one would predict that ECP is present in the granule matrix. Localization of ECP by immunoelectron microscopy revealed that it is localized to the granule matrix (20,21).

Functions

Toxicity to Parasites

ECP is a potent toxin for schistosomula of *S. mansoni*; in a comparative test, ECP was approximately 10 times more active than MBP (93,94). The killing of schistosomula by ECP differed qualitatively from that produced by MBP; ECP produces complete fragmentation and disruption of schistosomula, whereas MBP produces distinctive ballooning and detachment of the tegumental membrane. The latter effect of MBP is reminiscent of the effect of eosinophils themselves on schistosomula, where one sees similar effects on the membrane (46). ECP is also toxic for newborn larvae of *T. spiralis* and microfilariae of *B. pahangi* and *B. malayi in vitro* (47,49). In *T. spiralis* newborn larvae, ECP is more toxic on a molar basis than MBP. ECP is also lytic for *T. cruzi* trypomastigotes, and the toxicity of ECP for the trypomastigotes was not inhibited by the placental ribonuclease inhibitor (51).

Effects on Bacteria

Although early studies of ECP failed to demonstrate antibacterial activity (95), a more recent investigation revealed marked bactericidal activity against *S. aureus* 502A and *E. coli* ML-35 (54). ECP caused both outer- and inner-membrane permeabilization of *E. coli* ML-35, but the bactericidal effects of ECP were lost when the medium contained 140 mM NaCl, 1 mM Ca^{2+} or 1 mM Mg^{2+} (54).

Effects on Coagulation and Fibrinolysis

ECP binds to heparin and neutralizes its anticoagulant activity; it also shortens the coagulation time of plasma in a dose-dependent manner (96,97). At high concentrations, ECP prolonged the clotting time and inhibited activation of Hageman factor by ellagic acid (76). ECP also altered fibrinolysis, as demonstrated by enhancement of urokinase-induced plasminogen activation (98).

Neurotoxicity

As discussed below, eosinophil extracts produce a neurotoxic reaction when injected into the cerebrospinal fluid of rabbits or the brains of guinea pigs, and ECP (both ECP1 and ECP2) is a potent neurotoxin (79,99,100).

Effect on Lymphocyte Proliferation

One report has shown that ECP causes dose-dependent inhibition of proliferation of human peripheral blood lymphocytes induced by phytohemagglutinin and by a one-way mixed lymphocyte reaction; in these experiments EDN behaved similarly to ECP (101).

Effect on Mammalian Cells

ECP stimulates the release of histamine from rat mast cells, but it does not cause histamine release from basophils (68). ECP also kills K562 tumor cells *in vitro* (102). Finally, ECP causes desquamation of respiratory epithelial cells *in vitro* (60).

Mechanisms of Toxicity

ECP damaged target cell membranes through the formation of pores or transmembrane channels, whereas, under these conditions, EDN and EPO did not exhibit channel-forming activity (103). Eosinophil cytoplasts (eosinophil vesicles devoid of granules and nuclei, but possessing an intact oxidase in their plasma membrane), in combination with low ECP concentrations, enhanced killing of *S. mansoni* schistosomula (104). Cytoplasts from a patient with chronic granulomatous disease were unable to act in synergy with ECP, suggesting that oxygen and its metabolites were important for the synergy. These experiments suggest that oxygen and its metabolites aid the killing of schistosomula by lowering the concentrations of ECP needed to inflict damage (104). The toxicity of ECP may be neutralized by serum α_2-macroglobulin; ECP forms a strong, noncovalent complex with α_2-macroglobulin (105). Yet another mechanism by which the toxicity of ECP may be neutralized is interaction with heparin (95,96).

Eosinophil-Derived Neurotoxin (EDN)

In 1933, Gordon described a neurotoxic reaction that occurs in experimental animals (106). The cause of this reaction, now referred to as the Gordon phenomenon, was traced to eosinophils (99,107,108) and, ultimately, to EDN. Patients with the idiopathic hypereosinophilic syndrome, and patients with cerebrospinal fluid eosinophilia, exhibit neurologic abnormalities (109–111); thus, it is possible that the neurotoxic eosinophil granule proteins are important in diseases of the nervous system in humans.

Biochemical Properties

EDN was isolated from eosinophil granules and a mass of approximately 18,600 Da was found (79,81,112). The partial N-terminal sequence of EDN revealed marked sequence homology to ECP with identity at 37 of 54 N-terminal residues (79). Despite this finding, major differences in the sequences exist that may explain differences in reactivity with polyclonal and monoclonal antibodies (79,81,88). EDN and ECP are homologous to pancreatic RNase (77), but EDN has about 100 times more RNase activity than ECP (84).

EDN cDNA has been cloned, and the deduced amino acid sequence specifies a 134 amino acid polypeptide with a mass of 15,500 Da and a 27 residue amino-terminal hydrophobic leader (113,114). This sequence is identical to that reported for human urinary RNase and to the amino-terminal sequence of human liver RNase (115, 116). Comparison of the amino acid and nucleotide sequences of EDN and other proteins with ribonucleolytic activity (i.e., bovine seminal RNase, human and rat pancreatic RNase, ECP, and human angiogenin), revealed extensive homology at half-cystine residues and at the amino acids of active sites. These results support the concept of an RNase gene superfamily consisting of secretory and nonsecretory RNase, angiogenin, EDN, and ECP. Finally, when angiogenin was injected into *Xenopus* oocytes, it inhibited protein synthesis, and this inhibition was correlated with degradation of endogenous oocyte tRNA. By contrast, EDN nonspecifically degraded oocyte RNA similarly to RNase A. Thus, angiogenin appears to be specific for tRNA, in contrast to the other RNases (117).

A human liver RNase has been identified and classified as nonsecretory (115,116). Human liver RNase is structurally related, but distinct, from human pancreatic RNase, a secretory enzyme (118). EDN is similar to human liver RNase, and these two RNases are indistinguishable from each other. Antibodies to EDN and liver RNase showed identical cross-reactivities in assays of nuclease inhibition and in a radioimmunoassay (119).

The human genomic DNAs for ECP and EDN have been isolated, and alignment of EDN (RNS2) and ECP (RNS3) gene sequences demonstrates remarkable nucleotide similarities in the noncoding sequences, introns, and flanking regions, as well as in the previously known coding regions (86,87). A single intron of 230 bases is present in the 5′ untranslated region of both RNS2 and RNS3, suggesting that the single intron in this region and the existence of an intronless coding region are features common to many members of the RNase gene superfamily. The RNS2 and RNS3 genes have been localized to the q24-q31 region of human chromosome 14 (86,87). Comparison of the phylogenetic relations of EDN and ECP suggests that the genes for these proteins arose as a consequence of a gene duplication event that took place approximately 25 million to 40 million years ago, and that a subset of anthropoid primates have both of these genes or closely related genes (86).

Eosinophil protein X (EPX) was originally thought to be a novel eosinophil granule protein with properties similar to those of EDN (120). Comparison of EDN and EPX revealed that they have similar molecular weights and RNase activity, produce the Gordon phenomenon, and are relatively weak helminthotoxins against early-stage schistosomula of *S. mansoni* (79,84,94,100,112,121, 122). Detailed comparison of EDN and EPX indicated that they have virtually identical properties and are probably the same protein (123).

Localization

Early studies suggested that EDN is present in the eosinophil granule because extracts of highly purified eosinophil granules produced the Gordon phenomenon (79,112). Subsequent immunoelectron microscopy analyses have shown that EDN is localized to the granule matrix (21).

Functions

Neurotoxicity

When EDN is injected intrathecally into rabbits or guinea pigs, it causes the Gordon phenomenon, a syndrome that begins with stiffness (most notably in the forelegs) and mild ataxia, followed by incoordination and marked ataxia so severe that the animals have difficulty remaining upright. The final phase of the Gordon phenomenon is associated with severe weakness and muscle wasting (99,106–108,112). Studies of the comparative neurotoxicity of EDN and ECP in rabbits revealed that these proteins are almost equal in potency (79). However, later studies of the neurotoxicity of ECP and EPX (presumed to be EDN) in guinea pigs revealed that ECP is 100 times more potent than EPX (100). Because EDN and EPX appear to be identical, this difference may be attributable to a species difference between guinea pigs and rabbits. None of the other eosinophil granule proteins, including EPO, MBP, and the CLC protein (lysophospholipase), produced the Gordon phenomenon (79,112).

As noted earlier, EDN and liver RNase were essentially indistinguishable by immunoassay and by the pattern of their RNase activities. These proteins were compared to determine if human liver RNase produces the Gordon phenomenon; both EDN and liver RNase were comparably neurotoxic when injected intrathecally into rabbits. Human pancreatic RNase was less neurotoxic, and bovine pancreatic RNase showed no effect. Treatment of EDN, liver RNase, and ECP with iodoacetic acid resulted in inactivation of their RNase activity and neurotoxicity. These results suggest that RNase activity is necessary, but not sufficient, to induce a neurotoxic reaction (119).

The histopathology of the Gordon phenomenon in rabbits has been thoroughly described (99,112). By light microscopy, the histologic abnormalities are concentrated in the cerebellum, pons, and spinal cord. A striking characteristic of the Gordon phenomenon is the disappearance of cerebellar Purkinje cells. In addition, the white matter of the cerebellum, pons, and spinal cord shows a marked spongiform change, whereas the gray matter remains essentially normal.

Toxicity to Parasites

EDN is considerably less toxic for parasites and for other targets than the other eosinophil granule proteins. For example, EDN was only weakly toxic to schistosomula of *S. mansoni*, whereas EPX (presumably EDN) was highly toxic to lung-stage schistosomula of *S. mansoni* (94,122). EDN was toxic to newborn larvae of *T. spiralis*, but tenfold higher concentrations of EDN, compared to ECP, were required for toxicity (47). In addition, EDN was toxic to microfilariae of *B. pahangi* and *B. malayi*, though considerably less so than purified MBP, ECP, or EPO (49). EDN was an active toxin for *T. cruzi* trypomastigotes and was more potent than ECP. Finally, the toxicity of EDN for *T. cruzi* trypomastigotes was inhibited by heparin, dextran sulfate, and human placental RNasin® (a ribonuclease inhibitor)(51); the latter result suggests that the toxicity of EDN depends on its possession of RNase activity.

Eosinophil Peroxidase (EPO)

Biochemical Properties

EPO differs from neutrophil or monocyte myeloperoxidase (MPO) in its absorption spectrum and its heme prosthetic groups (124–128). Human EPO has been purified and has a mass ranging from approximately 67,000 Da (judged by gel electrophoresis) to 77,000 Da (by gel filtration) (125–127,129–131). EPO consists of two subunits, a heavy chain with a mass of 50,000 Da to 58,000 Da, and a light chain with a mass of 10,500 Da to 15,500 Da in 1:1 stoichiometry. Although the production of specific antisera to EPO has been described (129,132), in our experience extensive cross-reactivity between EPO and MPO exists with most polyclonal antibodies. A recent study reported that antineutrophil cytoplasmic antibodies in patients with systemic vasculitis recognized MPO, but not EPO (133). By radioimmunoassay, the cell content of EPO in one report was 15 µg/10^6 eosinophils; another report found 12.2±0.9 µg/10^6 cells (24,129).

Analyses of the amino acid sequence of EPO revealed that the heavy chain and the light chain differ; the light chain sequence also differs from that of MBP even though they co-migrated on sodium dodecyl sulfate-polyacrylamide gel electrophoresis (SDS-PAGE) (134,135). EPO cDNA has an open reading frame of 2106 nucleotides coding for a 381 bp prosequence, a 333 bp sequence corresponding to the coding region of the EPO light chain, a 1392 bp sequence coding for the EPO heavy chain, and a 452 bp untranslated 3′ region (136). The masses of heavy and light EPO subunits are 12,712 Da and 53,011 Da, respectively; and their calculated isoelectric points are 10.8 and 10.7, respectively. Comparison of the EPO sequence with other peroxidases revealed a striking similarity among EPO, MPO, and thyroid peroxidase; for example, EPO and MPO have 68.3 percent amino acid identity. Overall, these results suggest the existence of a peroxidase multigene family including EPO, MPO, and the thyroid peroxidase (137,138). The primary structure of bovine lactoperoxidase from cow's milk shows clear-cut similarities to human MPO, EPO, and thyroid peroxidase (139). Bovine lactoperoxidase consists of a single peptide chain of 612 amino acid residues and is homologous to the corresponding peptide sequences of MPO, EPO, and thyroid peroxidase. The human EPO gene has been cloned with MPO cDNA as a probe; it is similar to the human MPO gene, consisting of 12 exons and 11 introns spanning approximately 12 kb (140). Regarding transcriptional regulation of EPO, recent reports have clarified the existence of positively and negatively acting elements in the promoter region of EPO gene (141,142).

In the presence of H_2O_2, EPO oxidizes halides to form reactive hypohalous acids (124,143); for example, chloride is oxidized to form hypochlorous acid: $H_2O_2 + Cl^- + H^+ \rightarrow HOCl + H_2O$. Analyses of EPO halide preference showed that eosinophils preferentially utilize bromide over chloride (144–146). Therefore, it seemed that EPO, in the presence of normal body fluids, could use Br^- to form a toxic oxidant, hypobromous acid. Another report, however, indicated that the pseudohalide, thiocyanate, at a concentration of 1 µM, is a potent inhibitor of the reactivity of EPO with bromide or iodide, both present at 100 µM (147). EPO also catalyzed the covalent incorporation of thiocyanate into proteins, despite high bromide concentrations in these buffers. Even subphysiologic concentrations of thiocyanate (i.e., 3.3-10.0 µM,) nearly completely blocked the bromide-dependent toxicity of EPO for ^{51}Cr-labeled aortic endothelial cells. Therefore, the peroxidactic product of the EPO-thiocyanate interaction, namely hypothiocyanous acid, a weak, primarily sulfhydryl-reactive oxidant best known as a bacteriostatic agent

in saliva and milk, appears to be the major oxidant produced by EPO in physiologic fluids.

Localization

EPO has been localized to the matrix of the crystalloid-containing granules (20). Peroxidase activity has been detected in both the uterus and intestinal tissues. Because intestinal epithelial cells contain only small amounts of peroxidase, and because the peroxidase isolated from the intestine is similar to that obtained from the eosinophil, it seems likely that the intestinal peroxidase is derived from the eosinophil (148). Rat peritoneal mast cells have been shown to have peroxidase activity in their granules; the EPO that has been incorporated and bound to granule components in mast cells accounts for this activity (149).

Deficiency

EPO is absent in eosinophils of certain human kindreds, and among Yemenite Jews this deficiency appears to be inherited in an autosomal recessive mode (150–152). EPO deficiency has not been associated with any distinctive clinical symptoms, and it has been proposed as a marker in population genetics (153). An assay useful for discriminating EPO from neutrophil MPO has been described and used to detect individuals with EPO deficiency (154). The eosinophils of these individuals show an increased granule core volume/total granule volume ratio owing to contraction of the volume of the matrix; two other eosinophil matrix proteins, ECP and EDN, appear to be present in normal amounts in the EPO-deficient granules (155). Finally, EPO deficiency occurs in individuals in certain areas of northeastern Italy with a frequency of approximately one case in 14,000 (156). Although the molecular basis of the defect is unknown, a recent study suggests that a mutation in the EPO gene causes the production of an unstable EPO that degrades during eosinophil maturation (157).

Functions

Toxic effects of EPO/H_2O_2/Halide system

Tests of the activity of MPO from neutrophils and monocytes in the presence of H_2O_2 and halide showed that this system kills bacteria, viruses, mycoplasma, and fungi (158–161). Because eosinophils generate H_2O_2 and have an active halogenation capability, killing of microorganisms by the EPO/H_2O_2/halide system has been studied (124,162,163). These studies have shown that the EPO/H_2O_2/halide system kills not only a variety of microorganisms (e.g., E. coli, schistosomula of S. mansoni, microfilariae of *B. pahangi* and *B. malayi*, trypanosoma, toxoplasma, and mycobacteria), but mast cells and tumor cells as well (49,51,164–170). Studies of cultured human pneumocytes and nasal epithelial cells indicate that both the EPO/H$_2$O$_2$/Br$^-$ system and MBP cause toxicity to the cultured cells (171–173). Thus, the EPO/H$_2$O$_2$/halide system can mediate toxicity toward numerous targets using either iodide or bromide. However, in view of the finding that thiocyanate is the preferred substrate for EPO, these findings require reevaluation to determine if hypothiocyanaous acid exerts a toxic effect on the aforementioned targets, and if thiocyanate is the only substrate in biologic systems.

In the absence of H$_2$O$_2$ and halide (e.g., iodide), EPO is also toxic to some targets. For example, *B. pahangi* microfilariae were killed by EPO in the absence of H$_2$O$_2$ and iodide at concentrations as low as 1.7×10^{-5}M; however, in the same experiment the EPO/H$_2$O$_2$/I$^-$ system was effective in killing *B. pahangi* at EPO concentrations as low as 5×10^{-9}M, a 30,000-fold difference (49). Evidence that EPO is truly acting as a toxin (and not as a peroxidase) for *B. pahangi* microfilariae was shown by the inability of catalase to inhibit the toxic activity of EPO. In contrast, catalase totally inhibited the killing activity of the EPO/H$_2$O$_2$/I$^-$ system (49). Furthermore, bovine serum albumin (a hypohalous acid scavenger) inhibited EPO-mediated toxicity in the presence of H$_2$O$_2$/I$^-$; in contrast, it had relatively little effect on the toxicity of EPO by itself. Moreover, EPO in the absence of H$_2$O$_2$ and halide was a potent toxin for guinea pig tracheal epithelium, causing cessation of ciliary beating and the exfoliation and blebbing of epithelial cells (60). The latter results mimic the pathology of asthma and are similar to those caused by MBP. Lastly, EPO alters adherence of pneumocytes in culture, and it has been proposed that EPO may cause desquamation of epithelial cells *in vitro* (60,171).

Effects on Mast Cells and Their Granules

The granules of mast cells bind EPO, and the granule-EPO complex catalyzes the iodination of proteins and killing of microorganisms (174). The EPO/H$_2$O$_2$/I$^-$ system also induced rat mast cell degranulation and histamine release (169). Whereas EPO/H$_2$O$_2$/I$^-$ was noncytotoxic at low EPO concentrations, at higher concentrations ultrastructural evidence of mast cell damage was evident. Of interest is the observation that the EPO-mast cell granule complex is more effective than free EPO in terms of the ability to stimulate mast cell secretion.

Effects of EPO Bound to Effector Cells

Binding of EPO to microbial organisms (e.g., *S. aureus, T. cruzi, and T. gondii*) markedly enhanced their killing by mononuclear phagocytes (167,175,176). Fur-

thermore, tumor cells adsorb EPO, and this binding potentiates their lysis by H$_2$O$_2$ (177). Interestingly, tumor cells coated by EPO were spontaneously lysed by activated macrophages (which have the ability to release H$_2$O$_2$), and, thus, a synergy exists between EPO and H$_2$O$_2$ in the destruction of the tumor cells. These findings, as well as the observation that MBP is toxic to tumor cells, suggest that the eosinophil has the ability to limit the spread of tumors (102). Experiments demonstrating that EPO bound to pneumocytes resulted in cell lysis, whereas EPO in solution did not, also indicate the importance of EPO binding to targets.

Comparison of the toxicity of the EPO (from horse eosinophils)/H$_2$O$_2$/halide system to the toxicity of a group of eosinophil granule proteins, utilizing *S. mansoni* schistosomula and *E. coli* as targets, showed that the EPO/H$_2$O$_2$/halide system is at least 100-fold more potent than the cationic toxins, and that toxicity is more rapid (178). These results are consistent with comparable studies of human eosinophil granule proteins utilizing *B. pahangi* and *B. malayi* as targets (49).

Effect of EPO on Leukotrienes

Incubation of the EPO/H$_2$O$_2$/halide system with leukotriene C$_4$ or D$_4$ (LTC$_4$, LTD$_4$) rapidly decreased the biologic activity of the leukotrienes on smooth muscle (179). Similarly, the EPO/H$_2$O$_2$/halide system decreased the chemotactic activity of LTB$_4$ (179). Deleting any of the components of the EPO system decreased the degradation of leukotriene activity. Another analysis of the effect of the EPO/H$_2$O$_2$/halide on LTC$_4$ showed that LTC$_4$ is converted to isomers of LTB$_4$, possessing less than 1/100 of the chemotactic activity of LTB$_4$ (180). Therefore, the EPO/H$_2$O$_2$/halide system may regulate the concentrations of leukotrienes during inflammation and immediate hypersensitivity reactions. In these experiments, however, the halides employed were either iodide or bromide; and one must again exercise caution when extrapolating these results to disease situations in view of the preference of EPO for thiocyanate (147).

Other Effects of EPO

EPO is a potent platelet stimulant and does not require the peroxidase activity in this reaction (73). It is able to inhibit the formation of the cell-bound alternative pathway C3b convertase, an activity shared by ECP and MBP (65).

Effect of EPO in Pathologic Situations

EPO bound to rat heart and endothelial cells in the presence of H$_2$O$_2$/Br$^-$ caused cytolysis of the endothelial cells (181). This system was utilized as a model of eosinophilic endocarditis by binding EPO to the endothelial cells and perfusing the left ventricle with a buffer containing bromide and H_2O_2. Under these conditions, acute congestive heart failure occurred, suggesting that EPO plays an important role in the pathophysiology of the cardiomyopathy associated with the hypereosinophilic syndrome (181). Studies of mice infected with *Toxocara canis* have disclosed that EPO is deposited in the pulmonary parenchyma and the myocardium, and that this deposition may lead to peroxidactic cardiopulmonary damage (182). *T. canis*-infected rats showed a decrease in cardiac performance associated with an increase in blood eosinophils. By 14 days after infection, cardiac work had declined approximately 25%; as the eosinophilia dropped, cardiac function improved. These data support the hypothesis that eosinophilia can lead to cardiac dysfunction (183).

ASSOCIATION OF EOSINOPHIL BASIC PROTEINS WITH HYPERSENSITIVITY DISEASES

Do the Eosinophil's Basic Proteins Have Pathogenic Functions In Vitro?

As described previously, eosinophil basic proteins have been shown *in vitro* to provoke several pathogenic functions. MBP shows toxicity to bronchial epithelial cells, pneumocytes, and nasal epithelium (55,56,59,60,171–173,184,185). In addition to MBP, ECP and EPO also show cytotoxic effects on respiratory epithelium, causing desquamation of epithelial cells (60). In fact, MBP induced an increased responsiveness to acetylcholine in experiments using an *in situ in vivo* tracheal smooth muscle preparation, presumably by causing dysfunction of epithelial cells (186–188). MBP stimulates basophils, rat mast cells, platelets and eosinophils, inducing mediator release such as histamine, serotonin, superoxide anion and/or IL-8. ECP and EPO could also stimulate some of these effects (66,68,73,75). MBP and EPO are reported to bind to muscarinic M2, but not M3, receptors, causing an increase in bronchial hyperresponsiveness by overstimulation of the vagal nerve (189,190).

Do the Eosinophil's Basic Proteins Induce Inflammation In Vivo?

Purified MBP has been instilled into airways of experimental animals to test whether it can reproduce features of asthma. The results indicated that MBP induces bronchial hyperresponsiveness in guinea pigs and primates (191,192). Furthermore, a recent study shows that ECP and EPO, as well as MBP, increase vascular permeability in *ex vivo* experiments (193).

Do the Basic Proteins Localize at Inflammatory Sites in Hypersensitivity Diseases?

MBP levels are increased in sputum specimens or bronchoalveolar lavage fluids (BAL) from patients with asthma, and MBP is deposited at sites of tissue damage in patients dying from bronchial asthma (42,56,194). Clearly, eosinophils release their granule proteins into the inflamed tissues. In addition, the severity of bronchial hyperresponsiveness observed in patients with asthma, in experimental models in primates, and in guinea pigs has been directly correlated with either blood or bronchial eosinophilia or quantities of basic proteins in bronchoalveolar lavage fluids (194–201).

Do Specific Inhibitors for the Basic Proteins Inhibit Symptoms in Hypersensitivity Diseases?

Specific antagonists or synthesis inhibitors for these basic proteins are not available. However, polyglutamic acid and heparin do neutralize the functions of MBP; these anionic polymers can inhibit the killing of K562 induced by MBP (202). Interestingly, polyglutamic acid can inhibit both the bronchial hyperresponsiveness induced by MBP in primates and the increase in vagal responsiveness induced by antigen provocation in guinea pigs (102,190).

Overall, these findings provide support for the hypothesis that the eosinophil basic proteins make important contributions to the pathophysiology of a variety of hypersensitivity diseases, including bronchial asthma (1–3).

ACKNOWLEDGMENTS

Portions of this chapter have been taken in part and used with permission from G.J. Gleich et al. The eosinophil. In: JI Gallin, IM Goldstein, R Snyderman, eds: *Inflammation: basic principles and clinical correlates.* 2nd ed. New York: Raven Press, 1992; and from Sur S, et al. Eosinophils: biochemical and cellular aspects. In: E Middleton Jr et al, eds: *Allergy: principles and practice.* 4th ed. St. Louis: Mosby, 1993; and from Gleich GJ, et al. Eosinophils. In: Frank MM, et al., eds. Samter's Immunologic Diseases, 5th edition. Boston: Little, Brown, 1995.

REFERENCES

1. Gleich GJ, Loegering DA, Frigas E, Filley WV. The eosinophil granule major basic protein: biological activities and relationship to bronchial asthma. *Monogr Allergy* 1983;18:277–283.
2. Gleich GJ, Ottesen EA, Leiferman KM, Ackerman SJ. Eosinophils and human disease. *Int Arch Allergy Appl Immunol* 1989;88:59–62.
3. Gleich GJ, Adolphson C. Bronchial hyperreactivity and eosinophil granule proteins. *Agents Actions Suppl* 1993;43:223–230.
4. Leiferman KM, Ackerman SJ, Sampson HA, Haugen HS, Venencie PY, Gleich GJ. Dermal deposition of eosinophil-granule major basic

protein in atopic dermatitis. Comparison with onchocerciasis. *N Engl J Med* 1985;313:282–285.

5. Gleich GJ, Kita H, Adolphson CR. Volume 1: eosinophils. In: Frank MM, Austen KF, Claman HN, Unanue ER, eds. *Samter's immunologic diseases*. Boston: Little Brown, 1995;205–245.

6. Gleich GJ, Loegering DA, Maldonado JE. Identification of a major basic protein in guinea pig eosinophil granules. *J Exp Med* 1973;137:1459–1471.

7. Gleich GJ, Loegering DA, Kueppers F, Bajaj SP, Mann KG. Physicochemical and biological properties of the major basic protein from guinea pig eosinophil granules. *J Exp Med* 1974;140:313–332.

8. Gleich GJ, Loegering DA, Mann KG, Maldonado JE. Comparative properties of the Charcot-Leyden crystal protein and the major basic protein from human eosinophils. *J Clin Invest* 1976;57:633–640.

9. Wasmoen TL, Bell MP, Loegering DA, Gleich GJ, Prendergast FG, McKean DJ. Biochemical and amino acid sequence analysis of human eosinophil granule major basic protein. *J Biol Chem* 1988;263:12559–12563.

10. Lewis DM, Loegering DA, Gleich GJ. Isolation and partial characterization of a major basic protein from rat eosinophil granules. *Proc Soc Exp Biol Med* 1976;152:512–515.

11. Oxvig C, Gleich GJ, Sottrup-Jensen L. Localization of disulfide bridges and free sulfhydryl groups in human eosinophil granule major basic protein. *FEBS Lett* 1994;341:213–217.

12. Barker RL, Gleich GJ, Pease LR. Acidic precursor revealed in human eosinophil granule major basic protein cDNA. *J Exp Med* 1988;168:1493–1498.

13. McGrogan M, Simonsen C, Scott R, et al. Isolation of a complementary DNA clone encoding a precursor to human eosinophil major basic protein. *J Exp Med* 1988;168:2295–2308.

14. Metzger H. Molecular aspects of receptors and binding factors for IgE. *Adv Immunol* 1988;43:277–312.

15. Patthy L. Homology of cytotoxic protein of eosinophilic leukocytes with IgE receptor FcεRII: implications for its structure and function. *Mol Immunol* 1989;26:1151–1154.

16. Popken-Harris P, Thomas L, Oxvig C, et al. Biochemical properties, activities, and presence in biologic fluids of eosinophil granule major basic protein. *J Allergy Clin Immunol* 1994;94:1282–1289.

17. Aoki I, Shindoh Y, Nishida T, et al. Sequencing and cloning of the cDNA of guinea pig eosinophil major basic protein. *FEBS Lett* 1991;279:330–334.

18. Aoki I, Shindoh Y, Nishida T, et al. Comparison of the amino acid and nucleotide sequences between human and two guinea pig major basic proteins. *FEBS Lett* 1991;282:56–60.

19. Barker RL, Loegering DA, Arakawa KC, Pease LR, Gleich GJ. Cloning and sequence analysis of the human gene encoding eosinophil major basic protein. *Gene* 1990;86:285–289.

20. Egesten A, Alumets J, von Mecklenburg C, Palmegren M, Olsson I. Localization of eosinophil cationic protein, major basic protein, and eosinophil peroxidase in human eosinophils by immunoelectron microscopic technique. *J Histochem Cytochem* 1986;34:1399–1403.

21. Peters MS, Rodriguez M, Gleich GJ. Localization of human eosinophil granule major basic protein, eosinophil cationic protein, and eosinophil-derived neurotoxin by immunoelectron microscopy. *Lab Invest* 1986;54:656–662.

22. Lewis DM, Lewis JC, Loegering DA, Gleich GJ. Localization of the guinea pig eosinophil major basic protein to the core of the granule. *J Cell Biol* 1978;77:702–713.

23. Ackerman SJ, Kephart GM, Habermann TM, Greipp PR, Gleich GJ. Localization of eosinophil granule major basic protein in human basophils. *J Exp Med* 1983;158:946–961.

24. Abu-Ghazaleh RI, Dunnette SL, Loegering DA, et al. Eosinophil granule proteins in peripheral blood granulocytes. *J Leukoc Biol* 1992;52:611–618.

25. Dvorak AM, Klebanoff SJ, Henderson WR, Monahan RA, Pyne K, Galli SJ. Vesicular uptake of eosinophil peroxidase by guinea pig basophils and by cloned mouse mast cells and granule-containing lymphoid cells. *Am J Pathol* 1985;118:425–438.

26. Dvorak AM, Ishizaka T, Galli SJ. Ultrastructure of human basophils developing *in vitro*. Evidence for the acquisition of peroxidase by basophils and for different effects of human and murine growth factors on human basophil and eosinophil maturation. *Lab Invest* 1985;53:57–71.

27. Butterfield JH, Weiler D, Peterson EA, Gleich GJ, Leiferman KM. Sequestration of eosinophil major basic protein in human mast cells. *Lab Invest* 1990;62:77–86.

28. Padawar J. The mast cell and immediate hypersensitivity. In: Bach MK, ed. *Immediate hypersensitivity*. New York: Marcel Dekker, 1979;301–307.

29. El-Cheikh MC, Dutra HS, Borojevic R. Eosinophil granulocyte proliferation and differentiation in schistosomal granulomas are controlled by two cytokines. *Lab Invest* 1991;64:93–97.

30. Maddox DE, Butterfield JH, Ackerman SJ, Coulam CB, Gleich GJ. Elevated serum levels in human pregnancy of a molecule immunochemically similar to eosinophil granule major basic protein. *J Exp Med* 1983;158:1211–1226.

31. Wasmoen TL, Coulam CB, Leiferman KM, Gleich GJ. Increases of plasma eosinophil major basic protein levels late in pregnancy predict onset of labor. *Proc Natl Acad Sci U S A* 1987;84:3029–3032.

32. Coulam CB, Wasmoen T, Creasy R, Siiteri P, Gleich G. Major basic protein as a predictor of preterm labor: a preliminary report. *Am J Obstet Gynecol* 1987;156:790–796.

33. Wagner JM, Bartemes K, Vernof KK, et al. Analysis of pregnancy-associated major basic protein levels throughout gestation. *Placenta* 1993;14:671–681.

34. Maddox DE, Kephart GM, Coulam CB, Butterfield JH, Benirschke K, Gleich GJ. Localization of a molecule immunochemically similar to eosinophil major basic protein in human placenta. *J Exp Med* 1984;160:29–41.

35. Bonno M, Oxvig C, Kephart GM, et al. Localization of pregnancy-associated plasma protein-A and colocalization of pregnancy-associated plasma protein-A messenger ribonucleic acid and eosinophil granule major basic protein messenger ribonucleic acid in placenta. *Lab Invest* 1994;71:560–566.

36. Bonno M, Kephart GM, Carlson CM, Loegering DA, Vernof KK, Gleich GJ. Expression of eosinophil-granule major basic protein messenger ribonucleic acid in placental X cells. *Lab Invest* 1994;70:234–241.

37. Wasmoen TL, McKean DJ, Benirschke K, Coulam CB, Gleich GJ. Evidence of eosinophil granule major basic protein in human placenta. *J Exp Med* 1989;170:2051–2063.

38. Oxvig C, Sand O, Kristensen T, Gleich GJ, Sottrup JL. Circulating human pregnancy-associated plasma protein-A is disulfide-bridged to the proform of eosinophil major basic protein. *J Biol Chem* 1993;268:12243–12246.

39. Dembele-Duchesne M-J, Badia E, Etienne-Julan M, Capony JP. Identification and tissue localization of an eosinophil 17 kDa protein accumulating in rat uterus upon estradiol treatment. *J Steroid Biochem Mol Biol* 1991;38:321–330.

40. Duchesne M-J, Badia E. Immunohistochemical localization of the eosinophil major basic protein in the uterus horn and cervix of the rat at term and after parturition. *Cell Tissue Res* 1992;270:79–86.

41. Gallagher R, Collins S, Trujillo J, et al. Characterization of the continuous, differentiating myeloid cell line (HL-60) from a patient with acute promyelocytic leukemia. *Blood* 1979;54:713–733.

42. Filley WV, Holley KE, Kephart GM, Gleich GJ. Identification by immunofluorescence of eosinophil granule major basic protein in lung tissues of patients with bronchial asthma. *Lancet* 1982;2:11–16.

43. Gonzalez EB, Swedo JL, Rajaraman S, Daniels JC, Grant JA. Ultrastructural and immunohistochemical evidence for release of eosinophilic granules *in vivo*: cytotoxic potential in chronic eosinophilc pneumonia. *J Allergy Clin Immunol* 1987;79:755–762.

44. Butterworth AE, Sturrock RF, Houba V, Mahmoud AAF, Sher A, Rees PH. Eosinophils as mediators of antibody-dependent damage to schistosomula. *Nature* 1975;256:727–729.

45. Butterworth AE, Vadas MA, Wassom DL, et al. Interactions between human eosinophils and schistosomula of Schistosoma mansoni. II. The mechanism of irreversible eosinophil adherence. *J Exp Med* 1979;150:1456–1471.

46. Butterworth AE, Wassom DL, Gleich GJ, Loegering DA, David JR. Damage to schistosomula of Schistosoma mansoni induced directly by eosinophil major basic protein. *J Immunol* 1979;122:221–229.

47. Hamann KJ, Barker RL, Loegering DA, Gleich GJ. Comparative toxicity of purified human eosinophil granule proteins for newborn larvae of Trichinella spiralis. *J Parasitol* 1987;73:523–529.

48. Wassom DL, Gleich GJ. Damage to Trichinella spiralis newborn larvae by eosinophil major basic protein. *Am J Trop Med Hyg* 1979;28:860–863.

49. Hamann KJ, Gleich GJ, Checkel JL, Loegering DA, McCall JW, Barker RL. *In vitro* killing of microfilariae of Brugia pahangi and Brugia malayi by eosinophil granule proteins. *J Immunol* 1990;144:3166–3173.

50. Kierszenbaum F, Ackerman SJ, Gleich GJ. Inhibition of antibody-dependent eosinophil-mediated cytotoxicity by heparin. *J Immunol* 1982;128:515.

51. Molina HA, Kierszenbaum F, Hamann KJ, Gleich GJ. Toxic effects produced or mediated by human eosinophil granule components on Trypanosoma cruzi. *Am J Trop Med Hyg* 1988;38:327–334.

52. Villalta F, Kierszenbaum F. Role of inflammatory cells in Chagas disease. I. Uptake and mechanism of destruction of intracellular (amastigote) forms of *Trypanosoma cruzi* by human eosinophils. *J Immunol* 1984;132:2053–2058.

53. Kierszenbaum F, Villalta F, Tai PC. Role of inflammatory cells in Chagas disease. III. Kinetics of human eosinophil activation upon interaction with parasites *(Trypanosoma cruzi)*. *J Immunol* 1986;136:662–666.

54. Lehrer RI, Szklarek D, Barton A, Ganz T, Hamann KJ, Gleich GJ. Antibacterial properties of eosinophil major basic protein and eosinophil cationic protein. *J Immunol* 1989;142:4428–4434.

55. Gleich GJ, Frigas E, Loegering DA, Wassom DL, Steinmuller D. Cytotoxic properties of the eosinophil major basic protein. *J Immunol* 1979;123:2925–2927.

56. Frigas E, Loegering DA, Solley GO, Farrow GM, Gleich GJ. Elevated levels of the eosinophil granule major basic protein in the sputum of patients with bronchial asthma. *Mayo Clin Proc* 1981;56:345–353.

57. Durham SR, Loegering DA, Dunnette S, Gleich GJ, Kay AB. Blood eosinophils and eosinophil-derived proteins in allergic asthma. *J Allergy Clin Immunol* 1989;84:931–936.

58. Gleich GJ, Adolphson CR. The eosinophilic leukocyte: structure and function. *Adv Immunol* 1986;39:177–253.

59. Frigas E, Loegering DA, Gleich GJ. Cytotoxic effects of the guinea pig eosinophil major basic protein on tracheal epithelium. *Lab Invest* 1980;42:35–43.

60. Motojima S, Frigas E, Loegering DA, Gleich GJ. Toxicity of eosinophil cationic proteins for guinea pig tracheal epithelium *in vitro*. *Am Rev Respir Dis* 1989;139:801–805.

61. Robinson BW, Venaille T, Blum R, Mendis AH. Eosinophils and major basic protein damage but do not detach human amniotic epithelial cells. *Exp Lung Res* 1992;18:583–593.

62. Lewis DM, Loegering DA, Gleich GJ. Antiserum to the major basic protein of guinea pig eosinophil granules. *Immunochemistry* 1976;13:743–746.

63. Rent R, Ertel N, Eisenstein R, Gewurz H. Complement activation by interaction of polyanions and polycations. I. Heparin-protamine induced consumption of complement. *J Immunol* 1975;114:120–124.

64. Weiler JM, Gleich GJ. Eosinophil granule major basic protein regulates generation of classical and alternative-amplification pathway C3 convertases *in vitro*. *J Immunol* 1988;140:1605–1610.

65. Weiler JM, Edens RE, Gleich GJ. Eosinophil granule cationic proteins regulate complement. I. Activity on the alternative pathway. *J Immunol* 1992;149:643–648.

66. O Donnell MC, Ackerman SJ, Gleich GJ, Thomas LL. Activation of basophil and mast cell histamine release by eosinophil granule major basic protein. *J Exp Med* 1983;157:1981–1991.

67. Thomas LL, Zheutlin LM, Gleich GJ. Pharmacological control of human basophil histamine release stimulated by eosinophil granule major basic protein. *Immunology* 1989;66:611–615.

68. Zheutlin LM, Ackerman SJ, Gleich GJ, Thomas LL. Stimulation of basophil and rat mast cell histamine release by eosinophil granule-derived cationic proteins. *J Immunol* 1984;133:2180–2185.

69. Okayama Y, el Lati SG, Leiferman KM, Church MK. Eosinophil granule proteins inhibit substance P-induced histamine release from human skin mast cells. *J Allergy Clin Immunol* 1994;93:900–909.

70. Patella V, de Crescenzo G, Marino I, Genovese A, Adt M, Gleich GJ, Marone G. Eosinophil granule proteins activate human heart mast cells. *J Immunol* 1996; 157:1219–1225.

71. Moy JN, Gleich GJ, Thomas LL. Noncytotoxic activation of neutrophils by eosinophil granule major basic protein. Effect on superoxide anion generation and lysosomal enzyme release. *J Immunol* 1990;145:2626–2632.

72. Moy JN, Thomas LL, Whisler LC. Eosinophil major basic protein enhances the expression of neutrophil CR3 and p150,95. *J Allergy Clin Immunol* 1993;92:598–606.

73. Rohrbach MS, Wheatley CL, Slifman NR, Gleich GJ. Activation of platelets by eosinophil granule proteins. *J Exp Med* 1990;172:1271–1274.

74. Rankin JA, Harris P, Ackerman SJ. The effects of eosinophil-granule major basic protein on lung-macrophage superoxide anion generation. *J Allergy Clin Immunol* 1992;89:746–752.

75. Kita H, Abu-Ghazaleh RI, Sur S, Gleich GJ. Eosinophil major basic protein induces degranulation and IL-8 production by human eosinophils. *J Immunol* 1995;154:4749–4758.

76. Ratnoff OD, Gleich GJ, Shurin SB, Kazura J, Everson B, Embury P. Inhibition of the activation of Hageman factor (factor XII) by eosinophils and eosinophilic constituents. *Am J Hematol* 1993;42:138–145.

77. Slungaard A, Vercellotti GM, Tran T, Gleich GJ, Key NS. Eosinophil cationic granule proteins impair thrombomodulin function. A potential mechanism for thromboembolism in hypereosinophilic heart disease. *J Clin Invest* 1993;91:1721–1730.

78. Abu-Ghazaleh RI, Gleich GJ, Prendergast FG. Interaction of eosinophil granule major basic protein with synthetic lipid bilayers: a mechanism for toxicity. *J Membr Biol* 1992;128:153–164.

79. Gleich GJ, Loegering DA, Bell MP, Checkel JL, Ackerman SJ, McKean DJ. Biochemical and functional similarities between human eosinophil-derived neurotoxin and eosinophil cationic protein: homology with ribonuclease. *Proc Natl Acad Sci U S A* 1986;83:3146–3150.

80. Olsson I, Persson AM, Winqvist I. Biochemical properties of the eosinophil cationic protein and demonstration of its biosynthesis *in vitro* in marrow cells from patients with an eosinophilia. *Blood* 1986; 67:498–503.

81. Ackerman SJ, Loegering DA, Venge P, et al. Distinctive cationic proteins of the human eosinophil granule: major basic protein, eosinophil cationic protein, and eosinophil-derived neurotoxin. *J Immunol* 1983; 131:2977–2982.

82. Barker RL, Loegering DA, Ten RM, Hamann KJ, Pease LR, Gleich GJ. Eosinophil cationic protein cDNA. Comparison with other toxic cationic proteins and ribonucleases. *J Immunol* 1989;143:952–955.

83. Rosenberg HF, Ackerman SJ, Tenen DG. Human eosinophil cationic protein. Molecular cloning of a cytotoxin and helminthotoxin with ribonuclease activity. *J Exp Med* 1989;170:163–176.

84. Slifman NR, Loegering DA, McKean DJ, Gleich GJ. Ribonuclease activity associated with human eosinophil-derived neurotoxin and eosinophil cationic protein. *J Immunol* 1986;137:2913–2917.

85. Sorrentino S, Glitz DG. Ribonuclease activity and substrate preference of human eosinophil cationic protein (ECP). *FEBS Lett* 1991; 288:23–26.

86. Hamann KJ, Ten RM, Loegering DA, et al. Structure and chromosome localization of the human eosinophil-derived neurotoxin and eosinophil cationic protein genes: evidence for intronless coding sequences in the ribonuclease gene superfamily. *Genomics* 1990;7:535–546.

87. Mastrianni DM, Eddy RL, Rosenberg HF, et al. Localization of the human eosinophil Charcot-Leyden crystal protein (lysophospholipase) gene (CLC) to chromosome 19 and the human ribonuclease 2 (eosinophil-derived neurotoxin) and ribonuclease 3 (eosinophil cationic protein) genes (RNS2 and RNS3) to chromosome 14. *Genomics* 1992;13:240–242.

88. Tai PC, Spry CJ, Peterson C, Venge P, Olsson I. Monoclonal antibodies distinguish between storage and secreted forms of eosinophil cationic protein. *Nature* 1984;309:182–184.

89. Keshavarzian A, Saverymuttu SH, Tai PC, et al. Activated eosinophils in familial eosinophilic gastroenteritis. *Gastroenterology* 1985;88:1041–1049.

90. Spry CJ, Tai PC, Barkans J. Tissue localization of human eosinophil cationic proteins in allergic diseases. *Int Arch Allergy Appl Immunol* 1985;77:252–254.

91. Jahnsen FL, Brandtzaeg P, Halstensen TS. Monoclonal antibody EG2 does not provide reliable immunohistochemical discrimination between resting and activated eosinophils. *J Immunol Methods* 1994;175:23–36.

92. Rosenberg HF, Tiffany HL. Characterization of the eosinophil granule proteins recognized by the activation-specific antibody EG2. *J Leukoc Biol* 1994;56:502–506.

93. McLaren DJ, McKean JR, Olsson I, Venge P, Kay AB. Morphological studies on the killing of schistosomula of *Schistosoma mansoni* by human eosinophil and neutrophil cationic proteins *in vitro*. *Parasite Immunol* 1981;3:359–373.

94. Ackerman SJ, Gleich GJ, Loegering DA, Richardson BA, Butterworth AE. Comparative toxicity of purified human eosinophil granule cationic proteins for schistosomula of *Schistosoma mansoni*. *Am J Trop Med Hyg* 1985;34:735–745.

95. Olsson I, Venge P, Spitznagel JK, Lehrer RI. Arginine-rich cationic proteins of human eosinophil granules: comparison of the constituents of eosinophilic and neutrophilic leukocytes. *Lab Invest* 1977; 36:493–500.

96. Venge P. Cationic proteins of human eosinophils and their role in the inflammatory reaction. In: Mahmoud AAF, Austen KF, eds. *The eosinophil in health and disease.* New York: Grune and Stratton, 1980;131–146.

97. Venge P, Dahl R, Hallgren R. Enhancement of factor XII dependent reactions by eosinophil cationic protein. *Thromb Res* 1979;14:641–649.

98. Dahl R, Venge P. Enhancement of urokinase-induced plasminogen activation by the cationic protein of human eosinophil granulocytes. *Thromb Res* 1979;14:599–608.

99. Durack DT, Sumi SM, Klebanoff SJ. Neurotoxicity of human eosinophils. *Proc Natl Acad Sci U S A* 1979;76:1443–1447.

100. Fredens K, Dahl R, Venge P. The Gordon phenomenon induced by the eosinophil cationic protein and eosinophil protein X. *J Allergy Clin Immunol* 1982;70:361–366.

101. Peterson CG, Skoog V, Venge P. Human eosinophil cationic proteins (ECP and EPX) and their suppressive effects on lymphocyte proliferation. *Immunobiology* 1986;171:1–13.

102. Barker RL, Gundel RH, Gleich GJ, et al. Acidic polyamino acids inhibit human eosinophil granule major basic protein toxicity. Evidence of a functional role for ProMBP. *J Clin Invest* 1991;88:798–805.

103. Young JD, Peterson CG, Venge P, Cohn ZA. Mechanism of membrane damage mediated by human eosinophil cationic protein. *Nature* 1986;321:613–616.

104. Yazdanbakhsh M, Tai PC, Spry CJ, Gleich GJ, Roos D. Synergism between eosinophil cationic protein and oxygen metabolites in killing of schistosomula of *Schistosoma mansoni*. *J Immunol* 1987; 138:3443–3447.

105. Peterson CG, Venge P. Interaction and complex-formation between the eosinophil cationic protein and alpha 2-macroglobulin. *Biochem J* 1987;245:781–787.

106. Gordon MH. Remarks on Hodgkins disease: a pathogenic agent in the glands, and its application in diagnosis. *Brit Med J* 1933;1:641.

107. Turner JC, Jackson HJ, Parker FJ. The etiologic relation of the eosinophil to the Gordon phenomenon in Hodgkin's disease. *Am J Med Sci* 1938;195:27.

108. King LS. Encephalopathy following injections of bone marrow extract. *J Exp Med* 1939;70:303.

109. Moore PM, Harley JB, Fauci AS. Neurologic dysfunction in the idiopathic hypereosinophilic syndrome. *Ann Intern Med* 1985;102: 109–114.

110. Snead OC, Kalavsky SM. Cerebrospinal fluid eosinophilia: a manifestation of a disorder resembling multiple sclerosis in childhood. *J Pediatr* 1976;89:83–84.

111. Yii C-Y. Clinical observations on eosinophilic meningitis and meningoencephalitis caused by *Angiostrongylus cantonensis* on Taiwan. *Am J Trop Med Hyg* 1976;25:233–249.

112. Durack DT, Ackerman SJ, Loegering DA, Gleich GJ. Purification of human eosinophil-derived neurotoxin. *Proc Natl Acad Sci U S A* 1981;78:5165–5169.

113. Hamann KJ, Barker RL, Loegering DA, Pease LR, Gleich GJ. Sequence of human eosinophil-derived neurotoxin cDNA: identity of deduced amino acid sequence with human nonsecretory ribonucleases. *Gene* 1989;83:161–167.

114. Rosenberg HF, Tenen DG, Ackerman SJ. Molecular cloning of the human eosinophil-derived neurotoxin: a member of the ribonuclease gene family. *Proc Natl Acad Sci U S A* 1989;86:4460–4464.

115. Beintema JJ, Hofsteenge J, Iwama M, et al. Amino acid sequence of the nonsecretory ribonuclease of human urine. *Biochemistry* 1988; 27:4530–4538.

116. Sorrentino S, Tucker GK, Glitz DG. Purification and characterization of a ribonuclease from human liver. *J Biol Chem* 1988;263: 16125–16131.

117. Saxena SK, Rybak SM, Davey RT Jr, Youle RJ, Ackerman EJ. Angiogenin is a cytotoxic, tRNA-specific ribonuclease in the RNase A superfamily. *J Biol Chem* 1992;267:21982–21986.

118. Weickmann JL, Elson M, Glitz DG. Purification and characterization of human pancreatic ribonuclease. *Biochemistry* 1981;20:1272–1278.

119. Sorrentino S, Glitz DG, Hamann KJ, Loegering DA, Checkel JL, Gleich GJ. Eosinophil-derived neurotoxin and human liver ribonuclease. Identity of structure and linkage of neurotoxicity to nuclease activity. *J Biol Chem* 1992;267:14859–14865.

120. Peterson CG, Venge P. Purification and characterization of a new cationic protein—eosinophil protein-X (EPX)—from granules of human eosinophils. *Immunology* 1983;50:19–26.

121. Gullberg U, Widegren B, Arnason U, Egesten A, Olsson I. The cytotoxic eosinophil cationic protein (ECP) has ribonuclease activity. *Biochem Biophys Res Comm* 1986;139:1239–1242.

122. McLaren DJ, Peterson CG, Venge P. Schistosoma mansoni: further studies of the interaction between schistosomula and granulocyte-derived cationic proteins *in vitro*. *Parasitology* 1984;88:491–503.

123. Slifman NR, Venge P, Peterson CG, McKean DJ, Gleich GJ. Human eosinophil-derived neurotoxin and eosinophil protein X are likely the same protein. *J Immunol* 1989;143:2317–2322.

124. Klebanoff SJ, Jong EC, Henderson WRJ. The eosinophil peroxidase: purification and biological properties. In: Mahmoud AAF, Austen KF, eds. *The eosinophil in health and disease.* New York: Grune and Stratton, 1980;99–114.

125. Wever R, Plat H, Hamers MN. Human eosinophil peroxidase: a novel isolation procedure, spectral properties and chlorinating activity. *FEBS Lett* 1981;123:327–331.

126. Olsen RL, Little C. Purification and some properties of myeloperoxidase and eosinophil peroxidase from human blood. *Biochem J* 1983;209:781–787.

127. Bolscher BG, Plat H, Wever R. Some properties of human eosinophil peroxidase, a comparison with other peroxidases. *Biochim Biophys Acta* 1984;784:177–186.

128. Sibbett SS, Klebanoff SJ, Hurst JK. Resonance Raman characterization of the heme prosthetic group in eosinophil peroxidase. *FEBS Lett* 1985;189:271–275.

129. Carlson MG, Peterson CG, Venge P. Human eosinophil peroxidase: purification and characterization. *J Immunol* 1985;134:1875–1879.

130. Olsen RL, Syse K, Little C, Christensen TB. Further characterization of human eosinophil peroxidase. *Biochem J* 1985;229:779–784.

131. Olsson I, Persson AM, Stromberg K, Winqvist I, Tai PC, Spry CJ. Purification of eosinophil peroxidase and studies of biosynthesis and processing in human marrow cells. *Blood* 1985;66:1143–1148.

132. Salmon SE, Cline MJ, Schultz J, Lehrer RI. Myeloperoxidase deficiency: Immunologic study of a genetic leukocyte defect. *N Engl J Med* 1970;282:250–253.

133. Sullivan S, Salapow MA, Breen R, Broide DH. Eosinophil peroxidase differs from neutrophil myeloperoxidase in its ability to bind antineutrophil cytoplasmic antibodies reactive with myeloperoxidase. *Int Arch Allergy Immunol* 1994;105:150–154.

134. Ten RM, Pease LR, McKean DJ, Bell MP, Gleich GJ. Molecular cloning of the human eosinophil peroxidase. Evidence for the existence of a peroxidase multigene family. *J Exp Med* 1989;169:1757–1769.

135. Weller PF, Ackerman SJ, Smith JA. Eosinophil granule cationic proteins: major basic protein is distinct from the smaller subunit of eosinophil peroxidase. *J Leukoc Biol* 1988;43:1–4.

136. Saito H, Hatake K, Dvorak AM, et al. Selective differentiation and proliferation of hematopoietic cells induced by recombinant human interleukins. *Proc Natl Acad Sci U S A* 1988;85:2288–2292.

137. Johnson KR, Nauseef WM, Care A, et al. Characterization of cDNA clones for human myeloperoxidase: predicted amino acid sequence and evidence for multiple mRNA species. *Nucleic Acids Res* 1987; 15:2013–2028.

138. Kimura S, Kotani T, McBride OW, et al. Human thyroid peroxidase: complete cDNA and protein sequence, chromosome mapping and identification of two alternately spliced mRNAs. *Proc Natl Acad Sci U S A* 1987;84:5555–5559.

139. Cals MM, Mailliart P, Brignon G, Anglade P, Dumas BR. Primary structure of bovine lactoperoxidase, a fourth member of a mammalian heme peroxidase family. *Eur J Biochem* 1991;198:733–739.

140. Sakamaki K, Tomonaga M, Tsukui K, Nagata S. Molecular cloning and characterization of a chromosomal gene for human eosinophil peroxidase. *J Biol Chem* 1989;264:16828–16836.

141. Yamaguchi Y, Tenen DG, Ackerman SJ. Transcriptional regulation of the human eosinophil peroxidase genes: characterization of a peroxidase promoter. *Int Arch Allergy Immunol* 1994;104:30–31.

142. Yamaguchi Y, Zhang DE, Sun Z, et al. Functional characterization of the promoter for the gene encoding human eosinophil peroxidase. *J Biol Chem* 1994;269:19410–19419.

143. Bos AJ, Wever R, Hamers MN, Roos D. Some enzymatic characteristics of eosinophil peroxidase from patients with eosinophilia and from healthy donors. *Infect Immun* 1981;32:427–431.

144. Weiss SJ, Test ST, Eckmann CM, Roos D, Regiani S. Brominating oxidants generated by human eosinophils. *Science* 1986;234:200–203.

145. Mayeno AN, Curran AJ, Roberts RL, Foote CS. Eosinophils preferentially use bromide to generate halogenating agents. *J Biol Chem* 1989;264:5660–5668.

146. Thomas EL, Bozeman PM, Jefferson MM, King CC. Oxidation of bromide by the human leukocyte enzymes myeloperoxidase and eosinophil peroxidase. Formation of bromamines. *J Biol Chem* 1995;270:2906–2913.

147. Slungaard A, Mahoney JR, Jr. Thiocyanate is the major substrate for eosinophil peroxidase in physiologic fluids. Implications for cytotoxicity. *J Biol Chem* 1991;266:4903–4910.

148. De SK, De M, Banerjee RK. Localization and origin of the intestinal peroxidase—effect of adrenal glucocorticoids. *J Steroid Biochem Mol Biol* 1986;24:629–635.

149. Rickard A, Lagunoff D. Eosinophil peroxidase accounts for most if not all of the peroxidase activity associated with isolated rat peritoneal mast cells. *Int Arch Allergy Immunol* 1994;103:365–369.

150. Presentey BZ. A new anomaly of eosinophilic granulocytes. *Tech Bull Regist Med Technol* 1968;38:131–134.

151. Presentey BZ. Morphologic observations and genetic follow-up of a familial anomaly of eosinophils. *Am J Clin Pathol* 1969;51:458–462.

152. Presentey BZ. Partial and severe peroxidase and phospholipid deficiency in eosinophils: cytochemical and genetic considerations. *Acta Heamatol* 1970;44:345–354.

153. Presentey BZ, Joshua H. Peroxidase and phospholipid deficiency in human eosinophilic granulocytes—a marker in population genetics. *Experientia* 1982;38:628–629.

154. Menegazzi R, Zabucchi G, Zuccato P, Cramer R, Piccinini C, Patriarca P. Oxidation of homovanillic acid as a selective assay for eosinophil peroxidase in eosinophil peroxidase-myeloperoxidase mixtures and its use in the detection of human eosinophil peroxidase deficiency. *J Immunol Methods* 1991;137:55–63.

155. Zabucchi G, Soranzo MR, Menegazzi R, et al. Eosinophil peroxidase deficiency: morphological and immunocytochemical studies of the eosinophil-specific granules. *Blood* 1992;80:2903–2910.

156. Cappelletti P, Doretto P, Signori D, Bizzaro N. Eosinophilic peroxidase deficiency. Cytochemical and ultrastructural characterization of 21 new cases. *Am J Clin Pathol* 1992;98:615–22.

157. Romano M, Patriarca P, Melo C, Baralle FE, Dri P. Hereditary eosinophil peroxidase deficiency: immunochemical and spectroscopic studies and evidence for a compound heterozygosity of the defect. *Proc Natl Acad Sci U S A* 1994;91:12496–12500.

158. Klebanoff SJ. Iodination of bacteria: a bactericidal mechanism. *J Exp Med* 1967;126:1063–1078.

159. Belding ME, Klebanoff SJ, Ray CG. Peroxidase-mediated virucidal systems. *Science* 1970;167:195–196.

160. Jacobs AA, Low IE, Paul BB, Strauss RR, Sbarra AJ. Mycoplasmacidal activity of peroxidase-H₂O₂-halide systems. *Infect Immun* 1972;5:127–131.

161. Lehrer RI. Antifungal effects of peroxidase systems. *J Bacteriol* 1969;99:361–365.

162. Baehner RL, Johnston RBJ. Metabolic and bactericidal activities of human eosinophils. *Br J Haematol* 1971;20:277–285.

163. Klebanoff SJ, Durack DT, Rosen H, Clark RA. Functional studies on human peritoneal eosinophils. *Infect Immun* 1977;17:167–173.

164. Jong EC, Henderson WR, Klebanoff SJ. Bactericidal activity of eosinophil peroxidase. *J Immunol* 1980;124:1378–1382.

165. Jong EC, Mahmoud AA, Klebanoff SJ. Peroxidase-mediated toxicity to schistosomula of Schistosoma mansoni. *J Immunol* 1981;126:468–471.

166. Nogueira NM, Klebanoff SJ, Cohn ZA. T. cruzi: sensitization to macrophage killing by eosinophil peroxidase. *J Immunol* 1982;128:1705–1708.

167. Locksley RM, Wilson CB, Klebanoff SJ. Role of endogenous and acquired peroxidase in the toxoplasmacidal activity of murine and human mononuclear phagocytes. *J Clin Invest* 1982;69:1099–1111.

168. Klebanoff SJ, Shepard CC. Toxic effect of the peroxidase-hydrogen peroxide-halide antimicrobial system on Mycobacterium leprae. *Infect Immun* 1984;44:534–536.

169. Henderson WR, Chi EY, Klebanoff SJ. Eosinophil peroxidase-induced mast cell secretion. *J Exp Med* 1980;152:265–279.

170. Jong EC, Klebanoff SJ. Eosinophil-mediated mammalian tumor cell cytotoxicity: role of the peroxidase system. *J Immunol* 1980;124:1949–1953.

171. Ayars GH, Altman LC, Gleich GJ, Loegering DA, Baker CB. Eosinophil- and eosinophil granule-mediated pneumocyte injury. *J Allergy Clin Immunol* 1985;76:595–604.

172. Agosti JM, Altman LC, Ayars GH, Loegering DA, Gleich GJ, Klebanoff SJ. The injurious effect of eosinophil peroxidase, hydrogen peroxide, and halides on pneumocytes in vitro. *J Allergy Clin Immunol* 1987;79:496–504.

173. Ayars GH, Altman LC, McManus MM, et al. Injurious effect of the eosinophil peroxide-hydrogen peroxide-halide system and major basic protein on human nasal epithelium in vitro. *Am Rev Respir Dis* 1989;140:125–131.

174. Henderson WR, Jong EC, Klebanoff SJ. Binding of eosinophil peroxidase to mast cell granules with retention of peroxidatic activity. *J Immunol* 1980;124:1383–1388.

175. Ramsey PG, Martin T, Chi E, Klebanoff SJ. Arming of mononuclear phagocytes by eosinophil peroxidase bound to Staphylococcus aureus. *J Immunol* 1982;128:415–420.

176. Nogueira NM, Klebanoff SJ, Cohn ZA. Trypanosoma cruzi: sensitization to macrophage killing by eosinophil peroxidase. *J Immunol* 1982;128:1705–1708.

177. Nathan CF, Klebanoff SJ. Augmentation of spontaneous macrophage-mediated cytolysis by eosinophil peroxidase. *J Exp Med* 1982;155:1291–1308.

178. Klebanoff SJ, Agosti JM, Jorg A, Waltersdorph AM. Comparative toxicity of the horse eosinophil peroxidase-H₂O₂-halide system and granule basic proteins. *J Immunol* 1989;143:239–244.

179. Henderson WR, Jorg A, Klebanoff SJ. Eosinophil peroxidase-mediated inactivation of leukotrienes B4, C4, and D4. *J Immunol* 1982;128:2609–2613.

180. Goetzl EJ. The conversion of leukotriene C4 to isomers of leukotriene B4 by human eosinophil peroxidase. *Biochem Biophys Res Comm* 1982;106:270–275.

181. Slungaard A, Mahoney JR, Jr. Bromide-dependent toxicity of eosinophil peroxidase for endothelium and isolated working rat hearts: a model for eosinophilic endocarditis. *J Exp Med* 1991;173:117–126.

182. Dimayuga E, Stober M, Kayes SG. Eosinophil peroxidase levels in hearts and lungs of mice infected with Toxocara canis. *J Parasitol* 1991;77:461–466.

183. Schaffer SW, Dimayuga ER, Kayes SG. Development and characterization of a model of eosinophil-mediated cardiomyopathy in rats infected with Toxocara canis. *Am J Physiol* 1992;262:H1428–1434.

184. Hisamatsu K, Ganbo T, Nakazawa T, et al. Cytotoxicity of human eosinophil granule major basic protein to human nasal sinus mucosa in vitro. *J Allergy Clin Immunol* 1990;86:52–63.

185. Devalia JL, Sapsford RJ, Rusznak C, Davies RJ. The effect of human eosinophils on cultured human nasal epithelial cell activity and the influence of nedocromil sodium in vitro. *Am J Respir Cell Mol Biol* 1992;7:270–277.

186. Flavahan NA, Slifman NR, Gleich GJ, Vanhoutte PM. Human eosinophil major basic protein causes hyperreactivity of respiratory smooth muscle. Role of the epithelium. *Am Rev Respir Dis* 1988;138:685–658.

187. Brofman JD, White SR, Blake JS, Munoz NM, Gleich GJ, Leff AR. Epithelial augmentation of trachealis contraction caused by major basic protein of eosinophils. *J Appl Physiol* 1989;66:1867–1873.

188. White SR, Ohno S, Munoz NM, et al. Epithelium-dependent contraction of airway smooth muscle caused by eosinophil MBP. *Am J Physiol* 1990;2593.

189. Jacoby DB, Gleich GJ, Fryer AD. Human eosinophil major basic protein is an endogenous allosteric antagonist at the inhibitory muscarinic M2 receptor. *J Clin Invest* 1993;91:1314–1318.

190. Fryer AD, Jacoby DB. Function of pulmonary M2 muscarinic receptors in antigen-challenged guinea pigs is restored by heparin and poly-L-glutamate. *J Clin Invest* 1992;90:2292–2298.

191. Desai SN, Van G, Robson J, Letts LG, Gundel RH, Gleich GJ, Piper PJ, Noonan TC. Human eosinophil major basic protein (MBP) augments bronchoconstriction induced by IV agonists in guinea pigs. *Agents Actions* 1993;39:C132–135.

192. Gundel RH, Letts LG, Gleich GJ. Human eosinophil major basic protein induces airway constriction and airway hyperresponsiveness in primates. *J Clin Invest* 1991;87:1470–1473.

193. Minnicozzi M, Duran WN, Gleich GJ, Egan RW. Eosinophil granule proteins increase microvascular macromolecular transport in the hamster cheek pouch. *J Immunol* 1994;153:2664–2670.

194. Wardlaw AJ, Dunnette S, Gleich GJ, Collins JV, Kay AB. Eosinophils and mast cells in bronchoalveolar lavage in subjects with mild asthma. Relationship to bronchial hyperreactivity. *Am Rev Respir Dis* 1988;137:62–69.

195. Durham SR, Kay AB. Eosinophils, bronchial hyperreactivity and late-phase asthmatic reactions. *Clin Allergy* 1985;15:411–418.

196. Iijima M, Adachi M, Kobayashi H, Takahashi T. Relationship between airway hyperreactivity and various atopic factors in bronchial asthma. *Arerugi* 1985;34:226–233.

197. Taylor KJ, Luksza AR. Peripheral blood eosinophil counts and bronchial responsiveness. *Thorax* 1987;42:452–456.

198. Mapp CE, Plebani M, Faggian D, et al. Eosinophil cationic protein (ECP), histamine and tryptase in peripheral blood before and during inhalation challenge with toluene diisocyanate (TDI) in sensitized subjects. *Clin Exp Allergy* 1994;24:730–736.

199. Wever AM, Wever Hess J, Hensgens HE, Hermans J. Serum eosinophil cationic protein (ECP) in chronic asthma. Relationship to spirometry, flow-volume curves, PC20, and exacerbations. *Respir Med* 1994;88:613–621.

200. Gundel RH, Gerritsen ME, Gleich GJ, Wegner CD: Repeated antigen inhalation results in a prolonged airway eosinophilia and airway hyperresponsiveness in primates. *J Appl Physiol* 1990;68:779–786.

201. Pretolani M, Ruffie C, Joseph D, et al. Role of eosinophil activation in the bronchial reactivity of allergic guinea pigs. *Am J Respir Cell Mol Biol* 1994;149:1167–1174.

202. Barker RL, Gundel RH, Gleich GJ, et al. Acidic polyamino acids inhibit human eosinophil granule major basic protein toxicity. *Blood* 1991;88:798–805.

Asthma, edited by P.J. Barnes, M.M. Grunstein, A.R. Leff, and A.J. Woolcock.
Lippincott–Raven Publishers, Philadelphia © 1997

▪ 46 ▪

Proteases

George H. Caughey and Jay A. Nadel

Mast Cell and Basophil Proteases
   Tryptase: the Major Protein of Mast Cells
   Chymase and Cathepsin G: Chymotrpysin-like
     Proteases of a Subset of Human Mast Cells
Neutrophil Proteases
   Elastase
   Cathepsin G
   Proteinase-3
   Matrix Metalloproteinases
Lymphocyte Proteases
   Matrix Metalloproteinases
   Granzymes
Epithelial Proteases
   Neutral Endopeptidase

Virus-activating Proteases
   Gland Cell Matrix
     Metalloproteinases
   Plasminogen Activators
Endothelial Proteases
   Angiotensin Converting Enzyme
   Plasminogen Activators
Plasma-Derived Proteases
   Plasma Kallikrein
   Thrombin
Allergen-Associated Proteases
   Dust Mites
   Pollen

Proteases are implicated in the generation of many of the major pathological features of asthma, including cough, bronchoconstriction, mucus hypersecretion, airway edema, inflammatory cell recruitment and migration, and subendothelial fibrosis. This chapter discusses cell surface and extracellular proteases that are known or suspected to be involved in the regulation of airway secretion and caliber, and in the pathogenesis of asthma. Although intracellular proteases, such as those involved in antigen processing and presentation, are important, they are beyond the purview of this chapter.

MAST CELL AND BASOPHIL PROTEASES

Mast cells and basophils long have been associated with allergic airway inflammation (1–3). In this context, mast cells are well-known as a source of preformed and

newly formed inflammatory mediators, such as histamine, prostaglandin $(PG)D_2$, and peptidyl leukotrienes. They are more recently recognized—but less widely appreciated—as a storehouse of proteases, which, when secreted, potentially contribute in a variety of ways to the pathogenesis of asthma (4). Although human basophils release histamine and can be stimulated to release cytokines and active metabolites of arachidonic acid, they are not nearly as well-characterized as a source of proteases. Basophils make small amounts of immunoreactive tryptase, which is present in substantially greater concentrations in mast cells. The basophil tryptase may be the source of tosyl-L-arginine methyl ester (TAME)-hydrolyzing and kallikrein activity reported to be released from stimulated basophils (5,6). However, because of the difficulty in obtaining large numbers of highly purified basophils, the identity and cell origin of these activities remains to be established definitively.

Tryptase: The Major Protein of Mast Cells

Of the several proteases manufactured and released by mast cells (Fig. 1), tryptase has received the most attention because of its abundance, its value as an *in vivo* marker of

   G. H. Caughey: Department of Medicine, Cardiovascular Research Institute, University of California at San Francisco, San Francisco, California 94143-0911.
   J. A. Nadel: Departments of Medicine and Physiology, Cardiovascular Research Institute, University of California at San Francisco, San Francisco, California 94143-0130.

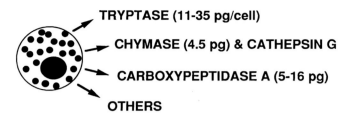

FIG. 1. Major proteases stored in human mast cell secretory granules.

mast cell activation, and its actions compatible with roles in asthmatic inflammation. Tryptase is a trypsin-like, granule-associated serine protease expressed by virtually all human mast cells, which are distributed widely in lung and airway tissues, and comprise ~5% of nucleated cells in suspensions of enzymatically dispersed lung parenchyma (7,8). Small amounts of tryptase are also expressed by a fraction of basophils at concentrations of protein and messenger ribonucleic acid (mRNA) that are substantially less than 1% of those in mast cells (9,10). Thus, mast cells are the major source of tryptase in human lungs and airways. Mast cells are not all identical in their expression of tryptase and other secretory granule proteases. Subsets of human mast cells have been identified and classified according to their content of tryptase and chymotrypsin-like enzymes (see following) (11). The mast cell tryptase and chymotrypsin-like protease (MC_{TC}) subset, which contains both types of enzymes, predominates in dermis and other connective tissues. MC_{TC} mast cells contain ~35 pg of tryptase per cell (7). Another subset (MC_T) predominates at other sites, notably gut mucosa and alveolar interstitium, and, to a lesser extent, bronchi. An MC_T cell contains ~11 pg of tryptase but no detectable chymotrypsin-like enzymes. By comparison, a human neutrophil contains only ~1 pg of its major granule proteases, elastase and cathepsin G (12). Tryptase is the single most abundant and specific protein product of mast cells, and, indeed, appears to be the most highly expressed protease of any granulated cell of bone-marrow origin (13). It is secreted by exocytosis from stimulated mast cells with other preformed mediators, including histamine and heparin (14–16). In association with heparin, human tryptase is stable, resisting inactivation by circulating protease inhibitors (17,18). Because of its abundance, mast cell specificity, and stability following secretion, tryptase is a useful marker of mast cell activation *in vivo* (19).

Biochemical Properties of Tryptases

In secreted form, human tryptase is a glycosylated, heparin-bound tetramer of noncovalently linked, catalytically active subunits (20,21). The tetramer itself is large (~150 kDa), and when associated with heparin proteoglycan, it is even larger. Because of its size, the tryptase tetramer-proteoglycan complex released from a degranulating mast cell diffuses more slowly away from the site of release than a small mediator, such as histamine. This is the probable basis of the observation that, following the acute, massive mast cell degranulation associated with bee sting anaphylaxis, the peak of tryptase immunoreactivity in the bloodstream appears later and lasts longer than that of histamine (22). In the absence of heparin, the tryptase tetramer rapidly dissociates into inactive monomers. The conformational change associated with the tetramer-to-monomer conversion is only transiently reversible. This disassociation and structural change may be the means by which tryptase activity is controlled after extracellular release *in vivo*. It is not yet clear how many tryptase genes are present in the human genome and, of these, which are expressed in mast cells of the lung and airway. Analysis of human tryptase complementary deoxyribonucleic acids (cDNAs), genes, and genomic DNA blots suggests that there are at least two distinct, but closely related, tryptase genes per haploid genome (23–25). Tryptase preparations exhibit heterogeneous electrophoretic banding, most or all of which is due to variable glycosylation (14,17). The two major human tryptase isoforms or glycoforms differ, somewhat, in substrate hydrolysis rate and specificity (26). Because human tryptase cDNAs vary in the number of predicted glycosylation sites, tryptase heterogeneity may result, in part, from the expression of more than one tryptase gene (25).

The Tryptase Gene Family

Several human tryptase cDNAs and a gene have been characterized (23–25). α-Tryptase, which was identified initially by screening a cDNA library prepared from human lung mast cells, is 92% to 93% identical in amino-acid sequence to tryptases I, II/β and III (β-tryptases), which are 97% to 99% identical to each other, and were identified originally from a library prepared from skin cells (23,25). In most individuals, the transcription of β-tryptases appears to predominate over that of α-tryptases in both lung and skin, although basophils transcribe mainly the latter (10). Some β-tryptases may be allelic variants, rather than the products of distinct gene loci (25). Current data are consistent with a minimum of two, different expressed human tryptase genes. It is not known whether there are functionally significant differences between the products of different human tryptase genes.

Tryptases in Asthma

The physiologic roles of tryptases in the lungs and airways remain to be established with certainty. However, *in vivo* and *in vitro* studies provide ample grounds for the hypothesis that tryptases play a role in lung disease, especially asthma (13,27–29) (Table 1). Bronchoalveolar

TABLE 1. *Possible roles in pathogenesis of asthma*

MAST CELL
Tryptase
- Inactivation bronchorelaxant peptides (VIP and PHM)
- Enhancement of histamine-induced bronchoconstriction
- Degradation and remodeling of extracellular matrix
- Stimulation of airway smooth muscle and fibroblast growth
- Recruitment of inflammatory cells
- Activation of eosinophils

Chymase
- Stimulation of gland cell secretion
- Inactivation of bronchorelaxant peptides
- Degradation and remodeling of extracellular matrix
- Infliction of epithelial damage
- Enhancement of tissue edema

Cathepsin G
- Degradation and remodeling of basement membrane and extracellular matrix
- Stimulation of gland cell secretion
- Infliction of epithelial damage

BASOPHILS
"Basophil Kallikrein"
- Enhancement of cough and bronchoconstriction via kinin generation

NEUTROPHILS
Elastase
- Stimulation of gland cell secretion
- Degradation and remodeling of basement membrane and extracellular matrix
- Infliction of epithelial damage

Cathepsin G
- (See under MAST CELL)

Proteinase-3
- ?Similar to elastase

Matrix Metalloproteases (neutrophil collagenase/MMP-8 and gelatinase B/MMP-9)
- Degradation and remodeling of basement membrane and extracellular matrix

LYMPHOCYTES
Matrix metalloproteinases (gelatinase A/MMP-2 and B/MMP-9)
- Migration of lymphocytes into tissues
- Degradation and remodelling of basement membrane and extracellular matrix

Granzymes
- ?Epithelial damage

EPITHELIAL/GLAND CELLS
Neutral endopeptidase
- Inactivation of inflammatory neuropeptides (tachykinins)

Viral protein-hydrolyzing proteases
- Activation of respiratory viruses

Gelatinase A (MMP-2)
- Growth and differentiation of airway submucosal glands

Plasminogen activators
- Tissue remodelling

ENDOTHELIAL PROTEASES
Angiotensin converting enzyme
- Generation of angiotensin II
- Inactivation of bradykinins (control of cough)

Plasminogen activators
- Tissue remodelling

PLASMA
Plasma kallikrein
- Enhancement of cough and bronchoconstriction via kinin generation

Thrombin
- Stimulation of airway fibroblast and smooth muscle growth

ALLERGENS
Dust mite and pollen proteases
- Degranulation of mast cells by cross-linking $Fc_\varepsilon RI$-bound allergen-specific IgE
- Enhancement of cough and bronchoconstriction via kinin generation
- Infliction of epithelial damage

---

lavage tryptase concentrations increase in asthmatics following endobronchial allergen challenge, suggesting that tryptase is released from activated airway mast cells in atopic asthma (30,31). Several lines of *in vitro* evidence indicate that tryptases influence bronchomotor tone. In isolated dog bronchi, for example, tryptase increases both the magnitude and sensitivity of histamine-induced bronchoconstriction (32). These phenomena, when present in patients, are hallmarks of asthma. Tryptases also may promote bronchoconstriction by degrading bronchoactive neuropeptides. Vasoactive intestinal peptide (VIP) and peptide histidine-methionine (PHM) are potent smooth

muscle relaxants (33). Both are readily hydrolyzed by tryptase, which may be responsible for the reported decrease in airway VIP immunoreactivity in asthmatics (34–36). However, it remains to be established whether the loss of VIP occurs *in vivo* or postmortem, and some investigators fail to confirm the decrease (37,38). Nonetheless, the concept that tryptases are involved in VIP degradation is supported by a guinea-pig model of allergic inflammation (39,40). In perfused lungs of guinea pigs chronically challenged with aerosolized ovalbumin, VIP is degraded by a serine protease similar or identical to tryptase (39,40). Furthermore, chronically inflamed lungs are more sensitive than normal lungs to the contractile effects of substance P (which is less efficiently hydrolyzed by neutral endopeptidase), and are less sensitive to the relaxant effects of VIP (which is degraded more efficiently by the tryptic enzyme/tryptase).

Tryptase-Stimulated Growth of Airway Smooth Muscle and Fibroblasts

Recent *in vitro* data implicate tryptase as a growth factor for airway smooth muscle cells *in vitro* (41). This activity of tryptase, if it also is manifest *in vivo*, provides one possible explanation of the airway smooth muscle hypertrophy or hyperplasia that is a pathological feature of asthmatic human airways (Fig. 2). Of additional interest, VIP is reported to inhibit airway smooth muscle growth (42). Thus, tryptase-mediated degradation of VIP may free smooth muscle from growth inhibition by this peptide, providing another means for tryptase to promote increases in smooth muscle mass. Tryptase also may contribute to the development of lung and airway fibrosis. Mast cells increase in numbers and mingle with proliferating fibroblasts in healing wounds and in fibrotic tissues of lung and skin (43–45). Furthermore, mediators (including tryptase) are released from mast cells in patients with pulmonary fibrosis associated with sarcoidosis and other interstitial lung diseases (46,47). A role for mast cells in pulmonary fibrosis is further supported by studies of mice exposed to bleomycin, ionizing radiation, or asbestos (48–51). Other studies specifically link mast cell tryptase to fibroblast growth. Tryptase induces fibroblast DNA synthesis and proliferation, acting synergistically with other mitogens such as epidermal growth factor and fibroblast growth factor (52,53). Therefore, the interaction of tryptase with other fibroblast mitogens may contribute to the "basement membrane thickening" (i.e., subepithelial fibrosis) seen in the airway mucosa of many persons with asthma.

Other Activities of Tryptase

Tryptase also cleaves and destroys the procoagulant proteins fibrinogen and high-molecular-weight kininogen (54). Therefore, in combination with heparin, tryptase may act as a local anticoagulant, facilitating the passage of leukocytes into airway loci of inflammation at sites of mast cell activation. The most rapidly hydrolyzed, identified natural peptide substrate of human tryptase is calcitonin gene-related peptide (CGRP) (35). It is likely that tryptase limits neurogenic, CGRP-mediated vasodilation in the dermis; in this context, its activity is anti-inflammatory (55). In human airway, where CGRP's roles are

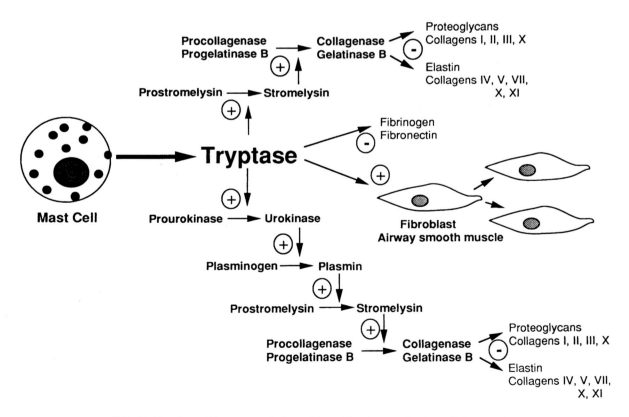

FIG. 2. Tryptase-driven remodeling of basal lamina and extracellular matrix.

less clear, the importance and consequences of tryptase-mediated inactivation of CGRP are uncertain. In contrast to its inactivation of some proteins and peptides, tryptase activates certain proteinases, e.g., single-chain urokinase and stromelysin; the latter, in turn, activates interstitial collagenase (56,57). By these means, tryptase may be involved in airway tissue remodeling (Fig. 2).

Antitryptases as Drugs

The properties of tryptases enumerated earlier have led to consideration of tryptases as targets for therapeutic inhibition. Recently, inhibitors of tryptases were reported to reduce early- and late-phase bronchoconstriction in *Ascaris*-challenged sheep (58). Confirmation of the hypothesis that tryptase contributes to bronchoconstriction in humans must await the results of human trials of tryptase inhibitors for asthma (59).

Chymase and Cathepsin G: Chymotrypsin-like Proteases of a Subset of Human Mast Cells

Chymase and cathepsin G are active extracellular serine proteases that are packaged along with histamine and tryptase in mast-cell secretory granules (29,60). Human chymase, the gene of which has been cloned and sequenced, is principally a product of mast cells, although human cardiac endothelial cells may synthesize small amounts (11,61,62). Cathepsin G, however, is found in neutrophils and monocytes as well as mast cells; its expression in mast cells is confined to those that also express chymase (60,63–66). As noted previously, the presence or absence of chymotrypsin-like enzymes distinguishes human mast cell subsets. The MC_{TC} subset of mast cells contain ~4.5 pg of chymase per cell (7). The concentration of cathepsin G in these cells is not known; however, the enzyme is detected as a major band in electrophoresed crude extracts of purified MC_{TC} mast cells (66). Although virtually 100% of human dermal mast cells contain chymase, only 7% of lung parenchymal mast cells contain the enzyme; however, the percentage is higher in bronchial and bronchiolar subepithelium (11). In human bronchi, the percentage of mast cells containing chymotrypsin-like activity varies according to the proximity of the cells to particular airway structures (67). For example, 73% of mast cells within 20 μm of submucosal glands contain chymase activity, whereas only 14% of mast cells within 20 μm of bronchial smooth muscle contain activity. The bronchi also occasionally harbor mast cells that appear to contain chymase without tryptase (MC_C mast cells), which comprise 12% of bronchial mast cells, although such cells are rare or nonexistent in many other tissues (68). Thus, human lungs and airways exhibit tissue-specific variation in expression of chymotrypsin-like mast cell enzymes.

Chymase and cathepsin G are catalytically, structurally and genetically related. The catalytic domains of human chymase and cathepsin G share 51% amino-acid identity. Both enzymes are glycosylated, chymotrypsin-like, cationic proteins with a high affinity for heparin (69,70). For a group of proteinases whose members are considered to have diverged only recently in protein evolution, the level of sequence similarity among mammalian chymases and related leukocyte granule proteases is surprisingly low (20,71). Thus, their biologic roles may be dissimilar. Nonetheless, features shared by all of these proteases include the presence of only three disulfide bonds, of a "signature" octapeptide (residues 9–16), and of an acidic two-residue propeptide terminating in glutamic acid, implying a shared pathway of activation from precursors (72,73). Indeed, recent evidence suggests that chymase and cathepsin G are activated by the same enzyme, dipeptidyl peptidase I, which is present in mast cells and myelomonocytic cells (74,75). This peptidase, however, does not activate mast cell tryptase and carboxypeptidase. The human chymase gene is related to that of cathepsin G and also is similar that of a number of other granule-associated serine proteases, including neutrophil elastase, and the T-lymphocyte granzymes (61,76,77). Perhaps surprisingly, the organization of the chymase gene is strikingly different from that of the human mast cell tryptase I gene, suggesting that the two mast cell proteases do not share a recent ancestor in protein evolution (25). The human chymase and cathepsin G genes are tightly linked on the long arm of chromosome 14 (14q11.2) (78). Both genes also are adjacent to related serine protease genes encoding granzymes B and H, which are expressed in cytotoxic T-lymphocytes and natural killer cells (76). The co-localization of these genes raises the possibility that a locus control element orchestrates high-level, lineage-specific expression. In addition, each gene in the cluster probably has its own sequences that control expression. Although chymase and cathepsin G expression normally is confined to a subset of human mast cells, it is possible that levels of expression change in lung and airway disease.

Chymase and cathepsin G increase vascular permeability and hydrolyze airway peptides. Several observations suggest roles for chymase and cathepsin G. For example, chymase modulates *in vivo* vascular permeability changes causing wheal formation in the skin of atopic dogs, and cathepsin G enhances transendothelial albumin flux in monolayers of endothelial cells (79,80). These observations invite speculation that similar events take place in nasal and tracheobronchial tissues of atopic individuals. In addition, chymase and cathepsin G are active peptidases, albeit with restricted target ranges. When profiled against a battery of peptidyl-4-nitroanilides, both chymase and cathepsin G are highly selective in hydrolyzing certain substrates, especially compared to chymotrypsin (81). Dog chymase, which is highly similar to the human enzyme, cleaves the Tyr^{22}-Leu^{23} bond of vasoactive intestinal peptide and the Phe[7]-Phe[8] bond of substance P, and, thus, may modulate the actions of these bronchoactive neuropeptides (20,34,59,61,73). Human cathepsin G also is active in this regard (81,82). Chymase and cathepsin G both inactivate kinins and activate angiotensin I to angiotensin II, hydrolyzing the Phe[8]-His[9] bond (70,83,84). Indeed, chymase accounts for more than 75% of converting enzyme activity in human ventricular myocardium (70). Recent *in vivo* data suggest that chymase-mediated production of angiotensin II is a determinant of ventricular performance in baboons (85). Thus, chymase and cathepsin G may generate extravascular vasoconstricting peptides in heart, lung, and other tissues. The significance of angiotensin II generation in bronchial tissues is speculative at present, but could include modulation of blood flow, smooth muscle growth, and other effects.

Chymase and cathepsin G stimulate gland cell secretion and degrade serous cell proteoglycans. Chymase and cathepsin G are noncytotoxic secretagogues for cultured airway submucosal gland cells (86,87). The extent of degranulation caused by these proteases is dramatically greater than that caused by histamine and isoproterenol, achieving ~80% exocytosis of granule proteoglycan. In conjunction with the observation that the percentage of mast cells that contain chymotrypsin-like activity in the immediate vicinity of bronchial submucosal glands is the greatest of any airway location, the previously mentioned findings support a role for chymase and cathepsin G in the physiological regulation of gland secretion and, possibly, in the hypersecretion associated with bronchitis and asthma (67). Both enzymes also are proteoglycanases, since they digest the chondroitin sulfate released from serous gland cells (86–88).

Chymase and cathepsin G hydrolyze epithelial glycocalyx and matrix proteins and participate in tissue remodeling. When incubated with cultured airway epithelial cells, chymase removes components of the surface glycocalyx (89). Both chymase and cathepsin G degrade various constituents of extracellular matrix (90,91). Indirectly, chymase released from activated mast cells may stimulate airway smooth muscle, fibroblast growth, and matrix production by solubilizing extracellular matrix-bound latent transforming growth factor (TGF)-β1 (92). However, because chymase appears to be incapable of activating TGF-β1 from its latent form, other proteases (e.g., plasmin) probably need to be recruited to help in the activation process to allow chymase-liberated latent TGF-β to stimulate mesenchymal cells in the vicinity of degranulating mast cells (92,93). A potential mast cell-initiated mechanism for generating active plasmin was suggested recently by the observation that human mast cell tryptase activates pro-urokinase to urokinase, which in turn cleaves plasminogen to generate active plasmin (56). In this manner, co-released chymotrypsin- and trypsin-like mast cell proteases may cooperate to repair the acute damage to extracellular matrix caused by their release into airway tissues (Fig. 3). In simple terms, what these proteases break they may help to fix. Recently, chymases have been shown to activate various matrix metalloproteinases (Fig. 4) with activation preferences different from those of tryptase noted earlier (94,95). Cathepsin G may act in this capacity to a lesser extent (96). The consequences of chymase and cathepsin G release in the immediate milieu of a degranulating airway mast cell, therefore, could range from generation of vasoactive peptides and infliction of epithelial damage, to stimulation of gland secretion and solubiliza-

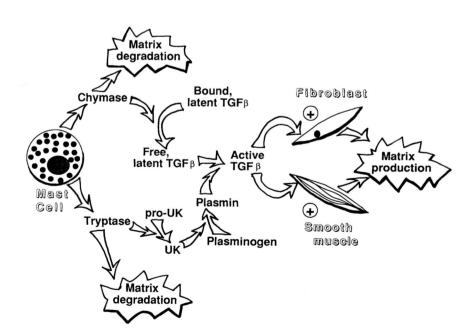

FIG. 3. A pathway for transforming growth factor (TGF)-β-mediated repair of extracellular matrix damaged by mast cell proteases.

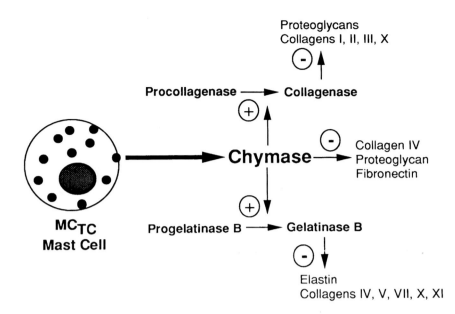

FIG. 4. Chymase-driven remodeling of basal lamina and extracellular matrix.

tion of extracellular matrix. *In vivo* tests of the importance of these identified activities await the availability of selective inhibitors suitable for use in animal models of asthma and in human subjects. However, species differences in the number of chymotrypsin-like mast-cell protease genes—and in their levels of expression, mast-cell subset distribution, and enzymatic and physical properties—are striking, especially between humans and rodents (4). Because of these differences, caution must be exercised in applying insights gained from the results of studies in mast cell-deficient or chymase "knockout" mice, to explanations of the role of this class of enzymes in human asthma.

NEUTROPHIL PROTEASES

Neutrophils are a cellular component of asthmatic inflammation (2). In mild asthma, the numbers of neutrophils in airway tissues are not particularly impressive. However, they are a more sizable contingent of inflammatory cells in severe (and, especially, fatal) asthma. The aspects of asthma pathology that are most likely to be influenced by neutrophil proteases, according to current evidence, are gland secretion and epithelial damage. These aspects are the focus of the discussions that follow.

Elastase

Human neutrophil elastase (HNE; EC3.4.21.37) is a serine protease found in the azurophilic granules of human neutrophils. It has long been known to degrade numerous connective tissue macromolecules such as elastin, fibronectin, collagen, and proteoglycan. Because neutrophils are present at sites of inflammation, HNE has

been implicated in tissue destructive diseases such as adult respiratory distress syndrome and emphysema (97,98). Neutrophil elastase is the best-studied neutrophil enzyme. Azurophilic granules form in promyelocytes and are stored until exocytosed from mature neutrophils (99). In normal blood, there is no evidence of activity of elastase. This could be due, in part, to the excess of anti-elastase activity normally present in blood. However, when neutrophils are isolated *in vitro*, it still is not easy to release substantial amounts of elastase, even when stimulated with chemoattractants (100). Nevertheless, the sputum of patients with cystic fibrosis (CF) may contain elastase concentrations exceeding 10^{-6} M and sputum from subjects with chronic bronchitis and bronchiectasis may contain high concentrations of active elastase (101–105). These high elastase concentrations could be due to "activation" of neutrophils, but are most likely due to the release of elastase from dying neutrophils.

Elastase cleaves cell surface receptors and inhibits ciliary beating. In addition to degradation of matrix materials, neutrophil elastase has some surprising effects in airways. In CF, blood neutrophils express low levels of complement receptors CR1 and CR2, and this is increased upon stimulation. In contrast, neutrophils recovered from bronchoalveolar lavage showed little CR1 expression in CF, an effect that was reproduced by administration of elastase and prevented by elastase inhibitors in activated blood neutrophils (106). These findings suggest that neutrophils at inflammatory sites have maximally upregulated expression of their complement receptors but that CRI is then cleaved by elastase proteolysis. Thus, high levels of free elastase may interfere with efficient phagocytosis and contribute to difficulty in eradicating lung infections. Elastase also inhibits ciliary beating and cleaves receptors on T cells and B cells (107,108).

Elastase is a potent gland and goblet cell secretagogue. One of the most surprising and striking effects of neutrophil elastase in airways is its secretagogue activity. Elastase causes secretion in airway submucosal gland cells and in goblet cells in various species, including humans, with a threshold of approximately 10^{-10} M and a maximum secretory effect of approximately 2,000-fold above baseline (87,109). This is an order of magnitude greater than the responses to classic secretagogues such as histamine. When sputum from patients with hypersecretion was co-cultured with airway gland cells, hypersecretion occurred even when the sputum was diluted several thousand-fold (110). The secretagogue activity was decreased markedly after pretreatment with a selective elastase inhibitor (104,110). These findings implicate neutrophil proteases as potentially important causes of hypersecretion in chronic obstructive airway diseases. In some cases, "trapping" of neutrophils in obstructive plugs could lead to the death of neutrophils and release of elastase.

However, this is not likely to be the only mechanism of hypersecretion for the following reasons. First, elastase has a high molecular weight and is not likely to cause secretion of glands (located deep in airway tissue) when elastase is present in the airway lumen. Second, in acute asthma, there is evidence of neutrophil recruitment but less evidence for high concentrations of free elastase in the lumen. In mild asthma, there is little evidence to implicate neutrophil-induced hypersecretion. β-adrenergic agonists and corticosteroids generally provide inexpensive, effective therapy for mild asthma. However, neutrophils may play a major role in some patients with acute asthma.

The evidence suggests that neutrophils do not release elastase "by themselves." It is suggested that neutrophils "have a large hardware, little software." By that is meant that neutrophils, when they leave the circulation, respond to signals in tissues that they traverse. It is hypothesized that tissue signals induce second messengers in neutrophils, causing exocytosis, perhaps only in the neutrophil pseudopod as it advances in tissue. Further, it is proposed that the signal could come from the surface of the gland or goblet cell ("adhesion molecule?"), perhaps by interacting with a neutrophil chemoattractant (e.g., interleukin [IL]-8) or other inflammatory mediator. It is important to remember that neutrophil granules contain approximately 10^{-3} M elastase. Therefore, at sites of release of elastase, especially if the release occurs at sites of tight adhesion of the neutrophil and secretory cell, the stimulus could be great. If this hypothesis is correct, it suggests multiple interventions that could be therapeutically useful.

Neutrophils and secreted elastase may contribute to acute asthma. Approximately 75% of the cost of treating all asthmatics is incurred by 10% of the patients. These patients have severe asthma, punctuated by repeated admissions to emergency wards and intensive care units where the hospitalization is the major expense. These are the patients at risk of dying! When asthmatics die, postmortem studies show obstruction of the peripheral airways by mucous plugs (111). This peripheral plugging may be mostly due to degranulation of goblet cells in the superficial epithelium and, thus, associated with few symptoms. In acute asthma, neutrophils often appear in the airways. Furthermore, antigen administration causes early neutrophil recruitment into the airways (eosinophils predominate at later stages of the response). Similarly, viral infection causes neutrophil recruitment into the airway tissue and lumen. Thus, acute hypersecretion, the main presumed cause of incapacitation and death, could be due to neutrophil elastase. Inhibitors of elastase could be life saving in these acute asthmatics. Appropriate clinical trials are needed to evaluate this therapeutic effect.

Cathepsin G

Key properties of this chymotryptic protease are considered elsewhere in this chapter in connection with its expression in the mast cell and so, are not repeated here. In neutrophils, cathepsin G is packaged with elastase in azurophil granules. Its levels in the neutrophil are similar to those of elastase (63). Monocytes also contain cathepsin G, but in much lesser amounts, probably as a remnant of protease manufacture at an earlier stage of myelomonocytic cell differentiation (112). Virtually across the board, cathepsin G is weaker than chymase in hydrolyzing identified targets of chymotrypsin-like enzymes, and is substantially weaker than either chymase or elastase as a secretagogue (87,104). Because cathepsin G is catalytically sluggish in cleaving substrates against which it has been tested, possibly its "true," preferred targets remain to be identified. In this regard, the recent evidence that cathepsin G or a closely related enzyme controls neutrophil migration in response to chemoattractants is intriguing because it suggests the possibility of novel cathepsin G substrates, perhaps on the surface of the migrating neutrophil itself (113).

Proteinase-3

This azurophil granule-associated serine protease has not been studied as intensively as its close cousin, neutrophil elastase. However, several of its properties suggest that it deserves consideration as an agent capable of inflicting damage to airway epithelium and subepithelium. Like elastase, it destroys many connective tissue proteins and causes emphysema, if delivered into the lungs of hamsters (114,115). Its amino-acid sequence, gene organization, chromosomal location, and levels of neutrophil expression are similar to those of elastase (116,117). However, it differs from elastase in resisting inactivation by the principal serine protease inhibitor of bronchial secretions, secretory leukocyte protease inhibitor, which it degrades (118). Thus, airway epithelia appear to be less well-defended against potentially deleterious effects of proteinase-3 than they are against those of neutrophil elastase. Proteinase-3 also is the major target of cytoplasmic antineutrophil cytoplasmic antibodies (c-ANCA) present in various vasculitides, notably Wegener's granulomatosis (119). Whether proteinase-3 and antibodies raised against this enzyme are causally related to the upper and lower airway and lung parenchymal pathology that is part of the Wegener's granulomatosis picture, is not clearly established, although it appears likely (120). At present, a role for proteinase-3 in epithelial damage and other manifestations of asthmatic inflammation is plausible, but speculative.

Matrix Metalloproteinases

Neutrophils secrete two major varieties of matrix metalloproteinase, an interstitial collagenase (MMP-8) and a gelatinase (gelatinase B; 92-kDa gelatinase; MMP-9). These enzymes degrade various proteins of basement membrane and extracellular matrix, and may mediate epithelial damage and other manifestations of the capacity of neutrophils for tissue destruction (121). 92-kDa gelatinase activity is particularly prominent in secretions obtained by bronchoalveolar lavage from persons with bronchitis and bronchiectasis, and the level of activity is reported to correlate with disease severity (122). Whether metalloproteinases secreted by neutrophils and other inflammatory cells help to produce the less dramatic forms of epithelial damage and tissue remodeling typical of asthma, is at present unknown.

LYMPHOCYTE PROTEASES

Increased numbers of activated lymphocytes are present in the airway mucosa of asthmatics. In atopic asthma, there is an excess of CD4+ lymphocytes producing the "TH2" spectrum of cytokines (e.g., IL-4 and IL-5), linked with the pathogenesis of allergic inflammation in the lung, nasal passages, and other tissues. This accumulation or increased traffic of lymphocytes in asthmatic airway tissue is the result of migration between vascular endothelial cells and penetration through the endothelial basement membrane (basal lamina). Recent evidence suggests that certain secreted proteases are critical for lymphocyte migration into extralymphoid tissues and for target cell killing by cytolytic, CD8+ T cells.

Matrix Metalloproteinases

Although a great deal is known and has been written about the roles of adhesion molecules in mediating the attachment of T lymphocytes to endothelium and extracellular matrix, comparatively little attention has been paid to the means by which lymphocytes pass through endothelial barriers into tissues. In this regard, recent intriguing evidence indicates that human T cells secrete basement membrane-degrading metalloproteinases (i.e., gelatinases A and B), which hydrolyze key components of the multi-layer network of collagens, proteoglycans, and glycoproteins upon which the barrier function of the basal lamina depends (123). Because incubation of T cells with a metalloproteinase inhibitor renders lymphocytes unable to penetrate artificial basement membranes, it is likely that T cells use one or more of these proteases to traverse the basal lamina. Other hydrolases, such as heparanase, may play an equal or greater role (124). Nonetheless, it is tempting to speculate that inhibitors of metalloproteinases, by preventing T-cell migration to tissue sites of inflammation, may ameliorate diseases such as asthma, which are mediated, in part, by T cells.

Granzymes

The granule-associated serine proteases of cytolytic T lymphocytes and natural killer cells are termed "granzymes." Although the members of this group of proteases are structurally and phylogenetically closely related (and are also cousins of cathepsin G, chymases, neutrophil elastase and proteinase-3), their substrate specificities vary dramatically (13,20). Granzyme A is tryptic, hydrolyzing peptide targets after basic residues, whereas granzyme B prefers to hydrolyze after aspartate, a specificity which is unique, or at least highly unusual, among serine proteases. Other lymphocyte granzymes exhibit a specificity for methionine, or may be chymotrypsin-like, hydrolyzing targets after aromatic residues. As noted earlier in this chapter, the gene encoding human granzyme B is clustered with those of chymase and cathepsin G (78). Like the latter chymotrypsin-like enzymes, granzyme B is activated intracellularly by dipeptidyl peptidase I (75). Although mice produce granzymes (especially relatives of granzyme B) in somewhat bewildering variety, the human granzyme repertoire appears to be much smaller (125). The most extensively characterized human granzymes are A and B, both of which are proposed to play a role in T-lymphocyte and natural killer-cell killing of target cells (i.e., cells expressing foreign antigens, such as tumor cells and infected cells), into which the enzymes are thought to gain entry through perforin-generated pores. Once inside the target cell, these enzymes appear to help launch or carry out an apoptosis program (126). The natural substrates of these enzymes are not known. Although granzymes (like the mast cell serine proteases discussed previously) reside in secretory granules, it is unlikely that their effects are as far-ranging or as damaging to airway tissues. This is because they have very narrow substrate preferences and are released focally in the context of intimate contact with target cells, with little chance to harm bystander cells. Even though considerable evidence suggests that granzymes are important and, possibly, critical, for host immunocompetence, their roles in the pathophysiology of asthma, if any, remain to be determined.

EPITHELIAL PROTEASES

Unlike mast cells, neutrophils, and lymphocytes, which secrete proteases into the extracellular space, epithelial cells are perhaps best known as a source of the plasma membrane-anchored ectoenzyme, neutral endopeptidase, a major determinant of the severity of tachykinin-mediated neurogenic inflammation. However, other epithelial proteases, such as those hydrolyzing respiratory viruses, may modulate the spread and extent of epithelial damage caused by viral infections, which are probably the most frequent precipitant of asthma exacerbations requiring hospitalization.

Neutral Endopeptidase

This enzyme (also known as enkephalinase, metalloendopeptidase, E.C. 3.4.24.11) was first discovered in the brush border epithelium of the kidney (127). Neutral endopeptidase (NEP) is a glycosylated Zn metallopeptidase and an integral membrane protein consisting of 749 amino-acid residues with a short cytoplasmic domain, a hydrophobic domain which anchors the enzyme to the plasma membrane, and a large extracellular domain containing the active site (128,129). NEP preferentially cleaves peptides on the amino side of hydrophobic residues (Phe, Leu, Met). It hydrolyzes peptide bonds of substance P and neurokinin A, thus yielding inactive fragments lacking the carboxyl-terminal region necessary for the binding to tachykinin receptors. NEP cleaves a variety of substrates including substance P, neurokinin A, bradykinin, and other peptides. Despite the broad spectrum of activities, some specificity is observed *in vivo*, conveyed partly by the location of the enzyme in tissue; it is normally attached to the surfaces of cells and the active site faces the external milieu. This structural arrangement allows the enzyme to cleave selected peptides in the environment near the cells to which the active site of the enzyme is attached, and these locations effectively limit its activity. In airways, NEP is located on basal cells near the sensory nerve terminals. Thus, NEP can cleave sensory neuropeptides (e.g., substance P) near their sites of release from sensory nerves. In addition, NEP is located on the surfaces of cells which are targets of peptide action (e.g., glands and airway smooth muscle), so NEP can also cleave and inactivate peptides at sites of their action.

NEP may limit asthmatic responses by cleaving inflammatory peptides. Evidence for the presence of NEP is provided by inhibiting NEP activity. Selective inhibitors of NEP increase various responses to sensory nerve stimulation and to the delivery of various peptides such as substance P and kinins to airways. The responses, plasma extravasation, bronchoconstriction, leukocyte adhesion, and cough, are exaggerated following pretreatment with NEP inhibitors. Knowledge of the role of NEP in human disease is hampered by the paucity of human studies with inhibitors of NEP. Studies in animals suggest a possible role in asthma. For example, aerosolized hypertonic saline triggers bronchospasm in asthmatics and cough (130, 131). Inhalation of aerosols of hypertonic saline in rats causes plasma extravasation and bronchoconstriction, and these responses are prevented by pretreatment with inhibitors of neurokinin receptors; NEP inhibitors exaggerate the responses (132,133). Bradykinin, a 9-amino-acid peptide formed from a plasma precursor, has been implicated in various diseases. Vascular extravasation caused by bradykinin in rats are potentiated by selective NEP inhibitors, suggesting that NEP modulates actions of bradykinin. Thus, in airways, NEP limits inflammatory responses by cleaving various inflammatory peptides (e.g., substance P, kinins). Therefore, a decrease of NEP activity (e.g., by drugs that inhibit NEP activity or by pathophysiologic states that decrease NEP activity in tissue) would be expected to exaggerate responses. Further evidence for the possible role of NEP in inflammation derives from studies of inhaled irritants. Inhalation of cigarette smoke or toluene diisocyanate exaggerate neurogenic inflammatory responses in animals by decreasing NEP activity, and respiratory viral infections produce the same effects (134). Thus, a decrease in NEP activity could be a cause of exaggerated responses in disease.

Aerosolized or upregulated NEP may reduce asthmatic responses. Human NEP cDNA has been cloned and recombinant human NEP is available. Aerosolized recombinant NEP inhibits cough produced by exogenously delivered and by endogenously released neuropeptides (135). Clinical studies with recombinant NEP will be required to determine the therapeutic usefulness of NEP in inhibiting inflammatory responses in asthma. For example, cough is an early and persistent problem in asthma, and current therapy of cough is unsatisfactory. If peptides such as substance P or bradykinin are important in inducing cough, NEP could provide effective therapy. Corticosteroids upregulate the synthesis of some enzymes, including NEP (136). Pretreatment with corticosteroids prevents neurogenic plasma extravasation in rats by increasing NEP activity (137). Thus, upregulation of endogenous NEP is another strategy for therapeutic intervention of inflammation caused by peptides.

Virus-Activating Proteases

Airway epithelial cells can be a source of respiratory virus-activating proteases. In the inflamed airway of asthmatics, variations in epithelial levels of virus-activating proteases may influence the extent and clinical severity of viral infection. Most viruses affecting tissues within as well as outside of the respiratory tract require the actions of one or more proteases for biogenesis and infectivity (138–140). Some viral genomes, such as those of human immunodeficiency virus, encode their own proteases, which are essential for proper posttranslational processing of key viral proteins (141). Other viruses co-opt host proteases for this task or use a combination of viral and host proteases. Among respiratory viruses, influenza virus and respiratory syncytial virus (RSV) are tropic for respiratory epithelial cells and greatly increase their ability to infect host cells when proteolytically cleaved by a host protease (138,142). The host proteases involved in this phenomenon have been studied most extensively in rodents. For example, a trypsin-like serine protease, named "tryptase Clara" (no apparent close relation to mast cell tryptase) has been localized to nonciliated epithelial cells in bronchioles of the rat (143,144). This enzyme cleaves surface proteins of influenza A virus and of related Sendai virus, enhancing infectivity; that is because in these viruses, protein cleavage is required before fusion with host cell membranes can occur. Antibodies against tryptase Clara inhibit activation and cycles of Sendai virus replication in the lungs of infected rats, suggesting that the enzyme is a determinant of viral pathogenicity (143). Because respiratory virus infections worsen asthmatic cough and bronchospasm (or does asthmatic airway inflammation worsen respiratory viral infection?), virus-activating airway epithelial proteases should be regarded as potential virulence factors for asthma.

Gland Cell Matrix Metalloproteinases

Growth of submucosal glands in the course of normal airway tissue development and disease progression in the airways of persons with bronchitis or asthma, requires epithelial gland precursor cells to penetrate the basement membrane and invade the extracellular matrix of the submucosa. This penetration is likely to require the action of proteases capable of hydrolyzing structural proteins of basement membrane and extracellular matrix. Tournier et al. (145) have identified a 72-kDa matrix metalloproteinase (gelatinase A) that is secreted by bovine tracheal gland cells but not by surface epithelial cells. Inhibition of this enzyme prevents gland cells from invading solid collagen substrates. Furthermore, immunocytochemical analysis of airway tissue sections identify gelatinase A specifically in certain glandular acini of bovine tracheal epithelium. Thus, this enzyme and related matrix metal-

loenzymes may assist gland growth and differentiation in airway diseases, including asthma.

Plasminogen Activators

Plasminogen activators (PAs), that hydrolyze plasminogen to yield active, fibrin-degrading plasmin, are recognized for their natural and therapeutic role in the removal of intravascular clots of fibrin. They are also expressed at extravascular sites, including the airway and alveolar lumen, where they are thought to function in a similar fashion to break down extravascular fibrin. The two main varieties of PA are tissue-type (t-PA) and urinary-type (u-PA). The former is principally a product of endothelial cells in the lungs and throughout the body (146). The latter is expressed mainly by extravascular cells, including airway epithelial cells (147,148). Although both PAs dissolve fibrin clots, extravascular u-PA differs in major ways from intravascular t-PA (149). Because PA-activated plasmin has fairly broad specificity (at least *in vitro*), degrading not only fibrin but various basement membrane proteins—and activating collagenase and TGF-β—the action of PAs may be a key step on the road to repair of tissue injury. Furthermore, certain airway cells, such as macrophages, express cell surface u-PA receptors which serve to collect secreted u-PA, localize its activity to the cell surface, and co-opt its functions into the service of the cell expressing the receptor (150,151). Other suggested functions of u-PA include stimulation of airway cell growth and facilitation of recruitment and migration of inflammatory cells (152,153). Because PAs are secreted as inactive zymogens, they must be activated by proteolysis to create a two-chain form of the enzymes. In allergic airway inflammation, one possible activator of u-PA is mast cell tryptase, which has been demonstrated *in vitro* to generate active, two-chain u-PA (56). Lung and airway epithelial cells also may regulate PA activity through production of PA inhibitors. Thus, although a complete picture of their production, activation, and inhibition is not yet available, airway PAs may contribute in several ways to the inflammation and tissue remodeling associated with asthma and other inflammatory airway diseases.

ENDOTHELIAL PROTEASES

Angiotensin Converting Enzyme (ACE)

Like NEP, ACE is a zinc metalloproteinase, which is membrane-bound and anchored to the cell by a single hydrophobic membrane-spanning region. Two ACE isoenzymes have been described. The larger form (150-180 kDA) is present in high concentrations in the vascular endothelium of the lungs and airways (154). Human endothelial ACE cDNA encodes a 1306-amino-acid polypeptide and is anchored to the cell surface by a hydrophobic region near its C-terminal domain (155). It contains two highly symmetrical extracellular domains, each containing putative Zn-binding sequences (155). The selectivity depends, in part, on the ability of the peptidase to cleave and thus, inactivate specific peptides. Because ACE is bound to the luminal surface of endothelial cells, it acts preferentially on the vasculature and so, mainly modulates vascular responses (e.g., vasomotion, vascular permeability, leukocyte adhesion) (156). Like NEP, ACE cleaves substance P and inactivates it. Unlike NEP, ACE inhibitors do not appear to affect bronchoconstrictor or secretagogue effects of substance P or of neurogenic inflammation; but they potently exaggerate neurogenic vascular effects.

The role of ACE in asthma is unknown. ACE inhibitors used therapeutically for the treatment of cardiovascular disease cause cough. This side effect is severe enough to cause withdrawal of the drug in a significant number of patients. This suggests that ACE plays a role in metabolizing peptides that, when inhibited, allows uncleaved peptides such as bradykinin to stimulate cough receptors. This effect also suggests clues concerning the mechanisms producing cough in asthma. Cleavage of cough-producing peptides by locally delivered drugs could provide effective therapy for this troublesome symptom.

Plasminogen Activators

Pulmonary vascular endothelium appears to be a source of both t-PA and u-PA (146). The former probably is involved primarily in the lysis of intravascular thrombi or of emboli that lodge in the pulmonary vascular bed. In the vessels of the bronchi, supplied mainly by the systemic arterial circuit, the role of t-PA in lysing emboli presumably is less important. The part played by u-PA in the airways is considered earlier, in the discussion of epithelial plasminogen activators.

PLASMA-DERIVED PROTEASES

Plasma is a rich soup of active proteases and their proenzymes, which participate in events such as hemostasis, fibrinolysis, and complement fixation. Transudation of plasma from the vascular space into airway tissues, (a feature of airway inflammation in general and asthma in particular), makes these proteases available to interact with airway cells. Two potentially key enzymes, plasma kallikrein and thrombin, are discussed here.

Plasma Kallikrein

In humans, there are two kinins: bradykinin and lysyl-bradykinin. Both are small peptides (9 and 10 amino

acids, respectively) with a host of biologic activities consistent with a role in inflammatory diseases, including asthma (5). Bradykinin differs from lysylbradykinin only by the lack of the amino-terminal arginine attached to the latter. Kinins are liberated in vivo from much larger precursors (kininogens) by the action of kininogenases (in particular, kallikreins) and are inactivated by several peptidases (collectively termed kininases). The major kininogenase in the circulation is "plasma" kallikrein, a serine protease which is structurally very different from "tissue" kallikrein, and is the product of a separate gene. The latter enzyme is produced in a variety of exocrine glands and has been localized to the serous cells of submucosal glands in human trachea (157). Both types of kallikrein are potential, but not proven, generators of the kinins that appear in human allergic reactions (158,159). The principal substrate of plasma kallikrein is thought to be the high-molecular-weight kininogen (HMWK) with which it is complexed in plasma. In the edematous airway tissue associated with chronic airway inflammation and asthma, extravascular plasma kallikrein and HMWK may generate kinins outside of vessels in the vicinity of kinin-vulnerable structures, such as surface epithelium, submucosal glands, blood vessels, and tachykinin-releasing nerves. Like most other serine proteases, (with mast cell tryptase a notable exception), plasma kallikrein is secreted (from hepatocytes) as an inactive zymogen (prekallikrein) which must be proteolytically cleaved to become catalytically active. In vivo, the activation of plasma kallikrein is thought to be mediated by factor XIIa in the setting of contact of the prekallikrein/HMWK complex and XIIa with a negatively charged surface, such as basement membrane. At present, the identity of the enzyme(s) contributing to kinin formation in allergic airway disease—and, indeed, the importance of kinins in general to the pathogenesis of asthma—is something of a mystery. However, the demonstration of inhibition of antigen-induced hyperresponsiveness in sheep by a first-generation, peptide-based kinin receptor antagonist is intriguing in this regard (160). The development of later-generation kinin receptor antagonists with increased stability, bioavailability, potency, and selectivity in humans, and the development and testing of kallikrein inhibitors, can be expected to shed new light on the issue of the importance of kinins and kallikreins in asthma.

Thrombin

Although a vast literature attests to the importance of intravascular thrombin in hemostasis and thrombosis, comparatively little consideration has been given to activation and actions caused by thrombin in extravascular tissues like airways (161). One of the most extensively studied and interesting nonhemostatic attributes of thrombin is growth factor activity. Catalytically active thrombin stimulates proliferation of a variety of cells *in vitro*, including fibroblasts and some types of smooth muscle cells. This mitogenic effect appears to be mediated through a thrombin receptor present on the surface of susceptible cells (162). This receptor is activated by thrombin-mediated cleavage (163). The mitogenic effects of thrombin on fibroblasts are superficially similar to those of mast-cell tryptase, for both are trypsin-like serine proteases with some overlapping substrate preferences. However, tryptase does not act by cleaving the thrombin receptor, as indicated by the following: a) identification of cells that respond to tryptase and not to thrombin (and vice versa); b) use of different intracellular signaling pathways by the two enzymes; and c) synergy between tryptase and thrombin or thrombin-receptor peptide in promoting DNA synthesis (53,164). Therefore, the two enzymes probably are independent growth factors. Both enzymes are potent fibroblast mitogens *in vitro*, and may, therefore, play a role in generating the subepithelial fibrosis observed in the biopsied bronchi of many asthmatics. Thrombin stimulates growth of cultured airway smooth muscle cells from humans (but not from dogs); therefore, thrombin may be a factor that increases smooth muscle mass in asthma (41,165). Although the *in vivo* importance of the proposed role of thrombin as an airway mitogen remains to be demonstrated, one aspect of the phenomenon now is clear: to achieve its potential as a growth factor, thrombin must be catalytically active (162). In certain types of lung pathology, such as that associated with scleroderma or with bleomycin- or endotoxin-inflicted injury, activated thrombin is abundant in bronchoalveolar lavage fluid. Such widespread activation is generally thought to require injury to the vascular endothelium (161). It is not yet apparent how thrombin can be generated from prothrombin in airway tissues in the presumed absence of major vascular injury and activation of the coagulation cascade. Nonetheless, in asthma, which is characterized by increased leakage of albumin and other circulating proteins into airway tissues, sufficient amounts of thrombin may be activated from extravasated thrombin to influence airway cell populations.

ALLERGEN-ASSOCIATED PROTEASES

The aeroallergens associated with allergic asthma include dust mite feces, animal dander, pollens, and fungi. Sensitization to these antigens is thought to require traversal of the airway epithelial barrier, uptake and hydrolysis by antigen presenting cells (e.g., dendritic cells), followed by mixed histocompatibility complex (MHC) II-restricted presentation to T cells. Conditions that damage epithelium improve the prospect of inhaled allergen penetrating the mucoepithelial barrier and contacting antigen-presenting cells, and thereby increase the likelihood that sensitization

will occur and that the inflammatory reaction on re-exposure will be severe. Such conditions classically include infection with epithelium-damaging respiratory viruses. In recent years, as several of the major aeroallergens have been characterized, it has become apparent that some allergens are not merely passive participants in the process, but themselves damage epithelium, thereby facilitating their own traversal of the mucosal barrier. Given the ability of neutrophil and mast cell proteases to inflict epithelial damage, it perhaps should come as no surprise that some of the best allergens are active proteases.

Dust Mites

At least two of the major allergens of dust mite feces are proteases. The group I antigen, *Der p*I, of the house mite *Dermatophagoides pteronyssinus*, is a cysteine protease that augments permeability of cultured epithelial cell sheets to albumin (166). In the same species, the group III antigen, *Der p*III, is a trypsin-like protease (167). An apparently similar trypsin-like serine protease (Df-protease) from a different house mite, *D. farinae*, has kallikrein activity, liberating kinins from plasma low- and high-molecular-weight kininogen (168). These mite proteases, therefore, may promote airway inflammation by means other than, or in addition to, degranulating mast cells and basophils via cross-linking mite antigen-specific IgE bound to Fc$_\varepsilon$RI receptors.

Pollen

A protease with distinct properties has been isolated from extracts of mesquite pollen, a major allergen in the southwestern United States (169). The mesquite enzyme, which appears to be a serine protease, although perhaps not of the trypsin family, has little if any ability to hydrolyze proteins. However, it cleaves after arginine residues of a number of active peptides, including atrial natriuretic peptide, VIP, and angiotensin II. Therefore, this peptidase, along with a chymotrypsin-like enzyme present in the same extracts, may modify the climate of various airway microenvironments by hydrolyzing bioactive peptides (169).

CONCLUSIONS

Considered as a whole, the experimental data summarized in this chapter strongly implicate proteases in the pathogenesis of asthmatic airway inflammation. Of course, the case for involvement is more compelling for some proteases than for others. No protease can be said (based on current evidence) to be indispensable to the development of human asthma. The suggestions that specific proteases are important in this regard must be regarded as a set of unproven hypotheses. This will remain the state-of-the-art conclusion until effective, selective inhibitors of the proteases (or of their products) are developed and tested in humans with asthma. Fortunately, several such pharmaceutical products are being tested or readied for testing. These include inhibitors of specific proteases (e.g., tryptase, matrix metalloproteinases, neutral endopeptidase, renin, kallikrein), antagonists of protease-generated peptides (e.g., bradykinin, angiotensin II), and either antagonists or agonists of protease-degraded peptides (e.g., tachykinins and VIP). As the results of trials with these products are revealed in the next few years, one can expect a clarification of the now somewhat muddy waters in this clinically important tributary of protease biology.

ACKNOWLEDGMENTS

This work is supported in part by grants HL-24136 and HL-54774 from the National Institutes of Health.

REFERENCES

1. Kaliner M. Asthma and mast cell activation. *J Allergy Clin Immunol* 1989;83:510–520.
2. Djukanovic R, Roche WR, Wilson JW, et al. Mucosal inflammation in asthma. *Am Rev Respir Dis* 1990;142:434–457.
3. Schulman ES. The role of mast cells in inflammatory responses in the lung. *Crit Rev Immunol* 1993;13:35–70.
4. Caughey GH, ed. *Mast cell proteases in immunology and biology.* New York: Marcel Dekker, 1995.
5. Proud D. Kinins and mast cell-related diseases. In: Kaliner MA, Metcalfe DD, eds. *The mast cell in health and disease.* New York: Marcel Dekker, 1993;415–441.
6. Newball HH, Berninger RW, Talamo RC, Lichtenstein LM. Anaphylactic release of a basophil kallikrein-like activity. I. Purification and characterization. *J Clin Invest* 1979;64:457–465.
7. Schwartz LB, Irani A-M A, Roller K, Castells MC, Schechter NM. Quantitation of histamine, tryptase, and chymase in dispersed human T and TC mast cells. *J Immunol* 1987;138:2611–2615.
8. Schulman ES, MacGlashan DW, Peters SP, Schleimer RP, Newball HH, Lichtenstein LM. Human lung mast cells: purification and characterization. *J Immunol* 1982;129:2662–2670.
9. Castells MC, Irani A-M A, Schwartz LB. Evaluation of human peripheral blood leukocytes for mast cell tryptase. *J Immunol* 1987;138:2184–2189.
10. Xia H-Zd, Kepley CL, Sakai K, Chelliah J, Irani A-M A, Schwartz LB. Quantitation of tryptase, chymase, FcεRIa, and FcεRIg mRNAs in human mast cells and basophils by competitive reverse transcription-polymerase chain reaction. *J Immunol* 1995;154:5472–5480.
11. Irani AA, Schechter NM, Craig SS, DeBlois G, Schwartz LB. Two types of human mast cells that have distinct neutral protease compositions. *Proc Natl Acad Sci U S A* 1986;83:4464–4468.
12. Sinha U, Sinha S, Janoff A. Characterization of sheep α-1-antiproteinase inhibitor. Important differences from the human protein. *Am Rev Respir Dis* 1988;137:558–563.
13. Caughey GH. Serine proteases of mast cell and leukocyte granules: a league of their own. *Am J Respir Crit Care Med* 1994;150:S138–S142.
14. Schwartz LB, Lewis RA, Seldin D, Austen KF. Acid hydrolases and tryptase from secretory granules of dispersed human lung mast cells. *J Immunol* 1981;126:1290–1294.
15. Goldstein SM, Leong J, Schwartz LB, Cooke D. Protease composition of exocytosed human skin mast cell protease-proteoglycan complexes: tryptase resides in a complex distinct from chymase and carboxypeptidase. *J Immunol* 1992;148:2475–2482.
16. Caughey GH, Lazarus SC, Viro NF, Gold NM, Nadel JA. Tryptase and chymase: comparison of extraction and release in two dog mastocytoma lines. *Immunology* 1988;63:339–344.
17. Smith TJ, Hougland MW, Johnson DA. Human lung tryptase. Purification and characterization. *J Biol Chem* 1984;259:11046–11051.
18. Schwartz LB, Bradford TR. Regulation of tryptase from human lung mast cells by heparin. Stabilization of the active tetramer. *J Biol Chem* 1986;261:7372–7379.
19. Schwartz LB, Metcalfe DD, Miller JS, Earl H, Sullivan T. Tryptase levels as an indicator of mast-cell activation in systemic anaphylaxis and mastocytosis. *N Engl J Med* 1987;316:1622–1626.
20. Caughey GH. Mast cell chymases and tryptases: Phylogeny, family relations and biogenesis. In: Caughey GH, ed. *Mast cell proteases in immunology and biology.* New York: Marcel Dekker, 1995;305–329.
21. Craig SS, Schechter NM, Schwartz LB. Ultrastructural analysis of human T and TC mast cells identified by immunoelectron microscopy. *Lab Invest* 1988;58:682–691.
22. Schwartz LB, Yunginger JW, Miller J, Bokhari R, Dull D. Time course of appearance and disappearance of human mast cell tryptase in the circulation after anaphylaxis. *J Clin Invest* 1989;83:1551–1555.
23. Miller JS, Westin EH, Schwartz LB. Cloning and characterization of complementary DNA for human tryptase. *J Clin Invest* 1989;84:1188–1195.
24. Miller JS, Moxley G, Schwartz LB. Cloning and characterization of a second complementary cDNA for human tryptase. *J Clin Invest* 1990;86:864–870.
25. Vanderslice P, Ballinger SM, Tam EK, Goldstein SM, Craik CS, Caughey GH. Human mast cell tryptase: multiple cDNAs and genes reveal a multigene serine protease family. *Proc Natl Acad Sci U S A* 1990;87:3811–3815.
26. Little SS, Johnson DA. Human mast cell tryptase isoforms: separation and examination of substrate-specificity differences. *Biochem J* 1995;307:341–346.
27. Schwartz LB. Mast cell tryptase: properties and roles in human allergic responses. In: Caughey GH, ed. *Mast cell proteases in immunology and biology.* New York: Marcel Dekker, 1995;9–23.
28. Schwartz LB. 1992. Cellular inflammation in asthma: neutral proteases of mast cells. *Am Rev Respir Dis* 145:S18–S21.
29. Caughey GH. 1991. The structure and airway biology of mast cell proteinases. *Am J Respir Cell Mol Biol* 1991;4:387–394.
30. Kalenderian R, Raju L, Roth W, Schwartz LB, Gruber B, Janoff A. Elevated histamine and tryptase levels in smokers' bronchoalveolar lavage fluid. Do lung mast cells contribute to smokers' emphysema? *Chest* 1988;94:119–123.
31. Wenzel SE, Fowler AD, Schwartz LB. Activation of pulmonary mast cells by bronchoalveolar allergen challenge. *In vivo* release of histamine and tryptase in atopic subjects with and without asthma. *Am Rev Respir Dis* 1988;137:1002–1008.
32. Sekizawa K, Caughey GH, Lazarus SC, Gold WM, Nadel JA. Mast cell tryptase causes airway smooth muscle hyperresponsiveness in dogs. *J Clin Invest* 1989;83:175–179.
33. Richardson JB, Beland J. Nonadrenergic inhibitory nerves in human airways. *J Appl Physiol* 1976;41:764–771.
34. Franconi GM, Graf PD, Lazarus SC, Nadel JA, Caughey GH. Mast cell chymase and tryptase reverse airway smooth muscle relaxation induced by vasoactive intestinal peptide in the ferret. *J Pharmacol Exp Ther* 1989;248:947–951.
35. Tam EK, Caughey GH. Degradation of airway neuropeptides by human lung tryptase. *Am J Respir Cell Mol Biol* 1990;3:27–32.
36. Ollerenshaw S, Jarvis D, Woolcock A, Sullivan C, Scheibner T. Absence of immunoreactive vasoactive intestinal polypeptide in tissues from the lungs of patients with asthma. *N Engl J Med* 1989;320:1244–1248.
37. Howarth PH, Djukanovic RD, Wilson JW, Holgate ST, Springal DR, Polak JM. Mucosal nerves in endobronchial biopsies in asthma and non-asthma. *Int Arch Allergy Appl Immunol* 1991;94:330–333.
38. Lilly CM, Bai TR, Shore SA, Hall AE, Drazen JM. Neuropeptide content of lungs from asthmatic and nonasthmatic patients. *Am J Respir Crit Care Med* 1995;151:548–553.
39. Lilly CM, Kobzik L, Hall AE, Drazen JM. Effects of chronic airway inflammation on the activity and enzymatic inactivation of neuropeptides in guinea pig lungs. *J Clin Invest* 1994;93:2667–2674.
40. Lilly CM, Stamler JS, Gaston B, Meckel C, Loscalzo J, Drazen JM. Modulation of vasoactive intestinal peptide pulmonary relaxation by

NO in tracheally superfused guinea pig lungs. *Am J Physiol* 1993; 265:L410–L415.

41. Brown JK, Tyler CL, Jones CA, Ruoss SJ, Hartmann T, Caughey GH. Tryptase, the dominant secretory granular protein in humans mast cells, is a potent mitogen for cultured dog tracheal smooth muscle cells. *Am J Respir Cell Mol Biol* 1995;13:227–236.

42. Maruno K, Absood A, Said SI. VIP inhibits basal and histamine-stimulated proliferation of human airway smooth muscle cells. *Am J Physiol* 1995;268:L1047–1051.

43. Claman HN. Mast cells and scleroderma. Reply. *JAMA* 1990;263:949.

44. Kawanami O, Ferrans VJ, Fulmer JD, Crystal RG. Ultrastructure of pulmonary mast cells in patients with fibrotic lung disorders. *Lab Invest* 1979;40:717–734.

45. Trabucchi E, Radaelli E, Marazzi M, et al. The role of mast cells in wound healing. *Int J Tissue React* 1988;10:367–372.

46. Casale TB, Trapp S, Zehr B, Hunninghake GW. Bronchoalveolar lavage fluid histamine levels in interstitial lung diseases. *Am Rev Respir Dis* 1988;138:1604–1608.

47. Walls AF, Bennett AR, Godfrey RC, Holgate ST, Church MK. Mast cell tryptase and histamine concentrations in bronchoalveolar lavage fluid from patients with interstitial lung disease. *Clin Sci* 1991;81: 183–188.

48. Wagner MM, Edwards RE, Moncrieff CB, Wagner JC. Mast cells and inhalation of asbestos in rats. *Thorax* 1984;39:539–544.

49. Watanabe S, Watanabe K, Ohishi T, Aiba M, Kageyama K. Mast cells in the rat alveolar septa undergoing fibrosis after ionizing radiation. *Lab Invest* 1974;31:555–567.

50. Takizawa H, Ohta K, Hirai K, et al. Mast cells are important in the development of hypersensitivity pneumonitis. A study with mast-cell-deficient mice. *J Immunol* 1989;143:1982–1988.

51. Goto T, Befus D, Low R, Bienenstock J. Mast cell heterogeneity and hyperplasia in bleomycin-induced pulmonary fibrosis in rats. *Am Rev Respir Dis* 1984;130:797–802.

52. Ruoss SJ, Hartmann T, Caughey GH. Mast cell tryptase is a mitogen for cultured fibroblasts. *J Clin Invest* 1991;88:493–499.

53. Hartmann T, Ruoss SJ, Raymond WW, Seuwen K, Caughey GH. Human tryptase as a potent, cell-specific mitogen: role of signalling pathways in synergistic responses. *Am J Physiol* 1992;262:L528–L534.

54. Maier M, Spragg J, Schwartz LB. Inactivation of human high molecular weight kininogen by human mast cell tryptase. *J Immunol* 1983; 130:2352–2356.

55. Walls AF, Brain SD, Desai A, Jose PJ, Hawkings E, Church MK, Williams TJ. Human mast cell tryptase attenuates the vasodilator activity of calcitonin gene-related peptide. *Biochem Pharmacol* 1992; 43:1243–1248.

56. Stack MS, Johnson DA. Human mast cell tryptase activates single-chain urinary-type plasminogen activator (pro-urokinase). *J Biol Chem* 1994;269:9416–9419.

57. Gruber BL, Marchese MJ, Suzuki K, Schwartz LB, Okada Y, Nagase H, Ramamurthy NS. Synovial procollagenase activation by human mast cell tryptase. Dependence upon matrix metalloproteinase 3 activation. *J Clin Invest* 1989;84:1657–1662.

58. Clark JM, WM Abraham, CE Fishman, et al. Tryptase inhibitors block allergen-induced airway and inflammatory responses in allergic sheep. *Am J Respir Crit Care Med* 1995;152:2076–2083.

59. Caughey GH, Leidig F, Viro NF, Nadel JA. Substance P and vasoactive intestinal peptide degradation by mast cell tryptase and chymase. *J Pharmacol Exp Ther* 1988;244:133–137.

60. Schechter NM, Irani AM, Sprows JL, Abernethy J, Wintroub B, Schwartz LB. Identification of a cathepsin G-like proteinase in the MCTC type of human mast cell. *J Immunol* 1990;145:2652–2661.

61. Caughey GH, Zerweck EH, Vanderslice P. Structure, chromosomal assignment, and deduced amino acid sequence of a human gene for mast cell chymase. *J Biol Chem* 1991;266:12956–12963.

62. Urata H, Boehm KD, Philip A, et al. Cellular localization and regional distribution of an angiotensin II-forming chymase in the heart. *J Clin Invest* 1993;91:1269–1281.

63. Campbell EJ, Silverman EK, Campbell MA. Elastase and cathepsin G of human monocytes. Quantification of cellular content, release in response to stimuli, and heterogeneity in elastase-mediated proteolytic activity. *J Immunol* 1989;143:2961–2968.

64. Hanson RD, Connolly NL, Burnett D, Campbell EJ, Senior RM, Ley TJ. Developmental regulation of the human cathepsin G gene in myelomonocytic cells. *J Biol Chem* 1990;265:1524–1530.

65. Whitaker-Menezes D, Schechter NM, Murphy GF. Serine proteinases are regionally segregated within mast cell granules. *Lab Invest* 1995;72:34–41.

66. Benyon RC, Enciso JA, Befus AD. Analysis of human skin mast cell proteins by two-dimensional gel electrophoresis: identification of tryptase as a sialylated glycoprotein. *J Immunol* 1993;151: 2699–2706.

67. Matin R, Tam EK, Nadel JA, Caughey GH. Distribution of chymase-containing mast cells in human bronchi. *J Histochem Cytochem* 1992; 40:781–786.

68. Weidner N, Austen KF. Heterogeneity of mast cells at multiple body sites-fluorescent determination of avidin binding and immunofluorescent determination of chymase, tryptase, and carboxypeptidase content. *Pathol Res Pract* 1993;189:156–162.

69. Sayama S, Iozzo RV, Lazarus GS, Schechter NM. Human skin chymotrypsin-like proteinase chymase. Subcellular localization to mast cell granules and interaction with heparin and other glycosaminoglycans. *J Biol Chem* 1987;263:6808–6815.

70. Urata H, Kinoshita A, Misono KS, Bumpus FM, Husain A. Identification of a highly specific chymase as the major angiotensin II-forming enzyme in the human heart. *J Biol Chem* 1990;265:22348–22357.

71. Jenne DE, Masson D, Zimmer M, Haefliger J-A, Li W-H, Tschopp J. Isolation and complete structure of the lymphocyte serine protease granzyme G, a novel member of the granzyme multigene family in murine cytolytic T lymphocytes. Evolutionary origin of lymphocyte proteases. *Biochemistry* 1989;28:7953–7961.

72. Caughey GH, Viro NF, Lazarus SC, Nadel JA. Purification and characterization of dog mastocytoma chymase. Identification of an octapeptide conserved in chymotryptic leukocyte proteases. *Biochim Biophys Acta* 1988;952:142–149.

73. Caughey GH, Raymond WW, Vanderslice P. Dog mast cell chymase: Molecular cloning and characterization. *Biochemistry* 1990;29: 5166–5171.

74. Dikov MM, Springman EB, Yeola Z, Serafin WE. Processing of pro-carboxypeptidase A and other zymogens in murine mast cells. *J Biol Chem* 1994;269:25897–25904.

75. McGuire MJ, Lipsky PE, Thiele DL. Generation of active myeloid and lymphoid granule serine proteases requires processing by the granule thiol protease dipeptidyl peptidase I. *J Biol Chem* 1993;268: 2458–2467.

76. Hanson RD, Hohn PA, Popescu NC, Ley TJ. A cluster of hematopoietic serine protease genes is found on the same chromosomal band as the human α/δ T-cell receptor locus. *Proc Natl Acad Sci U S A* 1990; 87:960–963.

77. Hohn PA, Popescu NC, Hanson RD, Salvesen G, Ley TJ. Genomic organization and chromosomal localization of the human cathepsin G gene. *J Biol Chem* 1989;264:13412–13419.

78. Caughey GH, Schaumberg TH, Zerweck EH, et al. The human mast cell chymase gene (CMA1): mapping to the cathepsin G/granzyme gene cluster and lineage-restricted expression. *Genomics* 1993;15:614–620.

79. Rubinstein I, Nadel JA, Graf PD, Caughey GH. 1990. Mast cell chymase potentiates histamine-induced wheal formation in the skin of ragweed-allergic dogs. *J Clin Invest* 1990;86:555–559.

80. Peterson MW. Neutrophil cathepsin G increases transendothelial albumin flux. *J Lab Clin Med* 1989;113:297–308.

81. Powers JC, Tanaka T, Harper JW, et al. Mammalian chymotrypsin-like enzymes. Comparative reactivities of rat mast cell proteases, human and dog skin chymases, and human cathepsin G with peptide 4-nitroanilide substrates and with peptide chloromethyl ketone and sulfonyl fluoride inhibitors. *Biochemistry* 1985;24:2048–2058.

82. Skidgel RA, Hackman HL, Erdos EG. Metabolism of substance P and bradykinin by human neutrophils. *Biochem Pharmacol* 1991;41: 1335–1344.

83. Reilly CF, Schechter NB, Travis J. Inactivation of bradykinin and kallidin by cathepsin G and mast cell chymase. *Biochem Biophys Res Commun* 1985;127:443–449.

84. Wintroub BU, Schechter NB, Lazarus GS, Kaempfer CE, Schwartz LB. Angiotensin I conversion by human and rat chymotryptic proteinases. *J Invest Dermatol* 1984;83:336–339.

85. Hoit BD, Shao Y, Kinoshita A, Gabel M, Husain A, Walsh RA. Effects of angiotensin II generated by an angiotensin converting enzyme-independent pathway on left ventricular performance in the conscious baboon. *J Clin Invest* 1995;95:1519–1527.

86. Sommerhoff CP, Caughey GH, Finkbeiner WE, Lazarus SC, Basbaum

CB, Nadel JA. Mast cell chymase. A potent secretagogue for airway gland serous cells. *J Immunol* 1989;142:2450–2456.

87. Sommerhoff CP, Nadel JA, Basbaum CB, Caughey GH. Neutrophil elastase and cathepsin G stimulate secretion from cultured bovine airway gland serous cells. *J Clin Invest* 1990;85:682–689.

88. Sommerhoff CP, Ruoss SJ, Caughey GH. Mast cell proteoglycans modulate the secretagogue, proteoglycanase, and amidolytic activities of dog mast cell chymase. *J Immunol* 1992;148:2859–2866.

89. Varsano S, Basbaum CB, Forsberg LS, Borson DB, Caughey G, Nadel JA. Dog tracheal epithelial cells in culture synthesize sulfated macromolecular glycoconjugates and release them from the cell surface upon exposure to extracellular proteinases. *Exp Lung Res* 1987;13:157–184.

90. Vartio T, Seppa H, Vaheri A. Susceptibility of soluble and matrix fibronectins to degradation by tissue proteinases, mast cell chymase and cathepsin G. *J Biol Chem* 1981;256:471–477.

91. Briggaman RA, Schechter NM, Fraki J, Lazarus GS. Degradation of the epidermal-dermal junction by proteolytic enzymes from human skin and human polymorphonuclear leukocytes. *J Exp Med* 1984;160:1027–1042.

92. Taipale J, Lohi J, Saarinen J, Kovanen PT, Keski-Oja J. Human mast cell chymase and leukocyte elastase release latent transforming growth factor-beta1 from the extracellular matrix of cultured human epithelial and endothelial cells. *J Biol Chem* 1995; 270:4689–4696.

93. Pennington, DW. Dog mastocytoma cells produce transforming growth factor beta1. *J Clin Invest* 1992;90:35–41.

94. Saarinen J, Kalkkinen N, Welgus HG, Kovanen PT. Activation of human interstitial procollagenase through direct cleavage of the Leu83-Thr84 bond by mast cell chymase. *J Biol Chem* 1994;269:18134–18140.

95. Fang KC, Raymond WW, Lazarus SC, Caughey GH. Dog mastocytoma cells synthesize a 92-kDa gelatinase activated by mast cell chymase. *J Clin Invest* 1996;97:1589–1596.

96. Morodomi T, Ogata Y, Sasaguri Y, Morimatsu M, Nagase H. Purification and characterization of matrix metalloproteinase 9 from U937 and HT1080 fibrosarcoma cells. *Biochem J* 1992;285:603–611.

97. Lee CT, Fein AM, Lippmann M, Holtzman H, Kimbel P, Weinbaum G. Elastolytic activity in pulmonary lavage fluid from patients with adult respiratory distress syndrome. *N Engl J Med* 1981;304:192–196.

98. Janoff A. Elastase and emphysema. current assessment of the protease-antiprotease hypothesis. *Am Rev Respir Dis* 1985;132:417–433.

99. Egesten A, Breton-Gorius J, Guichard J, Gullberg U, Olsson I. The heterogeneity of azurophil granules in neutrophil progranulocytes: Immunogold localization of myeloperoxidase, cathepsin G, elastase, proteinase 3, and bactericidal/permeability increasing protein. *Blood* 1994;83:2985–2994.

100. Jorens PG, Richman-Eisenstat JBY, Housset BP, et al. Interleukin-8 induces neutrophil accomulation but not protease secretion in the canine grachea. *Am J Physiol* 1992;263:L708–L713.

101. Jackson AH, Hill SL, Afford SC, Stockley RA. Studies of sputum sol-phase proteins and elastase activity in patients with cystic fibrosis. *Eur J Respir Dis* 1984;65:114–124.

102. Suter S, Schaad UB, Tegner H, Ohlsson K, Desgrandchamps D, Waldvogel FA. Levels of free granulocyte elastase in bronchial secretions from patients with cystic fibrosis: effect of antimicrobial treatment against Pseudomonas aeruginosa. *J Infect Dis* 1986;153:902–909.

103. Stockley RA, Burnett D. α1-antitrypsin and leukocyte elastase in infected and noninfected sputum. *Am Rev Respir Dis* 1979;120:1081–1086.

104. Fahy JV, Schuster A, Ueki I, Boushey HA, Nadel JA. Mucus hypersecretion in bronchiectasis. The role of neutrophilproteases. *Am Rev Respir Dis* 1992;146:1430–1433.

105. Stockley RA, Hill ASL, Morrison HW, Starkie CM. Elastolytic activity of sputum and its relation to purulence and to lung function in patients with bronchiectasis. *Thorax* 1984;39:408–413.

106. Konstan MW, Berger M. Infection and inflammation of the lung in cystic fibrosis. In: Davis PB, ed. *Cystic fibrosis*. New York: Marcel Dekker, 1993;219–276.

107. Smallman LA, Hill SL, Stockley RA. Reduction of ciliary beat frequency *in vitro* by sputum from patients with bronchiectasis: A serine protease efect. *Thorax* 1984;39:663–667.

108. Döring G. Polymorphonuclear leukocyte elastase: its effects on the pathogenesis of *Pseudomonas aeruginosa* infection in cystic fibrosis. *Thorax* 1989;45:881–884.

109. Schuster A, Ueki I, Nadel JA. Neutrophil elastase stimulates tracheal

110. Schuster A, Fahy FV, Ueki I, Nadel JA. Cystic fibrosis sputum induces a secretory response from airway gland serous cells that can be prevented by neutrophil protease inhibitors. *Eur Respir J* 1995;8:10–14.

111. Dunnill MS, Massarella GR, Anderson JA. A comparison of the quantitative anatomy of the bronchi in normal subjects, in status asthmaticus, in chronic bronchitis, and in emphysema. *Thorax* 1969;24:176–179.

112. Grisolano JL, Sclar GM, Ley TJ. Early myeloid cell-specific expression of the human cathepsin G gene in transgenic mice. *Proc Natl Acad Sci U S A* 1994;91:8989–8993.

113. Lomas DA, Stoone SR, Llewellyn-Jones C, et al. The control of neutrophil chemotaxis by inhibitors of cathepsin G and chymotrypsin. *J Biol Chem* 1995;270:23437–23443.

114. Kao RC, Wehner NG, Skubitz KM, Gray BH, Hoidal JR. Proteinase 3. A distinct human polymorphonuclear serine proteinase that produces emphysema in hamsters. *J Clin Invest* 1988;82:1963–1973.

115. Rao NV, Wehner NG, Marshall BC, Gray WR, Gray BH, Hoidal JR. Characterization of proteinase-3 (PR-3), a neutrophil serine proteinase. Structural and functional properties. *J Biol Chem* 1991;266:9540–9548.

116. Sturrock AB, Franklin KF, Rao G, Marshall BC, Rebentisch MB, Lemons RS, Hoidal JR. Structure, chromosomal assignment, and expression of the gene for proteinase-3. *J Biol Chem* 1992;267:21193–21199.

117. Zimmer M, Medcalf RL, Fink TM, Mattmann C, Lichter P, Jenne DE. Three human elastase-like genes coordinately expressed in the myelomonocyte lineage are organized as a single genetic locus on 19pter. *Proc Natl Acad Sci U S A* 1992;89:8215–8219.

118. Rao NV, Marshall BC, Gray BH, Hoidal JR. Interaction of secretory leukocyte protease inhibitor with proteinase-3. *Am J Respir Cell Mol Biol* 1993;8:612–616.

119. Ludemann J, Utecht B, Gross WL. Anti-neutrophil cytoplasm antibodies in Wegener's granulomatosis recognize an elastolytic enzyme. *J Exp Med* 1990;171:357–362.

120. Falk RJ, Terrell RS, Charles LA, Jennette JC. Anti-neutrophil cytoplasmic autoantibodies induce neutrophils to degranulate and produce oxygen radical *in vitro*. *Proc Natl Acad Sci U S A* 1990;87:4115–4119.

121. Weiss SJ. Tissue destruction by neutrophils. *N Engl J Med* 1989;320:365–376.

122. Sepper R, Konttinen YT, Sorsa T, Koski H. Gelatinolytic and type IV gelatinolytic activity in bronchiectasis. *Chest* 1994;106:1129–1133.

123. Leppert D, Waubant E, Galardy R, Bunnett NW, Hauser SL. T cell gelatinases mediate basement membrane transmigration *in vitro*. *J Immunol* 1995;154:4379–4389.

124. Lider O, Mekori YA, Miller T, et al. Inhibition of T lymphocyte heparanase by heparin prevents T cell migration and T cell-mediated immunity. *Eur J Immunol* 1990;20:493.

125. Jenne DE, Tschopp J. Granzymes, a family of serine proteases released from granules of cytolytic T lymphocytes upon T cell receptor stimulation. *Immunol Rev* 1988;103:53–71.

126. Heusel JW, Wesselschmidt RL, Shresta S, Russell JH, Ley TJ. Cytotoxic lymphocytes require granzyme B for the rapid induction of DNA fragmentation and apoptosis in allogeneic target cells. *Cell* 1994;76:977–987.

127. Kerr MA, Kenny AJ. The purification and specificity of a neutral endopeptidase from rabbit kidney brush border. *Biochem J* 1974;137:477–488.

128. Devault A, Lazure C, Nault C, et al. Amino acid sequence of rabbit neutral endopeptidase 24.11 (enkephalinase) deduced from complementary DNA. *EMBO J* 1987;1317–1322.

129. Roques BP, Noble F, Dauge V, Fournie-Zalwki MC, Beaumont A. Neutral endopeptidase 24.11: structure, inhibition, and experimental and clinical pharmacology. *Pharmacol Rev* 1993;45:87–146.

130. Smith CM, Anderson SD. Hyperosmolarity as the stimulus to asthma induced by hyperventilation? *J Allergy Clin Immunol* 1986;77:729–736.

131. Eschenbacher WL, Boushey HA, Sheppard D. Alteration in osmolarity of inhaled aerosols causes bronchoconstriction and cough, but absence of a permanent anion causes cough alone. *Am Rev Respir Dis* 1984;129:211–215.

submucosal gland secretion that is inhibited by ICI 200,355. *Am J Physiol* 1992;262:L86–L91.

132. Umeno E, McDonald DM, Nadel JA. Hypertonic saline increases vascular permeability in the rat trachea by producing neurogenic inflammation. *J Clin Invest* 1990;85:1905–1908.

133. Yoshihara S, Geppetti P, Hara M, et al. Cold-air induced bronchoconstriction is mediated by tachykinin and kinin release in guinea pigs. *Eur J Pharm* 1996;296:291–296.

134. Nadel JA. 1996. Peptidase modulation of neurogenic inflammation. In: Geppetti P, Holzer P, eds. *Neurogenic inflammation.* Boca Raton: CRC Press, Inc. 1996;115–127.

135. Kohrogi H, Nadel JA, Malfroy B, et al. Recombinant human enkephalinase (neutral endopeptidase) prevents cough induced by tachykinins in awake guinea pigs. *J Clin Invest* 1989;84:781–786.

136. Borson DB, Gruenert DC. Glucocorticoids induce neutral endopeptidase in transformed human tracheal epithelial cells. *Am J Physiol* 1991;260:L83–L89.

137. Piedimonte G, McDonald DM, Nadel JA. Glucocorticoids inhibit neurogenic plasma extravasation and prevent virus-potentiated extravasation in the rat trachea. *J Clin Invest* 1990;86:1409–1415.

138. Garten W, Bosch FX, Linder D, Rott R, Klenk H-D. Proteolytic activation of the influenza virus hemagglutinin: the structure of the cleavage site and the enzymes involved in cleavage. *Virology* 1981;115:361–374.

139. Mangel WF, McGrath WF, Toledo DL, Anderson CW. Viral DNA and a viral peptide can act as cofactors of adenovirus virion proteinase activity. *Nature* 1993;361:274–275.

140. Matthews DA, Smith WW, Ferre RA, et al. Structure of human rhinovirus 3C protease reveals a trypsin-like polypeptide fold, RNA-binding site, and means for cleaving precursor polyprotein. *Cell* 1994;77:761–771.

141. Rose JR, Craik CS. Structure-assisted design of nonpeptide human immunodeficiency virus-1 protease inhibitors. *Am J Respir Crit Care Med* 1994;150:S176–S182.

142. Dubovi EJ, Geratz JD, Tidwell RR. Enhancement of respiratory syncytial virus-induced cytopathology by trypsin, thrombin, and plasmin. *Infect Immun* 1983;40:351–358.

143. Tashiro M, Yokogoshi Y, Tobita K, Seto JT, Rott R, Kido H. Tryptase Clara, an activating protease for Sendai virus in rat lungs, is involved in pneumopathogenicity. *J Virol* 1992;66:7211–7216.

144. Sakai K, Kawaguchi Y, Kishino Y, Kido H. Electron immunohistochemical localization in rat bronchiolar epithelial cells of tryptase Clara, which determines the pneumotropism and pathogenicity of Sendai virus and influenza virus. *J Histochem Cytochem* 1993;41:89–93.

145. Tournier J-M, Polette M, Hinnrasky J, Beck J, Werb Z, Basbaum C. Expression of gelatinase A, a mediator of extacellular matrix remodeling, by tracheal gland serous cells in culture and *in vivo*. *J Biol Chem* 1994;269:25454–25464.

146. Takahashi K, Kiguchi T, Sawasaki Y, et al. Lung capillary endothelial cells produce and secrete urokinase-type plasminogen activator. *Am J Respir Cell Mol Biol* 1992;7:90–94.

147. Marshall BC, Xu, Q-P, Rao NV, Brown BR, Hoidal JR. Pulmonary epithelial cell urokinase-type plasminogen activator: induction by interleukin-1β and tumor necrosis factor-α. *J Biol Chem* 1992;267:11462–11469.

148. Marshall BC, Sageser DS, Rao NV, Emi M, Hoidal JR. Alveolar epithelial cell plasminogen activator: characterization and regulation. *J Biol Chem* 1990;265:8198–8204.

149. Sitrin RG. Plasminogen activation in the injured lung: pulmonology does not recapitulate hematology. *Am J Respir Cell Mol Biol* 1992;6:131–132.

150. Chapman HAJ, Reilly JJ, Kobzik L. Role of plasminogen activator in

151. Chapman HA, Bertozzi P, Sailor LZ, Nusrat AR. Alveolar macrophage urokinase receptors localize enzyme activity to the cell surface. *Am J Physiol* 1990;259:L432–L438.

152. Rabbani SA, Mazar AP, Bernier SM, Haq M, Bolivar I, Henkin J, Goltzman D. Structural requirements for the growth factor activity of the amino-terminal domain of urokinase. *J Biol Chem* 1992;267:14151–14156.

153. Boyle MDP, Chiodo VA, Lawman MJP, Gee AP, Young M. Urokinase: a chemotactic factor for polymorphonuclear leukocytes *in vivo*. *J Immunol* 1987;139:169–174.

154. Patchett AA, Cordes EH. The design and propeties of N-carboxyalkyldipeptide inhibitors of angiotensin converting enzyme. *Adv Enzyme Regul* 1985;57:1–84.

155. Soubrier F, Alhenc-Gelas F, Hubert C, et al. Two putative active centers in human angiotensin I-converting enzyme revealed by molecular cloning. *Proc Natl Acad Sci U S A* 1988;85:9386–9390.

156. Caldewell PRB, Seegal BC, Hsu KC, Das M, Soffer RL. Angiotensin-converting enzyme: vascular endothelial localization. *Science* 1976;191:1050–1051.

157. Proud D, Vio CP. Localization of immunoreactive tissue kallikrein in human trachea. *Am J Respir Cell Mol Biol* 1993;8:16–19.

158. Naclerio RM, Proud D, Togias AG, et al. Inflammatory mediators in late antigen-induced rhinitis. *N Engl J Med* 1985;313:65–70.

159. Baumgarten CR, Nichols RC, Naclerio RM, Lichtenstein LM, Norman PS, Proud D. Plasma kallikrein during experimentally induced allergic rhinitis: role in kinin formation and contribution to TAME-esterase activity in nasal secretions. *J Immunol* 1986;137:977–982.

160. Soler M, Sielczac M, Abraham, WM. A bradykinin antagonist blocks antigen-induced airway hyperresponsiveness and inflammation in sheep. *Pulmonary Pharmacol* 1990;3:9–15.

161. Bar-Shavit R, Benezra M, Sabbah V, Bode W, Vlodavsky I. Thrombin as a multifunctional protein: induction of cell adhesion and proliferation. *Am J Respir Cell Mol Biol* 1992;6:123–130.

162. McNamara CA, Sarembock IF, Gimple LW, Fenton IJW, Coughlin SR, Owens GK. Thrombin stimulates proliferation of cultured rat aortic smooth muscle cells by a proteolytically activated receptor. *J Clin Invest* 1993;91:94–98.

163. Vu T-K H, Hung DT, Wheaton VI, Coughlin SR. Molecular cloning of a functional thrombin receptor reveals a novel proteolytic mechanism of receptor activation. *Cell* 1991;64:1057–1068.

164. Hartmann T, Ruoss SJ, Caughey GH. Modulation of thrombin and thrombin receptor peptide mitogenicity by human lung mast cell tryptase. *Am J Physiol* 1994;267:L113–L119.

165. Tomlinson PRT, Wilson JW, Stewart AG. Inhibition by salbutamol of the proliferation of human airway smooth muscle cells grown in culture. *Br J Pharmacol* 1994;111:641–647.

166. Herbert CA, King CM, Ring PC, et al. Augmentation of permeability in the bronchial epithelium by the house dust mite allergen *Der* p1. *Am J Respir Cell Mol Biol* 1995;12:369–378.

167. Stewart GA, Ward LD, Simpson RJ, Thompson PJ. The group III allergen from house mite Dermatophagoides pteronyssinus is a trypsin-like enzyme. *Immunology* 1992;75:29–35.

168. Maruo K, Akaike T, Inada Y, Ohkubo I, Ono T, Maeda H. Effect of microbial and mite proteases on low and high molecular weight kininogens. *J Biol Chem* 1993;268:17711–17715.

169. Matheson N, Schmidt J, Travis J. Isolation and properties of an angiotensin II-cleaving peptidase from mesquite pollen. *Am J Respir Cell Mol Biol* 1995;12:441–448.

Asthma, edited by P.J. Barnes, M.M. Grunstein,
A.R. Leff, and A.J. Woolcock.
Lippincott–Raven Publishers, Philadelphia © 1997.

▪ 47 ▪

Reactive Oxygen Species

William M. Abraham

Cellular sources of ROS
Chemistry
Superoxide anion
Hydrogen Peroxide
Hydroxyl Radical

Anti-oxidants
    Nonenzymatic Scavengers
    Evidence for Increased ROS Production in Asthma
Mechanisms
Changes in anti-oxidant markers

The production of reactive oxygen species (ROS), which include superoxide anion (O_2^-), hydrogen peroxide (H_2O_2), hydroxyl radical ($OH\cdot$), and hypohalous acids, is an important host defense function of phagocytic cells. However, overproduction of these ROS has been implicated as a causal factor in a variety of diseases, including asthma. Thus, ROS have been shown to release mediators, cause bronchoconstriction, induce airway hyperresponsiveness, increase mucus secretion, inhibit ciliary activity, and slow mucus clearance (1–11). Recent studies have demonstrated that antioxidants can protect against some of these pathophysiological events (7,8,12). Collectively, these findings suggest that ROS contribute to the airway dysfunction in asthma. This chapter reviews the current information that supports this hypothesis.

CELLULAR SOURCES OF ROS

The airways of asthmatic subjects and experimental animals can remain inflamed for prolonged periods of time following a single antigen challenge, and this inflammatory state is associated with airway hyperresponsiveness (13–15). Many investigators have examined the relationship between airway inflammation, as assessed by either bronchial biopsy or bronchoalveolar lavage (BAL), and airway responsiveness in an attempt to identify a specific cell and/or mediator responsible for this abnormality. The

findings indicate, however, that numbers of eosinophils, epithelial cells, metachromatic cells (mast cells/basophils), and macrophages each can be correlated with airway hyperresponsiveness (16–22). Such observations suggest that the airway hyperresponsiveness, which is a characteristic of asthma, may be a multicellular process, rather than a single cell process. In searching for mediators common to the aforementioned cells, it becomes apparent that given the appropriate stimulus neutrophils, eosinophils, macrophages, epithelial cells, and possibly mast cells can generate ROS through various mechanisms. These mechanisms include the metabolism of arachidonic acid by the cyclooxygenase and 5-lipoxygenase enzymes, resulting in the formation of prostaglandins (PGs) and leukotrienes (LTs) (23–28). The concentrations of both PGs and LTs are greatly elevated during exacerbations of the disease and activation of this metabolic pathway, in addition to ROS generated by activated phagocytes, could result in a significant oxidant load that may contribute to the inflammatory response in asthmatic airways.

CHEMISTRY

The major pathways by which ROS are formed by the proposed effector cells of the asthmatic inflammatory response are outlined. The chemistry of ROS formation and the actions of the various anti-oxidant compounds have been the subject of extensive reviews (23,29–31). The information that is provided here is meant only as a cursory review for the subsequent discussion of the role of ROS in the airways.

W. M. Abraham: Department of Medicine, University of Miami School of Medicine, Mount Sinai Medical Center, Miami Beach, Florida 33140.

SUPEROXIDE ANION

The primary step in the production of ROS by stimulated phagocytic cells (neutrophils, eosinophils and macrophages) is the respiratory burst, which is catalyzed by membrane-bound nicotinamide adenine dinucleotide phosphate (NADPH) oxidase (23,29,32). In this reaction, a reduced pyridine nucleotide – NADPH – acts as an electron donor for the one electron reduction of O_2 to O_2^- through the reaction:

$$NADPH + 2O_2 \rightarrow NADP^+ + H^+ + 2O_2^-.$$

The O_2^- produced either can react spontaneously to produce H_2O_2 or the reaction can be catalyzed by superoxide dismutase (SOD), in which case it proceeds at 10^4-times its normal rate (23,33,34). Spontaneous dismutation occurs optimally at pH 4.8 where O_2^- and HO_2^- (perhydroxyl radical) are present in equal concentrations. This reaction slows considerably at alkaline pH because O_2^- predominates. However, the rate constant for SOD-catalyzed dismutation is not effected appreciably by pH changes from 5.0–10.0, and so is particularly effective at normal or alkaline pH where spontaneous dismutation is low (23,35).

Although O_2^- is a highly reactive species, its relative toxicity has been questioned (36–38). For the purposes of this discussion, however, O_2^- appears to contribute to the adverse pulmonary effects that characterize asthma, because in many instances these abnormalities can be inhibited by treatment with exogenous SOD (2,5,7,12,39,40). The toxicity of O_2^- is, in part, derived from its selective target specificity. It will directly inactivate catalase, glutathione peroxidase and glyceraldehyde 3-phosphate dehydrogenase, all important enzymes in the regulation of a cell's redox state (41). Furthermore, because O_2^- is a strong reducer, it readily donates electrons to metals such as Fe^{2+}, thereby contributing to the formation of OH· by the Fenton reaction (23,30,42–44). Thus, a considerable fraction of O_2^- produced could be released into the extracellular space where, in combination with metal ions and H_2O_2, OH· can be formed which then could initiate lipid peroxidation, DNA damage, and, ultimately, cell death.

Superoxide also can react rapidly with nitric oxide (NO·) in aqueous solutions and in gas phase to form peroxynitrite anion ($OONO^-$), a strong oxidizing agent. This reaction occurs rapidly in aqueous conditions at physiologic pH (45). In the presence of high O_2^- production, the conditions in the lung favor $OONO^-$ production which, because of its strong oxidant capabilities, could be another important mechanism for lipid peroxidation (45).

HYDROGEN PEROXIDE

Hydrogen peroxide is formed by stimulated phagocytes, primarily by the dismutation of O_2^-. The reactivity of H_2O_2 is low, and so it readily passes through cell membranes and other complex biologic fluids (46). Thus, unlike O_2^-, whose range of activity is limited, the toxic effects of H_2O_2 can occur at sites distant to where it was produced. The fate of H_2O_2 can vary. In the presence of granulocytic peroxidases (e.g. myeloperoxidase [neutrophils] or eosinophil peroxidase) and halides [chlorine (Cl^-), bromine (Br^-), iodine (I^-), or thiocyanate (SCN^-), H_2O_2 can be used as a substrate in the formation of hypohalous acids through the following reaction (23,47):

$$H_2O_2 + X^- + H^+ + HOX \rightarrow + H_2O$$

$$(X^- = CL^-, Br^-, I^- \text{ or } SCN^-)$$

For myeloperoxidase, Cl^- is the halide of choice, whereas for eosinophil peroxidase the rate of formation of hypohalous acid varies from $I^- > Br^- > Cl^-$ (48–52). These are important biocidal compounds that serve host defense functions. Probably more important for inflammation of the asthmatic airway, however, is the conversion of H_2O_2 to OH· (see below), which, as indicated above, can cause lipid peroxidation and cell death (23,30,42–44).

Although the primary source of ROS is thought to originate from phagocytes, recent data indicate that epithelial cells generate and release H_2O_2 towards the airway lumen. This basal release can be stimulated by platelet activating factor (PAF) or phorbol myrisitate acetate (PMA) and involves the activation of protein kinase C (26). Thus, epithelial cells could add to the ROS load following antigen or other inflammatory stimuli. In addition, the reactivity of H_2O_2 can be increased in the presence of serine proteases. This may be important to the overall inflammatory response in asthma given the potential interaction with mast cell tryptase (53,54).

HYDROXYL RADICAL

The OH· is formed nonenzymatically via the metal catalyzed Fenton reaction which, in addition to metal ions (eg Fe^{2+}) requires both O_2^- and H_2O_2 (23,30,42–44).

$$Fe^3 + O_2^- \rightarrow Fe^{2+} + O_2$$

$$\underline{Fe^{2+} + H_2O_2 \rightarrow Fe^{3+} + OH· + OH^-}$$

$$\text{Net Rx } O_2^- + H_2O_2 \rightarrow O_2 + OH· + OH^-$$

The OH· is extremely reactive and toxic, but the requirement for metal limit its sites of formation. Sources of iron include transferrin, ferritin, hemaglobin, or possibly an "intracellular mobile iron poole" (55–59). The OH· is one of the most relevant initiators of lipid peroxidation. Lipid peroxidation occurs because the carbon hydrogen bonds of polyunsaturated fatty acids are weakened by an adjacent double bond, which renders these hydrogens susceptible to extraction by free radicals. The removal of the hydrogen by the radical leaves the carbon bearing a single unparied electron.

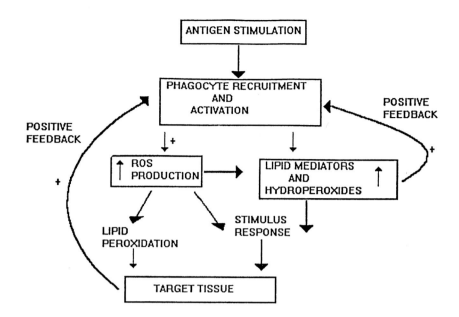

FIG. 1. Possible pathways by which reactive oxygen species (ROS) initiate and propagate the inflammatory response in asthma. Phagocytes recruited to the airways by chemotactic factors released during the initial stages of airway anaphylaxis release lipid mediators and ROS. The ROS can increase the formation of lipid radicals which then can cause additional phagocyte recruitment and activation.

$$R \cdot + LH \rightarrow RH + L \cdot$$

The resulting lipid radical (L·) then reacts with molecular oxygen to form a lipid peroxyl radical (LOO·) which is itself a strong oxidizing agent. This lipid peroxyl radical can then extract a second hydrogen, forming a lipid hydroperoxide (LOOH) and a new lipid radical.

$$LOO \cdot + LH \rightarrow LOOH + LOO \cdot$$

As this process continues, it can convert many of the membrane phospholipids to hydroperoxides which are unstable and readily break down. Such perturbations have been proposed to contribute to the generation of PAF from cell membranes via the deacylation of alkyl-acyl glycerophosphocholine which is a phospholipase-A_2-dependent reaction (60,61). This reaction also releases arachidonic acid. That these mediators are generated and contribute to airway inflammatory responses is consistent with the general protective actions of PAF antagonists, cyclooxygenase inhibitors, and thromboxane antagonists on ROS-induced responses (2, 62–67). Thus, exposure of cells to OH· can initiate a positive feedback loop that results in the destruction of membrane phospholipids (30,31). Such a mechanism could help explain the apparent self-perpetuating airway inflammation and resultant increases in airway responsiveness in the asthmatic airway (Fig. 1).

ANTIOXIDANTS

The major antioxidant defense mechanisms that protect cells against ROS, include SOD, catalase, and glutathione peroxidase (42,68–72). Most human cells have both cytosolic and mitochondrial forms of SOD (42). Superoxide dismutase is also found in extracellular spaces throughout the lung where it may function to protect matrix elements from oxidant stress (73). Specifically, extracellular SOD was located in the extracellular matrix, especially in areas containing high amounts of type I collagen, but not in areas rich in elastin. The areas of location were primarily around larger vessels and airways, rather than alveoli and capillaries (73).

As indicated previously, SOD catalyzes the dismutation of O_2^- to H_2O_2:

$$2O_2^- + 2H^+ \rightarrow H_2O_2 + O_2$$

The effectiveness of SOD as an antioxidant, however, depends on the cellular conditions. In the presence of free iron, SOD, because it increases the production of H_2O_2, can enhance the production of OH· via the Fenton reaction (see earlier). If, however, the iron is compartmentalized, then the H_2O_2 can be reduced by catalase or glutathione peroxidase.

Catalase is a 240-kDa tetrameric heme protein that undergoes alternate divalent oxidation and reduction in the presence of H_2O_2 and catalyses the reaction:

$$H_2O_2 \rightarrow 2\,H_2O + O_2$$

Because of the conformation of its active site, catalase is not effective in metabolizing larger molecules such as lipid hydroperoxides that arise from lipid peroxidation (42). Catalase appears localized to perioxisomes and microsomes, and is more efficient at scavenging higher levels of H_2O_2, whereas glutathione peroxidase is localized to the cytosol and the mitochondria, and is more efficient at scavenging low levels of H_2O_2 (42).

Glutathione peroxidase, in addition to reducing H_2O_2, can remove LOOH (42). Glutathione peroxidase is an

85-kD tetrameric protein which contains four atoms of selenium (42). Interestingly, asthmatics have been reported to have reduced blood levels of selenium and glutathione peroxidase (74–76). The action of glutathione peroxidase requires reduced glutathione (GSH) to catalyze the reaction:

$$LOOH + 2GSH \rightarrow GSSG + LOH + H_2O$$

which forms oxidized glutathione (GSSG). Under normal

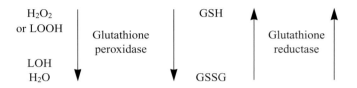

Nonenzymatic Scavengers

Mucus has long been known to act as a scavenger for ROS (79). Part of this anti-oxidant activity may be due to the nonspecific scavenging activity of albumin or mucus glycoproteins. Recently, Salate et al. (80) have shown that airway peroxidase (APO), a glycoprotein with a molecular weight ~80 kDa, is a specific anti-oxidant contained in mucus. These investigators showed that APO is a major scavenger of H_2O_2, with preliminary estimates indicating that APO may comprise as much as 1% of the mucus anti-oxidant capacity. The investigators were careful to show that the scavenging activity ascribed to APO was not due to: (a) the conversion of H_2O_2 to $OH\cdot$ by Fe^{2+} through the Fenton reaction; (b) cell associated enzymes; (c) the presence of cell-derived catalase; or (d) the presence of neutrophil myeloperoxidase. Thus, in addition to the nonspecific anti-oxidant capacities of albumin and mucus glycoconjugates in general, the mucus layer also contains specific anti-oxidant enzymes. However, little is known about the regulation of this APO under normal or inflamed conditions.

Evidence for Increased ROS Production in Asthma

Part of the evidence for increased ROS generation in asthma comes from the study of isolated cells, where investigators have compared the spontaneous and stimulated ROS generation by granulocytes obtained from normal and asthmatic subjects. The majority of studies show that cells from asthmatic patients have greater spontaneous release and stimulated release than cells from normal subjects. Although these data are suggestive, they provide circumstantial evidence for a role of ROS in asthma. More concrete evidence stems from observations where the increased ROS generation seen in cells from asthmatic patients has been correlated with decrements in lung function. Although differences in ROS production observed between asthmatics and normals is relatively independent of the stimulating agent used (e.g., PMA,

conditions cells maintain a high GSH:GSSG ratio and so may explain attempts to use GSH as a marker of oxidant stress (77,78). The high GSH:GSSG ratio ensures the availability of GSH for protection against hydroperoxides. To maintain GSH, GSSG is reduced back by glutathione reductase in conjunction with glucose-6-phosphate dehydrogenase from the hexose monophosphate shunt which supplies NADPH-reducing equivalents.

This process is outlined below:

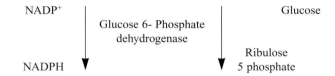

FMLP, or zymosan), comparisons of ROS production by eosinophils and neutrophils within the same group appears to be stimulus-dependent. Thus, eosinophils generate significantly more ROS than do neutrophils in response to PMA, zymosan, or the divalent ionophore A23178 (81). When FMLP was used as the stimulus, eosinophils generated less ROS than neutrophils, unless cytochalasin B was added (81).

Comparisons of circulating cells and airway cells have provided data demonstrating differences between ROS production by asthmatics and normals. Chanez and co-workers (82) found that peripheral blood eosinophils from patients with symptomatic asthma showed enhanced potential for activation by PAF or PMA when compared with patients with allergic rhinitis or asymptomatic asthma. Schauer et al.(83) obtained similar results in children. Eosinophils from asthmatic children showed enhanced O_2^- production (69%) compared to eosinophils from healthy controls (83). The eosinophil O_2^- production was also greater than that seen in neutrophils from the same patients or normals. However, these investigators found that preincubation with PAF or GM-CSF enhanced the O_2^- production from normal eosinophils, but not from eosinophils from asthmatic children, suggesting that cells from asthmatics were already primed for ROS release (83). Sedgwick et al. (24) compared the O_2^- production to various stimuli (PMA, A23187, FMLP, and zymosan) in peripheral eosinophils and neutrophils from normal and asthmatic subjects. Comparisons of the eosinophils from the asthmatic patients were also separated by density. The results depended on the stimulus used, as well as the cell type being studied. When cells were stimulated by A23187, O_2^- generation was similar in the three sets of eosinophils (normals, asthmatic normodense, and asthmatic hypodense), but greater than that seen in both groups (asthmatic and normal) of neutrophils. Eosinophils from asthmatic patients had greater PMA-stimulated O_2^- production than eosinophils obtained from normal subjects, but there was no difference between the normodense and hypodense eosinophils from the asthmatic patients (24). The eosinophils from both normals and asthmatics produced more ROS than the corresponding neutrophils. Responses to FMLP were similar in both eosinophils and neutrophils from both groups (24).

Mononuclear phagocytes release ROS and also participate in the airway inflammation associated with asthma. Comparisons of basal (unstimulated) O_2^- release from blood monocytes in suspension from normals and asthmatic subjects were not different from each other (84). However, as with the eosinophils and neutrophils, the response to PMA stimulation was greater in the monocytes from asthmatics compared to normals. When adherent monocytes from the two groups were studied, the monocytes from the asthmatics showed increased ROS production both when unstimulated and after PMA-stimulation (84). Thus, monocytes, like eosinophils and neutrophils, appear primed for ROS release. Furthermore, it appears that processes, such as adherence, augment this difference (84).

In some cases, the ROS production by peripheral cells has been linked to the severity of airway symptoms experienced by the patients. Kanasawa et al. (85) found that O_2^- production by neutrophils from asthmatic patients was greater after stimulation with PMA (71%) and FMLP (96%) than that found in neutrophils from normal patients. Furthermore, the O_2^- production from the more severe asthmatics (defined by contiuous use of inhalers) was approximately 45% greater than in the milder asthmatics (defined by intermittent inhaler use). The investigators also found a significant positive correlation between PMA-stimulated O_2 production and disease duration in years (r=0.6, P<0.05, n=11), and an inverse correlation with FEV$_1$ (r=0.7, P<0.05) (85). These studies confirmed earlier reports in patients with both asthma and chronic obstructive airway disease. In asthmatic patients, Meltzer et al. (86) found a correlation between the peripheral blood generation of O_2^- induced by FLMP and the severity of their bronchial hyperresponsiveness to methacholine, whereas in patients with chronic airflow obstruction, Postma and co-workers (87) found O_2^- production by PMNs was correlated with the degree of airway responsiveness to histamine. In 28 patients with chronic airflow obstruction, a correlation was found between the production of O_2^- by peripheral PMNs stimulated with phorbol ester and the degree of airway hyperresponsiveness (88). The relationship was significant whether the patients were smokers (r=0.59, n=14, P<0.01) or ex-smokers (r=0.79, n=14, P<0.01) . Alveolar macrophages, obtained by BAL from subjects challenged with cotton bract extract released increased amounts of O_2^- and thromboxane A$_2$ (TxA$_2$), compared to BAL cells from saline-challenged controls (89). Although, the in vitro parameters of BAL cell activation did not correlate with the degree of extract-induced bronchoconstriction, there was a relationship between the pulmonary response and the concentration of TxA$_2$ in BAL.

Jajour and Calhoun studied the O_2^- production by airspace cells in 56 patients with asthma as compared to 49 normal controls (90). These investigators found that in asthma patients with FEV$_1$<80%, unfractionated airspace cells had a 90% higher spontaneous O_2^- release than normal subjects, or a 71% greater spontaneous release than asthmatic patients with FEV$_1$>80%. Comparisons of the PMA-stimulated O_2^- production showed that both the moderate (37%) and mild asthmatic (71%) groups produced more than normals. Finally, there was an inverse correlation between spontaneous O_2^- production and %-predicted FEV$_1$. Interestingly, there was even a stronger correlation between spontaneous O_2^- release and % neutrophils in the BAL, whereas both eosinophils and neutrophils both correlated with PMA-induced O_2^- release, an observation which suggests that these granulocytes might be important contributors to this event (90). Cluzel et al. (91) showed that alveolar macrophages from asthmatic subjects had higher baseline and stimulated chemiluminesence compared to alveolar macrophages from normals; they also found a significant correlation between the maximal response of the cells and the clinical severity of the patient's asthma.

Calhoun and Bush (92) showed that both baseline and PMA-stimulated chemiluminesence of adherent cells was increased in subjects with mild asthma, 48 or 72 hours after aerosol antigen challenge. These investigators extended their findings by examining the O_2^- production by unfractionated airspace cells and pure alveolar macrophages immediately (12 minutes) after and 48 hours after segmental antigen challenge (25). Segmental provocation was performed with low, medium, and high doses of antigen. In samples obtained immediately after challenge, there were no differences in spontaneous O_2^- release either between saline- (control) challenged segments or the antigen- challenged segments. Furthermore, there were no differences in the spontaneous release among the cells obtained from the three antigen doses. The same results were obtained in the 48-hour specimens (25). When the unfractionated cells were stimulated with PMA, there was no difference in the response of the samples obtained immediately after challenge. The 48-hour samples from the antigen-challenged segments, however, produced approximately 2 to 3 times more O_2^- than did corresponding cells from the saline-challenged segment; but again, there was no difference in the O_2^- production among the three antigen doses. No differences were seen when zymosan was used as the stimulating agent.

When the same tests were performed in purified macrophages, the investigators found that spontaneous release was increased in the 48- hour samples, as was the response to PMA (25). The investigators also showed that there were differences in macrophage ROS release, depending on which percoll density fraction they used to isolate these cells, with the greatest production being found at a density of 1.075 mg/ml. Thus, high density macrophages obtained after antigen challenge which show increased nonspecific esterase staining, interleukin-1 secretion, and enhanced tumor cell cytotoxicity, had greater oxidative potential (25).

Sanders and colleagues (93) lavaged airways 19 hours after segmental bronchoprovocation to determine the relative ROS generation by the granulocytic and mononuclear cells recruited to the airway. For these studies, ROS were detected by electron paramagnetic resonance (EPR) spectroscopy with the spin trap 5,5-di-methyl-1-pyrroline-N-oxide and density gradient centrifugation was used for cell isolation (93). As in the other studies, there was no spontaneous ROS release from cells obtained from saline-challenged segments. However, cells from the antigen-challenged sites produced a prominent EPR signal, which was inhibitable by SOD, indicating the formation of O_2^-. Subsequently, the authors found that the granulocytic cells, which were predominately eosinophils, were the major source of the ROS. Interestingly, the investigators found a significant correlation between the levels of ROS produced by the BAL cells and the levels of albumin found in the BAL fluid (r=0.69, P=0.03, n=8). One interpretation of these data is that ROS contribute to the altered airway permeability associated with allergic inflammation (93). Examination of O_2^- production by cells obtained by BAL from patients with nocturnal asthma provides more direct clinical evidence for the contribution of ROS to airway dysfunction in asthma (94). In this study, BAL was performed at 4:00 P.M. and 4:00 A.M. in asthma patients with and without nocturnal worsening. Although there were no differences in the total number of cells or the cell differential between these groups, air-space cells from subjects that developed nocturnal asthma as demonstrated by a fall in FEV_1, showed a threefold greater increase in O_2^- production than did those patients who had no nocturnal component. Furthermore, there was a significant (P<0.01) correlation (r=0.71, n=15) between the change in O_2^- production between 4:00 P.M. and 4:00 A.M. and the change in FEV_1. These observations suggest that increased ROS generation can contribute to bronchial obstruction (94).

MECHANISMS

Although the aforementioned studies suggest a relationship between increased ROS generation and airway obstruction and/or airway hyperresponsiveness, the mechanisms involved have not been clearly identified. Possible explanations include direct effect of ROS on mast cells, stimulation of sensory nerves, increased epithelial permiablity, and/or the secondary generation of inflammatory lipid mediators.

Reactive oxygen species have been shown to cause smooth muscle contraction and enhance smooth muscle responsiveness, *in vitro*. Generation of O_2^- by xanthine oxidase caused a biphasic contraction of isolated guinea pig trachea, while H_2O_2 caused both contraction of rat-intrapulmonary bronchi and potentiation of the responses to electrical field stimulation (1,95). The H_2O_2-induced effects were thought to result from the liberation of 5-hydroxytryptamine because of H_2O_2-induced mast cell degranulation (96). In guinea pig trachealis muscle, LTD_4 potentiated the contractile response to histamine (97). As expected, this effect was blocked by the LT antagonist FPL-55712, but surprisingly the potentiation was also blocked by SOD. These results suggested that LTD_4 stimulated the release of O_2^- (97). The link between LTs and ROS was also found in H_2O_2-induced edema in isolated perfused rat lungs (98). The LT-ROS interaction may be an important factor in pathophysiology of asthma, because of the recent data implicating LTD_4 as a mediator of the late response (99–103). Interestingly, LTD_4 has also been shown to be a prerequisite for antigen-dependent TxA_2 synthesis in guinea pig lungs (104). Such results agree with studies demonstrating significant correlations between concentrations of LTC_4 and TxA_2, and airway hyperresponsiveness following antigen challenge. It might also explain why indomethacin blocks the airway hyperresponsiveness that follows the development of late airway responses (a LT-dependent response) in both man and sheep (105–107). These data would also be consistent with findings showing that indomethacin blocked contractions to low concentrations of H_2O_2 (108,109).

Two studies have suggested that ROS can stimulate tachykinin release, thereby modulating airway effects. Acute treatment with the OH· scavenger dimethylthiourea (DMTU), acute SOD + catalase, or tachykinin depletion was found to be effective in blocking hyperpnea-induced bronchoconstriction in guinea pigs, suggestive of OH· radical interaction with tachykinins (110). These results were substantiated when DMTU, but not SOD or catalase, was shown to mediate capsaicin-induced bronchoconstriction in guinea pigs (111). These studies also indicate that depending on the stimulus, hyperresponsiveness can be mediated by a specific radical species.

Airway epithelial cells are damaged by exposure to ROS (10). Thus, epithelial damage could result in the loss of epithelial relaxant factors and/or increased permeability which could contribute to ROS-induced increases in airway hyperresponsiveness. Hulsmann et al. (112) found that modulation of the sensitivity to contractile agonists by the epithelium increased with increasing airway size. This modulatory role was abolished by treating the epithelium with H_2O_2. However, the loss of epithelial protective effect was not due to a change in the barrier function served by the epithelium because when treated and intact tissues were perfused with histamine, both tissues showed similar histamine loss. Light microscopic examination of the H_2O_2-treated tissues showed selective damage to the columnar epithelium, with relative preservation of basal cells. Furthermore, it did not appear that the increased responsiveness of the H_2O_2-treated tissues were related to alterations in β-adrenergic receptor function, because the relaxant response to salbutamol was unaffected. These data are consistent with previous findings in guinea pig trachea where direct incubation with H_2O_2 had no effect on the response isoproterenol (109). However, there is a discrepancy between the functional data and receptor binding data which indicated that H_2O_2 caused a reduction in β-adrenergic receptor number (113). Nevertheless, it appears that ROS-induced hyperresponsiveness may not be related to a breakdown in the epithelial barrier, but rather to alternate mechanisms possibly involving the formation of lipid mediators such as is seen in vascular smooth muscle (114).

Exposure of cultured tracheal explants *in vitro* to H_2O_2-inhibited ciliary beat frequency (10). The inhibition appeared to be mediated through activation of protein kinase C, since H-7, a cell-permeable protein kinase inhibitor, prevented the cilioinhibition. That ROS are cilioinhibitory is consistent with the ability of catalase to block decreases in tracheal mucus velocity *in vivo* (11).

Although the airway epithelium is sensitive to ROS, and because epithelial shedding and damage are thought to be a characteristic feature of asthma, it is reasonable to hypothesize that ROS are primary agents initiating epithelial damage. However, the epithelium itself may be a potent source of ROS. Recent studies using primary cell cultures maintained in an air liquid interface showed that epithelial cells released H_2O_2 from their apical surface (26). This release could be enhanced considerably by stimulating the cells with PAF or PMA. These *in vitro* studies correlate well with studies *in vivo*. Allergic sheep that develop antigen-induced late bronchial responses also develop hyperresponsiveness 24h after antigen challenge. Morphometric studies done during this period showed a quantitative increase in O_2^- production in and around the airway epithelium (115). The localization of the O_2^- reaction product to the airway epithelium was surprising, considering the 2.4-fold increase in eosinophils and 2.0-fold increase in mast cells in the submucosa. The reaction was blocked by SOD *in vitro*, or *in vivo*, by treating the animals before antigen challenge with a combination of a 5-lipoxygenase inhibitor (Zileuton) and a PAF antagonist (WEB-2086), agents which had previously been shown to prevent antigen-induced airway inflammation and hyperresponsiveness (116,117).

As indicated previously, the mechanisms by which ROS can lead to changes in bronchial tone and/or airway hyperresponsiveness may involve lipid peroxidation of cell membranes and the secondary generation of inflammatory mediators. In cats and sheep, inhalation of xanthine-xanthine oxidase, which produces O_2^-, caused bronchoconstriction and airway hyperresponsiveness (2,5).

Both the bronchoconstriction and the airway hyperresponsiveness were blocked by pretreatment of the animals with inhaled SOD, catalase, or the combination of SOD and catalase. Subsequent studies in sheep showed that the xanthine-xanthine oxidase-induced bronchoconstriction and hyperresponsiveness could be blocked by anti-inflammatory agents that affect arachidonate metabolism, thereby adding strength to the argument that lipid peroxidation was occurring (2). Thus, the xanthine-xanthine oxidase-induced bronchoconstriction and airway hyperresponsiveness could be blocked by pretreatment with the cyclooxygenase inhibitor, indomethacin, the PAF antagonist, WEB-2086, and the glucocorticosteroid, methylprednisolone succinate. These results suggest that the ROS generated by inhalation of xanthine-xanthine oxidase induced the generation of arachidonic acid metabolites, which were, in turn, responsible for the bronchoconstriction and airway hyperresponsiveness. Subsequent studies showing that pretreatment with catalase did not block PAF-induced bronchoconstriction or PAF-induced airway hyperresponsiveness, supported the hypothesis that the ROS initiated the generation of lipid mediators. Such a hypothesis would be consistent with the findings of Sporn et al. (118) who showed that alveolar macrophages released arachidonic acid metabolites in a dose-dependent manner upon stimulation with H_2O_2, and that the response was inhibitable by indomethacin.

The strongest evidence supporting ROS involvement in antigen-induced airway pathophysiology comes from studies showing that ROS scavengers can abrogate these antigen-induced events. Lansing and co-workers showed that catalase given as an aerosol immediately before antigen challenge, and then every 30 minutes after challenge, blocked antigen-induced airway hyperresponsiveness, but not the immediate antigen-induced bronchoconstriction in allergic sheep. These results suggested that ROS were not a major factor in the immediate bronchoconstriction, but contributed to the subsequent events leading to airway hyperresponsiveness. Thus, it was not surprising that the airway hyperresponsiveness still could be blocked if catalase was given 1h and 2h after antigen challenge (7). Interestingly, although catalase prevented the airway hyperresponsiveness, it did not block the inflammatory cell recruitment to the lung. However, when catalase was only given 2h after antigen challenge, just prior to the determination of airway responsiveness, it was ineffective (Fig. 2). The time course of the protective effects of catalase described in these studies is consistent with the previous evidence indicating that ROS initiate the generation of inflammatory mediators. The results in sheep are supported by studies in dogs which showed that antigen-induced airway hyperresponsiveness was associated with increases in both the spontaneous and PMA-induced O_2^- production by BAL cells (119). The increased O_2^- production appeared dependent on the increased percentage of neutrophils in the BAL. The increase in neutrophil

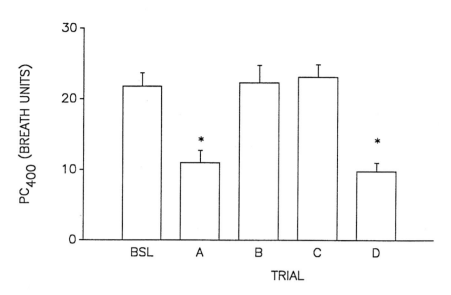

FIG. 2. Effect of aerosolized catalase, given before and after antigen challenge, on the provocative concentration of carbachol that produced a 400% increase in specific lung resistance (PC400) in allergic sheep. In the control trial (A) antigen challenge-induced airway hyperresponsiveness (indicated by a fall in the PC400). When catalase was given before antigen challenge, and then every 30 minutes after antigen challenge for 2 hours, the PC400 remained unchanged from baseline (BSL), e.g., there was no airway hyperresponsiveness (trial B). If the catalase was given 1 and 2 hours after challenge (trial C), the response was the same. If catalase was given only 2 hours after challenge (trial D), there was no protection and the animals developed airway hyperresponsiveness. (From Lansing MW, Ahmed A, Cortes A, Sielczak MW, Wanner A, Abraham WM. Oxygen radicals contribute to antigen-induced airway hyperresponsiveness in conscious sheep. *Am Rev Respir Dis* 1993;147:321–326, with permission.)

ROS production could be related to the upregulation of MAC-1 (CD11b/CD18) on these cells, and subsequent adhesion to ICAM-1, either on endothelial cells or epithelial cells (120,121). Twice daily intraperitoneal administrations of polyoxyethylene SOD or γ-glutamylcysteine ethyl ester, a prodrug of glutathione, blocked airway hyperresponsiveness in guinea pigs which had been challenged with ovalbumin for 10 consecutive days (8). In the protected animals, there was a concomitant protection against the ovalbumin-induced reduction in beta adrenoreceptors and the reduction in adenylate cyclase activity. Ovalbumin challenge also caused increases in xanthine oxidase activity in lung tissue, BAL, and serum, which were attenuated in the treated animals (8). Collectively, these studies indicate that ROS might contribute to the underlying mechanisms of airway hyperresponsiveness following antigen challenge by the generation of inflammatory lipid mediators.

CHANGES IN ANTI-OXIDANT MARKERS

Given that inflammatory cells from patients with asthma generate increased amounts of ROS, one might expect that anti-oxidant defenses might respond to the increased oxidant load. In keeping with this hypothesis, such observations have been made in serum from patients with adult respiratory distress syndrome (ARDS) who developed sepsis (122). The serum from these patients scavenged more H_2O_2 *in vitro* and had more catalase activity than patients without sepsis. Vachier et al. (84) found SOD levels to be decreased in adherent monocytes from asthmatic patients, when compared to monocytes

from normals before and after PMA stimulation. Likewise, platelet gluathione peroxidase which functions as an anti-oxidant by supplying reducing equivalents in the form of electrons to reduce peroxides was significantly lower (~15%, p<0.01) in 20 patients with intrinsic asthma than in controls (74). Animal studies have shown that GSH levels can increase during oxidant stress, and in patients with mild asthma, bronchial and alveolar GSH levels were increased relative to normal subjects (42,77). Interestingly, the higher the GSH levels in the alveolar fluid, the higher (i.e. the less reactive) the $PC_{20}FEV_1$ in the asthmatic patients (7). In the same study, SOD and catalase were not different between the groups. Thus, the ability to increase antioxidant defenses can be important in reducing asthma symptoms. Late airway responses in rats were associated with the induction of MnSOD, but not Cu/Zn SOD in bronchial epithelial cells (12). Treatment with recombinant human-SOD prevented the induction of MnSOD and almost completely suppressed the late airway response in these animals. A similar response was seen in primary human epithelial cell cultures which were exposed to influenza virus and interferon gamma (123). The exposures resulted in an increase in MnSOD mRNA expression. However, there was no change in Cu/Zn SOD gene expression. These data are suggestive for upregulation of MnSOD and a reduction of Cu/Zn SOD during inflammatory events.

Another mechanism by which ROS can increase pulmonary inflammation and maintain airway hyperreactivity, is by inactivating protease inhibitors. Proteins with sulfur containing amino acids (cysteine and methionine) are susceptible to oxidative stress. Oxidation of these sulfur-containing proteins may result in inactivation. Such a mechanism is proposed for α_1-protease inhibitor (α_1-PI). Lipid peroxidation products formed after exposure to oxidant gases can inactivate α_1-PI (124). This can occur in addition to ROS produced by activated granulocytes. The result is a decreased α_1-PI activity in the airways. Evidence for such a mechanism in asthma comes from experimental studies showing that after antigen challenge, the activity of α_1-PI is decreased and the airway hyperreactivity increased (125–127). Further studies indicated that the decrease in α_1-PI activity was associated with markers of increased ROS production. In these studies, antigen challenge which produced a late bronchial obstruction, 4 to 8 hours after challenge and airway hyperresponsiveness 24 hours after challenges, was associated with increased granulocyte recruitment, an increased recovery of albumin in BAL, indicating an active inflammatory response, and a concomitant increase in BAL catalase activity (Fig. 3), probably a response to the increased oxidant load such as was seen in patients with ARDS and sepsis (122). Interestingly, the airway hyperresponsiveness could be reversed by treatment with exogenous α_1-PI (125). These data are consistent with the reports of decreased α_1-PI levels in asthmatic patients (128,129).

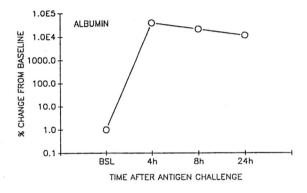

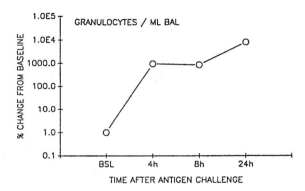

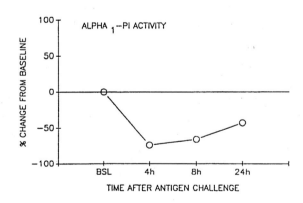

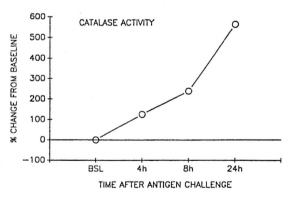

FIG. 3. Response patterns of albumin, granulocytes (eosinophils and neutrophils), alpha-1 protease (PI) activity, and catalase activity in bronchoalveolar lavage (BAL) from sheep before and after antigen challenge. Immediately after airway challenge with Ascaris suum, the sheep responded with 336±56% (mean ±SE, n=6) increase in specific lung resistance over baseline (BSL, =0%). Subsequently (4 to 8 hours after challenge), the animals developed a late bronchial response with specific lung resistance increasing 190±21% over baseline. On the following day, the animals developed airway hyperresponsiveness as indicated by a fall in PC400 to carbachol. Consistent with these pathophysiologic airway responses were elevated markers of inflammation, including increased numbers of granulocytes and albumin in BAL. Concomitant with these markers was increased catalase activity and a decrease in alpha-1-PI activity suggestive of an increased oxidant load in the airways. These data are supported by morphological evidence of increased ROS production in the airways after antigen challenge. Values are mean ±SE for six sheep. (Adapted from Liberman H, Mariassy AT, Sorace D, Suster S, Abraham WM. Morphometric estimation of superoxide generation in allergen-induced airway hyperresponsiveness. *Lab Invest* 1995;72:348–354.)

CONCLUSIONS

The findings reviewed here provide strong support that ROS contribute to the pathophysiology of asthma. Their role would appear to be one of an intermediary by initiating the release of lipid mediators and by inactivating protective mechanisms. Thus, one could propose a recurrent cycle of recruitment and stimulation of inflammatory cells, leading to the continued release of ROS. If such a scenario existed, then antioxidant therapy could, in fact, be useful in the treatment of this disease.

REFERENCES

1. Szarek JL, Schmidt NL. Hydrogen peroxide-induced potentiation of contractile responses in isolated rat airways. *Am J Physiol* 1990;258:L232–L237.
2. Lansing MW, Mansour E, Ahmed A, et al. Lipid mediators contribute to oxygen radical-induced airway responses in sheep. *Am Rev Respir Dis* 1991;144:1291–1296.
3. Rosales C, Juliano RL. Signal transduction by cell adhesion receptors in leukocytes. *J Leukoc Biol* 1995;57:189–198.
4. Prasad K, Gupta JB. Influence of hydroxyl radical on rabbit airway smooth muscle chronically exposed to H_2O_2 *in vivo*. *Am J Physiol* 1993;264:L566–L574.
5. Katsumata U, Miura M, Ichinose M, Kimura K, Takahashi T, Inoue H, Takishima T. Oxygen radicals produce airway constriction and hyperresponsiveness in anesthetized cats. *Am Rev Respir Dis* 1990;141:1158–1161.
6. Forteza R, Lauredo IT, Burch R, Abraham WM. Extracellular metabolites of *Pseudomonas aeruginosa* produce bronchoconstriction by different mechanisms. *Am J Respir Cell Mol Biol* 1994;149:687–693.
7. Lansing MW, Ahmed A, Cortes A, Sielczak MW, Wanner A, Abraham WM. Oxygen radicals contribute to antigen-induced airway hyperresponsiveness in conscious sheep. *Am Rev Respir Dis* 1993;147:321–326.
8. Ikuta N, Sugiyama S, Takagi K, Satake T, Ozawa T. Implication of Oxygen Radicals on Airway Hyperresponsiveness after Ovalbumin Challenge in Guinea Pigs. *Am Rev Respir Dis* 1992;145:561–565.
9. Rogers DF. Airway goblet cells: responsive and adaptable front-line defenders. *Eur Respir J* 1994;7:1690–1706.
10. Kobayashi K, Salathe M, Pratt M, Cartagena N, Soloni F, Seybold Z, Wanner A. Mechanism of hydrogen peroxide-induced inhibition of sheep airway cilia. *Am J Respir Cell Mol Biol* 1992;6:667–673.
11. Seybold ZV, Abraham WM, Gazeroglu H, Wanner A. Impairment of airway mucociliary transport by Pseudomonas aeruginosa products. *Am Rev Respir Dis* 1992;146:1173–1176.
12. Matsuyama T, Ihaku D, Tanimukai T, Uyama O, Kitada O. Superoxide dismutase suppressed asthmatic response with inhibition of manganese superoxide induction in rat lung. *Nippon Kyobu Shikkan Gakkai Zasshi* 1993;31:139–145.
13. Marsh WR, Irvin CG, Murphy KR, Behrens BL, Larsen GL. Increases in airway reactivity to histamine and inflammatory cells in bronchoalveolar lavage after the late asthmatic response in an animal model. *Am Rev Respir Dis* 1985;131:875–879.
14. Abraham WM, Sielczak MW, Ahmed A, et al. α_4-integrins mediate antigen-induced late bronchial responses and prolonged airway hyperresponsiveness in sheep. *J Clin Invest* 1994;93:776–787.
15. O'Byrne PM, Dolovich J, Hargreave FE. State of art: late asthmatic responses. *Am Rev Respir Dis* 1987;136:740–751.
16. Beasley R, Roche WR, Roberts JA, Holgate ST. Cellular events in the bronchi in mild asthma and after bronchial provocation. *Am Rev Respir Dis* 1989;139:806–817.
17. Ferguson AC, Wong FWM. Bronchial hyperresponsiveness in asthmatic children: correlation with macrophages and eosinophils in broncholavage fluid. *Chest* 1989;96:988–991.
18. Wardlaw AJ, Dunette S, Gleich GJ, Collins JV, Kay AB. Eosinophils and mast cells in bronchoalveolar lavage in subjects with mild asthma, relationship to bronchial hyperreactivity. *Am Rev Respir Dis* 1988;137:62–69.
19. Kelly C, Ward C, Stenton CS, Bird G, Hendrick DJ, Walters EH. Number and activity of inflammatory cells in bronchoalveolar lavage fluid in asthma and their relation to airway responsiveness. *Thorax* 1988;43:684–692.
20. Kirby J, Hargreave FE, Gleich GJ, O'Byrne PM. Bronchoalveolar cell profiles of asthmatic and nonasthmatic subjects. *Am Rev Respir Dis* 1987;136:379–383.
21. Lozewicz S, Wells C, Gomez E, Ferguson H, Richman P, Devalia J, Davies RJ. Morphological integrity of the bronchial epithelium in mild asthma. *Thorax* 1990;45:12–15.
22. Jeffery PK, Wardlaw AJ, Nelson FC, Collins JV, Kay AB. Bronchial biopsies in asthma: an ultrastructural, quantitative study and correlation with hyperreactivity. *Am Rev Respir Dis* 1989;140:1745–1753.
23. Klebanoff SJ. Phagocytic cells: products of oxygen metabolism. In: Gallin JI, Goldstein IM, Synderman R, eds. *Inflammation basic principles and clinical correlates*. New York: Raven Press, Ltd., 1988:391–444.
24. Sedgwick JB, Geiger KM, Busse WW. Superoxide generation by hypodense eosinophils from patients with asthma. *Am Rev Respir Dis* 1990;142:120–125.
25. Calhoun WJ, Reed HE, Moest DR, Stevens CA. Enhanced superoxide production by alveolar macrophages and air-space cells, airway inflammation, and alveolar macrophage density changes after segmental antigen bronchoprovocation in allergic subjects. *Am Rev Respir Dis* 1992;145:317–325.
26. Kinnula VL, Adler KB, Ackley NJ, Crapo JD. Release of reactive oxygen species by guinea pig tracheal epithelial cells *in vitro*. *Am J Physiol* 1992;262:L708–L712.
27. Barnes PJ. Reactive oxygen species and airway inflammation. *Free Radic Biol Med* 1990;9:235–243.
28. Kontos HA. Oxygen radicals from arachidonate metabolism in abnormal vascular responses. *Am Rev Respir Dis* 1987;136:474–477.
29. Weiss SJ. Tissue destruction by neutrophils *N Engl J Med* 1989;320:365–376.
30. Farber JL, Kyle ME, Coleman JB. Biology of disease: mechanisms of cell injury by activated oxygen species. *Lab Invest* 1990;62:670–679.
31. Kehrer JP. Free radicals as mediators of tissue injury and disease. *Crit Rev Toxicol* 1993;23:21–48.
32. Baggiolini M, Boulay F, Badwey JA, Curnutte JT. Activation of neutrophil leukocytes: chemoattractant receptors and respiratory burst. *FASEB J* 1993;7:1004–1010.
33. Behar D, Czapski G, Rabani J, Dorfman LM, Schwartz HA. The acid dissociation constant and decay kinetics of the perhydroxyl radical. *J Phys Chem* 1970;74:3209–3213.
34. Bielski BHJ, Allen AO. Mechanism of the disproportionation of superoxide radicals. *J Phys Chem* 1977;81:1048–1050.
35. Rabani J, Klug D, Fridovich I. Decay of the HO_2 and O_2 radicals catalyzed by superoxide dismutase: a pulse radiolytic investigation. *Isr J Chem* 1972;10:1095–1106.
36. Fee JA. Is superoxide toxic? *Dev Biochem* 1980;11B:41–48.
37. Fridovich I. Superoxide radical: an endogenous toxicant. *Annu Rev Pharmacol Toxicol* 1983;23:239–257.
38. Sawyer DT, Valentine JS. How super is superoxide. *Acc Chem Res* 1981;14:393–400.
39. Markey BA, Phan SH, Varani J, Ryan US, Ward PA. Inhibition of cytotoxicity by intracellular superoxide dismutase supplementation. *Free Radic Biol Med* 1990;9:307–314.
40. Takakura Y, Masuda S, Tokuda H, Nishikawa M, Hashida M. Targeted delivery of superoxide dismutase to macrophages via mannose receptor-mediated mechanism. *Biochem Pharmacol* 1994;47:853–858.
41. Duan X, Buckpitt AR, Plopper CG. Variation in antioxidant enzyme activities in anatomic subcompartments within rat and rhesus monkey lung. *Toxicol Appl Pharmacol* 1993;123:73–82.
42. Heffner JE, Repine JE. Pulmonary strategies of antioxidant defense. *Am Rev Respir Dis* 1989;140:531–554.
43. Cees J, Doelman A, Bast A. Oxygen radicals in lung pathology. *Free Radic Biol Med* 1990;9:381–400.
44. Halliwell B. Oxygen Radicals and Tissue Injury. In: *Proceedings of Brook Lodge symposium*. The FASEB Journal, 1988:1–143.
45. Gaston B, Drazen JM, Loscalzo J, Stamler JS. The biology of nitrogen oxides in the airways. *Am J Respir Cell Mol Biol* 1994;149:538–551.
46. Frimer AA, Forman A, Borg DC. H_2O_2-diffusion through lysosomes. *Isr J Chem* 1983;23:442–445.
47. Winterbourn CC. Myeloperoxidase as an effective inhibitor of hy-

droxyl radical production: implications for the oxidative reactions of neutrophils. *J Clin Invest* 1986;78:545–550.

48. Migler R, DeChatelet LR, Bass DA. Human eosinophilic peroxidase: role in bacterial activity. *Blood* 1978;51:445–456.

49. Jorg A, Pasquier J, Klebanoff SJ. Purification of horse eosinophil peroxidase. *Biochem Biophys Acta* 1982;701:185–191.

50. Jong EC, Mahmoud AAF, Klebanoff SJ. Peroxidase-mediated toxicity to schistosomula of *Schistosoma mansoni. J Immunol* 1981;126: 468–471.

51. Bozeman PM, Learn DB, Thomas ED. Assay of the human leukocyte enzymes myeloperoxidase and eosinophil peroxidase. *J Immunol Methods* 1990;126:125–133.

52. Mayeno AN, Curran AJ, Roberts RL, Foote CS. Eosinophil preferentially use bromide to generate halogenating agents. *J Biol Chem* 1988; 264:5660–5668.

53. Sedgwick JB, Calhoun WJ, Gleich GJ, et al. Immediate and late airway response of allergic rhinitis patients to segmental antigen challenge: characterization of eosinophil and mast cell mediators. *Am Rev Respir Dis* 1991;144:1274–1281.

54. Broide DH, Gleich GJ, Cuomo AJ, Coburn DA, Federman EC, Schwartz LB, Wasserman SI. Evidence of ongoing mast cell and eosinophil degranulation in symptomatic asthma airway. *J Allergy Clin Immunol* 1991;88:637–648.

55. Yoshino S, Blake DR, Hewitt S, Morris C, Bacon PA. Effect of blood on the activity and persistance of antigen-induced inflammation in the rat air pouch. *Ann Rheum Dis* 1985;44:485–490.

56. Biemond P, Van Eijk HG, Swaak AJG, Koster JF. Iron mobilization from ferritin by superoxide derived from stimulated polymorphonuclear leukocytes: possible mechanisms in inflammation diseases. *J Clin Invest* 1984;73:1576–1579.

57. Gutteridge JMC. Iron promoters of the Fenton reaction and lipid peroxidation can be released from hemoglobin by peroxides. *FEBS Lett* 1986;201:291–295.

58. Baker MS, Gebicki JM. The effect of pH on yields of hydroxyl radicals produced from superoxide by potential biological iron chelators. *Arch Biochem Biophys* 1986;246:581–588.

59. Floyd RA. Direct demonstration that ferrous iron complexes of di- and triphosphate nucleotide catalyse hydroxyl free radical formation from hydrogen peroxide. *Arch Biochem Biophys* 1983;225:263–270.

60. Braquet P, Touqui L, Shen TY, Vargaftig BB. Perspectives in platelet activating factor research. *Pharm Rev* 1987;39:98–133.

61. Sporn PHS, Murphy TM, Peters-Golden M. Glucocorticoids fail to inhibit arachidonic acid metabolism stimulated by hydrogen peroxide in the alveolar macrophage. *J Leukoc Biol* 1990;48:81–88.

62. Aizawa H, Chung KF, Leikauf GD, et al. Significance of thromboxane generation in ozone-induced airway hyperresponsiveness in dogs. *J Appl Physiol* 1985;59:1918–1923.

63. Alloatti G, Montrucchio G, Camussi G. Role of platelet activating factor (PAF) in oxygen radical-induced cardiac dysfunction. *J Pharmacol Exp Ther* 1994;269:766–771.

64. O'Byrne PM, Walters EH, Gold BD, et al. Indomethacin inhibits the airway hyperresponsiveness but not the neutrophil influx induced by ozone in dogs. *Am Rev Respir Dis* 1984;130:220–224.

65. Shacter E, Lopez RL, Pati S. Inhibition of the myeloperoxidase-H_2O_2-Cl$^-$ system of neutrophils by indomethacin and other nonsteroidal anti-inflammatory drugs. *Biochem Pharmacol* 1991;41:975–984.

66. Semb AG, Vaage J. Oxygen free radical-induced injury in isolated rat hearts: effects of ibuprofen and BW 755c. *Scand J Clin Lab Invest* 1991;51:377–384.

67. Abraham WM, Baugh LE. Animal models of asthma. In: Busse WW, Holgate ST, eds. *Asthma and rhinitis.* Boston: Blackwell Scientific Publications, Inc. 1995;961–977.

68. Diesseroth A, Dounce AL. Catalase: physical and chemical properties, mechanisms of catalysis, and physiological role. *Physiol Rev* 1970;50:319–375.

69. Reid TJ, III, Murthy MRN, Sicignano A, Tanaka N, Musick WDL, Rossman MG. Structure and heme environment of beef liver catalase at 2.5 A resolution. *Proc Natl Acad Sci U S A* 1981;78:4767–4771.

70. Chance B, Sies H, Boveris A. Hydroperoxide metabolism in mammalian organs. *Physiol Rev* 1979;59:527–605.

71. Ross D, Norbeck K, Moldeus P. The generation and subsequent fate of glutathionyl radicals in biological systems. *J Biol Chem* 1985;260: 15028–15032.

72. McCord JM, Fridovich I. Superoxide dismutase: an enzymic function for erythrocuprein (hemocuprein). *J Biol Chem* 1969;244:6049–6055.

73. Oury TD, Chang LY, Marklund SL, Day BJ, Crapo JD. Immunocytochemical localization of extracellular superoxide dismutase in human lung. *Lab Invest* 1994;70:889–898.

74. Hasselmark L, Malmgren R, Unge G, Zetterstrom O. Lowered platelet gluthathione peroxidase activity in patients with intrinsic asthma. *Allergy* 1990;45:523–527.

75. Stone J, Hinks LJ, Beasley R, Holgate ST, Clayton BE. Selenium status of patients with asthma. *Clin Sci* 1989;77:495–500.

76. Flatt A, Pearce N, Thomson CD, Sears MR, Robinson MF, Beasley R. Reduced selenium in asthmatic subjects in New Zealand. *Thorax* 1990;45:95–99.

77. Smith LJ, Houston M, Anderson J. Increased levels of glutathione in bronchoalveolar lavage fluid from patients with asthma. *Am Rev Respir Dis* 1993;147:1461–1464.

78. Cantin AM, Hubbard RC, Crystal RG. Gluthione deficiency in the epithelial lining fluid of the lower respiratory tract in idiopathic pulmonary fibrosis. *Am Rev Respir Dis* 1989;139:370–372.

79. Gong D, Turner B, Bhaskar KR, Lamont JT. Lipid binding to gastric mucin: protective effect against oxygen radicals. *Am J Physiol* 1990; 259:G681–G686.

80. Salathe M, Guldimann P, Conner GE, Wanner A. Hydrogen peroxide-scavenging properties of sheep airway mucus. *Am J Respir Cell Mol Biol* 1995;151:1543–1550.

81. Sedgwick JB, Vrtis RF, Gourley MF, Busse WW. Stimulus-dependent differences in superoxide anion generation by normal human eosinophils and neutrophils. *J Allergy Clin Immunol* 1988;81:876–883.

82. Chanez P, Dent G, Yukawa T, Barnes PJ, Chung KF. Generation of oxygen free radicals from blood eosinophils from asthma patients after stimulation with PAF or phorbol ester. *Eur Respir J* 1990;3:1002–1007.

83. Schauer U, Leinhaas C, Jäger R, Rieger CHL. Enhanced superoxide generation by eosinophils from asthmatic children. *Int Arch Allergy Appl Immunol* 1991;96:317–321.

84. Vachier I, Damon M, Le Doucen C, Crastes de Paulet A, Chanez P, Michel FB, Godard P. Increased oxygen species generation in blood monocytes of asthmatic patients. *Am Rev Respir Dis* 1992;146:1161–1166.

85. Kanazawa H, Kurihara N, Hirata K, Takeda T. The role of free radicals in airway obstruction in asthmatic patients. *Chest* 1991;100: 1319–1322.

86. Meltzer S, Goldberg B, Lad P, Easton J. Superoxide generation and its modulation by adenosine in the neutrophils of subjects with asthma. *J Allergy Clin Immunol* 1989;83:960–966.

87. Postma DS, Renkema TEJ, Noordhoek JA, Faber H, Sluiter HJ, Kauffman H. Association between nonspecific bronchial hyperreactivity and superoxide anion production by polymorphonuclear leukocytes in chronic air-flow obstruction. *Am Rev Respir Dis* 1988;137:57–61.

88. Renkema TE, Postma DS, Noordhoek JA, Faber H, Sluiter HJ, Kauffman HF. Association between nonspecific bronchial hyperreactivity and superoxide anion production by polymorphonuclear leukocytes in chronic airflow obstruction. *Agents Actions* 1989;26:52–54.

89. Cooper JAD, Merrill WW, Rankin JA, Sibille Y, Buck MG. Bronchoalveolar cell activation after inhalation of a bronchoconstricting agent. *J Appl Physiol* 1988;64:1615–1623.

90. Jarjour NN, Calhoun WJ. Enhanced production of oxygen radicals in asthma. *J Lab Clin Med* 1994;123:131–136.

91. Cluzel M, Damon M, Chanez P, Bousquet J, Crastes de Paulet A, Michel FB, Godard P. Enhanced alveolar cell luminol-dependent chemiluminescence in asthma. *J Allergy Clin Immunol* 1987;80:195–201.

92. Calhoun WJ, Bush RK. Enhanced reactive oxygen species metabolism of airspace cells and airway inflammation follow antigen challenge in human asthma. *J Allergy Clin Immunol* 1990;86:306–313.

93. Sanders SP, Zweier JL, Harrison SJ, Trush MA, Rembish SJ, Liu MC. Spontaneous oxygen radical production at sites of antigen challenge in allergic subjects. *Am J Respir Crit Care Med* 1995;151:1725–1733.

94. Jarjour NN, Busse WW, Calhoun WJ. Enhanced production of oxygen radicals in nocturnal asthma. *Am Rev Respir Dis* 1992;146:905–911.

95. Nishida Y, Suzuki S, Miyamoto T. Basic contraction of isolated guinea pig tracheal chains by superoxide radical. *Inflammation* 1985; 9:333–337.

96. Henderson WR, Chi EY, Klebanoff SS. Eosinophil peroxidase-induced mast cell secretion. *J Exp Med* 1986;152:265 (abstr).

97. Weiss EB, Bellino JR. Leukotriene-associated toxic oxygen metabolites induce airway hyperreactivity. *Chest* 1986;89:5:709–716.

98. Burghuber OC, Strife RJ, Zirrolli J, et al. Leukotriene inhibitors attenuate rat lung injury induced by hydrogen peroxide. *Am Rev Respir Dis* 1985;131:778–785.

99. Abraham WM, Delehunt JC, Yerger L, Marchette B. Characterization of a late phase pulmonary response following antigen challenge in allergic sheep. *Am Rev Respir Dis* 1983;128:839–844.

100. Abraham WM, Burch RM, Farmer SG, Sielczak MW, Ahmed A, Cortes A. A bradykinin antagonist modifies allergen-induced mediator release and late bronchial responses in sheep. *Am Rev Respir Dis* 1991;143:787–796.

101. Sladek K, Dworski R, Fitzgerald GA, Buitkus KL, Block FJ, Marney SR, Sheller JR. Allergen-stimulated release of thromboxane A_2 and leukotriene E_4 in humans. *Am Rev Respir Dis* 1990;141:1441–1445.

102. Rasmussen JB, Eriksson L-O, Margolskee DJ, Tagari P, Williams VC, Andersson K-E. Leukotriene D_4 receptor blockade inhibits the immediate and late bronchoconstrictor responses to inhaled antigen in patients with asthma. *J Allergy Clin Immunol* 1992;90:193–201.

103. Findlay SR, Barden JM, Easley CB, Glass M. Effect of the oral leukotriene antagonist, ICI 204,219, on antigen-induced bronchoconstriction in subjects with asthma. *J Allergy Clin Immunol* 1992;89:1040–1045.

104. Cheng JB, Pillar JS, Conklyn MJ, Breslow R, Shirley JT, Showell HJ. Evidence that peptidoleukotriene is a prerequisite for antigen-dependent thromboxane synthesis in IgG1-passively sensitized guinea pig lungs. *J Pharmacol Exp Ther* 1990;255:664–671.

105. Abraham WM. The interaction among granulocyte lipid mediators and the generation of oxygen radicals in antigen-induced airway hyperresponsiveness. In: Dahlen SE, Hedqvist P, Samuelsson B, Taylor WA, Fritsch J, eds. *Advances in prostaglandin, thromboxane, and leukotriene research*. New York: Raven Press, 1994;131–140.

106. Kirby JG, Hargreave FE, Cockcroft DW, O'Byrne PM. The effect of indomethacin on allergen-induced asthmatic responses. *J Appl Physiol* 1989;66:578–583.

107. Lanes S, Stevenson JS, Codias E, Hernandez A, Sielczak MW, Wanner A, Abraham WM. Indomethacin and FPL-57231 inhibit antigen-induced airway hyperresponsiveness in sheep. *J Appl Physiol* 1986;61:864–872.

108. Stewart RM, Weir EK, Mongomery MR, Niewoehner DE. Hydrogen peroxide contracts airway smooth muscle: a possible endogenous mechanism. *Respir Physiol* 1981;45:333–342.

109. Rhoden KJ, Barnes PJ. Effect of hydrogen peroxide on guinea-pig tracheal smooth muscle *in vitro*: role of cyclo-oxygenase and airway epithelium. *Br J Pharmacol* 1989;98:325–330.

110. Fang ZX, Lai Y-L. Oxygen radicals in bronchoconstriction of guinea pigs elicited by isocapnic hyperpnea. *J Appl Physiol* 1993;74:627–633.

111. Lai Y-L. Oxygen radicals in capsaicin-induced bronchoconstriction. *J Appl Physiol* 1990;68:568–573.

112. Hulsmann AR, Raatgeep HR, Den Hollander JC, Stijnen T, Saxena PR, Kerrebijn KF, De Jongste JC. Oxidative epithelial damage produces hyperresponsiveness of human peripheral airways. *Am J Respir Crit Care Med* 1994;149:519–525.

113. Van der Vliet A, Bast A. Hydrogen peroxide reduces β-adrenoceptor function in the rat small intestine. *Eur J Pharmacol* 1991;199:153–156.

114. Katusic ZS, Schugel J, Cosentino F, Vanhoutte PM. Endothelium-dependent contractions to oxygen-derived free radicals in the canine basilar artery. *Am J Physiol* 1993;264:H859–H864.

115. Liberman H, Mariassy AT, Sorace D, Suster S, Abraham WM. Morphometric estimation of superoxide generation in allergen-induced airway hyperresponsiveness. *Lab Invest* 1995;72:348–354.

116. Soler M, Sielczak MW, Abraham WM. A PAF-antagonist blocks antigen-induced airway hyperresponsiveness and inflammation in sheep. *J Appl Physiol* 1989;67:406–413.

117. Abraham WM, Ahmed A, Cortes A, et al. The 5-lipoxygenase inhibitor zileuton blocks antigen-induced late airway responses, inflammation and airway hyperresponsiveness in allergic sheep. *Eur J Pharmacol* 1992;217:119–126.

118. Sporn PHS, Peters-Golden M, Simon RH. Hydrogen-peroxide-induced arachidonic acid metabolism in the rat alveolar macrophage. *Am Rev Respir Dis* 1988;137:49–56.

119. Stevens WHM, Inman MD, Wattie J, O'Byrne PM. Allergen-induced oxygen radical release from bronchoalveolar lavage cells and airway hyperresponsiveness in dogs. *Am J Respir Crit Care Med* 1995;151:1526–1531.

120. Shappell SB, Toman C, Anderson DC, Taylor AA, Entman ML, Smith CW. Mac-1 (CD11b/CD18) mediates adherence-dependent hydrogen peroxide production by human and canine neutrophils. *J Immunol* 1990;144:2702–2711.

121. Lo SK, Janakidevi K, Lai L, Malik AB. Hydrogen peroxide-induced increase in endothelial adhesiveness is dependent on ICAM-1 activation. *Am J Physiol Lung Cell Mol Physiol* 1993;264:L406–L412.

122. Leff JA, Parsons PE, Day CE, Moore EE, Moore FA, Oppegard MA, Repine JE. Increased serum catalase activity in septic patients with the adult respiratory distress syndrome. *Am Rev Respir Dis* 1992;148:985–989.

123. White JE, Tsan M-F. Induction of pulmonary Mn superoxide dismutase mRNA by interleukin-1. *Am J Physiol Lung Cell Mol Physiol* 1994;266:L664–L671.

124. Mohsenin V. Lipid peroxidation and antielastase activity in the lung under oxidant stress: role of antioxidant defenses. *J Appl Physiol* 1991;70:1456–1462.

125. Forteza R, Botvinnikova Y, Ahmed A, Cortes A, Gundel RH, Wanner A, Abraham WM. The interacton of α1-protease inhibitor and tissue kallikrein in controlling allergic ovine airway hyperresponsiveness. *Am J Respir Crit Care Med* 1996;154:36–42.

126. Forteza R, Burch RM, Abraham WM. Increased tissue kallikrein activity, kinins and decreased α1-proteinase inhibitor activity are linked to ozone-induced airway hyperresponsiveness. *Am J Respir Crit Care Med* 1994;149:158(Abstract).

127. Forteza R, Botvinnikova Y, Ahmed A, Cortes A, Gundel R, Abraham WM. Aerosol α1-proteinase inhibitor (Prolastin) blocks antigen-induced airway hyperresponsiveness in sheep. *Am J Respir Crit Care Med* 1995;151:A563(Abstr).

128. Christiansen SC, Proud D, Cochrane CG. Detection of tissue kallikrein in the bronchoalveolar lavage fluid of asthmatic subjects. *J Clin Invest* 1987;79:188–197.

129. Christiansen SC, Zuraw BL, Proud D, Cochrane CG. Inhibition of human bronchial kallikrein in asthma. *Am Rev Respir Dis* 1989;139:1125–1131.

Asthma, edited by P.J. Barnes, M.M. Grunstein,
A.R. Leff, and A.J. Woolcock.
Lippincott–Raven Publishers, Philadelphia © 1997.

▪ 48 ▪

Complement Fragments

Norma P. Gerard

Activation of complement is one of the first lines of defense against foreign organisms and substances (1). The complement system consists of more than 16 characterized serum protein components that interact in cascade fashion, analogous to coagulation, generating a multitude of biologically active products whose targets are both local (membrane attack complex) and systemic (anaphylatoxins, products of C3b) (2). Because of the participation of complement in inflammatory reactions in the lung as well as other organs, its role in developing pathophysiological responses, including asthma, has been the subject of considerable research. Indeed, early studies of *in vivo* responses to complement in experimental animals demonstrated release of histamine in guinea pigs following injection of activated serum, with the greatest amount being released from the lung (3–5). Many target cells are activated by complement, responding with release of additional mediators, and activation of intracellular signalling pathways. These activities, in concert with the opsonic function of C3b and the lytic action of the membrane attack complex (MAC), result in effective clearance of foreign molecules and cells, as well as modulation of the immune response (reviewed in 6,7).

THE COMPLEMENT ACTIVATION PATHWAYS

Like the coagulation cascade, complement activation through either the classical or alternative pathway involves multiple proteolytic and molecular association events. Classical pathway activation is initiated by immune complexes containing particular complement-fixing antibodies (immunoglobulins (Ig)G or M), or independently of antibodies, by mitochondrial membranes, deoxyribonucleic acid (DNA), C-reactive protein, or particular viruses (Fig. 1) (8–17). Interaction of C1 with immune complexes containing IgG or IgM results in a conformational change in this heterotrimer that confers proteolytic activity with specificity for the fourth and second components of complement (C4 and C2, respectively) (18,19). C1 cleaves them to release the soluble peptides, C4a and C2b, and allows for association of C4b and C2a (C4b2a) (20,21). This complex creates a new protease, C3 convertase, that cleaves the third component of complement, C3, releasing a ~7kDa peptide, the C3a anaphylatoxin, and leaving C3b. C3b then associates with C4b2a to make C4b2a3b, or C5 convertase (22–25). The action of C5 convertase results in generation of the low-molecular-weight C5a anaphylatoxin and C5b, promoting its association with C6, C7, C8, and C9, to form the MAC (25,26).

Activation through alternative pathway is initiated by the recognition by C3 of relatively nonspecific foreign substances, generally weak nucleophiles contained in certain microbial polysaccharides (2,27) (Fig. 2). Hydrolysis

N.P. Gerard: Department of Medicine, Beth Israel Hospital, Harvard Medical School, Boston, Massachusetts 02215.

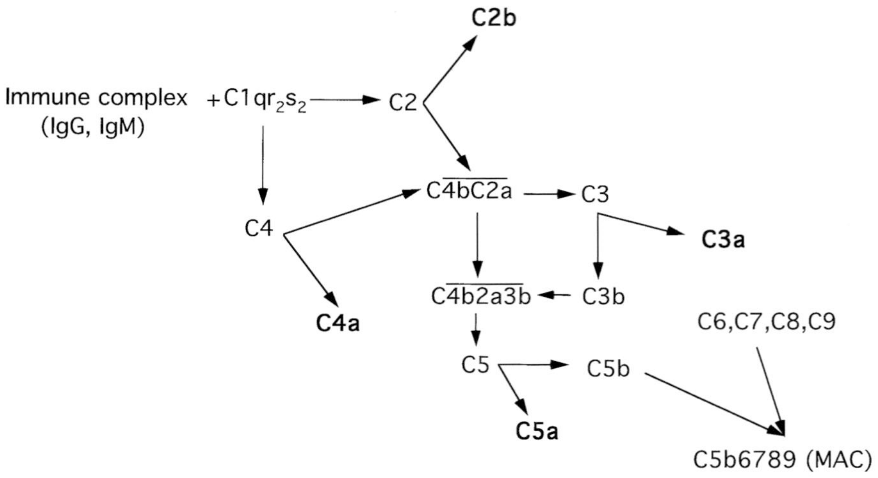

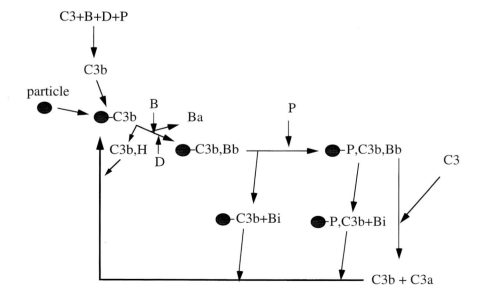

Fig. 1. Classical pathway of complement activation. Complexes of antigen with IgG or IgM bind C1, causing a conformational change which activates it to a protease with specificity for C4 and C2, generating the biologically active products C4a and C2b. C4b and C2a associate to form C3 convertase (C4b2a), cleaving C3 to C3a anaphylatoxin and C3b. C3b joins C4b2a to make C5 convertase (C4b2a3b). Cleavage of C5 releases the C5a anaphylatoxin, and C5b promotes association with C6, C7, C8, and C9 to form the membrane attack complex (MAC).

of an internal thiolester in this protein promotes association of factor B to form a C3 convertase, C3b,Bb, and, with the stabilizing action of properdin, this complex functions essentially identically to the C3 convertase generated by association of C4b and C2a in classical pathway activation (28–30). Addition of a second C3b molecule to the complex consisting of the activating surface, C3b,Bb and properdin, converts it to a C5 convertase capable of releasing C5a anaphylatoxin. At this step (formation of C5 convertase), the two pathways converge to generate the MAC, which inserts itself spontaneously to form a lytic pore or hole in the offending cell or organism. With either pathway, activation of complement involves amplification due to the enzymatic nature of the early steps of the cascade, making the system exquisitely sensitive to foreign perturbation for host defense.

BIOLOGY OF THE COMPLEMENT ACTIVATION PRODUCTS

Anaphylatoxins

Complement activation by either alternative or classical pathways is associated with the proteolytic generation of low-molecular-weight products with biological actions distinct from that of the MAC (reviewed in 31). These are listed in Table 1 along with some of their characteristic properties. Biochemical characterization of the anaphylatoxins, C3a, C4a, and C5a during the 1970s shows they are peptides of 74 to 77 amino acids, that are structurally stabilized by formation of intramolecular disulfide bonds (24,31). The biological activity of these peptides *in vivo* is primarily regulated by the action of serum carboxypep-

Fig. 2. Alternative pathway of complement activation. Physiological activation of the alternative pathway is initiated by binding of C3b (constitutively generated by interaction of C3 with factor B, factor D and properdin in the fluid phase) to an activating particle (e.g., bacterial wall polysaccharide), permitting association of factor B, and stabilization by properdin in competition with inactivation by factor H. Particle-bound C3b, Bb, properdin acts as a C3 convertase, generating more C3b and C3a to amplify the pathway.

Table 1. *Biologically Active Products of Complement Activation*

Product	Source	Molecular weight	Activity
C5a	C5	~7,000	Smooth muscle contraction, vascular leak, activation of PMNs, eosinophils, mast cells, macrophages, basophils, upregulation of CR3 (CD11b/CD18)
C3a	C3	~7,000	Smooth muscle contraction, vascular leak, PMN, eosinophil activation
C4a	C4	~7,000	Smooth muscle contraction, vascular leak
C2b	C2	~4,000	Smooth muscle contraction, vascular leak
iC3b, C3dg, C3d	C3	~180,000	Initiation of the primary immune response
iC5b67	C5, C6, C7	~400,000	Inhibitor of chemotaxis

tidase through removal of critical C-terminal arginine residues. In humans C5a removal of arginine 74 reduces its activity for smooth muscle contraction ~1000-fold, with 20- to 100-fold reduction in neutrophil chemotactic potential. In other species, particularly porcine, the effects of C-terminal arginine removal are less profound and complicated by the presence or absence of carbohydrate residues (32). Serum carboxypeptidase action on C3a and C4a appears to completely abrogate smooth muscle contractile activity, although C3a des Arg modulates expression of cytokines with equal potency as C3a (33,34).

Animal models designed to investigate the role of complement activation in disease demonstrate potentially adverse proinflammatory effects of anaphylatoxin generation in virtually every organ system (35–101). In the lung, anaphylatoxin generation has been associated with airway hyperresponsiveness following sinusitis, allergic asthma, chronic airway disease, idiopathic pulmonary fibrosis, chronic obstructive pulmonary disease, cystic fibrosis, influenza infection, endotoxin shock, and adult respiratory distress syndrome (35–48,102,103). Mechanistically, the common scenario underlying each clinical condition is infiltration of leukocytes, edema formation, and activation of the leukocytes for release of granule enzymes and toxic oxygen metabolites, and resultant tissue destruction.

C5a

As the inflammatory response is considered to include margination and infiltration of leukocytes, release of granule-bound proteolytic enzymes and activated oxygen- and nitrogen-derived radicals, changes in blood flow, increased vascular permeability, and contraction of smooth muscle, C5a is capable of all these functions. Thus, the C5a anaphylatoxin is a complete pro-inflammatory molecule. At subnanomolar to nanomolar levels, C5a elicits chemotaxis of all myeloid lineages (neutrophils, eosinophils, basophils, macrophages, and monocytes), causes an increase in vascular permeability that is markedly potentiated by prostaglandins and circulating leukocytes, and induces the expression of endothelial adhesion molecules (104–109).

Greater nanomolar concentrations induce release of intracellular granules and activation of NADPH oxidase for the respiratory burst. This breadth of bioactivity is in contrast to other inflammatory mediators. Chemotactic cytokines of the α- and β-chemokine families (interleukin [IL]-8, monocyte chemotactic protein [MCP]-1, RANTES, eotaxin, etc.) are both more selective in the cell types they chemoattract and more limited in their ability to activate signal transduction pathways (110–115). Bacterial formylated peptides (prototypically f-Met-Leu-Phe), leukotriene B_4, and platelet-activating factor have a similar profile of biological actions as C5a, with varying relative potencies on cell and tissue types. Histamine, bradykinin, and the peptidoleukotrienes are relatively potent at vascular and smooth muscle effects, but poor chemoattractants. Thus, under situations where complement is activated, a potent pro-inflammatory mediator is released into the fluid phase with pleiotropic effects.

Since activation of the complement system is considered a protective mechanism, an effect of this nature is demonstrated by comparing the sensitivity of a naturally occurring strain of mice genetically deficient in C5, the precursor for C5a, to lethal infection by *Pseudomonas aeruginosa* with that of wild type animals (116). Mortality was consistently higher in C5-deficient animals following intrapulmonary instillation of live bacteria, and the data indicated that in the absence of C5, the mice were unable to clear the organisms, suggesting a protective role for the protein. Because of the C5 deficiency, however, mice could generate neither C5a anaphylatoxin nor C5b to act as a nidus for assembly of the MAC, and the studies were unable to resolve the relative contribution of each. More recent studies have taken advantage of the ability to genetically manipulate the mouse and delete the C5a-receptor so that only the effects of the C5a-C5a-receptor pair are eliminated (see following).

Complement activation normally is initiated by alternative pathway fixation to bacterial, viral, or fungal surfaces, or by interaction of C1 with immune complexes in the classical pathway. Limited proteolysis of C5 can also yield biologically active C5a-like molecules in the absence of complement activation (117,118). Local synthesis of extravascular C5 also may be a significant source of anaphylatoxin (119,120). Neuroinflammatory C5a may depend on local complement protein production, and/or activation by extracellular protein aggregates such as beta-amyloid (86,87). The inflammatory response of astrocytes and microglia may be mediated by C5a-induced chemotaxis and cellular activation (68,69,121,122). More complex interactions of anaphylatoxins and complement in the immune system are currently under investigation; some may be mediated by C5a-stimulated production of IL-6 (123–125).

C3a

Like C5a, C3a is capable of inducing smooth muscle contraction and increasing vascular permeability (126–130). Threshold concentrations required are ~100-fold greater than for C5a, and the mechanism, at least in the guinea pig lung, appears to depend on the release of cyclooxygenase metabolites, as opposed to histamine and leukotrienes (129). C3a-mediated histamine release in other tissues has also been documented (131). This anaphylatoxin has been shown to act on neutrophils, but its effects are much less well-studied than those of C5a. Early evidence for chemotactic responses to the peptide were controversial, in part because of technical difficulties in obtaining chemically pure peptide, free of contaminating C5a (132). Despite this problem, several early reports indicated specific binding of C3a to polymorphonuclear neutrophils (PMNs), and activation of the cells to aggregate and release lysosomal enzymes (133–135). Current literature documents C3a interacting with a neutrophil receptor, distinct from the C5a-receptor, that is expressed at greatly reduced levels (~20% as many sites/cell) (136). Signalling is pertussis toxin-sensitive, mediates Ca^{++} influx, activation of phospholipase C, and production of reactive oxygen species; but, unlike C5a, C3a appears incapable of activating phosphatidylinositol 3-kinase (137–139). Evidence that C3a activates eosinophils suggested that PMN preparations containing as little as ~2% eosinophils may be responsible for the contradictory findings, since products derived from activated eosinophils are capable of activating the PMNs (140–142).

A new biological role shared by C3a and C3a desArg was recently reported by Takabyashi et al. (34) for regulation of cytokine synthesis in peripheral blood mononuclear cells (PBMC). Both peptides suppressed endotoxin-induced TNF-α and IL-1β in nonadherent PBMC in a concentration-dependent manner. In contrast, the peptides enhanced endotoxin-induced cytokine production in adherent cells, and both C3a and C3a desArg were equally potent. Thus, contributions of C3a (and C3a des-Arg) to inflammatory responses are potential consequences of complement activation in addition to the effects of C5a. The spectrum of target cells appears more limited than those for C5a, although the ~20-fold greater abundance of C3 relative to C5, may result in proportionately more C3a production. Both IL-1 and IL-4 increase the synthesis of C3, suggesting a positive feedback loop in inflammatory reactions (143,144). Also contrasting with C5a, whose activities are merely reduced by the removal of the C-terminal arginine residue by serum carboxypeptidase, removal of this homologous amino acid from C3a results in abrogation of all known functions except the newly described modulation of cytokine production, effectively giving the peptide a relatively short half-life *in vivo* (33).

C4a

The low-molecular-weight product of C4 cleavage, C4a, is also capable of inducing local erythema following intradermal injection and smooth muscle contraction on isolated tissues (130,145). Pharmacologically, it appears to interact with a receptor that is distinct from those for C3a and C5a (130,145). However, because its potency is roughly 1000-fold lower than C5a, the physiological relevence for inflammation of C4a release as an independent molecule is questionable.

C2 Kinin (C2b)

C2b

Hereditary angioneurotic edema is characterized by an acute noninflammatory, nonpainful edema of the skin and mucosa and is associated with a deficiency in the inhibitor of the first component of complement, C1INH (146–150). The resulting unregulated proteolytic activity of C1 leads to cleavage of C2 and C4. Further cleavage of C2 by plasmin can then release a 38 amino-acid peptide, C2b, or C2 kinin, that enhances permeability of postcapillary venules (147,149) (Table 1). A synthetic peptide corresponding to the C-terminal 17 amino acids of C2b appears to embody C2-kinin activity, since it also causes increased permeability in human and guinea pig skin and smooth muscle contraction in rat uterus and guinea pig lung (151–153). Pharmacologically, the C2b-receptor is distinct from the anaphylatoxin receptors since its responses are independent of histamine and prostanoids. Although the 17 residue peptide required relatively high concentrations (mM) to demonstrate activity, longer peptides were more active, and likely more closely approximate the physiological entity responsible for the pathophysiological consequences of angioedema (153).

Products of C3b

As described earlier, C3b binds through an internal thioester to weak nucleophiles as are found on polysaccharides commonly displayed on the surface of microorganisms. In this form, it can either interact with the alternative pathway components as shown in Figure 2, or it can interact with its receptor, complement receptor 1 (CR1) found on B lymphocytes, macrophages, and follicular dendritic cells (154,155) (Table 1). There, C3b is inactivated by factor I, a protease that cleaves it sequentially to iC3b and C3dg (156,157). These products bind complement receptor 2, CR2, on mature B cells, a subpopulation of T cells and follicular dendritic cells (158). C3dg can be cleaved further by enzymes like plasmin to generate C3d, which also interacts with CR2, and C3g. The interaction of iC3b, C3dg, and/or C3d with CR2 in the context of CD19 and TAPA-1 on B lymphocytes has been demonstrated to enhance the primary immune response (reviewed in 159). iC3b bound to activating surfaces also interacts with CR3, the neutrophil integrin consisting of CD11b/CD18 (135,160).

Intermediates in the Membrane Attack Complex

Although not strictly a "fragment" generated during activation of complement, the hemolytically inactive terminal complex component iC5b67, consisting of C5b, C6, and C7 has been shown to stimulate responses in neutrophils. This complex occurs upon fluid phase decay of hemolytically active C5b67 to an inactive form, and has the ability to induce chemotaxis that is sensitive to pertussis toxin, causes Ca^{++} flux, and inhibits C5a and f-Met-Leu-Phe-induced superoxide production (161,162). Hemolytically active C5b67 can interact directly with intracellular G proteins through its ability to insert in the cell membrane (163). By contrast, transfection experiments in COS cells demonstrate that iC5b67 does not interact directly with G proteins, nor does it inhibit C5a-mediated signal transduction (162). These data support the proposal that iC5b67 interacts with a distinct receptor on neutrophils, signalling with a potentially anti-inflammatory effect, which may contribute to the resolution of the acute inflammatory response (162).

RECEPTORS FOR THE COMPLEMENT FRAGMENTS

C5a-Receptor

Early studies established the presence of a high-affinity receptor for C5a on PMN leukocytes, with a Kd of ~1 nM, and relatively abundant expression of 100,000 to 200,000 sites per cell (164–166). Through the use of bifunctional crosslinking agents, [^{125}I]-labeled C5a was covalently bound to its receptor in PMN membranes, and SDS polyacrylamide gel electrophoresis identified a predominant molecular species at ~52kDa. Correcting for

the contribution of the ligand indicated the C5a-receptor molecular weight was ~42kDa (167–171). Human eosinophils also express a form of the C5a-receptor that exists in both high (Kd ~30 pM; 15,000 sites/cell) and low-affinity states (Kd ~100 nM; 375,000 sites/cell) (171). This receptor, crosslinked to [^{125}I]-labeled C5a also appears to have a higher molecular weight than the PMN receptor, suggesting the potential for C5a-receptor subtypes. Pharmacological studies indicate that the product of serum carboxypeptidase action on C5a, C5a$_{des Arg}$, should also interact with the C5a-receptor (32). Characterization of this ligand receptor interaction is complex, however, and limited data available indicate that C5a$_{des Arg}$ modulates binding to the receptor in a manner distinct from that of C5a (172).

Molecular cloning of the C5a-receptor from a U937 cell complementary DNA (cDNA) library indicates that it is a member of the seven transmembrane-segment superfamily of G-protein coupled receptors (173,174). Following transfection into COS or HEK293 cells, the cloned C5a-receptor cDNA expresses binding sites for C5a with a Kd of ~1nM. The deduced amino-acid sequence has ~34% homology with the f-Met-Leu-Phe receptor (175). Initial structure function studies of the C5a ligand indicated two discrete regions of the peptide that are required for high-affinity binding and potent signal transduction (reviewed in 125). The conformation of the ligand imposed by the critical disulfide bonds provides a core domain essential for high-affinity binding. Chemical and exopeptidase cleavages also demonstrate that the ligand C-terminal region encodes the receptor activating sequence, Met-Gln-Leu-Gly-Arg (176,177). Further studies using site-directed mutagenesis identified distinct receptor contact points within the ligand N-terminal region and the disulfide core (178).

Mirroring the duality of ligand interaction sites, evidence for distinct binding and activation sites in the C5a-receptor has been derived from mutagenesis and monoclonal antibody studies. The extracellular N-terminal region of the receptor provides one domain required for high affiinity ligand interaction, or "docking" (179–182). Interaction with a monoclonal anti-peptide antibody raised against the N-terminal sequence completely blocks ligand binding and activation (179). Treatment with a spider venom metalloproteinse indicates that specific celavage of the receptor blocks binding of intact C5a, but not C-terminal C5a analogs, further supporting the predicted existence of a second interaction site (182). Similarly, the alpha chemokines IL-8 and melanocyte growth-stimulating activity (MGSA)/Groα also recognize acidic N-terminal receptor sequences, and the selectivity for ligand binding can be switched by constructing chimeric receptors in which the N-terminal domains are switched (183,184). Site-directed mutagenesis of the human C5a-receptor additionally identify cysteine residues within transmembrane sequences four and five (TM4 and TM5) as involved in binding and signal transduction, and suggest it is an important interaction site with the ligand C-terminus (185). In addition, the relative orientation of the transmembrane domains appears important for maintainence of ligand binding, not only for the C5a-receptor, but for other members of this receptor family. Mutation of a leucine residue to proline in the third extracellular loop completely blocked ligand binding with no effect on expression of the receptor (185).

The C5a-receptor is encoded by a single copy gene with an unusual organization (173,186). The genes for most other members of the seven transmembrane segment G protein coupled receptor superfamily are typically intronless, although exceptions exist, as in the tachykinin receptors (187–190). An intron of ~9 kb separates the initiating methionine codon of the C5a-receptor gene from the exon (exon 2) containing the remainder of the receptor coding sequence. Approximately 35 bp of 5'-untranslated sequence and the Met-1 codon comprise exon 1. The 5'-flanking sequence appears to contain a promoter, several regulatory motifs, and a silencing element(s) which may regulate gene expression, similar to the NADPH-oxidase gp97phox (186,191). Although this genomic organization is unusual among the majority of seven transmembrane segment G-protein coupled receptors, it appears to be common to other leukocyte receptors, including those for interleukin 8, platelet activating factor, and f-Met-Leu-Phe (192–196). The significance of this organization is unclear at present, but may reflect a common genomic structure that regulates receptor expression in leukocytes. Receptor subtypes such as demonstrated on the human eosinophil may result either from post-translational modification (e.g., cell type-specific glycosylation) or potentially from alternative splicing of exon 1 (171). [Alternatively spliced variant cDNAs have not been identified, NP Gerard, C Gerard, unpublished.] Interestingly, the C5a-receptor gene was localized to human chromosome 19q13.3-13.4 along with the f-Met-Leu-Phe receptor and two f-Met-Leu-Phe receptor homologues, suggesting they may have evolved by gene duplication (192). One of the f-Met-Leu-Phe receptors has been claimed as a lipoxin receptor, although independent confirmation of this finding is wanting (197).

Targeted disruption of the murine C5a-receptor gene provides selective elimination of C5a-C5a receptor interactions (198,199). In models of immune complex injury in the lung, elimination of the anaphylatoxin receptor was protective (199). Homozygous C5a-receptor deficient mice had fewer BAL neutrophils and reduced vascular permeability compared with C5a-receptor sufficient littermates. In contrast, the same C5a-receptor deficient mice infected by intrapulmnoary instillation with Pseudomonas aeruginosa were much more sensitive than C5a-receptor sufficient littermates (198). The lethality following administration of 3×10^7 bacteria within 48 h

was >90% for the C5a-receptor deficient animals, compared with less than 10% for wild type mice. Although sensitive mice do not become septic, quantitation of the organisms recovered from the lungs indicates they continue to multiply. The data suggest that, at least in the lung, phagocytic cells require anaphylatoxin activation in order to clear such organisms. The analogy with cystic fibrosis patients who develop airway colonization by pseudomonas is striking; while they are not genetically deficient in C5a- or C5a-receptor, they appear functionally deficient (198).

C3a-Receptor

Based on the pertussis toxin sensitivity of cellular responses to C3a, it was predicted that its receptor should also be a member of the seven transmembrane segment G-protein coupled family of receptors (137–139). On guinea pig platelets, Scatchard analyses indicate high- and low-affinity binding sites with K_d's of 1.7 and 10 nM, respectively (136). On human PMNs, a single receptor class is observed, with an affinity of 30 nM. Crosslinking experiments using [^{125}I]-labeled guinea pig C3a and guinea pig platelets, identified three specific proteins of apparent molecular weights in the range of 83-103kDa (136). The analogous experiment performed using the human peptide on human PMNs did not identify a specific protein, potentially because of the reduced affinity on this cell type.

Crass et al. (200) used expression cloning to identify a cDNA encoding a functional C3a-receptor from dibutyryl-cAMP differentiated U937 cells. The same cDNA, designated AZ3B, was previously cloned by homology to the f-Met-Leu-Phe receptor and reported as an orphan receptor (201). Its deduced amino-acid sequence has 37% sequence identity to the C5a-receptor, with the unusual feature of a large second extracellular loop structure of 172 amino acids (the C5a-receptor has a 32 amino-acid second extracellular loop). Independent work demonstrates the ability of C5a to signal at this receptor when expressed in Xenopus oocytes, however, ligand binding studies did not corroborate this function (202). Although this work is still relatively preliminary, data indicate that the C3a- receptor is now molecularly characterized.

Receptors for C4a and C2b

As discussed previously, pharmacological analyses using desensitization studies indicate that both C4a and C2b have receptors that are distinct from those for C3a and C5a (130,153). Characterization of these proteins has apparently not been pursued since the impotence of the peptides (at least for smooth muscle contraction) suggests their affinities are low enough to preclude the use of standard techniques.

CR1

Like other regulators of complement activation (RCA) that target the C3 and C5 convertases, CR1 (CD35) is encoded on human chromosome 1 at q32. It is a single membrane-spanning protein with a relatively wide cell type distribution including erythrocytes, neutrophils, monocytes, macrophages, eosinophils, B lymphocytes, follicular dendritic cells, glomerular podocytes, Kupfer cells, Schwann cells, and some T lymphocytes (154,155,157). Also characteristic of the other members of the RCA complex, the extracellular domain of CR1 is composed of a series of short consensus repeats (SCR) of 60 to 70 amino acids, has a hydrophobic transmembrane sequence, and short cytoplasmic tail. The SCR domain contains distinct binding sites for one C4b and two C3b molecules, and serves as a cofactor for the serine protease, factor I, inactivating them to iC4b, iC3b, and C3dg (203,204). Thus, CR1 interrupts both the classical and alternative pathways of complement activation by interfering with formation of the C3 and C5 convertases. Allotypic variations in this protein, in which several SCRs are deleted, are associated with lupus and may result from a loss of the ability to bind immune complexes coated with complement fragments (205).

Because of its potency in inhibiting both complement activation pathways, CR1 was targeted as a potential theraputic agent. The cDNA encoding CR1 was modified by mutagenesis to delete the membrane spanning and cytoplasmic sequences, and used to make a recombinant soluble form of CR1, sCR1 (156,206). In experimental models of immune complex injury in the rat, sCR1 was shown to reduce alveolitis and vasculitis by as much as 70%. Cardiac allograft and xenograft rejection was delayed as much as 10-fold, depending on the dose of CR1. Nonantibody-mediated complement injury was also blocked by sCR1 in models of ischemia/referfusion injury and ARDS caused by thermal trauma. The use of complement-blocking substances like sCR1 may, therefore, have great value in certain clinical settings, particularly in organ transplantation.

CR2

Interaction of C3b with CR1 and factor I initiates another important function of the complement system: activation of the primary immune response. Like CR1, CR2 (CD21) derives from the RCA locus of chromosome 1 and consists of extracellular SCR units, a single membrane-spanning domain, and short cytoplasmic tail. Expressed on B lymphocytes, CR2 functions analogously to the T-cell receptor on T lymphocytes by reducing the threshold for antigen receptor stimulation. CR2 interacts with iC3b, C3dg and C3d, to which complement-activating molecules are bound via the internal thioester (155). CR2 also binds Epstein-Barr virus via the major viral envelope protein, gp350/220, and this interaction allows the virus particle to enter the cell. A short region of sequence homology between C3b and gp350/220 is responsible for viral interaction with CR2, and is an example of molecular mimicry frequently encountered in pathogens (155,158).

In the presence of membrane immunoglobulin (mIg), ligation of CR2 initiates signal transduction in B lymphocytes through an increase in $[Ca^{++}]_i$, activation of phospholipase C, phosphatidylinositol 3-kinase, tyrosine kinases, and DNA synthesis (reviewed in 159). Activation of the membrane-bound complex consisting of CR2, CD19 and TAPA-1 results in synergistic activation of the B cell signal transduction pathway, ultimately leading to clonal proliferation and antibody production (207). B cells stimulated with anti-IgM and anti-CD19 incorporated ^{3}H-thymidine into DNA with a threshold at 100-fold lower concentration, compared with cells stimulated with anti-IgM and irrelevant control antibody. Complement activation and C3b binding to the foreign surface, through interaction with CR2, mediates B cell activation in a mechanism that provides for greatly increased sensitivity for antibody production (159,207).

CR3

CR3 is a heterodimer of the single membrane spanning proteins, CD11b and CD18, and functions as a leukocyte integrin. CR3 binds iC3b attached to complement-activating surfaces, in addition to recognizing substances like zymosan, β-glucans, E. coli, and fibrinogen. In cooperation with Fcγ-receptors, CR3 triggers production of leukotriene B$_4$ and platelet-activating factor, and stimulates antibody-dependent phagocytosis, chemotaxis, activation of the respiratory burst, and tyrosine phosphorylation of the cytoskeletal protein paxillin (160,208,209). Indeed, CR3, through the function of its cytoplasmic domains, appears to be utilized by proteins like Fcγ- receptors that are anchored to the cell membrane by glycosylphosphatidylinositol linkages as a mechanism to mediate intracellular functions (210).

CR3 also communicates with receptors for chemotactic molecules including C5a, f-Met-Leu-Phe, and α-chemokines like IL-8, since interaction with their ligands causes profound upregulation of the integrin's expression on the neutrophil surface (160). Indeed, this function is often considered the first step of the inflammatory response, in which the chemoattractant-activated neutrophils begin to adhere to the endothelium through increased expression of CR3, slowing them in preparation for migration into extravascular spaces.

COMPLEMENT ACTIVATION IN ASTHMA

The T lymphocyte and eosinophil have become dominant themes in recent studies on the pathophysiology of asthma. While atopic mechanisms are clearly relevant in many asthmatic phenotypes, the root causes of the underlying chronic inflammation found in all forms of reactive airways disease remain unclear. In addition to eosinophils and lymphocytes, neutrophils have also been observed in asthmatic airways (211). There may be multiple redundant pathways leading to the underlying inflammatory events in asthma, of which atopy is a significant but nonexclusive subset.

Because of the proinflammatory and immunological consequences of complement activation, it is attractive to invoke this system in association with asthma. Numerous reports document activation of complement in this condition, and it is almost certainly involved (211–217). However, given the complexity and redundancy of the inflammatory response, the actual role of the complement proteins in the pathophysiologic findings associated with asthma remain somewhat difficult to sort out. Historically, measurement of complement activation relied on consumption of plasma C3, a relatively insensitive indicator. As described earlier, the advent of more sensitive methods, e.g., specific ELISAs and radioimmunoassays for activation products, $C5a/C5a_{desArg}$ or $C3a/C3a_{desArg}$, have provided a more representative picture of complement association in disease (222–225). Several studies provide examples of relevant findings. In one study, it was found that short-term exercise was associated with classical pathway activation (212). Both normal and asthmatic subjects had elevated C3a and C4a levels compared with nonexercising controls. Baseline levels of C3 and C4 were decreased significantly in runners relative to nonexercising controls, suggesting that regular aerobic exercise results in downregulation of complement protein production (212). Another study assessed two indices of complement activation, C3d and the C3d/C3 ratio in 73 adults (213). Asthmatics had significantly higher C3d and C3d/C3 levels compared with normals, and a subset additionally had decreased plasma C4, suggesting classical pathway activation. These findings are supported by Van de Graaf et al. (214), who reported more than twofold higher levels of C3a in bronchoalveolar lavage (BAL) fluid from asthmatic subjects, and compared with normals or patients infected with pneumocystis. The T-cell cytokine IL-4 has been shown to enhance the production of C3 by as much as fivefold in the human type II pneumocyte A549 cell line; this supports a cooperative role for T cells in complement production, as well as inflammatory disease (143).

Measurement of C3 levels in BAL fluid 6 h after challenge with antigen or diluent control, demonstrated no significant change in seven patients with antigen-induced single early reactions or in seven patients with dual (early and late phase) reactions (211). The percentage of monocyte complement rosettes increased significantly in late-phase responders, but not in early-phase responders. Unfortunately, changes in C3 levels may be so small as to be undetected in signal-to-noise ratios; monocyte complement rosettes are likely a more sensitive reflection of complement activation. Grassi et al. (215) additionally measured normal baseline levels of C3 and C4 in 32 atopic patients with rhinitis, asthma, or rhinitis and asthma; serum IgE concentrations were greater than in controls.

Arm et al. (216) demonstrated that neutrophils from patients following experimentally provoked asthma demonstrate increased complement receptor activity as measured by rosetting of C3b-coated erythrocytes. Maximal increases in granulocyte CR1 and CR3 of 28.2±7.5 and 33.4±9.5%, respectively, were observed at 3h after asthma induced by antigen. CR1, but not CR3, was elevated 32.0±7.3% at 1h after exercise-induced asthma. A similar increase in CR1 was observed following histamine challenge in asthmatic subjects with no change in CR3. These data suggest increased expression of CR1 on granulocytes following experimental provocation of asthma. Expression of granulocyte CR3 is also increased after bronchoprovocation with antigen, but not with histamine or exercise (216). Lundahl et al. (217) also observed significantly higher expression of CR1 in asthmatics compared with controls, as well as greater variability in expression. Additional data support a role for complement activation in bronchial asthma, and find no differences in allele frequencies for C3, or deficiencies in the complement regulatory proteins, C1 inhibitor, factor H, or factor I (218).

Given the immune and inflammatory processes associated with asthma, a role for complement activation fragments remains to be excluded. Exposure by inhalation to a complement-activating substance results in alternative pathway activation, or, in the presence of existing complement fixing antibodies, classical pathway activation. Formation of C3 and C5 convertases releases the anaphylatoxins C3a and C5a. Their pro-inflammatory activities cause mast cell activation with release of histamine, leukotrienes, platelet-activating factor, and other substances capable of bronchospasm and edema formation. C5a and, potentially, C3a elicit the influx of PMNs and eosinophils through chemotactic activity, upregulating expression of CR3 (CD11b/CD18). These cells release granule enzymes and toxic oxygen products that cause relatively indiscriminate tissue destruction. C3b formed during alternative pathway activation, besides participating in C5 convertase to make anaphylatoxin, C5b and the MAC, presents the foreign agent to B cells via CR2 and initiates a primary immune response. Involvement of chemokines and cytokines in these processes may additionally contribute to the cellular influx and airway hyperresponsiveness associated with asthma.

CONCLUSIONS

Overwhelming evidence indicates activation of complement in inflammatory diseases of the airways, including asthma. The biological profiles of complement fragments, particulary the C5a anaphylatoxin, are consistent with contributing to the pathophysiology of disease. While the absence of antagonists precludes evaluation of complement activation in humans, animal models, including targeted deletion of the C5a-receptor gene in mice, leave no question as to the role of this molecule in host defense. Additional products of complement activation, the C3a anaphylatoxin and the hemolytically inactive C5b67 complex, additionally possess anti-inflammatory properties, reflecting the homeostatic function of the complement system.

REFERENCES

1. Osler AG, Hawrisiak MM, Ovary Z, Siqueria M, and Bier OG. Studies on the mechanisms of hypersensitivity phenomena. II. The participation of complement in passive cutaneous anaphylaxis of the albino rat. *J Exp Med* 1957;106:811–834.
2. Muller-Eberhard HJ. Molecular organization and function of the complement system. *Annu Rev Biochem* 1988;57:321–347.
3. Hahn F, Oberdorf A. Antihistaminica and anaphylaktoid reaktionen. *Z Immunitaetsforsch Exp Ther* 1950;107:528–538.
4. Hahn F. Zur anaphylatoxinfrge. *Naturwissenshaften (Berlin)* 1954;41:465–470.
5. Hahn F. Anaphylatoxin, actions and role of anaphylaxis. In: Schacter M., ed. *Polypeptides which affect smooth muscles and blood vessels. Proc Symp* Bristol: Permagon Press, 1960;275–292.
6. Perlmutter DH, Strunk RC, and Colten HR. Complement. In: Crystal RG, West JB, et al., eds. *The lung: scientific foundations.* New York: Raven Press, 1991;511–525.
7. Muller-Eberhard HJ. The membrane attack complex of complement. *Ann Rev Immunol* 1986;4:503–528.
8. Burton DR, Boyd J. Brampton AD, Easterbrook-Smith SB, Emanuel EJ, Novotny J, Rademacher TW, van Schravendijk MR, Sternberg MJ, and Dwek AA. The C1q receptor site on immunoglobulin G. *Nature* 1980;288:338–343.
9. Hurst MM, Volanakis JE, Hester RB. The structural basis for for binding of complement by immunoglobulin *M J Exp Med* 1974;140:1117–1121.
10. Pinckard RN, O'Rourke RA, Crawford MH, et al. Complement localization and mediation of ischemic injury in baboon myocardium. *J Clin Invest* 1980;66:1050–1056.
11. Storrs SB, Kolb WP, Pinckard RN, and Olson MS. Characterization of the binding of purified human C1q to heart mitochondrial membranes. *J Biol Chem* 1981;256:10924–10929.
12. Welsh RM, Cooper NR, Jensem FC, and Oldstone MBA. Human serum lyses RNA tumor viruses. *Nature* 1975;257:612–614.
13. Cooper NR, Jensen FC, Welsh RM, and Oldstone MBA. Lysis of RNA tumor viruses by human serum: direct antibody-independent triggeringof the classical complement pathway. *J Exp Med* 1976;144:970–984.
14. Bartholemew RM, Esser AF. Mechanism of antibody-independent activation of the first component of complement (C1) on retroviral membranes. *Biochemistry* 1980;19:2847–2853.
15. Bartholomew RM, Esser AF, Muller-Eberhard HJ. Lysis of oncornaviruses by human serum. Isolation of the viral complement (C1) receptor and identification as p15E. *J Exp Med* 1978;147:844–853.
16. Kaplan MH, Volanakis JE. Interaction of C-reactive protein complexes with the complement system. I. Consumption of human complement associated with the reaction of C-reactive protein with pneumococcal C-polysaccharide and with choline phosphatides, lecithin and sphingomyelin. *J Immunol* 1974;112:2135–2147.
17. Richards RL, Gewurz H, Osmand AP, and Alving CR. Interactions of C-reactive protein and complement with liposomes. *Proc Natl Acad Sci U S A* 1977;74:5672–5676.
18. Colomb MG, Arlaud GJ, Villers CL. Activation of C1. *Philos Trans R Soc Lond* 1984;140:283–292.
19. Schumaker VN, Zavodszky P, Poon PH. Activation of the first component of complement. *Ann Rev Immunol* 1987;5:21–42.
20. Campbell RD, Dodds AW, Porter RR. The binding of human complement component C4 to antibody-antigen aggregates. *Biochem J* 1980;189:67–80.
21. Cooper NR. Enzymatic acitivty of the second component of complement. *Biochemistry* 1975;14:4245–4251.
22. Jensen JA. Anaphylatoxin in its relation to the complement system. *Science* 1967;155:1122–1123.
23. Lepow IH, Dias da Silva W, Eisele JW. Nature and biological properties of human anaphylatoxin. In: Austen KF, Becker EL, eds. *Biochemistry of the acute allergic reactions.* Oxford: Blackwell, 1968;265–282.
24. Hugli TE. Human anaphylatoxin (C3a) from the third component of complement. *J Biol Chem* 1975;250:8293–8301.
25. Hugli TE. Biochemistry and biology of anaphylatoxins. *Complement* 1986;3:111–127.
26. Bhakdi S, Tranum-Jensen J. Membrane damage by complement. *Biochim Biophys Acta* 1983;737:343–372.
27. Lachmann PJ, Thompson RA. Reactive lysis: The complement-mediated lysis of unsensitized cells. II. The characterization of activated reactor as C56 and the participtation of C8 and C9. *J Exp Med* 1970;131:643–657.
28. Thomas ML, Janatova J, Gray WR, Tack BF. Third component of human complement: localization of the internal thiolester bond. *Proc Natl Acad Sci U S A* 1982;79:1054–1058.
29. Hall RE, Blaese RM, Davis AE III, Decker JM, Tack BF, and Colten HR. Cooperative interaction of factor B and other complement components with mononuclear cells in the antibody-independent lysis of xenogeneic erythrocytes. *J Exp Med* 1982;156:834–843.
30. Pangburn MK. The alternative pathway. In: Ross GD, ed. *Immunobiology of the complement system.* New York: Academic Press, 1986;45–62.
31. Hugli TE. The structural basis for anaphylatoxin and chemotactic functions of C3a, C4a, and C5a. *Crit Rev Immunol* 1981;4:321–366.
32. Gerard C, Hugli TE. Identification of the classical anaphylatoxin as the des-Arg form of the C5a molecule: evidence of a modular role for the oligosaccharide unit in human des-Arg 74-C5a. *Proc Natl Acad Sci USA* 1978;78:1833–1837.
33. Stimler NP, Brocklehurst WE, Bloor CM, Hugli TE. Anaphylatoxin-mediated contraction of guinea pig lung strips: a non-histamine tissue response. *J Immunol* 1981;126:2258–2261.
34. Takabayashi T, Vannier E, Clark BD, Margolis NH, Dinarello CA, Burke JF, Gelfand JA. A new biologic role for C3a and C3a desArg. Regulation of TNF-α and IL-1β synthesis. *J Immunol* 1996;156:3455–3460.
35. Corrigan CJ, Kay AB. The roles of inflammatory cells in the pathogenesis of asthma and chronic destructive pulmonary disease. *Am Rev Respir Dis* 1991;143:1165–1168.
36. Brugman SM, Larsen GL, Henson PM, Honor J, and Irvin CG. Increased lower airways responsiveness associated with sinusitis in a rabbit model. *Am Rev Respir Dis* 1993;147:314–320.
37. Irvin CG, Berend N, Henson PM. Airways hyperreactivity and inflammation produced by aerosolization of human C5a des Arg. *Am Rev Respir Dis* 1986;134:777–783.
38. Metcalf JP, Thompson AB, Grossman GL, et al. GC-globulin functions as a co-chemotaxin in the lower respiratory tract. A potential mechanism for lung neutrophil recruitment in cigarette smokers. *Am Rev Respir Dis* 1991;143:844–849.
39. Ozaki T, Hayashi H, Tani K, Ogushi F, Yasuoka S, Ogura T. Neutrophil chemotactic factors in the respiratory tract of patients with airways diseases or idiopathic pulmonary fibrosis. *Am Rev Respir Dis* 1992;145:85–91.
40. Bjornson AB, Mellencamp MA, Schiff GM. Complement is activated in the upper respiratory tract during influenza virus infection. *Am Rev Respir Dis* 1991;143:1064–1066.
41. Barton PA, Warren JS. Complement component C5 modulates the systemic tumor necrosis factor response in murine endotoxic shock. *Infect Immun* 1993;61:1474–1481.
42. Stevens JH, O'Hanley P, Shapiro JM, et al. Effects of anti-C5a antibodies on the adult respiratory distress syndrome in septic primates. *J Clin Invest* 1986;77:1812–1816.
43. Hangen DH, Stevens JH, Satoh PS, Hall EW, O'Hanley PT, Raffin TA. Complement levels in septic primates treated with anti-C5a antibodies. *J Surg Res* 1989;46:195–199.
44. Gardinali M, Padalino P, Vesconi S, et al. Complement activation and

polymorphonuclear neutrohil leukocyte elastase in sepsis. Correlation with severity of disease. *Arch Surg* 1992;127:1219–1224.

45. Gallinaro R, Cheadle WG, Applegate K, Polk HC Jr. The role of the complement system in trauma and infection. *Surg Gynecol Obstet* 1992;174:435–440.

46. Bengtsson A, Redl H, Paul E, Schlag G, Mollnes TE, Davies J. Complement and leukocyte activation in septic baboons. *Circ Shock* 1993; 39:83–88.

47. Zilow G, Joka T, Obertacke U, Rother U, Kirshfink M. Generation of anaphylatoxin C3a in plasma and bronchoalveolar lavage fluid in trauma patients at risk for the adult respiratory distress syndrome. *Crit Care Med* 1992;20:468–473.

48. Langlois PF, Gawryl MS, Zeller J, Lint T. Accentuated complement activation in patient plasma during the adult respiratory distress syndrome: a potential mechanism for pulmonary inflammation. *Heart Lung* 1989;18:71–84.

49. Pemberton M, Anderson G, Vetvicka V, Justus DE, Ross GD. Microvascular effects of complement blockade with soluble recombinant CR1 on ischemia/reperfusion injury of skeletal muscle. *J Immunol* 1993;150:5104–5113.

50. Lindsay TF, Hill J, Ortiz F, et al. Blockade of complement activation prevents local and pulmonary albumin leak after lower torso ischemia-reperfusion. *Ann Surg* 1992;46:47–57.

51. Tomasdottir H, Henriksson BA, Bengston JP, Stenqvist O, Persson H. Complement activation during liver transplantation. *Transplantation* 1993;55:799–802.

52. Mollness TE, Redl H, Hoagsen K, et al. Complement activation in septic baboons detected by neoepitope-specific assays for C3b/IC3b/C3c, C5a and the terminal C5b-9 complement complex (TCC). *Clin Exp Immunol* 1993;91:295–300.

53. Heideman M, Norder-Hansson B, Bengtson A, Mollnes TE. Terminal complement complexes and anaphylatoxin in septic and ischemic patients. *Arch Surg* 1988;123:188–192.

54. Baars JW, Hack CE, Wagstaff J, et al. The activation of polymorphonuclear neutrophils and the complement system during immunotherapy with recombinant interleukin-2. *Br J Cancer* 1992;65:96–101.

55. Chenoweth DE, Cooper SW, Hugli TE, Stewart RW, Blackstone EH, Kerklin JW. Complement activation during cardiopulmonary bypass: evidence for generation of C3a and C5a anaphylatoxins. *N Engl J Med* 1981;304:497–503.

56. Gillinov A, Marc MD, Devaleria PA, et al. Complement inhibition with soluble complement receptor type 1 in cardiopulmonary bypass. *Ann Thorac Surg* 1993;55:619–624.

57. Mollnes TE, Videm V, Gotze O, Harboe M, Oppermann M. formation of C5a during cardiopulmonary bypass: inhibition by precoating with heparin. *Ann Thorac Surg* 1991;55:92–97.

58. Moore FD Jr, Warner KG, Assousa S, Valeri CR, Khuri SF. The effects of complement activation during cardiopulmonary bypass. Attenuation by hypothermia, heparin, and hemodilution. *Ann Surg* 1988;216:677–683.

59. Tamiya T, Yamasaki M, Maeo Y, Yamashiro T, Ogoshi S, Fujimoto S. Complement activation in cardiopulmonary bypass, with special reference to anaphylatoxin production in membrane and bubble oxygenator. *Ann Thorac Surg* 1992;46:47–57.

60. Videm V, Fosse E, Mollnes TE, Garred P, Svennevig JL. Time for new concepts about measurement of complement activation by cardiopulmonary bypass? *Ann Thorac Surg* 1992;54:725–731.

61. Ito BR, Roth DM, Chenoweth DE, Lefer AM, Engler RL. Thromboxane is produced in response to intracorony infusions of complement C5a in pigs. Cyclooxygenase blockade does not reduce the myocardial ischemia and leukocyte accumulation. *Circ Res* 1989;65:1220–1232.

62. Crawford MH, Grover FL, Kolb WP, et al. Complement and neutrophil activation in teh pathogenesis of ischemic myocardial injury. *Circulation* 1988;78:1449–1458.

63. Yasuda M, Takeuchi K, Hiruma B, et al. The complement system in ischemic heart disease. *Circ* 1990;81:156–163.

64. Ito BR, Roth DM, Engler RL. Thromboxane A2 and peptidoleukotrienes contribute to the myocardial ischemia and contractile dysfunction in response to intracoronary infusion of complement C5a in pigs. *Circ Res* 1990;66:596–607.

65. Stahl GL, Amsterdam EA, Summons JD, Longhurst JC. Role of thromboxane A2 in the cardiovascular response to intracoronary C5a. *Circ Res* 1990;66:1106–1111.

66. Shandelya AML, Kuppuasamy P, Weisfeldt ML, Zweier JL. Evaluation of the role of polymorphonuclear leukocytes on contractile function in myocardial reperfusion injury. Evidence for plasma-mediated leukocyte activation. *Circulation* 1993;87:536–546.

67. Montalescot G, Drobinski G, Maclouf J, et al. Evaluation of thromboxane production and complement activation during myocardial ischemia in patients with angina pectoris. *Circulation* 1991;84:2054–2062.

68. Martin SE, Chenoweth DE, Engler RL, Roth DM, Longhurst JC. C5a decreases regional coronary blood flow and myocardial function in pigs. Implications for a granulocyte mechanism. *Circ Res* 1988;63:483–491.

69. Dreyer EJ, Michael LH, Nguyen T, et al. Kinetics of C5a release in cardiac lymph of dogs experiencing coronary artery ischemia reperfusion injury. *Circ Res* 1992;71:1518–1524.

70. Engler RL, Roth DM, Del Balzo U, Ito BR. Intracoronary C5a induces myocardial ischemia by mechanisms independent of the neutrophil: Leukocyte filters desensitize the myocardium to C5a. *FASEB J* 1991;5:2983–2991.

71. Del Balzo U, Sakuma I, Levi R. Cardiac dysfunction caused by recombinant human C5a anaphylatoxin: mediation by histamine, adenosine and cyclooxygenase arachidonate metabolites. *J Pharmacol Exp Ther* 1990;253:171–179.

72. Del Balzo U, Polley MJ, Levi R. Cardiac anaphylaxis. Complement activation as an amplification system. *Circ Res* 1989;65:847–857.

73. Mugge A, Heistad DD, Densen P, et al. Activation of leukocytes with complement C5a is associated with prostanoid-dependent constriction of large arteries in atherosclerotic monkeys *in vivo*. *Atherosclerosis* 1992;95:211–222.

74. Platt JL, Damasso AP, Lindman BJ, Ihrcke NS, Bach FH. The role of C5a and antibody in the release of heparan sulfate from endothelial cells. *Eur J Immunol* 1991;21:2887–2890.

75. Marceau F, deBlois D, Laplante C, et al. Contractile effect of the chemotactic factors f-Met-Leu-Phe and C5a on the human isolated umbilical artery. Role of cyclooxygenase products and tissue macrophages. *Circ Res* 1990;67:948–951.

76. Weisman HF, Bartow T, Leppo MK, et al. Soluble human receptor type 1: *in vivo* inhibitor of complement suppressing post-ischemic myocardial inflammation and necrosis. *Science* 1990;249:146–151.

77. Ahrenstedt O, Knutson L, Nilsson-Ekdahl K, Odlind B, Hallgren R. Enhanced local production of complement components in the small intestines of patients with Crohn's disease. *N Engl J Med* 1990;322:1345–1349.

78. Halstensen TS, Das KM, Brandtzaeg P. Epithelial deposits of immunoglobulin G1 and activated complement colocalize with the m(r) 40 kD putative autoantigen in ulcerative colitis. *Gut* 1993;34:650–677.

79. Varade WS, Forristal J, West CD. Patterns of complement activation in idiopathic membranoproliferative glomerulonephritis, types I, II, and III. *Am J Kidney Dis* 1990;16:196–206.

80. Jose PJ, Moss IK, Maini RN, Williams TJ. Measurement of the chemotactic complement fragment C5a in rheumatoid synovial fluids by radioimmunoassay: role of C5a in the acute inflammatory phase. *Ann Rheum Dis* 1990;49:747–752.

81. Abbink JJ, Kamp AM, Nuijens JH, Erenberg AJ, Swaak AJ, Hack CE. Relative contribution of contact and complement activation to inflammatory reactions in arthritic joints. *Ann Rheum Dis* 1992;51:1123–1128.

82. Matzner Y, Ayesh S, Hochner-Celminker D, Ackerman Z, Ferne M. Proposed mechanism of the inflammatory attacks in familial Mediterranean fever. *Arch Intern Med* 1990;140:1289–1291.

83. Schattner A, Hahn T, Israel R. A proposed mechanism of the inflammatory attacks in familial Mediterranean fever. *Arch Intern Med* 1992;142:421.

84. Hopokins P, Belmont HM, Buyon J, Phillips M, Weissman G, Abramson SB. Increased levels of plasma anaphylatoxin in systemic lupus erythematosis predict flares of the disease and may elicit vascular injury in lupus cerebritis. *Arthritis Rheum* 1988;31:632–641.

85. Jarvis JN, Pousak T, Krenz M, Iobidze M, Taylor H. Complement activation and immune complexes in juvenile rheumatoid arthritis. *J Rheumatol* 1993;20:114–117.

86. Rogers J, Cooper NR, Webster S, et al. Complement activation by beta-amyloid in Alzheimer disease. *Proc Natl Acad Sci U S A* 1992;89:10016–10020.

87. Rogers J, Schultz J, Brachova L, et al. Complement activation and beta-amyloid-mediated neurotoxicity in Alzheimer's disease. *Res Immunol* 1992;143:624–630.

88. Davis WD, Brey RL. Antiphospholipid antibodies and complement activation in patients with cerebral ischemia. *Clin Exp Rheumatol* 1992;10:455–460.

89. Williams CA, Berkman A, Cattell WS, Kerper L. Binding specificity and presynaptic action of anaphylatoxin C5a in rat brain. *Brain Behav Immun* 1989;3:28–38.

90. Yamada T, McGeer PL, McCeer EG. Lewy bodies in Parkinson's disease are recognized by antibodies to complement proteins. *Acta Neuropathol (Berl)* 1992;84:100–104.

91. Schur PH. Complement and lupus erythematosus. *Arthritis Rheum* 1982;25:793–798.

92. Porcel JM, Vergani D. Complement and lupus: old concepts and new directions. *Lupus* 1992;1:343–349.

93. Bergh K, Iverson OJ, Lysvand H. Surprisingly high levels of anaphylatoxin C5a des Arg are extractable from psoriatic scales. *Arch Dermatol Res* 1993;285:131–134.

94. Tagami H. The role of complement-derived mediators in inflammatory skin diseases. *Arch Dermatol Res* 1993;284:S2–9.

95. Faccioli LH, Nourshargh S, Moqbel R, et al. The accumulaton of ^{111}In-eosinophils induced by inflammatory mediators *in vivo*. *Immunology* 1991;73:222–227.

96. Swerlick RA, Yancey KB, Lawley TJ. Inflammatory properties of human C5a and C5a des Arg in mast cell-depleted human skin. *J Invest Dermatol* 1989;93:417–422.

97. Lehmann P. Inflammatory properties of human C5a and C5a des Arg in mast cell-depleted human skin. *J Invest Dermatol* 1990;94:499.

98. Lim HW, He D, Esquenazi-Behar S, Yancey KB, Soter NA. C5a, cutaneous mast cells and inflammation: *in vitro* and *in vivo* studies in a murine model. *J Invest Dermatol* 1991;97:305–311.

99. Collins PD, Jose PJ, Williams TJ. The sequential generation of neutrophil chemoattractant proteins in acute inflammation in the rabbit. *In vivo* relationship between C5a and proteins characteristic of IL-8/neutrophil activating protein. *J Immunol* 1991;146:677–684.

100. Vanderpuye OA, Labarrer CA, McIntyre JA. The complement system in human reproduction. *Am J Reprod Immunol* 1992;27:145–155.

101. Haeger M, Unander M, Norder-Hansson B, Tylman M, Bengtsson A. Complement, neutrophil, and macrophage activation in women with severe preeclampsia and the syndrome of hemolysis, elevated liver enzymes, and low platelet count. *Obstet Gynecol* 1992;79:19–26.

102. Berger M, Sorensen RU, Tosi MF, Dearborne DG, Doring G. Complement receptor expression on neutrophils at an inflammatory site, the Pseudomonas-infected lung in cystic fibrosis. *Clin Invest* 1989; 84:1302–1313.

103. Fick RB, Robbins RA, Squier SU, Schoderbek WE, Russ WD. Complement activation in cystic fibrosis respiratory fluids: *in vivo* and *in vitro* generation of C5a and chemotactic activity. *Pediatr Res* 1986; 20:1258–1268.

104. Mourshargh S, Williams TJ. Evidence that a receptor-operated event on the neutrophil mediates neutrophil accumulation *in vivo* and pretreatment of ^{111}In-neutrophils with pertussis toxin *in vitro* inhibits their accumulation *in vivo*. *J Immunol* 1990;145:2633–2638.

105. Werfel T, Oppermann M, Schulz M, Krieger G, Weber M, Gotze O. Binding of fluorescein-labeled anaphylatoxin C5a to human peripheral blood, spleen, and bone marrow leukocytes. *Blood* 1992;79: 151–160.

106. Schulman ES, Post TJ, Henson PM, Giclas PC. Differential effects of the complement peptides C5a and C5a des Arg. *J Clin Invest* 1988;81: 918–923.

107. Yancey KB, Lawley TJ, Derskookian M, Harvath L. Analysis of the interaction of human C5a and C5a des Arg with human monocytes and neutrophils: Flow cytometric and chemotaxis studies. *J Clin Dermatol* 1989;92:184–189.

108. MacGlashan D Jr, Warner J. Stimulus-dependent leukotriene release from human basophils: A comparative study of C5a and f-Met-Leu-Phe. *J Leukoc Biol* 1991;49:29–40.

109. Foreman KE, Vaporciyan AA, Bonish BK, et al. C5a-induced expression of P-selectin in endothelial cells. *J Clin Invest* 1994;94: 1147–1155.

110. Baggiolini M, Walz A, Kunkel SL. Neutrophil-activating peptide-1/Interleukin-8, a novel cytokine that activates neutrophils. *J Clin Invest* 1989;84:1045–1049.

111. Oppenheim JJ, Zachariae CO, Mukaida N, Matsushima K. Properties of the novel pro-inflammatory supergene "intercrine" cytokine family. *Ann Rev Immunol* 1991;9:617–648.

112. Rollins BJ, Yoshimura T, Leonard EJ, Pober JS. Cytokine-activated human endothelial cells synthesize and secrete a monocyte chemoattractant, MCP-1/JE. *Am J Pathol* 1990;136:1229–1233.

113. Schall TJ, Bacon K, Toy KJ, Goeddel DV. Selective attraction of monocytes and T lymphocytes of the memory phenotype by the cytokine RANTES. *Nature* 1990;437:669–671.

114. Alam R, Stafford S, Forsythe P, et al. RANTES is a chemotactic and activating factor for human eosinophils. *J Immunol* 1993;150: 3442–3448.

115. Post TW, Bozic CR, Rothenberg ME, Luster AD, Gerard NP, Gerard C. Molecular characterization of two murine eosinophil beta-chemokine receptors. *J Immunol* 1995;155:5299–5305.

116. Larson GL, Mitchell BC, Harper TB, Henson PM. The pulmonary response of C5 sufficient and desicient mice to Pseudomonas aeruginosa. *Am Rev Respir Dis* 1982;126:306–311.

117. Wetsel RA, Kolb WP. Expression of C5a-like biological activities by the fifth component of human complement (C5) upon limited digestion with noncomplement enzymes without release of polypeptide fragments. *J Exp Med* 1983;157:2029–2048.

118. Wingrove JA, DiScipio RG, Chen Z, Potempa J, Travis J, Hugli TE. Activation of complement components C3 and C5 by a cysteine proteinase (gingipain-1) from porphyromonas (bacteroides) gingivalis. *J Biol Chem* 1992;267:18902–18907.

119. Strunk RC, Eidlen DM, Mason RJ. Pulmonary alveolar type II epithelial cells synthesize and secrete proteins of the classical and alternative complement pathways. *J Clin Invest* 1988;81:419–426.

120. Katz Y, Strunk RC. Synovial fibroblast-like cells synthesize seven proteins of the complement system. *Arthritis Rheum* 1988;3: 1365–1370.

121. Yao J, Harvath L, Gilbert DL, Colton CA. Chemotaxis by a CNS macrophage, the microglia. *J Neurosci Res* 1990;27:36–42.

122. Armstrong RC, Harvath L, Dubois-Dalcq ME. Type 1 astrocytes and oligodendrocyte-type 2 astrocyte glial progentiors migrate toward distinct molecules. *J Neurosci Res* 1990;27:400–407.

123. Morgan EL, Sanderson S, Scholz W, Noonan D, Weigel W, Hugli, TE. Identification and characterization of the effector region within human C5a responsible for stimunlation of IL-6 synthesis. *J Immunol* 1992;148:3937–3942.

124. Tomlinson S. Complement defense mechanisms. *Curr Opin Immunol* 1993;5:83–89.

125. Gerard C, Gerard NP. C5a anaphylatoxin and its seven transmembrane-segment receptor. *Ann Rev Immunol* 1994;12:775–808.

126. Cochrane CG, Muller-Eberhard HJ. The derivation of two distinct anaphylatoxin activities from the third and fifth components of human complement. *J Exp Med* 1968;127:371–386.

127. Hugli TE. Human anaphylatoxin (C3a) from the third component of complement. *J Biol Chem* 1975;250:8293–8301.

128. Stimler NP, Hugli TE, Bloor CM. Pulmonary injury induced by C3a and C5a anaphylatoxins. *Am J Pathol* 1980;100:327–348.

129. Stimler NP, Bloor CM, Hugli TE. C3a-induced contraction of guinea pig lung parenchyma: role of cyclooxygenase metabolites. *Immunopharmacology* 1983;5:251–257.

130. Stimler NP, Bloor CM, Hugli TE. Immunopharmacology of complement anaphylatoxins in the lung. In: Lenfant C. *Immunopharmacology of the lung*. New York: Marcel Dekker, 1983;401–434.

131. Greef K, Benfey BG, Bokelman UA. Anaphylaktische reaktionen am isolierten herzvorhofpraparat des meerschweinchens und ire beeinflussung durch antihistaminica, BOL, dihydroergotamin und reserpin. *Naunyn-Schmiedebergs Arch Exp Pathol Pharmak* 1959;236: 421–434.

132. Hugli TE, Gerard C, Kawahara M, et al. Isolation of three anaphylatoxins from complement-activated human serum. *Mol Cell Biochem* 1982;41:6346–6351.

133. Damerau B, Grunefeld E, Vogt W. Chemotactic effects of the complement-drived peptides C3a, C3ai and C5a (classical anaphylatoxin) in rabbit and guinea pig polymorphonuclear leukocytes. *Arch Pharmacol* 1978;305:181–184.

134. Glovsky MM, Hugli TE, Ishizaka T, Lichtenstein LM, EricksonBW. Anaphylatoxin-induced histamine release with human leukocytes. *J Clin Invest* 1979;64:804–811.

135. Showell HJ, Glovsky MM, Ward PA. C3a-induced lysosomal enzyme

secretion from human neutrophils: lack of inhibition by f-Met-Leu-Phe antagonists and inhibition by arachidonic acid antagonists. *Int Archs Allergy Appl Immunol* 1982;67:227–232.

136. Gerardy-Schahn R, Ambrosius D, Saunders D, et al. Characterization of C3a receptor-proteins on guinea pig platelets and human polymorphonuclear leukocytes. *Eur J Immunol* 1989;19:1095–1102.

137. Klos A, Bank S, Gietz C, et al. C3a receptor on dibutyryl-cAMP-differentiated U937 cells and human neutrophils: the human C3a receptor characterized by functional responses and ^{125}I-C3a binding. *Biochemistry* 1992;31:11274–11282.

138. Norgauer J, Dobos G, Kownatzki E, et al. Complement fragment C3a stimulates Ca— influx in neutrophils by a pertussis-toxin-sensitive G protein. *Eur J Biochem* 1993;217:289–294.

139. Elsner J, Oppermann M, Czech W, Kapp A. C3a activates the respiratory burst in human polymorphonuclear leukocytes via pertussis toxin-sensitive G-proteins. *Blood* 1994;83:3324–3331.

140. Goers JW, Glovsky MM, Hunkapiller MW, Farnsworth V, Richards JH. Studies on C3a$_{hu}$ binding to human eosinophils: characterization of binding. *Int Arch Allergy Appl Immunol* 1984;74:147–151.

141. Elsner J, Oppermann M, Czech W, et al. C3a activates reactive oxygen radical species productin and intracellular calcium transients in human eosinophils. *Eur J Immunol* 1994;24:518–522.

142. Daffern PJ, Pfeifer PH, Ember JA, Hugli TE. C3a is a chemotaxin for human eosinophils but not for neutrophils. I. C3a stimulation of neutrophils is secondary to eosinophil activation. *J Exp Med* 1995;181:2119–2127.

143. Khirwadkar K, Zilow G, Opperman M, Kabelitz D, Rother K. Interleukin-4 augments production of the third complement component by the alveolar epithelial cell line A549. *Int Arch Allergy Immunol* 1993;100:35–41.

144. Coulpier M, Andreev S, Lemercier C, et al. Activation of the endothelium by IL-1 alpha and glucocorticoids results in a major increase of complement component C3 and factor B production and generation of C3a. *J Clin Exp Immunol* 1995;101:142–149.

145. Gorski JP, Hugli TE, Muller-Eberhard HJ. C4a: the third anaphylatoxin of the human complement system. *Proc Natl Acad Sci U S A* 1979;76:5299–5302.

146. Donaldson VH, Rosen FS, Bing DH. Role of the second component of complement C2 and plasmin in kinin release in HAE plasma. *Trans Assoc Am Physicians* 1977;90:174–183.

147. Donaldson VH, Rosen FS. Action of complement in hereditary angioneurotic edema: the role of C1 esterase. *J Clin Invest* 1964;43:2204–2211.

148. Davis AE. C1 inhibitor and hereditary angioneurotic edema. *Ann Rev Immunol* 1988;6:595–628.

149. Donaldson VH, Rosen FS, Bing DH. Kinin-generation in hereditary angioneurotic edema (HAE) plasma. *Adv Exp Med Biol* 1983;156:183–191.

150. Strang CJ, Cholin S, Davis AE, et al. Angioedema induced by a peptide derived from complement component C2. *J Exp Med* 1988;168:1685–1698.

151. Strang CJ, Spragg JJ, Cholin S, Davis AE. Kinin-like activity of a peptide derived from complement component C2. *Fed Proc* 1987;46:1196.

152. Cholin S, Strang CJ, Spragg JJ, Rosen FS, Davis AE. Synthetic peptides derived from the second component of complement: spasmogenicity and enhanced vasopermeability. *FASEB J* 1988;2:871.

153. Cholin S, Gerard NP, Strang CJ, Davis AE. Biologic activity of a C2-derived peptide: demonstration of a specific interaction with guinea pig lung tissues. *J Immunol* 1989;142:2401–2404.

154. Klickstein LB, Bartow TJ, Miletic V, Rabson LD, Smith JA, Fearon DT. Identification of distinct C3b and C4b recognition sites in the human C3b/C4b receptor (CR1, CD35) by deletion mutagenesis. *J Exp Med* 1988;168:1699–1717.

155. Ahearn JM, Fearon DT. Structure and function of the compelment receptors, CR1 (CD35), and CR2 (CD21). *Adv Immunol* 1989;46:183–219.

156. Weisman HF, Bartow T, Leppo MK, et al. Soluble human complement receptor type 1: *in vivo* inhibitor of complement suppressing post-ischemic myocardial inflammation and necrosis. *Science* 1990;249:146–151.

157. Kalli KR, Hsu PH, Bartow TJ, et al. Mapping of the C3b-binding site of CR1 and construction of a (CR1)2-F(ab')2 chimeric complement inhibitor. *J Exp Med* 1991;174:1451–1460.

158. Moore MD, Cooper NR, Tack BF, Nemerow GR. Molecular cloning of the cDNA encoding the Epstein-Barr virus/C3d receptor (complement receptor type 2) of human B lymphocytes. *Proc Natl Acad Sci U S A* 1987;84:9194–9198.

159. Fearon DT, Carter RH. The CD19/CR2/TAPA-1 complex of B lymphocytes: linking natural to acquired immunity. *Ann Rev Immunol* 1995;13:127–149.

160. Springer TA, Anderson DC. The importance of the Mac-1, LFA-1 glycoprotein famiily in monocyte and granulocyte adherence, chemotaxis and migration into inflammatory sites: insights from an experiment of nature. In: D. Evered, J. Nugent, and M. O'Connor, eds. *Biochemistry of macrophages*. Pitman, London: Ciba Foundation Symposium 118, 1986;102–126.

161. Wang C, Barbashov S, Jack RM, Weller PF, Barrett T, Nicholson-Weller A. Hemolytically inactive C5b67: an agonist of polymorphonuclear leukocytes. *Blood* 1995;85:2570–2578.

162. Wang C, Gerard NP, Nicholson-Weller A. Signaling by hemolytically inactive C5b67, and agonist of polymorphonuclear leukocytes. *J Immunol* 1996;156:786–792.

163. Niculescu F, Rus H, Shin ML. Receptor-independent activation of guainine nucleotide-binding regulatory proteins by terminal complement complexes. *J Biol Chem* 1994;269:4417–4423.

164. Chenoweth DE, Hugli TE. Demonstration of specific C5a receptors on intact human polymorphonuclear leukocytes. *Proc Natl Acad Sci U S A* 1978;75:3943–3947.

165. Chenoweth DE, Goodman MG, Weigel WO. Demonstration of a specific receptor for C5a anaphylatoxin on murine macrophages. *J Exp Med* 1982;156:68–78.

166. Van Epps D, Chenoweth DE. Analysis of the binding of fluorescent C5a and C3a to human peripheral blood leukocytes. *J Immunol* 1984;132:2862–2867.

167. Rollins TE, Springer MS. Identification of the polymorphonuclear leukocyte C5a receptor. *J Biol Chem* 1985;60:7157–7160.

168. Johnson RJ, Chenoweth DE. Labeling the granulocyte C5a receptor with a unique photoreactive probe. *J Biol Chem* 1985;260:7161–7164.

169. Johnson RJ, Chenoweth DE. Synthesis of a new photoreactive C5a analog that permits identification of the ligand binding component of the granulocyte C5a receptor. *Biochem Biophys Res Commun* 1987;148:1330–1337.

170. Huey R, Hugli TE. C5a receptor. *Meth Enzymol* 1987;150:615–627.

171. Gerard NP, Hodges MK, Drazen JM, Weller PF, Gerard C. Characterization of a receptor for C5a anaphylatoxin on human eosinophils. *J Biol Chem* 1989;263:520–526.

172. Barker MD, Jose PJ, Williams TJ, Burton DR. The chemoattractant des-Arg74-C5a regulates the expression of its own receptor on a monocyte-like cell line. *Biochem J* 1986;288:911–917.

173. Gerard NP, and Gerard C. The chemotactic receptor for human C5a anaphylatoxin. *Nature* 1991;349:614–617.

174. Boulay F, Mery L, Tardif M, Brouchon L, Vignais P. Expression cloning of a receptor for C5a anaphylatoxin on differentiated HL-60 cells. *Biochemistry* 1991;30:2993–2999.

175. Boulay F, Tardif M, Brouchon L, Vignais P. The human N-formyl-peptide receptor. Characterization of two cDNA isolates and evidence for a new subfamily of G-protein coupled receptors. *Biochemistry* 1990;29:11123–11133.

176. Kawai M, Quincy DA, Lane B, Mollison KW, Luly JR, Carter GW. Identification and synthesis of a receptor binding site of human anaphylatoxin C5a. *J Med Chem* 1991;34:2068–2071.

177. Gerard C, Chenoweth DE, Hugli TE. Molecular aspects of the serum chemotactic factors. *J Reticuloendothel Soc* 1979;26:711–718.

178. Mollison KW, Mandecki W, Zuiderweg ERP, et al. Identification of the receptor-binding residues in the inflammatory complement protein C5a by site-directed mutagenesis. *Proc Natl Acad Sci U S A* 1989;86:292–296.

179. Oppermann M, Raedt U, Hebell T, Schmidt B, Zimmermann B, Gotze O. Probing the human receptor for C5a anaphylatoxin with site-directed antibodies. Identification of a potential ligand binding site on the NH2-terminal domain. *J Immunol* 1993;151:3785–3794.

180. Mery L, Boulay F. The NH2-terminal region of the C5aR but not that of the FPR is critical for both protein transport and ligand binding. *J Biol Chem* 1994;269:3457–3463.

181. DeMartino JA, Van Riper G, Siciliano SJ, et al. The amino terminus of the human C5a receptor is required for high affinity C5a binding

and for receptor activation by C5a but not C5a analogs. *J Biol Chem* 1994;269:14446–14450.

182. Siciliano SJ, Rollins TE, DeMartino JA, et al. Two-site binding of C5a by its receptor: an alternative binding paradigm for G-protein coupled receptors. *Proc Natl Acad Sci U S A* 1994;91:1214–1218.

183. LaRosa GJ, Thomas KM, Kaufmann ME, et al. Amino terminus of the interleukin-8 receptor is a major determinant of receptor subtype specificity. *J Biol Chem* 1992;267:25402–25406.

184. Gayle RB, Sleath PR, Srinivason S, et al. Importance of the amino terminus in the interleukin-8 receptor in ligand interactions. *J Biol Chem* 1993;268:7283–7289.

185. Kolakowski LF, Lu B, Gerard C, Gerard NP. Probing the "message:address" sites for chemoattractant binding to the C5a receptor. Mutagenesis of hydrophilic and proline residues within the transmembrane segments. *J Biol Chem* 1995;270:18077–18082.

186. Gerard NP, Lu B, He X-P, Eddy RL, Shows TB, Gerard C. Human chemotaxis receptor genes cluster at 19q13.3-13.4. Characterization of the human C5a receptor gene. *Biochemistry* 1993;32:1243–1250.

187. Dixon RA, Kobilka BK, Strader CD, et al. Cloning of the gene and cDNA for mammalian beta-adrenergic receptor and homology with rhodopsin. *Nature* 1986;321:75–79.

188. Libert F, Parmentier M, Lefort A, et al. Selective amplification and cloning of four new members of the G protein-coupled receptor family. *Science* 1989;244:569–572.

189. Gerard NP, Garraway LA, Eddy RL, Shows TB, Iijima H, Pacquet JL. Human substance P receptor (NK-1): organization of the gene, chromosome localization, and functional expression of cDNA clones. *Biochemistry* 1991;30:10640–10646.

190. Gerard NP, Eddy RL, Shows TB, Gerard C. The human neurokinin A (substance K) receptor. Molecular cloning of the gene, chromosome localization, and isolation of the cDNA from tracheal and gastric tissues. *J Biol Chem* 1990;265:20455–20462.

191. Skralnik DG, Strauss EC, Orkin SH. CCAAT displacement protein as a repressor of the myelomonocytic-specific gp91-phox gene promoter. *J Biol Chem* 1991;266:16736–16744.

192. Lu B, Gerard NP, Eddy RL, Shows TB, Gerard C. Mapping of genes for the human C5a receptor (C5aR), human FMLP receptor (FPR) and two FMLP receptor homologue orphan receptors (FPRH1, FPRH2) to chromosome 19. *Genomics* 1992;13:437–448.

193. Perez HD, Holmes R, Kelly E, McClary J, Chou Q, Andrews WH. Cloning of the gene coding for a human receptor for formyl peptides. Characterization of a promoter region and evidence for polymorphic expression. *Biochemistry* 1992;31:11595–11599.

194. Murphy PM, Tiffany HL, McDermott D, Abuja SK. Sequence and organization of the human N-formyl peptide receptor-encoding gene. *Gene* 1993;133:285–290.

195. Chase PB, Halonen M, Regan JW. Cloning of a human platelet-activating factor receptor gene: evidence for an intron in the 5'-untranslated region. *Am J Respir Cell Mol Biol* 1993;8:240–244.

196. Haviland DL, Borel AC, Fleischer DT, Haviland JC, Wetsel RA. Structure, 5'-flanking sequence, and chromosome location of the human N-formyl peptide receptor gene. A single-copy gene comprised of two exons on chromosome 19q13.3 that yields two distinct transcripts by alternative polyadenylation. *Biochemistry* 1993;32:4168–4174.

197. Fiore S, Maddox JF, Perez HD, Serhan CN. Identification of a human cDNA encoding a functional high affinity lipoxin A4 receptor. *J Exp Med* 1994;180:253–260.

198. Hoepkin U, Lu B, Gerard NP, Gerard C. The C5a chemoattractant receptor mediates mucosal defense to infection. *Nature* 1996;383:86–89.

199. Bozic CR, Lu B, Hophen UE, Gerard C, Gerard NP. Neurogenic amplification of immune complex inflammation. *Science* 1996;273:1722–1725.

200. Crass T, Raffetseder U, Grove M, Kohl J, Klos A, Bautsch W. Expression cloning of an inductor of the human C3a anaphylatoxin receptor in 293 cells. *Mol Immunol* 1996;33(Suppl 1):34 (abstr).

201. Roglic A, Prossnitz ER, Cavanagh SL, Pan Z, Zou A, Ye RD. cDNA cloning of a novel G protein-coupled receptor with a large extracellular loop structure. *Biochim Biophys Acta* 1996;1305:39–43.

202. Ames RS, Nuthulaganti P, Bergsma DJ, et al. Identification of an orphan G-protein coupled receptor which functions as a C5a receptor in Xenopus oocytes. *Mol Immunol* 1996;33(Suppl 1):37 (abstr).

203. Klickstein LB, Wong WW, Smith JA, et al. Human C3b/C4b receptor (CR1): demonstration of long homologous repeating domains that are composed of the short consensus repeats characteristic of C3/C4 binding proteins. *J Exp Med* 1987;165:1095–1112.

204. Klickstein LB, Bartow TJ, Miletic V, Rabson LD, Smith JA, Fearon DT. Identification of distinct C3b and C4b recognition sites in the human C3b/C4b receptor (CR1, CD35) by deletion mutagenesis. *J Exp Med* 1988;168:1699–1717.

205. Wong WW, Farrell SA. Proposed structure of the F' allotype of human CR1: loss of a C3b binding site may be associated with altered function. *J Immunol* 1991;146:656–662.

206. Kalli KR, Hsu P, Fearon DT. Therapeutic uses of recombinant complement protein inhibitors. *Springer Seminars on Immunopathol* 1994;15:417–431.

207. Carter RH, Fearon DT. CD19: lowering the threshold for antigen receptor stimulation of B lymphocytes. *Science* 1992;256:105–107.

208. Graham IL, Anderson DC, Holers VM, Brown EJ. Complement receptor 3 (CR3, Mac-1, integrin α M β 2, CD11b/CD18) is required for for tyrosine phosphorylation of paxillin in adherent and nonadherent neutrophils. *J Cell Biol* 1994;127:1139–1147.

209. Arnaut MA. Structure and function of the leukocyte adhesion molecules CD11b/CD18. *Blood* 1990;75:1037–1050.

210. Krauss JC, Poo H, Xue W, Mayo-Bond L, Todd RF III, Petty HR. Reconstitution of antibody-dependent phagocytosis in fibroblasts expressing Fc gamma receptor IIIB and the compelment receptor typr 3. *J Immunol* 1994;153:1769–1777.

211. Diaz P, Gonzalez MC, Galleguillos FR, et al. Leukocytes and mediators in bronchoalveolar lavage during allergen-induced late-phase asthmatic reactions. *Am Rev Respir Dis* 1989;139:1383–1389.

212. Smith JK, Chi DS, Krish G, Reynolds S, Cambron G. Effect of exercise on complement acitivity. *Ann Allergy* 1990;65:304–310.

213. Michel O, Sergysels R, and Duchateau J. Complement activation in bronchial asthma evaluated by the C3d/C3 index. *Ann Allergy* 1986;57:405–408.

214. van de Graaf EA, Jansen HM, Bakker MM, et al. ELISA of complement C3a in bronchoalveolar lavage fluid. *J Immunol Meth* 1992;147:241–250.

215. Grassi GG, Zanon P, Fietta A, DeRose V, Mangiarotti P, Grassi C. Evaluation of the host defense system in asthmatic patients. *Respiration* (Suppl 50) 1986;250:83–91.

216. Arm JP, Walport MJ, Lee TH. Expression of complement receptors type 1 (CR1) and type 3 (CR3) on circulating granulocytes in experimentally provoked asthma. *J Allergy Clin Immunol* 1989;83:649–655.

217. Lundahl J, Skedinger M, Hed J, Johansson SG, Zetterstrom O. Lability in complement receptor mobilization of granulocytes in patients with bronchial hyperreactivity. *Clin Exp Allergy* 1992;22:834–838.

218. Kirschfink M, Castro FF, Rother U, Nakhosteen JA, Deppisch R, Schmitz-Schumann M. Complement activation and C3 allotype distribution in patients with bronchial asthma. *Int Arch Allergy Immunol* 1993;100:151–155.

219. Tabayashi T, Vannier E, Clark BD, et al. A new biologic role for C3a and C3a desARg. Regulation of TNF-α and IL-1β synthesis. *J Immunol* 1996;156:3455–3460.

220. Podak ER, Biesecker G, Kolb W, and Muller-Eberhard HJ. The C5b-6 complex; reaction with C7, C8, C9. *J Immunol* 1978;121:484–490.

221. Pangburn MK, Muller-Eberhard HJ. The alternative pathway of complement. *Springer Semin Immunopathol* 1984;7:163–192.

222. Franke AE, Andrews GC, Stimler-Gerard NP, Gerard C, Showell HJ. Human C5a anaphylatoxin: Gene synthesis, expression, and recovery of biologically active material from *E. coli*. *Methods Enzymol* 1988;162:653–668.

223. Fukuoka Y, Yasui A, Tachibana T. Active recombinant C3a of human anaphylatoxin produced in *Escherichia coli*. *Biochem Biophys Res Commun* 1991;175:1131–1138.

224. Wagner JL, Hugli TE. Radioimmunoassay for anaphylatoxins; a sensitive method for determining complement activation products in biological fluids. *Anal Biochem* 1984;136:75–88.

225. Oppermann M, Schulze M, Gotze O. A sensitive enzyme immunoassay for the quantitation of human C5a/C5a(des Arg) anaphylatoxin using a monoclonal antibody with specificity for a neoepitope. *Complement Inflamm* 1991;8:13–24.

Asthma, edited by P.J. Barnes, M.M. Grunstein,
A.R. Leff, and A.J. Woolcock.
Lippincott–Raven Publishers, Philadelphia © 1997.

▪ 49 ▪

Proinflammatory Cytokines

Johan C. Kips and Romain A. Pauwels

Source and Structure
Proinflammatory Cytokines Present in Asthmatic
    Airways
Cellular Origin of Proinflammatory Cytokines
    in Asthma
    Macrophages
    T Lymphocytes

Mast Cells
Eosinophils
Epithelial Cells
Function of the Proinflammatory Cytokines
    Il-1β and TNF-α
Therapeutic Implications

It has become increasingly clear over the past few years that the chronic mucosal airway inflammation of asthma is regulated by a highly complex network of mutually interacting cytokines. Within this network, the exact contribution of each cytokine remains to be fully established. The possible role of lymphokines such as interleukin (IL)-4 and IL-5, or chemokines such as IL-8, monocyte chemoattractant protein-1 (MCP-1) or RANTES, have been emphasized; other potentially important cytokines include Tumor necrosis factor-alpha (TNF-α), IL-1β, and IL-6. These cytokines are frequently grouped as "proinflammatory" cytokines. As for the majority of cytokines, a large degree of redundancy exists within this group. In this overview, a few of the effects of these cytokines that could be of importance in asthma are highlighted.

SOURCE AND STRUCTURE

Tumor necrosis factor-alpha TNF-α is a 17 kDa, 157 amino acid long polypeptide, obtained by proteolytic cleavage from a 233 amino acid precursor (1). Human TNF is a trimeric molecule, with a structure described as a "β-jelly roll" (2). The gene coding for TNF is localized on the short arm of human chromosome 6 (3). TNF binds

with equal affinity to two different TNF receptors, the p55-60 and the p75-80 receptor (4,5). Most cell types express both receptors, and it has been proposed that both interact in the signal transduction leading to activation of various pathways, including NF-κB induction (6). As for all proinflammatory cytokines, the major source of TNF-α are macrophages/monocytes. However, a large number of other cell types, including T cells, mast cells, granulocytes, fibroblasts, muscle cells, and epithelial cells also can produce TNF in response to a wide array of stimuli (7). These include microbial products such as endotoxin and other cytokines such as IL-1, interferon γ (IFN-γ), and granulocyte-macrophage colony-stimulating factor (GM-CSF).

The two forms of IL-1, IL-1α, and IL-1β consist of approximately 150 amino acids. They are synthetized as 270 amino acid long propeptides. IL-1β is the prominent form of IL-1. Activated human peripheral blood mononuclear cells contain 25- to 50-fold more messenger ribonucleic acid (mRNA) for IL-1β than for IL-1α (8). Whereas IL-1α remains largely cell bound, IL-1β is mainly secreted. Secretion of mature IL-1β requires intracellular cleavage of pro-IL-1β by a specific protease, the IL-1 converting enzyme (9). The structure of IL-1 is characterized by 12 β pleated sheets. The genes coding for IL-1α and IL-1β are localized on the long arm of the chromosome 2 (10). IL-1α and IL-1β are distinct gene products, but bind to the same receptors and have common biological effects. Two cell surface IL-1 receptors have been identified. The type I IL-1R mediates the bio-

J. C. Kips and R. A. Pauwels: Department of Respiratory Diseases, University Hospital Ghent, B-9000 Ghent, Belgium.

logical effects of IL-1. The type II receptor acts as decoy; the extracellular portion is similar to the type I IL-1R, but the cytoplasmic domain is different. The type II IL-1R appears not to deliver biological signals, thus, acting negatively to regulate the actions of IL-1 (11). The biological effect of IL-1 can also be inhibited by competitive binding, predominantly to the type I IL-1R of a naturally occuring antagonist, the IL-1 receptor antagonist (IL-1RA) (12).

In addition to monocytes, other cell types that can synthetize IL-1 include T cells, endothelial cells, Langerhans cells, neutrophils, and smooth muscle cells. IL-1 production can be induced by a variety of stimuli, including microbial products such as endotoxin, but also C5a, TNF-α, TGF-β, or IL-1 itself. Factors inhibiting the release of IL-1 from macrophages include prostaglandins, acting through inhibition of protein translation, and cytokines such as IL-4 and IL-10. IL-10 inhibits transcription of IL-1α, IL-1β, in addition to TNF-α and IL-6 (13). IL-4 also inhibits IL-1 production, and at the same time, induces production of the IL-1RA (14,15).

IL-6 consists of 184 amino acids. The structure is similar to the four α-helix bundles found in a variety of cytokines (16). The gene coding for IL-6 is found on the short arm of chromosome 7 (17). The IL-6 receptor consists of the gp80 and the gp130 chain (Fig. 1); gp80 binds IL-6 and then associates with the nonligand binding gp130. This leads to the transduction of a signal accross the plasma membrane through gp130 (18,19). The main source of IL-6 includes monocytes, T lymphocytes, and fibroblasts. IL-6 is released in response to a wide range of stimuli such as viruses, LPS, TNF, IL-1, and IFN-γ (16).

PROINFLAMMATORY CYTOKINES PRESENT IN ASTHMATIC AIRWAYS

Using *in situ* hybridization, bronchoalveolar lavage (BAL) from atopic asthmatics has been reported to contain increased numbers of cells expressing mRNA for a variety of cytokines, including TNF-α and IL-1β, when compared to nonsmoking, nonatopic controls (20,21).

Since gene expression does not necessarily imply protein synthesis, these data have to be complemented with studies that either measure the synthetized protein in BAL fluid or demonstrate its presence by immunohistochemical means in biopsies. TNF and IL-1β are among the cytokines found in increased amounts in BAL fluid from symptomatic, as compared to asymptomatic, asthmatics (22,23). Positive immunohistochemical staining for TNF-α has been reported in bronchial biopsies from patients with mild atopic or occupational asthma (24,25).

CELLULAR ORIGIN OF PROINFLAMMATORY CYTOKINES IN ASTHMA

Different cell types present in asthmatic airways can account for the production of these cytokines (Table 1).

Macrophages

Macrophages are a well-established source of IL-1β, TNF-α, and IL-6 (21,26). The capacity to synthetize these cytokines seems to be upregulated in asthma. It has been shown that the immunoglobulin E (IgE)-dependent TNF-α and the IL-6 release from macrophages recovered from BAL is enhanced during an allergen-induced late asthmatic reaction (26). Similar data were obtained with peripheral blood monocytes (27). Others have reported that macrophages and monocytes from asthmatics produce greater amounts of TNF-α, IL-1, IL-8, and GM-CSF in response to LPS (28).

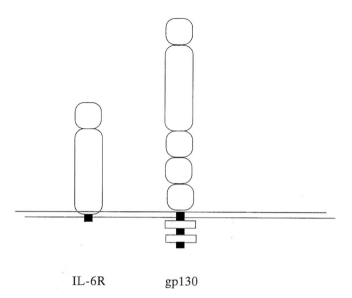

IL-6R   gp130

FIG. 1. Structure of interleukin-6 (IL-6) receptor.

TABLE 1. *Potential cellular sources of proinflammatory cytokines in asthma*

TNF-α	macrophages, mast cells, T lymphocytes, eosinophils, neutrophils, epithelial cells, fibroblasts, smooth muscle cells
IL-1β	macrophages, T lymphocytes, eosinophils, neutrophils, epithelial cells, fibroblasts, smooth muscle cells
IL-6	macrophages, T lymphocytes, eosinophils, fibroblasts, smooth muscle cells

TNF-α, tumor necrosis factor-α; IL-1β, interleukin-1β; IL-6, interleukin-6.

T Lymphocytes

CD4[+] T-helper (TH) lymphocytes are known to produce a range of cytokines. Within TH lymphocytes, a distinction has been made initially in mice, and, subsequently, also in humans, between TH1 and TH2 lymphocytes (29,30). Both subsets have the capacity to synthetize IL-1, IL-3, TNF, and GM-CSF. In addition, TH1 lymphocytes produce IL-2, TNF-β, and IFN-γ, whereas only TH2 lymphocytes produce IL-4, IL-5, IL-6, IL-10, and IL-13. The overall pattern of cytokine production in asthmatic airways is compatible with activation of TH2 lymphocytes (31). Moreover the majority of IL-4/IL-5 mRNA in BAL has been colocalized to CD4[+] T lymphocytes (32). It, therefore, seems reasonable to assume that TH2 cells also might be an important source of IL-1, TNF-α, and IL-6 in asthmatic airways.

Mast Cells

Human mast cells can produce various cytokines, including TNF-α (33–35). An important difference with T lymphocytes is that mast cells have the capacity to store cytokines in their granules. IgE-dependent mast cell stimulation leads to the immediate release of cytokines from these cells, whereas TNF production by stimulated T cells requires *de novo* synthesis. From immunohistochemical studies, it would indeed appear that the mast cell is the major source of preformed TNF-α in asthmatic airways (24).

Eosinophils

Human eosinophils have the capacity to release a large number of cytokines including IL-1α, IL-6, and TNF-α (36,37).

Epithelial cells

Structural tissue components such as epithelial cells and fibroblasts have the capacity to synthetize a range of cytokines. Asthmatic bronchial epithelial cells in culture have, for example, been shown to synthetize TNF-α, IL-1β, and IL-6 (38,39).

FUNCTION OF THE PROINFLAMMATORY CYTOKINES

IL-1β and TNF-α

IL-1β and TNF-α are extremely pleiotropic cytokines that could intervene at various stages in the pathogenesis of asthma (Table 2).

TABLE 2. *Effects of tumor necrosis factor-α (TNF-α)/ interleukin-1β (IL-1β) relevant to asthma*

Enhancement of sensitization to aeroallergens
Increase in bronchial responsiveness
Activation of inflammatory cells
Release of inflammatory mediators
Upregulation of adhesion molecules
Increased production of cytokines (e.g., GM-CSF, IL-8)
Increased expression of inducible NO synthase

GM-CSF, granulocyte-macrophage colony-stimulating factor; IL-8, interleukin-8.

Both IL-1β and TNF-α might play an important role in the initial sensitization process that underlies development of atopic asthma.

Sensitization to aeroallergens involves activation of T lymphocytes by dendritic cells that are currently considered a major antigen-presenting cell in the airways (40). It would appear that in atopic asthma this process leads to the preferential development of TH2 cells. The differentiation of TH0 into TH1 or TH2 is influenced by various cytokines present in the local micro-environment; a major role is attributed to IL-12 and IL-4 (41). IL-1 might also be involved in this process, since IL-1β is an important cofactor in the further growth of TH2, but not TH1 cells (42). Factors inducing the local production of IL-1β might, therefore, contribute to the development of TH2 cells. One of the potential cellular sources of IL-1β in the airways are epithelial cells, and it has been shown that NO_2 at concentrations that can be reached indoors induces the production of IL-1β in cultured airway epithelial cells (39). It has been hypothesized that this mechanism could provide a link between indoor pollution and increased prevalence of atopic disorders.

Stimulation of T-helper cells by antigen-presenting cells is suppressed by resident alveolar macrophages (43). This suppressive effect is inhibited by GM-CSF, especially in synergy with TNF-α (44). Therefore, increased TNF-α production could again constitute a mechanism by which pro-inflammatory stimuli early in childhood could enhance sensitization.

TNF-α and IL-1β also might play an important part within the cytokine network that regulates the airway inflammation in asthma, thus, contributing to several aspects of the disease (Fig. 2).

Nonspecific bronchial hyperresponsiveness is a key feature of asthma (45). Recently, IL-1β has been reported to increase airway responsiveness to bradykinin in Brown Norway rats (46). Similarly, aerosolized or intravenously administered TNF-α has been shown in *in vivo* animal studies conducted in rats and sheep to cause bronchial hyperresponsiveness (47,48). Inhalation of TNF-α has been confirmed to increase bronchial responsiveness in normal subjects (49). The mechanisms underlying the increase in responsiveness remain to be

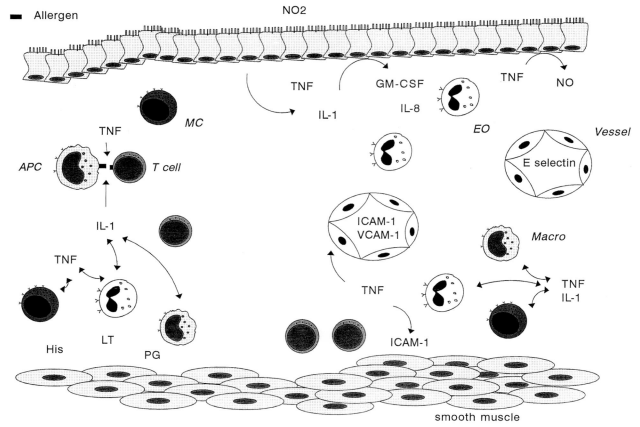

FIG. 2. Schematic representation of possible tumor necrosis factor-α (TNF-α) / interleukin-1β (IL-1β)-mediated effects in asthmatic airways.

investigated, but different pathways can be postulated. This includes the release of various inflammatory mediators including platelet activating factor (PAF), prostaglandins and leukotrienes, and the activation of other inflammatory cells, such as eosinophils, neutrophils, macrophages, and lymphocytes (50–57). Moreover, it has been reported that TNF-α can upregulate the expression of adhesion molecules such as intercellular adhesion molecule (ICAM-1) and vascular cell adhesion molecule (VCAM-1) on smooth muscle cells (58–60). This enhances interaction with inflammatory cells, which can lead to increased DNA synthesis in smooth muscle cells (61); whether this alters smooth muscle contractility is not known.

TNF-α and IL-1β are also potent inducers of NO synthesis (62). Increased expression of the inducible NO synthase (iNOS) in the bronchial epithelium of asthmatics has been reported, and exhaled air from asthmatics contains increased levels of NO (63–65). The net effect of increased NO production in astmatic airways is not yet resolved. NO could act as a bronchodilator and a functional antagonist to bronchoconstriction (66,67). In addition, endogenously produced NO can constitute a compensatory mechanism, modulating the increase in responsiveness induced by exogenous stimuli, or diminish the baseline degree of responsiveness (68–70). However NO might not only have beneficial effects, since it could also enhance airway inflammation, thus, possibly contributing to increased airway responsiveness (71).

Another important feature of TNF-α and IL-1β is their potential to induce an influx of inflammatory cells into the bronchial mucosa, partly through a direct chemotactic effect, but especially through increased expression of adhesion molecules on endothelial and epithelial cells (72–76). Immunohistochemical studies have confirmed enhanced expression of ICAM-1, E-selectin and VCAM-1 in the bronchial mucosa of asthmatics (77–79). It has been shown in humans that the granulocyte influx, which occurs during the late-phase allergic skin reaction, is accompanied by increased expression of E-selectin, which can be attributed to the release of TNF-α and IL-1β from resident skin mast cells (34,80). Other *in vitro* studies suggest that the upregulation of ICAM-1 observed during the late asthmatic response in the airways is mediated by TNF release from macrophages (81). The potential importance of these adhesion molecules and their counterligands on inflammatory cells in the pathogenesis of asthma, has been illustrated in animal models of allergic airway inflammation (82,83). Endogenously released

TNF-α has been shown to contribute to allergen-induced airway eosinophilia and hyperresponsiveness (84).

Another factor that could contribute to the proinflammatory effects of TNF-α and IL-1β is their capacity to induce the synthesis of other cytokines such as GM-CSF and chemokines including IL-8 and RANTES (85–88). Among its many effects, GM-CSF can stimulate the production, maturation, and activation of granulocytes, including eosinophils (89–91). The GM-CSF receptor consists of a ligand-specific α subunit and a β subunit, which is shared with the IL-3 and IL-5 receptor (92,93). Although the subunit in itself is nonligand binding, it is essential for the formation of high affinity receptors and for signal transduction (94,95). TNF and IL-1 have been shown to upregulate this common subunit on hematopoietic cell lines (96). IL-8 is a CXC chemokine, and is an important chemoattractant towards neutrophils (97). In addition, IL-8 also has chemotactic effect for IL-3- or IL-5-primed eosinophils (98). It has recently been confirmed *in vivo* that IL-1 can induce eosinophil accumulation in rat skin and that this effect can be inhibited by an anti-human IL-8 antibody (99).

Through the release of these cytokines, and in combination with upregulation of adhesion molecules, endogenous release of IL-1 and/or TNF may contribute to the recruitment of inflammatory cells, into the bronchial mucosa. Increased production or release of TNF-α and IL-1β might be also an important element in the exacerbation of disease severity induced by a variety of stimuli such as allergens, air pollutants, or viral infections. Indeed, human pulmonary macrophages and mast cells can release TNF-α through an IgE-dependent mechanism (26,33). NO$_2$, an important indoor and outdoor pollutant, has been shown to enhance IL-1β and TNF-α production in cultured airway epithelial cells, whereas TNF-α could also be involved in the influenza virus-induced IL-8 expression in human airway epithelial cells (39,100). The relative importance of this TNF-α/IL-1β pathway within the whole cytokine network responsible for disease modulation obviously remains to be further established.

An issue of increasing concern is the process of airway remodeling, which encompasses the structural airway changes observed in chronic asthma. The factors responsible for the different factors of airway remodeling such as subepithelial fibrosis, smooth muscle hypertrophy, and hyperplasia or neovascularization, are only beginning to emerge. The potential importance of several growth factors and profibrogenic cytokines such as platelet-derived growth factor (PDGF), GM-CSF, TGF-β, endothelin. or IGF has been emphasized (101–103). Again TNF-α and IL1β might be key elements in the induction of this process (Table 3). TNF-α has been reported to stimulate fibroblast proliferation and to increase type I collagen mRNA production in murine dermal fibroblasts (104, 105). TNF also is known to alter metabolic functions of vascular smooth muscle cells and at low concentrations,

TABLE 3. *Possible effects of tumor necrosis factor-α (TNF-α) / interleukin-1β (IL-1β) in airway remodelling*

Stimulation of fibroblast proliferation
Increased production of type I collagen
Stimulation of DNA synthesis in smooth muscle
Increased expression of growth factors (e.g., PDGF, HB-EGF, HBGF-2)

PDGF, platelet-derived growth factor; HB-EGF, heparin binding epithelial growth factor; HBGF-2, basic fibroblast growth factor

to stimulate DNA synthesis in cultured airway smooth muscle cells (106,107). Moreover, TNF can increase expression of adhesion molecules such as ICAM-1 and VCAM-1 on the surface of vascular and aiway smooth muscle cells (60,108). It has been shown that T lymphocytes adhere to airway smooth muscle cells through these integrins, and that this interaction induces DNA synthesis in the smooth muscle cells (60). In addition to these direct effects on fibroblast and smooth muscle cells, TNF also might induce the production of other potent growth factors. TNF has been shown to increase in endothelial cells the transcription of genes coding for growth factors such as PDGF and heparin binding epithelial growth factor like protein (HB-EGF)(109,110). Both PDGF and HB-EGF are known to be potent fibroblast and smooth muscle mitogens (111–113). IL-1β has also been reported to induce the production of growth factors including PDGF and basic fibroblast growth factor (HBGF-2)(114,115).

Finally, TNF stimulates bronchial epithelial cells to produce tenascin, an extracellular matrix glycoprotein that has been shown to be present in increased amounts in biopsies from asthmatics (116).

Interleukin-6

Another proinflammatory cytokine present in asthmatic airways is IL-6 (22). Epithelial cells and macrophages appear to be the predominant source (26,117). An allergen-specific upregulation of IL-6 production by alveolar macrophages and peripheral blood mononuclear cells in atopic asthmatics has been reported (26, 118). IL-6 is a pleiotropic cytokine, whose effects in asthma seem even less clear than those of IL-1 and TNF. IL-6 has growth regulatory effects on a variety of cells, is involved in T-cell activation, growth, and differentiation, and is a terminal differentiation factor of B cells, inducing immunoglobulin secretion (16). IL-6 has also been identified as an important cofactor in the IL-4 dependent IgE-synthesis (119). On the other hand, IL-6 might also have important anti-inflammatory effects. For example, IL-6 has been reported to inhibit the production of IL-1 and TNF from macrophages *in vitro* and to inhibit the endotoxin-induced TNF production and neutrophil influx into the airways in an *in vivo* animal model (120–122). Using IL-6 transgenic mice, it has been reported that IL-6 induces a lymphocytic infiltration around large and mid-sized airways, but, at the same time, diminishes airway responsiveness (123). Hence, IL-6 could represent an endogenous negative feedback mechanism, limiting the effect of other pro-inflammatory cytokines.

THERAPEUTIC IMPLICATIONS

As TNF and IL-1 clearly could be implicated at various stages in the pathogenesis of airway inflammation in asthma, antagonizing the effect or inhibiting the production of proinflammatory cytokines could be of therapeutic benefit.

This might, at least in part, explain the beneficial effect of some of the currently available broad acting "anti-inflammatory" compounds used in the treatment of asthma. Corticosteroids are known to inhibit the production of a range of cytokines, including TNF-α and IL-1 (1,124). Recently, biopsy studies have shown that treatment with inhaled steroids supresses production of proinflammatory cytokines in the bronchial epithelium of atopic asthmatics (125). That cromoglycate inhibits TNF-α release from mast cells is suggested by the observation *in vitro* that pre-incubation of skin explants with cromoglycate or neutralizing antibodies to TNF-α abrogates the induction of E-selectin on dermal venules, associated with mast cell degranulation (126). Nedocromil has been reported to inhibit *in vitro* the IL-1-induced production of GM-CSF and IL-8 in human bronchial epithelial cells (127,128).

It is known that the release of TNF-α by mononuclear cells is regulated by cyclic $3'$ $5'$ adenosine monophosphate (cAMP) regulated. An increase in the intracellular concentration of cAMP reduces the release of TNF-α by downregulating the expression of the TNF-α gene (129–131). Since phosphodiesterase (PDE) inhibitors increase the intracellular cAMP concentrations, it is not suprising that theophylline suppresses *in vitro* the release of TNF from monocytes and alveolar macrophages (132,133). More selective PDE inhibitors currently are being developed, and it has been confirmed in *in vivo* animal models that mixed PDEIII/IV or PDE IV inhibitors suppress endotoxin or antigen-induced TNF release in the airways (134,135). Increasing intracellular cAMP concentrations not only inhibit the release of TNF-α, but might also suppress TNF-α-mediated effects on various cells. For example, it recently has been reported that the TNF-α-induced expression of adhesion molecules on human vascular and airway smooth muscle cells is inhibited by an increase in cAMP concentrations (60,136).

An alternative approach to inhibiting the effect of pro-inflammatory cytokines is by developing cytokine receptor antagonists. One of the potential candidates in this regard is the IL-1RA. IL-1RA is a naturally occurring cytokine produced predominantly by monocytes and alveolar macrophages, which competes with IL-1α and IL-1β for binding to the IL-1 cell surface receptor (12,137). TH2 cytokines such as IL-4 and IL-10 have been shown to increase IL-1RA production by mononuclear cells (137, 138). Among its effects, IL-1RA has been shown *in vitro* to inhibit allergen-induced IgE-synthesis and production of IL-6, GMCSF, and TNF-α (139). IL-1RA also inhibits synthesis of IL-8 and MIP-1α in mixed lymphocyte cultures (140). *In vivo* animal data indicate that IL-1RA can suppress allergen-induced airway eosinophilia and airway hyperresponsiveness in guinea pigs (141,142).

CONCLUSIONS

Several cytokines, interacting in a complex network are probably involved in the pathogenesis of asthma. Among them, the proinflammatory cytokines IL-1β and TNF-α could play a major part, since they are able to interfere with the sensitization process, the acute inflammatory changes, as well as the chronic structural changes in long-standing asthma. Further development of specific inhibitors will provide more insight into their precise role and might, at the same time, prove to be of considerable therapeutic benefit.

REFERENCES

1. Beutler B, Cerami A. The biology of cachectin/TNF - a primary mediator of the host response. *Annu Rev Immunol* 1989;7:625–655.
2. Jones EY, Stuart DI, Walker NPC. Structure of tumor necrosis factor. *Nature* 1989;338:225–228.
3. Nedwin GE, Naylor SL, Sakagushi AY, et al. Human lymphotoxin and tumor necrosis factor genes: structure homology and chromosomal localization. *Nucleic Acids Res* 1985;13:6361–6371.
4. Loetscher H, Pan YCE, Lahm HW, et al. Molecular cloning and expression of the human 55kda tumor necrosis factor receptor. *Cell* 1990;61:351–359.
5. Schall TJ, Lewis M, Koller KJ, et al. Molecular cloning and expression of a receptor for human tumor necrosis factor. *Cell* 1990;61: 361–370.
6. Tartaglia LA, Goeddel DV. Two TNF receptors. *Immunol Today* 1992; 13:151–153.
7. Aggarwal BB. Tumor necrosis factor. In: Gutterman JV, Aggarwal BB, eds. *Human cytokines: handbook for basic and clinical researchers.* New York: Blackwell, 1992;270–285.
8. Dinarello CA. Interleukin-1 and interleukin-1 antagonism. *Blood* 1991;77:1627–1652.
9. Kostura MJ, Tocci MJ, Limjuco MJ, et al. Identification of a monocyte specific pre-interleukin-1β convertase activity. *Proc Natl Acad Sci U S A* 1989;86:5227–5231.
10. Webb AC, Collins KL, Auron PE, et al. Interleukin-1 gene (IL-1) assigned to long arm of chromosome 2. *Lymphokine Res* 1986;5:77–85.
11. Sims JE, Dower SK. Interleukin-1 receptors. In: Nicola NA, ed. *Guidebook to cytokines and their receptors.* Oxford: Oxford University Press, 1994;23–26.
12. Arend WP. Interleukin-1 receptor antagonist. *Adv Immunol* 1993;54: 167–227.
13. de Waal Malefyt R, Abrams J, Bennett B, Figdor CG, de Vries JE. Interleukin-10 (IL-10) inhibits cytokine synthesis by human monocytes: an autoregulatory role of IL-10 produced by monocytes. *J Exp Med* 1991;174:1209–1220.

14. Donnelly RP, Fenton MJ, Kaufman JD, Gerrard TL. IL-1 expression in human monocytes is transcriptionally and posttranscriptionally regulated by IL-4. *J Immunol* 1991;146:3431–3436.

15. Vannier E, Miller LC, Dinarello CA. Coordinated antiinflammatory effects of interleukin-4: interleukin-4 suppresses interleukin-1 production but up-regulates gene expression and synthesis of interleukin-1 receptor antagonist. *Proc Natl Acad Sci U S A* 1992;89:4076–4080.

16. Akira S, Taga T, Kishimoto T. Interleukin-6 in biology and medicine. *Adv Immunol* 1993;54:1–78.

17. Sehgal PB, Zilberstein A, Ruggieri RM, et al. Human chromosome 7 carries the 2 interferon gene. *Proc Natl Acad Sci U S A* 1987;84:3633–3637.

18. Yamasaki K, Taga T, Hirata Y, et al. Cloning and expression of the human interleukin-6 (BSF-2/IFN 2) receptor. *Science* 1988;241:825–828.

19. Hibi M, Murakami M, Saito M, Hirano T, Taga T, Kishimoto T. Molecular cloning and expression of an IL-6 signal transducer, gp130. *Cell* 1990;63:1149–1157.

20. Sun Ying, Robinson DS, Varney V, et al. TNF-alpha mRNA expression in allergic inflammation. *Clin Exp Allergy* 1991;21:745–750.

21. Borish L, Mascall JJ, Dishuck J, Bearn WR, Martin JR, Rosenwasser LJ. Detection of alveolar macrophage-derived IL-1β in asthma. *J Immunol* 1992;149:3078–3082.

22. Broide DH, Lotz M, Cuomo A, Coburn DA, Federman EC, Wasserman SI. Cytokines in symptomatic asthma airways. *J Allergy Clin Immunol* 1992;89:958–967.

23. Jarjour NN, Busse WW. Cytokines in bronchoalveolar lavage fluid of patients with nocturnal asthma. *Am J Respir Crit Care Med* 1995;152:1474–1477.

24. Bradding P, Roberts JA, Britten KM, et al. Interleukin-4, -5, and -6 and tumor necrosis factor-α in normal and asthmatic airways: evidence for the human mast cell as a source of these cytokines. *Am J Respir Cell Mol Biol* 1994;10:471–480.

25. Maestrelli P, Di Stefano A, Occari P, et al. Cytokines in the airway mucosa of subjects with asthma induced by toluene diisocyanate. *Am J Respir Crit Care Med* 1995;151:607–612.

26. Gosset P, Tsicopoulos A, Wallaert B, et al. Increased secretion of tumor necrosis factor-α and interleukin-6 by alveolar macrophages consecutive to the development of the late asthmatic reaction. *J Allergy Clin Immunol* 1991;88:561–571.

27. Gosset P, Tsicopoulos A, Wallaert B, Joseph M, Capron A, Tonnel AB. Tumor necrosis factor-α and interleukin-6 production by human mononuclear phagocytes from allergic asthmatics after IgE-dependent stimulation. *Am Rev Respir Dis* 1992;146:768–774.

28. Hallsworth MP, Soh CPC, Lane SJ, Arm JP, Lee TH. Selective enhancement of GM-CSF, TNN-α, IL-1β and IL-8 production by monocytes and macrophages of asthmatic subjects. *Eur Respir J* 1994;7:1096–1102.

29. Mosmann R, Coffman RL. TH1 and TH2 cells: different patterns of lymphokine secretion lead to different functional properties. *Ann Rev Immunol* 1989;7:145–173.

30. Del Prete G, Maggi E, Romagnani S. Biology of disease. Human TH1 and TH2 cells: functional properties, mechanisms of regulation, and role in disease. *Lab Invest* 1994;70:299–306.

31. Robinson DR, Hamid Q, Ying S, et al. Predominant TH2-like bronchoalveolar T-lymphocyte population in atopic asthma. *N Engl J Med* 1992;326:298–304.

32. Ying S, Durham SR, Corrigan JC, Hamid Q, Kay AB. Phenotype of cells expressing mRNA for TH2-type (Interleukin-4 and Interleukin-5) and TH1-type (Interleukin-2 and Interferon-γ) cytokines in bronchoalveolar lavage and bronchial biopsies from atopic asthmatic and normal control subjects. *Am J Respir Cell Mol Biol* 1995;12:477–487.

33. Okhawara Y, Yamauchi K, Tanno Y, et al. Human lung mast cells and pulmonary macrophages produce tumor necrosis factor-α after IgE receptor triggering. *Am J Respir Cell Mol Biol* 1992;7:385–392.

34. Walsh LJ, Trinchieri G, Waldorf HA, Whitaker D, Murphy GF. Human dermal mast cells contain and release tumor necrosis factor- alpha, which induces endothalial leukocyte adhesion molecule 1. *Proc Natl Acad Sci U S A* 1991;88:4220–4224.

35. Benyon RC, Bissonette EY, Befus AD. Tumor necrosis factor-alpha-dependent cytotoxicity of human skin mast cells is enhanced bu anti-TNF antibodies. *J Immunol* 1991;147:2253–2258.

36. Weller PF, Rand TH, Barrett T, Elovic A, Wong DT, Finberg RW. Accessory cell function of human eosinophils: HLA-DR dependent, MHC-restricted antigen- presentation and interleukin-Iα formation. *J Immunol* 1993;150:2554–2562.

37. Costa JJ, Matossian K, Beil WJ, Wong DTW et al. Human eosinophils can express the cytokines TNF-α and MIP1-α. *J Clin Invest* 1993;91:2673–2684.

38. Cromwell O, Hamid Q, Corrigan CJ, et al. Expression and generation of interleukin-8, IL-6 and granulocyte-macropahge colony-stimulating factor by bronchial epithelial cells and enhancement by IL-1β and tumour necrosis factor-α. *Immunology* 1992;77:330–337.

39. Devalia JL, Campbell AM, Sapsford RJ, et al. Effect of nitrogen dioxide on synthesis of inflammatory cytokines expressed by human bronchial epithelial cells *in vitro*. *Am J Respir Cell Mol Biol* 1993;9:271–278.

40. Hance AJ. Pulmonary immune cells in health and disease: dendritic cells and Langerhans' cells. *Eur Respir J* 1993;6:1213–1220.

41. Trinchieri G. Interleukin-12 and its role in the generation of TH1 cells. *Immunol Today* 1993;14:335–338.

42. Greenbaum LA, Horowitz JB, Woods A, Pasqualini T, Reich EP, Bottomly K. Autocrine growth of CD4- T cells. Differential effects of IL-1 on helper and inflammatory T cells. *J Immunology* 1988;140:1555–1560.

43. Holt PG, Oliver J, Bilyk N, et al. Downregulation of the antigen presenting cell function(s) of pulmonary dendritic cells *in vivo* by resident alveolar macrophages. *J Exp Med* 1993;177:397–407.

44. Bilyk N, Holt PG. Inhibition of the immunosuppressive activity of resident pulmonary alveolar macrophages by granulocyte-macrophage colony-stimulating factor. *J Exp Med* 1993;177:1773–1777.

45. Boushey HA, Holtzman MJ, Sheller JR, Nadel JA. Bronchial hyperreactivity. *Am Rev Respir Dis* 1980;121:389–413.

46. Tsukagoshi H, Sakamoto T, Xu W, Barnes PJ, Chung KF. Effect of interleukin-1 on airway hyperresponsiveness and inflammation in sensitized and nonsensitized Brown-Norway rats. *J Allergy Clin Immunol* 1994;93:464–469.

47. Kips JC, Tavernier J, Pauwels RA. Tumor necrosis factor (TNF) causes bronchial hyperresponsiveness in rats. *Am Rev Respir Dis* 1992;145:332–336.

48. Wheeler AP, Jesmok G, Brigham KL. Tumor necrosis factor's effect on lung mechanics, gas exchange and airway reactivity in sheep. *J Appl Physiol* 1990;68:2542–2549.

49. Thomas PS, Yates DH, Barnes PJ. TNF-α increases airway responsiveness and sputum neutrophilia in normal human subjects. *Am J Respir Crit Care Med* 1995;152:76–80.

50. Dayer JM, Beutler B, Cerami A. Cachectin/tumour necrosis factor stimulates collagenase and prostaglandin E_2 production by human synovial cells and dermal fibroblasts. *J Exp Med* 1985;162:2163–2168.

51. Huber M, Beutler B, Keppler D. Tumor necrosis factor stimulates leukotriene production *in vivo*. *Eur J Immunol* 1988;18:2085–2088.

52. Sun XM, Hsueh W. Bowel necrosis induced by tumor necrosis factor in rats is mediated by platelet activating factor. *J Clin Invest* 1988;1328–1331.

53. Silberstein DS, David JR. Tumor necrosis factor enhances eosinophil toxicity to *Schistosoma mansoni* larvae. *Proc Natl Acad Sci U S A* 1986;83:1055–1059.

54. Klebanoff SJ, Vadas MA, Harlan JM, et al. Stimulation of neutrophils by tumor necrosis factor. *J Immunol* 1986;136:4220–4225.

55. Shalaby MK, Aggarwal BB, Rinderknecht E, Svedersky LP, Finkle BS, Palladino MA. Activation of human polymorphonuclear neutrophil functions by interferon-γ and tumor necrosis factor. *J Immunol* 1985;135:2069–2073.

56. Bachwich PR, Chensue SW, Larrick LW, Kunkel SL. TNF stimulates interleukin-1 and prostaglandin E_2 production in resting macrophages. *Biochem Biophys Res Commun* 186;136:94–101.

57. Scheurich P, Thoma P, Ucer U, Pfizenmaier K. Immuno- regulatory activity of recombinant human tumor necrosis factor (TNF)-alpha: induction of TNF receptors on human T cells and TNF-alpha-mediated enhancement of T cell responses. *J Immunol* 1987;138:1786–1790.

58. Smith CW, Entman ML, Lance CL, et al. Adherence of neutrophils to canine cardiac myocytes *in vitro* is dependent on intercellular adhesion molecule-1. *J Clin Invest* 1991;88:1216–1223.

59. Warner JC, Libby P. Human vascular smooth muscle cells. Target for and source of tumor necrosis factor. *J Immunol* 1989;142:100–109.

60. Panettieri RA, Lazaar AL, Puré E, Albelda SM. Activation of cAMP-dependent pathways in human airway smooth muscle cells inhibits

TNF-α-induced ICAM-1 and VCAM-1 expression and T lymphocyte adhesion. *J Immunol* 1995; 154:2358–2365.

61. Lazaar AL, Albelda SM, Pilewski JM, Brennan B, Puré E, Panettieri RA. T lymphocytes adhere to airway smooth muscle cells via integrins and CD44 and induce smooth muscle cell DNA synthesis. *J Exp Med* 1994;180:807–816.

62. Moncada S, Palmer RMJ, Higgs EA. Nitric oxide: physiology, pathophysiology and pharmacology. *Pharmacol Rev* 1991;43:109–142.

63. Hamid Q, Springall DR, Riveros-Moreno V. Inducible nitric oxide synthase in asthma. *Lancet* 1993;342:1510–1513.

64. Kharitonov SA, Yates D, Robbins RA, Logan-sinclair R, Shinebourne EA, Barnes PJ. Increased nitric oxide in exhaled air of asthmatic patients. *Lancet* 1994;343:133–135.

65. Persson MG, Zetterström O, Agrenius V, Ihre E, Gustafsson LE. Single breath nitric oxide measurements in asthmatic patients and smokers. *Lancet* 1994;343:146–147.

66. Högman M, Frostell C, Arnberg H, Hedenstierna G. Inhalation of nitric oxide modulates methacholine-induced bronchoconstriction in the rabbit. *Eur Respir J* 1993;6:177–180.

67. Dupuy PM, Shore AS, Drazen JM, Frostell C, Hill WA, Zapol WM. Bronchodilator action of inhaled nitric oxide in guinea pigs. *J Clin Invest* 192;90:421–428.

68. Kips JC, Lefebvre RA, Peleman RA, Joos GF, Pauwels RA. The effect of a nitric oxide synthase inhibitor on the modulation of airway responsiveness in rats. *Am J Respir Crit Care Med* 1995;151:1165–1169.

69. Nijkamp FP, Van Der Linden HJ, Folkerts G. Nitric oxide synthesis inhibitors induce airway hyperresponsiveness in the guinea pig *in vivo* and *in vitro*. *Am Rev Respir Dis* 1993;148:727–734.

70. Tsukagoshi H, Robbins RA, Barnes PJ, Chung KF. Role of nitric oxide and superoxide anions in interleukin-1β-induced airway hyperresponsiveness to bradykinin. *Am J Respir Crit Care Med* 1994;150:1019–1025.

71. Kuo HP, Liu S, Barnes PJ. The effect of endogenous nitric oxide on neurogenic plasma exudation in guinea-pig airways. *Eur J Pharmacol* 1992;221:385–388.

72. Ming WJ, Bersani L, Mantovani A. Tumor necrosis factor is chemotactic for monocytes and polymorphonuclear leukocytes. *J Immunol* 1987;138:1469–1474.

73. Pober JS, Gimbrone MA, Lapierre LA, et al. Overlapping patterns of activation of human endothelial cells by interleukin-1, tumor necrosis factor and immune interferon. *J Immunol* 1986;137:1893–1896.

74. Bevilacqua MP, Pober JS, Mendrick DL, Cotran RS, Gimbrone MA. Identification of an inducible endothelial leukocyte adhesion molecule. *Proc Natl Acad Sci U S A* 1987;84:9238–9242.

75. Osborn L, Hession C, Tizard R, et al. Direct expression cloning of vascular cell adhesion molecule-1, a cytokine-induced endothelial protein that binds to lymphocytes. *Cell* 1989;59:1203–1211.

76. Godding V, Stark JM, Sedgwick JB, Busse WW. Adhesion of activated eosinophils to respiratory epithelial cells is enhanced by tumor necrosis factor-α and interleukin-1. *Am J Respir Cell Mol Biol* 1995;13:555–562.

77. Montefort S, Gratziou C, Goulding D, Polosa R, Haskard DO, Howarth PH, Holgate ST, Carroll MP. Bronchial biopsy evidence for leukocyte infiltration and upregulation of leukocyte-endothelial cell adhesion molecules 6 hours after local allergen challenge of sensitized asthmatic airways. *J Clin Invest* 1994;93:1411–1421.

78. Bentley AM, Durham SR, Robinson DS, Menz G, Storz C, Cromwell O, Kay AB, Wardlaw AJ. Expression of endothelial and leukocyte adhesion molecules intercellular adhesion molecule-1, E-selectin and vascular cell adhesion molecule-1 in the bronchial mucosa in steady state and allergen-induced asthma. *J Allergy Clin Immunol* 1993;92:857–868.

79. Fukuda T, Fukuskima Y, Numao T, et al. Role of interleukin-4 and vascular cell adhesion molecule-1 in selective eosinophil migration into the airways in allergic asthma. *Am J Respir Cell Mol Biol* 1996;14:84–94.

80. Leung DYM, Pober JS, Cotran RS. Expression of endothelial leukocyte adhesion molecule-1 in elicited late phase allergic reactions. *J Clin Invest* 1991;87:1805–1809.

81. Lassalle P, Gosset P, Delneste Y, et al. Modulation of adhesion molecule expression on endothelial cells during the late asthmatic reaction: role of macrophage-derived tumour necrosis factor-alpha. *Clin Exp Immunol* 1993;94:105–110.

82. Wegner CD, Gundel RH, Reilly P, Haynes N, Letts LG, Rothlein R. Intercellular adhesion molecule A (ICAM-1) in the pathogenesis of asthma. *Science* 1990;247:456–459.

83. Pretolani M, Ruffié C, Lapae Silva JR, Joseph D, Lobb RR, Vargaftig BB. Antibody to very late activation antigen 4 prevents antigen-induced bronchial hyperreactivity and cellular infiltration in the guinea pig airways. *J Exp Med* 1994;180:795–805.

84. Watson ML, Smith D, Bourne AD, Thompson RC, Westwich J. Cytokines contribute to airway dysfunction in antigen challenged guinea pigs: inhibition of airway hyperreactivity, pulmonary eosinophil accumulation, and tumor necrosis factor generation by pretreatment with an interleukin-1 receptor antagonist. *Am J Respir Cell Mol Biol* 1993;8:365–369.

85. Broudy VC, Kaushansky K, Segal GM, Harlan JM, Adamson JW. Tumor necrosis factor type-α stimulates human endothelial cells to produce granulocyte-macrophage colony-stimulating factor. *Proc Natl Acad Sci U S A* 1986;83:7467–7471.

86. Strieter RM, Chensue SW, Basha MA, et al. Human alveolar macrophage gene expression of interleukin-8 by tumor necrosis factor-alpha, lipopolysaccharide and interleukin-1β. *Am J Respir Cell Mol Biol* 1990;2:321–326.

87. Marini M, Soloperto M, Mezzetti M, Fasoli A, Mattoli S. Interleukin-1 binds to specific receptors on human bronchial epithelial cells and upregulates granulocyte-macrophage colony-stimulating factor synthesis and release. *Am J Respir Cell Mol Biol* 1991;4:519–524.

88. Wang JH, Devalia JL, Xia C, Sapsford RJ, Davies RJ. Expression of RANTES by human bronchial epithelial cells *in vitro* and *in vivo* and the effect of corticosteroids. *Am J Respir Cell Mol Biol* 1996;14:27–35.

89. Metcalf D, Begley CG, Johnson Gr, Nicola NA, Vadas MA, Lopez AF, Williamson DJ, Wong GG, Clark SC, Wang EA. Biologic properties *in vitro* of a recombinant human granulocyte-macrophage colony-stimulating factor. *Blood* 1986;67:37–45.

90. Lopez AF, Williamson J, Gamble JR, et al. Recombinant human granulocyte-macrophage colony-stimulating factor stimulates *in vitro* mature human neutrophil and eosinophil function, surface receptor expression and survival. *J Clin Invest* 1986;78:1220–1228.

91. Silberstein DS, Owen WF, Gasson JC, et al. Enhancement of human eosinophil cytotoxicity and leukotriene synthesis by biosynthetic (recombinant) granulocyte-macrophage colony-stimulating factor. *J Immunol* 1986;137:3290–3294.

92. Kitamura T, Sato N, Arai K, Miyajima A. Expression cloning of the human IL-3 receptor cDNA reveals a shared subunit for IL-3 and GM-CSF receptors. *Cell* 1991;66:1165–1174.

93. Tavernier J, Devos R, Cornelis S, et al. A human high affinity interleukin-5 receptor (IL-5R) is composed of an IL-5 specific α-chain and a chain shared with the receptor for GM-CSF. *Cell* 1991;66:1175–1184.

94. Devos R, Plaetinck G, Van der Heyden J, et al. Molecular basis of a high affinity murine interleukin-5 receptor. *EMBO J* 1991;10:2133–2137.

95. Sakamaki K, Miyajima I, Kitamura T, Miyajima A. Critical cytoplasmic domains of the common beta subunit of the human GM-CSF, IL-3 and IL-5 receptors for growth signal transduction and tyrosine phosphorylation. *EMBO J* 1992;11:3541–3549.

96. Watanabe Y, Kitamura T, Hayashida K, Miyajima A. Monoclonal antibody against the common subunit (c) of the human interleukin-3 (IL-3), IL-5 and granulocyte-macrophage colony-stimulating factor receptors shows upregulation of c by IL-1 and tumor necrosis factor-α. *Blood* 1992;80:2215–2220.

97. Baggiolini M, Dewald B, Mooser B. Interleukin-8 and related chemotactic cytokines-CXC and CC chemokines. *Adv Immunol* 1993;55:97–179.

98. Warringa RAJ, Schweizer RC, Maikoe T, Kuijper PHM, Bruijnzeel PLB, Koenderman L. Modulation of eosinophil chemotaxis by interleukin-5. *Am J Respir Cell Mol Biol* 1992;7:631–636.

99. Sanz MJ, Weg VB, Bolanowski MA, Nourshargh S. IL-1 is a potent inducer of eosinophil accumulation in rat skin. *J Immunol* 1995;154:1364–1373.

100. Choi AMK, Jacoby DB. Influenza virus A infection induces interleukin-8 gene expression in human airway epithelial cells. *FEBS Lett* 1992;309:327–329.

101. Holgate ST. Asthma: past, present and future. *Eur Respir J* 1993;6:1507–1520.

102. Stewart AG, Tomlinson PR, Wilson J. Airway wall remodeling in asthma: a novel target for the development of anti-asthma drugs. *Trends Pharmacol Sci* 1993;14:275–279.

103. Nicod LP. Cytokines 1. Overview. *Thorax* 1993;48:660–667.

104. Rogalsky V, Todorov G, Den T, Ohnuma T. Increase in protein kinase C activity is associated with human fibroblast growth inhibition. *FEBS Lett* 1992;304:153–156.

105. Gordon JR, Galli SJ. Promotion of mouse fibroblast collagen gene expression by mast cells stimulated via the Fc$_\epsilon$RI. Role for mast cell-derived transforming growth factor-β and tumor necrosis factor-α. *J Exp Med* 1994;180:2027–2037.

106. Warner SJC, Libby P. Human vascular smooth muscle cells. Target for and source of tumor necrosis factor. *J Immunol* 1989;142:100–109.

107. Stewart AG, Tomlinson PR, Fernandes DJ, Wilson JW, Harris T. Tumor necrosis factor-α modulates mitogenic responses of human cultured airway smooth muscle. *Am J Respir Cell Mol Biol* 1995;12:110–119.

108. Couffinhal T, Duplaa C, Labat L, et al. Tumor necrosis factor-alpha stimulates ICAM-1 expression in human vascular smooth muscle cells. *Arterioscler Thromb* 1993;13:407–414.

109. Kume N, Gimbrone MA. Lysophosphatidylcholine transcrip- tionally induces growth factor gene expression in cultured human endothelial cells. *J Clin Invest* 1994;93:907–911.

110. Yoshizumi M, Kourembanas DH, Temizer RP, Cambria P, Quertermous T, Lee M. Tumor necrosis factor increases transcription of the heparin-binding epidermal growth factor-like growth factor gene in vascular endothelial cells. *J Biol Chem* 1992;267:9467–9469.

111. Hirst SJ, Barnes PJ, Twort CHL. Quantifying proliferation of cultured human and rabbit airway smooth muscle cells in response to serum and platelet-derived growth factor. *Am J Respir Cell Mol Biol* 1992;7:574–581.

112. Higashiyama S, Abraham JA, Miller J, Fiddes JC, Klagsbrun M. A heparin-binding growth factor secreted by macrophage-like cells that is related to EGF. *Science* 1991;251:936–939.

113. Marikovsky M, Breuing K, Liu PY, et al. Appearance of heparin-binding EGF-like growth factor in wound fluid as a response to injury. *Proc Natl Acad Sci U S A* 1993;90:3889–3893.

114. Gay CG, Winkles JA. Interleukin-1 regulates heparin-binding growth factor 2 gene expression in vascular smooth muscle cells. *Proc Natl Acad Sci U S A* 1991:88:296–300.

115. Raines EW, Dower SK, Ross R. Interleukin-1 mitogenic activity for fibroblasts and smooth muscle cells is due to PDGF-AA. *Science* 1989;243:393–394.

116. Härkönen E, Virtanen I, Linnala A, Laitinen LL, Kinnula VL. Modulation of fibronectin and tenascin production in human bronchial epithelial cells by inflammatory cytokines *in vitro*. *Am J Respir Cell Mol Biol* 1995;13:109–115.

117. Mattoli S, Mattoso VL, Soloperto M, Allegra L, Fasoli A. Cellular and biochemical characteristics of bronchoalveolar lavage fluid in symptomatic nonallergic asthma. *J Allergy Clin Immunol* 1991;87:794–802.

118. McHugh SM, Wilson AB, Dreighton J, Lachmann PJ, Ewan PW. The profiles of interleukin (IL)-2, IL-6 and interferon-γ production by peripheral blood mononuclear cells from house-dust-mite-allergic patients: a role for IL-6 in allergic disease. *Allergy* 1994;49:751–759.

119. Vercelli D, Jabara HH, Arai K, Yokata T, Geha RS. Endogenous IL-6 plays an obligatory role in IL-4 induced human IgE synthesis. *Eur J Immunol* 1989;19:1419–1426.

120. Schindler R, Mancilla J, Endres S, Ghorbani R, Clark SC, Dinarello CA. Correlation and interaction in the production of IL-6, IL-1 and TNF in human blood mononuclear cells: IL-6 suppresses IL-1 and TNF. *Blood* 1990;75:40–47.

121. Ulich TR, Guo K, Remisk D, del Castillo J, Yin S. Endotoxin-induced cytokine gene expression *in vivo*. *J Immunol* 1991;146:2316–2323.

122. Ulich TR, Yin S, Guo K, Eunhee Y, Remick D, Castillo J. Intratracheal injection of endotoxin and cytokines. *Am J Pathol* 1991;138:1097–1101.

123. DiCosmo BF, Geba GP, Picarella D, Elias JA, Rankin JA, Stripp BR, Whitsett JA, Flavell RA. Airway epithelial cell expression of interleukin-6 in transgenic mice. Uncoupling of airway inflammation and bronchial hyperreactivity. *J Clin Invest* 1994;94:2028–2035.

124. Vecchiarelli A, Siracusa A, Cenci E, Puliti M, Abbritti G. Effect of corticosteroid treatment on interleukin-1 and tumour necrosis factor secretion by monocytes from subjects with asthma. *Clin Exp Allergy* 1992;22:365–370.

125. Wang JH, Trigg CJ, Devalia JL, Jordan S, Davies RJ. Effect of inhaled beclomethasone dipropionate on expression of proinflammatory cytokines and activated eosinophils in the bronchial epithelium of patients with mild asthma. *J Allergy Clin Immunol* 1994;94:1025–1034.

126. Klein LM, Lavker RM, Matis WL, Murphy GF. Degranulation of human mast cells induces an endothelial antigen central to leukocyte adhesion. *Proc Natl Acad Sci U S A* 1989;86:8972–8976.

127. Marini M, Soloperto M, Zheng Y, Mezzetti M, Mattoli S. Protective effect of nedocromil sodium on the IL-1 induced release of GM-CSF from cultured human bronchial epithelial cells. *Pulm Pharmacol* 1992;5:61–65.

128. Vittori E, Sciacca F, Colotta F, Mantovani A, Mattoli S. Protective effect of nedocromil sodium on the interleukin-1 induced production of interleukin-8 in human bronchial epithelial cells. *J Allergy Clin Immunol* 1992;90:76–84.

129. Taffet SM, Singhel KJ, Overholtzer JF, Shurtleff SA. Regulation of tumor necrosis factor expression in a macrophage-like cell line by lipopolysaccharide and cyclic AMP. *Cell Immunol* 1989;120:291–300.

130. Strieter RM, Remick DG, Ward PA, et al. Cellular and molecular regulation of tumor necrosis factor-α production by pentoxifylline. *Biochem Biophys Res Commun* 1988;155:1230–1236.

131. Renz H, Gong JH, Schmidt A, Nain M, Gemsa D. Release of tumor necrosis factor-α from macrophages. Enhancement and suppression are dose-dependently regulatd by prostaglandin E$_2$ and cyclic nucleotides. *J Immunol* 1988;141:2388–2393.

132. Endres S, Fulle HI, Sinha B, et al. Cyclic nucleotides differentially regulate the synthesis of tumour necrosis factor-α and interleukin-1 by human mononuclear cells. *Immunology* 1991;72:56–60.

133. Spatafora M, Chiappara G, Merendino AM, D'Amico D, Bellia V, Bonsignore G. Theophylline suppresses the release of tumour necrosis factor-α by blood monocytes and alveolar macrophages. *Eur Respir J* 1994;7:223–228.

134. Kips JC, Joos GF, Peleman RA, Pauwels RA. The effect of zardaverine, an inhibitor of phosphodiesterase isoenzymes III and IV, on endotoxin-induced airway changes in rats. *Clin Exp Allergy* 1993;23:518–523.

135. Turner CR, Andresen CJ, Smith WB, Watson JW. Effects of rolipram on responses to acute and chronic antigen exposure in monkeys. *Am J Respir Crit Care Med* 1994;149:1153–1159.

136. Pober JS, Slowik MR, De Luca LG, Ritchie AJ. Elevated cyclic AMP inhibits endothelial cell synthesis and expression of TNF-induced endothelial leukocyte adhesion molecule-1, and vascular cell adhesion molecule-1, but not intercellular adhesion molecule-1. *J Immunol* 1993;150:5114–5123.

137. Galve-de Rochemonteix B, Nicod LP, Chicheportiche R, Lacraz S, Baumberger C, Dayer J-M. Regulation of interleukin-1RA, Interleukin-1α, and interleukin-1β production by human alveolar macrophages with phorbol myristate acetate, lipopolysaccharide and Interleukin-4. *Am J Respir Cel Mol Biol* 1993;8:160–168.

138. Kline LN, Fisher PA, Monick MM, Hunninghake GW. Regulation of interleukin-1 receptor antagonist by Th1 and Th2 cytokines. *Am J Physiol* 1995;269:L92–L98.

139. Sim TC, Hilsmeier KA, Reece LM, Grant JA, Alam R. Interleukin-1 receptor antagonist protein inhibits the synthesis of IgE and proinflammatory cytokines by allergen-stimulated mononuclear cells. *Am J Respir Cell Mol Biol* 1994;11:473–479.

140. Lukacs N, Kunkel SL, Burdick MD, Lincoln PL, Strieter RM. Interleukin-1 receptor antagonist blocks chemokine production in the mixed lymphocyte reaction. *Blood* 1993;82:3668–3674.

141. Watson ML, Smith D, Bourne AD, Thompson RC, Westwick J. Cytokines contribute to airway dysfunction in antigen-challenged guinea pigs: inhibition of airway hyperreactivity, pulmonary eosinophil accumulation and tumor necrosis factor generation by pretreatment with an interleukin-1 receptor antagonist. *Am J Respir Cell Mol Biol* 1993;8:365–369.

142. Selig W, Tocker J. Effect of interleukin-1 receptor antagonist on antigen induced pulmonary responses in guinea pigs. *Eur J Pharmacol* 1992;213:331–336.

Asthma, edited by P.J. Barnes, M.M. Grunstein,
A.R. Leff, and A.J. Woolcock.
Lippincott–Raven Publishers, Philadelphia © 1997.

■ 50 ■

Lymphokines

Kaiser G. Lim and Peter F. Weller

Asthma is a disease characterized by intermittent reversible airway obstruction and bronchial hyperresponsiveness to nonspecific inhaled stimuli. Pathologically, there is usually a distinct eosinophilic and mononuclear infiltration with epithelial cell damage, goblet cell hyperplasia, and mucosal inflammation. Asthma was previously thought to be solely a hypersensitivity immune reaction with immunoglobulin (Ig) E-triggered release of mast cell mediators. This mechanism proved inadequate to explain the inflammation observed, nor could it account for some forms of asthma. Unlike extrinsic asthma, intrinsic asthma and occupational asthma are two clinical subsets of asthma where elevation of IgE to specific antigens is not seen (1). This differentiation of asthma is clinical. Histologically, there is no difference between the three in terms of inflammatory cell infiltrate (2,3). An increased numbers of activated eosinophils and T lymphocytes, but not neutrophil and monocyte/macrophages, have been observed in all three types of asthma.

In asthma, an increase in the number of activated T lymphocytes is a more consistent finding than an absolute increase in number of total T cells (4–7). The presence of activated T cells has been demonstrated in blood, bronchial biopsies, and bronchoalveolar lavage (BAL) from allergic asthmatics (4,8–10). In allergen bronchial challenges of sensitized atopic asthmatics, a selective increase in CD4+ cells in BAL fluid with active recruitment from peripheral blood, was observed during the late phase response (9,11). A higher proportion of peripheral blood CD4+ lymphocytes of patients with acute severe asthma had increased expression of interleukin (IL)-2R, HLA-DR, and VLA-1 (8). These activation markers decreased after corticosteroid therapy with clinical improvement (12,13). The increased number of activated T cells correlated with airway eosinophilia and with disease severity (8,10,12). The activation of T lymphocyte and the production of cytokine mediators with the subsequent recruitment of effector eosinophils, may be the common pathway in the pathogenesis of asthma. The activation of T cells with differential secretion of lymphokines may be involved in the pathogenesis of different types of asthma. Lymphokines originally were described as soluble factors generated by activated lymphocytes in response to specific antigen. With the advent of more sensitive detection methods, the cellular sources of so-called "lymphokines" have expanded considerably. *Cytokine* is the preferred term used to describe a group of lower molecular weight soluble proteins which act as chemical communicators between cells. Interleukins are molecular messengers acting between leukocytes and are considered a subset of cytokines.

While there is considerable redundancy and overlapping effects among the different cytokines, they seldom occur in isolation. It is clear that there are no circumstances *in vivo* in which cytokines are produced individually. Rather, they are produced together with other cytokines in patterns characteristic of particular diseases. Mosmann et al. (14) have identified two cytokine secretion profiles in murine CD4+ T lymphocytes or T helper

K. G. Lim and P. F. Weller: Department of Medicine, Beth Israel Deaconess Medical Center, Harvard Medical School, Boston, Massachusetts 02215.

(TH) lymphocytes. In murine systems, TH1 cells produce normal or increased levels of IL-2, interferon-γ (IFN-γ), and tumor necrosis factor-β (TNF-β), and favor macrophage activation that results in delayed-type hypersensitivity (DTH), antibody-dependent cell cytotoxicity, and production of opsonizing antibodies especially IgG_{2a}. TH2 response favors production of murine IgE and IgG_1 isotypes, mucosal immunity through production of growth, differentiation factors for mast cells and eosinophils, and facilitation of IgA synthesis. The TH2 response is associated with downregulation of TH1 response and the production of IL-3, IL-4, IL-5, IL-6, IL-10, and /or IL-13. The physical occurrence of these cytokines together in gene clusters such as IL-3, IL-4, IL-5, granulocyte-macrophage colony-stimulating factor (GM-CSF), IL-6, and IL-13 on chromosome 5 has been well-documented (15). The challenge now is to unravel the regulatory mechanisms involved. Differential regulation of cytokine production, expression, and secretion is required to tailor the immune response (16).

From experiments using cytokines as agonists, by blocking studies, by overexpression and deletion of cytokines in transgenic mice, the role and contribution of each cytokine in disease states is being unraveled. Simple *in vitro* systems have demonstrated potential roles for particular cytokines in asthma; but to integrate the total effects of cytokines found in asthma requires correlating kinetics of humoral and cellular immune responses with the pathophysiology during initiation, amplification, resolution, and repair stages of the disease, a formidable task, indeed. Rather than enumerating the cytokines present in asthma, and matching this with its experimentally derived function, this chapter provides a framework with which to understand the dynamic cellular response and cytokine interaction in the pathophysiology of asthma.

TH2 PATTERN IN ATOPY AND IN ASTHMA

Romagni et al. (17) have provided evidence that a similar TH1 and TH2 pattern that exists in mice, exists in humans. In atopic individuals, allergen-specific T cell clones have a TH2-like pattern of cytokine production, while nonallergenic antigen-specific T cell clones from the same patient have a TH1-like pattern of cytokine production. In human T-cell subsets, this phenotypic differentiation is not a categorical dichotomy. Cytokine profiles with production of both TH1 and TH2 cytokines also are observed, prompting the designation of TH0. More recently, it has been demonstrated using *in situ* hybridization, that the infiltrating cells in allergen-induced late-phase skin reactions express messenger ribonucleic acid (mRNA) for the IL-3, IL-4, IL-5, and GM-CSF gene cluster (TH2), but not for IL-2 or IFN-γ (15,18,19). Similar results were obtained by analyzing mRNA expression of BAL cells from asthmatic individuals, suggesting

that asthma is associated with TH2-type T cells (20). Allergen-specific CD4+ T-cell clones obtained from bronchial biopsies of patients with grass-pollen-induced asthma, exhibited a TH2 profile and were able to induce IgE production by autologous B cells in the presence of the specific allergen (21). Clinical improvement in asthma symptoms after treatment with corticosteroids, also is accompanied by down-modulation of the number of BAL cells positive for IL-4 and IL-5 mRNA with an increase in the number of IFN- mRNA-positive cells (22). It is important to realize that there are other cell sources of these so-called TH1 and TH2 cytokines in addition to CD4+ T cells. CD8+ T lymphocytes, leukocytes, and nonhematopoietic cells, are also capable of producing many of the TH1 and TH2 cytokines. Murine CD8+ CTL's have been shown to be capable of becoming CD8/CD4 double negative, and secreting IL-4, IL-5, IL-6, and IL-10, particularly after being cultured in a type 2 (e.g., IL-4) dominant environment (23–25). Murine CD8+ T cells, specific for viral peptides from a respiratory pathogen, could shift from TH1-type cytokine production to IL-5 production, and induce pulmonary eosinophilia after a TH2-cytokine (IL-4) milieu was induced by immunization with ovalbumin and alum adjuvant (26).

A similar mechanism may occur in humans to account for the exacerbations of asthma with viral respiratory infections. The mechanism responsible for the differentiation of naive TH cells into the TH1- or TH2-phenotype has not yet been clarified completely. Initially, it was thought that the selection was related to the character of the antigen-presenting cell type (27). It is now known that the prevailing cytokine milieu is a primary determinant of which TH phenotype develops (28). Macrophages produce IL-12 to stimulate NK cells to produce IFN-γ. The latter would then favor the development of TH1 cells. IL-4 promotes development of TH2 cells and inhibits development of cells with a TH1-cytokine phenotype (29,30). The bulk of experimental data would indicate that the availability of IL-4 and the absence of IFN-γ and IL-12 at the time of antigen stimulation, are both essential for the development of TH2 response. It should be emphasized that T cells require priming by IL-4 in order to differentiate into IL-4 secreting cells (31,32). Therefore, IL-4 production by mast cells and basophils, or even eosinophils, may be important in initiating the TH2 response in asthma (33–37).

CYTOKINES RELEVANT IN ASTHMA

T lymphocytes have limited stores of preformed cytokines and must synthesize cytokines *de novo* upon cell stimulation. Hence, immunochemical methods of cellular localization may fail to detect cytokines. In this context, the detection of cytokine transcripts has been most insightful. By enzyme-linked immunoadsorbent assay (ELISA), there were detectable levels of TNF-α, IL-1β, IL-2, IL-4, IL-5, IL-6, GM-CSF, Lymphocyte Chemoattractant Factor (LCF or IL-16), and IFN-γ in the BAL fluid of asthmatics (38–42). By *in situ* hybridization, increased proportions of BAL T cells from atopic asthmatic subjects were shown to express mRNA for TNF-α, IL-2, IL-3, IL-4, IL-5, and GM-CSF when compared with those of nonatopic control subjects (20,43,44). In this study, IL-4 and IL-5 probes hybridized to BAL T cells after immunomagnetic separation of BAL cells (20). In a model of inhalational allergen challenge, an increase in mRNA for IL-2, IL-4, IL-5, and GM-CSF, but not for IFN-γ was demonstrated in bronchial biopsies in atopic asthma (45). IL-5 mRNA was detected in the bronchial biopsies of symptomatic asthmatics, but not in asymptomatic or normal subjects (44).

While the majority of the cytokine transcripts appear to be in T lymphocytes, other cellular sources may be important, as well. More than 70% of IL-4 and IL-5 mRNA cells were activated T cells; the remaining IL-4 and IL-5 mRNA-positive signals were noted in mast cells and activated eosinophils (46). Mast cells and basophils are potential sources of IL-4 to prime the T cells. Mast cells in mucosal biopsies from atopic asthmatics were positive for IL-3, IL-4, IL-5, IL-6, and TNF-α by immunohistochemistry (47,48). Human basophils synthesize IL-4 *de novo* following stimulation of the high affinity IgE receptor (FcεRI) (34). Eosinophil cytokine production of GM-CSF has been detected by *in situ* hybridization of nasal polyposis, while immunoreactive GM-CSF and IL-5 in eosinophils were detected after endobronchial allergen challenge in asthmatics (49). Primary airway epithelial cell cultures from normal, allergic, and/or asthmatic individuals have been shown to elaborate IL-16 (LCF), GM-CSF, IL-6, and IL-8 (50, 51). Production of extracellular matrix like fibronectin by epithelial cells can contribute to prolonging eosinophil survival through GM-CSF secretion by eosinophils (52). Airway-derived fibroblasts are a source of GM-CSF, IL-6, and IL-8 (53). IL-1 upregulated gene expression and production of GM-CSF, IL-6, and IL-8 from airway-derived fibroblasts, but did not have a similar effect on airway-derived epithelial cells (53). Cytokine gene expression and production by airway epithelial cells and fibroblasts were sensitive to corticosteroids. The cellular sources of IL-1β were monocytes and dendritic cells in atopic patients, and monocytes in nonatopic asthmatics (48). The actual contributions *in vivo* of each of these potential cytokine sources remain to be elucidated. Whether they act as autocrine mediators or have additional paracrine functions is an important question. The redundancy and overlapping nature of the cytokine network and cytokine sources will impact on any therapeutic strategy directed at altering the cytokine milieu.

DIFFERENCES IN THE CYTOKINE PROFILE OF EXTRINSIC, INTRINSIC, AND OCCUPATIONAL ASTHMA

The functional differentiation of activated T lymphocytes into subsets may help explain the similar histology and nosology observed in the different subtypes of asthma (10,41,54,55). Peripheral blood T lymphocytes from both extrinsic and intrinsic asthmatics, secrete factors that prolong eosinophil survival *in vitro* (10). A majority of the activity has been due to IL-5 and, to a lesser extent, GM-CSF. A significant difference was detected in the cytokine profile of BAL fluid obtained from extrinsic and intrinsic asthmatics. Extrinsic asthmatics have increased levels of IL-4 and IL-5, while intrinsic asthmatics had elevated levels of IL-2, IFN-γ, and IL-5 (10). In both types of asthma, the presence of IL-5 may account for the eosinophil recruitment and activation seen histologically. Activation and degranulation of eosinophils with the release of eosinophil granular proteins and lipid mediators, may contribute significantly to the epithelial damage, bronchial hyperresponsiveness, and bronchospasm observed in asthma. The elevated IL-4 in extrinsic asthma may be responsible for the increased IgE concentrations observed in these patients. The IL-2, IFN-γ, and IL-5 cytokine pattern observed in intrinsic asthma clearly does not fall into the TH1- or TH2-cytokine subsets. IL-2 alone can induce the expression of IL-5 mRNA in T cells without detectable levels of mRNA for IL-4 and GM-CSF (56). Indeed, the eosinophilia observed during treatment with systemic IL-2 is mediated by IL-5 (57). Although IgE and IgG$_4$ isotype switching and production are enhanced by IL-4 and inhibited by IFN-γ, low levels of IFN-γ will suppress only IgE, but not IgG$_4$ (58). By immunohistochemistry in samples obtained from atopic and nonatopic, CD4$^+$ T lymphocytes from atopic symptomatic asthmatics subjects expressed IL-3, IL-4, IL-5, and GM-CSF, while CD4$^+$ T cells from nonatopic symptomatic patients predominantly expressed IL-2, IL-3, IL-5, and GM-CSF immunoreactivity (48). IL-4 was not detected in the nonatopic subjects (48). This suggests that in extrinsic asthmatics, IL-4 present may influence B cell immunoglobulin isotype switching to produce IgE; hence, the stronger association of the latter with IgE concentrations. The presence of IL-5 in both types of asthma could explain the common pathway of eosinophil recruitment and activation resulting in a similar clinical picture. More work is required to establish whether extrinsic asthmatics and intrinsic asthmatics can truly be differentiated into an IL-4- or IL-2-mediated pattern, respectively. Virchow et al. (59) recently did not detect IL-4 in BAL fluid after antigen challenge in a group of extrinsic asthmatics.

Occupational asthma induced by toluene diisocyanate is accompanied by increased levels of TNF-α and IL-1β (60). The majority of T cells cloned from bronchial samples obtained from two subjects actively exposed to toluene diisocyanate were CD8[+] T cell (80%) (61). All the CD8 clones produce IFN-γ, and 44% produce IL-5, but only 6% secreted IL-4. Three months after the cessation of exposure, growing T cells could not be recovered from bronchial biopsies (61).

DYSREGULATION OF IL-4 IN ATOPICS

There are data to suggest that dysregulation of IL-4 may be involved in atopy. In atopic subjects, there is a tendency for IL-4 production by T lymphocytes upon antigen specific stimulation. The majority of allergen-specific CD4[+] T-cell clones derived from atopic donors, express a TH2/TH0 phenotype with high production of IL-4 and very little IFN-γ when stimulated nonspecifically with phorbol ester and anti-CD3 mAb (62). CD4[+] T cells from atopic subjects are able to produce IL-4 and IL-5, even in response to bacterial antigens like purified protein derivative for tuberculosis (PPD) or streptokinase: antigens that usually evoke responses with a restricted TH1 profile from nonatopic subjects (63). Der p I-specific T-cell clones derived from cord blood of newborns with nonatopic parents, showed a prevalent TH1 profile, whereas if both parents were atopic, newborn CD4[+] T-cell clones exhibited a TH0 or TH2 profile (64). The fact that allergen-specific T-cell clones derived from patients with severe atopy produce very high amounts of IL-4, IL-5, IL-3, and GM-CSF, suggests that dysregulation of the cytokine gene cluster on chromosome 5 may be, in some fashion, responsible for the atopic phenotype (63).

Studies using local bronchial instillation of antigen in atopic, but nonasthmatic, subjects showed eosinophil infiltration, a late-phase response, and an increase in IL-4 and IL-5 after challenge (42,65). In a group of steroid-resistant asthmatics, there was a significantly greater number of BAL cells expressing IL-2 and IL-4 mRNA, compared to steroid-responsive asthma (66). After a week of corticosteroid-treatment, the corticosteroid-responsive group had a significant reduction in the number of IL-4 and IL-5 mRNA-positive cells and an increase in IFN-γ mRNA-positive cells. The corticosteroid-unresponsive group had no significant change in the number of cells expressing mRNA for IL-4 or IL-5. IL-2 expression in both groups was unchanged. This suggests a dysregulation of IL-4, IL-5, and IFN-γ gene expression in corticosteroid-resistant asthma (66).

A great deal of progress has been made in the last decade on the cellular and molecular regulation of IgE antibody synthesis. The main regulatory cytokines involved are IL-4 and IFN-γ. IgE synthesis occurs in the presence of IL-4 and IL-13, in conjunction with the engagement of CD40 on the cell surface of B cells (36,67–71). This is an antigen-specific or cognate T cell-B cell interaction. The physical interaction between activated T cells expressing CD40L and secretion of IL-4 are required for B cell im-

munoglobulin isotype switching to IgE and IgG₄. The existence of a noncognate or nonantigen-specific B cell isotype switching occurs when activated human basophils express CD40L and secrete IL-4 to interact with B cells leading to IgE synthesis (36). IgE occurs only in mammals and IgE-secreting B cells are abundant in the skin, lungs, and gut (72). IgE elicits an inflammatory immune response to antigens that results in inflammation, pruritus, coughing, bronchoconstriction, and mucus secretion seen in asthma. Epidemiologically, asthma is associated with serum IgE concentrations and skin-test reactivity to allergens (73). When serum IgE concentrations were standardized according to age and sex, 28% of those with the greatest IgE concentrations reported having asthma, while those with low concentrations reported no asthma. IgE concentrations were significantly greater in the serum and BAL fluid of allergic asthmatics than in those of control subjects (74). Likewise, airway hyperresponsiveness, which closely correlated with the clinical assessments of the presence and severity of asthma, appears to be closely linked to the serum total IgE concentration (75). Others, however, have not detected an association between airway hyperresponsiveness and serum IgE levels (76–79). A lack of correlation between titers of serum allergen-specific IgE and symptoms in untreated patients with seasonal allergic rhinitis also has been reported (80).

Cookson et al. (81) provided evidence for a genetic linkage between generalized atopic IgE responses and a locus on human chromosome 11q. Further studies have suggested the candidate to be a mutation in the β subunit of the high affinity IgE receptor FCεRI (82,83). The FcεRI, in addition to mediating peripheral and systemic anaphylaxis, has a regulatory effect on IgE production through IL-4 production by mast cells (84). There are data to support the speculation that mutation in β subunit of the FCεRI could result in modulation of FcεRI signaling, either rendering the receptor more sensitive to ligands, or by enhancing IL-4 production in response to crosslinkage (85). The markers around the IL-4 locus on chromosome 5q31 have been linked to a gene controlling total serum IgE concentrations but not to antigen specific IgE antibody concentration (37). The study suggests that IL-4 or a nearby gene in 5q31.1 regulates IgE production in a nonantigen specific fashion. The upregulation and enhanced release of IL-4 from non-T cell sources may be enough to prime naive T cells to switch to a TH2-cytokine profile. This generalized upregulation of IL-4 with noncognate B cell stimulation by mast cells and basophils may result in a polyclonal upregulation of IgE. The resulting IgE produced will not be directed against common environmental allergens but not to antigen specific IgE antibody concentration (37). The study suggests that IL-4 or a nearby gene in 5q31.1 regulates IgE production in a nonantigen specific fashion. More work is required to establish the relationship and mechanism between the dysregulation of IL-4 production and mutation of the β subunit of the FCεRI.

A clue to the apparent inconsistent link between IgE and asthma may come from the study of an IgE transgenic knockout mouse model. In this animal model, the absence of IgE did not protect mice from developing anaphylactic response. This suggests the existence of non-IgE pathways for hypersensitivity reactions in mast cells and basophil (86). This is important since mast cell activation and degranulation by IgE is considered one of the inciting events in asthma. When IL-4- and IL-6- secreting non-B/non-T cells from spleens of immunized mice were preincubated with antigen-specific IgE and/or IgG$_2$ and IgG$_3$, they released IL-4 and IL-6 upon antigen challenge (87). Whether IgG's can replace IgE in mediating anaphylaxis is an important question since Fc$_\varepsilon$RI and Fc$_\gamma$RIII share the same gamma subunit (88). The β subunit of the Fc$_\varepsilon$RI can associate with the Fc$_\gamma$RIII on murine mast cells (89). Functional reconstitution studies with a mastocytoma cell line indicate that Fc$_\gamma$RIII composed of Fc$_\gamma$RIII α subunit and Fc$_\varepsilon$RIβ and γ subunits has the capacity for signal transduction (89). Crosslinking of Fc$_\gamma$RIII initiated phosphorylation of protein tyrosines, elevation in intracellular calcium, hydrolysis of phosphoinositides, the release of arachidonic acid metabolites, and hexosaminidase in a quantitatively smaller, but qualitatively indistinguishable manner from those stimulated by Fc$_\varepsilon$RI (90). These studies suggest that through the association of alternative ligand recognition subunits (Fc$_\gamma$RIII α subunit, Fc$_\varepsilon$RI α subunit), a common signal transduction complex (β and γ_2 subunits) may mediate similar biochemical and effector functions in response to IgG and IgE. The effects of Fc$_\varepsilon$RI-α, β, γ and subunit knockout mouse models in atopy and asthma are currently unknown.

INDIVIDUAL CYTOKINES

Interleukin-4

Interleukin-4 (IL-4) is a cytokine, recognized initially to be derived from T cells and mast cells, with multiple effects on B cells, T cells, and many nonlymphoid cells including monocytes, endothelial cells, and fibroblasts. IL-4 plays a dominant role in the differential development of TH0 into TH2 and has a pivotal role in the regulation of IgG$_4$ and IgE synthesis by human B cells (28). IL-4 appears to share this property with IL-13. IL-4 upregulates vascular cell adhesion molecule-1 that mediates VLA-4-dependent selective recruitment of T cells and eosinophils. It induces the expression of the low affinity IgE receptor (CD23) on macrophages, fibroblast chemotaxis, ICAM-1 expression, and stimulates the synthesis of extracellular matrix proteins such as type I and type III procollagen and fibronectin (53). Cells that have been identified as possible sources of IL-4 are mast cells, basophils, T cells, bone marrow stromal cells, and eosinophils (35,91–93). IL-4 potentiates the antigen-induced

proliferation and cytokine production of TH2, but not of TH1 T-cell clones (30). Transgenic mice overexpressing IL-4 develop allergic-like inflammatory disease and altered T-cell development (94).

The possibility that cytokines may recruit selectively certain subsets of responding cells is accompanied by evidence of selective downregulation and tailoring of the function of other cell types. IL-4 can inhibit the IgG-triggered, but not IgE-dependent, human eosinophil degranulation by reducing the expression of IgG receptor (95). The proportion of BAL cells expressing mRNA for IL-4 and IL-5 correlated with measures of airflow obstruction and bronchial hyperresponsiveness (96). IL-4 is a potent inhibitor of proinflammatory cytokine (TNF-α, IL-1, MIP-1α, IL-6, and IL-8) production from monocytes (97–100). There is evidence that IL-4 may downregulate the effects of IL-1 by inducing the expression of IL-1 receptor type II receptor that acts as a decoy to inhibit IL-1 activity (101). IL-4 also inhibits human macrophage colony formation and monocyte-derived hydrogen peroxide production (102,103).

In recent years, other cells have been found to produce IL-4. Mast cells and basophils express CD40L and directly support IgE synthesis by B cells (34). Mast cells in mucosal biopsies from atopic asthmatics were positive for IL-3, IL-4, IL-5, IL-6, and TNF-α by immunohistochemistry (47,48). Human basophils synthesize IL-4 *de novo* following Fc$_\varepsilon$RI engagement (34). By immunohistochemistry, eosinophils in nasal polyposis and asthma were positive for IL-4 and capable of releasing it (35).

Interleukin-5

Interleukin-5 (IL-5) is the only disulphide-linked homodimeric glycoprotein in the hematopoeitic cytokine family (104). IL-3, IL-5, and GM-CSF are all capable of stimulating eosinophil production (105,106). This overlap in function may be explained by the fact that IL-3, IL-5, and GM-CSF receptors share the same β subunit, which is necessary for signaling and high affinity binding (107,108). They exhibit cross inhibition in receptor binding assays *in vitro* due to limiting numbers of β chain (109). The alpha chain is unique to each cytokine and forms a low affinity bond with their respective cytokine (110). Once the cytokines bind to their respective alpha chain, residues in the amino-terminal alpha-helix of the cytokine are targeted to the β component of the receptor (111,112). This apparent redundancy of function between IL-3, IL-5, and GM-CSF may be an *in vitro* phenomenon and each one may have a unique and essential role *in vivo* (113). In patients with filarial infection, subjects with and without eosinophilia had the same levels of IL-3 and GM-CSF. The subjects with eosinophilia had cells that produced high concentrations of IL-5 (114). Although IL-3 and GM-CSF may increase bone marrow eosinophil production, the actual increase is small compared to the effect on other granulocyte lineages, like neutrophils and macrophages (115). Only IL-5 is selective for eosinophil progenitors. In fact, transgenic animals overexpressing IL-3 and GM-CSF survive only a few weeks, and death is caused by massive tissue infiltration by myeloid cells. By contrast, IL-5 transgenics develop eosinophilia but remain healthy (116–119). In asthma, IL-5 is the major cytokine responsible for prolonging eosinophil survival (120).

The molecular biology of the IL-5 receptor is intriguing since two soluble isoforms have been obtained from a butyrate-induced eosinophilic HL-60 cells and cord blood eosinophils (108,121,122). The soluble form is inhibitory in an eosinophil differentiation assay with IL-5, raising the possibility that eosinophil production may be regulated by switching between a membrane bound and a soluble form of the IL-5 receptor (R). The soluble IL-5R alpha subunit binds the IL-5 dimer in a 1:1 molar ratio (123). The membrane-bound and the soluble isoforms are all derived from the same genetic locus by differences at the splicing level (122). The presence of soluble receptor variants belonging to the hematopoietin receptor family has now been detected in IL-4R, IL-5R), IL-6R, IL-7R, and GM-CSF receptor alpha chain (108,124–127). Soluble receptors for IL-1R (128), IL-2R alpha (129) and TNF-α R (130) have also been identified. These soluble receptors may act as regulatory elements to downregulate the immune response (101).

IL-3 and GM-CSF both increase the number of IL-5 responsive eosinophil colony-forming cells while IL-5 promotes the generation of mature eosinophils from these precursors. IL-3-, IL-5- and GM-CSF-induced eosinophils to degranulate *in vitro* and to alter the centrifugal density, a phenotypic marker of activation (131–133). Hypodense eosinophils are a feature of asthma and hypodense eosinophils have enhanced leukotriene production, superoxide generation, and Ig-dependent cytotoxicity (134–137). IL-3, IL-5, TNF-α, and GM-CSF have all been shown to increase CD11b/CD18 expression on eosinophils (138). This is accompanied by increased eosinophil adhesion to endothelial cells (139). IL-3, IL-5, and GM-CSF are only weakly chemotactic themselves, but they prime the eosinophil to increase its response to PAF, LTB$_4$, and IL-8 (140–142). IL-3, IL-5, and GM-CSF prolong the survival of the eosinophil *in vitro*. The mechanism by which IL-5 and GM-CSF enhance survival is by preventing programmed cell death (143,144). GM-CSF-induced inhibition of programmed cell death is associated with increases in tyrosine phosphorylation (144). IL-5 enhances IL-4-induced IgE production by normal human B cells (145). Recombinant human IL-5 when administered repeatedly onto nasal mucosa of subjects with Japanese cedar pollinosis, induced the influx of eosinophils and increased the number of shed epithelial cells and the amount of ECP and secretory IgA in nasal lavage fluid (146).

Interleukin-6

Interleukin-6 (IL-6) first was identified as a T cell-derived factor acting on B cells to induce immunoglobulin secretion (147). IL-6 production, subsequently, was found not to be restricted to T cells (147). While IL-6 does not promote B cell proliferation, it acts on mitogen-activated B cells to induce IgM, IgG, and IgA production (148,149). The concentration of IL-6 required for this function is in the nanogram per milliliter range. Anti-IL-6 antibody completely inhibited immunoglobulin production (147). IL-6 stimulated the proliferation of peripheral T cells activated with lectins or anti-TCR antibodies (150–152). IL-6 upregulates the production of and response to IL-2 (153,154). IL-6 can replace the requirement for antigen-presenting cell (APC) -derived costimulatory signals for IL-2 secretion and proliferation (155, 156). IL-6 also induces acute-phase protein synthesis in hepatocytes (147).

Interleukin-16 (Lymphocyte Chemoattractant Factor)

LCF, a 56 kda homotetrameric cytokine, is a CD8$^+$ lymphocyte-derived product that requires CD4 for bioactivity (40). LCF induces migration of CD4$^+$ lymphocytes, monocytes, and eosinophils but not neutrophils (157, 158). In addition, LCF induces the expression of IL-2R on responding lymphocyte population (157). Bronchial epithelial cells cultured with histamine was found to elaborate LCF and induce CD4$^+$ T-cell migration (50). There is a selective secretion of LCF from CD8$^+$ T cells and from airway epithelium within hours following histamine stimulation *in vitro*. While it is hypothesized that there is a selective recruitment of CD4$^+$ cells after antigen stimulation of asthmatic airways, the cytokine mediators involved have not been well-established. IL-2, IL-16 (LCF), RANTES and MIP1-α all have been found to influence lymphocyte migration (159–162). RANTES and LCF are particularly interesting since they both are potent chemoattractants for CD4$^+$ cells. IL-2, IL-16 (LCF), RANTES, and MIP-1α have been identified in BAL fluid of asthmatics (40,163). In a recent study of lymphocyte chemoattractants present in the early phase of airway inflammation after antigen challenge, IL-16 (LCF) and MIP1-α, but not RANTES, bioactivity and protein were detected (40, manuscript submitted). LCF was the major lymphocyte chemoattractant in this study after antigen challenge (40). This suggests a possible mechanism by which antigen-activated IgE sensitized mast cells can initiate the immune response by recruiting T lymphocytes and eosinophils into the site of inflammation. Further studies are needed to evaluate the role of LCF in recruiting CD4$^+$ T lymphocytes and eosinophils into asthmatic airways.

CONCLUSIONS

Asthma is a heterogeneous clinical disease with many inciting variables, leading to the common manifestation of bronchospam, bronchial hypersensitivity, and airway inflammation. In asthma, cytokines are part of this veritable Forgon's knot of allergens, cellular, humoral immune responses, and genetic susceptibility. By understanding the roles that cytokines play and their regulatory pathways, we hope to develop novel and effective therapeutic approaches in the future.

REFERENCES

1. Rackemann, F. A working classification of asthma. *Am J Med* 1947; 3:601–606.
2. Fabbri L, Danielli D, Crescioli S, et al. Fatal asthma in a subject sensitised to toluene diisocyanate. *Am Rev Respir Dis* 1988;137:1494–1498.
3. Bentley AM, Menz G, Storz C, et al. Identification of T lymphocytes, macrophages, and activated eosinophils in the bronchial mucosa in intrinsic asthma. Relationship to symptoms and bronchial responsiveness. *Am Rev Respir Dis* 1992;146:500–506.
4. Azzawi M, Bradley B, Jeffrey PK, et al. Identification of activated T lymphocytes and eosinophils in bronchial biopsies in stable atopic asthma. *Am Rev Resp Dis* 1990;142:1407–1413.
5. Bradley BL, Azzawi M, Jacobson M, et al. Eosinophils, T-lymphocytes, mast cells, neutrophils, and macrophages in bronchial biopsy specimens from atopic subjects with asthma: comparison with biopsy specimens from atopic subjects without asthma and normal control subjects and relationship to bronchial hyperresponsiveness. *J Allergy Clin Immunol* 1991;88:661–677.
6. Graham D, Luksza A, Evans C. Bronchoalveolar lavage in asthma. *Thorax* 1985;40:717.
7. Wardlaw AJ, Dunnette S, Gleich GJ, et al. Eosinophils and mast cells in bronchoalveolar lavage in subjects with mild asthma. Relationship to bronchial hyperreactivity. *Am Rev Resp Dis* 1988; 137:62–69.
8. Corrigan CJ, Hartnell A and Kay AB. T-lymphocyte activation in acute severe asthma. *Lancet* 1988;1:1129–1132.
9. Gerblich AA, Campbell AE, Schuyler MR. Changes in T-lymphocyte subpopulations after antigenic bronchial provocation in asthmatics. *N Engl J Med* 1984;310:1349–1352.
10. Walker C, Kaegi MK, Braun P and Blaser K. Activated T cells and eosinophilia in bronchoalveolar lavages from subjects with asthma correlated with disease severity. *J Allergy Clin Immunol* 1991;88: 935–942.
11. Metzger WJ, Zavala D, Richerson HB, et al. Local allergen challenge and bronchoalveolar lavage of allergic asthmatic lungs. *Am Rev Respir Dis* 1987;135:433–440.
12. Corrigan CJ. Kay, AB. CD4 T-lymphocyte activation in acute severe asthma. Relationship to disease severity and atopic status. *Am Rev Respir Dis* 1990;141:970–977.
13. Corrigan CJ, Haczku A, Gemou-Engesaeth V, et al. CD4 T-lymphocyte activation in asthma is accompanied by increased serum concentration of IL-5. *Am Rev Respir Dis* 1993;147:540–547.
14. Mosmann T, Coffman R. Heterogeneity of cytokine secretion pattern and functions of helper T cells. *Adv Immunol* 1989;46:11–24.
15. Chandrasekharappa SC, Rebelsky MS, Firak TA, Le BM, Westbrook CA. A long-range restriction map of the interleukin-4 and interleukin-5 linkage group on chromosome 5. *Genomics* 1990;6:94–99.
16. Paul W, Seder R. Lymphocyte responses and cytokines. *Cell* 1994;76: 241–251.
17. Wierenga E, Snoek M, De Groot C, et al. Evidence for compartmentalisation of functional subsets of CD4+ T lymphocytes in atopic patients. *J Immunol* 1990;144:4651–4656.
18. Van-Leeuwen B, Martinson M, Webb G, Young I. Molecular organization of the cytokine gene cluster, involving the human IL-3, IL-4, IL-5 and GM-CSF genes on human chromosome. *Blood* 1989;73: 1142.
19. Kay A, Ying S, Varney V, et al. Messenger RNA expression of the cy-

20. tokine gene cluster IL-3, IL-4, IL-5 and GM-CSF in allergen induced late-phase cutaneous reactions in atopic subjects. *J Exp Med* 1991; 173:775–778.
20. Robinson DS, Hamid Q, Ying S, et al. Predominant TH2-like bronchoalveolar T-lymphocyte population in atopic asthma. *N Engl J Med* 1992;326:298–304.
21. Del Prete G, De Carli M, Maestrelli M, Ricci L, Fabri L, Romagnani S. Allergen exposure induces activation of allergen-specific TH2 cells in the airway mucosa of patients with allergic respiratory disorders. *Eur J Immunol* 1993;23:1445–1449.
22. Robinson D, Hamid Q, Ying S, et al. Prednisolone treatment in asthma is associated with modulation of bronchoalveolar lavage cell IL-4, IL-5 and IFN- cytokine gene expression. *Am Rev Respir Dis* 1993;148:401–406.
23. Connors M, Giese N, Kulkarni A, Firestone C, Morse HI, Murphy B. Enhanced pulmonary histopathology induced by respiratory syncytial virus (RSV) challenge of formali-inactivated RSV-immunized BALB/c mice is abrogated by depletion of interleukin-4 and interleukin-10. *J Virol* 1994;68:5321–5325.
24. Erard F, Wild M, Garcia-Sanchez J, Le Gros G. Switch of CD8 T cells to noncytolytic CD8-CD4- cells that make TH2 cytokines anf help B cells. *Science* 1993;260:1802–1805.
25. Seder R, Boulay J, Finkelman Fea. CD8+ T cells can be primed *in vitro* to produce IL-4. *J Immunol* 1992;148:1652–1656.
26. Coyle A, Erard F, Bertrand C, Walti S, Pircher H, Le Gros G. Virus-specific CD8+ cells can switch to IL-5 production and induce airway eosinophilia. *J Exp Med* 1995;181:1229–1233.
27. Chang T, Shea C, Urioste S, Thompson R, Boom W and Abbas A. Heterogeneity of helper/inducer T lymphocytes. III. Responses of IL-2 and IL-4-producing (TH1 and TH2) clones to antigens presented by different accessory cells. *J Immunol* 1990;145:2803–2808.
28. Seder R, Paul W, Davis M, Fazekas De St. Groth B. The presence of interleukin-4 during *in vitro* priming determines the lymphokine producing potential of CD4+ T cell from T cell receptor transgenic mice. *J Exp Med* 1992;176:1091–1098.
29. Swain S, Huston G, Tonkonogy S, Weinberg A. TGF- and IL-4 cause helper T cell precursors to develop into dictinct effector helper cells that differ in lymphokine secretion pattern and cell surface phenotype. *J Immunol* 1991;147:2991–3000.
30. Swain S, Weinberg A, English M, Huston G. IL-4 directs the development of TH2-like helper effectors. *J Immunol* 1990;145:3796–3806.
31. Romagnani S. Induction of TH1 and TH2 response: A key role for the "natural" immune response? *Immunol Today.* 1992;13:379–381.
32. Le Gros G, Ben-Sasson S, Seder R, Finkelman F, Paul W. Generation of IL-4 producing cells *in vivo* and *in vitro*: IL-2 and IL-4 are required for *in vitro* generation of IL-4 producing cells. *J Exp Med* 1990;172: 921–929.
33. Bradding P, Feather IH, Howarth PH, et al. Interleukin-4 is localized to and released by human mast cells. *J Exp Med* 1992; 176:1381–1386.
34. Brunner T, Heusser C, Dahinden C. Human peripheral blood basophils primed by IL-3 produce IL-4 in response to IgE receptor stimulation. *J Exp Med* 1993;177:605–611.
35. Nonaka M, Nonaka R, Woolley K, et al. IL-4 is localized to eosinophils *in vivo* and released by peripheral blood eosinophils. *J Immunol* (in press).
36. Gauchat J, et al. Induction of human IgE synthesis in B cells by mast cells and basophils. *Nature* 1993;365:340–343.
37. Marsh D, Neely J, Breazeale D, et al. Linkage analysis of IL-4 and other chromosome 5q31.1 markers and total serum immunoglobulin E concentrations. *Science* 1994;264:1152–1156.
38. Broide, DH, Lotz, M, Cuomo, AJ, Coburn, DA, Federman, EC and Wasserman, SI. Cytokines in symptomatic asthma airways. *J Allergy Clin Immunol* 1992;89:958–94.
39. Borish L, Mascali JJ, Dishuck J, Beam WR, Martin RJ, Rosenwasser LJ. Detection of alveolar macrophage-derived IL-1β in asthma. *J Immunol* 1992;149:3078–3082.
40. Cruikshank W, Melissa F, Teran L, Center D. Early detection of a CD4- lymphocyte and eosinophil chemoattractant in bronchoalveolar lavage fluid from asthmatics following antigen challenge. *Am J Respir* 1994;149:A954.
41. Walker C, Bode E, Boer L, Hansel TT, Blaser K, Virchow,J. Allergic and nonallergic asthmatics have distinct patterns of T-cell activation and cytokine production inperipheral blood and bronchoalveolar lavage. *Am Rev Respir Dis* 1992;146:109–115.

42. Sedgwick JB, Calhoun WJ, Gleich GJ, et al. Immediate and late airway response of allergic rhinitis patients to segmental antigen challenge. Characterization of eosinophil and mast cell mediators. *Am Rev Resp Dis* 1991;144:1274–1281.

43. Ying S, Robinson S, Varney V, et al. TNF-α mRNA expression in allergic inflammation. *Clin Exp Allergy* 1991;21:745.

44. Hamid Q, Azzawi S, Ying S, et al. Expression of mRNA for interleukin-5 in mucosal bronchial biopsies from asthma. *J Clin Invest* 1991;87:1541.

45. Bentley AM, Meng Q, Robinson DS, Hamid Q, Kay AB, Durham, SR. Increases in activated T lymphocytes, eosinophils, and cytokine mRNA expression for interleukin-5 and granulocyte-macrophage colony-stimulating factor in bronchial biopsies after allergen challenge in atopic asthmatics. *Am J Respir Cell Mol Biol* 1993;8:35–42.

46. Ying S, Durham S, Corrigan C, Hamid Q, Kay A. Phenotype of cells expressing mRNA for TH2-type (IL-4 and IL-5) and TH1-type (IL-2 and IFN-γ) cytokines in bronchoalveolar lavage and bronchial biopsies from atopic and normal control subjects. *Am J Respir Cell Mol Biol* 1995;12:477–487.

47. Bradding P, Roberts JA, Britten KM, et al. Interleukin-4, -5, -6 and Tumor necrosis factor-α in normal and asthmatic airways: evidence for the human mast cell as a source of these cytokines. *Am J Respir Cell Mol Biol* 1994;10:471–480.

48. Ackerman V, Marini M, Vittori E, Bellini A, Vassali G, Mattoli S. Detection of cytokines and their cell sources in bronchial biopsy specimen from asthmatic patients. *Chest* 1994;105:687–696.

49. Broide DH, Paine MM, Firestein GS. Eosinophils express interleukin 5 and granulocyte-macrophage colony-stimulating factor mRNA at sites of allergic inflammation in asthmatics. *J Clin Invest* 1992;90:1414–1424.

50. Bellini A, Yoshimura H, Vittori E, Marini M, Mattoli S. Bronchial epithelial cells of patients with asthma release chemoattractant factors for T lymphocytes. *J Allergy Clin Immunol* 1993;92:412–424.

51. Marini M, Vittori E, Hollemborg J, Mattoli S. Expression of the potent inflammatory cytokines, granulocyte-macrophage colony-stimulating factor, interleukin-6 and interleukin-8, in bronchial epithelial cells of patients with asthma. *J Allergy Clin Immunol* 1992; 89:1001–1009.

52. Anwar ARF, Moqbel R, Walsh GM, Kay AB, Wardlaw AJ. Adhesion to fibronectin prolongs eosinophil survival. *J Exp Med* 1993;177:839–843.

53. Denburg D, Gauldie J, Dolovich J, Ohtoshi T, Cox G, Jordana M. Structural cell-derived cytokines in allergic inflammation. *Int Arch Appl Immunol* 1991;94:127–132.

54. Walker C, Virchow JCJ, Bruijnzeel PL, Blaser K. T-cell subsets and their soluble products regulate eosinophilia in allergic and nonallergic asthma. *J Immunol* 1991;146:1829–1835.

55. Walker C. The immunology of extrinsic and intrinsic asthma. *Agents Actions Suppl* 1993;43:97–106.

56. Bohjanen PR, Okajima M, Hodes RJ. Differential regulation of interleukin 4 and interleukin 5 gene expression: a comparison of T-cell gene induction by anti-CD3 antibody or by exogenous lymphokines. *Proc Natl Acad Sci U S A* 1990;87:5283–5287.

57. Macdonald D, Gordon AA, Kajitani H, Enokihara H, Barrett AJ. Interleukin-2 treatment-associated eosinophilia is mediated by interleukin-5 production. *Br J Haematol* 1990;76:168–173.

58. Ishizaka A, et al. The inductive effect of interleukin-4 on IgG4 and IgE synthesis in human peripheral blood lymphocytes. *Clin Exp Immunol* 1990;79:392.

59. Virchow JJ, Walker C, Hafner D, et al. T cells and cytokines in bronchoalveolar lavage fluid after segmental allergen provocation in atopic asthma. *Am J Respir Crit Care Med* 1995;151:969–968.

60. Maestrelli P, Di Stefano A, Occari P, et al. Cytokines in the airway mucosa of subjects with asthma induced by toluene diisocyanate. *Am J Respir Crit Care Med* 1995;151:607–612.

61. Maestrelli P, Del Prete G, De Carli M, et al. CD8 T-cell clones producing IL-5 and IFN-γ in bronchial mucosa of patients with asthma induced by toluene diisocyanate. *Scand J Work Environ Health* 1994; 20:376–381.

62. Parronchi P, Macchia D, Piccini M, et al. Allergen- and bacterial antigen-specific T-cell clones estabished from atopic donors show a different profile of cytokine production. *Proc Natl Acad Sci U S A* 1991; 88:4538–4542.

63. Parronchi P, Decarli M, Manetti R, et al. Aberrant Interleukin (IL)-4 and IL-5 production *in vitro* by CD4+ helper T cells from atopic subjects. *Eur J Immunol* 1992;22:1615–1620.

64. Piccini M, Mecacci F, Sampognaro S, et al. Aeroallergen sensitization can occur during fetal life. *Int Arch Allergy Immunol* 1993;102: 301–303.

65. Zangrilli J, Shaver J, Cirelli R, et al. Garlisli, C, Falcone, A, Cuss, F, Fish, J and Peters, S. sVCAM levels after segmental antigen challenge corrleate with eosinophil influx, IL-4 and IL-5 production, and the late phase response. *Am J Respir Crit Care Med* 1995;151:1346–1353.

66. Leung D, Martin R, Szefler S, et al. Dysregulation of IL-4, IL-5 and IFN-γ gene expression in steroid-resistant asthma. *J Exp Med* 1995; 181:33–40.

67. Punnonen J, Aversa G, Cocks B, et al. IL-13 induces IL-4 independent IgG4 and IgE synthesis and CD23 expression by human B cells. *Proc Natl Acad Sci U S A* 1993;90:3730–3734.

68. Gauchat J, Lebman D, Coffman R, Gascan H, De Vries J. Structure and expression of germline ε transcripts in human B cells induced by interleukin-4 to switch to IgE production. *J Exp Med* 1990; 172:463–471.

69. Jabara H, Fu S, Geha R, Vercelli D. Synergism between anti-CD40 monoclonal antibody and interleukin-4 in the induction of IgE synthesis by highly purified B cells. *J Exp Med* 1990;172:1861–1866.

70. Romagnani S. Regulation and deregulation of human IgE synthesis. *Immunol Today* 1990;11:316–321.

71. Maggi E, Romagnani S. Role of T cells and T-cell derived cytokines in the pathogenesis if allergic diseases. *Ann N Y Acad Sci* 1994;725: 2–12.

72. Sutton B, Gould H. The human IgE network. *Nature* 1993;366:421–428.

73. Burrows B, Martinez F, Halonen M, Barbee R, Cline M. Association of asthma with serum IgE levels and skin-test reactivity to allergens. *N Engl J Med* 1989;320:271–277.

74. Crimi E, Scordamaglia A, Crimi P, Zupo S, Barocci S. Total and specific IgE in serum, bronchial lavage, and bronchoalveolar lavage of asthmatic patients. *Allergy* 1983;38:553–559.

75. Sears MR, et al. Relation between airway responsiveness and serum IgE in children with asthma and in apparently normal children. *N Engl J Med* 1991;325:1067–1071.

76. Muranaka M, Suzuki S, Miyamoto T, Takeda K, Okumura H. Bronchial reactivities to acetylcholine and IgE levels in asthmatic subjects after longterm remissions. *J Allergy Clin Immunol* 1974; 54:32–40.

77. Bryant D, Burns M. The relationship between bronchial histamine reactivity and atopic status. *Clin Allergy* 1976;6:373–381.

78. Lam S, Tan F, Chan H, Chan-Yeung M. Relationship between types of asthmatic reaction, nonspecific bronchial reactivity, and specific IgE antibodies in patients with red cedar asthma. *J Allergy Clin Immunol* 1983;72:134–139.

79. Woolcock A, Colman M, Jones M. Atopy and bronchial reactivity in Australian and Melanesian populations. *Clin Allerg* 1978;8:155–164.

80. Nickelsen J, Georgitis J, Reisman R. Lack of correlation between titers of serum allergen-specific IgE and symptoms in untreated patients with seasonal allergic rhinitis. *J Allergy Clin Immunol* 1986;77: 43–48.

81. Cookson W, Sharp P, Faux J, Hopkin J. Linkage between immunoglobulin E responses underlying asthma and rhinitis and chromosome 11q. *Lancet* 1989;1:1292–1295.

82. Sandford A, Shirakawa T, Moffatt M, et al. Localization of atopy and beta subunit of high-affinity IgE receptor on chromosome 11q. *Lancet* 1993;341:332–334.

83. Shirakawa T, Li A, Dubowitz M, et al. Association between atopy and variants of the beta subunit of the high affinity immunoglobulin E receptor. *Nat Genet* 1994;7:125–130.

84. Paul W, Seder R, Plaut M. Lymphokine and cytokine production by FcₑRI+ cells. *Adv Immunol* 1992;53:1–29.

85. Ravetch J. Atopy and Fc receptors: mutation is the message? *Nat Genet* 1994;7:117–118.

86. Oettgen H, Martin T, Wynshaw-Boris A, et al. Active anaphylaxis in IgE-deficient mice. *Nature* 1994;370:367–370.

87. Aoki I, Kinzer C, Shirai A, Paul W, Klinman D. IgE receptor-positive non-B/non-T cells dominate the production of IL-4 and IL-6 in immunized mice. *Proc Natl Acad Sci U S A* 1995;92:2534–2538.

88. Ra C, Jouvin M, Blank U, Kinet J. A macrophage Fcγ receptor and the mast cell receptor for IgE share an identical subunit. *Nature* 1989; 341:752.

89. Kurosaki T, Gander I, Wirthmueller U, Ravetch J. The β subunit of the FcεRI is associated with the FcγRIII on mast cells. *J Exp Med* 1992; 175:447–451.

90. Alber G, Kent U, Metzger H. Functional comparison of FcεRI, FcγRII, and FcγRIII in mast cells. *J Immunol* 1992;149:2428–2436.

91. Ohara J, Paul W. Receptors for B-cell stimulatory factor-1 expressed on cells of haematopoietic lineage. *Nature* 1987;325:537–540.

92. Park L, Friend D, Grabstein K, Urdal D. Characterization of the high-affinity cell-surface receptor for murine B-cell-stimulating factor 1. *Proc Natl Acad Sci U S A* 1987;84:1669–1673.

93. Park L, Friend D, Sassenfeld H, Urdal D. Characterization of the human B-cell stimulatory factor-1 receptor. *J Exp Med* 1987;166:476–488.

94. Tepper RI, Levinson DA, Stanger,BZ, et al. IL-4 induces allergic-like inflammatory disease and alters T cell development in transgenic mice. *Cell* 1990;62:457–467.

95. Baskar P, Silberstein DS, Pincus SH. Inhibition of IgG-triggered human eosinophil function by IL-4. *J Immunol* 1990;144:2321–2326.

96. Robinson D, Ying S, Bentley A, et al. Relationships among numbers of bronchoalveolar lavage cells expressing mRNA for cytokines, asthma symptoms and airway methacholine responsiveness in atopic asthma. *J Allergy Clin Immunol* 1993;92:397.

97. Standiford T, Kunkel S, Liebler J, et al. Gene expression of MIP-1α from human blood monocytes and alveolar macrophages is inhibited by interleukin-4. *Am J Respir Cell Mol Biol* 1993;9:192–198.

98. Standiford T, Strieter R, Chensue S, et al. IL-4 inhibits the expression of IL-8 from stimulated human blood monocytes. *J Immunol* 1990; 145:1435–1439.

99. Gauchat D, Gauchat J, Bettens F, de Weck A, Stadler B. Cytokine gene expression in atopics: effect of IL-4 on IL-1β and IL-6 mRNA levels. *Eur Cytokine Netw* 1990;1:85–90.

100. Hart P, Vitti G, Burgess D, Whitty G, Piccoli D, Hamilton J. Potential antiinflammatory effects of IL-4: suppression of human monocyte TNF-α, IL-1 and PGE₂. *Proc Natl Acad Sci U S A* 1989;86:3803–3807.

101. Colotta F, Re F, Muzio M, et al. Interleukin-1 type II receptor: a decoy target for IL-1 that is regulated by IL-4. *Science* 1993;261:472–475.

102. Jansen J, Wientjens G, Fibbe W, Willemze R, Kluin-Nelemans H. Inhibition of human macrophage colony formation by IL-4. *J Exp Med* 1989;170:577–582.

103. Lehn M, Weisner W, Engelhorn S, Gillis S, Remold H. IL-4 inhibits H₂O₂ production and anti-leishmanial capacity of human cultured monocytes mediated by IFN-γ. *J Immunol* 1989;143:3020–3024.

104. Sanderson CJ. Interleukin-5, eosinophils, and disease. *Blood* 1992;79:3101–3109.

105. Clutterbuck EJ, Hirst EM, Sanderson CJ. Human interleukin-5 (IL-5) regulates the production of eosinophils in human bone marrow cultures: comparison and interaction with IL-1, IL-3, IL-6, and GM-CSF. *Blood* 1989;73:1504–1512.

106. Clutterbuck EJ, Sanderson CJ. Regulation of human eosinophil precursor production by cytokines: a comparison of recombinant human interleukin-1 (rhIL-1), rhIL-3, rhIL-5, rhIL-6, and rh granulocyte-macrophage colony-stimulating factor. *Blood* 1990;75:1774–1779.

107. Tominaga A, Takaki S, Koyama N, et al. Transgenic mice expressing a B-cell growth and differentiation factor gene (interleukin-5) develop eosinophilia and autoantibody production. *J Exp Med* 1991;173:429–437.

108. Tavernier J, Devos R, Cornelius S, et al. A human high affinity interleukin-5 receptor (IL-5R) is composed of an IL-5-specific alpha-chain and a beta-chain shared with the receptor for GM-CSF. *Cell* 1991;66:1175–1184.

109. Nicola N, Metcalf, D. Subunit promiscuity among hemopoietic growth factor receptors. *Cell* 1991;67:1.

110. Bazan, J. Structural design and molecular evolution of a cytokine receptor superfamily. *Proc Natl Acad Sci* 1990;87:6934.

111. Scanafelt A, Miyajima A, Kitamura T,Kastelein, R. The amino-terminal helix of GM-CSF and IL-5 governs high affinity binding to their receptors. *EMBO J* 1991;13:4105–4112.

112. Lopez A, Shannon M, Hercus T, et al. Residue 21 of human GM-CSF is critical for biological activity and for high not low affinity binding. *EMBO J* 1992;11:909–916.

113. Coffman RL, Seymour BWP, Hudak S, Jackson J, Rennick D. Antibody to interleukin-5 inhibits helminth-induced eosinophilia in mice. *Science* 1989;245:308–310.

114. Limaye AP, Abrams JS, Silver JE, Ottesen EA, Nutman TB. Regulation of parasite-induced eosinophilia: selectively increased interleukin-5 production in helminth-infected patients. *J Exp Med* 1990; 172:399–402.

115. Ganser A, Lindemann A, Seipelt G, et al. Effects of recombinant human IL-3 in patients with normal hematopoiesis and with bone marrow failure. *Blood* 1990;76:666.

116. Johnson G, Gonda T, Metcalf D, Hariharan I, Cory S. A lethal myeloproliferative syndrome in mice transplanted with bone marrow cells infected with a retrovirus expressing GM-CSF. *EMBO J* 1989; 8:441.

117. Chang J, Metcalf D, Lang R, Gonda T, Johnson G. Nonneoplastic hematopoietic myeloproliferative syndrome induced by dysregulated multi-CSF (IL-3) expression. *Blood* 1989;73:1489.

118. Dent LA, Strath M, Mellor AL, Sanderson CJ. Eosinophilia in transgenic mice expressing interleukin-5. *J Exp Med* 1990;172:1425–1431.

119. Lang R, Metcalf D, Cuthbertson R, et al. Transgenic mice expressing a hematopoietic growth factor gene (GM-CSF) develop accumulations of macrophages, blindness, and a fatal syndrome of tissue damage. *Cell* 1987;51:675.

120. Ohnishi T, Kita H, Weiler D, et al. IL-5 is the predominant eosinophil-active cytokine in the antigen-induced pulmonary late-phase reaction. *Am Rev Resp Dis* 1993;147:901–907.

121. Murata Y, Takaki S, Migita M, Kikuchi Y, Tominaga A, Takatsu K. Molecular cloning and expression of the human interleukin-5 receptor. *J Exp Med* 1992;175:341–351.

122. Tavernier J, Tuypens T, Plaetinck G, Verhee A, Fiers W, Devos R. Molecular basis of the membrane-anchored and two soluble isoforms of the human interleukin-5 receptor a subunit. *Proc Natl Acad Sci U S A* 1992;89:7041–7045.

123. Devos R, Guisez Y, Cornelis S, et al. Recombinant soluble human IL-5 receptor molecules: crosslinking and stoichiometry of binding to IL-5. *J Biol Chem* 1993; 268:6581–6587.

124. Mosley B, Bechmann M, March C, et al. The murine IL-4 receptor: molecular cloning and characterization of secreted and membrane forms. *Cell* 1989;59:335–348.

125. Novick D, Engelmann H, Wallach D, Rubinstein M. Soluble cytokine receptors are present in normal human urine. *J Exp Med* 1989;170:1409–1414.

126. Goodwin R, Friend D, Ziegler et al. Cloning of the human and murine IL-7 receptors: demonstration of a soluble form and homology to a new receptor superfamily. *Cell* 1990;60:941–951.

127. Raines M, Liu L, Quan S, Joe V, DiPersio J, Golde D. Identification and molecular cloning of a soluble human GM-CSF receptor. *Proc Natl Acad Sci* 1991;88:8203–8207.

128. Symons J, Duff G. A soluble form of the IL-1 receptor produced by a human B cell line. *FEBS Lett* 1990;272:133–136.

129. Marcon L, Fritz M, Kurman C, Jensen J, Nelson D. Soluble Tac peptide is present in the urine of normal individuals and at elevated levels in patients with adult T cell leukemia. *Clin Exp Immunol* 1988;73:29–33.

130. Loetscher H, Steinmatz M, Lesslauer W. Tumour necrosis factor: receptors and inhibitors. *Cancer Cells* 1991;3:221–226.

131. Fujisawa T, Abu-Ghazaleh R, Kita H, Sanderson CJ, Gleich GJ. Regulatory effect of cytokines on eosinophil degranulation. *J Immunol* 1990;144:642–646.

132. Owen WF Jr, Rothenberg MF, Silberstein DS, et al. Regulation of human eosinophil viability, density, and function by granulocyte-macrophage colony-stimulating factor in the presence of 3T3 fibroblasts. *J Exp Med* 1987;166:129–141.

133. Rothenberg ME, Owen WF Jr, Silberstein DS,et al. Human eosinophils have prolonged survival, enhanced functional properties, and become hypodense when exposed to human interleukin-3. *J Clin Invest* 1988;81:1986–1992.

134. Kajita T, Yui Y, Mita H, et al. Release of leukotriene C₄ from human eosinophils and its relation to the cell density. *Int Arch Allergy Appl Immunol* 1985;78:406–410.

135. Pincus SH, Schooley WR, DiNapoli AM, Broder S. Metabolic heterogeneity of eosinophils from normal and hypereosinophilic patients. *Blood* 1981;58:1175–1181.

136. Owen WF, Rothenberg ME, Petersen J, et al. Interleukin-5 and phenotypically altered eosinophils in the blood of patients with the idiopathic hypereosinophilic syndrome. *J Exp Med* 1989;170:343–348.

137. Hodges MK, Weller PF, Gerard NP, Ackerman SJ, Drazen JM. Heterogeneity of leukotriene C₄ production by eosinophils from asthmatic and normal subjects. *Am Rev Resp Dis* 1988;138:799–804.

138. Thorne KJI, Richardson BA, Mazza G, Butterworth AE. A new method for measuring eosinophil activating factors, based on the expression of CR3 alpha-chain (CD11b) on the surface of the activated eosinophils. *J Immunol Methods* 1990;133:47–54.

139. Walsh GM, Wardlaw AJ, Hartnell A, Sanderson CJ, Kay AB. Interleukin-5 enhances the *in vitro* adhesion of human eosinophils, but not neutrophils, in a leukocyte integrin (CD11/18)-dependent manner. *Int Arch Allergy Appl Immunol* 1991;94:174–178.

140. Wang JM, Rambaldi A, Biondi A, Chen ZG, Sanderson CJ, Mantovani A. Recombinant human interleukin-5 is a selective eosinophil chemoattractant. *Eur J Immunol* 1989;19:701–705.

141. Warringa RA, Koenderman L, Kok PT, Kreukniet J, Bruijnzeel PL. Modulation and induction of eosinophil chemotaxis by granulocyte-macrophage colony-stimulating factor and interleukin-3. *Blood* 1991; 77:2694–2700.

142. Warringa RA, Schweizer RC, Maikoe T, Kuijper PH, Bruijnzeel PL, Koendermann L. Modulation of eosinophil chemotaxis by interleukin-5. *Am J Respir Cell Mol Biol* 1992;7:631–636.

143. Stern M, Meagher L, Savill J, Haslett C. Apoptosis in human eosinophils. Programmed cell death in the eosinophil leads to phagocytosis by macrophages and is modulated by IL-5. *J Immunol* 1992;148:3543–3549.

144. Yousefi S, Green D, Blaser K, Simon H. Protein-tyrosine phosphorylation regulates apoptosis in human eosinophils and neutrophils. *Proc Natl Acad Sci U S A* 1994;91:10868–10872.

145. Pene J, Rousset F, Briere F, et al. Interleukin-5 enhances interleukin 4-induced IgE production by normal human B cells. The role of soluble CD23 antigen. *Eur J Immunol* 1988;929–935.

146. Terada N, Konno A, Tada H, Shirotori K, Ishikawa K, Togawa K. The effect of recombinant human interleukin-5 on eosinophil accumulation and degranulation in human nasal mucosa. *J Allergy Clin Immunol* 1992;90:160–168.

147. Akira S, Taga T, Kishimoto T. Interleukin-6 in biology and medicine. *Adv Immunol* 1993;54:1–78.

148. Beagley K, Eldridge J, Lee F, et al. Interleukins and IgA synthesis: human and murine interleukin-6 induce high rate of IgA secretion in IgA-committed B cells. *J Exp Med* 1989;169:2133–2148.

149. Muraguchi A, Hirano T, Tang B, et al. The essential role of B cell stimulatory factor 2 (BSF-2/IL-6) for the terminal differentiation of B cells. *J Exp Med* 1988;167:332–344.

150. Garman R, Jacobs K, Clark S, Raultet D. B-cell-stimulatory factor 2 (β2 interferon) functions as a second signal for IL-2 production by mature murine T cells. *Proc Natl Acad Sci U S A* 1987;84:7629–7633.

151. Lotz M, Jirik F, Kabouridis R, Tsoukas C, Hirano T, Kishimoto T. BSF-2/IL-6 is a co-stimulant for human thymocytes and T lymphocytes. *J Exp Med* 1988;167:1253–1258.

152. Uyttenhove C, Coulie P, Van Snick J. T cell growth and differentiation induced by interleukin-HP1/IL-6, the murine hybridoma, plasmacytoma growth factor. *J Exp Med* 1988;167:1417–1427.

153. Noma T, Mizuta T, Rosen A, Hirano T, Kishimoto T, Honjo T. Enhancement of the IL-2 receptor expression on T cells by multiple B-lymphotropic lymphokines. *Immunol Lett* 1987;15:249–253.

154. Le J, Frederickson G, Reis L, et al. IL-2-dependent and IL-2-independent pathways of regulation of thymocyte function by IL-6. *Proc Natl Acad Sci U S A* 1988;85:509–514.

155. Kasahara Y, Miyawaki T, Kato K, et al. Role of IL-6 for differential response of naive and memory CD4+ T cells in CD2-mediated activation. *J Exp Med* 1990;172:1419–1424.

156. Lorre K, Van Damme J, Verwilghem J, Baroja M, Ceuppens J. IL-6 is an accessory signal in the alternative CD2-mediated pathway of T-cell activation. *J Immunol* 1990;144:4681–4687.

157. Cruikshank WW, Berman JS, Theodore AC, Bernardo J, Center DM. Lymphokine activation of T4⁺ lymphocytes and monocytes. *J Immunol* 1987;138:3817–3823.

158. Rand TH, Cruikshank WW, Center DM, Weller PF. CD4-mediated stimulation of human eosinophils: lymphocyte chemoattractant factor and other CD4-binding ligands elicit eosinophil migration. *J Exp Med* 1991;173:1521–1528.

159. Kornfeld H, Berman JS, Beer DJ, Center DM. Induction of human T-cell motility by interleukin-2. *J Immunol* 1985;134:3887–3890.

160. Berman JS, Beer DJ, Cruikshank WW, Center DM. Chemoattractant lymphokines specific for the helper/inducer T-lymphocyte subset. *Cell Immunol* 1985;95:105–112.

161. Schall TJ, Bacon K, Toy KJ, Goeddel DV. Selective attraction of monocytes and T lymphocytes of the memory phenotype by cytokine RANTES. *Nature* 1990;347:669–671.

162. Taub DD, Conlon K, Lloyd AR, Oppenheim JJ, Kelvin DJ. Preferential migration of activated CD4+ and CD8+ T cells in response to MIP-1α and MIP-1. *Science* 1993;260:355–358.

163. Alam R, York J, Boyars M, et al. The detection of the mRNA for MCP-1, MCP-3, RANTES, MIP-1α and IL-8 in bronchoalveolar lavage cells, and the measurement of RANTES and MIP-1α in the lavage. *American Thoracic Society.* 1994;149:A951.

Asthma, edited by P.J. Barnes, M.M. Grunstein, A.R. Leff, and A.J. Woolcock.
Lippincott–Raven Publishers, Philadelphia © 1997.

▪ 51 ▪

Chemokines

Kian Fan Chung

Discovery And Structure	T lymphocytes
C-X-C Chemokines	Basophils
C-C Chemokines	Monocytes
Sources	**Chemokine Receptors**
Regulation	Specific Receptors
Chemokines As Chemoattractants And Cell Activators	Shared Receptors
Neutrophils	Promiscuous Receptors
Eosinophils	**Potential Role in Asthma**

Chemotactic cytokines or chemokines, an entirely new class of leukocyte chemoattractants (*chemo*attractant cy-to*kine*), consist of a superfamily of small secreted factors with little similarity in structure and function to traditional immune cytokines such as tumor necrosis factors (TNF), interferons (IFN) and the interleukins (IL). Up to 18 human chemokines have been identified so far by cloning or biochemical purification and amino acid sequencing. Chemokines have sequences that have been conserved, indicating a common ancestral gene, and share four conserved cysteine residues which form disulphide bonds in the tertiary structures. This superfamily of chemokines has been classified into 2 branches according to the position of the first two cysteines in the conserved motif (Table 1) (Fig. 1). The C-X-C branch (where X is an amino acid) also known as α-chemokines is characterized by the separation of the first two cysteines in the primary structure by an amino acid, while in the C-C branch (or β-chemokines), the two cysteines are directly adjacent. In general, this distinction also allows some separation of their activities, such that most C-X-C chemokines are chemoattractant for neutrophils and most C-C chemokines are monocyte, but not neutrophil, chemoattractants. The discovery of lymphotactin, which does not attract neutrophils or monocytes, but is active as

a chemoattractant for lymphocytes, has led to the description of another branch, the C branch (1). Lymphotactin lacks the first and third cysteines in the four-cysteine motif, but shares much similarity in amino acid sequence to the C-C chemokines.

TABLE 1. *Human Chemokine Superfamily*

C-X-C chemokines
  Epithelial-derived neutrophil attractant-78 (ENA-78)
  Interleukin-8 (IL-8) or neutrophil-activating protein-1
    (NAP-1)
  Stromal cell-derived factor-1α & β (SDF-1α & β)
  Granulocyte chemotactic protein-2 (GCP-2)
  Melanocyte growth stimulatory activity (MGSA/GROα,
    β or γ)
  Platelet factor-4 (PF-4)
  IP-10
  Monokine-induced by interferon-γ (MIG)
  Platelet basic protein
    Thromboglobulin
    Connective tissue protein-III (CTAP-III)
    Neutrophil-activating protein-2 (NAP-2)
C-C chemokines
  RANTES (Regulated on activation, normal T-cell
    expressed, and secreted)
  C10
  HC-14
  I-309/T-cell activation gene 3 (TCA3)
  Macrophage inflammatory protein-1α & β (MIP-1α & β)
  Monocyte chemoattractant protein-1, 2 & 3 (MCP-1, 2 & 3)
C chemokine
  Lymphotactin

K. F. Chung: Department of Thoracic Medicine, Imperial College School of Medicine at The National Heart and Lung Institute; and Royal Brompton Hospital, London SW3 6LY United Kingdom.

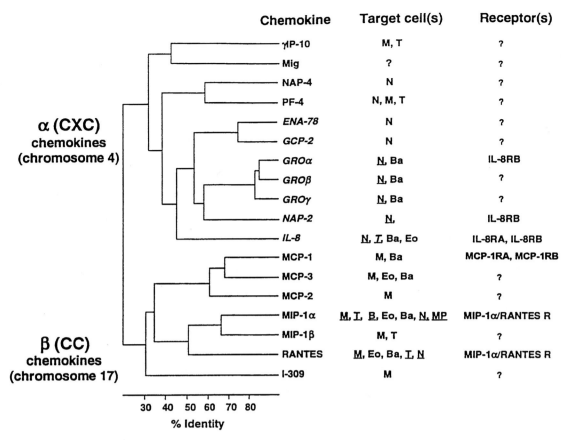

FIG. 1. Graphical representation of the amino-acid sequence relationship between known human C-X-C and C-C chemokines, with the percentage identity between any two sequences estimated by the position of their common branch point, as measured against the scale. Target cells in the middle column are based on the basis of functional and/or binding assays. Underlined targets indicate that the mRNA for the corresponding cloned receptor is detectable. Abbreviations: for chemokines, see Table 1; M, monocyte/macrophage; T, T lymphocyte; N, neutrophil; Ba, basophil; Eo, eosinophil; B, B lymphocyte; MP, myeloid-progenitor cells and/or precursor cell lines; IL-8RA, interleukin 8 receptor type A. (From Ahuja SK, Gao JL, Murphy PM. Chemokine receptors and molecular mimicry. *Immunol Today* 1994;15:282, with permission.)

DISCOVERY AND STRUCTURE

C-X-C Chemokines

Platelet-factor 4 (PF-4) stored in platelet granules is the first member of C-X-C chemokines to be described in 1955, and its amino acid sequence was published in 1977. IL-8, another C-X-C chemokine, is the most intensively studied member of the chemokine superfamily, and also is referred to as neutrophil-activating protein-1 (NAP-1); its major actions are as a neutrophil chemoattractant and activator. The sequence of an IL-8 complementary deoxyribonucleic acid (cDNA) clone first was described in 1987, using differential hybridization to identify genes expressed in activated human lymphocytes (2). This was followed later by the partial amino acid sequences of identical neutrophil chemotactic factors described as monocyte-derived neutrophil-activating peptide, and monocyte-derived neutrophil chemotactic factor, which were identical to the deduced sequence of the IL-8 cDNA clone (3,4). The gene encoding IL-8 was cloned and sequenced in 1989 (5). Several other C-X-C chemokines, similar to IL-8, were discovered in rapid succession including neutrophil-activating protein-2 (NAP-2), arising from N-terminal processing of platelet basic protein, GROα, GROβ and GROγ, epithelial cell derived neutrophil-activating protein (ENA-78) and granulocyte chemotactic protein-2 (GCP-2) (6–10). A secreted protein produced by lipopolysaccharide (LPS)-stimulated murine macrophages called macrophage-inflammatory protein-2 (MIP-2) was found to be a chemoattractant for human neutrophils and is closely related to GRO (11). Another cDNA clone, KC, identified a transcript induced in murine fibroblasts with its predicted amino acid sequence similar to murine MIP-2 (12). Because GRO was more closely related to KC than to MIP-2, it was suggested that KC, rather than MIP-2, was the murine homologue of GRO. Another C-X-C chemokine, cytokine-induced neutrophil chemoattractant (CINC), first was purified from an epithelial clone of normal rat kidney line stimulated by IL-1β or TNF-α with neutrophil chemoattractant activity; its closest reported human homologue is GRO/Melanocyte growth stimulatory activity (MGSA) (13).

C-C Chemokines

The first human C-C chemokine gene called LD78 was discovered by differential hybridization cloning of human tonsillar lymphocytes (14). cDNA isoforms of a closely related chemokine, Act-2, also were described (15), and two similar proteins, macrophage-inflammatory protein 1α (MIP-1α) and MIP-1β , were purified from culture media of endotoxin-stimulated mouse macrophages (16). Because the close identity of the amino acid sequence between the murine and human proteins (75% identity) suggested that these two molecules were homologues, the terms human MIP-1α and MIP-1β have replaced LD78 and Act-2, respectively. Both MIP-1α and MIP-1β genes can be coordinately expressed after stimulation of T cells (e.g., with anti- CD-3), B cells or of monocytes and macrophages (e.g., with lipopolysaccharide) (14,16–21). MIP-1 gene is rapidly induced in human monocytes following adherence to endothelial cells and to other substrates (22). In murine fibroblasts, platelet-derived growth factor induced two genes, one of which proved to be a murine homologue of GRO gene (KC), and the other designated JE (23). The human homologue of JE was found to encode a monocyte chemoattractant and activating factor, which led to the identification of monocyte chemoattractant protein-1 (MCP-1). MCP-1 is the best characterized CC chemokine, having been purified and cloned from different sources (15,24,25).

The other C-C chemokines, I-309, Regulated on Activation, Normal T-Cell Expressed, and Secreted (RANTES) and HC-14 were purified and cloned as products of activated T cells (18,26,27). Substractive hybridization was used to find genes expressed uniquely in T cells, and this led to the discovery of RANTES cDNA encoding a polypeptide of 91 amino acids with an 8kd secreted protein. RANTES gene is expressed in IL-2-dependent T-cell lines. In peripheral blood mononuclear cells, low, but detectable, concentration of RANTES transcripts can be measured in unstimulated cells, and there is an increase in mRNA 5 to 7 days after antigen or stimulation with phytohemaggltinin (26). HC-14, discovered from IFN-stimulated monocytes, now called MCP-2, also has been isolated from osteosarcoma cell cultures (28). These cultures also have yielded MCP-3, which has been cloned and expressed (29,30).

SOURCES

In general, monocytes and tissue macrophages are a rich source of C-X-C and C-C chemokines, usually associated with *de novo* synthesis. Monocytes respond to a large variety of proinflammatory agents including IL-1, IL-1, TNF, granulocyte-macrophage colony-stimulating factor (GM-CSF), IL-3, lipopolysaccharide, and immune complexes to release IL-8. IL-8 also has been induced following adherence of monocytes to plastic and by changes in ambient oxygen (31,32). GROα, GROβ, and GROγ are expressed and secreted by monocytes and macrophages (7,33,34).

Lymphocytes are sources of some C-C chemokines, particularly RANTES (18,26,35). I-309, MIP-1α, and MIP-1β (17,18,35–38,) but are less prominent than mononuclear phagocytes as C-X-C chemokine producers. Neutrophils produce IL-8 in response to IL-1, TNF-α, adherence, and GM-CSF, GROα and GROβ on adherence to fibronectin, and, in addition, the C-X-C chemokine, MIP-1α (7,39–41). Eosinophils release IL-8 after stimulation with calcium ionophore, A23187, but not with TNF, or IL-1, and eosinophils of patients with hypereosinophilic syndrome express mRNA for MIP-1α (42,43).

Epithelial cells stimulated with IL-1 or TNF produce IL-8, GROα, GROβ, and GROγ, ENA-78, MCP-1 and RANTES, but not MIP-1 (7,9,40,44–50). IL-8 expression by epithelial cells is increased by respiratory syncitial virus infections and on exposure to neutrophil elastase (51,52). MCP-1 and RANTES immunoreactivity has been reported in human airway epithelium (50,53). RANTES also has been shown to be produced by human vascular endothelial cells.

REGULATION

The transcriptional control of IL-8 gene remains the most studied. Several transcriptional regulatory elements can bind to the region preceding the first exon, including NF-B, NF-IL-6, AP-1, glucocorticoid element and an octamer-binding motif(5). NF-IL-6 and NF- B-like factors may act as *cis*-acting elements in IL-8 mRNA expression (54). IL-8 mRNA expression after stimulation with IL-1 or TNF-α is rapid, and results at least partly from transcriptional activation, as shown by nuclear run-off assays (46,55–57). A secondary phase of IL-8 mRNA expression following an early rapid increase induced by IL-1 has been observed with cultured human airway epithelial cells. Enhancement of expression can be induced by cycloheximide, presumably by co-induction of inhibitors of synthesis of negative regulatory elements (56,57). The stability of IL-8 mRNA may be influenced by RNA instability elements, AUUUA, found in the 3′ untranslated region (58,59). IL-8 expression can be inhibited in blood monocytes and in airway epithelial cells by glucocorticoids, and IFN-γ , IL-4, and IL-10 can inhibit IL-8 production from blood monocytes (60–63). Most of the effect of glucocorticoids on IL-8 mRNA occurs through inhibition of transcription (61).

The RANTES gene has several transcriptional consensus elements for DNA binding in its immediate upstream region, including NF-B, NF-IL-6, AP-1, and AP-3 (64). Many of these potential regulatory sites were originally described in promoters, expressed specifically in T cells and myeloid or erythroid cells, whereas other elements first were described as consensus sites for factors responsive to specific second messenger stimulation. This large number of potential regulatory sites raises the possibility of a wide range of transcriptional controls for RANTES expression in different tissues. For the MIP-1α genes, cis regulatory elements include GRE and CK-1 (65).

Comparison of RANTES and MIP-1α expression illustrates the differences in cellular sites and regulation of expression. MIP-1α, but not RANTES mRNA expression and protein release, can be induced from blood monocytes and alveolar macrophages by IL-1 and lipopolysaccharide (20,66). IL-1 and LPS-induced expression and protein release of MIP-1 were inhibited by glucocorticoids, effects that occurred through inhibition of transcription (20). No GRE sites have been found in the upstream of the transcription initiation site of the human MIP-1α gene, and it is possible that the effect of glucocorticoids could be exerted by interacting at other regulatory sites, or with other transcription factors such as AP-1 (67). The inhibitory effect of glucocorticoids was largely reversed by cycloheximide, suggesting the intermediary effect of a protein. Part of the inhibition of MIP-1α mRNA, resulted from a small increase in mRNA breakdown, probably related to repeating nucleotide motifs in the 3′untranslated region of the MIP-1α mRNA (17). In cultured human airway epithelial cells, RANTES, but not MIP-1α mRNA and protein, can be induced by a mixture of cytokines, TNF-α , IL-1β, and IFN-γ, even though each individual cytokine was ineffective (50). This suggests that there is true synergy between these cytokines in inducing the expression of RANTES. Although there does not appear to be a GRE consensus element on the upstream region of the RANTES gene, glucocorticoids also potently inhibit the induced expression and release of RANTES (50).

The effect of T-helper-2 (TH2)-derived cytokines, IL-4, IL-10 and IL-13, on the induced expression of MIP-1α and RANTES also shows interesting differences. All of these cytokines inhibit the induction of MIP-1α mRNA and protein release from blood monocytes and alveolar macrophages. Blood monocytes are more sensitive to the inhibitory effects of IL-10 than are alveolar macrophages, while their sensitivities to the inhibitory effects of IL-4 are similar (66,68). In monocytes, IL-4, IL-10, and IL-13 induced inhibition of MIP-1α mRNA, mainly at the level of mRNA transcription with some additional effect on mRNA stability, particularly for IL-4 and IL-10,

all requiring de novo protein synthesis as assessed with cycloheximide (66,68,69). Conversely, in human airway epithelial cells, only IL-4 showed significant inhibitory effects on the induction of RANTES mRNA expression and protein release (50). These studies suggest that endogenously-released Th-2 cytokines may control the effects of chemokine expression and release.

CHEMOKINES AS CHEMOATTRACTANTS AND CELL ACTIVATORS (FIG. 1)

Migration of leukocytes from the vascular compartment into tissues, occurs through the sequence of adhesion to the endothelial cell through the expression of integrins, diapedesis, and migration, in response to a chemoattractant gradient. Chemokines may play a major role in activating migrating leukocytes and endothelial cells to increase adhesiveness and in establishing a chemotactic gradient. Interaction between chemokines and negatively-charged proteoglycans may provide a solid phase for maintainence of a persistent chemotactic gradient following only a brief burst of chemokine release (70). The activity of IL-8 as a neutrophil chemoattractant has been shown to be potentiated by its binding to heparan sulfate or heparin, although the IL-8 activating activity is reduced (71). MIP-1β, immobilized by binding to proteoglycans, binds to endothelium to trigger adhesion of T-cells, particularly CD8[+] T-cells to vascular cell adhesion molecule (VCAM-1) (72). MIP-1β has been localized to lymph node endothelium and could act as a tethered ligand on endothelial cells, thus providing the required signals for activation of lymphocyte integrins for adhesion to endothelium and migration.

Neutrophils

IL-8, which has been most studied among the C-X-C chemokines, induces shape change, a transient rise in intracellular free calcium concentrations ($[Ca^{++}]_i$), exocytosis with release of enzymes and proteins from intracellular storage organelles, and respiratory burst through activation of NADPH-oxidase. As such, it behaves like a classical chemoattractant (73). IL-8 also up-regulates the expression of two integrins (CD11b/CD18 and CD11c/CD18) during exocytosis of specific granules (74,75). IL-8 activates neutrophil 5-lipoxygenase, with the formation of LTB4 and 5-HETE, and also induces the production of platelet-activating factor (76,77).

Eosinophils

IL-8 induces $[Ca^{++}]_i$ elevation, shape change, and release of eosinophil peroxidase from eosinophils of hypereosinophilic syndrome patients, and can induce eosinophil chemotaxis of primed eosinophils (78,79), However, eosinophils are more responsive to C-C rather than C-X-C chemokines. RANTES is a powerful eosinophil chemoattractant, being as effective as C5a and 2 to 3 times more potent than MIP-1α (80,81). RANTES up-regulates the expression of CD11b/CD18 on eosinophils (82). RANTES and MIP-1α induce exocytosis of eosinophil cationic protein from cytochalasin B-treated cells, although RANTES is relatively weak in this effect (80). When injected in the skin of dogs, RANTES induced an infiltration of eosinophils and monocytes (83). RANTES, but not MIP-1α, also elicited a respiratory burst from eosinophils (80). MCP-3 was found to be an effective chemoattractant for eosinophils as RANTES (84).

T Lymphocytes

Although in the original description of IL-8, chemotactic activity for human T lymphocytes was described *in vitro* with induction of lymphocyte infiltration on intradermal injection in rats, more recent studies show that IL-8 has a small chemotactic activity for either CD4+ or CD8+ T lymphocytes (85,86). Intradermal injection of IL-8 in humans does not attract lymphocytes (87,88). Conversely, RANTES is a chemoattractant for memory T cells *in vitro* (89). Human MIP-1α and MIP-1β are also chemoattractants for distinct subpopulations of lymphocytes with MIP-1α towards CD8+ and MIP-1β towards CD4+ T-lymphocytes (90). RANTES attracts both phenotypes and acts on resting and activated T-lymphocytes, while MIP-1α and MIP-1β are effective on anti-CD3 stimulated cells only (91). Again, MIP-1β , but not MIP-1α , has been reported to be chemotactic for resting T-cells and enhances the adherence of CD8+, but not CD4+, cells to VCAM-1 (72).

MCP-1 induces T-cell migration (92). Natural killer cells migrate vigorously in response to RANTES, MIP-1α, and MCP-1 (93). Human recombinant IP-10 is a chemoattractant for human monocytes and promotes T-cell adhesion to endothelial cells (94). The C chemokine lymphotactin also shares T-lymphocyte chemoattractant activity (1). The selective chemoattractant activities for different subsets of lymphocytes suggest that specific members of the chemokine family may be involved in different immune and inflammatory responses.

Basophils

IL-8 induces the release of histamine and sulfidopeptide leukotrienes from human blood basophils with enhanced release of IL-3, IL-5, or GM-CSF pretreatment (95–97). C-C chemokines are more powerful stimulants of basophils. MCP-1 is as potent as C5a in stimulating exocytosis in human basophils, with release of high concentrations of histamine (98–100). In the presence of IL-3,

IL-5, or GM-CSF, there is enhanced release of histamine and production of leukotriene C4 (98,100). RANTES and MIP-1α are less effective releasers of histamine from basophils. MIP-1β is inactive on basophils (101). RANTES is the most effective basophil chemoattractant, while MCP-1 is more effective as an inducer of histamine and leukotriene release (99,101,102).

Monocytes

C-X-C chemokines generally are not active on monocytes; IL-8 being able to induce a small release of $[Ca^{++}]_i$ and respiratory burst activity (103). By contrast, C-C chemokines MCP-1, RANTES, I-309, HC14 (or MCP-2), and MCP-3 attract monocytes *in vitro*, and MCP-1, MCP-2, and MCP-3 induce a selective infiltration of monocytes in animal skin (28,89,104–109). All C-C chemokines stimulate $[Ca^{++}]_i$ release (101,108,110). MCP-1 also induces a respiratory burst, an expression of 2-integrins (CD11b/CD18 and CD11c/CD18), and the production of IL-1 and IL-6 (106,109,111). Growth of tumor cell lines cultured in the presence of human blood lymphocytes is inhibited by the addition of MCP-1 (25).

CHEMOKINE RECEPTORS

The chemokine receptors form a family of structurally and functionally related proteins, and are members of the superfamily of heptahelical, rhodopsin-like, G-protein-coupled receptors. Thus, the responses of basophils, eosinophils, and monocytes to C-C chemokines are prevented by pretreatment of these cells with *Bordetella pertussis* toxin, which specifically inhibits GTP-binding proteins indicating the coupling to G proteins (101,107). C-X-C chemokines' effects on neutrophils also induce G protein activation (112). For chemokine receptors that have been cloned so far, the following general classification can be made.

Specific receptors

Specific receptors bind to only one chemokine such as the IL-8 receptor A (IL-8RA) and the MCP-1 receptor, although for the MCP-1, receptor binding characteristics to the closely related MCP-2 and MCP-3 are not known (113,114). IL-8RA has been cloned from a neutrophil cDNA that has been isolated from cDNA pools, using its ability to confer IL-8 binding sites to COS cells, and the deduced sequence is 77% identical to that of IL-8 RB (113). A cDNA encoding an MCP-1 receptor has been isolated from a human cell line, and its 3 kb RNA has been found in monocytes, but not in neutrophils or lymphocytes (115).

Shared receptors

These receptors bind to more than one chemokine within either class of C-X-C or C-C chemokine and are exemplified by the IL-8 receptor B (IL-8RB) and the C-C chemokine receptor-1 (C-C CKR-1, also called the RANTES/MIP-1 receptor). IL-8RB can be activated by C-X-C chemokines containing the sequence Glu-Leu-Arg in the N-terminal domain, including IL-8, GRO, and NAP-2, but not by C-C chemokines (116,117). The C-C CKR-1 receptor, which binds to several C-C chemokines, has been cloned from monocyte cDNA and has also been detected in neutrophils, and B and T lymphocytes (118.119).

Promiscuous receptors

This class binds chemokines of both C-X-C and C-C classes of which there is only one example described to date, the erythrocyte chemokine receptor (120,121). The role for this receptor on red blood cells is unclear, but it has been suggested that this is a mechanism by which chemokines may be removed. The ECKR has been identified as the Duffy blood group antigen expressed on red cells, where it acts as a ligand through which *Plasmodium vivax* enters red blood cells (122).

Another class of chemokine receptors include virally-encoded receptors, such as one encoded by a cytomegalovirus open reading frame CMV US28, and one from the herpes saimiri virus HSV ECRF3, which probably are shared C-C and C-X-C receptors, respectively (118,123). It is possible that these receptors have been transduced by viruses during evolution, and the relevance of this is not clear.

POTENTIAL ROLE IN ASTHMA

The chronic inflammatory response in asthma is characterized by a submucosal infiltration of eosinophils, T lymphocytes, activated moncytes/macrophages, and mast cells (124–127). Activated T-cells have been identified as CD4$^+$ T-cells, expressing the TH-2 profile of cytokines with IL-3, IL-4, and IL-5 (128,129). Some of these T cells also express CD45-RO, supporting their role as memory T cells (130). Following allergen challenge, there is an increase in the number of EG2-positive cells, indicating activated eosinophils and an increase of CD4$^+$ T cells (131–133). In addition, there is recruitment of neutrophils, and in the nose, basophil recruitment also is observed (134–136). Although eosinophils are most prominent in the airways of patients dying of severe asthma, a predominant neutrophil infiltration of the airway submucosa has been observed in some cases of asthma deaths of sudden onset (137,138). The role of chemotactic cytokines as major chemoattractants in asthma remains to be determined. The potential role of chemokines in asthma is supported by observations that many cell types present in the asthmatic airway have the potential of generating chemokines, in particular monocytes/macrophages, T cells, and airway epithelium.

An early report has shown enhanced co-expression of IL-8 and GM-CSF in bronchial epithelial cells of patients with asthma, which is of particular interest because GM-CSF, IL-3, and IL-5 can increase the responses of basophils and eosinophils to chemokines (79,98,100,139). In addition, IL-8 appears to possess chemotactic activity for primed eosinophils (79). Human IL-8 is able to induce accumulation of peritoneal guinea-pig eosinophils in guinea-pig skin, and a human anti-IL-8 antibody inhibited IL-1-induced accumulation of eosinophil in rat skin (140,141). Enhanced release of IL-8 has been demonstrated from alveolar macrophages obtained from mild asthmatics, compared to those from normal subjects (142). High concentrations of IL-8 are not specific for asthma because these have been reported in sputum samples obtained from patients with chronic bronchitis and bronchiectasis (143).

Chemokines in bronchoalveolar lavage fluid can be detected, even at low levels after the fluid has been concentrated. Concentration of MIP-1α and RANTES in bronchoalveolar lavage fluid are different between normal and mild asthmatic patients. It is possible that the preferential binding of these chemokines to proteoglycans may make it difficult to detect chemokines in such fluids in asthma, although increased concentrations of IL-8, MCP-1, and MIP-1α have been shown in patients with interstitial lung disease and pulmonary sarcoidosis (144,145). Using a semi-quantitative reverse-transcriptase polymerase-chain reaction, RANTES, but not MIP-1α mRNA expression, has been shown to be increased in bronchial biopsies of patients with mild asthma (146). No differences in MIP-1α mRNA expression were observed in alveolar macrophages obtained from normal and asthmatic subjects. Although RANTES expression by immunohistochemistry can be demonstrated in the epithelium of the airway mucosa, there does not appear to be differences between normals and asthmatics. However, the C-C chemokine, MCP-1, has been shown to be overexpressed in asthmatic epithelium (53).

A new chemokine, eotaxin, which is a major eosinophil chemoattractant, has been identified and cloned from bronchoalveolar lavage fluid of allergen-challenged sensitized guinea-pigs (147,148). Its human homologue has not been reported yet.

CONCLUSIONS

Although chemokines are structurally related, they form a diverse group of potent chemoattractants and cell activators, and affect a wide range of cells. The central role of chemokines appears to be related to the trafficking of leukocytes, and it is likely, therefore, that they would be involved in immunological and inflammatory processes as part of the normal or pathological response. Much needs to be done to determine the role of chemokines in the pathogenesis of asthma. It is unclear at present why there are so many chemokines with overlapping and similar functions between the different members. The nature of the chemokine signal transduction remains to be elucidated. While blocking antibodies and pharmacological approaches will be developed to neutralize the effects of chemokines, it is not known whether specific inhibition against one or several chemokines will lead to a therapeutic effect.

REFERENCES

1. Kelner GS, Kennedy J, Bacon KB, et al. Lymphotactin: a cytokine that represents a new class of chemokine. *Science* 1994;266:1395–1399.
2. Schmid J, Weissmann C. Induction of mRNA for a serine protease and a beta-thromboglobulin-like protein in mitogen-stimulated human leukocytes. *J Immunol* 1987;139:250–256.
3. Schroder JM, Mrowietz U, Morita E, Christophers E. Purification and partial biochemical chracterisation of a human monocyte-derived, neutrophil-activating peptide that lacks interleukin-1 activity. *J Immunol* 1987;139:3474–3483.
4. Yoshimura T, Matsushima K, Tanaka S, Robinson EA, Appella E, Leonard EJ. Purification of a human monocyte-derived neutrophil chemotactic factor that has peptide sequence similarity to other host defense cytokines. *Proc Natl Acad Sci U S A* 1987;84:9233–9237.
5. Mukaida N, Shiroo M, Matsushima K. Genomic structure of the human monocyte-derived neutrophil chemotactic factor IL-8. *J Immunol* 1989;143:1366–1371.
6. Walz A, Baggiolini M. Generation of the neutrophil-activating peptide NAP-2 from platelet basic protein or connective tissue-activating peptide III through monocyte proteases. *J Exp Med* 1990;171:449–454.
7. Haskill S, Peace A, Morris J, et al. Identification of three related human GRO genes encoding cytokine functions. *Proc Natl Acad Sci U S A* 1990;87:7732–7736.
8. Geiser T, Dewald B, Ehrengruber MU, Clark-Lewis I, Baggiolini M. The interleukin-8-related chemotactic cytokines GROα, GROβ, and GROγ activate human neutrophil and basophil leukocytes. *J Biol Chem* 1993;268:15419–15424.
9. Walz A, Burgener R, Car B, Baggiolini M, Kunkel SL, Strieter RM. Structure and neutrophil-activating properties of a novel inflammatory peptide (ENA-78) with homology to interleukin-8. *J Exp Med* 1991;174:1355–1362.
10. Proost P, De Wolf-Peeters C, Conings R, Opdenakker G, Billiau A, VanDamme J. Identification of a novel granulocyte chemotactic protein (GCP-2) from human tumor cells. *In vitro* and *in vivo* comparison with natural forms of GRO, IP-10, and IL-8. *J Immunol* 1993;150:1000–1010.
11. Wolpe SD, Cerami A. Macrophage inflammatory proteins 1 and 2: members of a novel superfamily of cytokines. *FASEB J* 1989;3:2565–2573.
12. Oquendo P, Alberta J, Wen DZ, Graycar JL, Derynck R, Stiles CD. The platelet-derived growth factor-inducible KC gene encodes a secretory protein related to platelet α-granule proteins. *J Biol Chem* 1989;264:4133–4137.
13. Watanabe K, Kinoshita S, Nakagawa H. Purification and characterization of cytokine-induced neutrophil chemoattractant produced by epithelioid cell line of normal rat kidney (NRK-52E cell). *Biochem Biophys Res Commun* 1989;161:1093–1099.
14. Obaru K, Fukuda M, Maeda S, Shimada K. A cDNA clone used to study mRNA inducible in human tonsillar lymphocytes by a tumor promoter. *J Biochem* 1986;99:885–894.
15. Miller MD, Krangel MS. Biology and biochemistry of the chemokines: a family of chemotactic and inflammatory cytokines. *Crit Rev Immunol* 1992;12:17–46.
16. Wolpe SD, Davatelis G, Sherry B, et al. Macrophages secrete a novel heparin-binding protein with inflammatory and neutrophil chemokinetic properties. *J Exp Med* 1988;167:570–581.
17. Zipfel PF, Balke J, Irving S, Kelly K, Siebenlist U. Mitogenic activation of human T cells induces two closely related genes which share structural similarities with a new family of secreted factors. *J Immunol* 1989;142:1582–1590.
18. Miller MD, Hata S, de Waal Malefyt R, Krangel MS. A novel polypeptide secreted by activated human T lymphocytes. *J Immunol* 1989;143:2907–2916.
19. Lipes MA, Napolitano M, Jeang KT, Chang NT, Leonard WJ. Identification, cloning, and characterization of an immune activation gene. *Proc Natl Acad Sci U S A* 1988;85:9704–9708.
20. Berkman N, Jose P, Williams T, Barnes PJ, Chung KF. Corticosteroid inhibition of macrophage inflammatory protein-1α expression in human monocytes and alveolar macrophages. *Am J Physiol* 1995;269:L443–L452.
21. VanOtteren GM, Standiford TJ, Kunkel SL, Danforth JM, Burdick MD, Strieter RM. Expression and regulation of macrophage inflammatory protein-1 by murine alveolar and peritoneal macrophages. *Am J Respir Cell Mol Biol* 1994;10:8–15.
22. Sporn SA, Eierman DF, Johnson CE, Morris J, Martin G, Ladner M. Monocyte adherence results in selective induction of novel genes sharing homology with mediators of inflammation and tissue repair. *J Immunol* 1990;144:4434–4441.
23. Cochran BH, Reffel AC, Stiles CD. Molecular cloning of gene sequences regulated by platelet-derived growth factor. *Cell* 1983;33:939–947.
24. Yoshimura T, Yuhki N, Moore SK, Appella E, Lerman MI, Leonard EJ. Human monocyte chemoattractant protein-1 (MCP-1). Full-length cDNA cloning, expression in mitogen-stimulated blood mononuclear leukocytes, and sequence similarity to mouse competence gene JE. *FEBS Lett* 1989;244:487–493.
25. Matsushima K, Larsen CG, DuBois GC. Purification and characterisation of a novel monocyte chemotactic and activating factor produced by a human myelomonocytic cell line. *J Exp Med* 1989;169:1485–1490.
26. Schall TJ, Jongstra J, Dyer BJ, Jorgensen J, Clayberger C, Davis MM. A human T cell-specific molecule is a member of a new gene family. *J Immunol* 1988;141:1018–1025.
27. Chang HC, Hsu F, Freeman GJ, Griffin JD, Reinherz EL. Cloning and expression of a γ-interferon-inducible gene in monocytes: a new member of a cytokine gene family. *Int Immunol* 1989;1:388–397.
28. Van Damme J, Proost P, Lenaerts J-P, Opdenakker G. Structural and functional identification of two human, tumor-derived monocyte chemotactic proteins (MCP-2 and MCP-3) belonging to the chemokine family. *J Exp Med* 1992;176:59–64.
29. Minty A, Chalon P, Guillemot JC, et al. Molecular cloning of the MCP-3 chemokine gene and regulation of its expression. *Eur Cytokine Netw* 1993;4:99–104.
30. Opdenakker G, Froyen G, Fiten P, Proost P, Van Damme J. Human monocyte chemotactic protein-3 (MCP-3): molecular cloning of the cDNA and comparison with other chemokines. *Biochem Biophys Res Commun* 1993;191:535–542.
31. Kasahara K, Strieter RM, Chensue SW, Standiford TJ, Kunkel SL. Mononuclear cell adherence induces neutrophil chemotactic factor/interleukin-8 gene expression. *J Leukoc Biol* 1991;50:287–295.
32. Metinko AP, Kunkel SL, Standiford TJ, Strieter RM. Anoxia-hyperoxia induces monocyte-derived interleukin-8. *J Clin Invest* 1992;90:791–798.
33. Schroder JM, Persoon NL, Christophers E. Lipopolysaccharide-stimulated human monocytes secrete, apart from neutrophil-activating peptide 1/interleukin-8, a second neutrophil-activating protein. NH2-terminal amino acid sequence identity with melanoma growth stimulatory activity. *J Exp Med* 1990;171:1091–1100.
34. Iida N, Grotendorst GR. Cloning and sequencing of a new GRO transcript from activated human monocytes: expression in leukocytes and wound tissue *Mol Cell Biol* 1990;10:5596–5599.
35. Schall TJ, O'Hehir RE, Goeddel DV, Lamb JR. Uncoupling of cytokine mRNA expression and protein secretion during the induction phase of T cell anergy. *J Immunol* 1992;148:381–387.
36. Miller MD, Wilson SD, Dorf ME, Seuanez HN, O'Brien SJ, Krangel

MS. Sequence and chromosomal location of the I-309 gene. Relationship to genes encoding a family of inflammatory cytokines. *J Immunol* 1990;145:2737–2744.

37. Lipes MA, Napolitano M, Jeang KT, Chang NT, Leonard WJ. Identification, cloning and characterisation of an immune activation gene. *Proc Natl Acad Sci U S A* 1988;85:9704–9708.

38. Ziegler SF, Tough TW, Franklin TL, Armitage RJ, Alderson MR. Induction of macrophage inflammatory protein-1 gene expression in human monocytes by lipopolysaccharide and IL-7. *J Immunol* 1991; 147:2234–2239.

39. Strieter RM, Kasahara K, Allen RM, Standiford TJ, Rolfe MW, Becker FS, Chensue SW, Kunkel SL. Cytokine-induced neutrophil-derived interleukin-8. *Am J Pathol* 1992;141:397–407.

40. Galy AH, Spits H. IL-1, IL-4, and IFN- differentially regulate cytokine production and cell surface molecule expression in cultured human thymic epithelial cells. *J Immunol* 1991;147:3823–3830.

41. Kasama T, Strieter RM, Standiford TJ, Burdick MD, Kunkel SL. Expression and regulation of human neutrophil-derived macrophage inflammatory protein 1. *J Exp Med* 1993;178:63–72.

42. Braun RK, Franchini M, Erard F, Rihs S, De Vries IJ, Blaser K, Walker C. Human peripheral blood eosinophils produce and release interleukin-8 on stimulation with calcium ionophore. *Eur J Immunol* 1993;23:956–960.

43. Costa JJ, Matossian K, Resnick MB, et al. Human eosinophils can express the cytokines tumor necrosis factor- and macrophage inflammatory protein-1. *J Clin Invest* 1993;91:2673–2684.

44. Elner VM, Strieter RM, Elner SG, Baggiolini M, Lindley I, Kunkel SL. Neutrophil chemotactic factor (IL-8) gene expression by cytokine-treated retinal pigment epithelial cells. *Am J Pathol* 1990;136: 745–750.

45. Standiford TJ, Kunkel SL, Basha MA, et al. Interleukin-8 gene expression by a pulmonary epithelial cell line. A model for cytokine networks in the lung. *J Clin Invest* 1990;86:1945–1953.

46. Kwon O, Au BT, Collins PD, et al. Tumour necrosis factor-induced interleukin-8 expression in pulmonary cultured human airway epithelial cells. *Am J Physiol* 1994;267:L398–L405.

47. Anisowicz A, Zajchowski D, Stenman G, Sager R. Functional diversity of gro gene expression in human fibroblasts and mammary epithelial cells. *Proc Natl Acad Sci U S A* 1988;85:9645–9649.

48. Standiford TJ, Kunkel SL, Phan SH, Rollins BJ, Strieter RM. Alveolar macrophage-derived cytokines induce monocyte chemoattractant protein-1 expression from human pulmonary type II-like epithelial cells. *J Biol Chem* 1991;266:9912–9918.

49. Elner SG, Strieter RM, Elner VM, Rollins BJ, Del Monte MA, Kunkel SL. Monocyte chemotactic protein gene expression by cytokine-treated human retinal pigment epithelial cells. *Lab Invest* 1991;64: 819–825.

50. Berkman N, Robichaud A, Krishnan VL, et al. RANTES is expressed by human airway epithelium *in vitro* and *in vivo*. *Am J Respir Crit Care Med* 1995;151:A191.

51. Choi AMK, Jacoby DB. Influenza virus A infection induces interleukin-8 gene expression in human airway epithelial cells. *FEBS Lett* 1992;309:327–329.

52. Nakamura H, Yoshimura K, McElvaney NG, Crystal RG. Neutrophil elastase in respiratory epithelial lining fluid of individuals with cystic fibrosis induces interleukin-8 gene expression in a human bronchial epithelial cell line. *J Clin Invest* 1992;89:1478–1484.

53. Sousa AR, Lane SJ, Nakhosteen JA, Yoshimura T, Lee TH, Poston RN. Increased expression of the monocyte chemoattractant protein-1 in bronchial tissues from asthmatic subjects. *Am J Resp Cell Mol Biol* 1994;10:142–147.

54. Mukaida N, Mahé Y, Matsushima K. Cooperative interaction of nuclear factor kB and cis-regulatory enhancer binding protein-like factor bonding elements in activating the interleukin-8 gene by pro-inflammatory cytokines. *J Biol Chem* 1990;265:21128–21133.

55. Sica A, Matsushima K, Van Damme J, et al. IL-1 transcriptionally activates the neutrophil chemotactic factor/IL-8 gene in endothelial cells. *Immunology* 1990;69:548–553.

56. Mukaida N, Matsushima K. Regulation of IL-8 production and the characteristics of the receptor for IL-8. *Cytokine* 1992;4:41–53.

57. Mukaida N, Harada A, Yasumoto K, Matsushima K. Properties of pro-inflammatory cell type-specific leukocyte chemotactic cytokines, interleukin 8 (IL-8) and monocyte chemotactic and activating factor (MCAF). [Review]. *Microbiol Immunol* 1992;36:773–789.

58. Matsushima K, Morishita K, Yoshimura T, et al. Molecular cloning of a human monocyte-derived neutrophil chemotactic factor (MDNCF) and the induction of MDNCF mRNA by interleukin 1 and tumor necrosis factor. *J Exp Med* 1988;167:1883–1893.

59. Shaw G, Kamen R. A conserved AU sequence from the 3′ untranslated region of GM-CSF mRNA mediates selective mRNA degradation. *Cell* 1986;46:659–667.

60. Seitz M, Dewald B, Gerber N, Baggiolini M. Enhanced production of neutrophil-activating peptide-1/interleukin-8 in rheumatoid arthritis. *J Clin Invest* 1991;87:463–469.

61. Kwon OJ, Au BT, Collins PD, Baraniuk JN, Adcock IM, Chung KF, Barnes PJ. Inhibition of interleukin-8 expression by dexamethasone in human cultured airway epithelial cells. *Immunology* 1994;81:389–394.

62. Standiford TJ, Strieter RM, Chensue SW, Westwick J, Kasahara K, Kunkel SL. IL-4 inhibits expression of IL-8 from stimulated human monocytes. *J Immunol* 1990;145:1435–1439.

63. de Waal Malefyt R, Abrams J, Bennett B, Figdor CG, De Vries JE. Interleukin 10 (IL-10) inhibits cytokine synthesis by human monocytes: an auto regulatory role of IL-10 produced by monocytes. *J Exp Med* 1991;179:1209–1220.

64. Nelson PJ, Kim HT, Manning WC, Goralski TJ, Krensky AM. Genomic organization and transcriptional regulation of the RANTES chemokine gene. *J Immunol* 1993;151:2601–2612.

65. Widmer U, Manogue KR, Cerami A, Sherry B. Genomic cloning and promoter analysis of macrophage inflammatory protein (MIP)-2, MIP-1α, and MIP-1β, members of the chemokine superfamily of proinflammatory cytokines. *J Immunol* 1993;150:4996–5012.

66. Standiford TJ, Kunkel SL, Liebler JM, Burdick MD, Gilbert AR, Strieter RM. Gene expression of macrophage inflammatory protein-1α from human blood monocytes and alveolar macrophages is inhibited by interleukin-4. *Am J Respir Cell Mol Biol* 1993;9:192–198.

67. Nakao M, Nomiyama H, Shimada K. Structures of human genes coding for cytokine LD78 and their expression. *Mol Cell Biol* 1990;10: 3646–3658.

68. Berkman N, Roesems G, Jose PJ, Barnes PJ, Chung KF. Production of macrophage inflammatory protein-1a by human alveolar macrophages is more resistant to inhibition by interleukin-10 as compared to peripheral blood monocytes. *Am J Respir Crit Care Med* 1995;151: A549.

69. Berkman N, Roesems G, Jose PJ, Barnes PJ, Chung KF. Interleukin-13 inhibits expression of macrophage-inflammatory protein-1 from human blood monocytes and alveolar macrophages. *Am J Resp Crit Care Med* 1995;151:A826.

70. Witt DP, Lander AD. Differential binding of chemokines to glycosaminoglycan subpopulations. *Curr Opin Cell Biol* 1994;4:394–400.

71. Webb LM, Ehrengruber MU, Clark-Lewis I, Baggiolini M, Rot A. Binding to heparan sulfate or heparin enhances neutrophil responses to interleukin-8. *Proc Natl Acad Sci U S A* 1993;90:7158–7162.

72. Tanaka Y, Adams DH, Hubscher S, Hirano H, Siebenlist U, Shaw S. T-cell adhesion induced by proteoglycan-immobilized cytokine MIP-1 beta [see comments]. *Nature* 1993;361:79–82.

73. Baggiolini M, Wymann MP. Turning on the respiratory burst. [Review]. *Trends Biochem Sci* 1990;15:69–72.

74. Detmers PA, Lo SK, Olsen-Egbert E, Walz A, Baggiolini M, Cohn ZA. Neutrophil-activating protein 1/interleukin-8 stimulates the binding activity of the leukocyte adhesion receptor CD11b/CD18 on human neutrophils. *J Exp Med* 1990;171:1155–1162.

75. Detmers PA, Powell DE, Walz A, Clark-Lewis I, Baggiolini M, Cohn ZA. Differential effects of neutrophil-activating peptide 1/IL-8 and its homologues on leukocyte adhesion and phagocytosis. *J Immunol* 1991;147:4211–4217.

76. Schroder JM. The monocyte-derived neutrophil activating peptide (NAP/interleukin-8) stimulates human neutrophil arachidonate-5-lipoxygenase, but not the release of cellular arachidonate. *J Exp Med* 1989;170:847–863.

77. Bussolino F, Sironi M, Bocchietto E, Mantovani A. Synthesis of platelet-activating factor by polymorphonuclear neutrophils stimulated with interleukin-8. *J Biol Chem* 1992;267:14598–14603.

78. Kernen P, Wymann MP, von Tscharner V, et al. Shape changes, exocytosis, and cytosolic free calcium changes in stimulated human eosinophils. *J Clin Invest* 1991;87:2012–2017.

79. Warringa RA, Koenderman L, Kok PT, Kreukniet J, Bruijnzeel PL.

Modulation and induction of eosinophil chemotaxis by granulocyte-macrophage colony-stimulating factor and interleukin-3. *Blood* 1991; 77:2694–2700.

80. Rot A, Krieger M, Brunner T, Bischoff SC, Schall TJ, Dahinden CA. RANTES and macrophage inflammatory protein Ia induce the migration and activation of normal human eosinophil granulocytes. *J Exp Med* 1992;176:1489–1495.

81. Kameyoshi Y, Dorschner A, Mallet AI, Christophers E, Schroder Jens-M. Cytokine RANTES released by thrombin-stimulated platelets is a potent attractant for human eosinophils. *J Exp Med* 1992; 176:587–592.

82. Alam R, Stafford S, Forsythe P, et al. RANTES is a chemotactic and activating factor for human eosinophils. *J Immunol* 1993;150:3442–3447.

83. Meurer R, Van Riper G, Feeney W, et al. Formation of eosinophilic and monocytic intradermal inflammatory sites in the dog by injection of human RANTES but not human monocyte chemoattractant protein 1, human macrophage inflammatory protein 1 , or human interleukin-8. *J Exp Med* 1993;178:1913–1921.

84. Dahinden CA, Geiser T, Brunner T, et al. Monocyte chemotactic protein 3 is a most effective basophil- and eosinophil-activating chemokine. *J Exp Med* 1994;179:751–756.

85. Larsen CG, Anderson AO, Appella E, Oppenheim JJ, Matsushima K. The neutrophil-activating protein (NAP-1) is also chemotactic for T lymphocytes. *Science* 1989;243:1464–1466.

86. Bacon KB, Camp RD. Interleukin (IL)-8-induced *in vitro* human lymphocyte migration is inhibited by cholera and pertussis toxins and inhibitors of protein kinase C. *Biochem Biophys Res Commun* 1990; 169:1099–1104.

87. Swensson O, Schubert C, Christophers E, Schroder JM. Inflammatory properties of neutrophil-activating protein-1/interleukin-8 (NAP-1/IL-8) in human skin: a light- and electronmicroscopic study. *Journal of Investigative Dermatology* 1991;96:682–689.

88. Leonard EJ, Yoshimura T, Tanaka S, Raffeld M. Neutrophil recruitment by intradermally injected neutrophil attractant/activation protein-1. *Journal of Investigative Dermatology* 1991;96:690–694.

89. Schall TJ, Bacon K, Toy KJ, Goeddel DV. Selective attraction of monocytes and T lymphocytes of the memory phenotype of cytokine RANTES. *Nature* 1990;347:669–671.

90. Schall TJ, Bacon K, Camp RD, Kaspari JW, Goeddel DV. Human macrophage inflammatory protein α (MIP-1α) and MIP-1 chemokines attract distinct populations of lymphocytes. *J Exp Med* 1993; 177:1821–1826.

91. Taub DD, Conlon K, Lloyd AR, Oppenheim JJ, Kelvin DJ. Preferential migration of activated CD4+ and CD8+ T cells in response to MIP-1 and MIP-1. *Science* 1993;260:355–357.

92. Carr MW, Roth SJ, Luther E, Rose SS, Springer TA. Monocyte chemoattractant protein 1 acts as a T-lymphocyte chemoattractant. *Proc Natl Acad Sci USA* 1994;91:3652–3656.

93. Maghazachi AA, Al Aarkaty A, Schall TJ. C-C chemokines induce the chemotaxis of NK and IL-2 activated NK cells: role for G proteins. *J Immunol* 1994;153:4969–4977.

94. Taub DD, Lloyd AR, Conlon K, Wang JM, Ortaldo JR, Harada A, Kelvin DJ, Oppenheim JJ. Recombinant human interferon-inducible protein 10 is a chemoattractant for human monocytes and T lymphocytes and promotes T cell adhesion to endothelial cells. *J Exp Med* 1993;177:1809–1814.

95. White MV, Yoshimura T, Hook W, Kaliner MA, Leonard EJ. Neutrophil attractant/activation protein-1 (NAP-1) causes human basophil histamine release. *Immunol Lett* 1989;22:151–154.

96. Dahinden CA, Kurimoto Y, De Weck AL, Lindley I, Dewald B, Baggiolini M. The neutrophil-activating peptide NAF/NAP-1 induces histamine and leukotriene release by interleukin 3-primed basophils. *J Exp Med* 1989;170:1787–1792.

97. Bischoff SC, Baggiolini M, De Weck AL, Dahinden CA. Interleukin 8-inhibitor and inducer of histamine and leukotriene release in human basophils. *Biochem Biophys Res Commun* 1991;179:628–633.

98. Kuna P, Reddigari SR, Rucinski D, Oppenheim JJ, Kaplan AP. Monocyte chemotactic and activating factor is a potent histamine-releasing factor for human basophils. *J Exp Med* 1992;175:489–493.

99. Alam R, Forsythe PA, Stafford S, Lett-Brown MA, Grant JA. Macrophage inflammatory protein-1 activates basophils and mast cells. *J Exp Med* 1992;176:781–786.

100. Bischoff SC, Krieger M, Brunner T, Dahinden CA. Monocyte chemotactic protein 1 is a potent activator of human basophils. *J Exp Med* 1992;175:1271–1275.

101. Bischoff SC, Krieger M, Brunner T, et al. RANTES and related chemokines activate human basophil granulocytes through different G protein-coupled receptors. *Eur J Immunol* 1993;23:761–767.

102. Kuna P, Reddigarl SR, Schall TJ, Rucinski D, Viksman MY, Kaplan AP. RANTES, A monocyte and T lymphocyte chemotactic cytokine releases histamine from human basophils. *J Immunol* 1992;149:636–642.

103. Walz A, Meloni F, Clark-Lewis I, von Tscharner V, Baggiolini M. [Ca2-]i changes and respiratory burst in human neutrophils and monocytes induced by NAP-1/interleukin-8, NAP-2, and GRO/MGSA. *J Leukoc Biol* 1991;50:279–286.

104. Yoshimura T, Robinson EA, Tanaka S, Appella E, Leonard EJ. Purification and amino acid analysis of two human monocyte chemoattractants produced by phytohemagglutinin-stimulated human blood mononuclear leukocytes. *J Immunol* 1989;142:1956–1962.

105. Yoshimura T, Robinson EA, Appella E, Matsushima K, Showalter SD, Leonard EJ. Three forms of monocyte-derived neutrophil chemotactic factor (MDNCF) distinguished by different lengths of the amino-terminal sequence. *Mol Immunol* 1989;26:87–93.

106. Rollins BJ, Walz A, Baggiolini M. Recombinant human MCP-1/JE induces chemotaxis, calcium flux, and the respiratory burst in human monocytes. *Blood* 1991;78:1112–1116.

107. Sozzani S, Luini W, Molino M, et al. The signal transduction pathway involved in the migration induced by a monocyte chemotactic cytokine. *J Immunol* 1991;147:2215–2221.

108. Miller MD, Krangel MS. The human cytokine I-309 is a monocyte chemoattractant. *Proc Natl Acad Sci U S A* 1992;89:2950–2954.

109. Zachariae CO, Anderson AO, Thompson HL, Appella E, Mantovani A, Matsushima K. Properties of monocyte chemotactic and activating factor (MCAF) purified from a human fibrosarcoma cell line. *J Exp Med* 1990;171:2177–2182.

110. McColl SR, Hachicha M, Levasseur S, Neote K, Schall TJ. Uncoupling of early signal transduction events from effector function in human peripheral blood neutrophils in response to recombinant macrophage inflammatory proteins α-1 and β-1. *J Immunol* 1993;150: 4550–4560.

111. Jiang Y, Beller DI, Frendl G, Graves DT. Monocyte chemoattractant protein-1 regulates adhesion molecule expression and cytokine production in human monocytes. *J Immunol* 1992;148:2423–2428.

112. Kupper RW, Dewald B, Jakobs KH, Baggiolini M, Gierschik P. G-protein activation by interleukin-8 and related cytokines in human neutrophil plasma membranes. *Biochem J* 1992;282:429–434.

113. Holmes WE, Lee J, Kuang WJ, Rice GC, Wood WI. Structure and functional expression of a human interleukin-8 receptor. *Science* 1991;253:1278–1280.

114. Charo IF, Myers SJ, Herman A, Franci C, Connolly AJ, Coughlin SR. Molecular cloning and functional expression of two monocyte chemoattractant protein 1 receptors reveals alternative splicing of the carboxyl-terminal tails. *Proc Natl Acad Sci U S A* 1994;91:2752–2756.

115. Murphy PM. The molecular biology of leukocyte chemoattractant receptors. [Review]. *Annu Rev Immunol* 1994;12:593-633.

116. Murphy PM, Tiffany HL. Cloning of complementary DNA encoding a functional human interleukin-8 receptor. *Science* 1991;253:1280–1283.

117. Lee J, Horuk R, Rice GC, Bennett GL, Camerato T, Wood WI. Characterization of two high affinity human interleukin-8 receptors. *J Biol Chem* 1992;267:16283–16287.

118. Neote K, Digregorio D, Mak JY, Horak R, Schall TJ. Molecular cloning, functional expression and signaling characteristics of a C-C chemokine receptor. *Cell* 1993;72:415–425.

119. Gao JL, Kuhns DB, Tiffany HL, et al. Structure and functional expression of the human macrophage inflammatory protein 1/RANTES receptor. *J Exp Med* 1993;177:1421–1427.

120. Neote K, Mak JY, Kolakowski LF, Jr, Schall TJ. Functional and biochemical analysis of the cloned Duffy antigen: identity with the red blood cell chemokine receptor. *Blood* 1994;84:44–52.

121. Neote K, Darbonne W, Ogez J, Horuk R, Schall TJ. Identification of a promiscuous inflammatory peptide receptor on the surface of red blood cells. *J Biol Chem* 1993;268:12247–12249.

122. Horuk R, Colby TJ, Darbonne WC, Schall TJ, Neote K. The human erythrocyte inflammatory peptide (chemokine) receptor. Biochemical

characterization, solubilization, and development of a binding assay for the soluble receptor. *Biochemistry* 1993;32:5733–5738.

123. Ahuja SK, Murphy PM. Molecular piracy of mammalian interleukin-8 receptor type B by herpesvirus saimiri. *J Biol Chem* 1993;268:20691–20694.

124. Bousquet J, Chanez P, Lacoste JY, et al. Eosinophilic inflammation in asthma. *N Engl J Med* 1990;323:1033–1039.

125. Djukanovic R, Wilson JW, Britten KM, et al. Quantitation of mast cells and eosinophils in the bronchial mucosa of symptomatic atopic asthmatics and healthy control subjects using immunohistochemistry. *Am Rev Respir Dis* 1990;142:863–871.

126. Bentley AM, Menz G, Storz C, et al. Identification of T lymphocytes, macrophages and activated eosinophils in the bronchial mucosa of intrinsic asthma. Relationship to symptoms and bronchial hyperresponsiveness. *Am Rev Respir Dis* 1992;146:500–506.

127. Poston R, Chanez P, Lacoste JY, Litchfield P, Lee TH, Bousquet J. Immunohistochemical characterization of the cellular infiltration of asthmatic bronchi. *Am Rev Respir Dis* 1992;145:918–921.

128. Hamid Q, Azzawi M, Ying S, et al. Expression of mRNA for interleukins in mucosal bronchial biopsies from asthma. *J Clin Invest* 1991;87:1541–1546.

129. Robinson DS, Hamid Q, Ying S, et al. Predominant TH2-like bronchoalveolar T-lymphocyte population in atopic asthma. *N Engl J Med* 1992;326:298–304.

130. Robinson DS, Bentley AM, Hartnell A, Kay AB, Durham SR. Activated memory T helper cells in bronchoalveolar lavage fluid from patients with atopic asthma: relation to asthma symptoms, lung function, and bronchial responsiveness. *Thorax* 1993;48:26–32.

131. Bentley AM, Meng Q, Robinson DS, Hamid Q, Kay AB, Durham SR. Increasesin activated T lympohcytes, eosinophils and cytokine mRNA expression for interleukin-5 and granulocyte-macrophage colony-stimulating factor in bronchial biopsies after allergen inhalation challenge in atopic asthmatics. *Am J Respir Cell Mol Biol* 1993;8:35–42.

132. Robinson D, Hamid Q, Bentley A, Sun Y, Kay AB, Durham SR. Activation of CD4+ T cells, increased TH2-type cytokine mRNA expression, and eosinophil recruitment in bronchoalveolar lavage after allergen inhalation challenge in patients with atopic asthma. *J Allergy Clin Immunol* 1993;92:313–324.

133. Broide DH, Firestein GS. Endobronchial allergen challenge: demonstration of cellular source of granulocyte-macrophage colony-stimulating factor by *in situ* hybridization. *J Clin Invest* 1991;88:1048–1053.

134. Boschetto P, Fabbri LM, Zocca E, et al. Prednisone inhibits late asthmatic reactions and airway inflammation induced by toluene diisocyanate in sensitized subjects. *J Allergy Clin Immunol* 1987;80:261–267.

135. Diaz P, Gonzalez MC, Galleguillos FR, et al. Leucocytes and mediators in bronchoalveolar lavage during allergen-induced late-phase asthmatic reactions. *Am Rev Respir Dis* 1989;139:1383–1389.

136. Bascomb R, Wachs M, Naclerio RM, Pipkorn U, Galli SJ, Lichtenstein LM. Basophil influx occurs after nasal antigen challenge: effect of topical corticosteroid therapy. *J Allergy Clin Immunol* 1988;81:580–589.

137. Dunnill MS. The pathology of asthma with special reference to changes in the bronchial mucosa. *J Clin Pathol* 1960;13:27–33.

138. Sur S, Crotty TB, Kephart GM, et al. Sudden-onset fatal asthma: A distinct entity with few eosinophils and relatively more neutrophils in the airway submucosa? *Am Rev Respir Dis* 1993;148:713–719.

139. Marini M, Vittori E, Hollemburg J, Mattoli S. Expression of the potent inflammatory cytokines granulocyte-macrophage colony stimulating factor, interleukin-6 and interleukin-8 in bronchial epithelial cells of patients with asthma. *J Allergy Clin Immunol* 1992;82:1001–1009.

140. Collins PD, Weg VB, Faccioli LH, Watson ML, Moqbel R, Williams TJ. Eosinophil accumulation induced by human interleukin-8 in the guinea-pig *in vivo. Immunology* 1993;79:312–318.

141. Sanz MJ, Weg VB, Bolanowski MA, Nourshargh S. IL-1 is a potent inducer of eosinophil accummulation in rat skin. Inhibition of response by platelet activating factor antagonist and an anti-human IL-8 antibody. *J Immunol* 1995;154:1364–1373.

142. Hallsworth MP, Soh CPC, Lane SJ, Arm JP, Lee TH. Selective enhancement of GM-CSF, TNF , IL-1 and IL-8 production by monocytes and macrophages of asthmatic subjects. *Eur Respir J* 1994;7:1096–1102.

143. Richman-Eisenstat JB, Jorens PG, Hebert CA, Ueki I, Nadel JA. Interleukin-8: an important chemoattractant in sputum of patients with chronic inflammatory airway diseases. *Am J Physiol* 1993;264:L413–L418.

144. Car BD, Meloni F, Luisetti M, Semenzato G, Gialdroni-Grassi G, Walz A. Elevated IL-8 and MCP-1 in the bronchoalveolar lavage fluid of patients with idiopathic pulmonary fibrosis and pulmonary sarcoidosis. *Am J Respir Crit Care Med* 1994;149:655–659.

145. Standiford TJ, Rolfe MW, Kunkel SL, et al. Macrophage inflammatory protein-1α expression in interstitial lung disease. *J Immunol* 1993;151:2852–2863.

146. Berkman N, O'Connor BJ, Barnes PJ, Chung KF. Expression of RANTES but not of MIP-1α mRNA from endobronchial biopsies is greater in asthmatics than in normal controls. *Eur Respir J* 1994;7:468s.

147. Jose PJ, Griffiths-Johnson DA, Collins PD, et al. Eotaxin: a potent eosinophil chemoattractant cytokine detected in a guinea pig model of allergic airways inflammation. *J Exp Med* 1994;179:881–887.

148. Griffiths-Johnson DA, Collins PD, Rossi AG, Jose PJ, Williams TJ. The chemokine, eotaxin, activates guinea-pig eosinophils *in vitro* and causes their accumulation into the lung *in vivo. Biochem Biophys Res Commun* 1993;197:1167–1172.

Asthma, edited by P.J. Barnes, M.M. Grunstein,
A.R. Leff, and A.J. Woolcock.
Lippincott–Raven Publishers, Philadelphia © 1997.

▪ 52 ▪

Growth Factors

Jason Kelley

This chapter discusses the physiology of the mitogenic growth factors involved in asthma and related airway disorders. The airway walls of patients with asthma are thickened by an increase in the amount of both smooth muscle cells and connective tissue elements. While there exists at this time only a small amount of information about the potential roles of growth factors in asthma and airways disorders, it is clear that much of the current knowledge regarding growth factor control of cells of epithelial cells, smooth muscle cells, and fibroblasts in other tissues and disorders is relevant to the pathogenesis of asthma.

Connective tissue is integral to the normal functioning of the large and small airways of the lung. Indeed, lung contains more connective tissue as a proportion of total weight than any other organ of the body (1). It has become clear in recent years that significant remodeling takes place in the asthmatic lung in response to exogenous, inflammatory, and biomechanical signals (2). In pathological states, excess amounts of connective tissue can be deposited at several levels in the airway: large and small airways as well as in alveolar capillary membranes and airspaces. The deleterious physiological effects of increased mass of airway smooth muscle, adventitia, and submucosal elements have been quantitated in patients with asthma and chronic obstructive pulmonary disease

(COPD) (3). With greater smooth muscle thickness, the development of greater tension and, thus, more constriction of the lumen is facilitated. Recent reviews on the subject of airway cells and remodeling have appeared (See Chapters 16, 17, 66, also ref. 4).

BASIC BIOLOGY OF GROWTH FACTORS

The peptide growth factors are pleiotropic molecules produced ubiquitously, which modulate the proliferation of a range of target cells. The strict definition of a growth factor (versus other cytokines) remains problematic: many, if not all, cytokines modulate growth of some cells directly or indirectly. It is also important to note that the activities triggered by growth factors in appropriate target cells are not limited to proliferation. They also include such changes in phenotype as cellular hypertrophy, cytoskeletal reorganization, change in shape, and migration. Historically, cytokines first recognized for their mitogenic activity have been given names highlighting that role. Although this chapter focuses on the growth-promoting cytokines as they relate to asthma, it is important to remember that these cytokines act in a milieu intermittently rich in pro-inflammatory cytokines and chemokines. This complexity of interactions between mesenchymal growth factors and other cytokines has led to the concept of cytokine networks (5,6). Moreover, growth factors are produced in abundance by migratory inflam-

J. Kelley: Department of Medicine, University of Vermont College of Medicine, Burlington, Vermont 05405.

matory cells, as well as by resident structural cells of the lungs, making distinctions between different types of cytokines difficult. Growth factors are relatively small proteins with molecular weights in the range 6-40 kDa. Many growth factors are often dimers or multimers of one or several closely related gene products. The subunits are usually covalently linked by disulfide bonds. The individual growth factor peptides lose their ability to bind to their receptors when chemically separated, and thereby lose their biological activity. Historically, investigators had for decades sought for solid evidence of secreted molecules with mitogenic activity. The discovery of the mitogenic growth factors became feasible when cells could be cultured in a defined medium, free of serum and other complex biological fluids which support a high background of cell replication. Observable phenotypic changes of cultured cell lines could then be detected and the accountable proteins isolated. Upon purification of adequate amounts of growth factor, the amino acid and nucleic acid sequences could be deduced. The discovery of hundreds of cytokines began in the mid-1970s with the simultaneous characterization of interleukin-1 and platelet-derived growth factor.

Clarification of nucleic acid sequence of individual cytokines facilitated the generation of recombinant growth factors proteins for use as biologically active probes. Complementary deoxyribonucleic acid (cDNA) constructs have been hybridized to ribonucleic acid (RNA), as well as tissue sections, for quantitation and localization of gene expression. The cDNA constructs also allowed rapid searching of cDNA and genomic libraries for related peptides. This strategy has brought to light whole growth factor gene families. Several hundred distinct cytokines discovered to date can be classified as members of one of the cytokine superfamilies.

PLATELET-DERIVED GROWTH FACTOR

Platelet-derived Growth Factor (PDGF) is a potent mitogenic protein with activity in the low picomolar range (7). It is a cationic glycoprotein with molecular weight ranging from 28 to 34 kDa. PDGF was discovered originally as a soluble factor present in serum. Its origin was traced to platelet α granules, which had been allowed to lyse during blood collection and clot formation. Like many mitogenic cytokines, it is now recognized to have several molecular forms. Thus, the several PDGF proteins are members of a family of related, but distinct gene products which act on cells through an array of related cognate high affinity receptors. The cellular targets of PDGF action include smooth muscle cells and fibroblasts, some endothelial and epithelial cells, and other cells.

Classic studies of Pledger et al. (8) indicated that serum-derived PDGF acts during the very early hours of the cell cycle. After serum-depletion, PDGF makes BALB/c 3T3 cells competent to begin their transition from dormancy (G_0) into the first stage of the cell cycle (G_1). Later-acting serum factors including insulin-like growth factor (IGF-I), promote the further progression through the later stages of this transition. Although studies of cell cycle kinetics based the BALB/c 3T3 cells were instrumental in dissecting events in the cell cycle, subsequent studies cast doubt on the precise timing of PDGF action as it applies to other less prototypic mammalian cell lines (9).

Subsequent sequencing of proteins associated with the mitogenic activity purified from platelet α granules revealed the presence of two distinct, but related, peptide chains, PDGF-A and PDGF-B (10,11). Both were shown to be dimers linked covalently by four disulfide bonds. These PDGF peptides can, therefore, exist in any of three dimerized forms composed of pairs of A and B chains: PDGF-AA, -AB, and -BB. The dimerized forms of PDGF exhibit variable mitogenic potency on target cells which, in turn, depends on the specific receptor subtypes present (See following and also references 12–15). The PDGF-A chain gene is found on chromosome 7 in humans; PDGF-B chain is identical to the c-*sis* oncogene product; its gene is localized on chromosome 22 (16).

OTHER ACTIONS OF PDGF FAMILY CYTOKINES

At the whole tissue level, PDGF has been shown to be involved in granulation tissue deposition. When placed on experimentally induced skin wounds, PDGF can overcome impaired wound healing in such disorders as diabetes (17). Like many other mitogenic cytokines, PDGF has potency as a chemotaxin for mesenchymal cells (18). It also may act as an inducer of extracellular matrix, albeit with far less potency than transforming growth factor-β (TGF-β). PDGF has also been shown to promote fibroblast mediated wound contraction (19).

A role for PDGF as an immune-modulator has emerged only recently as PDGF receptors have been defined on T-cells and other inflammatory cells. The T cell lymphokines modulated in response to PDGF include enhanced interleukin (IL)-2, but reductions in the production of IL-4, IL-5, and IFN-γ. It appears PDGF that acts primarily through a PDGF β receptor subunit on lymphocytes to influence the behavior of T cells at concentrations < 1 ng/ml (20). In addition to its direct role on immune cells, PDGF can also induce both tumor necrosis factor-α (TNF-α) and IL-1 production by other cell types such as smooth muscle cells and fibroblasts (21,22).

PDGF RECEPTORS

PDGF receptors are glycoproteins integrally located within cell membranes of mesenchymal cells and other susceptible cells. Responsiveness of cells to PDGF depends on the presence of the appropriate cell surface receptor. Growth factors resemble other signalling molecules in binding to specific surface receptors exhibited on target cells. Membrane receptors are linked to a specific array of intracellular signalling pathways which transduce the signal in the cytoplasm or nucleus. Growth factor receptors of the lungs exhibit classic extracellular, transmembrane, and intracellular domains (23). The extracellular domain of the receptor binds the growth factor ligand, whereupon the intracellular portion engages a specific signalling pathway. All lung cells can be presumed to express a diverse population of high affinity growth factor receptors; this receptor array characterizes the phenotypic response of the cell to its environment. This array can be assumed to change during the life of the cell, as well as in response to immediate internal and external stimulation.

In general, growth factors act extracellularly in transcellular signalling, binding and activating receptors present in cell membranes. However, interactions between PDGF and its receptors also have been shown to take place within intracellular sites (24,25).

Exposure of cells to one particular growth factor may modulate later responses to other cytokines. Alteration of the specific population of receptors present on the cell surface (receptor trans-modulation) often ensues. For example, exposure of mesenchymal cells to PDGF modulates the binding of epidermal growth factor to its receptor (26). There also are multiple examples of growth factors upwardly modulating their own receptors, enhancing the sensitivity of cells to them. The potential for such a seemingly unchecked positive feedback loop goes against the basic precepts of tissue and cell homeostasis, but is usually balanced by the simultaneous induction of opposing negative signals.

Several forms of PDGF receptors have been described, which differ in their specificity for the various molecular isotypes of PDGF, allowing the three dimeric ligands to exert different mechanisms of action (12–15,27). High affinity binding of PDGF requires association of two receptor subunits: an α subunit that can bind either a PDGF-B or a PDGF-A chain, and a β subunit that can bind only the PDGF-B unit. The α and β receptor subunits can be distinguished by binding specificity, as well as by blocking or activating antibodies. Upon exposure to active PDGF, these subunits rapidly form reversible complexes on the cell surface.

The interaction of PDGF ligand with cell surface receptor results in dimerization of pairs of high affinity receptor subunits (28). Immediately following binding of ligand and receptor, intrinsic receptor tyrosine kinase and auto-phosphorylation of tyrosine residues on the intra-cytoplasmic domain of the receptor take place (29,30).

Modulation of receptor population density controls cell phenotype with regard to mitogenic potential in response to PDGF (31). PDGF-BB generally has been found to be a more potent mitogen than the AA dimer by virtue of its greater density on most cells. Counterbalancing its greater potency is the finding that PDGF-BB is less well-secreted than PDGF-AA, potentially limiting its role as a mitogen. Transfection of cell lines devoid of PDGF receptors with cDNAs for PDGF receptor genes conferred on them the ability to move chemotactically in a PDGF concentration-gradient (32). The alteration in phenotype is dependent on the receptor type transfected: receptor-negative cells transfected with the β receptor subunit gene become responsive specifically to PDGF-BB; cells expressing only the α receptor subunit are equally responsive to all three dimeric ligands.

Given their importance to cell growth, it is not surprising that expression of PDGF receptors is regulated very closely; the α and β protein components of the PDGF receptor appear to respond independently to control signals. Exposure of 3T3 cells to TGF-β down-regulates their binding of different PDGF isotypes (33). PDGF-AA binding is markedly down-regulated as compared to PDGF-BB. The loss of PDGF-AA binding is accompanied by selective loss of ability to undergo mitosis in response to PDGF-AA. Such differential regulation clearly has implications for processes of pathologic remodeling in lung and other tissues.

It had not been clear whether PDGF-AB could bind to cells expressing only PDGF β receptor and, if so, whether PDGF-AB could act as an agonist. To answer this question, Seifert et al. turned to cell lines from Patch mutant mouse embryos. This strain harbors a mutational deletion of the PDGF α receptor gene but no alteration in expression or activity of PDGF β receptors (34). Comparison between the binding and response properties of wild type and mutant cell lines allowed definition of the contribution that PDGF α receptors make to the ability of these cells to respond to PDGF-AB. PDGF-AB binds to PDGF α receptor-negative cells and induces PDGF β receptor dimerization, phosphorylation on tyrosine, and, ultimately, DNA synthesis.

CONNECTIVE TISSUE GROWTH FACTOR

Recently, investigators have called into question whether the PDGF peptides as described earlier truly account for the mitogenic activity for smooth muscle cells and fibroblasts that is released by many cell types other than platelets (35,36). There is no longer any debate that PDGF dimers are active as mitogens and chemotactic agents. However, most of the early studies ascribed mitogenic activity to PDGF merely on the basis of circumstantial arguments alone. When the levels of mitogenic activity changed in concert with varying PDGF messenger RNA (mRNA) levels, this was interpreted to indicate that observed mitogenic activity resulted from PDGF protein secretion. Missing from these analyses have been rigorous biochemical isolation and sizing techniques, or, ultimately, *in vitro* translation and identification of protein.

A series of studies have pointed out the existence of several novel growth factors which, although structurally only minimally related to PDGF in amino acid sequence, nevertheless appear to act through the PDGF receptor system (37,38). These growth factors differ from PDGF in having unique coding sequences distinct from the various PDGFs. They do share antigenic determinants with the classic forms of PDGF and can be considered mimitopes of the PDGFs.

Two such peptide growth factors have now been described. The first mitogen appears to be a unique product of monocytes (37,38). A monomer, it lacks the characteristic inter- and intra-chain disulfide bonds of PDGF and behaves as a 16 kDa peptide under nonreducing conditions. It is of interest that peptide mitogens of this molecular weight have been found in lavage fluid from subjects with adult respiratory distress syndrome (ARDS), suggesting a role for this growth factor in the progressive fibrotic remodeling that often complicates this disorder (39).

Grotendorst et al. also have described a peptide of molecular weight 34 to 38 kDa, which is somewhat larger than expected for the largest forms of authentic PDGF. The monomeric growth factor they have isolated and described has been given the name connective tissue growth factor (CTGF) (40). Grotendorst's group originally detected CTGF in wound exudate fluid where it was found in association with the previously mentioned 16 to 17 kDa monocyte peptide (38). Large molecular weight CTGF has also been found in culture medium from skin fibroblasts, in which setting they are uniquely inducible by TGF-β (41). Indeed, it has been argued rather persuasively that CTGF rather than PDGF-AA is the primary mitogenic peptide induced by TGF-β stimulation of mesenchymal cells. In this regard, it is interesting to note that CTGF supports normal wound healing in the absence of detectable authentic PDGF, suggesting that its efficacy closely parallels that of PDGF (38).

To substantiate the role of CTGF in lung remodeling, Walsh et al. studied its presence in bleomycin-induced injury/remodeling in the rat lung (42). Lung epithelial lining fluid harvested by lavage contains at least two PDGF-like peptides, which appear in a characteristic temporal sequence. Mitogenic peptides were purified partially in epithelial lining fluid with mitogenic activity and analyzed by immuno-blotting to determine their molecular weight and immunologic identity. Blots were probed with polyclonal antibodies to PDGF isoforms. Antibodies capable of detecting PDGFs and CTGF stained peptides of two distinct size classes (38 to 40 kDa and 29 kDa) in the alveolar fluid from all the rats with lung injury induced by bleomycin, but not from control rats. The 38 to 40 kDa peptide was detected only with anti-PDGF-BB antibody,

suggesting that CTGF more closely resembles this form of PDGF.

The 29 kDa peptide was detected only with anti-PDGF-AA antibody. This peptide is likely authentic PDGF-AA. The amounts of CTGF and PDGF-AA varied independently with time after exposure to bleomycin: the larger CTGF peptide reached maximal amounts 3 to 6 days after lung injury. The 29 kDa PDGF-AA was present at all times following injury, but with little or no variation over time. In parallel with these immunoassays for PDGF-like molecules, abundant mitogenic activity for fibroblasts was demonstrated in the concentrated epithelial lining fluid following bleomycin. The amount of growth promoting activity paralleled temporally the amount of the 38 to 40 kDa peptide detected by immuno-blotting. Anti-PDGF-BB (but not anti-PDGF-AA) antibodies blocked most of this activity. These findings strongly suggest that the most important mitogenic activity for fibroblasts and smooth muscle cells released into the remodeling lung is CTGF, rather than PDGF. The cellular sources of this CTGF remain uncertain. Quite possibly it may derive in large part from airway epithelium, which is prominently injured during intra-tracheal instillation of bleomycin.

In patients with ARDS, crude and partially purified lavage fluid contains PDGF-like peptides (39). However, the sizing of the mitogenic activity detected exhibits anomalous molecular weights, distinct from PDGF. PDGF-B-like activity also increases in the lungs within days of acute injury in both clinical studies and experimental models. There is an increase in the steady-state level of PDGF-B mRNA and PDGF-like protein in the lungs of rats exposed to hyperoxia, with increased c-*sis*/PDGF-B gene expression after exposure of rats to adaptive hyperoxia (43,44). PDGF-B mRNA levels rise within 3 days and stay up for at least a week. Given that the elevation in steady state mRNA levels precedes evidence of mesenchymal cell proliferation, it can be assumed to be one of the proliferative stimuli in this model.

MACROPHAGE PRODUCTION OF MITOGENIC CYTOKINES

Despite its identification as a platelet product, PDGF is a key signalling molecule produced by multiple nucleated cells. Monocyte-macrophages are known to produce and secrete a large number of growth factors (For review see ref. 45). Initial studies of the unpurified mitogenic activities released by monocyte-macrophages detected an aggregate activity originally described as "macrophage-derived growth factor." However, when individual growth factors could be isolated and distinguished it became apparent that monocyte-macrophages produce a number of specific mitogenic, pro-inflammatory, anti-inflammatory, and chemokinetic growth factors including PDGF (46).

Subsequent studies suggested that PDGF accounts for much of the fibroblast growth promoting activity produced by human alveolar macrophages (47). PDGF-B mRNA can be detected in lung macrophages from various sources, including cultured monocytes induced to differentiate *in vitro* (48–50). Like platelet PDGF, macrophage-derived PDGF acts both as a mitogen and chemotactic factor for mesenchymal cells (51,52).

There is growing evidence for the importance of PDGF-B in human pulmonary remodeling. Alveolar macrophages from patients with pulmonary fibrosis exhibit an increased steady state amount of PDGF-B mRNA, as well as an increased rate of transcription of PDGF and spontaneous secretion of PDGF protein (53–55). *In situ* hybridization techniques have been applied to the study of fibrotic lungs in order to localize PDGF-B gene expression (36). Cells appearing to express PDGF mRNA most vigorously appeared to be macrophages and type II cells. At the same time, there are local increases of PDGF-B-containing protein as demonstrated by immuno-staining. Vignaud et al. (56) further have demonstrated that PDGF-B is prominent in interstitial macrophages in lung biopsies from patients with lung fibrosis. This is true even in areas with little overt evidence of fibrosis, suggesting that PDGF accumulation precedes focal remodeling. If true, this suggests a major causative role for locally deposited PDGF in the process of lung fibrosis.

The stimuli responsible for inducing macrophage PDGF-B gene expression in the setting of chronic inflammation and fibrosis are largely speculative. Lymphocytes are prominent cells in these acute and chronic inflammatory responses. This has sparked investigations of production of the lymphokine interferon-γ (IFN-γ). IFN-γ is a product of T cells of the TH1 subtype and its presence has been reported in some patients with spontaneous pulmonary fibrosis (57,58). IFN-γ clearly induces increased steady state levels of PDGF-B mRNA in lung macrophages (50). Moreover, antigen-stimulated lymphocytes release one or more factors which cause macrophages to expand their PDGF-B mRNA pool.

Parallel findings have been noted during the course of experimental pulmonary fibrosis induced by bleomycin instillation. As indicated earlier, lavage derived T cells from rats previously exposed to bleomycin release fibroblast mitogens, notably CTGF (59). From this observation, we have posited that antigen-stimulated TH1-lymphocyte activation mediates release of IFN-γ.

Few studies have directly examined the potential roles of growth factors in asthma. Aubert et al. (60) have studied the expression of PDGF and its receptors in lungs from asthmatics, contrasting them to those from patients with COPD and cigarette smoking patients with normal lung function. The histologic material used for this study was post-mortem lung specimens and several lung resection specimens. Using immuno-histochemical techniques, they localized PDGF to tissue monocyte-macro-

phages; however, the macrophages found free in alveoli did not exhibit PDGF production. The number of PDGF-positive cells was no greater in the 12 asthmatic subjects' lungs than in the two other clinical groups studied. The PDGF receptor β subunit, the hemi-receptor selectively able to respond to PDGF-BB, was expressed only on a few (nonmacrophage) interstitial cells and some of the basal cells of the bronchial epithelium. The mRNA levels of PDGF β receptor showed a positive correlation of PDGF-B and a greater abundance of PDGF-B and β receptor mRNA in the asthmatics, as compared to the COPD patients. The investigators concluded from these largely negative, but important, observations that PDGF and its receptor are expressed in human lungs but that their density does not correlate well with the structural airway changes of asthma. Tempering these conclusions was the finding that amounts of extractable mRNA for both the PDGF-B ligand and the PDGF β receptor subunit, were greater in the asthmatic lungs than in the control lungs. Moreover, the study was weighted heavily toward severe asthma, since most of the lungs came from victims of fatal asthma attacks. Hence, a potential role for PDGF early in the course of airway remodeling cannot be excluded from these data.

RELEASE OF GROWTH FACTORS BY LUNG STRUCTURAL CELLS

Inflammatory cells moving into the injured lung are not the only sources of mitogenic cytokines. Resident structural cells also produce PDGF and other mitogens. Epithelial cells of the airways are likely a major source of growth modulating cytokines involved in airway development, homeostasis, and remodeling (4). Fibroblasts cultured from rat lungs secrete *in vitro* a PDGF-like mitogenic cytokine, which, in turn, causes proliferation of lung fibroblasts (61). The growth factor(s) responsible for this activity act in the aggregate as a competence factor for murine BALB/c 3T3 cells as demonstrated in the classic cell cycle assay for PDGF (8). Anti-PDGF antibodies added to the fibroblast cultures block most of this proliferogenic activity. At the same time, northern blots of whole cell RNA isolated from cultured fibroblasts detect mRNA for the PDGF-A chain in those cultures that are secreting PDGF-like mitogenic activity. In contrast, no PDGF-B chain gene expression was apparent in the lung fibroblast lines examined.

FIBROBLAST GROWTH FACTORS AND KERATINOCYTE GROWTH FACTOR

The fibroblast growth factors (FGFs) are a family of structurally related polypeptides characterized by a high affinity for heparin (62,63). FGF family members originally were divided into two groups based on their differing affinities for heparin. Acidic FGFs can be eluted from immobilized heparin at lower salt concentrations than the basic FGF. The FGFs are among the most potent known inducers of neovascularization. They have prominent roles as mitogens for endothelial cells and induce synthesis of plasminogen activator.

Basic FGF is the product of a single gene; cDNAs and genomic clones of basic FGFs from a number of species have been identified and sequenced (64). The amino acid sequence of basic FGF varies very little across mammalian species, implying a strong evolutionary selection pressure. Basic FGF mRNA is notably unstable and the protein appears to be stored in tissues within cells and bound to extracellular matrix. Indeed, secreted basic FGF has been found to be associated with extracellular matrix, which may represent a major pool of this growth factor (65). Endothelial cell-derived heparan sulfate binds basic FGF and protects it from proteolytic digestion by plasmin, without limiting its access to its high-affinity receptor (66). Numerous cell types, in addition to endothelial cells, exhibit specific high-affinity receptors for basic FGF. Lung is rich in FGF receptors, as determined by immunohistochemical localization studies of acidic and basic FGFs in postnatal developing and adult rat lungs (67). Immuno-peroxidase staining of adult rat airways indicates that acidic FGF is present on ciliated cells, nonciliated cells of bronchioles, smooth muscle cells, type II alveoli pneumocytes, and interstitial and epithelial cells of alveolar septal regions. Staining of sections with antibody to basic FGF is confined to alveolar and vascular basement membrane regions but is also found on external laminae of smooth muscle cells.

Keratinocyte growth factor (KGF), a more recently described member of the fibroblast growth factor family, carries the alternate designation FGF-7. KGF is expressed in stromal fibroblasts and acts specifically on cells of epithelial origin as a paracrine growth modulator (68). KGF is a member of the FGF family, which is particularly rich in cysteine residues. KGF has received interest as a therapeutic agent because of its potency in wound healing (69). The function of KGF in normal and wounded skin has been assessed using dominant-negative KGF receptor transgenes expressed in keratinocytes. Upon skin injury of transgenic mice, inhibition of KGF receptor signalling reduces the proliferation rate of epidermal keratinocytes, delaying re-epithelialization of experimentally induced wounds (70). Human fibroblasts appear to express biologically active KGF on the outer surface of their plasma membranes, one of a growing number of examples of cell surface growth factor activity (71).

VASCULAR ENDOTHELIAL GROWTH FACTOR

Vascular endothelial growth factor (VEGF) is an approximately 43-kDa protein that induces endothelial pro-

liferation and angiogenesis. VEGF also induces abnormal capillary permeability, which activity resulted in its alternate name, vascular permeability factor (VPF). VEGF mRNA is expressed in the lungs and multiple other tissues. Of tissues surveyed, VEGF expression appears to be greatest in the lungs of normal rats (72). In the lung parenchyma, intense hybridization of VEGF mRNA is homogeneously distributed, with mRNA in virtually every alveolar cell. VEGF may be produced by smooth muscle cells in response to hypoxia (73). It almost certainly plays an important role in the physiology of vasculature in health and diseases, and by extension, the vessels of airways, and, perhaps, even airways themselves (74). However, a role for VEGF in airways disorders has not yet been determined.

HEPATOCYTE GROWTH FACTOR

Hepatocyte growth factor (HGF), a plasminogen-like protein, is a recently discovered cytokine that has both mitogenic and chemotactic effects on a wide variety of cells (75). HGF has been found to be identical to so-called "Scatter Factor," a cytokine discovered as a stimulant of epithelial and vascular endothelial cell motility. HGF is produced by mesenchymal cells and acts on a wide variety of epithelial cells, as a mitogen, a motogen (stimulator of cell motility), and a morphogen (promotor of multicellular architecture). HGF is also moderately potent as a tumor cytotoxic factor in *in vitro* assay systems (76). HGF mRNA and HGF protein are rapidly and markedly increased in the liver, and excess amounts of HGF protein can be detected in the plasma of rats with various types of liver injuries. During liver injury, hepatocyte HGF receptors are markedly down-regulated due to HGF-binding and subsequent internalization. Interestingly, the basal levels of HGF mRNA of the lung and other tissues markedly increases after administration of hepatotoxins to rats (77). HGF mediates its effects by activation of a membrane-spanning tyrosine kinase, identified as the met protooncogene product. Like other growth factors, HGF clearly participates in a complex cytokine network. TGF-β1 and also glucocorticoids downregulate HGF gene expression (78).

To determine if human lung fibroblasts are an important source of soluble growth factors for alveolar type II cells, Panos et al. (79) investigated the effect of fibroblast-conditioned medium on freshly isolated adult rat alveolar type II cell proliferation. They recognized that mesenchymal cells are important in the restoration of alveolar architecture following lung injury. Stimulation of type II cell DNA synthesis by crude fibroblast conditioned medium was observed only in the presence of serum. The responsible activity could be eliminated by various protein denaturing protocols and binding to heparin. It was additive with high concentrations of acidic fibroblast growth factor, epidermal growth factor, and insulin. Neutralizing antibody studies demonstrated that the primary mitogens isolated represent a mixture of HGF and KGF. These were confirmed by immunoblotting and Northern blot analysis. Moreover, human recombinant KGF and HGF induce type II cell DNA synthesis. The investigators concluded that adult human lung fibroblasts produce at least two soluble heparin-binding growth factors, KGF and HGF. In combination, they promote DNA synthesis and proliferation of type II cells in primary culture. HGF and KGF may be important in protecting airway epithelium in asthma and related disorders as well as during normal lung growth and after lung injury.

TRANSFORMING GROWTH FACTOR-β

Multiple growth factors assuredly play important roles as mediators of remodelling of small and large airways. The several transforming growth factors (TGF-βs) are pleiotropic growth modulators that are conspicuous for their ability to modulate a wide array of cellular behaviors. At least 5 closely-related TGF-β molecules, each distinct gene products, now have been described. The TGF-βs have been shown to be the most potent direct regulators of extracellular matrix gene expression (For reviews, see refs. 80–82). In addition to stimulating expression of matrix genes, TGF-β down-regulates expression of a variety of matrix degrading enzymes, such as the metalloproteinases. The net result of TGF-β action, then, is connective tissue accumulation.

TGF-β1, the prototype of the family and the most abundant member in most mammalian systems, is a 25 kDa dimeric molecule. It induces proliferation of certain target cells such as smooth muscle cells and fibroblasts through indirect mechanisms involving production of PDGF-like molecules and CTGF (41). This most likely explains why cell proliferation in response to TGF-β exhibits a bimodal concentration response relationship. TGF-β stimulates proliferation at low concentrations, but suppresses it in a higher concentration range (83). It appears to induce proliferation of connective tissue cells at low concentrations by stimulating secondary PDGF-AA or CTGF secretion. Released growth factor in turn acts in an autocrine fashion. At high concentrations, TGF-β mitogenic activity is dampened by down-regulation of PDGF α receptor, blocking the action of PDGF-AA.

Generally, the TGF isotypes (when acting alone) restrict proliferation of epithelial and endothelial cells. They also regulate multiple aspects of connective tissue turnover, and modulate the immune and hematopoietic systems. Upon binding of TGF-β to one of its several cognate receptors, genes for a host of connective tissue matrix proteins become up-regulated (84). At least one of the matrix proteins, decorin, appears to be a potent inactivator of TGF-β (85). Thus, an extracellular feedback loop may be active in response to TGF-β. Moreover, other cytokines contribute indirectly to the fibrogenic process; they may serve as chemo-attractants for inflammatory cells, promote maturation or proliferation in situ of cells involved in extracellular matrix production, or act via other mechanisms. TGF-β exhibits the novel property of being able to induce its own expression (86). Auto-induction appears to be mediated through an AP-1 nuclear complex (87). It has been suggested that through this mechanism, exogenous TGF-β arriving at the cell membrane can expand its effect through enhanced local TGF-β gene expression.

In concert with PDGF, TGF-β stimulates granulation tissue formation in adult skin, promotes scar formation in wounds, and enhances the strength of the maturing wound. In contrast, TGF-β appears to play little or no role in the healing of fetal wounds. The lack of a role for TGF-β may explain why fetal wounds heal with little or no scar formation (88).

A wide variety of pulmonary cells have been shown to produce TGF-β. Among them are macrophages, mast cells, human pulmonary endothelial cells exposed to bleomycin, and polymorphonuclear leukocytes (89–92). Kelley et al. previously have documented that rat lung fibroblasts produce and secrete TGF-β (93). The three major TGF-β isotypes present in mammalian tissues (Types 1 to 3) are present in developing murine lung, and appear to play critical roles in morphogenesis (94). Immunohistochemical techniques have been used to detect TGF-β protein in bronchial epithelium. TGF-β mRNA transcripts for each are present in fibroblasts and smooth muscle cells of the airway wall. Direct evidence for the specific involvement of TGF-βs in peri-bronchial fibrosis has been slow in coming. However, TGF-βs clearly have been implicated in diseases involving focal fibrotic derangement of multiple tissues including skin, liver, and heart.

Macrophages have a significant storage pool of TGF-β (95); moreover, mRNA levels do not parallel TGF-β protein secretion rates in macrophages following acute stimulation (89). This property may explain why this growth factor is so readily stained in immunohistochemistry studies of macrophages. As might be expected, macrophage TGF-β production and secretion are strongly modulated by prior or simultaneous exposure to other cytokines. For example, PDGF induces expression of TGF-β in cultured rat macrophages (96).

Many aspects of TGF-β biology indicate it to be a potently anti-inflammatory cytokine capable of down-regulating lymphocyte functions. A TGF-β1 deficient mouse strain recently has been developed in which inflammatory responses result in strikingly rapid mortality with particular involvement of heart and lung (97). The excess TGF-β present is detected easily by immunohistochemistry in models of inflammation, and remodeling process such as that induced by experimental bleomycin administration (98). Abundant quantities of TGF-β are present, with peak levels 7 days following bleomycin instillation. TGF-β1 could be detected in airway epithelial cells and subadjacent matrix elements. Macrophages stain intensely simultaneously with the peak tissue levels of extractable TGF-β (3 to 10 days).

Several studies have demonstrated the co-localization of expression of matrix genes and TGF-β in remodeling tissues in humans and animal models. In a study focusing on advanced remodeling associated with spontaneous pulmonary fibrosis, Khalil et al. (99) confirmed in human subjects that airway epithelial cells are a major source of TGF-β. At a different anatomic level, the sites of production of TGF-β1 mRNA in lung biopsy samples of patients with pulmonary fibrosis have been delineated by in situ hybridization (100). In biopsies from cases of chronic pulmonary fibrosis, TGF-β1 mRNA localizes to areas of the most intense macrophage aggregation. These areas are also rich in mRNA for fibronectin but not type I procollagen. Attempts to detect cytokine protein using immunohistochemical techniques failed to demonstrate commensurate increases in stainable TGF-β1 protein in macrophage aggregates. Areas such as alveolar buds populated predominantly by fibroblasts are relatively devoid of TGF-β mRNA, but contain mRNAs for procollagen I and fibronectin in abundance. Such fibroblast rich areas also stain positively for TGF-β protein. In this study, only the TGF-β1 isotype was studied. It is quite possible that other isotypes are importantly involved in the process, as has been demonstrated in other disorders such as systemic sclerosis (101).

Kulozik et al. (101) have shown by in situ hybridization that there is co-localization of TGF-β2 mRNA and procollagen α1(I) expression around dermal blood vessels in patients with the inflammatory stage of systemic sclerosis. There is no expression of either gene in the dermis of patients with the fibrotic stage of the same disorder or in other control patients. Thus, TGF-β2, but not TGF-β1 appears to play a role in this process in skin.

Recent evidence suggests that major inter-individual differences in growth factor responsiveness occur, possibly on a genetic basis. This evidence derives from a novel study of women at risk for development of either hepatic veno-occlusive disease or idiopathic interstitial pneumonitis after bone marrow transplantation, the latter provided as therapy for advanced breast cancer (103). Baseline plasma TGF-β concentrations measured even before transplantation could be used to predict the likelihood of developing fibrotic complications after bone marrow transplantation. Pre-transplantation TGF-β levels were significantly greater in patients in whom hepatic disease or pneumonitis developed, than in the controls or the patients without these conditions. One interpretation of these data is that human populations vary in terms of their risk of developing fibrotic disorders. Those with high endogenous TGF-β levels are at particular risk at times when events such as transplantation are undertaken.

Whether patients with a predisposition to fibrotic complications are more likely to develop bronchial wall remodeling when afflicted by inflammatory airways diseases has not been studied.

TGF-β is a key differentiation factor during development of airway epithelium (103). However, few investigations of a potential role of TGF-β in airway remodeling in obstructive lung diseases are available. Aubert et al. (104) contrasted TGF-β expression in lungs from asthmatic patients, patients with chronic obstructive pulmonary disease, and nonobstructed cigarette smokers (104). TGF-β1 expression was probed by Northern blot analysis using a cDNA probe for TGF-β1 and by immunohistochemical analyses using antibodies specific for the intracellular and extracellular forms of TGF-β1. TGF-β1 mRNA was seen in all samples and there were no differences between the three groups. TGF-β1 precursor protein was immunolocalized throughout the airway wall, including the epithelium and in alveolar macrophages. Mature TGF-β1 was seen primarily within the connective tissue of the airway wall. These patterns of expression of both precursor and mature forms of TGF-β1 were alike in lungs from asthmatic patients, those with COPD, and control subjects. Thus, while TGF-β mRNA and protein are abundantly expressed in human lungs, there are no clear differences in expression between the airways of asthmatic subjects and those of smokers with and without COPD. The authors of this report have pointed out that the lack of differences in amounts of detectable TGF-β1 does not exclude a potential role for this fibrogenic growth factor in airway remodeling. More than most other growth factors, TGF-β undergoes post-translational intra- and extra-cellular modifications before it becomes active. It is quite possible that the activating enzymes involved in these steps are more active in peri-bronchial areas of the asthmatic lung, allowing for greater activity of the normally abundant amounts of TGF-β in these zones.

TRANSFORMING GROWTH FACTOR-β RECEPTORS

TGF-β signal transduction is mediated through two receptor subunits, type I (also known as ALK-5) and type II TGF-β receptors; although several other TGF-β binding proteins can be found on cell surfaces. The type I receptor has been found to have multiple subtypes, a feature not shared by the single type II receptor protein (105, 106). Other cell surface TGF-β binding moieties, such as the low affinity binding betaglycan originally termed the "type III receptor" do not appear to transduce biological signals directly. TGF-β cannot engage its active heteromeric protein kinase receptor alone. This limitation is overcome by the action of betaglycan which presents TGF-β to the kinase subunit of the signalling receptor, thereby forming a high affinity ternary complex (107).

The type I receptor mediates responsiveness of human fibroblasts to TGF-β (108). Activation by TGF-β requires the participation of both subunit receptors, both with serine-threonine kinase domains critical for function (46,109,110). The two receptor subunits dimerize into an active signalling complex on the cell membrane in response to ligand. However, at this time, little positive information is available about the signalling pathways through which the TGF-β receptors signal the nucleus. Although TGF-β receptors are nearly ubiquitous on cultured cells, their amount and activity are subject to regulation (111).

TRANSFORMING GROWTH FACTOR-β MODULATION OF OTHER GROWTH FACTORS

As indicated earlier, TGF-β auto-induces its own expression and also induces the potent smooth muscle cell mitogen CTGF. A number of the other protean actions of TGF-β appear to be mediated indirectly through induction of secondary cytokines. TGF-β has the potential to modulate the expression of multiple growth factors. TGF-β treatment of quiescent cultures of several cell lines results in the induction of vascular endothelial growth factor (VEGF) mRNA and protein (112). VEGF induction occurs regardless of whether TGF-β stimulates or inhibits the growth of the target cell line. In this study, exposure of endothelial cells to TGF-β did not induce VEGF. Because VEGF is known to be a potent angiogenic factor for endothelial cells, these results suggest that the angiogenic effect of TGF-β on endothelial cells may be mediated, in part, through the paracrine induction of VEGF in other surrounding cells. TGF-β1 and also glucocorticoids down-regulate HGF gene expression (113).

The endothelins are low molecular weight peptides, which are the most potent known constrictors of smooth muscle (See Chapter 60). Endothelins also are known to be potent smooth muscle cell mitogens. Recent studies indicate that endothelin release is under the control of TGF-β but not other cytokines (114). TGF-β was found to be a potent stimulator of endothelin secretion in bovine endothelial cells from large, medium, and small vessels. Of various cytokines tested, TGF-β is unique in inducing endothelins; TNF-α and IFN-τ have only minor effects on endothelin production by large vessel endothelial cells and none from retinal microvessels. IL-1β, IL-6, and IL-8 do not affect endothelin secretion at all. Further, TGF-β appears to be the major component in serum capable of inducing endothelin gene expression and may play a role as a physiological regulator of endothelin production by vascular endothelial cells (115). Despite the limited repertoire of cytokines capable of inducing endothelin secretion, it appears that endothelial cells contain stores of endothelin that can be released rapidly by mechanical stimuli such as cell stretching (116).

Growth Factors and Airway Infections

Bacteria and viruses have been implicated in airway reactivity and remodeling (See Chapter 89 and ref. 117). Growth factor production by lung cells recently has been shown to be capable of modulation by infectious agents. Human lung fibroblasts cultivated from biopsy specimens were assayed for production of IL-6 and granulocyte-macrophage colony stimulating factor (GM-CSF) (118). Fibroblasts used for this study were isolated from lung allografts, as well as from recipient lungs obtained at time of transplant and from normal lung tissue removed during tumor resection. Several early passage fibroblast lines from transplant recipients were observed to contain mycoplasma-like organisms. Concentrations of secreted IL-6 and GM-GSF were increased 50-fold in infected fibroblast lines, as compared to control (uninfected) cells. Use of antibiotics to remove mycoplasma from infected cultures reduced the production of these cytokines. The authors concluded that other growth factors are likely to be similarly modulated by infectious agents. Whether such upregulation of cytokines occurs *in situ* in episodes of infection in asthmatics has not been examined.

REFERENCES

1. Kelley J. Collagen. In: Massaro D, ed. *Lung cells biology*. New York: Marcel Dekker Inc, 1989;821–866.
2. Roche WR, Beasley R, Williams JH, Holgate ST. Subepithelial fibrosis in the bronchi of asthmatics. *Lancet* 1989;I:520–524.
3. Lambert RK, Wiggs BR, Kuwano K, Hogg JC, Pare PD. Functional significance of increased airway smooth muscle in asthma and COPD. *J Appl Physiol* 1993;74:2771–2781.
4. Jetten AM. Growth and differentiation factors in tracheobronchial epithelium. *Am J Physiol* 1991;260:L361–373.
5. Kohase M, May LT, Tamm I, Vilcek J, Sehgal PB. A cytokine network in human diploid fibroblasts: interactions of β-interferons, tumor necrosis factor, platelet derived growth factor, and interleukin-1. *Molec Cell Biol* 1987;7:273-280.
6. Kelley J. State of the art: cytokines of the lung. *Amer Rev Respir Dis* 1990;141:765–788.
7. Raines EW, Bowen-Pope DF, Ross R. Platelet-derived growth factor. In Peptide Growth Factors and their Receptors. In: Sporn MB, Roberts AB, eds. *Handbook of experimental pharmacology*. Vol.95. Heidelberg: Springer-Verlag, 1990;173–262.
8. Pledger WJ, Stiles CD, Antoniades HN, Scher D. An ordered sequence of events is required before BALB/c-3T3 cells become committed to DNA synthesis. *Proc Natl Acad Sci U S A* 1977;74:4481–4490.
9. Shimokado K, Raines EW, Madtes DK, Barrett TB, Benditt EP, Ross R. A significant part of macrophage-derived growth factor consists of at least two forms of PDGF. *Cell* 1985;43:277–286.
10. Doolittle RF, Hunkapiller MW, Hood LE, Devare SG, Robbins KC, Aaronson SA, Antoniades HN. Simian sarcoma virus onc gene, v-*sis*, is derived from the gene (or genes) encoding a platelet-derived growth factor. *Science* 1983;221:275–277.
11. Johnsson A, Heldin C-H, Wasteson A, Westermark B, Deuel TF, Huang JS et al. The c-*sis* gene encodes a precursor of the B-chain of platelet-derived growth factor. *EMBO J* 1984;3:921–928.
12. Hart CE, Forstrom JW, Kelly JD, Seifert RA, Smith RA, Ross R, et al. Two classes of PDGF receptor recognize different isoforms of PDGF. *Science* 1988; 240:1529–1531.
13. Gronwald RGK, Grant FJ, Haldeman BA, Hart CE, O'Hara PJ, Hage FS et al. Cloning and expression of a cDNA coding for the human platelet-derived growth factor receptor: evidence for more than onereceptor class. *Proc Natl Acad Sci U S A* 1988;85:3435–3439.

14. Claesson-Welsh L, Hammacher A, Westermark B, Heldin C-H, Nister M. Identification and structural analysis of the A type receptor for platelet-derived growth factor. *J Biol Chem* 1989;264:1742–1747.

15. Claesson-Welsh L, Eriksson A, Westermark B, Heldin C-H. CDNA cloning and expression of the human A type PDGF receptor establishes similarity to the B type receptor. *Proc Natl Acad Sci USA* 1989; 86:4917–4921.

16. Swan DC, McBride DW, Robbins KC, Keithley DA, Reddy EP, Aaronson SA. Chromosomal mapping of the simian sarcoma virus onc gene analog in human cells. *Proc Natl Acad Sci USA* 1982;79: 4691–4695.

17. Grotendorst GR, Martin GR, Pencev D, Sodek J, Harvey AK. Stimulation of granulation tissue formation by platelet-derived growth factor in normal and diabetic rats. *J Clin Invest* 1985;76:2323–2329.

18. Deuel TF, Senior RM, Huang JS, Griffin GL. Chemotaxis ofmonocyes and neutrophils to platelet-derived growth factor. *J Clin Invest* 1982;69:1046–1049.

19. Clark RAF, Folkvord JM, Hart CE, Murray MJ, McPherson JM. Platelet isoforms of platelet-derived growth factor stimulate fibroblasts to contract collagen matrices. *J Clin Invest* 1989;84:1036–1040.

20. Daynes RA, Dowell T, Araneo BA. Platelet-derived growth factor is a potent biologic response modifier of T cells. *J Exp Med* 1991;174: 1323–1333.

21. Paulsson Y, Austgulen R, Hofsli E, Heldin C-H, Westermark B, Nissen-Meyer J. Tumor necrosis factor-induced expression of platelet-derived growth factor A-chain messenger RNA in fibroblasts. *Exp Cell Res* 1989;180:490–496.

22. Raines EW, Dower SK, Ross R. Interleukin-1 mitogenic activity for fibroblasts and smooth muscle cells is due to PDGF-AA. *Science* 1989;243:393–396.

23. Shepherd VL. Cytokine receptors of the lung. *Amer J Resipir Cell Molec Biol* 1991;5:403–410.

24. Keating MT, Williams LT. Autocrine stimulation of intracellular PDGF receptors in v-*sis*-transformed cells. *Science* 1988;239:914–916.

25. Bejcek BE, Li DI, Deuel T. Transformation by v-*sis* occurs by an internal autoactivation mechanism. *Science* 1989;245:1496–1499.

26. Zachary I, Rozengurt E. Modulation of epidermal growth factor receptor by mitotic ligands: effects of bombesin and the role of protein kinase C. *Cancer Surv* 1985;4:729–765.

27. Seifert RA, Hart CE, Phillips PE, Forstrom JW, Ross R, Murray MJ, Bowen-Pope DF. Two different subunits associate to create isoform-specific platelet-derived growth factor receptors. *J Biol Chem* 1989; 264:8771–8778.

28. Kelly JD, Haldeman BA, Grant FJ, Murray MJ, Seifert RA, Bowen-Pope DF, et al. Platelet-derived growth factor (PDGF) stimulates PDGF receptor subunit dimerization and intersubunit transphosphorylation. *J Biol Chem* 1991;266:8987–8992.

29. Williams LT. Signal transduction by the platelet-derived growth factor receptor. *Science* 1989;243:1564–1570.

30. Nishimura R, Li W, Kashishian A, et al. Two signaling molecules share a phosphotyrosine-containing binding site in the platelet-derived growth factor receptor. *Mol Cell Biol* 1993;13:6889–6896.

31. Ferns GA, Sprugel KH, Seifert RA, et al. Relative platelet-derived growth factor receptor subunit expression determines cell migration to different dimeric forms of PDGF. *Growth Factors* 1990;3:315–324.

32. LaRochelle WJ, Giese N, May-Siroff M, Robbins KC, Aaronson SA. Molecular localization of the transforming and secretary properties of PDGF A and PDGF B. *Science.* 1990;248:1541–1544.

33. Gronwald RGK, Seifert RA, Bowen-Pope DF. Differential regulation of expression of two platelet-derived growth factor receptors by transforming growth factor-β. *J Biol Chem* 1989;264:8120–8125.

34. Seifert RA, van Koppen A, Bowen-Pope DF. PDGF-AB requires PDGF receptor α-subunits for high-affinity, but not for low-affinity, binding and signal transduction. *J Biol Chem* 1993;268:4473–4480.

35. Sariban E, Sitaras NM, Antoniades HN, Kufe DW, Pantazis P. Expression of platelet-derived growth factor (PDGF)-related transcripts and synthesis of biologically active PDGF-like proteins by human malignant epithelial cell lines. *J Clin Invest* 1988;92:1157–1164.

36. Antoniades HN, Bravo MA, Avila RE, et al. Platelet-derived growth factor in idiopathic pulmonary fibrosis. *J Clin Invest* 1990;86:1055–1064.

37. Pencev D, Grotendorst GR. Human peripheral blood monocytes secrete a unique form of PDGF. *Oncogene Res* 1988;3:333–342.

38. Matsuoka J, Grotendorst GR. Two peptides related to platelet-derived growth factor are present in human wound fluid. *Proc Natl Acad Sci U S A* 1989;86:4416–4420.

39. Snyder LS, Hertz MI, Peterson MS, Harmon KR, Marinelli WA, Henke CA et al. Acute lung injury. Pathogenesis of intraalveolar fibrosis. *J Clin Invest* 1991;88:663–673.

40. Bradham DM, Igarashi A, Potter RL, Grotendorst GR. Connective tissue growth factor: a cysteine-rich mitogen secreted by human vascular endothelial cells is related to the SRC-induced immediate early gene product CEF-10. *J Cell Biol* 1991;114:1285–1294.

41. Soma Y, Grotendorst GR. TGF-S stimulates primary human skin fibroblast DNA synthesis via an autocrine production of PDGF-related peptides. *J Cell Physiol* 1989;140:246–253.

42. Walsh J, Absher M, Kelley J. Variable expression of plateletderived growth factor (PDGF) family proteins in acute lung injury. *Am J Respir Cell Molec Biol* 1993;9:637–644.

43. Han RNN, Buch S, Freeman BA, Post M, Tanswell AK. Platelet-derived growth factor and growth-related genes in rat lung. II. Effect of exposure to 859S 02. *Am J Physiol* 1992;262:L140–146.

44. Fabisiak JP, Evans JN, Kelley J. Increased expression of PDGF-B (c-*sis*) MRNA in rat lung precedes DNA synthesis and tissue repair during chronic hyperoxia. *Am J Respir Cell Molec Biol* 1989;1:181–189.

45. Shaw RJ, Kelley J. Monocyte-Macrophages. In: Phan SH, Thrall RS, eds. *Pulmonary fibrosis*. New York: Marcel Dekker Inc, 1994;405–444.

46. Rappolee DA, Mark D, Banda MJ, Werb Z. Wound macrophages express TGF-α and other growth factors *in vivo*: analysis by MRNA typing. *Science* 1988;241:708–712.

47. Martinet Y, Bitterman PB, Mornex J-F, Grotendorst GR, Crystal RM. Activated human monocytes express the c-*sis* protooncogene and release a mediator showing PDGF-like activity. *Nature* 1986;319:158–160.

48. Pantazis P, Lanfrancone L, Pelicci PG, Dalla-Favera R, Antoniades HN. Human leukemia cells synthesize and secrete proteins related to platelet-derived growth factor. *Proc Natl Acad Sci U S A* 1986;83: 5526–5530.

49. Mornex J, Martinet Y, Yamauchi K, et al. Spontaneous expression of the cis-gene and release of platelet-derived growth factorlike molecule by human alveolar macrophages. *J Clin Invest* 1986;78:61–66.

50. Shaw RJ, Doherty DE, Ritter AG, Benedict SH, Clark AF. Adherence-dependent increase in human monocyte PDGF(B) MRNA is associated with increases in c-*fos*, c-*jun*, and EGR2 MRNA. *J Cell Biol* 1990;111:2139–2148.

51. Beckmann MP, Betsholtz C, Heldin C-H, et al. Comparison of biological properties and transforming potential of human PDGF-A and PDGF-B chains. *Science* 1988;241:1346–1349.

52. Nister M, Hammacher A, Mellstrom K, et al. A glioma-derived PDGF A chain homodimer has different functional activities from a PDGF AB heterodimer purified from human platelets. *Cell* 1988;52:791–799.

53. Shaw RJ, Benedict SH, Clark RA, King TE, Jr. Pathogenesis of pulmonary fibrosis in interstitial lung disease. Alveolar macrophage PDGF(B) gene activation and upregulation by interferon-gamma. *Am Rev Respir Dis* 1991;143:167–173.

54. Nagaoka I, Trapnell BC, Crystal RG. Upregulation of platelet-derived growth factor-A and -B gene expression in alveolar macrophages of individuals with idiopathic pulmonary fibrosis. *J Clin Invest* 1990;85: 2023–2027.

55. Martinet Y, Rom WN, Grotendorst GR, Martin GR, Crystal RG. Exaggerated spontaneous release of platelet-derived growth factor by alveolar macrophages from patients with idiopathic pulmonary fibrosis. *N Enql J Med* 1987;317:202–209.

56. Vignaud J-M, Allam M, Martinet N, Pech M, Plenat F, Martinet Y.Presence of platelet-derived growth factor in normal and fibrotic lung is specifically associated with interstitial macrophages, while both interstitial macrophages and alveolar epithelial cells express the c-*sis* oncogene. *Am J Respir Cell Mol Biol* 1991;5:531–538.

57. Kay AB. Origin of type 2 helper T cells. *N Encrl J Med* 1994;330: 567–569.

58. Robinson BW, Rose AH. Pulmonary gamma interferon production in patients with fibrosing alveolitis. *Thorax* 1990;45:105–108.

59. Kovacs EJ, Kelley J. Lymphokine regulation of macrophagederived growth factor secretion following pulmonary injury. *Am J Pathol* 1985;121:261–268.

60. Aubert JD, Hayashi S, Hards J, Bai TR, Pare PD, Hogg JC. Platelet-

derived growth factor and its receptor in lungs from patients with asthma and chronic airflow obstruction. *Am J Physiol* 1994;266: L655–663.

61. Fabisiak JP, Absher M, Evans JN, Kelley J. Spontaneous production of PDGF A-chain homodimer by rat lung fibroblasts *in vitro*. *Am J Physiol* 1992;263:L185–l93.

62. Gospodarowicz D, Ferrara N, Schweigerer L, Neufeld G. Structural characterization and biological functions of fibroblast growth factor. *Endocrin Rev* 1987;8:95–114.

63. Rifkin DB, Moscatelli D. Recent developments in the cell biology of basic fibroblast growth factor. *J Cell Biol* 1989;109:1–6.

64. Abraham JA, Whang JL, Tumolo A, Mergia A, Fiddes JC. Human basic fibroblast growth factor: nucleotide sequence, genomic organization, and expression in mammalian cells. *Cold Spring Harb Symp Quant Biol* 1986;51 Pt 1:657–668.

65. Baird A, Ling N. Fibroblast growth factors are present in the extracellular matrix produced by endothelial cells *in vitro*: implications for a role of heparinase-like enzymes in the neovascularization response. *Biochem Biophys Res Comm* 1987; 142:428–35.

66. Saksela 0, Moscatelli D, Sommer A, Rifkin DB. Endothelial cell-derived heparan sulfate binds basic fibroblast growth factor and protects it from proteolytic degradation. *J Cell Biol* 1988; 107:743–51.

67. Sannes PL, Burch KK, Khosla J. Immunohistochemical localization of epidermal growth factor and acidic and basic fibroblast growth factors in postnatal developing and adult rat lungs. *Am J Respir Cell Mol Biol* 1992;7:230–237.

68. Sotozono C, Kinoshita S, Kita M, Imanishi J. Paracrine role of keratinocyte growth factor in rabbit corneal epithelial cell growth. *Exp Eye Res* 1994;59:385–391.

69. Tsuboi R, Sato C, Kurita Y, Ron D, Rubin JS, Ogawa H. Keratinocyte growth factor (FGF-7) stimulates migration and plasminogen activator activity of normal human keratinocytes. *J Invest Dermatol* 1993; 101:49–53.

70. Werner S, Smola H, Liao X, et al. The function of KGF in morphogenesis of epithelium and reepithelialization of wounds. *Science* 1994;266:819–822.

71. Yaeger PC, Stiles CD, Rollins BJ. Human keratinocyte growth promoting activity on the surface of fibroblasts. *J Cell Physiol* 1991;149: 110–116.

72. Monacci WT, Merrill Mi, Oldfield EH. Expression of vascular permeability factor/vascular endothelial growth factor in normal rat tissues. *Am J Physiol* 1993;264:C995–1002.

73. Shweiki D, Itin A, Soffer D, Keshet E. Vascular endothelial growth factor induced by hypoxia may mediate hypoxia-initiated angiogenesis. *Nature* 1992;359:843–845.

74. Kourembanas S, Bernfield M. Hypoxia and endothelial-smooth muscle cell interactions in the lung. *Am J Respir Cell Mol Biol* 1994;11: 373–374.

75. Chan A, Rubin J, Bottaro D, Hirschfield D, Chedid M, Aaronson SA. Isoforms of human HGF and their biological activities. *EXS* 1993;65: 67–79.

76. Higashio K, Shima N. Tumor cytotoxic activity of HGF-SF. *EXS* 1993;65:351–368.

77. Kitamura N, Miyazawa K, Uehara Y, et al. Gene expression and regulation of HGF-SF. *EXS* 1993;65:49–65.

78. Matsumoto K, Tajima H, Okazaki H, Nakamura T. Negative regulation of hepatocyte growth factor gene expression in human lung fibroblasts and leukemic cells by transforming growth factors-β1 and glucocorticoids. *J Biol Chem* 1992;267:24917–24920.

79. Panos RJ, Rubin JS, Csaky KG, Aaronson SA, Mason RJ. Keratinocyte growth factor and hepatocyte growth factor/scatter factor are heparin-binding growth factors for alveolar type I cells in fibroblast-conditioned medium. *J Clin Invest* 1993;92:969–977.

80. Kelley J. Transforming growth factor-β. In: Kelley J, ed. *Cytokines of the lung.* New York:Marcel Dekker Inc, 1992;101–137.

81. Border WA, Ruoslahti E. Transforming growth factor-β in disease: the dark side of tissue repair. *J Clin Invest* 1992;90:1–7.

82. McCartney-Francis NL, Wahl SM. Transforming growth factor-β: a matter of life and death. *Leukocyte Biol* 1994;55:401–409.

83. Battegay EJ, Raines EW, Seifert RA, Bowen-Pope DF, Ross R. TGF-β induces bimodal proliferation of connective tissue cells via complex control of an autocrine PDGF loop. *Cell* 1990;63:51S524.

84. Rossi R, Karsenty G, Roberts AB, Roche NS, Sporn MB, de Crombrugghe B. A nuclear 1 binding site mediates the transcriptional activation of a type I collagen promoter by transforming growth factor-β. *Cell* 1988;52:405–414.

85. Border WA, Noble NA, Yamamoto T, et al. Natural inhibitor of transforming growth factors protects against scarring in experimental kidney disease. *Nature* 1992;360:361–364.

86. Kelley J, Shull S, Walsh JJ, Cutroneo KR, Absher M. Autoinduction of transforming growth factor-β (TGF-β) in human lung fibroblasts. *Am J Respir Cell Molec Biol* 1993;8:417–424.

87. Kim SJ, Angel P, Lafyatis R, et al. Autoinduction of transforming growth factor-β1 is mediated by the AP-1 complex. *Molec Cell Biol* 1990;10:1492–1497.

88. Shah M, Foreman DM, Ferguson MWJ. Control of scarring in adult wounds by neutralising antibody to transforming growth factor-β. *Lancet* 1992;339:213–214.

89. Assoian RK, Fleurdelys BE, Stevenson HC, et al. Expression and secretion of type β transforming growth factor by activated human macrophages. *Proc Natl Acad Sci U S A* 1987;84:6020–6024.

90. Pennington DW, Lopez AR, Thomas PS, Peck C, Gold WM. Dog mastocytoma cells produce transforming growth factors-β1. *J Clin Invest* 1992;90:35–41.

91. Phan SH, Gharaee-Kermani M, Wolber F, Ryan US. Stimulation of rat endothelial cell transforming growth factor-β production by bleomycin. *J Clin Invest* 1991;87:148–154.

92. Grotendorst GR, Smale G, Pencev D. Production of transforming growth factor-β by human peripheral blood monocytes and neutrophils. *J Cell Physiol* 1989;140:396–402.

93. Kelley J, Fabisiak JP, Hawes K, Absher M. Cytokine signalling in lung: transforming growth factor-β secretion by lung fibroblasts. *Am J Physiol* 1991;260:L123–128.

94. Pelton RW, Johnson MD, Perkett EA, Gold LI, and Moses HL. Expression of transforming growth factor-β1, -β2, and -β3 MRNA and protein in the murine lung. *Am J Respir Cell Mol Biol* 1991;5:522–530.

95. Grotendorst GR, Smale G, Pencev D. Production of transforming growth factor-β by human peripheral blood monocytes and neutrophils. *J Cell Physiol* 1989;140:396–402.

96. Pierce GF, Mustoe TA, Lingelbach J, et al. Platelet-derived growth factor and transforming growth factor-β enhance tissue repair activities by unique mechanisms. *J Biol Chem* 1989;109:429–440.

97. Kulkarni AB, Huh CG, Becker D, Geiser A, Lyght M, Flanders KC, et al. Transforming growth factor-β1 null mutation in mice causes excessive inflammatory response and early death. *Proc Natl Acad Sci U S A* 1993;90:770–774.

98. Khalil N, Bereznay O, Sporn M, Greenberg AH. Macrophage production of transforming growth factor-β and fibroblast collagen synthesis in chronic pulmonary fibrosis. *J Exp Med* 1989;170:727–737.

99. Khalil N, O'Connor RN, Unruh HW, et al. Increased production and immunohistochemical localization of transforming growth factor-β in idiopathic pulmonary fibrosis. *Am J Respir Cell Mol Biol* 1991;5: 155–162.

100. Broekelmann TJ, Limper A.H, Colby TV, McDonald JA. Transforming growth factor-β, is present at sites of extracellular matrix gene expression in human pulmonary fibrosis. *Proc Natl Acad Sci USA* 1991; 88:6642–6646.

101. Kulozik M, Hogg A, Lankat-Buttgereit 3, and Krieg T. Colocalization of transforming growth factor-β2 with -α1 (I) procollagen MRNA in tissue sections of patients with systemic sclerosis. *J Clin Invest* 1990; 86:917–922.

102. Anscher MS, Peters WP, Reisenbichler H, Petros WP, Jirtle RL. Transforming growth factor-β as a predictor of liver and lung fibrosis after autologous bone marrow transplantation for advanced breast cancer. *N Engl J Med* 1993;328:1592–1598.

103. Masui T, Wakefield LM, Lechner JF, LaVeck MA, and Sporn MB. Type β transforming growth factor is the primary differentiationinducing serum factor for normal human bronchial epithelial cells. *Proc Natl Acad Sci U S A* 1986;83:2438–2442.

104. Aubert JD, Dalal BI, Bai TR, Roberts CR, Hayashi S, Hogg JC. Transforming growth factor-β1 gene expression in human airways. *Thorax* 1994;49:225–232.

105. Franzen P, ten Dijke P, Ichijo H, Yamashita H, Schulz P, Heldin CH, et al. Cloning of a TGF-β type I receptor that forms a heteromeric complex with the TGF-β type II receptor. *Cell* 1993;75:681–692.

106. Attisano L, Carcamo J, Ventura F, Weis FM, Massague J, Wrana JL. Identification of human activin and TGF-β type I receptors that form

heteromeric kinase complexes with type II receptors. *Cell* 1993;75: 671–680.

107. Lopez-Casillas F, Wrana JL, Massague J. Betaglycan presents ligand to the TGF-β signaling receptor. *Cell* 1993;73:1435–1444.

108. ten Dijke P, Yamashita H, Ichijo H, Franzen P, Laiho M, Miyazono K, et al. Characterization of type I receptors for transforming factor-β and activin. *Science* 1994;264:101–104.

109. Lin HY, Moustakas A, Knaus P, Wells RG, Henis YI, Lodish HF. The soluble exoplasmic domain of the type II transforming growth factor (TGF)-β receptor. A heterogeneously glycosylated protein with high affinity and selectivity for TGF-β ligands. *J Biol Chem* 1995;270: 2747–2754.

110. Ebner R, Chen RH, Lawler S, Zioncheck T, Derynck R. Determination of type I receptor specificity by the type II receptors for TGF-β or activin. *Science* 1993;262:900–902.

111. Fine A, Panchenko MP, Smith BD, Yu Q, and Goldstein RH. Discordant regulation of transforming growth factor-β receptors by prostaglandin E₂. *Biochim Biophys Acta* 1995;1261:19–24.

112. Pertovaara L, Kaipainen A, Mustonen T, Orpana A, Ferrara N, Saksela O, Alitalo K. Vascular endothelial growth factor is induced in response to transforming growth factor-β in fibroblastic and epithelial cells. *J Biol Chem* 1994;269:6271–6274.

113. Matsumoto K, Tajima H, Okazaki H, Nakamura T. Negative regulation of hepatocyte growth factor gene expression in human lung fibroblasts and leukemic cells by transforming growth factor-β 1 and glucocorticoids. *J Biol Chem* 1992;267:24917–24920.

114. Kanse SM, Takahashi K, Lam HC, Rees A, Warren JB, Porta M et al. Cytokine stimulated endothelin release from endothelial cells. *Life Sci* 1991;48:1379–1384.

115. Brown MR, Vaughan J, Jimenez LL, Vale W, Baird A. Transforming growth factor-β: role in mediating serum-induced endothelin production by vascular endothelial cells. *Endocrinology* 1991;129:2355–2360.

116. Macarthur H, Warner TD, Wood EG, Corder R, Vane JR. Endothelin-1 release from endothelial cells in culture is elevated both acutely and chronically by short periods of mechanical stretch. *Biochem Biophys Res Commun* 1994;200:395–400.

117. Bardin PG, Johnston SL, Pattemore PK. Viruses as precipitants of asthma symptoms. II. Physiology and mechanisms. *Clin Exp Allergy* 1992;22:809–822.

118. Fabisiak JP, Weiss RD, Powell GA, Dauber JH. Enhanced secretion of immune-modulating cytokines by human lung fibroblasts during *in vitro* infection with *Mycoplasma fermentans*. *Am J Respir Cell Mol Biol* 1993;8:358–364.

Asthma, edited by P.J. Barnes, M.M. Grunstein,
A.R. Leff, and A.J. Woolcock.
Lippincott–Raven Publishers, Philadelphia © 1997.

■ 53 ■

Nitric Oxide

Richard A. Robbins

Because of its capacity to relax vascular smooth muscle, there has been great interest in the physiological and pathophysiological effects of nitric oxide (NO). Recent investigations now have implicated NO in a large number of physiological and pathophysiological processes (1,2). Suggested roles for NO include regulation of smooth muscle tone, neurotransmission, host defense, and cytotoxicity, which have all either been demonstrated or proposed to be disordered in asthma. This chapter reviews the recent advances in the understanding of NO, emphasizing those most potentially relevant to asthma.

The endothelial-dependent relaxation of blood vessels has been recognized for a number of years (3). However, the identity of this endothelial-derived relaxing factor (EDRF) remained baffling because of its exceedingly short half-life; that is, until two groups independently reported that EDRF was analogous to NO (4,5). Simultaneously, two groups investigating the mechanisms of murine macrophage-induced cytotoxicity attributed this activity to NO (6,7). Together, these initial investigations laid the foundation on which many of the more recent advances have occurred.

FORMATION OF NITRIC OXIDE

NO is formed when the guanido group of the essential amino acid L-arginine is cleaved, producing NO and L-citrulline (1,2) (Fig. 1). The reaction is catalyzed by a group of enzymes called nitric oxide synthase (NOS) and several co-factors. The reaction is stereospecific, meaning that only L-arginine, but not D-arginine, is cleaved by NOS forming L-citrulline.

Although arginine transport into the cell is probably necessary for continued NO production, NOS activity appears to be the major rate-limiting step of NO formation (2). NOS exists in several forms, which accounts for much of the variation in NOS activity (8). In the vasculature, a constitutive NOS (cNOS) exists, which is a calcium-dependent enzyme (9,10). The enzyme migrates as a monomer of 135 kD gel electrophoresis and has a high degree of homology with cytochrome P-450 reductase (11,12). cNOS accounts for the baseline production of the small, picomolar amounts of NO from endothelial cells, but also has been identified in a variety of nonendothelial cells and may account for the baseline production of NO by these cells (13–22).

Brain NOS (bNOS, also called neural NOS or nNOS) is another constitutively expressed NOS and is similar in many aspects to cNOS; bNOS is found predominantly in neural tissue (8,23). Both cNOS and bNOS are calcium-dependent and produce picomolar amounts of NO. The

R. A. Robbins: Departments of Medicine and Physiology, Louisiana State University Medical Center; and Overton Brooks Veterans Affairs Medical Center, Shreveport, Louisiana 71101.

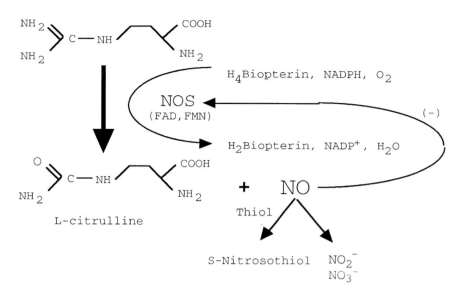

L-arginine

L-citrulline

H₄Biopterin, NADPH, O₂

NOS (FAD,FMN)

H₂Biopterin, NADP⁺, H₂O

(-)

+ NO

Thiol

S-Nitrosothiol   NO₂⁻ NO₃⁻

FIG. 1. Diagrammatic representation of the L-arginine-nitric oxide pathway. The guanido group of L-arginine is cleaved generating nitric oxide (NO) and L-citrulline. The reaction is catalyzed by nitric oxide synthase (NOS) and several cofactors, including nicotinamide adenine dinucleotide phosphate (NADPH), tetrahydrobiopterin (H4 biopterin), and the flavones (FAD, FMN). NO can inhibit its production by inhibiting NOS. Although the half-life of NO in biologic systems is short, thiol formation with later release of NO may result in NO effects long after production.

similarity is not surprising since the proteins are approximately 60% homologous (8–11,23).

An inducible form of NOS (iNOS) has been detected in a variety of tissues and organs in addition to vascular endothelium (6,7,18,22,24–29). In contrast to cNOS or bNOS, iNOS is not expressed in most tissues but is induced by bacterial lipopolysaccharide (LPS) or cytokines such as tumor necrosis factor (TNF)-α, interleukin-1 (IL-1), and γ interferon (IFN-γ) (2,8). Although its mechanism of activation appears different, iNOS appears to be approximately 50% homologous with cNOS or bNOS (26,30,31). Induction of iNOS can result in the formation of much larger, nanomolar amounts of NO than the picomolar amount, which results from cNOS or bNOS (2).

Several co-factors are necessary for NOS activity, including flavones (FAD,FMN), tetrahydrobiopterin, and NADPH (2,8,32) (Fig.1). bNOS colocalizes with NADPH diaphorase, and it now appears that bNOS and NADPH diaphorase are, in fact, the same enzyme (33). This activity is useful in that nitroblue tetrazolium can be used to localize bNOS activity (34). Nitroblue tetrazolium does not appear to be specific for bNOS and can be used to localize NOS activity due to cNOS and, possibly, iNOS (22).

cNOS is a calcium-dependent enzyme and is activated by Ca⁺⁺ and/or calmodulin (2,8). Therefore, stimuli that increase intracellular calcium increase cNOS activity; this causes an increase in NOS activity within seconds (34). cNOS activity also may be regulated more slowly by increasing or decreasing synthesis of the enzyme. In the endothelium, sheer stress greater than 24 hours, increases cNOS, messenger ribonucleic acid (mRNA), and protein (36). Downregulation of cNOS to levels below baseline constitutive expression also may occur. Hypoxia down-

regulates cNOS in pulmonary endothelium presumably as a mechanism to shunt blood to better ventilated areas of the lungs (37–39). Interestingly, in contrast to iNOS (see following), TNF, or LPS actually decrease cNOS (36,41).

bNOS appears to be regulated similarly to cNOS, predominantly through Ca⁺⁺ and calmodulin (2,8,23); bNOS transfected into kidney 293 cells is phosphorylated and, consequently, inhibited by protein kinase C (42). However, both cNOS and bNOS have a cyclic AMP-dependent protein kinase phosphorylation site; but phosphorylation of bNOS by this kinase has no effect on catalytic activity (35). Therefore, the significance of such phosphorylation is unclear.

In contrast to cNOS and bNOS, iNOS was thought to be a calcium-independent enzyme; however, a recent study suggests that human iNOS may be partially calcium-dependent. The activity of hepatocyte iNOS cloned into human embryonic kidney cells, demonstrates a decrease in activity with calcium chelators suggesting a partial calcium dependence (26). The major regulator of iNOS activity appears to be transcriptional regulation of iNOS. Stimuli such as LPS or cytokines such as TNF, IL-1, and IFN-γ, increase iNOS mRNA, which correlates with iNOS protein expression and function (25,43,44). The observation that combinations of cytokines with or without LPS appear to be more potent in augmenting iNOS mRNA than individual cytokines or LPS alone, suggests that the transcriptional regulation of iNOS may be complex (25,43,44). *In vitro* it takes several hours to increase iNOS mRNA and, once induced, the RNA has a half-life of several hours (43). Corticosteroids, transforming growth factor-β (TGF-β), IL-10 monocyte chemotactic protein-1, IL-4, interleukin-8, and a cigarette smoke extract recently have been reported to inhibit cytokine- or LPS-induced increases in iNOS (43–56).

METABOLISM OF NITRIC OXIDE

NO is a highly reactive gas with an estimated half-life of seconds in biological tissues (57). NO reacts rapidly with O_2^- to form peroxynitrite ($OONO^-$) (58–60). Peroxynitrite, a strong oxidizing agent, spontaneously forms hydroxyl anions ($OH\cdot$) and nitrite (NO_2^-) through several intermediate reactions (60,61). The former facilitates lipid peroxidation, and, therefore, might be important in both host defense or tissue damage resulting from NO formation (58–62). Nitrite is stable for several hours in water and plasma, but is rapidly converted to nitrate in whole blood (2,63).

NO may react with a number of heme- and nonheme-containing metaloproteins (57,64,65). Binding of NO to the porphyrin ring of guanylyl cyclase results in activation of the enzyme, leading to formation of cyclic guanosine monophosphate (cGMP) (66). The increase in cGMP leads to relaxation of vascular smooth muscle accounting for the reduction in blood pressure induced by NO (2,66). In addition, NO can react with a number of other proteins including hemoglobin, myoglobin, cytochrome C, catalase, succinate dehydrogenase, lipoxygenase, ascorbate oxidase, ceruloplasmin, and tyrosinase, and in some instances, modify function of these proteins (67).

Sulfur-containing compounds may react with NO forming S-nitrosothiols (RS-NO) (57). This has been one proposed mechanism for attenuating the toxicity of NO and peroxynitrite (57,68). However, the formation of these compounds is a reversible reaction, and NO can be released from the nitrosothiol with a change in redox state, pH, or thiol content (69). Therefore, these reactions might be considered an NO repository and might be important in situations where NO might have an effect longer than a few seconds (70). The relevance of this concept in lung disorders such as asthma is suggested by the observation that a variety of nitrosothiols have been found in the lung under physiologic conditions, including S-nitroso-albumin, S-nitroso-glutathione, S-nitrosocysteine, and S-nitroso homocysteine (71–76).

Peroxynitrite formed from NO and superoxide can react with proteins by adding a nitro group (NO_2) to the ortho position of the hydroxyl group of tyrosine, forming 3-nitro-tyrosine (77–79). The formation of 3-nitro-tyrosine may have a biologic effect on the protein structure and function. For example, nitration of surfactant protein A by peroxynitrite has been associated with decreased function (80). Nitration of tyrosine also has been shown to inhibit cytochrome P450 and inactivate the immunoglobulin-binding portion of the first component of complement (C1q) (81,82). Tyrosine nitration has also been shown to inhibit protein phosphorylation, which may interfere with intracellular signal transduction (83). The occurrence of protein nitration in the lung has been demonstrated in lung sections of patients and animals with acute lung injury, implying that nitration and altered protein function might occur in other lung disorders (77).

NO can react with deoxyribonucleic acid (DNA) and through this mechanism, might be able to affect protein formation (84,85). *In vitro*, NO can deaminate deoxynucleosides, deoxynucleotides, and intact DNA (84). These reactions have been shown to result in the formation of C-τT transitions in bacteria, with resultant mutagenesis (84). Presumably, these same reactions could occur in humans. NO could also react with the primary amines of amino acids in proteins, resulting in alteration of protein structure and sequence (84).

The previous observations suggest that the oxidant chemistry of NO is extremely complex. These reactions suggest potential mechanisms that allow NO to alter the basic composition and/or structure of cellular lipids, proteins, and DNA. Thus, the potential for increased levels of NO altering lung cellular function in disorders such as asthma seems likely.

PHARMACOLOGY OF NITRIC OXIDE

Both synthetic and naturally occurring inhibitors of NOS have been described. Most inhibitors have substitutions at the guanido group of arginine and compete for the active site on NOS with arginine (2). As with arginine, only the L-forms are active (2). Asymmetric dimethylarginine and N^G-monomethyl-L-arginine (L-NMMA) are both inhibitors of NOS, and are present in plasma and urine (2,86). These compounds accumulate in renal failure and have been hypothesized to block the action of EDRF, thus causing hypertension (2,86).

A number of NOS inhibitors have been synthesized and are used to block the action of NOS in the laboratory. These not only include the naturally occurring L-NMMA, but also L-N^G-nitroarginine methyl ester (L-NAME), N^G-nitro-L-arginine (L-NOARG), N^G-iminoethyl-L-ornithine (L-NIO), L-N^G-nitroarginine-p-nitroanilide (L-NAPNA), L-canavanine, hydroxycobalamin, and aminoguanidine (87). In addition to inhibiting NOS, L-NMMA and L-NIO inhibit arginine transport into the cell, suggesting an additional mechanism for inhibition of NO production (88). Hydroxycobalamin appears to be a more selective inhibitor of endothelial cNOS than bNOS, and, conversely, L-NAPNA appears to be more selective for bNOS than endothelial cNOS (89,90). Aminoguanidine has been reported to have 10- to 100-fold greater inhibitory activity for iNOS than cNOS, proposing that it might have potential therapeutically in those situations when selective inhibition of iNOS is desirable (91).

Glucocorticoids inhibit iNOS induction, but not constitutively expressed cNOS (43–46). The mechanism of action appears to be the reduction of iNOS mRNA transcription, and not by a direct effect on the enzyme (43–46). More recently, cyclosporin A and FK506 have been reported also to decrease NO production (92). The mechanism of action of cyclosporin and FK506 may be, at least in part, a direct inhibitory effect on NOS activity, perhaps as a result of binding to calmodulin (93,94).

A variety of compounds are known to release NO. Two of the more common are nitroglycerin and sodium nitroprusside, which act predominantly by releasing NO (95). In addition, a number of synthetic donors, including S-nitroso-N-acetylpenicillamine (SNAP) and spermine-NO (SPERNO), have been synthesized for use in laboratory investigations (96,84).

PHYSIOLOGY OF NITRIC OXIDE

Vasodilatation

Vasodilatation of the microcirculation influences edema formation and leukocyte accumulation. NO has a well-established role in the endothelial-dependent control of vascular tone (2). In addition, there is evidence suggesting that NO-mediated vasodilatation may potentiate edema. NO appears to mediate the edema resulting from injection of substance P or LPS and the edema resulting from ultraviolet light irradiation in rat skin (97–99). L-NMMA attenuates the edema formation during the late allergic response in the skin, suggesting that NO is important in edema formation (100).

NO also may cause vascular relaxation by neural stimulation (2,35). In addition to its direct vasodilatory properties, NO can mediate endothelium-independent vascular smooth muscle relaxation in cerebral and other arteries, as well as the penile corpus cavernosum (101–103). The mechanism for these responses is suggested by the demonstration that the NO-mediated vascular relaxation is sensitive to tetrodotoxin which blocks the voltage-dependent Na^+ channels responsible for propagation of action potentials in nerves. Depolarization of nerves resulting in an increased cytosolic Ca^{++} concentration, stimulates bNOS in nerve terminals which, in turn, results in production of NO and stimulation of guanylyl cyclase in vascular smooth muscle, causing relaxation (35).

Inflammation

The role of NO in an inflammatory response is unclear and, at times, contradictory. NO enhances the chemotaxis of neutrophils, monocytes, and eosinophils by a cGMP-dependent mechanism (104–107). However, NO appears to inhibit adhesion of leukocytes to vascular endothelium and bronchial epithelium (108,109).

NO has been suggested to mediate both acute and chronic inflammatory reactions. Inhibition of NO formation attenuates acute joint inflammation in rats with adjuvant arthritis and the inflammatory responses in the lung and skin after immune-complex mediated lung or dermal injury (110–112). A role for NO also has been suggested for ileitis because NOS inhibitors ameliorate the disorder (113). Nitrite is increased in joint fluid aspirated from patients with rheumatoid arthritis suggesting increased NO formation (114).

However, other experimental evidence has led to the hypothesis that NO suppresses inflammation. Lymphocytes can release nitric oxide, and murine macrophage release of NO can reduce lymphocyte activation (115–119). These observations have recently been expanded to examine the potential for T helper type 1 (TH1) and T helper type 2 (TH2) cells to produce NO (120). Murine TH1, but not TH2, cells can be activated by specific antigens or the T cell mitogen, conclavin A, to produce large amounts of NO. Furthermore, NO inhibited the secretion of interleukin-2 and INF by TH1 cells, but had no effect on interleukin-4 production by TH2 cells. These observations suggest that NO exerts a self-regulatory effect on TH1 cells.

Bronchodilatation and Bronchoconstriction

NO-mediated bronchodilatation may occur by several mechanisms (Fig. 2). NO donors such as nitroglycerin or sodium nitroprusside long have been known to relax smooth muscle, including airway smooth muscle, in vitro (121,122). NO administered as a gas relaxes tracheal muscle and reduces methacholine-induced bronchoconstriction (96,123,124). Interestingly, these effects appear to be more marked in epithelium denuded strips, suggesting that the epithelium may serve as a barrier, preventing access of NO to the bronchial smooth muscle (125). These observations recently have been extended to humans. NO administration (80 ppm) produced a modest improvement of approximately 50% in airway conductance in asthmatics (126). However, NO administration does not appear to alter bronchial tone in normal volunteers (126,127).

There is increasing evidence that NO may function as the neurotransmitter of the inhibitory nonadrenergic, noncholinergic (iNANC) bronchodilator response (Fig. 2). bNOS has been localized to airway nerves in the guinea pig, ferret, and human airways which innervate airway vessels, smooth muscle, and submucosal glands. bNOS has also been detected in the parasympathetic, sympathetic, and sensory ganglia supplying the airways (127–130). NO appears to account for a portion of iNANC response in pig, guinea pig, cat, and horse airways. However, NO neurotransmission accounts for nearly all the human iNANC response (131–140). This may have functional significance because NANC nerves are the only known neural bronchodilator mechanism in human airways (141).

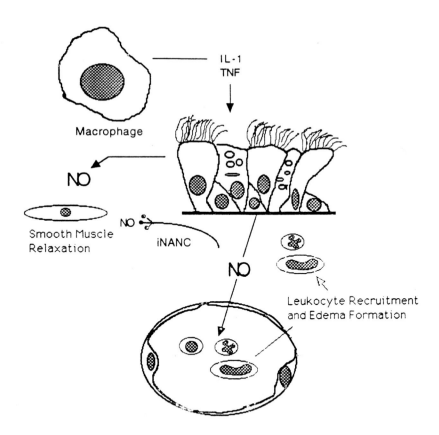

FIG. 2. Schematic representation of possible roles for NO in the lung. Stimulation of alveolar macrophages results in release of cytokines and NO. The cytokines stimulate bronchial epithelium, causing additional NO production. The NO can be released into the airway and detected in the exhaled air or interact with smooth muscle or blood vessels. The NO together with the NO-dependent inhibitory nonadrenergic, noncholinergic (iNANC) pathway results in bronchodilatation. NO interaction with blood vessels and leukocytes may result in edema formation and enhanced recruitment of inflammatory cells.

In contrast to the direct relaxing action on smooth muscle or relaxation induced by neurotransmission, the potential exists for NO to potentiate bronchial narrowing (Fig. 2). NO is a potent bronchial vasodilator in animal airways (142). Blood vessel dilatation and edema of airways have been proposed to play a major role in the airway obstruction of asthma. Paré et al. (143,144), through the use of mathematical modeling, have demonstrated that small amounts of airway edema can result in significant airway narrowing, resulting in airway obstruction. Although controversial, it seems likely that blood vessel dilatation and edema formation contribute to the airway narrowing in asthma, and that NO might contribute to this narrowing. NO inhibitors reduce neurogenic plasma exudation in guinea pig airways (145).

Host Defense

Murine macrophages release NO which posses antimicrobial activity (6,7,146). The NO released by macrophages also may be cytotoxic for tumor cells (147,148). These cytotoxic effects appear to be dependent on the combination of NO with enzymes of the respiratory cycle and DNA synthesis in the target cells, and suggest that NO production by macrophages may be an important mechanism in host defense against microorganisms or tumor cells (84,148–150). Neutrophils also produce NO,

suggesting that these cells may also participate in host defenses by a similar mechanism (14). Recent evidence reveals that there may be interspecies variation in the capacity of macrophages to produce NO. Human macrophages derived by culturing peripheral blood monocytes do not consistently produce detectable nitrite levels in response to most stimuli used to activate macrophages (151). The capacity of human macrophages recovered by bronchoalveolar lavage (BAL) to produce NO may also be limited; nitrite concentrations are less than 1 μM in 24 hour-culture- supernatant fluids, even after stimulation (RA Robbins, unpublished observations).

NO also is generated by respiratory tract epithelial cells (21,22,43,44,152). Although it is controversial whether iNOS is constitutively expressed by these cells or must be induced, macrophage-derived cytokines such as TNF, IL-1, and IFN-γ can induce iNOS mRNA transcription, resulting in a several-fold increase in NO production (22, 43,44,152). This suggests that macrophages may participate indirectly in NO production by releasing cytokines which stimulate resident epithelial cells to release NO.

Removing particulate matter and microorganisms by modulating the mucociliary escalator represents another mechanism by which NO may enhance host defense. NO increases ciliary beat frequency above baseline (153). Isoproterenol increases ciliary beat frequency within minutes, and NOS inhibitors attenuate this increase (153). TNF and IL-1 also increase ciliary beat frequency;

NOS inhibitors also decrease this cytokine-mediated effect (154). These observations would be consistent with an early effect occurring predominantly through a cNOS mechanism, and a later effect caused by an iNOS mechanism. The later cytokine-mediated increase provides further evidence that macrophage release of cytokines may enhance NO production by bronchial epithelial cells.

NITRIC OXIDE IN ASTHMA

Exhaled Nitric Oxide Concentration

NO has been detected in the exhaled air of normal humans and animals (155,156). Several studies have now documented that exhaled NO concentrations are increased in asthma (157–159) (Fig. 3). These observations recently have been extended to demonstrate that exhaled NO concentrations are not increased after the early allergic reaction, or acutely after methacholine inhalation (160,161). By contrast, exhaled NO concentrations are increased in asthmatics several hours after antigen chal-

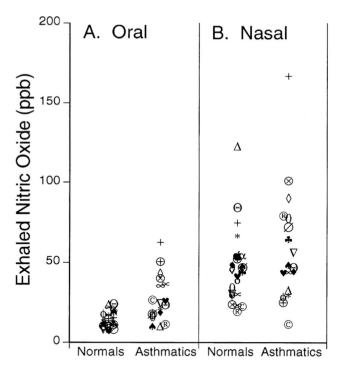

FIG. 4. Exhaled NO levels measured by collecting exhaled air through the mouth (*Panel A*) or through the nose (*Panel B*). Both normal and asthmatic subjects had increased NO levels when measured through the nose ($p<0.01$, both comparisons) but the NO oxide was increased in asthmatics only when measured through the mouth ($p<0.05$).

lenge, and correspond to the time of the late asthmatic reaction (161,162). These observations are most consistent with induction of cytokines during the late asthmatic reaction leading to an increase in iNOS transcription and an increase in exhaled NO.

NO production in the upper respiratory tract with inhalation and subsequent exhalation has been proposed to account for a large portion of exhaled NO (163). Recent studies have confirmed that greater concentrations of NO are measured when exhaled air is collected from the nose, rather than from the mouth (164) (Fig. 4). However, several lines of evidence suggest that autoinhalation likely does not account for the increased orally exhaled NO in asthmatics. First, there is no difference between nasally exhaled NO concentrations in normals and asthmatics (Fig. 4, p is greater than 0.05). Second, noseclips were worn is some studies during both inhalation and exhalation, thus, preventing autoinhalation of NO from the nose (157). Third, inhalation of up to 1000 ppm of NO does not effect exhaled NO concentrations (SA Kharitonov and RA Robbins, personal observations). Fourth, immunohistochemistry has demonstrated iNOS on the respiratory epithelial cells in asthma (152). However, these observations would not exclude autoinhalation of NO reacting with the lower respiratory tract cells, or proteins in the lower respiratory tract, and altering their function.

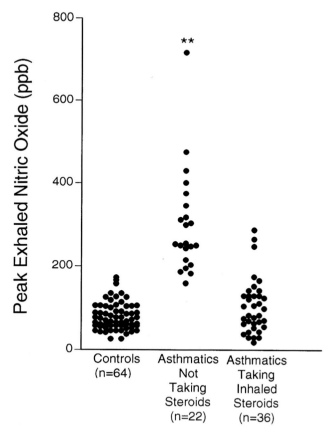

FIG. 3. Peak exhaled nitric oxide levels in normal nonasthmatic, nonsmoking controls, subjects with asthma not taking corticosteroids, and subjects with asthma taking inhaled corticosteroids. ** $p<0.01$ compared to controls and asthmatic subjects receiving corticosteroids.

Cellular Sources and Mechanisms for Increased Nitric Oxide Production in Asthma

The cellular sources for the increase in exhaled NO seen in asthmatics is not known definitely and, likely, is heterogenous. However, several lines of evidence suggest that airway epithelial cells are likely major contributors. The high concentration of NO in the exhaled air, combined with the highly reactive nature of nitric oxide in biological tissues, suggests that the source resides within the airways. Inhalation of the NOS inhibitors, L-NAME or aminoguanidine, reduces exhaled NO levels in asthmatics (165). Immunohistochemical studies indicate that a major source of the increased nitric oxide may the bronchial epithelium which strongly stains for iNOS in asthmatics (152).

Although macrophage production of NO in the lower respiratory tract of asthmatics requires further study, macrophages in the lower respiratory tract of asthmatics may modulate NO production by releasing cytokines such as TNF and IL-1 (166,167). These cytokines can, in turn, stimulate increased iNOS mRNA transcription in the airway epithelium, resulting in increased NO production (43,44) (Fig. 2).

Pharmacology of Nitric Oxide in Asthma

Inhaled corticosteroids decrease exhaled NO levels in asthmatics, but not in normal, nonasthmatic subjects (142,168). This is consistent with the effects of corticosteroids on iNOS mRNA transcription (43,44). β_2-adrenergic agonists do not alter exhaled NO concentrations in asthma (169); this is also consistent with their lack of effect on NO production by bronchial epithelial cells (RA Robbins, unpublished observations).

Functional Role of Lower Respiratory Tract Nitric Oxide in Asthma

The role that increased NO might be playing in the lower respiratory tract of asthmatics is unclear, although multiple mechanisms have been suggested (Fig. 2). One potential effect of NO released by the bronchial epithelium, is bronchial smooth muscle relaxation resulting in bronchodilatation. NO causes a direct bronchodilator effect by relaxing airway smooth muscle (121). However, when given by inhalation, concentrations of NO less than or equal to 80 ppm do not dilate normal human airways and NO is a weak bronchodilator in asthmatics (126). Although bronchial epithelium releases a bronchodilatory substance, this is not likely to be NO (170).

As noted earlier, there is increasing evidence that NO functions as the neurotransmitter in the inhibitory nonadrenergic, non-iNANC response. It appears that this is the only neural bronchodilatory pathway in humans, and,

therefore, this mechanism assumes increased functional significance in airway disorders such as asthma (141). Airway responses to iNANC responses are reduced in cystic fibrosis, an airway disorder associated with substantial airway inflammation (171). However, in the same study, airways obtained from subjects with mild asthma had the same response as airways obtained from subjects without apparent airway disease (171). The mechanism by which airway inflammation might be associated with a decrease in the NO-dependent iNANC response is unknown, but the observation that superoxide anions released from inflammatory cells enhance the breakdown of NO suggests a possible functional mechanism (172).

Increased NO may enhance airway edema formation and augment bronchoconstriction. Increased endogenous NO mediates neurogenic plasma exudation in guinea-pig airways (145). Inhibitors of NO decrease microvascular permeability of guinea pig airways in response to inhalation of histamine, platelet activating factor, substance P, A23187, or ovalbumin in sensitized animals (173). Edema formation is reduced by NO inhibitors during the late allergic reaction in the skin (174). In contrast, a recent study suggests the opposite effect, e.g., that NO inhibitors applied topically to guinea pig airway epithelium actually decrease airway plasma exudation (175).

NO may play a role in the airway inflammation, epithelial cell cytotoxicity, and shedding of airway epithelial cells into the airway lumen in asthma. Although NO is not chemotactic for eosinophils, it enhances eosinophil migration in response to a chemotactic stimulus (107). This suggests that enhanced bronchial epithelial cell production of NO may enhance an influx of eosinophils into the airways in asthma. Studies with pertussis toxin, which has previously been used in creating an animal model of asthma, have demonstrated that NO can play a role in epithelial cytotoxicity (176,177). Pertussis toxin-induced release of IL-1β ,in turn, induces epithelial cell production of NO. The increased production of NO is cytotoxic for the epithelial cells. Macrophage release of IL-1 (167) and bronchial epithelial cell production of NO (152) both have been demonstrated in asthma, suggesting that this mechanism might account, at least in part, for the epithelial cytotoxicity and shedding observed in asthma.

CONCLUSIONS

Nitric oxide has a number of physiological effects on the lung which are of potential importance in asthma. NO can modulate airway smooth muscle tone, bronchial edema, and bronchial inflammation, and is known to be increased in the exhaled air of asthmatics. Although the source of the increased exhaled NO is unknown, immunohistochemical studies suggest that increased airway epithelial cell expression of iNOS accounts for much of the increase in NO production. Macrophages from asthmatics are known to release increased amounts of IL-1β, which can, in turn, stimulate increased mRNA transcription of iNOS in airway epithelial cells. The functional significance of the increased NO production in asthma is unknown, but studies suggest that the bronchodilatory effect of NO is rather modest in humans. However, NO may enhance airway edema formation and enhance lower respiratory tract inflammation. Corticosteroids decrease exhaled NO in asthmatics, suggesting another mechanism by which corticosteroid therapy may improve asthma. Further definition of the role of NO in asthma likely will require the administration of specific NO inhibitors and observation of the physiologic effects.

REFERENCES

1. Culotta E, Koshland DE. NO news is good news. *Science* 1992; 258: 1862–1863.
2. Moncada S, Higgs A. The L-arginine-nitric oxide pathway. *N Engl J Med* 1993;329:2002–2012.
3. Furchgott RF, Zawadski JV. The obligatory role of endothelial cells in the relaxation of arterial smooth muscle by acetylcholine. *Nature* 1980;288:373–376.
4. Palmer RMJ, Ferrige AG, Moncada S. Nitric oxide release accounts for the biological activity of endothelium-derived relaxing factor. *Nature* 1987;327:524–526.
5. Ignarro LJ, Buga, CM, Wood KS, Byrns RE, Chaudhuri G. Endothelium derived relaxing factor produced and released from artery and vein is nitric oxide. *Proc Natl Acad Sci U S A* 1987;84:9265–9269.
6. Hibbs JB, Taintor RR, Vaurin Z. Macrophage cytotoxicity: role of L-arginine deimunase activity and imino nitrogen oxidation to nitrite. *Science* 1987;235:473–476.
7. Iyengar R, Stuehr DJ, Marletta MA. Macrophage synthesis of nitrite, nitrate and N-nitrosamines; precursors and role of the respiratory burst. *Proc Natl Acad Sci U S A* 1987;84:6369–6373.
8. Förstermann U, Schmidt HHHW, Pollock JS, Sheng H, Mitchell JA, Warner TD, Masaki N, Murad F. Isoforms of nitric oxide synthase: characterization and purification from different cell types. *Biochem Pharmacol* 1991;10:1849–1857.
9. Lamas S, Marsden PA, Li GK, Tempst P, Michel T. Endothelial nitric oxide synthase: molecular cloning and characterization of a distinct constitutive enzyme isoform. *Proc Natl Acad Sci U S A* 1992;89: 6348–6352.
10. Janssens SP, Shimouchi A, Quertermous T, Bloch DB, Block KD. Cloning and expression of a cDNA encoding human endothelium-derived relaxing factor/nitric oxide synthase. *J Biol Chem* 1992;267: 14519–14522.
11. Pollock JS, Förstermann U, Mitchell JA, et al. Purification and characterization of particulate endotheium-derived relaxing factor synthase from cultured and native bovine aortic endothelial cells. *Proc Natl Acad Sci U S A* 1991;88:10480–10484.
12. Bredt DS, Hwang PM, Glatt CE, Lowenstein C, Reed RR, Snyder SH. Cloned and expressed nitric oxide synthase structurally resembles cytochrome P-450 reductase. *Nature* 1991;351:714–718.
13. Salvemini D, Masini C, Anggard E, Mannaioni PF, Vane J. Synthesis of nitric oxide-like factor from L-arginine by rat serosal mast cells: stimulation of guanylate cyclase and inhibition of platelet aggregation. *Biochem Biophys Res Commun* 1990;169:596–601.
14. Yui Y, Hattori R, Kosuga K, et al. Calmodulin-independent nitric oxide synthase from rat polymorphonuclear neutrophils. *J Biol Chem* 1991;266:3369–3371.
15. Hiki K, Yui Y, Hattori R, Eizawa H, Kosuga K, Kawai C. Three regulation mechanisms of nitric oxide synthase. *Eur J Pharmacol* 1991; 206:163–164.
16. Radomski NW, Moncada S. Biological role of nitric oxide in platelet function. In: Moncada S, Higgs EA, Berrazueta JR, eds. *Clinical releavance of nitric oxide in the cardiovascular system.* Madrid: EDI-COMPLET, 1991;45–56.

17. Smith JA, Shah AM, Lewis MJ. Factors released from endocardium of the ferret and pig modulate myocardial contraction. *J Physiol* 1991; 439:1–14.
18. DeBelder AJ, Radomski MW, Why HJF, et al. Nitric oxide synthase activities in human myocardium. *Lancet* 1993;341:84–85.
19. Terada Y, Tomita K, Nonoguchi H, Marumo F. Polymerase chain reaction localization of constitutive nitric oxide synthase and solbule guanylate cyclase messenger RNAs in microdissected rat nephron segments. *J Clin Invest* 1992;90:659–665.
20. Brown JF, Tepperman BL, Hanson PJ, Whittle BJR, Moncada S. Differential distribution of nitric oxide synthase between cell fractions isolated from the rat gastric mucosa. *Biochem Biophys Res Commun* 1992;184:680–685.
21. Robbins RA, Hamel FG, Floreani AA, et al. Bovine bronchial epithelial cells metabolize L-arginine to L-citrulline: possible role of nitric oxide synthase. *Life Sci* 1993;52:709–716.
22. Kobzik L, Bredt DS, Lowenstein CJ, et al. Nitric oxide syntase in human and rat lung: immunochemical and histochemical localization. *Am J Respir Cell Mol Biol* 1993;9:371–377.
23. Bredt DS, Snyder SH. Isolation of nitric oxide synthetase, a calmodulin-requiring enzyme. *Proc Natl Acad Sci U S A* 1990;87:682–685.
24. Jorens PG, van Overveld FJ, Vermeire PA, Bult H, Herman AG. Synergism between interleukin-1β and the nitric oxide synthase inducer interferon-τ in rat lung fibroblasts. *Eur J Pharmacol* 1992;224:7–12.
25. Nakayama DR, Geller DA, Lowenstein CJ, Davies P, Pitt BR, Simmons RL, et al. Cytokines and lipopolysaccharide induce nitric oxide synthase in cultured rat pulmonary artery smooth muscle. *Am J Respir Cell Mol Biol* 1992;7:471–476.
26. Geller DA, Lowenstein CJ, Shapiro RA, et al. Molecular cloning and expression of inducible nitric oxide synthase from human hepatocytes. *Proc Natl Acad Sci U S A*;90:3491–3495.
27. McCall TB, Broughton-Smith NK, Palmer RMJ, Whittle BJR, Moncada S. Synthesis of nitric oxide from L-arginine by neutrophils. Release and interaction with superoxide anions. *Biochem J* 1989;169: 596–601.
28. Eizirik DL, Björklund A, Welsh N. Interleukin-1-induced expression of nitric oxide synthase in insulin-producing cells is preceded by c-*fos* induction and depends on gene transcription and protein synthesis. *FEBS Lett* 1993;317:62–66.
29. Stadler J, Stefanovic-Racic M, Billiar TR, et al. Articular chondrocytes synthesize nitric oxide in response to cytokines and lipopolysaccharide. *J Immunol* 1991;147:3915–3920.
30. Xie Q-W, Cho HJ, Claycay J, Mumford RA, Swiderek KM, Lee TD, et al. Cloning and characterization of inducible nitric oxide synthase from mouse macrophages. *Science* 1992;256:225–228.
31. Lyons CR, Orloff GJ, Cunningham JM. Molecular cloning and functional expression of an inducbile nitric oxide sythase from a murine macrophage cell line. *J Biol Chem* 1992;172:1246–1252.
32. Kwon NS, Nathan CF, Stueh DS. Reduced biopterin as a cofactor in the generation of nitrogen oxides by murine macrophages. *J Biol Chem* 1989;264:20496–20501.
33. Hope BT, Michael GJ, Knige KM, Vincent SR. Neuronal NADPH-disphorase is a nitric oxide synthase. *Proc Natl Acad Sci U S A* 1991; 88:2811–2814.
34. Hope BT, Vincent SR. Histochemical characterisation of neuronal NADPH-disphorase. *J Histochem Cytochem* 1989;37:653–661.
35. Knowles RG, Moncada S. Nitric oxide as a signal in blood vessels. *Trends Biochem Sci* 1992;17:399–402.
36. Nishida K, Harrison DG, Navas JP, et al. Molecular cloning and characterization of the constitutive bovine aortic endothelial cell nitric oxide synthase. *J Clin Invest* 1992;90:2092–2101.
37. Liu SF, Crawley DE, Barnes PJ, Evans TW. Endothelium-derived nitric oxide inhibits pulmonary vasoconstriction in isolated blood perfused rat lungs. *Am Rev Respir Dis* 1991;143:32–37.
38. Persson MG, Gustafsson LE, Wiklund NP, Moncada S, Hedqvist P. Endogenous nitric oxide as a probable modulator of pulmonary circulation and hypoxic pressor response *in vivo. Acta Physiol Scand* 1990;140:449–457.
39. Adnos S, Raffestin B, Eddamibi S, Braquet P, Chabrier PE. Loss of endothelium-dependent relaxant activity in the pulmonary circulation of rats exposed to chronic hypoxia. *J Clin Invest* 1991;87:155–162.
40. Buga GM, Griscavage JM, Rogers NE, Ignarro LJ. Negative feedback regulation of endothelial cell function by nitric oxide. *Circ Res* 1993; 73:808–812.

41. Myers PR, Wright TF, Tanner MA, Adams HR. EDRF and nitric oxide production in cultured endothelial cells: direct inhibition by E.coli endotoxin. *Am J Physiol* 1992;262:H710–H718.

42. Bredt DS, Ferris CD, Snyder SH. Nitric oxide synthase sites. Phosphorylation by cyclic AMP-dependent protein kinase, protein kinase C, and calcium/calmodulin protein kinase; identification of flavin and calmodulin binding sites. *J Biol Chem* 1992;267:10976–10981.

43. Robbins RA, Springall DR, Warren JB, et al. Inducible nitric oxide synthase is increased in murine lung epithelial cells by cytokine stimulation. *Biochem Biophys Res Commun* 1994;198:835–843.

44. Robbins RA, Barnes PJ, Springall DR, et al. Expression of inducible nitric oxide in human lung epithelial cells. *Biochem Biophys Res Commun* 1994;203:209–218.

45. DiRosa M, Radomski M, Carnuccio R, Moncada S. Glucocorticoids inhibit the induction of nitric oxide synthase in macrophages. *Biochem Biophys Res Commun* 1990; 172:1246–1252.

46. Radomski MW, Palmer RMJ, Moncada S. Glucocorticoids inhibit the expression of an inducible, but not the constitutive nitric oxide synthase in vascular endothelial cells. *Proc Natl Acad Sci U S A* 1990;87: 10043–10049.

47. Junquero DC, Schini VB, Scott-Burden TS, Vanhoutte PM. Transforming growth factor-β_1 inhibits L-arginine-derived relaxing factor(s) from smooth muscle cells. *Am J Physiol* 1992; 262 (Heart Circ Physiol 31):H1788–H1795.

48. Ding A, Nathan CF, Graycar J, Derynck R, Steuhr DJ, Srimal S. Macrophage deactivating factor and transforming growth factors β-1, β-2 and β-3 inhibit induction of macrophage nitrogen oxide synthase by interferon-gamma. *J Immunol* 1990;145:940–944.

49. Pfeilschifter J, Vosbeck K. Transforming growth factor β₂ inhibits interleukin 1β- and tumour necrosis factor-α-induction of nitric oxide synthase in rat renal mesangial cells. *Biochem Biophys Res Commun* 1991;175:372–379.

50. Liew FY, Li Y, Severn A, Millot S, Schmidt J, Salter M, Moncada S. A possible novel pathway of regulation of murine T helper type-2 (TH2) cels of a TH1 cell activity via the modulation of the induction of nitric oxide synthase on macrophages. *Eur J Immunol* 1991;21: 2489–2494.

51. Cunha FQ, Moncada S, Liew FY. Interleukin-10 (IL-10) inhibits the induction of nitric oxide synthase by interferon-γ in murine macrophages. *Biochem Biophys Res Commun* 1992;182:1155–1159.

52. Heck DE, Laskin DL, Gardner RC, Laskin DJ. Epidermal growth factor suppresses nitric oxide and hydrogen peroxide production by keratinocytes: potenital role for nitric oxide in the regulation of wound healing. *J Biol Chem* 1992;267:21277–21280.

53. McCall TB, Palmer RMJ, Moncada S. Interleukin-8 inhibits the induction of nitric oxide synthase in rat peritoneal macrophages. *Biochem Biophys Res Commun* 1992;186:680–685.

54. Rojas A, Delgado R, Claria L, Palacios M. Monocyte chemotactic protein-1 inhibits the induction of nitric oxide synthase in J774 cells. *Biochem Biophys Res Commun* 1993;196:274–279.

55. McCall TB, Palmer RMJ, Moncada S. Interleukin-8 inhibits the induction of nitric oxide synthase in rat peritoneal neutrophils. *Biochem Biophys Res Commun* 1992;186:680–685.

56. Kharitonov SA, Yates DH, Robbins RA, Keatings VM, Robichaud A, Barnes PJ. Cigarette smoking decreases exhaled nitric oxide. *Am J Respir Crit Care Med* 1994;149:A199.

57. Stamler JS, Singel DJ, Loscalzo J. Biochemistry of nitric oxide and its redox-activated forms. *Science* 1992;258:1898–1902.

58. Beckman JS, Beckman TW, Chen J, Marshall PA, Freeman BA. Apparent hydroxyl radical production by peroxynitrite: implications for endothelial injury from nitric oxide and superoxide. *Proc Natl Acad Sci U S A* 1990;87:1620–1624.

59. Blough NV, Zafiriou OC. Reaction of superoxide with nitric oxide to form peroxynitrite in alkaline aqueous solution. *Inorganic Chemistry* 1985;24:3502–3504.

60. Saran M, Michel C, Bors W. Reaction of NO with O₂⁻: implications for the action of endothelium-derived relaxing factor (EDRF). *Free Radical Res* 1990;10:221–226.

61. Radi R, Beckman JS, Bush KM, Freeman BA. Peroxynitrite-induced membrane lipid peroxidation: the cytotoxic potential of superoxide and nitric oxide. *Arch Biochem Biophys* 1991;288:481–487.

62. Radi R, Beckman JS, Bush KM, Freeman BA. Peroxynitrite oxidation of sulfhydyls: the cytotoxic potential of superoxide and nitric oxide. *J Biol Chem* 1991;266:4244–4250.

63. Kelm M, Feelisch M, Grude R, Motz W, Strauer BE. Metabolism of enodthelium-derived nitric oxide in human blood. In: Mocada S, Marletta MA, Hibbs JB Jr, Higgs EA, eds. *The biology of nitric oxide.* Vol. 1. London: Portland Press, 1992;319–322.

64. Marletta MA, Tayeh MA, Hevel JM. Unraveling the biological significance of nitric oxide. *Biofactors* 1990;2:219–225.

65. McCleverty JA. Reactions of nitric oxide coordinated to transitition metal. *Chem Rev* 1979;79:53–76.

66. Waldman SA, Murad F. Biochemical mechanisms underlying vascular smooth muscle relaxation: the guanylate cyclase-cyclic GMP system. *J Cardiovasc Pharmacol* 1988;12:(Suppl 5):S115–S118.

67. Henry Y, Ducrocq C, Drapier J-C, Servent D, Pellat C, Guissani A. Nitric oxide: a biological effector: electron paramagnetic resonance detection of nitrosyl-iron-protein complexes in whole cells. *Eur Biophys J* 1991;20:1–15.

68. Kanner J, Harel S, Granit R. Nitric oxide as an antioxidant. *Arch Biochem Biophys* 1991;289:130–136.

69. Mirvish S. Formation of N-nitroso compounds; chemistry, kinetics and *in vivo* occurrence. *Toxicol Appl Pharmacol* 1975;31:325–351.

70. Gaston B, Drazen JM, Loscalzo J, Stamler JS. The biology of nitrogen oxides in the airways. *Am J Respir Crit Care Med* 1994;149:538–551.

71. Stamler JS, Jaraki O, Osborne J, et al. Nitric oxide circulates in mammalian plasma primarily as an S-nitroso adduct of serum albumin. *Proc Natl Acad Sci U S A* 1992;89:7674–7677.

72. Stamler JS, Simon DI, Osborne JA, et al. S-nitrosylation of proteins with nitric oxide; synthesis and chacterization of biologically active compounds. *Proc Natl Acad Sci U S A* 1992;89:444–448.

73. Lascalzo J. N-acetylcysteine potentiates inhibition of platelet aggregation by nitroglycerine. *J Clin Invest* 1985;76:703–708.

74. Wei EP, Kontos HA. H₂O₂ and endothelium-dependent cerebral arteriolar dilation. *Hypertension* 1990;16:162–169.

75. Myers PR, Minor RL, Guerra R, Bates JN, Harrison DG. Vasorelaxant properties of the endothelium-derived relaxing factor more closely resemble S-nitrosocysteine than nitric oxide. *Nature* 1990; 345:161–163.

76. Stamler JS, Simon DI, Jaraki O, et al. S-nitrosylation of tissue-type plasminogen activator confers vasodilatory and antiplatelet properties on the enzyme. *Proc Natl Acad Sci U S A* 1992;89:8087–8091.

77. Haddad IY, Pataki G, Hu P, Galliani C, Beckman JS, Matalon S. Quantitaion of nitrotyrosine levels in lung sections of patients and animals with acute lung injury. *J Clin Invest* 1994;94:2407–2413.

78. Haddad IY, Crow J, Yoazu Y, Beckman JS, Matalon S. Concurrent generation of nitric oxide and superoxide damages surfactant protein A (SP-A). *Am J Physiol* 1994;267:L242–L249.

79. Ishiropooulos H, Zhu L, Chen J, et al. Peroxynitrite-mediated tyrosine nitration catalyzed by superoxide dismutase. *Arch Biochem Biophys* 1992;298:431–437.

80. Haddad IY, Ishiropoulos H, Holm BA, Beckman JS, Baker JR, Matalon S. Mechanisms of peroxynitrite induced injury to pulmonary surfactant. *Am J Physiol* 1993;265:L555–L564.

81. Janing GR, Kraft R, Blank J, Ristau O, Rabe H, Ruckpaul K. Chemical modification of cytochrome P-450 LM4. Identification of functionally linked tyrosine residues. *Biochim Biophys Acta* 1987;916: 512–523.

82. McCall MN, Easterbrook-Smith SB. Comparison of the role ot tyrosine reisudes in human IgG and rabbit IgG in binding complement cubcomponent C1q. *Biochem J* 1989;257:845–851.

83. Martin BL, Wu D, Jakes S, Graves DJ. Chemical influences on the specificity of tyrosine phosphorylation. *J Biol Chem* 1990;265:7108–7111.

84. Wink DA, Kasprzak KS, Maragos CM, et al. DNA deaminating ability and genotoxicity of nitric oxide and its progenitors. *Science* 1991; 254:1001–1003.

85. Nguyen T, Brunson D, Crespi CL, Penman BW, Wishok JS, Tannenbaum SR. DNA damage and mutation in human cells exposed to nitric oxide *in vitro*. *Proc Natl Acad Sci U S A* 1992;89:3030–3034.

86. Vallance P, Leone A, Calver A, Collier J, Moncada S. Accumulation of an endogenous inhibitor of nitric oxide synthesis in chronic renal failure. *Lancet* 1992;339:572–575.

87. Rees DD, Palmer RMJ, Schulz R, Hodson MF, Moncada S. Characterization of three inhibitors of endothelial nitric oxide synthase *in vitro* and *in vivo*. *Br J Pharmacol* 1990;101:746–752.

88. Bogle RG, Moncada S, Pearson JD, Mann GE. Identification of in-

hibitors of nitric oxide synthase that do not interact with the endothelial cell L-arginine transporter. *Br J Pharmacol* 1992;105:768–770.

89. Rajanayagam MAS, Li C-G, Rand MJ. Differential effects of hydroxcobalamin on NO-mediated relaxations in rat aorta and ancoccygeus muscle. *Br J Pharmacol* 1993;108:3–5.

90. Baddedge RC, Moore PK, Gathen Z, Hart SL. L-N^G-nitroarginine p-nitroanilide (l-NAPNA): a selctive inhibitor of nitric oxide synthase in the brain. *Br J Pharmacol* 1993;107:194P.

91. Misko TP, Moore WM, Kasten TP, Nickols GA, Corbett JA, Tilton RG, et al. Selective inhibtion of inducible nitric oxide synthase by aminoguanidine. *Eur J Pharmacol* 1993;233:119–125.

92. Conde M, Andrade J, Bedoya FJ, Santa Maria C, Sobrino F. Inhibitory effect of cyclosporin A and FK506 on nitric oxide production by cultured macrophages. Evidence or a direct effect on nitric oxide syntase activity. *Immunology* 1995;84:476–481.

93. Conde M, Andrade J, Bedoya FJ, Santa Maria C, Sobrino F. Inhibitory effect of cyclosporin A and FK506 on nitric oxide production by cultured macrophages. Evidence or a direct effect on nitric oxide syntase activity. *Immunology* 1995;84:476–481.

94. Colombani PM, Ross A, Hess AD. Cyclosporin A binding to calmodulin: a possible site of action on T lymphocytes. *Science* 1985;228:337–339.

95. Feelisch M. The ciochemical pathways of nitric oxide formation from nitrovasodilators; appropriate choice of exogenous NO donors and aspects of preparation and handling of aqueous NO solutions. *J Cardiovasc Pharmacol* 1991;17:Suppl3:S25–S33.

96. Dupuy G, Shore SA, Drazen JM, Frostell C, Hill WA, Zapol WM. Bronchodilator action of inhaled nitric oxide in guinea pigs. *J Clin Invest* 1992;90:421–428.

97. Hughes SR, Williams TJ, Brain SD. Evidence that endogenous nitric oxide modulates edema formation induced by substance P. *Eur J Pharmacol* 1990;191:481–484.

98. Pons F, Williams TJ, Warren JB. Nitric oxide, but not interleukin-1, mediates the local blood flow response to lipopolysaccharide in rabbit skin. *Eur J Pharmacol* 1993;239:23–30.

99. Warren JB, Loi RK, Couglan ML. Involvement of nitric oxide synthase in the delayed vasodilator response to ultraviolet light irradiation of rat skin *in vivo*. *Br J Pharmacol* 1993;109:802–806.

100. Townley RG, Romero FA, Robbins RA. Inhibition of nitric oxide synthase (NOS) decreases edema formation during the late allergic skin response. *Am J Respir Crit Care Med* 1995;151:A127.

101. Toda N, Okamura T. Modification by L-N^G-monomethyl-arginine (L-NMMA) of the response to nervestimulation in isolated dog mesenteric and cerebral arteries. *Jpn J Pharmacol* 1990;52:170–173.

102. Gaw AJ, Aberdeen J, Humphrey PPA, Wadsworth RM, Burnstock G. Relaxation of sheep cerebral arteries by vasoactive intestinal polypeptide and neurogenic stimulation: inhibition by L-N^G-monomethyl-arginine in endothelium-denuded vessels. *Br J Pharmacol* 1991;102:567–572.

103. Rajfer J, Aronson WJ, Bush PA, Dorey FJ, Ignarro LJ. Nitric oxide as a mediator of relaxation of the corpus cavernosum in response to nonadrenergic, noncholinergic neurotransmission. *N Engl J Med* 1992;326:90–94.

104. Kaplan SS, Billiar T, Curran RD, Zdziarski UE, Simmons RL, Basford RE. Attenuation of chemotaxis with N^G-monomethyl-L-arginine: a role for cyclic GMP. *Blood* 1989;74:1885–1887.

105. Belenky SN, Robbins RA, Rennard SI, Gossman GL, Nelson KJ, Rubinstein I. Inhibitors of nitric oxide synthase attenuate neutrophil chemotaxis *in vitro*. *J Lab Clin Med* 1993;122:388–394.

106. Belenky SN, Robbins RA, Rubinstein I. Nitric oxide synthase inhibitors attenuate human monocyte chmotaxis *in vitro*. *J Leukoc Biol* 1993;53:498–503.

107. Robbins RA, Romero FA, Nelson KJ, Hill GE, Townley RG. Inhibitors of nitric oxide attenuate human eosinophil chemotaxis. *Am J Respir Crit Care Med* 1995;151:A238.

108. Kubes P, Suzuki M, Granger DN. Nitric oxide: an endogenous modulator of leukocyte adhesion. *Proc Natl Acad Sci U S A* 1991;33:289–292.

109. Robbins RA, Nelson KJ, Gossman GL, Spurzem JM, Sisson JH, Romberger DJ, Rennard SI, Rubinstein I. Modulation of neutrophil adhesion to bronchial epithelial cells by nitric oxide. *Am Rev Respir Dis* 1993;147:A435.

110. Isalenti A, Ianaro A, Moncada S, Di Rosa M. Modulation of acute inflammation by endogenous nitric oxide. *Eur J Pharmacol* 1992;211:177–182.

111. Ialenti A, Moncada S, Di Rosa M. Modulation of adjuvant arthritis by endogenous nitric oxide. *Br J Pharmacol* 1993;110:701–706.

112. Mulligan MS, Hevel JM, Marletta MA, Ward PA. Tissue injury caused by deposition of immune complexes is L-arginine dependent. *Proc Natl Acad Sci U S A* 1991;88:6338–6342.

113. Miller MJS, Sadowska-Krowicka H, Chotinauruemol S, Kakkis JL, Clark DA. Amelioration of chronic ileitis by nitric oxide synthase inhibition. *J Pharmacol Exp Ther* 1993;264:11–16.

114. Farrell Aj, Blake DR, Palmer RMJ, Moncada S. Increased concentrations of nitrite in synovial fluid and serum samples suggest increased nitric oxide synthesis in rheumatic diseases. *Ann Rheum Dis* 1992;51:1219–1222.

115. Kirk SJ, Regan MC, Barbul A. Cloned murine T lymphocytes synthesize a molecule with biological characteristics of nitric oxide. *Biochem Biophys Res Commun* 1990;173:660–665.

116. Hoffman RA, Lanrehr JM, Billiar TR, Curran RD, Simmons RL. Alloantigen-induced activation of rat splenocytes is regulated by the oxidative metabolism of L-arginine. *J Immunol* 1990;145:2220–2226.

117. Albina JE, Abate JA, Henry WL Jr. Nitric oxide production is required for murine resident peritoneal macrophages to suppress mitogen-stimulated T cell proliferation; role of IFN-γ in the induction of the nitric oxide-synthesizing pathway. *J Immunol* 1991;147:144–148.

118. Langrehr JM, Hoffman RA, Billiar TR, Lee KKW, Schraut WH, Simmons RL. Nitric oxide synthesis in the *in vivo* allograft response; a possible regulatory mechanism. *Surgery* 1991;110:335–342.

119. Mills CD. Molecular basis of suppressor macrophages; arginine metabolism via the nitric oxide synthetase pathway. *J Immunol* 1991;146:2719–2723.

120. Taylor-Robinson AW, Liew FY, Severn A, et al. Regulation of the immune response by nitric oxide differentially produced by T helper type 1 and T helper type 2 cells. *Eur J Immunol* 1994;24:980–984.

121. Gruetter CA, Childers CC, Bosserman MK, Lemke SM, Ball JG, Valentovic MA. Comparison of relaxation induced by glyceryl trinitrate, isosobide dinitrate and sodium nitroprusside in bovine airways. *Am Rev Respir Dis* 1989;139:1192–1197.

122. Kishen R, Bleuvry BJ. Some actions of sodium nitroprusside and glyceryl trinitrate on guinea pig isolated trachealis muscle. *J Pharm Pharmacol* 1985;37:502–504.

123. Masaki Y, Munakata M, Ukita H, Houma Y, Kawakami Y. Nitric oxide (NO) can relax canine airway smooth muscle. *Am Rev Respir Dis* 1989;139:A350.

124. Högman M, Frostell C, Arnberg H, Hedenstierna G. Inhalation of nitric oxide modulates methacholine-induced bronchoconstriction in the rabbit. *Eur Respir J* 1993;6:177–180.

125. Munakata M, Masaki Y, Saxuma I, Ukita H, Obuka Y, Homma Y, et al. Pharmacological differentiation of epithelium-derived relaxing factor from nitric oxide. *J Appl Physiol* 1990;69:665–670.

126. Högman M, Frostell CG, Hedenström H, Hedenstierna G. Inhalation of nitric oxide modulates adult human bronchial tone. *Am Rev Respir Dis* 1993;148:1474–1478.

127. Hulks G, Warren PM, Douglas NJ. The effect of inhaled nitric oxide on bronchomotor tone in the normal human airway. *Am Rev Respir Dis* 1993;147:A515.

128. Fischer A, Mundel P, Mayer B, Preissler U, Philippin B, Dummer W. Nitric oxide synthase in guinea-pig lower airway innervation. *Neurosci Lett* 1993;149:157–160.

129. Dey RD, Dalal G, Pinkstaff CA, Mayer B, Kummer W, Said SI. Nitric oxide synthase and vasoactive intestinal peptide are colocalized in neurons of the ferret tracheal plexus. *Am Rev Respir Dis* 1993;147:A288.

130. Fischer A, Hoffman B, Hauser-Kronberger C, Mayer B, Kummer W. Nitric oxide synthase in the innervation of the human respiratory tract. *Am Rev Respir Dis* 1993;147:A662.

131. Tucker JF, Brane SR, Charalambons L, Hobbs AJ, Gibson A. L-N^G-nitroarginine inhibits nonadrenergic, noncholinergic relaxations of guinea pig trachea. *Br J Pharmacol* 1990;100:663–664.

132. Li CG, Rand MJ. Evidence that part of the NANC relaxant response of guinea-pig trachea to electrical field stimulation is mediated by nitric oxide. *Br J Pharmacol* 1991;102:91–94.

133. Kannan MS, Johnson DE. Functional innervation of pig tracheal smooth muscle: neural and nonneural mechanisms of relaxation. *J Pharmacol Exp Ther* 1992;260:1180–1184.

134. Kannan MS, Johnson DE. Nitric oxide mediates the neural nonadrenergic, noncholinergic relaxation of pig tracheal smooth muscle. *Am J Physiol* 1993;262:L511–L514.

135. Fischer JT, Anderson JW, Waldron MA. Nonadrenergic noncholinergic neurotransmission of feline trachealis: VIP or nitric oxide? *J Appl Physiol* 1993;74:31–39.

136. Yu M, Robinson E, Wang Z. Regional distribution of nitroxidergic and adrenergic nerves in equine airway smooth muscle. *Am Rev Respir Dis* 1993;147:A286.

137. Belvisi MG, Stretton CD, Barnes PJ. Nitric oxide is the endogenous neurotransmitter of bronchodilator nerves in human airways. *Eur J Pharmacol* 1992;210:221–222.

138. Belvisi MG, Stretton CD, Miura M, Verlenden GM, Tadjarimi S, Yacoub MH, et al. Inhibitory NANC nerves in human tracheal smooth muscle: a quest for the neurotrasmitter. *J Appl Physiol* 1992;73:2505–2510.

139. Ellis JL, Undem BJ. Inhibtion by L-N^G-nitro-L-arginine of nonadrenergic noncholinergic mediated relaxations of human isolated central and peripheral airways. *Am Rev Respir Dis* 1992;146:1543–1547.

140. Bai TR, Bramley AM. Effect of an inhibitor of nitric oxide synthase on neural relaxation in human bronchi. *Am J Physiol* 1993;8:425–430.

141. Lammers JWJ, Barnes PJ, Chung KF. Nonadrenergic, noncholinergic airway inhibitory nerves. *Eur Respir J* 1992;5:239–246.

142. Alving K, Fornhem C, Wietzberg E, Lundber JM. Nitric oxide mediates cigarette-smoke-induced vasodilatory responses in the lung. *Acta Physiol Scand* 1992;146:407–408.

143. Paré PD, Wiggs BR, James A, Hogg JC, Bosken C. The comparative mechanics and morphology of airways in asthma and in chronic obstructive pulmonary disease. *Am Rev Respir Dis* 1992;143:1189–1193.

144. Wiggs BR, Bosken C, Paré PD, James A, Hogg JC. A model of airway narrowing in asthma and in chronic obstructive pulmonary disease. *Am Rev Respir Dis* 1992;145:1251–1258.

145. Kuo H-P, Liu S, Barnes PJ. The effect of endogenous nitric oxide on neurogenic plasma exudation in guinea pig airways. *Eur J Pharmacol* 1992;221:177–182.

146. Marletta MA, Yoon PS, Iyengar R, Leaf CD, Wishnok JS. Macrophage oxidation of L-arginine to nitrite and nitrate; nitric oxide is an intermediate. *Biochemistry* 1988;27:8706–8611.

147. Fast DJ, Shannon BJ, Herriott MJ, Kennedy MJ, Rummage JA, Leu RW. Staphylococcal exotoxins stimulate nitric oxide-dependent murine macrophage tumoricidal activity. *Infect Immun* 1991;59:2987–2993.

148. Hibbs JB Jr, Taintor RR, Vavrin Z, et al. Synthesis of nitric oxide from a terminal guanidino nitrogen atom of L-arginine: a molecular mechanism regulating cellular proliferation that targets intracellular iron. In: Moncada S, Higgs EA, eds. *Nitric oxide from L-arginine: a bioregulatory system*. Amsterdam: Excerpta Medica, 1990;189–223.

149. Ignarro LJ. Heme-dependent activation of guanylate cyclase by nitric oxide: a novel signal transduction mechanism. *Blood Vessels* 1991;28:67–73.

150. Lepoivre M, Flaman J-M, Henry Y. Early loss of the tyrosyl radical ribonucleotide reductase of adenocarcinoma cells producing nitric oxide. *J Biol Chem* 1992;267:22994–223000.

151. Padgett EL, Pruett SB. Evaluation of nitrite production by human monocyte-derived macrophages. *Biochem Biophys Res Commun* 1992;186:775–781.

152. Hamid Q, Springall DR, Riveros-Moreno V, et al. Induction of nitric oxide synthase in asthma. *Lancet* 1993;342:1510–1513.

153. Jain B, Rubinstein I, Robbins RA, Leise KL, Sisson JH. Modulation of airway epithelial cell ciliary beat frequency by nitric oxide. *Biochem Biophys Res Commun* 1993;191:83–88.

154. Jain B, Robbins RA, Rubinstein I, Sisson JH. TNF-α and IL-1β modulate airway epithelial ciliary activity by a nitric oxide-dependent mechanism. *Clin Res* 1994;42:115A.

155. Gustafsson LE, Leone AM, Persson MG, Wiklund NP, Moncada S. Endogenous nitric oxide is present in the exhaled air of rabbits, guinea pigs and humans. *Biochem Biophys Res Commun* 1991;181:852–857.

156. Borland C, Cox Y, Higenbottam T. Measurement of exhaled nitric oxide in man. *Thorax* 1993;48:1160–1162.

157. Kharitonov SA, Yates D, Robbins RA, Logan-Sinclair R, Shinebourne EA, Barnes PJ. Increased nitric oxide in exhaled air of asthmatic patients. *Lancet* 1994; 343:133–135.

158. Alving K, Wietzberg E, Lundberg JM. Increased amount of nitric oxide in exhaled air of asthmatics. *Eur Respir J* 1993;6:1368–1370.

159. Persson MG, Zetterström O, Agrenius V, Ihre E, Gustafsson LE. Single-breath nitric oxide measurements in asthmatic patients and smokers. *Lancet* 1994;343:146–147.

160. Kharitonov SA, Evans DJ, Barnes PJ, O Connor BJ. Bronchial provocation challenge with histamine or adenosine 5′-monophosphate (AMP) does not alter exhaled nitric oxide in asthma. *Am J Respir Crit Care Med* 1995;151:A129.

161. Kharitonov SA, Evans DJ, Barnes PJ, O Connor BJ. Allergen-induced late asthmatic reactions are associated with elevation of nitric oxide in exhaled air. *Am J Respir Crit Care Med* 1995;151:A698.

162. Deykin A, Massaro AF, McGarry WP III, McFadden CA, Drazen JM, Israel E. Exhaled nitric oxide following allergen challenge in atopic patients with asthma. *Am J Respir Crit Care Med* 1995;151:A699.

163. Gerlach H, Rossaint R, Pappert D, Knorr M, Falke KJ. Autoinhalation of nitric oxide after endogenous synthesis in nasopharynx. *Lancet* 1994;343:518–519.

164. Robbins RA, Floreani AA, Von Essen SG, Sisson JH, Hill GE, Rubinstein I, Townley RG. Measurement of exhaled nitric oxide by three different techniques. *Am J Respir Crit Care Med* 1996;153:1631–1635.

165. Yates DH, Kharitonov SA, Worsdell M, Thomas PS, Barnes PJ. Exhaled nitric oxide is decreased after inhalation of a specific inhibitor of inducible nitric oxide synthase in asthmatic but not in normal subjects. *Am J Respir Crit Care Med* 1995;151:A699.

166. Ohna I, Ohkawara Y, Yamauchi K, Tanno Y, Takishima T. Production of tumor necrosis factor with IgE receptor triggering from sensitized lung tissue. *Am J Respir Cell Mol Biol* 1990;3:285–289.

167. Borish L, Mascali JJ, Dishuck J, Beam WR, Martin RJ, Rosenwasser LJ. Detection of alveolar macrophage-derived IL-1β in asthma: inhibition with corticosteroids. *J Immunol* 1992 149:3078–3082.

168. Yates DH, Kharitonov SA, Robbins RA, Thomas PS, Barnes PJ. Effect of a nitric oxide synthase inhibitor and a glucocorticosteroid on exhaled nitric oxide. *Am J Resp Crit Care Med* 1995;152:892–892.

169. Yates DH, Kharitonov SA, Scott DM, Worsdell M, Barnes PJ. Short and long acting β$_2$-agonists do not alter exhaled nitric oxide in asthma. *Am J Respir Crit Care Med* 1995;151:A129.

170. Fernandes LB, Preuss JMH, Paterson JW, Goldies RG. Epithelium-derived inhibitory factor in human bronchus. *Eur J Pharmacol* 1990;187:331–336.

171. Belvisi MG, Ward JK, Tadjarimi S, Yacoub MH, Barnes PJ. Inhibitory NANC nerves in human airways: differences in disease and after extrinsic denervation. *Am Rev Respir Dis* 1993;147:A286.

172. Rubanyi GM, Vanhoutte PM. Oxygen derived free radicals, endothelium and responsiveness of vascular smooth muscle. *Am J Physiol* 1986;250:H815–H821.

173. Sherwood J, Kretner W. Microvascular permaeability of guinea pig airways is modulated by nitric oxide formation. *FASEB J* 1994;8:A383.

174. Townley RG, Romero FA, Robbins RA. Inhibition of nitric oxide synthase (NOS) decreases edema formation during the late allergic skin response. *Am J Respir Crit Care Med* 1995;151:A127.

175. Erjefält JS, Erjefält I, Sundler F, Persson CGA. Mucosal nitric oxide may tonically suppress airways plasma exudation. *Am J Respir Crit Care Med* 1994;150:227–232.

176. Townley RG, Trapani IL, Szentivanyi A. Sensitization to analphylaxis and to some its pharmacological mediators by blockade of the beta adrenergic receptors. *J Allergy* 1967;39:177–197.

177. Heiss LN, Lancaster JR Jr, Corbett JA, Goldman WE. Epithelial autotoxicity of nitric oxide: role in the respiratory cytopathology of pertussis. *Proc Natl Acad Sci U S A* 1994;91:267–270.

Asthma, edited by P.J. Barnes, M.M. Grunstein,
A.R. Leff, and A.J. Woolcock.
Lippincott–Raven Publishers, Philadelphia © 1997.

▪ 54 ▪

Endothelins

Douglas W.P. Hay and Roy G. Goldie

The endothelium and its many biologically active constituents play a vital homeostatic role in the cardiovascular system (1,2). A major focus of research on endothelial cell biology in the 1980s was on relaxant substances released from the endothelium, in particular, endothelium-derived relaxing factor (EDRF), which was shown subsequently to be nitric oxide or a nitric oxide-containing moiety (3). During this time there was minimal information on endothelium-derived vasoconstrictor substances. However, evidence was provided that thromboxane and superoxide, released from the endothelium, and a protease-sensitive substance (i.e., peptide) produced by cultured bovine aortic endothelial cells, contracted vascular smooth muscle (4–6). In 1988, Yanagisawa and co-workers (7) described the isolation, purification, cloning, expression, and pharmacological characterization of a potent vasoconstrictor 21-amino-acid peptide, designated endothelin, which was released from porcine aortic endothelial cells (7). This material was demonstrated to be a member of a mam-

malian family of vasoconstrictor peptides, the endothelins (ETs), designated ET-1, ET-2 and ET-3, which are encoded by three similar but distinct genes, localized to chromosomes 6, 1 and 20, respectively (8–11). ET-1 is the original porcine/human ET; ET-2 differs by two amino-acid substitutions from ET-1, and ET-3 differs by six amino acids. The ETs possess a close structural and functional homology to a group of snake toxins, the sarafotoxins, which are found in the venom of the Middle Eastern burrowing asp, *Atractaspis engaddensis* (12–14).

Since the discovery of ET-1 a large amount of research has been performed on the biology of the ETs and, in particular, their potential physiological and pathophysiological roles. There have been approximately 5,200 publications on these mediators at the time of this writing. ETs cause an array of biologic activities in various cells and tissues (12–14). For example, there is increasing research and information describing diverse effects of the ETs, in particular ET-1, in the pulmonary system. In this chapter, a review of the present understanding of the influence of the ETs in various cells in the lung will be provided, with special attention to evidence for a pathophysiological role of the ETs in asthma. Thus, the focus will be on information in human cells and tissues [note that most studies in the lung have utilized ET-1].

D. W. P. Hay: Department of Pulmonary Pharmacology, SmithKline Beecham Pharmaceuticals, King of Prussia, Pennsylvania 19406.

R. G. Goldie: Department of Pharmacology, University of Western Australia, Nedlands, Western Australia 6907, Australia.

SYNTHESIS, DISTRIBUTION, RELEASE, METABOLISM, UPTAKE AND CLEARANCE

Synthesis

ET-1 synthesis involves an unusual, two-step, proteolytic process (7) (Fig. 1). In humans, the initial stage results in the formation of a 38-amino-acid residue intermediate, designated "big endothelin," from a 212-residue preproendothelin, via the activity of an endopeptidase(s), which is specific for the paired dibasic amino-acid residues (8,12–15). Big endothelin also is formed from preproendothelin under the catalytic influence of furin, a mammalian convertase involved in the processing of precursors (16). Big endothelin then undergoes a previously unknown type of cleavage between Trp[73] and Val[74], via the activity of a putative endopeptidase with chymotrypsin-like activity, called "endothelin-converting enzyme (ECE)" (7,8,12–15). ET does not appear to be stored preformed but is generated by *de novo* synthesis (12,14,17).

The contractile potency of big ET-1 in isolated blood vessels is at least 100-fold less than ET-1, suggesting that the formation of ET-1 is critical for optimal biologic activity of the ET system (18,19).

There are results from various systems suggesting the existence of several ECE-like enzymatic activities, both cytosolic and membrane-associated. However, most of the evidence indicates that the physiologically relevant ECE is a membrane-bound, neutral metalloprotease, which is sensitive to phosphoramidon (14,17). There is considerable information from *in vitro* studies in the lung that supports this postulate. A phosphoramidon-sensitive (IC$_{50}$ = 0.5 μM) neutral protease, which converts big ET-1 to ET-1, was detected in rat lung; the ratio in the membrane vs. the cytosol was 4:1 (20). ECE has also been partially solubilized and purified from porcine lung, and purified to homogeneity from rat lung microsome (21,22). The purified enzyme (m.w. =130 kDa) specifically catalyzed the conversion of big ET-1 to ET-1 by a mechanism that was inhibited by phosphoramidon and metal chelators (22). Sucrose-gradient ultracentrifugation analysis suggests that a significant portion of the ECE activity is associated with the Golgi apparatus, where it co-exists with endogenous ET-1 (23). Two distinct forms of ECE called ECE-1 and ECE-2 have been described recently. Both enzymes are found in bovine aortic endothelial cells and are sensitive to phosphoramidon. ECE-1 is cell membrane-bound, and ECE-2 is associated with the trans-Golgi network and is approximately 250 times more sensitive to phosphoramidon than ECE-1 (24,25). ECE-1 may convert both intracellular and exogenously applied big ET-1 and ECE-2 may control only the intracellular conversion of big ET-1, perhaps in vesicles derived from trans-Golgi network (26). An ECE, sensitive to phosphoramidon and thiorphan, has been isolated from human bronchiolar smooth muscle cells (27). There is also evidence *in vivo* and from studies isolated-using perfused lungs that the ECE in airways is phosphoramidon-sensitive (28–30).

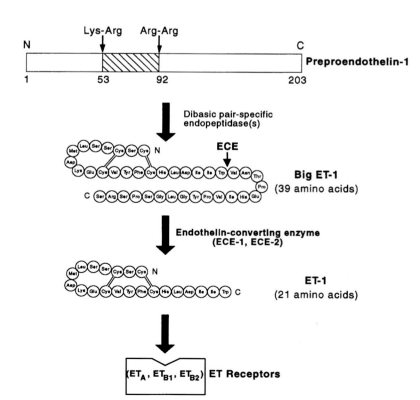

FIG. 1. Endothelin-1 (ET-1) biosynthetic pathway. (Adapted from Yanagisawa M, Kurihara H, Kimura S, Tomobe Y, Kobayashi M, Mitsui Y, et al. A novel potent vasoconstrictor peptide produced by vascular endothelial cells. *Nature* 1988; 332:411–415.)

Several other types of ECE activity other than the previously mentioned membrane-bound, phosphoramidon-sensitive form have been demonstrated. For example, an aspartic protease with ECE activity in rat lung was proposed and evidence was presented for a novel, serine protease enzyme in the soluble fraction of porcine lung, which cleaved big ET-1 at the bond between Val^{22} and Asn^{23} (31). This enzyme was sensitive to diisopropylfluorophosphate and called ET-Val-generating endopeptidase (32). A lung mast cell-derived chymase was speculated to produce extracellular processing of big ET-1 to ET-1 in the perfused rat lung (33). The physiological significance of these putative ECEs in the pulmonary system is unknown.

Distribution

ETs are distributed widely in mammals, including humans. Concentrations in the lung are among the highest detected (34–37). The cellular origins of ET in the pulmonary system include the endothelium, epithelium, endocrine cells, as well as some inflammatory cells (38–42).

ET-1 messenger ribonucleic acid (mRNA) was measured in human lung homogenates and ir-ET and mRNA for the three ET isoforms has been demonstrated in human airway epithelial and endocrine cells (42,43). Immunoreactivity was observed predominantly in pulmonary endocrine cells and, to a lesser extent, in the airway epithelium (in about 50% of human adults) (42). ET concentrations (immunoreactivity and mRNA) in vascular endothelial cells are highest in the developing lung, decrease before birth, and are minimal in adults. Therefore, it has been speculated that ET is involved in growth regulation (42). The expression and release of ET-1 also has been demonstrated from human macrophages, an inflammatory cell found in relatively high numbers in the lung (41).

Release

Consistent with the detection of ET mRNA and ir-ET in airway epithelium and the presence of ECE in the lung, ET-1 is released basally from cultured porcine, canine and human bronchial epithelial cells, and from cultured guinea-pig and rabbit tracheal epithelial cells (44–48). The release of ET from cultured tracheal epithelial cells is increased by endotoxin, thrombin, and various cytokines (46–50). For example, interleukin (IL)-1α, IL-1β, and tumor necrosis factor (TNF)-α enhanced the expression of prepro ET-1 mRNA and ET-1 release from human cultured bronchial epithelial cells (50). The regulatory role of the cytokines on ET-1 synthesis and release may be of relevance in inflammation and tissue repair associated with many pulmonary disorders.

Metabolism

Based on the ability of the epithelium to inhibit ET-1-induced contractile responses in guinea-pig trachea through a mechanism which was sensitive to phosphoramidon, an inhibitor of neutral endopeptidase (NEP), it was hypothesized that ET-1 is metabolized by epithelium-derived NEP (51). The epithelium is a rich source of NEP, for which the ETs were demonstrated subsequently to be good substrates (52–54). There is additional functional data to support a modulatory role of epithelium-derived NEP on ET-1-induced contraction in guinea-pig trachea, including attenuation of ET-1-induced contraction by recombinant human NEP (55,56). In a pig lung membrane fraction, NEP was demonstrated to be the principal metabolic pathway for ET-1 (57). Furthermore, *in vivo* studies in guinea pigs have demonstrated that phosphoramidon potentiates ET-1-induced bronchoconstriction (58). In human bronchus, there is conflicting information on the influence of NEP on the metabolism of the ETs. Thus, one study indicated that NEP is involved in the breakdown of ET-3 but not ET-1, whereas other studies concluded that phosphoramidon-sensitive NEP attenuates contraction induced by ET-1, and also ET-2 and ET-3 (59–61).

Collectively, the data indicate that two phosphoramidon-sensitive enzymes have opposing effects in the control of ET-1 levels in airways: one (ECE) is involved in the synthesis of ET-1 from big ET-1, and another (NEP) is involved in ET-1 metabolism. Although NEP appears to be the major enzyme involved in the degradation of ET-1 in the airways, it was suggested that cathepsin G, rather than NEP, is involved in ET-1 metabolism by activated human polymorphonuclear neutrophils (62).

Uptake and Clearance

There are significant species differences in the contribution of the pulmonary circulation to the uptake and clearance of ET. In rats, the accumulation of intravenously administered ET-1 was largely in the lungs (up to 82%), predominantly to alveolar capillary endothelium (63–66). Substantial removal of ET-1 by the pulmonary circulation (> 50% in a single passage) also occurred in guinea-pig and rat-isolated perfused lungs (67). In rabbits significant uptake of ET-1 was demonstrated by the pulmonary, but not the coronary, circulation (68). By contrast, no clearance in the lungs was observed during infusion of ET-1 in pigs, (36). Uptake of [^{125}I]-ET-1 in rat-perfused lungs (80% of which occurred after a single passage), was inhibited by BQ-788, the ET$_B$ receptor antagonist, suggesting a role for this ET receptor subtype in this phenomenon (69). Conflicting data have been reported in humans. Thus, in two studies in humans, it was estimated that the lung is the main organ responsible for the removal of ET-1, accounting for approximately 50% of the elimination after intravenous infusion. In contrast, another study concluded that ET was not extracted by the pulmonary system in humans (70–72).

RECEPTORS

Background

Based upon the quantitative and qualitative differences in the pharmacological profiles of the ET isoforms in various systems, it soon became apparent that the many biologic effects of the ETs were mediated through ET receptor subtypes (12–14,73–76). A few years ago biochemical, molecular, and functional studies clearly demonstrated the existence of two mammalian ET receptors, designated ET_A and ET_B. Subsequent research produced evidence for additional receptors, designated provisionally as subtypes of the ET_A and ET_B receptors, as well as an ET_C receptor. For example, binding studies in rat brain and atrium provided evidence for two subtypes of ET_B receptors, called ET_{B1}, which were designated as super high-affinity sites (in the pM range) and ET_{B2}, high-affinity sites (77). It was hypothesized that ET_{B1} receptors were involved in the vasodilator effects of the ETs, whereas ET_{B2} receptors mediated the vasoconstriction (77–79). However, there remains considerable uncertainty about ET receptor classification (80). In the following sections, information is presented concerning our present understanding of ET receptors, with particular emphasis on the results of studies in lung, which has been widely used for research on ET receptor classification, isolation, and purification.

Biochemical and Molecular Biologic Studies

Biochemical studies provided initial evidence for more than one ET receptor in lung. Cross-linking, affinity labeling studies in rat lung membranes suggested the presence of two ET receptors, one (44kDa) which had greater affinity for ET-1 and ET-2 than ET-3, and another (32kDa) which had a greater affinity for ET-3 (81). Ligand binding and affinity labeling studies in porcine lung also provided evidence for two distinct ET receptor subtypes, an ET-1-specific receptor (ET_A) and an ET_B receptor that has similar affinities for all members of the ET/sarafotoxin family (82).

The cloning and expression of complementary deoxyribonucleic acid (cDNA) of ET_A and ET_B receptors has been achieved in several systems, including lung (14, 73,74,83–85). An additional ET receptor subtype, ET_C, which possesses selectivity for ET-3, has been cloned from *Xenopus laevis* dermal melanophores, but not from any mammalian system, although there is evidence for its presence in rat cultured anterior pituitary cells and rat PC12 phaeochromocytoma cells (14,86–88). ET receptors

belong to the superfamily of G-protein-coupled, seven transmembrane domain spanning receptors (14,73,74, 83–85,88). The human ET_A and the ET_B receptors have been cloned, and the ET_A receptor has been localized to chromosome 4 (85,89–93). High or moderate distribution of mRNA for ET_A and ET_B receptors in human tissues has been detected in various tissues including lung (85,91,93).

The solubilization of ET_A and ET_B receptors from rat lung and the isolation and purification of the ET_B receptor from bovine lung have been demonstrated (94–97).

Functional Studies

Considerable functional data exist supporting the presence of multiple ET receptors in the pulmonary system. Initially, indirect evidence, based on a comparison of the contractile activities of various ligands and also cross-desensitization experiments, provided evidence for distinct ET receptors in guinea-pig airways and guinea-pig pulmonary artery (98–101). Subsequently, direct support for ET receptor subtypes in the pulmonary system has been provided utilizing subtype-selective ligands. These include sarafotoxin S6c, (Ala^{1,3,11,15})-ET-1, IRL 1620 and BQ-3020 (ET_B-receptor agonists), BQ-123 and FR 139317 (peptide ET_A-receptor antagonists) and RES-701-1 (peptide ET_B- receptor antagonists of microbial origin) (102–108). Using such compounds as well as recently identified nonpeptide compounds, e.g. bosentan and SB 209670, it was demonstrated that ET_A receptors predominantly mediated ET-induced contraction in guinea-pig and human pulmonary artery, whereas in guinea-pig trachea and bronchus and in human bronchus, the ET_B receptor population is largely responsible for ET-induced contraction (109–114).

However, within a tissue, different receptors may exist and subserve distinct roles. For example, in human bronchus in contrast to the contractile response (largely ET_B-mediated), ET-induced airway smooth muscle mitogenesis and prostanoid release appear to involve ET_A receptor activation (115–117).

Functional studies indicate regional differences in the relative distribution of ET_A and ET_B receptors in guinea-pig airways. Although both ET_A and ET_B receptors contribute to contraction in guinea pig bronchus and trachea, ET_B receptor-mediated response predominates over ET_A receptor-induced contraction in guinea pig bronchus, whereas ET_A and ET_B receptors contribute equally to the ET-1-induced contraction in guinea-pig trachea and parenchyma, as occurs in rat teachea (113,118,119). *In vivo* experiments indicate that ET-induced bronchoconstriction in guinea-pigs involves ET_B receptor activation (120).

The classification of ET receptors is incomplete. Thus, although there is increasing evidence from functional and binding studies for the existence of additional subtypes of

ET receptors, further research is required to elucidate the distribution and physiological and pathophysiological significance of these putative receptors (78,80,121,122). It is noteworthy that to date only two mammalian receptors, ET_A and ET_B, have been identified by molecular biologic techniques, and there are limitations to receptor classification using only the results of functional studies (123). A complicating factor in ET receptor classification is that ET-1 binds to ET_A and ET_B receptors in a pseudo-irreversible manner, and there are ET ligand-dependent as well as species-dependent differences in the kinetic characteristics of ET-receptor agonists and antagonists (123–131). In addition, the potency of ET-receptor antagonists may depend on the ET ligand (78,118,122,132).

Receptor Localization

Appreciable quantities of high-affinity ET-1 binding sites are detected in various regions of the respiratory tract of humans and several animal species (133–139). In human bronchial tissues, labeling of [125I]-ET-1 was localized predominantly to airway and vascular smooth muscle, with little or no binding to cartilage, connective tissues, the submucosal layer (including glandular cells), or the epithelium (134,136). Similar results were observed in mouse, rat, and guinea-pig tracheal sections, although in sheep trachea, large amounts of specific binding sites for ET-1 in cells associated with submucosal glands and in the submucosa immediately below the epithelium (lamina propria) were detected (136,139). In human, rat, and guinea-pig airways, significant binding was associated with alveolar septae and parasympathetic ganglia and with paravascular nerves and nerves in the connective tissues (134–136,138). A single, specific, high-affinity binding site for [125I]-ET-1 was demonstrated on cultured human bronchial smooth muscle cells (K_d of 0.11 nM and B_{max} = 22.1 fmol/10^6 cells) (45).

There is conflicting information as to the presence of ET receptors in airway epithelium. Thus, in contrast to some of the earlier studies, binding sites in airway epithelium have been reported. For example, in guinea-pig tracheal epithelium diffuse binding was noted, although it was markedly less than that in the smooth muscle and especially in the submucosal region (133). Significant labeling of [125I]-ET has been detected in rat airway epithelium, feline tracheal epithelial cells (two sites), and rat alveolar type II cells (63,140,141). In situ hybridization studies indicate strongly positive staining for ET_B receptor probes in ciliated and nonciliated rat and rabbit bronchial epithelial cells (142). Specific binding sites for [125I]-ET-1, which appear to be of the ET_A receptor subtype, were demonstrated in cultured canine tracheal epithelial cells (143). The location of ET receptors on the same cells that synthesize ET suggests that there may be autocrine regulation of its secretion (142).

Both ET_A and ET_B receptors are abundant in mammalian lung, including humans. Autoradiography and binding studies reveal that there was no difference in the proportions of ET_B and ET_A receptors in human bronchial smooth muscle from both nonasthmatic and asthmatic lung about 88% ET_B: 12% nonET_B). However, functionally there was evidence of receptor desensitization in asthmatic tissues (shift to the right in sarafotoxin S6c concentration-response curves), perhaps as a result of excessive ET release and receptor activation over an extended period (144). There are species differences in the relative amounts of ET receptor subtypes and their regional distribution (Table 1). For example, using immunohistochemical and immunoprecipitation techniques with an ET_B-specific antiserum, it was calculated that about 70% of the ET receptors in bovine lung were of the ET_B subtype (144,145). In rat pulmonary tissues, binding studies indicated that the proportions of ET_A:ET_B receptors in bronchus are about 70:30, whereas in lung parenchyma the reverse ratio was observed (146). Autoradiographic analysis confirmed the predominance of the ET_A receptor in the bronchi, as well as the pulmonary vasculature, and of the ET_B receptor in the parenchyma (146). Similarly, autoradiography demonstrated the presence of the ET_A and ET_B receptors in similar amounts in rat tracheal smooth muscle (147), whereas in ovine tracheal smooth muscle, an almost homogeneous population of ET_A receptors appears to exist (147–149). Functionally, both ET_A and ET_B receptors are present in guinea-pig trachea (with the amounts of ET_A receptors decreasing from proximal to distal regions), whereas in bronchus, ET_B receptors predominate (113).

In pig airways, the ratio of ET_A:ET_B receptors, assessed using inhibition of [125I]-ET-1 binding with BQ-123 and sarafotoxin S6c, was 30:70 in the trachea and 70:30 in the bronchus (150). The relative regional distribution of ET_A and ET_B receptors in human lung has not been reported.

Binding studies in rat lung membranes indicated that the ratio of ET_A:ET_B receptors was 60:40 and 70:30 (151,152). In porcine lung, appreciable binding of the ET_B-selective radioligand, [125I]-BQ-3020, was demonstrated in paren-

TABLE 1. *Relative proportions of ET_A and ET_B receptors in pulmonary tissues*

Species	Tissues	Approximate Ratio ET_A: ET_B	References
Human	Bronchus	10:90	144
	Pulmonary artery	90:10	154,155
Sheep	Trachea	100:0	139
Pig	Trachea	30:70	150
	Bronchus	70:30	
Rabbit	Pulmonary artery	20:80	155
Rat	Trachea	50:50	147
Mouse	Trachea	40:60	185

ET, endolithin

chyma, parasympathetic ganglia, pulmonary and submucosal plexuses, with minimal binding to circular smooth muscle layers or airway epithelium (153).

In human pulmonary artery, functional and radioligand binding studies indicate that the predominant receptor is of the ET_A subtype, although mRNA encoding both ET_A and ET_B receptors has been demonstrated (113,114,154, 155). In rabbit pulmonary artery, both ET_A and ET_B receptors are present, with the ET_B receptor being the major subtype that mediates the contractile response (155, 156). The relative proportions of ET_A:ET_B receptors in membrane preparations of human and rabbit pulmonary artery are 93:7 and 23:77, respectively (155).

SIGNAL TRANSDUCTION

Although it was originally proposed by Yanagisawa and co-workers (7) that ET-1 produced contractions in porcine coronary artery by stimulating voltage-dependent, membrane Ca^{2+} channels, most subsequent studies have indicated that ET-induced responses in the majority of systems result from activation of the phosphatidylinositol pathway and release of intracellular Ca^{2+} (14,74,157–166). Thus, ET-1 stimulates the formation of inositol phosphates and diacylglyerol/protein kinase, the two second messengers formed from the metabolism of phosphatidylinositol, and enhances intracellular concentrations of Ca^{2+} (14,74,161–164). In addition, purported protein kinase C inhibitors decreased ET-1-induced responses (14,74,161,165,166).

Most of the information on signal transduction mechanisms in the lung comes from contraction studies in airway and pulmonary vascular smooth muscle. In the first study exploring the effects of ET-1 in the pulmonary system, contraction induced by ET-1 in guinea-pig trachea was reduced by nicardipine, the dihydropyridine, voltage-dependent Ca^{2+} channel inhibitor, supporting the original hypothesis that ET-1 is an endogenous Ca^{2+} agonist (7,167). Further studies revealed that ET-1-induced contraction in this tissue is mediated predominantly by stimulation of phosphatidylinositol turnover and intracellular Ca^{2+} release, with only a minor contribution of extracellular Ca^{2+} influx through voltage-dependent membrane channels. For example, ET-1-induced contraction is resistant to incubation in Ca^{2+}-free physiological buffer or Ca^{2+} channel inhibitors. ET-1 stimulates phosphatidylinositol turnover in guinea-pig trachea with a potency comparable to that which elicits the contractile response (168–171). A similar mechanism appears to be responsible for ET-induced contraction in guinea-pig isolated pulmonary arteries and veins (171). *In vivo* ET-1-induced bronchoconstriction in guinea pigs is not markedly influenced by Ca^{2+} channel inhibitors (172,173). ET-1, but not ET-3, increased PI turnover in human bronchus; unlike ET-1, ET-3-induced contractions are mediated by the influx of extracellular Ca^{2-} (174). ET-1

also increased phosphatidylinositol turnover in rat trachea and bovine bronchus (147,175). Interestingly, ET-3 did not enhance phosphatidylinositol pathway in bovine bronchus, and, unlike responses produced by ET-1, ET-3-induced contractions were markedly decreased by nifedipine (175). This would suggest that agonist-dependent differences exist in the mechanisms responsible for contractions produced by ET ligands. In relation to this, a previous report presented evidence, based on autoradiographic, biochemical and functional studies, that ET_A and ET_B receptors contribute to the ET-1-induced contraction in rat tracheal smooth muscle via different second messenger pathways involving stimulation of phosphatidylinositol turnover and activation of extracellular Ca^{2+} influx (via non-L-type membrane channels), respectively (147). Furthermore, in rat lung ET_A receptor activation may be linked to stimulation of phosphoinositol metabolism and arachidonic-acid release, whereas ET_B receptors were only associated with the former pathway (152).

Pretreatment with protein kinase C inhibitors had no effect on contractions induced by ET-1 in guinea-pig trachea or bovine bronchus, but decreased responses in rabbit trachea, suggesting that there are species differences in the contribution of protein kinase C to ET-1-induced responses (169,175,176). ET-1 stimulated cyclic adenosine 3'5'-monophosphate (cAMP) formation and the phosphatidylinositol pathway in cultured embryonic bovine tracheal cells (177). It has been proposed that there may be a role for Na^+/H^+ exchange in ET-1-induced contraction in guinea-pig airways (178).

Most studies indicated that ET-1-induced contraction in human airways is mediated through release of intracellular Ca^{2+} rather than influx with extracellular Ca^{2+} via voltage-sensitive channels, although it was reported that part of the response in human bronchus was mediated by the latter mechanism (135,179–181). In cultured human bronchial smooth muscle, ET-1 elicits a biphasic rise in intracellular Ca^{2+} via stimulation of the phosphatidylinositol pathway, and influx of extracellular Ca^{2+} via a dihydropyridine-insensitive membrane channel (182).

The evidence indicates that ET-induced contraction of human and animal isolated airways appears to be largely due to stimulation of PI turnover and mobilization of intracellular Ca^{2+}, although the relative contribution of these signal transduction pathways may depend on the ET receptor subtype, the ET ligand, and the species.

BIOLOGIC EFFECTS IN THE PULMONARY SYSTEM

In light of the abundance of the ETs and their receptors in mammalian lung (*vide supra*) it is perhaps not surprising that several activities of the ET ligands, primarily ET-1, have been demonstrated. The most widely studied effect of ET-1 is contraction of airway smooth muscle. However, there are accumulating data on actions of the ETs other than contractile effects, several of which may be relevant to a potential pathophysiological role (Table 2) (Fig. 2).

In Vitro Studies

Contractile Activity

Airway Smooth Muscle

The ETs are among the most potent contractile agonists in isolated mammalian airway smooth muscle preparations identified to date. For example, ET-1 potently contracts human bronchial smooth muscle, with $EC_{50}s$ in the 1-30 nM range (135,136,138,167–169,183). A correlation exists between the density of ET-1 binding sites and the contractile effects induced by ET-1 in human, rat, and guinea-pig preparations (136). In human bronchus (normal and asthmatic), evidence suggests that ET_B receptor activation is responsible predominantly for ET-1-induced contraction (113,118). Similar findings are observed in guinea-pig bronchus and rabbit bronchus, although in guinea pig trachea, there is a significant contribution of ET_A receptors to the response (113,132,184). In rat and mouse trachea, which have equivalent proportions of ET_A and ET_B receptors, ET-1 induces contraction by stimulation of both receptor subtypes (119,185).

In human bronchus ET-1 appears to be more potent than ET-2 or ET-3, perhaps partly because of differences in susceptibility to metabolism by NEP (59,61,135,138, 177). ET-1-induced contraction of human bronchus, fer-

ret, and bovine airways is not modulated by cyclooxygenase products, whereas in guinea-pig trachea there is conflicting information on the ability of cyclooxygenase products to modulate ET-1-induced contraction (117,136, 138,168–170,175,179,183,186,187).

In human bronchus, ET-1-induced contraction appears to occur via a direct mechanism which does not involve a contribution from acetylcholine, PAF, histamine, peptidoleukotrienes, or tachykinins (117). However, in guinea-

TABLE 2. *Potentially relevant effects induced by ET-1 in human pulmonary cells and tissues*

Locus	Effect	Predominant ET Receptor Subtype	References
Airway smooth muscle	Contraction	ET_B	113,144
Airway smooth muscle	Proliferation	ET_A	116
Airway smooth muscle	Prostanoid release	ET_A	117
Pulmonary vascular smooth muscle	Contraction	ET_A	113,114,155
Pulmonary vascular smooth muscle	Proliferation	ET_A	227
Nasal mucosa	Lactoferrin and glycoprotein release	?	220
Nasal mucosa	Prostanoid release	?	222

ET, endolithin

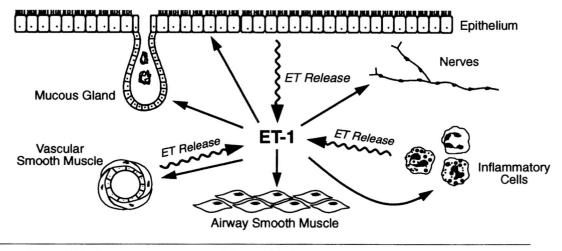

Sites of ET release:
- Epithelium
- Endothelium
- Inflammatory cells
- Endocrine cells

Effects of ET in lung:
- Smooth muscle contraction
- Mitogenesis
- Inflammatory cell chemotaxis
- Mediator release
- Microvascular permeability
- Neuromodulation
- Smooth muscle relaxation
- Mucous secretion
- Ciliary beating
- Cl⁻ secretion

FIG. 2. Summary of loci for release; potential sites of action and effects of ET-1 in the lung.

pig trachea there is conflicting evidence for indirect pathways, involving the release of mediators such as PAF, peptidoleukotriene and histamine, mediating ET-1-induced contraction (169,187–191). ET-1 stimulates the release of various prostanoids, in particular PGD_2, from guinea-pig trachea and human bronchus (117,188). Although based on the lack of effect of cyclooxygenase inhibitors—they do not contribute significantly to the contractile response—the possibility exists that they influence ET-induced effects other than bronchospasm.

Pulmonary Vascular Smooth Muscle

ETs potently contract isolated human pulmonary artery and vein (135,137,138). The response to ET-1 in human pulmonary artery is due predominantly to ET_A-receptor activation, i.e., responses were potently antagonized by BQ-123, whereas S6c, the ET_B-selective agonist, had no effect on vascular smooth muscle tone (113,114). However, in human small pulmonary resistance arteries (150 to 200 μm, i.d.), evidence was presented for a significant role of ET_B receptors in mediating ET-1 induced contraction (192). Furthermore, ET_B receptors mediate contraction in porcine pulmonary vein and artery and rabbit pulmonary artery (121,193,194). In guinea-pig pulmonary artery ET-1 and ET-2, on the one hand, and ET-3, on the other, have been proposed to elicit contraction via distinct receptors (195). ET-1 potently contracted rat pulmonary artery (EC_{50} = 1.3 nM) and pulmonary vein (EC_{50} = 0.6 nM) (196).

The relative contribution of ET_A and ET_B receptors to ET-1-induced contraction may depend on the level of the pulmonary vasculature. For example, ET_B-agonists generally are effective contractile agents in small arteries and veins but not major pulmonary arteries (121,197). Pulmonary veins are generally more sensitive to ET-1 than are pulmonary arteries (197–200).

In isolated rat lungs, ET-1 elicits an increase in pulmonary artery pressure when basal tone is low, whereas with elevated tone ET-1 may produce pulmonary vasodilation (201–203). In rat isolated lungs the pulmonary vasoconstrictor response to ET-1 does not involve cyclooxygenase products, but appears to be inhibited by released NO (200,204). In contrast, in guinea-pig perfused lungs cyclooxygenase inhibitors attenuate ET-1-induced pulmonary vasoconstriction (67).

Relaxant Activity

Airway Smooth Muscle

Although normally a potent contractile agonist in guinea-pig trachea, ET-1 has been shown to produce a transient relaxant response in this tissue (118,205,206). In studies utilizing isolated tracheal spiral preparations,

under either basal or precontracted conditions, ET-1-induced relaxation was epithelium-dependent and in precontracted tissues it was postulated that the ET-1-induced relaxation was due to release of NO from epithelial cells (118,206). However, the relaxation induced by ET-1 in guinea-pig trachea *in situ* was not influenced by removal of the epithelium or by cyclooxygenase inhibitors (205). Under basal tone, ET-1-induced relaxation, which occurred before a sustained contractile response, was inhibited by the ET_A-receptor antagonists, BQ-123 or FR 139317, and not produced by IRL 1620, the ET_B-selective agonist. It was proposed to be due to activation of ET_A receptors on epithelial cells (118). ET-1- and ET-3-induced relaxation of guinea-pig trachea may also involve charybdotoxin-sensitive K^+ channels (207). ET-1 ($\leq 10^{-9}$ M) also produces an epithelium-dependent relaxation in isolated rabbit trachea which was associated with enhanced release of prostaglandin (PG)I_2 and PGE_2, and is decreased, but not abolished, by indomethacin (10 μM), suggesting a role for epithelium-derived prostanoid and nonprostanoid relaxants (176).

Pulmonary Vascular Smooth Muscle

In various isolated or perfused vascular smooth muscles, the ETs and sarafotoxins elicit an endothelium-dependent relaxation via NO release (75,208–210). In precontracted rat pulmonary arteries, ET-1 did not elicit relaxation, whereas in porcine pulmonary artery both ET-1 and ET-3 were potent relaxants via a mechanism which was not affected by an ET_A-receptor antagonist, BQ-153, suggesting ET_B receptor activation underlies this phenomenon (193,202). In rat lungs, the vasodilation response to ET-1 or ET-3 was potentiated by cyclooxygenase inhibition or a thromboxane receptor antagonist but was not affected by N^a-monomethyl-L-arginine (L-NMMA) or methylene blue, suggesting that ET-1- or ET-3-induced vasodilation is due to the release of inhibitory prostanoids rather than NO (202,211).

Airway Epithelium

The epithelium is important in the pathophysiology of several lung disorders, notably asthma and cystic fibrosis (212–214). The airway epithelium is a significant site of release of the ETs, and ET receptors are also present (*vide supra*). There have only been a few reports describing the effects of the ETs on the airway epithelium.

ET-1 increased the negativity of transepithelial potential difference in ferret trachea (215). Furthermore, ET-1 (0.1 nM–1 μM), but not ET-2 or ET-3, stimulated the potential difference and short-circuit current in canine tracheal epithelium, resulting in a selective increase in Cl^- secretion, with no effect on Na^+ absorption; the mechanism was partially dependent on the release of cyclooxygenase products (216). ET-1 increased, through an indomethacin-sensitive mechanism, short-circuit current in canine tracheal epithelium (EC_{50} = 2.2 nM), and also stimulated mucosal net ^{36}Cl flux, with no effect on ^{22}Na flux, enhanced [^3H]-arachidonate release from membrane phospholipids and increased intracellular Ca^{2+} and cAMP accumulation (217). ET-1 potently increased ciliary beat frequency (EC_{50} = 3 nM) in canine cultured tracheal epithelium, as well as enhancing short circuit current and Cl^- secretion, by a mechanism involving the release of prostanoids (218). Relatively high concentrations of ET-1 (0.1 μM–10 μM) stimulated the release of several prostanoids from [^3H]-arachidonic acid-labeled cultured feline tracheal epithelial cells (140).

ET-1 potently (EC_{50} = 0.7 nM) enhanced phosphatidylcholine secretion (2-fold maximum with 10 nM) from rat alveolar type II cells via a mechanism involving an influx of extracellular Ca^{2+} through voltage-dependent membrane channels and the diacyglycerol/protein kinase C system (141). It was speculated that endothelium-derived ET-1 may regulate surfactant secretion (141).

Mucous Glands

ET-1 is located in human nasal mucosal tissue, primarily in the endothelium and venous sinusoids and [^{125}I]-ET-1 binding sites are demonstrated in submucosal glands, venous sinusoids, and small muscular arterioles (219,220). ET-1 stimulated serous and mucous cell secretion although high concentrations of ET-1 (0.1 μM - 10 μM) were required (220). There is conflicting information from studies in animals investigating the influence of ET-1 on mucous gland secretion. Thus, ET-1 (1 nM–1 μM) increased glycoconjugate secretion from feline tracheal isolated glands, but decreased secretion from tracheal explants (221). In ferret trachea, ET-1 alone was without effect on serous cell secretion, and inhibited phenylephrine- or methacholine-induced secretion (215). ET-1 increased prostanoid production in human cultured nasal mucosa, but again high peptide concentrations were required (≥ 0.1 μM) (222).

Smooth Muscle and Fibroblast Proliferation

Airways remodeling, including increased airway smooth muscle mass, is a feature of chronic asthma. In the initial publication, ET-1 (EC_{50} = ca. 1 nM) produced a small (2.3 fold) mitogenic response in cultured human *bronchial* smooth muscle cells, which was not inhibited by salbutamol (115,223). However, a subsequent study revealed no significant influence of ET-1 on proliferation of cultured human *tracheal* smooth muscle (116). In this study ET-1, but not sarafotoxin S6c, potentiated proliferation induced by the powerful mitogen, EGF. The potentiating influence

(approximately a 3- to 3.5-fold increase) is blocked by BQ-123, but not BQ-788, suggesting that it is due to ET_A receptor activation. ET-1 potently but modestly increased proliferation in guinea pig, rabbit, and ovine cultured tracheal smooth muscle cell (223–225). In ovine smooth muscle, ET-1 (0.1 and 1 μM) transiently enhanced by about 2.5-fold the expression of the proto-oncogene c-*fos* mRNA (225). Expression of c-*fos* was demonstrated in bronchial biopsies from 8 out of 12 asthmatic patients but not in any of the 10 nonasthmatic specimens (226). Perhaps surprisingly, the c-*fos* expression was localized to the airway epithelium rather than the smooth muscle.

Proliferative activity of the ETs also was demonstrated in pulmonary vasculature, which may be important in the etiology of pulmonary hypertension, specifically the characteristic vascular remodeling. ET-1 and ET-3 produced concentration-dependent mitogenesis of human pulmonary artery smooth muscle cells via an ET_A-receptor-mediated mechanism (sensitive to BQ-123) (227). ET-1 (1 nM - 3 nM) generally stimulated DNA synthesis and proliferation of pig pulmonary artery smooth muscle cells, although under some conditions there was a paradoxical inhibitory effect (228).

ET also is mitogenic for Swiss 3T3 fibroblasts (229). This may be relevant to the structural changes observed in the airway wall in asthma, which include increased numbers of fibroblasts and enhanced thickness of the collagen layer (230). ET-1 and also ET-3 induced chemotaxis and replication of fibroblasts obtained from rat pulmonary arteries; the effects on replication were small (maximum of 30% above control), and occurred at higher concentrations (> 10 nM) than those that induced chemotaxis (1 pM–0.1 μM) (231). By contrast, ET-1 (1-1000 ng/mL) was observed to be weakly mitogenic (measured as [^3H]-thymidine incorporation) in porcine and bovine pulmonary artery smooth muscle cells and not thought to contribute markedly to remodeling, which is a feature of hypoxic pulmonary hypertension (232).

Mediator Release

It is clear that a significant component of ET-1-induced bronchoconstriction in guinea pigs *in vivo* is mediated by release of thromboxane (120,172,173,233). ET-1 stimulates thromboxane A_2 release from perfused guinea-pig lung, although the cellular source of thromboxane A_2 is unknown. There is conflicting information on the ability of ET-1 to stimulate mediator release from inflammatory cells (67). ET-1 (1 nM - 10 nM) stimulated thromboxane and PGD_2, but not histamine, release from cells obtained from bronchoalveolar lavages (BALs) in canine airways (234). An initial study revealed that ET_A receptor activation of murine bone-marrow-derived mast cells was without effect on histamine release (235). However, a later report revealed significant release of histamine, as well as 5-HT and

LTC$_4$, by ET-1 only when marine bone- marrow-derived mast cells were incubated with IL-4; IL-4 seems to act by being involved in the differentiation of mature mast cells to a phenotype that is sensitive to ET-1 (236). ET-1 had no effect on the release of histamine or the peptidoleukotrienes from guinea-pig trachea or human bronchus, but stimulated the release of various prostanoids (117, 188). In contrast, it was reported that ET-1 potently (EC$_{50}$ = 0.05 nM) and effectively stimulated histamine release from guinea-pig pulmonary but not peritoneal mast cells (237). ET-1 intravenous (i.v.) increased the levels of 15-HETE in BAL fluid and the generation of oxygen radicals in BAL cells in rats (238). In addition, ET-1 (10 nM) stimulated 15-lipoxygenase activity in lung homogenates. High concentrations of ET-1 ($\geq$ 0.1 µM) stimulated prostanoid release from human cultured nasal mucosa (222).

Microvascular Permeability

Edema may be an important feature of asthma. ET-1 (10 nM) enhances microvascular permeability in perfused rat lungs via a mechanism which requires the presence of both leukocytes and plasma components (239). Various studies in guinea-pig and rat-perfused lungs indicate that ET-1 induces pulmonary edema with conflicting information about the contribution of prostanoids (196,201,240–242). In rat-perfused lungs ET-1- or ET-3-induced hydrostatic edema formation was insensitive to BQ-123, suggesting it is not mediated via ET$_A$-receptor mediated mechanism (243). However, another study demonstrated that in conscious rats ET-1 elicited an increase in microvascular permability in part by activation of ET$_A$ receptors (244). Similarly, bolus i.v. administration of ET-1 increased albumin extravasation in guinea-pig airways via ET$_A$ receptor activation (245). It was hypothesized that in rat and guinea-pig lung, ET-1 causes lung edema predominantly via a hydrostatic mechanism, rather than by directly increasing vascular permeability (196,240). In blood-perfused, rather than physiological salt solution-perfused lungs, ET-1 produced little edema (196,246).

Inflammatory Cell Function

One study has reported that ET-1 (1 nM–1 µM) stimulates human blood monocyte chemotaxis, although another revealed that ET-1 did not induce or influence human peripheral blood monocyte chemotaxis, adhesion, or superoxide production (247,248). ET-1 increased arachidonic acid and thromboxane release from guinea-pig alveolar macrophages (maximum effect at 1 nM), and high concentrations (1 µM) increased superoxide production, intracellular Ca^{2+} levels, and protein phosphorylation in human alveolar macrophages (249,250). Other reports indicate ET-1-induced release of inflammatory cell products (234,237,238). ET-1 potently stimulated the release of

TNF-α, IL-1β, and IL-6 from human monocytes (251). Infusion of ET-1 produced adhesion of leukocytes to the endothelium in pulmonary vessels and sequestration of these cells in the pulmonary capillaries (252).

ET-1 potentiated superoxide production from alveolar macrophage induced by formyl-met-leu-phe (FMLP) or platelet-activating factor (PAF), via an ET$_A$-mediated mechanism (245).

Modulation of Neurotransmission

Neuronal dysfunction has been proposed to play an important role in the etiology of pulmonary diseases including asthma (253). Both stimulatory and inhibitory effects of the ETs on neurotransmission in the peripheral nervous system have been observed. For example, ET-1 inhibited adrenergic and cholinergic neuroeffector transmission in various tissues including guinea-pig pulmonary artery, apparently by prejunctional inhibition of neurotransmitter release (254–257). ET-1 also stimulates neurotransmission in some preparations by postjunctional mechanisms (254–257).

Research on the effects of the ETs on neurotransmission in the lung has been very limited and is a potentially important area of study. In rabbit bronchus ET-3 (10 or 100 nM) increased responses (about 2- and 3-fold, respectively) produced by parasympathetic stimulation but not those due to exogenous acetylcholine, suggesting that the potentiation was via a prejunctional mechanism (258). ET ligands, including ET-1, potentiated cholinergic nerve-induced concentration in mouse airways, again through which a prejunctional mechanism appeared to be mediated by ET$_B$ receptor activation (259). In contrast, in sheep trachea, ET-1 inhibited postganglianic nerve-induced contraction, apparently by stimulation of prejunctional ET$_B$ receptors (259). ET receptors, predominantly of the ET$_B$ subtype, were localized to cell bodies, processes, and varicosities of adrenergic and cholinergic intramural autonomic neurons found in primary cultures of guinea-pig tracheal smooth muscle (260). Stimulation of these receptors elicited a tetrodotoxin (TTX)-sensitive elevation in (Ca^{2+})$_i$ and associated contraction of adjacent smooth muscle cells, which contrasts with the lack of effect of TTX on ET-1-induced contractions in isolated guinea-pig trachea (168,188). It was proposed that adrenergic neurons, unlike cholinergic neurons, may have significant quantities of ET$_A$ receptors (260). [^{125}I-]ET-1 binding sites have been associated with parasympathetic ganglia, paravascular nerves, and nerves in the connective tissues in mammalian lung (134,136,138).

In Vivo Studies

Actions on Bronchoconstrictor Tone

Although studies describing the effects of direct ET administration to human airways in vivo have not been reported, the pulmonary effects of intravenous infusion of ET-1 have been explored. In one study, ET-1 (4 pmol/kg/min for 20 min) increased pulmonary vascular resistance by 67%, whereas in another, 60-minute infusion of ET-1 at a lower rate (0.4 pmol/kg/min) was without significant effect in the human pulmonary circulation (70,71).

Various studies have explored the pulmonary effects of the ETs in animals. Many of these preclinical studies have been conducted in guinea pigs, although ET-1 also produces bronchospasm in several species, including dog, rat, and sheep (261–263). In guinea pigs, i.v. or aerosol administration of ET-1 produces maintained bronchoconstriction which is mediated to a significant extent via the release of secondary mediators, predominantly thromboxane but also including PAF (172,173, 233). The extent to which secondary mediators contribute to ET-1-induced bronchoconstriction depends on the route of administration (172,173,233,241). The cellular source of these substances has not been elucidated. However, the bronchospasm induced by i.v. administration of ET-1 in guinea pigs is not associated with a change in the number of circulating polymorphonuclear cells (PMNs) or platelets, suggesting that the response was independent of these cells (264). Bronchospasm produced by ET-1 was potentiated by hexamethonium or propranolol, suggesting a modulatory influence of the autonomic nervous system (172,173). ET-1-induced bronchospasm appears to be mediated by stimulation of both ET_A and ET_B receptors (265,266).

Potentiation in the responsiveness of aerosol-sensitized and antigen-exposed guinea pigs to the bronchoconstrictor effects of ET-1 has been demonstrated, perhaps as a result of an alteration in the proteolytic activity (i.e., NEP) in the airway epithelium, which metabolizes ET-1 (58,267).

Actions on Vasomotor Tone

The ETs produce vasodilation or vasoconstriction in the cardiovascular system, and have been demonstrated to elicit a transient systemic vasodilation preceding a sustained elevation in pressure after intravenous bolus administration (7,8,74,201). The profile of the hemodynamic response in the pulmonary and other regions will depend on the level of tone in the vessel and the relative distribution of the ET receptor subtypes. ET_A receptors predominate in the vascular smooth muscle and result in vasoconstriction, whereas ET_B receptors are distributed on endothelial cells and smooth muscle cells, and can produce vasodilation (perhaps via the release of NO/EDRF) or vasoconstriction (14,73; *vide supra*).

ET-1 causes pulmonary vasodilation in newborn lamb under conditions when tone is elevated or during pulmonary hypertension induced by alveolar hypoxia; the effect appears to involve NO and ATP-sensitive K^+ -channels, but not prostaglandins (268). In cats, i.v. ET-1 elicited both pulmonary and systemic vasodilation; the former but not the latter was decreased by the ATP-sensitive K^+-channel antagonist, glibenclamide (269,270). In the rat pulmonary circulation, ET-1 produced vasoconstriction and vasodilation: the vasodilation may involve NO and ATP-sensitive K^+-channels (201,202). Intravenous ET-1 was reported to be a potent constrictor of canine airway circulation (271). ET-1-induced vasoconstriction in rat perfused lungs is inhibited by BQ-123 (1 μM) whereas ET-1-induced vasodilation or hydrostatic edema is unaffected suggesting that the latter are mediated by non-ET_A receptor pathways (243).

Hypoxia (10% O_2 for 3 weeks) abolished, in a reversible manner, the pulmonary vasodilation normally elicited by ET-1 or ET-3 in rat perfused lungs (205). In control tissues the vasodilation appears to be caused by activation of ATP-sensitive K^+-channels and ET_B receptors (insensitive to BQ-123). The mechanism of chronic hypoxia is not known although it does not appear to result from alterations in ET_A and ET_B receptor-binding characteristics or a change in the responsiveness of the K^+ channels (205). Similarly, in neonatal pigs, ET-1 induced pulmonary vasodilation was mediated via a non-ET_A, probably ET_B, receptor subtype and involved the release of NO but not prostanoids or ATP-sensitive K^+ channels (272).

Other In Vivo Effects

Airway hyperresponsiveness is a feature of asthma, and most studies in guinea pigs have failed to demonstrate the ability of ET-1, administered by aerosol or i.v. routes (bolus or infusion), to produce this phenomenon (173, 273–275). However, in one study a low concentration of aerosolized ET-1 (1pM), which was without direct effect on pulmonary function, potentiated the bronchospasm produced by histamine (276). In sheep inhaled ET-1 elicited airway hyperresponsiveness to carbachol (277).

In guinea pig i.v. ET-1 did not increase lung permeability, produce epithelial damage or elicit inflammatory cell influx into the alveolar or vascular walls or the bronchial epithelium (173). Similarly, aerosolized ET-1 had no influence on the levels of eosinophils in guinea pig lung samples (4 or 24 hours after exposure), and infusion of ET-1 (2 nmol/day) through the jugular vein to guinea pigs for 6 days did cause histologic changes and infiltration of inflammatory cells in the lung (274,275).

POTENTIAL PATHOPHYSIOLOGICAL ROLE

Background

As outlined earlier, there is increasing information from preclinical research to indicate various effects of the ETs in the pulmonary system, although some of the actions are observed only with high concentrations of the ETs. The significance of these diverse and, in some cases, conflicting results to a potential role of the ETs in the pathophysiology of lung diseases remains to be determined. Before ETs can be proposed confidently as being involved in the pathophysiology of pulmonary disorders, standard criteria have to be fulfilled: a) pathways for the synthesis, release and metabolism of the ETs must be present in the airways; b) the ETs must mimic several, if not all, of the features of the disease(s); c) the concentrations of the ETs must be increased in disease states, with a correlation between ET amounts and disease severity; and d) drugs that inhibit the release and/or antagonize the actions of the ETs must attenuate the symptoms of the disease(s). For asthma and pulmonary hypertension, several of the aspects of the criteria outlined in a) and, to a lesser extent, b) and c) have been fulfilled, although some of the information is preliminary and requires further investigation. Several studies have demonstrated increased levels and expression of ET in various lung disease (Table 3).

Asthma

Since the first publication on ET-1 in the pulmonary system in 1988 which described the potent contractile effects of ET-1 in guinea-pig trachea, many studies have confirmed that ET-1 is a potent contractile agonist in mammalian airways, including human bronchus (113, 117,135–138,167,179). Based solely on this ability to produce bronchoconstriction of isolated airways, ET-1 was proposed, perhaps rather prematurely, as an important mediator in asthma. Thus, asthma is recognized as being not just bronchospasm, but a chronic inflammatory disorder with several distinct pathologies. These features include airway hyperreactivity, mucus hypersecretion, mucus gland and airway smooth muscle cell hyperplasia, subepithelial fibrosis, inflammatory cell infiltration and activation, increased bronchial microvascular permeability and edema, and epithelial cell damage and desquamation (278). There is some data from preclinical research

TABLE 3. *Human pulmonary diseases in which increased expression, elevated BAL levels and/or increased plasma levels have been detected*

Disease	References
Asthma	279-287
Pulmonary Hypertension	293-301
ARDS/Acute Lung Injury	319,320
Lung Tumors	317
Acute Respiratory Failure	321
Cryptogenic Fibrosing Alveolitis	322
Interstitial Lung Diseases	282
Idiopathic Lung Fibrosis	323
Pulmonary Fibrosis	322

BAL, bronchoalveolar lavage fluid; ARDS, adult respiratory distress syndrome.

on the effects of ETs on many of these characteristics of asthma (Table 2, *vide supra*).

The most convincing evidence for a role of the ETs in asthma is found in several recent studies which suggest that there is increased synthesis and release of ET in the airways of asthmatic subjects, compared with nonasthmatic individuals. In the first study in humans, Nomura and co-workers (279) reported that there was elevation (nearly 6-fold) in the concentrations of ir-ET in BAL fluid obtained from one individual during a status asthmaticus attack (279). Subsequently, more comprehensive studies have demonstrated elevated concentrations of ET (> 3-fold) in BALs of asthmatic subjects compared to nonasthmatic individuals or patients with chronic bronchitis or chronic extrapulmonary diseases (280–282). Based upon the similarities in the ET concentrations in the peripheral venous blood among the three groups of patients, it was proposed that the increased BAL concentrations of ET caused by enhanced local synthesis and release in the bronchial mucosa, and not due to changes in microvascular permeability (280). Furthermore, ET concentrations decreased to control values, concomitant with an improvement in lung function, after 15-day treatment with inhaled β-agonists and oral corticosteroids (280). There is a significant increase in BAL ET levels in nonsteroid-treated asthmatics, but not in steroid-treated patients, compared with nonasthmatic individuals (281). There was a significant negative correlation between ET amounts and % predicted forced expiratory flow in one second (FEV_1) in the nonsteroid-treated asthmatics, but not in the steroid-treated group of patients. A correlation did not exist between BAL ET concentrations and bronchial reactivity in any of the three groups (281). It also has been demonstrated that bronchial epithelial cells obtained by bronchoscopy from six asthmatic patients expressed preproendothelin-1 mRNA and released significant quantities of ET-1, whereas cells from five control, nonasthmatic individuals and five chronic bronchitic patients contained little or no preproET-1 mRNA and did not release ET-1 (283). ET-1 expression is increased by IL-1 and histamine in bronchial epithelial cells obtained by bronchoscopy from asthmatics compared with nonasthmatics (284). Release of ET-1 also is increased from peripheral blood mononuclear cells obtained from asthmatics compared to those nonasthmatics (285). Immunotherapy decreased ET-1 release by cultured mononuclear cells (285). Circulatory blood levels of ET-1 are also increased in asthmatic individuals (285,286).

A comprehensive immunohistochemical analysis of ET-1 expression in endobronchial biopsies from 17 asthmatic patients and 11 atopic and nonatopic healthy controls revealed a substantial increase in the incidence of the expression of ET in airway epithelium, and also the vascular endothelium, of asthmatics (detected in 11 out of 17) compared with nonasthmatic controls (detected in 1 out of 11) (287). However, in the asthmatic individuals, a correlation was not observed between positive staining for ET-1 and parameters such as degree of airflow obstruction, level of bronchial responsiveness, atopy, or corticosteroid therapy. There was a significant inverse correlation between the fall in FEV_1 overnight and BAL ET-1 levels in patients with nocturnal asthma (288). A correlation existed between BAL levels of ET and changes in baseline FEV_1 and responses to methacholine challenge in asthmatics (281,286).

In patients with nocturnal asthma, a significant decrease in BAL ET-1 concentrations in the nighttime asthmatic group compared to the day-time asthmatic group or nighttime control group was demonstrated; there was no difference in plasma ET levels between nonasthmatics and asthmatics and also between day-time and night-time asthmatic groups (288). It was speculated that ET-1 may be more tightly bound to the airway smooth muscle and epithelial ET receptors, which may be upregulated overnight during exacerbations of asthma.

No difference was detected in the proportions, densities, and distributions of ET receptor subtypes in central or peripheral airways from asthmatic and nonasthmatic airways, suggesting no significant change in ET receptor properties in asthma, at least at the level of the airway smooth muscle (144,289). Interestingly, a decrease in sensitivity of bronchial smooth muscle to the contractile effects of sarafotoxin S6c was demonstrated in diseased preparations, suggesting that receptor desentization may be occurring as a result of increased release and exposure to ET.

Pulmonary Hypertension

Although the mechanisms underlying pulmonary hypertension remain uncertain, it is recognized to be a progressively deteriorating condition characterized by an increase in vascular tone and enhanced mitogenesis of smooth muscle cells. This produces a significant increase in pulmonary vascular resistance, which can result in right-heart failure and death. Another feature is enhanced recruitment of myofibroblasts into the intima and "remodeling" of pulmonary arteries, characterized by hyperplasia and hypertrophy of smooth muscle cells (290–292).

ET-1 long has been speculated to play a role in the etiology of pulmonary hypertension. This is based upon the ability of ET-1 to produce the two features of the disease, namely vasoconstriction and enhanced proliferation of vascular smooth muscle cells, as well as reports of an elevation in ET levels. In fact, pulmonary hypertension was the first pulmonary disorder in which increased concentrations of ET were demonstrated; there was about a 6-fold increase in plasma ET concentrations in 4 patients with pulmonary hypertension compared to controls (n=14) (293). Several subsequent reports in children and adults confirmed the enhanced plasma ET levels in this disease (both primary and secondary categories), and in several in-

stances a correlation was noted between ET amounts and the disease severity (294–300). The increase in plasma ET levels in arterial vs. venous blood was greater in patients with pulmonary hypertension compared to those with secondary hypertension (294). Pulmonary hypertension is a frequent cause of mortality in children with cardiopulmonary disease. Children with pulmonary hypertension have elevated blood levels of ET compared to those with chronic cardiac disease or those with lung disease not associated with pulmonary hypertension (296).

Tissue ET-1, assessed by immunoreactivity and mRNA, was also markedly enhanced in patients with various causes of pulmonary hypertension compared to controls; ET-1-like immunoreactivity predominated in endothelial cells of pulmonary arteries with medial thickening and fibrosis (301). A correlation was demonstrated between ir-ET-1 and pulmonary vascular resistance in patients with plexogenic pulmonary arteriopathy, but not those with secondary pulmonary hypertension. The mechanism responsible for the increase in ET release in pulmonary hypertension is unknown but may be a consequence of altered hemodynamic conditions; for example, shear stress increases ET production from cultured endothelial cells (302).

The ETs potently constrict isolated pulmonary blood vessels from various species including humans and *in vivo* studies demonstrate potent vasoconstrictor properties in the pulmonary vasculature (135,136,138,269,303). The ETs also potently produce mitogenesis in human pulmonary artery smooth muscle cells, via ET_A-receptor activation, which may be relevant to the characteristic vascular remodeling and smooth muscle cell proliferation associated with many forms of pulmonary hypertension (227,290–292).

It remains to be determined clinically whether ET contributes directly to the pathogenesis of the disorder or whether the elevated levels of ET are merely markers of the disease, for example, an indicator of endothelial cell damage or dysfunction.

There is support from animal models and isolated tissues for a role for ET-1 in the genesis and maintenance of pulmonary hypertension. For example, ET-1 mRNA expression increased in rats with idiopathic pulmonary hypertension (304). In monocrotaline-induced pulmonary hypertension in rats, plasma ET-1 concentrations increased progressively, preceeding the development of pulmonary hypertension (305). Infusion of BQ-123, the ET_A-receptor antagonist, reduced the progression of pulmonary hypertension and right ventricular hypertrophy and prevented the characteristic pulmonary arterial medial thickening. There are several reports of BQ-123, the ET_A-receptor antagonist, or bosentan, the mixed ET_A-/ET_B-receptor antagonist, reducing the many features of hypoxia-induced pulmonary hypertension in rats, including increased pulmonary artery pressure, right ventricular hypertrophy, and pulmonary artery muscularization

(305–308). Similarly, in a Beagle dog model of monocrotaline-induced pulmonary hypertension, the ET_A-receptor antagonist FR 139317 decreased pulmonary artery pressure, but not systemic arterial pressure, whereas RES-701-1, an ET_B-receptor antagonist, increased pulmonary arterial pressure (309). ET-1, and also ET-3, induced chemotaxis and replication of fibroblasts obtained from rat pulmonary arteries, suggesting a role in vascular remodeling; however, high concentrations of the ETs were needed to elicit modest effects (231). Furthermore, ET-1 (1 nM–3 nM) stimulated DNA synthesis and proliferation of pig pulmonary artery smooth muscle cells (228). However, based on the weakly mitogenic effect of ET-1 in canine and porcine pulmonary artery smooth muscle cells and lack of effect of hypoxia on ET secretion from porcine endothelial cells, Hassoun and co-workers (232) concluded that ET-1 does not contribute significantly to the remodeling seen in hypoxic pulmonary hypertension. ET-1 does not mediate acute hypoxic pulmonary vasoconstriction in newborn lamb (310). Furthermore, hypoxia decreased ET-1 release and ET-1 mRNA expression in bovine pulmonary microvascular endothelial and pulmonary artery cells (311). These data do not support a role for enhanced release of ET-1 in regulating the characteristic hypoxia-induced proliferation of pulmonary vascular smooth muscle cells and fibroblasts in the pulmonary circulation. However, two-day exposure to hypoxia increased ET-1 mRNA, ET-1 peptide and ET_A receptor mRNA, but not ET_B receptor mRNA, in rat lung, and ET-1 mRNA was increased in pulmonary artery but not aorta (312). Normobaric hypoxia enhances ET-1 gene expression in the rat and hypoxia and ischemia increase ET-1 release in rat and guinea-pig lung (313–315).

Other Pulmonary Disorders

ET-1 mRNA and ir-ET-1 have been detected in human nasal mucosa, and binding sites for ET-1 have been demonstrated in various loci in the nasal mucosa including submucosal glands, venous sinusoids, and small muscular arterioles (219,220). *In vitro* studies suggest that ET-1 stimulates serous and mucous cell secretion and prostanoid release, although high concentrations were required (≥ 0.1 μM) (220,222). There is a recent report describing the effects of intranasal administration of ET-1 to humans (316). Riccio and colleagues (316) demonstrated that in both symptomatic allergic and nonallergic individuals, ET-1 (0.3-10 μg) produced concentration-related bilateral increases in secretion weights, lysozyme secretion, symptoms of rhinorrhea, and symptoms of itch and sneezing; it was without effect on histamine release, albumin secretion or symptoms of nasal congestion. Interestingly, with several of the parameters (sneezing, symptoms of rhinorrhea, bilateral secretion weights, contralateral lysozyme secretion), the effects of

ET-1 were significantly more pronounced in allergic individuals. These data suggest that allergic inflammation in allergic rhinitic individuals enhances the responsiveness of the nasal mucosa to ET-1, especially in relation to symptoms attributed to neural reflex responses, and also provides preliminary evidence in support of a role for ET-1 in upper airway diseases.

ET immunoreactivity and mRNA were detected in most surgical specimens of various lung tumours, in particular squamous cell carcinoma and adenocarcinoma, and it was hypothesized that ET may be involved in their growth and/or differentiation (317). Recently, specific [^{125}I]-ET-1 binding was demonstrated in various pulmonary tumors, localized to blood vessels and in stromal tissues surrounding the tumor (318). In humans, expression was greatest in the developing lung and lowest in adult lung, and it was speculated that ET may be important in promoting or regulating cellular growth in lung development (42).

Adult respiratory distress syndrome (ARDS) encompasses several forms of acute lung injury that result in compromized pulmonary gas exchange, abnormal lung mechanics, and often pulmonary hypertension. Arterial and venous plasma ET levels are increased during clinical exacerbations of ARDS and decline with improvement in the patient's condition (319,320).

Plasma ET-1 concentrations in patients with acute respiratory failure (10.7 ± 5.0 pg/mL; n=13) were about 7-fold higher than those in control individuals (1.5 ± 0.5 pg/mL, n=16), with a correlation between ET-1 levels and several haemodynamic and respiratory parameters, including mean pulmonary arterial pressure and airway resistance (321).

An increase in the BAL ET concentrations was detected in 10 patients with idiopathic lung fibrosis (mean = 12.4 pg/mL) and 9 patients with miscellaneous interstitial lung disease (mean = 2.9 pg/mL) compared with 5 normal individuals (< 0.8 pg/mL) and 5 patients with chronic extrapulmonary disease (1.15 pg/mL) (282). A markedly increased expression of ET-1, most notably in airway epithelium and type II pneumocytes, was detected in lung tissue from patients with cryptogenic fibrosing alveolitis (CFA)—a fatal condition of unknown cause that is characterized by inflammation, type II pneumocyte and fibroblastic proliferation, and collagen deposition—compared with control tissue or tissues from patients with focal fibrosis (322). A correlation existed between the expression of ET-1 and the histologic parameters of the disease. ET-1 expression has also been demonstrated in alveolar epithelial cells of patients with pulmonary fibrosis, but minimally in patients with pulmonary hypertension without fibrosis (301). Amounts of ET-1 in BALs were elevated in patients with systemic sclerosis, who often develop fibrosis (323). Interestingly, BAL fluid samples enhanced fibroblast proliferation *in vitro* via a mechanism sensitive to BQ-123 or ET-1 antisera, suggesting it was mediated by ET-1 via an ET_A receptor-induced mechanism. Preliminary data in two patients with cystic fibrosis and one with CFA detected ir-proET-1 and ir-proET-3, but not ir-proET-2, in airway epithelium, whereas immunoreactivity for the three isoforms was localized in submucosal glands (324).

In patients with chronic obstructive pulmonary disease with chronic hypoxia, there was a negative correlation between PaO_2 and circulating ET-1 levels and a positive correlation between pulmonary arterial pressure and ET-1 amounts (325).

Animal Studies

Preclinical research in animal models has provided additional evidence in support of a role of ET in pulmonary disorders. In a rat model of lung inflammation produced by intratracheal administration of Sephadex beads, there was a 3.5-fold increase in lung ET-1 content, which was abolished by the glucocorticoid, budesonide (326). An increase in ET levels in sheep plasma and pulmonary lymph, concomitant with pulmonary vasconstriction, was detected during endotoxin shock, perhaps as a result of endothelial cell injury (327). Furthermore, enhanced plasma, BAL or tissue concentrations of ET have been demonstrated in various other models including: anaphylaxis in ovalbumin-induced actively and passively sensitized guinea-pigs, a model of postobstructive pulmonary vasculopathy in dogs (produced by chronic ligation of one pulmonary artery resulting in bronchial collateral vessel proliferation and pulmonary arterial abnormalities), a rat model of oleic acid-induced respiratory distress syndrome (increase preceded maximum hypoxia), a rat model of acute pulmonary alveolar hypoxia (correlation between the severity of hypoxia and ET levels), warm ischemia/reperfusion injury in rat lung, and during acute rejection of lung allografts in dogs (328–333). In the latter increased ETs levels in BALs in rejected lung allografts were reduced to control values by immunosuppresive therapy.

Interestingly, mice made deficient in ET-1 ("knockout mice") died of respiratory failure at birth (334). The anoxia-induced death was thought to be due, in part, to a dysfunction in the central control of respiration or in the respiratory muscle, and it was speculated that ET-1 may play a critical role in neural regulation of the respiratory system (334).

CONCLUSIONS

There remains considerable uncertainty regarding the precise role of ETs in the pathophysiology of pulmonary disorders. However, since the first publication describing the potent contractile effects of ET-1 in the guinea-pig isolated trachea in 1988, there has been increasing information indicating multiple potentially pertinent effects of the ETs, in particular ET-1, in different cells in the respiratory

tract (48). The accumulating evidence in support of a significant influence of ET-1 in lung pathophysiology, especially asthma and pulmonary hypertension, is intriguing and merits further investigation. Thus, several of the standard criteria for an important mediator have been fulfilled (e.g., pathways for systems and metabolism, mimicry of disease features, and elevation of levels in disease states). Overall, the strongest scientific rationale and evidence for a pathophysiological role for ET-1 are in pulmonary vascular diseases such as pulmonary hypertension. However, the unequivocal determination of the pathophysiological role of the ETs in pulmonary disorders requires the clinical testing of potent and selective receptor antagonists for the various ET receptor subtypes and/or ECE inhibitors; these studies may be performed in the near future with the potent and selective nonpeptide receptor antagonists that have recently been identified.

Many important issues and questions remain to be addressed. For example, preclinical research has focused to a significant extent on the contractile effects of the ETs. Although this is an important characteristic of many lung diseases, including asthma and pulmonary hypertension, future studies should be directed more toward comprehensive elucidation of the effects of ET on parameters other than bronchoconstriction, e.g., influence on nerves, inflammatory cell function, and the effects of chronic exposure on smooth muscle and fibroblast proliferation and other structural components of the lung. It remains to be clarified whether the most appropriate therapeutic agent(s) for the various pulmonary diseases is an ET_A-selective, ET_B-selective or perhaps a combined ET_A-/ET_B-selective antagonist. In addition, future research may identify additional ET receptor subtypes. Determination of the ET receptor subtypes mediating the diverse effects of the ETs in the lung will be important to this selection process; it is likely that the required profile will likely depend on the specific disorder. What are the beneficial effects of the ETs in the lung and which receptor subtype(s) mediates these influences? Will there be an advantage of an ECE inhibitor over an ET receptor subtype-selective antagonist? It is thought that the former strategy, because of its inherent lack of selectivity compared with subtype-selective receptor antagonists, could have liabilities, in particular associated with inhibition of the potential beneficial effects of the ETs, which may be due to activation of a specific receptor subtype. Preclinical research will be critical to address these and other pivotal questions and to assist the clinicians in the selection of the most appropriate novel therapeutic strategy for individual pulmonary disorders in which the ETs have been implicated.

ACKNOWLEDGMENTS

The authors thank Dotti Lavan for typing this material. RGG is a Senior Principal Research Fellow with the National Health and Medical Research Council of Australia.

REFERENCES

1. Furchgott RF, Vanhoutte PM. Endothelium-derived relaxing and contracting factors. *FASEB J* 1989;3:2007–2018.
2. Lüscher TF. Endothelium-derived relaxing and contracting factors: potential role in coronary artery disease. *Eur Heart J* 1989;10: 847–857.
3. Moncada S, Palmer RMJ, Higgs, EA. Nitric oxide: Physiology, Pathophysiology, and Pharmacology. *Pharmacol Rev* 1991;43:109–142.
4. Hickey KA, Rubanyi G, Paul RJ, Highsmith RF. Characterization of a coronary vasoconstrictor produced by cultured endothelial cells. *Am J Physiol* 1985;248:C550–C556.
5. Gillespie MN, Owasoyo JO, McMurtry IF, O'Brien RF. Sustained coronary vasoconstriction provoked by a peptidergic substance released from endothelial cells in culture. *J Pharmacol Exp Ther* 1986; 236:339–343.
6. O'Brien RF, Robbins RJ and McMurtry IF. Endothelial cells in culture produce a vasoconstrictor substance. *J Cell Physiol* 1987;132: 263–270.
7. Yanagisawa M, Kurihara H, Kimura S, Tomobe Y, Kobayashi M, Mitsui Y et al. A novel potent vasoconstrictor peptide produced by vascular endothelial cells. *Nature* 1988;332:411–415.
8. Inoue A, Yanagisawa M, Kimura S, Kasuya Y, Miyauchi T, Goto K et al. The human endothelin family: three structurally and pharmacologically distinct isopeptides predicted by three separate genes. *Proc Natl Acad Sci U S A* 1989;86:2863–2867.
9. Bloch DK, Friedrich SP, Lee M-E, Eddy RL, Shows TB, Quertermous T. Structural organization and chromosomal assignment of the gene encoding endothelin. *J Biol Chem* 1989;264:10851–10857.
10. Bloch KD, Hong CC, Eddy RL, Shows TB, Quertermous T. cDNA cloning and chromosomal assignment of the endothelin 2 gene: vasoactive intestinal contractor peptide in rat endothelin 2. *Genomics* 1991;10:236–242.
11. Bloch KD, Eddy RL, Shows TB, Quertermous T. cDNA cloning and chromosomal assignment of the gene encoding endothelin 3. *J Biol Chem* 1989;264:18156–18161.
12. Yanagisawa M, Masaki T. Endothelin, a novel endothelium-derived peptide. Pharmacological activities, regulation and possible roles in cardiovascular control. *Biochem Pharmacol* 1989;38:1877–1883.
13. Yanagisawa M, Masaki T. Molecular biology and biochemistry of the endothelins. *Trends Pharmacol Sci* 1989;10:374–378.
14. Masaki T, Yanagisawa M, Goto K. Physiology and pharmacology of endothelins. *Medicinal Res Rev* 1992;12:391–421.
15. Itoh Y, Yanagisawa M, Ohkubo S, Kimura C, Kosaka T, Inoue A et al. Cloning and sequence analysis of cDNA encoding the precursor of a human endothelium-derived vasoconstrictor peptide, endothelin: identity of human and porcine endothelin. *FEBS Letts* 1988;231: 440–444.
16. Denault JB, Claing A, D Orleans-Juste P, Sawamura T, Kido T, Masaki T et al. Processing of proendothelin-1 by human furin convertase. *FEBS Lett* 1995;362:276–280.
17. Opgenorth TJ, Wu-Wong JR, Shiosaki K. Endothelin-converting enzymes. *FASEB J* 1992;6:2653–2659.
18. Kashiwabara T, Inagaki Y, Ohta H, Iwamatsu A, Nomizu M, Morita A et al. Putative precursors of endothelin have less vasoconstrictor activity *in vitro* but a potent pressor effect *in vivo*. *FEBS Letts* 1989;247: 73–76.
19. Kimura S, Kaysuya Y, Sawamura T, Shinmi O, Sugita Y, Yanagisawa M et al. Conversion of big endothelin-1 to 21-residue endothelin-1 is essential for expression of full vasoconstrictor activity: structure-activity relationships of big endothelin-1. *J Cardiovasc Pharmacol* 1989;13(Suppl 5):S5–S7.
20. Takaoka M, Shiragami K, Fujino K, Miki K, Miyake Y, Yasuda M et al. Phosphoramidon-sensitive endothelin converting enzyme in rat lung. *Biochem Internat* 1991;25:697–704.
21. Sawamura, T., Shinmi, O., Kishi, N, Sugita, Y, Yanagisawa M, Goto K et al. Characterization of phosphoramidon-sensitive metalloproteinases with endothelin-converting enzyme activity in porcine lung membrane. *Biochim Biophys Acta* 1993;1161:295–302.
22. Takahashi M, Matsushita Y, Iijima Y, Tanzawa K. Purification and characterization of endothelin-converting enzyme from rat lung. *J Biol Chem* 1993;268:21394–21398.
23. Gui G, Xu D, Emoto N, Yanagisawa M. Intracellular localization of membrane-bound endothelin-converting enzyme from rat lung. *J Cardiovasc Pharmacol* 1993;22(Suppl 8):S53–S56.
24. Xu D, Emoto N, Giaid A, Slaughter C, Kaw S, deWit D, et al. ECE-1: a membrane-bound metalloprotease that catalyzes the proteolytic activation of big endothelin-1. *Cell* 1994;78:473–485.
25. Emoto N, Yanagisawa M. Endothelin-converting enzyme-2 is a membrane-bound, phosphoramidon-sensitive metalloprotease with acidic pH optimum. *J Biol Chem* 1995;270:15262–15268.
26. Harrison VJ, Barnes K, Turner AJ, Wood E, Corder R, Vane JR. Identification of endothelin-1 and big endothelin-1 in secretory vesicles isolated from bovine aortic endothelial cells. *Proc Natl Acad Sci U S A* 1995;92:6344–6348.
27. Bihovsky R, Levinson BL, Loewi RC, Erhardt PW, Polokoff MA. Hydroxamic acids as potent inhibitors of endothelin-converting enzyme from human bronchiolar smooth muscle. *J Med Chem* 1995;38: 2119–2129
28. Ishikawa S, Tsukada H, Yuasa H, Fukue M, Wei S, Onizuka M et al. Effects of endothelin-1 and conversion of big endothelin-1 in the isolated perfused rabbit lung. *J Appl Physiol* 1992;72:2387–2392.
29. Pons F, Touvay C, Lagente V, Mencia-Huerta JM, Braquet P. Involvement of a phosphoramidon-sensitive endopeptidase in the processing of big endothelin-1 in the guinea-pig. *Eur J Pharmacol* 1992;217: 65–70.
30. Vemulapalli S, Rivelli M, Chiu PJS, del Prado M, Hey JA. Phosphoramidon abolishes the increases in endothelin-1 release induced by ischemia-hypoxia in isolated perfused guinea pig lungs. *J Pharmacol Exp Therap* 1992;262:1062–1069.
31. Wu-Wong JR, Budzik GP, Devine EM, Opgenorth TJ. Characterization of endothelin converting enzyme in rat lung. *Biochem Biophys Res Comm* 1990;171:1291–1296.
32. Watanabe T, Yokosawa H. The generation of big-endothelin (1-22) (endothelin-valine) from big-endothelin in the soluble fraction of porcine lung. *Biochem Internat* 1992;27:1–8.
33. Wypij DM, Nichols JS, Novak PJ, Stacy DL, Berman J, Wiseman JS. Role of mast cell chymase in the extracellular processing of big-endothelin-1 to endothelin-1 in the perfused rat lung. *Biochem Pharmacol* 1992;43:845–853.
34. Kitamura K, Tanaka T, Kata J, Eto T, Tanaka K. Regional distribution of immunoreactive endothelin in porcine tissue: abundance in inner medulla of kidney. *Biochem Biophys Res Comm* 1989;161:348–352.
35. Matsumoto H, Suzuki N, Onda H, Funjo M. Abundance of endothelin-3 in rat intestine, pituitary gland and brain. *Biochem Biophys Res Comm* 1989;164:74–80.
36. Pernow J, Hemsén A, Lundberg JM. Tissue specific distribution, clearance and vascular effects of endothelin in the pig. *Biochem Biophys Res Comm* 1989;161:647–653.
37. Yoshimi H, Hirata Y, Fukuda Y, Kawano Y, Emori T, Kuramochi M et al. Regional distribution of immunoreactive endothelin in rats. *Peptides* 1989;10:805–808.
38. Rozengurt N, Springall DR, Polak JM. Localization of endothelinlike immunoreactivity in airway epithelium of rats and mice. *J Pathol* 1989;707:5–8.
39. Rennick RE, Loesch A, Burnstock G. Endothelin, vasopressin, and substance P like immunoreactivity in cultured and intact epithelium from rabbit trachea. *Thorax* 1992;47:1044–1049.
40. MacCumber MW, Ross CA, Glaser BM, Snyder SH. Endothelin: visualization of mRNAs by *in situ* hybridization provides evidence for local action. *Proc Natl Acad Sci U S A* 1989;86:7285–7289.
41. Ehrenreich H, Anderson RW, Fox CH, Rieckmann P, Hoffman GS, Travis WD et al. Endothelins, peptides with potent vasoactive properties, are produced by human macrophages. *J Exp Med* 1990;172: 1741–1748.
42. Giaid A, Polak JM, Gaitonde V, Hamid QA, Moscoso G, Legon S et al. Distribution of endothelinlike immunoreactivity and mRNA in the developing and adult human lung. *Am J Respir Cell Mol Biol* 1991;4: 50–58.
43. Nunez DJR, Brown MJ, Davenport AP, Neylon CB, Schofield JP, Wyse RK. Endothelin-1 mRNA is widely expressed in porcine and human tissues. *J Clin Invest* 1989;85:1537–1541.
44. Black PM, Ghatei MA, Takahashi K, Bretherton-Watt D, Krausz T, Dollery CT et al. Formation of endothelin by cultured airway epithelial cells. *FEBS Letts* 1989;255:129–132.
45. Mattoli S, Mezzetti M, Riva G, Allegra L, Fasoli A. Specific binding of endothelin on human bronchial smooth muscle cells in culture and

secretion of endothelinlike material from bronchial epithelial cells. *Am J Respir Cell Mol Biol* 1990;3:145–151.

46. Ninomiya H, Uchida Y, Ishii Y, Nomura A, Kameyama M, Saotome M et al. Endotoxin stimulates endothelin release from cultured epithelial cells of guinea-pig trachea. *Eur J Pharmacol* 1991;203: 299–302.

47. Endo T, Uchida Y, Matsumoto H, Suzuki N, Nomura A, Hirata F et al. Regulation of endothelin-1 synthesis in cultured guinea pig airway epithelial cells by various cytokines. *Biochem Biophys Res Comm* 1992;186:1594–1599.

48. Rennick RE, Milner P, Burnstock G. Thrombin stimulates release of endothelin and vasopressin, but not substance P, from isolated rabbit tracheal epithelial cells. *Eur J Pharmacol* 1993;230:367–370.

49. Franco-Cereceda A, Rydh M, Lou Y-P, Dalsgaard C-J, Lundberg JM. Endothelin as a putative sensory neuropeptide in the guinea pig: different properties in comparison with calcitonin gene-related peptide. *Regul Peptides* 1991;31:253–265.

50. Nakano J, Takizawa H, Ohtoshi T, Shoji S, Yamaguchi M, Ishii A et al. Endotoxin and pro-inflammatory cytokines stimulate endothelin-1 expression and release by airway epithelial cells. *Clin Exp Allergy* 1994;24:330–336.

51. Hay DWP. Guinea-pig tracheal epithelium and endothelin. *Eur J Pharmacol* 1989;171:241–246.

52. Johnson AR, Asthon J, Schulz WW, Erdös EG. Neutral metalloendopeptidases in human lung tissue and cultured cells. *Am Rev Respir Dis* 1985;132:564–568.

53. Vijayaraghavan J, Scicli AG, Carretero OA, Slaughter C, Moomaw C, Hersh LB. The hydrolysis of endothelins by neutral endopeptidase 24.11 (enkephalinase). *J Biol Chem* 1990;265:14150–14155.

54. Fagny C, Michel A, Léonard I, Berkenboom G, Fontaine J, Deschodt-Lanckman M. *In vitro* degradation of endothelin-1 by endopeptidase 24.11 (enkephalinase) *Peptides* 1991;12:773–778.

55. Noguchi K, Fukuroda T, Ikeno,Y, Hirose H, Tsukada Y, Nishikibe M et al. Local formation and degradation of endothelin-1 in guinea pig airway tissues. *Biochem Biophys Res Comm* 1991;179:830–835.

56. Di Maria GU, Katayama M, Borson DB, Nadel JA. Neutral endopeptidase modulates endothelin-1-induced airway smooth muscle contraction in guinea-pig trachea. *Regul Peptides* 1992;39:137–145.

57. Murphy LJ, Greenough KJ, Turner AJ. Processing and metabolism of endothelin peptides by porcine lung membranes. *J Cardiovasc Pharmacol* 1993;22 (Suppl 8):S94–S97.

58. Boichot E, Pons F, Lagente V, Touvay C, Mencia-Huerta JM, Braquet P. Phosphoramidon potentiates the endothelin-1-induced bronchopulmonary response in guinea-pigs. *Neurochem Internat* 1991;18: 477–479.

59. McKay KO, Black JL, Armour CL. Phosphoramidon potentiates the contractile response to endothelin-3, but not endothelin-1 in isolated airway tissue. *Br J Pharmacol* 1992;105:929–932.

60. Candenas M-L, Naline E, Sarria B, Advenier C. Effect of epithelium removal and of enkephalin inhibition on the bronchoconstrictor response to three endothelins of the human isolated bronchus. *Eur J Pharmacol* 1992;210:291–297.

61. Yamaguchi T, Kohrogi H, Kawano O, Ando M, Araki S. Neutral endopeptidase inhibitor potentiates endothelin-1-induced airway smooth muscle contraction. *J Appl Physiol* 1992;73:1108–1113.

62. Fagny C, Michel A, Nortier J, Deschodt-Lanckman M. Enzymatic degradation of endothelin-1 by activated human polymorphonuclear neutrophils. *Regul Peptides* 1992;42:27–37.

63. Koseki C, Imai M, Hirata Y, Yanagisawa M, Masaki,T. Autoradiographic distribution in rat tissues of binding sites for endothelin: a neuropeptide? *Am J Physiol* 1989;256:R858–R866.

64. Shiba R, Yanagisawa M, Miyauchi T, Ishii Y, Kimura S, Uchiyama Y et al. Elimination of intravenously injected endothelin-1 from the circulation of the rat. *J Cardiovasc Pharmacol* 1989;13 (Suppl. 5): S98–S101.

65. Sirviö M-L, Metsärinne K, Saijonmaa O, Fyhrquist F. Tissue distribution and half-life of ^{125}I-endothelin in the rat: importance of pulmonary clearance. *Biochem Biophys Res Comm* 1990;167: 1191–1195.

66. Furuya S, Naruse S, Nakayama T, Nokihara K. Effect and distribution in rat kidney and lung examined by electron microscopic radioautography. *Anat Embryol* 1992;185:87–96.

67. De Nucci G, Thomas R, D'Orleans-Juste P, Antunes E, Walder C, Warner TD, et al. Pressor effects of circulating endothelin are limited by its removal in the pulmonary circulation and by the release of prostacyclin and endothelium-derived relaxing factor. *Proc Natl Acad Sci U S A* 1988;85:9797–9800.

68. Rimar S, Gillis CN. Differential uptake of endothelin-1 by the coronary and pulmonary circulations. *J Appl Physiol* 1992;73:557–562.

69. Fukuroda T, Fujikawa T, Ozaki S, Ishikawa K, Yano M, Nishikibe M. Clearance of circulating endothelin-1 by ET$_B$ receptors in rats. *Biochem Biophys Res Commun* 1994;199:1461–1465.

70. Wagner OF, Vierhapper H, Gasic S, Nowotny P, Waldhäusl W. Regional effects and clearance of endothelin-1 across pulmonary and splanchnic circulation. *Eur J Clin Invest* 1992;22:277–282.

71. Weitzberg E, Ahlborg G, Lundberg JM. Differences in vascular effects and removal of endothelin-1 in human lung, brain, and skeletal muscle. *Clin Physiol* 1993;13:653–662.

72. Ray SG, McMurray JJ, Morton JJ, Dargie, HJ. Circulating endothelin is not extracted by the pulmonary circulation in man. *Chest* 1992;102: 1143–1144.

73. Sakurai T, Yanagisawa M, Masaki T. Molecular characterization of endothelin receptors. *Trends Pharmacol Sci* 1992;13:103–108.

74. Masaki T, Kimura S, Yanagisawa M, Goto K. Molecular and cellular mechanism of endothelin regulation. Implications for vascular function. *Circulation* 1989;80:219–233.

75. Warner TD, de Nucci G, Vane JR. Rat endothelin is a vasodilator in the isolated perfused mesentery of the rat. *Eur J Pharmacol* 1989; 159:325–326.

76. Yanagisawa M, Inoue A, Ishikawa T, Kasuya Y, Kimura S, Kumagaye S-I et al. Primary structure, synthesis and biological activity of rat endothelin, an endothelin-derived vasoconstrictor peptide. *Proc Natl Acad Sci U S A* 1988;85:6964–6967.

77. Sokolovsky M, Ambar I, Galron R. A novel subtype of endothelin receptors. *J Biol Chem* 1992;267:20551–20554.

78. Warner TD, Allcock GH, Mickley EJ, Corder R, Vane JR. Comparative studies with the endothelin receptor antagonists BQ-123 and PD 142893 indicate at least three endothelin receptors. *J Cardiovasc Pharmacol* 1993;22 (Suppl 8):S117–S120.

79. Warner TD, Allcock GH, Corder R, Vane JR. Use of the endothelin antagonists BQ-123 and PD 142893 to reveal three endothelin receptors mediating smooth muscle contraction and the release of EDRF. *Br J Pharmacol* 1993;110:777–782.

80. Bax WA, Saxena PR. The current endothelin receptor classification: time for reconsideration? *Trends Pharmacol Sci* 1994;15:379–386.

81. Masuda Y, Miyazaki H, Kondoh M, Watanabe H, Yanagisawa M, Masaki T et al. Two different forms of endothelin receptors in rat lung. *FEBS Letts* 1989;257:208–210.

82. Takayanagi R, Ohnaka K, Takasaki C, Ohashi M, Nawata H. Multiple subtypes of endothelin receptors in porcine tissues: characterization by ligand binding, affinity labeling and regional distribution. *Regul Peptides* 1991;32:23–37.

83. Arai H, Hori S, Aramori I, Ohkubo H, Nakanishi S. Cloning and expression of a cDNA encoding and endothelin receptor. *Nature* 1990; 348:730–732.

84. Sakurai T, Yanagisawa M, Takuwa Y, Miyazaki H, Kimura S, Goto K et al. Cloning of a cDNA encoding a non-isopeptide-selective subtype of the endothelin receptor. *Nature* 1990;348:732–735.

85. Sakamoto A, Yanagisawa M, Sakurai T, Takuwa Y, Yanagisawa H, Masaki T. Cloning and functional expression of human cDNA for the ET$_B$ endothelin receptor. *Biochem Biophys Res Comm* 1991;178: 656–663.

86. Martin E.R, Brenner BM, Ballermann BJ. Heterogeneity of cell surface endothelin receptors. *J Biol Chem* 1990;265:14044–14049.

87. Samson WK, Skala KD, Alexander BD, Huang F-L S. Pituitary site of action of endothelin: selective inhibition of prolactin release *in vitro*. *Biochem Biophys Res Comm* 1990;169:737–743.

88. Karne S, Jayawickreme CK, Lerner MR. Cloning and characterization of an endothelin-3 specific receptor (ET$_C$ Receptor) from Xenopus laevis dermal melanophores. *J Biol Chem* 1993;268: 19126–19133.

89. Adachi M, Yang Y-Y, Furuichi Y, Miyamoto C. Cloning and characterization of cDNA encoding human A-type endothelin receptor. *Biochem Biophys Res Comm* 1991;180:1265–1272.

90. Cyr C, Huebner K, Druck T, Kris R. Cloning and chromosomal localization of a human endothelin ETA receptor. *Biochem Biophys Res Comm* 1991;181:184–190.

91. Hosoda K, Nakao K, Arai-H, Suga S-i, Ogawa Y, Mukoyama M et al.

Cloning and expression of human endothelin-1 receptor cDNA. *FEBS Letts* 1991;287:23–26.

92. Nakamuta, M, Takayanagi R, Sakai Y, Sakamoto S, Hagiwara H, Mizuno et al. Cloning and sequence analysis of a cDNA encoding human non-selective type of endothelin receptor. *Biochem Biophys Res Comm* 1991;177:34–39.

93. Ogawa Y, Nakao K, Arai H, Nakagawa O, Hosoda K, Suga S-i et al. Molecular cloning of a non-isopeptide-selective human endothelin receptor. *Biochem Biophys Res Comm* 1991;178:248–255.

94. Kondoh M, Miyazaki H, Uchiyama Y, Yanagisawa M, Masaki T, Murakami K. Solubilization of two types of endothelin receptors, ET_A and ET_B, from rat lung with retention of binding activity. *Biomed Res* 1991;12:417–423.

95. Kozuka M, Ito T, Hirose S, Lodhi KM, Hagiwara H. Purification and characterization of bovine lung endothelin receptor. *J Biol Chem* 1991;266:16892–16896.

96. Hagiwara H, Nagasawa T, Lodhi KM, Kozuka M, Ito T, Hirose S. Affinity chromatographic purification of bovine lung endothelin receptor using biotinylated endothelin and avidin-agarose. *J Chromat* 1992;597:331–334.

97. Hick S, Heidemann I, Soskic V, Müller-Esterl W, Godovac-Zimmermann J. Isolation of the endothelin B receptor from bovine lung. Structure, signal sequence, and binding site. *Eur J Biochem* 1995;234:251–257.

98. Maggi CA, Giuliani S, Patacchini R, Rovero P, Giachetti A, Meli A. The activity of peptides of the endothelin family in various mammalian smooth muscle preparations. *Eur J Pharmacol* 1989;174:23–31.

99. Maggi CA, Giuliani S, Patacchini R, Santicioli P, Rovero P, Giachetti A. The C-terminal hexapeptide, endothelin-(16-21), discriminates between different endothelin receptors. *Eur J Pharmacol* 1989;166:121–122.

100. Maggi CA, Giuliani S, Patacchini R, Santicioli P, Giachetti A, Meli A. Further studies on the response of the guinea-pig isolated bronchus to endothelins and sarafotoxin S6b. *Eur J Pharmacol* 1990;176:1–9.

101. Cardell LO, Uddman R, Edvinsson L. Evidence for multiple endothelin receptors in the guinea-pig pulmonary artery and trachea. *Br J Pharmacol* 1992;105:376–380.

102. Williams Jr DL, Jones KL, Pettibone DJ, Lis EV, Clineschmidt BV Sarafotoxin S6c: an agonist which distinguishes between endothelin receptor subtypes. *Biochem Biophys Res Comm* 1991;175:556–561.

103. Ihara M, Saeki T, Fukuroda T, Kimura S, Ozaki S, Patel AC et al. A novel radioligand [^{125}I]BQ-3020 selective for endothelin (ET_B) receptors. *Life Sci* 1992;51:PL47–PL52.

104. Saeki T, Ihara M, Fukuroda T, Yamagiwa M, Yano M. (Ala^{1,3,11,15})Endothelin-1 analogs with ET_B agonistic activity. *Biochem Biophys Res Comm* 1991;179:286–292.

105. Takai M, Umemura I, Yamasaki K, Watakabe T, Fujitani Y, Oda K et al. A potent and specific agonist, Suc-(Glu^9,Ala^{11,15})-Endothelin-1(8-21), IRL 1620, for the ET_B receptor. *Biochem Biophys Res Comm* 1992;184:953–959.

106. Ihara M, Noguchi K, Saeki T, Fukuroda T, Tsuchida S, Kimura S et al Biological profiles of highly potent novel endothelin antagonists selective for the ET_A receptor. *Life Sci* 1991;50:247–255.

107. Sogabe K, Nirei H, Shoubo M, Nomoto A, Henmi K, Notsu Y et al. A novel endothelin receptor antagonist: studies with FR 139317. *Jap J Pharmacol* 1992;58:105P.

108. Tanaka T, Tsukuda E, Nozawa M, Nonaka H, Ohno T et al. RES-701-1, a novel, potent, endothelin type B receptor-selective antagonist of microbial origin. *Molec Pharmacol* 1994;45:724–730.

109. Clozel M, Breu V, Burri K, et al. Pathophysiological role of endothelin revealed by the first orally active endothelin receptor antagonist. *Nature* 1993;365:759–761.

110. Ohlstein EH, Nambi P, Douglas SA, Edwards RM, Gellai M, Lago A et al. SB 209670, a rationally designed potent nonpeptide endothelin receptor antagonist. *Proc Natl Acad Sci U S A* 1994;91:8052–8056.

111. Hay, DWP. Pharmacological evidence for distinct endothelin receptors in guinea-pig bronchus and aorta. *Br J Pharmacol* 1992;106:759–761.

112. Cardell LO, Uddman R, Edvinsson L. A novel ET_A-receptor antagonist, FR 139317, inhibits endothelin-induced contractions of guinea-pig pulmonary arteries, but not trachea. *Br J Pharmacol* 1993;108:448–452.

113. Hay DWP, Luttmann MA, Hubbard WC, Undem BJ. Endothelin receptor subtypes in human and guinea-pig pulmonary tissues. *Br J Pharmacol* 1993;110:1175–1183.

114. Buchan KW, Magnusson H, Rabe KF, Sumner MJ, Watts IS. Characterisation of the endothelin receptor mediating contraction of human pulmonary artery using BQ123 and Ro 46-2005. *Eur J Pharmacol* 1994;260:221–225.

115. Tomlinson PR, Wilson JW, Stewart AG. Inhibition by salbutamol of the proliferation of human airway smooth cells grown in culture. *Br J Pharmacol* 1994;111:641–647.

116. Panettieri RA Jr., Goldie RG, Rigby PJ, Eszterhas AJ, Hay DWP. Endothelin-1-induced potentiation of human airway smooth muscle proliferation: an ET_A receptor-mediated phenomenon. *Brit J Pharmacol* 1996 (*in press*).

117. Hay DWP, Hubbard WC, Undem BJ. Endothelin-induced contraction and mediator release in human bronchus. *Br J Pharmacol* 1993;110:392–398.

118. Battistini B, Warner TD, Fournier A, JR. Characterization of ET_B receptors mediating contractions induced by endothelin-1 or IRL 1620 in guinea-pig isolated airways: effects of BQ-123, FR139317 or PD 145065. *Br J Pharmacol* 1994;111:1009–1016.

119. Henry PJ. Endothelin-1 (ET-1)-induced contraction in rat isolated trachea: involvement of ET_A and ET_B receptors and multiple signal transduction systems. *Br J Pharmacol* 1993;110:435–441.

120. Noguchi K, Noguchi Y, Hirose M, Niskikibe M, Ihara M, Ishikawa K, et al. Role of endothelin ET_B receptors in bronchoconstrictor and vasoconstrictor responses in guinea-pigs. *Eur J Pharmacol* 1993;233:47–51.

121. Sudjarwo SA, Hori M, Takai M, Urade Y, Okada T, Karaki H. A novel subtype of endothelin B receptor mediating contraction in swine pulmonary vein. *Life Sci* 1993;53:431–437.

122. Yoneyama T, Hori M, Makatani M, Yamamura T, Tanaka T, Matsuda Y, et al. Subtypes of endothelin ET_A and ET_B receptors mediating tracheal smooth muscle contraction. *Biochem Biophys Res Commun* 1995;207:668–674.

123. Kenakin TP, Bond RB, Bonner TI. Definition of pharmacological receptors. *Pharmacol Rev* 1992;44:351–362.

124. Nambi P, Pullen M, Spielman W. Species differences in the binding characteristics of [^{125}I]IRL-1620, a potent agonist specific for endothelin-B receptors. *J Pharmacol Exp Ther* 1994;268:202–207.

125. Waggoner WG, Genova SL, Rash VA. Kinetic analyses demonstrate that the equilibrium assumption does not apply to [^{125}I]endothelin-1 binding data. *Life Sci* 1992;51:1869–1876.

126. Wu-Wong JR, Chiou WJ, Magnuson SR, Opgenorth TJ. Endothelin receptor agonists and antagonists exhibit different dissociation characteristics. *Biochim Biophys Acta* 1994;1224:288–294.

127. Ihara M, Saeki T, Fukuroda T, Kimura S, Ozaki S, Patel AC et al. A novel radioligand [^{125}I]BQ-3020 selective for endothelin (ET_B) receptors. *Life Sci* 1992;51:PL47–PL52.

128. Watakabe T, Urade Y, Takai M, Umemura I, Okada T. A reversible radioligand specific for the ET_B receptor: [^{125}I]Tyr13-Suc-[Glu^9,Ala^{11,15}]-endothelin-1(8-21), [^{125}I]IRL 1620. *Biochem Biophys Res Commun* 1992;185:867–873.

129. Ihara M, Yamanaka R, Ohwaki K, Ozaki S, Fukami T, Ishikawa K et al. [^{3}H]BQ-123, a highly specific and reversible radioligand for the endothelin ET_A receptor subtype. *Eur J Pharmacol* 1995;274:1–6.

130. Peter MG, Davenport AP. Selectivity of [^{125}I]-PD151242 for human, rat and porcine endothelin ET_A receptors in the heart. *Br J Pharmacol* 1995;114:297–302.

131. Wu-Wong JR, Chiou WJ, Dixon DB, Opgenorth TJ. Dissociation characteristics of ET_A receptor agonist and antagonists. *J Cardiovasc Pharmacol* 1995;26:S280–S384.

132. Kizawa Y, Nakajima Y, Nakano J, Uno H, Sano M, Murakami H. Pharmacological profiles of contractile endothelin receptors in guinea pig hilar bronchus. *Receptor* 1994;4:269–276.

133. Tschirhart EJ, Drijfhout JW, Pelton JT, Miller RC, Jones CR. Endothelins: functional and autoradiographic studies in guinea pig trachea. *J Pharmacol Exp Therap* 1991;258:381–387.

134. Power RF, Wharton J, Zhao Y, Bloom SR, Polak JM. Autoradiographic localization of endothelin-1 binding sites in the cardiovascular and respiratory systems. *J Cardiovas Pharmacol* 1989;13 (Suppl. 5):S50–S56.

135. Hemsén A, Franco-Cereceda A, Matran R, Rudehill A, Lundberg JM. Occurrence, specific binding sites and functional effects of endothelin in human cardiopulmonary tissue. *Eur J Pharmacol* 1990;191:319–328.

136. Henry PJ, Rigby PJ, Self GJ, Preuss JM, Goldie RG. Relationship between endothelin-1 binding site densities and constrictor activities in human and animal airway smooth muscle. *Br J Pharmacol* 1990;100: 786–792.

137. Brink C, Gillard V, Roubert P, Mencia-Huerta JM, Chabrier PE, Braquet P et al. Effects and specific binding sites of endothelin in human lung preparations. *Pulmon Pharmacol* 1991;4:54–59.

138. McKay KO, Black JL, Diment LM, Armour CL. Functional and autoradiographic studies of endothelin-1 and endothelin-2 in human bronchi, pulmonary arteries, and airway parasympathetic ganglia. *J Cardiovasc Pharm* 1991;17(Suppl 7):S206–S209.

139. Goldie RG, Grayson, PS, Knott, PG, Self, GJ, Henry, PJ. Predominance of endothelin$_A$ (ET$_A$) receptors in ovine airway smooth muscle and their mediation of ET-1-induced contraction. *Br J Pharmacol* 1994;112:749–756.

140. Wu T, Rieves RD, Larivee P, Logun C, Lawrence MG, Shelhamer JH. Production of eicosanoids in response to endothelin-1 and identification of specific endothelin-1 binding sites in airway epithelial cells. *Am J Respir Cell Mol Biol* 1993;8:282–290.

141. Sen M, Grunstein MM, Chander A. Stimulation of lung surfactant secretion by endothelin-1 from rat alveolar type II cells. *Am J Physiol* 1994;266:L255–L262.

142. Durham SK, Goller NL, Lynch JS, Fisher SM, Rose PM. Endothelin receptor B expression in the rat and rabbit lung as determined by *in situ* hybridization using nonisotopic probes. *J Cardiovasc Pharmacol* 1993;22 (Suppl 8):S1–S3.

143. Ninomiya H, Yu X-Y, Uchida Y, Hasegawa S, Spannhake EW. Specific binding of endothelin-1 to canine tracheal epithelial cells in culture. *Am J Physiol* 1995;268:L424–L431.

144. Goldie RG, Henry PJ, Knott PG, Self GJ, Luttmann M, Hay DWP. Endothelin-1 receptor subtype density, distribution and function in human isolated asthmatic airways. *Am J Respir Crit Care Med* 1995; 152;1653–1658.

145. Hagiwara H, Nagasawa, T, Yamamoto T, Lodhi KM, Ito T, Takemura N et al. Immunochemical characterization and localization of endothelin ET$_B$ receptor. *Am J Physiol* 1993;264:R777–R783.

146. Nakamichi K, Ihara M, Kobayashi M, Saeki T, Ishikawa K, Yano M. Different distribution of endothelin receptor subtypes in pulmonary tissues revealed by the novel selective ligands BQ-123 and [Ala^{1,3,11,15}]ET-1. *Biochem Biophys Res Comm* 1992;182:144–150.

147. Henry PJ. Endothelin-1 (ET-1)-induced contraction in rat isolated trachea: involvement of ET$_A$ and ET$_B$ receptors and multiple signal transduction systems. *Br J Pharmacol* 1993;110:435–441.

148. Noguchi K, Ishikawa K, Yano M, Ahmed A, Cortes A, Hallmon J et al. An endothelin (ET)$_A$ receptor antagonist, BQ-123, blocks ET-1 induced bronchoconstriction and tracheal smooth muscle (TSM) contraction in allergic sheep. *Am Rev Respir Dis* 1992;145:A858.

149. Goldie RG, Grayson PS, Henry PJ. Endothelin-1 (ET-1)-induced contraction of ovine tracheal smooth muscle is mediated via ET$_A$ receptors. *Am Rev Respir Dis* 1993;147:A182.

150. Goldie RG, D Aprile AC, Cvetkovski R, Rigby PJ, Henry PJ. Influence of regional differences in ET$_A$ and ET$_B$ receptor subtype proportions on endothelin-1-induced contractions in porcine isolated trachea and bronchus. *Br J Pharmacol* 1996;117:736–742.

151. D'Orléans-Juste P, Télémaque S, Claing A, Ihara M, Yano M. Human big-endothelin-1 and endothelin-1 release prostacyclin via the activation of ET$_1$ receptors in the rat perfused lung. *Br J Pharmacol* 1992; 105:773–775.

152. Cioffi CL, Neale RF Jr, Jackson RH, Sills, MA. Characterization of rat lung endothelin receptor subtypes which are coupled to phosphoinositide hydrolysis. *J Pharmacol Exp Ther* 1992;262:611–618.

153. Kobayashi M, Ihara M, Sato N, Saeki T, Ozaki S, Ikemoto F et al. A novel ligand, [125I]BQ-3020, reveals the localization of endothelin ETB receptors. *Eur. J. Pharmacol.* 1993;235:95–100.

154. Davenport AP, O Reilly G, Kuc RE. Endothelin ET$_A$ and ET$_B$ mRNA and receptors expressed by smooth muscle in the human vasculature: majority of the ET$_A$ sub-type. *Br J Pharmacol* 1995;114:1110–1116.

155. Fukuroda T, Kobayashi M, Ozaki S, Yano M, Miyauchi T, Onizuka M et al. Endothelin receptor subtypes in human versus rabbit pulmonary arteries. *J Appl Physiol* 1994;76:1976–1982.

156. LaDouceur DM, Flynn MA, Keiser JA, Reynolds E, Haleen SJ. ET$_A$ and ET$_B$ receptors coexist on rabbit pulmonary artery vascular smooth muscle mediating contraction. *Biochem Biophys Res Commun* 1993;196:209–215.

157. Resink T, Scott-Burden T, Bühler FR. Endothelin stimulates phospholipase C in cultured vascular smooth muscle cells. *Biochem Biophys Res Comm* 1988; 157:1360–1368.

158. Van Renterghem C, Vigne P, Barhanin J, Schmid-Alliana A, Frelin C, Lazdunski M. Molecular mechanism of action of the vasoconstrictor peptide endothelin. *Biochem Biophys Res Comm* 1988;157:977–985.

159. Griendling KK, Tsuda T, Alexander RW. Endothelin stimulates diacylglycerol accumulation and activates protein kinase C in cultured vascular smooth muscle cells. *J Biol Chem* 1989;264:8237–8240.

160. Muldoon LL, Rodland KD, Forsythe ML, Magun BE. Stimulation of phosphatidylinositol hydrolysis, diacylglycerol release, and gene expression in response to endothelin, a potent new agonist for fibroblasts and smooth muscle cells. *J Biol Chem* 1989;264:8529–8536.

161. Ohlstein EH, Horohonich S, Hay DWP. Cellular mechanisms of endothelin in rabbit aorta. *J Pharmacol Exp Ther* 1989;250:548–555.

162. Marsden PA, Danthuluri NR, Brenner BM, Ballermann BJ, Brock TA. Endothelin action of vascular smooth muscle involves inositol trisphosphate and calcium mobilization. *Biochem Biophys Res Comm* 1989;158:86–93.

163. Xuan, Y-T, Whorton AR, Watkins WD. Inhibition by nicardipine on endothelin-mediated inositol phosphate formation and Ca^{2-} mobilization in smooth muscle cell. *Biochem Biophys Res Comm* 1989;160: 758–764.

164. Takuwa N, Takuwa Y, Yanagisawa M, Yamashita K, Masaki T. A novel vasoactive peptide endothelin stimulates mitogenesis through inositol lipid turnover in Swiss 3T3 fibroblasts. *J Biol Chem* 1989;264: 7856–7861.

165. Sugiura M, Inagami T, Hare GMT, Johns JA. Endothelin action: inhibition by a protein kinase C inhibitor and involvement of phosphoinositols. *Biochem Biophys Res Comm* 1989;158:170–176.

166. Pitkänen M, Mäntymaa P, Ruskoaho H. Staurosporine, a protein kinase C inhibitor, inhibits atrial natriuretic peptide secretion induced by sarafotoxin, endothelin and phorbol ester. *Eur J Pharmacol* 1991; 195:307–315.

167. Uchida Y, Ninomiya H, Saotome M, Nomura A, Ohtsuka M, Yanagisawa M et al. Endothelin, a novel vasoconstrictor peptide, as potent bronchoconstrictor. *Eur J Pharmacol* 1988;154: 227–228.

168. Maggi CA, Patacchini S, Meli A. Potent contractile effect of endothelin in isolated guinea-pig airways. *Eur J Pharmacol* 1989;160:179–182.

169. Hay DWP. Mechanism of endothelin-induced contraction in guinea-pig trachea: comparison with rat aorta. *Br J Pharmacol* 1990;100: 383–392.

170. Sarriá B, Naline E, Morcillo E, Cortijo J, Esplugues J, Advenier C. Calcium dependence of the contraction produced by endothelin (ET-1) in isolated guinea-pig trachea. *Eur J Pharmacol* 1990;187: 445–453.

171. Cardell LO, Uddman R, Edvinsson L. Analysis of endothelin-1-induced contractions of guinea-pig trachea, pulmonary veins and different types of pulmonary arteries. *Acta Physiol Scand* 1990;139: 103–111.

172. Lagente V, Chabrier PE, Mencia-Huerta JM, Braquet P. Pharmacological modulation of the bronchopulmonary action of the vasoactive peptide, endothelin, administered by aerosol in the guinea-pig. *Biochem Biophys Res Comm* 1989;158:625–632.

173. Macquin-Mavier I, Levame M, Istin N, Harf A. Mechanisms of endothelin-mediated bronchoconstriction in the guinea pig. *J Pharmacol Exp Therap* 1989;250:740–745.

174. Nally JE, McCall R, Young LC, Wakelam MJO, Thomson NC, McGrath JC. Mechanical and biochemical responses to endothelin-1 and endothelin-3 in human bronchi. *Eur J Pharmacol* 1994;288:53–60.

175. Nally JE, McCall R, Young LC, Wakelam MJO, Thomson NC, McCrath JC. Mechanical and biochemical responses to endothelin-1 and endothelin-3 in bovine bronchial smooth muscle. *Br J Pharmacol* 1994;111:1163–1169.

176. Grunstein MM, Chuang ST, Schramm CM, Pawlowski NA. Role of endothelin 1 in regulating rabbit airway contractility. *Am J Physiol* 1991;L75–L82.

177. Oda K, Fujitani Y, Watakabe T, Inui T, Okada T, Urade Y, et al. Endothelin stimulates both cAMP formation and phosphatidylinositol hydrolysis in cultured embryonic bovine tracheal cells. *FEBS Letts* 1992;299:187–191.

178. Battistini B, Filep JG, Cragoe EJ Jr., Fournier A, Sirois P. A role of Na$^-$/H$^-$ exchange in contraction of guinea-pig airways by endothelin-1 *in vitro*. *Biochem Biophys Res Comm* 1991;175:583–588.

179. Advenier C, Sarria B, Naline E, Puybasset L, Lagente V. Contractile activity of three endothelins (ET-1, ET-2 and ET-3) on the human isolated bronchus. *Br J Pharmacol* 1990;100:168–172.

180. McKay, KO, Black JL, Armour CL. The mechanism of action of endothelin in human lung. *Br J Pharmacol* 1991;102:422–428.

181. Hay DWP, Luttmann MA, Goldie RG. Calcium (Ca^{2+}) translocation mechanisms mediating endothelin-1 (ET-1)- and sarafotoxin S6c (S6c)-induced contractions in isolated human bronchus. *Am J Respir Crit Care Med* 1994;149:A1083.

182. Mattoli S, Soloperto M, Mezzetti M, Fasoli A. Mechanisms of calcium mobilization and phosphoinositide hydrolysis in human bronchial smooth muscle cells by endothelin 1. *Am J Respir Cell Mol Biol* 1991;5:424–430.

183. Hay DWP, Henry PJ, Goldie RG. Endothelin and the respiratory system. *Trends Pharmacol Sci* 1993;14:29–32.

184. Hay DWP, Luttmann MA, Beck G, Ohlstein EH. Comparison of endothelin B (ET_B) receptors in rabbit isolated pulmonary artery and bronchus. *Br J Pharmacol* 1996;118:1209–1217.

185. Henry PJ, Goldie RG. ET_B but not ET_A receptor-mediated contraction to endothelin-1 attenuated by respiratory tract viral infection in mouse airways. *Br J Pharmacol* 1994;112:1188–1194.

186. Lee H-K, Leikauf GD, Sperelakis N. Electromechanical effects of endothelin on ferret bronchial and tracheal smooth muscle. *J Appl Physiol* 1990;68:417–420.

187. Filep JG, Battistini B, Sirois P. Endothelin induces thromboxane release and contraction of isolated guinea-pig airways. *Life Sci* 1990;47:1845–1850.

188. Hay DWP, Hubbard WC, Undem BR. Relative contributions of direct and indirect mechanisms mediating endothelin-induced contraction of guinea-pig trachea. *Br J Pharmacol* 1993;110:955–962.

189. Battistini B, Sirois P, Braquet P, Filep JG. Endothelin-induced constriction of guinea-pig airways: role of platelet-activating factor. *Eur J Pharmacol* 1990;186:307–310.

190. Filep JG, Battistini B, Sirois P. Pharmacological modulation of endothelin-induced contraction of guinea-pig isolated airways and thromboxane release. *Br J Pharmacol* 1991;103:1633–1640.

191. Ninomiya H, Uchida Y, Saotome M, Nomura A, Ohse H, Matsumoto H et al. Endothelins constrict guinea pig tracheas by multiple mechanisms. *J Pharmacol Exp Therap* 1992;262:570–576.

192. MacLean MR, McCulloch KM, Baird M. Endothelin ET_A- and ET_B-receptor-mediated vasoconstriction in rat pulmonary arteries and arterioles. *J Cardiovasc Pharmacol* 1994;23:838–845.

193. Fukuroda T, Nishikibe M, Ohta Y, Ihara M, Yano M, Ishikawa K et al. Analysis of responses to endothelins in isolated porcine blood vessels by using a novel endothelin antagonist, BQ-153. *Life Sci* 1991;50:107–112.

194. White DG, Cannon TR, Garratt H, Mundin JW, Sumner MJ, Watts IS. Endothelin ET_A and ET_B receptors mediate vascular smooth-muscle contraction. *J Cardiovasc Pharmacol* 1993;22(Suppl 8):S144–S148.

195. Cardell LO, Uddman R, Edvinsson L. Two functional endothelin receptors in guinea-pig pulmonary arteries. *Neurochem Internat* 1991;18:571–574.

196. Rodman DM, Stelzner TJ, Zamora MR, Bonvallet ST, Oka M, Sato K et al. Endothelin-1 increases the pulmonary microvascular pressure and causes pulmonary edema in salt solution but not blood-perfused rat lungs. *J Cardiovasc Pharmacol* 1992;20:658–663.

197. Zellers TM, McCormick J, Wu Y. Interaction among ET-1, endothelium-derived nitric oxide, and prostacyclin in pulmonary arteries and veins. *Am J Physiol* 1994;267:H139–H147.

198. Wang Y, Coceani F. Isolated pulmonary resistance vessels from fetal lambs. Contractile behavior and responses to indomethacin and endothelin. *Circ Res* 1992;71:320–330.

199. Lippton HL, Ohlstein EH, Summer WR, Hyman AL. Analysis of responses to endothelins in the rabbit pulmonary and systemic vascular beds. *J Apply Physiol* 1991;70:331–341.

200. Toga H, Ibe BO, Raj JU. *In vitro* responses of ovine intrapulmonary arteries and veins to endothelin-1. *Am J Physiol* 1992;263:L15–L21.

201. Raffestin B, Adnot S, Eddahibi S, Macquin-Mavier I, Braquet P, Chabrier PE. Pulmonary vascular response to endothelin in rat. *J Appl Physiol* 1991;70:567–574.

202. Hasunuma K, Rodman DM, O'Brien RF, McMurtry IF. Endothelin 1 causes pulmonary vasodilation in rats. *Am J Physiol* 1990;259:H48–H54.

203. Eddahibi S, Adnot S, Carville C, Blouquit Y, Raffestin B. L-arginine restores endothelium-dependent relaxation in the pulmonary circulation of chronically hypoxic rats. *Am J Physiol* 1992;263:L194–L200.

204. Adnot S, Raffestin B, Eddahibi S, Braquet P, Chabrier PE. Loss of endothelium-dependent relaxant activity in the pulmonary circulation of rats exposed to chronic hypoxia. *J Clin Invest* 1991;87: 155–162.

205. White SR, Hathaway DP, Umans JG, Tallet J, Abrahams C, Leff AR. Epithelial modulation of airway smooth muscle response to endothelin-1. *Am Rev Respir Dis* 1991;144:373–378.

206. Filep JG, Battistini B, Sirois P. Induction by endothelin-1 of epithelium-dependent relaxation of guinea-pig trachea *in vitro*: role for nitric oxide. *Br J Pharmacol* 1993;109:637–644.

207. Hadj-Kaddour K, Michel A, Chevillard C. Endothelin-1 and endothelin-3 relax isolated guinea-pig trachea through different mechanisms. *J Cardiovasc Pharmacol* 1995;26:S115–S116.

208. Karaki H, Sudjarwo SA, Hori M, Sakata K, Urade Y, Takai M et al. ET_B receptor antagonist, IRL 1038, selectively inhibits the endothelin-induced endothelium-dependent vascular relaxation. *Eur J Pharmacol* 1993;231:371–374.

209. Cocks TM, Broughton A, Dib M, Sudhir K, Angus JA. Endothelin is blood vessel selective: studies on a variety of human and dog vessels *in vitro* and on regional blood flow in the conscious rabbit. *Clin Exp Pharmacol Physiol* 1989;16:243–246.

210. Clozel M, Gray GA, Breu V, Löffler B-M, Osterwalder R. The endothelin ET_B receptor mediates both vasodilation and vasoconstriction *in vivo*. *Biochem Biophys Res Comm* 1992;186:867–873.

211. Eddahibi S, Springall D, Mannan M, Carville C, Chabrier P-E, Levame M et al. Dilator effect of endothelins in pulmonary circulation: changes associated with chronic hypoxia. *Am J Physiol* 1993;265:L571–L580.

212. Johnson DE. Pulmonary neuroendocrine cells. In: Farmer SG, Hay DWP, eds. *Physiology, pathophysiology, and pharmacology.* New York: Marcel Dekker, 1991:335–397.

213. O'Byrne PM. The airway epithelium and asthma. In: Farmer SG and Hay DWP, editors. *Physiology, pathophysiology, and pharmacology.* New York: Marcel Dekker, 1991:171–186.

214. Stutts, MJ, Knowles MR, Chinet T, Boucher RC. Abnormal ion transport in cystic fibrosis airway epithelium. In: Farmer SG and Hay DWP, editors. *Physiology, pathophysiology, and pharmacology.* New York: Marcel Dekker, 1991:301–334.

215. Webber SE, Yurdakos E, Woods AJ, Widdicombe JG. Effects of endothelin-1 on tracheal submucosal gland secretion and epithelial function in the ferret. *Chest* 1992;101:63S–67S.

216. Satoh M, Shimura S, Ishihara H, Nagaki M, Sasaki H, Takishima T. Endothelin-1 stimulates chloride secretion across canine tracheal epithelium. *Respiration* 1992;59:145–150.

217. Plews PI, Abdel-Malek ZA, Doupnik CA, Leikauf GD. Endothelin stimulates chloride secretion across canine tracheal epithelium. *Am J Physiol* 1991;261:L188–L194.

218. Tamaoki J, Kanemura T, Sakai N, Isono K, Kobayashi K, Takizawa T. Endothelin stimulates ciliary beat frequency and chloride secretion in canine cultured tracheal epithelium. *Am J Respir Cell Mol Biol* 1991;4:426–431.

219. Casasco A, Benazzo M, Casasco M, Cornaglia AI, Springall DR, Calligaro A et al. Occurrence, distribution and possible role of the regulatory peptide endothelin in the nasal mucosa. *Cell Tissue Res* 1993;274:241–247.

220. Mullol J, Chowdhury BA, White MV, Ohkubo K, Rieves RD, Baraniuk J et al. Endothelin in human nasal mucosa. *Am J Respir Cell Mol Biol* 1993;8:393–402.

221. Shimura S, Ishihara H, Satoh M, Masuda T, Nagaki N, Sasaki H et al. Endothelin regulation of mucus glycoprotein secretion from feline tracheal submucosal glands. *Am J Physiol* 1992;262:L208–L213.

222. Wu T, Mullol J, Rieves RD, Logun C, Hausfield J, Kaliner MA et al. Endothelin-1 stimulates eicosanoid production in cultured human nasal mucosa. *Am J Respir Cell Mol Biol* 1992;6:168–174.

223. Stewart AG, Grigoriadis G, Harris T. Mitogenic actions of endothelin-1 and epidermal growth factor in cultured airway smooth muscle. *Clin Exper Pharmacol Physiol* 1994;21:277–285.

224. Noveral JP, Rosenberg SM, Anbar RA, Pawlowski NA, Grunstein MM. Role of endothelin-1 in regulating proliferation of cultured rabbit airway smooth muscle cells. *Am J Physiol* 1992;263:L317–L324.

225. Glassberg MK, Ergul A, Wanner A, Puett D. Endothelin-1 promotes mitogenesis in airway smooth muscle cells. *Am J Respir Cell Mol Biol* 1994;10:316–321.

226. Demoly P, Basset-Seguin N, Chanez P, et al. C-*fos* proto-oncogene expression in bronchial biopsies of asthmatics. *Am J Respir Cell Mol Biol* 1992;7:128–133.

227. Zamora MA, Dempsey EC, Walchak SJ, Stelzner TJ. BQ123, an ET_A recepetor antagonist, inhibits endothelin-1-mediated proliferation of human pulmonary artery smooth muscle cells. *Am J Respir Cell Mol Biol* 1993;9:429–433.

228. Janakidevi K, Fisher MA, Del Vecchio PJ, Tiruppathi C, Figge J, Malik AB. Endothelin-1 stimulates DNA synthesis and proliferation of pulmonary artery smooth muscle cells. *Am J Physiol* 1992;263: C1295–C1303.

229. Takuwa Y, Kasuya Y, Takuwa N, Kudo M, Yanagisawa M, Goto K et al. Endothelin receptor is coupled to phospholipase C via a pertussis toxin-insensitive guanine-nucleotide binding regulatory protein in vascular smooth muscle cells. *J Clin Invest* 1990;85:653–658.

230. Brewster CEP, Howarth PH, Djukanovic R, Wilson J, Holgate ST, Roche WR. Myofibroblasts and subepithelial fibrosis in bronchial asthma. *Am J Respir Cell Mol Biol* 1990;3:507–511.

231. Peacock AJ, Dawes KE, Shock A, Gray AJ, Reeves JT, Laurent GJ. Endothelin-1 and endothelin-3 induce chemotaxis and replication of pulmonary artery fibroblasts. *Am J Respir Cell Mol Biol* 1992;7: 492–499.

232. Hassoun PM, Thappa V, Landman MJ, Fanburg BL. Endothelin 1: mitogenic activity on pulmonary artery smooth muscle cells and release from hypoxic endothelial cells. *Proc Soc Exp Biol Med* 1992;199: 165–170.

233. Payne AN, Whittle BJR. Potent cyclo-oxygenase-mediated bronchoconstrictor effects of endothelin in the guinea-pig *in vivo*. *Eur J Pharmacol* 1988;158:303–304.

234. Ninomiya H, Yu XY, Hasegawa S, Spannhake EW. Endothelin-1 induces stimulation of prostaglandin synthesis in cells obtained from canine airways by bronchoalveolar lavage. *Prostaglandins* 1992;43: 401–411.

235. Ehrenreich H, Burd PR, Rottem M, Hültner L, Hylton JB, Garfield M et al. Endothelins belong to the assortment of mast cell-derived and mast cell-bound cytokines. *New Biologist* 1992;4:147–156.

236. Egger D, Geuenich S, Denzlinger C, Schmitt E, Mailhammer R, Ehrenreich H et al. IL-4 renders mast cells functionally responsive to endothelin-1. *J Immunol* 995;154:1830–1837.

237. Uchida Y, Ninomiya H, Sakamoto T, Lee JY, Endo T, Nomura A et al. ET-1 released histamine from guinea pig pulmonary but not peritoneal mast cells. *Biochem Biophys Res Comm* 1992;189: 1196–1201.

238. Nagase T, Fukuchi Y, Jo C, Teramoto S, Uejima Y, Ishida K et al. Endothelin-1 stimulates arachidonate 15-lipoxygenase activity and oxygen radical formation in the rat distal lung. *Biochem Biophys Res Comm* 1990;168:485–489.

239. Helset E, Kjæva J, Hauge A. Endothelin-1-induced increases in microvascular permeability in isolated, perfused rat lungs requires leukocytes and plasma. *Circul Shock* 1993;39:15–20.

240. Horgan MJ, Pinheiro JMB, Malik AB. Mechanism of endothelin-1-induced pulmonary vasoconstriction. *Circul Res* 1991;69:157–164.

241. Pons F, Touvay C, Lagente V, Mencia-Huerta JM, Braquet P. Comparison of the effects of intra-arterial and aerosol administration of endothelin-1 (ET-1) in the guinea-pig isolated lung. *Br J Pharmacol* 1991;102:791–796.

242. Ercan ZS, Kiling M, Yazar Ö, Korkusuz P, Türker RK. Endothelin-1-induced oedema in rat and guinea-pig isolated perfused lungs. *Arch int Pharmacodyn* 1993;323:74–84.

243. Bonvallet ST, Oka M, Yano M, Zamora MR, McMurtry IF, Stelzner TJ. BQ123, an ET_A receptor antagonist, attenuates endothelin-1-induced vasoconstriction in rat pulmonary circulation. *J Cardiovasc Pharmacol* 1993;22:39–43.

244. Filep JG, Sirois MG, Földes-Filep É, Rousseau A, Plante GE, Fournier A et al. Enhancement by endothelin-1 of microvascular permeability via the activation of ET_A receptors. *Br J Pharmacol* 1993; 109:880–886.

245. Filep JG, Fournier A, Földes-Filep . Acute pro-inflammatory actions of endothelin-1 in the guinea-pig lung: involvement of ET_A and ET_B receptors. *Brit J Pharmacol* 1995;115:227–236.

246. Barnard JW, Barman SA, Adkins WK, Longenecker GL, Taylor AE. Sustained effects of endothelin-1 on rabbit, dog, and rat pulmonary circulations. *Am J Physiol* 1991;261:H479–H486.

247. Achmad TH, Rao GS. Chemotaxis of human blood monocytes toward endothelin-1 and the influence of calcium channel blockers. *Biochem Biophys Res Comm* 1992;189:994–1000.

248. Bath PMW, Mayston SA, Martin JF. Endothelin and PDGF do not stimulate peripheral blood monocyte chemotaxis, adhesion to endothelium, and superoxide production. *Exper Cell Res* 1990;187: 339–342.

249. Millul,V, Lagente V, Gillardeaux O, Boichot E, Dugas B, Mencia-Huerta J-M et al. Activation of guinea pig alveolar macrophages by endothelin-1. *J Cardiovasc Pharmacol* (Suppl 7) 1991;S233–S235.

250. Haller H, Schaberg T, Lindschau C, Lode H, Distler A. Endothelin increases $[Ca^{2+}]_i$, protein phosphorylation, and O_2^- production in human alveolar macrophages. *Am J Physiol* 1991;261:L478–L484.

251. Helset E, Sildnes T, Seljelid R, Konoski ZS. Endothelin-1 stimulates human monocytes *in vitro* to release TNF-α, IL-1β and IL-6. *Mediators Inflamm* 1993;2:417–422.

252. Helset E, Ytrehus K, Tveita T, Kjaeve J, Jorgensen L. Endothelin-1 causes accumulation of leukocytes in the pulmonary circulation. *Circ Shock* 1994;44:201–209.

253. Barnes PJ. The role of neurotransmitters in bronchial asthma. *Lung* 1990:168:57–65(Suppl).

254. Tabuchi Y, Nakamaru M, Rakugi H, Nagano M, Mikami H, Ogihara T. Endothelin inhibits presynaptic adrenergic neurotransmission in rat mesenteric artery. *Biochem Biophys Res Commun* 1989;161: 803–808.

255. Wiklund NP, Öhlén A, Cederqvist B. Adrenergic neuromodulation by endothelin in guinea pig pulmonary artery. *Neurosci Letts* 1989;101: 269–273.

256. Wiklund NP, Wiklund CU, Öhlén A, Gustafsson LE. Cholinergic neuromodulation by endothelin in guinea pig ileum. *Neurosci Letts* 1989; 101:342–346.

257. Wiklund NP, Öhlén A, Wiklund CU, Hedqvist P, Gustafsson LE. Endothelin modulation of neuroeffector transmission in rat and guinea pig vas deferens. *Eur J Pharmacol* 1990;185:25–33.

258. McKay KO, Armour CL, Black JL. Endothelin-3 increases transmission in the rabbit pulmonary parasympathetic nervous system. *J Cardiovasc Pharmacol* 1993;22(Suppl 8):S181–S184.

259. Henry PJ, Goldie RG. Endothelin-1, via activation of an ET_B receptor, inhibits cholinergic nerve-mediated contractions in sheep trachea. *J Cardiovasc Pharmacol* 1995;26:S117–S119.

260. Takimoto M, Inui T, Okada T, Urade Y. Contraction of smooth muscle by activation of endothelin receptors on autonomic neurons. *FEBS Letts* 1993;324:27–82.

261. Uchida Y, Hamada M, Kameyama M, Ohse H, Nomura A, Hasegawa S et al. ET-1 induced bronchoconstriction in the early phase but not late phase of anesthetized dogs is inhibited by indomethacin and ICI 198615. *Biochem Biophys Res Comm* 1992;183:1197–1202.

262. Matsuse T, Fukuchi Y, Suruda T, Nagase T, Ouchi Y, Orimo H. Effect of endothelin-1 on pulmonary resistance in rats. *J Appl Physiol* 1990; 68:2391–2393.

263. Abraham WM, Ahmed A, Cortes A, Spinella MJ, Malik AB, Anderson TT. A specific endothelin-1 antagonist blocks inhaled endothelin-1-induced bronchoconstriction in sheep. *J Appl Physiol* 1993;74: 2537–2542.

264. Touvay C, Vilain B, Pons F, Chabrier P-E, Mencia-Huerta JM, Braquet P. Bronchopulmonary and vascular effect of endothelin in the guinea pig. *Eur J Pharmacol* 1990;176:23–33.

265. Noguchi K, Noguchi Y, Hirose H, Nishikibe M, Ihara M, Ishikawa K, et al. Role of endothelin ET_B receptors in bronchoconstrictor and vasoconstrictor responses in guinea-pigs. *Eur J Pharmacol* 1993;233: 47–51.

266. Nagase T, Fukuchi Y, Matsui H, Aoki T, Matsuse T, Orimo H. *In vivo* effects of endothelin A- and B-receptor antagonists in guinea pigs. *Am J Physiol* 1995;268:L846–L850.

267. Boichot E, Lagente V, Mencia-Huerta JM, Braquet P. Effect of phosphoramidon and indomethacin on the endothelin-1 (ET-1) induced bronchopulmonary response in aerosol sensitized guinea pigs. *J Vasc Med Biol* 1990;2:206.

268. Wong J, Vanderford PA, Fineman JR, Chang R, Soifer SJ. Endothelin-1 produces pulmonary vasodilation in the intact newborn lamb. *Am J Physiol* 1993;265:H1318–H1325.

269. Minkes RK, Bellan JA, Saroyan RM, Kerstein MD, Coy DH, Murphy WA, et al. Analysis of cardiovascular and pulmonary responses to endothelin-1 and endothelin-3 in the anesthetized cat. *J Pharmacol Exp Therap* 1990;253:1118–1125.

270. Lippton HL, Cohen GA, McMurtry IF, Hyman AI. Pulmonary vasodilation to endothelin isopeptides *in vivo* is mediated by potassium channel activation. *J Appl Physiol* 1991;70:947–952.

271. Barman SA, Ardell JL, Taylor AE. Effect of endothelin-1 on canine airway blood flow. *J Cardiovasc Pharm* 1993;22 (Suppl 8): S274–S277.

272. Pinheiro JMB, Malik AB. Mechanisms of endothelin-1-induced pulmonary vasodilation in neonatal pigs. *J Physiol* 1993;469:739–752.

273. Lagente V, Boichot E, Mencia-Huerta J, Braquet P. Failure of aerosolized endothelin (ET-1) to induce bronchial hyperreactivity in the guinea pig. *Fundam Clin Pharmacol* 1990;4:275–280.

274. Boichot E, Carré C, Lagente V, Pons F, Mencia-Huerta JM, Braquet P. Endothelin-1 (ET-1) and bronchial hyperresponsiveness in the guinea-pig. *J Cardiovasc Pharmacol* 1991;17 (Suppl 7):S329–S331.

275. Pons F, Boichot E, Lagente V, Touvay C, Mencia-Huerta JM, Braquet P. Role of endothelin in pulmonary function. *Pulmon Pharmacol* 1992;5:213–219.

276. Kanazawa H, Kurihara N, Kirata K, Fujiwara H, Matsushita H, Takeda T. Low concentration endothelin-1 enhanced histamine-mediated bronchial contractions of guinea pigs *in vivo*. *Biochem Biophys Res Comm* 1992;187:717–721.

277. Noguchi K, Ishikawa K, Yano M, Ahmed A, Cortes A, Abraham WM. Endothelin-1 contributes to antigen-induced airway hyperresponsiveness. *J Appl Physiol* 1995;79:700–705.

278. Kay AB. Asthma and inflammation. *J Allergy Clin Pharmacol* 1991; 87:893–910.

279. Nomura A, Uchida Y, Kameyama M, Saotome M, Oki K, Hasegawa S. Endothelin and bronchial asthma. *Lancet* 1989;2(8665):747–748.

280. Mattoli S, Soloperto M, Marini M, Fasoli A. Levels of endothelin in the bronchoalveolar lavage fluid of patients with symptomatic asthma and reversible airflow obstruction. *J Allergy Clin Immunol* 1991;88: 376–384.

281. Redington AE, Springall DR, Ghatei MA, Lau LCK, Bloom SR, Holgate ST, et al. Endothelin in bronchoalveolar lavage fluid and its relation to airflow obstruction in asthma. *Am J Respir Cric Care Med* 1995;151:1034–1039.

282. Sofia M, Mormile M, Faraone S, Alifano M, Zofra S, Romano L, Carratú L. Increased endothelinlike immunoreactive material on bronchoalveolar lavage fluid from patients with bronchial asthma and patients with interstitial lung disease. *Respiration* 1993;60:89–95.

283. Vittori E, Marini M, Fasoli A, De Franchis R, Mattoli S. Increased expression of endothelin in bronchial epithelial cells of asthmatic patients and effect of corticosteroids. *Am Rev Respir Dis* 1992;146: 1320–1325.

284. Ackerman V, Carpi S, Bellini A, Vassalli G, Marini M, Mattoli S. Respiratory pathophysiologic responses. Constitutive expression of endothelin in bronchial epithelial cells of patients with symptomatic and asymptomatic asthma and modulation by histamine and interleukin-1. *J Allergy Clin Immunol* 1995;96:618–627.

285. Chen WY, Yu J, Wang JY. Decreased production of endothelin-1 in asthmatic children after immunotherapy. *J Asthma* 1995;32:29–35.

286. Aoki T, Kojima T, Ono A, Unishi G, Yoshijima S, Kameda-Hayashi N et al. Circulating endothelin-1 levels in patients with bronchial asthma. *Ann Allergy* 1994;73:365–369.

287. Springall DR, Howarth PH, Counihan H, Djukanovic R, Holgate ST, Polak JM. Endothelin immunoreactivity of airway epithelium in asthmatic patients. *Lancet* 1991;337:697–701.

288. Kraft M, Beam WR, Wenzel SE, Zamora MR, O'Brien RF, Martin RJ. Blood and bronchoalveolar lavage endothelin-1 levels in nocturnal asthma. *Am J Respir Crit Care Med* 1994;149:947–952.

289. Knott PG, Daprile AC, Henry PJ, Hay DWP, Goldie RG. Receptors for endothelin-1 in asthmatic human peripheral lung. *Br J Pharmacol* 1995;114:1–3.

290. Reid, L. The pulmonary circulation: remodeling in growth and disease. *Am Rev Respir Dis* 1979;119:531–547.

291. Wagenvoort CA. Grading of pulmonary vascular lesions—a reappraisal. *Histopathol* 1981;5:595–598.

292. Heath D, Smith P, Gosney J, Mulcahy D, Fox K, Yacoub M et al. The pathology of the early and late stages of primary pulmonary hypertension. *Br Heart J* 1987;58:204–213.

293. Cernacek P, Stewart DJ. Immunoreactive endothelin in human plasma: marked elevations in patients in cardiogenic shock. *Biochem Biophys Res Comm* 1989;161:562–567.

294. Stewart DJ, Levy RD, Cernacek P, Langleben D. Increased plasma endothelin-1 in pulmonary hypertension: marker or mediator of disease? *Ann Intern Med* 1991;114:464–469.

295. Yoshibayashi M, Nishioka K, Nakao K, Saito Y, Matsumura M, Ueda T et al. Plasma endothelin concentrations in patients with pulmonary hypertension associated with congenital heart defects. *Circulation* 1991;84:2280–2285.

296. Allen SW, Chatfield BA, Koppenhafer SA, Schaffer MS, Wolfe RR, Abman SH. Circulating immunoreactive endothelin-1 in children with pulmonary hypertension. *Am Rev Respir Dis* 1993;148,519–524.

297. Cacoub P, Dorent R, Maistre G, Nataf P, Carayon A, Piette JC, et al. Endothelin-1 in primary pulmonary hypertension and the Eisenmenger Syndrome. *Am J Cardiol* 1993;71,448–450.

298. Chang H, Wu G-J, Wang S-M, Hung C-R. Plasma endothelin levels and surgically correctable pulmonary hypertension. *Ann Thorac Surg* 1993;55:450–458.

299. Rosenberg AA, Kennaugh J, Koppenhafer SL, Loomis M, Chatfield BA, Abman SH. Elevated immunoreactive endothelin-1 levels in newborn infants with persistent pulmonary hypertension. *J Pediatr* 1993; 123–124.

300. Cody RJ, Haas GJ, Binkley PF, Capers Q, Kelley R. Plasma endothelin correlates with the extent of pulmonary hypertension in patients with chronic congestive heart failure. *Circulation* 1992;85:504–509.

301. Giaid A, Yanagisawa M, Langleben D, Michel RP, Levy R, Shennib H et al. Expression of endothelin-1 in the lungs of patients with pulmonary hypertension. *N Engl J Med* 1993;328:1732–1739.

302. Yoshizumi M, Kurihara H, Sugiyama T, Takaku F, Yanagisawa M, Masaki T et al. Hemodynamic shear stress stimulates endothelin production by cultured endothelial cells. *Biochem Biophys Res Comm* 1989;161:859–864.

303. Lippton HL, Hauth TA, Summer WR, Hyman AL. Endothelin produces pulmonary vasoconstriction and systemic vasodilation. *J Appl Physiol* 1989;66:1008–1012.

304. Stelzner TJ, O'Brien RF, Yanagisawa M, Sakurai T, Sato K, Webb S et al. Increased lung endothelin-1 production in rats with idiopathic pulmonary hypertension. *Am J Physiol* 1992;262:L614–L620.

305. Miyauchi T, Yorikane R, Sakai S, Sakurai T, Okada M, Nishikibe M et al. Contribution of endogenous endothelin-1 to the progression of cardiopulmonary alterations in rats with monocrotaline-induced pulmonary hypertension. *Circul Res* 1993;73:887–897.

306. Bonvallet ST, Zamora MR, Hasunuma K, Sato K, Hanasato N, Anderson D et al. BQ123, an ET$_A$-receptor antagonist, attenuates hypoxic pulmonary hypertension in rats. *Am J Physiol* 1994;266: H1327–H1331.

307. DiCarlo VS, Chen S-J, Meng QC, Durand J, Yano M, Chen Y-F et al. ET$_A$-receptor antagonist prevents and reverses chronic hypoxia-induced pulmonary hypertension in rat. *Am J Physiol* 1995;269: L690–L697.

308. Eddahibi S, Raffestin B, Clozel M, Levame M, Adnot S. Protection from pulmonary hypertension with an orally active endothelin receptor antagonist in hypoxic rats. *Am J Physiol* 1995;268:H828–H835.

309. Okada M, Yamashita C, Okada K. Endothelin receptor antagonists in a beagle model of pulmonary hypertension-contribution to possible potential therapy. *J Am Coll Cardiol* 1995;25:1213–1217.

310. Wong J, Vanderford PA, Winters JW, Chang R, Soifer SJ, Fineman JR. Endothelin-1 does not mediate acute hypoxic pulmonary vasoconstriction in the intact newborn lamb. *J Cardiovasc Pharmacol* 1993; 22 (Suppl 8):S262–S266.

311. Wiebke JL, Montrose-Rafizadeh C, Zeitlin PL, Guggino WB. Effect of hypoxia on endothelin-1 production by pulmonary vascular endothelia cells. *Biochim Biophys Acta* 1992;1134:105–111.

312. Li H, Elton TS, Chen YF, Oparil S. Increased endothelin receptor gene expression in hypoxic rat lung. *Am J Physiol* 1994;266:L553–L560.

313. Elton TS, Oparil S, Taylor GR, Hicks PH, Yang RH, Jin H et al. Normobaric hypoxia stimulates endothelin-1 gene expression in the rat. *Am J Physiol* 1992;263:R1260–R1264.

314. Vemulapalli S, Rivelli M, Chiu PJ, del Prado M, Hey JA. Phosphoramidon abolishes the increases in endothelin-1 release induced by ischemia-hyposia in isolated perfused guinea pig lungs. *J Pharmacol Exp Ther* 1992;262:1062–1069.

315. Shirakami G, Nakao K, Saito Y, Magaribuchi T, Jougasaki M, Mukoyama et al. Acute pulmonary alveolar hypoxia increases lung and plasma endothelin-1 levels in conscious rats. *Life Sci* 1991;48: 969–976.

316. Riccio MM, Reynolds CJ, Hay DWP, Proud D. Effects of intranasal

administration of endothelin-1 to allergic and nonallergic individuals. *Am J Respir Crit Care Med* 1995;152:1757–1764.

317. Giaid A, Hamid QA, Springall DR, Yanagisawa M, Shinmi O, Sawamura T et al. Detection of endothelin immunoreactivity and mRNA in pulmonary tumours. *J Pathol* 1990;162:15–22.

318. Zhao YD, Springall DR, Hamid Q, Levene M, Polak JM. Localization and characterization of endothelin-1 receptor binding in the blood vessels of human pulmonary tumors. *J Cardiovasc Pharmacol* 1995; 26:S341–S345.

319. Druml W, Steltzer H, Waldhausl W, Lenz K, Hammerle A, Vierhapper H, et al. Endothelin-1 in adult respiratory distress syndrome. *Am J Respir Dis* 1993;148:1169–1173.

320. Langleben D, DeMarchie M, Laporta D, Spanier AH, Schlesinger RD, Stewart DJ. Endothelin-1 in acute lung injury and the adult respiratory distress syndrome. *Am J Respir Dis* 1993;148:1646–1650.

321. Mitaka C, Hirata Y, Nagura T, Tsunoda Y, Amaha K. Circulating endothelin-1 concentrations in acute respiratory failure. *Chest* 1993; 104:476–480.

322. Giaid A, Michel RP, Stewart DJ, Sheppard M, Corrin B, Hamid Q. Expression of endothelin-1 in lungs of patients with cryptogenic fibrosing alveolitis. *Lancet* 1993;341:1550–1554.

323. Cambrey AD, Harrison NK, Dawes KE, Southcott AM, Black CM, du Boi RM et al. Increased levels of endothelin-1 in bronchoalveolar lavage fluid from patients with systemic sclerosis contribute to fibroblast mitogenic activity *in vitro*. *Am J Respir Cell Mol Biol* 1994; 11:439–445.

324. Marciniak SJ, Plumpton C, Barker PJ, Huskisson NS, Davenport AP. Localization of immunoreactive endothelin and proendothelin in the human lung. *Pulmon Pharmacol* 1992;5:175–182.

325. Ferri C, Bellini C, De Angelis C, De Siati L, Perrone A, Properzi G et al. Circulating endothelin-1 concentrations in patients with chronic hypoxia. *J Clin Pathol* 1995;48:519–524.

326. Andersson SE, Zackrisson C, Hemsén A, Lundberg JM. Regulation of lung endothelin content by the glucocorticosteroid budesonide. *Biochem Biophys Res Comm* 1992;188:1116–1121.

327. Morel DR, Lacroix JS, Hemsen A, Steinig DA, Pittet J-F, Lundberg JM. Increased plasma and pulmonary lymph levels of endothelin during endotoxin shock. *Eur J Pharmacol* 1989;167:427–428.

328. Filep JG, Télémaque S, Battistini B, Sirois P, D'Orléans-Juste P. Increased plasma levels of endothelin during anaphylactic shock in the guinea-pig. *Eur J Pharmacol* 1993;239:231–236.

329. Giaid A, Stewart DJ, Michel RP. Endothelin-1-like immunoreactivity in postobstructive pulmonary vasculopathy. *J Vasc Res* 1993;30: 333–338.

330. Simmet T, Pritze S, Thelen KI, Peskar BA. Release of endothelin in the oleic acid-induced respiratory distress syndrome in rats. *Eur J Pharmacol* 1992;211:319–322.

331. Shirakami G, Nakao K, Saito Y, Magariibuchi T, Jougasaki M, Mukoyama M. et al. Acute pulmonary alveolar hypoxia increases lung and plasma endothelin-1 levels in conscious rats. *Life Sci* 1991;48: 969–976.

332. Okada M, Yamashita C, Okada M, Okada K. Contribution of endothelin-1 to warm ischemia/reperfusion injury of the rat lung. *Am J Resp Crit Care Med* 1995;152:2105–2110.

333. Scherstén H, Aarnio P, Burnett Jr JC, McGregor CGA, Miller VM. Endothelin-1 in bronchoalveolar lavage during rejection of allotransplanted lungs. *Transplant* 1994;57:159–161.

334. Kurihara Y, Kurihara H, Suzuki H, Kodama T, Maemura K, Nagai et al. Elevated blood pressure and craniofacial abnormalities in mice deficient in endothelin-1. *Nature* 1994;368:703–710.

▪ 6 ▪

Target Cells

Asthma, edited by P.J. Barnes, M.M. Grunstein,
A.R. Leff, and A.J. Woolcock.
Lippincott–Raven Publishers, Philadelphia © 1997.

▪ 55 ▪

Airway Smooth Muscle Structure

Richard W. Mitchell and Andrew J. Halayko

In the lung, smooth muscle is found in the airways, from the trachea to the terminal bronchioles. The smooth muscle contracts and relaxes; the level of tone determines the caliber of the airways and, thus, the resistance to the flow of air to and from the alveoli. Airway smooth muscle tone is a dynamic product of intrinsic neural, hormonal, and inflammatory cell influences and extrinsic chemical insults or therapies. Hyperresponsiveness and hypertrophy/hyperplasia of the smooth muscle layer within the resistance airways are hallmarks of asthma.

This chapter will describe the normal macroscopic and microscopic structure of airways and the airway smooth muscle of humans and animal models. It will illustrate also changes in ultrastructure, content, and activity of contractile, regulatory, and structural proteins that have been observed in asthma and in models of hyperresponsiveness and hypertrophy/hyperplasia. Furthermore, using immunohistochemical methods, phenotypic changes in airway smooth muscle cells will be described. Contraction, regulation of contraction, and airway smooth muscle hyperresponsiveness will be dealt with in Chapter 56.

R. W. Mitchell: Section of Pulmonary and Critical Care Medicine, Division of the Biological Sciences, The University of Chicago, Chicago, Illinois 60637.

A. J. Halayko: Department of Physiology, University of Manitoba, Winnipeg, Manitoba R3E 3J7 Canada.

SINGLE UNIT, MULTI-UNIT, AND INTERMEDIATE SMOOTH MUSCLE

Smooth muscle has been categorized into multi-unit, single-unit, and intermediate types based upon density of innervation and the ability of the tissue to propagate membrane depolarizing pulses and, thus, waves of contraction from cell to cell (1). Multi-unit smooth muscle has a rich neural network with individual myocytes being innervated (Fig. 1). There is little cell-to-cell communication based on the facts that a) there are few, if any, gap junctions (Fig. 2) or nexuses (low impedance areas of the sarcolemma that allow the propagation of electrical pulses from one smooth muscle cell to the next), b) the tissue has a high membrane resistance, and c) no action potentials can be observed (2). When artificially stretched, multi-unit smooth muscles do not demonstrate a rebound myogenic contractile response. The larger blood vessels contain multi-unit smooth muscle.

Single-unit smooth muscles demonstrate a sparse neural network, many gap junctions, and low electrical resistance, allowing the tissue to contract as a syncytium. Depolarizing electrical pulses (including action potentials) are easily transmitted throughout the tissue and the membrane potential displays oscillations (3). Single-unit smooth muscles demonstrate spontaneous contractile activity and myogenic responses, and can be found in the

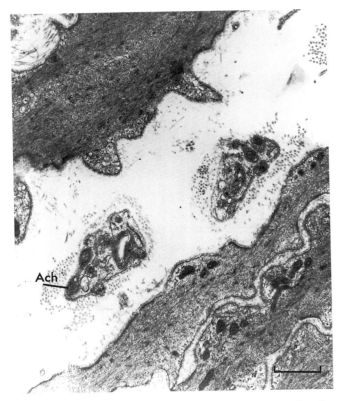

FIG. 1. Transmission electron micrograph demonstrating the presence of two nerve terminals located between two longitudinally sectioned canine tracheal smooth muscle cells. Cholinergic endings containing acetylcholine vesicles (Ach) are clearly visible in one of the axons.

intestines, ureters, the term-pregnant uterus, and smaller blood vessels.

Originally, the smooth muscle of the airways was characterized as the intermediate type (1). The smooth muscle of the upper airways is characteristically more multi-unit; tracheal smooth muscle has relatively few gap junctions, displays no action potentials or myogenic responses, but has a relatively sparse innervation (4). For these reasons, airway smooth muscle has been catego-

rized as the intermediate type. However, in the presence of K^+ channel blockers such as tetraethylammonium, canine tracheal smooth muscle has been shown to demonstrate a) membrane depolarization with the decreased permeability to K^+, resulting in a decreased electrical resistance and increased electrical conduction velocity through the tissue, b) spontaneous electrical activity, and c) myogenic contractile activity—characteristics of single-unit smooth muscle (5).

Like the smaller blood vessels, it has been speculated that the smaller bronchioles may demonstrate single-unit type electrical and contractile responses. It is known that the innervation of the airway smooth muscle decreases distally from the trachea, and sixth to seventh generation bronchi dissected from lung resections demonstrate spontaneous active tone and some myogenic response to quick stretch (6). It has been suggested, on the basis of *in vivo* human studies and *in vitro* studies using K^+ channel blockers, that, in airway hyperresponsive diseases such as asthma, the smooth muscle may change from a more multi-unit to a more single-unit type by a quantitative change in the excitability of the tissue (7).

GROSS ANATOMY

Tracheal Smooth Muscle

Smooth muscle of the trachea is found as a unified layer of thick bundles of cells from the larynx to the carina within the dorsally situated posterior membrane or paries membranaceus—a multi-layered tissue that spans the gap between the ends of the incomplete cartilagenous rings. These bundles of cells run parallel to each other and perpendicular to the long axis of the trachea. There is little or no branching. Between the bundles can be found collagen and elastin. Isolated strips of trachealis muscle have been demonstrated to be greater that 75% muscle with connective tissue, fibroblasts, and neural elements accounting for the major proportion of the balance of cellular and noncellular constituents (Fig. 3). Individual

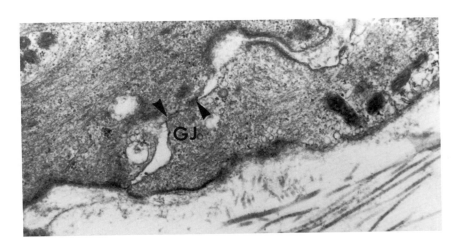

FIG. 2. High-power electron micrograph of canine trachealis showing the presence of a gap junction (*GJ*) between two myocytes. These cell-to-cell connections are associated with single-unit smooth muscles and, as such, they are infrequently seen in tracheal smooth muscle.

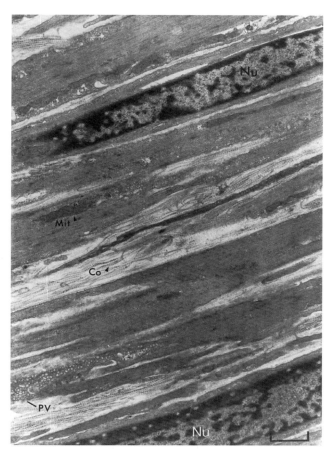

FIG. 3. Low-power electron micrograph of longitudinally sectioned canine tracheal smooth muscle. The picture illustrates that greater than 75% of the trachealis consists of smooth muscle cells. Longitudinally oriented collagen fibers (*Co*) can be seen in the extracellular spaces between cells. Note the parallel arrangement of myocytes. Nuclei (*Nu*) of two cells can be clearly seen. Mitochondria (*Mi*) and pinocytotic vesicles (*PV*) are also apparent on the muscle cells.

muscle cells are 3 to 5 microns wide, and may be greater than 1 mm in length (8). The cells are fusiform in shape and contain a centrally located, cigar-shaped nucleus.

With reference to the lumen of the airway, the trachealis muscle lies below the epithelium, basement membrane, and mucosa of the tunica fibrosa (Fig. 4). In humans, the muscle layer is internal to the tunica propria, and the muscle bundles insert by elastic tendons to the internal aspect of the perichondrium of the cartilage ring and the annual ligaments, which bind the tracheal rings together. In some species, like the dog, the trachealis bundles insert onto the external perichondrium.

Bronchial Smooth Muscle

Unlike the trachealis, bronchial smooth muscle does not insert directly onto the cartilagenous plaques that are found throughout the central airways (Fig. 5). Instead, the smooth muscle is found in branching bundles that interdigitate with the cartilage plaques, blood vessels, and other structures found within the bronchial wall. These bundles neither run circumferentially nor helically through the bronchi. However, despite this lack of a specific anatomic arrangement, the smooth muscle is capable of completely occluding the bronchial lumen (given an adequate stimulus) without appreciable reduction of the outer diameter of the airway (9).

Where greater than 75% of isolated trachealis strips is muscle, isolated bronchial preparations with cartilage plaques removed are only 30% smooth muscle cells (10) (Fig. 6). Under light microscopy, bronchial smooth muscle cells do not appear any different from those myocytes found in the trachea (Fig. 5). Also, within a bronchial smooth muscle bundle, the cells are arranged in parallel with each other; again, the airway myocytes are fusiform in shape and possess cigar-shaped nuclei. Figure 5 demonstrates that contracted airway smooth muscle cells do not appear as uniform as in relaxed preparations, have lost their fusiform shape, and appear as a wavy band of tissue.

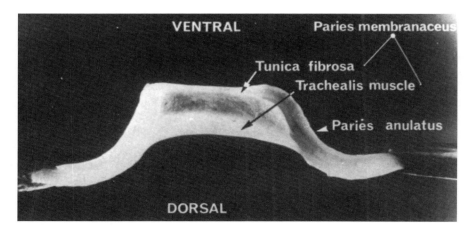

FIG. 4. Photograph of the cross section of a single canine tracheal ring which has been cut ventrally and everted, causing the trachealis and the tunica fibrosa to separate spontaneously. In the dog, the trachealis is attached to the external aspect of the cartilage; however, attachment in the human trachea is to the inner aspect of the cartilage. (From Stephens NL. Physical properties of contractile systems. In: Daniel EE, Paton DM, eds. *Methods in pharmacology*, vol 3. New York: Plenum Press, 1975;555–591, with permission.)

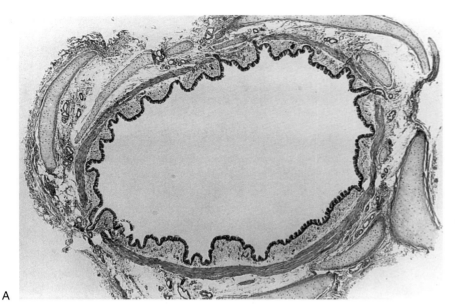

A

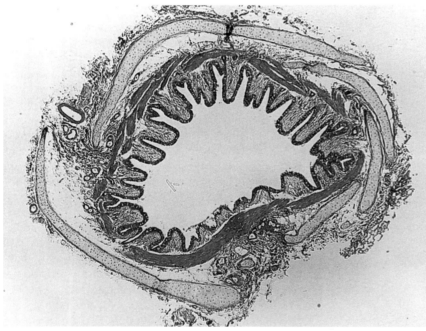

B

FIG. 5. Panels **A** and **B** are 5 μm sections (30X) of contiguous, canine bronchial rings (4 mm diameter) relaxed maximally with β-adrenergic receptor agonist (**A**) and contracted maximally with a muscarinic receptor agonist (**B**). The figure demonstrates that the smooth muscle does not insert onto the cartilagenous plaques of the airway. Epithelium, smooth muscle, secretory glands and cartilage plaques can be observed. In relaxed airways, the smooth muscle cells, which lie in parallel with each other, appear fusiform in shape with cigar-shaped nuclei. Contraction of the smooth muscle, which lies just under the epithelium and mucosa, significantly reduced the lumenal area of the bronchus, increasing the depth of the infolding of the epithelial and mucosal layers and displacing the surrounding lunate, cartilage plaques. Also, the smooth muscle cells do not appear as uniform as in panel **A**, have lost their fusiform shape, and appear as a wavy band of tissue.

External to the airway smooth muscle bundles of the trachea and bronchi, a connective tissue stroma is observed containing mast cells, blood vessels, fibroblasts, nerves, elastin and collagen. Serial sections show collagen spiralling around the muscle bundles. Amorphous and fibrous elastin are found within the interfascicular space. Collagen and elastin fibers intermesh with each other and with the lacy basement membrane associated with the sarcolemma (Fig. 7).

Innervation

The dominant neural input to the airways is the parasympathetic nervous system, which, when stimu-lated, causes contraction of the airway smooth muscle through the release of acetylcholine from the postganglionic *en passage* neural net observed in electron micrographs (11) (Fig. 8A). (There are no true neuromuscular junctions in airway smooth muscle. Neural nodes are found as neuronal outpouchings that contain neurotransmitter in vesicles.)

Sympathetic nerves are found in close association with parasympathetic fibers. In fact, electron micrographs demonstrate both clear (acetylcholine) and dense cored (norepinephrine) "synaptic" vesicles within the same neural nodes (Fig. 8B). The interaction of these two neural networks in airway smooth muscle is still poorly understood, but the effect of norepinephrine release and

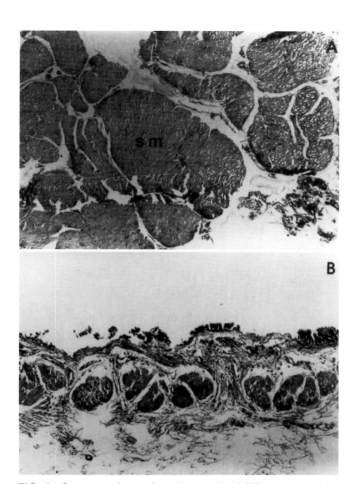

FIG. 6. Cross sections of canine tracheal (**A**) and bronchial main stem (fourth generation) smooth muscle (**B**) preparations as seen using light microscopy. Planimetry revealed that smooth muscle *(sm)* occupied 77% and 30% respectively of the total cross-sectional area of the muscle strips. (Tissues were stained with H&E staining; original magnification x 200.) (From Jiang H, Stephens NL. Contractile properties of bronchial smooth muscle with and without cartilage. *J Appl Physiol* 1990;69:120–126, with permission.)

subsequent activation of relaxant β-adrenergic receptors probably plays a minor role in the control of tone because of the dominance of the parasympathetic input (11). There also is evidence for α-adrenergic receptors on airway smooth muscle; these receptors are activated in the presence of increased basal active tone and cause further contraction. A definitive role for α-adrenergic receptors in the airways has yet to be determined.

Nonadrenergic, noncholinergic inhibitory (NANC_i) nerves are present in the airways, but vary considerably in their significance from species to species. Electrical field stimulation of guinea pig trachealis strips *in vitro* demonstrates significant relaxation of spontaneous tone or agonist-elicited contraction that is sensitive to tetrodotoxin, a Na+ channel blocker that inhibits neuronal transmission, but the electrically induced relaxations are not sensitive to β-adrenergic or muscarinic receptor blockade (12). Human bronchial ring preparations do not demonstrate significant relaxation to electrical stimulation, indicating a sparse NANC_i neural input. Recent studies of porcine trachealis muscle suggest that the neurotransmitter may be nitric oxide (NO).

Contraction also can be elicited through the release of substance P (SP) and neurokinin A (NKA) from sensory c-fibers found in the airways—a nonadrenergic, noncholinergic contractile (NANC_c) system found in many species (13). Release of these tachykinins causes a neurogenic inflammatory response in the airways, which includes increased vascular permeability, direct and indirect (neutrophil-mediated) inflammation and sloughing of the epithelium, and contraction of the airway smooth muscle. Tachykinins have been shown to be released by capsaicin, an extract which gives red peppers their characteristic hot flavor (14). Substance P and NKA contract airway smooth muscle directly and cause the release of other neurotransmitters, including acetylcholine from cholinergic nerves, to indirectly add to airway smooth

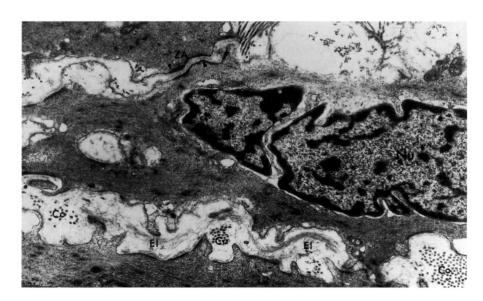

FIG. 7. High-power micrograph demonstrating that collagen fibers (*Co*), cut here in cross section, are seen to alternate with elastic filaments (*El*) running parallel with the longitudinal axis of the cells. An intermediate junction (*ZA*) is also visible between two myocytes.

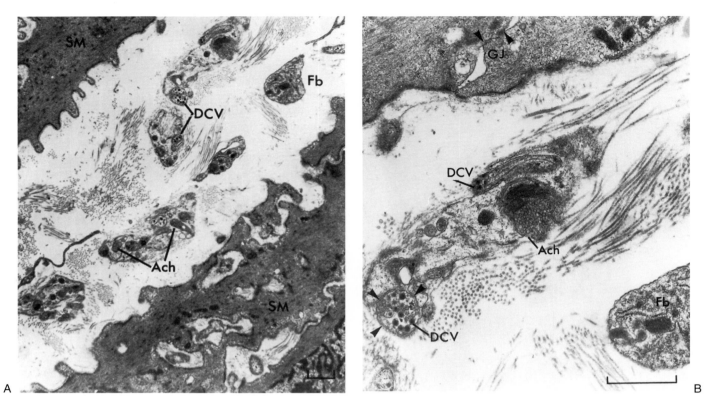

FIG. 8. Electron micrographs depicting innervation of canine tracheal smooth muscle by parasympathetic and sympathetic nerves. (**A**) Longitudinal muscle section showing several nerve terminals in the extracellular space between two smooth muscle (*SM*) bundles. Cholinergic vesicles (*Ach*) and dense core vesicles (*DCV*), which are characteristic of parasympathetic and sympathetic terminals respectively, can be seen. Fibroblasts (*Fb*) also can be observed between the cells. (**B**) High-power micrograph showing the presence of dense core vesicles (*DCV*) and cholinergic vesicles (*Ach*) in the same nerve terminal in canine tracheal smooth muscle. Muscle cells at the top of the picture show the presence of a gap junction (*GJ*); a fibroblast (*Fb*) is also visible.

muscle tone. Inhibition of neutral endopeptidase (NEP), an epithelium-associated enzyme that metabolizes the tachykinins, causes augmentation of contractile responses of airways to SP, NKA, and capsaicin. In the presence of NEP inhibitors or in the absence of epithelium (due to some inflammatory process), tachykinins released would be unopposed in causing constriction of the bronchioles.

ULTRASTRUCTURE

Sarcoplasmic Reticulum

There is a restricted reticular structure in airway smooth muscle. Rough endoplasmic reticulum is not very evident in electron micrographs of smooth muscle from mature airways, though it has been demonstrated that during early development, these reticular structures predominate (15). In fully-developed airway myocytes, smooth reticular tubules are in intimate contact with pinocytotic vesicles and with the caveoli associated with the sarcolemma (Fig. 9). The precise function of this reticular system is not fully understood. However, it is be-

lieved that, along with the caveoli, these structures are the source of intracellular calcium used in receptor-mediated contraction (16).

Caveoli

It has been estimated that each airway myocyte has 100,000 to 200,000 caveoli lining the inner aspect of the sarcolemma (17). They appear to be invaginations of the sarcolemma, and all are in contact with the extracellular space through a neck-like structure (Fig. 10). Intramembraneous structures are observed surrounding the necks of the caveoli. Although their exact function remains unclear, in endothelial cells, caveoli have been demonstrated to have pinocytotic activity and mechanisms for the active transport of ions and other small molecules across the sarcolemma (18,19). It has been estimated that caveoli increase the surface area of airway smooth muscle cells by 70%.

There is strong evidence that caveoli, along with the sarcoplasmic reticulum, store and release calcium for contraction. Using calcium-specific markers, it has been demonstrated that the major portion of the calcium used

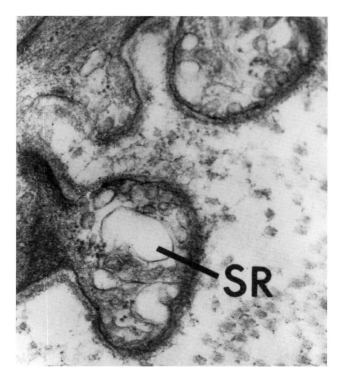

FIG. 9. High-power electron micrograph showing projections or outpouchings of the sarcolemma seen often in tracheal smooth muscle cells. Pinocytotic vesicles and caveoli are seen to line the projections, which also contain large areas of smooth sarcoplasmic reticulum (*SR*).

with contractions elicited in the presence of extracellular calcium), and b) decrease in amplitude with successive exposure (21).

Organelles

In addition to those cellular structures that are important in contraction-coupling, airway myocytes contain a nucleus with nuleoli, nuclear membrane, and nuclear pores. Close to the polar ends of the nucleus are found the major concentrations of mitochondria (Fig. 11A) and golgi bodies (Fig. 11B). The number of mitochondria is relatively small in comparison to skeletal muscle, and can account for approximately 10% of the adenosine triphosphate (ATP) produced by striated myocytes. However, this amount of high energy phosphate probably is sufficient to accommodate contraction of the relatively slow airway smooth muscle cell. Glycogen granules are concentrated near mitochondria. Lyposomes are rarely observed (Fig. 11C), but become more prominent when the myocytes are subjected to outside stresses such as hypoxia (22).

Sarcolemma-Associated Structures

Dense Bodies, Dense Bands, and Intermediate Fibers

Fundamental to the surface caveoli, the sarcolemma of airway myocytes displays the typical bilayer of eukaryotic cells. Contracted smooth muscle displays outpouchings of the sarcolemma (Fig. 12) that are relatively electron-translucent and contain pinocytotic vesicles and sarcoplasmic reticulum (23). Electron-dense areas of the sarcolemma are found adjacent to these evaginations.

in contraction is released from the cytoplasmic face of the sarcolemma (20). Repeated exposure to acetylcholine of canine tracheal smooth muscle in a calcium-free perfusate elicits receptor-linked contractions that a) demonstrate initial phasic contractile spikes followed by a maintained plateau (which is significantly reduced compared

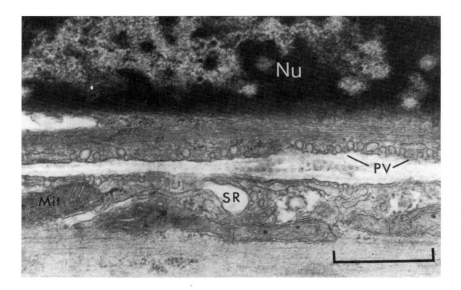

FIG. 10. A high-power micrograph demonstrating the presence of numerous caveoli (labeled *PV*) on the surface of canine tracheal smooth muscle cells. Other organelles which can be seen include sarcoplasmic reticulum (*SR*), a nucleus (*Nu*) and a mitochondrion (*Mi*).

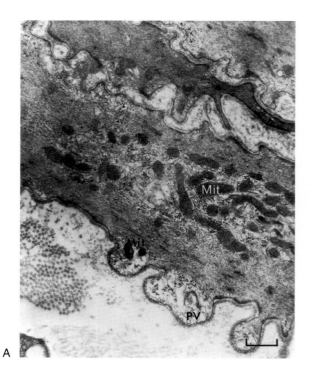

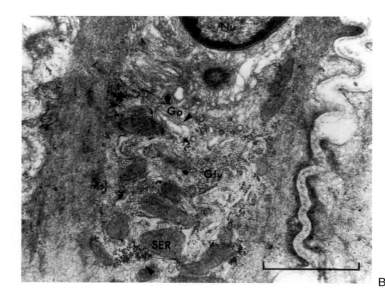

B

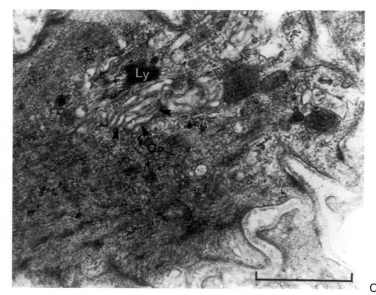

C

FIG. 11. Electron micrographs demonstrating the presence of cytoplasmic organelles in canine tracheal smooth muscle cells. (**A**) Typical arrangement of mitochondria (*Mit*) at the pole of the nucleus in areas devoid of thick and thin filaments. Note that mitochondria can occasionally be seen in sarcolemmal projections. Pinocytotic vesicles (*PV*) are also visible. (**B**) High-power micrograph showing organelles located at the pole of a nucleus: Golgi bodies (*Go*), clusters of glycogen particles (*Gly*) and smooth endoplasmic reticulum (*SER*). (**C**) A rarely seen lysosome (*Ly*), in close proximity to dilated cisternae of a Golgi apparatus (*Go*), can be seen in this high-power micrograph.

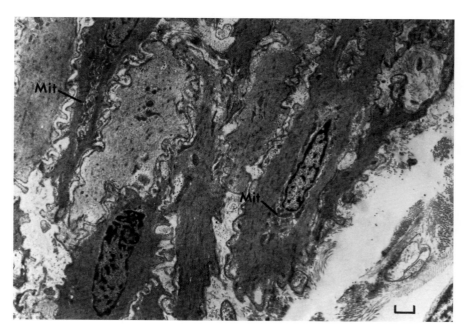

FIG. 12. Electron micrograph of a longitudinal section of partially contracted canine tracheal smooth muscle. Note the numerous outpouchings of the sarcolemma and the presence of symmetrical dense band areas between adjacent cells. Numerous organelles, including mitochondria (*Mit*), can be seen at the poles of the nuclei.

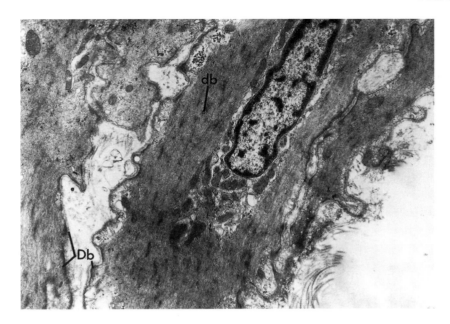

FIG. 13. Photomicrograph of a longitudinal section of canine tracheal smooth muscle demonstrating both membrane dense bands (*Db*) and cytoplasmic dense bodies (*db*). Note that the dense bodies are present in areas rich with myofilaments; this observation is consistent with the hypothesis that dense bodies function as attachment sites for contractile structures.

These dense bands (comprising approximately one-half of the cell surface area) are located along the entire surface of the sarcolemma (Fig. 13), and, inserting onto their intracellular aspect, can be found actin and intermediate filaments. The intermediate filaments are attached to a network of cytoplasmic dense bodies. The dense bands and dense bodies, held together by the intermediate filaments, form a lattice structure in which the contractile proteins, actin and myosin may interact more effectively to contract and shorten the smooth muscle. The protein composition of the dense bands and bodies is similar to the Z-bands of skeletal muscle, and these structures probably delineate smooth muscle sarcomeres.

Cell-to-Cell Junctions

The dense bands are sites of linkage between airway smooth muscle cells. Elastin and collagen make up these interconnections which allow for the transmission of force among adjacent myocytes. These interconnections are known as intermediate junctions or *zona adherens* and span 50 to 100 nm between cells (Fig. 14). Poles of the smooth muscle cells taper, but end in a foot-like structure that, through connective tissue again, attaches to the next myocyte, allowing for transmission of force along the muscle bundle.

In addition to these mechanical junctions, gap junctions that span only 2 to 3 nm are found between adjacent airway myocytes. The gap junction or nexus is an area of low electrical impedance and allows for electrical coupling among cells (Fig. 2). Multi-unit smooth muscle, like that found in the airways, possesses fewer nexuses than the highly electrically coupled smooth muscle of the gut. However, there appear to be a greater number of gap

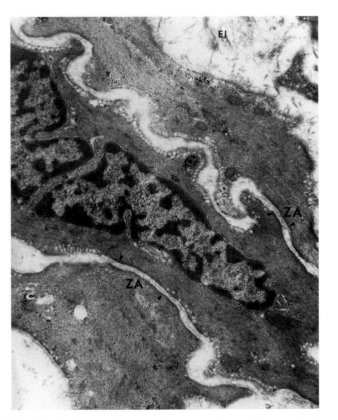

FIG. 14. A micrograph of canine tracheal smooth muscle depicting two intermediate types of *zona adherens* (*ZA*) between three cells. Electron dense material is observed on the cytoplasmic side of both cells involved in a junction. In addition, the characteristic single strand of basal lamina can be seen in the center of the cleft between two cells at the site of the junction.

junctions in the smooth muscle of bronchi than of the trachea, and their number may increase as the airways approach the periphery where innervation is more sparse (1). It has been demonstrated that the number of gap junctions in tracheal smooth muscle increases in preparations that are exposed to agents, such as tetraethylammonium, which cause spontaneous contractions of the normally quiescent canine airway (24). These tissues also showed an increased capacity to transmit electrical impulses along an airway smooth muscle bundle (5). Increased electrical and/or mechanical activity has been demonstrated for hyperresponsive airway smooth muscle from immune-sensitized guinea pigs and dogs, and in humans with asthma (6,7,25,26).

Contractile Proteins

In skeletal muscle, globular actin monomers are linked together to form the thin filament—a double-stranded, α-helical protein with a half-pitch rotation every 7 monomers (Fig. 15). One tropomyosin molecule is associated with every 7 actin monomers and, in association with one Ca^{2+}-sensitive troponin complex per 7

actin monomers, regulates the binding of myosin molecule heads to the actin filament (crossbridges). Also in skeletal muscle, actin filaments are anchored to Z-discs, which delineate each sarcomere and maintain the crystalline-like structure of the actin and myosin filaments in this tissue. In smooth muscle, actin is found in α-helices with associated tropomyosin like skeletal muscle, but troponin is absent (Fig. 15). Actin filaments are found passing through dense bodies in smooth muscle myocytes and anchoring to dense bands on the sarcolemmal membrane. This less-structured organization with dense bodies and dense bands probably is what allows smooth muscle to be able to shorten down to 25% of the normal resting body length compared to skeletal muscle, which can shorten maximally to 75% of original length (27). Although the gross structures of skeletal and smooth muscle differ, the similar interaction between actin and myosin is responsible for the qualitative similarities the two types of muscle display in their biophysical (mechanical) properties and relationships between length, stress, and velocity (9).

Myosin monomers contain six protein chains (Fig. 15). Two heavy chains form the crossbridge heads at one end

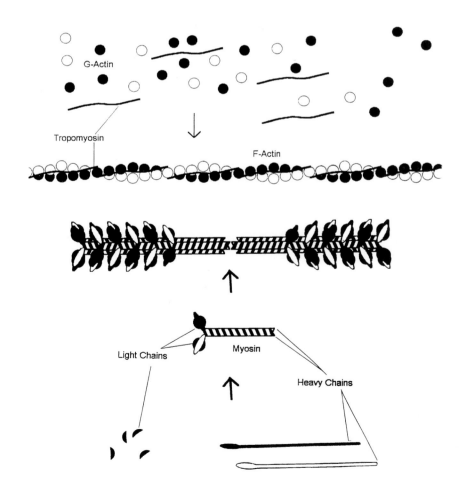

FIG. 15. Globular actin (*g-actin*) monomers are linked together to form the thin filament (*f-actin*)—a double-stranded, α-helical protein with a half-pitch rotation every 7 monomers. One tropomyosin molecule is associated with every 7 actin monomers. Myosin monomers contain 6 protein chains. Two heavy chains form the crossbridge heads at one end of the molecule; the other ends of the heavy chains are twisted into an helix that shapes the tail of the monomer. Four light chains are associated with the 2 heads of the heavy chains. The thick myosin filament is formed from monomers with the tails of the heavy chains entwined in such a way that there is a central bare region with the myosin heads projecting out distally from the center. The myosin heads can bind to actin filaments and the resulting actomyosin can hydrolyze ATP (actomyosin ATPase) in the presence of increased cytosolic calcium. The energy derived from the splitting of ATP to ADP and inorganic phosphate is used to cause an angular rotation of the myosin head while attached to actin and, thus, slide the two filaments past each other. (From Mitchell RW. Regulation of smooth muscle contraction. In: Leff AR., ed. *Pulmonary Pharmacology and Therapeutics.* New York: Mc-Graw-Hill, 1995;191–198.)

of the molecule; the other ends of the heavy chains are twisted into an helix that shapes the tail of the monomer. Four light chains are associated with the two heads of the heavy chains. The thick myosin filament is formed from monomers with the tails of the heavy chains entwined in such a way that there is a central bare region with the myosin heads projecting out distally from the center. The myosin heads can bind to actin filaments and the resulting actomyosin can hydrolyze adenosine triphosphate (ATP). The energy derived from the splitting of ATP to adenosine diphosphate (ADP) and inorganic phosphate (P_i) is used to cause an angular rotation of the myosin head while attached to actin and, thus, slide the two filaments past each other.

Contraction of airway smooth muscle, like skeletal muscle, is manifest by the interaction of the contractile proteins, α-actin and myosin. Calcium is required for contraction in both smooth and skeletal muscle. However, unlike skeletal muscle, regulation of contraction is myosin-, rather that actin-linked, and smooth muscle appears to lack a highly organized sarcomere structure. The deficiency of sarcomeres accounts for the lack of striations observed under light microscopy. Also, smooth muscle lacks troponin, a regulatory protein in skeletal muscle associated with the thin actin filament that, in the presence of calcium, allows the myosin heads to bind with actin and form crossbridges (actin-linked regulation). In smooth muscle, calcium for contraction binds with calmodulin, which begins a cascade of regulatory steps necessary before the interaction of actin and myosin.

Thick myosin and thin actin filaments can be seen in airway smooth muscle (Fig. 16). Myosin filaments are ~15ηm in diameter and are spaced laterally in airway myocytes at regular intervals (28,29). Crossbridges are seen to project from the thick filament similar to skeletal muscle; however, unlike skeletal muscle, there appears to be no central bare zone of the myosin filament nor are any

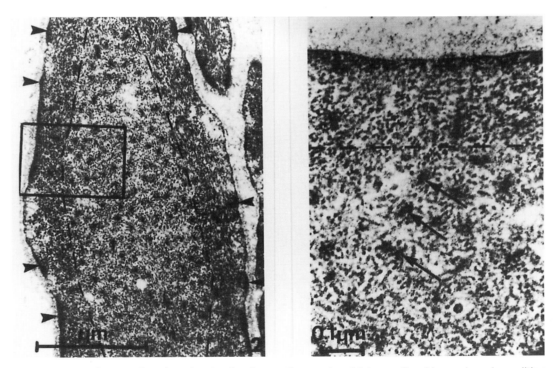

FIG. 16. Photomicrographs of canine tracheal smooth muscle which was fixed in a relaxed condition. Sections were made perpendicular to the orientation of the contractile filaments. **Left panel**: Thick filaments appear as uniform sized densities in the central cytoplasm. As demarcated by the dotted line, a thin cortical strip of denser filamentous material can be seen extending approximately 300nm into the cell. Arrowheads identify anchoring densities of the plasmalemma. The boxed region is shown at higher magnification in the right panel. **Right panel**: At this magnification thick filaments (*arrows*) can be seen to be surrounded by thin filaments in a symmetrical pattern (*see top arrow*). The increased density of the peripheral cortical strip (*demarcated by the dotted line*) can be seen beneath the plasmalemma; it shows a variable orientation of fibers and the presence of numerous intermediate (10-nm) filaments. (From Avner BP, Delongo J, Wilson S, Ladman AJ. A method for culturing canine tracheal smooth muscle cells *in vitro*: morphologic and pharmacologic observations. *Anat Rec* 1981; 200:357–370, with permission.)

sarcomeres evident (30,31). In general, the ratio of actin to myosin is much greater in smooth (10 to 15:1) compared to skeletal (6:1) muscle. Thin filaments have been observed in smooth muscle running through dense bodies and inserting onto dense bands (32).

Regulatory Proteins

Calmodulin, Myosin Light Chain Kinase, and Myosin Light Chain Phosphatase

In the cytosol, Ca^{2+} binds to calmodulin, a ubiquitous protein similar in molecular structure to the troponin-C found in skeletal muscle. Four Ca^{2+} ions bind to each calmodulin molecule, which increases the calmodulin affinity for the enzyme myosin light chain kinase (MLCK). The Ca^{2+}-calmodulin complex binds to MLCK; the Ca^{2+}-calmodulin-MLCK can now phosphorylate the light chains on the myosin heads. Phosphorylation of the light chains is necessary for the initiation of contraction of smooth muscle, but not for the maintenance of contraction in the presence of increased $[Ca^{2+}]_i$ (33,34). Myosin light chain phosphatases dephosphorylate the light chains and greatly reduce the activity of the actomyosin ATPase, slowing down the making and breaking of the crossbridges (35,36). These slowly cycling crossbridges (or latchbridges) require little energy to maintain contraction (37). Relaxation occurs with reduction in cytosolic $[Ca^{2+}]_i$ and deactivation of the actomyosin ATPase.

Calponin and Caldesmon

Calponin and caldesmon are constituent proteins associated with the actin filament and may provide a mechanism by which regulation of contraction of smooth muscle is thin filament-linked. A detailed description of the potential mechanisms by which these proteins regulate contraction in smooth muscle is found in Chapter 56.

Caldesmon is found in a ratio of 1 molecule for every ~20 actin monomers (38). It binds to actin, tropomyosin, and calmodulin. It has been demonstrated in vitro that, in the presence of caldesmon, the actin-activated ATPase activity of phosphorylated myosin is inhibited; this inhibition and the affinity of caldesmon for actin are reduced in the presence of the calcium-calmodulin complex.

Calponin is found in a ratio of 1:1 with tropomyosin in smooth muscle, and its amino-acid sequence has some similarity to that of the troponin found in skeletal muscle. Calponin is a calmodulin-binding protein that also binds to actin and inhibits actomyosin ATPase activity (39,40).

STRUCTURAL ALTERATIONS IN AIRWAY SMOOTH MUSCLE IN HYPERRESPONSIVE DISEASE

Airways Remodeling: Smooth Muscle Hyperplasia and Hypertrophy

Asthma is a chronic inflammatory disease characterized symptomatically by persistent airway hyperreactivity to allergic and nonallergic stimuli (41). Acute exacerbations of the disease are the result of airway obstruction resulting from spasm of airway smooth muscle and luminal plugging with excessive mucus secretions. Acute obstruction can be ameliorated with the use of β-adrenergic bronchodilators; however, in the chronic disease, a nonreversible component of hyperreactivity persists that is unresponsive to β-adrenergic agonist therapy. Severe airway inflammation is characteristic of patients who die of asthma; it also exists, though to a lesser degree, in patients with only mild forms of the disease (42–44). It now appears that remodeling and thickening of the airway wall, which occur as a result of chronic inflammation, may represent a basic mechanism underlying irreversible chronic airway hyperreactivity (45,46). Indeed, using computer modeling techniques, Wiggs et al. (46) have demonstrated that, for a particular degree of airway smooth muscle shortening, substantially greater airway resistance develops if airway wall thickening exists to the extent that has been measured in postmortem samples from asthmatic patients (45).

Fairly well-defined structural changes associated with airway wall thickening have been identified from autopsy samples of patients dying of status asthmaticus and from biopsy samples from subjects with milder disease (Fig. 17). These changes include infiltration with eosinophils and macrophages, edema, epithelial denudation, hyperplasia of mucus secreting glands, thickening of the basement membrane, subepithelial collagen deposition, subepithelial accumulation of myofibroblasts, and substantial thickening of the medial smooth muscle layers (42–45,47–54). The focus of the following sections will be on features of airway smooth muscle associated with medial thickening during airway remodeling.

Airway smooth muscle cell hyperplasia and hypertrophy appear to occur in remodeling airways (52,54,55). Ebina et al. (54) have described different patterns of medial thickening in human airways from patients who died in status asthmaticus. In one-half of the subjects, referred to as type I patients, increased smooth muscle mass was seen only in large bronchi. In the remainder, termed type II patients, smooth muscle thickening was evident from large bronchi to small bronchiolar segments. Muscle thickening in type I subjects resulted almost exclusively from cellular hyperplasia in large bronchi, whereas, in type II subjects, cellular hypertrophy occurred along the

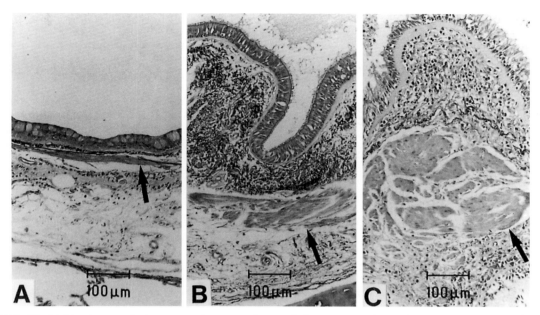

FIG. 17. Light micrograph demonstrating smooth muscle in cross sections of segmental bronchi of human airways taken at autopsy. Medial smooth muscle layers are denoted by *arrows*; elastica-Goldner staining. (**A**) A relaxed segmental bronchus from a nonasthmatic patient. (**B**) A constricted human segmental bronchus from a nonasthmatic subject. (**C**) A constricted bronchus in an asthmatic subject showing striking thickening of the smooth muscle layer. Also note evidence of epithelial sloughing, subepithelial fibrosis, and infiltration by inflammatory cells. (From Ebina M, Yaegashi H, Chibo R, Takahashi T, Motomiya M, Tanemura M. Distribution of smooth muscles along the bronchial tree: A morphometric study of ordinary autopsy lungs. *Am Rev Respir Dis* 1990;141:1322–1326, with permission.)

entire bronchial tree in addition to hyperplastic growth in large bronchi. Regional disparity in the modality of airway myocyte growth suggests that a) different mechanisms and/or stimuli might trigger smooth muscle growth in different areas of the lung and b) heterogeneous populations of airway myocytes may exist, which differ in distribution along the bronchial tree.

No conclusive evidence is at hand to clarify whether a change in the intrinsic contractility of airway smooth muscle might persist in chronic asthma. The contribution of the growth response of bronchial smooth muscle to the pathogenesis of asthma is considered to be merely that of a geometric obstruction to airflow via thickening of the airway wall. The possibility that cells of smooth muscle origin might be involved to a broader degree in the pathogenesis of asthma, through recruitment and modulation to functionally different phenotypes, has not been established. Figure 18 illustrates schematically an hypothesis suggesting that, in a fashion similar to vascular smooth muscle cells in atherogenesis, the phenotypes expressed by subsets of airway smooth muscle cells in asthmatic airways may play a critical role in determining the pathophysiology of chronic asthma (56). The hypothesis is based on a pre-supposition that airway remodeling, which includes thickening of the smooth muscle layer, could be the principal causative factor in

chronic airway hyperreactivity (45,46). This scheme does not, however, negate the possibility that other mechanisms, such as bronchoconstrictor hypersensitivity, defects in autonomic regulation, and altered nonadrenergic, noncholinergic neuropeptide release and processing, might have an additive effect on airway hyperresponsiveness.

Several studies exist concerning the isometric responsiveness of human asthmatic smooth muscle preparations to various spasmogens (57,58). However, these types of pharmacological investigations do not address potential differences in functionally important modalities of smooth muscle contractility such as auxotonic shortening capacity and relaxation. Bramley et al. (59) recently have reported striking increases in the capacity for muscle shortening and for force generation of mainstem bronchial airways smooth muscle from a mildly asthmatic patient, as compared to similar tissue obtained from nonasthmatics. There are several animal models of bronchial hyperresponsiveness in which the fundamental *in vitro* contractile properties of airways smooth muscle appear to be altered (60,61). Measurement of force-velocity relationships for airway smooth muscle from a canine model of allergic bronchial hyperresponsiveness, which mimics early asthma *prior to the onset of bronchial inflammation*, has revealed an intrinsic increase in muscle shortening veloc-

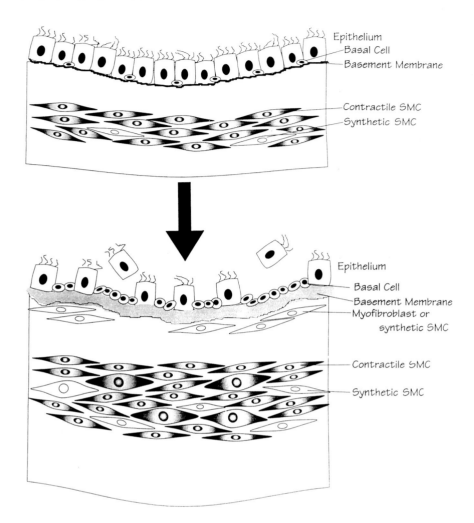

FIG. 18. Schematic diagram depicting proposed changes in airway smooth muscle cells which could occur in the course of airways remodeling in chronic asthma. In the healthy airway (*upper panel*), smooth muscle cells present a primarily contractile phenotype, although it is likely that a range in cellular phenotype exists and that topographical differences in their distribution also exist. In chronic asthmatic airways (*lower panel*), wall thickening develops, which includes smooth muscle cell hyperplasia and hypertrophy (denoted by larger cells). Subepithelial fibrosis and basement membrane thickening develop, while synthetic smooth muscle cell-like myofibroblasts, which synthesize and deposit collagen and extracellular matrix components, appear in the interstitium. These cells could be derived from subsets of smooth muscle cells that have migrated from the media. The airway wall thickening that occurs results in the increased airway resistance and contributes to the maintenance of chronic airways hyperreactivity. (From Halayko AJ, Stephens NL. Potential role for phenotypic modulation of bronchial smooth muscle cells in chronic asthma. *Can J Physiol Pharmacol* 1994;72: 1448–1457, with permission.)

ity and capacity. Similar changes have been measured for tracheal smooth muscle from an inbred rat model of hyperresponsiveness (60). The enhanced dynamic properties of smooth muscle from these animal models have been shown to be associated with increased levels of regulatory myosin light chain phosphorylation and myosin light chain kinase activity (62,63). In addition, the activity of acetylcholinesterase, which is likely secreted by the smooth muscle cells, is reduced (64).

Myofibroblasts are thought to contribute to subepithelial fibrosis via enhanced collagen deposition (47). There is debate as to the source or stem cell of the myofibroblast. Interestingly, the smooth muscle cell is considered a candidate (65). Modulation of the contractile smooth muscle cell phenotype toward a myofibroblast-like cell is associated with focal fibrous intimal thickening seen in atherosclerosis (66,67). Changes in cellular function of myocytes associated with intimal thickening include increased production of collagen, elastin, fibronectin, and glycosaminoglycans. These types of changes are in line with some of those described in fibrotic asthmatic bronchi (47,50).

Airway Smooth Muscle Cells in Culture

A wide range of cytokines, growth factors and other molecules capable of stimulating smooth muscle cell proliferation and hypertrophy are present in the asthmatic airway (68). Cultured airway myocytes provide a convenient model system to study:

1. the effects of specific mediators on smooth muscle cell proliferation and differentiation,
2. secondary signaling pathways which regulate contraction and proliferation,
3. membrane receptor and ion channel properties,
4. regulation of gene expression and posttranslational processing of functionally important smooth muscle proteins,
5. the effects of therapeutic interventions on the properties of airway myocytes.

The number of studies using primary cultures of tracheal and bronchial myocytes has risen dramatically in the past 10 years. Cells from human airway smooth muscle have been used by several investigators (69–71). In addition, numerous studies using airway myocyte primary cultures of canine, guinea pig, ovine, bovine and lepine origin have been reported (56,72–77).

The majority of protocols used for preparing airway myocytes for primary culture entail the use of acute enzymatic dissociation of cells from tissues (78). Airway tissues are usually isolated, cleaned of adventitia by dissection, then minced and the individual myocytes isolated using a digestion solution containing chiefly collagenase and elastase. Enzyme dispersal of cells is, in fact, a harsh treatment after which the cells often become rounded in shape and the number of viable cells may be compromised by as much as 50% (Fig. 19). Dispersed cells are easily grown on uncoated plastic tissue culture plates in a range of culture media supplemented with fetal bovine serum (FBS) and a variety of antibiotics. Once plated, myocytes begin adhering to the culture surface with 1 to 3 hours and become flattened in appearance over the subsequent 24 to 48 hours. Normal plating densities range from 1 to 10 x 10³ cells per cm². Little change in cell number occurs over the first 3 to 4 days after plating (79) (Fig. 20). During this time, few cell-to-cell contacts exist, as cell density is low; the cells display morphologic characteristics typical of cultured vascular smooth muscle cells, appearing spindle- or ribbon-shaped with a large, oval, central nucleus marked by distinct nucleoli, and having well-defined, perinuclear granules (80) (Figs. 20 and 21). Immunofluorescent staining for smooth muscle-specific marker proteins is often used to confirm the identity of the smooth muscle cells; for cultures obtained from tracheal sources, usually greater

than 95% of the attached cells are positive for smooth muscle-α-actin (sm-α-actin) and smooth muscle-specific myosin heavy chain (sm-MHC) (79) (Fig. 20). Approximately 4 days after initial seeding, cell number begins increasing and continues until confluence is reached, usually 7 to 10 days after initial seeding. The rate of increase in cell number diminishes drastically postconfluence due to contact inhibition. At confluence, the cells exist in several layers and the cultures exhibit a "hill-and-valley" pattern, which is typical of smooth muscle cells in culture (73,80) (Fig. 21).

Phenotypic Changes of Airway Myocytes in Primary Culture

Heterogeneous populations of myocytes are known to exist within and between different smooth muscles (81,82). Though smooth muscle cells exist in a range of phenotypes *in vivo*, two extremes in phenotype, contractile and synthetic, have been characterized (80). Contractile cells are rich in myofilamentous structure, are mitotically quiescent, and respond to contractile agonists. Synthetic cells have a reduced myofilamentous apparatus, synthesize and secrete collagen and glycosaminoglycans, are mitotically active, capable of migration, and have elevated activity of lysosomal hydrolases. The use of specific antibodies against cytoskeletal proteins has been used as a means of characterizing features of smooth muscle cell differentiation (65–67).

Principally, studies utilizing cultured airway smooth muscle cells have addressed questions relating to mech-

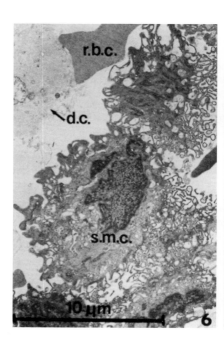
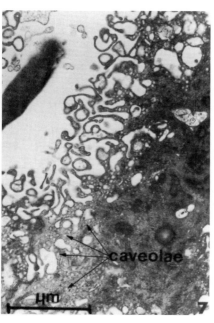

FIG. 19. Transmission electron micrographs of canine tracheal smooth muscle cells enzymatically dissociated for use in establishing primary cultures. **Left panel:** Constituents found in the tracheal digests include darkly staining, viable smooth muscle cells (*s.m.c.*), lightly staining smooth muscle cells (*d.c.*), which have lost membrane integrity and are inviable, and red blood cells (*r.b.c.*). **Right panel:** A higher magnification showing the morphology of an acutely dissociated, viable smooth muscle cell. In response to enzymatic dissociation the sarcolemma appears to be highly active, as evidenced by extreme degrees of folding associated with numerous caveolae and pinocytotic vesicles. Note also that enzymatic dispersal of the cells leads to loss of a definitive basal lamina on the cell surface. (From Avner BP, Delongo J, Wilson S, Ladman AJ. A method for culturing canine tracheal smooth muscle cells *in vitro*: morphologic and pharmacologic observations. *Anat Rec* 1981;200:357–370, with permission.)

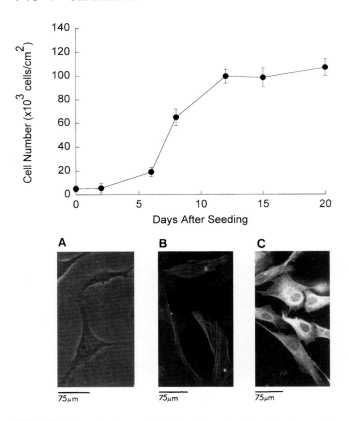

FIG. 20. Growth characteristics of canine tracheal smooth muscle cells in primary culture. The **top panel** illustrates a typical pattern for cells grown in culture medium (Dulbecco's Modified Eagles Medium) containing 10% foetal bovine serum; initial seeding density was 5 x 10³ cells/cm². Morphological characteristics of the cells 6 days after plating are shown in the lower panels using (**A**) phase contrast microscopy, (**B**) immunofluorescent staining using a primary anti-sm-α-actin antibody and a Texas Red-conjugated secondary antibody, and (**C**) immunofluorescent staining using a primary anti-sm-myosin heavy chain antibody and a FITC-conjugated secondary antibody. (From Halayko AJ, Salari H, Ma X, Stephens NL. Markers of phenotypic heterogeneity in airway smooth muscle cells. *Am J Physiol* 1995;270:L1040–L1051, with permission.)

anisms coupling extracellular stimuli and subcellular signaling pathways in the regulation of airway myocyte proliferation or contraction/relaxation (56, 83–86). Directly relating data obtained using cultured smooth muscle cells to *in vivo* circumstances is likely to be confounded by the tendency for phenotypic modulation of myocytes under normal culture conditions. It now is well established that in primary culture, serum-stimulated smooth muscle cells undergo spontaneous, reversible modulation from the contractile to the synthetic phenotype similar to the changes seen during injury repair and proliferative responses *in vivo* (80,87). Culture techniques have been used to exploit this phenomenon in order to characterize differences in protein expression and cellular function in smooth muscle cells expressing different phenotypes.

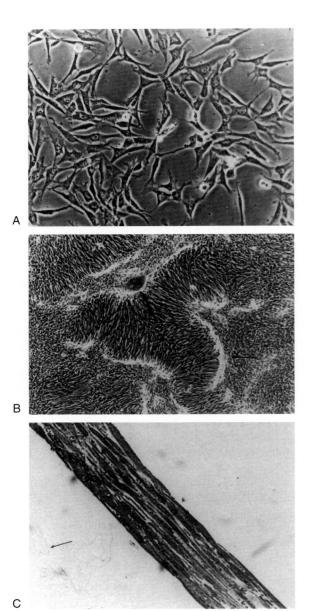

FIG. 21. Photomicrographs of canine tracheal smooth muscle cells in primary culture. (**A**) Phase contrast micrograph of cells taken 5 days after seeding. The bright, rounded cells seen are those in the process of cytokinesis; nondividing cells possess relatively large nuclei and are flat and fusiform in shape, though considerable heterogeneity in cell shape can be seen. The number of cell-to-cell contacts are minimal since cell density is low. (**B**) Phase contrast micrograph of a confluent culture taken 12 days after initial seeding. The cells grow in a characteristic "hill and valley" pattern; "hills" appear to be multi-layered nodules of cells whereas the surrounding cells in "valleys" appear to grow in an organized pattern with cells oriented in parallel to one another. (**C**) Cross section, seen by light microscopy, of a "valley" from a confluent culture. Note that the cells do not grow as a monolayer; multiple layers can be observed with intercellular matrix visible in some places. The small arrow at the left denotes the presence of plastic substrate to which the cells were attached (toluidine blue staining.) (From Tom-Moy M, Madison JM, Jones CA, de Lanerolle P, Brown JK. Morphologic characterization of cultured smooth muscle cells isolated from the tracheas of adult dogs. *Anat Rec* 1987;218:313–328, with permission.)

It appears that de-differentiation of airway smooth muscle cells occurs in culture. Data obtained using immunoblotting techniques have provided the most thorough and quantitative analysis of the changes occurring in protein expression of primary cultured airway myocytes (56,69,79). Assessment of the temporal changes occurring in the content of proteins, which compose and regulate the contractile apparatus and which are associated with the cytoskeleton in canine tracheal myocytes, indicated that the cells de-differentiate rapidly when cultured in the presence of FBS (79) (Fig. 22). These cells demonstrated phenotypic plasticity and the relative content of specific proteins was differentiation-state dependent. Similar studies have been described in numerous reports concerning vascular smooth muscle cells in culture, and have led to the establishment of specific contractile and cytoskeletal proteins as markers of smooth muscle phenotype (88,89). Freshly dispersed, contractile airway myocytes are relatively rich in proteins associated with the contractile apparatus (79). These proteins include sm-MHC, sm-α-actin, calponin, desmin, β-tropomyosin, myosin light chain kinase (MLCK) and *h*-caldesmon (Fig. 23). Conversely, the content of these proteins is diminished by as much as 5-fold in proliferating tracheal myocytes. Proliferating myocytes are, however, enriched in:

1. the nonsarcomeric isoforms of nonmuscle myosin heavy chain (nm-MHC),
2. the nonmuscle *l*-caldesmon isoform,
3. protein kinase C (which is involved with the regulation of pathways mediating cell division),
4. CD44, an integral membrane receptor for extracellular matrix components (Fig. 23).

Re-expression of sm-MHC and sm-α-actin occurs in postconfluent cultures, which indicates that airway myocytes possess plasticity of phenotypic expression and are capable of reversion to a mature phenotype from a proliferative phenotype in culture.

Few studies have assessed the contractile performance of cultured airway myocytes. Notwithstanding the tendency for cultured airway myocytes to lose their contractile proteins rapidly in culture, the adherent nature of the cells in culture precludes assessment of myocyte shortening because the plastic substrate to which they are attached presents a load which cannot be overcome. Receptor expression and coupling have been examined in cultured airway smooth muscle cells (78). The profile of agonist receptors and their intracellular messenger pathways differ considerably between intact airway smooth muscle and cultured myocytes. There is a marked decrease in the inositol phosphate response to muscarinic receptor stimulation (90). The receptor subtypes mediating Ca^{2+} and inositol phosphate responses to some agonists appear to be the same in cultured cells and intact tissue. This has been established for histamine H_1-

receptor subtype in cultured human tracheal myocytes (91). Subcultured human airway smooth muscle cells also are known to express functionally coupled receptors that are linked to adenylyl cyclase (92,93). Cultured airway myocytes appear to express different profiles of receptor subtypes depending on culture conditions. Therefore, *in vitro* culture of airway smooth muscle cells does provide a useful tool in the study of gene expression for the structural and regulatory proteins involved in excitation-contraction coupling.

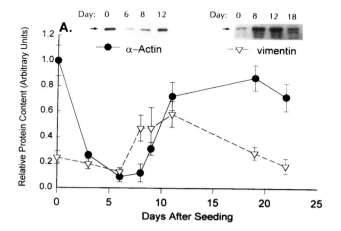

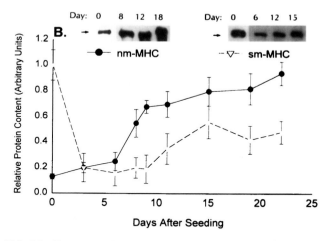

FIG. 22. Temporal changes in the relative abundance of specific smooth muscle proteins in cultured tracheal smooth muscle cells as assayed by immunoblotting. Specific protein content was estimated using laser densitometry; values plotted were normalized to the amount of total crude protein applied to gels in the assays. **(A)** Changes with time in primary culture of the abundance of the contractile protein, sm-α-actin (43kDa), and the intermediate filament protein, vimentin (57kDa). **(B)** Changes with time in primary culture of the abundance of the isoforms of myosin associated with contractile, thick filaments (sm-MHC, 200-204kDa) and the nonmuscle isoforms of myosin, nm-MHC (196-198kDa). (From Halayko AJ, Salari H, Ma X, Stephens NL. Markers of phenotypic heterogeneity in airway smooth muscle cells. *Am J Physiol* 1995;270:L1040–L1051, with permission.)

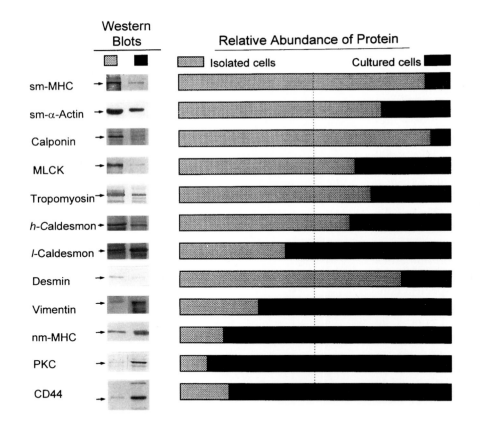

FIG. 23. Comparison, using immunoblotting and densitometry, of the relative abundance of specific smooth muscle proteins in freshly isolated canine tracheal myocytes with that in tracheal smooth muscle cells in primary culture for 7 days. Prior to immunoblotting the proteins were separated by gel electrophoresis; the apparent Mr, in kDa, for each protein were as follows: sm-MHC (200 to 204), sm-α-actin (43), calponin (34), MLCK (138), β-tropomyosin (36), h-caldesmon (150), l-caldesmon (80), desmin (53), vimentin (54), nm-MHC (196-198), α/β-PKC (79) and CD44 (85-90). (From Halayko AJ, Salari H, Ma X, Stephens NL. Markers of phenotypic heterogeneity in airway smooth muscle cells. *Am J Physiol* 1995;270:L1040–L1050, with permission.)

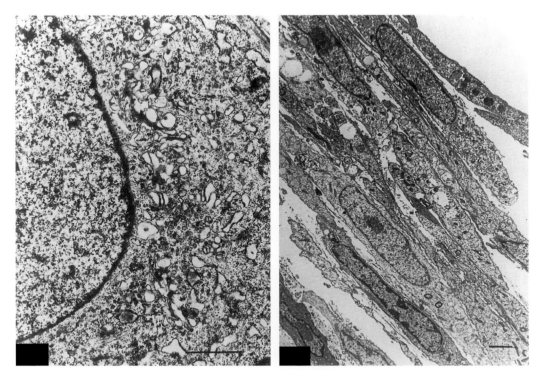

FIG. 24. Ultrastructural morphology of cultured canine tracheal smooth muscle cells as seen by transmission electron microscopy. **Left panel**: High-power micrograph of a cell in a subconfluent culture showing a dense accumulation of Golgi apparatus and free ribosomes near the nucleus. Note also the absence of myofilaments in the cytoplasm. These characteristics are consistent with the process of de-differentiation known to occur in smooth muscle cells in culture. **Right panel**: Low-power micrograph of a cross section of "valley"-situated cells in a confluent culture. Note the multi-layered, parallel arrangement of myocytes, the presence of extracellular matrix and a lack of myofilaments in the cytoplasm. (From Tom-Moy M, Madison JM, Jones CA, de Lanerolle P, Brown JK. Morphologic characterization of cultured smooth muscle cells isolated from the tracheas of adult dogs. *Anat Rec* 1987;218:313–328, with permission.)

Ultrastructure of Airway Myocytes in Culture

Primary cultures of airway myocytes have been used as a model system for the proliferative response of airway smooth muscle cells associated with airway remodeling in chronic asthma. Ultrastructural characterization of cultured airway smooth muscle cells in different developmental states may provide insight into the functional changes which may occur in cells in *in vivo*. Morphologic changes of vascular smooth muscle cells associated with growth and development in culture and *in vivo* have been well-documented (80,94). No systematic study of the morphologic changes in airway myocytes in hyperreactive airway disease has been reported. However, immunocytochemical and electron microscopic analysis of cultured airway myocytes have been completed (69,72,73,79). These studies

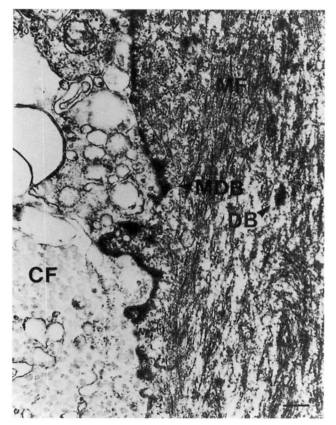

FIG. 25. High-power electron micrograph of a canine tracheal smooth muscle cell from a hill region of a confluent primary culture. These cells exhibit many ultrastructural characteristics common to differentiated myocytes in intact tissue. The cytoplasm is relatively electron dense, containing numerous myofilaments (*MF*) and few other organelles. Cytoplasmic dense bodies (*DB*) and dense bands associated with the sarcolemma (*MDB*) are visible. Extracellular collagen fibrils (*CF*) can also be seen. (From Tom-Moy M, Madison JM, Jones CA, de Lanerolle P, Brown JK. Morphologic characterization of cultured smooth muscle cells isolated from the tracheas of adult dogs. *Anat Rec* 1987;218: 313–328, with permission.)

reveal that the changes known to occur in the cytostructural morphology of vascular myocytes in primary culture also occur in cultured airway myocytes (80).

Organelles

The most comprehensive analyses of the ultrastructural properties of cultured airway myocytes have been performed by transmission electron microscopy of tracheal myocytes of canine origin (72,73). These studies reveal that:

1. the cultured cells take on the morphologic appearance of smooth muscle cells of the so-called synthetic phenotype,
2. even in long-term cultures, however, several morphologic features unique to smooth muscle cells *in vivo* are maintained,
3. considerable ultrastructural heterogeneity exists between cells in culture.

Within several days of primary culture in media supplemented with FBS, cytoplasmic organelles associated with cells that express the synthetic phenotype increase in number (Fig. 24). These organelles include chiefly Golgi apparatus, sarcoplasmic reticulum, free ribosomes, and mitochondria; this increase in density is associated with a concomitant disappearance of myofilaments in the cells. In support of the contention that these cells are synthetic in nature, considerable deposition of extracellular matrix, in the form of collagen fibrils and other amorphous materials, develops between adjacent cells (Figs. 24 and 25). In postconfluent cultures these features are most striking, though not exclusively, in cells growing in "valleys."

Morphologic features of cells from intact tissues, including the presence of cytoplasmic dense bodies and membranous dense bands, are preserved in most cultured cells (Figs. 25 and 26). Myofilaments are also present in peripheral cytoplasmic domains of most cells, though the cytoplasmic volume fraction occupied by these structures is greatly diminished compared to cells of intact tissues (Figs. 25 and 26). These features are often most easily seen in cells growing in the "hills" of confluent cultures. Cultured cells possess an extensive array of cytoskeletal, intermediate filaments, which can be visualized easily using immunofluorescent staining techniques (Fig. 26).

Cell-to-Cell Junctions

Sites of cell-to-cell attachment, known as *zona adherens*, are a common feature of airway myocytes *in vivo*. These contacts are disrupted during enzymatic dispersal of tissues in the preparation of airway smooth muscle cells for primary culture. Few cell-to-cell contacts can be seen in newly plated primary cultures since spaces between cells are very large. However, consider-

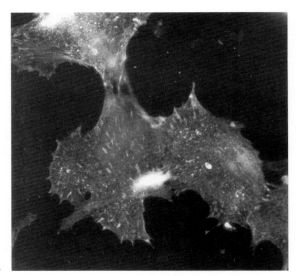
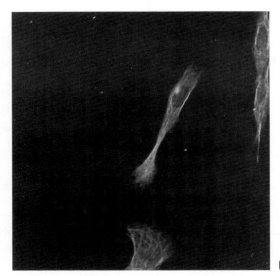

A   B

FIG. 26. Demonstration of dense bodies and intermediate filaments in cultured canine tracheal smooth muscle cells using indirect immunohistochemical techniques. **(A)** Recently divided myocytes, 6 days after plating, stained for α-actinin, a structural protein constituent of dense bodies. Dense bodies appear as bright foci of staining within the cell cytoplasm. Bright staining can be seen at the site of sharp filopodia along the sarcolemmal edges; these are sites of cell attachment to the culture plate and likely correspond to membrane-dense focal adhesion plaques. Extremely bright peri-nuclear α-actinin staining can also be seen and is a common feature of cultured airway smooth muscle cells. **(B)** Tracheal smooth muscle cells, stained for vimentin using a commercial monoclonal antibody, four days after plating in primary culture. Vimentin is a stuctural protein constituent of intermediate filaments. The cells demonstrate an extensive intermediate filament network surrounding the nucleus which extends throughout the whole cytoplasm.

able cell-to-cell contact, in the form of intermediate junctions and gap junctions, begin to reform as cultures near confluent densities (Fig. 27). Studies done using cultured rat aortic smooth muscle cells demonstrate that in multi-layered, confluent smooth muscle cell cultures, gap junctions connected cells to lateral and vertical neighbors (95). The numbers of gap junctions seen between cultured airway myocytes are similar in both "hill" and "valley" cells, and appear as classical multilayered structures as revealed by transmission electron microscopy (Fig. 28). The gap junctions in canine tracheal myocyte cultures provide functional metabolic coupling between cells. Low-molecular fluorescent tracer solutions microinjected into a single myocyte of confluent primary cultures spread to neighboring cells within several minutes (Fig. 29).

Cytocontractile Structures

Thick and thin filaments comprise the myofilamentous cytocontractile apparatus in smooth muscle cells. Thick filaments have been visualized, using transmission electron microscopy, in both acutely dissociated and cultured canine tracheal myocytes (Fig. 30). The orientation of

thick filaments in these preparations is more variable than that seen in cells of intact tissue. This may be an effect of disrupting the normal integrity of the shape of the myocyte upon enzymatic dispersal. Thin filaments are also seen in areas of the cytoplasm occupied by thick filaments. The volume fraction of the cytoplasm occupied by myofilamentous structure becomes reduced dramatically in de-differentiated cells in culture (94); these filaments are localized to the periphery of myocytes. The effects of cyclic mechanical strain on the volume fraction of myofilaments in canine tracheal smooth muscle cells cultured on flexible silastic membranes have been examined. The concentration of myofilaments is increased in stretched cells (95).

Localization of contractile proteins in cultured canine tracheal smooth muscle cells, using immunofluorescent staining techniques, shows the presence of filamentous structures oriented along the long axis of the cells. Thick filaments are composed of sarcomeric myosin. The sarcomeric myosin heavy chain subunit in smooth muscle is referred to as sm-MHC; two isoforms of sm-MHC are expressed in airway smooth muscle cells (62). Nonsarcomeric, nm-MHC, forms of myosin heavy chain are also expressed in airway smooth muscle cells (79). Immunostaining of cultured tracheal myocytes with an-

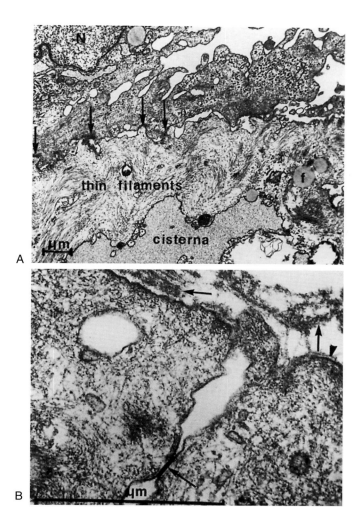

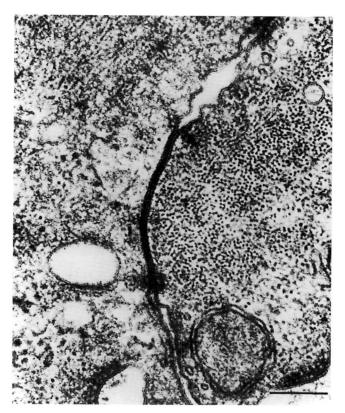

Fig. 28. A high-power electron micrograph of a gap junction between two cultured canine tracheal smooth muscle cells. At least five layers can be distinguished in the junction structure; scale bar = 0.1 μm. (From Tom-Moy M, Madison JM, Jones CA, de Lanerolle P, Brown JK. Morphologic characterization of cultured smooth muscle cells isolated from the tracheas of adult dogs. *Anat Rec* 1987;218: 313–328, with permission.)

FIG. 27. Transmission electron micrographs of canine tracheal smooth muscle cells from long-term (2-month) cultures demonstrating cell-to-cell contacts. (**A**) Two cells can be seen sharing several mechanical attachment sites, or intermediate junctions (*arrows*). The nucleus (*N*) of one cell can be clearly seen, while in another cell peripherally localized thin filaments, dilated cisternae of the endoplasmic reticulum and some cytoplasmic fat droplets (*f*) are visible. (**B**) A higher power micrograph depicting a nexus formed between two adjacent cells (*lower arrow*). The arrowhead demarcates the fuzzy basal lamina of a cell which appears to communicate directly with extracellular matrix components (*upper arrows*) via fibrous connections. (From Avner BP, Delongo J, Wilson S, Ladman AJ. A method for culturing canine tracheal smooth muscle cells *in vitro*: morphologic and pharmacologic observations. *Anat Rec* 1981;200:357–370, with permission.)

tibodies recognizing either sm-MHC or the A isoform of nm-MHC demonstrates the localization of these proteins into filaments within the cytoplasm of the cells (96,97) (Fig. 31). Structures which are positive for sm-MHC can be seen in tracheal myocytes through three subcultures. However, the intensity of staining is greatest in confluent plates and diminishes with each passage. Conversely, nm-MHC staining increases during the course of the initial primary culture, and that level is maintained in subcultures thereafter. In addition, staining of filamentous structures using an antibody which recognizes the A isoform of nm-MHC appears to be intermittent (Fig. 31C), suggesting that this isoform may be localized only within specific segments of the filaments. Filamentous structures similar to those seen with sm-MHC staining can be seen if cells are immunostained with antibodies that recognize either sm-α-actin or caldesmon (Fig. 32). Actin is the primary constituent of thin filaments, and caldesmon is a thin filament-associated regulatory protein; dual staining of cells for actin and caldesmon confirms that the proteins co-localize to the same cytoskeletal structures. It is not clear whether the structures visualized by these methods in de-differentiated, cultured airway myocytes represent contractile structures or if they constitute cytoskeletal structures involved with changes in cell shape and cytokinesis.

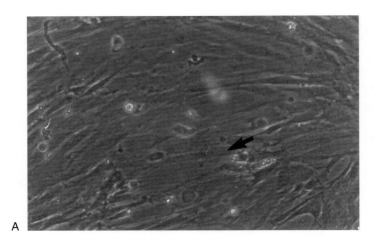

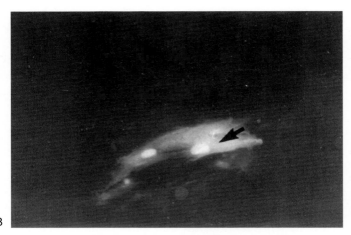

FIG. 29. Demonstration of functional cell-to-cell coupling between canine tracheal smooth muscle cells in primary culture using the fluorescent tracer Lucifer Yellow. The tracer is a water-soluble, low M_r (~500 Da), blue-violet excited, green fluorescent anionic dye. (**A**) Phase contrast micrograph of a 10-day old confluent primary culture. Each cell in the field appears to be in contact with one or more of the others. The arrow denotes a cell into which a saline solution containing Lucifer Yellow was microinjected. (**B**) A fluorescent micrograph of the same field seen in panel A but taken 15 minutes after microinjection of Lucifer Yellow into a single myocyte. The microinjected myocyte (*arrow*) demonstrates abundant fluorescence and, in addition, two cells, laying immediately above and to the left of the injected cell, also possess considerable fluorescence. This observation indicates that dye translocation through functional cell-to-cell junctions, perhaps gap junctions, occurs between the injected cell and the cells adjacent to it. Also, note the presence of mild fluorescence in the cells below the injected cell, suggesting that functional coupling may also exist between those cells.

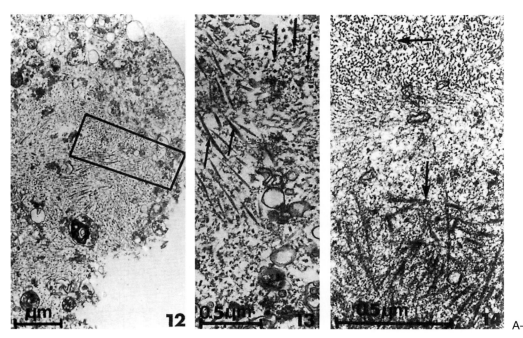

FIG. 30. A series of electron micrographs illustrating the presence and arrangement of myosin thick filaments in both cultured and acutely dissociated canine tracheal myocytes. (**A**) Low- power micrograph of a canine tracheal myocyte dispersed from an 8-day primary culture. The cell membrane was mechanically disrupted so that thick and thin myofilaments could be observed; the rectangle drawn defines the area seen under higher power in the middle panel. (**B**) Thick myosin filaments are clearly seen in the cultured cell cytoplasm as demarcated by the *arrows*. Note that the filaments are oriented in various planes; filaments at the top run perpendicular to the plane of the section whereas filaments at the left run longitudinally in the same plane as the section. (**C**) The filamentous disposition of a myocyte freshly dispersed from a canine trachealis. Note the presence of thick filaments in the lower half of the picture *(vertical arrow)* and thin filaments in the upper part of the panel *(horizontal arrow)*. (From Avner BP, Delongo J, Wilson S, Ladman AJ. A method for culturing canine tracheal smooth muscle cells *in vitro*: morphologic and pharmacologic observations. *Anat Rec* 1981;200:357–370, with permission.)

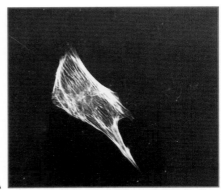

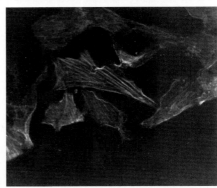

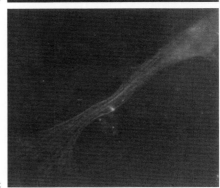

FIG. 31. Indirect immunofluorescence staining, using FITC-conjugated secondary antibodies, of myosin isoforms expressed in canine tracheal smooth muscle cells in primary culture. Cells were grown in media supplemented with 10% fetal bovine serum. (**A**) A cell stained 5 days after initial plating for smooth muscle myosin heavy chain (sm-MHC). The primary antibody employed recognized both the 200kDa and 204kDa isoforms of sm-MHC. Numerous myosin-labeled myofilaments are present and are oriented along the long axis of the myocyte; note that the number of filaments appears to be greater at the perimeters of the cell (magnification x 250). (**B**) Cells stained 7 days after initial plating using a primary antibody against the 196 kDa non-muscle myosin heavy chain isoform (nmA-MHC). Filaments running the full length of the long axis of the cells can be seen (magnification x 200). (**C**) Higher magnification (magnification x 400) of seven-day old myocytes stained for nmA-MHC. Note that the filaments stain in a regular, periodic pattern, suggesting that they may be organized into discrete, repeating units.

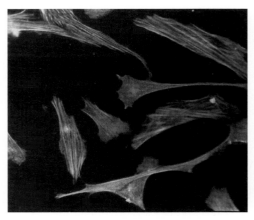

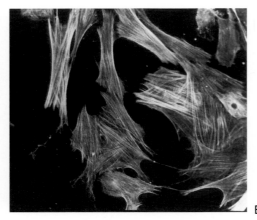

FIG. 32. Indirect immunofluorescence staining, using FITC-conjugated secondary antibodies, of smooth muscle-α-actin and h-caldesmon in canine tracheal myocytes in primary culture. Cells were grown in media supplemented with 10% fetal bovine serum. (**A**) A cell stained for sm-α-actin 5 days after initial plating. Note that all cells stain positively; actin myofilaments can be clearly seen which run the full length of the long axis of the cells (magnification x 200). (**B**) Cells similar to those in plate A but stained for the actin filament-associated protein, h-caldesmon. Caldesmon-positive filaments demonstrate a similar orientation and size as those seen when cells are stained for sm-α-actin.

REFERENCES

1. Burnstock G. Purinergic nerves. *Pharmacol Rev* 1972;24:509–581.
2. Kirkpatrick CT. Excitation and contraction in bovine tracheal smooth muscle. *J Physiol (Lond)* 1975;244:263–281.
3. Abe Y, Tomita T. Cable properties of smooth muscle. *J Physiol (Lond)* 1968;196:87–100.
4. Stephens NL. State of the Art. Airway smooth muscle. *Am Rev Resp Dis* 1987;135:960–975.
5. Kroeger EA, Stephens NL. Effect of tetraethylammonium on tonic airway smooth muscle. Initiation of phasic electrical activity. *Am J Physiol* 1975;228:633–636.
6. Ito Y, Suzuki H, Aizawa H, Hokada H, Hirose T. The spontaneous electrical and mechanical activity of human bronchial smooth muscle: its modulation by drugs. *Br J Pharmacol* 1989;98:1249–1260.
7. Akasaka K, Konno K, Ono Y. Electromyographic study of bronchial smooth muscle in bronchial asthma. *Tohoku J Exp Med* 1975;117:55–64.
8. Suzuki H, Morita K, Kuriyama H. Innervation and properties of the smooth muscle of the dog trachea. *Jpn J Physiol* 1976;26:303–320.
9. Stephens NL, Jiang H. Basic physiology of airway smooth muscle. In: Busse WW, Holgate ST, eds. *Asthma and rhinitis.* Boston: Blackwell Scientific, 1995;1087–1115.
10. Jiang H, Stephens NL. Contractile properties of bronchial smooth muscle with and without cartilage. *J Appl Physiol* 1990;69:120–126.
11. Barnes PJ. Cholinergic control of airway smooth muscle. *Am Rev Respir Dis* 1987;136:S42–S45.
12. Ndukwu IM, Solway J, Arbetter K, Uzendoski K, Leff AR, Mitchell RW. Immune senitization augments epithelium-dependent spontaneous tone in guinea pig trachealis. *Am J Physiol* 1994;266:L485–L492.
13. Martling CR. Sensory nerves containing tachykinins and CGRP in the lower airways. Functional implications for bronchoconstriction, vasodilation, and protein extravasation. *Acta Physiol Scand Suppl* 1987;563:1–57.
14. Holzer P, Bucsics A, Lembeck F. Distribution of capsaicin-sensitive nerve fibres containing immunoreactive substance P in cutaneous and visceral tissues of the rat. *Neurosci Lett* 1982;31:253–257.
15. Yamauchi A, Burnstock G. Post-natal development of smooth muscle cells in the mouse vas deferens. A fine structure study. *J Anat* 1969;104:1–5.
16. Somlyo AP, Devine CE, Somlyo AV. Sarcoplasmic reticulum, mitochondria and filament organization in vascular smooth muscle. In: Betz E, ed. *Vascular smooth muscle. A symposium.* Heidelberg: Springer-Verlag, 1972;119–121.
17. Gabella G, Blundell D. Effect of stretch and contraction on caveolae of smooth muscle cells. *Cell Tissue Res* 1978;190:255–271.
18. Bruns RR, Palade G. Studies on blood capillaries. II. Transport of ferritin molecules across the wall of mouse capillaries. *J Cell Biol* 1968;37:277–299.
19. Jennings MA, Marchesi VT, Florey H. The transport of particles across the walls of small blood vessels. *Proc R Soc [B]* 1962;156:14–19.
20. Sugi H, Daimon T. Translocation of intracellularly stored calcium during the contraction-relaxation cycle in guinea pig taenia coli. *Nature* 1977;269:436–438.
21. Stephens NL, Kroeger EA. Ultrastructure, biophysics and biochemistry of airway smooth muscle. In: Nadel JA, ed. *Physiology and pharmacology of the airways.* New York: Marcel Dekker, 1980;31–121.
22. Stephens NL, Nathaniel V, Kepron W, Mitchell RW, Seow CY, Kong SK. Theory: anatomy and physiology of respiratory smooth muscle tone. In: Jenne JW, Murphy S, eds. *Drug therapy for asthma. Research and clinical practice.* New York: Marcel Dekker, 1987;1–65.
23. Fay FS. Structural and functional features of isolated smooth muscle cells. In: Hatano S, Ishikawa H, Sato H, eds. *Cell motility: molecules and organization.* Tokyo: University of Tokyo Press, 1976;185–197.
24. Kannan MS, Daniel EE. Formation of gap junctions by treatment *in vitro* with potassium conductance blockers. *J Cell Biol* 1978;78:338–348.
25. Ndukwu IM, Solway J, Arbetter K, Uzendoski K, Leff AR, Mitchell RW. Immune sensitization augments epithelium-dependent spontaneous tone in guinea pig trachealis. *Am J Physiol* 1994;266:L485–L492.
26. Mitchell RW, Kroeger EA, Kepron W, Stephens NL. Local parasympathetic mechanisms for ragweed-sensitized canine trachealis hyperresponsiveness. *J Pharmacol Expt Ther* 1987;243:907–914.
27. Stephens NL. Physical properties of contractile systems. In: Daniel EE, Paton DM, eds. *Methods in pharmacology,* vol 3. New York: Plenum Press, 1975;555–591.
28. Rice RV, McManus GM, Devine CE, Somlyo AP. A regular organization of thick filaments in mammalian smooth muscle. *Nature* 1971;231:242–243.
29. Somlyo AP, Devine CE, Somlyo AV, Rice RV. Filament organization in vertebrate smooth muscle. *Phil Trans R Soc Lond [B]* 1973;265:223–229.
30. Lowy J, Poulsen FR, Vibert PJ. Myosin filaments in vertebrate smooth muscle. *Nature* 1970;225:1053–1054.
31. Shoenberg CF, Haseltone J. Filaments and ribbons in vertebrate smooth muscle. *Nature* 1974;249:152–154.
32. Somlyo AV, Bond M, Berner PF, Ashton FT, Holtzer H, Somlyo AP, Butler TM. The contractile apparatus of smooth muscle: an update. In: Stephens NL, ed. *Vascular smooth muscle. A symposium.* New York: Marcel Dekker, 1984;1–20.
33. Kamm KE, Stull JT. Activation of smooth muscle contraction: relation between myosin phosphorylation and stiffness. *Science* 1986;232:80–82.
34. Dillon PF, Aksoy MO, Driska SP, Murphy RA. Myosin phosphorylation and the cross-bridge cycle in arterial smooth muscle. *Science* 1981;211:495–497.
35. Cohen P. The structure and regulation of protein phosphatases. *Ann Rev Biochem* 1989;58:453–508.
36. Pato MD, Kerc E. Regulation of smooth muscle phosphatase-II by divalent cations. *Mol Cell Biochem* 1991;101:31–41.
37. Wendt IR, Gibbs CL. Energy expenditure of longitudinal smooth muscle of rabbit urinary bladder. *Am J Physiol* 1987;252:C88–C96.
38. Hartshorne DJ. Biochemistry of the contractile process in smooth muscle. In: Johnson LR, ed. *Physiology of the gastrointestinal tract.* 2nd ed. New York: Raven, 1987;423–482.
39. Takahashi K, Hiwada K, Kokubu T. Vascular smooth muscle calponin. A novel troponin T-like protein. *Hypertension Dallas* 1988;11:620–626.
40. Winder SJ, Walsh MP. Smooth muscle calponin. Inhibition of actomyosin Mg ATPase and regulation by phosphorylation. *J Biol Chem* 1990;265:10148–10155.
41. Barnes PJ, Rodger IW, Thomson NC. Pathogenesis of asthma. In: Barnes PJ, Rodger IW, Thomson NC, eds. *Asthma: basic mechanisms and clinical management.* London: Academic Press Ltd, 1988;415–444.
42. Dunnill MS. The pathology of asthma with special reference to the changes in the bronchial mucosa. *J Clin Pathol* 1960;13:27–33.
43. Laitinen LA, Heino M, Laitinen A, Kava T, Hashtela T. Damage of the epithelium and bronchial reactivity in patients with asthma. *Am Rev Respir Dis* 1985;131:599–606.
44. Beasley R, Roche WR, Roberts JA, Holgate ST. Cellular events in the bronchi in mild asthma and after bronchial provocation. *Am Rev Respir Dis* 1989;139:806–817.
45. James AL, Paré PD, Hogg JC. The mechanisms of airway narrowing in asthma. *Am Rev Respir Dis* 1989;139:242–246.
46. Wiggs BR, Bosken C, Paré PD, James A, Hogg JC. A model of airway narrowing in asthma and in chronic obstructive pulmonary disease. *Am Rev Resp Dis* 1992;145:1251–1258.
47. Roche WR, Beasley R, Williams JH, Holgate ST. Subepithelial fibrosis in bronchi of asthmatics. *Lancet* 1989;1:520–524.
48. Djukanovic R, Roche WR, Wilson JW, Beasley CRW, Twentyman OP, Howarth PH, Holgate ST. Mucosal inflammation in asthma. *Am Rev Respir Dis* 1990;142:434–457.
49. Cutz E, Levison H, Cooper DM. Ultrastucture of airways in children with asthma. *Histopathol* 1978;2:407–421.
50. Brewster CEP, Howarth PH, Djukanovic R, Wilson J, Holgate ST, Roche WR. Myofibroblasts and subepithelial fibrosis in bronchial asthma. *Am J Respir Mol Biol* 1990;3:507–511.
51. Dunnill MS, Masserella GR, Anderson JA. A comparison of the quantitative anatomy of the bronchi in normal subjects, in status asthmaticus, in chronic bronchitis and in emphysema. *Thorax* 1969;24:176–179.
52. Hossain S. Quantitative measurement of bronchial muscle in men with asthma. *Am Rev Respir Dis* 1973;107:99–109.
53. Ebina M, Yaegashi H, Chibo R, Takahashi T, Motomiya M, Tanemura M. Distribution of smooth muscles along the bronchial tree: a morphometric study of ordinary autopsy lungs. *Am Rev Respir Dis* 1990;141:1322–1326.

54. Ebina M, Takahashi T, Chiba T, Motomiya M. Cellular hypertrophy and hyperplasia of airway smooth muscles underlying bronchial asthma, a 3-D morphometric study. *Am Rev Respir Dis* 1993;148:720–726.

55. Panettieri RA Jr, Murray RK, Bilgen G, Eszterhas AJ, Martin JG. Repeated allergen inhalations induce DNA synthesis in airway smooth muscle and epithelial cells *in vivo: Chest* 1995;107 (Suppl 3):94S–95S.

56. Halayko AJ, Stephens NL. Potential role for phenotypic modulation of bronchial smooth muscle cells in chronic asthma. *Can J Physiol Pharmacol* 1994;72:1448–1457.

57. Schellenberg RR, Foster A. *In vitro* response of human asthmatic airway and pulmonary vascular smooth muscle. *Int Arch Allergy Appl Immunol* 1984;75:237–241.

58. deJongste JC, Mons H, Bonta IL, Kerribijn KF. *In vitro* responses of airways from an asthmatic patient. *Eur J Respir Dis* 1987;71:23–29.

59. Bramley AM, Thomson RJ, Roberts CR, Schellenberg RR. Hypothesis: excessive bronchoconstriction in asthma is due to decreased airway elastance. *Eur Respir J* 1994;7:337–341.

60. Stephens NL, Jiang H, Xu J, Kepron W. Airway smooth muscle mechanics and biochemistry in experimental asthma. *Am Rev Respir Dis* 1991;143:1182–1188.

61. Stephens NL, Jiang H, Halayko AJ. The role of airway smooth muscle in asthma: possible relation to the neuroendocrine system. *Anat Rec* 1993;236:152–163.

62. Kong S-K, Halayko AJ, Stephens NL. Increased myosin phosphorylation in sensitized canine tracheal smooth muscle. *Am J Physiol* 1990;259:L53–L56.

63. Jiang H, Rao K, Halayko AJ, Liu X, Stephens NL. Ragweed sensitization-induced increase of myosin light chain kinase content in canine airway smooth muscle. *Am J Respir Cell Mol Biol* 1992;7:567–573.

64. Mitchell RW, Kelly E, Leff AR. Reduced activity of acetylcholinesterase in canine tracheal smooth muscle homogenates after active immune-sensitization. *Am J Respir Cell Mol Biol* 1991;5:56–62.

65. Sappino AP, Schürch W, Gabbiani G. Differentiation repertoire of fibroblastic cells: expression of cytoskeletal proteins as markers of phenotypic modulations. *Lab Invest* 1990;63:144–161.

66. Campbell JH, Tachas G, Black MJ, Cockerill G, Campbell GR. Molecular biology of vascular hypertrophy. *Basic Res Cardiol* 1991;86(Suppl 1):3–11.

67. Babaev VR, Bobryshev YV, Stenina OV, Tararak, EM, Gabbiani G. Heterogeneity of smooth muscle cells in atheromatous plaque of human aorta. *Am J Pathol* 1990;136:1031–1042.

68. Hirst, SJ, Twort CHC. The proliferative response of airway smooth muscle. *Clin Expt Allergy* 1992;22:907–915.

69. Panettieri RA, Murray RK, DePalo LR, Yadvish PA, Kotlikoff MI. A human airway smooth muscle cell line that retains physiological responsiveness. *Am J Physiol* 1989;256:C329–C335.

70. Twort CH, Van Breeman C. Human airway smooth muscle in cell culture: control of the intracellular calcium store. *Pulm Pharmacol* 1989;2:45–53.

71. Hall IP, Widdop S, Townsend P, Daykin K. Control of cyclic AMP content in primary cultures of human tracheal smooth muscle cells. *Br J Pharmacol* 1992;107:422–428.

72. Avner BP, Delongo J, Wilson S, Ladman AJ. A method for culturing canine tracheal smooth muscle cells *in vitro*: morphologic and pharmacologic observations. *Anat Rec* 1981;200:357–370.

73. Tom-Moy M, Madison JM, Jones CA, de Lanerolle P, Brown JK. Morphologic characterization of cultured smooth muscle cells isolated from the tracheas of adult dogs. *Anat Rec* 1987;218:313–328.

74. Pyne S, Pyne NJ. Bradykinin stimulates phospholipase D in primary cultures of guinea pig tracheal smooth muscle. *Biochm Pharmacol* 1993;45:595–603.

75. Farmer SG, Ensore JE, Burch RM. Evidence that cultured airway smooth muscle cells contain bradykinin B2 and B3 receptors. *J Am Respir Cell Mol Biol* 1991;4:273–277.

76. Lew DB, Nebigil C, Malik KU. Dual regulation by cAMP of β-hexosaminidase-induced mitogenesis in bovine racheal myocytes. *Am J Repir Cell Mol Biol* 1992;7:614–619.

77. Chopra LC, Twort CHC, Cameron IR, Ward JPT. Inositol (1,4,5) triphosphate and guanosine 5'-O-(3-thiotriphosphate) induced Ca^{2+} release in cultures airway smooth muscle. *Br J Pharmacol* 1991;104:901–906.

78. Hall IP, Kotlikoff M. Use of cultured airway myocytes for study of airway smooth muscle. *Am J Physiol* 1995;268:L1–L11.

79. Halayko AJ, Salari H, Ma X, Stephens NL. Markers of airway smooth muscle cell phenotype. *Am J Physiol* 1996;270:L1040–L1051.

80. Chamley-Campbell JH, Campbell GR, Ross R. The smooth muscle cell in culture. *Physiol Rev* 1979;59:1–61.

81. Frid MG, Moiseeva EP, Stenmark KR. Multiple phenotypically distinct smooth muscle cell populations exist in the adult and developing bovine pulmonary arterial media *in vivo. Circ Res* 1994;75:669–681.

82. Daemen MJAP, De Mey JGR. Regional heterogeneity of arterial structural changes. *Hypertension* 1995;25:464–473.

83. Panetteri RA, Yadvish PA, Kelly AM, Rubenstein NA, MI Kotlikoff. Histamine stimulates proliferation of airway smooth muscle and induces c-fos expression. *Am J Physiol* 1990;259:L365–L371.

84. Hirst SJ, Barnes PJ, Twort CHC. Quntifying proliferation of cultured human and rabbit airway smooth muscle cells in response to serum and platelet derived growth factor. *Am J Respir Cell Mol Biol* 1992;7:574–581.

85. Smith PG, Janiga KE, Bruce MC. Strain increases airway smooth muscle cell proliferation. *Am J Respir Cell Mol Biol* 1994;10:85–90.

86. Kelleher MD, Abe MK, Chao T-SO, Jain M,Green JM, Solway J, Rosner MR, Hershenson MB. Role of MAP kinase activation in bovine tracheal smooth muscle mitogenesis. *Am J Physiol* 1995;268:L894–L901.

87. Bowers CW, Dahm LM. Maintenance of contractility in dissociated smooth muscle: low density cultures in a defined medium. *Am J Physiol* 1993;264:C229–C236.

88. Shanahan CM, Weissberg PL, Metcalfe JC. Isolation of gene markers of differentiated and proliferating vascular smooth muscle cells. *Circ Res* 1993;73:193–204.

89. Sartore S, Scatena M, Chiavegato A, Faggin E, Giuriato L, Pauletto P. Myosin isoform expression in smooth muscle cells during physiological and pathological vascular remodelling. *J Vasc Res* 1994;31:61–81.

90. Yang CM, Chou S-P, Sung T-S, Chien H-J. Regulation of functional muscarininc receptor expression in tracheal smooth muscle cells. *Am J Physiol* 1991;261:C1123–C1129.

91. Daykin KS, Widdop S, Hall IP. Control of histamine induced inositol phospholipid hydrolysis in cultured human tracheal smooth muscle cells. *Eur J Pharmacol Mol Pharmacol Sect* 1993;246:135–140.

92. Hall IP, Widdop S, Townsend P, Daykin K. Control of cyclic AMP content in primary cultures of human tracheal smooth muscle cells. *Br J Pharmacol* 1992;107:422–428.

93. Widdop SK, Daykin K, Hall IP. Expression of muscarinic M2 receptors in cultured airway smooth muscle cells. *Am J Respir Cell Mol Biol* 1993;9:541–546.

94. Campbell JH, Campbell GR. Chemical stimuli of the hypertrophic response in smooth muscle. In: Siedel CL, Weisbrodt NW, eds. *Hypertrophic response in smooth smooth muscle.* Boca Raton: CRC Press Inc, 1987;153–192.

95. Blennerhassett MG, Kannan MS, Garfield RE. Functional characterization of cell-to-cell coupling in cultured rat aortic smooth muscle. *Am J Physiol* 1987;252:C555–C569.

96. Gröschel-Stewart U, Schreiber J, Mahlmeister C, Weber K. Production of specific antibodies to contractile proteins and their use in immunofluorescence microscopy: I, Antibodies to smooth and striated chicken myosins. *Histochemistry* 1976;46:229–236.

97. Takahashi M, Kawamoto S, Adelstein RS. Evidence for inserted sequences in the head region of nonmuscle myosin specific to the nervous system. *J Biol Chem* 1992;267:17864–17871.

98. Mitchell RW. Regulation of smooth muscle contraction. In: Leff AR. ed. *Pulmonary pharmacology and therapeutics.* New York: McGraw-Hill, 1995;191–198.

Asthma, edited by P.J. Barnes, M.M. Grunstein, A.R. Leff, and A.J. Woolcock.
Lippincott–Raven Publishers, Philadelphia © 1997.

▪ 56 ▪

Airway Smooth Muscle Contraction

Newman L. Stephens, Jizhong Wang, and Andrew J. Halayko

Elucidation of the pathogenesis of asthma continues to be the *primum movens* of the vast amount of research being conducted today on airway smooth muscle. Though the role of airway smooth muscle (ASM) in normal respiration is still the subject of debate, there is no doubt that the respiratory distress of asthma stems from abnormal contraction of airway smooth muscle (1,2,3). In recent times, the exciting notion that asthma is essentially a chronic inflammatory disease has caught the imagination of the respiratory research community. The notion has advanced *pari passu* with the concept that limitation of airflow in the asthmatic attack is predominantly due to the mechanical effect of a thickened airway media, lamina propria, and epithelium; a geometrical limitation as it were. Nevertheless, it must be pointed out that the great effectiveness of β_2 agonists in combating the attack, points to the still important role of airway smooth muscle contraction in chronic asthma.

The *secundum movens*, to coin a neologism, is provided by the impact of cell and molecular biology on ASM re-

search. Though sadly lagging behind frontier research in these areas, and tailing advances made in vascular smooth muscle research (from whom a good many ideas have been borrowed) ASM research seems to have achieved a lift-off status. The impetus for this has come from the belated realization that after all the pressure-and-flow measurements have been completed, and functional disorders identified at organ level, it is some disorder in the structure and function of a molecule that is responsible for respiratory pathophysiology in general, and for asthma, in particular. Contributing further to this trend is the near-miraculous precision and user friendliness of the techniques employed in molecular biology. Some of the current limitations to a more extensive application of these techniques in asthma research seem to be the esoteric jargon one has to become *au fait* with, and inertia.

The following review is, to some extent, biased by attempts to present recent developments in the field, some of which are controversial and others wherein developments are occurring so rapidly that today's dogma becomes tomorrow's debris.

N. L. Stephens and A. J. Halayko: Department of Physiology, University of Manitoba, Winnipeg, Manitoba R3E 3J7 Canada.
    J. Wang: Department of Information Services, St. Boniface General Hospital, Winnipeg, Manitoba R3E 3J7 Canada.

STRUCTURE

It comes as a surprise to modern students of ASM structure that most of the definitive and competent work in this area was completed almost 50 years ago and led to concepts of function that were amazingly prescient.

In the last 20 years, pulmonary structure has been revisited, the new characteristic has been the use of controlled conditions such as the histological study of the lung at known volumes and transpulmonary pressures, and the use of stratified random sampling techniques (5–13). Perhaps the giant among the measurers is Weibl (12). Pare's group (13) and Horsfall (15) have been major contributors to the field of model building. Only selected areas of structure are dealt with here, and that, only because of their relevance to function. The subject of ASM structure is dealt with more exhaustively elsewhere in this book.

Interdependence

It is fairly firmly established that lung parenchyma exerts a tethering effect on intrapulmonary airways and the traction exerted on the latter regulates the volume of these airways and, thus, the distribution of global and regional ventilation (16–22). At increasing lung volumes, the wider airways facilitate ventilation. Bronchoconstriction would also be limited by the increasing load placed on the airway muscle by the progressively increasing stretch of the lung parenchyma.

This concept has led to the very reasonable corollary that the increased bronchoconstriction typically seen in an asthmatic attack results from the known increased compliance of the lung parenchyma, with a resultant decrement in the afterload on the shortening ASM. Uncoupling of the elastic forces of the parenchyma from the ASM, either by collection of peribronchial inflammatory exudate, or a transudate resulting from the increased permeability of the blood vessels of the bronchial wall, would also facilitate asthmatic bronchospasm.

Alternative Hypothesis: Studies of Isolated Bronchial Cylinders

However, there is some evidence that at least in normal isolated canine airways, air smooth muscle can constrict independent of any connection to the adventitia and cartilages (23). Video-imaging of isolated cylindrical segments of 5th to 6th generation bronchi shows on quantitative analysis, that when the bronchi are maximally contracted by carbachol (10^{-3}M), their external tissue layers show no change in perimetric length while the muscular layer shortens so considerably, that the lumen is almost occluded. Figure 1 shows a video-photograph of the bronchial segment seen end-on. The outermost and innermost perimeters were measured as well as the luminal areas. Figure 2 shows the same segment at the end of a contraction produced by 10^{-3}M carbachol. The average outermost perimeter (N=6) shows no significant change, while the luminal area shows a large and significant change. From these data it seemed clear that the adventitia and cartilages

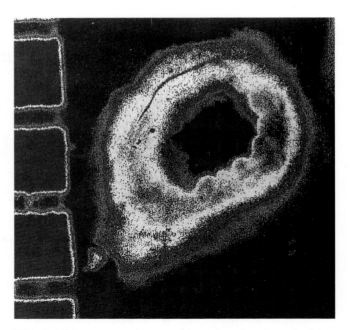

FIG. 1. Video camera image of bronchus (*end-on view*) before stimulation.

do not limit bronchial smooth muscle shortening. The load on the muscle must be the connective tissue joining the muscle to the superjacent cartilage. This tissue must be fairly compliant to permit luminal occlusion. Early reports had suggested that the smooth muscle is directly attached to cartilage (13,29). We have however failed to confirm this and in several sections from different dog lungs seldom see any direct connection. (See Fig. 3). The only direct connection seen is at airway bifurcations (4). The compliance of the connective tissue mentioned earlier crucially regulates bronchoconstriction.

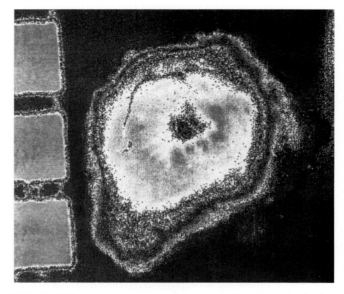

FIG. 2. Video camera image of bronchus (*end-on view*) after maximal constriction.

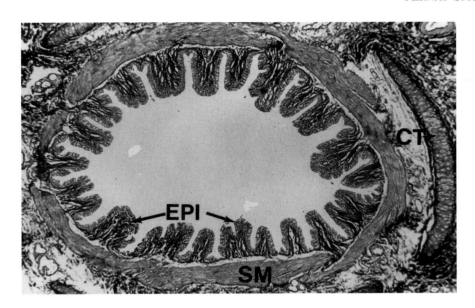

FIG. 3. Histologic section of fifth order canine bronchus before removal of cartilage. Smooth muscle layer *(SM)* is located immediately subjacent to the epithelium *(EPI)* and does not attach to the superjacent cartilage directly. *CT* is loose connective tissue attaching muscle to cartilage. H&E staining;magnification x 200.

The Origin of the Load on ASM: Parenchyma Versus Mural-Connective Tissue

In terminal and respiratory bronchioles which are devoid of cartilage, it is claimed that lung parenchyma is directly attached to the airway. Figure 4 taken from Von Hayek (4) seems to show this in human material quite well. However, when the airway is constricted, then between the end of the alveolar septae and the external bronchiolar wall, a fairly large area of stippling is seen, which presumably represents connective tissue cut transversely. Along with others, we have seen a similar pattern in canine small airways (Fig. 5). Our tentative explanation is that there are concentric layers of connective tissue which fuse with the bronchiolar adventitia. When bronchoconstriction occurs these are either pulled inwards by the constricting muscle, or, alternatively, outwards by the lung septae. In the former case this suggests the load—

probably of an auxotonic nature—on the muscle is imposed by this connective tissue and not the septae.

BIOPHYSICS (MECHANICS) OF ASM CONTRACTION

Biophysics consists of study of the electrical properties of the muscle cell membrane and of the mechanical properties of the contractile apparatus. Here we will deal only with the latter (See also chapter 57).

Length-Tension (LT) Relationships

These are the time-honored tools for measuring the static properties of resting and active muscle. The methods for eliciting length-tension (LT) curves from smooth muscle are identical to those for striated muscle. However recent advances, *vide infra*, suggesting a new way of elic-

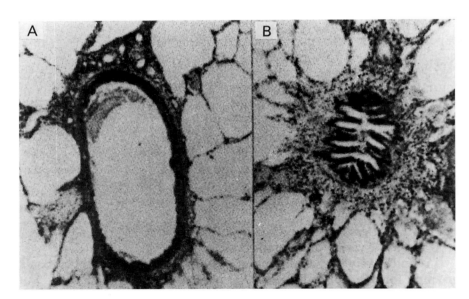

FIG. 4. Cross-sections through a relaxed (**A**), magnification x 160 and contracted bronchiole; same lung fixed *in situ* (**B**), magnification x 40. Note the peri-bronchial space which increases on bronchoconstriction. Note (after allowing for difference in magnification) with contraction there is no great distortion of alveolar sacs, but a marked increase of loose connective tissue is seen just arrived the airway. (From Von Hayek H. *The human lung.* New York: Hafner, 1960;127–226, with permission.)

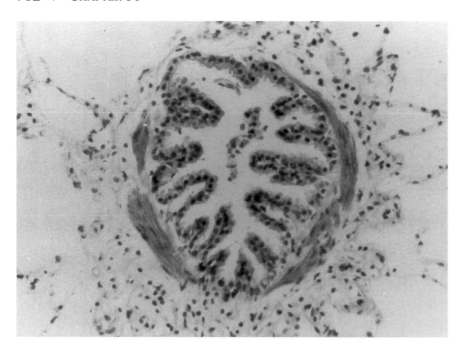

FIG. 5. Transverse section of contracted canine bronchiole; magnification x 120. Same findings as in Figure 4.

iting data for the delineation of LT curves in smooth muscle will have to be considered (24).

Perhaps this is the place to point out that the method used most for studying ASM function *in vitro* has been, with few exceptions, to measure, isometric force. In most cases the objective has been to measure the pharmacological properties of control and sensitized smooth muscle (25). Once again it must be said that dose-response curves are not acceptable as indicators of mechanism of drug action unless they apply to all modalities of smooth muscle function. They must, therefore, apply equally well to both isometric force development and to isotonic or auxotonic shortening; yet, one seldom sees reports of isotonic dose-response curves.

The argument has been used that isometric curves provide insight into shortening mechanisms to the extent that crossbridges are cycling in both modes of contraction. However, in shortening, the number of cycling bridges varies with load while in isometric contraction, a maximum number (50% of the total in striated muscle; percentage for smooth muscle unknown) of bridges cycle. Moreover, the energetics of the two modes of contraction are quantitatively different. Thus, the limitations of the isometric mode of study are obvious.

It is also clear that some internal shortening of the contractile element does occur in smooth muscle, owing to the extension of the series elastic component. However, based on our older studies, this cannot be more that $0.07 l_o$ (where l_o represents optimal muscle length) and more recent unpublished work from our laboratory indicates it is less than $0.03 l_o$ (26). As the lightly loaded muscle shortens isotonically by $0.65 l_o$, it is clear that only a very small portion of shortening is available for study in an isometric contraction.

One must conclude that the most valid studies are those of shortening, since it is via that modality that ASM operates *in vivo* to regulate airway conductance. Currently the most meaningful studies are clinical ones, in which conductance is directly measured. However, there are a host of variables that modulate the magnitude of conductance and limit any conclusions that one would like to make regarding contractility of the ASM.

LT Curves of Tracheal and Bronchial Smooth Muscle (TSM and BSM)

Tracheal Smooth Muscle LT Curves

Figure 6 depicts LT curves for canine tracheal smooth muscle. The muscle strip is dissected and mounted for isometric study according to methods developed by us (1,2,27). Appropriate equilibration is crucial for maintaining steady state for 6 to 8 hours, to allow for sufficient time to acquire valid data.

The resting tension curve represents the passive properties of the muscle, namely, those of the muscle's parallel elastic component. In TSM the curve indicates considerable tissue compliance, with the resting tension at muscle optimal length (l_o) being equal to $0.05 P_o$ where P_o is the maximum active tension developed by the supramaximally stimulated muscles. At lengths equal to $1.10 l_o$, the curve indicates considerably increased stiffness. The reason for this behavior of the resting muscle has not yet been investigated in the TSM. By analogy with vascular smooth muscle, it is likely that the more compliant part of the curve ($0.3 l_o$ to $1.0 l_o$) results from the physi-

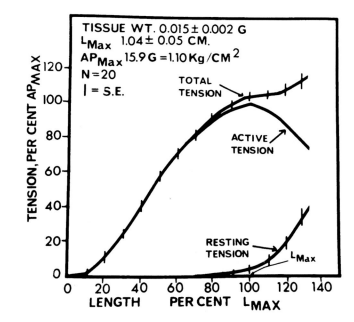

FIG. 6. Mean LT curves (SEs shown) for canine trachealis. Note, full curve not shown.

cal properties of elastin. Collagen, which is stiffer, does not contribute to muscle stiffness, because it is slack. At lengths greater than l_o collagen straightens out and contributes the major share of resting tension.

The properties of the resting muscle are usually assessed by measuring the length-tension curves over lengths where tension is greater than 0. For the trachealis this covers a length varying from 0.2 to 1.3 l_o. Employing heroic measures even 1.4 l_o can be studied. One can liken the resting muscle to an elastic spring and term it "the parallel elastic component" (PEC).

It is clear that when the muscle is at slack length where resting tension is 0, the PEC spring can be compressed further if the muscle can be adequately shortened. Under these conditions the compressed spring acts as an internal resistance which limits further shortening, thus, generating the notion of an internal resistor (See following). Its role in ASM has not been adequately studied.

The active tension curve shows the expected length-tension relationship originally demonstrated in cardiac muscle where it was termed the "Frank-Starling low" The maximum stress (P_o/muscle cross-sectional area) developed by TSM is in the low normal range for all muscles in general, both smooth and striated.

The total tension curve is the sum of the resting and active tensions and shows the expected configuration for a muscle whose resting tension curve shows considerable muscle compliance.

The slope of the curves ($\Delta P/\Delta L$, where ΔP = change in tension and ΔL = change in length) represents the stiffness of the muscle. As expected the activated muscle is considerably stiffer than the resting muscle, which ac-

counts for the increased load-bearing capacity of the activated muscle. In comparing the static mechanical properties of different muscles, normalization is required. This is achieved by expressing tension in stress units (*vide supra*) and length change in strain units ($\Delta l/l_o$ where l_o = optimal length). A *caveat* must be entered at this point, that because of hysteresis effects, initial muscle length is not easy to measure. For example, a smooth muscle that is stretched to beyond 25% of its length requires an hour to recover from stress-relaxation effects.

The integral of the length-tension curve represents the work done by the muscle over the length range examined. It represents an easy way of determining muscle work, but it must be remembered that this represents a theoretical maximum.

One other parameter that can also be derived is the maximum shortening capacity (Δl_{max}) for any given starting length of the muscle. The horizontal line in Figure 12 represents this. Since shortening is load-dependent the only way to assess shortening capacity is at zero load. This can be achieved by zero-load clamping with an appropriate muscle lever system. The shortening capacity derived from LT curves is an overestimate, since no actual shortening (in which additional energy is consumed and shortening is consequently limited) is involved. Our data indicate that TSM can shorten by 90% of l_{max} as judged from LT curves. However if shortening is measured with the muscle set at l_o and carrying an isotonic load (0.05 P_o) equal to the resting tension at l_o, then a value of 65% is obtained (23,27–29). *In vivo* shortening is auxotonic and so the relationships will be different (See following).

Bronchial Smooth Muscle Length-Tension Curves

Tracheal smooth muscle curves have been used as models for curves of airway smooth muscle (including bronchial) in general. However the physiologically and pathophysiologically relevant curves are those of central bronchi (3rd to 5th generation) since regulation of ventilation occurs at this location as does the development of bronchospasm of the early asthmatic attack. With respect to regulation of regional distribution of ventilation and to the late asthmatic attack, bronchiolar smooth muscle curves are important; these need to be delineated.

We have published LT curves for BSM taken from 5th generation canine bronchi and described a technique (23,27,28) whereby strips of muscle can be obtained. The cartilaginous plaques from the strips have been carefully dissected away to ensure that ASM mechanical function remains intact. Figure 3 shows a transverse section of the bronchus. The epithelium, lamina propria, muscle layer and cartilage plaques are clearly seen. Figure 7 shows a similar transverse section from which the cartilage plaques have been removed. The membrane of the muscle cells adjacent to the erstwhile cartilage appears intact.

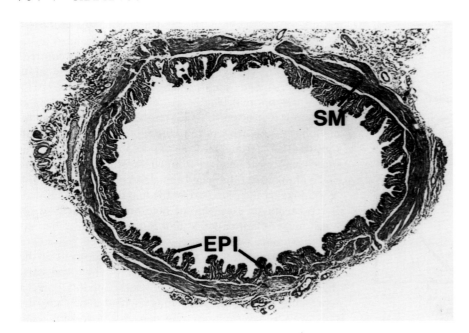

FIG. 7. Section from same airway as shown in Figure 3 but after careful removal of cartilage after which muscle is unimpaired. Haematoxylin and eosin stain; magnification x 200. *EPI*, epithelium; *SM*, smooth muscle layer.

Furthermore, mechanical studies show that when the plaques have been removed maximum shortening capacity (Δl_{max}) and velocity (V_o) increase while P_o remains unchanged (28).

Figure 8 shows LT curves from BSM strips prepared as just described. Length-tension curves for TSM taken from the same animals are also shown. The resting tension curves show no significant difference, indicating that the two have the same compliance. The marked difference is in P_o. This when expressed in stress units is almost 5 times greater in the TSM. The reason for this is seen in Figure 9A which shows a light microscopic transverse section of TSM. Quantitative morphometry indicated 80% of the tissue was made up of smooth muscle.

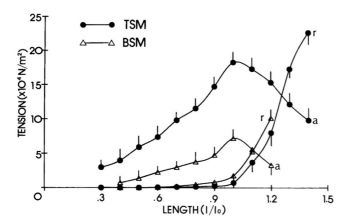

FIG. 8. Superimposed length-tension curves of TSM and BSM. Tensions are expressed as x10⁴N/m² of histologically indentified muscle tissue. Lengths are corrected by dividing strip length by l_0. Active (*a*) tensions of the 2 groups differed, whereas resting tensions (*r*) were similar.

Figure 9B shows a similar picture for 5th- generation bronchi. Morphometry indicated that on the average (N = 9) the muscle content of the bronchial wall was only 25%. This shows quite forcefully that normalizing force (P_o) with respect to tissue cross-sectional are—it must be pointed out that this is the usual practice—is quite inadequate. When P_o is normalized with respect to muscle cell cross-sectional area (e.g, it is expressed as muscle stress and not tissue stress), then the difference between the P_o's of the TSM and BSM is only 25%.

It might be further argued that it is only the contractile proteins in the tissue cross-section that are relevant to force development, and that since not all the protein in the cross-section of the muscle cell is contractile, but also includes regulatory and cytoskeletal proteins, normalization with respect to only the amount of contractile protein in the cross-section is required. We have made estimates of contractile protein using densitometry of Western blots of myosin-heavy chains and of actin. Using this as the normalization parameter did not yield any increase in developed stress.

We conclude that normalization of force developed by ASM must be very carefully carried out. This is especially important when force development among airways of different sizes or different animals or in the same animal at different ages, is being compared (30–32).

Segmental LT Curves

It is well-established for striated muscle that when an isometric muscle contracts, though the ends of the tissue do not move, the segments within the muscle or muscle strip move quite considerably with respect to one another (33). Hence, what is occurring at the crossbridge is not

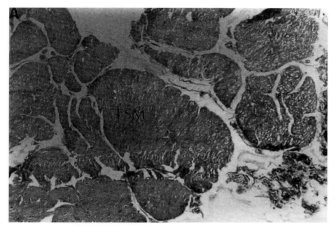

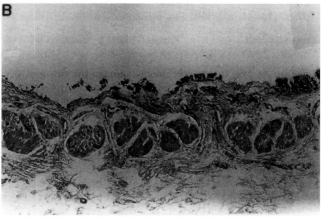

FIG. 9. Cross-sections of *TSM* (A, x 210) and *BSM* (B, x 200). Smooth muscle tissue occupied 77 and 30% of total cross-sectional area of strips for TSM and BSM, respectively.

reflected at the ends of the muscle. The isometric LT curves of the whole muscle or strip do provide information as to what is occurring *in vivo*. From the mechanical behavior of the muscle in the bronchial wall, one can predict the intraluminal pressure and wall stiffness. However to interpret these findings in terms of crossbridge mechanisms one needs to delineate the LT properties of individual segments. This can be achieved by marking the surface of the ASM strip with carbon granules to delimit segments or by passing very fine steel microelectrodes (1μ in diameter) through the belly of the muscle (1). The signals generated by these devices can be monitored to show how much of a given segment shortens. Force is transmitted uniformly throughout the muscle and, hence, the force at the ends of a segment is the same as that at the ends of the muscle strip. Length-tension curves can be obtained for the segment by measuring the force at the muscle ends and the steady state length of the segment at end contraction (2). Alternatively, using a spot-follower of the type developed by Gordon et al. (33), one can obtain signals from the markers delimiting the segment to activate a servo system which holds the segment length

constant and provides data for accurately measuring segmental length-tension relationships.

It must be pointed out that the segmental data for smooth muscle are not the same as for a single fiber of striated muscle where the length of a sarcomere is monitored more exactly using either X-ray diffraction or laser diffraction techniques, and the sarcomere LT curve still shows Frank-Starling behavior.

Pratusewich et al. (24) found to their surprise that such active tension versus length curves were quite unlike those reported for smooth muscle in the literature, in that active tension was independent of length from 0.3 l_o to 1.3 l_o (23,27,34–37). Figure 10A shows such a curve for a TSM segment obtained in our laboratory.

Pratusewich and co-workers also found that at any length, other than what was termed "l_o" on the basis of whole TSM strip active tension curves, active tension was reduced as seen in conventional curves. However if stimulation was repeated about 5 times, at these new lengths, active tension progressively increased until a value equal to P_o was obtained, and in this way, the length independence of P_o was demonstrated. No further increase in P_o was seen after the fifth stimulation, and the force developed was termed "adapted force."

A practical difficulty is that when maximum active tension is length-independent it becomes meaningless to talk of l_o. The experiments are, therefore, conducted by setting the length of the equilibrated muscle at an arbitrary initial length (l_i) at which the resting tension just achieves zero. Successive length increments are described as proportions of l_i. When length is thus defined, the range of lengths over which active tension independence is seen extends from l_i to $4l_i$.

Before one can provide an explanation for this extremely unusual behavior, additional data adduced by Pratusewich, et al. must be cited. They found that over the length range mentioned previously, V_o (zero load velocity) increased linearly with length. Compliance behaved similarly although the slope of V_o versus l curve was steeper than that of compliance versus l (See Fig. 10B, panels b and c).

Their explanation for their force, velocity, and compliance findings, was that the number of contractile units in series varies directly with the adapted muscle length. Temporary force depression after a length change would occur if the change transiently moved the filaments from their optimum overlap. The relative length independence of the adapted force was explained by the reforming of the filament lattice to produce optimum force development with commensurate changes of velocity and compliance.

The foundation for the earlier explanation was that smooth muscle filaments are plastic and display evanescence. This was suggested by several researchers who felt that thick filaments form during contraction and depolymerize during relaxation (38–40). This, in turn, was based on the fact that low pH or high [Ca^{2+}] in the preparative solutions produced more abundant, thick filaments. Since

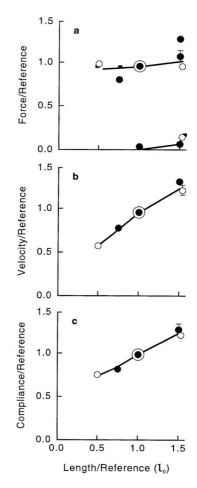

FIG. 10. A: Segmental length-tension curves of canine tracheal smooth muscle. **B:** Isometric force (a), velocity scale factor (b) and compliance (c) plotted as a function of central segment length. The lower set of points in (a) represents rest force.

these two conditions are present in the muscle cell during contraction, grounds for the proposal exist. Sobieszek and Small (38) have also shown there is more myosin incorporated into thick filaments during activation than at rest. Birefrengensce data published by Gillis et al. (39) also show that new structures form in smooth muscle during contraction. Trybus et al. (40,41) found that the unphosphorylated myosin molecule exists in a 10s configuration that is not conducive to filament formation because of steric hindrance. However, phosphorylation of the carboxyl-terminal of the heavy chain converts the 10s into a 6s configuration that facilitates synthesis of thick filaments (42). While all of this is highly speculative, at least it shows along what channels future investigations should be directed to provide a mechanism for the exciting new finding of length-independence of active tension in smooth muscle segments. It may be pointed out, inter alia, that we have confirmed Pratusewich's finding in our laboratory with respect to canine tracheal smooth muscle (unpublished observations).

The question remaining is how does one relate the segmental LT curves to those of the whole muscle, and both of these to what happens *in vivo*. Given the present state of knowledge, the segmental curve (in spite of the limitation that smooth muscle does not possess an ordered sarcom-

eric structure, but nevertheless demonstrates only mini-sarcomeres) provides the best evidence relating to crossbridge mechanics. In the whole *in vitro* muscle strip which is so dissected as to contain parallel fibers, because of segmental asynchrony the mechanical data do not provide direct information relating to crossbridges, but provide information on the modification of crossbridge activity by segmental asynchrony, the latter acting as an additional series elastic component. *In vivo,* this is further complicated by the fact that fibers are not arranged in parallel array around the airway, and this geometric heterogeneity further modifies crossbridge activity. One could conclude then that what is physiological and occurring in the body is assessed by making measurements such as of pressure-volume-flow. However, to deduce the underlying subcellular mechanism responsible for pathophysiological changes, data obtained from the muscle strip subsegment are necessary.

Assessment of Maximum Shortening Capacity ($\Delta l max$)

Because ventilation is regulated by airway conductance *in vivo*, the important parameter to measure in *in vitro* experiments of ASM function is some suitable index of shortening. Several factors determine the extent of ASM shortening; some of these are the initial length of the mus-

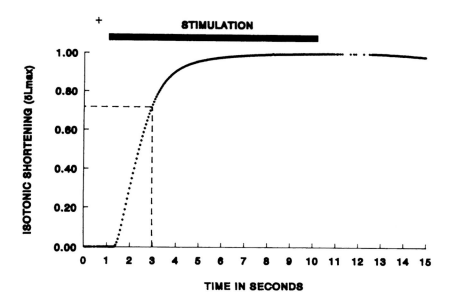

FIG. 11. Isotonic shortening with load = 0.1 Po. Record of shortening versus time elicited from a muscle shortening isotonically with a light preload. It is clear that better than 75% of total shortening is complete within 2 seconds of stimulation.

cle, the force developed, which depends on the contractility of the muscle, the magnitude, nature, and history of the load imposed, and the internal resistance to shortening. Any two of these can be studied provided the others are held constant or reasonably assumed to be constants.

It must be pointed out that studies of shortening are important not only for their relevance to shortening, but also that in disease models and likely in human respiratory disorders also, shortening is the first entity to manifest a change. Isometric force, which is the most often measured purely because it is easy to do so, shows changes much later. Hence, if one is interested in elucidating the cause of a disorder it follows that the earliest manifestation of changed function must be sought.

A conventional method to measure shortening is to do so in a muscle whose initial length is optimal, i.e., one at which force and shortening are maximal, and the load imposed is isotonic, thus, enabling shortening to be measured in the absence of any load variation. With the muscle supramaximally activated, the maximum shortening (Δl_{max}) under a load equivalent to that required to stretch the muscle to its optimal length is measured. As this load is equal to that imposed on the muscle *in vivo*, the shortening represents maximal physiological shortening. Figure 11 shows a record of such shortening as a function of time.

One very important additional datum is that 75% of the total shortening is achieved within 2 to 3 seconds. With respect to regulating airway conductance, therefore, little is possible between 3 to 10 seconds (10 seconds representing contraction time). We have found, for example, that ragweed pollen-sensitized canine ASM shortens more than control (1,27). However, this increased shortening develops within the first 2 seconds. The additional shortening developing between 2 and 10 seconds is not different between the two muscles. Meaningful studies of ASM shortening should, therefore, be conducted in the first 2 to 3 seconds. Interestingly, this is the period when the muscle is in

its rapidly shortening phase, phosphorylation of the 20kDa myosin light chain (MLC_{20}) is at a maximum, and force developing ability is low. Thereafter, the muscle is in its very slowly shortening phase, MLC_{20} phosphorylation is low, and force development is at a maximum. This, the steady state, when the vast majority of measurements (isometric) are made by investigators in the field, provides very little mechanistic information relevant to the muscle's shortening ability or its contractility.

The measured Δl_{max}, *in vitro*, for canine ASM is 65% of l_o (13,23,29).

Maximum shortening capacity can also be deduced from static length-tension curves as indicated by the horizontal line in Figure 12. This turns out to be almost 85%

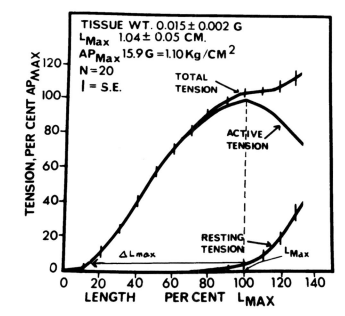

FIG. 12. Mean LT curves (SEs shown) for canine trachealis; maximum shortening capacity shown as Δl_{max}.

of l_o, the difference being that in making these measurements no actual muscle shortening occurs, whereas in isotonic shortening reduction in energy limits shortening.

The question of the nature and history of loading and their influence on Δl_{max} will be dealt with further on.

The Δl_{max} thus far described is a measure of physiological shortening, but is still load-dependent in that the muscle is lightly loaded to stretch it to l_o. True shortening ability should be measured under zero load when it becomes a measure of true shortening capacity. This is akin to measuring velocity (V_o) under zero-loaded conditions. Using the zero load clamp technique, maximum shortening capacity was measured and found to be approximately 15% greater than Δl_{max}. For reasons we do not currently know, airway smooth muscle does not tolerate zero-load shortening and, at best, the maneuver can only be repeated 3 or 4 times.

In summarizing this section then, we conclude that the best *in vitro* index of change in *in vivo* airway resistance is maximum shortening ability, and it is the shortening occurring in the first 2 seconds that is of critical importance.

Derivation of Work from LT Curves

It is clear that integration of the LT curve (force or tension x length) provides a measure of work (force x distance), and the work performed by the active muscle in shortening a given distance is obtained by integration of the active tension curve between the appropriate bounds. This parameter of work has not yet found any significant application in study of ASM function. Changes in working capacity induced by environmental changes (e.g., changes in temperature, pH, osmolarity, and oxygenation state) can be assessed by eliciting appropriate length-tension curves.

Another reason as to why work curves derived from LT data are infrequently used is that they represent essentially static measures. In reality, shortening is carried out at different velocities both *in vivo* and *in vitro*. Better analysis of the energetics of smooth muscle contraction is obtained by integrating force-velocity curves. This provides a measure of power (equivalent to force x velocity) (See following).

Force-Velocity (FV) Relationships

The superiority of studying FV relationships in understanding the mechanics of smooth muscle contraction has already been pointed out. The validity of analyzing these curves and assigning physiological meaning to the various muscle constants derived from such analysis, has still to be established.

The displaced rectangular hyperbolic equation derived by Hill (43) to fit skeletal muscle, isotonic force-velocity data is as follows: $(P + a)(v + a) = (P_o + a)b$ where P = force developed by the muscle, V = velocity of shortening for a given load, P_o = maximum force developed by the muscle, and a and b are constants with units for force

and velocity respectively. The maximum velocity of shortening, which is the unloaded shortening velocity, is represented by V_o and is equal to $P_o b/a$.

Hill has himself shown that the a constant is not a true constant and varies with load. The equation, therefore, at best only serves to describe the curve and does not permit analysis of its constants in terms of crossbridge kinetics. However, the case for smooth muscle may be different. Woledge et al. (44) have shown that for the amphibian illofibulares muscle a does behave as a true load-independent constant. This muscle is mechanically a very slow muscle as is smooth muscle, and we have used this similarity to argue that the a constant for smooth muscle may also be a true constant. If this is conceded, then smooth muscle FV constants can be interpreted in terms of numbers of crossbridges and rates of their cycling. The experiment to prove that a is constant for smooth muscle has never been conducted; given its importance this is puzzling.

Figure 13 shows FV curves for canine tracheal smooth muscle. They confirm that, just as in striated muscle muscle, the relationship is hyperbolic. The value of maximum stress (P_o/muscle cross-sectional area) is at the lower end of the normal range for all muscles. Murphy (45) has pointed out that smooth muscle surprisingly develops the same maximum stress as striated muscle, surprising because it possesses only one-fifth the myosin (and, therefore, of force-generating crossbridges) of striated muscle.

The maximum velocity of shortening (V_o) of smooth muscle is between 30- to 50-fold less than that of skele-

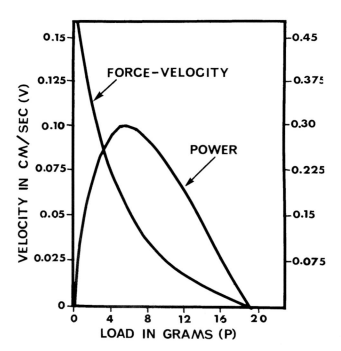

FIG. 13. Force-velocity and power curve shown for canine trachealis. The right hand ordinate (product of load and velocity) refers to the power curve.

tal muscle. This results from the slower actin-activated myosin Mg^{2+}-ATPase activity of the former. Teleologically, this makes sense, since smooth muscle has no need for very rapid movements.

The value a is an index of numbers of crossbridges in the cross-sectional areas of the muscle, and, thus, of the strength of the muscle. Put in another way, the thicker the muscle the stronger it is. Recent data suggest this is an over-simplification because the force developed in smooth muscle depends on the nature of the crossbridge. It appears that force development and load-bearing capacity in smooth muscle are a function of so-called "latchbridges" (46).

Value b is an index of the kinetic properties of myosin ATPase, as is V_o (equivalent to P_ob/a); a/b is an index of internal resistance to shortening as reported by Seow and Stephens (47); and $a \times b$ is an index of maintenance energy. These constants show the values expected of them for slow smooth muscle.

Figure 13 shows a power curve for airway smooth muscle. It demonstrates the expected peak at 0.33 P_o. Power curves have not been used much in analysis of smooth muscle contraction since the rate of energy consumption can be measured directly by biochemical measurements of cellular ATP, adenosine diphosphate (ADP), and creatine phosphate (CrP).

The force-velocity analysis of smooth muscle contraction is based on the procedure used for striated muscle. In the latter it is justified, to some extent, by the presence of a highly orderly array of contractile units organized in sarcomeres. No such array has been clearly designed for smooth muscle. However, recent evidence suggests that quasi-sarcomeric structures (or "mini-sarcomeres" as they are called) do exist in smooth muscle. Somlyo et al. (48) and Fay et al. (49) have shown that dense bodies (cytoplasmic) and bands (sarcolemmal) which are analogous to z discs, are arranged in considerable order and seem to delimit sarcomeric arrays. This then is the structural substrate used to justify analysis of smooth muscle force-velocity data in terms of crossbridges.

The concept of contractility has often been used in describing smooth muscle mechanics without due appreciation of the rigorousness of the concept. Maximum force development has been incorrectly used as an index of contractility. Since muscle, whether striated or smooth, both develops force (isometrically) or shortens (isotonically or auxotonically) at different velocities, it is clear that contractility should encompass all these functions. For this reason muscle contractility is defined as the simultaneous relation between force, velocity, and length. Since the state of activation of the muscle can also vary with time, the latter has also to be defined. Considered in this way, the fourth parameter involved in contractility is time. Instantaneous force-velocity-length-time relationship is, thus, the correct index of contractility. One cannot infer that because force developing ability is at a max-

imum, shortening and velocity are also at a maximum. A simple example is the effect of temperature. As temperature falls so does maximum velocity of shortening, while force development is unaffected. In closing this paragraph it must be pointed out that the concept of contractility was generally applied to whole muscles (frog sartorius) or to strips of muscle (canine trachealis). Now with the striking advances made with respect to the development of the motility assay combined with the use of laser traps, it is possible to determine contractility at single crossbridge level (50,51).

Deviation of FV curve from Hyperbolic Configuration at Loads Approaching Po

It has been shown in striated muscle that the FV curve is not a simple hyperbola as defined by Hill (43,52,53). We, therefore, determined whether airway smooth muscle behaved similarly, by eliciting FV data using quick-release methods.

Figure 14 shows FV curves obtained by quick release from canine tracheal smooth muscle. Releases were made at the peak of the isometric plateau e.g., at the end of the contraction time which for this muscle is 10 seconds. Deviation of velocities at high loads (100 to 130mN/mm) is evident. As the airway smooth muscle's parallel elastic component (PEC) is stretched slightly at optimal muscle length, l_o, at which such experiments are generally carried out, there is a small external recoil force on the contractile elements (CE) that has the same direction of shortening as that of the CE, with the same magnitude of resting tension. So the conventional V_o is the maximum velocity of shortening of the muscle, rather than its CE; the latter could be expected to be less than V_o. To eliminate the effect of this recoil of the PEC, we reduced the initial muscle length to ~ 0,80 l_o, such that resting tension was zero. A non-hyperbolic relationship was still obtained.

We focused on finding an equation to also fit those directly measured data points that did not conform to a hyperbola. The rationale in developing the equation was that a plot of the linearized transform of Hill's equation should yield a straight line over the entire range of loads at which velocities were measured. Figure 15 shows that in the low-load, high-velocity portion of the curve, a peak value was reached at 70% to 80% P_o. Values decreased thereafter, as load increased in the high-load low-velocity portion. From the fact that this relationship proved to be parabolic, an equation was derived to achieve the best fit to the experimental data by use of the principle of least squares:

$$V = \beta(Po - P) / [(\alpha + P)(\gamma - P)$$

where V is velocity, α, β, γ and P_o are constants; α and β/γ are approximations to Hill's a and b constants and $\gamma > P_o$.

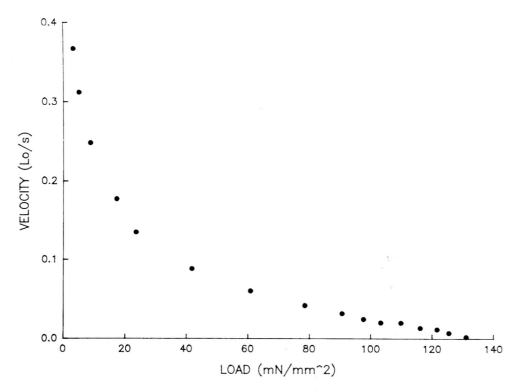

FIG. 14. Conventional force-velocity curve elicited by quick-release technique 2 s after onset of stimulation. Note deviation of velocities at high load.

Figure 16 shows curves fitted to the data points by Hill's equation and our modified equation. A goodness of fit test confirmed that a better fit was achieved by using the modified equation.

The physiological significance of the γ constant should be shown to be important if the new equation is to do anything other than provide an empirical fit. As P approaches γ, V, calculated from the modified equation, approaches in-

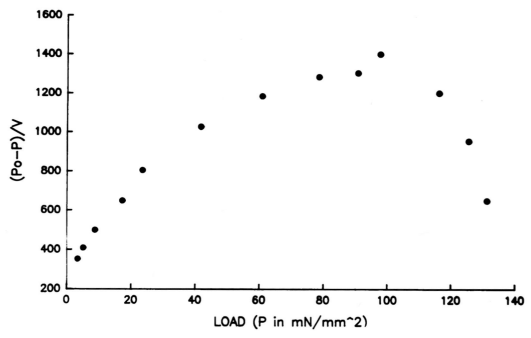

FIG. 15. Plot of the linearized transform of Hill's equation for canine trachealis.

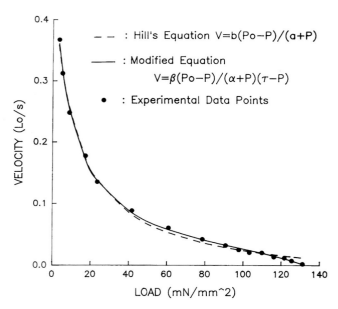

FIG. 16. Comparison of Hill's equation and modified equation to experimental data points taken from Figure 14. A better fit is achieved by using modified force-velocity equation, especially at high load end of curve; a, b, α, β, and γ are constant.

finity, which suggests that γ can be interpreted as the maximum force the crossbridges can bear. Skeletal muscle can bear a load of 1.6 P_o before the crossbridge attachment is mechanically broken and rapid lengthening occurs.

Stochastic Modelling of Smooth Muscle Crossbridge Activity Using Monte Carlo Methods and the 5-State Model

No work has so far been conducted on modelling of ASM contraction, apart from communications from Hai and Murphy (54) and Paul (55).

In 1957 AF Huxley (56) developed the sliding filament theory of contraction and formulated methods for determination of crossbridge distribution at different velocities assuming linear attachment and detachment. The key point in his model was that the crossbridge of the myosin molecule was bound to a binding site on actin; the binding was regulated by attachment and detachment rate constants. The tension arose from the distortion of a hypothetical spring representing the attachment site. Using this approach, he was able to predict the relation between force and velocity, and between rate of energy liberation and tension.

Since then Eisenberg and Greene (57) proposed a biochemical model based on ATP utilization for skeletal muscles as did Lymn and Taylor (58). Brokaw (59) developed a stochastic protocol to evaluate the time course of force development, early force recovery after rapid length changes, and the behavior of force development during constant velocity stretches/releases. Hai and Murphy (54) proposed a 4-state crossbridge model for vascular smooth muscle based on phosphorylation of the 20,000 Dalton myosin light chain (LC2O). By solving numerically four differential equations simultaneously, this model gave a solution for the relation between stress and phosphorylation. Later, they (54) linked their mode to Huxley's strain-dependent model to yield a conventional force-velocity relation.

In our pilot study we added a weakly-binding state (which is very important in the discussion of muscle contraction) to Hai's 4-state model, from which it was conspicuously absent (57,60). This provided us with a more flexible and complete five-state model. We also assumed that weakly-bound crossbridges would act as internal resistors during muscle shortening. Due to the intrinsically stochastic nature of crossbridge attachment, (theoretically, ordinary differential equation can only describe a mean behavior of the system), we adopted Brokaw's stochastic procedure and modified it to our particular needs.

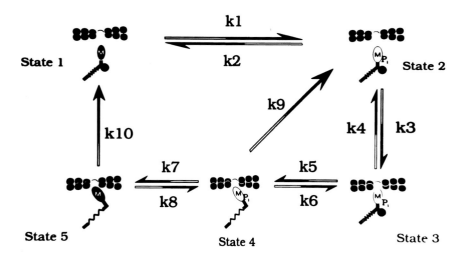

FIG. 17. Schematic of five state model for smooth muscle crossbridges, starting from top left and proceeding clockwise: unattached, unphosphorylated (A + M·ADP·Pi; state 1), unattached, phosphorylated (A + M_p·ADP·Pi; state 2), attached and phosphorylated with a hydrolyzed ATP bound (A·M_p·ADP·Pi, weakly binding; state 3), attached and phosphoorylated (A·M_p, strongly binding; state 4), and attached and recently dephosphorylated (A·M, latch or slowly cycling; state 5).

In Figure 17 crossbridges are shown as possessing five states:

1. free unphosphorylated with a hydrolyzed ATP attached to the head of the myosin heavy chain (M·ATP·Pi, state 1);
2. free phosphorylated with an attached hydrolyzed ATP (Mp·ADP·Pi. state 2)
3. attached and phosphorylated with a hydrolyzed ATP bound to myosin (A·M$_p$·ADP, Pi, weakly binding state 3)
4. attached and phosphorylated without bound ATP (A·Mp$_i$ strongly binding, state 4))
5. recently dephosphorylated (A·M latchbridge, state 5).

The five states were linked by ten rate functions (Figure 18): $k_1(t)$ and $k_8(t)$ represented phosphorylation of a resting crossbridge and a latchbridge respectively; k_2 and k_7 represented the activity of myosin light chain phosphatase or dephosphorylation of myosin light chain (MLC); $k_3(x,t)$ and $k_4(x,t)$ were rate functions representing crossbridge association and dissociation with a strain x at time t; k_5 was a rate constant representing the transfer from the weakly to strongly binding states or ADP and Pi release, k_6 was a rate constant representing simply the reverse transition; k_9 and k_{10} were rate constants representing crossbridge dissociation or ATP hydrolysis of a latchbridge and a strongly bound crossbridge respectively; t represented time, x represented extension of an attached bridge; $N_i(t)$ represented number of crossbridges in state i (i=1,...,5) at time t. The kinetically based model can also be described by five linear differential state equations shown in Figure 18.

We assumed that $k_1 = k_8$ and $k_2 = k_7$, due to the lack of direct evidence showing they were different (54). Additional constraints were not sensitive. Because V$_o$ decreased with time, we postulated that the fraction of latchbridges which cycled slowly and acted as internal resistances in a rapidly shortening muscle, increased with

time. The measured numerical value of this reduction enabled us to assume $k_{10} = 1.5$ kg. For crossbridge transformation from weak binding to strong binding, we chose $k_5 = 60k_6$ to fit the experimental evidence that crossbridge attachment or stiffness preceded force generation for both smooth and striated muscle (61–64,66).

For rate functions $k_3(x,t)$ and $k_4(x,t)$ we adopted Brokaw's (59) functions since he had shown reasonable duplication of steady-state behavior of frog sartorius muscle at 0°C:

$$k_3(x,t) = \begin{cases} 65x/h & t < T_s, 0 < x \leq h \\ [(65x)]/he \wedge \gamma(T_s - t) & t \geq T_s, 0 < x \leq h \\ 0 & \textbf{\textit{otherwise}} \end{cases}$$

$$k_4(x,t) = \begin{cases} 1.5x/h & 0 \leq x \\ 150 & x < 0 \end{cases}$$

where Ts was the stimulus duration, h was the maximum power stroke of a crossbridge and given a value of 10nm. The constant γ in equation (6) had a value of 2 for canine ASM.

A constant x_o was used to represent the initial relevant position of the filaments before stimulation. A length control variable provided a measure of displacement between the filaments in terms of the current position of the origin of the binding site sequence, relative to the origin of the crossbridge sequence, which enabled us to control muscle length during simulations so we could simulate length change experiments, as in isovelocity, and isotonic and auxotonic shortening.

The probability function for myosin phosphorylation (P$_{ph}$) was given by:

$$Pph(t) = K_1(t)/K_1(t) + K_2(t)(1 - e^{-(K_1(t) + K_2(t))\Delta t})$$

and the probability of myosin dephosphorylation (P dephos) was given by:

$$P_{dephos}(t) = K_2(t)/K_1(t) + K_2(t)(1 - e^{-K_1(t) + K_2(t)\Delta t})$$

$$\frac{dN_1(t)}{dt} = -k_1N_1(t) + k_2N_2(t) + k_9N_5(t) \tag{S1}$$

$$\frac{dN_2(t)}{dt} = -(k_2 + k_3)N_2(t) + k_1N_1(t) + k_4N_3(t) + k_{10}N_4(t) \tag{S2}$$

$$\frac{dN_3(t)}{dt} = k_3N_2(t) - (k_4 + k_5)N_3(t) + k_6N_4(t) \tag{S3}$$

$$\frac{dN_4(t)}{dt} = k_5N_3(t) - (k_6 + k_7 + k_{10})N_4(t) + k_8N_5(t) \tag{S4}$$

$$\frac{dN_5(t)}{dt} = k_7N_4(t) - (k_8 + k_9)N_5(t) \tag{S5}$$

FIG. 18. Five determinative linear differential equations which describe the 5 state model shown in Figure 17.

The probabilities (P_f) that a crossbridge was attached to actin with extension x during a short time period t and that it was detached (P_g) could be fairly easily derived.

The probability of weak binding crossbridges converting to strong binding bridge P_s was given by:

$$P_s(x,t) = K_5 / (K_5 + K_6)(1 - e^{-(K_5 - K_6)\Delta t})$$

that for strong binding reverting to weak binding (P_w) was given by:

$$P_w(x,t) = K_6 / (K_5 + K_6)(1 - e^{-(K_5 - K_6)\Delta t})$$

The probability of detachment from strong binding state (P_{SATP}) was given by:

$$P_{SATP} = 1 - e^{K_{10}\Delta t}$$

and that of detachment from latch state (P_{lATP}) was given by

$$P_{lATP} = 1 - e^{K9\Delta t}$$

Based on Huxley's theory (56,65) the average force per crossbridge ($P(t)$) for a population N_c's is given by:

$$P(t) = \Sigma[K_L \, x(N_L)] + \Sigma[K_S x(N_S)]$$

where K_S and K_L were the force constants of the strongly binding and latch crossbridges. $x(N_L)$ and $x(N_S)$ represented the extensions for latch and strongly binding crossbridges respectively. Since V_o of normally cycling crossbridges for canine tracheal smooth muscle was 50% faster than that of latchbridges we reasonably assumed $K_L = 1.5 K_S$ (67).

To determine the distance shortened Dx in Dt under certain internal and external loads, we assumed the internal resistance came from three sources: compression of the cytoskeleton or parallel elastic component (PEC), weakly binding crossbridges which could not move at all, and latchbridges which moved very slowly. Muscle length was represented by the length control variable. Applying the force balance and energy balance equations, the energy balance equation for each latchbridge and each weakly binding crossbridge was obtained.

Using the previously mentioned approach we could simulate the following relationships:

1. Length-tension relationship. Figure 19 shows active tension versus length (using normalized units) curves. These closely resemble those obtained experimentally.
2. The isometric myogram. This is shown in Figure 20; it closely simulates the experimentally elicited curve. The contraction time for the simulated myogram (7 to 8s) was close to that for the experimental curve (8 to 10s).
3. Force transients. Figure 21 shows force transients after a 2nm quick release and 2 nm quick stretch with a time step of 500µs. The force, as expected, after a quick drop or rise due to the elastic SEC recovered, reflecting the reattachment of crossbridges at the new length. The early recovery time of quick release, however, was shorter than that of quick stretch. In the quick release, two fast force transients followed

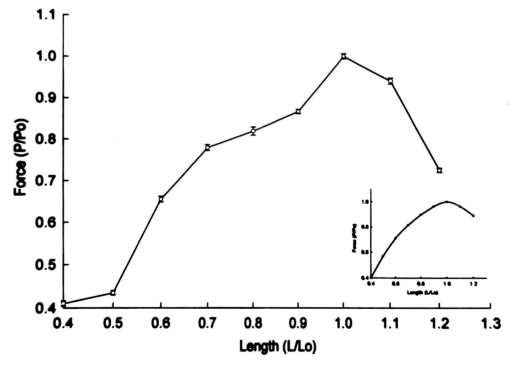

FIG. 19. A simulated conventional length-active tension curve is shown. The inset shows an isometric LT curve from canine trachealis (From Stephens NL, Kroeger E, Mehta JA. Force-velocity characteristics of respiratory airway smooth muscle. *J Appl Physiol* 1969;26(6):685–692.)

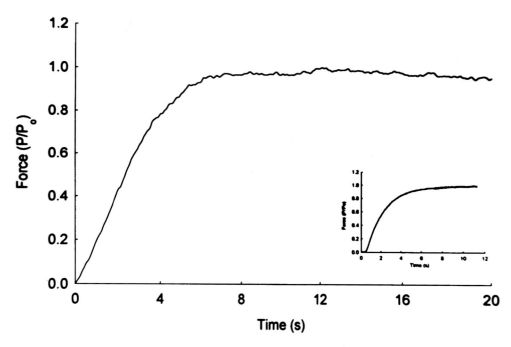

FIG. 20. Time course of isometric force development. Simulated isometric myogram. The inset shows experimental myogram from canine trachealis.

by a slow transient were seen with some variability due to stochastic fluctuations arising from our model stimulation.

T1 and T_2 curves akin to those reported for skeletal muscle by Huxley et al. (65) were also simulated by our model and are shown in Figure 22. The T_1 curve showed a linearity referred to small stretches and releases; the T_2 curve was flatter than that of skeletal muscle (65).

4. Isotonic shortening. This is another meaningful parameter to be examined. The model simulated conventional force-velocity curves as shown in Figure 23.

The maximum shortening velocity, V_o, was 20.6 nm/s or 0.009 l_o/s, for n = 10.

5. Stiffness. Since muscle stiffness is an index of the number of attached bridges, we could, in reverse, estimate stiffness by counting the number of attached bridges. Figure 24 shows force initially lagged stiffness which corresponded to experimental data reported by us (64). Stiffness reached its saturated value about 3 to 4 seconds after onset of stimulation, during which force increased and then remained at a plateau value without further increase in number of attached bridges. The fraction of latch to normally cycling

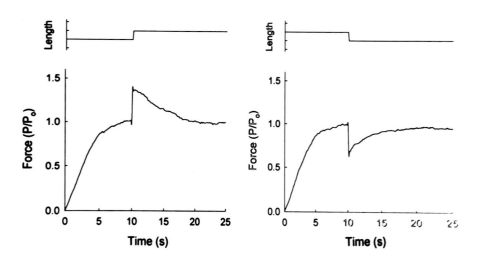

FIG. 21. Froce transients to rapid length changes. Transient analysis simulation. The early tension recovery time is shorter in release than in stretch which corresponds to AF Huxley's experimental finding in a striated muscle sarcomere. Note that the typical four phases in force recovery can be seen.

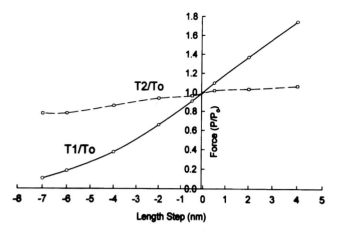

FIG. 22. T_1 and T_2 curves of smooth muscle. Plots of the instantaneous tension at the end of the length step (T_1) and at the plateau following early tension recovery (T_2) against the amplitude of the length step. T_1/T_0 curve showed a linearity referred to small stretches and releases which demonstrated the same tendency as that of vascular smooth muscle; T_2/T_0 curve was flatter than that of striated muscle reported by Huxley (1971). No experimental evidence has been reported for the T_2/T_0 curve in smooth muscle.

bridges increased with time which corresponded to the force elevation after stiffness reached its peak.

6. Myosin light chain phosphorylation. Summing crossbridges in phosphorylated state (states, 2,3 and 4) yielded a value for the fraction of phosphorylated

bridges. The phosphorylation level reached its peak at 4 seconds, as expected, and gradually decreased to a lower steady level in the later phase. Figure 25 shows the time course of force development and of phosphorylation.

The previous simulation shows that our modified five-state model, based on the phosphorylation of the 20 kDa myosin light chain (MLC_{20}) and utilization of ATP for crossbridge cycling, satisfactorily predicted the fundamental mechanical behavior of smooth muscle.

Even though the regulatory mechanisms in smooth muscle were different from those in striated muscle, biochemical and biophysical studies indicated that smooth muscle contraction could also be understood in terms of the sliding filament/crossbridge rotation paraadigm. Crossbridge attachment in smooth muscle, as in striated, is dependent on random interaction between binding sites in thin and thick filaments, and the binding occurs within the range of crossbridge power strokes. The likelihood of attachment is influenced by local biochemical environment and the nature of the crossbridges themselves. The state equations (S1-S5), therefore, symbolized a mean behavior of crossbridges, and thus provide, in a sense, a deterministic view of muscle contraction. They do not incorporate any parameters dealing with the known randomness of crossbridge cycling. Theoretically, a system of stochastic differential equations should be applied. This is most conveniently carried out with a computer. Computer simulation of a stochastic model of contraction

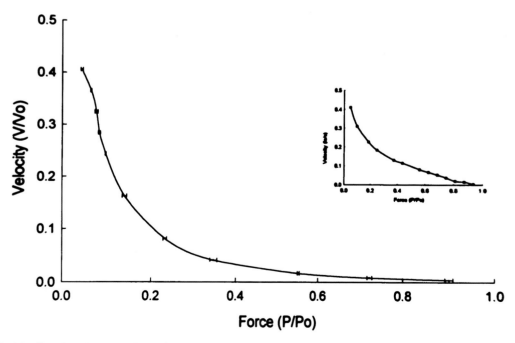

FIG. 23. Simulated conventional force-velocity curve for smooth muscle. The V_0 is in the low normal range for airway smooth muscle. The inset shows an experimentally obtained curve from canine tracheal smooth muscle.

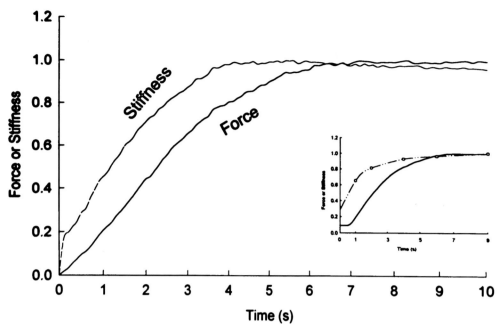

FIG. 24. Time courses of force and stiffness. The left-most curves represent simulation. The insert shows experimentally obtained curves by Seow and Stephens and Kamm and Stull (1986).

makes the latter more realistic and natural. In a real smooth muscle preparation, a large compliance and the large number of crossbridges smooth out the fluctuation so that only mean response curves can be seen. Compared with the analytical technique used by Hai and Murphy (54), the stochastic technique we developed, apart from its reality and conformation to what really happens at a crossbridge, is far more flexible to fit newly found experimental data by simply changing values and/or forms of state-transformation functions, regardless of their mathematical complexity.

Normally Cycling and Latchbridges in Smooth Muscle

Perhaps the greatest advances in understanding the mechanics of smooth muscle contraction was made by Dillon and Murphy's group (61) who reported in isolated hog carotid artery strips that unloaded, (i.e. zero load), shortening velocity (V_o) elicited by quick-release techniques, showed a progressive reduction during the duration of an isometric tetanus. This does not occur in striated muscle. Since Murphy's report, a host of smooth muscle preparations (carotid artery, saphenous vein canine bronchial, and tracheal smooth muscle have been shown to possess similar characteristics (35,66). Murphy explained this behavior on the basis of his experimental demonstration that phosphorylation of the regulatory myosin light chain (MLC_{20}) showed a similar decrease with time. He suggested that the rapid velocity of short-

ening that developed early in contraction was due to maximal phosphorylation of MLC_{20}. Later in contraction both shortening velocity and phosphorylation dropped considerably while force production and load-bearing capacity increased. He felt that the cycling of some of the bridges had slowed considerably. These acted as a relative brake on normally cycling crossbridges and produced the considerably reduced V_o he had found. Because of this behavior he termed these "latchbridges."

Ever since he coined the term, a great deal of controversy has developed. Seigman's group (35) believe that no brake-like latchbridges exist and that the reduced V_o is due to progressive showing of all bridges. Merkel et al. (68) reported that unlike time-dependent increases in shortening velocity and glycogen phosphorylase activity, agonist-induced myosin phosphorylation was not markedly transient. Furthermore, regardless of the contractile agonist used, no correlation was found between myosin phosphorylation and shortening velocity when these parameters were compared at corresponding time points. They concluded that myosin phosphorylation is not the sole determinant of shortening velocity in canine trachealis. In analyzing this conclusion, one must keep in mind that the status of MLC_{20} phosphorylation depends on the intactness and activity of MLC_{20} phosphatase. Any loss would result in spurious maintained phosphorylation. Moreland et al. (69) reported an apparent dissociation between MLC_{20} phosphorylation and maximum velocity of shortening in KCl depolarized swine carotid artery. The controversy has spread to other areas. For example, others have shown that MLC_{20} phosphorylation is

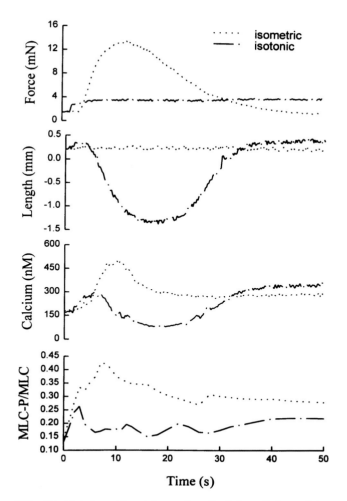

FIG. 25. Relationship of force, length, intracellular calcium and stoichiometry of myosin light chain phosphorylation during isometric and isotonic contractions. Note the lower calcium and phosphorylation levels in isotonic contractions.

not a *sine qua non* for contraction, and the latter can develop even in the absence of any increase in intracellular calcium (70,71). The latter has been explained by the development of increased sensitivity to calcium (72). Some of the mechanisms responsible for this may be a decrease in MLC phosphatase activity or a change in the function of an inhibitor protein (73).

Contraction in the absence of phosphorylation is unusual and is induced by rather unphysiological molecules such as phorbol esters. Under physiological circumstances, all would agree to the importance of phosphorylation of MLC_{20} in initiating contraction.

Another explanation for the maintained phase of force production is that it is due to a mechanism not related to contractile proteins. Parks and Rasmussen (74) found phosphorylation of several proteins during late contraction. These seemed to be cytoskeletal proteins. They felt that the sustained force developed stemmed from cytoskeletal mechanisms. The consensus at this time is that marked changes (4-fold) in V_o do occur during the course

of an isometric contraction, but the causative role of dephosphorylation in late contraction is far from decided. A recent report by Moreland et al. (working with skinned vascular smooth muscle), in which the time course of MLC_{20} phosphorylation was measured, provides new evidence that latchbridges do exist (69). Unfortunately, measurements of shortening velocity were not reported; presumably these experiments are under way.

Time Course of Isotonic Shortening

Importance of "2 Second" Shortening

Sufficient cognizance has not been taken of the importance of the time course of shortening of ASM in analyzing the mechanical properties of shortening muscle which is a fairly serious shortcoming in view of its unique role in determining total muscle shortening.

Figure 11 shows the time course of isotonic shortening (under light preload) of canine TSM *in vitro*. It is clear that shortening is not a linear function of time, but what is not apparent unless one specifically looks for it, is that 75% of the total shortening of the muscle is complete in 2 seconds which represents 20% of the total contraction time. In the remaining 8 seconds, only 25% additional shortening is achieved. One may speculate that in the first 2 seconds normally cycling crossbridges are active and produce the bulk of the shortening. In the remaining time latchbridges slow down the normally cycling bridges and, thus, produce little shortening. This behavior is seen when the muscle is lightly loaded. In most instances this represents a load equivalent to that which just stretches the muscle to its optimal length and which is likely to be the physiological load on the muscle. Under zero loading conditions brought about by electronic muscle levers which can abruptly change the load to zero, the shortening occurring in the first two seconds is even greater. This represents true shortening ability of the muscle since it is now load-independent. This shortening is patently not physiological but provides insight into subcellular mechanisms of shortening. When the load increases to 0.25 P_o or more, the magnitude of this early shortening is reduced.

One application of this finding is seen in ragweed pollen-sensitized airway smooth muscle. In this muscle we have reported that the total shortening of the sensitized muscle is greater than that of the muscle from the littermate control. This entire difference emerges in the first 2 seconds and the additional shortening developed in the following 8 seconds is identical for the muscles. This shows the importance of studying the entire time course of shortening and not just the maximal steady state value. While the latter does show the difference by incorporating the preponderant early shortening, it provides no insight into mechanisms. With respect to regulation of airway conductance, the meaningful parameter to study is that of shortening. Isometric studies yield very little information about conductance. The information they yield relates mainly to the stiffness properties of the airways, which, other than modifying somewhat the nature of the propagated pressure pulse, do not affect conductance. While recognition of the role of steady state shortening measurements is important, it is, nevertheless, inadequate. To elucidate mechanisms, attention must be focused on the shortening occurring in the first 2 seconds in airway smooth muscle.

"2 Second Shortening" Parameter Changes Indicate the Meaningful Biochemical Changes to Investigate

Another consideration stemming from the 2 second shortening parameter is that the regulatory biochemical mechanism is the activity of myosin light chain kinase which phosphorylates the 20kDa myosin light chain and initiates and controls the activity of normally cycling crossbridges. It is this which focused our research on myosin light chain kinase content and activity in sensitized ASM which shortened more than control muscle. We were gratified to detect increased content and total activity of the enzyme.

It must also be pointed out that shortening in the late phase of contraction is regulated by slowly cycling or latchbridges. The enzyme of relevance is myosin light chain phosphatase since it is this that dephosphorylates the light chain and produces the latch state.

Relevance of V_o to Δl_{max}

This discussion is speculative and based on data from the author's laboratory; it needs confirmation. *A priori* it may seem that Δl_{max} would not be regulated by V_o, since the contraction time (10s) of this muscle would be perfectly adequate for maximum shortening to occur, no matter how slow the V_o. However, as just pointed out, smooth muscle is unique in that 75% of its total shortening is complete within 2 seconds. This indicates that were

V_o not of adequate magnitude, shortening would not be complete in the available time. It appears also that the shortening deficit generated in the first 10 seconds cannot be made up in the remainder of the contraction time.

Loading History-Dependent Shortening of Airway Smooth Muscle: The Role of Isotonic and Auxotonic Loading

Since *in vivo* the load against which ASM shortens, progressively increases because of the connective tissues to which the muscle cells are tethered, shortening is auxotonic. We, therefore, tested the hypothesis that shortening of canine ASM is a function, not only of the magnitude of the load, but also of its history.

To test this, an electronic loader system was built allowing us to study shortening under four shortening-dependent loading modes. Canine tracheal smooth muscle was supramaximally stimulated electrically and shortened under the following loading modes: (1) Linear: $R = K \times \Delta L$; (2) Logarithmic: $R = K \times Log(A \times \Delta L + 1)$; (3) Sigmoidal: $R = K \times EXP[A - (b/\Delta L)]$; (4) Exponential: $R = EXP(\Delta L \times K) - 1$ where ΔL is length change, R is the load generated by the loader, K is an adjustable constant, and A and b are fixed constants of the loader.

Figure 26 shows that the magnitude of shortening is not only a function of the magnitude of the load imposed, but, as importantly, a function of the history of loading. It can be seen in the upper panel that the maximum force developed in response to magnitude of loading is the same for sigmoidal, exponential, linear, and logarithmic loading modes. However, the greatest shortening is seen in exponential loading mode and the smallest in logarithmic loading mode. The proposed mechanism for this behavior is that smooth muscle crossbridges cycle faster in the early contraction phase and, therefore, produce more shortening than that of the slower cycling crossbridges in the later phase.

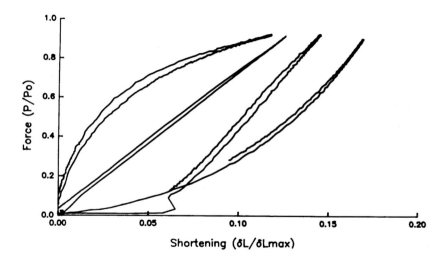

FIG. 26. Auxotonic shortening-force plot under different loading modes. Length-tension curves of trachealis shortening under logarithmic, linear (elastic), and sigmoidal loading modes. Even though the maximal load was the same for all loading modes, it is clear that maximum shortening differs. The least shortening is seen where heaviest loads (logarithmic) are applied early in contraction. The curves reading from left to right are logarithmic, linear, sigmoidal, and exponential.

Figure 11 shows data from a pilot study of lightly pre-loaded ($0.05P_o$) isotonic shortening of tracheal smooth muscle, whose stimulus duration was 10 seconds. About 75% of maximum shortening was complete within the first 3 seconds. It is clear that loading in this phase would have the greatest repercussion on total muscle shortening. Since loading is greatest in this period under logarithmic mode, shortening would be the least, while it would be greatest for exponential loading mode. Inhibition of shortening in the early phase by heavy load cannot be adequately compensated for by later phase shortening because of the lower crossbridge cycling rate and the negative feedback loop formed by connective tissue and muscle.

This novel behavior is unique and has physiological importance because shortening *in vivo* is auxotonic. Once again it must be emphasized that to elucidate mechanisms of allergic bronchoconstriction, measurements of auxotonic shortening and velocity must be made early in contraction.

The Series Elastic Component of Airway Smooth Muscle

Overview

Smooth muscle contraction both at strip and single cell level is brought about by activation of the so-called "contractile element" (CE). The time course of this activation has been delineated by quick-stretch and quick-release experiments (23,28,66). It is also well-known that the force or shortening generated by the CE is not transmitted instantaneously to the outside world. but after a well-defined time lag. This lag is due to the fact that, in conceptual terms, transmission occurs via an elastic structure, the series elastic component (SEC). Hence, activity measured at the ends of a strip of muscle or cell is not a direct index of what is happening with respect to magnitude and rate of shortening at the all-important, energy-consuming, working contractile element. To study the CE, the length and stiffness of the SEC must be known. We have reported such data for canine tracheal smooth muscle in 1971 (26). At that time, it was reported that when developing force equal to P_o, the SEC in skeletal muscle was stretched by 1.5% to 3% of initial muscle length, 8% to 10% in cardiac, and 7.5% in TSM (26,75,76). Since then, as equipment and methodology have improved, these values have all become smaller. For example we now find that the SEC elongation is 3% in TSM (unpublished observations). Seow and Ford using the same preparation, but with higher resolution and recision lever systems obtain a value of 2% (personal communication).

It must be kept in mind that the SEC elongation stems from two sources, one is from the actomyosin crossbridges themselves and the other from cell attachments such as small tendinous segments, other connections at-taching the muscle strip or cell to the muscle lever and dead muscle tissue. The last named can contribute the bulk of the stray compliance and is usually present at the sites of ligature application. Major focus is, of course, on the crossbridge component.

For smooth muscle, just as for striated, it is generally agreed that SEC stiffness is an index of the numbers of attached crossbridges (63,75–77). A recent nuance is that there are two states of such attachment—the weakly attached and the strongly attached states (57).

Stiffness Versus Time

The SEC stiffness of TSM at resting and rigor states, as well as at different points in time in an isometric contraction, needs to be delineated since it would provide a read-out of the time course of crossbridge recruitment. In smooth muscle this is particularly important because crossbridges change their properties (latchbridges develop) and, perhaps, their numbers.

To determine stiffness at different time points it is very important to ensure that all estimates based on quick-release techniques must be made at the same specific stress level. A family of stress-strain curves for the SEC of TSM was obtained by quick-releasing the muscle at different points in time during contraction. Figure 27 shows sample experimental records from which the length and force change data of the SEC can be obtained; a family of stress-strain curves was calculated

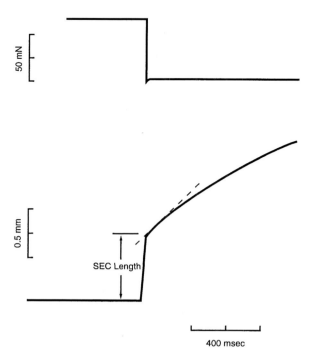

FIG. 27. Length and force versus time records for electrically stimulated canine trachealis. The perturbation represents quick release to a lower load.

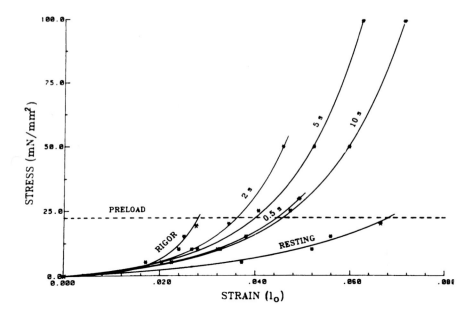

FIG. 28. Stress-strain curves of the SEC from a single experiment. The equation $\sigma = (E_o/A)(e^{AE} - 1)$ was used to fit the experimental data. Labels on curves indicate state of muscle under which they were obtained. Time (in seconds) on curves indicate time when muscle was released. Stimulation started at time 0. Dashed line indicates stress level (preload) at which stiffness values of SECs were compared. Constant stress-stiffness values were obtained by measuring slopes of stress-strain curves at intersections of dashed line (preload) and curves; l_o, optimum muscle length.

and is shown in Figure 28. At the points on these curves intersected by the constant preload line, the slopes of the line were obtained and provide the constant-stress stiffness. The equation used to fit the data points was:

$$d\sigma/de = E_o + A\sigma$$

where σ is muscle stress, de is the strain of SEC, $d\sigma/de$ is stiffness, E_o is the initial elastic modulus and A is the slope of the linear stiffness-stress curve.

Stiffness of the SEC is broken down into two components: the initial elastic modules E_o, which is stress-independent; $A\sigma$ which depends on stress. Both components are shown in Figure 29. To compare the stiffness of the SEC, the magnitude of the stress in the SEC has to be specified. However, because E_o is relatively small and remains constant throughout contraction, the only parameter that determines the stiffness at any stress level is the constant A, which, therefore, is an index of stiffness that ex-

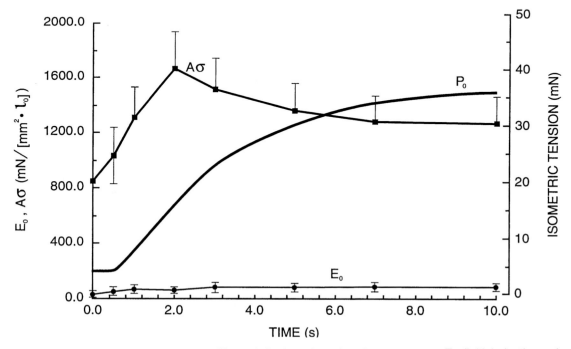

FIG. 29. Series elastic component stiffness is broken down into 2 components: Eo (initial elastic modulus, stress independent) and Aσ (stress dependent, where A is a slope and σ is a stress) is plotted to illustrate the time relationship of stages in contractile l_o, optimum muscle length.

cludes the effect of stress in the SEC. The behavior of A as a function of time is shown in Figure 29; it represents the time variation of SEC stiffness. Here the value of A is multiplied by a constant stress value of $22.2 mN/mm^2$ (10% of P_o) so that the relative values of E_o and $A\sigma$ can be compared. A typical isometric tension-time curve is also shown to indicate the time course of contraction.

The stiffness curve in the figure is of considerable interest in that it shows that a peak value occurs very early in the contraction (at 2 seconds), and thereafter, a slow decline occurs in the ensuing 8 seconds. This behavior could not have been demonstrated without the technique of measuring stiffness at different times but at constant stress. Were it not for this, stiffness would have increased progressively with time. There is only one other similar report in the literature but in that, the complete time course of stiffness was not described (62).

The behavior of the stiffness curve indicates that the maximum number of cycling crossbridges was seen early in the contraction. This is very likely, since crossbridges are in a normally cycling phase, and, therefore, a maximum number can be made. Later in contraction, the number of cycling bridges is reduced. Dillon et al. (46) and Kamm and Stull (62) found that shortening velocity and phosphorylation of the 20 kDa myosin light chain showed the same time course as the stiffness curves we report here. Therefore, the late decrease in stiffness signifying reduced number of cycling crossbridges, supports the idea that the late development of maximum isometric force (See Figure 28) must originate in time-dependent alteration in the properties of the crossbridges, which is compatible with the development of the latchbridge state.

Stiffness Versus Length

In vivo, as the bronchus actively constricts, changes in stiffness of the wall, probably resulting from changes in stiffness of its smooth muscle, would be modified by changes in muscle length; *a priori* one could conceive that as length decreased, stiffness would also decrease resulting in mechanical instability of the bronchial wall.

Therefore, we measured the stiffness of the SEC of canine tracheal smooth muscle during isotonic shortening by applying small force perturbations to the muscle and measuring the resulting length responses (77). The force perturbation was a train of 10-Hz rectangular force waves varying from 0 to 10% of P_o, i.e. $\Delta P=10\%P_o$. Sample records from a single experiment are shown in Figure 30. Stiffness of the SEC was estimated from the ratio $\Delta P/\Delta L$. The change in SEC stiffness with respect to change in muscle length was further studied by obtaining the stress-strain curves of the SEC at different muscle lengths using the load-clamping method. The clamps were applied at a fixed time after stimulation. Length of the muscle 10s after contraction was controlled by the magnitude of the isotonic load. It was found, somewhat surprisingly, that the appar-

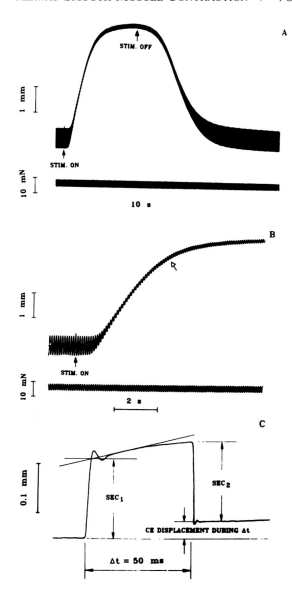

FIG. 30. Records of input force perturbations (*lower trace*) and resulting length perturbations (*upper trace*) during active shortening and relaxation of canine trachealis. **A:** Force perturbations were produced by rapidly (10Hz) changing force level in lever from 0 to 4 mN repetitively (*rectangular force wave*). Amplitude of force wave was ~10% of P_o. Onset and termination of electrical stimulation are indicated on traces. Shortening is indicated in upward direction. **B:** portion of traces in A are here displayed at different time scale. Rectangular shape of force wave is visible here. Line through middle of upper trace was displacement curve of the muscle under a preload of 2mN (mean value of force levels of rectangular force wave). **C:** Magnification of a small portion of length perturbation around area indicated by area in B. SEC length was obtained by averaging lengths of SEC, and SEC2 and subtraction compliance of thread and lever from averaged value. Data were recorded with a sampling frequency of 4,000 Hz to show details of trace.

ent SEC stiffness increased as length decreased. This stiffness increase palpably cannot be due to increase in number of attached crossbridges, but is perhaps due to the gradual diminution of the SEC length itself during muscle shortening. As a matter of fact, length-tension curves for this muscle clearly show that the number of active crossbridges decreases at lengths less than optimal (l_o).

One explanation for our finding, that stiffness increases as muscle length decreases, is that part of the structure that constitutes the SEC becomes shorter when muscle shortens. To turn this around, one could conclude that the diminution of the length of SEC is the cause of the apparent increase in SEC stiffness.

The Parallel Elastic Component (PEC)

The concept of the existence of a PEC is based on the observation that a resting muscle can maintain its length indefinitely without energy expenditure greater than its basal energy consumption rate (i.e., it does this without activating a cycling crossbridge mechanism). This property is based on the existence of a substantial elastic structure in parallel with the fibers in whole muscles. The passive tension may, therefore, be high at long muscle lengths and, even near the *in situ* length in some muscles; examples of the latter are cardiac muscle and some varieties of smooth muscles.

Figure 31 depicts the Voigt model for muscle. The CE and its in-series SE constitute the 2-component model of AV Hill. The PEC is in parallel with the CE. At rest, or when the tension in the muscle is just at zero, the weight of the muscle is borne by the PEC and the SEC. In the Maxwell model it would be borne entirely by the PEC. As stretch is induced, resting tension increases because of

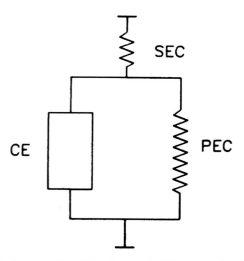

FIG. 31. Schematic of Voigt model. CE, ontractile element; PEC, parallel elastic component; SEC, series elastic component.

the elastic properties of PEC. However, when the SEC is activated it eventually develops a tension greater than that in the SEC at which time load bearing passes from the PEC-SEC combination to the CE-SEC combination. Conventional passive length-tension curves display the mechanical properties of the PEC.

Though well-investigated in cardiac muscle, relatively little attention has been paid to the behavior of the PEC when the muscle actively shortens such that its resting tension is zero. At zero tension the spring representing the PEC would be at its equilibrium position. Any further shortening of the muscle, such as brought about by activation of the CE, would compress the PEC spring which would internally load the CE, thus reducing the maximum velocity of shortening. This constitutes the internal resistance to shortening, and the hypothetical structure (perhaps the cytoskeleton and/or the extracellular matrix) subserving it is the internal resistor. In cardiac muscle, recoil of the internal resistor which is compressed during systole, helps in filling the atria and ventricles during diastole. We feel that the internal resistor is of some importance in smooth muscle function also. At the very least it says that shortening is not the sole function of force developed but is also regulated by the elastic properties of the internal resistor (IR).

The evidence for the existence of an internal resistor is straightforward. If one stretches an active muscle to beyond its optimal length (l_o) and then releases it, it returns to l_o. Conversely, if one allows a stimulated muscle to shorten maximally and then removes the stimulus, the muscle re-elongates to its original length. It is as if there was an intracellular elastic resistance to shortening and stretching. In shortening mode the IR undergoes compression and stores potential energy. When the stimulus is turned off, the resistor re-expands and restores the muscle to its original length.

We developed a method to delineate the length-tension curve of the IR. Consideration of Figure 31 indicates that when a load is applied to an activated muscle it is transferred to the muscle's CE via the spring-like SEC. The maximal CE velocity would be an inverse function of the load. If the external load is suddenly changed to zero with an electronically applied, so-called "zero load clamp," the muscle will shorten at maximum velocity. As stated previously, as the shortening increased the PEC would relax from its slightly stretched state at l_o. With further CE shortening, the parallel component would be compressed further, thus, applying an internal load on the CE whose velocity would be reduced.

It is possible to measure maximum velocities (zero load) of shortening at different CE lengths. Figure 32 shows a series of shortening records in which the maximally stimulated muscle shortened isotonically. At any given time the CE length was a function of magnitude of the load. At the moment shown in the records zero load clamps were applied. A rapid transient emanating from

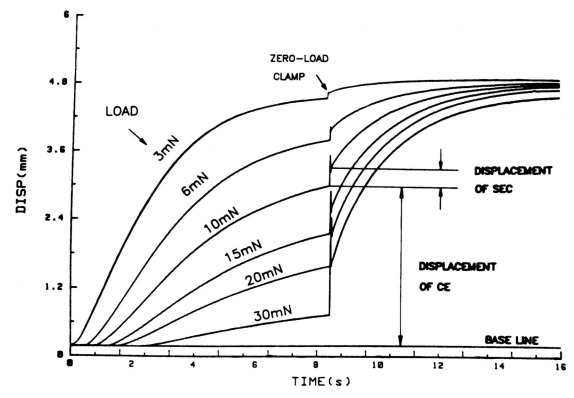

FIG. 32. Experimental records of shortening versus time of a strip of canine trachealis set at optimal length initially. The contractile element was obtained by subtracting the displacement of the contractile element and the series elastic component from the optimal muscle length. The maximum velocity (V_o) for each length was obtained by measuring the slope of the shortening curve 100 msec after the zero load clamp. The time chosen is arbitrary.

the SEC was seen in each trace, followed by a slower transient that represented CE shortening. The maximum velocity attained by the CE was plotted against the calculated CE length. Velocity-CE length curves derived from the data are shown in Figure 33. The curvilinear relationship is clearly seen and a quadratic function best fitted the data. In terms of physiological significance it is evident that for the first 25%, shortening velocity is almost independent of length.

Conventional force-velocity curves were obtained from the same muscle by quick-release techniques at the same time at which the studies of the IR were conducted. Figure 34 shows superimposition of the V_o versus CE length curve and the force-velocity curve. From analysis of these curves tension-extension data for the IR, i.e., for the PEC in compression mode, can be obtained. At a selected velocity, V_1, the corresponding load point P_1 can be read off the force-velocity curve. This represents the load on the CE produced by extension of the SEC resulting from the external load. Reading the velocity-length curve (note the abscissa represents both length and load) for the PEC one determines the length (l_1) at which V_1 develops. Several P_i, l_i points are plotted to yield the tension-extension curve of Figure 35.

The previously mentioned data represent the first report of a method to characterize the elastic properties of airway smooth muscle's internal resistor (See following for discussion of its application to studies of asthma).

Airway Smooth Muscle Relaxation: The Role of Isotonic Studies

Very little work has been carried out with respect to smooth muscle relaxation. It may sound strange to be dealing with relaxation in a section devoted to smooth muscle contraction. The justification is that reduced relaxation could contribute to increased contraction by providing a higher base line force or shortening muscle length. Shibata et al. (78) reported that isometric relaxation was prolonged in caudal artery strips from spontaneously hypertensive rats. What they measured was the half-time of force decay after the stimulus was turned off. Isometric relaxation studies are of limited value since they only tell us about changes in wall stiffness and almost nothing about changes in vascular resistance. The meaningful variable to measure is that of isotonic relaxation. The major component of resistance decrease during

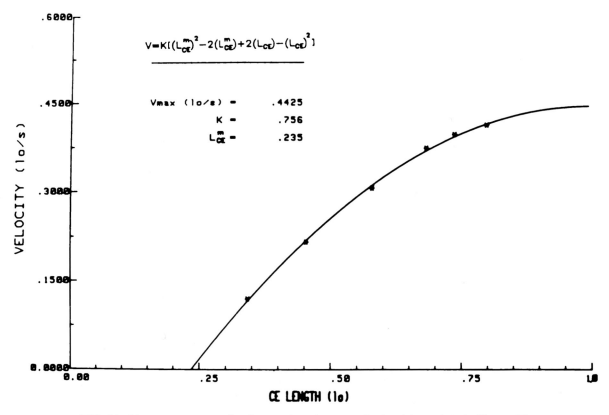

FIG. 33. V_0 versus contractile element length curve obtained from data in Figure 32.

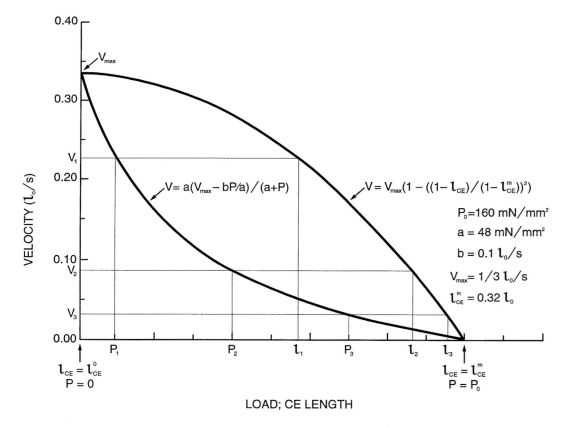

FIG. 34. Curves of Figure 33 superimposed on a force-velocity curve for the same muscle. Note the abscissa represents load for the force-velocity curve and CE length for the length-velocity phase plane.

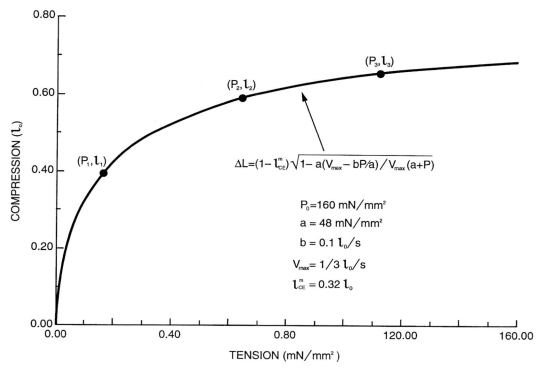

FIG. 35. Tension-compression curve for the PEC obtained from Figure 34.

bronchoconstriction is controlled by isotonic or auxotonic relaxation of the airway smooth muscle. With one exception, neither in smooth nor striated muscle has this been carried out *in vitro* (79). In striated muscle only isometric relaxation was studied even though isotonic relaxation traces were published in those papers (80,81).

Development of a Relaxation Index

Surprisingly, no such index has been published and it behooved us to develop one.

At l_o, the muscle strip under a variety of loads was supramaximally stimulated so as to elicit maximum isotonic shortening. The stimulus was turned off at peak shortening and the muscle strips were allowed to elongate. Since relaxation depends on load, state of activation, and the length of the muscle's CE at the onset of relaxation, in order to describe the mechanical characteristics of relaxation, a specific parameter which accounts for these variables was developed. To do this, we selected the half-time for relaxation. This represents the time needed for the muscle to re-elongate from peak of shortening to half of its Δl (shortening in length) under the load (Figure 36) borne by the muscle. Since this parameter was load-dependent, it was plotted against load. A regression equation was fitted to the curve and from this the load-independent half-relaxation time was computed.

Although the half-time gave us a load-independent index, it must be pointed out that for each of the relaxation curves in Figure 36, because of the different loads on the muscle, the initial lengths of the CE at the onset of relaxation were also different. This produced a second source of variability in the index of relaxation for which adjustment had to be made. To eliminate the effect of the varying initial CE lengths the muscle was allowed to shorten from l_o bearing the preload ($0.05\ P_o$) required to set it at that length. At a desired time point, a series of load clamps were applied (Figure 37) . The application of the load clamp at the same point in time for each contraction ensured that the muscle strip started to relax at the same CE length, even under different loads. The relaxation trajectories for the different load clamps are shown in the upper panel of Figure 36. The fast transients represent re-elongation of the series elastic component of the muscle, whereas the slow transients represent re-elongation of CE from the same initial length. The half-times for these slow transients under their respective loads were fitted with an exponential function (a coefficient of determination, R^2, of 0.9888 and $P < 0.01$ indicated a good fit of the curve), and the zero load half-time was extrapolated from the plot as shown in Figure 36. The coefficient of the equation gave the relaxation index, $T_{1/2,CE}$, which is load- and initial contractile element length-independent.

Figure 38 shows values of $T_{1/2,CE}$ obtained from bronchial smooth muscle after 1 and 10s of stimulation.

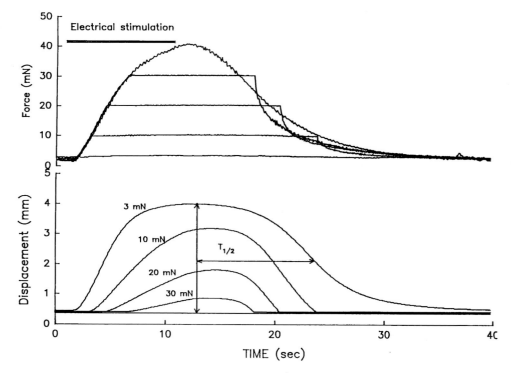

FIG. 36. Isotonic relaxation of bronchial smooth muscle after 10 seconds of electrical stimulation. Force (*upper panel*) and displacement (*lower panel*) are shown as functions of time. The muscle strip was allowed to shorten and relax under different loads. The time needed for muscle to re-elongate to one-half of its shortening from l_o was designated as the half-relaxation time ($t_{1/2}$) for that load.

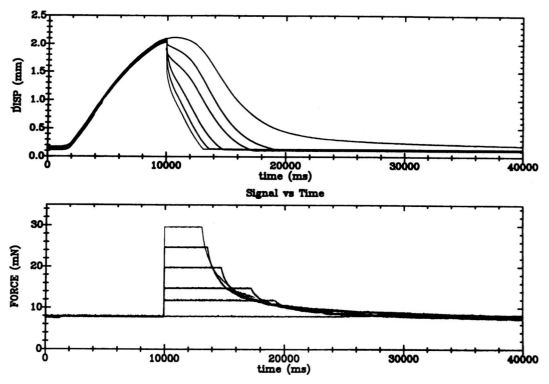

FIG. 37. Isotonic load clamp—signal vs. time. Force and displacement versus time records of a muscle strip allowed to shorten under a light preload and at a specific point in time quickly clamped to different heavier loads. Thereafter, muscle strips relax faster. Values of $t_{1/2CE}$ for these relaxation curves were obtained and plotted against their respective loads from a single experiment.

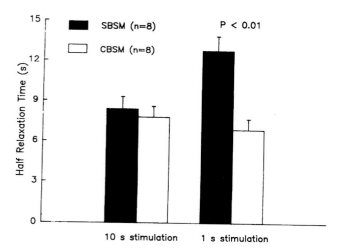

FIG. 38. Mean half-relaxation time ($t_{1/2CE}$) in sensitized and control bronchial smooth muscle (SBSM and CBSM). Value of $T_{1/2CE}$ in SBSM was similar to that of CBSM after 10s stimulation. However, after 1s stimulation it was almost doubled in SBSM than CBSM, indicating alterations in properties of early normally cycling crossbridges.

This half-time for re-elongation of the muscle is, we feel, the best index of relaxation, since it is independent of load, which when operative, would result in rapid relaxation, and of the initial length of the muscle's contractile element.

We were also interested in the mechanisms underlying smooth muscle relaxation. Muscle relaxation has been described as inactivation of the active state of the muscle (81). This was estimated by quickly releasing the relaxing muscle strip load to zero (zero load clamps) at different time points in isometric relaxation and in isotonic relaxation. Figure 39 shows records of zero

load clamps applied during isometric relaxation (Fig. 39A) and during isotonic relaxation (Fig. 39B). The zero load shortening velocity of the contractile element (the slow transients of the quick release in the figure) is a good index of crossbridge cycling rate and, thus, of active state (36,50,66).

Analysis of the transients elicited during isometric relaxation showed that within 5 seconds of onset of relaxation, the maximum slope of the slow transient (maximum velocity of shortening, V_o) had achieved its lowest value. This was not different from that shown by load clamps applied to a passive muscle. We concluded that active state no longer existed after 5 seconds.

Figure 40 demonstrates that isotonic relaxation consists of an initial slow phase (likely due to waning of the muscle's active state) that we have termed "phase i," the convexity of which is upward, followed by a linear phase, (phase ii), and then a final slow phase (phase iii, the convexity of which is downward). Phase i represents the balance between the elongating effect of the load and the retarding effect of residual activation. Phase ii represents the continued elongation effected by the load on a muscle the activation of which is also absent. Whether passive recoil of the compressed internal resistor reported by us (97) also contributes to the relaxation is a possibility that needs further study. Phase iii is surprising. The velocity transients show that V_o drops progressively, but 20 seconds after onset of relaxation increases spontaneously. This is a novel finding and indicates spontaneous re-activation of the muscle. Figure 39B once again shows that the state of activation of the crossbridges in isometric relaxation decayed gradually to basal values as judged by the behavior of V_o shown in panel B. Spontaneous reactivation in phase iii is seen. The function of this terminal

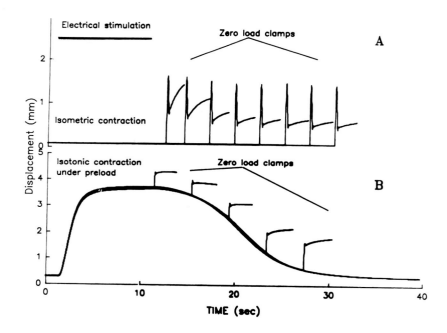

FIG. 39. Zero-load velocities (V_o) during isometric and isotonic relaxation. **A:** isometrically contracted muscle strip was quickly released from afterload to zero load at different points in time during relaxation. V_o (slope of slow transient after quick release) decreases with time after turning off the stimulator. **B:** zero load clamps were applied at various points after isotonic contraction. V_o decreases at 1st 5s and then started to increase without any external stimulation, indicating a spontaneous reactivation of crossbridge cycling.

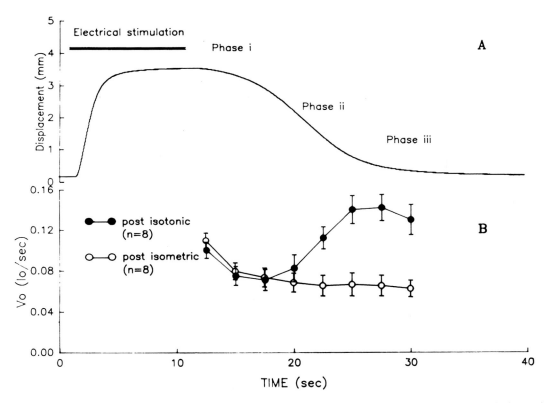

FIG. 40. Inactivation of bronchial smooth muscle's active state during isotonic relaxation. **A**: isotonic shortening recording showing three phases during relaxation. **B**: zero-load velocities (V_o) from quick release during isotonic relaxation (shown in Figure 39B). During phase 1, V_o decreased gradually while the relaxation became faster in Figure 40A. In phase 3, V_o increased spontaneously, accompanied by slowing of relaxation.

slowing is unknown, but the slowing of the elongation of the relaxing airway wall may serve to minimize turbulence of air currents.

Whatever the purpose of this spontaneous reactivation, its presence is substantiated by an increase in spontaneous myosin light chain (20kDa) phosphorylation, (Figure 41) and in intracellular Ca^{2+} concentration measured by the Fura 2 technique (Figure 42 in phase iii of relaxation. It is interesting that spontaneous reactivation is not seen in isometric relaxation. This led us to think that the spontaneous reactivation of phase iii is due to re-elongation of the muscle which would be by approximately 30% during isometric relaxation, but only 7% during isometric relaxation: the 7% being determined by the internal record of the muscle's series elastic component. (See following for the results of studies of isotonic relaxation in ragweed pollen-sensitized ASM.)

BIOCHEMISTRY OF AIRWAY SMOOTH MUSCLE CONTRACTION

Most of the work conducted on ASM biochemistry has stemmed from a desire to elucidate the mechanisms underlying the increased shortening capacity and veloc-

ity seen in ragweed pollen-sensitized canine tracheal smooth muscle which was used as a model of human asthma.

Myofibrillar and Actomyosin (AM) ATPase

As in striated muscle, actin-activated myosin Mg^{2+} ATPase activity results in maximal cycling velocity (V_o) of unloaded actomyosin crossbridges. This velocity is regulated by the load on the muscle, the relationship between the two being hyperbolic. Because of these relationships V_o is used as an index of actin-activated Mg^{2+} ATPase activity (actomyosin ATPase activity).

While actomyosin ATPase is measured *in vitro* using purified proteins and appropriate substrates, it is simpler to measure this activity in myofibrils. Furthermore, the latter is a more physiological preparation than purified actomyosin since the thick and thin filaments retain the same relationship to each other as in the intact cell.

The work we have conducted on myofibrillar ATPase activity is deferred to a later section wherein all the biophysical and biochemical changes that occur in allergic bronchospasm are described. At this time we pass on to a consideration of a new and exciting technique that per-

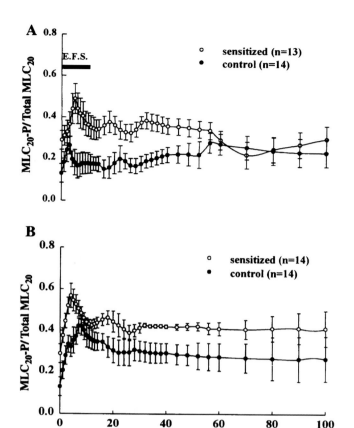

FIG. 41. Time course of 20 kDa myosin light-chain phosphorylation. **A:** isotonic curves for sensitized and control. **B:** isometric curves for sensitized and control. Sensitized tissues showed higher phosphorylation level during isotonic and isometric contraction. MLC_{20}-P, phosphorylated 20-kDa myosin light chain; EFS, electrical field stimulation.

mits the measurement of this biochemical enzyme activity in terms of biophysical parameters.

The Motility Assay

Insight into the mechanism of smooth muscle contraction at molecular level has taken a quantum leap with the development of the motility assay (50,51). This technique has permitted a narrowing of the enormous gap that existed between our understanding of the mechanism of striated muscle contraction and that of smooth muscle.

It now allows us to study the mechanics of the contractile interaction between a single molecule of actin and subunits of single myosin molecules, and almost to achieve the holy grail of deciphering the final energy transduction step. Though technically laborious, the assay provides more reliable results than study of single airway smooth muscle cells. The latter is more of an art than a science and bedevilled with technical problems. The motility assay has surpassed single cell study techniques, at least with respect to study of the contractile machinery.

Admittedly, the motility assay has its greatest applications and returns in elucidating basic molecular mechanisms of contraction. However, it should prove of use in comparing acto-myosin intermolecular interactions between molecules from healthy and diseased animals.

Though at this point in time it seems unlikely, for example in asthma, that pathogenesis stems from change in the structure and/or function of the myosin molecule, nevertheless that possibility cannot be ignored. The motility assay should be able to provide a definitive answer. We have obtained some very preliminary evidence to show that the increased maximum actomyosin ATPase

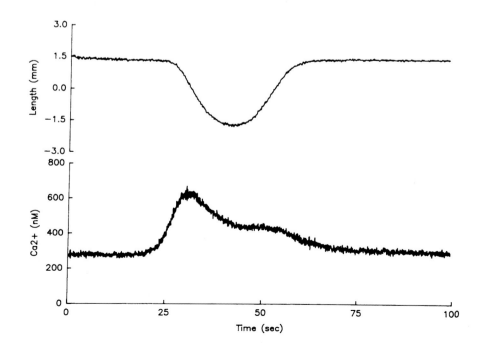

FIG. 42. Upper trace is a record of isotonic shortening in a lightly loaded muscle. Shortening is depicted downwards. The stimulus was turned off at peak shortening. The lower trace represents the corresponding Fura-2 (Ca^{2+}) concentration late in relaxation.

activity we have reported in ASM from a canine model of allergic bronchospasm, is associated with an increased content of a newly discovered myosin-heavy chain isoform which contains a unique 7 amino acid insert in its amino-terminal end (84,85). This insert-containing isoform contains almost treble the ATPase activity of the other isoforms. Its activity could account for the increased crossbridge cycling velocity seen in allergic bronchospasm, were it present in increased amounts. The motility assay carried out with the insert-containing isoform from control and sensitized airway smooth muscle could confirm that the increased content of the isoform was indeed responsible for increased crossbridge cycling rate. Such studies are under way.

At the risk of being redundant, let me review some of the biochemical underpinnings of the motility assay.

Actin and myosin are the two major proteins directly involved in muscle contraction. Their interaction has been extensively studied using a variety of biophysical and biochemical methods. In ASM, as in smooth muscles in general, the calcium- and calmodulin-dependent phosphorylation of the 20-kDa light chain (MLC_{20}) subunit of myosin by myosin light chain kinase (MLCK) is required for the initiation of contraction (61,62,83). *In vitro* this phosphorylation results in a substantial increase in actin-activated MgATPase activity. The *in vitro* motility assay system allows for direct visualization of the movement of fluorescently labelled actin filaments over a surface of myosin heads attached to a glass coverslip (8,86). A number of studies suggests that these assays correlate very reliably with the unloaded shortening velocity (V_{max} or V_o) of muscle fibers (88).

In practical terms, smooth muscle myosin is prepared as described by Umemoto et al. (50). MLCK is prepared from turkey gizzard and calmodulin from bovine brain (85,89,90). Rabbit skeletal muscle actin is prepared by the method of Spudich and Watt (91) as modified from Eisenberg and Kelley (92).

For the motility assay myosin must be phosphorylated at serine 19 on the 20kDa light chain (1 mol of Pi/mol of light chain).

The motility assay is carried out at 25°C (93–95). F-actin is labelled with tetramethylrhodamine-phalloidin. Phosphorylated myosin (0.1 to 0.3 mg/ml) is introduced into a flow chamber which is bound on the upper surface by a coverslip coated with nitrocellulose film. Myosin binds to the glass; the unbound myosin is then washed away. Then 1 volume of 5 to 10nM fluorescently labelled actin filaments are allowed to bind to the myosin-coated surface in the absence of ATP. The movement of fluorescently labelled actin filaments is initiated by adding assay buffer containing 1 mM ATP. The movement of fluorescently labelled actin filaments is recorded with a standard microscope outfitted with epi-illumination optics and a tetramethylrhodamine filter set, a 100x objective, an image intensifier coupled with a video camera and video recorder.

The data are analyzed using a computer-assisted tracking system described by Sheetz et al. (88).

Results published by Umemoto and Sellers (50) show that phosphorylated smooth muscle myosin filaments bound to the surface of a nitrocellulose-coated coverslip translocated fluorescently labelled actin filaments at the same rate as the myosin-coated beads moved in a *Nitella*-based assay.

The velocity of actin transduction was half maximal at an ATP concentration of about 50μm. Above 0.1 mM ATP it was constant.

With respect to the effect of ionic concentration, it was found that increasing ionic strength between 0 and 90 mM KCl increased velocity 4-fold. In the motility assay using phosphorylated smooth muscle myosin, it was difficult to see motility above 100mM KCl since few filaments attached under those conditions.

In contrast to what is seen in the *Nitella* based assay, the movement of fluorescently labelled actin over the smooth muscle myosin-coated surface was not significantly effected by $MgCl_2$ over a range of 3 to 20 mM.

Calcium from 10^{-8} to 10^{-4} M had no effect on the velocity of actin filaments. Phosphorylated smooth muscle myosin propelled actin filaments of smooth muscle and skeletal muscle actin at the same rate. Phosphorylated smooth muscle and cytoplasmic myosin monomers also moved actin filaments, demonstrating that myosin filament formation is not required for movement.

Interestingly the addition of tropomyosin increased the velocity of both skeletal and smooth muscle actin filaments.

AIRWAY SMOOTH MUSCLE CONTRACTION IN ALLERGIC BRONCHOCONSTRICTION

The role of the contractile machinery of airway smooth muscle cell in the pathogenesis of asthma occupies a strange place in asthma research.

In the early days, any primary role of airway smooth muscle in regulating airway narrowing was totally ignored. In asthma, it was felt that the smooth muscle and its contractility were perfectly normal and bronchospasm was due to increased concentrations of agonists liberated as the result of the allergic response. However, the fact that a variety of different stimuli precipitated bronchospasm, indicated that change in the contractility of the muscle itself could be the cause of the bronchospasm.

The previous notion has not had sufficient attention paid to it, and current thinking is that asthma has its origins in chronic inflammation. The limitation to airflow is said to be due to thickening of the tunica media; the thickening itself being the result of ASM hypertrophy or hyperplasia. Thus, chronic inflammation, wall edema, and muscle hypertrophy and hyperplasia all combine to produce airflow limitation.

Our own approach has been to look for the primary cause of asthma which we feel would be best identified in the very early stages of disease. To this end we have developed a canine model of airway hyperreactivity by sensitizing the animal with intraperitonial injections of ragweed pollen (96). Their non-injected litter mates served as controls; thus, these animals have only been sensitized but never challenged. Nevertheless, the ASM demonstrated an increased shortening capacity and velocity (1,2). What is even more remarkable is that careful histological studies showed no evidence of smooth muscle hypertrophy or hyperplasia, nor was there any evidence of inflammation. Biochemical studies of the ASM showed no increase in total protein, messenger ribonucleic acid (mRNA), and deoxyribonucleic acid (DNA) contents.

It is clear, therefore, that changes in mechanical properties occur prior to any structural or biochemical changes. Time studies will be carried out to determine whether these mechanical changes alter as inflammation, hypertrophy, and hyperplasia develop with repeated challenges.

We conclude that sensitization per se, induces marked changes in contractile function. What the mechanism is, is not known.

In what follows, the biophysical and biochemical changes that we have found in canine sensitized ASM will be described.

Biophysical Changes

Changes in Shortening Capacity

Figure 43 shows length-tension curves from sensitized tracheal smooth muscle (STSM) and muscle from litter

mate controls (CTSM). They demonstrate that STSM shortens more than CTSM by 15% of optimal muscle length (l_o). This translates into a 50% increase in airway resistance, and could account for allergic bronchospasm with limitation of air flow. In arriving at this conclusion, the assumption made is that shortening is isotonic. The physiologically relevant shortening is that developing at a resting load 10% of P_o, since it is this load that maintains the muscle at its *in vivo*, optimal length.

Our studies have revealed the interesting finding that 75% to 80% of the total isotonic shortening is completed within 2 to 3 seconds of onset of tetanic stimulation. This was shown in Figure 11. We have also found that the increased shortening of the sensitized muscle is achieved within 2 seconds; no further increment in shortening occurs thereafter. The significance of this finding is, as we indicated before, that studies of ASM shortening should be conducted between 0 to 2 seconds of stimulation, and not at a steady state, which develops at 8 to 10 seconds. Furthermore, we must also conclude that the major proportion of shortening must be regulated by normally cycling crossbridges which, in turn, are regulated by phosphorylation of the 20kDa myosin light chain. Myosin light chain kinase is, therefore, the important enzyme determining the shortening capacity of ASM.

We have conducted studies on smooth muscle from 4th to 6th generation bronchi from sensitized and control dogs and obtained findings almost exactly the same as for the tracheal smooth muscle (2).

Changes in Shortening Velocity

Figure 44 shows conventional force-velocity curves obtained from records of afterloaded isotonic shortening

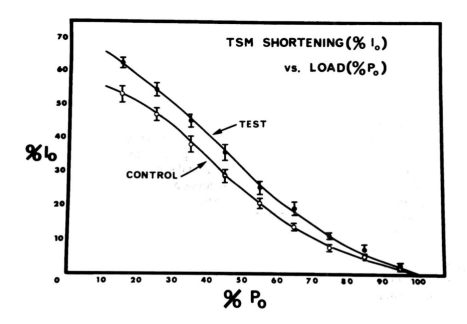

FIG. 43. Length-tension curves for control and sensitized (test) tracheal smooth muscles, expressed in percentized units.

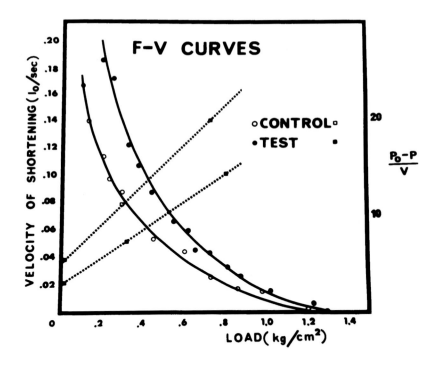

FIG. 44. Force-velocity curves for control and sensitized (test) canine tracheal smooth muscle. The linearized transforms $(P_o-P)/V$ versus load are also plotted. They demonstrate the hyperbolic nature of the parent curves.

in sensitized and control muscles. The sensitized muscle shows a faster shortening velocity than the control. Because of the normalization for force there is, of course, no difference in the ability to develop maximum isometric force (P_o), However even when P_o is expressed in stress units (force/cross-sectional area) no difference is seen. This points out the importance of measuring isotonic shortening parameters in studying smooth muscle. In our early model of allergic bronchospasm, had we merely measured isometric force development we would have concluded that sensitization had produced no effect and the sensitized muscle was normal. It was the shortening parameters, maximum shortening capacity (Δl_{max}), and velocity (V_o), that demonstrated change had occurred in the 3-dimensional contractility surface of the muscle.

Furthermore, in elucidating the cause of allergic spasm, the relevant measure is that of Δl_{max}; P_o provides no insight into bronchospasm. At best, the latter only tells us about the magnitude and time course of wall stiffness. Since in an isometric contraction there is some internal shortening due to the elongation of the muscle's series elastic component, it may be inferred that the force record is providing some information about crossbridge cycling during this small degree of shortening. However, the extent of this shortening is only 7.5% and in the light of recent work (Seow and Ford; personal communication) may actually be only 2% in canine tracheal smooth muscle (26). This is entirely too small a range to relate to the range of shortening of ASM *in vivo* (about 65% of l_o), and it would be undoubtedly more rel-

evant to measure shortening directly by isotonic or auxotonic methods.

The other shortcoming of using isometric methods is that they provide no index of the bioenergetics of smooth muscle contraction and cannot tell us about the long-term performance of the muscle since the ability of the muscle to continue contracting depends on energy supply. It has been shown that the energy consumption for an isotonic contraction is greater than that for an isometric (the Fenn effect) in both striated and smooth muscle, and hence, the shortening performance of a muscle is of key importance.

No clear cut answer exists but is likely related to the fact that technically, isometric studies are much easier to conduct than isotonic.

A final question relates to the significance of carrying out studies of velocity of shortening in allergic bronchospasm, since it is the extent of smooth muscle shortening that determines the extent of bronchoconstriction, and a priori velocity should not be an important determinant. However, in airway smooth muscle 75% of the total muscle shortening is completed within the first 2 seconds of contraction. This being so, velocity becomes an important determinant of total shortening. Were velocity too slow, then in the 2 seconds available, adequate shortening would not be achieved.

Increased Compliance of the Internal Resistor

The total extent of shortening of a muscle depends on the force generated, which is determined by the load on the muscle and the internal resistance to shortening. That a resistor exists has been most rigorously investigated for cardiac muscle (80). In fact, it is the elastic recoil of this resistor that is responsible for diastolic filling of the heart.

A method for measuring the compliance of the normal resistor was described above (97).

A similar analysis was carried out for records obtained from sensitized canine trachealis. The two curves are shown in Figure 45. They reveal that the internal resistor (or parallel elastic component) of the sensitized tracheal muscle is more compliant than that of the control. This could account for the increased bronchoconstriction of allergic bronchoconstriction.

What the mechanism is for the increased compliance of the internal resistor in the sensitized trachealis is unknown. While collagen and elastin and other structures in the extracellular and extra-fascicular spaces are strong contenders, there are others that should be considered. At cellular level the cytoskeleton could play a very important role.

It is now recognized that the cytoskeleton is a very important component of any cell, and especially of the smooth muscle cell. Furthermore, it forms an exquisitely organized network around and through the sarcomeres of striated muscle (98). In skeletal muscle the major components of the system are nebulin, titin, and desmin. Horowits et al. (99) reported that changes induced in neb-

ulin and titin by low doses of ionizing radiation of skinned skeletal muscle cells, resulted in reduced ability of the cells to both generate passive tension in response to calcium. These experiments highlight the importance of the cytoskeleton in muscle contraction.

Titin and nebulin have not been found in smooth muscle. However, this may be because appropriate polyacrylamide gels have not been utilized. The lowest concentration used was about 3.5% and the very large molecular weight proteins may have found it impossible to enter the gel. Studies using 2% polyacrylamide need to be carried out.

Conversely, there are a large number of low molecular weight cytoskeletal proteins in smooth muscle such as filamin, α and β desmin, vimentin, vinculin, plectin, α-actinin, and synemin (74). In addition, 4 low molecular weight (18,000 to 30,000 Dalton) cytosolic proteins, and a separate 23,000 Dalton protein, have been reported by the same authors. While some or all of these could contribute to the structure of the internal resistor, it may be mentioned *en passant* that Rasmussen (74) has shown that these proteins are phosphorylated late in the contraction. He has developed a theory that the sustained phase of contraction is not maintained by slowly cycling or latch crossbridges, but by these proteins. Relaxation is brought about by a gelsolin-induced solation.

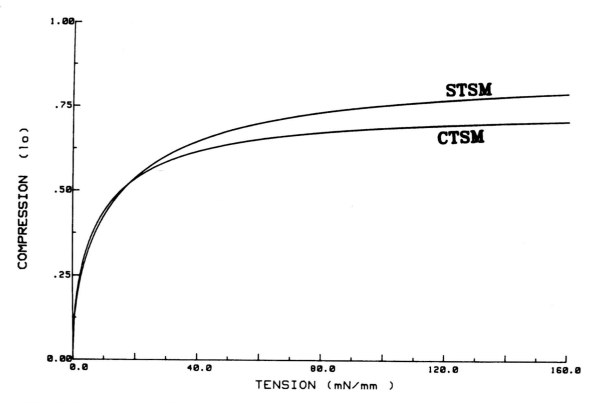

FIG. 45. Tension-compression curves for the internal resistor of sensitized *(STSM)* and control *(CTSM)* canine trachealis.

Biochemical Changes

Role of Extracellular Collagen and Intracellular Cytoskeletal Proteins Desmin and Vimentin in the Increased, Shortening Capacity (Δl_{max}) of Sensitized Airway Smooth Muscle

By analogy with vascular smooth muscle, it has been felt that asthmatic airway smooth muscle cells undergoing hyperplasia *in situ* could secrete collagen and, thus, change the compliance properties of the airway wall. To investigate this, alterations of biophysical and biochemical properties of cytoskeleton and extracellular collagen in tracheal smooth muscle (TSM) were studied. Our studies showed that smooth muscle passive elastic properties were not significantly altered by removal of cytoskeleton with guanidine HCl and -mercaptoethanol; collagenase digestion reduced smooth muscle force development, but did not affect its Δl_{max} and passive elastic properties in both sensitized and control dogs. There were no significant differences in the amount of cytoskeletal intermediate filament proteins, desmin, and vimentin between sensitized and control TSM. The contents of total collagen, collagen type I, and collagen cross-linking in sensitized TSM were significantly greater than in control; collagen in sensitized TSM was more resistant to collagenase attack; and only a very small amount of collagen type III was found in these tissues. We conclude that increased Δl_{max} in sensitized canine TSM is not the result of alterations in passive cytoskeletal and extracellular collagen structures (100). It is likely the latter, even though stiffer, is not strained over physiological length changes.

Increased Myofibrillar ATPase Activity in Sensitized Airway Smooth Muscle

Given our finding that V_o was increased in sensitized ASM, we measured myofibrillar ATPase activity since this is the enzyme that is located in the amino terminal end of the myosin heavy chain close to the ATP binding site, and regulates velocity of crossbridge cycling.

Table 1 shows data from experiments on 7 control and 7 sensitized airway smooth muscle cells. It shows that ATPase is significantly higher in the latter (101).

Because in heart muscle, change in velocity of shortening is ascribed to change in the distribution of myosin

TABLE 1. *ATPase activity of canine tracheal smooth muscle myofibrils*

	ATPase Activity of Myofibrils (mMPi mg mosin $^{-1}$ min^{-1})
STSM, n = 7	499.29 ± 11.49
CTSM, n = 7	345.00 ± 6.81

STSM, sensitized tracheal smooth muscle; CTSM,muscle from litter mate controls.

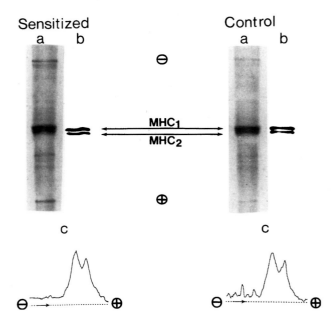

FIG. 46. Stained SDS-polyacrylamide gels (*a*) loaded with crude extracts from sensitized and control tracheal smooth muscle. Western blots (*b*) using myosin heavy chain antibodies are shown immediately to the right of the gels. Densitometric tracings (*c*) are provided further on.

heavy chain isozymes and similar results have been obtained from uterine and urinary bladder smooth muscle, we determined whether any change in distribution of myosin heavy chain isozymes was present in sensitized ASM (102–105).

SDS polyacrylamide gels of crude extracts of control and sensitized muscles are shown in Figure 46. The bands depicting smooth muscle myosin heavy chains 1 and 2 (of molecular weight 204 kDa and 200 kDa respectively) are seen. Western blots using specific antibodies are shown just to the right of these gels and densitometric traces are provided below. Mean results from six experiments showed that although the two myosin heavy chain isozymes are present, they do not change their distribution. At the time these experiments were conducted, a third isozyme with a unique 7 amino acid insert in its NH2-terminal had not been discovered. Nagai et al. (84) and Kelley et al. (85) were the first to report its occurrence. As stated earlier, Kelley et al. are currently collaborating with us, and have obtained preliminary evidence (unpublished observations) to show that the content of this isoform is not increased in sensitized ASM.

Increased MLC20 Phosphorylation in Sensitized Airway Smooth Muscle

In smooth muscle it is now well-established that the regulatory troponin system is absent and that regulation is brought about by phosphorylation of the 20kDa myosin light chain. A linear relationship between this phosphorylation and actomyosin ATPase has been shown to exist (106).

We have reported previously that both in isotonic and isometric contraction, MLC_{20} phosphorylation is greater in sensitized airway smooth muscle compared to the control. Figure 40 showed the data. The typical phasic response in phosphorylation is also seen, as is the presence of oscillations.

These data confirm that increased myofibrillar ATPase activity is associated with increased phosphorylation of the regulatory, 20 kDa, myosin light chain.

Increased Myosin Light Chain Kinase (MLCK) Total Activity in Sensitized Airway Smooth Muscle

The increased phosphorylation of MLC_{20} described earlier can result from increased activity of the responsible enzyme, MLCK, or from reduced activity of myosin light chain phosphatase.

MLCK Content

MLCK Content in tissue homogenates of sensitized tracheal smooth muscle (STSM) and of bronchial smooth muscle (SBSM) was measured employing quantitative 7.5% SDS-polyacrylamide, mini-gel electrophoresis (Figure 47). The protein loads for both groups were the same (5,10 and 15μg in respective lanes). The contents of MLCK were determined by two-dimensional laser densitometry of the gels; a chicken gizzard MLCK standard was run concomitantly. The intensity of the laser scanning signal was linearly correlated with the loading of MLCK standards, ranging from 0 to 4 μg. The identity of the bands was confirmed by Western blotting using monoclonal anti-smooth muscle MLCK antibody.

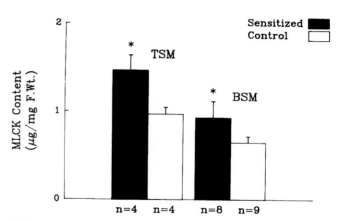

FIG. 47. Myosin light chain kinase contents for control and sensitized tracheal smooth muscles. The contents were greater in sensitized muscles. **P <0.001; *P <0.05. FWT, fresh weight of tissue.

Figure 47 shows a significant increase in MLCK content in STSM and SBSM which is responsible for the higher level of MLC_{20} phosphorylation (97).

MLCK Specific Activity

In addition to assaying total content, the specific activity of the enzyme must also be known. The rate of incorporation of radioactive inorganic phosphorus $\gamma^{32}Pi$ into MLC_{20} by MLCK was estimated as an index of MLCK activity by measuring the time course of MLC_{20} phosphorylation.

The rate of $\gamma^{32}Pi$ incorporated per minute into MLC_{20} was found to be significantly higher in STSM and SBSM than in controls. See Figure 48.

The *specific* MLCK activity expressed as the rate of $\gamma^{32}Pi$ incorporation into MLC_{20} in nanomoles of Pi per

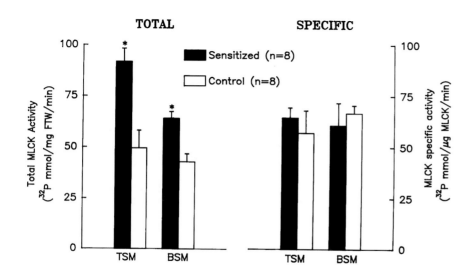

FIG. 48. Total specific MLCK activity in sensitized and control TSM and BSM. *Left panel:* The incorporation rate of ^{32}P into MLC (MLCK activity) in TSM and BSM was significantly higher than in control. *Right panel:* When expressed as the incorporation rate of ^{32}P into MLC/μgMLCK/min, i.e., specific activity of MLCK the difference between sensitized and control muscles disappeared. FWT, fresh weight of tissue.

microgram MLCK per minute (normalized with respect to the amount of MLCK in the tissues) showed no difference between sensitized and control groups.

We conclude that increased myosin MLCK content accounts for the increased total MLCK activity in sensitized ASM. As discussed previously, increased myofibrillar ATPase activity of sensitized TSM could have resulted from altered intrinsic properties of MLCK. Cleveland mapping of MLCK did not disclose any notable change in the primary structure of sensitized ASM, eliminating this possibility. In addition, the specific activity of MLCK from sensitized TSM and BSM was the same as that for the control (*vide supra*).

Myosin Light Chain Phosphatase

Though increased MLCK activity likely accounts for the increased phosphorylation of MLC_{20} from sensitized ASM the possibility existed that the increased phosphorylation may be the result of reduced activity of myosin light chain phosphatase.

We have developed a myosin phosphatase assay to compare the enzyme's activity in crude TSM homogenates from control and sensitized muscle (108).

Phosphorylation of the 20 kDa of the 20 myosin light chain was initiated with Mg^{2-}-ATP; maximum levels were reached within 40s. Peak phosphorylation levels were stable for at least 3 minutes. The relative stoichiometry of 20 KD myosin light chain phosphorylation was estimated by chemiluminescent immunoblot assay. Smooth muscle phosphatase activity was estimated by the rate of decline in peak light chain phosphorylation, while myosin light chain kinase was inhibited indirectly

with trifluoperazine, or EGTA, or directly by a synthetic peptide inhibitor. Okadaic acid, an inhibitor of phosphatase activity, curbed the decline in light chain phosphorylation seen after myosin light chain kinase inhibition, indicating that the light chain dephosphorylation observed was the result of smooth muscle phosphatase activity. Addition of okadaic acid to the samples led to a 30% to 40% increase in peak myosin light chain phosphorylation in all samples. This indicates that similar populations of phosphatases were present in the homogenates of both control and sensitized tissues. Peak light chain phosphorylation levels were 20% higher in tracheal homogenates from sensitized animals; however, no difference in phosphatase activity was measured between control and sensitized samples. These results indicate that in ASM from hyperresponsive, ragweed pollen-sensitized dogs, increased maximum velocity of shortening, consequent to the increased myosin light chain phosphorylation, is not contributed to by any change in myosin light chain phosphatase activity, but is mainly the result of the increased myosin light chain kinase activity.

Studies of Calmodulin and Intracellular Ca^{2+} Transients

Even though MLCK is the most important rate-limiting enzyme among the regulatory proteins in smooth muscle, and its increased content could account for the increased MLC_{20} phosphorylation of sensitized TSM, it was necessary to determine whether changes in MLCK triggers (Ca^{2+} and calmodulin) were contributory. To this end we conducted the following studies:

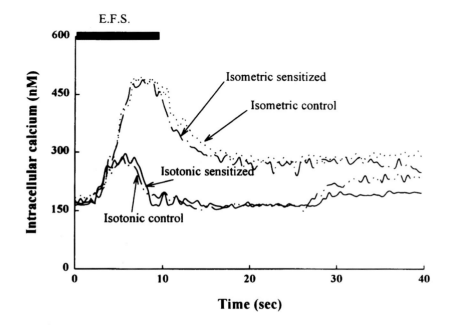

FIG. 49. Typical Ca^{2+} transients during EFS of sensitized and control TSM. No difference was found between sensitized and control. Isotonic shortening records in both sensitized and control groups showed lower Ca^{2+} transients than those of isometrics. Ca^{2+} concentration was normalized using standard Ca^{2+} solution from Molecular Probes.

Study of intracellular Ca²⁺ transients

These transients were measured using Fura 2 in control and sensitized TSMs during both isometric and isotonic contraction, the muscles being stimulated electrically (109). Submaximal (80% of maximal) current density was used as this eliminated electrolytic bubbling of the perfusing solutions in the quartz curvette (volume = 500 μl) containing the muscles for the study. Figure 49 shows the typical intracellular Ca²⁺ transients.

There was no difference between control and sensitized groups, although, the isotonic Ca²⁺ transients in both these groups were significantly lower during contraction, while the resting levels were the same, as if shortening induced certain modifications in Ca²⁺-releasing mechanisms. The peak of the isotonic Ca²⁺ level conformed with the highest unloaded shortening velocity of smooth muscle at 4 to 6 s after onset of electrical stimulation. However, the maximum shortening was achieved only after the intracellular Ca²⁺ started to decline while the stimulus was maintained. The values of the calcium transients during isometric contraction were about three times as high as those of isotonic values.

Studies of Calmodulin

Since the 4Ca²⁺·calmodulin complex is the regulatory subunit of MLCK it became necessary to study calmodulin.

The relative calmodulin content was estimated using 15% acrylamide SDS-PAGE. Western blotting, employing specific calmodulin antibody, was conducted and the visualized bands were scanned and analysed with a LKB Ultroscan XL laser densitometer connected to a computer.

With respect to calmodulin activity the assay was based on the ability of calmodulin to activate 3′-, 5′-cyclic nucleotide phosphodiesterase, which converts adenosine 3′-, 5′-cyclic monophosphate (cAMP) to AMP. The 5 phosphate was subsequently cleaned from the newly formed AMP by the addition of 5 nucleotidase. Because calmodulin is heat resistant, the TSM and BSM homogenates were heated to 95°C for 3 minutes (to denature other proteins), and then rapidly cooled to 4°C. The reaction was initiated by adding cAMP to assay tubes containing aliquots of tissue homogenate and phosphodiesterase (25°C). The reaction was stopped with trichloroacetic acid at 40 minutes, by which time activity had peaked. The concentration of P_i was measured using the malachite green method (110,111). The activity of calmodulin was expressed as Pi per mg of muscle tissue and per microgram of total tissue protein.

The results obtained from these experiments are shown in Figure 50. Calmodulin activities normalized with respect to the weight of the tissue and to the amount of protein in the tissue are shown in Figure 50A,B. There was no significant difference between sensitized and control

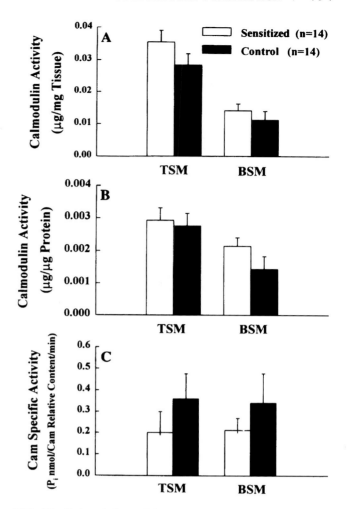

FIG. 50. Calmodulin activity of sensitized and control TSM and BSM. **A**: total calmodulin activity expressed per milligram of FTW. **B**: activity expressed per microgram of total proteins in tissue. Both showed no difference in sensitized airway smooth muscle calmodulin activity from their control counterparts. **C**: calmodulin (Cam) specific activity in sensitized muscles was not different from that in controls.

groups. Since our interest was to compare sensitized and control groups, the absolute value of calmodulin content was not of major concern. Instead, the relative calmodulin content was obtained for both groups by scanning the calmodulin bands on 15% SDS-polyacrylamide gels. There was no difference in relative calmodulin content between the two groups. Calmodulin activity was normalized (Fig. 50C) with respect to relative calmodulin content to obtain specific calmodulin activity, but no difference was found between sensitized and control smooth muscles.

These studies of intracellular Ca²⁺ transients revealed no difference between control and sensitized tracheal smooth muscles. Hence, it is processes downstream to this that must be involved in the increased MLC_{20} phosphorylation we found in sensitized TSM.

In preliminary studies (112) we have found that the binding stoichiometry of Ca^{2+} to calmodulin is greater in sensitized muscle. We have no explanation for this since calmodulin content and activity (with respect to activation of phosphodiesterase) were not changed with sensitization. Cleveland mapping showed no difference in the pattern of peptide fragments. Perhaps differences in tyrosine phosphorylation of the molecule could be responsible; these were not resolvable by the techniques we employed. We are conducting studies to determine tyrosine phosphorylation of calmodulin from control and sensitized muscles.

We have also conducted studies which show that the binding of the $4Ca^{2+}$ calmodulin complex to the catalytic subunit of myosin light chain kinase was not changed with sensitization.

Our final studies were directed towards determining whether the increased MLCK content we found in sensitized TSM was due to changes in gene expression. Using suitable probes we carried out agarose gel analysis of MLCK-mRNA from control and sensitized TSMs. We found no difference in MLCK-mRNA content of control and sensitized TSM. Nor did we find any difference in the stability of the messages. We concluded that increased MLCK content is not the result of changes in gene transcription, but of gene translation or post-translational modification.

This section may be summarized by stating that increased velocity of shortening of canine ASM develops with sensitization alone of the animal. It develops in the absence of any challenge and of any change in the total protein, DNA, and mRNA content of the sensitized muscle, and any evidence of inflammation. Because of the unique history of shortening of ASM in which 75% of total shortening occurs within 20% (2 seconds) of the total shortening time (10 seconds), increased velocity of shortening is an important factor contributing to the increased total shortening of the sensitized muscle. The most probable cause of the increased velocity is the increased total activity and content of myosin light chain kinase, stemming from a change in gene translation.

CONCLUSIONS

In this chapter attention has been focused on the ASM as a shortening machine because in the final analysis that is what it is. Its ability to stiffen actively and provide tone to the airway has been deliberately ignored as we found no change in this parameter in sensitized airway smooth muscle. The mechanical properties of this machine have been described using the classical relationships laid down by skeletal muscle research, regarding the analysis of length-tension and force-velocity curves, and of rapid mechanical transients. The major differences from skeletal muscle are the heterogeneity of crossbridges in the smooth muscle. These are bridges active in early contraction (normally cycling) that subserve shortening velocity and are regulated by a phosphorylation mechanism, and those active later on which shorten very slowly but produce the major part of the force of which the muscle is capable. They develop when the regulatory light chain is dephosphorylated by myosin light chain phosphatase activity and have been termed latch bridges. The term however is, as of this moment, controversial. What we consider important in terms of regulation of in vitro muscle shortening (bronchoconstriction in vivo) is the fact that most of this regulation occurs very early in the contraction and is clearly a function of myosin light chain (20 kDa) phosphorylation by myosin light chain kinase. Hence, studies of ASM shortening (or bronchoconstriction in vivo) should be conducted early in the contraction. The vast majority of studies are usually conducted at the plateau of an isometric response. These are inadequate for two reasons. Isometric studies provide no insight into mechanisms of ASM shortening; they only tell us about wall stiffness. Furthermore, at the plateau of the isometric force response, the favored point for measurement since it represents a steady state, only latchbridges or slowly cycling bridges are active. Hence in terms of subcellular, crossbridge mechanisms, such measurements provide little insight.

The properties of ASM just dealt with, represent a slightly older generation of research. Current emphasis has shifted to study of the mechanical interactions between single actin and myosin molecules on the biophysical front with the use of the motility assay. From a biochemical control point of view the study of myosin heavy chain isozymes has considerably advanced our understanding of how ASM contraction is regulated.

ACKNOWLEDGMENTS

The expert wordprocessing of this manscript by J. Olfert is gratefully acknowledged.

The work described in this chapter was supported by operating grants from the Medical Research Council of Canada, Inspiraplex, Canada and the Manitoba Lung Association.

REFERENCES

1. Antonissen LA, Mitchell RW, Kroeger EA, Kepron W, Tse KS, Stephens NL. Mechanical alterations of airway smooth muscle in a canine asthmatic model. *J Appl Physiol* 1989;46:681–687.
2. Jiang H, Rao K, Halayko AJ, Kepron W, Stephens NL. Mechanical alterations in sensitized (S) canine bronchial smooth muscle (BSM). *FASEB J* 1990;4:A444.
3. De Jongste JC, Mons H, Bonta IL, Kerribijn KF. *In vitro* responses of airways from an asthmatic patient. *Eur J Respir Dis* 1987;1:23.
4. Von Hayek H. *The human lung.* New York: Hafner, 1960;127–226.
5. Kannan MS, Daniel EE. Structural and functional study of control of canine tracheal smooth muscle. *Am J Physiol* 1980;238:C27–C33.

6. Jones TR, Kannan MS, Daniel EE. Ultrustructural study of guinea pig tracheal smooth muscle and its innervation. *Can J Physiol Pharmacol* 1980;58:974–983.

7. Cameron AR, Bullock CG, Kirkpatrick CT. The ultrastructure of bovine tracheal muscle. *J Ultrastruct Res* 1982;81:290–305.

8. Dunnill MS, Bassarella GR, Anderson JA. A comparison of the quantitative anatomy of the bronchi in normal subjects, in status asthmaticus in chronic bronchitis and in emphysema. *Thorax* 1969; 24:176–179.

9. Hogg JC. Airway hyperreactivity, relationship to disease states. In: Coburn RF, ed. *Airway smooth muscle in health and disease.* New York: Plenum, 1989;267–276.

10. Thurlbeck WM, Hogg JC. Pathology of asthma. In: Middleton & Reed CE, Ellis FF, Atkinson Jr NF, Yunginer Jr TW, eds. *Allergy: principles and practice.* 3rd ed. St. Louis: CV Mosby, 1988;1008–1017.

11. Ebina M, Yaegashi H, Takahashi T, Motomiya M, Tanenura M. Distribution of smooth muscles along the bronchial tree. *Am Rev Resp Dis* 1990;141:1322–1326.

12. Weibl ER. *Morphometry of the human lung.* Berlin: Springer-Verlag, 1963.

13. Wiggs BR, Paré P. A model of the mechanics of narrowing. *J Appl Physiol* 1990;69:848.

14. Eidelman DH, Irvin CG. Airway mechanics in asthma. In: Busse WW, Holgate ST, eds. *Asthma and rhinitis.* Cambridge: Blackwell Scientific, 1995;1033–1043.

15. Horsfield K, Cumming G. Morphology of the bronchial tree in man. *J Appl Physiol* 1968;24:373.

16. Macklem PT. Bronchial hyperresponsiveness. *Chest* 1985;87:1585–1595.

17. Sly PD, Brown KA, Bates JHT, Macklem PT, Milic-Emili J, Martin JG. Effect of lung volume on interrupted resistance in cats challenged with methacholine. *J Appl Physiol* 1988;64:360–366.

18. Colebatch HJH, Mitchell CA. Constriction of isolated living liquid-filled dog and cat lungs with histamine. *J Appl Physiol* 1971;30(5):691–702.

19. Hildebrandt J. Pressure-volume data of cat lung interpreted by a plasto-elastic, linear viscoelastic models. *J Appl Physiol* 1970;28(3):365–372.

20. Romero PV, Ludwig MS. Maximal methacholine-induced constriction in rabbit lung: interactions between airways and tissue. *J Appl Physiol* 1991;70(3):1044–1050.

21. Ding DJ, Martin JG, Macklem PT. Effects of lung volume on maximal MCh-induced bronchoconstriction in normal humans. *J Appl Physiol* 1987;62:1324–1330.

22. Macklem PT. Mechanical factors determining maximum bronchoconstriction. *Eur Respir* 1989;J2 (suppl 6):5165–5195.

23. Stephens NL, Jiang H. Basic physiology of airway smooth muscle. In; Busse WT, Holgate ST, eds. *Asthma and rhinitis.* Cambridge: Blackwell Scientific Publications, 1995;1087–1115.

24. Pratusewich V, Seow CY, Ford LE. Plasticity in canine airway smooth muscle. *J General Physiol* 1994;13:35–44.

25. Bramley AM, Thompson RJ, Roberts CR, Schellenberg RR. Hypothesis: excessive bronchoconstriction in asthma is due to diseased airway elastance. *Eur Resp J* 1994;7:337-341.

26. Stephens NL, Kromer U. Series elastic component of tracheal smooth muscle. *Am J Physiol* 1971;220:1890–1895.

27. Jiang H, Rao K, Halayko AJ, Kepron W, Stephens NL. Bronchial smooth muscle mechanics of a canine model of allergic airway hyperresponsiveness. *J Appl Physiol* 1992;72(1):39–45.

28. Jiang H, Stephens NL. Contractile properties of bronchial smooth muscle with and without cartilage. *J Appl Physiol* 1990;69(1):120–126.

29. James AL, Paré PD, Moreni RH, Hogg JC. Quantitative measurement of smooth muscle shortening in isolated pig trachea. *J Appl Physiol* 1987;63:1360–1365.

30. Shioya T, Pollack ER, Munoz WM, Leff AR. Distribution of airway responses in major airway resistance airways of the dog. *Am J Pathol* 1987;129(1):102–117.

31. Mapp EE, Chitano P, DeMarzo P, et al. Response to acetylcholine and myosin content of isolated canine airways. *J Appl Physiol* 1989;67(4):1331–1335.

32. Armour CL, Black JL, Verend N, Woolcock AJ. The relationship between bronchial hyperresponsiveness to methacholine and airway smooth muscle structure and reactivity. *Respir Physiol* 1984;58:223–233.

33. Gordon AM, Huxley AF, Julian FJ. Tension development in highly stretch vertebrate muscle fibres. *J Physiol* 1966;184:143–169.

34. Meiss RA. Graded activation in rabbit mesatubarium smooth muscle. *Am J Physiol* 1975;229:455–465.

35. Seigman MG, Butler TM, Mooers SU, Davies RE. Calcium-dependent resistance to stretch and stress relaxation in resting smooth muscle. *Am J Physiol* 1976;231:1504–1508.

36. Johansson B. Active state in the smooth muscle of the rat portal vein. *Circ Res* 1973;32:246–257.

37. Meiss RA. Dynamic stiffness of rabbit mesaturbarium smooth muscle: effect of isometric length. *Am J Physiol* 1978;234(Cell Physiol 3):C14–C26.

38. Sobieszek A, Small JV. The assembly of ribbon-shaped structures in low ionic strength extracts from vertebrate smooth muscle. *Philosoph Transacns of the Roy Soc Lond B* 1973;265:203–212.

39. Gillis JM, Cao ML, Godfraind-deBecker A. Density of myosin filaments in the rat anococcygeus muscle at rest and in contraction. *J Muscle Res Cell Motil* 1991;9:18–29.

40. Trybus KM. Assembly of cytoplasmic and smooth muscle myosins. *Curr Opin Cell Biol* 1991;3:105–111.

41. Trybus KM and Lowey S. The regulatory light chain is required for folding of smooth muscle myosin. *J Biol Chem* 1988;263:16485–16492.

42. Hartshorne D, Semenkowski RE. Regulation of smooth muscle actomyosin. *Annu Rev of Physiol* 1980;43:519–530.

43. Hill AV. The heat of shortening and the dynamic constants of muscle. *Proc Soc Lond B Biol Sci* 1938;126:136–195.

44. Woledge RC, Curtin NA, Homsher E. *Energetic aspects of muscle contraction.* Orlando: Academic Press, 1985;27–117.

45. Murphy RA. The mechanics of vascular smooth muscle. In: Bohr DF, Somlyo AP, Sparks HV, eds. *Handbook of vascular smooth muscle.* Bethesda: Amererican Physiological Society, 1980;325.

46. Dillon PF, Aksoy AAO, Driska SP, Murphy RA. Myosin phosphorylation and the crossbridge cycle in arterial smooth muscle. *Science* 1981;211:495–497.

47. Seow CY, Stephens NL. Force-velocity curves for smooth muscle: Analysis of internal factors reducing velocity. *Am J Physiol* 1980;251:C362–C368.

48. Somlyo AV, Lemanski FT, Vallierres J, Somlyo AP. Filament organization and dense bodies in vertebrate smooth muscle. In: Stephens NL, ed. *The biochemistry of smooth muscle.* Baltimore: University Park Press, 1977;445–471.

49. Fay FS, Fogarty K. The organization of the contractile apparatus in single isolated smooth muscle cells. In: Stephens NL, ed. *Smooth muscle contraction.* New York: Marcel Dekker, 1984;75–90.

50. Umemoto S, Sellers JR. Characterization of *in vitro* motility assays using smooth muscle and cytoplasmic myosins. *J Biol Chem* 1990;265(25):14864–14869.

51. Spudich JA. How molecular motors work. *Nature* 1994;372:515–518.

52. Edman KAP, Mulieri LA, Scubon-Muliere B. Non-hyperbolic force-velcity relationship in single muscle fibres. *Acta Physiol Scand* 1976;98:143–156.

53. Lannergren J. The force-velocity relation of isolated twitch and slow muscle fibres of *xenopus laevis. J Physiol (Lond)* 1978;238:501–521.

54. Hai C, Murphy RA. Crossbridge phosphorylation and regulation of latch state in smooth muscle. *Am J Physiol* 1988;254 (Cell Physiol 23):C99–C106.

55. Paul R. Smooth muscle energetics:testing theories of crossbridge regulation. In: Sperelakis N, Wood JD, eds. *Frontiers in smooth muscle research.* New York: Wiley-Liss, 1990;29–38.

56. Huxley AF. Muscle strucutre and theories of contraction. *Progr Biophys Biophy Chem* 1957;7:255–318.

57. Eisenberg E, Greene LE. The relation of muscle biochemistry to muscle physiology. *Annu Rev Physiol* 1980;42:293–309.

58. Lymn RW, Taylor EW. Mechanisms of adenosine triphosphate hydrolysis by actomyosin. *Biochemistry* 1980;10:4617–4624.

59. Brokaw DJ. Computer simulation of movement-generating crossbridges. *Biophys J* 1976;16:1013–1027.

60. Brenner B, Schoenberg M,, Chabovich JM, Green LE, Eisenberg E. Evidence for crossbridge attachment in relaxed muscle at low ionic strength. *Proc Natl Acad Sci U S A* 1982;79:7288–7391.

61. Dillon PF, Murphy RA. Tonic force maintenance with reduced shortening velocity in arterial smooth muscle. *Am J Physiol* 1982;242:C102–C108.

62. Kamm KE, Stull JT. Activation of smooth muscle contraction: relation between myosin phosphorylation and stiffness. *Science* 1986; 232:80–92.

63. Bagni MA, Cecchi G, Schoenberg M. A model of force production that explains the lag between crossbridge attachment and force after electrical stimulation of striated muscle fibres. *Biophys* 1988;J54: 1105–1114.

64. Seow CY, Stephens NL. Time dependence of series elasticity in tracheal smooth muscle. *J Appl Physiol* 1987;62(4):1556–1561.

65. Huxley AF, Simmons RM. Proposed mechanism of force generation in striated muscle. *Nature* 1971;233:533–538.

66. Stephens NL, Kagan ML, Packer CS. Time dependence of shortening velocity in tracheal smooth muscle. *Am J Physiol* 1986;251: C435–C442.

67. Wang Z, Seow CY, Stephens NL. Mechanical alterations in sensitized canine saphenous vein. *J Appl Physiol* 1986;69(1):171–178.

68. Merkel L, Gerthoffer WT, Torphy TJ. Dissociation between myosin phosphorylation and shortening velocity in canine tracheal. *Am J Physiol* 1990;258(3 Pt 1):C524–C532.

69. Moreland RS, Glea J, Moreland S. Calcium dependent regulation of vascular smooth muscile contraction. *Adv Exp Med Biol* 1991;308: 81–94.

70. Collins EM, Walsh MP, Morgan KG. Contraction of single vascular smooth muscle cells by phenylephrine at constant [Ca^{2+}]$_i$. *Am J Physiol* 1992;262:H754–H762.

71. Morimoto S and Ogawa Y. Ca^{2+} insensitive contraction of skinned smooth muscle. *Am J Physiol* 1994;268:C24–C29.

72. Gerthoffer WT, Murphy KA, Gunst SJ. Aequorin luminescence, myosin phosphorylation, and active stress in tracheal smooth muscle. *Am J Physiol* 1989;257(6 Pt 1):C1062–C1068.

73. Somlyo AP, Kitazawa T, Himpens B, et al. Modulation of Ca^{2+} sensitivity and of the time course of contraction in smooth muscle: a major role of protein phosphatases? In: Verlevede N, diSalvo J, eds. *Advances in protein phosphatases* 5. Leuven University Press, 1989;181–185, 1989.

74. Parks S, Rasmussen H. Carbachol-induced protein phosphorylation changes in bovine tracheal smooth muscle. *J Biol Chem* 1986;261: 15734–15739.

75. Ford LE, Huxley AF, Simmons RM. The relation between stiffness and filament overlap in stimulated frog muscle fibres. *J Physiol (Lond)* 1981;311:219–249.

76. Sonnenblick EH. Series elastic and contractile elements in heart muscle. *Am J Physiol* 1966;207:1330–1338.

77. Seow CY, Stephens NL. Changes of tracheal smooth muscle stiffness during an isotonic contraction. *Am J Physiol* 1989;256:C341–C350.

78. Shibata S, Cheng JR. Relaxation of vascular smooth muscle in spontaneously hypertensive rats. *Blood Vessels* 1977;14:247–248.

79. Packer CS, Stephens NL. Mechanics of canal artery relaxation in control and hypertensive rats. *Can J Physiol Pharmacol* 1985;633: 2109–2123.

80. Brutsaert DL, deClerck NM, Goethals MA, Housmans PR. Relaxation of ventricular cardiac muscle. *J Physiol (Lond)* 1978;283:469–480.

81. Jewell BR, Wilkie DR. The mechanical properties of relaxing muscle. *J Physiol (Lond)* 1960;152:30–47.

82. Jiang H, Stephens NL. Isotonic relaxation of sensitized bronchial smooth muscle. *Am J Physiol* 1992; 6:L344–L350.

83. Sobieszek A, Bremel R. Preparation and properties of vertebrate smooth muscle myofibrils and actomyosin. *Eur J Biochem* 1975;55: 49–60.

84. Nagai R, Kuro-o M, Babij P, Periasamy M. Identification of two types of smooth muscle myosin heavy chain isoforms by cDNA cloning and immunoblast analysis. *J Biol Chem* 1989;264(17):9734–9737.

85. Kelley CA, Takahashi M, Yu JH, Adelstein RS. An insert of 7 amino acids confers functional differences between smooth muscle myosin from intestines and v asculations. *J Biol Chem* 1993;268:12848–12854.

86. Kron SJ, Spudich JA. Fluorescent actin filaments move on myosin fixed to a glass surface. *Proc Natl Acad Sci U S A* 1986;83:6272–6276.

87. Harada Y, Noguchi A, Kishino A, Yanagide T. Sliding movement of single actin filaments on one-headed myosin filaments. *Nature* 1987;326:805–808.

88. Sheetz MP, Chasan R, Spucich JA. ATP-dependent movement of myosin *in vitro*: Characterization of quantitative assay. *J Cell Biol* 1984;99:1867–1871.

89. Adelstein RS, Klee CB. Purification and characterization of smooth muscle myosin light chain kinase. *J Biol Chem* 1981;256:7501–7509.

90. Klee CB. Calmodulin: Structure-function relationships. In: Cheung W, ed. *Calcium and cell function*. New York: Academic Press, 1980;59–78.

91. Spudich JA, Watt S. Regulation of rabbit skeletal muscle contraction. (1) Biochemical studies of intereaction of tropomyosin-tropinin complex with actin and protelytic fragments of myosin. *J Biol Chem* 1971; 246:4866–4871.

92. Eisenberg E, Kelley WW. Troponin-tropomyosin complex - column chromatography -separation and activity of 3 active troponin components with and without tropomyosin present. *J Biol Chem* 1974;249: 4742–4748.

93. Toyoshima YY, Kron SG, McNally SM, Wiebling EM, Toyoshima KR and Spudich JA. Myosin subragment-1 is sufficient ot move actin filaments *in vitro*. *Nature* 1987;328:536–539.

94. Kishimo A, Yanagida T. Force measurements by micro-manipulation of a single actin filament by glass needles. *Nature* 1988;334:74–76.

95. Sheetz MP, Block SM, Spudich JA. Myosin movements *in vitro*: a quantitative assay usng oriented actin cables from Nitella. *Methods Enzymol* 1986;134:531–544.

96. Kepron W, James JM, Kirk B, Sehon AH, Tse KS. A canine model for reaginic hypersensitivity and allergic hypersensitivity. *J Allergy Clin Immunol* 1977;59:64–68.

97. Stephens NL, Kong SK, Seow CY. Mechanisms of increased shortening of sensitized airway smooth muscle. In: Armour CL, Black JL, eds. *Mechanisms in asthma*. New York: Alan R. Liss, 1988;231–254.

98. Wang K, Ramirez-Mitchell R. A network of transverse and longitudinal intermediate filaments is associated with sarcomeres of adult vertebrate skeletal muscle. *J Cell Biol* 1983;96:562–570.

99. Horowits R, Kempher ES, Bisher ME, Podolski RJ. A phyiosslogical role for itin and nebulin (titin) in skeletal muscle. *Nature* 1986;323: 160–164.

100. Ma X, Stephens NL. The contribution of the cytoskeleton and extracellular matrix to increased shortening capacity in sensitized canine tracheal smooth muscle. *Resp Physiol* 1996 (*in press*).

101. Kong KS, Halayko AJ, Stephens NL. Increased myosin phosphorylation in sensitized canine tracheal smooth muscle. *Am J Physiol* 1990;256:L53–L56 .

102. Hoh JFY, McGrath PA, Hale PT. Electrophoretic analysis of multiple forms of rat cardiac myosin-effect of hypophysectomy and thyroxine replacement. *J Mol Cell Cardiol* 1978;10:1053–1076.

103. Schwartz K, LeCarpentier Y, Martin JL, Lonpre AM, Mercadier JJ, Swynghedauw B. Myosin isoenzymic distribution correlated with speed of myocardial contraction. *J Mol Cell Cardiol* 1981;13: 1071–1075.

104. Hewett TE, Martin AF, Paul RJ. Correlations between myosin heavy chain isoforms and mechanical parameters in rat myometrium. *J Physiol (Lond)* 1993;460:351–364.

105. Malmquist U, Arner A, Uvelius B. Contractile and cytoskeletal proteins in smooth muscle during hypertrophy and its reversal. *Am J Physiol* 1991;260:C1085–C1093.

106. Aksoy MO, Murphy RA, Kamm KE. Role of Ca^{2+} and myosin light chain phsophorylation in regulation of smooth muscle. *Am J Physiol* 1982;242:C109–C116.

107. Jiang H, Rao K, Halayko AJ, Liu X, Stephens NL. Ragweed sensitization-induced increase of myosin light chain kinase content in canine airway smooth muscle. *Am J Respir Cell Mol Biol* 1992;7:567–573.

108. Liu X, Halayko AJ, Liu G, Rao K, Jiang H, Stephens NL. Myosin light chain phosphatase activity in ragweed pollen-sensitized canine tracheal smooth muscle. *Am J Respir Cell Mol Biol* 1994;11:676–681.

109. Jiang H, Rao K, Liu X, Liu G, Stephens NL. Intra-cellular Ca^{2+}, myosin phosphorylation and calmodulin activity in sensitized airway smooth muscles. *Am J Physiol* 1955;268:L739–L746.

110. Lanzetta PA, Alvarez LJ, Reinach PS, Candia OA. An improved assay for nanomole amounts of inorganic phosphate. *Anal Biochem* 1979; 100:95–97.

111. Arner B, Moosmyer M. Rapid determination of inorganic phosphate in biological systems by a highly sensitive photometric method. *Anal Biochem* 1975;65:305–309.

112. Liu G, Stephens NL. Increased Ca^{2+} - calmodulin complex in ragweed pollen sensitized canine tracheal smooth muscle. *Amer J Resp and Critical Care Medicine* 1995;151(4),Part 2:A288.

Asthma, edited by P.J. Barnes, M.M. Grunstein,
A.R. Leff, and A.J. Woolcock.
Lippincott–Raven Publishers, Philadelphia © 1997.

▪ 57 ▪

Molecular Biology of Potassium Channels in Airway Smooth Muscle

Michael I. Kotlikoff

Potassium Channels in Airway Smooth Muscle
Voltage-Dependent Potassium Channels
  Molecular Structure
  Molecular Physiology

Calcium-Activated Potassium Channels
  Molecular Structure
  Molecular Physiology
Conclusions and Therapeutic Significance

The importance of membrane potassium conductances for the maintenance of normal electrical behavior in smooth muscle has long been known (1) By controlling the membrane potential of airway myocytes and intrinsic nerves in the airways, potassium channels are critical determinants of resting bronchial tone. Additionally, the active regulation of potassium channels during contraction and relaxation evoked by endogenous hormones/neurotransmitters or exogenous drugs, suggests that these proteins play a prominent role in bronchospasm and its treatment. Recent studies at the single-channel and whole-cell level have established that voltage-dependent, delayed rectifier potassium channels are critical determinants of cell membrane potential and resting muscle tone in airway smooth muscle (2,3). Voltage-dependent potassium (K_V) channels are encoded by a large family of genes that has been well-characterized following the initial cloning of the *Drosophila Shaker* locus, the gene encoding a major class of voltage-dependent potassium channels (4,5). The expression of these channels in heterologous cell systems provides the ability to study the pharmacology and molecular regulation of these channels under relatively simple conditions, and may lead to the development of subtype-selective channel agonists that are useful in the treatment of bronchospasm. Important progress on the structure and molecular regulation of calcium-acti-

vated potassium (K_{Ca}) channels has also been made recently. Following the cloning and expression of the *Drosophila* channel dslo, and the mammalian homologues, information about the structural relationship between this channel and the voltage-dependent channels has rapidly emerged (6–8). The large single-channel conductance of this channel and ease with which it can be measured in re-expression or bilayer systems will likely result in rapid progress, with respect to information about the structural elements of those proteins that underlie key aspects of regulation.

This chapter will summarize information with respect to the structure and function of voltage-dependent and calcium-activated potassium channels. It is likely that information at the molecular level about the structure and regulation of these important proteins will result in specific hypotheses and targeted experiments that will provide insight into the consequences of channel regulation, and the development of channel-specific assay systems for the discovery of improved bronchoactive drugs.

POTASSIUM CHANNELS IN AIRWAY SMOOTH MUSCLE

In airway smooth muscle (ASM), potassium channels play important roles in setting the resting membrane potential, generating and propagating rhythmic slow waves, determining the passive electrical properties of the cell membrane, and limiting electrical responses to excitatory

---

M. I. Kotlikoff: Department of Animal Biology, School of Veterinary Medicine, University of Pennsylvania, Philadelphia, Pennsylvania 19104-6064.

stimuli. ASM generally behaves as an electrically quiescent tissue that depolarizes during activation in a graded fashion, without prominent spike depolarizations, although there are prominent slow waves in some tissues (9–13). The tissue displays a large increase in potassium conductance following depolarization (10,11,14). Several early studies clearly indicated that these properties were due to the potassium conductance of the tissue and provided important information with respect to the specific channels underlying these properties. Thus, in the presence of substances known to block potassium channels, prominent spike depolarizations and increases in tonic force are initiated (9,10,14). The pharmacology emerging from many of these early studies indicated that high concentrations (greater than 30 mM) of tetraethylammonium (TEA) were required to produce this effect, suggesting that channels other than K_{Ca} or K_{ATP} (ATP-sensitive potassium channels), which are quite sensitive to TEA block, were involved. It now appears that specific proteins encoded by the delayed-rectifier gene family underlie the outward rectification and determine the resting membrane potential in the airway myocyte, as well as other smooth muscle cells (2,15–17). Recent measurements in human bronchial rings indicate that a 4-aminopyridine-sensitive, but charybdotoxin and glybenclamide-insensitive (i.e., not K_{Ca} or K_{ATP}) potassium channel underlies bronchial tone (3,18). Moreover, potassium channels are also important determinants of the release of neurotransmitters and neuropeptides from airway nerves (19,20). Antagonism of potassium channels facilitates neurotransmitter release and contraction, whereas channel agonists stabilize the airways (21).

In addition to a prominent role in maintaining the resting membrane potential and indirectly controlling the cytosolic calcium concentration of myocytes under nonstimulated conditions, potassium channels are prominently involved in excitation-contraction coupling processes initiated by contractile agents. Cholinergic contraction of ASM is associated with the inhibition of potassium channels and disruption of this inhibitory linkage markedly reduces functional responses of muscle segments in vitro (22,23). Conversely, various agents that relax ASM hyperpolarize the tissue by activating potassium channels (12,24–26). The physiologically important linkage between muscarinic contractile agonists and inhibition of calcium-activated potassium channels on the one hand, and β_2-adrenergic bronchodilation and activation of these channels on the other, suggests that these proteins play a fundamental role in hormone/neurotransmitter-mediated excitation-contraction (E-C) coupling (27,28).

Over the past decade, a substantial expansion of our knowledge about potassium channels has occurred, facilitated by the development of smooth muscle disaggregation techniques, single-cell and single-channel patch-clamp methods, intracellular imaging methods, and the cloning and re-expression of numerous potassium channels. Specific channels mediating drug or hormone actions have been elucidated in some cases, leading to an awareness of the importance of specific channel subtypes in mediating hormone or drug actions (e.g., ATP-sensitive potassium channels) (22,29–37). While in many cases the specific mechanism by which these actions occur and the channel subtypes responsible for the function is still not completely known, these proteins represent an important and accessible target for the development of selective and potent inhibitors of bronchospasm.

VOLTAGE-DEPENDENT POTASSIUM CHANNELS

Molecular Structure

Delayed rectifier potassium currents that activate with characteristic kinetics and inactivate to varying degrees are voltage-gated, calcium-insensitive channels that belong to the now well-characterized family of channel proteins that have been identified following the cloning of the *Shaker locus* in *Drosophila* (2,4,38–40). The discovery of the mammalian homologues to the *Drosophila Shaker* proteins has led to the cloning and re-expression of these genes, and has established the relationship between potassium channels and other voltage-dependent, cation-selective channels. The cloned K channels vary substantially in terms of biophysical properties, pharmacology, and modulation by cellular second messengers. They include the more traditional rapidly activating and inactivating "A"-type currents and more slowly activating delayed rectifier currents. The differential expression of individual gene products in some but not all smooth muscles almost certainly underlies much of the substantial diversity observed between tissues. Additionally, within each class of channels, subtypes are expressed that may differ in biophysical properties, and splice variants within each subtype, adding substantially to the potential diversity of this large gene family (41).

The cloning of the *Shaker locus* immediately suggested a surprising similarity to the previously cloned pore-forming subunits of sodium and calcium channels. Whereas obvious homology existed in numerous areas, the predicted size of the peptide encoded by *Shaker* was roughly one-fourth of that of the other voltage-gated cation channels (656 residues). Since the other channels were known to encode four highly homologous domains, it was likely that the *Shaker* gene encoded one of these domains and that the channel was assembled as a tetramer. Strong evidence now indicates that potassium channels are in fact tetramers, and that they can be constructed as heteromultimers from distinct potassium channel subunits (42–47).

Following the cloning of *Shaker*, three other similar *Drosophila* genes were cloned termed *Shab, Shal, and*

Shaw, and now Kv1, Kv2, Kv3, and Kv4 subfamilies, respectively (48,49). The subsequent cloning of numerous mammalian homologues of these genes has revealed that they comprise the four major subfamilies of voltage-dependent potassium channels, and that each subfamily is comprised of multiple, distinct potassium channel genes. Within subfamilies, related channel genes show approximately 70% homology, whereas members of different subfamilies show roughly 40% amino acid identity (50). All of these genes encode proteins with a generally similar predicted structure (Fig. 1). The N-terminal and C-terminal regions are hydrophilic, whereas the central region shows significant structural similarity to sodium and calcium channels with six transmembrane-spanning hydrophobic stretches. Like the other voltage-gated cation-selective channels, the fourth hydrophobic domain, S4, contains the likely voltage sensor with a basic residue at every third position; a hydrophobic linker region between the predicted membrane spanning S5 and S6 domains, is the likely pore region, which shows almost signature homology between potassium channels (51).

To date, only members of the *Shaker* family have been reported in smooth muscle. Roberds and Tamkun (52) reported the expression of Kv1.5 and Kv1.2 messenger ribonucleic acids (mRNAs) by Northern analysis of RNA prepared from intact aortas. Hart el al. (53) cloned and reexpressed Kv1.2 channels from canine colonic smooth muscle, and the same laboratory has recently reported the cloning and reexpression of Kv1.5 channels from vascular and visceral smooth muscles (54). We have recently reported the expression of Kv1.1, 1.2, and 1.5 mRNAs in ASM (3). Since smooth muscle tissues contain numerous cell types, expression of these transcripts was confirmed in cultured human myocytes. As described further on, functional evidence indicates that the major regulator of membrane potential in ASM is Kv1.5.

Kv1.5 channels were first cloned from rat brain by Swanson et al. (55) and, subsequently, from human pancreatic cells and human ventricle (56,57). Studies of tissue-specific expression indicated that Kv1.5 mRNA was prominently expressed in atrium, ventricle, aorta, and skeletal muscle, although expression was not determined in the lung (52). Like other *Shaker* homologues, cloned Kv1.5 genes are encoded by distinct, intronless genes. Alternative mRNA splicing has been shown to result in the expression of at least two alternately spliced Kv1.5 isoforms (58). Gene splicing within the 5′ and 3′ exonic sequence results in truncated mRNAs. At least one of these mRNAs expresses functional potassium channels, although the physiological importance of these transcripts is not known. The human Kv1.5 gene maps to chromosome 12 (58).

The expression of these complementary deoxyribonucleic acids (cDNAs) in oocytes or human embryo kidney (HEK) cells produced a rapidly activating, partially inactivating potassium current, quite similar to voltage-dependent potassium currents observed in airway and other smooth muscle cells (2,15,38,59,60). The currents were more resistant to tetraethylammonium (TEA) block than previously cloned *Shaker* homologues, which also compares well with recordings in airway myocytes. In fact, there is no peptidyl toxin or other potassium channel blocker with high affinity (K_d less than 10 μM) or high specificity for Kv1.5 (60). Interestingly, the expression of Kv1.5 channels has been shown to be regulated by hormones; a cyclic 3′ 5′ adenosine monophosphate (cAMP) response element and a glucocorticoid response element are present in the 5′ noncoding region of the gene (61). In GH3 cells, steroids specifically increase Kv1.5 mRNA and channel protein expression within hours (62). Elevations of cAMP also regulate gene transcription in a complex and tissue-specific manner. cAMP increases Kv1.5 transcript in cardiac cells, but decreases message in GH3 cells (61). At present, little is known about the transcriptional regulation of Kv1.5 genes in smooth muscle. However, the presence of these regulatory elements raises obvious questions with respect to the potential for effects on ASM excitability associated with the treatment of asthma with glucocorticoids or β-adrenergic agents.

In addition to the *Drosophila* homologues that correspond in structure to other voltage-gated cation channels, a class of delayed rectifier proteins with markedly different structure has been identified in heart and brain. Unlike larger (40 to 100 kD) Kv proteins, I_{sK} RNA encodes a small molecular weight protein (predicted size 15 kD) that bears little homology to other known proteins. The

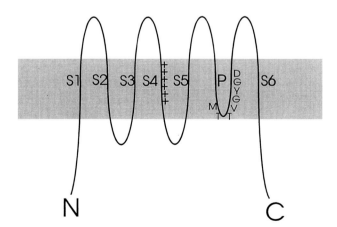

FIG. 1. Molecular structure of mammalian Kv1 potassium channels. The diagram shows the putative structure of a potassium channel monomer with six membrane spanning segments (S1-S6). The pore forming (P) linker between S5 and S6 is shown with the signature 8 amino acids that characterize potassium selective ions channels. + symbols indicate the basic residues (arginine or lysine) at every third position comprising the voltage sensor within the S4 segment. Multimeric potassium channels are assembled from four identical (homomultimeric channels) or different (heteromultimeric channels) peptide monomers.

channel was initially identified by expression cloning, and is now known to be expressed in several tissues (63–66). While this channel has not been investigated in ASM, it has been shown to be induced in uterine smooth muscle by exposure to estrogens (64,66). I_{sK} proteins produce slowly activating, sustained potassium currents. Such currents could partially underlie the noninactivating current component that has been identified in smooth muscle (38,40). The current-voltage relationship (activates positive to -50 mV) and the pharmacology (relatively TEA insensitive, blocked by clofillium) of I_{sK} suggest that this channel could be a physiologically relevant potassium conductance in ASM. Interestingly, I_{sK} currents are modulated by cellular second messengers; increases in calcium and cAMP augment the current, whereas PKC phosphorylation results in current inhibition (67). Future experiments will need to determine whether I_sK channels are expressed in ASM and, if so, whether they have a physiological role in ASM contractility.

Molecular Physiology

Potassium currents have been measured by numerous laboratories in airway myocytes. Early studies were complicated by the incomplete separation of voltage-dependent from calcium-activated potassium currents, and by the fact that the degree of K_{Ca} current availability was largely dependent on the calcium buffering conditions chosen. The development of nondialyzed whole-cell recording methods that utilize pore-forming antibiotics, such as nystatin, provided the ability to examine the availability of specific potassium currents under near- physiological conditions (68). Experiments revealed that a low noise, slowly inactivating current was the predominant current over the range of physiological potentials (2). Application of 4-aminopyridine, but not charybdotoxin, depolarized current-clamped myocytes held at physiological membrane potentials. These experiments suggested that under resting conditions, a 4-aminopyridine-sensitive, voltage-dependent potassium current controls the resting membrane potential, and that calcium-activated potassium channels contribute little net current in this potential range. Importantly, these findings hold in myocytes dispersed from human tracheobronchial segments (18). Depolarizing voltage steps from a holding potential of -80 mV-evoked outward potassium currents that activated with voltage-dependent kinetics and inactivated in a time and voltage-dependent manner, similar to previously reported delayed rectifier currents in nonhuman smooth muscle cells (2,15,38,40). These currents have been characterized pharmacologically by the application of charybdotoxin, dendrotoxin, and 4-aminopyridine. Dendrotoxin I is a 60 amino acid peptide toxin isolated from the black mamba snake. The peptide selectively blocks Kv1.1 and Kv1.2 channels at nanomolar concentrations, and can, thus, be used to distinguish these channels from the far less sensitive Kv1.5 channels. In nystatin-permeabilized, voltage-clamp experiments, these currents have been shown to be predominately insensitive to charybdotoxin and dendrotoxin, but sensitive to 4-aminopyridine, results consistent with the primary potassium current in ASM being Kv1.5 (3). Based on the biophysical and pharmacological data obtained in single cells, we reasoned that selective inhibition of potassium conductances should have predictable results on tone in human airway tissue. To test this hypothesis, force measurements were made in human bronchial smooth muscle rings, under conditions of selective channel blockade. Dendrotoxin, charybdotoxin, and glybenclamide were without effect on the resting tone of human bronchial smooth muscle, whereas 4-aminopyridine increased tone in a concentration-dependent manner, with a potency virtually identical to the block of Kv1.5 channels (3). These data suggest that Kv1.5 channels play a major role in determining basal tone in human airways.

CALCIUM-ACTIVATED POTASSIUM CHANNELS

Molecular Structure

K_{ca} channels are distributed in numerous tissues throughout the mammalian body and appear to comprise a family of genes encoding numerous biophysically distinct channel proteins. A prominent member of the family of calcium-activated potassium channels is the large conductance K_{Ca} channel (also termed BK or maxiK), which was easily observed at the single-channel level in early patch-clamp experiments (69). This channel is now recognized as a ubiquitous channel found in high copy number in smooth muscle and other tissues. The discovery of potent and selective peptide inhibitors of BK channels has proven quite valuable in selectively inhibiting this channel, as well as providing a means of isolating the channel protein (70,71).

As with the cloning of voltage-dependent potassium channels, a key step in the determination of the molecular structure of K_{Ca} channel proteins was the cloning of the gene locus associated with a *Drosophila* mutant of the previously identified *slo* phenotype (6). Mutations of the *slo* locus resulted in the loss of a calcium-activated potassium current that was sensitive to charybdotoxin (72–74). The *slo* locus was mapped and cloned, and the gene was shown to have substantial homology to voltage-dependent potassium channels, particularly in defining regions such as the S4 voltage sensor and the H5 pore region (6). Subsequent experiments demonstrated that the injection of numerous mRNAs differing in only a few codons, directed expression of large-conductance calcium-activated potassium channels in *Xenopus* oocytes (75). Cloning and expression of the mouse homologue followed swiftly (7,8). The human gene maps to chromosome 10 (8).

The gene encodes a protein of roughly 1200 amino acids that is highly homologous with the pore-forming α subunit of other voltage-gated potassium channels, but which contains an extended C terminal region. The six transmembrane segments characteristic of all voltage-dependent cation channels are present, and the putative H5 pore region is highly homologous with other potassium channels. Alternative splice sites are present in the N terminal and C terminal regions, and multiple splice variants have been detected in *Drosophia*, mouse, and human mRNAs (7,8,75,76). Expression of the α subunit produces a functional channel with the appropriate conductance (272 pS in 156 mM K (7)), that is blocked by the peptidyl scorpion toxins (charybdotoxin and iberiotoxin) that bind to the external surface of the channel pore. Channel activity is augmented by increasing calcium concentration at the cytoplasmic membrane surface; however, expressed channels require substantially higher concentrations of calcium at the cytosolic surface than channels recorded in patches from smooth muscle. The calcium-binding site on the protein is believed to be contained within the extended C terminal segment, since replacing this region with that of the drosophila protein confers the calcium sensitivity of the latter protein (77). A second subunit has been purified and cloned from smooth muscle and coexpression of this smaller subunit markedly increases calcium sensitivity, resulting in an nP_o/calcium relationship similar to that observed in membrane patches from smooth muscle cells (78–80). Both the α and β subunits contain several consensus PKA phosphorylation sites, although the site(s) associated with physiological regulation have not been determined.

Molecular Physiology

Large conductance, K_{Ca} channels have been measured in airway myocytes in numerous laboratories since the first reports by McCann and Welsh (81) in canine tracheal myocytes. There is substantial agreement about its single-channel characteristics, pharmacology, and distribution (22,38,81–86). Additionally, the channel has been isolated from canine and bovine trachealis membranes, and reconstituted in planar lipid bilayers (87). Under conditions of symmetrical potassium, this channel has a conductance of over 220 pS and open-state probability is markedly increased as the cytosolic calcium concentration is increased. Channel activity is also significantly dependent on cytoplasmic pH, with higher concentrations of hydrogen ions decreasing open-state probability at any given voltage or calcium concentration (83).

Substantial evidence indicates that modulation of K_{Ca} channel activity is an important component of cellular signaling pathways associated with contractile and relax-

ant agents in smooth muscle (22,23,27,29,31,88–93). An important demonstration of the unique role of these channels in β-adrenergic relaxation of ASM was provided by Jones et al. (27) and later by Miura et al. (28) in human airway smooth muscle. Using the highly specific peptidyl toxin, charybdotoxin (CHTX), both groups observed that the efficacy of β-adrenergic hormones is markedly diminished when K_{Ca} channels are prevented from opening with 100 or 200 nM CHTX. This suggests, particularly at low hormone concentrations, that the ability of β-adrenergic hormones to relax ASM depends to a surprising degree on their ability to open K_{Ca} channels. Conversely, numerous laboratories have shown that contractile agonists inhibit K_{Ca} channel opening, suggesting that this channel is an important regulatory target during excitation-contraction coupling (29,94–97).

The molecular mechanisms linking β-adrenergic receptors to K_{Ca} channel activation have recently been reviewed (98). Evidence exists for the activation of K_{Ca} channels (augmentation of open-state probability) by cAMP-dependent protein kinase, cyclic guanosine momnohosphate (cGMP)-dependent protein kinase, cGMP-dependent dephosphorylation, and the GTP-activated stimulatory G protein, G_S (31,32,87,93,99,104–106). A clear consensus on the physiological importance of discrete signaling pathways has not emerged.

Substantial agreement does exist from numerous laboratories indicating that K_{Ca} channels are inhibited during excitation-contraction coupling in smooth muscle. The marked rise in $[Ca^{++}]_i$ accompanying contraction would increase cellular potassium conductance, resulting in hyperpolarization and decreased cell-cell coupling in the absence of an inhibitory feedback mechanism limiting K_{Ca} activity. Some of the earliest patch-clamp recordings in smooth muscle demonstrated a prolonged inhibition of K_{Ca} channel activity during cholinergic excitation of smooth muscle (94). These findings have been reproduced in several laboratories and the molecular pathway coupling receptor stimulation to channel inactivation explored. Cole and Sanders (95) demonstrated at the whole-cell level that cholinergic inhibition of K_{Ca} channels was G protein-dependent, and that a pertussis-toxin-sensitive G protein mediated this inhibitory coupling. Similarly, Toro et al. (97) demonstrated G-protein-dependent inhibition in planar lipid bilayers, suggesting a membrane-delimited coupling between receptor and channel. Work in this laboratory examined this coupling and provided further evidence for such a membrane-delimited G protein action by demonstrating muscarinic inhibition in outside-out patches from airway myocytes and the pertussis sensitivity of this coupling. Moreover, functional experiments provided evidence that the inhibitory linkage between the muscarinic receptor and K_{Ca} channels is necessary for normal force development (23). Disruption of receptor/channel linkage using pertussis toxin or M_2-selective receptor antagonists resulted in a marked inhibition of cholinergic contraction, and normal force development was restored by inhibiting channel activity with charybdotoxin. It should be noted, however, that several studies have suggested acetylcholine inhibits K_{Ca} channels indirectly by blocking calcium release from intracellular stores (85,107). Recent evidence indicates that it is likely that the spontaneous outward currents (STOCs), that are due to the spontaneous opening of K_{Ca} channels, are linked to quantal release of SR calcium near the plasma membrane, and that this tonic SR release is abolished in the presence of caffeine (108).

CONCLUSIONS AND THERAPEUTIC SIGNIFICANCE

Studies to date have begun to provide information about the specific potassium channel proteins expressed in ASM, the role of these proteins in excitation-contraction coupling, and the molecular processes that couple hormone action with alterations in channel function. Important functional roles have been ascribed to Kv1.5, delayed rectifier channels, and BK, calcium-activated channels. Given the demonstration of expressed mRNAs for additional channels, it is likely that future studies will provide insight into the function of these channels. Table 1 provides a list of potassium channel blockers. Evidence suggests that Kv1.5 channels are importantly involved in the determination of resting membrane potential in ASM. These channels are open under resting conditions, and channel blockade results in depolarization. At present, the extent to which these potassium channels are also modulated by agents that alter the contractile state of smooth muscle is unknown. No channel agonists for delayed rectifiers currently exist, but the molecular characterization of this family of channel proteins, as well as the ability to easily re-express the channels, is likely to facilitate the development of such drugs. Activation of these channels would also be likely to hyperpolarize and relax ASM, since only a small fraction of the maximum conductance is available at hyperpolarized potentials. Large-conductance calcium-activated potassium channels are important hormone targets, whose open probability is modulated by agents that alter smooth muscle tone. The demonstration

that β-adrenergic agonists act, at least partially, by opening these channels, presents interesting therapeutic possibilities for the use of K_{Ca} agonists as bronchodilators (27,31,32). This would provide the ability to bypass the β-adrenergic receptor, stimulating an important final target protein directly. While such agents might be expecting to be less effective than β-agonists to the extent that β-receptors activate other functional target proteins, they might avoid problems related to receptor desensitization and β-adrenergic side effects. Of course, issues of the specificity of the channel agonist would be vital in the development of selective bronchodilators for any potassium channel openers. The enormous potential diversity associated with the formation of splice variants and heterotetramers may provide optimism that unique tissue-specific channels subtypes may be exploited.

TABLE 1. The pharmacology and funciton of potassium channels expressed in human airway smooth muscle

Potassium Channels	Inhibitors	Function
K_v 1.1	Dendrotoxin	Unknown
K_v 1.2	Dendrotoxin, Charybdotoxin	Unknown
K_v 1.5	4-AP (not specific)	Resting E_m
K_{Ca}	Iberiotoxin, Charybdotoxin	Hormone responses

REFERENCES

1. Casteels R. Smooth Muscle: An assessment of current knowledge. In: Bulbring E, Brading AF, Jones AW, Tomita T, eds. *Membrane potential in smooth muscle cells.* London: Arnold, 1981;105–126.
2. Fleischmann BK, Washabau RJ, Kotlikoff MI. Control of resting membrane potential by delayed rectifier potassium currents in ferret airway smooth muscle cells. *J Physiol (London)* 1993;468:625–638.
3. Adda S, Fleischmaun BK, Freedman BD, Yu M-F, Hay DWP, Kotlikoff MI. Expression and function of voltage-dependent potassium channel genes in human airway smooth muscle. *J Biol Chem* 1996;271:13239–13243.
4. Papazian DM, Schwarz TL, Tempel BL, Jan YN, Jan LY. Cloning of genomic and complementary DNA from *Shaker,* a putative potassium channel gene from Drosophila. *Science* 1987;237:749–753.
5. Kamb A, Iverson LE, Tanouye MA. Molecular characterization of *Shaker,* a Drosophilia gene that encodes a potassium channel. *Cell* 1987;50:405–413.
6. Atkinson NS, Robertson GA, Ganetzky B. A component of calcium-activated potassium channels encoded by the *Drosophilia slo locus. Science* 1991;253:551–553.
7. Butler A, Tsunoda S, McCobb DP, Wei A, Salkoff L. *mSLO,* a complex mouse gene encoding "maxi" calcium-activated potassium channels. *Science* 1993;261:221–224.
8. Pallanck L, Ganetzky B. Cloning and characterization of human and mouse homologues of the Drosophilia calcium-activated potassium channel gene, slowpoke. *Hum Mol Genet* 1994;3:1239–1243.
9. Coburn RF. The airway smooth muscle cell. *Fed Proc* 1977;36:2692–2697.
10. Kirkpatrick CT. Excitation and contraction in bovine tracheal smooth muscle. *J Physiol (Lond)* 1975;244:263–281.
11. Kroeger EA, Stephens NL. Effect of tetraethylammonium on tonic airway smooth muscle: initiation of phasic electrical activity. *Am J Physiol* 1975;228:633–636.
12. Honda K, Satake T, Takagi K, Tomita T. Effects of relaxants on electrical and mechanical activities in the guinea-pig tracheal muscle. *Br J Pharmacol* 1986;87:665–671.
13. Small RC. Electrical slow waves and tone of guinea-pig isolated trachealis muscle: effects of drugs and temperature changes. *Br J Pharmacol* 1982;77:45–54.
14. Kannan MS, Jager LP, Daniel EE, Garfield RE. Effects of 4-aminopyridine and tetraethylammonium chloride on the electrical activity and cable properties of canine tracheal smooth muscle. *J Pharmacol Exp Ther* 1983;227:706–716.
15. Beech DJ, Bolton TB. Two components of potassium current activated by depolarization of single smooth muscle cells from the rabbit portal vein. *J Physiol (Lond)* 1989;418:293–309.
16. Robertson BE, Nelson MT. Aminopyridine inhibition and voltage dependence of K^+ currents in smooth muscle cells from cerebral arteries. *Am J Physiol* 1994;36:C1589–C1597.

17. Volk KA, Matsuda JJ, Shibata EF. A voltage-dependent potassium current in rabbit coronary artery smooth muscle cells. *J Physiol (Lond)* 1991;439:751–768.

18. Fleischmann BK, Hay DWP, Kotlikoff MI. Control of basal tone by delayed rectifier potassium channels in human airways. *Am Rev Respir Dis* 1994;149:A1080.

19. Barnes PJ. Modulation of neurotransmission in airways. *Physiol Rev* 1992;72:699–729.

20. Lou YP, Lundberg JM. Different effects of the K- channel blockers 4-aminopyridine and charybdotoxin on sensory nerves in guinea-pig lung. *Pharmacol and Toxicol* 1993;72:139–144.

21. Black JL, Barnes PJ. Potassium channels and airway function: new therapeutic prospects. [Review]. *Thorax* 1990;45:213-218.

22. Kume H, Kotlikoff MI. Muscarinic inhibition of single K_{Ca} channels in smooth muscle cells by a pertussis-sensitive G protein. *Am J Physiol* 1991;261:C1204–C1209.

23. Kume H, Mikawa K, Takagi K, Kotlikoff MI. Role of G proteins and K_{Ca} channels in the muscarinic and -adrenergic regulation of tracheal smooth muscle. *Am J Physiol* 1995;12:L221–L229.

24. Allen SL, Beech DJ, Foster RW, Morgan GP, Small RC. Electrophysiological and other aspects of the relaxant action of isoprenaline in guinea-pig isolated trachealis. *Br J Pharmacol* 1985;86:843–854.

25. Allen SL, Cortijo J, Foster RW, Morgan GP, Small RC, Weston AH. Mechanical and electrical aspects of the relaxant action of aminophylline in guinea-pig isolated trachealis. *Br J Pharmacol* 1986;88:473–483.

26. Weston AH, Abbott A. New class of antihypertensive acts by opening K+ channels. *TIPS* 1987;8:283–284.

27. Jones TR, Charette L, Garcia ML, Kaczorowski GJ. Selective inhibition of relaxation of guinea-pig trachea by charybdotoxin, a potent Ca++-activated K+ channel inhibitor. *J Pharmacol Exp Ther* 1990;255:697–706.

28. Miura M, Belvisi MG, Stretton D, Yacoub MH, Barnes PJ. Role of potassium channels in bronchodilator response in human airways. *Am Rev Respir Dis* 1992;146:132–136.

29. Cole WC, Carl A, Sanders KM. Muscarinic suppression of Ca2—dependent K current in colonic smooth muscle. *Am J Physiol* 1989;257:C481–C487.

30. Komori S, Bolton TB. Role of G-proteins in muscarinic receptor inward and outward currents in rabbit jejunal smooth muscle. *J Physiol (Lond)* 1990;427:395–419.

31. Kume H, Graziano MP, Kotlikoff MI. Stimulatory and inhibitory regulation of calcium-activated potassium channels by guanine nucleotide-binding proteins. *Proc Natl Acad Sci USA* 1992;89:11051–11055.

32. Kume H, Takai A, Tokuno H, Tomita T. Regulation of Ca2+-dependent K+ channel activity in tracheal myocytes by phosphorylation. *Nature* 1989;341:152–154.

33. Nelson MT, Huang Y, Brayden JE, Hescheler J, Standen NB. Arterial dilations in response to calcitonin gene-related peptide involve activation of K+ channels. *Nature* 1990;344:770–773.

34. Nelson MT, Standen NB, Brayden JE, Worley JF. Noradrenaline contracts arteries by activating voltage-dependent calcium channels. *Nature* 1988;336:382–385.

35. Sims SM, Singer JJ, Walsh JV. Antagonistic adrenergic-muscarinic regulation of M current in smooth muscle cells. *Science* 1988;239:190–193.

36. Standen NB, Quayle JM, Davies NW, Brayden JE, Huang Y, Nelson MT. Hyperpolarizing vasodilators activate ATP-sensitive K+ channels in arterial smooth muscle. *Science* 1989;245:177–180.

37. Vivaudou MB, Clapp LH, Walsh JVJ, Singer JJ. Regulation of one type of Ca++ current in smooth muscle cells by diacylglycerol and acetylcholine. *FASEB J* 1988;2:2497–2504.

38. Boyle JP, Tomasic M, Kotlikoff MI. Delayed rectifier potassium channels in canine and porcine airway smooth muscle cells. *J Physiol (Lond)* 1992;447:329–350.

39. Kotlikoff MI. Airway smooth muscle in health and disease. In: Coburn RF, eds.*Ion channels in airway smooth muscle.* New York: Plenum Publishing, 1989;169–180.

40. Kotlikoff MI. Potassium currents in canine airway smooth muscle cells. *Am J Physiol* 1990;259:L384–L395.

41. Schwarz TL, Tempel BL, Papazian DM, Jan YN, Jan LY. Multiple potassium-channel components are produced by alternative splicing at the Shaker locus n Drosophila. *Nature* 1988;331:137–142.

42. Ruppersberg JP, Schroter KH, Sakmann B, Stocker M, Sewing S, Pongs O. Heteromultimeric channels formed by rat brain potassium channel proteins. *Nature* 1990;345:535–537.

43. MacKinnon R. Determination of the subunit stoichiometry of a voltage-activated potassium channel. *Nature* 1991;350:232–235.

44. Po S, Roberds S, Snyders DJ, Tamkun MM, Bennett PB. Heteromultimeric assembly of human potassium channels. Molecular basis of a transient outward current? *Circ Res* 1993;72:1326–1336.

45. Isacoff EY, Jan YN, Jan LY. Evidence for the formation of heteromultimeric potassium channels in Xenopus oocytes. *Nature* 1990;345:530–534.

46. Christie MJ, North RA, Osborne PB, Douglass J, Adelman JP. Heteropolymeric potassium channels expressed in Xenopus oocytes from cloned subunits. *Neuron* 1990;4:405–411.

47. MacKinnon R, Aldrich RW, Lee AW. Functional stoichiometry of Shaker potassium channel inactivation. *Science* 1993;262:757–759.

48. Wei A, Covarrubias M, Butler A, Baker K, Pak M, Salkoff L. K+ current diversity is produced by an extended gene family conserved in Drosophila and mouse. *Science* 1990;248:599–603.

49. Chandy KG, Douglas J, Gutman GA, et al. Simplified gene nomenclature. *Nature* 1991;352:26.

50. Jan LY, Jan YN. Structural elements involved in specific K+ channel functions. *Annu Rev Physiol* 1992;54:537–555.

51. Heginbotham L, Abramson T, MacKinnon R. A functional connection between the pores of distantly related ion channels as revealed by mutant K+ channels. *Science* 1992;258:1152–1155.

52. Roberds SL, Tamkun MM. Cloning and tissue-specific expression of five voltage-gated potassium channel cDNAs expressed in rat heart. *Proc Natl Acad Sci U S A* 1991;88:1798–1802.

53. Hart PJ, Overturf KE, Russell SN, Carl A, Hume JR, Sanders Km, Horowitz B. Cloning and expression of Kv1.2 class delyed rectifier K+ channel from canine colonic smooth muscle. *Proc Natl Acad Sci USA* 1993;90:9659–9663.

54. Overturf KE, Russell SN, Carl A, Vogalis F, Hart PJ, Hume JR, Sanders KM, et al. Cloning and characterization of a Kv1.5 delayed rectifier K+ channel from vascular and visceral smooth muscles. *Am J Physiol* 1994;36:C1231–C1238.

55. Swanson R, Marshall J, Smith JS, Williams JB, Boyle MB, Folander K, Luneau CJ, et al. Cloning and expression of cDNA and genomic clones encoding three delayed rectifier potassium channels in rat brain. *Neuron* 1990;4:929–939.

56. Philipson LH, Hice RE, Shaefer K, LaMendola J, Bell GI, Nelson DJ, Steiner DF. Sequence and functional expression in Xenopus oocytes of a human insulinoma and islet potassium channel. *Proc Natl Acad Sci U S A* 1991;88:53–57.

57. Tamkun MM, Knoth KM, Walbridge JA, Kroemer H, Roden DM, Glover DM. Molecular cloning and characterization of two voltage-gated K+ channel cDNAs from human ventricle. *FASEB J* 1991;5:331–337.

58. Attali B, Lesage F, Ziliani P, Guillemare E, Honore E, Waldmann R, Hugnot J-P, et al. Multiple mRNA isoforms encoding the mouse cardia Kv1.5 delayed rectifier K+ channel. *J Biol Chem* 1993;268:24283–24289.

59. Fedida D, Wible B, Wang Z, Fermini B, Faust F, Nattel S, Brown AM. Identity of a novel delayed rectifier current from human heart with a cloned K+ channel current. *Circ Res* 1993;73:210–216.

60. Grissmer S, Nguyen AN, Aiyar J, Hanson DC, Mather RJ, Gutman GA, Karmilowicz MJ, et al. Pharmacological characterization of five cloned voltage-gated K+ channels, types Kv1.1, 1.2, 1.3, 1.5, and 3.1, stably expressed in mammalian cell lines. *Mol Pharmacol* 1994;45:1227–1234.

61. Mori Y, Matsubara H, Folco E, Siegel A, Koren G. The trancription of mammalian voltage-gated potassium channel is regulated by cAMP in a cell-specific manner. *J Biol Chem* 1993;268:26482–26493.

62. Takimoto K, Fomina A, Gealy R, Trimmer JS, Levitan ES. Dexamethasone rapidly induces Kv1.5 K+ channel gene transcription and expression in clonal pituitary cells. *Neuron* 1993;11:359–369.

63. Takumi T, Ohkubo H, Nakanishi S. Cloning of a membrane protein that induces a slow voltage-gated potassium current. *Science* 1988;242:1042–1045.

64. Folander K, Smith JS, Antanavage J, Bennett C, Stein RB, Swanson R. Cloning and expression of the delayed-rectifier I_{sK} channel from neonatal rat heart and kiethylstilbestrol-primed rat uterus. *Proc Natl Acad Sci U S A* 1990;87:2975–2979.

65. Honore E, Attali B, Romey G, Heurteaux C, Ricard P, Lesage F, Lazdunski M, et al. Cloning, expression, pharmacology and regulation of a delayed rectifier K$^+$ channel in mouse heart. *EMBO J* 1991;10: 2805–2811.

66. Pragnell M, Snay KJ, Trimmer JS, MacLuskey NJ, Naftolin F, Kaczmarek LK, Boyle MB. Estrogen induction of a small putative K$^+$ channel mRNA in rat uterus. *Neuron* 1990;4:807–812.

67. Swanson R, Hice RE, Folander K, Sanguinetti MC. The I$_{sK}$ protein, a slowly activating voltage-dependent K$^+$ channel. *Neuroscience* 1993; 5:117–124.

68. Horn R, Marty A. Muscarinic activation of ionic currents measured by a new whole-cell recording method. *J Gen Physiol* 1988;92:145–159.

69. Blatz AL, Magleby KL. Calcium-activated potassium channels. *Trends Neurosci* 1987;10:463–467.

70. Galvez A, Gimenez-Gallego G, Reuben JP, et al. Purification and characterization of a unique, potent, peptidyl probe for the high conductance calcium-activated potassium channel from venom of the scorpion Buthus tamulus. *J Biol Chem* 1990;265:11083–11090.

71. Miller C, Moczydlowski E, Latorre R, Phillips M. Charybdotoxin, a protein inhibitor of single Ca2+-activated K$^+$ channels from mammalian skeletal muscle. *Nature* 1985;313:316–318.

72. Elkins T, Ganetzky B, Wu CF. A *Drosophila* mutation that eliminates a calcium-dependent potassium current. *Proc Natl Acad Sci U S A* 1986;83:8415–8419.

73. Komatsu A, Singh S, Rathe P, Wu CF. Mutational and gene dosage analysis of calcium-activated potassium channels in *Drosophila*: correlation of micro- and macroscopic currents. *Neuron* 1990;4:313–321.

74. Singh S, Wu CF. Complete separation of four potassium currents in *Drosophila. Neuron* 1989;2:1325–1329.

75. Adelman JP, Shen K-Z, Kavanaugh MP, et al. Calcium-activated potassium channels expressed from cloned complementary DNAs. *Neuron* 1992;9:209–216.

76. Lagrutta A, Shen K-Z, North RA, Adelman JP. Functional differences among alternatively spliced variants of *Slowpoke*, a *Drosophila* calcium-activated potassium channel. *J Biol Chem* 1994;269:20347–20351.

77. Wei A, Solaro C, Lingle C, Salkoff L. Calcium sensitivity of BK-type KCa channels determined by a separable domain. *Neuron* 1994;13: 671–681.

78. Garcia-Calvo M, Knaus H-G, McManus OB, Giangiacomo KM, Kaczorowski GJ, Garcia ML. Purification and reconstitution of the high-conductance, calcium-activated potassium channel from tracheal smooth muscle. *J Biol Chem* 1994;269:676–682.

79. Knaus HG, Garcia-Calvo M, Kaczorowski GJ, Garcia ML. Subunit composition of the high conductance calcium-activated potassium channel from smooth muscle, a representative of the *mSlo* and *slowpoke* family of potassium channels. *J Biol Chem* 1994;369:3921–3924.

80. McManus OB, Helms LMH, Pallanck L, Ganetzky B, Swanson R, Leonard RJ. Functional role of the subunit of high-conductance calcium-activated potassium channels. *Neuron* 1995;14:645–650.

81. McCann JD, Welsh MJ. Calcium-activated potassium channels in canine airway smooth muscle. *J Physiol (Lond)* 1986;372:113–127.

82. Green KA, Foster RW, Small RC. A patch-clamp study of K—channel activity in bovine isolated tracheal smooth muscle cells. *Br J Pharmacol* 1991;102:871–878.

83. Kume H, Takagi K, Satake T, Tokuno H, Tomita T. Effects of intracellular pH on Ca2+-activated potassium channels in rabbit tracheal smooth muscle cells. *J Physiol* 1990;424:445–457.

84. Muraki K, Imaizumi Y, Kawai T, Watanabe M. Effects of tetraethylammonium and 4-aminopyridine on outward currents and excitability in canine tracheal smooth muscle cells. *Br J Pharmacol* 1990;100: 507–515.

85. Saunders H-M, Farley JM. Pharmacological properties of potassium currents in swine tracheal smooth muscle. *J Pharmacol Exp Ther* 1992;260:1038–1044.

86. Stockbridge LL, French AS, Man SFP. Subconductance states in calcium-activated potassium channels from canine airway smooth muscle. *Biochim Biophys Acta* 1991;1064:212–218.

87. Savaria D, Lanoue C, Cadieux A, Rousseau E. Large conducting potassium channel reconstituted from airway smooth muscle. *Am J Physiol* 1992;262:L327–L336.

88. Anwer K, Toro L, Oberti C, Stefani E, Sanborn BM. Ca2+-activated K$^+$ channels in pregnant rat myometrium: modulation by a β-adrenergic agent. *Am J Physiol* 1992;263:C1049–C1056.

89. Anwer K, Oberti C, Perez GJ, Perez-Reyes N, McDougall JK, Monga M, Sanborn BM, et al. Calcium-activated K$^+$ channels as modulators of human myometrial contractile activity. *Am J Physiol* 1993;265: C976–C985.

90. Brayden JE, Nelson MT. Regulation of arterial tone by activation of calcium-dependent potassium channels. *Science* 1992;256:532–535.

91. Perez G, Toro L. Differential modulation of large-conductance KCa channels by PKA in pregnant and nonpregnant myometrium. *Am J Physiol* 1994;266:C1459–C1463.

92. Scornik FS, Codina J, Birnbaumer L, Toro L. Modulation of coronary smooth muscle KCa channels by Gs alpha independent of phosphorylation by protein kinase A. *Am J Physiol* 1993;265:H1460–H1465.

93. Kume H, Hall I, Washabau RJ, Takagi K, Kotlikoff MI. β-adrenergic agonists regulate K$_{Ca}$ channels in airway smooth muscle by cAMP dependent and independent mechanisms. *J Clin Invest* 1994;93:371–379.

94. Benham CD, Bolton TB. Spontaneous transient outward currents in single visceral and vascular smooth muscle cells of the rabbit. *J Physiol* 1986;381:385–406.

95. Cole WC, Sanders KM. G proteins mediate suppression of Ca2+- activated K current by acetylcholine in smooth muscle cells. *Am J Physiol* 1989;257:C596–C600.

96. Sims SM, Vivaudou MB, Hillemeier C, Biancani P, Walsh JVJ, Singer JJ. Membrane currents and cholinergic regulation of K+ 7current in esophageal smooth muscle cells. *Am J Physiol* 1990;258:G794–G802.

97. Toro L, Amador M, Stefani E. ANG II inhibits calcium-activated potassium channels from coronary smooth muscle in lipid bilayers. *Am J Physiol* 1990;258:H912–H915.

98. Kotlikoff MI, Kamm KE. Molecular mechanisms of ββ-adrenergic relaxation of airway smooth muscle. *Annu Rev Physiol* 1996;58:115–141.

99. Ewald DA, Williams A, Levitan IB. Modulation of single Ca+-dependent K$^+$-channel activity by protein phosphorylation. *Nature* 1985; 315:503–506.

100. Sadoshima J, Akaike N, Kanaide H, Nakamura M. Cyclic AMP modulates Ca-activated K channel in cultured smooth muscle cells of rat aortas. *Am J Physiol* 1988;255:H754–H759.

101. Carl A, Kenyon JL, Uemura D, Fusetani N, Sanders KM. Regulation of Ca2+-activated K$^+$ channels by protein kinase A and phosphatase inhibitors. *J Physiol* 1991;261:C387–C392.

102. Williams DL, Jr., Katz GM, Roy-Contancin L, Reuben JP. Guanosine 5′-monophosphate modulates gating of high-conductance Ca2+-activated K$^+$ channels in vascular smooth muscle cells. *Proc Natl Acad Sci U S A* 1988;85:9360–9364.

103. Robertson BE, Schubert R, Hescheler J, Nelson MT. cGMP-dependent protein kinase activates Ca-activated K channels in cerebral artery smooth muscle cells. *Am J Physiol* 1993;265:C299–C303.

104. Alioua A, Huggins JP, Rousseau E. PKG-Iα phosphorylates the α-subunit and upregulates reconstituted GK$_{Ca}$ channels from tracheal smooth muscle. *Am J Physiol* 1995;268:L1057–L1063.

105. White RE, Schonbrunn A, Armstron DL. Somatostatin stimulates Ca2+-activated K$^+$ channels through protein dephosphorylation. *Nature* 1991;351:570–573.

106. White RE, Lee AB, Shcherbatko AD, Lincoln TM, Schonbrunn A, Armstrong DL. Potassium channel stimulation by natriuretic peptides through cGMP-dependent dephosphorylation. *Nature* 1993;362:263–266.

107. Benham CD, Bolton TB, Lang RJ. Acetylcholine activates an inward current in single mammalian smooth muscle cells. *Nature* 1985;316: 345–347.

108. Stehno-Bittel L, Sturek M. Spontaneous sarcoplasmic reticulum calcium release and extrusion from bovine, not porcine, coronary artery smooth muscle. *J Physiol (Lond)* 1992;451:49–78.

Asthma, edited by P.J. Barnes, M.M. Grunstein,
A.R. Leff, and A.J. Woolcock.
Lippincott–Raven Publishers, Philadelphia © 1997.

▪ 58 ▪

Airway Smooth Muscle in Asthma

Judith L. Black

THE IMPORTANCE OF THE SMOOTH MUSCLE IN AIRWAY NARROWING

It is clear that airway smooth muscle contraction plays a pivotal role in the airway narrowing that accompanies both the acute asthmatic episode and the events associated with the late asthmatic response. The evidence for this is indirect but nevertheless compelling. The contraction can be due to the effects of neurotransmitters released from nerves in the vicinity of the airway smooth muscle, the action of inflammatory mediators released from mast cells and other inflammatory cells, either resident or recruited into the airways, or as a result of provocative agents such as histamine and methacholine inhaled under diagnostic conditions. Moreover, the bronchospasm is reversed or prevented by pharmacological agents, the activity of which is associated with either relaxation of airway smooth muscle (β- adrenoceptor agonists), prevention of release of mediators from inflammatory cells (cromoglycate and nedocromil) or direct antagonism of released neurotransmitters (ipratropium bromide), or inhaled provoking agonists (1).

Finally, since the array of stimuli which can produce airway narrowing in an asthmatic subject is so diverse as to include allergens like house dust mite, animal dander, molds and pollens, cold air, exercise and nonisotonic solutions and drugs such as propranolol and aspirin, it is difficult to imagine any event other than increased contraction of the smooth muscle which could constitute an etiological factor common to all these stimuli.

It is convenient to consider the smooth muscle in asthma as being abnormal in its reactivity—either pharmacological, or biochemical, abnormal in amount, or that a combination of these factors is responsible for the exaggerated airway narrowing that accompanies the stimuli listed earlier.

An Abnormality in Smooth Muscle Mass

As early as 1922, Huber and Koessler (2) noted that in the bronchi of patients dying of asthma, there was an increase in the thickness of the smooth muscle in the airway wall. They quantified the muscle by measuring muscle thickness and normalized it to the outside diameter of the airway. Subsequently, others have confirmed this increase, in patients dying in status asthmaticus and those dying of complications of asthma (3). In a study of the postmortem pathology of 24 children aged 5 months to 14 years, in 20 of these, there was an observation of an increase in the musculature of the bronchial walls (4). The authors

J.L. Black: Department of Pharmacology, University of Sydney, Sydney, New South Wales 2006, Australia.

termed this increase "hypertrophy" although no objective measurements were made. Dunnill and co-workers (5) compared the pathology of the airways in bronchi of normal subjects, those dying in status asthmaticus, and patients with chronic bronchitis and with emphysema. They found that the mean muscle area in asthmatic airway walls was nearly 3 times that of the muscle in the walls of nonasthmatic bronchi. This was confirmed by Heard and Hossain (6) and Hossain (7), who studied specific bronchi from the lower lobe of the left lung of asthmatic subjects and nonasthmatic controls. Again, they found an increase in smooth muscle mass and attempted to distinguish between hypertrophy and hyperplasia. Since then, opportunities have arisen to report on the nature of the smooth muscle in the airways of asthmatics not only dying of asthma, but also those with long-standing asthma who had died of other causes. These reports have given rise to the concept that the changes in pathology in fatal asthma may be considerably different from those associated with nonfatal asthma, and not just in terms of the degree of severity of change. The issue of the uniformity of the changes throughout the respiratory tree has also received attention. Indeed, Carroll et al. (8) studying 11 cases of fatal asthma, 13 cases of nonfatal asthma, and 11 subjects who were used as controls reported that the smooth muscle area was increased in all airways except the smallest studied (internal diameter 0.6mm). This study confirmed the findings of an earlier report in which the smooth muscle area was increased in the airway walls of 6 asthmatic subjects postmortem compared with 6 controls dying of nonrespiratory causes. In this case, airways examined were less than 2mm in internal diameter and contained no cartilage (9). Ebina et al. (10) conducted a detailed study of the airway tree in postmortem tissue from asthmatic subjects, those with chronic obstructive pulmonary disease (COPD), and nonasthmatic controls. They reported two types of changes in the airway smooth muscle: type 1 in which thickening occurred in the larger airways and type 2 in which increase in muscle mass involved the whole length of the respiratory tree. Hogg (11) has commented on the consequences of structural changes occurring in different areas of the airways. An increase in airway smooth muscle mass results in a thicker airway wall. For a similar degree of airway smooth muscle shortening, this thicker wall will result in an increased narrowing of the lumen, and since, in the bronchioles, the muscle encircles the lumen, then perhaps "the pathology in the peripheral airways is the key to asthma (11)."

However, an increase in airway smooth muscle may not be an absolute *sine qua non* in asthma. Sobonya (12) studied the lungs of six asthmatic subjects who died with, but not of, asthma, and, although there was significant thickening of the basement membrane, the area of muscle was not greater than that measured in control subjects. However, on close examination of these data, it is apparent that only very small airways were studied (mean diameter 0.59 mm), and when the amount of muscle in the walls of the bronchi was expressed as a percentage of bronchial wall area, there was, in fact, an increase in the asthmatic subjects.

Lambert et al. (13) have created a mathematical modeling system in which they are able to examine the impact of theoretical changes in each of the various components of the airway wall on airway closure. Their studies allowed them to conclude that an increase in smooth muscle mass may be the single most important contributing factor to exaggerated airway narrowing. For a given maximal muscle stress, greater muscle thickness allows the development of increased tension and, thus, greater narrowing of the airway lumen. Others have proposed that the increased narrowing that is evident in the asthmatic airway is the result of a decrease in those forces that serve to keep the airway open. Thus, infiltration of subepithelial layers of the bronchial wall with inflammatory cells, the appearance of dilated small blood vessels and the formation of edema, especially in the outer layers of the wall, will cause a lack of the tethering forces or preload on the smooth muscle, thereby allowing relatively unopposed closure in response to a provoking stimulus.

AN INCREASE IN SMOOTH MUSCLE MASS—HYPERTROPHY OR HYPERPLASIA?

In the earliest reports of the pathologic description of the asthmatic lung, an increase in the amount of smooth muscle in the airway wall was a relatively consistent finding. Often, a distinction was not made between a hypertrophic response, i.e., an increase in the individual size of airway smooth muscle cells, and a hyperplastic response, i.e., an increase in the actual number of smooth muscle cells, and, in fact, the terms were used interchangeably. However, Heard and Hossain (6) did count individual muscle fibers and smooth muscle cell nuclei, and reported that these were increased three-fold in bronchi examined from five men with fatal asthma. All these early reports were obtained from postmortem tissue and usually asthma was the cause of death. Carroll et al. (8), although noting an increase in the muscle mass in almost all areas of the respiratory tree, nevertheless did not comment on whether the increased area was due to hypertrophy or hyperplasia. In a study designed to distinguish between hypertrophy and hyperplasia, Ebina et al. (14) concluded that in type 1 asthmatics, i.e., those with muscle thickening in the larger airways, the increase was due to hyperplasia. The predominant change in those with thickening throughout the whole respiratory tree (type 2) was hypertrophy, which was most marked in the smaller airways, whereas hyperplasia appeared to be localized to bronchi. The significance of these findings, however, in terms of both underlying causation and clinical relevance remains unclear.

If the smooth muscle increase is due to hyperplasia, then any number of inflammatory or contractile mediators could be causative factors. These could be released from mast cells like histamine, from serum or plasma associated with tissue edema, such as platelet-derived growth factor, from epithelial cells such as endothelin and various cytokines, or from components of the matrix such as the epidermal growth factors and fibroblast growth factors (15–17). Alternatively, excessive growth of airway smooth muscle could result from the withdrawal of factors which normally would serve to inhibit cell growth such as prostaglandin E_2 or heparin (18) (Fig. 1).

There is, in fact, direct evidence for the effect of infiltrated inflammatory cells on smooth muscle cell growth (19). Stimulation of human airway smooth muscle cells with the cytokine tumor necrosis factor (TNF)-α causes upregulation of the expression of the adhesion molecules intercellular adhesion molecule (ICAM-1) and vascular cell adhesion molecule (VCAM)-1. In addition, adhesion of activated T cells to muscle cells produces an increase in deoxyribonucleic acid (DNA) synthesis in the muscle. Thus, there is a direct link between the infiltration of inflammatory cells into the environment of smooth muscle and an increase in its growth.

If the increase in smooth muscle mass is due to hypertrophy, then the cause of this requires elucidation. Whereas hyperplasia is likely to be a result of the inflammatory me-

diators which are almost certainly bathing the smooth muscle of the asthmatic airway, very few of these produce hypertrophy as opposed to hyperplasia. The possibility exists that a hypertrophic response could result from mechanical strain or a pressure or volume stimulus such as would occur with frequent bronchoconstriction and bronchodilatation in the airways of asthmatic subjects. In a group of premature neonates subjected to assisted ventilation, postmortem examination revealed gross hypertrophy of the airway smooth muscle, presumably in response to the increased pressure associated with mechanical ventilation (20). There is additional evidence to support the hypothesis that mechanical stress will promote hypertrophy (21). Canine airway smooth muscle cells in culture were subjected to a stretch relaxation stimulus. The amount of stretch applied was such as to be compatible with the physiological range of tracheal distension during deep inhalation in adult humans. There was an increase in cell number and an increase in tritiated thymidine incorporation, indicative of DNA synthesis. The protein content of stretched cells also increased, as did the myofilament concentration, indicating that stretch produces expression of a contractile, rather than a synthetic, phenotype of smooth muscle cell. Whether these results can be extrapolated to human airway smooth muscle cells requires investigation.

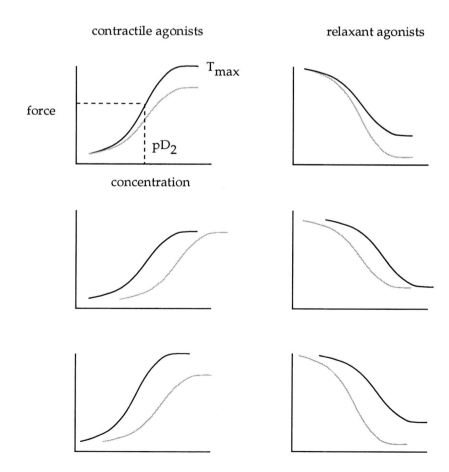

FIG. 1. Schematic representation of *in vitro* hyperresponsiveness. This could occur as a result of an increase in contraction, which could be exhibited as an increase in the maximal force (T_{max}), or an increase in the pD_2—the negative log of the concentration of the agonist which produces half the maximal response—or a combination of these factors. Alternatively, the relaxation response could be diminished, exhibited either as a decrease in the maximal relaxation force, or a decrease in the pD_2. The bold line in each panel represents the hyperresponsive condition.

If asthma is associated with an abnormality in the proliferation of smooth muscle, then it may be that, like coronary artery disease, this is associated with alterations in protooncogenes such as c-myc- and c-myb-mediated signal transduction. Recently, the frequent presence of increased amounts of wild-type p53 protein has been noted in re-stenosed human coronary artery segments, and this is correlated with the presence of the human cytomegalovirus and its protein IE84. The latter prevents p53 from activating a gene in human smooth muscle cell culture and may block the inhibitory effect of p53 on cell-cycle progression (22). This would lead to excessive proliferation and, in the airways, increased narrowing.

IS THERE AN ABNORMALITY IN MUSCLE PHARMACOLOGICAL REACTIVITY IN ASTHMA?

Since asthma is almost exclusively a human disease and since differences between animal species are well-documented and inconsistent in terms of the parameter under investigation, meaningful data to test the hypothesis that abnormalities in airway smooth muscle exist in asthma can be obtained only from the study of human tissue. Again, extrapolation from tissue obtained from nonasthmatic subjects to the asthmatic situation may be invalid. Nevertheless, the study of human airway smooth muscle remains the best method of obtaining relevant information regarding airway smooth muscle reactivity *in vitro*.

Methods for the Study of Human Isolated Lung *In Vitro*

Source of Tissue

Numerous types of preparations have been used to provide useful data about the function of human airway smooth muscle. The tissue source may be from autopsy specimens, obtained up to 14h postmortem or thoracotomies performed on those requiring resection of isolated peripheral lung lesions—usually carcinoma (23). Tissue obtained at autopsy has the advantage of being relatively free of macroscopic disease and can be obtained in large amounts. In addition, it provides an opportunity to study airway preparations from various locations in the respiratory tree, including the trachea. Tissue obtained in the course of surgical resection usually originates from subjects who are most often current or heavy ex-smokers (24,25). More recently, tissue has become available as a result of lung or heart/lung transplantation—mostly excised and, thus, markedly diseased lungs—in addition to an occasional nondiseased donor lung which could not be used for technical reasons for transplantation. These specimens are invaluable, since they provide not only a large tissue sample, but one in which disease processes do not constitute a confounding variable for *in vitro* reactivity. However, for the purpose of studying most pharmacological responses *in vitro*, tissue associated with a variety of disease states can be used since these have been recently characterized in terms of pharmacological responses (26). Tissue obtained from patients transplanted for α1 antitrypsin deficiency is unsuitable for the study of cholinergic responses, but that from patients with most other pulmonary diseases displays a pattern of *in vitro* reactivity not significantly different from disease-free lung. Cryopreservation of human lung at -190°C, in a mixture of fetal bovine serum and dimethylsulfoxide, enables preservation of a variety of functional responses for up to 3 weeks postretrieval. However, cryopreserved tissue is unsuitable for the study of contractile responses to antigen, since these responses are lost after cryopreservation (27).

Types of Tissue Preparation

Airway smooth muscle function can be studied with the use of a number of different tissue preparations. Slices of lung tissue, chains of tracheal or bronchial rings, strips of lung parenchyma, and bronchial strips and spirals have all been widely used (28). Recent additions to these available options is the strip or bundle of muscle fibers which is particularly useful for studying muscle function in the absence of confounding influences such as the epithelium, which can be dissected away under microscopy. In addition, these preparations can be adapted for the study of skinned fibers in which the cell membrane is also absent. Isolated airway smooth muscle cells can also be prepared from a variety of tissue sources, and a number of laboratories are studying the growth of these cells in primary culture (29–31). These cell preparations can also be frozen in liquid nitrogen and thawed for subsequent culture.

Is There an Alteration in Pharmacological Reactivity?

Functional Studies

If such an abnormality does exist, it could take the form of an exaggerated contraction, or a decrease in the ability of the muscle to relax to relevant pharmacological exogenous or endogenous stimuli. This could be manifest in an increase in the maximal contractile force produced in response to a contractile agonist, a decrease in the maximal relaxation to a relaxant agonist, or an increase or decrease in the potency of these, respectively. Thus, a segment of asthmatic bronchus could either exhibit an increased T_{max} (maximal tension) or an increased pD_2 (the negative log of the concentration of contractile agonist producing one-half the maximal response) or a decreased Tmax or decreased pD_2 to a relaxant agent (Fig. 2).

PDGF, EGF, ET-1, Histamine, thrombin, IL1.

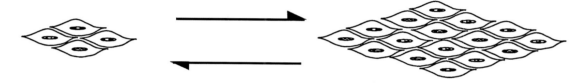

TNF$_\alpha$, PGE$_2$, heparin, ß agonists, dexamethasone, VIP, NO.

FIG. 2. The effects of various inflammatory mediators and other compounds on airway smooth muscle growth. Platelet-derived growth factor (PDGF), epidermal growth factor (EGF), endothelin-1 (ET-1), histamine, thrombin, and interleukin 1 (IL-1) cause cell proliferation, whereas tumor necrosis factor-α (TNF-α) prostaglandin E$_2$ (PGE$_2$) heparin, β-agonists, dexamethasone, vasoactive intestinal peptide (VIP) and nitric oxide (NO) inhibit growth.

Given that an abnormality in pharmacological reactivity exists, then it would be reasonable to expect that tissue from subjects who exhibit altered reactivity *in vivo,* i.e., airway hyperresponsiveness, should display features of this abnormality when studied *in vitro.* Results of the studies conducted to date are conflicting. Most of these have relied on the use of tissue resected at thoracotomy, the indication for which was a single, peripherally located malignant lesion. These patients, for the most part, were not true asthmatics but, rather, patients with COPD associated with chronic smoking who exhibited a degree of reversibility to their airway narrowing and a measurable degree of airway hyperresponsiveness to inhaled provocative stimuli. The majority of findings demonstrated no signs of hyperresponsiveness *in vitro,* at least to contractile stimuli (32–38). Whether this reflects the fact that these patients did not suffer from true asthma is not clear. The other possible explanation is that in removing the tissue from its usual milieu *in situ,* one has removed some additional factor which is responsible for the tissue hyperresponsiveness.

Studies on Asthmatic Tissue

Contraction

There are a small number of reports of asthmatic airway smooth muscle function. They have been drawn from different patient populations with respect to differences in severity of disease and drug therapy prior to tissue retrieval. Although single case studies report increases in contractility, in a series of eight patients with mild asthma undergoing thoracotomy for reasons unrelated to their asthma, and a group of patients who had fatal asthma, no differences in contractile responses were seen (39–42). Values for the potency of contractile agents such as histamine were comparable in different studies, even though there were marked differences in patient characteristics.

For instance, those studied by Goldie and co-workers (42) died in status asthmaticus, whereas the asthma of the patients in the study by Whicker and colleagues (41) was sufficiently mild as to permit lung resection. In both of these studies, histamine sensitivity in asthmatic subjects was decreased. In the reports of isolated cases of one or two subjects in which increases in maximal contraction were in fact observed, there was also no increase in sensitivity to histamine noted (39,40). Unlike the findings in these studies, however, Cerrina and colleagues (43) did report that, in a group of asthmatic subjects, there was, in fact, an increase in the sensitivity to histamine-induced contraction. This, however, was not mirrored in the response to other contractile agents, such as acetylcholine or prostaglandin F$_{2\alpha}$. This underlines the differences between *in vitro* and *in vivo* findings in asthmatic subjects, in whom airway hyperresponsiveness is demonstrable to a wide range of bronchoconstricting agents *in vivo.*

As for histamine, there is no demonstrable increase in sensitivity to cholinergic agonists in tissue from asthmatic subjects when *in vitro* responses are elicited. Whicker and colleagues (41) and Goldie and colleagues (42) again reported, if anything, a decrease in potency of these agonists.

Others have studied a wider range of contractile agonists such as the leukotrienes and prostaglandins. Dahlen et al. (44) found that tissue sensitivity to leukotrienes was no different in asthmatics and nonasthmatics, and prostaglandin-induced *in vitro* responses also failed to distinguish between patient groups. In another study, which examined tissue from mild-to-moderate asthmatic subjects, an increased sensitivity in the contractile response to adenosine was observed (45).

The situation in terms of the extent or height of the maximal contraction in asthmatic tissue *in vitro* is different from that examining tissue sensitivity or agonist potency. In a series of patients with fatal asthma, responses to histamine and acetylcholine in strips of tracheal smooth muscle were increased, compared to tissue from subjects without asthma (46). In a subsequent study, however, the same authors then examined the reactivity of subsegmental bronchi from the same patients (47). In contrast to their findings in tracheal tissue, new responses to histamine and acetylcholine were not different from those in control tissues, taken from nonasthmatic subjects. The discrepancy in the findings can perhaps be explained on the basis of regional differences in smooth muscle reactivity and ultrastructure and/or differential rates of tissue autolysis after death (48). The authors of this study suggest that tracheal responses would be less affected by tissue autolysis than those elicited from tissues deeper in the airways.

Relaxation

Rather than an increase in smooth muscle reactivity forming the basis for airway hyperresponsiveness, it is theoretically possible that a decrease in the ability of asthmatic smooth muscle to relax could account for exaggerated airway narrowing. It is here that some degree of consistency has been noted in *in vitro* studies. In at least two separate studies of tissue from asthma deaths, an impaired relaxation reponse to β-adrenoceptor stimulation with a β-agonist, isoprenaline, has been observed (42,46). However, not all studies concur with this finding. In a group of asthma subjects whose disease was mild, isoprenaline-induced relaxation responses were not, in fact, impaired (41). Moreover, in one of the studies which did demonstrate a defect in isoprenaline-mediated responses, responses to another β-agonist, salbutamol, were not decreased (42). Thus, it is difficult to conceptualize how a putative defect in β-adrenoceptor function could be selective for only one agonist.

Some recent evidence does suggest an abnormality in β-adrenoceptor function. Autoantibodies to β adrenoceptors have been reported in 5% of normal subjects and 40% of asthmatic subjects; these may functionally antagonize the receptor. Genetic variation in the receptor structure confers differences in the ability of β-agonists to promote desensitization or downregulation of β-receptors in human airway smooth muscle cells. This may account for variability in responses to β-agonists in patients with asthma (49,50).

Relaxation responses can be elicited in airway tissue by means other than β-adrenoceptor stimulation. Three studies have examined the effect of theophylline in asthmatic airway tissue. Two found that responses were no different from those in nonasthmatic tissue, whereas in one study, a significantly decreased response was observed (41,42,46). This would indicate that a general impairment of the relaxation pathway, rather than a specific abnormality of β-receptor function was an etiological factor.

Recent reports have provided convincing evidence for the identity of the endogenous neurotransmitter mediating relaxation in human airway tissue. It seems likely that nitric oxide (NO) is released after nerve stimulation in human airway tissue *in vitro* and is responsible for the relaxation effects observed in the presence of atropine to block contractile responses (51). However, this same group also provided evidence that in asthmatic airways this process is not impaired, in that there was no difference between NO-mediated relaxation responses in asthmatic and nonasthmatic tissue.

Thus, it is unlikely that, based on evidence from *in vitro* studies of human airway smooth muscle reactivity, a generalized impairment of relaxation responses underlies the abnormality in asthma. Nor is it likely that this is accounted for by a defect in the β-adrenoceptor. Whereas it is widely accepted that administration of β-adrenoceptor antagonists to asthmatic subjects can induce profound bronchoconstriction, a nonasthmatic subject cannot be converted into an asthmatic by administration of these drugs.

Thus, there are very few studies which have closely examined airway smooth muscle reactivity in verified asthmatic subjects. This situation could possibly be addressed in the future if asthmatic biopsy tissue is available with sufficient muscle content to conduct length-tension studies. It may be that patients with severe asthma, for whom there is no therapeutic alternative, may come to lung transplantation, in which case their lungs could become available for *in vitro* studies. Under these circumstances, valuable information would be acquired to provide weight to support or disprove the hypothesis that the smooth muscle is abnormal.

Radioligand Binding Studies/Autoradiography

Studies of this type provide us with a direct assessment of the numbers of receptors present in a given structure and also the affinity of the receptors. Autoradiographic visualization of receptors also allows us to localize a particular receptor to a particular component of a nonhomogeneous structure such as a segment of bronchus. Thus, the latter technique enables the localization of specific receptors to, for instance, the airway smooth muscle within the bronchial wall. The possibility exists that changes in receptor characteristics or receptor number may play a role in the etiology of airway hyperresponsiveness. There are, in fact, little data to support the hypothesis that any change in receptor number or affinity for any ligand occurs in asthmatic airway tissue. The receptors which have attracted most interest are the adrenoceptors and the muscarinic. Szentivanyi et al. (52) proposed that a defect in the β-adrenoceptor was a major contributing factor to the development of asthma. In one of the few studies of receptor numbers in asthmatic airway tissue, he found that in airway parenchymal tissue, the total number of binding sites for dihydroalprenolol (a β-receptor ligand) was decreased in asthma, compared to nondiseased tissue. At the same time, he reported an increase in the number of α-adrenoceptor binding sites. Similar observations have been made when tissue from subjects with chronic obstructive lung disease, as opposed to asthma, was examined. This, therefore, casts doubts on the significance of the understanding of the abnormality in asthma specifically. Bai and colleagues (53) examined the expression of β₂-adrenergic receptor mRNA in peripheral lung of asthmatic subjects. There were no consistent differences between expression in normal lung, that from patients with COPD, and those with asthma, although highest expression was noted in resected lungs from asthmatics. When β-receptor number on the bronchial smooth muscle was studied, although, in functional studies, decreased responsiveness to relaxation with isoprenaline was noted; there was, in fact, a three-fold increase in β-receptor number as well as affinity (54). Although there is one report of a decrease in cholinergic receptor number in patients with COPD, this was not confirmed subsequently (55,56). Recently, work conducted in guinea-pig airways has suggested that a change in muscarinic receptors may play a role in asthma pathogenesis. There is solid evidence for the existence of inhibitory M₂-receptors located on the postganglionic cholinergic nerve ending which terminates on the airway smooth muscle in both animals and humans (57). Stimulation of these receptors results in a decrease of release of endogenous acetylcholine. Thus, a dysfunction in these receptors could possibly result in a cholinergically mediated hyperresponsive airway. Recent studies suggest that viruses or eosinophil-derived products can selectively target M₂-receptors and decrease their function (58). Whereas these receptors are known to exist in humans, whether or not they are susceptible to the changes described in guinea pigs remains to be explored.

The endogenous vasoactive peptide endothelin has been the subject of much investigation for its possible role in asthma pathogenesis. Endothelin is produced not only in endothelial cells, but also in airway epithelial cells, at least in culture (59). Levels of endothelin are increased in the blood and bronchoalveolar lavage fluid of asthmatic subjects during an acute asthmatic exacerbation, and return to levels seen in nonasthmatic subjects when the lung function improves. The immunohistochemical detection of the message for endothelin has indicated that this is increased in the epithelium of asthmatic subjects (60). Receptors for endothelin have been detected on human airway smooth muscle and the smooth muscle of both the pulmonary and bronchial vasculature. Moreover, autoradiographically demonstrable binding sites for endothelin have been visualized on airway parasympathetic ganglia. In addition, endothelin is a powerful contractor of human airway smooth muscle, has been shown to modulate neurotransmission, and has mitogenic and comitogenic properties for airway smooth muscle in culture (61–65). This body of evidence would suggest that endothelin may have an etiological role in

asthma. However, if this is the case, then it is likely not to be on the basis of altered endothelin receptor number. Knott and associates (66) have recently reported that the number of binding sites for endothelin is not different in asthmatic lung from that in nonasthmatic lung. This, however, does not rule out the potential relevance of an abnormality in endothelin-receptor function, or simply the production of an excess of endogenous endothelin.

The relevance and interpretation of the results of studies investigating receptor characteristics is not clear. Often the relationship between receptor number and pharmacological response is not strong (67). This may indicate that not all receptors are functional and, indeed, some receptors may be "spare," or not directly linked to a physiological response. These spare receptors could be recruited under a variety of pathologic and experimental circumstances.

Thus, the evidence for a receptor abnormality for any known agonist being implicated in a dysfunction of airway smooth muscle, which could account for airway hyperresponsiveness, is lacking, and given the breadth and diversity of studies conducted so far, is unlikely to be forthcoming.

WHAT ARE THE REASONS WHY NO ABNORMALITY IN PHARMACOLOGICAL REACTIVITY IS DEMONSTRABLE *IN VITRO?*

Mechanical Factors

It is important that when airway preparations are studied *in vitro,* optimal conditions are established. This includes the determination of the optimal length (L₀) at which a tissue is studied. This is derived from a series of experiments in which the length of the preparation is correlated to the tension. This generates a length-tension curve. An increase in the length increases the tension which consists of the resting tension developed as a result of stretch applied to the elastic components of the tissue, and the active tension developed in the course of contraction by the contractile apparatus. This curve has a maximum value and at values higher than this length, tension either does not increase further, or alternatively decreases (68). Ideally, length-tension curves should be established for every tissue in every experiment performed. During this procedure, the length of the preparation is gradually increased by means of equilibration to increasing preloads or weights applied, and then the preparation is maximally stimulated by the application of either an electrical stimulus or a pharmacological agent such as acetylcholine. However, this is a time-consuming process and it is possible that its execution would affect tissue viability. Fortunately, L₀ may be estimated from studies in other tissues of comparable size and, on this basis, optimal lengths can be extrapolated to human tissue preparations of comparable size (69). Thus, it is unlikely that the lack of a demonstrable hyperresponsiveness *in vitro* is due to the fact that tissues are not studied at optimal length.

Type of Measurement

In situ, asthmatic airway smooth muscle not only develops force, but also undergoes shortening. Thus, for accurate measurement of change in muscle response, estimates of length, force, and velocity should be made simultaneously. In practice, however, responsiveness of muscle is estimated as either a change in force or a change in length. Thus, either isometric or isotonic measurements are made respectively. A comparison of results obtained with the two methods has been made by de Jongste et al. (70) These authors found that, in fact, there was a small difference in sensitivity to methacholine between preparations, but that maximal force and shortening are linearly related. When relaxant responses were compared, no significant differences were observed. Therefore, failure to observe smooth muscle hyperresponsiveness *in vitro* is unlikely to be related to the type of measurement used.

The Epithelium as a Barrier to Diffusion

Another possible explanation for the inability to demonstrate airway muscle hyperresponsiveness *in vitro* may be related to the natural barrier function of the epithelium *in situ*. Mitchell and Omari and colleagues (71, 72) have provided firm evidence that perfused segments of bronchus, as opposed to bronchial rings, are more representative of the *in vivo* situation than the more commonly used bronchial rings. In the latter preparation, drugs applied to the tissue can gain access to the smooth muscle via both the luminal and serosal route. However, when asthmatic subjects demonstrate hyperresponsiveness to inhaled agonists *in vivo*, the provocative agents gain access primarily via the lumen. If in a normal individual, the epithelium presents a barrier to the diffusion of inhaled agents and diminishes access to the smooth muscle, and if, as has been proposed, epithelial function is perturbed in asthma, then inhaled agents will have increased access to the smooth muscle and, thus, cause airway hyperresponsiveness. Whether smooth muscle dysfunction will be demonstrable *in vitro* with the use of closed, bilaterally cannulated perfused segments of human bronchus, is currently under investigation (Fig. 3).

"MODELS" OF AIRWAY HYPERRESPONSIVENESS

Although insufficient data are available to demonstrate a smooth muscle abnormality *in vitro*, certain "models of hyperresponsiveness" do enable the observation of altered reactivity. If one postulates that when the muscle is removed from its environment, the factor(s) responsible for the abnormality is now absent, then it is reasonable to assume that it is possible to "add back" these factors. There are several ways in which these can be achieved, and, even though they are artificial situations, they provide valuable information about smooth muscle reactivity.

Neurally Mediated Mechanisms

When most airway preparations are studied *in vitro*, the majority of neural pathways are disconnected. This situation is difficult to rectify, given the type of specimens of human tissue available . Although animal-isolated airway preparations can be studied with an intact branch of the vagus nerve attached, these are difficult to obtain for human tissue (73). However, postganglionic cholinergic fibers are still intact and their stimulation via the application of an electrical field results in the release of endogenous neurotransmitter and a contractile response. In many animal airway preparations, it has been easy to demonstrate a neurally mediated hyperresponsiveness, e.g., an augmentation of the contractile response to field stimula-

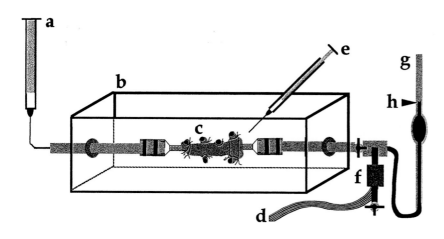

Fig. 3. Schematic representation of experimental apparatus designed to examine the *in vitro* pharmacological reactivity of perfused, intact segments of human bronchus. *a*, mucosal drug administration; *b*, organ bath; *c*, segment of bronchus; *d*, to computer; *e*, serosal drug administration; *f*, pressure transducer; *g*, column; *h*, pressure head.

tion by neuropeptides such as substance P (74). This, however, was much more difficult to demonstrate in human tissue. Substance P or neurokinin A applied to electrically stimulated airway tissue failed to show an augmentation of the contractile response. However, in the presence of a potassium (K^+) channel blocker-4 aminopyridine-neurokinin A did produce an increase in the contractile response (75). This raises the question of the role of the K^+ channels in keeping human airway smooth muscle cells electrically quiescent or rectified (76). Moreover, it highlights the importance of the potential for an abnormality of the K^+ channel to render a cell hyperresponsive or electrically active. Indeed, others have reported that blockade of the K^+ channel appears to increase smooth muscle activity and, conversely, agonists at the K^+ channel decrease tone in human airway smooth muscle (77).

Products of Inflammatory Cells

Another way in which it has been possible to demonstrate hyperresponsiveness in human airways *in vitro* has been via the addition of products of relevant inflammatory cells to the airway and the observation of a subsequently augmented response to agonist or nerve stimulation. If populations of neutrophils or eosinophils from healthy human volunteers are stimulated with calcium ionophore, the supernatants derived from these cells will augment the response to both histamine and electrical field stimulation (78,79). Subsequently, these results were confirmed in a series of experiments in which contractile responses were induced in human bronchi by the addition of eosinophils activated by platelet activating factor (PAF) (80). Moreover, PAF, a product of macrophages, as well as platelets, augments the contractile response of human bronchi to histamine (81). The cytokine tumor necrosis factor α, produced by a variety of lung inflammatory cells, also potentiates the contractile response to electrical field stimulation (82). Thus, these findings provide a direct link between the products of inflammatory cells and smooth muscle hyperresponsiveness. Whether these products or their effects are the link that is missing when tissue is studied *in vitro*, and therefore explains why, in previous studies, hyperresponsiveness has not been demonstrable, remains to be clarified.

Passive Sensitization

One of the most consistent features of asthma is its association with allergy (83). Exactly how the allergic process is linked to the pathologic changes which are the hallmark of asthma, is the subject of intensive investigation and is covered elsewhere in this volume. In recent years, we have addressed the question of how the allergic process affects smooth muscle function by examin-

ing the effect of passive sensitization on human airway smooth muscle. Tissue is obtained from a patient who is not sensitized, i.e., is either known to be skin-test negative to a range of common allergens or, most importantly, in whom the bronchus *in vitro* does not exhibit a contractile response to the application of common allergens. All tissues tested from a particular patient react in a reproducible manner to antigen stimulation and in a quantal fashion—either a contraction is elicited or it is not. Bronchial rings are then divided into two groups. One-half of the rings are incubated overnight in serum from a highly atopic asthmatic patient. The total serum immunoglobulin (Ig)E is in excess of 1000 IU/mL and the radioallergosorbent test (RAST) is 4^+ to dermatophagoides (d.) pteronyssinus. The remaining tissues are incubated in the serum of an individual who has no history of allergic disease, is skin-test negative to a complete range of antigens, and whose total serum IgE does not exceed 20 IU/mL. After the 12-hour incubation, reactivity to a range of contractile and relaxant agonists is studied. After these responses have been obtained, the allergic status of all tissues is tested by the application of allergen. All tissues which have been incubated in allergic serum contract to d. pteronyssinus, whereas those incubated in nonallergic serum exhibit no such response. Tissue response is homogeneous for any given patient, in that all tissues test either negative or positive for antigen at this stage. These experiments have given rise to the following important information. In passively sensitized tissue, contractile responses to histamine, K^+,

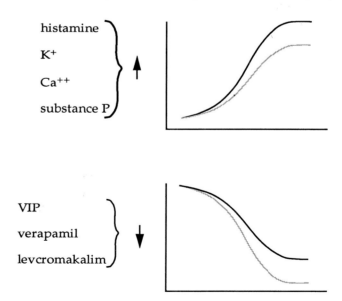

FIG. 4. Representation of the effects of passive sensitization on contraction and relaxation responses in human bronchi. Contractile responses to histamine, K^+, Ca^{++} and substance P are increased, while relaxation responses to vasoactive intestinal peptide (VIP) the calcium channel antagonist verapamil and the K^+ channel agonist levcromakalim are reduced. The bold line indicates the passively sensitized tissues.

and substance P, but not carbachol, were increased (84–86). These heightened contractile responses have been noted, not only with regard to force generation, but also with respect to increased velocity of shortening and shortening capacity (87). Relaxation responses are also altered by passive sensitization. Responses to vasoactive intestinal polypeptide (VIP), the calcium channel antagonist verapamil, and the K^+ channel opener levcromakalim were decreased (88). By contrast, responses to neither the β-adrenoceptor agonist isoprenaline, nor an adenylate cyclase activator, nor cAMP were affected (89) (Fig. 4).

The mechanisms underlying these changes require investigation and here some guidance may be available from studies in animal tissue. In the guinea pig, Souhrada and Souhrada (90) have provided evidence that the relevant immunoglobulin in this species, namely IgG_1, binds directly to the smooth muscle cell, thereby altering its electrical and biochemical properties. The sequelae of this are increases in calcium and sodium influx, potentiation of electrogenic Na/K-ATPase, and potentiation of protein kinase C. (90–92).

IS THERE A BIOCHEMICAL ABNORMALITY IN AIRWAY SMOOTH MUSCLE REACTIVITY?

Investigation of the biochemical/signal transduction events associated with airway smooth muscle contraction has revealed that the following series of steps takes place. Stimulation of a cell surface receptor results in a rise in intracellular calcium, either from entry into the cell via a voltage-dependent or voltage-independent calcium channel, or by means of a release of calcium from intracellular stores. This causes calcium to bind to calmodulin to form a calcium-calmodulin complex. This results in the activation of myosin light-chain kinase which phosphorylates the 20kDa light chain of myosin. Phosphorylated myosin then interacts with actin and the ATP hydrolyzed causes the sliding of thick and thin filaments. The contraction that results can be reversed when myosin light chain is dephosphorylated by endogenous phosphatases and myosin light chain kinase (MLCK) is deactivated. However, a two-stage model of smooth muscle contraction has also been proposed in which the initial events are as described previously and the immediate contractile response is mediated by MLCK. A second, sustained phase of contraction may also occur associated with activation of protein kinase C (PKC) after the formation of diacylglycerol from membrane phospholipids. Activated PKC phosphorylates a series of structural and regulatory components of the filamin-actin-desmin fibrillar domain. PKC also may phosphorylate MLC at different sites from those phosphorylated by MLCK (93) (Fig. 5). Although there is

some controversy surrounding the extent of PKC involvement in airway smooth muscle contraction, there is recent evidence obtained in functional length-tension studies to suggest that it is involved in the contraction of human airway smooth muscle to agonists such as histamine (94). Not only does PKC have a role in the regulation of tone in airway smooth muscle, but it is also implicated in cell growth and hypertrophy (95,96). Activation of PKC by phorbol esters stimulates proliferation of human airway smooth muscle in culture and, conversely, inhibition of PKC by relatively specific inhibitors inhibits growth of muscle cells (97,98). Proliferating cells exhibit greater PKC activity than quiescent cells and, during proliferation, relatively more PKC is found in the particulate cell fraction, indicating that PKC has been activated and translocated to the cell membrane (95). PKC was originally designated a single enzyme with dependence on calcium and phospholipids, but recently, it has emerged that PKC is, in fact, a family of isoenzymes which have different biochemical characteristics, substrates, and co-factor requirements. The various isoforms, which differ in their tissue distribution and function, have been divided into three groups: group A, the conventional or calcium-dependent isoforms, which are α, βI, βII, and γ; group B, the calcium-independent or novel isoforms -δ, ε, η and θ; and group C, the atypical isoforms γ, μ, ι, and ζ. Little was known of the isoform pattern of expression of PKC in airway smooth muscle until a recent report that addressed this question in canine airway smooth muscle (99). Of the conventional isoforms, PKC βI and βII, but not PKC α, were expressed as well as PKC δ, ε, and θ. The lung specific isoform, PKCη, was not detected, but there was expression of PKC ζ. The fact that multiple isoforms of PKC are expressed in airway smooth muscle would suggest a complex role for this enzyme in both contraction and replication.

The delineation of these pathways opens up a new area for investigation of possibilities for abnormalities in these mechanisms which could account for smooth muscle dysfunction. It is apparent that, for instance, if MLCK were to be overactive in airway smooth muscle, then an increase in contractility could occur. Conversely, if a deficiency in the activity in one of the phosphatases which remove phosphate groups from MLC were to occur, again excessive contraction could result. Indeed, there is some evidence to support this possibility in experiments conducted in dogs. Animals which are sensitized to ragweed from birth display airway hyperresponsiveness. This has been associated with the finding that there is an increase in the MLC phosphorylation in the bronchial smooth muscle (100,101). This increase could either have been the result of excessive MLCK, or deficient phosphatase activity, and, in fact, the former and not the latter, proved

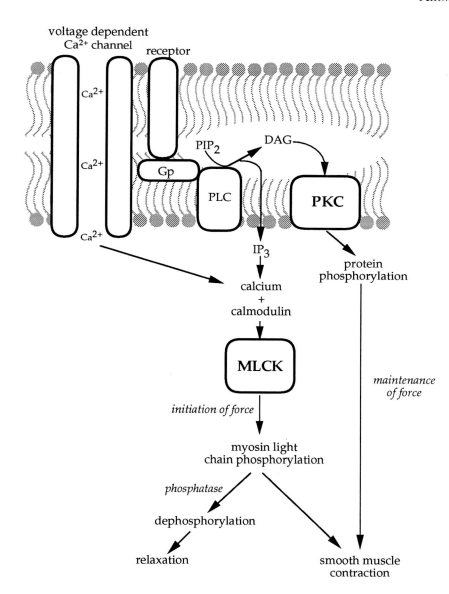

FIG. 5. Schematic representation of the signal transduction pathways to demonstrate the roles for protein kinase C (PKC) and myosin light chain kinase (MLCK) in airway smooth muscle contraction. Gp, G protein; DAG, diacyl glycerol; PIP$_2$, phosphatidylinositol 4,5 biphosphate; IP$_3$ phosphatidylinositol 3,4,5 triphosphate; PLC phospholipase C.

to be the case. These studies provide a direct link, albeit in animals, between a muscle biochemical abnormality and airway hyperresponsiveness. Whether these data can be obtained from human airway tissue remains to be established.

Similarly, it is possible that an overexpression of one isoform of PKC, at the expense of others, could result in either excessive contraction of airway smooth muscle and/or an excessive growth of airway smooth muscle. Once the pattern of expression of PKC isoforms has been identified in human airway smooth muscle, then it would theoretically be possible to investigate whether the pattern of expression and activity is altered in association with disease states. For this to be feasible, however, specific substrates for the different isoforms would be re-quired, and these are as yet not available. Once this line of investigation is further explored, specific therapeutic targeting with selective PKC isoform inhibitors may become a possibility.

ACKNOWLEDGMENTS

The work in this chapter has been supported by grants from The National Health and Medical Research Council of Australia, The Asthma Foundation of New South Wales, and Community Health and Antituberculosis Association. Thanks are extended to Brent McParland for Figure 3 and to Dr. Peter Johnson for general assistance with the chapter and for Figures 1, 2, 4, and 5.

REFERENCES

1. Finney MJB, Anderson SD, Black JL. Terfenadine and nonisotonic aerosols. *Am Rev Respir Dis* 1990;141:1151–1157.
2. Huber H, Koessler K. The pathology of bronchial asthma. *Arch Intern Med* 1922;30:689–760.
3. Messer JW, Peters GA, WA. B. Causes of death and pathological findings in 304 cases of bronchial asthma. *Dis Chest* 1960;38: 616–624.
4. Richards W, Patrick JR. Death From Asthma in Children. *Am J Dis Child* 1965;110:4–21.
5. Dunnill M, Massarella G, Anderson J. A comparison of the quantitative anatomy of the bronchi in normal subjects, in status asthmaticus, in chronic bronchitis and in emphysema. *Thorax* 1969;24:176–179.
6. Heard B, Hossain S. Hyperplasia of bronchial muscle in asthma. *J Pathol* 1973;110:319–331.
7. Hossain S. Quatitative measurement of bronchial muscle in men with asthma. *Am Rev Respir Dis* 1973;107:99–109.
8. Carroll N, Elliot J, Morton A, James A. Structure of large and small airways in fatal and non fatal asthma. *Am Rev Respir Dis* 1993;147: 405–410.
9. Saetta M, Di Stefano A, Rosina C, Thiene G, Fabbri L. Quantitative structural analysis of peripheral airways and arteries in sudden fatal asthma. *Am Rev Respir Dis* 1991;143:138–143.
10. Ebina M. Hyperreactive site in the airway tree of asthmatics thickened bronchial muscles—morphometry. *Am Rev Respir Dis* 1990;5: 1327–1332.
11. Hogg J. Pathology of asthma. *J Allergy Clin Immunol* 1993;92:1–5.
12. Sobonya R. Quantitative structural alterations in long-standing allergic asthma. *Am Rev Respir Dis* 1984;130:289–296.
13. Lambert R, Wiggs B, Kuwano K, Hogg J, Pare P. Functional significance of increased airway smooth muscle in asthma and COPD. *J Appl Physiol* 1993;74:2771–2781.
14. Ebina M, Takahashi T, Chiba T, Motomiya M. Cellular hypertrophy and hyperplasia of airway smooth muscles underlying bronchial asthma:a 3-D morphometric study. *Am Rev Respir Dis* 1993;148: 720–726.
15. Panettieri R, Yadvish P, Kelly A, Rubenstein N, Kotlikoff M. Histamine stimulates proliferation of airway smooth muscle and induces *c-fos* expression. *Am J Physiol* 1990;259:L365–L371.
16. Hirst SJ, Barnes PJ, Twort CHC. Quantifying proliferation of cultured human and rabbit airway smooth muscle cells in responses to serum and platelet-derived growth factor. *Am J Respir Cell Mol Biol* 1992; 7:574–581.
17. Noveral J, Rosenberg S, Anbar R, Pawlowski N, Grunstein M. Role of endothelin-1 in regulating proliferation of cultured rabbit airway smooth muscle cells. *Am J Physiol* 1992;263:L317–L324.
18. Johnson P, Carey D, Armour C, Black J. PGE₂ and heparin are antiproliferative mediators for human airway smooth muscle cells in culture. *Am J Physiol* 1995;in press.
19. Lazaar AL, Albelda SM, Pilewski JM, Brennan B, Pure E, Panettieri RA. T lymphocytes adhere to airway smooth muscle cells via integrins and CD44 and induce smooth muscle cell DNA synthesis. *J Exp Med* 1994;180:807–816.
20. Hislop A, Haworth S. Airway size and structure in the normal fetal and infant lung and the effect of premature delivery and artifical ventilation. *Am Rev Respir Dis* 1989;140:1717–1726.
21. Smith P, Janiga K, Bruce M. Strain increases airway smooth muscle cell proliferation. *Am J Respir Cell Mol Biol* 1994;10:85–90.
22. Somlyo AP, Somlyo AV. Signal transduction and regulation in smooth muscle. *Nature* 1994;372:231–236.
23. Goldie R, Paterson J, Wale J. Pharmacological responses of human and porcine lung parenchyma, bronchi and pulmonary artery. *Br J Pharmacol* 1982;76:515–521.
24. Brink C, Grimaud C, Guillot C, Orehek J. The interaction between indomethacin and contractile agents on human isolated airway muscle. *Br J Pharmacol* 1980;60:383–388.
25. Black J, Turner A, Shaw J. α-adrenoceptors in human peripheral lung. *Eur J Pharmacol* 1981;72:83–86.
26. Armour C, McKay K, Johnson P, Glanville A, Black J. Does the disease state of the patient influence the responsiveness of human airways studied *in vitro*? *J Appl Physiol* 1996;80:2211–2218.
27. Johnson P, McKay K, Armour C, Black J. The maintenance of func-

28. tional activity in human isolated bronchus after cryopreservation. *Pulm Pharmacol* 1995;8:43–48.
29. Sollman T, Gilbert A. Microscopic observations of bronchiolar reactions. *J Pharmacol Exp Ther* 1937;61:272–285.
30. Hall I, Widdop S, Townsend P, Daykin K. Control of cyclic AMP levels in primary cultures of human tracheal smooth muscle. *Br J Pharmacol* 1992;107:422–428.
31. Panettieri R, Kotlikoff M. A human airway smooth muscle cell line that retains physiological responsiveness. *Am J Physiol* 1989;256: C329–C335.
32. Stewart A, Tomlinson P, Fernandes D, Wilson J, Harris T. Tumor necrosis factor a modulates mitogenic responses of human cultured airway smooth muscle. *Am J Resp Cell Mol Biol* 1995;12:110–119.
33. de Jongste J, Sterk P, Willems L, Mons H, Timmers M, Kerrebijn K. Comparison of maximal bronchoconstriction *in vivo* and airway smooth muscle responses *in vitro* in nonasthmatic humans. *Am Rev Respir Dis* 1988;138:321–326.
34. Armour C, Lazar N, Schellenberg R, Taylor S, Chan N, Hogg J, Pare P. A comparison of *in vivo* and *in vitro* human airway reactivity to histamine. *Am Rev Respir Dis* 1984;129:907–910.
35. Armour C, Black J, Berend N, Woolcock AJ. The relationship between bronchial hyperresponsiveness to methacholine and airway smooth muscle structure and reactivity. *Respir Physiol* 1984;58:223–233.
36. Vincenc K, Black J, Yan K, Armour C, Donnelly P, Woolcock A. Comparison of *in vivo* and *in vitro* responses to histamine in human airways. *Am Rev Respir Dis* 1983; 128:875–879.
37. Roberts J, Raeburn D, Rodger I, Thomson N. Comparison of *in vivo* airway responsiveness and *in vitro* smooth muscle sensitivity to methacholine in man. *Thorax* 1984;39: 837–843.
38. Roberts J, Rodger I, Thomson N. Airway responsiveness to histamine in man: effect of atropine on *in vivo* and *in vitro* comparison. *Thorax* 1985;40:261–267.
39. Roberts J, Rodger I, Thomson N. *In vivo* and *in vitro* human airway responsiveness to leukotriene D₄ in patients without asthma. *J Allergy Clin Immunol* 1987;80:688–694.
40. Schellenberg R, Foster A. *In vitro* responses of human asthmatic airway and pulmonary vascular smooth muscle. *Int Arch Allergy Appl Immunol* 1984;75:237–241.
41. de Jongste J, Mons H, Bonta I, Kerribijn K. Human asthmatic airway responses *in vitro*—a case report. *Eur J Respir Dis* 1987;71:23–29.
42. Whicker S, Armour C, Black J. Responsiveness of bronchial smooth muscle from asthmatic patients to relaxant and contractile agonists. *Pulm Pharmacol* 1988;1:25–31.
43. Goldie R, Spina D, Henry P, Lulich K, Paterson J. *In vitro* responsiveness of human asthmatic bronchus to carbachol, histamine, β-adrenoceptor agonists and theophylline. *Br J Clin Pharmacol* 1986; 22:669–676.
44. Cerrina J, Labat C, Haye-Legrande I, Raffestin B, Benveniste J, Brink C. Human isolated bronchial muscle preparations from asthmatic patients: effects of indomethacin and contractile agonists. *Prostaglandins* 1989;37:457–470.
45. Dahlen S-E, Hedqvist P, Hammarström S, Samuelsson B. Leukotrienes are potent constrictors of human bronchi. *Nature* 1980; 288:484–486.
46. Björck T, Gustafsson L, Dahlen S. Isolated bronchi from asthmatics are hyperresponsive to adenosine, which apparently acts indirectly by liberation of leukotrienes and histamine. *Am Rev Respir Dis* 1992; 145:1087–1091.
47. Bai T. Abnormalities in airway smooth muscle in fatal asthma. *Am Rev Respir Dis* 1990;141:552–557.
48. Bai T. Abnormalities in airway smooth muscle in fatal asthma. A comparison between trachea and bronchus. *Am Rev Respir Dis* 1991;143: 441–443.
49. Daniel E, Kannan M, Davis C, Posey-Daniel V. Ultrastructural studies of the neuromuscular control of human tracheal and bronchial muscle. *Respir Physiol* 1986;63:109–128.
50. Turki J, Liggett SB. Receptor-specific functional properties of β2-adrenergic receptor autoantibodies in asthma. *Am J Respir Cell Mol Biol* 1995;12:531–539.
51. Green SA, Turki J, Bejarano P, Hall IP, Liggett SB. Influence of β2-adrenergic receptor genotypes on signal transduction in human airway smooth muscle cells. *Am J Respir Cell Mol Biol* 1995;13:25–33
52. Belvisi MG, Stretton D, Yacoub M, Barnes PJ. Nitric oxide is the en-

dogenous neurotransmitter of bronchodilator nerves in human. *Eur J Pharmacol* 1992;210:221–222.

52. Szentivanyi A, Heim O, Schultze P. Changes in adrenoceptor densities in membranes of lung tissue and lymphocytes from patients with atopic disease. *Ann N Y Acad Sci* 1979;332: 295–298.

53. Bai TR, Zhou D, Aubert JD, Lizee G, Hayashi S, Bondy GP. Expression of beta 2-adrenergic receptor mRNA in peripheral lung in asthma and chronic obstructive pulmonary disease. *Am J Respir Cell Mol Biol* 1993;8:325–333.

54. Bai T, Mak J, Barnes P. A comparison of β-adrenergic receptors and *in vitro* relaxant responses to isoproterenol in asthmatic airway smooth muscle. *Am J Respir Cell Mol Biol* 1992;6:647–651.

55. Raaijmakers J, Wassink G, Kreukniet J, Terpstra G. Adrenoceptors in lung tissue: characterization, modulation, and relations with pulmonary function. *Eur J Respir Dis* 1984;65; Suppl 135:215–220.

56. Joad J, Casale T. (³H)quinuclidinyl benzilate binding to the human lung muscarinic receptor. *Biochem Pharmacol* 1988;37:973–976.

57. Minette P, Barnes P. Prejunctional inhibitory muscarinic receptors on cholinergic nerves in human and guinea-pig airways. *J Appl Physiol* 1988;64:2532–2538.

58. Fryer A, Jacoby D. Function of pulmonary M2 muscarinic receptors in antigen-challenged guinea pigs is restored by heparin and poly-L-glutamate. *J Clin Invest* 1992;90:2292–2298.

59. Black P, Ghatei M, Takahashi K, Bretherton-Watt D, Krausz T, Dollery C, Bloom S. Formation of endothelin by cultured airway epithelial cells. *FEBS Lett* 1989;255:129–132.

60. Springall D, Howarth P, Counihan H. Endothelin immunoreactivity in airway epithelium in asthmatic patients. *Lancet* 1991; 337:697–701.

61. McKay K, Black J, Diment L, Armour C. Functional and autoradiographic studies of endothelin-1 and endothelin-2 in human bronchi, pulmonary arteries, and airway parasympathetic ganglia. *J Cardiovasc Pharmacol* 1991;17:s206–s209.

62. McKay K, Black J, Armour C. Phosphoramidon potentiates the contractile response to endothelin-3, but not endothelin-1 in isolated airway tissue. *Br J Pharmacol* 1992;105:929–932.

63. McKay K, Armour C, Black J. Endothelin-3 increases transmission in the rabbit pulmonary parasympathetic nervous system. *J Cardiovasc Pharmacol* 1993;22:S181.

64. Stewart AG, Grigoriadis G, Harris T. Mitogenic actions of endothelin-1 and epidermal growth factor in cultured airway smooth muscle. *Clin Exp Pharmacol Physiol* 1994;21:277–285.

65. Johnson P, Carey D, Armour C, Black J. Endothelin-1 and platelet derived growth factor are co-mitogenic on human airway smooth muscle cells in culture. *Am J Respir Crit Care Med* 1995;151:A48.

66. Knott P, D'Aprile A, Henry P, Hay D, Goldie R. Receptors for endothelin-1 in asthmatic human peripheral lung. *Br J Pharmacol* 1995; 114:1–3.

67. Van Koppen C, Siero H, Rodrigues de Miranda J, Beld A, Ariens E. Simultaneous assay of muscarinic and β-adrenergic receptors using a double isotope technique. *Biochem Biophys Res Comm* 1984;120: 665–669.

68. Stephens N, Kroeger E, Mehta J. Force-velocity characteristics of respiratory airway smooth muscle. *J Appl Physiol* 1969;26:685–692.

69. Mitchell R, Kelly E, Leff A. Effect of *in vitro* preconditioning on tracheal smooth muscle responsiveness. *Am J Physiol* 1991;260: L168–L173.

70. de Jongste JC, Mons H, Van Strik R, Bonta IL, Kerrebijn KF. Comparison of human bronchiolar smooth muscle responsiveness *in vitro* with histological signs of inflammation. *Thorax* 1987;42: 870–876.

71. Mitchell HW, Willet KE, Sparrow MP. Perfused bronchial segment and bronchial strip: narrowing vs. isometric force by mediators. *J Appl Physiol* 1989;66:2704–2709.

72. Omari TI, Sparrow MP, Mitchell HW. Responsiveness of human isolated bronhial segments and its relationship to epithelial loss. *Br J Clin Pharmacol* 1993;35:357–365.

73. Skoogh B, Svedmyr N. β2 adrenoceptor stimulation inhibits ganglionic transmission in ferret trachea. *Pulm Pharmacol* 1989;1: 167–172.

74. Tanaka D, Grunstein M. Mechanisms of substance P-induced contraction of rabbit airway smooth muscle. *J Appl Physiol* 1984;57: 1551–1557.

75. Black JL, Johnson PRA, Alouan L, Armour CL. Neurokinin A with

76. Marthan R, Martin C, Amedee T, Mironneau J. Calcium channel currents in isolated smooth muscle cells from human bronchus. *J Appl Physiol* 1989;66:1706–1714.

77. Black JL, Armour CL, Johnson PRA, Alouan LA, Barnes PJ. The action of a potassium channel activator, BRL 38227 (Lemakalim), on human airway smooth muscle. *Am Rev Respir Dis* 1990;142: 1384.

78. Hallahan AR, Armour CL, Black JL. Products of neutrophils and eosinophils increase the responsiveness of human isolated bronchial tissue. *Eur Respir J* 1990;3:554–558.

79. Hughes J, McKay K, Johnson P, Tragoulias S, Black J, Armour CL. Neutrophil-induced human bronchial hyperresponsiveness *in vitro*-pharmacological modulation. *Clin Exp Allergy* 1993;23:251–256.

80. Rabe KF, Munoz NM, Vita AJ, Morton BE, Magnussen H, Leff AR. Contraction of human bronchial smooth muscle caused by activated human eosinophils. *Am J Physiol* 1994;267:L326–L334.

81. Johnson P, Black J, Armour C. Investigation of the platelet activating factor induced contraction of human isolated bronchus. *Eur Resp J* 1992;5:970–974.

82. Armour C, Anticevich S, Hughes JM, Black JL. Tumour necrosis factor-alpha (TNF-α) increases responsiveness of human airways. *Am J Respir Crit Care Med* 1995;151:A396.

83. Burrows B, Martinez F, Halonen M, Baerbee R, Cline M. Association of asthma with serum IgE levels and skin-test reactivity to allergens. *New Engl J Med* 1989;320:271–277.

84. Black J, Marthan R, Armour C, Johnson P. Sensitization alters contractile responses and calcium influx in human airway smooth muscle. *J Allergy Clin Immunol* 1989;84:440–447.

85. Marthan R, Crevel H, Guenard H, Savineau J. Responsiveness to histamine in human sensitized airway smooth muscle. *Respir Physiol* 1992;90:239.

86. Ben-Jebria A, Marthan R, Rossetti M, Savineau J-P. Effect of passive sensitization on the mechanical activity of human isolated bronchial smoth muscle induced by substance P, neurokinin A and VIP. *Br J Pharmacol* 1993;109:131.

87. Mitchell RW, Ruhlmann E, Magnussen H, Leff AR, Rabe KF. Passive sensitization of human bronchi augments smooth muscle shortening velocity and capacity. *Am J Physiol* 1994;267:L218–L222.

88. Ben-Jebria A, Marthan R, Rossetti M, Savineau J. Effect of passive sensitisation on the mechanical activity of human isolated bronchial smooth muscle induced by substance P, neurokinin A and VIP. *Br J Pharmacol* 1993;109:131.

89. Villanove X, Marthan R, Black J. Sensitization and relaxation in human airways. *Am Rev Respir Dis* 1993;148:107.

90. Souhrada M, Souhrada J. Potentiation of Na⁺—electrogenic pump of airway smooth muscle by sensitization. *Respir Physiol* 1982;47: 69–81.

91. Souhrada M, Souhrada J, . The role of protein kinase-C in sensitization and antigen response of airway smooth muscle. *Am Rev Respir Dis* 1989;140:1567–1572.

92. Souhrada M, Souhrada JF. Immunological changes of airways smooth muscle reactivity. In: Raeburn D, Giembycz MA, eds. *Airways smooth muscle: development and regulation of contractility.* Basel: Birkhauser Verlag, 1994;219–258.

93. Kamm K, Hsu L, Kubota Y, Stull J. Phosphorylation of smooth muscle myosin heavy and light chains: effects of phorbol dibuyrate and agonists. *J Biol Chem* 1989;264:21223.

94. Yang K, Black J. The involvement of protein kinase C in the contraction of human airway smooth muscle. *Eur J Pharmacol* 1995;275: 283–289.

95. Adamo S, Caporale C, Aguanno S, et al. Proliferating and quiescent cells exhibit different subcellular distribution of protein kinase C activity. *FEBS Lett* 1986;195: 352–356.

96. Newby A, Assender J, Evans M, Lim K, Bennett M, Evans G. Transduction pathways for growth stimulatory and inhibitory actions of vasoactive agents. *Exp Nephrol* 1994;2: 94–100.

97. Panettieri R, Cohen M, Bilgen G. Airway smooth muscle proliferation is inhibited by microinjection of the catalytic subunit of cAMP dependent protein kinase. *Am Rev Respir Dis* 1993;147:A252.

98. Hirst S, Webb B, Giembycz M, Barnes P, Twort C. Inhibition of fetal calf serum-stimulated proliferation of rabbit cultured tracheal smooth

muscle cells by selective inhibitors of protein kinase c (and protein tyrosine kinase). *Am J Respir Cell Mol Biol* 1995; 12:149–161.

99. Donnelly R, Yang K, Bishr Omary M, Azhar S, Black J. Expression of multiple isoenzymes of protein kinase C in airway smooth muscle. *Am J Respir Cell Mol Biol* 1995;13:253–256.

100. Jiang H, Rao K, Halayko AJ, Liu X, Stephens NL. Ragweed sensitization-induced increase in myosin light chain kinase content in canine airway smoth muscle. *Am J Respir Cell Mol Biol* 1992;7:567.

101. Liu X, Halayko A, Liu G, Rao K, Jiang H, Stephens N. Myosin light chain phosphatase activity in ragweed pollen-sensitized canine tracheal smooth muscle. *Am J Respir Cell Mol Biol* 1994;11:676–681.

Asthma, edited by P.J. Barnes, M.M. Grunstein, A.R. Leff, and A.J. Woolcock. Lippincott–Raven Publishers, Philadelphia © 1997.

▪ 59 ▪

Airway Smooth Muscle Hyperplasia and Hypertrophy

Reynold A. Panettieri, Jr. and Michael M. Grunstein

The principal dysfunctional features of the airways in asthma include exaggerated narrowing to bronchoconstrictor agonists and attenuated relaxation to beta-adrenoceptor stimulation. These physiological perturbations are associated with inflammation and re-modeling of the airways, the latter including an increase in airway smooth muscle (ASM) cell mass, disruption of the airway epithelium, and changes in the airway tissue extracellular matrix. While the complex mechanistic interplay between these altered functional and structural features of the asthmatic airway remains to be identified, in recent years a host of studies have provided compelling evidence in support of two fundamental concepts: (1) that the actions of various infiltrating inflammatory cells including mast cells, eosinophils, lymphocytes, and neutrophils, significantly contribute to the initiation and perpetuation of the changes in airway structure and function in asthma, primarily via the release of various pro-inflammatory mediators and growth factors; and (2) that the structural re-modeling of the airways, notably including an increase in ASM cell mass, importantly contributes to the enhanced airway constrictor responsiveness and airflow limitation in asthma. Both these basic concepts are addressed in various sections throughout this text, with the present chapter focused on much of the information gained to date on the cellular and molecular mechanisms regulating ASM growth. The chapter begins with overviews of the key structural and pathophysiological changes in the asthmatic airway, followed by discussion of the extracellular stimuli and receptors coupled to ASM cell hyperplasia and/or hypertrophy, and ends with overviews of the intracellular second messenger and downstream effector systems implicated in regulating smooth muscle cell growth.

R. A. Panettieri, Jr.: Department of Medicine, Pulmonary and Critical Care Division, University of Pennsylvania Medical Center, Philadelphia, Pennsylvania 19104-4283.
M. M. Grunstein: Division of Pulmonary Medicine, The Children's Hospital of Philadelphia, University of Pennsylvania School of Medicine, Philadelphia, Pennsylvania 19104.

PATHOLOGY OF THE AIRWAYS IN ASTHMA

Although asthma typically induces reversible airway obstruction, in some asthmatics, airflow obstruction can become irreversible (1–3). Such obstruction may be a consequence of persistent structural changes in the airway wall due to the frequent stimulation of ASM by contractile agonists, inflammatory mediators, and growth factors. Increased smooth muscle mass, which has been attributed to increases in myocyte number and in myocyte size, is a well-documented pathologic finding in the airways of patients with chronic severe asthma (4–8). Little information is available, however, with respect to factors that promote ASM cell proliferation or the cellular mechanisms that regulate airway myocyte growth.

Many studies have characterized the stimulation of smooth muscle growth in response to mitogenic agents such as polypeptide growth factors, inflammatory mediators, and cytokines (9–15). Other trophic factors, such as alterations in extracellular matrix and mechanical stress, have also been identified (16). In recent studies, the observation that contractile agonists induce smooth muscle cell proliferation may be a critical link between the chronic stimulation of muscle contraction and myocyte proliferation (9,17,18). Although the mechanisms by which agonists induce cell proliferation are unknown, similarities exist between signal transduction processes activated by these agents, and those of known growth factors. Interestingly, growth factors also stimulate smooth muscle contraction (11,12). These diverse extracellular stimuli appear to induce cell growth, at least in part, by activating certain common intracellular signal transduction pathways. The identification of critical regulatory sites in these pathways may provide new therapeutic approaches to alter the airway remodeling seen in patients with chronic severe asthma.

Apart from myocyte hyperplasia, other chronic adaptive changes in ASM may contribute to increasing ASM mass. Alterations in contractile protein expression may increase myocyte size and also contribute to increasing smooth muscle mass. In addition, altered secretion of extracellular matrix by myocytes may induce sub-basement membrane collagen deposition that significantly contributes to airway remodeling. To date, few studies have addressed whether extracellular matrix secretion or alterations in ASM contractile protein expression are important in altering ASM cell function.

PATHOPHYSIOLOGY RELATED TO INCREASED ASM CELL MASS IN ASTHMA

Emerging evidence suggests that the structural changes of the airways in asthma importantly contribute to their altered function in this disease. In this regard, recent theoretical models based on morphometric analyses of asthmatic airways collectively demonstrate that the mechanism of excessive airway narrowing may be attributed to intrinsic changes in the ASM, a reduction in the load acting against the contracting ASM, and/or altered airway wall geometry (19–23). Accordingly, the increase in ASM cell mass, coupled to inflammation-induced perturbations of the surrounding extracellular matrix, may give rise to increased ASM contractility together with a reduction in the load acting on the ASM due to peribronchial inflammation (23–25). This process may result in disruption of normal airway/parenchymal interdependence. As the latter phenomenon serves to maintain the integrity of volume-dependency of airway caliber and patency, disruption of this interdependence may, at least in part, contribute to fixed airways obstruction and gas trapping, as well as to the exaggerated degree of airway narrowing observed in asthmatic subjects in response to bronchoconstrictor agonists (23,24).

An increase in smooth muscle cell mass may be intrinsically related to altered contractility of the ASM, as evidenced by the finding of a positive correlation between the volume of airway smooth muscle and its degree of isometric force of contraction to *in vitro* administration of constrictor agonists (26). Moreover, in considering the mechanics of airway narrowing in asthma, James et al. (19) have provided a compelling argument that airway wall thickening importantly determines the enhanced magnitude of airway constrictor responsiveness seen in asthmatic individuals. In their analysis using morphometric data, these authors calculated that the enhanced airway wall area in asthmatic bronchi, in part, attributed to an increase in ASM cell mass, allows for a relatively greater increase in airways resistance in response to a given degree of ASM shortening. This computational analysis was subsequently extended by Lambert et al. (22) to demonstrate that among the morphological changes seen in asthmatic airways, including adventitial and submucosal thickening and smooth muscle hyperplasia, the latter most importantly contributes to the increase in airway resistance in response to bronchoconstrictor agonists.

Given the previously mentioned considerations regarding the important pathophysiological consequences of an increase in ASM cell mass in asthma, the ensuing sections of this chapter provide a review of the emerging knowledge on the cellular and molecular transmembrane signaling mechanisms that regulate ASM cell proliferation.

EXTRACELLULAR STIMULI TRANSDUCE GROWTH SIGNALS BY ACTIVATING RECEPTORS COUPLED TO SECOND MESSENGER SYSTEMS

The binding of mitogens to their receptors promotes the generation of early signals in the membrane cytosol and the nucleus that leads to cell growth. Since the initiation of deoxyribonucleic acid (DNA) synthesis occurs 10 to 15 hours after the addition of mitogens, it is expected that knowledge of these early events will provide clues regarding the primary regulatory mechanisms.

Smooth muscle cell proliferation is stimulated by mitogens that fall into two broad categories: (a) those that activate receptors with intrinsic tyrosine kinase activity (RTK); and (b) those that mediate their effects through receptors coupled to heterotrimeric guanosine triphosphate (GTP)-binding proteins (G proteins) and activate nonreceptor-linked tyrosine kinases found in the cytoplasm (Fig. 1). Although both pathways increase cytosolic cal-

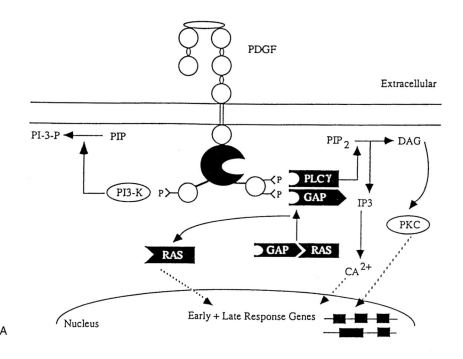

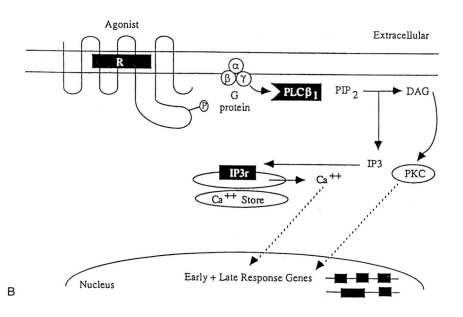

FIG. 1. Characterization of smooth muscle cell mitogens: An overview. **A:** Some growth factors stimulate cell surface receptors with intrinsic tyrosine kinase activity (RTK). **B:** Others activate receptors coupled to heterotrimeric G proteins. Activation of either receptor increases cytosolic calcium through activation of specific phospholipase C isozymes (PLC) that hydrolyze phosphatidylinositol 3,4-bisphosphate (PIP$_2$) to phosphatidylinositol 3,4,5-trisphosphate IP3 and diacylglycerol (DAG). These second messengers then activate other cytosolic tyrosine kinases as well as serine and threonine kinases such as protein kinase C (PKC). Stimulation of RTK-dependent receptors also activates phosphatidylinositol 3-phosphate kinase (PI 3-kinase); however, the role of 3′-inositol phosphates in signaling smooth muscle cell growth remains unknown. (From Panettieri RA. In: Raeburn D, Giembycz MA, eds. *Airways smooth muscle: development and regulation of contractility.* Basel: Birkhauser Verlag, 1994;42, with permission.)

cium through activation of phospholipase C (PLC), different PLC isoenzymes appear to be involved. Activated PLC hydrolyzes phosphatidylinositol bisphosphate (PIP$_2$) to phosphatidylinositol trisphosphate (IP$_3$) and diacylglycerol (DAG) (27). These second messengers activate other cytosolic tyrosine kinases, as well as serine and threonine kinases (protein kinase C and G) that have pleotrophic effects including the activation of protooncogenes (28,29). Protooncogenes, which are a family of cellular genes (c-onc) that control normal cellular growth and differentiation, were characterized initially from viral genes (v-onc) that induced cellular transformation in eukaryotic cells. The protein products of protooncogenes play a critical role in transducing growth signals from the cell surface to the nucleus and in regulating gene transcription.

Growth Factor Receptors with Intrinsic Receptor Tyrosine Kinase Activity.

Growth factors are defined as polypeptides that stimulate cell proliferation through binding to specific high-affinity cell membrane receptors (30). Growth factor receptors with intrinsic tyrosine kinase activity (RTK) play a central role in the regulatory mechanisms controlling cell growth and proliferation. In smooth muscle, epidermal growth factor (EGF), basic fibroblast growth factor (FGF), platelet-derived growth factor (PDGF), insulin-like growth factor-1 (IGF-1), and colony stimulating factor-1 (CSF-1) induce cell proliferation by binding to receptors with RTK activity (18,31–34). Importantly, these growth factors are among the most potent smooth muscle mitogens.

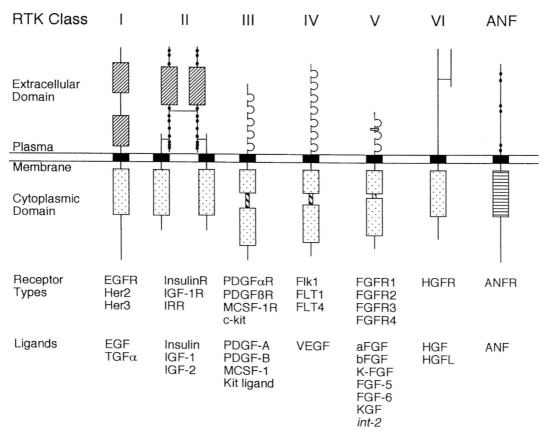

FIG. 2. Pulmonary receptor tyrosine kinases (RTKs). Representative receptors and specific ligands for each RTK class are listed below the schematized receptors. Stippled boxes symbolize the tyrosine kinase domain(s), separated by slashed kinase insert regions in Class III, IV, and V receptors; slashed extracellular boxes symbolize cysteine-rich regions and dots represent conserved cysteine residues; semicircles symbolize immunoglobulin-like domains, with an interspersed acid box domain depicted by the open box in the Class V receptors; the striped cytoplasmic box of the ANF receptor symbolizes its guanylyl cyclase domain. Principal abbreviations: EGF, EGFR, epidermal growth factor and receptor; TGF-α, transforming growth factor-α; IGF-1, IGF-2, IGF-1R, insulin-like growth factor types 1 and 2 and receptor; IRR, insulin-related receptor; PDGF, PDGFR, platelet-derived growth factor and receptor; MCSF-1, MCSF-1R, macrophage colony-stimulating growth factor-1 and receptor; VEGF, vascular endothelial growth factor; aFGF, bFGF, FGFR, acidic and basic fibroblast growth factors and receptor; KGF, keratinocyte growth factor; HGF, hepatocyte growth factor and receptor; ANF, ANFR, atrial natriuretic factor and receptor. (From Schramm CM, Grunstein MM. In: Leff AR, ed. *Pulmonary and Critical Care Pharmacology and Therapeutics.* New York: McGraw-Hill, 1996, with permission.)

Receptor tyrosine kinases share a molecular topology and possess a large extracellular ligand-binding region, a single hydrophobic transmembrane segment, a cytoplasmic portion that contains the tyrosine kinase catalytic domain, and a carboxy-terminal regulatory region (35) (Fig. 2). Structural similarities among growth factor receptors have led to their classification into seven broad groups. Firstly, the EGF receptor, the hepatocyte growth factor receptor (c-met), as well as the teterameric-containing insulin and insulin growth factor-1 receptors, contain cysteine-rich segments in their extracellular domain. Sec-

ondly, PDGF, CSF-1, and FGF mediate their effects through receptors that contain regulatory regions that are inserted in the cytoplasmic kinase portion and contain extracellular immunoglobulin-like domains (35,36). The third group is represented by the nerve growth factor receptor, which has also been identified as the oncoprotein trk, and contains neither cysteine-rich nor immunoglobulin-like regions. Finally, a variety of hematopoietic growth factor receptors, as well as glycoprotein cytokine receptors, belong to another group that transduce their signals by recruiting tyrosine kinases from the cytosol

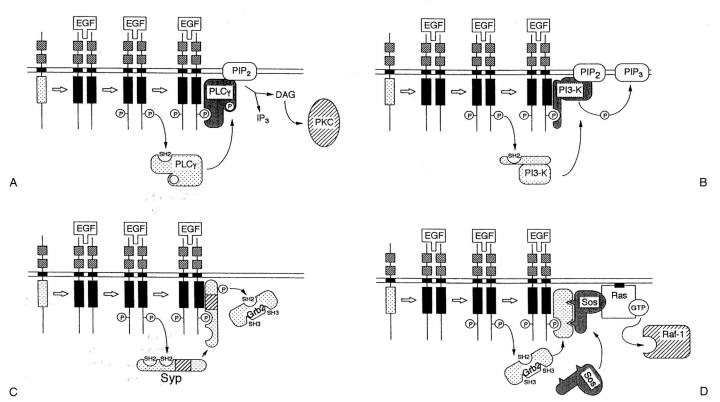

FIG. 3. Paradigms of signal transduction through receptor tyrosine kinases. **A:** Activation by tyrosine phosphorylation, as shown for epidermal growth actor (EGF) activation of phospholipase Cγ (PLCγ). EGF induces dimerization and autophosphorylation of the epidermal growth factor receptor (EGFR). The SH2 domain of inactive PLCγ interacts with the autophosphorylated (P) EGFR, resulting in phosphorylation and activation of PLCγ, which then hydrolyses membrane phosphatidylinositol 4,5-bisphosphate (PIP_2) to form inositol 1,4,5-trisphosphate (IP_3) and diacylglycerol (DAG). DAG, in turn, can activate protein kinase C (PKC). **B:** Activation by conformational change, as shown for EGF-induced activation of phosphatidylinositol 3-kinase (PI3-K). The SH2 domain of the p85 component of PI3-K (long bar) interacts with the autophosphorylated EGFR, resulting in a transformational change in and consequent activation of the p110 subunit of PI3-K, which can then phosphorylate PIP_2 to form phosphatidylinositol 3,4,5-trisphosphate (PIP_3). **C:** Activation by association and possible phosphorylation, as shown for EGF-induced activation of the cytoplasmic protein tyrosine phosphatase Syp. One of two SH2 domains of Syp interacts with the autophosphorylated EGFR, bringing its protein tyrosine phosphatase domain *(striped area)* into contact with the RTK. Activated Syp is capable of interacting with the SH2 domain of the Ras-associated adaptor protein, Grb2. **D:** Activation by localization, as shown for EGF activation of Ras. The SH2 domain of Grb2 interacts with the autophosphorylated EGFR, and the SH3 domains of Grb2 interact with Ras guanine nucleotide releasing factor, Sos. The translocation of Sos to the inner surface of the cell membrane brings it into contact with the membrane-associated GTPase, Ras. The activated (GTP-bound) Ras can then associate with the regulatory domain of the serine/threonine kinase Raf-1. (From Schramm CM, Grunstein MM. In: Leff AR, ed. *Pulmonary and Critical Care Pharmacology and Therapeutics.* New York: McGraw-Hill, 1996, with permission.)

and by creating a signaling complex. The interleukin-2 receptor, as well as interleukin-3 receptor, are included in this group and appear to induce cell proliferation by coupling the ligand-activated receptor to nonreceptor kinases p56lck and Lyn kinase of the src family, respectively (See refs. 14,15,82 for review).

Activation of the receptor tyrosine kinase is necessary for transduction of the growth factor-mediated responses. Although the precise mechanism by which the ligand activates the RTK is unknown, studies suggest that ligand binding to the receptor may induce oligomerization of receptor monomers or may form a receptor-ligand complex that is then internalized (see ref. 42 for review). The next step, autophosphorylation of tyrosine residues on the receptor, is critically important in transduction of the extracellular signal. Autophosphorylation of the receptor removes inhibitory substrates and creates high-affinity sites containing phosphotyrosine residues. The substrates that bind to these autophosphorylated tyrosine residues contain particular binding sites, termed "SH2 domains." SH2 domains refer to an amino acid motif that is homologous with the protein product of the Src oncogene (p60src), the first member identified in this family of protein substrates (154,155).

Substrates with SH2 domains are responsible for coupling activated growth factor receptors to intracellular signaling pathways involved in the control of a variety of cell functions including cell proliferation, cytoskeletal protein remodeling, and gene expression. Proteins with one or more SH2 domains include the GTPase-activating protein (GAP) of p21ras, phospholipase-τ_1, phosphatidylinositol 3-kinase (PI 3-kinase), Ras, and other cytoplasmic kinases (Fig. 3). Specificity of the growth factor response is determined not only by the SH2 recognition sites of the substrates, but also by the three amino acid residues immediately C-terminal to the phosphotyrosine to which the SH2 domains bind. Studies, however, suggest that formation of receptor-SH2 complexes is important in some, but not all, responses of cells to growth factors.

Many proteins that possess SH2 domains also contain a distinct sequence of approximately 50 amino acid residues termed "the SH3 domain." Evidence suggests that SH3 domains may modulate protein-protein interactions through the recognition of short peptide sequences that do not require phosphorylation. SH3 domains appear to regulate the interaction of the growth factor receptors with small Ras-like guanine nucleotide-binding proteins. Ultimately, the physical association of these proteins having SH2 and SH3 domains with that of RTK may require their translocation from the cytosol to the membrane. This translocation may result in an increased affinity of the receptor to become tyrosine phosphorylated (85).

Signaling complexes based on the formation of SH2/SH3 interactions are then followed by activation of downstream effector proteins which involve, for example, Src nonreceptor tyrosine kinases, small GTP-binding proteins

of the Ras family, serine/threonine kinases of Raf, and mitogen-activated protein kinase (MAP) families (40–43) (Fig. 3). These intracellular enzymes are the products of oncogenes and protooncogenes whose function is to regulate expression of a large and diverse group of proteins involved in complex cellular functions, such as cell proliferation and growth (See refs. 122,123 for review). Importantly, protooncogenes encode proteins involved in virtually every step of the growth factor signaling cascade. Current challenges are directed at identifying protooncogenes that are both necessary and sufficient to induce cell proliferation such that new therapeutic approaches can be developed to alter expression of these genes and to inhibit smooth muscle cell growth (156–158).

RTK-Dependent Growth Factors that Induce Airway Smooth Muscle Cell Proliferation.

Airway inflammation, which is a hallmark of asthma, is represented by recruitment of various inflammatory cells to the airways including macrophages, mast cells, basophils, platelets, epithelial cells, eosinophils, and T lymphocytes. These cells have been suggested as important immune effector cells involved in modulating airway responsiveness (1). Many of these cells secrete a variety of known smooth muscle cell mitogens, which may mediate their effects in a RTK-dependent manner, and potentially induce ASM cell growth (Table 1). In addition to direct stimulation of myocyte proliferation, these mitogens can stimulate myocyte growth in an autocrine manner. In vascular smooth muscle, stimulation of cells with PDGF or interleukin-1 induces myocytes to secrete PDGF and interleukin-1 that may further enhance the proliferative response (see review, 159). Smooth muscle cell hyperplasia is likely a consequence of the chronic stimulation of myocytes with a variety of cytokines and mitogens, rather than a single growth factor. To date, there are, however, no in vivo studies that have conclusively identified specific growth factors or mitogens that induce ASM cell hyperplasia.

Since few studies have characterized ASM cell hyperplasia or hypertrophy in chronic animal models of asthma, investigators have used models of cultured ASM cells to study myocyte proliferation (30–35,44,45). As a model, ASM in culture has several advantages over whole organ or strip studies. The availability of large populations of pure airway myocytes without contamination from neuronal or epithelial cells, allows for the precise control of extracellular conditions and provides the ability to reversibly synchronize the cells in G_0 (resting phase) of the cell cycle. Monolayers of cells eliminate variability in diffusion of agonists through tissue that may alter cellular concentrations. In addition, a human model eliminates interpretative difficulties from interspecies variations. Although extrapolation from cultured models

TABLE 1. *Potential airway smooth muscle cell mitogens*[a]

Mitogen	Cell Source	Signaling Pathway[b]	Autocrine Stimulation[c]
Epidermal growth factor	Macrophage, epithelium	RTK	Unknown
Insulin-like growth factor-1	Macrophage, smooth muscle, fibroblast	RTK	Yes
Platelet derived growth factor	Macrophage, epithelium, platelet, endothelium	RTK	Yes
Fibroblast growth factor	Endothelium, smooth muscle, fibroblast	RTK	Yes
Interleukin-1	Macrophage, T- and B- lymphocyte, endothelium, smooth muscle, fibroblast, glial cell	RTK	Yes
Colony stimulating factor	Macrophage, T- lymphocyte, endothelium, basophil, mast cell	RTK	Yes
Histamine	Basophil, mast cell	G protein	No
Serotonin	Platelet, neural cells	G protein	No
Thrombin	Serum protein	G protein	No
Endothelin-1	Epithelium, endothelium	G protein	No
Thromboxane A_2	Macrophage, platelet, smooth muscle, mast cell, basophil, eosinophil, and others	G protein	Yes
β-Hexosaminidase	Macrophages, eosinophils, mast cell	Unknown	Unknown
Leukotriene D_4	Macrophage, platelet, smooth muscle, mast cell, eosinophil, and others	G protein	Yes

[a]The mitogens that are listed have been reported to induce cultured airway or vascular smooth muscle cell proliferation. To date, there are no studies that have reported growth factors that induce airway smooth muscle *in vivo*.

[b]Smooth muscle cell mitogens are coupled either to receptors with intrinsic tyrosine kinase activity (RTK) or to receptors coupled to guanine nucleotide binding regulatory proteins (G proteins).

[c]Autocrine stimulation refers to mitogen-induced smooth muscle secretion of growth factors.

to *in vivo* conditions may be problematic, human ASM models have been developed which demonstrate morphological and functional compatibility with *in vivo* conditions (31,32).

Recently, EGF in human cells and PDGF in guinea pig, human, and bovine cells have been characterized as ASM cell mitogens (30–32,35). These growth factors likely mediate their effects through intrinsic RTK activity. In comparison to contractile agonists, which mediate their effects through G proteins, EGF and PDGF are more potent with half maximal concentrations in the nanomolar range. Typically, treatment of human ASM cells with 100 ng/ml EGF for 48 hours stimulates DNA synthesis with 33.5 ± 8.2 fold increases in [3H]-thymidine incorporation and induces cell proliferation with 30% ± 2.4% increases in cell number as compared with that of unstimulated, quiescent ASM cells (32,42). In addition, EGF also induces messenger ribonucleic acid (mRNA) expression of c-*fos*, a protooncogene whose induction is one of the earliest markers of proliferation and differentiation in mesenchymal-derived cells (88).

Other growth factors found to stimulate ASM cell proliferation are the insulin-like growth factors, IGF-I and IGF-II, which are ubiquitous peptides that mediate cell proliferation and differentiation by acting via RTK-dependent type-1 and type-2 IGF receptors (33,34). Interestingly, cultured rabbit ASM cells were found to release IGF-II, as well as the IGF-binding protein (IGFBP), IGFBP-2, which largely acts to inhibit the promitogenic action of IGFs by limiting their bioavailability to cell surface IGF receptors (33,34). The latter inhibitory action of

IGFBP-2 was further found to be down-regulated by treatment of rabbit ASM cells with the proinflammatory eicosanoid, leukotriene D_4 (LTD$_4$), which acts to release an IGFBP-2 protease and, hence, facilitates the ASM cell proliferative response to IGFs (33). Taken together, these findings suggest that, apart from any direct action of a growth factor on cell proliferation, the ASM cell growth response may be significantly modulated by activation of an autocrine network involving the IGF axis (i.e., IGFs, IGFBPs, and proteases) which may up- or down-regulate the net proliferative response to the mitogen.

The downstream signaling events that modulate RTK-dependent proliferation of ASM cells have not been well-characterized. A recent study has examined the role of protein kinase C activation in modulating PDGF-induced ASM cell growth. In that study, cell proliferation induced by PDGF was markedly attenuated by pretreating the cells with protein kinase C inhibitors (160). Others have determined that pretreatment of rabbit ASM cells with genistein or lavendustin A, which are tyrosine kinase inhibitors, inhibited serum-, EGF- or PDGF-induced cell growth (161). Since these inhibitors lack specificity and block a variety of serine, threonine, or tyrosine kinases, further study is needed to identify specific kinases that regulate RTK-dependent airway myocyte growth.

Although tyrosine kinases are critically important in signaling growth factor responses, recent attention has also focused on the role of cytosolic calcium in modulating RTK-dependent growth in ASM cells. Using single cell fluorescence measurements of fura 2-loaded cells, studies show that EGF is far less potent in mobilizing increases in intracellular calcium as compared to bradykinin, serotonin, or endothelin-1 (RA Panettieri and RK Murray, unpublished observations). Interestingly, bradykinin, serotonin, or endothelin-1 are less effective in stimulating human ASM cell proliferation as compared to cells treated with EGF (32). Whether alterations in cytosolic calcium induced by RTK-dependent growth factors are necessary to induce ASM cell proliferation remains unknown. The role of calcium mobilization in regulating myocyte growth will be addressed later in this chapter.

Growth Factor Receptors Coupled to Heterotrimeric GTP-Binding Proteins (G Proteins)

The recent observations that agonists which induce smooth muscle cell contraction can also induce myocyte proliferation may have important pathophysiologic implications in diseases characterized by smooth muscle hyperplasia. A variety of contractile agonists have been identified as vascular and ASM cell mitogens (Table 1).

The majority of contractile agonist receptors share a common topography that consists of a seven-membrane spanning region and a site that couples the receptor to a heterotrimeric G protein (Fig. 1). In a similar manner to RTK-dependent growth factor receptors, those coupled to G proteins activate phosphoinositide (PI)-specific phospholipase C, that then hydrolyzes phosphoinositides to generate IP$_3$ and DAG. In the case of G protein-coupled receptors, a specific PI-PLC isotype, PLC-β1, is activated, rather than PLC-τ which is activated by RTK-dependent receptors.

Activation of protein kinase C by DAG is considered a pivotal event in regulating G protein-dependent cell proliferation (162). Activated protein kinase C in conjunction with increased cytosolic calcium induces intracellular alkalinization by promoting Na$^+$/H$^+$ exchange and by phosphorylating specific substrates that have been associated with cell proliferation. In addition, specific agonists also induce expression of the protooncogenes, c-*fos* and c-*myc*, whose activation regulates myriad cellular functions that include gene transcription and cell proliferation (88,163–165).

Despite certain similarities in stimulatory signal transduction pathways between RTK-dependent growth factors and contractile agonists, important disparities exist. Firstly, cell proliferation stimulated by most growth factors is mediated by receptor-linked tyrosine kinase activation; to date, no such activity has been described in cell proliferation induced by agonists. Secondly, contractile agonists that both induce cell proliferation and contraction, appear to do so by receptors coupled to different G proteins (18,32,37,38). Finally, RTK-dependent cell proliferation is both protein kinase C-dependent and -independent, whereas agonist-induced mitogenesis is thought to be protein kinase C-dependent (166). In addition to

differences between the proliferative mechanisms of these mitogens, substantial variability exists in the mitogenic capacity among contractile agonists. Firstly, some, but not all, contractile agonists stimulate smooth muscle cell proliferation, despite the fact that most of these agonists induce comparable levels of polyphosphoinositide hydrolysis, cytosolic calcium transients, protein kinase C activation, and c-*fos* mRNA expression (32,33). Secondly, the mitogenic effects of endothelin and serotonin on vascular smooth muscle appear to be coupled to pertussis toxin-sensitive G proteins that differ from the pertussis toxin-insensitive G proteins that mediate agonist-induced PI hydrolysis, cytosolic calcium release, or smooth muscle contraction (9,18). The differences in proliferative responses induced by growth factors and contractile agonists, and differential contractile agonist effects, imply that other regulatory components are involved. Potential regulatory sites for agonist-induced proliferation of smooth muscle cells will be considered separately.

INOSITOL LIPIDS IN THE REGULATION OF CELL PROLIFERATION

Phospholipase C Activation and Inositol Trisphosphate

The recognition of phosphatidylinositol 4,5-bisphosphate hydrolysis as a ubiquitous receptor-activated signaling mechanism in eukaryotic cells was one of the major achievements of the 1980s. Recent studies have focused on other aspects of phospholipid metabolism in signaling cell growth, including phosphatidylinositol 3,4,5-trisphosphate formation by inositol lipid 3-kinases and phospholipase D-catalyzed phosphotidylcholine hydrolysis. Although there is little doubt that inositol lipids are important in cell signaling, the precise mechanism by which these molecules modulate cell proliferation remains largely unknown.

To date, two phosphoinositide pathways have been characterized. In the canonical PI pathway, activation of phosphatidylinositol-specific phospholipase C hydrolyzes phosphatidylinositol 4,5-bisphosphate to inositol 1,4,5,-trisphosphate and diacylglycerol. In the 3-phosphoinositide pathway, activation of phosphatidylinositol 3-kinase (PtdIns 3-kinase), which involves protein tyrosine kinase-mediated recruitment, phosphorylates phosphatidylinositides at the D3 position of the inositol ring, leading to the formation of phosphatidylinositol 3-phosphate, phosphatidylinositol 3,4-bisphosphate and phosphatidylinositol 3,4,5-trisphosphate (PtdIns 3,4,5-P3) (77,80,83,84) (Fig. 4).

Receptors with intrinsic tyrosine kinase activity and those coupled to G proteins both activate specific phospholipase C isoforms. These phosphoinositidases are the

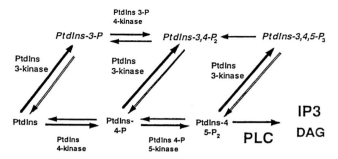

FIG. 4. Synthesis of phosphoinositides: The lipid products generated by the 3-phosphoinositide pathway are shown in italics to differentiate those involved in the canonical PI turnover pathway. The *solid arrows* indicate pathways known to occur *in vivo*. PLC, PtdIns-specific phospholipase C; DAG, diacylglycerol. (Modified from Kapeller R, Cantley LC. *Bioessays* 1994;16:565–576, with permission.)

critical regulatory enzymes in activation of the PI pathway. The γ family of phospholipase C contain src-homology SH2 and SH3 domains, and are regulated by tyrosine phosphorylation. The other PLC isoforms are controlled by G proteins and/or Ca^{+2}.

The regulation of the PLC-γ_l family has been elucidated in considerable detail. Kim et al. (85) have determined the relative contributions made to PLC-γ_l activation by three tyrosine residues that are phosphorylated when PLC-γ_l associates with the PDGF receptor in 3T3 cells. Substitution of Tyr771 with phenylalanine slightly enhanced the activation, but a similar substitution of Tyr1254 markedly decreased the extent to which the enzyme was activated by the PDGF receptor in these cells (85). An even stronger attenuation was caused by substituting Tyr783 with phenylalanine; the PLC-γ_l Tyr783Phe could associate with the PDGF receptor and was serinephosphorylated as a consequence, although no activation occurred. Thus, tyrosine residues 783 and, to a lesser degree, 1254 are those that contribute to the control of the activity of PLC-γ_l in intact cells (85). Interestingly, others have shown that mutant EGF and PDGF receptors, which fail to activate PLC-γ_l and increase cytosolic calcium *in vivo*, effectively induced gene expression and mitogenesis (86). Taken together, these studies suggest that formation of receptor-SH2 complexes is important in some, but not all, responses of cells to growth factors, and other parallel signaling pathways apart from PLC-γ_l activation may be necessary to mediate growth factor-induced mitogenesis.

In ASM cells, some growth factors which activate receptors with intrinsic tyrosine kinases have been identified. PDGF and EGF in human ASM cells and IGF-1 in bovine and rabbit ASM cells have been shown to induce myoctye proliferation (30–35). However, the role of PLC-γ_l activation in modulating ASM cell growth remains unknown.

In recent years, our understanding of the regulation of PLC by G proteins has grown remarkably. Although the role of PLC activation in mediating G protein-dependent cell growth is complex, G protein activation is critically important in transducing contractile agonist-induced cell growth. G proteins are composed of three distinct subunits, α, β, and γ: the latter two existing as a tightly associated complex (see ref.36 for review). Although α subunits were considered the functional components important in downstream signaling events, recent evidence suggests that $\beta\gamma$ subunits also play a critical role in modulating cell function (37). To date, there exist approximately a total of 15 distinct genes that encode mammalian $G\alpha$ subunits grouped into four classes (G_s, G_i, G_q, and G_{12}) based on their amino acid sequence (38). On the basis of the ADP-ribosylation of certain α subunits by pertussis toxin (PTX), G proteins may also be classified as PTX-sensitive and as PTX insensitive. The subunits $G_{i\alpha 1}$, $G_{i\alpha 2}$, $G_{i\alpha 3}$, $G_{o\alpha 1}$, and $G_{o\alpha 2}$ are PTX-sensitive; whereas all other α subunits are PTX-insensitive.

Advances in single cell microinjection techniques in combination with the development of neutralizing antibodies to specific $G\alpha$ subunits have enabled investigators to characterize the role of G protein activation in cell proliferation. Using these techniques, studies with 3T3 fibroblasts have determined that while both thrombin and bradykinin required G_q activation to mobilize cytosolic calcium to generate IP_3 and to induce mitogenesis, thrombin, but not bradykinin, appeared also to require G_{i2} in addition to G_q to stimulate cell growth (87). These studies determined that a single mitogen may require functional coupling to distinct subtypes of G proteins in order to stimulate cell growth. This also provides a mechanism to explain why some, but not all, agonists induce cell proliferation while mobilizing comparable levels of cytosolic calcium.

Recently, the role of PLC activation and inositol trisphosphate in mediating contractile agonist-induced ASM cell growth has been explored. Several contractile agonists, which mediate their effects through G protein-coupled receptors, induce ASM cell proliferation. Studies have determined that histamine and serotonin induce canine and porcine ASM cell proliferation (39,88). Endothelin-1, leukotriene D_4 and U-46619, a thromboxane A_2 mimetic, induce rabbit ASM cell growth, and thrombin induces mitogenesis in human ASM cells (30,32,40, 41). Although the mechanisms that mediate these effects are unknown, agonist-induced cell growth probably is modulated by activation of G proteins in a manner similar to that described in vascular smooth muscle.

Using human ASM cells, Panettieri et al. (32) recently examined whether contractile agonist-induced human ASM cell growth was dependent on PLC activation and inositol trisphosphate formation. These investigators examined the relative effects of bradykinin and thrombin on myocyte proliferation and PI turnover. Thrombin, but not bradykinin, stimulated ASM cell proliferation despite a 5-fold greater increase in [³H]-inositol phosphate formation in cells treated with bradykinin, as compared with those treated with thrombin. These investigators also determined that inhibition of PLC activation with U-73122 had no effect on thrombin- or EGF-induced myocyte proliferation. In addition, pertussis toxin completely inhibited thrombin-induced ASM cell growth but had no effect on PI turnover induced by either thrombin or bradykinin (32). Taken together, these studies suggest that thrombininduced human ASM cell growth by activation of a pathway that was pertussis toxin-sensitive and independent of phospholipase C activation or PI turnover.

In comparison to RTK-dependent growth factors, contractile agonists, with the exception of thrombin, appear to be less effective human ASM mitogens (42). In cultured human ASM cells, 100 μM histamine or serotonin induces 2- to 3-fold increases in [³H]-thymidine incorporation, as compared to that obtained from unstimulated cells. EGF, serum, or phorbol esters, which directly activate protein kinase C, induce 20- to 30-fold increases in [³H]-thymidine incorporation (39,43,44). Interestingly, histamine is as effective as serum in stimulating cell growth and c-*fos* expression in canine ASM cells (88). In rabbit ASM cells, endothelin-1 induces cell proliferation by activating phospholipase A₂, and by generating thromboxane A₂ and LTD₄ (40,41). In human ASM cells, however, endothelin-1, thromboxane A₂, and LTD₄ appear to have little effect on ASM cell proliferation, despite these agonists inducing increases in cytosolic calcium (32,43, 45). Clearly, interspecies variability exists with regard to contractile agonist-induced cell proliferation. These models, however, may prove useful in dissecting downstream signaling events that modulate the differential effects of contractile agonists on ASM cell proliferation.

3-Phosphorylated Inositol Lipids

Recently, these phospholipids have been recognized as a new class of second messengers (46,84,89). Based on a number of studies, PtdIns 3,4,5-P3 appears to be the critical signaling 3-phospholipid (Fig. 4). This assumption is supported by the time course of accumulation and the subsequent metabolism of the individual 3-phosphoinositides following agonist stimulation (47,77). Although the routes of metabolism of these lipids are poorly understood when compared to those of the canonical phosphoinositides, some important features have emerged. The 3-phosphoinositides are not substrates for any known phospholipase C30-32, and are not components of the canonical phosphoinositide turnover pathway. Rather, their rapid increase upon growth factor stimulation suggests that the lipids themselves may act as second messengers mediating PtdIns 3-kinase mitogenic signals (83). The recent identification that 3-phosphoinositides directly activate the ζ isoform of protein kinase C may

have important implications in understanding mechanisms that induce smooth muscle cell proliferation, since myocyte growth is thought to be protein kinase C-dependent (48).

Compelling evidence suggests a role for PtdIns 3-kinase and its lipid products in regulating various cellular functions that include mitogenesis (83). PtdIns 3-kinase, which consists of an 85 kD regulatory subunit (p85) and a 110 kD catalytic subunit (p110), is required for DNA synthesis induced by some, but not all, growth factors (49). In 3T3 fibroblasts, microinjection of cells with a neutralizing antibody to the p110 catalytic subunit of PtdIns 3 kinase was found to completely inhibit PDGF- and EGF-induced mitogenesis (49). The role of PtdIns 3-kinase activation in modulating cell proliferation, however, is cell type specific. In some cells, bombesin and LPA, which induce cell proliferation by activating receptors coupled to G proteins, stimulated cell growth in the absence of PtdIns 3-kinase activity (49,83). Taken together, these studies suggest that mitogens may activate different intracellular signaling pathways in a cell-specific manner.

Few investigators have examined the role of PtdIns 3-kinase activation in modulating human ASM cell proliferation. A recent study examined whether PtdIns 3-kinase mediated ASM cell growth or modulated calcium transients induced by contractile agonists. Thrombin-induced increases in cytosolic calcium were examined in fura-2 loaded cells pretreated with wortmannin, a PtdIns 3-kinase inhibitor (50). As shown in Figure 5A, inhibition of PtdIns 3-kinase did not alter calcium transients induced by thrombin (50). In parallel experiments, confluent ASM cells that were growth-arrested for 24 hours were pretreated with wortmannin and then stimulated with thrombin or EGF. DNA synthesis was then measured by [³H]-thymidine incorporation. In a dose-dependent manner, wortmannin inhibited thrombin and EGF-induced DNA synthesis, as shown in Figure 5B. Wortmannin had no effect on basal levels of [³H]-thymidine incorporation as compared to cells treated with diluent alone. If wortmannin was added 6 hours after the cells were stimulated with mitogens, then wortmannin did not inhibit cell proliferation. This data suggests that PtdIns 3-kinase may mediate early signaling events that modulate myocyte growth. Collectively, these studies suggest that PtdIns 3-kinase activation may play an important role in modulating ASM cell proliferation induced by growth factors and contractile agonists.

Diacylglycerol Synthesis from PI- and PC-PLC Activation

Although the hydrolysis of polyphosphoinositides, especially PIP₂, to DAG is critically important in agonist-induced activation of protein kinase C, recent evidence suggests that phosphatidylcholine (PC) hydrolysis is also a major source of DAG and may be as important in regu-

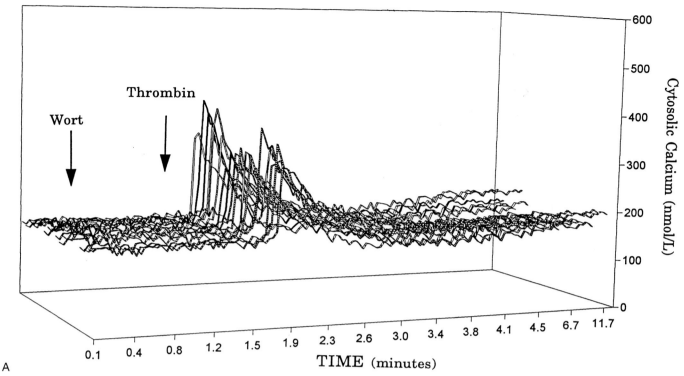

A

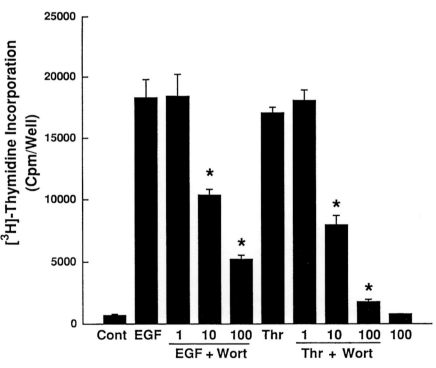

B

FIG. 5. Effects of PtdIns 3-kinase on cytosolic calcium mobilization and [³H]-thymidine incorporation in ASM cells. **A**: PtdIns 3-kinase inhibition does not modulate agonist-induced calcium transients. Monolayers were pretreated for 10 minutes with 100 nM wortmannin and then stimulated with 0.3 U/mL thrombin. The experiment is representative of five with similar results. **B**: Inhibition of PtdIns 3-kinase abolishes DNA synthesis induced by agonists and growth factors in ASM cells. Confluent, growth-arrested ASM cells were pretreated with 1.0, 10, or 100 nM wortmannin (Wort) for 10 minutes and then stimulated with either 1 U/ml thrombin, 100 ng/ml EGF, or diluent. [³H]-thymidine incorporation was then measured and compared with that obtained in cells treated with either thrombin (Thr), EGF, 100 nM wortmannin or diluent (Cont) alone. Data represent means ± SEM from six experiments, each containing four replicates for each condition (*$P<0.01$). (Date from Panettieri RA, Krymskaya V, Scott P, Plevin R, Al-Hafidh J, Eszterhas A, Chilvers ER. Thrombin induces human airway smooth muscle (ASM) cell proliferation by activation of a novel signaling pathway. *Am J Respir Crit Care Med* 1996; 153:A742.)

lating protein kinase C (PKC) activation (Fig. 6). PC hydrolysis produces a prolonged increase in cellular DAG, which has been hypothesized to induce sustained activation of PKC. The experimental evidence to support the role of agonist-induced PC hydrolysis in DAG synthesis

is derived from two observations: (1) the time course and magnitude of increases in DAG levels with receptor stimulation differ from those of IP₃ levels (51–54); and (2) the fatty acid composition of DAG often differs from the mass of DAG and/or phosphatidic acid that is produced,

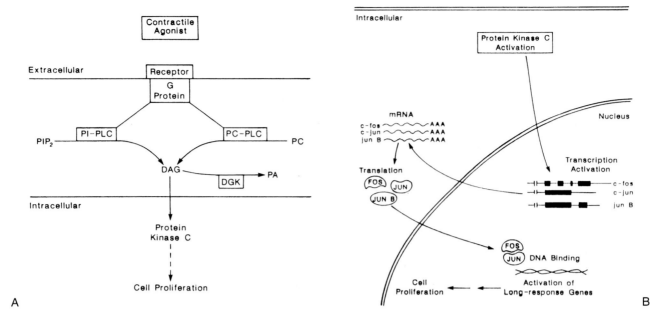

FIG. 6. A model to illustrate the proposed mechanisms that regulate airway smooth muscle proliferation induced by contractile agonists. **A:** Possible cell membrane-associated regulatory events. **B:** Possible nuclear regulatory events. Abbreviations are: G proteins, guanine nucleotide binding regulatory protein; PIP_2, phosphatidylinositol 4,5 bisphosphate; DAG, 1,2-diacylglycerol; PC, phosphatidylcholine; PI-PLC, phosphoinositol-specific phospholipase C; PC-PLC, phosphatidylcholine-specific phospholipase C; DGK, diacylglycerol kinase; PA, phosphatidic acid. For ease of presentation, the receptor is linked to one G protein; however, it is possible that different G proteins are involved. (Modified from Panettieri RA. In: Raeburn D, Giembycz MA, eds. *Airways smooth muscle: development and regulation of contractility.* Basel: Birkhauser Verlag, 1994;41–68, with permission.)

and markedly exceeds the decrease in the mass of inositol phospholipids (52–58). Since increases in DAG activate protein kinase C, the regulation of DAG formation is likely to play an important role in the regulation of cell proliferation.

The role of DAG formation in mediating mitogenesis has been supported by studies in 3T3 cells and hematopoietic cell lines (63) stimulated with permeable DAG analogs (59–61). Other investigators, using 3T3 cells, transfected with vectors that express the entire Ha-ras oncogene p21 protein or infected with Kirsten sarcoma virus, have observed that these cells undergo cellular transformation and have sustained increases in DAG, phosphatidylcholine, and phosphatidylethanolamine, but unchanged phosphoinositide levels (64). Increases in DAG levels with agonist stimulation may result not only from newly synthesized DAG, but also from its decreased degradation. Diacylglycerol kinase (DGK), which rapidly converts DAG to phosphatidic acid, plays a central role in the degradation of DAG (65–67). To date, studies have only characterized the regulatory role of this pathway in cells undergoing malignant transformation (68). Alteration in the activity of this kinase may also affect protein kinase C activation and potentially cell growth.

In vascular smooth muscle studies, investigators have determined that vasopressin, a vascular smooth muscle

mitogen, and phorbol esters appear to induce a sustained elevation of DAG, derived primarily from PC hydrolysis or from phospholipase D activation (58,69). This sustained elevation in DAG may then induce prolonged activation of protein kinase C and stimulate cell proliferation. Studies on ASM have not resolved the individual contribution of PI and PC hydrolysis to DAG synthesis.

Intracellular Calcium Modulates Mitogen-Induced Cell Proliferation

To a large extent, cellular processes regulated by alterations in the cytoplasmic concentration of ionized calcium are initiated by the release of this ion from sequestered intracellular stores. The most well-studied example is the release mediated by IP_3-gating of its receptor/ion channel. Compelling evidence, however, suggests that there are more calcium storage pools and release mechanisms than can be explained by the action of IP_3 alone. The exact nature of these pools and how they interact is an intensely investigated topic which has been extensively reviewed (74,75,90). In this section, the role of intracellular calcium signaling in regulating cell proliferation will be discussed as it pertains to smooth muscle cell growth.

Numerous studies have postulated the involvement of intracellular calcium signals in growth (91). Studies using the Ca^{+2} ionophore, A23187, have determined that increases in cytosolic calcium induce protooncogene expression and cell proliferation (76,78). The interpretation of these experiments, however, remains difficult since this molecule has pleiotrophic effects (79,81). Despite these drawbacks, much evidence supports the role of growth factor-induced cytosolic Ca^{+2} signals as being necessary for activation of G_0 to G_1 transition and mitogenesis in some cell types (82,92).

More recent studies suggest that the levels of Ca^{+2} remaining in Ca^{+2}-accumulating organelles may also have important consequences for signaling and growth regulation (93,94). Depletion of calcium stores within the endoplasmic reticulum by thapsigargin markedly inhibited growth factor-induced mitogenesis in a transformed smooth muscle cell line (93). Such effects may result from either an altered ability of the endoplasmic reticulum to generate specific Ca^{+2} signals necessary for cell growth or a modulation of key endoplasmic reticulum functions that are dependent on intraluminal Ca^{+2} to induce mitogenesis. Interestingly, the effects of thapsigargin on cell growth were independent of any observed effects on protein kinase C activation (93). Taken together, current evidence suggests that cytosolic Ca^{+2} mobilization or depletion of Ca^{+2} stores in response to growth factors, may be critical to modulate cell proliferation in some cells.

Although both growth factors and contractile agonists evoke calcium transients by stimulation of phospholipase C in smooth muscle cells, the role of Ca^{+2} in regulating smooth muscle cell growth remains controversial. Contractile agonists that both induce cell proliferation and contraction appear to do so by receptors coupled to different G proteins (9,18,32,95,96). Some, but not all, contractile agonists stimulate ASM cell proliferation, despite the fact that most of these agonists induce comparable levels of polyphosphoinositide hydrolysis, cytosolic calcium transients, and c-fos mRNA expression (10,29,39, 43). Thus, for example, while bradykinin and thrombin were both found to evoke comparable levels of cytosolic calcium in human ASM cells, thrombin, but not bradykinin, induced DNA synthesis in these cells (32). In other studies, Stewart et al. (30) determined that EGF stimulated human ASM cell proliferation at concentrations that were markedly less than those necessary to evoke calcium transients. These studies suggest that regulatory processes, apart from calcium mobilization, are important in mediating smooth muscle cell proliferation.

CYCLIC NUCLEOTIDES AND SMOOTH MUSCLE CELL GROWTH

Recognition that vascular smooth muscle proliferation is important in the pathogenesis of atherosclerosis has fo-

cused attention on identifying cellular and molecular mechanisms that inhibit smooth muscle cell growth. An understanding of these mechanisms is not only critical in preventing cell growth, but also in addressing whether the loss of inhibitory signals may induce myocyte proliferation. Activation of cyclic 3′ 5′ adenosine monophosphate (cAMP)- (A-kinase) or cyclic guanosine monophosphate (cGMP)- (G-kinase) dependent kinases, and alterations in extracellular matrix proteins, have been reported to inhibit myocyte proliferation (97). To date, several studies have determined that similar mechanisms inhibit ASM cell growth (42,44,88,98,99).

Cyclic AMP and Cell Proliferation

New insights into the mechanisms by which cAMP-dependent pathways inhibit cell growth have recently been described. The activation of A-kinase results in the inhibition of Raf-1 activation in mammalian cells (100, 101). Raf-1, a serine-threonine protein kinase, is an effector for Ras-GTP, and the interaction of Raf-1 with Ras-GTP induces Raf activation. Activation of Raf-1 phosphorylates and activates other serine threonine kinases, which ultimately activates the mitogen-activated protein kinase (MAPK) pathway. This pathway is thought to be critically important in modulating mitogen-induced cell proliferation of some cell types.

A-kinase is capable of phosphorylating Raf-1 at Ser43 in the amino-terminal regulatory domain of the kinase (101). Inhibition of Raf-1 activation by A-kinase was found to be independent of Ras-GTP loading stimulated by growth factors, PtdIns 3-kinase activation or PLC-γ_1 activity. A-kinase, therefore, selectively inhibited Raf activation, but not activation of other components of the signal-transduction pathway required for mitogenesis in 3T3 cells. It remains unclear as to whether this phosphorylation site is responsible for uncoupling Raf-1 from Ras-GTP-dependent activation. Despite these advances in our knowledge concerning A-kinase effects on cell growth, mitogenesis of some cell types appears to be independent of Raf-1 inhibition, suggesting substantial redundancy in signal transduction pathways that induce cell proliferation (102,103).

In vascular, as well as in ASM cells, activation of receptors coupled to G_s, which increases cytosolic cAMP levels and activates A-kinase, inhibits cell growth induced by growth factors (42,44,104–107). A-kinase activation, however, appears to selectively inhibit mitogens that induce ASM cell growth through PI-PLC- and protein kinase C-dependent pathways (107). Alternatively, mitogens that stimulate cell proliferation through activation of receptor-linked tyrosine kinases are less sensitive to this inhibition (44,107). Interestingly, these mitogens stimulate growth, in part, through protein kinase C-independent mechanisms. In smooth muscle, "cross-talk" between intracellular kinases appears crucial in coordinating cell proliferation.

In other cell lines, these distinctions have been questioned (108). Growth inhibition by protein kinase activation is markedly cell-specific. While elevations of intracellular cAMP inhibit cell growth in a wide variety of cell types, it acts as a potent mitogen in other cells, such as 3T3 cells or PC12 cells (105,106,109–112). Investigators using bovine ASM cells have reported that β-hexosaminidase, which transiently increases cytosolic cAMP levels, induces cell growth (113,114). In these studies, however, sustained increases in cytosolic cAMP levels also inhibited myocyte proliferation induced by β-hexosaminidase (114).

Using a human ASM cell line that retains a coupled β-adrenergic receptor-adenylate cyclase system, investigators have determined the role of A-kinase activation in modulating ASM cell proliferation induced by phorbol ester, EGF, or thrombin (62,107). Confluent growth-arrested cells were pretreated with forskolin, which directly activates adenylyl cyclase, and were then stimulated with PMA or EGF. Forskolin pretreatment inhibited PMA-induced DNA synthesis by 70%±3.2%, and that induced with EGF by 23%±5% (42,107). Receptor-specificity was confirmed by pretreating cells with either isoproterenol or isoproterenol and propranolol, and DNA synthesis was measured after stimulating the cells with PMA. In a receptor-specific manner, isoproterenol completely abolished protein kinase C-dependent DNA synthesis (107). Similarly, PGE$_2$, which also induces increases in cAMP levels and activates A-kinase, inhibited PMA- and EGF-induced DNA synthesis (RA Panettieri, unpublished observations). In rabbit ASM cells and in guinea pig ASM, activation of cAMP-dependent pathways also inhibited mitogen-induced ASM cell growth (98,99). Taken together, these studies suggest that DNA synthesis induced by growth factors or agonists are inhibited by pathways that activate A-kinase.

Identifying cellular mechanisms that inhibit cell growth may be relevant, not only with regard to preventing ASM cell proliferation, but also in terms of understanding the full spectrum of pathways that regulate cell growth. For example, further studies may clarify whether myocyte proliferation results from a loss of tonic inhibitory effects of A-kinase. Such studies may have important implications concerning the chronic use of therapeutic agents that manipulate these signal transduction pathways.

The Role of cGMP in Modulating Smooth Muscle Cell Growth

Atrial naturetic factor, as well as sodium nitroprusside and nitric oxide, are potent vasodilators that mediate their effects by increasing cytosolic cGMP levels and activat-

ing cyclic GMP-dependent kinase (G-kinase). Recently, investigators have reported that vascular smooth muscle cell proliferation induced by serum or by serotonin is inhibited by pretreating the cells with atrial naturetic peptide or with permeant cGMP analogs (115–117). In a preliminary study using guinea pig ASM cells, nitroprusside and dibutyryl cGMP, a permeable cGMP analog, also inhibited serum-induced cell proliferation (118). However, the downstream signaling events that mediate G-kinase inhibition of cell growth remains unknown.

In some cell types, cGMP may enhance the formation of cyclic adenosine diphosphate ribose (cADPR), a metabolite of NAD that can release Ca^{+2} by acting on the ryanodine receptor (119–121). In these cells, increases in cGMP induced cell proliferation. Clearly, further studies are needed to define the role of cGMP in modulating cell proliferation.

SECOND MESSENGERS MODULATE SMOOTH MUSCLE CELL GROWTH BY ACTIVATION OF DOWNSTREAM EFFECTORS

The previous discussion has focused on the second messenger systems that modulate ASM cell proliferation. While an exhaustive review of the sequential protein kinase cascades activated by mitogens extends beyond the scope of this chapter, it is important to review some recent advances in our understanding of downstream effector molecules that are activated by second messengers and that may play critical roles in transducing growth signals in smooth muscle cells.

Activation of Ras (p21ras)

The proteins encoded by ras genes serve as essential transducers of diverse physiological signals, and ras proteins, which are mutationally altered, can induce cell transformation. Although the ras gene was first identified in transforming retroviruses (v-ras), the identification that retroviral oncogenes (v-ras) were derived from normal cellular genes (c-ras) has led to the recognition that Ras activation plays a critical role in mediating normal cell growth and differentiation (122,123).

Ras, which migrates as a 21-kDa protein (p21ras), has served as a prototype for the superfamily of Ras-related proteins, a group of guanine nucleotide-binding proteins that share structural homology (122–124). The discovery that Ras proteins bind guanine nucleotides (GTP and GDP) with high affinity, and possess intrinsic GTPase activity, suggested a mechanism by which Ras activity is regulated. Ligand-bound receptors induce the active GTP-bound form of Ras by enhancing the ability of guanine nucleotide-exchange factors to accelerate the replacement of bound GDP with GTP. Ras proteins are then deactivated by interaction with GTPase-activating proteins (GAPs) that promote GTP hydrolysis by Ras (Fig. 3). In some cell types, active Ras promotes cell proliferation; in others, it arrests cell division and induces the expression of differentiated phenotypes (122). The role of Ras activation in mediating mitogen-induced smooth muscle cell proliferation remains unknown.

Recent studies have identified that activated Ras interacts with both Raf kinase and PtdIns 3-kinase, two important Ras effector proteins that modulate growth factor-induced proliferation of 3T3 and Rat-1 fibroblasts (123, 125). The initial step in Ras activation of Raf involves the binding of active GTP-Ras to Raf kinase (123). Ras binding alone does not activate the intrinsic kinase activity of Raf; rather, it localizes Raf to the plasma membrane where it is activated. Activated Raf then stimulates a cascade of other kinases including MAP kinase, whose activation in some cells is necessary to induce cell proliferation. A parallel pathway, however, by which activated Ras may induce cell growth involves PtdIns 3-kinase activation (125). Evidence suggests that Ras binds to PtsIns 3-kinase *in vitro* only when Ras is in the active state and the level of PtdIns 3-kinase generated *in vivo* can be increased or decreased, depending on whether activated or dominant negative Ras mutants are expressed (122,123, 125). Interestingly, Raf activation does not alter the level of these molecules, suggesting that PtdIns 3-kinase may be one component of a distinct parallel downstream pathway from Ras. To date, studies on ASM have not addressed the role that Ras activation may play in regulating mitogen-induced ASM proliferation.

Protein Kinase C Activation

Activation of PKC, either directly by phorbol esters or indirectly by mitogens, is an important signaling event for the proliferation of many cells, including smooth muscle (28,59,126–129). Activated PKC in conjunction with increased cytosolic calcium induces intracellular alkalinization by promoting Na^+/H^+ exchange, and by phosphorylating specific substrates that have been associated with cell proliferation. PKC represents a family of protein kinases, activated by calcium and diacylglycerol, that induces protein phosphorylation of serine and threonine residues of many proteins. One such protein with a molecular weight of 76,000 (p76) has been well- characterized, and its phosphorylation associated with mitogenesis (126,129–133). Cloning and molecular biology studies have revealed the existence of multiple isotypes of protein kinase C. To date, at least four calcium- and phosphatidyl serine-dependent PKC isotypes (α, βI-, βII-, γ-PKC) and four calcium-independent isotypes (δ-, ε-, ζ- and η-PKC) have been identified (134–137; Todo T, Nakamura H, Mobuyuki S, et al., personal communication, 1990). A recent study has determined that most of the previously mentioned PKC isotypes are found in ca-

nine ASM, except for η-PKC which was not present (138). Currently, there is little evidence to designate specific functions for each PKC isotype; however, their distribution appears to be tissue-specific.

The role of PKC activation in fibroblast and smooth muscle cell proliferation induced by contractile agonists has been demonstrated by downregulation of PKC following prolonged pretreatment with phorbol esters. In these cells, pretreatment diminished phorbol ester-induced p76 phosphorylation by 80% to 90%, abolished phorbol ester stimulation of cell proliferation in 3T3 cells and vascular smooth muscle cells, as well as markedly attenuating phorbol ester-induced c-*fos* expression (10,129, 130,139). However, the mitogenic responses of PKC-deficient 3T3 cells to PDGF, EGF, and FGF were not attenuated. Other studies have demonstrated that rabbit ASM cell proliferation induced by serum was inhibited by the selective PKC inhibitors, RO-318220 and RO-317549 (140–143). Taken together, these data suggest that PKC activation is necessary in transducing growth signals from receptors coupled to G proteins and from receptors with intrinsic tyrosine kinases in some cell types.

The dependence of receptor-activated mitogenesis on PKC appears to be growth factor- and cell-specific. For example, EGF- or IGF-1-induced proliferation of 3T3 cells was protein kinase C-independent, while PKC activation of human fibroblasts actually inhibited EGF-induced cell proliferation (141,142). Further, some but not all, contractile agonists that activate PKC induce vascular smooth muscle cell proliferation (10,144). These data suggest that PKC activation may be necessary, but not sufficient to induce G protein-dependent cell growth, and other signaling pathways must modulate the proliferative response.

Mitogen-Activated Protein Kinases (MAP Kinase)

MAP kinases, which are a family of 40 kD to 46 kD serine/threonine kinases, are activated early in response to extracellular signals, and appear to play an integral role in the signaling cascade initiated by diverse stimuli. A variety of mitogens activate MAP kinase *in vivo*, including PDGF, EGF, and nerve growth factor, all of which induce autophosphorylation of their receptors on tyrosine residues (145–147). Evidence also suggests that MAP kinase activation occurs in response to stimulation of receptors coupled to heterotrimeric G proteins (39,148). Although the precise signaling events that modulate MAP kinase activation remain unknown, a major pathway requires the sequential activation of Ras, Raf, and MAP kinase/Erk-activating kinase, also known as MAP kinase kinase (MAPKK). MAPKK has been shown to directly phosphorylate MAP kinase on both tyrosine and threonine residues (149,150). The phosphorylation of both these residues is required for maximal enzymatic activation of MAP kinase (149,150). Subsequently, the activated MAP kinase, which translocates from the cytoplasm to the nucleus, induces expression of the protooncogenes, c-*jun* and c-*myc*, which are necessary for cell proliferation (149,151,152). In Chinese hamster fibroblasts, transient expression of p44^{mapk} antisense RNA, or a p44^{mapk} kinase-deficient mutant, abolished growth factor-stimulated c-*fos* and c-*jun* expression, as well as cell proliferation (153). The integration of signal events activated by tyrosine and serine/threonine phosphorylation at the level of MAP kinase suggests that MAP kinase plays a central role in the downstream regulation of cell proliferation.

Recent studies have revealed that growth factors that stimulate receptors with intrinsic tyrosine kinases, and those that stimulate receptors coupled to G proteins, activate MAP kinases in bovine ASM cells (35,148). The investigators suggested that sustained activation of MAP kinase correlated with the proliferative response of bovine ASM cells to the putative mitogen. Others have also suggested that prolonged activation of MAP kinase is necessary to induce cell proliferation of CCL 39 cells stimulated with thrombin (149). Despite these studies, the role of MAP kinase in regulating cell proliferation remains controversial. It is likely that the role of MAP kinase activation as a requirement for growth factor-stimulated DNA synthesis will vary among different cell types, and more studies are needed to determine whether MAP kinase activation is necessary and sufficient to induce ASM cell growth.

CONCLUSIONS

Asthma, a common cause of pulmonary impairment, is a chronic disease characterized by airway hyperreactivity and airflow obstruction. Despite considerable research effort, asthma mortality rates continue to rise, and the primary defects that underlie airway hyperreactivity remain unknown, although an intrinsic abnormality of ASM has been postulated.

Although asthma typically induces reversible airway obstruction, in some asthmatics, airflow obstruction can become irreversible. Such obstruction may be a consequence of persistent structural changes in the airway wall due to the frequent stimulation of airway smooth muscle (ASM) by contractile agonists, inflammatory mediators, and growth factors. Increased smooth muscle mass, which has been attributed to increases in myocyte number, is a well-documented pathologic finding in the airways of patients with chronic severe asthma.

Although the mechanisms by which agonists induce cell proliferation is unknown, similarities exist between signal transduction processes activated by these agents and those of known growth factors. Diverse extracellular stimuli induce cell growth, in part, by activating common intracellular signal transduction pathways. The identification of critical regulatory sites in these pathways may provide new therapeutic approaches to alter the airway remodeling seen in patients with chronic severe asthma.

ACKNOWLEDGMENTS

Sources of Support: National Institutes of Health, HL02647 and HL31467; National Aeronautics and Space Administration.

REFERENCES

1. Barnes PJ. Inflammation. In: Weiss EB, Stein M, eds. *Bronchial asthma.* Boston: Little, Brown and Co, 1993;80–95.
2. Brown JP, Breville WH, Finucane KE. Asthma and irreversible airflow obstruction. *Thorax* 1984;39:131–136.
3. Peat JK, Woolcock AJ, Cullen K. Rate of decline of lung function in subjects with asthma. *Eur J Respir Dis* 1987;70:171–179.
4. Woolcock AJ. Asthma—what are the important experiments? State of the art/conference summary. *Am Rev Respir Dis* 1988;138:730–744.
5. Dunnill MS, Massarella GR, Anderson JA. A comparison of the quantitative anatomy of the bronchi in normal subject, in status asthmaticus, in chronic bronchitis and in emphysema. *Thorax* 1969;24:176–179.
6. Hossain S. Quantitative measurement of bronchial muscle in asthma. *Am Rev Respir Dis* 1973;107:99–109.
7. Huber HL, Koessler KK. The pathology of bronchial asthma. *Arch Intern Med* 1922;30:690–760.
8. Heard BE, Hossain S. Hyperplasia of bronchial muscle in asthma. *J Pathol* 1973;110:319–331.
9. Bobik A, Grooms A, Millar JA, Mitchell A, Grinpukel S. Growth factor activity of endothelin on vascular smooth muscle. *Am J Physiol* 1990;258:C408–C415.
10. Taubman MB, Berk BC, Izumo S, Tsuda T, Alexander RW, Nadal Ginard B. Angiotensin II induces c-*fos* mRNA in aortic smooth muscle. Role of Ca^{2-} mobilization and protein kinase C activation. *J Biol Chem* 1989;264: 526–530.
11. Berk BC, Brock TA, Webb RC, et al. Epidermal growth factor, a vascular smooth muscle mitogen, induces rat aortic contraction. *J Clin Invest* 1985;75:1083–1086.
12. Berk BC, Alexander RW, Brock TA, Gimbrone M, Webb R. Vasoconstriction: a new activity for platelet-derived growth factor. *Science* 1986;232:87–90.
13. Glenn K, Bowen-Pope DF, Ross R. Platelet-derived growth factor. III. Identification of a platelet-derived growth factor receptor by affinity labeling. *J Biol Chem* 1982;257:5172–5176.
14. Rozengurt E. Early signals in the mitogenic response. *Science* 1986; 234:161–166.
15. Sporn MB, Roberts AB. Peptide growth factors and inflammation, tissue repair, and cancer. *J Clin Invest* 1986;78:329–332.
16. Clowes AW, Clowes MM, Kocher O, Ropraz P, Chaponnier C, Gabbiani G. Arterial smooth muscle cells *in vivo*: relationship between actin isoform expression and mitogenesis and their modulation by heparin. *J Cell Biol* 1988;107:1939–1945.
17. Nemecek GM, Coughlin SR, Handley DA, Moskowitz MA. Stimulation of aortic smooth muscle cell mitogenesis by serotonin. *Proc Natl Acad Sci USA* 1986;83:674–678.
18. Kavanaugh WM, Williams LT, Ives HE, Coughlin SR. Serotonin-induced deoxyribonucleic acid synthesis in vascular smooth muscle cells involves a novel, pertussis toxin-sensitive pathway. *Mol Endocrinol* 1988;123:599–605.
19. James HL, Paré PD, Hogg JC. The mechanics of airway narrowing in asthma. *Am Rev Respir Dis* 1989;139:242–246.
20. Wiggs BR, Morono R, Hogg JC, Hillian C, Paré PD. A model of the mechanics of airway narrowing. *J Appl Physiol* 1990;69:849–860.
21. Wiggs BR, Bosken C, Paré PD, James A, Hogg JC. A model of airway narrowing in asthma and in chronic obstructive pulmonary disease. *Am Rev Respir Dis* 1992;145:1251–1258.

22. Lambert BR, Wiggs BR, Kuwano K, Hogg JC, Paré PD. Functional significance of increased airway smooth muscle in asthma and COPD. *J Appl Physiol* 1993;74:2771–2781.

23. Macklem PT. A theoretical analysis of the effect of airway smooth muscle load on airway narrowing. *Am J Respir Crit Care Med* 1996; 153:83–89.

24. Ding DJ, Martin JG, Macklem PT. Effects of lung volume on maximal methacholine-induced bronchoconstriction in normal humans. *J Appl Physiol* 1987;62:1324–1330.

25. Ishida K, Paré PD, Blogg T, Schellenberg RR. Effects of elastic loading on porcine trachealis muscle mechanics. *J Appl Physiol* 1990;69: 1033–1039.

26. Armour CL, Diment LM, Black JL. Relationship between smooth muscle volume and contractile response in airway tissue. Isometric versus isotonic measurement. *J Pharmacol Exp Ther* 1988;245:687–691.

27. Nishizuka Y. Turnover of inositol phospholipids and signal transduction. *Science* 1984;225:1365–1370.

28. Nishizuka Y. The role of protein kinase C in cell surface signal transduction and tumour promotion. *Nature* 1984;308:693–698.

29. Nambi P, Watt R, Whitman M, Aiyar N, Moore JP, Evan GI, Crooke S. Induction of c-*fos* protein by activation of vasopressin receptors in smooth muscle cells. *FEBS Lett* 1989;245:61–64.

30. Stewart AG, Grigoriadis G, Harris T. Mitogenic actions of endothelin-1 and epidermal growth factor in cultured airway smooth muscle. *Clin Exp Pharmacol and Physiol* 1994;21:277–285.

31. Hirst SJ, Barnes PJ, Twort CHC. Quantifying proliferation of cultured human and rabbit airway smooth muscle cells in response to serum and platelet-derived growth factor. *Am J Respir Cell Mol Biol* 1992; 7:574–581.

32. Panettieri RA, Hall IP, Maki CS, Murray RK. a-thrombin increases cytosolic calcium and induces human airway smooth muscle cell proliferation. *Am J Respir Cell Mol Biol* 1995;13:205–216.

33. Cohen P, Noveral JP, Bhala A, Nunn SE, Grunstein MM. Leukotriene D$_4$ facilitates airway smooth muscle cell proliferation via modulation of the IGF axis. *Am J Physiol* 1995;269:L151–L157.

34. Noveral JP, Bhala A, Hintz RL, Grunstein M, Cohen P. The insulin-like growth factor axis in airway smooth muscle cells. *Am J Physiol* 1994;267:L761–L765.

35. Kelleher MD, Abe MK, Chao T-SO, et al. Role of MAP kinase activation in bovine tracheal smooth muscle mitogenesis. *Am J Physiol* 1995;268:L894–L901.

36. Hepler JR, Gilman AG. G proteins. *Trends Biochem Sci* 1992;17: 383–387.

37. Sternweis PC. The active role of βγ in signal transduction. *Curr Opin Cell Biol* 1994;6:198–203.

38. Simon MI, Strathmann MP, Gautam M. Diversity of G proteins in signal transduction. *Science* 1991;252:802–808.

39. Panettieri RA, Eszterhas A, Murray RK. Agonist-induced proliferation of airway smooth muscle cells is mediated by alteration in cytosolic calcium. *Am Rev Respir Dis* 1992;145:A15.

40. Noveral JP, Rosenberg SM, Anbar RA, Pawlowski NA, Grunstein MM. Role of endothelin-1 in regulating proliferation of cultured rabbit airway smooth muscle cells. *Am J Physiol* 1992;263:L317–L324.

41. Noveral JP, Grunstein MM. Role and mechanism of thromboxane-induced proliferation of cultured airway smooth muscle cells. *Am J Physiol* 1992;263:L555–L561.

42. Panettieri RA. Airways smooth muscle cell growth and proliferation. In: Raeburn D, Giembycz MA, eds. *Airways smooth muscle: development and regulation of contractility*. Basel: Birkhauser Verlag, 1994;41–68.

43. Panettieri RA, Rubinstein NA, Kelly AM, Kotlikoff MI. The specificity of c-*fos* expression in the induction of airway smooth muscle proliferation by contractile agonists. *Am Rev Respir Dis* 1991;143: A934.

44. Panettieri RA, Cohen MD, Bilgen G. Airway smooth muscle cell proliferation is inhibited by microinjection of the catalytic subunit of cAMP dependent kinase. *Am Rev Respir Dis* 1993;147:A252.

45. Panettieri RA, Murray RK, DePalo LR, Yadvish PA, Kotlikoff M. A human airway smooth muscle cell line that retains physiological responsiveness. *Am J Physiol* 1989;256:C329–C335.

46. Stephens L, Cooke FT, Walters R, et al. Characterization of a phosphatidylinositol-specific phosphoinositide 3-kinase from mammalian cells. *Curr Opin Cell Biol* 1994;4:203–214.

47. Irvine RF. Inositol lipids in cell signalling. *Curr Opin Cell Biol* 1992; 4:212–219.

48. Nakarish H, Brewer KA, Exton JH. Activation of the zeta isoenzyme of protein kinase C by phosphotidylinositol 3,4,5-trisphosphate. *J Biol Chem* 1993;268:13–16.

49. Roche S, Koegl M, Courtneidge SA. The phosphatidylinositol 3-kinase is required for DNA synthesis induced by some, but not all, growth factors. *Proc Natl Acad Sci U S A* 1994;91:9185–9189.

50. Panettieri RA, Krymskaya V, Scott P, Plevin R, Al-Hafidh J, Eszterhas A, Chilvers ER. Thrombin induces human airway smooth muscle (ASM) cell proliferation by activation of a novel signaling pathway. *Am J Respir Crit Care Med* 1996;153:A742.

51. Exton JH. Mechanisms of alpha-1-adrenergic and related responses: Roles of calcium, phosphoinositides, calmodulin and guanine nucleotides and changes in protein phosphorylation. In: Elson EL, Frazier WA, Glaser L, eds. *Cell membranes: methods and reviews*. Vol 3. New York: Plenum, 1987;113–182.

52. Bocckino SB, Blackmore PF, Wilson PB, Exton JH. Phosphatidate accumulation in hormone-treated hepatocytes via a phospholipase D mechanism. *J Biol Chem* 1987;262:15309–15315.

53. Bocckino SB, Blackmore PF, Exton JH. Stimulation of 1,2-diacylglycerol accumulation in hepatocytes by vasopressin, epinephrine, and angiotensin II. *J Biol Chem* 1985;260:14201–14207.

54. Exton JH. Mechanisms of action of calcium-mobilizing agonists: Some variations on a young theme. *FASEB J* 1988;2:2670–2676.

55. Grillone LR, Clark MA, Godfrey RW, Stassen F, Crooke ST. Vasopressin induces V$_1$ receptors to activate phosphatidylinositol- and phosphatidylcholine-specific phospholipase C and stimulates the release of arachidonic acid by at least two pathways in the smooth muscle cell line, A-10. *J Biol Chem* 1988;263:2658–2663.

56. Takuwa N, Takuwa Y, Rasmussen H. A tumour promoter, 12-O-tetradecanoylphorbol 13-acetate, increases cellular 1,2-diacylglycerol content through a mechanism other than phosphoinositide hydrolysis in Swiss-mouse 3T3 fibroblasts. *Biochem J* 1987;243:647–653.

57. Daniel LW, Waite M, Wykle RL. A novel mechanism of diglyceride formation. 12-O-tetradecanoylphorbol-13-acetate stimulates the cyclic breakdown and resynthesis of phosphatidylcholine. *J Biol Chem* 1986;261:9128–9132.

58. Griendling KK, Rittenhouse SE, Brock TA, Ekstein LS, Gimbrone Jr MA, Alexander RW. Sustained diacylglycerol formation from inositol phospholipids in angiotensin II-stimulated vascular smooth muscle cells. *J Biol Chem* 1986;261:5901–5906.

59. Rozengurt E, Rodriguez-Pena A, Coombs M, Sinnett-Smith J. Diacylglycerol stimulates DNA synthesis and cell division in mouse 3T3 cells: Role of Ca^{2-}-sensitive phospholipid-dependent protein kinase. *Proc Natl Acad Sci U S A* 1984;81:5748–5752.

60. Kishimoto A, Takai Y, Mori T, Kikkawa U, Nishizuka Y. Activation of calcium and phospholipid-dependent protein kinase by diacylglycerol, its possible relation to phosphatidylinositol turnover. *J Biol Chem* 1980;255:2273–2276.

61. Davis RJ, Ganong BR, Bell RM, Czech MP. sn-1,2-dioctanoylglycerol. A cell-permeable diacylglycerol that mimics phorbol diester action on the epidermal growth factor receptor and mitogenesis,. *J Biol Chem* 1985;260:1562–1566.

62. Tomlinson PR, Wilson JW, Stewart AG. Inhibition by salbutamol of the proliferation of human airway smooth muscle cells grown in culture. *Br J Pharmacol* 1994;111:641–647.

63. Pai J-K, Siegel MI. Activation of phospholipase D by chemotactic peptide in HL-60 granulocytes. *Biochem Biophys Res Commun* 1988; 150:355–364.

64. Lacal JC, Moscat J, Aaronson SA. Novel source of 1,2-diacylglycerol elevated in cells transformed by Ha-ras oncogene. *Nature (London)* 1987;330:269–272.

65. Hokin MR, Hokin LE. The synthesis of phosphatidic acid from diglyceride and adenosine triphosphate in extracts of brain microsomes. *J Biol Chem* 1959;234:1381–1386.

66. Michell RH. Inositol lipids and their role in receptor function: history and general principles. In: Putney Jr JW, ed. *Phosphoinositides and receptor mechanisms*. New York: Alan R Liss Inc, 1986;1–24.

67. Irving HR, Exton JH. Phosphatidylcholine breakdown in rat liver plasma membranes. Roles of guanine nucleotides and P$_2$-purinergic agonists. *J Biol Chem* 1987;262:3440–3443.

68. Huang M, Chida K, Kamata N, Nose K, Kato M, Homma Y, Takenawa T, Kuroki T. Enhancement of inositol phospholipid metabolism

and activation of protein kinase C in ras-transformed rat fibroblasts. *J Biol Chem* 1988;263:17975–17980.

69. Konishi F, Kondo T, Inapami T. Phospholipase D in cultured rat vascular smooth muscle cells and its activation by phorbol ester. *Biochem Biophys Res Commun* 1991;179:1070–1076.

70. Cocco L, Gilmour RS, Ognibene A, Letcher AJ, Manzoli FA, Irvine RF. Synthesis of polyphosphoinositides in nuclei of Friend cells. Evidence for polyphosphoinositide metabolism inside the nucleus which changes with cell differentiation. *Biochem J* 1987;248:765–770.

71. Leach KL, Powers EA, Ruff VA, Jaken S, Kaufmann S. Type 3 protein kinase C localization to the nuclear envelope of phorbol ester-treated NIH 3T3 cells. *J Cell Biol* 1989;109:685–695.

72. Hocevar BA, Fields AP. Selective translocation of b_{11}-protein kinase C to the nucleus of human promyelocytic (HL60) leukemia cells. *J Biol Chem* 1991;266:28–33.

73. Divecha N, Banfic H, Irvine RF. The polyphosphoinositide cycle exists in the nuclei of Swiss 3T3 cells under the control of a receptor (for IGF-I) in the plasma membrane, and stimulation of the cycle increases nuclear diacylglycerol and apparently induces translocation of protein kinase C to the nucleus. *EMBO J* 1991;10:3207–3214.

74. Cheek TR. Calcium regulation and homeostasis. *Curr Opin Cell Biol* 1991;3:199–205.

75. Tsien RW, Tsien RY. Calcium channels, stores and oscillations. *Annu Rev Cell Biol* 1990;6:715–760.

76. Büscher M, Rahmsdorf HJ, Litfin M, Karin M, Herrlich P. Activation of the c-*fos* gene by UV and phorbol ester: different signal transduction pathways converge to the same enhancer element. *Oncogene* 1988;3:301–311.

77. Fry MJ. Structure, regulation and function of phosphoinositide 3-kinases. *Biochim Biophys Acta* 1994;1226:237–268.

78. Fisch TM, Prywes R, Roeder RG. c-*fos* sequence necessary for basal expression and induction by epidermal growth factor, 12-O-tetradecanoyl phorbol-13-acetate, and the calcium ionophore. *Mol Cell Biol* 1987;7:3490–3502.

79. Smith PL, McCabe RD. A23187-induced changes in colonic K and Cl transport are mediated by separate mechanisms. *Am J Physiol* 1984;247:G695–G702.

80. Varticovski L, Harrison-Findik D, Keeler ML, Susa M. Role of PI 3-kinase in mitogenesis. *Biochim Biophys Acta* 1994;1226:1–11.

81. Erlij D, Gersten L, Sterba G, Schoen HF. Role of prostaglandin release in the response of tight epithelia to Ca^{2-} ionophores. *Am J Physiol* 1986;250:C629–C636.

82. Rozengurt E. Growth factors and cell proliferation. *Curr Opin Cell Biol* 1992;4:161–165.

83. Kapeller R, Cantley L C. Phosphatidylinositol 3-kinase. *Bioessays* 1994;16:565–576.

84. Stephens LT, Jackson T, Hawkins P. Agonist stimulated synthesis of phosphatidylinositol (3,4,5)-trisphosphate: A new intracellular signalling system? *Biochim Biophys Acta* 1993;1179:27–75.

85. Kim HK, Kim JW, Zilberstein A, Margolis B, et al. PDGF stimulation of inositol phospholipid hydrolysis requires PLC-γ_1 phosphorylation on tyrosine residues 783 and 1254. *Cell* 1991;65:435–441.

86. Chen WS, Lazar CS, Lund KA, Welsh JB, et al. Functional independence of the epidermal growth factor receptor from a domain required for ligand-induced internalization and calcium regulation. *Cell* 1989;59:33–43.

87. Lamorte VJ, Harootunian AT, Spiegel AM, Tsien RY, Feransico JR. Mediation of growth factor induced DNA synthesis and calcium mobilization by G_q and G_{i2}. *J Cell Biol* 1993;121:91–99.

88. Panettieri RA, Yadvish PA, Kelly AM, Rubinstein NA, Kotlikoff MI. Histamine stimulates proliferation of airway smooth muscle and induces c-*fos* expression. *Am J Physiol* 1990;259:L365–L371.

89. Stephens L, Smrcka A, Cooke FT, Jackson TR, Sternweis PC, Hawkins PT. A novel phosphoinositide 3-kinase activity in myeloid-derived cells is activated by G protein bg subunits. *Cell* 1994;77:83–93.

90. Burgoyne R D, Cheek TR. Locating intracellular calcium stores. *Trends Biochem Sci* 1991;16:319–320.

91. Whitaker M, Patel R. Calcium and cell cycle control. *Development* 1990;108:525–542.

92. Lopez-Rivas A, Mendoza SA, Nanberg E, Sinnett-Smith J, Rozengurt E. Ca^{2+}-mobilizing actions of platelet-derived growth factor differ from those of bombesin and vasopressin in Swiss 3T3 mouse cells. *Proc Natl Acad Sci U S A* 1987;84:5768–5772.

93. Ghosh TK, Bian JH, Short AD, Rybak SL, Gill DL. Persistent intracellular calcium pool depletion by thapsigargin and its influence on cell growth. *J Biol Chem* 1991;266:24690–24697.

94. Schönthal A, Sugarman J, Brown JH, Hanley MR, Feramisco JR. Regulation of c-*fos* and c-*jun* protooncogene expression by the Ca^{2+}-ATPase inhibitor thapsigargin. *Proc Natl Acad Sci U S A* 1991;88:7096–7100.

95. Chambard JC, Paris S, L'Allemain G, Pouyssegur J. Two growth factor signaling pathways in fibroblasts distinguished by pertussis toxin. *Nature* 1987;326:800–803.

96. Vicentini LM, Villereal ML. Serum, bradykinin and vasopressin stimulate release of inositol phosphates from human fibroblasts. *Biochem Biophys Res Commun* 1984;123:663–670.

97. Pastan IH, Johnson GS, Anderson WB. Role of cyclic nucleotides in growth control. *Annu Rev Biochem* 1975;44:491–522.

98. Noveral JP, Grunstein, MM. Adrenergic receptor-mediated regulation of cultured rabbit airway smooth muscle cell proliferation. *Am J Physiol* 1994;267:L291–L299.

99. Florio C, Martin JG, Styhler A, Heisler S. Antiproliferative effect of prostaglandin E2 in cultured guinea pig tracheal smooth muscle cells. *Am J Physiol* 1994;266:L131–L137.

100. Sevetson BR, Kong X, Lawrence Jr JC. Increasing cAMP attenuates activation of mitogen-activated protein kinase. *Proc Natl Acad Sci U S A* 1993;90:10305–10309.

101. Wu J, Dent P, Jelinek T, Wolfman A, Weber MJ, Sturgill TW., Inhibition of the EGF-activated MAP kinase signaling pathway by adenosine 3′ 5′ -monophosphate. *Science* 1993;262:1065–1069.

102. Thomas SM, DeMarco M, D Arcangelo G, Halegoua S, Brugge JS. Ras is essential for nerve growth factor- and phorbol ester-induced tyrosine phosphorylation of MAP kinases. *Cell* 1992;68:1031–1040.

103. Rukenstein A, Rydel RE, Greene LA. Multiple agents rescue PC12 cells from serum-free cell death by translation- and transcription-independent mechanisms. *J Neurosci* 1991;11:2552–2563.

104. Jonzon B, Nilsson J, Fredholm BB. Adenosine receptor-mediated changes in cyclic AMP production and DNA synthesis in cultured arterial smooth muscle cells. *J Cell Physiol* 1985;124:451–456.

105. Loesberg C, Van Wijk R, Zandbergen J, Van Aken WG, Van Mourik JA, De Groot PG. Cell cycle-dependent inhibition of human vascular smooth muscle cell proliferation by prostaglandin E1. *Exp Cell Res* 1985;160:117–125.

106. Nilsson J, Olsson AG. Prostaglandin E1 inhibits DNA synthesis in arterial smooth muscle cells stimulated with platelet-derived growth factor. *Atherosclerosis* 1984;53:77–82.

107. Panettieri RA, Rubenstein NA, Feuerstein B, Kotlikoff MI. Beta-adrenergic inhibition of airway smooth muscle proliferation. *Am Rev Respir Dis* 1991;143:A608.

108. Magnaldo I, Pouyssegur J, Paris S. Cyclic AMP inhibits mitogen-induced DNA synthesis in hamster fibroblasts, regardless of the signaling pathway involved. *FEB* 1989;245:65–69.

109. Rozengurt E. Cyclic AMP: A growth-promoting signal for mouse 3T3 cells. *Adv Cyclic Nucleotide Res* 1981;14:429–442.

110. Speir ES, Epstein SE. Inhibition of smooth muscle cell proliferation by antisense oligodeoxynucleotide targeting the messenger RNA encoding proliferating cell nuclear antigen. *Circulation* 1992;86:538–547.

111. Rozengurt E, Legg A, Strang G, Courtenay-Luck N. Cyclic AMP: A mitogenic signal for Swiss 3T3 cells. *Proc Natl Acad Sci U S A* 1981;78:4392–4396.

112. Deuel TF. Polypeptide growth factors: roles in normal and abnormal cell growth. *Annu Rev Cell Biol* 1987;3:443–492.

113. Lew DB, Pattazzi MC. Mitogenic effect of lysosomal hydrolases on bovine tracheal myocytes in culture. *J Clin Invest* 1991;88:1969–1975.

114. Lew DB, Nebigil C, Malik KU. Dual regulation by cAMP of b-hexosaminidase-induced mitogenesis in bovine tracheal myocytes. *Am J Respir Cell Mol Biol* 1992;7:614–619.

115. Garg UC, Hassid A. Nitric oxide-generating vasodilators and 8-bromo-cyclic guanosine monophosphate inhibit mitogenesis and proliferation of cultured rat vascular smooth muscle cells. *J Clin Invest* 1989;83:1774–1777.

116. Itoh H, Pratt RE, Dzau VJ. Atrial naturetic polypeptide inhibits hypertrophy of vascular smooth muscle cells. *J Clin Invest* 1990;86:1690–1697.

117. Assender JW, Southgate KM, Hallet MB, Newby AC. Inhibition of

proliferation, but not of Ca^{2+} mobilization, by cyclic AMP and GMP in rabbit aortic smooth muscle cells. *Biochem J* 1992;288:527–532.

118. De S, Zelazny E, Souhrada JF, Souhrada M. Nitric oxide has an inhibitory effect on growth of airway smooth muscle (ASM) cells. *Am J Respir Crit Care Med* 1995;151:A49.

119. Galione A, White A, Willmott N, Turner M, Potter BV, Watson SP. cGMP mobilizes intracellular Ca^{2+} in sea urchin eggs by stimulating cyclic ADP-ribose synthesis. *Nature* 1993;365:456–459.

120. Galione A, McDougall A, Busa WB, Willmott N, Gillot I, Whitaker M. Redundant mechanisms of calcium-induced calcium release underlying calcium waves during fertilization of sea urchin eggs. *Science* 1993;261:348–352.

121. Lee HC, Aarhus R, Walseth TF. Calcium mobilization by dual receptors during fertilization of sea urchin eggs. *Science* 1993;261:352–355.

122. Lowy DR, Willumsen BM. Function and regulation of ras. *Annu Rev Biochem* 1993;62:851–891.

123. Feig LA, Schaffhausen B. The hunt for ras targets. *Nature* 1994;370:508–509.

124. Monia BP, Johnston JF, Ecker DJ, Zounes MA, Lima WF, Freier SM. Selective inhibition of mutant Ha-ras mRNA expression by antisense oligonucleotides. *J Biol Chem* 1992;267:19954–19962.

125. Rodriguez-Viciana P, Warne PH, Dhand R, et al. Phosphatidylinositol-3-OH kinase as a direct target of ras. *Nature* 1994;370:527–532.

126. Isacke CM, Meisenhelder J, Brown KD, Gould KL, Gould SJ, Hunter T. Early phosphorylation events following the treatment of Swiss 3T3 cells with bombesin and the mammalian bombesin-related peptide, gastrin-releasing peptide. *EMBO J* 1986;5:2889–2898.

127. Heldin C-H, Westermark B. Growth factors: mechanism of action and relation to oncogenes. *Cell* 1984;37:9–20.

128. Chen LB, Buchanan JM. Mitogenic activity of blood components. I. Thrombin and prothrombin. *Proc Natl Acad Sci U S A* 1975;72:131–135.

129. Kariya K, Kawahara Y, Tsuda T, Fukuzaki H, Takai Y. Possible involvement of protein kinase C in platelet-derived growth factor-stimulated DNA synthesis in vascular smooth muscle cell. *Atherosclerosis* 1987;63:251–255.

130. Rozengurt E, Rodriguez-Pena M, Smith KA. Phorbol esters, phospholipase C, and growth factors rapidly stimulate the phosphorylation of a M_r 80,000 protein in intact quiescent 3T3 cells. *Proc Natl Acad Sci U S A* 1983;80:7244–7248.

131. Albert KA, Walaas SI, Wang JK-T, Greengard P. Widespread occurrence of "87 kDa," a major specific substrate for protein kinase C. *Proc Natl Acad Sci U S A* 1986;83:2822–2826.

132. Blackshear PJ, Wen L, Glynn BP, Witters LA. Protein kinase C-stimulated phosphorylation in vitro of a M_r 80,000 protein phosphorylated in response to phorbol esters and growth factors in intact fibroblasts. Distinction from protein kinase C and prominence in brain. *J Biol Chem* 1986;261:1459–1469.

133. Blackshear PJ, Witters LA, Girard PR, Kuo JF, Quamo SN. Growth factor-stimulated protein phosphorylation in 3T3-L1 cells. Evidence for protein kinase C-dependent and -independent pathways. *J Biol Chem* 1985;260:13304–13315.

134. Sekiguchi K, Tsukuda M, Ogita K, Kikkawa U, Nishizuka Y. Three distinct forms of rat brain protein kinase C: Differential response to unsaturated fatty acids. *Biochem Biophys Res Commun* 1987;145:797–802.

135. Sekiguchi K, Tsukuda M, Ase K, Kikkawa U, Nishizuka Y. Mode of activation and kinetic properties of three distinct forms of protein kinase C from rat brain. *J Biochem (Tokyo)* 1988;103:759–765.

136. Jones SD, Hall DJ, Rollins BJ, Stiles CD. Platelet-derived growth factor generates at least two distinct intracellular signals that modulate gene expression. *Cold Spring Harbor Symposia on Quantitative Biology* 1988;53:531–536.

137. Majundar S, Kane LH, Rossi MW, et al. Protein kinase C isotypes and signal-transduction in human neutrophils: selective substrate specificity of calcium-dependent β PKC and novel calcium-independent η PKC. *Biochim Biophys Acta* 1993;1176:276–286.

138. Donnelly R, Yang K, Omary MB, Azhar S, Black JL. Expression of multiple isoenzymes of protein kinase C in airway smooth muscle. *Am J Respir Cell Mol Biol* 1995;13:253–256.

139. Greenberg ME, Hermanowski AL, Ziff EB. Effect of protein synthesis inhibitors on growth factor activation of c-*fos* and c-*myc* and actin gene transcription. *Mol Cell Biol* 1986;6:1050–1057.

140. Castellot J, Wong K, Herman B, et al. Binding and internalization of heparin by vascular smooth muscle cells. *J Cell Physiol* 1985;124:13–20.

141. Dicker P, Rozengurt E. Phorbol esters and vasopressin stimulate DNA synthesis by a common mechanism. *Nature* 1980;287:607–612.

142. Decker SJ. Effects of epidermal growth factor and 12-O-tetradecanoylphorbol-13-acetate on metabolism of the epidermal growth factor receptor in normal human fibroblasts. *Mol Cell Biol* 1984;4:1718–1724.

143. Hirst SJ, Webb BLJ, Giembycz MA, Barnes PJ, Twort CHC. Inhibition of fetal calf serum-stimulated proliferation of rabbit cultured tracheal smooth muscle cells by selective inhibitors of protein kinase C and protein tyrosine kinase. *Am J Respir Cell Mol Biol* 1995;12:149–161.

144. Berk BC, Aronov MS, Brock TA, Cragoe E, Gimbrone MA, Alexander RW. Angiotensin II stimulates Na^+/H^+ exchange in cultured vascular smooth muscle cells. Evidence for protein kinase C-dependent and -independent pathways. *J Biol Chem* 1988;262:5057–5064.

145. L'Allemain G, Sturgill TW, Weber MJ. Defective regulation of mitogen-activated protein kinase activity in a 3T3 cell variant mitogenically nonresponsive to tetradecanoyl phorbol acetate. *Mol Cell Biol* 1991;11:1002–1008.

146. Ahn NG, Seger R, Bratlien RL, Diltz CD, Tonks NK, Krebs EG. Multiple components in an epidermal growth factor-stimulated protein kinase cascade: *in vitro* activation of a myelin basic protein/microtubule-associated protein 2 kinase. *J Biol Chem* 1991;266:4220–4227.

147. Gotoh Y, Nishida E, Yamashita T, Hoshi M, Kawakami M, Sakai H. Microtubule-associated-protein (MAP) kinase activated by nerve growth factor and epidermal growth factor in PC12 cells: identity with mitogen-activated MAP kinase of fibroblastic cells. *Eur J Biochem* 1990;193:661–669.

148. Abe MK, Chao T-SO, Solway J, Rosner MR, Hershenson M. Hydrogen peroxide stimulates mitogen-activated protein kinase activation in bovine tracheal myocytes: implications for human airway disease. *Am J Respir Cell Mol Biol* 1994;11:577–585.

149. Blenis J. Signal transduction via the MAP kinases: proceed at your own RSK. *Proc Natl Acad Sci USA* 1993;90:5889–5892.

150. Vouret-Craviari V, Van Obberghen-Schilling E, Rasmussen UB, Pavirani A, Lecocq J-P, Pouyssegur J. Synthetic α-thrombin receptor peptides activate G protein-coupled signaling pathways but are unable to induce mitogenesis. *Mol Biol Cell* 1992;3:95–102.

151. Alvarez E, Northwood IC, Gonzalez FA, et al. Pro-Leu-Ser/Thr-Pro is a consensus primary sequence for substrate protein phosphorylation: Characterization of the phosphorylation of c-*myc* and c-*jun* proteins by an epidermal growth factor receptor threonine 669 protein kinase. *J Biol Chem* 1991;266:15277–15285.

152. Pulverer BJ, Kyriakis JM, Avruch J, Nikolakaki E, Woodgett JR. Phosphorylation of c-*jun* mediated by MAP kinases. *Nature* 1991;353:670–674.

153. Pages G, Lenormand P, L'Allemain GL, Chambard J-C, Meloche S, Pouyssegur J. Mitogen-activated protein kinases p42^{mapk} and p44^{mapk} are required for fibroblast proliferation. *Proc Natl Acad Sci U S A* 1993;90:8319–8323.

154. Cardenn DL, Gill GN. Receptor tyrosine kinases. *FASEB J* 1992;6:2332–2337.

155. Carpenter G. Receptor tyrosine kinase substrates: scr homology domains and signal transduction. *FASEB J* 1992;6:3283–3289.

156. Speir ES, Epstein SE. Inhibition of smooth muscle cell proliferation by antisense oligodeoxynucleotide targeting the messenger RNA encoding proliferating cell nuclear antigen. *Circulation* 1992;86:538–547.

157. Simons M, Rosenberg RD. Antisense nonmuscle myosin heavy chain and c-*myb* oligonucleotides suppress smooth muscle cell proliferation *in vitro*. *Circ Res* 1992;70:835–843.

158. Simons M, Edelman ER, Dekeverer JL, Langer R, Rosenberg RD. Antisense c-myb oligonucleotides inhibit arterial smooth muscle cell accumulation *in vivo*. *Nature* 1992;359:67–70.

159. Hajjar DP, Pomerantz KB. Signal transduction in atherosclerosis: integration of cytokines and the ekosanoid network. *FASEB J* 1992;6:2933–2941.

160. Hirst SJ, Barnes BJ, Twort CHC. Protein kinase inhibitors (PKC and PKA) and phorbol esters inhibit proliferation induced by serum in cultured rabbit airway smooth muscles. *Am Rev Resp Dis* 1993;147:A252 (abstr).

161. Delamere F, Townsend P, Knox A. Tyrosine kinases transduce serum and specific growth factor mediated mitogenesis in airway smooth muscle. *Am Rev Resp Dis* 1993;147:A254 (abstr).

162. Collins MKL, Rozengurt E. Binding of phorbol esters to high-affinity sites on murine fibroblastic cells elicits a mitogenic response. *J Cell Physiol* 1982;112:42–50.

163. Greenberg ME, Ziff EB, Greene LA. Stimulation of neuronal acetylcholine receptors induces rapid gene transcription. *Science* 1986;234:80–83.

164. Morgan JI, Curran T. Role of ion flux in the control of c-*fos* expression. *Nature* 1986;322:552–555.

165. Sheng M, Dougan ST, McFadden G, Greenberg ME. Calcium and growth factor pathways of c-*fos* transcriptional activation require distinct upstream regulatory sequences. *Mol Cell Biol* 1988;8:2787–2796.

166. Stumpo DJ, Blackshear PJ. Insulin and growth factor effects on c-*fos* expression in normal and protein kinase C-deficient 3T3-L1 fibroblasts and adipocytes. *Proc Natl Acad Sci U S A* 1983;83:9453–9457.

Asthma, edited by P.J. Barnes, M.M. Grunstein, A.R. Leff, and A.J. Woolcock. Lippincott–Raven Publishers, Philadelphia 1997.

▪ 60 ▪

Airway Mucus Secretion

Shahriyar Tavakoli, Stewart J. Levine, and James H. Shelhamer

Airway obstruction in asthma is due to mucosal edema, bronchial smooth muscle contraction, increased airway mucus secretion, and airway inflammation. Each of these features has been noted in severe asthma and each may also be present in mild-to-moderate asthma (1). The airway epithelium provides protection from a variety of external stimuli by secreting a complex liquid mixture (mucus) into the airway lumen. This mixture is composed of water, electrolytes, proteins, proteoglycans, glycoproteins, and lipids. Mucus can serve as protective barrier against airborne physicochemical insults and invasion of microorganisms. Airway mucus is composed of two thin layers, a liquid or sol phase and a more viscous gel phase, covering the conducting airways. The airway cilia are in contact with the sol phase of mucus and propel the gel layer toward the pharynx by the beating action of the cilia. When the quantity or nature of airway secretions is abnormal, mucociliary clearance may be altered. An excessive volume of airway secretions due to increased cellular secretion of mucus or due to increased exudation of plasma products may overwhelm this transport system leading to retained airway secretions and to airway ob-

struction. This chapter reviews airway mucin production in the context of airway inflammation. In this context, we will review factors which alter secretory cell exocytosis, stimuli of mucin gene expression, and stimuli of secretory cell hyperplasia and metaplasia.

SECRETORY CELLS

The airway mucosa is lined with a superficial, pseudostratified, ciliated columnar epithelium extending from the nares to the bronchioles. Interspersed among the ciliated cells are basal cells, neuroendocrine cells, and a secretory cell, the goblet cell. Goblet cells (mucus-secreting cells) are found in proximal airways and less often in bronchioles less than 1mm in diameter (2,3). The cytoplasm of goblet cells is filled with electron-lucent granules. These granules are bound with membranes which give the secretory granules a confluent, tightly packed configuration (4). Clara cells are mainly seen in the terminal bronchioles and protrude into the airway lumen. These cells have egg-shaped electron dense granules in humans; their function remains to be determined. The role of ciliated cells is to clear the airways of secreted products. They are also presumably a principal site for chloride flux. Transitional cells in the surface epithelium are also seen (5–8). Below the superficial epithelium, the submucosa contains submucosal glands,

S. Tavakoli, S.J. Levine, and J.H. Shelhamer: Department of Critical Care Medicine, Clinical Center, National Institutes of Health, Bethesda, Maryland 20892.

muscle, blood vessels, and cartilage. Submucosal glands can be found throughout the large airways, mainly in the cartilaginous portions (trachea and bronchi). In the proximal airway, submucosal gland cells outnumber goblet cells 40 to 1. These are complex tubuloacinar glands composed of a dilated collecting duct, with many secretory tubules coming off the collecting duct and ending in multiple serous and mucus cells, which form acinar structures. The collecting duct is lined with ciliated-pseudostratified columnar epithelium. The secretory tubules are lined by columnar epithelium, which controls the concentration of secretions by regulating water and electrolytes. The mucus cells of the acinar structure have a columnar shape with basally positioned nuclei and large amounts of electron-lucent granules (9). The serous cells of acinar structure appear by light microscopy as pyramidal in shape, with basally placed small, round nuclei. The cytoplasm is packed with electron-dense secretory granules. Serous cells secrete several nonglycoprotein products, such as lysozyme, lactoferrin, low-molecular-mass antiprotease, and an albuminlike protein, as well as high molecular-weight glycoconjugates or proteoglycans (10–13).

BIOCHEMICAL COMPOSITION OF MUCUS

Airway mucus has viscoelastic properties primarily due to the presence of mucus glycoproteins. Other constituents of airway secretions which may substantially affect the rheologic properties of respiratory mucus include DNA and polymerized actin released from inflammatory cells (14). Airway mucus is a heterogenous fluid composed of 84% to 95% water, 1% to 5% protein, 0.9% to 1.1% carbohydrate, and 0.8% to 3.1% lipid (15). However, this composition can change by an increase of local production of proteins such as lysozyme, lactoferrin, immunoglobulin (Ig)A, or IgE, and transduction of serum proteins such as α_1 antitrypsin, α_2 macroglobulin, haptoglobin, transferrin, IgM, IgG, and IgA (16–18). Increased local production of proteins can occur in a variety of diseases characterized by airway inflammation such as asthma, bronchitis, and cystic fibrosis.

Mucin glycoproteins are composed of a protein core encoded by several genes. Portions of this protein core are rich in serine, threonine, and proline. Numerous oligosaccharide side chains are linked via an O-glycosidic bond to serine or threonine residues on the protein core (19).

Mucin glycoproteins are characterized by a high content of carbohydrates (greater than 70% by weight). These exist in the form of oligosaccharide side chains of approximately 1 to 20 monosaccharides made up of fucose, galactose, N-acetylneuraminic, N-acetylglucosamine, and N-acetylgalactosamine. Some of the oligosaccharide side chains are sulfated. The estimated size of mucin glycoproteins ranges from 1.8 to 7 x 10^6 daltons (20,21). The structure of mucus glycoprotein (MGP) is dependent on the intra- and interchain disulfide bonds between cysteine residues. The acidic property of many of these mucins is due to the presence of sialic acid and sulfate (22).

MUCIN GENES

In recent years much progress has been made in identifying the genes encoding for airway mucins. Mucin genes have in common domains of repeating amino-acid sequences which are in general rich in serine, threonine, or proline residues. It is these tandem repeat regions which are heavily glycosylated via O-glycosidic bonds. Those mucin genes known to be expressed in the airway have been designated MUC-1, MUC-2, MUC-4 and MUC-5 (Table 1). This section will briefly review the human mucin genes that are expressed in human bronchial epithelial cells.

The human MUC-1 gene encodes a glycoprotein localized in the airway to the cell surface of bronchial and nasal epithelial cells (42). This gene has three specific regions. The amino terminal region may be of variable length depending on the splice variant (25,40). The second region makes up the vast portion of the protein and is composed of variable numbers of tandem-repeat sequences. Each sequence contains 20 amino acids (25–28, 39,40). The carboxy terminal portion containing 326 amino acids is divided into two segments: a transmembrane segment and a cytoplasmic tail (26,27). This glycoprotein is a membrane protein which has a mucin structure (25,26). It is not secreted but may be proteolytically cleaved to function as an airway mucin.

TABLE 1. *Human airway mucin genes and their tandem repeats*

Nomenclature	Tissue Type	Chromasomal Location	Repeat Sequence	Refs
MUC1	Mammary/Lung	1q21-24	PDTRPAPGSTAPPAHGVTSA	23-28
MUC2	Intestinal/tracheal	11p15.5	PTTTPITTTTTVTPTPTPTGTQT	29-34
MUC4	Tracheal	3q29	TSSVSTGHATSLPVTD	35
MUC5	Tracheal	11p15	TTSTTSAP	36-38

Table derived from information in listed references and from Rose MC. Mucin structure, function, and role in pulmonary diseases. *Am J Physiol* 1992;413–429, with permission; from Gum JR. Mucin gene and the proteins they encode: Structure, Diversity, and Regulation. *Am J Respir Cell Mol Biol* 1992;7:557–564, with permission; from Basbaum C, Welsh M. Mucus secretion and ion transport in airways. In: Murray J, Nadel J., eds. *Respiratory Medicine*, Philadelphia: WB Saunders Company, 1994; 323–344, with permission.

Human MUC-2 was first detected in the small intestine, colon, and airways (30–32). This mucin is made up of two repetitive domains (33). The central tandem repeat is the largest domain, containing 23 amino-acid residue tandem repeats, the number of which may vary with the type of allele (33,34). The most common MUC-2 allele contains close to 100 tandem-repeat units averaging 2,300 amino acids in length. These tandem-repeat amino acids are rich in threonine, 78% of which are glycosylated, and contain approximately 1,000 O-linked oligosaccharide chains (30,40,43). The carboxy terminal domain of MUC-2 is composed of 984 amino acids which can be divided into cysteine-rich (845 amino acids) and mucinlike (139 amino acids) subdomains. Upstream (toward the amino terminal end of the molecule) of the area of the tandem repeats, the molecule contains 1,270 amino residues divided into two subdomains: cysteine-rich and mucinlike. Both of the cysteine-rich subdomains have sequence similarities to prepro von Willebrand factor and, because of the cystein-rich domains, may be involved in the packaging of secretory granules and possibly in the determination of mucus viscoelasticity due to disulfide bond formation (29,40,44).

Human MUC-4 was identified by immunoscreening of a tracheobronchial complementary deoxyribonucleic acid (cDNA) library with antibodies directed against the peptide core of deglycosylated mucins. Only its tandem-repeat unit sequence is known. This tandem repeat consists of 16 amino acids, rich in serine and threonine. As with MUC-2, northern analysis of human tracheobronchial mRNA probed for the MUC-4 sequence gives a polydisperse signal (35).

Human MUC-5 has been sequenced from a nasal polyp cDNA library screened with nucleotide probes based on the amino-acid sequence of proteolytic fragments of a mucus gel from an asthmatic patient. MUC-5 has 5 tandem repeats and cysteine-rich domains which are similar to MUC-2 (38,45). As in MUC-2, the carboxyl terminal cysteine-rich domains of MUC-5 have sequence homology with human von Willebrand factor, again suggesting that these sequences are important for the structure of the secreted glycoprotein (38).

Finally, quantation of mucin messenger ribonucleic acid (mRNA) has been difficult because of the polydispersity of mRNA transcripts (32,46). In general, in the airway, MUC-5 is probably expressed in greater abundance than MUC-2 (46).

METHODS OF STUDY OF AIRWAY SECRETION

A variety of methods have been adopted to collect and quantitate airway secretion (Table 2). *In vivo* collection of respiratory secretions collected by spontaneous expectoration, induced expectoration, and bronchoscopic aspiration all have been used to study the rheologic, chemical,

TABLE 2. *Methods and strategies to study airway secretion*

Method	State	Measurement	Example Ref.
Collection			
Expectorated mucus	*In Vivo*	A,C	47,48
Spontaneous			
Induced			49
Whole trachea preparation	*In Vitro*	A,C	50
Micropipetting of submucosal glands	*In Vitro*	D	51,52
Culture of airway tissue			
Organ cultures	*In vitro*	A,C	53,54
Isolated submucosal glands		A,C	55,56
Primary cultures			
Surface tracheal epithelial cells	*In Vitro*	A,B,C	57-60
Submucosal gland cells	*In Vitro*	A,C	61,62
Cell lines	*In Vitro*	A,C	63,64

A, Quantition of radiolabeled macromolecules (i.e., respiratory glycoconjugate (RGC)); B, Quantition of mucus glycoprotein by size exclusion chromatography after hyaluronidase digestion (i.e., mucuslike glycoprotein); C, Quantition of secreted products by enzyme-linked immunosorbent assay (ELISA) (i.e., mucin, lysozyme, or lactoferrin).

and cellular characteristics of airway secretions. However, sputum contains saliva which may be a source of contaminating products. Other *in vivo* methods such as micropipette aspiration and the quantitation of tracheal hillocks have been used for the quantitation of respiratory secretion and secretory activity from submucosal glands, respectively (51,65). Isolation of tracheal segments from live animals has been utilized in the collection of tracheal secretions after electrical, pharmacologic, and physical stimulation (66). The formation of a tracheal pouch permits the study and collection of secretions on a long-term basis (67). *In vitro* culture methods have been utilized to study airway secretion from human and animal tissues. These include airway organ culture, primary cultures of cells from surface epithelium, submucosal glands, and airway epithelial cell lines. In addition, modified Ussing chambers have been used to study the secretion from tracheal and bronchial tissue. These cell culture methods permit the study of secretions from specific cell types that are independent of external hormonal and neuronal control. The detection and measurement of secretory products have been analyzed in several different ways. Radiolabeled precursors such as glucosamine, galactosamine, threonine, or sulfate may be incorporated into MGP and proteoglycans. The term "respiratory glycoconjugate" (RGC) represents the radiolabelled macromolecular products (MGP and proteoglycans) of submucosal gland cells and goblet cells. RGC quantitation is accomplished by scintillation counting of collected media after dialysis or precipitation with ethanol or trichloroacetic acid. Chromatography of radiolabeled glycoconjugates after proteoglycan-degrading enzyme digestion is a more specific way to quantitate mucinlike glycoprotein. Monoclonal and polyclonal antibodies have been used to detect cell-specific secretory products such as lactoferrin, lysozyme, and mucin glycoprotein (68–70). Mucin secretion from human explants, human tracheobronchial epithelial cells, and feline epithelial cell cultures have been quantified with monoclonal antibody based enzyme-linked immunosorbent assays (ELISAs).

NEURAL REGULATION OF MUCUS SECRETION

Airway mucus glycoprotein secretion from submucosal glands is controlled in part by the autonomic nervous system. The autonomic nervous system has three pathways: the cholinergic, the adrenergic, and the nonadrenergic-noncholinergic (NANC) pathways. These pathways may affect exocytosis of stored products. In addition, they control airway smooth muscle tone, vascular permeability, bronchial vasculature tone, bronchial blood flow, fluid and electrolyte secretion, and, to some degree, the liberation of the mediators from mast cells and inflammatory cells. The effect of various neurohormones and neuropeptides on airway mucin secretion is presented in Table 3.

The airways of humans and animals have a rich cholinergic innervation which mainly participates in the regulation of airway smooth muscle tone and secretion (71,72). Efferent fibers of the cholingeric nervous system originate in the vagal nuclei located in the brain stem. These fibers travel down the vagus nerve until they synapse with postganglionic fibers in ganglia within the airway wall, and subsequently innervate the submucosal gland and smooth muscle cells. In contrast, the goblet cells of the superficial epithelium are not innervated with cholinergic fibers (73,74). Stimulation of the vagus nerve results in increased mucus secretion (65,75). The presence of muscarinic receptors has been demonstrated on serous and mucous airway gland cells. These cells have equal proportions of muscrinic receptors (76,77). Muscarinic receptor-stimulation of human airway in vitro and isolated submucosal glands from feline and swine trachea induces mucus glycoprotein secretion (53,56,78,79). Three pharmacologic muscarinic receptor subtypes have been identified in the lung: M_1, M_2, and M_3 (80). Mak and Barnes (81) demonstrated by autoradiography that M_3-receptors outnumber M_1-receptors by a ratio of 2:1 over the submucosal glands in human airway. Similar findings have been reported in swine trachea (78). Mucus glycoprotein secretion, in response to cholinergic stimulation, such as methacholine, can be entirely inhibited by M_3-muscarinic receptor blockade (79,82). M_1-muscarinic receptor blockade with pirenzepine does not completely inhibit the mucus secretion from human bronchi or feline airways in culture (82,83). These findings suggest that the M_3- muscarinic receptor is the receptor primarily involved in submucosal gland exocytosis in response to cholinergic stimulation in the bronchial tree.

Adrenergic regulation of airway secretion occurs through epinephrine and norepinephrine release from the adrenal medulla and sympathetic nerves, respectively. These catecholamines are capable of activating both α- and β-receptors of airway cells. Glandular secretion via the adrenergic pathway occurs in response to impulses from the preganglionic neuron through the stellate ganglion to the postganglionic neuron and, finally, to the secretory cells of submucosal glands. Morphometric and histochemical analyses of cat and guinea pig trachea have shown that adrenergic nerve fibers are in the proximity of submucosal glands (84–86). Nevertheless, adrenergic innervation of lung varies among species. Human airway sympathetic innervation is more sparse than feline airway, which has a rich sympathetic innervation (71,87,88). Autoradiographic studies have demonstrated α-adrenoreceptor binding sites over secretory cells of submucosal glands (89). Phenylephrine increases the secretion of radiolabeled macromolecules from human bronchi in vitro and from feline airway in vivo (53,90). Respiratory glycoconjugate and mucus glycoprotein secretion occurs predominantly via α-1 adrenoreceptor stimulation. Serous cells compared to mucus cells have a greater density of α-1 adrenoreceptor binding sites (89,91,92). Therefore, stimulation of gland cells with phenylephrine may cause a less viscoelastic and more watery secretion (91,93,94). In some diseases associated with airway inflammation, such as chronic bronchitis, pneumonia, or endotoxin exposure, there is an increase of α-1 adrenoreceptor density (95,96).

β-adrenoreceptors have been demonstrated on submucosal gland cells of human airways and other species

TABLE 3. *Neuronal control of human airway mucin release*

Nervous System	Mediator	Receptor Location	Effect on Mucus Secretion
Cholinergic	ACh	SG	Increase
Adrenergic			
α-Adrenergic	NE	SG	Increase
β-Adrenergic	NE	SG	Varible
NANC			
Sensory	SP	SG and SE	Increase
	NKA		Increase*
	GRP	SG and SE	Increase
Parasympathetic	VIP	SG and SE	Variable
Other Peptides	Endothelin	SG	Increase

ACh, acetylcholine; NE, norepinephrine; SP, substance P; NKA, neurokinin A; GRP, gastrin releasing hormone; VIP, vasoactive intestinal peptide; SG, submucosal glands; SE, surface epithelium.

*Interreaction of NKA with NK-1 receptors rather than NK-2 receptors causes mucus secretion *in vitro*. See text for details.

(97,98). Stimulation of β-adrenoreceptors results in mucin glycoprotein secretion in a variety of species (99). Stimulation of β-adrenoreceptors on submucosal glands in experimental animals induces secretions with higher viscoelastic properties, suggesting selective stimulation of submucosal gland mucus cell activation, but no significant glandular contraction (55,94). However, varied responses have been reported in regards to mucin glycoprotein secretion from human tissue. For example, β-adrenergic stimulation of human airways in organ culture of human bronchi failed to induce RGC secretion (53,100).

Nonadrenergic Noncholinergic Innervation

The nonadrenergic noncholinergic (NANC) nervous system contains a variety of neuropeptides (see Chapter 73) which may be synthesized and released in the trachea and bronchi. Some peptides may co-exist with norepinephrine in sympathetic nerves or with acetylcholine in cholinergic nerve fibers. Stimulation of the NANC may cause mucus secretion from submucosal glands and perhaps goblet cells of the superficial epithelium. Vagal nerve stimulation of cats in vivo produces airway mucus secretion, which is only partially inhibited by the muscarinic antagonist atropine (101). Similarly, electrical stimulation of ferret trachea results in $^{35}SO_4$-labeled macromolecule secretion, which is not completely inhibited by cholinergic and adrenergic antagonists in combination (75). These studies suggest that other stimulants such as neuropeptides are involved in vagal stimulation of airway secretion. The effect of specific neuropeptides, such as the tachykinins (substance P and neurokinin A), gastrin-releasing peptide (GRP), and vasoactive intestinal peptide (VIP), will be discussed briefly in regards to their effect on airway secretion.

Substance P is localized to sensory neurons of conducting airways (102,103). Substance P is mainly concentrated in capsaicin-sensitive unmyelinated nerves in the airways. The substance P receptor (NK-1) is widely distributed on submucosal glands in human airway (104). Substance P stimulation of ferret trachea and isolated submucosal glands from feline trachea results in RGC secretion (105,106). This may be a result of substance P-stimulated exocytosis or of substance P-stimulated contraction of the myoepithelial cells surrounding the submucosal gland. Substance P may also stimulate goblet cell secretion (107,108). A second tachykinin, Neurokinin A, may also bind to tachykinin receptors on glandular cells but is relatively less potent than substance P (109). Neurokinin A acting through the NK2-receptor may be more potent in inducing vascular permeability and edema formation.

Gastrin-releasing peptide (GRP), a mammalian neuropeptide (Bombesin in amphibian), has been localized within autonomic ganglia in the airway (110). GRP coex-

ists with SP in some neuronal tissues and has also been found in macrophages and respiratory neuroendocrine cells (111). GRP receptors are present over submucosal glands and superficial epithelium of the human trachea (112). GRP added to feline trachea in vitro causes respiratory glycoconjugate secretion (113). Similar findings were observed from human nasal tissue in organ culture (110).

Vasoactive intestinal peptide (VIP) is a 28 amino-acid peptide found in significant quantity in airway tissue (114,115). VIP neurons are abundant in the nasal mucosa, upper respiratory tract, and proximal airways, but occur with a lesser density in peripheral airways (102,116). The pattern of distribution of VIP is the same as the distribution of cholinergic nerves (116,117). Autoradiographic studies have demonstrated VIP-binding sites in high density over bronchopulmonary vasculature, particularly in large airways, submucosal glands, and airway epithelium. The nasal mucosa also has VIP-binding sites predominantly on epithelial cells, submucosal glands, and arterial vessels, except sinusoidal vessels (111). VIP has been reported to have both stimulatory and inhibitory effects on airway secretion from submucosal glands. Peatfield et al. (118) and Gashi et al. (119) observed the secretion of S[35]-labeled macromolecules from ferret tracheal submucosal glands after VIP stimulation. On the other hand, Coles et al. (120) showed inhibition of radiolabeled glycoconjugate secretion from human bronchi in organ culture. These variations could be explained by species diversity or experimental model. In the upper airway, VIP induces the secretion of lactoferrin from serous cells in the human nasal mucosa explants in organ culture, but has no significant effect on mucus secretion in same culture tissue (121). In the airway, VIP may also have anti-inflammatory properties mediated by its effect on inflammatory cell function (122). VIP immunoreactivity has been shown in nerve fibers innervating smooth muscle cells of the bronchial tree and in single nerve fibers near the basal surface of epithelial cells, and in the vicinity of vessels and glands in nonasthmatic patients. In one study, no immunoreactivity was observed in asthmatic subjects (123). This raised the possibility that the loss of VIP effects contributes to clinical asthma.

Endothelin

Endothelins consist of three polypeptides: endothelin-1, 2, and 3. Endothelin-1 is made up of 21 amino acids. The airway epithelium in addition to the vascular endothelium may be a source of endothelin production (124,125). In addition to its vasoconstrictive and bronchoconstrictive properties, endothelin-1 induces mucin secretion from human bronchi in organ culture (126). Endothelin-1 stimulates the release of respiratory glycoconjugates from feline isolated tracheal submucosal glands (127). Endothelin-1 increases the release of eicosanoids from human nasal explants in culture, suggesting that some effects of endothelin in the airway may be related to endothelin stimulation of eicasnoid production and the subsequent effect of bioactive eicosanoids on epithelial secretory cells (128).

NEUROGENIC INFLAMMATION VIA AXONAL REFLEXES AND ANTIDROMIC REFLEXES

Neurogenic inflammation was first described by Jancscó and his colleagues (129) as an increase in vascular permeability, plasma extravasation, and edema. Neurogenic inflammation arises via axonal reflexes in which sensory nerve stimulation leads to the antidromic release of sensory neuropeptides. It has been speculated that neurogenic inflammation may explain, in part, mucus hypersecretion in respiratory diseases such as asthma (130). The airway epithelial damage in these conditions exposes sensory nerve C-fiber endings which can be activated by noxious stimuli or inflammatory mediators. This nerve stimulation leads to reflex antidromic conduction down collateral sensory endings where the release of neuropeptides, such as SP, NKA, and perhaps GRP, may occur. Consequently, these peptides may stimulate mucus secretion from both submucosal glands and surface epithelial goblet cells, induce vascular leakage, and activate inflammatory cells. Moreover, surface epithelium damage or shedding as may occur in the setting of bacterial or viral infection or in response to products of inflammatory cells may result in a decrease in tachykinin-degrading enzymes produced by epithelial cells such as neutral endopeptidase. This reduction in neutral endopeptidase could lead to an increase in the half life of tachykinins and prolong their effect on mucus secreting cells.

INFLAMMATORY STIMULI AND AIRWAY MUCUS SECRETION

A variety of products released during the inflammatory response may alter airway secretion by the stimulation of secretory cell exocytosis of secretory vesicles. Other stimuli may alter the capacity of secretory cells to respond to a secretory stimulus by altering the gene expression of secretory cell constituents, or by altering the number of secretory cells in the airway. This includes secretory cell hyperplasia in the large airways where secretory cells are normally located or secretory cell metaplasia in the portions of the airway where secretory cells are not normally present.

Stimuli of Secretory Cell Exocytosis

Mediators of the inflammatory response may be released from airway resident cells (epithelial cells, mast cells, and macrophages) and migratory inflammatory cells (neutrophils, eosinophils, and mononuclear cells and lymphocytes). Inflammatory mediators, such as lipid mediators and some cytokines, may serve as stimuli for exocytosis of products from secretory cells. They may also have a chemoattractant property for leukocytes which may release additional inflammatory mediators which have an effect on secretory cell exocytosis or induction of gene expression for secreted products. This section will review the effects of inflammatory mediators on secretory cells.

Lipid Mediators

Lipid mediators are products of the activation of phospholipase A_2, which releases free arachidonic acid and lyso-platelet activating factor (PAF) from membrane phospholipids. The metabolism of arachidonic acid (AA) through the cyclooxygenase pathway will lead to the formation of prostaglandins (PGs) and thromboxanes (TXs), and via lipoxygenase pathway to leukotrienes (LTs) and hydroxyeicosatetraenoic acids (HETEs). The acetylation of lyso-PAF forms PAF. These eicosanoid mediators may have a variety of effects on conducting airways, such as induction of mucus secretion, inflammatory cell recruitment, alteration of mucociliary transport and ion transport, changes in vascular permeability, and bronchoconstriction.

The liberation of eicosanoids is specific to each cell type in the airway (131). Human airway epithelial cells have been shown to release eicosanoids produced via both the lipoxygenase and cyclooxygenase pathways (132–136). Human airway epithelial cells generate primarily prostaglandin $(PGE)_2$ from the cyclooxygenase pathway and 15-HETE from the lipoxygenase pathway (137–139). The eicosanoids produced by airway cells and their effect on airway macromolecule secretion are presented in Table 4. A variety of eicosanoids may stimulate respiratory glycoconjuate (RGC) release from human and

TABLE 4. *Effect of lipid mediators on airway mucus secretion*

	Major Cellular Source	Mucus Secretion	Refs
Lipoxygenase products			
5-HETE	PMN, MAC	⇑⇑	136,139
15-HETE	Epi, EOS	⇑⇑	137,139
LTC$_4$/D$_4$	MC, EOS, MAC	⇑⇑⇑	140,141
Cyclooxygenase products			
PGE$_2$	Epi	⇓	137,139
PGF$_{2\alpha}$	Epi	⇑	139,142,143
PGD$_2$	MC	⇔	138
Platelet-activating factor	MC,MAC,Eos		
	PMN,Epi	⇑	144,145

PMN, polymorphonuclear leukocyte; MAC, macrophage; Epi, airway epithelial cell; EOS, eosinophil; MC, mast cell experimental animal airway cells (140,141,147). The eicosanoids that can induce macromolecule secretion from the most potent to the least potent are sulfidopeptide leukotrienes < HETES < LTB_4 < prostaglandins. A variety of *in vitro* studies using human airway tissue in culture would suggest a broad range in the lowest effective concentration of leukotrienes (picomolar), HETES (nanomolar), and prostaglandins (micromolar) for stimulation of airway macromolecule secretion (148). Studies of primary culture of superficial airway epithelial cells have not universally shown these cells to secrete macromolecles in response to eicosanoids. Guinea-pig tracheal epithelial cells stimulated with $PGF_{2\alpha}$ or 5- 12- and 15 HETE in combination secrete mucinlike glycoprotein (149,150). Studies in primary cultures of hamster epithelial cells stimulated with $PGF_{2\alpha}$, PGE_2, LTC_4, or LTD_4 failed to show mucus secretion (59). MGP secretion from the human airway in response to leukotrienes can be inhibited by the leukotriene receptor antagonist FPL 55712 (141). PGE_2 reduces baseline airway macromolecule secretion from human bronchi in culture. Finally, PAF may act on epithelial cells through a cell surface receptor to directly stimulate secretory cell exocytosis (150,151). PAF may also have an effect on these cells by inducing cellular production of eicosanoids with a subsequent autocrine stimulation of exocytosis. There are multiple sources for PAF in the airway, including resident noninflammatory and inflammatory cells. PAF may also serve as a chemoattractant in the recruitement and activation of inflammatory cells which may then lead to mucus secretion in response to their released products.

SPECIFIC INFLAMMATORY CELL PRODUCTS

The resident airway epithelial cells and recruited inflammatory cells play an important role in the modulation of airway inflammation by releasing inflammatory mediators, some of which may cause mucus hypersecretion (Table 5). This process may explain a variety of respiratory diseases such as asthma, in which mucus hypersecretion may be present. This section will review the products of specific inflammatory cells which may be relevant to this process.

Mast Cells

Mast cells can be found in the submucosa and within the lumen of the conducting airways (152). Bronchoalveolar lavage (BAL) of allergic asthmatic patients has demonstrated that the quantity of mast cells and mast cell products is increased especially after exposure to antigen (153,154). Mast cells are known to release various mediators that cause the early phase of the asthmatic reaction. RGC secretion is increased in cultured human airways after mast cell degranulation. This finding suggests that

TABLE 5. *Specific inflammatory cells products mediating mucus hypersecretion*

Mast cells
Histamine
Eicosanoids (PGD_2, LTB_4, LTC_4)
PAF
Chymase
TNF-α
Neutrophils
Elastase
Cathepsin G
LTB_4
Oxygen species
Eosinophils
ECP
LTC_4, LTD_4
PAF
Oxygen species
Aleveolar Macrophages
5HETE, LTB_4, LTC_4
MMS
PAF
Oxygen species
TNF-α, IL-1

PGD_2, prostaglandin D_2; TNF-α, tumor necorsis factor-α; IL, interleukin; PAF, platelet-activating factor; ECP, eosinophilic cationic protein; MMS, Macrophage mucous secretagogue.

mast cell degranulation may stimulate secretory cell exocytosis and increase mucus secretion (50). A variety of mast cell-derived mediators are capable of stimulating mucus secretion. Histamine has been shown to increase glycoconjugate secretion from human airway cultures and from cultured bovine airway gland serous cells. This histamine induced secretion can be inhibited by an H_2-receptor antagonist (53,155). Prostaglandin-generating factor of anaphylaxis (PGFA), one of the products of activated mast cells, has been shown to cause RGC secretion from human airway organ cultures (156). PGF-A induction of secretion requires eicosanoid metabolism in the airway. In addition, mast cells release PGD_2, LTB_4, LTC_4, and PAF, all of which are capable of stimulating mucus secretion from airway epithelial cells (157–159). The mast cell enzymes chymase and tryptase are stored in mast cell granules. Chymase has been reported to profoundly increase radiolabeled glycoconjugate release from both cultured bovine tracheal gland serous cells and canine tracheal epithelial cells (155,160). The majority of mast cells (70%) in the vicinity of submucosal glands contain chymase (161).

Neutrophils

Neutrophils exist in the normal human conducting airway and are recruited in a variety of airway diseases including the late phase of the asthmatic reaction (162,163). Neutrophils may stimulate mucus secretion mediated, in part, by cell-derived products such as lipid mediators (PAF, 5-HETE, and LTB_4); by the release of serine proteases such as elastase and cathepsin G; and by the production of oxygen metabolites. Human neutrophil elastase has been demonstrated to profoundly stimulate airway macromolecule secretion from epithelial cell cultures and from human airway organ cultures (160,164). Similar findings have been demonstrated with cathepsin G in feline tracheal epithelial cells and bovine serous cells (165,166). Neutrophils are able to liberate toxic oxygen metabolites and subsequently stimulate airway secretion. This effect is mediated, in part, by induced eicosanoid production (149).

Eosinophils

Eosinophils, like mast cells, can be recovered in the BAL from conducting airways of asthmatic patients (167,168). Eosinophils may stimulate secretion by releasing lipid mediators, such as LTC_4, and LTD_4 and PAF, and by the release of several protein constituents of the eosinophil granule. For example, eosinphil cationic protein (ECP) enhances mucus secretion in a dose-dependent fashion in both human and feline airway in organ culture. In contrast, major basic protein (MBP) does not directly induce mucus secretion. MBP has been reported to have a cytotoxic effect on epithelial cells and might have in indirect effect on secretion by the stimulation of exposed C-fiber endings, resulting from airway surface epithelial damage and shedding. Finally, other eosinophil granule products such as eosinophil peroxidase and eosinophil-derived neurotoxin (EDN) have no documented effect on airway secretion (169).

Macrophages

Macrophages are present in activated form in the airway mucosa of patients with chronic asthma and bronchitis. Increases in the numbers of macrophages have been demonstrated in BAL from asthmatic airways *in vivo* after allergen challenge (163). Alveolar macrophages exhibit an increase in the number of low-affinity IgE-receptors, an increased lipid mediator liberation, and an enhanced ability to produce proteases after being provoked with antigen or anti-IgE (170–173). Activated macrophages may alter airway mucus release via production of eicasanoids and produce a macrophage-specific product designated macrophage mucus secretegogue (MMS). Production of lipid mediators, specifically PGD_2, LTB_4, and LTC_4, as well as oxygen metabolites has been detected from a monocyte-macrophage cell line (174). These products may also have an effect on airway secretion as previously described. MMS is synthesized and secreted by the activated alveolar macrophage or by activated peripheral blood monocytes. MMS is present in the BAL fluid of patients with chronic airway inflamma-

tion. It directly stimulates secretory cells to release mucin-type glycoprotiens (175,176). Finally, macrophage-derived cytokines such as tumor necrosis factor (TNF)-α and interleukin (IL)-1β stimulate mucin secretion in human airway organ explants and from superficial epithelial cells (177,178).

SERUM DERIVED MEDIATORS

Alteration of vascular permeability as a result of the release of mast cell products leads to vascular leakage of serum proteins which may stimulate mucus-secreting cells. These include C_{3a} and bradykinin. A component of the alternative and classic complement pathways, C_{3a} has been demonstrated to increase RGC release from explants of human airway in organ culture (179). This process appears to function separately from mast cell activation or eicosanoid liberation. Bradykinin is produced by the proteolytic action of kallikrein and other proteases such as mast cell tryptase on tissue or plasma kininogens. Binding sites for bradykinin in the airway are found mainly over vessels and in much lower density over glands and epithelium (180). Bradykinin *in vitro* has a small stimulatory effect on respiratory glycoconjugate release from ferret trachea and from human nasal mucosa in organ culture. The effect of bradykinin on secretion may be indirect via the induction of eicosanoid metabolism or via sensory nerve activation.

EXOGENOUS PRODUCTS

A variety of exogenous substances may stimulate airway secretory cell exocytosis. Included in this group are bacterial products such as pseudomonas elastase and alkaline protease which stimulate respiratory macromolecule secretion from human, feline, and guinea-pig airway cultures (181,182). Rhamnolipid, another product of *Pseudomonas aeruginosa*, was also found to stimulate mucus secretion from human and feline airway organ cultures (183). Lipopolysaccharide (LPS), a cell wall component of gram-negative bacteria, stimulates the release of MGP from primary cultures of feline tracheal cells, human epithelial cells, and human airway in organ culture (184). This effect was found to peak at 48 hours. In a recent study, mucin concentration measurement in BAL from endotoxin-treated rats revealed that endotoxin increases the production of mucinlike molecules by rat airway epithelium (185). Finally, noxious chemical agents such as air pollutants (SO2, ozone), irritants (ammonia, charcoal dust, and barium sulfate), and tobacco smoke are all able to stimulate mucus secretion from airway epithelium (186–189). This response *in vivo* may occur via three mechanisms: a) a direct effect on the superficial epithelium, b) neuropeptide mediated antidromic reflex in response to stimulation of C-fiber ending, and c) activation of transspinal C-fiber reflexes leading to parasympathetic stimulation of glandular secretion. In addition, ozone has been found to activate phospholipases in guinea-pig tracheal epithelial cells in primary culture and to cause the release of PAF, which may have a direct effect on secretory cells or induce the additional production of lipid mediators (190).

STIMULI OF MUCIN GENE EXPRESSION

Induction of mucin gene expression may be a mechanism by which secretory cells may produce, store, and secrete increased amounts of airway mucins. It may also be a mechanism by which nonsecretory cells may change phenotype. Knowledge of the control of specific mucin genes in the airway epithelium is limited. Two cytokine products of activated mast cells, macrophages and activated lymphocytes, TNF-α, IL-1β, are capable of increasing MUC-2 mRNA levels. Both of these stimuli act through specific cytokine receptors and have an effect which lasts up to 24 to 48 hours (177,178). The pleiotrophic cytokine, IL6, also is capable of increasing MUC-2 gene expression in airway

epithelial cells, but with a much longer time to peak effect (24 to 48 hours) (191). The administration of endotoxin to rodents *in vivo* has been shown to increase PAS-positive material in secretory cells. Endotoxin treatment of human epithelial cells in culture has been shown not only to increase mucus secretion, but also to increase MUC-2 mRNA levels, suggesting that the increases in secreted product are a result of increased expression of one or more mucin genes. Finally, a 1 kDa protein product of *P. aeruginosa* has been found to induce increases in MUC-2 and MUC-5 steady-state mRNA levels in a human airway epithelial cell line (192).

STIMULI OF SECRETORY CELL HYPERPLASIA

Secretory cell hyperplasia and metaplasia is a pathologic response that occurs after exposure to stimuli such as inhalants (tobacco smoke and sulfur dioxide), neutrophil products, and endotoxin (185,193,194). Asthma, chronic bronchitis, and cystic fibrosis are the best examples of diseases associated with goblet cell hyperplasia. Goblet cell hyperplasia has been induced in the trachea of

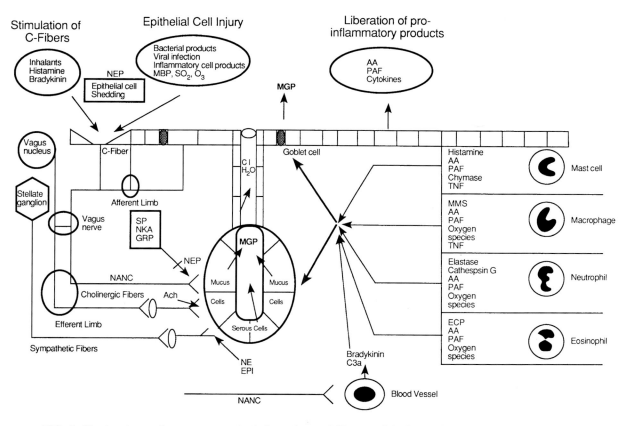

FIG. 1. Mechanisms of mucus exocytosis in asthma. *ACh*, acetylcholine; *EPI*, epinephrine; *NE*, norepinephrine; *NANC*, nonadrenergic, noncholinergic nervous system; *SP*, substance P; *GRP*, gastrin releasing peptide; *NKA*, neurokinin A; *AA*, arachidonic acid metabolites; *MGP*, mucus glycoprotein; *ECP*, eosinophil cationic protein; *MBP*, major basic protein; *PAF*, platelet activating factor; *TNF*, tumor necrosis factor; *SO₂*, sulfur dioxide; *O₃*, ozone; *C3ₐ*, fragment of the third component of complement.

rats and hamsters after intratracheal installation with neutrophil elastase. This effect was prevented by preadministration of dexamethasone and elastase inhibitors (chloromethylketone or elgin C) in rats and hamsters, respectively (194–197). Cathepsin G, another neutrophil serine esterase, has been shown to induce secretory cell metaplasia. Secretory cell hyperplasia in response to a variety of irritants, may be mediated by inflammatory cells or their products. It has been speculated that the lipid mediators, particularly eicosanoids released from inflammatory cells, may cause secretory cell hyperplasia in response to cigarette smoke. For example, glucocorticoids and indomethacin can inhibit secretory cell hyperplasia, secondary to tobacco smoke (198). Nevertheless, the exact nature of the mechanism for this process remains to be explained. Irritants such as ammonia, charcoal dust, and barium sulfate powder have been reported to induce secrectory cell hyperplasia (188,189,199). A mechanism more specific than the induction of chronic airway inflammation has yet to be suggested.

THE ASTHMATIC RESPONSE AND AIRWAY SECRETION

The inflammatory response arising in the airway of patients with bronchial asthma is frequently accompanied with mucus hypersecretion (200). The development of this condition is due to the complex network of mediators released during the inflammatory response. It is clear from the previous discussion that lipid mediators, peptides, proteinases, oxygen metabolites, and cell-specific products may directly or indirectly stimulate the release of mucins from secretory cells. Certainly in asthma, more than one mechanism may lead to mucus hypersecretion (Fig. 1).

CONCLUSIONS

The allergic asthmatic response may be initiated by the interaction in the airway of allergen and sensitized mast cells. This event results in the release of mast cell histamine, peptidyl leukotrienes, PGD_2 and platelet activating factor, all of which may directly cause secretory cell exocytosis. In addition, mast cell chymase is an extremely potent stimulus of exocytosis. Mast cell production of TNF-α may cause prolonged mucin secretion and induce mucin gene expression. Mast cell lipid and cytokine mediators will facilitate the migration and activation of eosinophils, and, to a lesser extent, neutrophils to the airway. Eosinophil peptidyl leukotrienes, PAF, and eosinophil cationic protein (ECP) may directly stimulate airway mucin secretion. Neutrophil elastase and cathepsin G may also profoundly stimulate secretory cell exocytosis. Eosinophil products such as ECP and major basic protein (MBP) and oxygen radicals from mast cells, eosinophils

and neutrophils, may damage the superficial epithelium. This damage may result in the exposure of subepithelial C-fibers and in a reduction of epithelial cell neutral endopeptidase production. These two events will result in the increased release of tachykinins from sensory nerves and in a reduced breakdown of these neuropeptides resulting in a prolonged effect. The release of mast cell histamine and leukotrienes, and sensory nerve release of Neurokinin A will result in increased vascular permeability allowing extravasation of plasma constituents. C_{3a} and bradykinin may both be activated by mast cell tryptase. The half life of bradykinin and its induction of eicosanoid production in the airway may also be prolonged by the reduction in airway neutral endopeptidase production. Increased levels of substance P may also contribute to the further recruitment and activation of inflammatory cells such as eosinophils, monocytes, and lymphocytes.

Increased numbers of alveolar macrophages are noted in bronchial lavage studies after antigen challenge. These cells may stimulate secretory cell exocytosis via the release of macrophage mucus secretagogue, lipid mediators, and oxygen species. They may also release TNF-α and IL-1 which, along with the TNF released from mast cells and lymphocytes, may induce mucin gene expression and an increase in stored mucin granule constituents available for release with a subsequent stimulus. Chronic airway inflammation in general, the presence of neutral elastase in particular, and chronic use of some β-adrenergic therapies may predispose to secretory cell hyperplasia or metaplasia and, therefore, an increase in the number of secretory cells available for activation. Thus, it seems likely that a variety of neural, structural, and inflammatory cell products interact in the asthmatic response to produce airway mucus hypersecretion, and through this hypersecretion, some of the morbidity of clinical asthma. It is hoped that an understanding of these mechanisms will allow for new therapeutic approaches to this chronic problem.

REFERENCES

1. Bradding P, Freezer N, Sheffer A, Holgate S. Asthma. In: Frank M, Austen K, Claman H, Unanue E, eds. *Samter's immunologic diseases.* Fifth Edition. Boston: Little, Brown and Company, 1995;1293–1327.
2. Jeffery P K. Embryology and growth. In: Brewis R, Gibson G, Geddes D, eds. *Respiratory medicine.* Toronto: Bailliere Tindall, 1990;3–20.
3. Lumsden AB, Mclean A, and Lamb D. Goblet and clara cells of human distal airways: Evidence for smoking-induced changes in numbers. *Thorax* 1984;39:844–853.
4. Neutra MR, and Schaeffer SF. Membrane interactions between adjacent mucus secretion granules. *J Cell Biol* 1977:74:983–991.
5. Jeffrey PK, and Reid L. Intraepithelial nerves in normal rat airways: A quantitative electron microscopic study. *J Anat* 1973:114: 33–45.
6. Jeffrey PK, and Reid L. New observations of rat airway epithelium: A quantitative electron microscopic study. *J Anat* 1975:120:295–320.
7. Jeffrey PK, and Reid L. The respiratory mucous membrane. In: Brain J, Proctor D, Reid L, eds. *Respiratory defense mechanisms.* New York, Marcel Dekker, 1977:193–246.
8. McDowell EM, Becci P J, Barrett LA, and Trump CF. Morphogenesis and classification of lung cancer. In: CC Harris, ed. *Pathogenesis and therapy of lung cancer* New York: Marcel Dekker, 1978;445–519.

9. Meyrick B, and Reid L. Ultrastructure of cells in the human bronchial submucosal glands. *J Anat* 1970;107:207.

10. Bowes D, Clark AE, and Corrin B. Ultrastructural localization of lactoferrin and glycoprotein in human bronchial glands. *Thorax* 1981; 36:108–115.

11. Kramps JA, Franken C, and Dijkman JH. ELISA for quantitative measurement of low-molecular-weight bronchial protease inhibitor in human sputum. *Am Rev Respir Dis* 1984;129:959–963.

12. Basbaum CB, Jany B, and Finkbeiner WE. The serous cell. *Annu Rev Physiol* 1990;52:97–113.

13. Perini JM, Marianne T, Lafitte JJ, Lamblin G, Roussel P, Mattuca M. Use of an antiserum against deglycosolated human mucins for cellular localization of their peptide precursors: antigenic similiarities between bronchial and intestinal mucins. *J Histochem Cytochem* 1989; 37:869–875.

14. Vasconcellos CA, Allen PG, Wohl ME, Drazen JM, Janmey PA, and Stossel TP. Reduction in viscosity of cystic fibrosis sputum *in vitro* by gelsolin. *Science* 1994;263:969–971.

15. Havez R, Roussel P. Bronchial mucus: physical and biochemical features. In: Weiss, EB, Segal MS, eds. *Bronchial asthma: mechanisms and therapeutics.* Boston: Little, Brown and Company, 1976; 409–422.

16. Brogen TD. The high molecular weight components of sputum. *Br J Exp Pathol* 1960;41:288–297.

17. Potter JL, Matthews LW, Lemm J, and Spector, S. Human pulmonary secretions in health and disease. *Ann NY Acad Sci* 1963;106:692–697.

18. Masson PL, Heremans JF, and Prignot J. Studies on the proteins of human bronchial secretions. *Biochem Biophys Acta* 1965;111: 466–478.

19. Roberts GP. Chemical aspects of respiratory mucus. Br Med Bull 1978;34:39–41.

20. Creeth JM, Bhaskar KR, Horton JR, Das I, Lopez-Vidriero MT, and Reid L. The separation and characterization of bronchial glycoproteins by density-gradient methods. *Biochem J* 1977;167: 557–569.

21. Woodward H, Horsey B, Bhavanandan VP, and Davidson EA. Isolation, purification, and properties of respiratory mucus glycoproteins. *Biochemistry* 1982;21:694–701.

22. Boat TF, Cheng PW, Iyer RN, Carlson DM, Polony I. Human respiratory tract secretions. *Arch Biochem Biophys* 1976;177:95–104

23. Siddiqui J Abe M, Hayes D, Shane E, Yunis E, Kufe D. Isolation and sequencing of a cDNA coding for the human DF3 brease carcinoma-associated antigen. *Proc Nat Acad Sci USA* 1988;85: 2320–2323.

24. Swallow D, Gendler S, Grifiths B, Corney G, Taylor-Papadimitriou J, Bramwell M. The human tumor-associated epithelial mucins are coded by an expressed hypervariable gene locus PUM. *Nature* 1987; 328:82–84.

25. Ligtenberg M, Kruishaar L, Buijs F, Van Meijer M, Litvinov S, and Hllkens J. Cell-associated episialin is a complex containing two proteins derived from a common precursor. *J Biol Chem* 1992;267: 6171–6177.

26. Genddler SJ, Lancaster CA, Taylor-Papadimitriou J et al. Molecular cloning and expression of human tumor-associated polymorphic epithelial mucin. J Biol Chem 1990;265:15286–15293.

27. Wreschner DH, Hareuveni M, Tsarfaty H et al. Human epithelial tumor antigen cDNA sequences. Differential splicing may generate multiple protein forms. *Eur J Biochem* 1990;189:463–473.

28. Lan MS, Khorrami A, Kaufman B, and Metzgar RS. Molecular characterization of a human pancreatic tumor mucin cDNA. *J Biol* Chem 1990;265:15294–15299.

29. Gum JR, Hicks JW, Toribara NW, Rothe EM, Lagace RE, and Kim YS. The human MUC2 intestinal mucin has cysteine-rich subdomains located both upstream and downstream of its central repetitive region. *J Biol Chem* 1992;267:21375–21383.

30. Gum JR, Byrd JC, Hicks JW, Toribara NW, Lamport DT, and Kim YS. Molecular cloning of human intestinal mucin cDNAs. Sequence analysis and evidence for genetic polymorphism. *J Biol Chem* 1989; 264:6480–6487.

31. Gerard C, Eddy RL, and Shows TB. The core polypeptide of cystic fibrosis tracheal mucin contains a tandem repeat structure. Evidence for a common mucin in airway and gastrointestinal tissue. *J Clin Invest* 1990;87: 77–82.

32. Jany B H, Gallup MW, Yan P, Gum JR, Kim YS, and Basbaum CB. Human bronchus and intestine express the same mucin gene. *J Clin Invest* 1991;87:77–82.

33. Toribara NW, Gum JR, and Culhane PJ. et al. MUC2 human small intestinal mucin gene structure. Repeated arrays and polymorphism. *J Clin Invest* 1991; 88:1005–1013.

34. Griffiths B, Matthews DJ, West L, Attwood J, Povey S, Swallow DM, Gum JR, and Kim YS. Assignment of the polymorphic intestinal mucin gene (MUC2) to chromosome 11p15. *Ann Hum Genet* 1990; 54:277–285.

35. Porchet N, Van Cong N, Duffose J, Audie J, Guyonnet-Duperat B, Gross M, Denis C, Degand P Bernheim A, Aubert J. Molecular cloning chromosomal localization of a nobel human tracheobronchial mucin cDNA containing tandemly repeated sequences of 48 base pairs. *Biochem Biophys Res Commun* 1991;175:414–422.

36. Van Cong N, Aubert P, Gross M, Porchet N, Degand P, Frezal J. Assignment of human tracheobronchial mucin gene(s) to 11p15 and tracheobronchial mucin related sequence to chromosome 13. *Hum Genet* 1990;86:167–172.

37. Aubert J, Prochet N, Crepin M, Duterque-Coquillaud M, Bergnes G, Mazzuca M, Debuire B, Petitprez D, Degand P. Evidence for different human tracheobronchial mucin peptides deduced from nucleotide cDNA sequences. *Am J Respir Cell Mol Biol* 1991;5:178–185.

38. Meerzaman D, Charles P, Daskal E, Polymeropoulos MH, Martin B.M, Rose M. C. Cloning and Analysis of cDNA encoding a major airway glycoprotein, human tracheobronchial mucin (MUC5). *J Biol Chem* 1994;269:12932–12939.

39. Rose MC. Mucin structure, function, and role in pulmonary diseases. *Am J Physiol* 1992;413–429.

40. Gum JR. Mucin gene and the proteins they encode: Structure, Diversity, and Regulation. *Am J Respir Cell Mol Biol* 1992;7:557–564.

41. Basbaum C, Welsh M. Mucus secretion and ion transport in airways. In: Murray J, Nadel J. 2eds. *Respiratory medicine*, Philadelphia: W.B. Saunders Company, 1994;323–344.

42. Hollingsworth MA, Batra SK, QiW, and Yankaskas J]R. MUC-1 mucin mRNA expression in cultured human nasal and bronchial epithelial cells. *Am J Respir Cell Mol Biol* 1992;6:516–520.

43. Byrd JC, Nardelli J, Siddiqui B, Kim Y. Isolation and characterization of colon cancer mucin from xenografts of LS174T cells. *Cancer Research* 1988;48:6678–6685.

44. Gum J, Hicks J, Toribara N, Siddiki B, Kim Y. Molecular cloning of human intestinal mucin (MUC2) cDNA. Identification of the amino terminus and overall sequence similarity to prepro-von Willebrand factor. *J Biol Chem* 1994;269:2440–2446.

45. Rose MC, Kaufman B, and Martin B. Proteolytic fragmentation and peptide mapping of human carboxyamidomethylated tracheobronchial mucin. *J Biol Chem* 1989;264:8193–8199.

46. Voynow JA, Rose MC. Quantitation of mucin mRNA in respiratory and intestinal epithelial cells. *Am J Respir Cell Mol Biol* 1994;11: 742–750.

47. Puchelle E, Tournier JM, Zahm JM, and Sadoul, P. Rheology of sputum collected by a simple technique limiting salivary contamination. *J Lab Clin Med* 1984;103:347–353.

48. Chase KV, Flux M, and Sachdev GP. Comparison of physicochemical properties of purified mucus glycoproteins isolated from respiratory secretions of cystic fibrosis and asthmatic patients. *Biochemistry* 1985;24:7334–7338.

49. Rahmoune H, Lamblin G, Lafitte JJ, Galabert C, Filliat M, and Roussel P. Chondroitin sulfate in sputum from patients with cystic fibrosis and chronic bronchitis. *Am J Resp Cell Mol Biol* 1991;5:315–320.

50. Robinson N, Widdicombe JG, and Xie CC. *In vitro* collection of mucus from the ferret trachea. *J Physiol* 1983;340:7–8.

51. Ueki I, German VF, and Nadel JA. Micropipette measurement of airway submucosal gland secretion: autonomic effects *Am Rev Respir Dis* 1980;121:351–357.

52. Leikauf GD, Ueki IF, and Nadel JA. Autonomic regulation of viscoelasticity of cat tracheal gland secretions. *J Appl Physiol* 1984;56: 426–430.

53. Shelhamer JH, Marom Z, and Kaliner M. Immunologic and neuropharmacologic stimulation of mucus glycoprotein release from human airways. *J Clin Invest* 1980;66:1400–1408.

54. Adler KB, Schwartz JE, Anderson WH, and Welton AF. Platelet activating factor stimulates secretion of mucin by explants of rodent airways in organ culture. *Exp Lung Res* 1987;13:25–43.

55. Shimura S, Sasaki T, Sasaki H, and Takishima T. Contractility of isolated single submucosal gland from trachea. *J Appl Physiol* 1986;60: 1237–1247.

56. Shimura S, Sasaki T, Ikeda K, Sasaki H, and Takishima T. VIP aug-

ments cholinergic-induced glucoconjugates secretion in tracheal submucosal glands. *J Appl Physiol* 1988;65:2537–2544.

57. Wu R. *In vitro* differentiation of airway epithelial cells. In: Schiff LJ, ed. *In vitro models of respiratory epithelium.* Boca Raton: CRC Press, 1986:1–26.

58. Wu R, Martin WR, Robinson CB, St. George JA, Plopper CG, Kurland G, Last JA, Cross CE, McDonaldRJ, and Boucher R. Expression of mucin synthesis and secretion in human tracheobronchial epithelial cells grown in culture. *Am J Respir Cell Mol Biol* 1990;3:467–478.

59. Kim KC, and Brody JS. Use of primary cell culture to study regulation of airway surface epithelial mucus secretion. In: Chandler EN, Ratcliffe NA, eds. *Mucus and related topics.* Cambridge: Company of Biologists Limited, 1989;231–239.

60. Rieves RD, Goff J, Wu T, Larivee P, Logun C, and Shelhamer J. H. Airway epithelial cell mucin release: Immunologic quantitation and response to platelet activating factor. *Am J Respir Cell Mol Biol.* 1992;6:158–167.

61. Culp DJ, Penney DP, and Marin MG. A technique for the isolation of submucosal gland cells from cat trachea. *J Appl Physiol* 1983;55:1035–1041.

62. Tournier JM, Merten M, Meckler Y, Hinnraski J, Fuchey C, and Puchelle E. Culture and characterization of human tracheal gland cells. *Am Rev Respir Dis* 1990;141:1280–1288.

63. Finkbeiner WE, Nadel JA, and Basbaum CB. Establishment and characterization of a cell line derived from bovine tracheal glands. *In vitro* 1986;22:561–567.

64. Goswami SK, Kivity S, and Marom Z. Erythromycin inhibits respiratory glycoconjugate secretion from human airways *in vitro. Am Rev Respir Dis* 1990;141:72–78.

65. Davis B, Nadel JA. New methods used to investigate the control of mucus secretion and ino transport in airways. *Environ Health Perspect* 1980;35:121–130.

66. Gallagher JT, Kent PW, Passatore M, Phipps RJ, and Richardson PS. The composition of tracheal mucus and the nervous control of its secretion in the cat. *Proc R Soc Lond* 1975;192:49–76.

67. Wardell JR, Chakrin LW, Payne BJ. The canine tracheal pouch: A model for use in respiratory mucus research. *Am Rev Resp Dis* 1970;101:741–754.

68. Baraniuk JN, Lundgren JD, Okayama M, Goff J, Mullol J, Merida M, Shelhamer JH, and Kaliner MA. Substance P and neurokinin A in human nasal mucosa. *Am J Respir Cell Mol Biol* 1991;4:228–236.

69. Logun C, Mullol J, Rieves D, Hoffman A, Johnson C, Miller R, Goff J, Kaliner M, and Shelhamer JH. Use of a monoclonal antibody enzyme-linked immunosorbent assay to measure human respiratory glycoprotein production *in vitro. Am J Respir Cell Mol Biol* 1991;5:71–79.

70. Lin H, Carlson D, St. George J, Plopper C, Wu R. An ELISA method for the quantitation of tracheal mucins from human and nonhuman primates. *Am J Respir Cell Mol Biol* 1989;1:41–48.

71. Richardson JB. Nerve supply to the lung. *Am Rev Resir Dis* 1979;785–802.

72. Nadel JA, and Davis B. Parasympathetic and sympathetic regulation of secretion from submucosal glands in airways. *Federation Proc* 1980;39:3075–3079.

73. Partanen M, Laitinen A, Hervonen A, Toivanen M, Laitinen LA. Catecholamine and acetylcholinesterase-containing nerves in human lower respiratory tract. *Histochemistry* 1982;76:175–188.

74. Sheppard MN, Kurian SS, Henzen-logmans SC, Michetti F, Cocchia D, Cole P, Rush RA, Marangos PJ, Bloom SR, Polak J. Neuronspecific enolase and S-100: new markers for delineating the innervation of the respiratory tract in man and other mammals. *Thorax* 1983;38:333–340.

75. Borson DB, Charlin M, Gold W, and Nadel JA. Neural regulation of $^{35}SO_4$- macromolecule secretion from tracheal glands of ferrets. *J Appl Physiol* 1984;57:457–466.

76. Barnes PJ, Nadel JA, Roberts JM, and Basbaum CB. Muscarinic receptors in lung and trachea: autoradiographic localization using [^{3}H]quinuclidinyl benzilate. *Eur J Pharmacol* 1983;86:103–106.

77. Basbaum CB, Grillo MA, and Widdicombe JH. Muscarinic receptors: Evidence for a nonuniform distribution in tracheal smooth muscle and exocrine glands. *J Neurosci* 1984;4:508–520.

78. Yang CM, Farley JM, and Dwyer TM. Muscarinic stimulation of submucosal glands in swine trachea. *J Appl Physiol* 1988;64:200–209.

79. Ishihara H, Shimura S, Satoh M, Masuda T, Nonaka H, Kase H,

Sasaki T, Sasaki H, Takishima T, and Tamura K. Muscarinic receptor subtypes in feline tracheal submucosal gland secretion. *Am J Physiol* 1992;259:L345–L350.

80. Barnes PJ. Muscarinic receptor subtypes: implications for lung disease. *Thorax* 1989;44:161–167.

81. Mak JCW, and Barnes PJ. Autoradiographic visualization of muscarinic receptor subtypes in human and guinea pig lung. *Am Rev Respir Dis* 1990;141:1559–1568.

82. Johnson CW, Rieves RD, Logun C, Shelhamer JH. Muscrinic stimulation of human submucosal gland secretion is mediated at least in part by M_1 receptor. *Clin Res* 1990;38:273A

83. Gater PR, Alabaster VA, and Piper I. A study of the muscarinic receptor subtype mediating mucus secretion in cat trachea *in vitro. Pulmonary Pharmacol* 1989;2:87–92.

84. Silva DG, and Ross G. Ultrastructural and fluorescence histochemical studies on the innervation of the tracheobronchial muscle of normal cats and cats treated with 6 hydroxydopamine. *J Ultrastruct Res* 1974;47:310–328.

85. Murlas C, Nadel JA, and Basbaum CB. A morphometric analysis of the autonomic innervation of cat tracheal glands. *J Auton Nerv Syst* 1980;2: 23–37.

86. Baluk P, Fujiwara T, and Matsuda S. The fine structure of the ganglia of the guinea-pig trachea. *Cell Tissue Res* 1985;239:51–60.

87. Richardson J, and Beland J. Nonadrenergic inhibitory nervous system in human airways. *J Appl Physiol* 1976;41:764–771

88. Barnes PJ. Neural control of human airways in health and disease. *Am Rev Respir Dis* 1986;134:1289–1314.

89. Barnes PJ, and Basbaum CB. Mapping of adrenergic receptors in the trachea by autoradiography. *Exp Lung Res* 1983;5:183–192.

90. Phipps RJ, Nadel JA, and Davis B. Effect of α-adrenergic stimulation on mucus secretion and on ion transport in cat trachea *in vitro. Am Rev Respir Dis* 1980;121:359–365.

91. Basbaum CB, Ueki I, Brezina L, and Nadel JA. Tracheal submucosal gland serous cells stimulated *in vitro* with adrenergic and cholinergic agonists. A morpho-metric study. *Cell Tissue Res* 1981;220:481–489.

92. Tom-Moy M, Basbaum CB, and Nadel JA. Localization and release of lysozyme from ferret trachea: effects of adrenergic and cholinergic drugs. *Cell Tissue Res* 1983;228:549–562.

93. Ueki I, and Nadel JA. Differences in total protein concentration in submucosal gland fluid: α-adrenergic vs. cholinergic. *Fed Proc* 1981;40:622–662.

94. Leikauf GD, Ueki IF, Nadel JA. Autonomic regulation of viscoelasticity of cat tracheal gland secretion. *J Appl Physiol* 1984;56:426–430.

95. Simonsson BG, Svedmyr N, Skoogh B-E, Andersson R, and Bergh NP. *In vivo* and *in vitro* studies on α-receptors in human airways. Potentiation with bacterial endotoxin. *Scand J Respir Dis* 1972;53:227–236.

96. Kneussl MP, and Richardson JB. α-adrenergic receptors in human and canine tracheal and bronchial smooth muscle. *J Appl Physiol* 1978;45:307–311.

97. Barnes PJ, Karliner JS, and Dollery CT. Human lung adreno-receptors studied by radioligand binding. *Clin Sci* 1980;58:457–461.

98. Engel G. Subclasses of β-adrenoreceptors- a quantitive estimation of β_1 and β_2 adrenoceptors in guinea pig and human lung. *Post grad Med* 1981;57 (Suppl 1):77–83.

99. Nadel JA, Widdicombe JH, and Peatfield AC. Regulation of airway secretions, ion transport, and water movement. In: Fishman AP, Fisher AB, eds. *Handbook of physiology.* Sec. 3, The Respiratory System. Vol. 1. Washington, D. C.: American Physiological Society, 1985:416–445.

100. Boat TF, Kleinerman JI. Human respiratory tract secretions effect of chlinergic and adrenergic agents on *in vitro* release of protein and mucous glycoprotein. *Chest* 1975;67:S325–S334.

101. Peatfield AC, and Richardson PS. Evidence for noncholinergic, nonadrenergic nervous control of mucus secretion into the cat trachea. *J Physiol (Lond)* 1983;342:335–345.

102. Uddman R, and Sundler F. Neuropeptides in the airways: A Review. *Am Rev Respir Dis* 1987;136(6 PT2)S3–S8.

103. Lunberg JM, Hökfelt T, Martling C-R, Saria A, and Cuello C. Substance P- immunoreactive sensory nerves in the lower respiratory tract of various mammals including man. *Cell Tissue Res* 1984;235:251–261.

104. Carstairs JR, and Barnes PJ, Autoradiographic mapping of substance P receptors in lung. *Eur J Pharmacol* 1986;127:295–296

105. Borson DB, Corrales R, Varsano S, Gold, WM, Viro N, Caughy G, Ramachandran J, Nadel JA. Enkephalinase inhibitors potentiate substance P- induced secretion of 35 SO4- macromolecules from ferret trachea. *Exp Lung Res* 1987;12:21–36.

106. Shimura S, Sasaki T, Okayama H, Sasaki T, and Takishima T. Neural control of contraction in isolated submucosal gland from feline trachea. *J Appl Physiol* 1987;62:2404–2409.

107. Tokuyama K, Kuo H-P, Rohde J, Barnes PJ, Rogers DF. Neural control of goblet cell secretion in guinea pig airways. *Am J Physiol* 1990; 259:L108–L115.

108. Kuo H-P , Rhode J, Tokuyama K, Barnes PJ, Rogers DF. Capsaicin and sensory neuropeptide stimulation of goblet cell secretion in guinea pig trachea. *J Physiol (Lond)* 1990;431:629–641

109. Regoli D, Drapeau G, Dion S, D'Orleans-Juste P. Pharmacological receptors for substance P and neurokinins. *Life Sci* 1987;40:109–117.

110. Baraniuk JN, Lundgren JD, OKayama M, Goff J, Peden D, Merida M, Shelhamer JH, Kaliner M. Gastrin- releasing peptide in human nasal mucosa. *J Clin Invest* 1990;85:998–1005

111. Baraniuk JN, and Kaliner M. Neuropeptides and nasal secretion. *Am J Physiol* 1991;261:L223–L235.

112. Baraniuk J, Lundgren J, Shelhamer J, Kaliner M. Gastrin-releasing peptide (GRP) binding sites in human tracheobronchial mucosa. *Neuropeptides* 1992;21:81–84.

113. Lundgren JD, Ostrowski N, Baraniuk JN, Shelhamer JH, Kaliner M. Gastrin-releasing peptide stimulates glycoconjugate release from feline tracheal explants. *Am J Physiol* 1990;258: L68–L74.

114. Barnes, P. J. Neuropeptides in human airways: Function and clinical implications. *Am Rev Respir Dis* 1987;136(Suppl) 77–83.

115. Said SI, Geumi A, and Hara N. Bronchodilator effect of VIP *in vivo*: protection against bronchoconstriction induced by histamine and prostaglandin F$_{2a}$. In: Said SI, ed. *Vasoactive intestinal peptide*. New York: Raven Press, 1982;185–191.

116. Lundberg JM, Änggård A, Fahrenkrug J, Hökfelt T, and Mutt V. Vasoactive intestinal polypeptide in cholinergic neurons of exocrine glands: Functional significance of coexisting transmitters for vasodilation and secretion. *Proc Natl Acad Sci* 1980;77:1651–1655.

117. Laitinen A, Partanen M, Hervonen A, Peto-Juikko M, and Laitinen LA. VIP-like immunoreactive nerves in human respiratory tract. Light and electron microscope study. *Histochemistry* 1985;82: 313–319.

118. Peatfield AC, Barnes PJ, Bratcher C, Nadel JA, Davis B. Vasoactive intestinal peptide stimulates tracheal sub mucosal gland in ferret. *Am Rev Respir Dis* 1983;128:89–93.

119. Gashi AA, Borson DB, Finkbeiner WE, Nadel JA, and Basbaum C. B. Neuropeptides degranulate serous cells of ferret tracheal glands. *Am J Physiol* 1986;251:C223–C229.

120. Coles SJ, Said SI, Reed L. Inhibition by Vasoactive Intestinal Peptide of glycoconjugate and lysozyme secretion by human airways *in vitro*. *Am Rev Respir Dis* 1981;124: 531–536.

121. Baraniuk JN, Okoyama M, Lundgren JD, Mullol M, Merida M, Shelhamer JH, and Kaliner MA. Vasoactive intestinal peptide (VIP) in human nasal mucosa. *J Clin Invest* 1990;86:825–831.

122. Said SI. VIP as a modulator of lung inflammation and airway constriction. *Am Rev Respir Dis* 1991;143:S22–S24.

123. Ollerenshaw S, Jarvis D, Woolcock A, Sullivan C, and Scheibner T. Absence of immunoreactive vasoactive intestinal polypeptide in tissue from the lungs of patients with asthma. *N Engl J Med* 1989;320: 244–248.

124. Black PN, Ghatei MA, Takahashi K, Bretherton-WattD, Krausz, T., Dollery CT, and Bloom SR. Formation of endothelin by cultured airway epithelial cells. *FEBS Lett* 1989;255:129–132.

125. Mattoli S, Mezzetti M, Riva G, Allegra L, and Fasoli A. Specific binding of endothelin on human bronchial smooth muscle cells in culture and secretion of endothelinlike material from bronchial epithelial cells. *Am J Resp Cell Mol Biol* 1990;3:145–151.

126. Johnson CW, Logun C, Wu T, and J Shelhamer. Endothelin-1 induced secretion of mucin type glycoprotein from human airways is enhanced by inhibitors of neutral endopeptidase and is independent of eicosanoid generation. *Am Rev Resp Dis* 1992;145:4A362.

127. Shimura S, Ishihara H, Satok M, Matsuda T, Nagaki N, Sasaki H, Takishima T. Endothelin regulation of mucus glocoprotein secretion from feline submucosal glands. *Am J Physiol* 1992;262:L208–L213.

128. Wu T, Mullol J, Rieves R, Logun C, Hausfield J, Kaliner M, Shelhamer J. Enndothelin-1 stimulates eicosanoid production in cultured human nasal mucosa. *Am J Respir Cell Mol Biol* 1990;6:168–174.

129. Janscó N. Role of the nerve terminals in the mechanism of inflammatory reactions. *Bull Millard Fillmore Hosp* 1960;7:53–77.

130. Barnes PJ. Asthma as an axon reflex. *Lancet* 1986;1:242–245.

131. Henderson WR, Jr. Eicosanoids and platelet-activating factor in allergic respiratory diseases. *Am Rev Respir Dis* 1991;143:S86–S90.

132. Holtzman MJ, Aizawa H, Nadel JA, and Goetzl EJ. Selective generation of leukotriene B$_4$ by tracheal epithelial cells from dogs. Biochem. *Biophys Res Commun* 1983;114:1071–1076.

133. Holtzman M. J. Arachidonic acid metabolism. Implications of biological chemistry for lung function and disease. *Am Rev Respir Dis* 1991; 143:188–203.

134. Sigal E, and Nadel JA. The airway epithelium and arachidonic acid 15-lipoxygenase. *Am Rev Respir Dis* 1991;143:S71–S74.

135. Bigby T, Goetzl EJ, and Holtzman MJ. Epithelial cells from canine trachea generate leukotriene B$_4$ in response to calcium ionophore. *Clin Res* 1985;33:76A.

136. Eling TE, Danilowicz RM, Henke DC, Sivarajah K, Yankaskas JR, and Boucher RC. Arachidonic acid metabolism by canine tracheal epithelial cells. Product formation and relationship to chloride secretion. *J Biol Chem* 1986;261:12841–12849.

137. Hunter J, Finkbeiner W, Nadel J, Goetzl E, Holtzman M. Predominant generation of 15-lipoxygenase metabolites of arachidonic acid by epithelial cells from human trachea. *Proc Natl Acad Sci U S A* 1985;82: 4633–4637.

138. Holtzman MJ, Hansrough JR, Rosen GD, TurkJ. Synthesis of the 1-ohexadecyl molecular species of platelet-activating factor by airway epithelial and vascular endothelial cells *Biochem Biophys Res Comm* 1976;177:357–364.

139. Churchill L, Chilton FH, Resau JH, Bascom R, Hubbard Wc, Proud D. Cyclooxygenase metabolism of endogenous arachidonic acid by cultured human tracheal epithelial cells. *Am Rev Resp Dis* 1989;140: 449–459.

140. Marom Z, Shelhamer JH, and Kaliner M. The effect of arachidonic acid, monohydroxyeicosatetraenoic acid and prostaglandins on the release of mucous glycoproteins from human airways *in vitro*. *J Clin Invest* 1981;67:1695–1702.

141. Marom Z, Shelhamer JH, Bach M K, Morton DR, and Kaliner M. Slow-reacting substances, leukotriene C$_4$ and D$_4$, increase the release of mucus from human airways *in vitro*. *Am Rev Respir Dis* 1982;126: 449–451.

142. Coles SJ, Neill KH, Reid LM, Austen KF, Nii Y, Corey EJ, Lewis RA. Effects of leukotrienes C4 and D4 on glycoprotein and lysozyme secretion by human bronchial mucosa. *Prostaglandins* 1983; 25:155–170.

143. Rich B, Peatfield AC, Willams IP, and Richardson PS. Effects of prostaglandingsE1, E2 and F$_{2a}$, on mucin secretion from human bronchi *in vitro*. *Thorax* 1984;39:420–423.

144. Lopez-Vidriero, MT, Das I, Smith P, Picot R, and Reid L. Bronchial secretion from normal human airways after inhalation of prostaglandin F$_{2a}$, acetyl choline, histamine, and citric acid. *Thorax* 1977;32:734–739.

145. Lundgren JD, Kaliner M, Logun C, Shelhamer JH. Platelet activating factor and tracheobronchial respiratory glycoconjugate release in feline and human explants: involvement of the lipoxygenase pathway. *Agent and actions* 1990;30:329–337.

146. Goswami Sk, Ohashi M, Stathas P, and Marom ZM. Platelet-activating factor stimulates secretion of respiratory glycoconjugate from human airways in culture. *J Allergy Clin Immunol* 1989;84:726–734.

147. Marom Z, Shelhamer JH, Sun F, and Kaliner M. Human airway monohydroxyeicosatetraenoic acid generation and mucus release. *J Clin Invest* 1983;72:122–127.

148. Lundgren JD, and Shelhamer JH. Pathogenesis of airway mucus hypersecretion. *J Allergy Clin Immunol* 1990;85:399–419.

149. Adler KB, Holden, Stauffer WJ, and Repine JE. Oxygen metabolites stimulate release of high-molecular-weigh glycoconjugates by cell and organ cultures of rodent respiratory epithelium via an arachidonic acid-dependent mechanism. *J Clin Invest* 1990;85:75–85.

150. Adler KB, Akley NJ, and Glasgow W. Platelet-activating factor provokes release of mucinlike glycoproteins from guinea pig respiratory epithelial cells via a lipoxygenase-dependent mechanism. *Am J Respir Cell Mol Biol* 1992;6:550–556.

151. Rieves RD, Goff J, Wu T, Larivee P, Logun C, and Shelhamer JH. Airway epithelial cell mucin release: immunologic quantitation and response to platelet-activating factor. *Am J Respir Cell Mol Biol* 1992; 6:158–167.

152. Crimi E, Chiaromaondia M, Milanese M, Rossi G, Brusasco V. Increased numbers of mast cells in the bronchial mucosa after the late-phase asthmatic resoponse to allergen. *Am Rev Respir Dis* 1991;144: 1282–1286.

153. Creticos P, Peters S, Adkinson N, Naclerio R, Hayes D, Norman P, Lichtenstein L. Peptide leukotriene release after antigen challenge in patients sensitive to ragweed. *N Engl J Med* 1984;310:1626–1630.

154. Brodie D, Gleich G, Guomo A, coburn D, Federman D, Schwartz L Wasserman S. Evidence of ongoing mast cell and eosinophil degranulation in symptomatic asthma airway. *J Allergy Clin Immunol* 1991; 88:637–648.

155. Sommerhoff CP, Caughey GH, Finkbeiner WE, Lazarus SC, Basbaum CB, and Nadel JA. Mast cell chymase: a potent secretagogue for airway gland serous cells. *J Immunol* 1989;142:2450–2456.

156. Marom Z, Shelhamer J, Steele L, Goetzl E, Kaliner M. Prostaglandin -generating factor of anaphylaxis induces mucous glycoprotein release and formation of lipoxygenase products of arachidonate from human airways. *Prostaglandins* 1984;28:79–91.

157. Wardlaw AJ, Dunnette S, Gleich GJ, Collins JV, and Kay AB. Eosinophils and mast cells in bronchoalveolar lavage in subjects with mild asthma: Relationship to bronchial hyperreactivity. *Am Rev Respir Dis* 1988;137:62–69.

158. Tomioka M, Ida S, Shindoh Y, Ishihara T, and Takishima T. Mast cells in bronchoalveolar lumen of patients with bronchial asthma. *Am Rev Respir Dis* 1984;129:1000–1005.

159. Schleimer RP, MacGlashan DW, Peters SP, Pinckard RN, Adkinson NF, and Lichtenstein LM. Characterization of inflammatory mediator release from purified human lung mast cells. *Am Rev Respir Dis* 1986;133:614–617.

160. Varsano S, Basbaum C, Forsberg L, Borson B, Caughey G, Nadel J. Dog tracheal epithelial cells in culture synthesize sulfated macromolecular glycoconjugates and release them from the cell surface upon exposure of extracellular proteinases. *Exp Lung Res* 1987;13: 157–184.

161. Caughey G. The structure and airway biology of mast cell proteinases. *Am J Resp Cell Mol Biol* 1991;4:387–394.

162. Rennard SI, Daughton D, Fujita J, Oehlerking MB, Dobson JR, Stahl MG, Robbins RA, and Thompson AB. Short-term smoking reduction is associated with reduction in measures of lower respiratory tract inflammation in heavy smokers. *Eur Respir J* 1990;3:752–759.

163. Metzger W, Zavala D, Richreson H, Mosely P, Iwamota P, Monick M, Sjoersma K, Hunninghake G. Local allergen challenge and bronchoalveolar lavage of allergic asthmatics lungs. Description of the model and local airway inflammation. *Am Rev Respir Dis* 1987;291: 1239.

164. Kim K, Wasano K, Niles R, Schuster J, Stone P, Snider G. Human neutrophil elastase releases cell surface mucin from primary cultures of hamster tracheal epithelial cells. *Proc Nat Acad Sci U S A* 1987;84: 9304–9308.

165. Rieves RD, Logun C, Lundgren JD, and Shelhamer JH. Characterization of glycoconjugates released from primary feline tracheal epithelial cell cultures. *Am Rev Respir Dis* 1989;139:A405.

166. Sommerhoff CP, Nadel JA, Basbaum CB, and Caughey GH. Neutrophil elastase and cathepsin G stimulate secretion from cultured bovine airway gland serous cells. *J Clin Invest* 1990;85:682–689.

167. Diaz P, Gonzalez MC, Galleguillos FR, Ancic P, Cromwell O, Shepherd D, Durham SR, Gleich GJ, Kay AB. Leukocytes and mediators in bronchoalveolar lavage during allergen-induced late phase asthmatic reactions. *Am Rev Resp Dis* 1989;139:1383–1389.

168. De monchy NGR, Kauffman HF, Venge P, Koëter GH, Jansen M, SLuiter HJ, Vries KD. Bronchoalveolar eosinophilia during allergen-induced late asthmatic reactions. *Am Rev Resp Dis* 1985;131: 373–376.

169. Lundgren JD, Davey RJ Jr, Lundgren B, Mullol J, Maron Z, Logun C, Baraniuk J, Kaliner MA, Shelhamer JH. Eosinophils and mucus airway secretion: Eosinophil cationic protein stimulates and major basic protein inhibits secretion from airway organ culture. *J Allergy Clin Immunol* 1991;87:689–698.

170. Fuller RW, Morris PK, Richmond R, Sykes D, Varndell IM, Kemeny DM, Cole PJ, Dollery CT, MacDermot J. Immunoglobulin E-dependent stimulation of human alveolar macrophages: Significance in type 1 hypersensitivity. *Clin Exp Immunol* 1986;65:416–426.

171. Godard P, Chaintreuil J, Damon M, Coupe M, Flandre O, Crasttes de Paulet A, Michel FB. Functional assessment of alveolar macrophages:

172. Joseph MA, Tonnel AB, Torpier G, Capron A, Arnoux B, Benveniste J. Involvement of immunoglobulin E in the secretory processes of alveolar macrophages from asthmatic patients. *J Clin Invest* 1983; 221–230.

173. Capron M, Jouault T, Prin L, Joseph M, Ameisen JC, Butterworth AE, Papin JP. Kusnierz JP, Capron A. Functional study of a monoclonal antibody to IgE FC receptor (Fc R2) of eosinophils, platelets, and macrophages. *J Exp Med* 1986;164:72–89.

174. Balter MS, Eschenbacher WL, and Peters-Golden M. Arachidonic acid metabolism in cultured alveolar macrophages from normal, atopic, and asthmatic subjects. *Am Rev Respir Dis* 1988;138: 1134–1142.

175. Marom Z, Shelhamer JH, Kaliner M. Human monocyte-derived mucus secretagogue. *J Clin Invest* 1985;75:191–198.

176. Marom Z, Shelhamer JH, Kaliner M. Human pulmonary macrophage-derived mucus secretagogue. *J Clin Invest* 1984;159: 844–860.

177. Levine SJ, Larivée P, Logun C, Angus CW, Ognibene FP, and Shelhamer JH. TNF-a induces mucin hypersecretion and MUC2 gene expression by human airway epithelial cells. *Am J Respir Cell Mol Biol* 1995;12:196–204.

178. Levine SJ, Logun C, Larivée P, and Shelhamer J H. IL-1β induces secretion of respiratory mucous glycoprotein from human airways *in vitro*. *Am Rev Dis* 1993;147: A437.

179. Marom Z, Shelhamer J, Berger M, Frank M, Kaliner M. Anaphylatoxin C3a enhances mucus glycoprotein release from human airways *in vitro*. *J Exp Med* 1985;161:657–668.

180. Mak JCW, Barnes PJ. Autoradiographic visualization of bradykinin receptors in human and guinea pig lung. *Eur J Pharmacol* 1991;194: 37–43.

181. Somerville M, Richardson PS, Rutman A, Wilson R, and Cole PJ. Stimulation of secretion into human and feline airways by Pseudomonas aeruginosa proteases. *J Appl Physiol* 1991;70: 2259–2267.

182. Adler KB, Hendley DD, and Davis GS. Bacteria associated with obstructive pulmonary disease elaborate extracellular products that stimulate mucin secretion by explants of guinea pig airways. *Am J Pathol* 1986;125:501–514.

183. Somerville M, Taylor GW, Watson D, Rendell NB, Rutman A, Todd H, Davies JR, Wilson R, Cole P, and Richardson PS. Release of mucus glycoconjugates by Pseudomonas aeruginosa rhamnolipids into feline trachea *in vivo* and human bronchus *in vitro*. *Am J Respir Cell Mol Biol* 1992;6:116–122.

184. Levine SJ, Larivee P, Logun C, and Shelhamer JH. Endotoxin induces respiratory mucous Glycoprotein secretion by feline tracheal epithelial cells. *Am Rev Resp Dis* 1992:145;4:A361.

185. Steiger D, Hotchkiss J, Bajaj L, Harkema J, and Basbaum C. Concurrent increases in the storage and release of mucinlike molecules by rat airway epithelial cells in response to bacterial enddotoxin. *Am J Respir Cell Mol Biol* 1995;12(3):307–314.

186. Lamb D, and Reid L. Mitotic rates, goblet cell increase and histochemical changes in mucus in rat bronchial epithelium during exposure to sulfur dioxide. *Br Med J* 1968;1:33–35.

187. Chapman RS, Calafiore DC, Hasselblad V. Prevalence of persistent cough and phlegm in young adults in relation to long-term ambient sulfur oxide exposure. *Am Rev Respir Dis* 1985;132:261–267.

188. Gallagher JT, Hall RL, Phipps RJ, Jeffrey PK, Kent PW, and Richardson PS. Mucus-glycoproteins (mucins) of the cat trachea: Characterization and control of secretion. *Biochem Biophys Acta* 1986;886: 243–254.

189. Peatfield AC, and Richardson PS. The action of dust in the airways on secretion into the trachea of the cat. *J Physiol* 1983;342: 327–334.

190. Wright DT, Adler KB, Akley NJ, Dailey LA, and Friedman M. Ozone stimulates release of platelet activating factor and activates phospholipases in guinea pig tracheal epithelial cells in primary culture. *Tox Appl Pharm* 1994;127:27–36.

191. Levine SJ, Larivée P, Logun C, and Shelhamer JH. IL-6 induces respiratory mucous glycoprotein secretion and MUC2 gene expression by human airway epithelial cells. *Am J Respir Crit Care Med* 1993; 149:A27.

192. Dohrman A, Young C, Gallup M, Ohmori H, Massion P, Nadel J, Escudier E, Chapelin C, Coste A, and Basbaum C. MUC2 mucin gene

expression is upregulated in human airways by products of Pseudomonas aeruginosa. *Am J Respir Crit Care Med* 1995;151: A160.

193. Lamb D, and Reid L. Goblet cell increase in rat bronchial epithelium after exposure to cigarette and cigar tobacco smoke. *Br Med J* 1969; 1:33–35.

194. Breuer R, Christensen TG, Lucey EC, Stone PJ, and Snider G. Quantitative study of secretory cell metaplasia induced by human neutrophil elastase in the large bronchi of hamsters. *J Lab Clin Med* 1985;105:635–640.

195. Snider GL, Stone PJ, Lucey EC, Breuer R, Calore JD, Seshadri T, Catanese A, Maschler R, and Schnebli H-P. Eglin-C, a polypeptide derived from the medicinal leech, prevents human neutrophil elastase-induced emphysema and bronchial secretory cell metaplasia in hamster. *Am Rev Respi Dis* 1985;132:1155–1161.

196. Breuer R, Lucey EC, Stone PJ, Christensen TG, and Snider GL. Pro-

teolytic activity of human neutrophil elastase and porcine pancreatic trypsin causes bronchial secretory cell metaplasia in hamsters. *Exp Lung Res* 1985;9:167–175.

197. Lundgren JD, Kaliner M, Logun C, Shelhamer JH. Dexamethasone reduces cat trachea goblet cell hyperplasia produced by human neutrophil products. *Exp Lung Res* 1988;14:853–863.

198. Rogers DF, and Jeffrey PK. Inhibition of cigarette smoke-induced airway secretory cell hyperplasia by indomethacin, dexamethasone, prednisolone, or hydrocortisone in the rat. *Exp Lung Res* 1986;10: 285–298.

199. Douglas, A. N. Quantitative study of bronchial mucous gland enlargement. *Thorax* 1980;35:198-201.

200. Fahy J, Steiger D, Liu J, Basbaum C, Finkbeiner W, Boushey H. Markers of mucus secretion and DNA levels in induced sputum from asthmatic and from healthy subjects. *Am Rev Respir Dis* 1993;147: 1132–1137.

Asthma, edited by P.J. Barnes, M.M. Grunstein,
A.R. Leff, and A.J. Woolcock.
Lippincott–Raven Publishers, Philadelphia © 1997.

▪ 61 ▪

Mucociliary Clearance

Adam Wanner

The principal physiological features of asthma are airway smooth muscle contraction, microvascular hyperemia and edema of the airway wall, and excessive luminal mucus. It is assumed that the accumulation of luminal mucus and the formation of mucus plugs result from the combination of mucus hypersecretion by the epithelium and impaired ciliary clearance of mucus from the airways. As a substitute for ciliary clearance, cough can serve as a backup mechanism for mucus clearance. However, the efficacy of cough clearance is frequently diminished because the requirements for optimal gas-liquid interaction are not met (1). These requirements include a high airflow velocity during the expiratory phase of the cough maneuver and low mucus viscosity (2,3). In patients with asthma, the presence of airflow obstruction reduces airflow velocity and mucus viscosity is increased (4,5). Furthermore, airflow velocity is too low for effective gas-liquid interaction in small bronchi (1).

Since cough efficacy is frequently inadequate in patients with asthma, the impairment of ciliary mucus clearance (mucociliary clearance) assumes an important pathophysiologic and clinical role (6). There is strong evidence suggesting that mucociliary dysfunction in asthma is related to airway inflammation. This chapter is divided into three sections. The first section is a description of the normal structure and function of the mucociliary apparatus. The second section deals with the effect of airway inflammation on mucociliary clearance. The last section is a discussion of what is currently known about mucociliary clearance in patients with asthma, and what its clinical implications might be.

THE NORMAL MUCOCILIARY APPARATUS

Normal clearance of mucus from the airways depends primarily on how well cilia interact with mucus. Morphologically and functionally, the mucociliary apparatus forms the basis of this interaction. To understand the factors which contribute to normal mucociliary interaction, and, hence, clearance, a working knowledge of the morphology and physiology of the mucociliary apparatus is useful. Relevant information has been obtained in animals and human subjects. With rare exceptions, the basic structure and function of the mucociliary apparatus is consistent among different species; this raises confidence in extrapolating animal observations to humans (7).

Morphology

The respiratory tract is lined by a ciliated epithelium extending from the proximal trachea to the terminal bronchioles (7). Most of the surface of the larynx is covered by mucus-secreting squamous epithelium; cilia are present only in the posterior commissure. In central airways,

A. Wanner: Division of Pulmonary and Critical Care Medicine, University of Miami School of Medicine, Miami, Florida 33101.

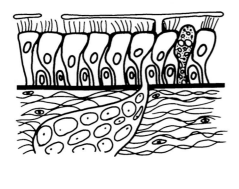
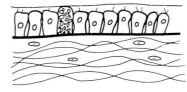
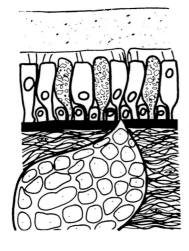
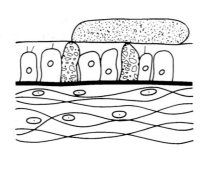

FIG. 1. In most mammals, including humans, the normal mucociliary apparatus of the central tracheobronchial tree *(upper left)* consists of ciliated surface epithelial cells, nonciliated surface epithelial cells containing secretory granules (goblet cells), submucosal gland cells, a periciliary fluid (sol), and a surface mucus layer (gel). The ratio of goblet cells to ciliated surface epithelial cells is approximately 1:5. In normal peripheral bronchioles *(upper right)* the epithelium is thin, the ciliation is sparse, there are no mucus-producing structures (goblet cells or submucosal glands), and there is no mucus. Granule-containing cells (Clara cells) do not produce mucins. In airway disease *(lower left and right)* there is typically decreased ciliation, goblet cell hyperplasia in central airways and metaplasia in peripheral bronchioles, submucosal gland hyperplasia and hypertrophy in central airways, excessive mucus in central airways, and luminal mucus in peripheral bronchioles. (From Wanner A. The role of mucociliarydysfunction in bronchial asthma, *Am J Med* 1979;67:477–485), with permission.)

the ratio of ciliated columnar cells to goblet cells is approximately 5:1. The absolute numbers of both decrease from the trachea to the peripheral airways (Fig. 1). Submucosal glands are only found in cartilaginous airways. In the most peripheral bronchi, goblet cells are also absent, and there is a smaller number of ciliated cells, which are characterized by fewer and shorter cilia than in the large bronchi (8).

In the trachea, most of the surface epithelium is ciliated, with focal areas as large as 1 mm in diameter, devoid of cilia (7). Small areas of squamous metaplasia may be found. The surface of each ciliated columnar cell contains approximately 200 cilia with an average length of 6 µm and a diameter of 0.1 to 0.2 µm. The cilia of human and other mammalian respiratory epithelial or cilia from lower animals are remarkably similar when compared by

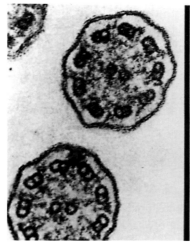
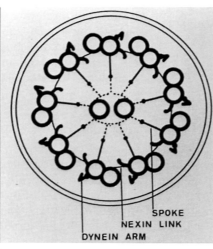

SPOKE
NEXIN LINK
DYNEIN ARM

FIG. 2. Schematic cross-section of a cilium *(right)* and transmission electronmicrograph of cilia *(left)* show microtubules and dynein arms responsible for ciliary bending. (From Mosbesrg B, et al. On the pathogenesis of obstructive lung disease, *Scand J Resp Dis* 1978;59:55–65.)

transmission and scanning electron microscopy (9). Each cilium contains longitudinal microtubules that represent contractile elements. Two microtubules form a central core and nine doublets of microtubules are arranged in a circular fashion in the periphery of the cilium. The peripheral microtubules join to one structure towards the tip of the cilium. A basal body in the apex of the cell corresponds to each cilium (Fig. 2). Dynein arms bridging the space between the microtubules are thought to play an important role in ciliary bending (*vide infra*).

With an increase in airway generations, there is a decrease in the number of goblet cells and submucosal glands (7). Submucosal glands are absent in noncartilaginous airways. In the most peripheral bronchioles, the surface epithelium is no longer pseudostratified, but characterized by flattened cells (Fig. 1). Distinct secretory cells which do not appear to release mucus substances (Clara cells), can be identified in most animals species (10).

The airway epithelium is covered by a surface liquid throughout its length. Lucas and Douglas (11) proposed a two-layer principle of the surface liquid. According to their concept, cilia are surrounded by a periciliary fluid layer (sol), and are covered by a mucous layer (gel) that interacts physically with the tips of the cilia. The presence of these two layers has been clearly demonstrated in several animal species (12). It is still being debated whether the mucous layer is a contiguous blanket covering the surface of the trachea or consists of discontinuous islands (13,14). The latter is more likely to apply in the unstimulated airway. While the periciliary fluid layer is present in peripheral airways as well, the mucous layer cannot be identified in them. Several investigators have identified a thin lipophilic layer which covers the periciliary fluid and is interposed between the periciliary fluid and mucus layer when the latter is present (15). The lipophilic layer contains phospholipids which may represent alveolar surfactant which has been transported in a cephalad direction; alternatively, the phospholipids could be a product of airway epithelial cells.

Function

Interaction of all parts of the mucociliary system (cilia, mucus, periciliary fluid) result in transport of mucus towards the larynx (Fig. 3).

Role of Cilia

The tip of the ciliary shaft terminates in a crown of short "claws" (3 to 7; 25- to 35-nm long) whose function is to engage the overlying mucous gel, either mechanically or biochemically, for mucus transport (16). The nine doublets of microtubules arranged along the perimeter of the cilium are responsible for ciliary bending (Fig. 2). This has been well worked out in several lower and higher

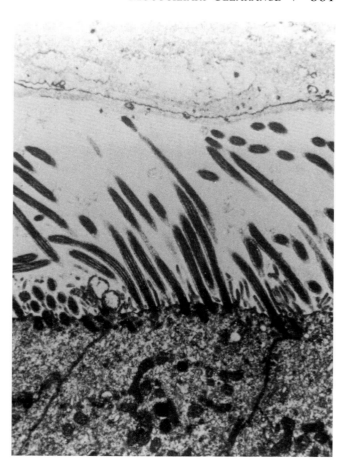

FIG. 3. Transmission electronmicrograph of tracheal epithelial surface. Cilia protrude into periciliary fluid and can interact with mucus floating on periciliary fluid. Osmophilic (lipid) film between periciliary fluid and mucus is clearly visible. (From Yoneda K. Mucous blanket of rat bronchus: an ultrastructural study. *Am Rev Respir Dis* 1976; 114:837–842.)

animals (17–20). The doublets are connected by strands of nexin, and one subfiber of each doublet possesses two dynein arms that project towards the next doublet, and a radial spoke that attaches to one of the two central microtubules. Dynein is an ATPase protein and is the site of energy usage in the cilia. It uses ATP to form molecular bridges between adjacent doublet microtubules, and to actively slide against each other. Active sliding of doublets on one side of the axoneme (attached to one of the central fibrils) bends the cilium in one direction, and active sliding of doublets on the other side (attached to the other central fibril) bends it in the opposite direction. Airway cilia move fluid and mucus by the mechanics of their beat cycle. During the effective stroke, (towards the nasopharynx for airway cilia), the cilium is straight and is perpendicular to the cell surface; it moves through an arc of approximately 110° and has a maximum tip velocity of 1000 μm per second. At the end of the effective stroke, when it is projecting forward, the cilium disengages from the mucus and "rests" to prevent backward flow of mucus. The cilium then bends and makes a recovery stroke close to the cell surface. Periciliary fluid, in which the recovery stroke occurs, probably just oscillates and is not transported; however, the mucous gel layer and periciliary fluid above the recovery stroke experience force only during the effective stroke, and so are moved in the direction of the beat. The force exerted by a cilium, and, therefore, the rate of fluid-mucus transport, increases with ciliary length and distance above the recovery stroke. Airway cilia do not beat in isolation but as part of a metachronal wave; adjacent cilia beat in succession, so that the wave of the effective stroke is propagated in the required direction of mucus transport. Ciliary coordination required for the metachronal wave may simply result from a mechanical interaction between adjacent cilia and may, therefore, be influenced by the number of cilia in contact with the mucus. Other mechanisms involving intercellular signaling have been suggested but thus far, not been convincingly demonstrated. Power is related to the number and rate of dynein microtubule interactions; in the absence of a load, this is directly related to beat frequency. Airway cilia appear to have two independent mechanisms for controlling beat frequency: One utilizing cyclic 3' 5'-adenosine monophosphate (cAMP) with increased cAMP leading to increased ATP production, and the other using changes in intracellular Ca^{2+} (maybe involving Ca^{2+}-calmodulin-dependent kinase systems). Indeed, intracellular Ca^{2+} may be the most important regulator of ciliary beat frequency (21).

In humans, it seems as if ciliary beat frequency is not different in large and small airways (15 to 18 Hz), but this has been measured on epithelial cells removed from the airway (22). In animal studies, *in situ*, ciliary beat frequency has been reported to be slower in peripheral airways than central airways (approximately 6 Hz in peripheral airways compared with 18 Hz in main bronchi) (23). Because tip velocity and force generated are related to beat frequency, such an increase could contribute to the increase in mucus transport from peripheral to central airways.

Periciliary Fluid

The periciliary fluid depth increases with increasing ciliary length from 3 to 4 μm in peripheral airways to 6 μm in central airways. It is assumed that the periciliary fluid is secreted in the distal airways and/or alveoli, and is gradually reabsorbed as it passes up the tracheobronchial tree to maintain an optimal depth (24). Airway epithelia of all species studied, including humans, can actively secrete Cl+ and actively absorb Na^+ (from the airway surface) (25); both processes are ATP-dependent. Under basal conditions, epithelia in human proximal airways, including the nose and large bronchi, are absorp-

tive. Na^+ absorption dominates and results in net absorption of sodium chloride (NaCl). Water (fluid) flow follows along the osmotic gradient generated by this salt absorption. Cl^- and fluid secretion serve to produce periciliary fluid in distal airways and to aid in hydration of mucus in all airways. Cl^- secretion can be stimulated by cAMP-dependent and Ca^{2+} calmodulin-dependent kinase systems that open Cl^- channels in the apical membranes of airway epithelial cells; thus, β-adrenoreceptor agonists stimulate airway Cl^- secretion by increasing intracellular cAMP. If Cl^- secretion is greater than Na^+ absorption, net ion transport is reversed, resulting in net secretion of NaCl and fluid.

Mucus

Mucus is only present in airways which are lined by mucous cell-containing epithelia; this excludes the bronchioles. It is produced by submucosal glands and goblet cells. Mucus first appears in bronchi as discrete rafts or flakes, and as airway surface area decreases, going proximal, these flakes coalesce and get larger. Mucous layer thickness (up to 10 to 15 μm) increases in more central airways, but unlike the periciliary fluid, mucus is not a continuous layer under normal conditions (14,15,26). While mucus is synthesized and secreted by mucous cells, transepithelial fluid can also influence the physical properties of mucus, especially by regulating its hydration. The mucus macromolecules and water interact mainly in the submucosal gland ducts and on the surface epithelium. Some hydration may also occur within secretory granules prior to exocytosis, at least in submucosal glands.

For mucus to be moved by cilia (against gravity in humans), it must possess certain structural and physical properties. These properties of mucus are determined by its chemical composition, mainly the macromolecules (glycoconjugates) and water. Mucus hydration probably occurs by a Gibbs-Donnan-like equilibrium by which the macromolecules essentially control their own hydration via pH and ionic concentration (27,28). The high molecular weight glycoconjugates form a three-dimensional network that both binds the water and traps it in interstices of the gel. However, the manner in which the glycoproteins bond to form the network is disputed. Most likely, glycopeptide units are linked end-to-end by disulfide bonds to produce very long (0.5-3 μm) glycoprotein molecules that are entangled and intertwined, with the coils held together by weak noncovalent bonds. Glycoprotein concentration and the three-dimensional structure and hydration of the mucus gel determine the physical properties of mucus and, in turn, its transportability by the cilia.

Airway mucus has viscous (liquid) and elastic (solid) properties (e.g., it is viscoelastic (29–32). Viscosity is important for providing mucus with long relaxation times (much longer than the time interval between successive ciliary beats, so that the mucus acts like a solid), and also enables the mucus to retain particles. However, elasticity is the more important determinant of mucus transport by cilia. Transport is related directly to the elastic recoil of mucus within wide limits, but indirectly to the viscosity of mucus (and of periciliary fluid). Other physical properties such as surface tension, "stickiness," and spinability (thread-forming ability) may be important in determining mucus transport as well. The phospholipids contained in the epithelial surface liquids could facilitate the engulfing and, hence, clearance of particulate matter which has deposited on the airway liquids.

Mucociliary Interaction

Theoretically, the depth and rheologic properties of both the mucous layer and periciliary fluid layer govern the interaction between cilia and mucus, and, hence, mucociliary transport (Fig. 3). Studies of the ultrastructure of mucus in the upper and central airways of animals have revealed a heterogeneous basic fiber network (33). The luminal surface of the mucous layer appears smooth, whereas the under-surface in contact with cilia is irregular, with the mucus penetrating a short distance between the ciliary shafts. This indentation along with the brush-like projections at the ciliary tips, may further facilitate the mechanical interaction between cilia and mucus. Conversely, the importance of this contact between cilia and mucus has been called into question. For example, in vitro experiments utilizing the frog palate have suggested that the direct contact between the cilia and the mucociliary is not necessary to transmit the shear forces to the mucus (34). For a surface liquid 60 μm deep, the flow characteristics within the mucous layer were similar throughout the entire depth.

Within a moderate range of deviation from "normal," and with ciliary beat frequency and wave velocity held constant, the mucus transport velocity is directly related to mucus elasticity and the depth of periciliary fluid, and inversely related to mucus viscosity and the depth of the mucous layer (35). Some of these factors have been tested experimentally. Thus, Stewart (36) found that up to a weight of 20 mg/mm², the ciliated epithelium is capable of transporting test particles without decreasing their velocity. The relationship between the rheology and transportability of mucus has also been demonstrated by determining the viscosity and elastic modulus of artificial mucus or of sputum from patients, and measuring the transport rate of the same material on the frog palate. There appears to be an ideal viscosity/elasticity ratio for optimal mucociliary interaction, with an increase in viscosity and a decrease in elasticity resulting in reduced transport rates (32,37). Similar observations have been recently made in the excised bovine trachea (38). From a

practical standpoint, both depth and rheologic properties of mucus appear to have a major influence on mucociliary interaction; in contrast, changes in the rheologic properties of periciliary fluid, a sol, appear to be less important than changes in its depth. It has been speculated that the mucous layer is absent in the unstimulated airway, and that mucus secretion and its transport require a chemical or mechanical stimulus (secretion-clearance coupling). This concept remains to be investigated.

Neural mechanisms have a role in the regulation of respiratory secretions. There is evidence that submucosal glands are innervated by the parasympathetic, sympathetic, nonadrenergic, and noncholinergic nervous systems with efferent fibers containing neurotransmitters (39–41). In contrast, the presence of efferent autonomic nerve endings is less certain in the surface epithelium containing goblet and ciliated cells. In humans, stimulation of cholinergic and alpha and β-adrenergic neurons results in an increased secretion of mucins from submucosal glands. Nonadrenergic, noncholinergic neural pathways have also been implicated in the regulation of airway mucus, and their action is possibly mediated by vasoactive intestinal peptide, which inhibits the secretion of mucus from normal human bronchus in vitro (42). Therefore, depletion of this neurotransmitter in the airway and, thus, removal of an inhibitory factor of mucus secretion have a role in the pathogenesis of airway disease characterized by mucus hypersecretion. The tachykinins, notably substance P, stimulate the contraction of gland ducts and cause degranulation of serous cells in ferrets (43,44). The secretory response of substance P can be markedly enhanced by inhibiting neutral endopeptidase, an observation that has led some investigators to suggest that infections may promote mucus release by reducing the levels of neutral endopeptidase, thus prolonging the effect of tachykinins (45,46).

Mucociliary transport rates increase from small towards large bronchi and the trachea; this, combined with some reabsorption of liquid along the tracheobronchial tree, is felt to prevent the excessive accumulation of airway liquid as the branches of the bronchial tree converge towards the trachea. Normal in vivo tracheal mucus transport rates have been reported to range between 2 and 20 mm/min (7). This wide variability is probably due more to differences in technique than to interspecies differences. In any case, the clearance of particulate matter from the trachea is remarkably fast. In an adult human with a tracheal length of 12 cm and a mucus transport rate of 10 ml/min, it would take a particle deposited at the carina 12 minutes to reach the larynx. Mucociliary clearance can also be assessed by determining the overall rate of mucus removal from the lower airways. This is typically measured by assessing the clearance of an inhaled radioaerosol which deposits in the tracheobronchial tree; the total radioactivity remaining in the lungs over time is measured externally by scintillation detection over the chest and back (47). Movement of individual particles is not measured, and so the results are expressed as a percentage of initial lung burden retained or cleared over time. Clearance has two exponential phases: (a) an initial phase complete in less than 24 hours with a half-life of 4 hours, which represents mucociliary clearance in the tracheobronchial tree; and (b) a later slower phase with a half-life of weeks or even months, which represents clearance in the alveoli by a nonmucociliary mechanism. Indirect evidence for this is the fact that people with primary ciliary dyskinesia do not show the fast phase of lung clearance (48).

If mucus and periciliary fluid are not to accumulate and cause obstruction, secretion and removal by ciliary activity must be balanced. Also, the depth of the periciliary layer must be well- regulated (to the height of the cilia, or just a little lower), because it is critical for optimal mucociliary interaction. Structural and functional defects of cilia (decrease in the number of cilia, decrease in ciliary beat frequency, discoordination of ciliary activity), changes in the depth of periciliary fluid, and increases in the depth and changes in the rheologic properties of mucus can all impair mucociliary clearance and lead to accumulation of mucus in the lower airways. One or more of these abnormalities have been observed in airway inflammation, including the inflammation characteristic of bronchial asthma.

EFFECT OF AIRWAY INFLAMMATION ON MUCOCILIARY CLEARANCE

Normal mucociliary clearance requires an optimal balance between the production and luminal clearance of the surface liquid covering the tracheobronchial tree. Therefore, the disruption of ciliary activity, quantitative and qualitative changes in periciliary fluid and mucus, or both could lead to impaired mucociliary interaction and clearance. Mucociliary clearance is impaired in patients with asthma. Judging by the available information, the impairment seems to result primarily from a defective secretory function, while primary ciliary abnormalities might have a secondary role. Asthma is characterized by airway inflammation. It is, therefore, useful to first review the effect of inflammation on mucociliary clearance. Most of the relevant data have been obtained in *in vitro* studies using animal or human tissues, and in *in vivo* animal studies.

Cilia

As it will be discussed later, the destruction of the ciliated surface epithelium is incomplete in patients with stable asthma, and more extensive damage with sloughing of the surface epithelium is usually only observed in patients with status asthmaticus (49). Furthermore, the ciliary apparatus has an impressive functional reserve (50).

The studies examining the effects of inflammation on cilia have, therefore, focused on ciliary activity. With a few notable exceptions, most inflammatory mediators have been shown to increase ciliary beat frequency, again a strong indication that primary dysfunction of ciliary activity is not likely to explain the asthma associated impairment of mucociliary clearance. Since several investigations of cilia have suggested that intracellular-free calcium ($[Ca^{2+}]i$) and cAMP are critical second messengers in the regulation of ciliary beat frequency, inflammatory mediators which raise the intracellular concentration of these messengers are those which are likely to stimulate ciliary activity (21,51–53). The more potent ciliostimulators are the sulfidopeptide leukotrienes, the prostaglandins E_1 and E_2, and the inflammatory peptides substance P and bradykinin (54–58). The effects of the sulfidopeptide leukotrienes might be mediated by a secondary prostaglandin E_1 generation which, in turn, increases intracellular cAMP and $[Ca^{2+}]i$ (55,56). In contrast, bradykinin seems to stimulate the ciliary activity by directly increasing $[Ca^{2+}]i$ and/or by releasing substance P and acetylcholine from nerve endings, at least in the rabbit maxillary sinus (58,59). The cyclooxygenase pathways and adenylate cyclase do not appear to be involved in this response. Interestingly, sulfidopeptide leukotrienes have been shown to decrease ciliary beat frequency of the human nasal cilia (60). It is not clear if the discrepancy between this study and other studies using tracheal epithelial cells is due to differences between the responsiveness of nadal and tracheal epithelial cells, or to technical differences. Histamine causes an increase in $[Ca^{2+}]i$ and ciliostimulation only at relatively high histamine concentrations ($>10^{-5}$ M) (54,56,61). Endothelin-1 has also been shown to stimulate ciliary beat frequency at high concentrations only (62). Several other inflammatory mediators including prostaglandin $F_{2\alpha}$ have been shown to be without effect on ciliary beat frequency (54).

Eosinophil granule major basic protein, adenosine, and reactive oxygen species are the best-studied inflammatory mediators which inhibit ciliary activity. Human eosinophil major basic protein decreases ciliary beat frequency at concentrations between 5×10^{-6} M and 10^{-5} M (63). This appears to be a clinically relevant observation since major basic protein concentration in the sputum of patients with bronchial asthma have been reported to range between 10^{-6} M and 10^{-5} M (64,65). The cilioinhibitory action of adenosine is accompanied by a decrease in intracellular cAMP concentration and a causal relationship between the two has been suggested (66). In contrast, the effects of reactive oxygen species generated by eosniophils and phagocytes in the inflamed airway seem to involve activation of protein kinase C and protein kinase C-dependent phosphorylation of a ciliary protein (67–70). The magnitude and duration of cilioinhibition by reactive

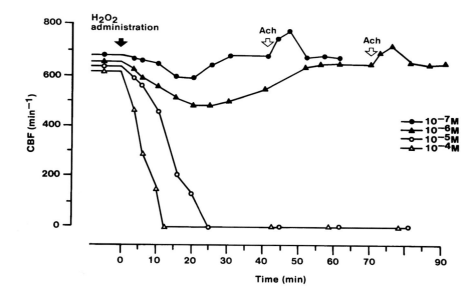

FIG. 4. Representative time courses of ciliary beat frequency (CBF) in sheep tracheal epithelium during and after exposure to different concentrations of hydrogen peroxide (H_2O_2), with acetylcholine (Ach) (10-5 M) responsiveness after exposure. Note H_2O_2 concentration-dependent differences in maximal decrease, recovery, and ACh responsiveness. (From Kobayashi, et al. Mechanism of hydrogen peroxide induced inhibition of sheep airway cilia, *Am J Respir Cell Mol Biol* 1992; 6:667–673.)

oxygen species is concentration dependent. For example, hydrogen peroxide (H_2O_2) causes transient cilioinhibition at $< 10^{-6}$ M and irreversible ciliostasis and evidence of cell disruption at $> 10^{-5}$ M (68) (Fig. 4). Human serum has also been shown to agglutinate and discoordinate ciliary activity, and this could be of clinical importance because bronchial asthma is associated with microvascular hyperpermeability and the appearance of serum components in airway secretions (71–73). The ciliotoxic serum factor has not been convincingly identified; in one study, immunoglobulin M was suspected (71).

Antigen challenge of cells and tissues obtained from allergic animals have been used to stimulate the effects of asthmatic inflammation on ciliary activity. In sheep, Maurer et al. (74) found that the ciliary beat frequency of epithelial cells obtained from the trachea of allergic animals increased on *in vitro* exposure to various concentrations of the specific antigen. This effect was completely blocked by cromolyn sodium and a specific sulfidopeptide leukotriene antagonist. Since the suspended tracheal cell preparation also contained luminal mast cells, the observation was interpreted as showing that the antigen-induced release of chemical mediators, including leukotrienes, caused transient ciliostimulation. The finding of Maurer et al. was subsequently verified by showing that the *in vitro* antigen exposure of tracheal explants obtained from allergic sheep increased ciliary beat frequency (75).

Periciliary Fluid

If one assumes that periciliary fluid is produced by the airway epithelium, quantitative information about the production of this fluid could be obtained by analyzing active epithelial ion and water transport. In canine, ovine, and equine tracheal preparations, various inflammatory substances have been shown to influence epithelial ion transport. For example, histamine, leukotriene C_4 and D_4, and bradykinin have been shown to increase chloride transport towards the luminal side of the epithelium (76–84). In some of these preparations, the enhanced net chloride secretion was associated with changes in net sodium absorption, while in others sodium absorption was not observed, possibly as a result of interspecies differences in ion transport properties. Human eosinophil major basic protein has also been shown to increase net chloride secretion in dog tracheal epithelium without a concomitant change in sodium transport; interestingly, the protein was only effective when applied to the mucosal side of the preparation (85). In the ferret trachea, ET-1 has been reported to increase transepithelial potential difference at concentrations ranging from 0.1 to 10 nM (86). It is not known whether this effect of ET-1 reflected chloride secretion, sodium absorption, or decreases in the size of paracellular pathways. Likewise, the stimulating effect of bradykinin on chloride secretion is greater when bradykinin is applied to the mucosal side than when it is applied to the serosal side of the epithelium (80). Possibly, the expression of the respective receptors is greater on the apical membrane than the basolateral membrane of the epithelial cells. At least in the canine tracheal epithelium, the effects of sulfidopeptide leukotrienes and bradykinin appear to involve prostaglandin biosynthesis as suggested by blocking experiments with indomethacin (80,81).

Phipps et al. (87) determined the effects of antigen challenge on epithelial fluxes of water, chloride, and sodium *in vitro* using pieces of trachea obtained from allergic sheep. Immediately after antigen challenge, there was a net ion and water absorption from the luminal side, followed by a transient increase net ion and water flux towards the lumen. Changes in sodium fluxes paralleled those of water fluxes, while there was an initial absorption of chloride from the luminal side with a subsequent transient increase in chloride secretion towards the lumen. Both phases of the response were prevented when the tissues were incubated with a sulfidopeptide leukotriene antagonist or a glucocorticosteroid, indicating the involvement of sulfidopeptide leukotrienes in the responses to antigen. Similar observations have been made in the rat trachea *in vitro*; in this species, the response to antigen was capsaicin- sensitive, suggesting the involvement of substance P (88). Thus, a variety of inflammatory mediators and antigen-induced mediator release seem to increase water secretion towards the airway lumen, possibly preceded by a transient water absorption. Water secretion appears to be of greater importance, and it is tempting to speculate from these observations that airway inflammation is associated with the addition of water to the periciliary fluid layer by epithelial ion and water transport.

Mucus

A variety of techniques have been used to quantitate mucus secretion in mucous cell cultures, tracheal explants, and *in vivo* using postmortem histologic assessments in response to exogenous inflammatory mediators or antigen-induced mediator release. Rats, rabbits, ferrets, dogs, sheep, cats, and human tissues and cells have all served as experimental models, and morphologic, vol-

umetric, and macromolecular labeling have been the principal methodologies used. Such studies are relevant to bronchial asthma because mucociliary interaction depends on the depth (weight) of the mucous layer.

Lipid mediators have been shown to be potent stimulators of mucus secretion. For example, Marom et al. (89, 90) showed that monohydroxyeicosatetraenoic acid, leukotriene C_4 and leukotriene D_4 stimulate glycoprotein secretion in human airway fragments. Similarly, 15-hydroxyeicosatetraenoic acid (15-HETE), but not 15-H(P)ETE or 5-HETE, have been reported to stimulate airway mucus secretion in dogs (91). Other lipid mediators such as platelet activating factor (PAF) and thromboxane A_2 are also mucus secretagogues, but these mediators are less potent than the lipoxygenase products (92,93). It is possible that there is an interaction among various lipid mediators; for example, the stimulating effects of platelet activating factor on mucin secretion in rodent airways may be an indirect effect which involves the biosynthesis of lipoxygenase products, and the effects of 15-HETE on mucus secretion in dogs can be partially blocked by indomethacin, thereby, implicating the generation of cyclooxygenase products (91,93). In the cat airway, the mucus secretagogue effect of platelet activating factor seems to involve protein kinase C as a second messenger system (94). Other inflammatory mucus secretagogues include: (a) the peptides bradykinin, endothelin-1, endothelin-2, and gastrin-releasing peptide with some of these effects being mediated by cyclooxygenase products; (b) the nucleotides adenosine, adenosine-diphosphate, and adenosine-triphosphate, probably acting via P_2-purinoceptor coupled to phospholipase C on either the apical or baso-

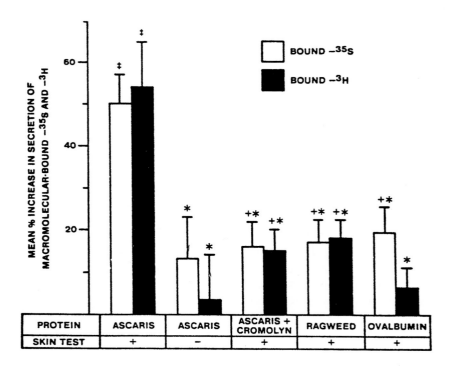

FIG. 5. Effect of challenge with various proteins on secretion of glycoprotein bound ^{35}S and [3]H (mean±SE), as % increase in 15 min output of radiolabel during protein 0 to 15 compared to control 0 to 15 in sheep tracheal tissues. Tissues from sheep allergic to Ascaris suum (skin test +) were challenged with *Ascaris suum* alone (25 μg protein.ml[-1]) and the control antigens ragweed (50 μg protein.ml[-1]), and ovalbumin (50 μg protein.ml[-1]); tissues from nonallergic sheep were challenged with *Ascaris suum* antigen alone (25 μg protein.ml[-1]). Effect significant †$P < 0.005$, ‡ $P < 0.001$: effect significantly different from effect of *Ascaris suum* alone, in allergic sheep tissues, * $P < 0.001$. (From Phipps RJ, Denas SM, Wanner A. Antigen stimulates glycoprotein secretion and alters ion fluxes in sheep trachea, *J Appl Physiol* 1983;55:1593–1602.)

lateral membrane of epithelial cells; and (c) human eosinophil major basic protein and eosinophil cationic protein (86,95–100). Finally, serum proteins (exceeding 13 kD in size), a macrophage derived mucus-like glycoconjugate secretagogue (68 kD), and proteases (especially human neutrophil elastase), also stimulate airway mucus secretion (101–103). Human neutrophil elastase and other neutrophil products can also cause goblet cell hyperplasia in rat and hamster airways (101–105). These effects appear to be more relevant in chronic bronchitis and cystic fibrosis where neutrophil recruitment into the airway is typically seen; in asthma, eosinophils predominate and neutrophils only seem to accumulate in severe asthma which has a sudden onset (106). Histamine has inconsistent effects on mucus secretion, and in the studies in which histamine was found to stimulate mucus secretion, high histamine concentrations were required for the effect to occur (5,40,107–110). In one of the studies, a marked stimulation of mucus glycoprotein release from human airways *in vitro* was found in response to histamine, and this effect was mediated primarily through H_2-histamine receptors (110).

The effects of allergic airway inflammation on mucus secretion have also been investigated. Yamatake et al. (111) demonstrated hypersecretion of respiratory tract fluid after inhalation challenge with specific antigen in allergic dogs. By using IgE-sensitized human airway fragments, Shelhamer et al. (110) found a 35% increase in radiolabeled glycoprotein secretion after the addition of antigen to the preparation. Similar observations were made by Phipps et al. (87). They studied the effects of purified *Ascaris suum* antigen on tracheal glycoprotein secretion *in vitro* by using pieces of trachea obtained from allergic sheep who had responded previously with bronchoconstriction to inhalation of *Ascaris suum* antigen. Glycoprotein secretion was assessed by adding ^{35}S-sulfate and ^{3}H-thrionine to the submucosal side of the tissue and monitoring the output of macromolecular-bound ^{35}S and ^{3}H on the luminal side. *Ascaris suum* antigen increased the secretion of bound ^{35}S by 57% and of bound ^{3}H by 78% (Fig. 5). A sulfidopeptide leukotriene receptor antagonist blocks these effects.

These experiments strongly suggest that airway inflammation is characterized by excessive secretion of mucus, and that several inflammatory products contribute to it.

Mucociliary Interaction

Given the demonstrated actions of inflammatory products on ciliary and secretory function in the airway, one might expect that selected exogenous chemical mediators or the combination of locally released inflammatory mediators after antigen challenge would affect mucociliary interaction and, hence, clearance. The first observations of this nature were made in *Ascaris suum* hypersensitive

dogs (112). In these animals, the inhalation of aerosolized *Ascaris suum* extract had differential effects on airway function and mucociliary transport. Although only 50% of the dogs responded with bronchospasm to inhalation of *Ascaris suum* antigen, tracheal mucociliary transport rates decreased in all animals by a mean of 70% within 30 to 45 minutes of antigen challenge, regardless of whether bronchospasm occurred; tracheal mucociliary transport rates were still decreased at the end of 2 hours. No changes in airway function or mucociliary transport were seen in control animals after inhaled ragweed, an antigen to which they were not sensitive. This observation also demonstrated that there is no interdependence between changes in airway mechanics and mucociliary transport. Subsequently, it was shown that sheep with *Ascaris suum* hypersensitivity exhibit airway responses to the inhalation of aerosolized *Ascaris suum* antigen that are similar to those in allergic dogs (113). Mucociliary transport was also reduced to 55% of baseline 1 hour (and to 51% of baseline 2 hours) after antigen challenge in these animals (114). The depression of mucociliary transport lasted up to a week after a single antigen challenge (115). Mucociliary impairment was not observed in the same animals when challenged with a control antigen (ragweed) and was completely prevented by prior inhalation of cromolyn sodium or the β-adrenergic agonist terbutaline sulfate, both of which presumably protect against development of allergic mucociliary dysfunction by inhibiting mast cell degranulation.

Several chemical mediators released during anaphylaxis may be responsible for the observed mucociliary dysfunction in these animals. In the allergic dog model, the question of whether histamine and leukotrienes have a role in mucociliary dysfunction, and whether the effects of these mediators on the mucociliary apparatus is direct or involves a cholinergic reflex, were addressed (112). Inhalation of histamine or acetylcholine aerosols in concentrations that produce a degree of bronchospasm comparable to that observed after antigen challenge, resulted in a transient increase in tracheal mucociliary transport rates, thereby, excluding these substances as mediators of the observed mucociliary impairment after antigen challenge. Conversely, inhalation of *Ascaris suum* antigen together with a sulfidopeptide leukotriene receptor antagonist produced a transient, nearly three-fold increase in tracheal mucus velocity, regardless of whether bronchospasm was elicited. The antagonist, when given alone or with a control antigen, had no effect on tracheal mucociliary transport rates, thereby, excluding a nonspecific stimulatory action. These results suggest that mucociliary dysfunction is related to the release of leukotrienes and does not involve a vagal reflex, at least in dogs. One might speculate that the stimulation of tracheal mucus transport rates by the combined administration of specific antigen and a sulfidopeptide leukotriene receptor antagonist was related to inhibition of the depressing effects of leukotrienes, thereby, unmasking the stimulatory effects of other mediators, such as histamine.

The role of sulfidopeptide leukotrienes in allergic mucociliary dysfunction in these animal models was further investigated in sheep (116). Aerosol challenge with leukotriene D_4 decreased tracheal mucus velocity in allergic and nonallergic sheep alike. In contrast, only the allergic animals exhibited bronchial smooth muscle responses following challenge with leukotriene D_4. The maximal decline in mucus clearance and the duration of the effect were similar to those observed after antigen challenge in allergic sheep. Considering that leukotriene D_4 stimulates the output of radiolabeled mucin and ciliary activity in the trachea of sheep *in vitro*, it is suspected that leukotriene D_4 induced-impairment of mucus transport is related to its secretory effects, rather than its ciliary (stimulatory) effects (117). This apparent dissociation between ciliostimulation and mucociliary impairment is further supported by the observations of Seybold et al. (75), that *in vitro* antigen challenge of tracheal explants obtained from allergic sheep increases ciliary beat frequency while slowing surface liquid transport velocity.

MUCOCILIARY CLEARANCE IN ASTHMA

As predicted by the *in vitro* and *in vivo* experimental data described earlier, airway mucociliary clearance has been shown to be impaired in patients with bronchial asthma. The mucociliary dysfunction of bronchial asthma is accompanied by histologic lesions of the mucociliary apparatus which link structural defects to functional defects.

Structural Lesions of Mucociliary Apparatus

In status asthmaticus, the mucosa is characterized by edema and disruption of epithelial cells, a decrease in the number of ciliated cells, and an increase in the number of goblet cells, along with goblet cell metaplasia in peripheral airways (118). Detachment of superficial epithelial cells can be seen in some areas. There is hyperplasia and hypertrophy of the submucosal glands. Widespread mucus plugging of the bronchi is usually seen. It should be pointed out that none of these lesions is pathognomonic for bronchial asthma; they can also been seen in chronic bronchitis.

The pathologic features of stable bronchial asthma and of asthma in remission probably differ only quantitatively from those of status asthmaticus (49). The destructive changes of the epithelium are not as evident, and the amount of luminal mucus is less in the former. However, spotty obstruction of smaller airways with mucus plugs has been clearly demonstrated, mainly in bronchi greater than 1 mm in diameter, but also in smaller peripheral airways (119) (Fig. 6). Thus, with respect to mucociliary

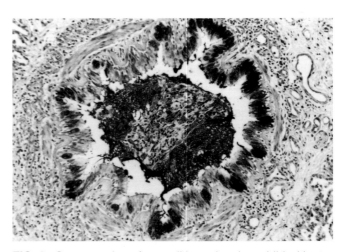

FIG. 6. Cross-section of a small bronchus in a child with stable bronchial asthma, exemplifying typical mucosal abnormalities: thickened basement membrane, increased number of goblet cells, submucosal gland hypertrophy, and a mucus plug obstructing the airway lumen. The mucus plug is undergoing organization by macrophages. (From Cutz E, et al. Ultrastructure of airways in children with asthma, *Histopathology* 1978; 2:407–421.)

function, the relevant pathologic findings in bronchial asthma are excessive mucus in large airways, the presence of mucus in small airways that in the normal lung do not contain mucus, and disruption of the ciliated epithelium. These epithelial changes are accompanied by varying degrees of inflammatory cell infiltration, further supporting the connection between inflammation and mucociliary dysfunction (49).

Airway Secretions

The expectoration of sputum and the pathological findings described previously suggest an increased quantity of airway secretions in asthma. These quantitative changes are coupled with qualitative changes (6). Glycoconjugates (especially glycoproteins) seem to determine the rheologic properties of mucus to a great extent. Increased concentrations of unusual polysaccharides and cross-linking between transudated serum protein and secretory IgA have been found in the sputum of patients with bronchial asthma (120–122). Changes in electrolyte concentrations including increases in calcium have also been reported, and serum proteins appear to accumulate in the sol phase of asthmatic sputum (121,123). These distinguishing biochemical characteristics of respiratory secretions in asthma could have an effect on their rheologic properties. Unfortunately, this has not been adequately studied. The best known observation was made on expectorated sputum that may not be representative of lower airway secretions (124). In that study, sputum from asthmatic patients tended to be more viscous than that from patients with other types of obstructive airway disease; a marked increase in viscosity at a low shear rate was particularly characteristic for sputum obtained from asthmatic patients. If mucus in the lower airways indeed possesses abnormal rheologic properties, this abnormality may well alter transport rates. One study demonstrated that sputum obtained from patients with asthma can all impair ciliary activity through biochemical, rather than rheologic factors (125). Ciliary beat frequency measured photoelectrically in a bronchial explant was reduced when expectorated sputum from allergic and nonallergic asthmatic patients was placed on the preparation. The cilioinhibitory of sputum was more pronounced during clinical exacerbations of asthma. Induced sputum obtained from patients with stable asthma has also been found to contain higher concentrations of mucin-like glycoprotein and extracellular DNA (reflection of disrupted epithelial or inflammatory cells) than induced sputum in normal subjects (126). Since lactoferrin was also found to be elevated, the authors suggested that these changes in the sputum of patients with asthma are a reflection of glandular hypersecretion, since lactoferrin has been shown to be a marker of glandular secretion (127).

Mucociliary Clearance

There is indirect evidence that inflammation has a role in the asthma associated impairment of mucociliary clearance. This has been shown by several investigators who used different experimental techniques and studied groups of asthmatic patients in different stages of their disease (Table 1). Mezey et al. (128) measured tracheal mucus velocity with discrete surface markers of mucus transport in asymptomatic patients with ragweed asthma. In those patients, mean tracheal mucus velocity was lower than in normal age-matched nonsmokers. In patients with mild (symptomatic) asthma, Bateman et al. (129) also observed impaired clearance, in this case, of an

TABLE 1. *Mucociliary Clearance in Asthma*

Clinical Severity of Asthma	Anatomical Site	Mucociliary Clearance (%)[a]	Reference
In remission	trachea	54	(128)
Stable			
Mild	lung	69	(129)
Moderate	lung	50	(131)
Severe	trachea	15	(132)
Acute exacerbation	lung	<5	(135)

[a]Group mean expressed as percent of age-matched controls. Tracheal clearance was measured by surface marker velocity, lung clearance with inhaled radioaerosols. The 60 minute retention value was taken to compare radioaerosol clearance between asthmatics and normal controls.

inhaled radioaerosol. In their study, patients who were in remission had normal radioaerosol clearance values when compared to controls. In patients with stable symptomatic asthma, Foster et al. (130) reported impaired tracheal and bronchial radioaerosol clearance. In another study by the same group of investigators, a decrease in central radioaerosol clearance was only seen in patients who had tidal flow limitation on their flow-volume curve (131). The authors suggested that dynamic compression of large airways could be causally related to airway epithelial damage and to disruption of ciliary clearance. Finally, in three elderly patients with adult-onset asthma, tracheal mucus velocity was found to be markedly reduced when compared to normal age-matched controls and indistinguishable from values seen in patients with chronic bronchitis (132).

The interpretation of these findings requires caution because of confounding factors which influence mucus clearance. For example, clearance of inhaled radioaerosol is a function of its deposition pattern since centrally deposited particles are cleared faster than peripherally deposited particles. If radioaerosol clearance is not normalized for deposition, the impairment of radioaerosol clearance in patients with bronchial asthma may be underestimated or missed because the patients may have preferential central aerosol deposition due to airflow obstruction. In addition, cough clearance is not always separated from ciliary clearance in such studies, and cough cannot always be suppressed for the duration of the study in patients with bronchial asthma. Finally, anti-asthma medication with mucociliary effect cannot always be withheld. These factors may explain why not all investigators have found an impairment of mucociliary clearance in patients with asthma (133,134).

As one might expect from the pathological lesions seen in patients who died in status asthmaticus, patients with acute exacerbations could be expected to have the greatest impairment of mucociliary clearance. Indeed, this was observed by Messina et al. (135). In their study, patients with acute exacerbations of bronchial asthma severe enough to require hospitalization, had severely impaired radioaerosol clearance in their airways. The patients were studied again after discharge from the hospital. At this time, their mean radioaerosol clearance values were markedly improved. During the acute exacerbation of their asthma, the patients were given supplemental oxygen and may have had an acute viral respiratory infection as a trigger of the exacerbation. Oxygen therapy and acute viral respiratory infections have been associated with mucociliary impairment (136,137). However, the authors did not attribute the difference in mucociliary clearance during and after hospitalization entirely to these confounders, but concluded that the acute worsening of airway inflammation had a critical role.

Some of the inflammatory mediators responsible for the mucociliary dysfunction of bronchial asthma have

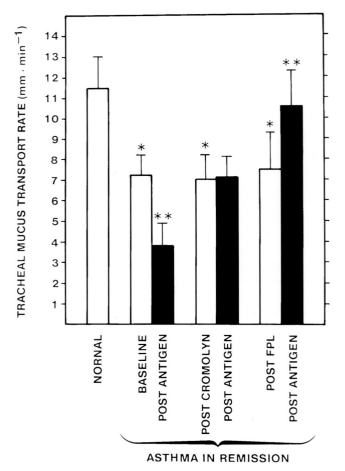

FIG. 7. Tracheal mucus velocity is lower in asymptomatic ragweed hypersensitive asthmatics (in remission) than in normal nonsmokers, and is further decreased 1 hour after inhalation challenge with ragweed extract. Mean of 6 (SE in brackets). * Significantly different from normals, ** significantly different from respective baseline. Cromolyn prevents the ragweed effect, and the leukotriene antagonist FPL 55712 converts an expected decrease of tracheal mucus velocity, after ragweed, into an increase. This suggests that a baseline mucociliary clearance is diminished in asymptomatic allergic asthmatics, and that antigen challenge produces an acute further decrease in tracheal mucus velocity that is related to chemical mediators of anaphylaxis, presumably leukotrienes. The acceleration of tracheal mucus transport by antigen in the presence of the leukotriene antagonist could reflect the stimulating effects of other chemical mediators, e.g., histamine. The net effect of all mediators released by antigen is a depression of tracheal mucus velocity *(3rd bar)*. (From Ahmed T, et al. Abnormal mucociliary transport in allergic patients with antigen-induced bronchospasm. *Am Rev Respir Dis* 1981;124:110–114; and from Mezey RJ, et al. Mucociliary transport in allergic patients with antigen-induced bronchospasm, *Am Rev Respir Dis* 1978; 118:677–684).

been identified. In the previously described asymptomatic patients with a history of ragweed asthma, bronchial challenge with ragweed extract reduced the mean tracheal mucociliary transport rate to 72% of baseline immediately after completion of bronchial challenge when mean specific airway conductance was reduced by 35% (128). One hour later, mean specific airway conductance had returned to its baseline value; however, the mean tracheal mucociliary transport rate was further reduced to 47% of baseline at this time (Fig. 7). These changes in mucus transport were prevented by pretreatment with cromolyn sodium by inhalation. Thus, in patients with allergic asthma and antigen-induced bronchospasm, the decrease in tracheal mucus transport appears to be independent of bronchospasm and to be related to airway anaphylaxis and the release of chemical mediators. In a subsequent study, Ahmed et al. (138) found that the administration of a sulfidopeptide leukotriene receptor antagonist in conjunction with antigen challenge converted the expected decrease in tracheal mucus velocity after ragweed challenge to an increase above baseline (Fig. 7). This effect was observed with both 0.5 and 1% solutions of the antagonist, and there was no difference between the two doses. This suggests that sulfidopeptide leukotrienes may be involved in acute allergic mucociliary dysfunction, similar to what was observed in allergic dogs (112). Again, the observed increase in tracheal mucus velocity when antigen challenge was combined with the sulfidopeptide leukotriene receptor antagonist suggests the unmasking of stimulatory inflammatory mediators. In keeping with this interpretation, it has been shown that inhaled histamine stimulates radioaerosol clearance in normal subjects (139). In addition to sulfidopeptide leukotrienes, other lipid mediators have also been investigated. For example, it has been reported that inhalation challenge with aerosolized 15(S)-HETE fails to alter radioaerosol clearance in normal subjects, while inhalation of aerosolized platelet activating factor (nebulized to dose 500 μg) impairs radioaerosol clearance (140,141). Based on the observed effects of pharmacological pretreatment, the platelet activating factor, induced mucociliary impairment was not felt to be mediated by prostaglandin biosynthesis, but possibly the activation of the lipoxygenase pathway.

Clinical Implications

These studies suggest that airway mucociliary clearance is impaired in bronchial asthma, that the degree of impairment varies with the severity of the disease, and that airway inflammation has a critical role in the pathogenesis of mucociliary dysfunction. A combination of epithelial hypersecretion and impaired mucociliary interaction leads to the accumulation of mucus in the airways. While cough can compensate for the impaired ciliary clearance in central airways, there is no known effective backup system for the impaired mucociliary mucociliary clearance in peripheral airways.

The theoretical consequences of asthma-associated mucociliary dysfunction are cough, airflow obstruction due to excessive airway secretions, and increased susceptibility to respiratory infection (1). These consequences have, thus far, not been experimentally demonstrated in human subjects. Nonetheless, clinicians frequently consider the beneficial mucociliary effects of anti-asthma medications, such as β-adrenergic agonists and methylxanthines, when administering them for the reversal of bronchospasm.

REFERENCES

1. Wanner A., Phipps RJ, Kim CS. Mucus Clearance: Cilia and Cough. In: Chernick V, Mellins RB, eds. *Basic mechanisms of pediatric respiratory disease: cellular and integrative.* Philadelphia: BC Decker, Inc., 1991;361–382.
2. Kim CS, Rodriguez CR, Eldridge MA, Sackner MA. Criteria for mucus transport in the airways by two-phase gas-liquid flow mechanism. *J Appl Physiol* 1986;60:901–907.
3. King M, Brock G, Lundell C. Clearance of mucus by simulated cough. *J Appl Physiol* 1985;58:1776–1782.
4. Lopez-Vidriero MT, Allegra L, Sackner MA, Puchelle, E.. The physical properties of mucus and their clinical significance. *Bull Europ Physiopath Resp* 1986;22:207–212.
5. Chakrin LW, Baker AP, Christian P, Wardell Jr, JR. Effect of cholinergic stimulation on the release of macromolecules by canine trachea *in vitro. Am Rev Respir Dis* 1973;108:69–76.
6. Wanner A. The role of mucociliary dysfunction in bronchial asthma. *Am J Med* 1979;67:477–485.
7. Wanner A. Clinical aspects of mucociliary transport. *Am Rev Respir Dis* 1977;116:73–125.
8. Serafini S, Michaelson ED, Wanner A. Mucociliary clearance in central and intermediate airways: effect of aminophyllin. *Bull Europ Physiopath Resp* 1976;12:415–418.
9. Roth LE, Shingenaka Y. The structure and formation of cilia and filaments in rumen protozoa. *J Cell Biol* 1964;20:249–270.
10. Breeze RG, Wheeldon EB. The cells of the pulmonary airways. *Am Rev Respir Dis* 1977;116:705–777.
11. Lucas AM, Douglas LC. Principles underlying ciliary activity in the respiratory tract. II. A comparison of nasal clearance in man, monkey and other mammals. *Arch Otolaryngol* 1934;20:518–541.
12. Nowell JA, Tyler WS. Scanning electron microscopy or the surface morphology of mammalian lungs. *Am Rev Respir Dis* 1971;103:313–328.
13. Barclay AE, Franklin KJ. The rate of excretion of India ink injected into the lungs. *J Physiol* 1937;90:482.
14. Van As, A. Pulmonary airway clearance mechanisms: a reappraisal. *Am Rev Respir Dis* 1977;115:721–726.
15. Yoneda K. Mucous blanket of rat bronchus: an ultrastructural study. *Am Rev Respir Dis* 1976;114:837–842.
16. Foliguet B, Puchelle E. Apical structure of human respiratory cilia. *Bull Europ Physiopath Resp* 1986;22:43–47.
17. Sleigh MA. *The biology of cilia and flagella.* Oxford: Pergamon Press Ltd, 1962.
18. Saavedra S, Penaud F. Studies on reactivated cilia. 1. The utilization of various nucleoside triphosphates during ciliary movement. *Exp Cell Res* 1975;90:439–443.
19. Satir, P. The present status of the sliding microtube model of ciliary motion. In: Sleigh MA, ed. *Cilia and flagella.* Oxford: Pergamon Press, 1974;131.
20. Usuki I. Effect of adenosine triphosphate on the ciliary activity and its histochemical demonstration in the oyster gill. *Sci Rep Res Inst Tohoku Univ (Biol)* 1959;25:65.
21. Salathe M, Bookman RJ. Coupling of $[Ca2+]i$ and ciliary beating in cultured tracheal epithelial cells. *J Cell Sci* 1995;108:431–440.
22. Yager JA, Ellmann H, Dulfano MJ. Human ciliary beat frquency at three levels of the tracheobronchial tree. *Am Rev Respir Dis* 1980; 121:661–665.
23. Iravani J, Van As A. Mucus transport in the tracheobronchial tree of normal and bronchitic rats. *J Pathol* 1972;106:81–93.
24. Boucher RC, Stutts MJ, Gatzy JT. Regional differences in bioelectric properties and ion flow in excised canine airways. *J Appl Physiol* 1981;51:706–719.
25. Phipps RJ, Abraham WM, Mariassy AT, et al. Developmental changes in the tracheal mucociliary system in neonatal sheep. *J Appl Physiol* 1989;67:824–832.
26. Sturgess JM. The mucous lining of major bronchi in the rabbit lung. *Am Rev Respir Dis* 1977;115:819–827.
27. Verdugo P, Tam PY, Butler J. Conformational structure of respiratory mucus studied by laser correlation spectroscopy. *Biorheology* 1983; 20:223–230.
28. Verdugo P. Hydration kinetics of exocytosed mucins in cultured secretory cells of the rabbit trachea: a new model. *Ciba Found Symp* 1984;109:212–225.
29. Litt M. Physicochemical determinants of mucociliary flow. *Chest* 1981;80(Suppl):846–849.
30. Puchelle E, Zahm JM, Girard F, et al. Mucociliary transport *in vivo* and *in vitro.* Relation to sputum properties in chronic bronchitis. *Eur J Resp Dis* 1980;61(5):254–264.
31. Puchelle E, Zahm JM, Duvivier C. Spinability of bronchial mucus. Relationship with viscoelasticity and mucous transport properties. *Biorheology* 1983;20:239–250.
32. King M, Viires N. Effect of methacholine chloride on rheology and transport of canine tracheal mucus. *J Appl Physiol* 1979;47:26–31.
33. Reissig M, Bang BG, Bang FB. Ultrastructure of the mucociliary interface in the nasal mucosa of the chicken. *Am Rev Respir Dis* 1978; 117:327–341.
34. Winet H, Yates GT, Wu TY, Head J. On the mechanics of mucociliary flows. III. Flow-velocity profiles in frog palate mucus. *J Appl Physiol* 1984;56:785–794.
35. Ross SM, Corrsin S. Results of an analytical model of mucociliary pumping. *J Appl Physiol* 1974;37:333–340.
36. Stewart WC. Weight-carrying capacity and excitability of excised ciliated epithelium. *Am J Physiol* 1948;152:1–5.
37. Dulfano MJ, Adler KB. Physical properties of sputum. VII: Rheologic properties and mucociliary transport. *Am Rev Respir Dis* 1975;112: 341–347.
38. Wills PJ, Garcia Suarez MJ, Rutman A, Wilson R, Cole PJ. The ciliary transportahility of sputum is slow on the mucus-depleted bovine trachea. *Am J Respir Crit Care Med* 1995;151:1255–1258.
39. Florey H, Carleton HM, Wells AQ. Mucus secretion in the trachea. *Br J Exp Pathol* 1932;13:269.
40. Sturgess JM, Reid, L. An organ culture study of the effect of drugs on the secretory activity of the human bronchial submucosal gland. *Clin Sci* 1972;43:533–543.
41. Webber SE, Widdicombe JG. The actions of methacholine, pheylephrine, salbutamol, and histamine on mucus secretion from the ferret *in vitro* trachea. *Agents and Actions* 1987;22:82.
42. Coles SJ, Said SI, Reid LM. Inhibition by vasoactive intestinal peptide of glyucoconjugate and lysozyme secretion by human airways *in vitro. Am Rev Respir Dis* 1981;124:531–536.
43. Coles SJ, Neill KH, Reid LM. Potent stimulation of glycoprotein secretion in canine trachea by substance P. *J Appl Physiol* 1984;57: 1323–1327.
44. Gashi AA, Borson DB, Finkbeiner WE, Nadel JA, Basbaum CB. Neuropeptides degranulate serous cells of ferret tracheal glands. *Am J Physiol* 1986;251:C223–C229.
45. Borson DB, Corrales R, Varsano S, et al. Enkephalinase inhibitors potentiate substance P-induced secretion of $^{35}SO_4$-macromolecules from ferret trachea. *Exp Lung Res* 1987;12:21–36.
46. McDonald DM. Respiratory tract infections increase susceptibility to neurogenic inflammation in the rat trachea. *Am Rev Respir Dis* 1988; 137:1432–1440.
47. Foster WM, Langenback EG, Bergofsky EH. Association in the mucociliary function of central and peripheral airways. *Am Rev Respir Dis* 1985;132:633–639.
48. Afzelius BA, Camner P, Mossberg B. Acquired ciliary defects compared to those seen in the immotile-cilia syndrome. *Eur J Respir Dis* 1983;64(suppl 127):5–10.

49. Mariassy AT, Wanner A. Morphologic Basis of Airflow Obstruction. In: Gershwin ME, ed. *Bronchial asthma: principles of diagnosis and treatment.* Totowa: The Humana Press, Inc., 1994;75–92.

50. Battista SP, Denine EP, Kensler CJ. Restoration of tracheal mucosa and ciliary particle transport activity after mechanical denudation in the chicken. *Toxicol Appl Pharmacol* 1972;22:59–69.

51. Verdugo P. Ca^{2+}-dependent hormonal stimulation of ciliary activity. *Nature* 1980;283:764–765.

52. Di Benedetto G, Magnus CJ, Gray PTA, Mehta A. Calcium regulation of ciliary beat frequency in human respiratory epithelium *in vitro. J Physiol* 1991;439:103–113.

53. Salathe M, Pratt MM, Wanner A. Cyclic AMP-dependent phosphorylation of a 26 kDa axonemal protein in ovine cilia isolated from small tissue pieces. *Am J Respir Cell Mol Biol* 1993;9:306–314.

54. Maurer DR, Schor J, Sielczak M, Wanner A, Abraham WM. Ciliary motility in airway anaphylaxis. *Cell Motility Suppl* 1982;1:67–70.

55. Wanner A, Sielczak M, Mella JF, Abraham WM. Ciliary responsiveness in allergic and nonallergic airways. *J Appl Physiol* 1986;60:1967–1971.

56. Dolata J. Prostaglandin E_1 enhances the histamine induced stimulation of the mucociliary activity in the rabbit maxillary sinus. *Eur Respir J* 1990;3:559–565.

57. Wong LB, Miller IF, Yeates DB. Stimulation of tracheal ciliary beat frequency by capsaicin. *J Appl Physiol* 1990;68:2574–2580.

58. Lindberg S, Mercke U. Bradykinin accelerates mucociliary activity in rabbit maxillary sinus. *Acta Otolaryngol* 1986;101:114–121.

59. Paradiso AM, Cheng EHC, Boucher RC. Effects of bradykinin on intracellular calcium regulation in human ciliated airway epithelium. *Am J Physiol* 1991;261:L63–L69.

60. Bisgaard H, Pedersen M. SRS-A leukotrienes decrease the activity of human respiratory cilia. *Clin Allergy* 1987;17:95–103.

61. Noah TL, Paradiso AM, Madden MC, McKinnon KP, Devlin RB. The response of a human bronchial epithelial cell line to histamine: Intracellular calcium changes and extracellular release of inflammatory mediators. *Am J Respir Cell Mol Biol* 1991;5:484–492.

62. Tamaoki J, Kanemura T, Sakai N, Isono K, Kobayashi K, Takizawa T. Endothelin stimulates ciliary beat frequency and chloride secretion in canine cultured tracheal epithelium. *Am J Respir Cell Mol Biol* 1991; 4:426–431.

63. Hisamatsu K, Ganbo T, Nakazawa T, et al. Cytotoxicity of human eosinophil granule major basic protein to human nasal sinus mucosa *in vitro. J Allergy Clin Immunol* 1990;86:52–63.

64. Frigas E, Loegering DA, Gleich GJ. Cytotoxic effects of the guinea pig eosinophil major basic protein on tracheal epithelium. *Laboratory Investigation* 1980;42:35–43.

65. Dor PJ, Ackerman SJ, Gleich GJ. Charcot-Leyden crystal protein and eosinophil granule major basic protein in sputum of patients with respiratory diseases. *Am Rev Respir Dis* 1984;130:1072–1077.

66. Tamaoki J, Kondo M, Takizawa T. Adenosine-mediated cyclic AMP-dependent inhibition of ciliary activity in rabbit tracheal epithelium. *Am Rev Respir Dis* 1989;139:441–445.

67. Jackowski JT, Szepfalusi ZS, Wanner DA, et al. Effects of Pseudomonas aeruginosa derived bacterial products on tracheal ciliary function: Role of oxygen radicals. *Am J Physiol* 1991;261:L61–L67.

68. Kobayashi K, Salathe M, Pratt M, et al. Mechanism of hydrogen peroxide induced inhibition of sheep airway cilia. *Am J Respir Cell Mol Biol* 1992;6:667–673.

69. Salathe M, Pratt MM, Wanner A. Protein kinase C-dependent phosphorylation of a ciliary membrane protein and inhibition of ciliary beating. *J Cell Sci* 1993;106:1211–1220.

70. Yukawa T, Read RC, Kroegel C, et al. The effects of activated eosinophils and neutrophils on guinea pig airway epithelium *in vitro. Am J Respir Cell Mol Biol* 1990;2:341–353.

71. Sanderson MJ, Sleigh MA. Serum proteins agglutinate cilia and modify ciliary coordination. *Pediatr Res* 1981;15:219–228.

72. Persson CGA. Leakage of macromolecules from the tracheobronchial microcirculation. *Am Rev Respir Dis* 1987;135:S71–S75.

73. Conover JH, Conod EJ, Hirsch-Horn K. Ciliary dyskinesia factor in immunological and pulmonary disease. *Lancet* 1973;1:1194.

74. Maurer DR, Sielczak M, Oliver W, Jr, Abraham WM, Wanner A. Role of ciliary motility in acute allergic mucociliary dysfunction. *J Appl Physiol* 1982;52:1018–1023.

75. Seybold ZV, Mariassy AT, Stroh D, Kim CS, Gazeroglu H, Wanner A. Mucociliary interaction *in vitro:* effects of physiological and inflammatory stimuli. *J Appl Physiol* 1990;68:1421–1426.

76. Phipps RJ, Denas SM. Epithelial water fluxes in sheep trachea. *Physiologist* 1982;25(5):224 (Abstract).

77. Marin MG, Davis B, Nadel JA. Effect of histamine on electrical and ion transport properties of tracheal epithelium. *Am J Physiol* 1977;42: 735–738 (Abstract).

78. Marom Z, Shelhamer JH, Steel L, Goetzl EJ, Kaliner M. Prostaglandin-generating factor of anaphylaxis induces mucous glycoprotein release and the formation of lipoxygenase products of arachidonate from human airways. *Prostaglandins* 1984;28:79–91.

79. Rangachari PK, Donoff B, Vavrek RJ, Stewart J.M. Luminal responses to bradykinin on the isolated canine tracheal epithelium: effects of bradykinin antagonists. *Regulatory Peptides* 1990;30:221–230.

80. Leikauf GD, Ueki IF, Nadel JA, Widdicombe JH. Bradykinin stimulates Cl secretion and prostaglandin E_2 release by canine tracheal epithelium. *Am J Physiol* 1985;248:F48–F55.

81. Leikauf GD, Ueki IF, Widdicombe JH, Nadel JA. Alteration of chloride secretion across canine tracheal epithelium by lipoxygenase products of arachidonic acid. *Am J Physiol* 1986;250:F47–F53.

82. Smith JJ, McCann JD, Welsh MJ. Bradykinin stimulates airway epithelial Cl^- secretion via two second messenger pathways. *Am J Physiol* 1990;258:L369–L377.

83. Rangachari PK, McWade D, Donoff B. Luminal receptors for bradykinin on the canine tracheal epithelium: functional subtyping. *Regulatory Peptides* 1988;21:237–244.

84. Tessier GJ, Traynor TR, Kannan MS, O'Grady SM. Mucosal histamine inhibits Na absorption and stimulates Cl secretion across equine tracheal epithelium. *Am J Physiol* 1991;261:L456–L461.

85. Jacoby DB, Ueki IF, Widdicombe JH, Loegering DA, Gleich GJ, Nadel JA. Effect of human eosinophil major basic protein on ion transport in dog tracheal epithelium. *Am Rev Respir Dis* 1988;137: 13–16.

86. Webber SE, Yurdakos E, Woods AJ, Widdicombe JG. Effects of endothelin-1 on tracheal submucosal gland secretion and epithelial function in the ferret. *Chest* 1992;101(Suppl):63S–67S.

87. Phipps RJ, Denas SM, Wanner A. Antigen stimulates glycoprotein secretion and alters ion fluxes in sheep trachea. *J Appl Physiol* 1983;55: 1593–1602.

88. Sestini P, Bienenstock J, Crowe SE, et al. Ion transport in rat tracheal epithelium *in vitro. Am Rev Respir Dis* 1990;141:393–397.

89. Marom Z, Shelhamer JH, Bach MK, Morton DR, Kaliner M. Slow-reacting substances, leukotrienes C_4 and D_4, increase the release of mucous from human airways *in vitro. Am Rev Respir Dis* 1982;126: 449–451.

90. Marom Z, Shelhamer JH, Kaliner M. Effects of arachidonic acid, monohydroxyeicosatetraeonic acid and prostaglandins on the release of mucous glycoproteins from human airways *in vitro. J Clin Invest* 1981;67:1695–1702.

91. Johnson HG, McNee ML, Sun FF. 15-hydroxyeicosatetraenoic acid is a potent inflammatory mediator and agonist of canine tracheal mucus secretion. *Am Rev Respir Dis* 1985;131:917–922.

92. Yanni JM, Smith WL, Foxwell MH. U46619 and carbocyclic thromboxane A_2-induced increases in tracheal mucous gel layer thickness. *Prostaglandins Leukot Essent Fatty Acids* 1988;32:45–49.

93. Adler KB, Schwarz JE, Anderson WH, Welton AF. Platelet activating factor stimulates secretion of mucin by explants of rodent airways in organ culture. *Exp Lung Res* 1987;13:25–43.

94. Larivee P, Levine SJ, Martinez, A, et al. Platelet activating factor induces airway mucin release via activation of protein kinase C: Evidence for translocation of protein kinase C to membranes. *Am J Respir Cell Mol Biol* 1994;11:199–205.

95. Baraniuk JN, Lundgren JD, Mizoguchi H, et al. Bradykinin and respiratory mucous membranes. Analysis of bradykinin binding site distribution and secretory responses *in vitro* and *in vivo. Am Rev Respir Dis* 1990;1141:706–714.

96. Wu T, Mullol J, Rieves RD, et al. Endothelin-1 stimulates eicosanoid production in cultured human nasal mucosa. *Am J Respir Cell Mol Biol* 1992;6:168–174.

97. Mullol J, Ohkubo K, Rieves RD, et al. Endothelin in human nasal mucosa. *J Allergy Clin Immunol* 1991;87:217 (Abstract).

98. Kim, K.C., Zheng, Q-X. and Van-Seuningen, I. Involvement of a signal transduction mechanism in ATP-induced mucin release from cultured airway goblet cells. *Am J Respir Cell Mol Biol* 1993;8: 121–125.

99. Davis CW, Dowell ML, Lethem M. Van Scott M. Goblet cell degran-

ulation in isolated canine tracheal epithelium: response to exogenous ATP, ADP, and adenosine. *Am J Physiol* 1992;262:C1313–C1323.

100. Lundgren JD, Davey RT, Jr, Lundgren B, et al. Eosinophil cationic protein stimulates and major basic protein inhibits airway mucus secretion. *J Allergy Clin Immunol* 1991;87:689–698.

101. Peatfield AC, Hall RL, Richardson PS, Jeffery PK. The effect of serum on the secretion of radiolabeled mucous macromolecules into the lumen of the cat trachea. *Am Rev Respir Dis* 1982;125:210–215.

102. Sperber K, Gollub E, Goswami S, Kalb TH, Mayer L, Marom Z. *In vivo* detection of a novel macrophage-derived protein involved in the regulation of mucus-like glycoconjugate secretion. *Am Rev Respir Dis* 1992;146:1589–1597.

103. Schuster A, Ueki I, Nadel JA. Neutrophil elastase stimulates tracheal submucosal gland secretion that is inhibited by ICI 2000,355. *Am J Physiol* 1992;262:L86–L91.

104. Lundgren JD, Kaliner M, Logun C, Shelhamer JH. Dexamethasone reduces rat tracheal goblet cell hyperplasia produced by human neutrophil products. *Exp Lung Res* 1988;14:853–863.

105. Breuer R, Christensen TG, Lucey EC, Stone PJ, Snider GL. Quantitative study of secretory cell metaplasia induced by human neutrophil elastase in the large bronchi of hamsters. *J Lab Clin Med* 1985;105:635–640.

106. Sur S, Crotty TB, Kephart GM, et al. Sudden-onset fatal asthma. A distinct entity with few eosinophils and relatively more neutrophils in the airway submucosa? *Am Rev Respir Dis* 1993;148:550–552.

107. Gawin AZ, Baraniuk JN, Kaliner M. Effects of histamine on guinea pig nasal mucosal secretion. *Am J Physiol* 1992;262:L590–L599.

108. Lopez-Vidriero MT, Das I, Smith AP, Picot R, Reid L. Bronchial secretion from normal human airways after inhalation of prostablandin F2a, acetylcholine, histamine and citric acid. *Thorax* 1977;32:734–739.

109. Parke DV. Pharmacology of mucus. *Br Med Bull* 1978;34:89.

110. Shelhamer JH, Marom Z, Kaliner M. Immunologic and neuropharmacologic stimulation of mucous glycoprotein release from human airways *in vitro*. *J Clin Invest* 1980;66:1400–1408.

111. Yamatake Y, et al. Allergy induced asthma with Ascaris suum administration to dogs. *Jpn J Pharmacol* 1977;27:285.

112. Wanner A, Zarzecki S, Hirsch J, Epstein S. Tracheal mucous transport in experimental canine asthma. *J Appl Physiol* 1975; 39:950–957.

113. Wanner A, Mezey RJ, Reinhart ME, Eyre P. Antigen-induced bronchospasm in conscious sheep. *J Appl Physiol* 1979;47:917–922.

114. Weissberger D, Oliver W, Jr, Abraham WM, Wanner A. Impaired tracheal mucous transport in allergic bronchoconstriction: Effect of terbutaline pretreatment. *J Allergy Clin Immunol* 1981;67:357–362.

115. Allegra L, Abraham WM, Chapman GA, Wanner A. Duration of mucociliary dysfunction following antigen challenge in allergic sheep. *J Appl Physiol* 1983;55:726–730.

116. Russi EW, Abraham WM, Chapman GA, Stevenson JS, Codias E, Wanner A. Effects of leukotriene D4 on mucociliary and respiratory function in allergic and nonallergic sheep. *J Appl Physiol* 1985;59:1416–1422.

117. Phipps RJ, Denas S, Wanner A. Leukotriene D4 stimulates secretion of glycoproteins, ions and water in sheep trachea. *Fed Proc* 1983;42:461 (Abstr).

118. Dunnill MS, Massarella GR, Anderson JA. A comparison of the quantitative anatomy of the bronchi in normal subjects, in status asthmaticus, in chronic bronchitis, and in emphysema. *Thorax* 1969;24:176–179.

119. Cutz E, Levison H, Cooper DM. Ultrastructure of airways in children with asthma. *Histopathology* 1978;2:407–421.

120. Gurgis HA, Townley RG. Biochemical study on sputum in asthma and emphysema. *J Allergy Clin Immunol* 11973;51:86.

121. Ryley HC, Brongan TD. Variation in the composition of sputum in chronic chest disease. *Br J Exp Pathol* 1968;49:625.

122. Savato G. Some histological changes in chronic bronchitis and asthma. *Thorax* 1968;23:168.

123. Hoffnianvou H, Ebelt H. Der elektrolytgehalt des sputums und des serums bein patientem mit asthma und chronischer bronchitis. *Allerg Asthmaforsch* 1968;14:227.

124. Charman J, Reid L. Sputum viscosity in chronic bronchitis, bronchiectasis, asthma, and cystic fibrosis. *Biorheology* 1972;9:185.

125. Dulfano MJ, Luk CK. Sputum and ciliary inhibition in asthma. *Thorax* 1982;37:646–651.

126. Fahy JV, Steiger DJ, Liu J, Basbaum CB, Finkbeiner WE, Boushey HA. Markers of mucus secretion and DNA levels in induced sputum from asthmatic and from healthy subjects. *Am Rev Respir Dis* 1993;147:1132–1137.

127. Thompson AB, Bohling T, Payvandi F, Rennard SI. Lower respiratory tract lactoferrin and lysozyme arise primarily in the airways and are elevated in association with chronic bronchitis. *J Lab Clin Med* 1990;115:148–158.

128. Mezey RJ, Cohn MA, Fernandez RJ, Januszkiewicz AJ, Wanner, A. Mucociliary transport in allergic patients with antigen-induced bronchospasm. *Am Rev Respir Dis* 1978;118:677–684.

129. Bateman JRM, Pavia D, Sheahan NF, Agnew JE, Clarke SW. Impaired tracheobronchial clearance in patients with mild stable asthma. *Thorax* 1983;38:463–467.

130. Foster WM, Langenback E, Bohning D, Bergofsky EH. Quantitation of mucus clearance in peripheral lung and comparison with tracheal and bronchial mucus transport velocities in man: adrenergics return depressed clearance and transport velocities in asthmatics to normal. *Am Rev Respir Dis* 1978;117(4):337 (Abstr).

131. O'Riordan TG, Zwang, J, Smaldone GC. Mucociliary clearance in adult asthma. *Am Rev Respir Dis* 1992;146:598–603.

132. Santa Cruz R, Landa J, Hirsch J. Tracheal mucous velocity in normal man and patients with obstructive lung disease. *Am Rev Respir Dis* 1974;109:458–463.

133. Mossberg B, Strandberg K, Philipson K, Camner P. Tracheobronchial clearance in bronchial asthma: Response to β-adrenoreceptor stimulation. *Scand J Resp Dis* 1976;57:119.

134. Svartengren M, Ericsson CH, Philipson K, Mossberg B, Camner P. Tracheobronchial clearance in asthma-discordant monozygotic twins. *Respiration* 1989;56:70–79.

135. Messina MS, O'Riordan TG, Smaldone GC. Changes in mucociliary clearance during acute exacerbations of asthma. *Am Rev Respir Dis* 1991;143:993–997.

136. Sackner MA, Hirsch JA, Epstein S, Rywlin AM. Effect of oxygen in graded concentrations upon tracheal mucous velocity: a study in anesthetized dogs. *Chest* 1976;69:164–167.

137. Camner P, Jarstrand C, Philipson K. Tracheobronchial clearance in patients with influenza. *Am Rev Respir Dis* 1973;108:131–135.

138. Ahmed T, Greenblatt DW, Birch S, Marchette B, Wanner A. Abnormal mucociliary transport in allergic patients with antigen-induced bronchspasm: Role of SRS-A. *Am Rev Respir Dis* 1981;124:110–114.

139. Mussatto DJ, Garrard CS, Lourenço RV. The effect of inhaled histamine on human tracheal mucus velocity and bronchial mucociliary clearance. *Am Rev Respir Dis* 1988;138:775–779.

140. Lai CKW, Polosa R, Pavia D, et al. Effect of inhaled 15-(s)-hydroxyeicosatetraenoic acid on tracheobronchial clearance in normal human airways. *Thorax* 1991;46:446–448.

141. Nieminen MM, Moilanen EK, Nyholm J-EJ, et al. Platelet-activating factor impairs mucociliary transport and increases plasma leukotriene B4 in man. *Eur Respir J* 1991;4:551–560.

Asthma, edited by P.J. Barnes, M.M. Grunstein, A.R. Leff, and A.J. Woolcock.
Lippincott–Raven Publishers, Philadelphia © 1997.

▪ 62 ▪

Epithelium as a Target

Steven R. White

The epithelial lining of airways is a complex structure with several roles in the protection and regulation of airway function. Previously considered an inert barrier to the outside environment, the epithelium is now recognized as having substantial contributions to make to bronchial airway function. It aids in the protection of airway cells and structures from the external environment and the regulation of fluid and ion transport across the airway and into the airway lumen. It is also a potential modulator of airway caliber and airway smooth muscle tone, and modulator of inflammatory cells and mediator secretion. The epithelium may be a specific target of inflammation in asthma, and damage to the epithelium, combined with perturbation of its function, may contribute substantially to airways inflammation, edema formation, mucous plugging, and bronchoconstriction in the asthmatic state. It is not clear whether damage to the epithelium is part of the beginning or end of the process that leads to asthma. The question remains: is the epithelial layer simply a target for other cells and for inflammation, or does it participate in the genesis of airways inflammation? This chapter fo-

cuses primarily on the epithelium as a target organ in asthma, and examines the morphologic and functional consequences of such targeting. The role of the epithelium as an effector as a direct response to damage also is examined.

NORMAL MORPHOLOGY OF THE AIRWAYS EPITHELIUM

The mucosal lining of central airways classically is considered a pseudostratified columnar epithelium attached to a basement membrane (Fig. 1). The height of the epithelial layer from the basement membrane to the lumenal surface is determined by the columnar epithelial cells, and is greatest in the central airways, with progressive diminution as airway caliber decreases (1). In human airways, the bronchiolar airways are lined with an epithelium that has a simple cuboidal appearance. The epithelial layer is pierced by the terminal process of nerve fibers whose cell bodies lie deep to the epithelium. Several epithelial cell types have been identified in mammalian proximal airways. Basal epithelial cells attach to the basement membrane but do not extend to the lumenal surface; this accounts for the pseudostratified appearance of the epithelium. These are mod-

S. R. White: Department of Medicine, Section of Pulmonary and Critical Care Medicine, Division of Biological Sciences, The University of Chicago, Chicago, Illinois 60637.

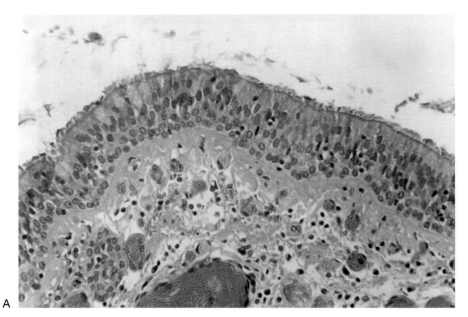

A

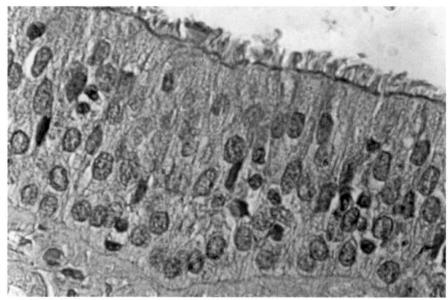

B

FIG. 1. Normal human tracheal epithelial layer, taken from an autopsy specimen of a 19-year-old man with no known history of airways disease. **A:** Low power view. Epithelial cells are normal in appearance and are tightly packed. Few inflammatory cells are present in the submucosa. Numerous small blood vessels are seen. The basement membrane is intact and thin, compared to the height of the epithelium. (Original magnification, ×100.) **B:** High power view. The stratified columar cells and basal cells are clearly seen. (Original magnification, ×400.) (Courtesy of Dr. Thamrong Chira, Cook County Medical Examiner's Office, Chicago, Illinois.)

erately differentiated cells that increase the surface area of the epithelial layer for attachment of columnar cells (2). In their role as attachment cells for the columnar epithelium, they increase in number as the height of the columnar cells increase (2). In rat airways larger than 2.5 mm in diameter, as much as 90% of the basal lamina is covered by basal cells (2,3). This location also means that the basal cell may take on additional functions such as maintenance of the basement membrane and communications between the columnar epithelium and underlying fibroblasts. The stem or regenerating cell of the central airway is controversial; in some studies the basal cell has been shown to be the progenitor cell, whereas in other studies secretory cells have been

demonstrated to serve this function (4–10). This is species specific.

There are several types of columnar epithelial cells identified by light and electron microscopy within the airways epithelium. Ciliated epithelial cells attach both to basal cells and to the basement membrane and extend to the lumen. Among the most numerous cells within the tracheobronchial epithelium, their primary function is to generate mucous flow and direct this flow in an appropriate direction. Motile cilia are attached to the apical surface; these consist of characteristic longitudinal tubules. The outer doublet tubules are composed of dynein, a specific protein with ATPase activity which provides the cilia with motility (11,12). Ciliated cells have 200 to 300

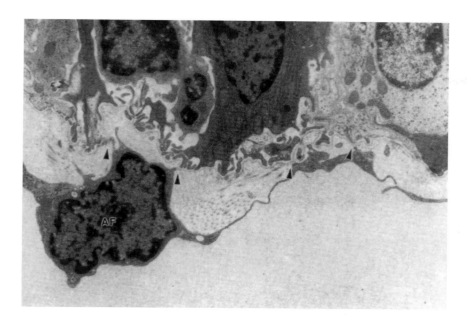

FIG. 2. Longitudinal section of an attenuated fibroblast (AF) in a cross-section of rat trachea viewed via transmission electron microscopy. These long, thin cells (up to 30 μm in length) contain abundant endoplasmic reticulum and are not oriented to a particular tissue plane. The fibroblasts rest immediately beneath the basement membrane and make contact with the basal lamina at various points *(arrows)*. These cells maintain the overlying basement membrane and may communicate with basal epithelial cells. (From Evan MF, Guha SC, Cox RA, Moller PC. Attenuated fibroblast sheath around the basement memebrane zone in the trachea. *Am J Respir Cell Mol Biol* 1993;8:188–192, with permission.)

cilia per cell which beat at 15 to 18 hertz (Hz). Ciliated epithelial cells also may regulate fluid and ion transport into the lumen through numerous microvilli and cytoplasmic processes on the apical surface.

A number of secretory columnar epithelial cell types also are present within different levels of the conducting airways. These include mucous goblet cells, Clara cells and serous cells. These cells are tall and contain numerous secretory granules, numerous mitochondria, and a high cytoplasm/nucleus ratio. Goblet cells, in concert with submucosal glands, produce and secrete airway mucus and maintain the mucociliary barrier which traps inhaled particles and pollutant gases. These are abundant in the central airways and less so in the more peripheral airways (13). Clara cells are found only in the bronchioles in humans and provide secretory material for the lumenal lining of airways (14–16). The Clara cell exhibits self-renewal and also can differentiate into ciliated cells, though in some species this ability to repopulate a small airway may be limited (17,18).

The basement membrane immediately beneath the epithelial layer acts as a scaffold and serves as a structural barrier to the passage of cells and macromolecules. In normal human airways, the true basement lamina (lamina lucida plus the lamina densa) is not discernible by light microscopy, being < 150 nm thick. Below this lies a reticular lamina which is visible on routine hematoxylin and eosin (H and E) stain of an airway in cross-section. The true lamina consists of type IV collagen, laminin, fibronectin, proteoglycans, entactin and nidogen (19). The lamina lucida contains the subbasal dense plates and anchoring filaments of hemidesmosomes from the overlying basal cells, while in the lamina densa anchoring fibrils extend into underlying connective tissue where they

attach to anchoring plaques (20,21). The lamina reticularis consists primarily of types III and V collagen, and fibronectin (19). Below this are cells called myofibroblasts, which have morphologic features of fibroblasts but which also have contractile filaments. These cells have long cytoplasmic processes stretching beneath the basement membrane and they contain numerous polyribosomes. It is not clear whether the overlying epithelium, the underlying submucosal myofibroblasts, or both contribute to the formation and maintenance of the basement membrane in the normal state, since both cell types are capable of secreting the various extracellular matrix proteins required. Recent studies demonstrate a specific sheath of fibroblasts immediately beneath the basement membrane (21) (Fig. 2). These cells may have a prominent role both in normal repair and in deranged deposition of matrix proteins in asthma.

The organization of the epithelial layer, particularly in how the various cells are attached both to each other and to the basement membrane, has been better defined recently. It is now clear that columnar epithelial cells generally do not attach to the basement membrane, but are instead, fixed to the epithelial layer through their attachment to the basal cells (2,22,23). Thus, the epithelial layer in central airways is best considered truly stratified, and not pseudostratified. Tight junctions, a complex adhesive structure binding columnar cells, maintain the integrity of the apical border of the epithelial layer (24–26) (Fig. 3). The number of strands comprising the tight junction belt is hypothesized to relate to epithelial permeability and correlates to the magnitude of the electrical potential difference that is generated as a result of epithelial ion transport (27). Below this are intermediate junctions which bind suprabasal cells; these have recently been

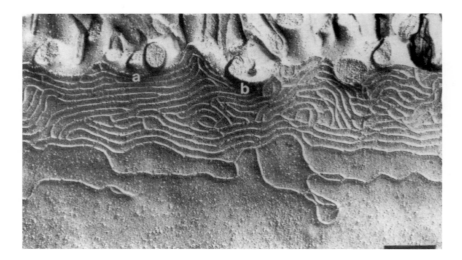

FIG. 3. Freeze-fracture photograph of a single tight junction in the epithelial layer of a normal human bronchus. The junction is between a ciliated and an indeterminate cell type. Both parallel (*a*) and network (*b*) strand arrangements are seen. Both types of strand arrangements may be seen in any tight junction and represent opposite extremes of a single junctional form. Bar=250 nm. (From Godfrey RWA, Severs NJ, Jeffrey PK. Freeze-fracture morphology and quantification of human bronchial epithelial tight junctions. *Am J Respir Cell Mol Biol* 1992;6:453–458, with permission.)

demonstrated to contain the adhesion molecule E-cadherin (28). Both tight and intermediate junctions serve to bind columnar epithelial cells and also serve to regulate paracellular transport. Desmosomes are typical structures found in the epithelium at many sites; these have a complex structure that includes a centralized plaque with outwardly radiating filaments into the cytoplasm of the bound cells. There is a particularly dense population of desmosomes binding columnar and basal cells (28). The desmosomal attachment sites of columnar cells to basal cells may be a point of attack in asthma, as will be discussed further on. Hemidesmosomes containing the specific integrin subunits α_6 and β_4 anchor the basal cells to

the underlying basement membrane (28,29). The laminin-binding integrin subunit α_6 is found in the basilar region, and the fibronectin-binding subunit α_v at the basolateral region of the epithelium in normal bronchial airways (30) (Fig. 4). That basal cells serve as the primary anchor for columnar cells is demonstrated by the paucity of primary attachment sites of columnar cells to the basement membrane and by the correlation between epithelium height, volume of keratin filaments, and total desmosome length in airway sections (29). Increasing epithelial height in larger airways is due to taller columnar cells, and is associated with increased adhesions of the basal cells to the basement membrane (2).

A

α_2

B

α_6

C

α_v

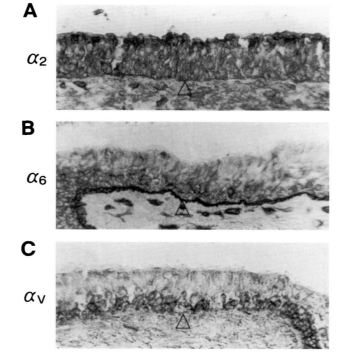

FIG. 4. Cellular distribution of the α_2 (**A**), α_6 (**B**), and α_v (**C**) integrins in the epithelium of normal human bronchial tissue. Serial frozen sections were stained, using immunohistochemical techniques with monoclonal antibodies directed against each subunit. Three patterns of distribution are seen: α_2 integrins are found diffusely at cell-cell and cell-substratum borders, α_6 integrins are found along the basilar border, and α_v integrins are found along the basolateral margins. Open arrowheads indicate the epithelial basement membrane. (Original magnification, ×213.) (From Damjanovich L, Albelda SM, Mete SA, Buck CA. Distribution of integrin cell adhesion receptors in normal and malignant lung tissue. *Am J Respir Cell Mol Biol* 1992;6:197–206, with permission.)

STRUCTURAL DAMAGE TO THE EPITHELIUM IN ASTHMA

Characteristic changes are found in the airways epithelium in asthma, even when the clinical state of the syndrome is judged to be mild. Constitutive structures are damaged and inflammatory cells are present. These structural changes can be correlated to certain physiologic changes in asthma.

Structural Changes in the Epithelium

Damage to the epithelial layer is commonly found in the central airways of asthmatic subjects and may be present even in the mildest asthmatic subjects (31–33). Histologic examination of airways of patients dying of status asthmaticus demonstrates severe inflammation, with infiltration of inflammatory cells, particularly eosinophils, but also mononuclear cells and lymphocytes (Fig. 5). Damage to and shedding of the epithelium is common; in severe cases complete sloughing of large sections of epithelium into the lumen is seen (Fig. 5). Typically, the columnar epithelium is shed, leaving behind a thin layer of basal cells. In patients dying of status asthmaticus, it can be difficult to find areas of normal epithelium. The airway lumen is clogged with mucus plugs and shed cells. Edema of the mucosa and lamina propria is common. Shed epithelial cells collect in the lumen and can be found in the sputum in the form of creola bodies and Curchmann's spirals (34).

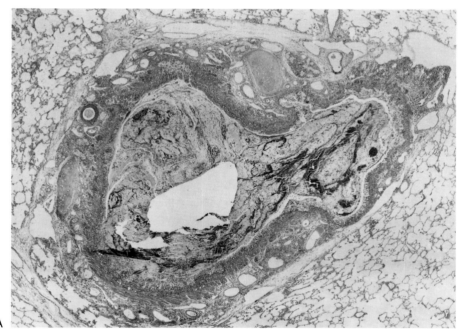

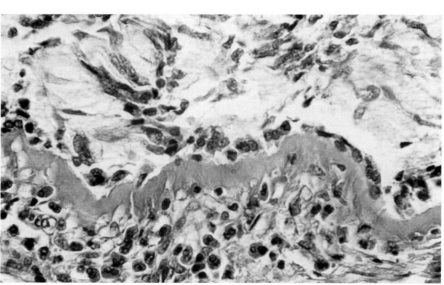

FIG. 5. Epithelial damage of the human central airways in severe asthma: representative photomicrographs. **A:** low power view of a central airway from an autopsy specimen of an asthmatic patient who died of status asthmaticus. Extensive plugging of the airway lumen, mucosal thickening and cellular infiltration of the epithelium and submucosa can be appreciated. Hematoxylin and eosin stain. (Original magnification, ×100.) **B:** High power view of a similar central airway from another asthmatic patient. The epithelium *(top)* is damaged and infiltrated with inflammatory cells. The basement membrane upon which the epithelium rests is markedly thickened. Eosinophils and mast cells are numerous throughout the epithelium and mucosa. Hematoxylin and eosin stain. (Original magnification, ×400.) (Courtesy of Dr. Cyril Abrahams, Department of Pathology, the University of Chicago.)

Chronic damage within the epithelium and lamina propria includes thickening of the basement membrane, deposition of collagen immediately beneath the basement membrane, and an increase in fibroblast activity, including secretion of growth factors (32).

In milder cases, the epithelium still may be strikingly abnormal (Fig. 6). Increased numbers of goblet cells are found in endobronchial biopsies of patients with newly-diagnosed asthma, and other epithelial structural abnormalities, such as a thickened basement membrane, can be seen (35). Columnar cells remain attached to each other, but may be separated from the basal cells by a plasma exudate or edema fluid (31). Airways inflammation and infiltration of multiple inflammatory cells types can be seen even in the mildest cases (35). However, not all subjects with mild asthma will demonstrate these changes. In at least one study, light and electron microscopy examination of bronchial biopsies from stable asthmatic subjects did not differ substantially from similar biopsies in control subjects lacking airway hyperreactivity (36). These studies suggest that epithelial damage occurs early in the asthmatic state, although changes in the epithelium in the setting of mild asthma may vary between patients and within a given patient over time.

The site of epithelial disruption in asthmatic central airways has been investigated recently. Generally, these studies have been undertaken with the use of endobronchial biopsies via fiberoptic bronchoscopy in asthmatic and control subjects. While these data have been extremely useful in understanding some of the mechanisms by which the epithelium is shed, the small size of these biopsies makes quantification of changes within the epithelium difficult. Sampling error and artifactual loss during the collection and preparation of the biopsy spec-

imens also makes interpretation more difficult. Nevertheless, these experiments have provided the best examination to date of the structure of the airways epithelium in mild-to-moderate asthma.

Basal cells tend to remain on the surface when the epithelium is partially denuded (31,37). In electron microscopy studies of bronchial biopsies from asthmatic patients, eosinophils and their granular proteins tend to be present in the intercellular spaces between basal cells and columnar cells (31). Beasley et al. (32) have shown that asthmatic subjects shed four-fold as many epithelial cells as do control subjects on bronchial washing. In the asthmatic subjects, epithelial cells tended to be shed as clusters, which were both larger and more numerous than in normal controls. By morphology, the great majority of these shed cells are columnar. A study from Montefort et al. (38) suggests that in asthmatic airways, columnar epithelial cells are preferentially shed while basal cells remain attached to the basement membrane. These studies suggest that a plane of cleavage may exist between the superficial columnar epithelial cells and the deeper basal cells. Such shedding could occur if the desmosomes binding the columnar to the basal cells were perturbed by, for example, neutral proteases released by eosinophils or other inflammatory cells. Evidence for this is found in a study by Frigas et al. (39), which demonstrated in an *in vitro* model of guinea pig tracheal epithelium that the concentration of the eosinophil granular cationic protein, major basic protein (MBP), required to detach columnar cells is lower than that required to detach basal cells from the basement membrane. Other insults to airway epithelium, such as smoke exposure and influenza virus, also elicit selective shedding of more superficial cells (40,41). A more recent study suggests that columnar cell shedding is due to selective disruption of adhesive mechanisms, as opposed to cell death (42). Taken together, these studies suggest the potential for partial or selective desquamation of the epithelium at the junction of the columnar and basal cell layers in asthma. Whether this is due to a specific insult on the desmosomal or other adhesive structures at this junction, or simply that these structures are more available to a given insult than the lower adhesive structures binding the basal cells to the basement membrane, is not clear.

Epithelial damage in asthmatic subjects can be correlated to the degree of airway hyperresponsiveness. In general, greater airway reactivity correlates to a greater degree of epithelial damage. In the previously referenced study by Beasley et al. (32), asthmatic subjects with greater numbers of shed epithelial cells and pathologic changes on endobronchial biopsy had an increased reactivity to histamine compared to normal controls. However, within the asthmatic cohort, the thickening of the basement membrane and presence of inflammatory cells in endobronchial biopsies were found, irrespective of the degree of reactivity to histamine. Jeffery et al. (33) dem-

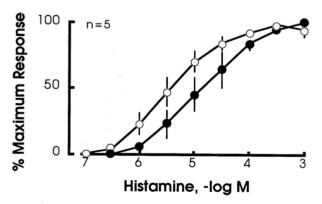

FIG. 6. Effects of epithelium removal on responsiveness of canine bronchial rings to histamine. Data are expressed as a percent maximal response. Rings without an epithelium *(open circles)* have a somewhat greater response to histamine than rings with an intact epithelium *(closed circles).* (From Flavahan NA, Aarhus LL, Rimele TF, Vanhoutte PM. Respiratory epithelium inhibits bronchial smooth muscle tone. *J Appl Physiol* 1985;58:834–838, with permission.)

onstrated that epithelial cell fragility and denudation was correlated to methacholine reactivity, and suggested that thickening of the reticular lamina begins early in asthma. This study also showed infiltration of the epithelial layer by lymphocytes. Laitinen et al. (31) demonstrated extensive epithelial damage in mild asthma with exposure of intraepithelial nerve fibers, which they hypothesized could then be stimulated by specific or nonspecific stimuli within the airway lumen. As noted earlier, the epithelium may not appear different in asthmatics, compared to normal volunteers, even though asthmatics have demonstrable airways hyperreactivity (36).

It is not clear whether the pathologic changes within the epithelium in asthma actually cause the airways hyperreactivity; such a correlation may simply demonstrate the similar degree of the structural and functional changes of the underlying insult in asthma. There is experimental evidence that the responsiveness of the airways smooth muscle to contractile agonists placed in the airway lumen correlates well with epithelial layer integrity (43). The close approximation of smooth muscle to epithelium suggests that a damaged, and thus more porous, epithelium may permit greater access, both of external toxins and inflammatory mediators to the smooth muscle.

Structural Changes to the Basement Membrane

Thickening of the basement membrane is a characteristic feature of chronic asthma. This thickening involves deposition of collagen immediately beneath the lamina reticularis and an increase in fibroblast activity (32). The epithelial cells may not be responsible for the deposition of new matrix. Roche et al. (44) have documented the absence of type IV collagen and laminin, and the presence of interstitial collagens (types I, III and V) and fibronectin in the thickened lamina reticularis in biopsy specimens obtained via fiberoptic bronchoscopy in asthmatic subjects. Subsequent study has demonstrated an association between subepithelial myofibroblasts and collagen deposition in a small cohort of volunteers with allergic asthma (45). These changes occur in the presence of other indices of inflammation in asthmatic airways, such as the presence of eosinophils and lymphocytes. Moreover, thickening of the basement membrane may be a manifestation of general atopy, as opposed to asthma *per se*. In a recent study, Djukanovic et al. (46) studied endobronchial biopsies collected from a cohort of stable, atopic asthmatic subjects, subjects with atopy but not asthma, and normal volunteers. The thickness of the basement membrane was greatest in the asthmatic subjects, but atopic, nonasthmatic subjects had a basement membrane that was thicker than that of the normal volunteers. These changes were paralleled both by the presence of eosinophils and by degranulation of mast cells within the mucosa, which were greatest in the asthmatic

subjects, intermediate in the atopic subjects, and lowest in the normal volunteers. The mechanism by which atopy alone, in the absence of overt airways disease, could cause such changes is not clear. It is not clear whether the induced changes in the basement membrane are the direct result of stimulation of the myofibroblasts (or epithelial cells) by inflammatory cells, or whether the effect is indirect and dependent on intermediate activation of other cells within the airway.

There is some evidence that the increased thickness of the basement membrane in asthma can be ameliorated, either with treatment or with removal of causative agents. Trigg et al. (47) examined a cohort of 25 nonsmoking mild asthmatic subjects previously treated only with inhaled β-adrenergic agonists. Subjects were treated either with inhaled beclomethasone, 1000 μg daily, or placebo for 4 months, after which responsiveness to histamine was determined and fiberoptic bronchoscopy was done to obtain lavage fluid and endobronchial biopsies. As expected, airway reactivity improved and fewer eosinophils were found in the airways mucosa. The thickness of type III collagen deposition was less in the steroid-treated group compared to subjects treated with placebo: 19.8 ± 3.4 vs. 29.7 ± 4.4 μm. In another series of studies, Saetta et al. (48,49) examined the effect of cessation of exposure to toluene diisocyanate (TDI), a known inducer of asthma in occupational settings, on the bronchial mucosa of subjects with TDI-induced asthma. Bronchial biopsies were collected at the time of entry into the study, and again 6 months after cessation of TDI exposure. The basement membrane was thickened at the time of diagnosis and entry into the study with increased deposition of type III collagen. The reticular layer decreased significantly in thickness over the 6 months after cessation of TDI exposure. This occurred in spite of a lack of change in the numbers of eosinophils and mast cells in the biopsy specimens and continued airways reactivity to either methacholine and/or TDI. These studies suggest that even a relatively short course of treatment for asthma, or cessation in that exposure which has initiated and sustained the asthmatic response, may begin the reversal of structural changes in the airway epithelial layer. Whether longer periods of treatment or cessation of exposure would lead to more profound beneficial structural changes within the epithelium, is not known.

Inflammatory Cells Eliciting Structural Damage of the Epithelium

Inflammatory cells target the airways epithelium in asthma. Such targeting is not necessarily exclusive nor specific, as reported elsewhere in this volume. One of the principal inflammatory cells involved in asthma, the eosinophil, can secrete a variety of mediators which damage the epithelium. Increased numbers of eosinophils are found within the bronchial mucosa, as ascertained by endobronchial biopsy in asthmatic subjects, and present in large numbers in sputum and in bronchoalveolar lavage fluid (BAL) obtained from asthmatic patients, as well. (50–53). One class of toxic products derived from eosinophils is the granular basic proteins as described in Chapter 45. The MBP of eosinophils, a highly cationic protein with a molecular weight of approximately 14,000 daltons, has been demonstrated within the airways of patients dying of severe asthma, even when eosinophils themselves cannot be identified (54,55). Another eosinophil cationic protein, eosinophil cationic protein (ECP), also is found in the bronchial mucosa of asthmatic subjects (51). These proteins can elicit damage to the epithelium. Both MBP and ECP are toxic to epithelial cell lines in culture and cause bleb formation and detachment of cells from culture substrate (39,56). These proteins may be responsible, in large part, for the effects of whole, activated eosinophils on epithelial cell exfoliation (57). Eosinophil proteins may also alter substantially the function of epithelial cells and, thus, may perpetuate the asthmatic state at several levels.

T cell lymphocytes have been associated with eosinophil infiltration in the bronchial mucosa of asthmatic subjects. In mildly asthmatic patients, intraepithelial lymphocytes may represent the major proportion of migratory inflammatory cells within the mucosa (33,35,50). In the previously cited study of newly diagnosed asthmatic subjects, lymphocytes outnumbered all other migratory inflammatory cells seen in endobronchial mucosal biopsies, and were present in numbers that were 5 times greater than in controls (35). Bronchial biopsies of subjects with either extrinsic or intrinsic asthma demonstrate the presence of CD3+ and CD4+ lymphocytes within the epithelial layer; such cells are virtually absent in control subjects (58). These lymphocytes may be activated (59,60). In the former study, bronchial biopsies were collected in subjects with isocyanate-induced asthma and in normal volunteers. The former group had increased numbers of CD25– cells in the mucosa compared to the latter; this marker represents cells bearing and interleukin-2 receptor and indicates the presence of activated lymphocytes. In another study, the ratio of T to B lymphocytes was markedly increased (6:1) in endobronchial biopsies of asthmatic subjects, compared to the ratios in biopsies of either normal subjects (2:1), or subjects with cystic fibrosis (1:1) (50). It is interesting to speculate that T lymphocytes, by virtue of their secretion of cytokine mediators, may elicit the migration and activation of eosinophils into the airways mucosa after a provoking stimulus with subsequent damage to epithelial cells. Taken together, these studies suggest that the damage to the epithelium as seen in asthma may be the direct result of the mediators secreted by several types of inflammatory cells.

Mast cells also target the airways epithelium. Mast cells are found with regularity in the epithelium, even in the mildest cases of asthma. These cells are more activated and degranulated, both as demonstrated in autopsy cases of severe asthma, and in more recent studies of airway morphology in mild atopic and nonatopic asthmatics (61–64). The accumulation of mast cells in the epithelium of asthmatic subjects may be independent of allergy status (63). While most major mast cell mediators such as histamine, tryptase, and leukotrienes are not known to be cytotoxic to the epithelium, these agents also have potent effects on epithelial cell function.

Other inflammatory cells have been implicated in the structural damage to the epithelium in asthma, though these reports have not suggested as strong a link between inflammatory cell products and subsequent damage to the epithelium as seen with eosinophils and mast cells. Neutrophils infiltrate the airway mucosa of some asthmatic subjects, but the role of neutrophils, both in the genesis of asthma and in epithelial cell damage, is unclear. Activated neutrophils damage alveolar epithelial cells *in vitro*, but to date, similar studies utilizing airway epithelial cells have not been done (65).

In summary, the structural damage to the airways epithelium may be extensive even in mild cases of asthma. Targeting of the epithelium by inflammatory cells and their mediators causes the shedding of the columnar epithelium, most likely by loosening its adhesive contacts with the basal epithelium. Sloughing of the epithelium contributes to lumenal plugging and impairment of the barrier between the airway and the external environment. Thickening of the basement membrane occurs though it is not clear that epithelial cells specifically contribute to this process. These structural abnormalities lead to substantial changes in epithelial layer function.

FUNCTIONAL DAMAGE TO THE EPITHELIUM IN ASTHMA

In addition to its function as a barrier to the outside environment, the epithelial lining of airways has a number of metabolic functions. These include regulation of fluid and ion transport (See Chapter 64), production, secretion, and movement of mucus (See Chapters 64 and 65), and presentation of antigen and foreign substances to immunologic cells within the airway. In recent years it has been postulated that the epithelium also regulates airway caliber by secretion of substances that alter smooth muscle reactivity (See Chapter 63). Airway edema and plasma exudation into airways also may alter airway function substantially, and alterations in epithelial permeability may, in part, account for airways edema. This section focuses on the functional consequences of damage to the epithelium in asthma, with specific reference to the epithelium as a target organ, and the initial response of the epithelium to such targeting.

Changes in Function that Alter Airway Tone

Damage to the airway epithelium may be associated with changes in airway responsiveness in asthma. Injury elicited by environmental insults or other stimuli may inhibit the ability of the epithelium to produce mediators which regulate airway responsiveness and caliber. Even after the resolution of an acute asthmatic exacerbation, continued targeting of the epithelium may both elicit production of factors which enhance reactivity and disrupt the production of factors which normally down-regulate reactivity.

Environmental insults to the epithelium may be associated with changes in airway reactivity. In normal subjects, bronchial reactivity may be increased during upper respiratory tract infection (66). Administration of live, attenuated influenza virus to normal subjects elicits bronchial responsiveness in those subjects who develop significant titers to the virus (67). These viruses damage the epithelium and cause shedding of the epithelial lining (40). In animal models, infection with either influenza or Sendai virus causes increased response to inflammatory peptides such as substance P (68,69). In these experiments, epithelial destruction was almost complete and suggested that loss of epithelial factors, perhaps the neutral endopeptidase that normally degrades substance P and similar peptides, accounted for the change in reactivity. Airway reactivity returns to normal in almost all human subjects after repair of the damaged epithelium is complete.

Ozone (O_3) is another environmental agent that may alter airway responsiveness by damaging the epithelium. Exposure to low concentrations (≤ 0.4 ppm) of ozone causes both bronchial hyperreactivity and increased epithelial permeability in human subjects (70–72). Exposure to 1.0 ppm O_3 in a canine model of airway responsiveness, elicited substantial changes in the response to both acetylcholine and histamine within 1 hour of exposure (71). Ozone-induced airway hyperreactivity may depend, in part, on induction of airway inflammation with loss of airway mucosal goblet cells, and an increase in intraepithelial mast cells over several hours, followed 4 to 8 hours later by infiltration of the epithelium and mucosa with neutrophils and other inflammatory cells (73). Increased responsiveness elicited by O_3 preceded infiltration of neutrophils into the airways. Depletion of neutrophils in a canine model prior to ozone exposure, inhibits both airway hyperresponsiveness and an influx of intra-epithelial neutrophils (74). However, neutrophil infiltration may not be essential (17). Though not as well-established as with O_3, other environmental toxic gases may work via similar mechanisms.

In addition to the changes in epithelial function that may occur in response to an inflammatory or environmental stimulus, some existing evidence suggests that the epithelium secretes endogenous factors which tonically regulate the state of bronchomotor tone. While the presence and physiological importance of such factors is not yet clear, epithelial-derived factors that influence smooth muscle function may serve as regulators of final airway caliber.

The vascular endothelium modulates the final diameter of blood vessels by secreting local factors that both relax and constrict vascular smooth muscle (75). This knowledge, along with the known perturbation of the epithelium in asthma, prompted a search for analogous epithelial-derived factors in airways (76). In initial experiments, rings or strips of airway smooth muscle were suspended in an organ bath and prepared for measurement of isometric force generation. In some smooth muscle rings/strips, the epithelium was removed by gentle abrasion or dissection, without damage to the underlying muscle; whereas in others, the epithelium was left intact. Subsequent contraction of each set of smooth muscle rings/strips demonstrated a leftward shift in the response to contractile agonists (e.g., acetylcholine, histamine) in those rings/strips in which the epithelium had been removed, generally without a change in the maximal response (Fig. 6). These results suggested that removal of the epithelium also removed a factor that had tonically relaxed the smooth muscle, the epithelial-derived relaxing factor (EpDRF). Since these initial descriptions, similar results have been demonstrated in a number of animal and human airways, different generations of airways, and to different contractile agonists: antigen stimulation in sensitized animals, β-adrenergic agonists, calcium channel blockers, leukotrienes, and a number of physiologic stimuli (78–87). In each, the results generally are similar; removal of the epithelium causes a shift in the response of airway smooth muscle that suggests the presence of an EpDRF. This change is modest in most studies; the shift in responsiveness between epithelium-intact and epithelium-denuded smooth muscle preparations *in vitro* is approximately 4.5-fold ($< 1/2$ log) for acetylcholine, and approximately 3.4-fold ($< 1/3$ log) for serotonin (88). *In vitro* preparations that limit the perfusion of agonist into the smooth muscle to transepithelial routes exclusively, may demonstrate somewhat greater shifts in responsiveness after removal of the epithelium, suggesting a physiologically-significant role for the epithelium in regulating smooth muscle contraction (89).

The identity of EpDRF has not been confirmed. A number of experiments have demonstrated that it is not similar to the relaxing factors produced by endothelial cells (e.g., nitric oxide), although at least two reports dispute this (90–94). Prostaglandins, including prostaglandins (PG) E_2 and I_2, are secreted by airway epithelial cells (95–97). While both PGE_2 and PGI_2 directly relax airway smooth muscle in several models, in some circumstances PGE_2 can elicit contraction (95,98–100). It has been suggested that PGE_2 modulates the epithelium-dependent relaxation elicited by arachidonic acid in airway smooth muscle *in vitro*; this can be antagonized by inhibition of cyclooxygenase (101,102). Conditioned media from cultured epithelial cells also inhibit the contraction of isolated canine tracheal smooth muscle; this effect likely is due to PGE_2 (103). However, given the direct and bimodal effects of exogenous PGE_2 on airway smooth muscle, the fact that PGE_2 derived from airway epithelial cells will also relax smooth muscle, does not necessarily implicate endogenous production of PGE_2 as the (or an) EpDRF. Inhibition of cyclooxygenase in animal models does not appear to alter the described effect of EpDRF (77,87,104). In addition, treatment of smooth muscle strips *in vitro* with a cyclooxygenase inhibitor can decrease the intrinsic (so called "spontaneous") tone in airway smooth muscle of some species, such as guinea pig, and render subsequent determination of an epithelium-dependent effect on smooth muscle problematic, as described further on (105).

Even if an EpDRF exists, the potential physiological significance of this epithelium-derived molecule is unclear. Even in the best *in vitro* experiments, the upregulation of airway smooth muscle reactivity generally is less than 1 log of agonist, and in many cases, less than one-half log (88). Recent observations suggest that mast cell damage and mediator release occurs after mechanical disruption of the epithelium, and that this mediator release may correlate with increased airway responsiveness (106,107). Mechanical removal of the epithelium as accomplished in *in vitro* preparations, might damage mast cells or sensory nerve dendrites within the epithelial layer. Damaged mast cells would release histamine, and damaged nerve dendritic processes would release tachykinins such as substance P and neurokinin A, which are potent bronchoconstrictors (108). These then could augment, nonspecifically, the response of airway smooth muscle to other contractile agonists within the inflammatory milieu, as opposed to a specific effect of an epithelial cell-derived mediator.

Recent studies have focused on the ability of EpDRF to cause physiological antagonism of airway contraction *in situ*. Using an *in situ* preparation of airway smooth muscle in which the circulation and innervation to the muscle remain intact, Brofman et al. (109) in dogs and White et al. (110) in guinea pigs have demonstrated that removal of the epithelium from tracheal smooth muscle does not augment subsequent force generation caused by acetylcholine. In a more recent study, Strek et al. (111) have examined the potential dependence of guinea pig trachealis contraction on the epithelium, both in an *in vivo* and an *in vitro* model. Simple removal of the epithelium *in vivo* did not alter the response of the trachealis to acetylcholine (Fig. 7). Further, the method of normalizing *in vitro* data may influence subsequent interpretation. As shown in Figure 8, normalizing data as a percent of maximal response apparently demonstrates a shift in re-

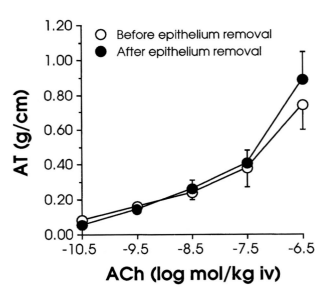

FIG. 7. Effect of removing the epithelium from the response of an isolated tracheal smooth muscle segment in guinea pigs to acetylcholine (ACh) *in vivo*. The *in vivo* preparation preserves circulation, innervation, and anatomical relationships. Concentration-response curves to ACh were generated before and 30 minutes after mechanical removal of the epithelium, and active tension (AT, in grams per cm length of the segment) was measured using a force transducer. There is little difference in the concentration-response curves, suggesting that there is little physiologic effect of an epithelial-derived relaxing factor *in vivo*.

sponsiveness typical for an EpDRF, while normalizing as a percent of the response to an external standard, such as electrical field stimulation, or expressing the data in raw (not normalized) grams force, demonstrates no such shift. In another study, Ndukwu et al. (105) demonstrated that removal of the epithelium from guinea pig tracheal smooth muscle strips *in vitro* attenuated substantially the intrinsic tone of the strip (Fig. 9). Subsequent responses to electrical field stimulation were similar in strips with and without an epithelium, once adjusted for the difference in intrinsic tone. This was true both in normal guinea pigs, and animals sensitized to albumin. These data suggest that if an EpDRF exists, it may not modulate airway tone within the physiologic range of airway reactivity in the living state.

In contrast, some data suggest that the epithelium might secrete contractile factors that modulate smooth muscle reactivity. Damage (e.g., early inflammation) to the epithelium in asthma might stimulate release of such pro-contractile factors, causing increased airway reactivity. One study from our research group (110) demonstrates that eosinophil MBP causes airway contraction that is dependent on the presence of an intact epithelial layer. This may be due to secretion of prostaglandins such as PGE_2 and $PGF_{2\alpha}$, both of which are secreted by airway epithelial cells in culture in response to treatment with

MBP (97). Conditioned medium from epithelial cells in culture can both contract or relax airways *in vitro*, depending on conditions (100,103). In both of these studies, prostaglandins were implicated as the responsible factor. However, other contractile factors may exist. Cationic proteins from eosinophils could elicit airways contraction via an interaction with the epithelium based on charge (110,112). These preliminary observations require further exploration.

In summary: factors could be released from epithelial cells in response to targeting by inflammatory cells in asthma. The potential for an EpDRF to regulate smooth muscle reactivity is enticing, given the close approximation of these two tissues. However, the specific identity of either relaxing or contractile factors derived from the epithelium is not clear, and the physiologic importance of these factors in regulating airway tone is controversial.

Changes in Function that Alter Fluid and Ion Transport in Airways

Tracheobronchial secretions atop the epithelium in airways float upon an underlaying layer of periciliary fluid, where they serve to trap inhaled particles and pollutant gases, and prevent direct contact with the underlying epithelial cells. The depth of the sol layer is about the same as the length of cilia throughout the tracheobronchial tree

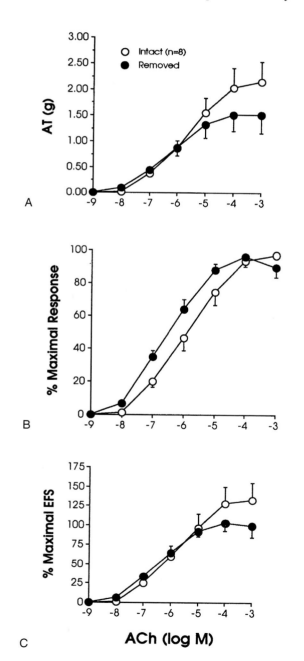

FIG. 8. Effect of removing the epithelium from the response of tracheal smooth muscle strips from guinea pigs to acetylcholine (ACh) *in vitro*. Standard methods for tissue isolation and measurement of force generation were used. **A:** active tension in grams force for strips with and without an epithelium treated with ACh. **B:** active tension as percent maximal response for the same strips. **C:** active tension as percent maximal response to electrical field stimulation (EFS) for the same strips. N=8 trachealis strips in each graph. While strips lacking an epithelium have an overall contraction that is less than strips with an intact epithelium as measured by active force generation or as a percent of an external standard (such as EFS), when normalized to an internal standard (percent maximal response), they appear to have a greater contraction (approximately 1/2 log shift in response). This must be true given the flattened peak response in the denuded strips as shown in **A**. Thus, apparent shifts in responsiveness due to removal of the epithelium (and, thus, the removal of an epithelial-derived relaxing factor), as shown in **B**, may represent an artifact of measurement. (From Strek ME, White SR, Munoz NM, et al. Physiological significance of epithelium removal in guinea pig tracheal smooth muscle. *Am Rev Respir Dis* 1993;147:1477–1482, with permission.)

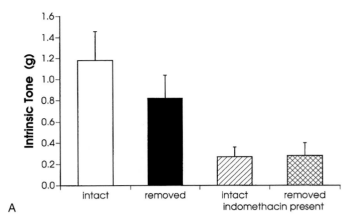

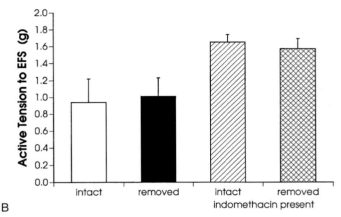

FIG. 9. Effect of epithelial removal and cyclooxygenase blockade on intrinsic (spontaneous) tone in guinea pig tracheal smooth muscle (GP-TSM) strips *in vitro*. **A:** intrinsic tone in normal animals. Removal of the epithelium attenuated intrinsic tone, and addition of the cyclooxygenase inhibitor indomethacin blocked intrinsic tone almost completely. **B:** cholinergic response (electrical field stimulation, or EFS) of the same GP-TSM strips after epithelium removal and treatment with indomethacin. Once adjusted for the difference in intrinsic tone as shown in **A**, there is no change in responsiveness to EFS (measured as active tension in grams) after removal of the epithelium compared to control. Treatment with indomethacin increases active tension somewhat, and this is not changed by removal of the epithelium. (Graph drawn from data in Ndukwu IM, Solway J, Arbetter K, Uzendoski K, Leff AR, Mitchell RW. Immune sensitization augments epithelium-dependent spontaneous tone in guinea pig trachealis. *Am J Physiol* 1994; 266:L485–L492, with permission.)

(113). Three factors affect mucociliary clearance: ciliary motion, secretion of mucins, and fluid secretion. Damage to the airway epithelium in asthma may impair each.

Airway diseases such as viral infection and asthma are associated with reduced ciliation of the surface epithelial cells, which in turn causes a reduction in tracheal mucous velocity (114). Ciliary function also can be depressed in asthma. Extracts from sputum obtained from asthmatic subjects decreases ciliary beat frequency in bronchial explants (115). Several inflammatory media-

tors found in asthmatic airways decrease ciliary beat frequency, such as eosinophil MBP and adenosine (39,116). Other mediators such as leukotriene C_4 and prostaglandins E_1 and E_2 increase ciliary beat frequency but reduce overall mucous transport rates (114). While ciliary motion may be enhanced after antigen challenge, the net effect of an acute exacerbation of asthma is ciliostasis, even when overt damage to ciliated epithelial cells is minimal (117). Finally, the effects of inflammatory mediators on ciliary function can be influenced by other factors which alter the internal regulation of ciliary movement. For example, inhibition of nitric oxide synthesis in epithelial cells can block the stimulation of ciliary movement normally elicited by isoproterenol or substance P (118). Targeting of ciliary function, therefore, can be either direct or indirect.

The viscosity and elasticity characteristics of tracheobronchial mucus are determined primarily by mucous glycoproteins which account for 2% of mucus by mass (95% being water) (119). Normal control of mucus composition and secretion is effected by several mechanisms. Neural regulation of mucus secretion is achieved via innervation by both cholinergic and adrenergic innervation of secretory cells and submucosal gland cells (120). Peptide mediators of afferent nerves within the airway epithelium, such as substance P and neurokinins, also stimulate secretion of mucous glycoproteins in mucus; this secretion is potentiated greatly by inhibitors of neutral endopeptidase, the enzyme responsible for neuropeptide metabolism within airway epithelium (121). Local control by epithelial cells also may occur, though this has not been described in detail.

Several cell types may target epithelial mucociliary clearance during an acute exacerbation of asthma. Mediators released from mast cells such as histamine, and prostaglandins and leukotrienes released from both mast cells and other inflammatory cells within the airway, may stimulate both fluid and mucous glycoprotein secretion (122–124). Cationic proteases also stimulate goblet cell mucin release (125) (Table 1). Inflammatory lipid mediators such as platelet activating factor (PAF) and hydroxyeicosatetraenoic acids can stimulate mucin secretion from epithelial cells in culture (126,127). Messina et al. (128) evaluated five asthmatic subjects during and immediately after an acute exacerbation of asthma with radiolabeled aerosol. They demonstrated that mucociliary clearance was decreased during an exacerbation of asthma, with rapid improvement of mucociliary clearance upon recovery from the exacerbation. While the exact mechanisms and interactions of mediators have yet to be defined, it is probable that impairment of the ability of epithelial cells within the airway is responsible. Alterations in mucociliary clearance may occur even when morphologic damage to the airway is absent or minimal, and may contribute to the increased volume and viscosity of secretions in mildly asthmatic patients.

TABLE 1. *Effects of proteases on mucin release and degradation[a]*

Protease (µg/ml)	Release	Degradation
Elastase (neutrophil)		
0	100 ± 5	0
10	199 ± 16[b]	50
100	185 ± 7[b]	75
Cathepsin G (neutrophil)		
0	100 ± 5	0
10	143 ± 8[b]	41
100	130 ± 6[b]	48
Cathepsin G (neutrophil)		
0	100 ± 5	0
10	112 ± 8	0
100	133 ± 8[b]	5

[a]Confluent cultures were labeled with [3H]glucosamine for 24 hr and chased for 30 min in the presence of varying concentrations of the listed proteases. Release data are mean ± SE and expressed as percent control; degradation data represent percent degradation of released mucins. N = 4 experiments.

[b]*p < 0.01 versus control

Changes in Function that Alter the Barrier to the Outside Environment

It is clear that disruption of the epithelial layer must lead to changes in the ability of the epithelium to exclude the external environment from the underlying airway. The airway epithelium normally maintains a tight barrier to the external environment, principally through the presence of the basement membrane and the tight adhesion of epithelial cells, both to each other and to the basement membrane. Small, charged, hydrophilic molecules may pass between the epithelial cells, and this is regulated locally (129). While much attention has been given recently to potential metabolic functions of the epithelium in regulating airway caliber and its perturbation in asthma, the barrier function still is of considerable importance.

Under normal physiologic conditions there is restricted intracellular transepithelial passage of plasma proteins (130). Edema and plasma exudation is an important manifestation of inflammation and is a characteristic pathologic finding in asthmatic airways (131,132). Movement of plasma proteins from the vascular compartment into the airway lumen may occur within minutes after a challenge to the airway (133). In airway inflammation intercellular passage of fluid and proteins would best account for the rapid lumenal accumulation of both (133). Extravasation of inflammatory molecules into the airway epithelium and lumen may perpetuate and augment the inflammatory response, leading to further epithelial cell damage and subsequent alterations in epithelial cell function. Events leading to airway edema and plasma exudation appear to be concentrated in the airway capillaries, and the role of the airway epithelium in permitting edema

accumulation in the mucosa remains incompletely defined (134).

Much of what is known about the functional consequences of changes in airway epithelial barrier function comes from study of changes in permeability caused by environmental toxins such as cigarette smoke and ozone, from studies of epithelia in cystic fibrosis, and from studies of airway epithelial and microvascular permeability and plasma exudation in asthma (See Chapter 64), and from *in vivo* measures of airway permeability in asthmatic subjects (131,132.134–142). These investigations generally demonstrate that, as expected, epithelial layer permeability in increased in asthmatic subjects or after exposure to an epithelial toxin. In some studies, such changes in permeability are associated with increases in airway reactivity (142) (Fig. 10). These data, coupled with changes in plasma exudation and edema, suggest that alterations in airway epithelial permeability may be associated with airway hyperresponsiveness and continued inflammation.

Exactly which cells and mediators target the epithelial barrier is not clear. Structural damage elicited by eosinophils as described earlier certainly could alter barrier function. It has been suggested that tight junctions or E-cadherin containing intermediate junctions are targeted by inflammatory mediators (42). Disruption of these sites would loosen cell-to-cell integrity, permit passage of plasma proteins to the lumen, and, conversely, passage of the external environment to the submucosa. One report demonstrates that histamine does not alter human

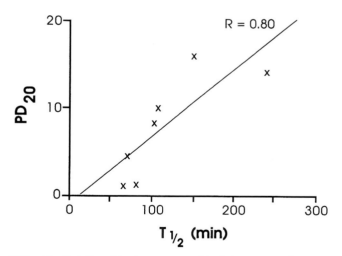

FIG. 10. Relationship between epithelial permeability and bronchial reactivity in asthmatic subjects. Permeability was demonstrated by clearance of ⁹⁹ᵐTc-DTPA aerosol and reactivity was assessed with aerosolized methacholine (at a different time). Bronchial mucosal permeability in asthmatic subjects was increased over that in normal subjects. (From Ilowite JS, Bennett WD, Sheetz MS, Groth ML, Nierman DM. Permeability of the bronchial mucosa to ⁹⁹ᵐTc-DTPA in asthma. *Am Rev Respir Dis* 1988;139:1139–1143, with permission.)

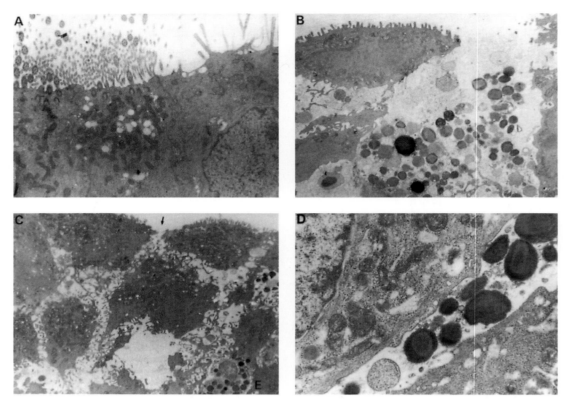

FIG. 11. Electron photomicrographs of the bronchial epithelium collected by biopsy in a cohort of asthmatic subjects. **A**: intact tight junctions in the epithelium of a subject with chronic asthma. (Original magnification, ×5400.) **B**: opened tight junction in the epithelium. Eosinophil granules are found in the widened intercellular space. (Original magnification, ×5400.) **C**: opened tight junction *(arrow)* and a widened intercellular space in a subject with chronic asthma. Eosinophils (E) are found in the space. (Original magnification, ×3400.) **D**: opened intercellular space in which many specific granules are seen. (Original magnification, ×18000.) These photomicrographs demonstrate the potential for inflammatory cells and granules to infiltrate between epithelial cells in asthma. It is not clear whether the tight junctions are damaged and widened by the eosinophils, or whether the openings precede eosinophil infiltration. (From Ohashi Y, Motojima S, Fukuda T, Makino S. Airway hyperresponsiveness, increased intracellular spaces of bronchial epithelium, and increased infiltration of eosinophils and lymphocytes in bronchial mucosa in asthma. *Am Rev Respir Dis* 1992;145:1469–1476, with permission.)

bronchial epithelial cell permeability and tight junction integrity, as assessed by movement of labeled mannitol and albumin across cultured cell membranes (143). In a study involving endobronchial biopsy of subjects with chronic asthma, Ohashi et al. (144) demonstrated a higher incidence of tight junction opening and a widening of epithelial intercellular spaces associated with infiltration of eosinophils into the airway (Fig. 11). Such openings would permit plasma extravasation. Exactly how inflammatory mediators alter these adhesive junctions requires further study.

Changes in Cytokine Secretion by Epithelial Cells

Airway epithelial cells produce a number of cytokines under normal conditions. These include interleukins (IL) 6 and 8, and the granulocyte-macrophage colony-stimulating factor (GM-CSF) (145–147). Both GM-CSF and IL-8 stimulate the migration of eosinophils into the airways, and GM-CSF secreted by epithelial cells in culture promotes eosinophil survival and activation (148–150). Cytokine secretion by epithelial cells can be stimulated by other cytokines, such as IL-1, and tumor necrosis factor-alpha in a variety of conditions (147,151). Epithelial cell targeting in asthma may stimulate cytokine secretion as well. Several studies have demonstrated recently that epithelial cells collected from asthmatic subjects secrete higher concentrations of IL-6, IL-8, and GM-CSF in culture when compared to epithelial cells collected from normal donors (152,153); the inference is that there is something about the asthmatic state that stimulates the epithelial cells. Treatment of epithelial cell lines in culture, or the epithelium *in vivo* with corticosteroids or nedocromil, suppresses both the production of IL-8 and GM-CSF, and the migration of eosinophils into the airways (148,151,153,154) (Figs. 12 and 13).

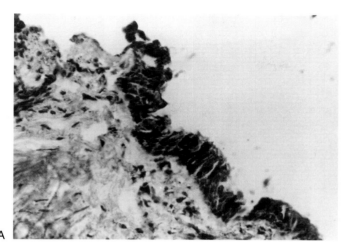
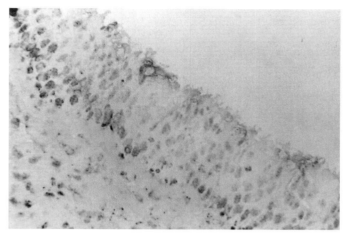

FIG. 12. A: presence of the cytokine granulocyte-macrophage colony-stimulating factor (GM-CSF) in a bronchial biopsy of an asthmatic subject. The cytokine is demonstrated with a polyclonal antibody using an immunoperoxidase method. The epithelium shows diffuse, intense staining by the dark reaction product. **B**: bronchial biopsy from a control subject treated in a similar fashion. No GM-CSF immunoreactivity is demonstrated. (From Sousa AR, Poston RN, Lane SJ, Nakhosteen JA, Lee TH. Detection of GM-CSF in asthmatic bronchial epithelium and decrease by inhaled corticosteroids. *Am Rev Respir Dis* 1993;147:1557–1561, with permission.)

The epithelium also can release chemotactic peptides for lymphocytes, monocytes, and neutrophils in response to injury (155–157). There is an overlap in responses to these factors; for example, as noted previously, eosinophils respond to several factors. Further, a single factor such as IL-8 can elicit migration of both eosinophils and neutrophils (148,157). Epithelial cells, thus, may have a role in eliciting migration of several different inflammatory cell types into the airway lumen via both common and specific pathways.

It is clear that in reference to cytokine secretion and regulation in asthma, the epithelium is both target and effector. Inflammatory cytokines released by other cells within the airway can stimulate the epithelium to release factors which promote inflammatory cell migration and activation. This targeting can be suppressed not only by treating the inflammatory cells directly, but also by modulating epithelial cell secretion of cytokines.

Changes in Expression of Adhesion Molecules by Epithelial Cells

Adhesion of inflammatory cells to various constitutive cells and structures in the airways is a necessary step in their migration from the capillaries to their final site of action. As discussed in chapter 38, there are multiple families of adhesion receptors and molecules found on airway cells, and each set has a specific function. The airways epithelium can express adhesion molecules that bind inflammatory cells such as eosinophils and neutrophils. The consequences are both structural and functional; the former because such expression may allow binding of inflammatory cells, and the latter because such expression may change the nature of the inflammatory process in airways. The cell adhesion protein intercellular adhesion molecule 1 (ICAM-1, or CD54), a member of the immunoglobulin superfamily,

FIG. 13. Percentage of airway epithelium stained with a polyclonal antibody for the cytokine granulocyte-macrophage colony-stimulating factor (GM-CSF) in bronchial biopsies of asthmatic subjects before and 8 weeks after inhalation of 1,000 μg beclomethasone (8 subjects, steroid group) or placebo (6 subjects). There is a decrease in GM-CSF immunoreactivity in the beclomethasone-treated group. *Closed circles* present the means for each group. From Sousa AR, Poston RN, Lane SJ, Nakhosteen JA, Lee TH. Detection of GM-CSF in asthmatic bronchial epithelium and decrease by inhaled corticosteroids. *Am Rev Respir Dis* 1993;147:1557–1561, with permission.)

is expressed constitutively by the airways epithelium of both humans and other primates, though ICAM-1 expression has been shown to be very low in human epithelial cells in another study (158–163). ICAM-1 expression can be induced by cytokines such as interferon-γ (IFN-γ) and tumor necrosis factor-α (TNF-α), and after infection with parainfluenza type-2 virus (159–161,164). Increased expression of ICAM-1 is associated with increased influx and binding of both neutrophils and eosinophils into airways (162,164). However, introduction of blocking antibodies for ICAM-1 only partially blocks influx and adhesion of neutrophils, suggesting that other adhesive mechanisms are involved as well (164).

Changes in the expression of ICAM-1 in asthmatic epithelium are controversial. Increased expression of ICAM-1 could lead to increased binding and influx of eosinophils, with subsequent damage to the mucosa. One study by Montefort et al. (165) suggested that while there was a basal, constitutive expression of ICAM-1 in the bronchial epithelium of asthmatic subjects, such expression was not increased when compared to similar biopsies obtained from normal volunteers. Expression of ICAM-1 was not altered by treatment with inhaled beclomethasone. In contrast, Vignola et al. (163), examining epithelial cells obtained from bronchial brushings from normal subjects and subjects with either asthma or chronic bronchitis, found that the expression of ICAM-1 was increased in epithelial cells from asthmatics. This study also demonstrated increased expression of the class II human leukocyte antigen HLA-DR on epithelial cells of asthmatics. Increased expression of both ICAM-1 and HLA-DR was correlated with clinical symptomatology (Fig. 14) and with airflow obstruction as measured by the FEV_1. Increased expression of HLA-DR might allow epithelial cells to present antigen to T cells, which in turn would be enhanced by the increased epithelial cell to T-cell binding, mediated by ICAM-1 (163). Blocking the actions of ICAM-1 may attenuate the influx of eosinophil into the airway. Wegner et al. (162) created a model of chronic allergic inflammation in cynomolgus monkeys by repeated aerosol challenge with *Ascaris* antigen. These monkeys had demonstrable airway hyperresponsiveness to methacholine and a histologic presentation in their central airways similar in a number of key aspects to that seen in chronic asthma. Using these animals, they demonstrated that pre-treatment with an antibody specific for ICAM-1 attenuated eosinophil infiltration in the bronchi and diminished the response to a subsequent challenge of aerosolized methacholine (162). While it was not clear that blocking ICAM-1 specific to epithelial cells was responsible, as opposed to the ICAM-1 expression on other constitutive cells within the airway, this study demonstrates the potential to modulate airways inflammation by altering the functional changes to the epithelium (and other cells).

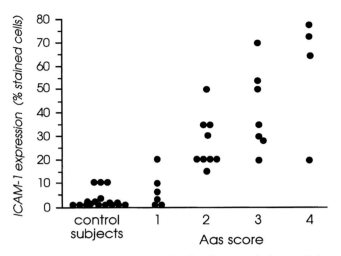

FIG. 14. Expression of the cell adhesion protein intercellular adhesion molecule 1 (ICAM-1) in epithelial cells obtained from bronchial brushings in subjects with asthma, compared to normal volunteers. ICAM-1 expression (presented as the percent stained cells) is very low in normal subjects, but is increased in asthmatic subjects. This increase is related to clinical severity as measured by the Aas scoring system. Both the differences between control and asthmatic subjects, and the differences based on severity, are statistically significant. (From Vignola AM, Campbell AM, Chanez P, et al. HLA-DR and ICAM-1 expression on bronchial epithelial cells in asthma and chronic bronchitis. *Am Rev Respir Dis* 1993; 148:689–694, with permission.)

As described earlier, the integrins constitute another class of adhesion molecules normally expressed by airway epithelial cells. There is little evidence to date of alterations in integrin expression in asthma.

Changes in Expression of Epithelial Neutral Endopeptidase

The effects of tachykinins and certain other peptides in the airways are limited by the degradation of these mediators by neutral endopeptidase (EC 3.4.24.11, NEP) present in high concentrations in airway epithelial cells (166). Sekizawa et al. (167) have demonstrated that NEP is present in greatest concentrations both in the brush border of the epithelium and in the submucosal glands (167). The enzyme also can be demonstrated in cultures of epithelial cells; in this setting, treatment of the cells with glucocorticoids increases the expression of NEP (168). Inhibition of NEP by agents, such as thiorphan or phosphoramidon, can potentiate the effects of peptide mediators in airways and, thereby, alter airway function. For example, treatment of rabbit tracheal epithelial cells in culture with thiorphan potentiates the increase in ciliary beat frequency observed after stimulation with either of the tachykinins neurokinin A or substance P (169). Numerous studies have demonstrated that inhibition of NEP increases the responsiveness of airway smooth muscle *in vitro* to tachykinins, and that this effect is lost when the epithelium is removed (170–172). Thus, a damaged epithelium rendered incapable of producing NEP may allow tachykinins and other mediators to elicit their effects on airways in a more pronounced and sustained way.

Neutral endopeptidase expression in airways epithelium can be decreased in several disease states. Viral infection causes a decrease in NEP expression in rat airways, and NEP activity can be decreased by as much as 50% in ferret tracheal segments after influenza infection (173,174). Such loss of NEP expression and activity could conceivably account for increased airways hyperreactivity by allowing tachykinins and other peptides continued activity. In support of this, when both infected and control ferret airways were treated with thiorphan in the latter study, the subsequent response to substance P was greater in the control tissues than in the infected tissues, so that in the presence of the NEP inhibitor, there was no difference in the response of the tracheal segments to substance P (174). Studies of NEP expression and activity in asthmatic subjects, however, are few. Diamant et al. (175) have examined the effect of thiorphan on responsiveness to inhaled leukotriene D_4 in asthmatic and normal subjects. Treatment with thiorphan did not alter leukotriene responsiveness in either group. Another study has demonstrated that, as expected, treatment of either normal or asthmatic subjects with thiorphan enhances the response to inhaled neurokinin A (176). It is not clear what the extent of the loss of NEP activity is in asthmatic subjects based on morphologic techniques. While it is attractive to hypothesize that a given degree of epithelial damage translates into a given degree of loss in NEP activity, and then a subsequent, certain degree of deleterious alteration in function caused by tachykinins and inflammatory mediators, (which also may be secreted to excess by their progenitor cells), this has not been proven.

Summary of Functional Damage to the Epithelium

The epithelium is both an initial target and an initial effector in the early stages of asthma. Both structural and functional damage to the epithelium impairs its ability to protect the airway from the external environment. Such damage also prevents the epithelium from modulating airway caliber, mucus transport, and fluid balance in the airway. A damaged epithelium may lose the ability to produce enzymes and factors required to protect the airway from inflammatory mediators. Damage to the epithelium stimulates the epithelium to produce factors which may, in turn, up-regulate the initial inflammation and allow such inflammation to become more established and more chronic.

REPAIR AND RESTORATION OF THE EPITHELIUM

Repair of the damaged airway epithelium occurs as an exacerbation of asthma resolves. However, the process by which the epithelium repairs itself is incompletely understood. It is probable that targeting of the epithelium by inflammatory cells not only damages the epithelial layer and disrupts its several functions, but also impedes the ability of the epithelium to initiate repair.

Normal Processes by Which the Epithelium Is Repaired After Injury

The regeneration of epithelia of mature adult tissues displays properties and structures that are similar to those of corresponding fetal tissues (177). Repair of airways epithelium also has similarities to the repair of other epithelial layers in the body, such as epidermis and cornea. Some recent studies have examined specifically the repair of the airways epithelium both *in vivo* and in culture, usually after the creation of a small wound by mechanical disruption of the mucosal or cell layer. In a series of studies, Keenan et al. (178) have demonstrated the sequence of epithelium regeneration in hamster trachea after mechanical injury (10,179,180). Within 12 hours after injury, secretory and basal cells adjacent to the wound flatten into a squamous morphology and migrate into the wound. Cell proliferation begins within 24 hours and produces a multilayered, metaplastic epithelium within 48 hours of the initial injury. Mitosis continues among the newly migrated cells, producing immature, indifferent cells which differentiate into functional, subtype cells by 96 to 120 hours after the initial injury. Submucosal mesenchymal proliferation also is seen during regeneration, and may become more important if the injury is large or causes disruption of the basement membrane (180). In a primary culture model of human nasal epithelium injury, Zahm et al. (181) demonstrated that both migration of single cells and movement of cell sheets is responsible for closure of a small wound in an epithelial cell monolayer created with a stylette (181). Treatment with inhibitors of either cytoskeletal rearrangement or protein synthesis blocked the repair process (181). Several nonciliated cell types have been implicated in different species as the stem cell for regeneration, as has been noted earlier in this chapter. It is not resolved completely which cell type is the stem cell in human central airways. What is clear is that the epithelium generally repairs itself quickly. In the studies by Zahm, closure of 100- to 200-μm diameter wounds was complete within 8 hours (Fig. 15). Even a large wound can be healed with relative quickness. In a sheep model in which injury to the tracheal epithelium was induced by cotton bract smoke, repair to a large (approximately 12

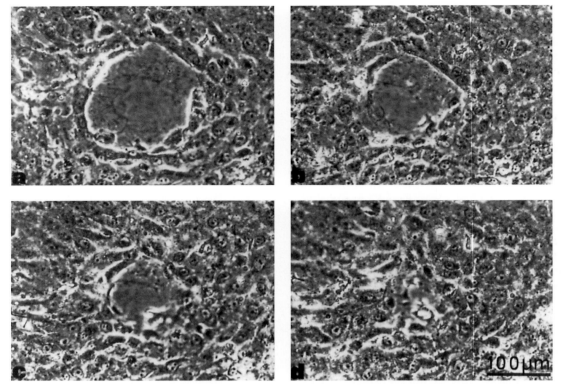

FIG. 15. Repair of a small wound in a respiratory epithelial cell monolayer in explant culture as demonstrated by sequential phase-contrast microscopy. The wound was created with a stylette at time 0. Times presented: **A**: 0 hours; **B**: 2 hours; **C**: 4 hours; **D**: 6 hours. Progressive closure of the wounded monolayer is noted. (From Zahm J-M, Chevillard M, Puchelle E. Wound repair of human surface respiratory epithelium. *Am J Respir Cell Mol Biol* 1991;5:242–248, with permission.)

cm length of the trachea) injury is virtually complete after 18 days (182).

Airway epithelial cells must not only fill a wound after injury, but must subsequently differentiate into all needed columnar and basal cell types. In the sheep model studies, basal and undifferentiated cells predominate at first and cover the injury site. Differentiation begins after undifferentiated cells fill the injury site (approximately day 8), and continues until the injury is completely repopulated (approximately day 18) (182) (Fig. 16). Similar patterns are seen in other airway repair models in the rat in both *in vivo* and tracheal graft models (183,184). In these, cells from the adjacent nonwounded epithelium flatten, migrate, and de-differentiate within the first 24 to 48 hours after injury. A pseudostratified epithelium is regenerated by 72 hours after the initial injury, and phenotypic markers of differentiated cells begin to appear at this time. Differentiation continues until the wound site is completely repaired (183).

A number of factors have been implicated in the repair of the epithelium, some of which may be secreted by epithelial cells themselves, and some of which are produced by neighboring cells in the airway such as fibroblasts, macrophages, and sensory nerves (185–190). Both proliferation and migration of epithelial cells may be mediated by the same factor or group of factors secreted by

a given cell line, giving rise to the concept of a mitoattractant. Growth factors such as insulin and insulin-like growth factors, epidermal growth factor, and retinoic acid are required for epithelial cell growth in culture (191–193). Other factors, such as exposure to air or to transforming growth factor-β (TGF-β), may signal epithelial cells to differentiate, as noted previously (185, 193–195). Changes in calcium concentration in culture media can promote either mucus-cell or squamous cell differentiation (196). The timing by which these and other factors are expressed at critical moments to direct repair has yet to be established; such timing provides a further point at which the repair process can be either disrupted or enhanced.

From these studies, a simple schematic for repair of an injured epithelium can be developed (Fig. 17). In this schema, injury to the epithelium, (which may also be accompanied by injury to other cells besides epithelial cells, such as afferent nerves and mesenchymal cells), leads rapidly to denudation and sloughing of injured and dead cells. Adjacent cells begin migrating into the denuded area; once in the damaged area, these cells flatten and spread over the surface. For small wounds, such spreading and migration may be sufficient to cover the site of injury. If the injury is large, proliferation of stem cells begins to generate the new cells necessary. Underlying mesenchymal cells repair damaged basement membrane as required. A multi-cell layer covers the injured site. Differentiation into a single layer then begins, followed later by appearance of specific cell types. Repair then may be mediated by both adjacent epithelial cells and by nonepithelial cells including fibroblasts, inflammatory cells, and sensory nerves. The process by which repair is coordinated at a cell and molecular level is not yet understood. This schema provides a starting point by which targeted damage to epithelial repair in asthma can be considered.

Targeting of Epithelium Repair in Asthma

Relatively few studies have been done to examine specifically the epithelial repair process in asthma, as opposed to the initial damage to the epithelium in asthma. One study by Demoly et al. (197) examined epithelial cell proliferation *in situ* via endobronchial biopsies in the airways of nonsmoking and smoking asthmatics, smokers with chronic bronchitis, and nonsmoking and smoking volunteer subjects. Asthmatic and bronchitic subjects were stable and had been free of recent exacerbations. Approximately one-half of the asthmatic subjects had been treated with high doses of inhaled corticosteroids.

Subjects who smoked had an increased proliferation index, regardless of disease state. In subjects with bronchitis, the increased proliferation index was correlated to the presence of squamous metaplasia. The epithelial proliferation index in nonsmoking asthmatic patients was no greater than control, even though the histologic appearance of the biopsies from asthmatic subjects demonstrated the characteristic changes seen in asthma, with an increased thickness of the basement membrane, mucosal eosinophilia, and partial shedding of the epithelium in approximately two-thirds of the samples. This study suggests that cell proliferation may not be required to maintain the epithelial layer, even in asthmatic subjects who have some degree of damage. Processes other than proliferation (e.g., differentiation from a pool of basal cells) may be sufficient to maintain the epithelium when the damage is mild. Alternately, epithelium repair could be suppressed in asthma even when the disease is mild if any degree of inflammation is present. Further studies are required to demonstrate which of these explanations explains better the continued presence of epithelial damage.

Chronic inflammation in the airway may target the epithelium in ways that abort repair. For example, fibroblasts can secrete TGF-β which suppresses proliferation (186). How this may occur in asthma is still open to investigation.

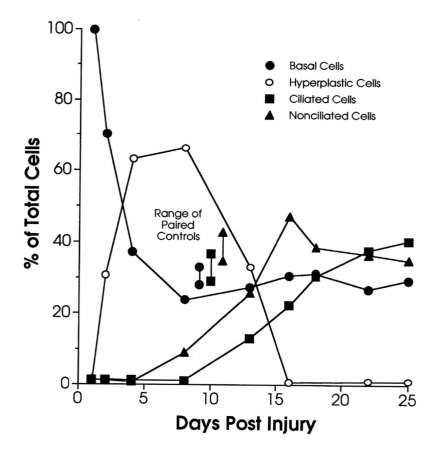

FIG. 16. Comparison of cell counts in sheep trachea at various times after smoke inhalation injury. In the beginning, basal cells and hyperplastic (less differentiated than basal cells) cells predominate. Ciliated and nonciliated columnar cells appear from approximately day 8, and reach control values by days 16 to 18. Differentiation of epithelial cells to needed cell types is a later stage in the repair process. The range of each normal cell type in paired controls (no injury) is shown. (From Barrow RE, Wang C-Z, Cox RA, Evans MJ. Cellular sequence of tracheal repair in sheep after smoke inhalation injury. *Lung* 1992; 170:331–338, with permission.)

immediately after injury

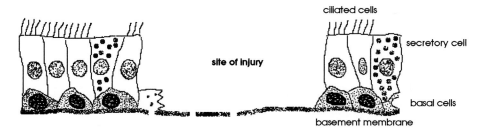

ciliated cells

site of injury

secretory cell

basal cells

basement membrane

6 – 72 hours after injury

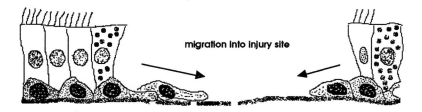

migration into injury site

1 – 8 days after injury

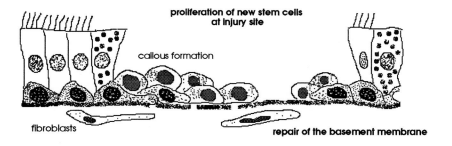

proliferation of new stem cells
at injury site

callous formation

fibroblasts

repair of the basement membrane

6 – 21 days after injury

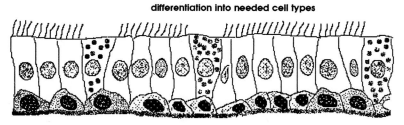

differentiation into needed cell types

FIG. 17. Schema of epithelial repair and restoration. The injury may be created by any trauma. Within hours of the original injury, surviving adjacent cells at the injury site begin to migrate and spread into the site of injury. If the wound is larger, stem cells begin to proliferate so that daughter cells continue the process of closure. These cells are less differentiated than the original cells at the site. Migration and proliferation continue until the original injury site is covered. A multi-layer callous is formed, after which the cells thin into a single layer and differentiate into the other required cell types, including various secretory cells and ciliated cells. Damage to the basement membrane is repaired by fibroblasts immediately beneath the lamina propria, though epithelial cells may contribute to this process.

In light of the above considerations, the sum total of injury to the epithelium in asthma then, includes more than just the direct effects of the initial damage to the mucosa. Targeted injury may delay repair of the epithelium, and this may exacerbate the impairment of the barrier and metabolic functions critical to restoration of airway homeostasis. It is not clear at what point direct damage leaves off and repair delay begins; both types of injury may be required to perpetuate epithelial injury in asthma.

CONCLUSIONS

Damage to the epithelium may have profound effects in asthma. Airway epithelial cells may be both a target of, and effector in, other cells of inflammation in asthma. Damage to the epithelium elicited by inflammatory cells and mediators may disrupt the barrier to the external environment and impair the regulation of fluid balance and mucus secretion in airways. Thickening of the basement membrane may lead to a more rigid airway and may promote disordered healing. Activation of other inflammatory cells, such as eosinophils and mast cells, may promote continued inflammation within the airway. Damaged epithelium may not respond appropriately to signals for normal repair and restoration. It has become clear that the epithelium is not an innocent bystander in the genesis of asthma, and does not remain passive during the early stages of airways injury. Epithelial-derived factors released as a result of damage elicited by other cells, may contribute substantially to the final state of airways inflammation. Further understanding of the pathways by which the epithelium contributes both to the homeostatic environment within airways, and to the inflammatory process, may suggest new and novel therapies for chronic asthma and other airways diseases.

ACKNOWLEDGMENTS

Supported in part by NHLBI grants HL-51853, HL-48696, HL-02484, and a grant from the American Lung Association.

REFERENCES

1. Evans MJ, Moller PC. Biology of airway basal cells. *Exp Lung Res* 1991;17:513–531.
2. Evans MJ, Cox RA, Shami SG, Wilson B, Plopper CG. The role of basal cells in attachment of columnar cells to the basal lamina of the trachea. *Am J Respir Cell Mol Biol* 1989;1:463–469.
3. Evans MJ, Cox RA, Burke AS, Moller PC. Differentiation of anchoring junctions in tracheal basal cells in the growing rat. *Am J Respir Cell Mol Biol* 1992;6:153–157.
4. Blenkinsopp WK. Proliferation of respiratory tract epithelium in the rat. *Exp Cell Res* 1967;46:144–154.
5. Breuer R, Zajicek G, Christensen TG, Lucey EC, Snider GL. Cell kinetics of normal adult hamster bronchial epithelium in the steady state. *Am J Respir Cell Mol Biol* 1990;2:51–58.
6. Brody AR, Hook GE, Cameron GS, Jetten AM, Butterick CJ, Nettesheim P. The differentiation capacity of Clara cells isolated from the lungs of rabbits. *Lab Invest* 1987;57:219–229.
7. Inayama Y, Hook GE, Brody AR, Jetten AM, Gray T, Mahler J, Nettesheim P. In vitro and in vivo growth and differentiation of clones of tracheal basal cells. *Am J Pathol* 1989;134:539–549.
8. Inayama Y, Hook GE, Brody AR, Cameron GS, Jetten AM, Gilmore LB, Gray T, Nettesheim P. The differentiation potential of tracheal basal cells. *Lab Invest* 1989; 58:706-717.
9. Johnson NF, Hubbs AF. Epithelial progenitor cells in the rat trachea. *Am J Respir Cell Mol Biol* 1990;2:579–585.
10. Keenan KP, Combs JW, McDowell EM. Regeneration of hamster tracheal epithelium after mechanical injury. I. focal lesions: quantitative morphologic study of cell proliferation. *Virchows Arch Cell Pathol* 1982;41:193–214.
11. Satir P, Dirksen ER. Function-structure correlations in cilia from mammalian respiratory tract. In: Fishman AP, Cherniack NS, Widdicombe JG, Geiger SR, eds. *Handbook of physiology: the respiratory system*, section 3, vol. 1. Bethesda: American Physiological Society, 1985:473–494.
12. Sleigh MA, Blake JR, Liron M. The propulsion of mucus by cilia. *Am Rev Respir Dis* 1988;137:726–731.
13. Lumsden AB, McLean A, Lamb D. Goblet and Clara cells of human distal airways: evidence for smoking-induced changes in numbers. *Thorax* 1984;39:844–855.
14. Smith MN, Greenberg SD, Spjut HJ. The Clara cell: a comparative ultrastructural study in mammals. *Am J Anat* 1979;155:15–30.
15. Widdicombe HG, Pack RJ. The Clara cell. *Eur J Respir Dis* 1982;63:202–220.
16. Harkema JR, Mariassy A, St. George J, Hyde DM, Plopper CG. Epithelial cells of the conducting airways: a species comparison. In: Farmer SG, Hay DWP, eds. *The airway epithelium: physiology, pathophysiology, and pharmacology*. New York: Marcel Dekker, 1991; 3–41.
17. Evans TW, Brokaw JJ, Chung KF, Nadel JA, McDonald DM. Ozone-induced bronchial hyperresponsiveness in the rat is not accompanied by neutrophil influx or increased vascular permeability in the trachea. *Am Rev Respir Dis* 1988;138:140–144.
18. Hook GER, Brody AR, Cameron GS, Jetten AM, Gilmore LB, Nettesheim P. Repopulation of denuded tracheas by Clara cells isolated from the lungs of rabbits. *Exp Lung Res* 1987;12:311–330.
19. Jeffery PK. Structural, immunologic, and neural elements of the normal human airway wall. In: Busse WW, Holgate ST, eds. *Asthma and rhinitis* Boston: Blackwell, 1995;80–106.
20. Kawanami O, Ferrans VJ, Crystal RG. Anchoring fibrils in the normal canine respiratory system. *Am Rev Respir Dis* 1979;120:595–611.
21. Evans MJ, Guha SC, Cox RA, Moller PC. Attenuated fibroblast sheath around the basement membrane zone in the trachea. *Am J Respir Cell Mol Biol* 1993;8:188–192.
22. Dales H. An ultrastructural study of the tracheal epithelium of the guinea pig with special reference to the ciliary structure. *J Anat* 1983;136:47–67.
23. Christensen TG, Breuer R, Hornstra LJ, Lucey EC, Snider GL. The ultrastructure of hamster bronchial epithelium. *Exp Lung Res* 1987;13:253–277.
24. Hogg JC, Inoue S. Freeze-etch study of the tracheal epithelium of normal guinea pigs with particular reference to intracellular junctions. *J Ultrastruct Res* 1977;61:89–99.
25. Walker DC, MacKenzie A, Wiggs BR, Hulbert WC, Hogg JC. The structure of tight junctions may not correlate with permeability. *Cell Tissue Res* 1984;235:607–613.
26. Godfrey RWA, Severs NJ, Jeffrey PK. Freeze-fracture morphology and quantification of human bronchial epithelial tight junctions. *Am J Respir Cell Mol Biol* 1992;6:453–458.
27. Claude P. Morphological factors influencing transepithelial permeability: a model for the resistance of the zonula occludens. *J Membr Biol* 1978;39:219–232.
28. Montefort S, Baker J, Roche WR, Holgate ST. The distribution of adhesive mechanisms in the normal bronchial epithelium. *Eur Respir J* 1993;6:1257–1263.
29. Evans MJ, Cox RA, Shami SG, Plopper CG. Junctional adhesion mechanisms in airway basal cells. *Am J Respir Cell Mol Biol* 1990;3:341–347.
30. Damjanovich L, Albelda SM, Mette SA, Buck CA. Distribution of in-

tegrin cell adhesion receptors in normal and malignant lung tissue. *Am J Respir Cell Mol Biol* 1992;6:197–206.

31. Laitinen LA, Heino M, Laitinen A, Kava T, Haaahtela T. Damage of the airway epithelium and bronchial reactivity in patients with asthma. *Am Rev Respir Dis* 1985;131:599–606.

32. Beasley R, Roche WR, Robets JA, Holgate ST. Cellular events in the bronchi in mild asthma and after bronchial provocation. *Am Rev Respir Dis* 1989;139:806–817.

33. Jeffery PK, Wardlaw AJ, Nelson FC, Collins JV, Kay AB. Bronchial biopsies in asthma. An ultrastructural, quantitative study and correlation with hyperreactivity. *Am Rev Respir Dis* 1989;140:1745–1753.

34. Naylor B. The shedding of the mucosa of the bronchial tree in asthma. *Thorax* 1962;17:69–72.

35. Laitinen LA, Laitinen A, Haaahtela T. Airway mucosal inflammation even in patients with newly diagnosed asthma. *Am Rev Respir Dis* 1993;147:697–704.

36. Lozewicz S, Weels C, Gomez E, Ferguson H, Richman P, Devalia J, Davies RJ. Morphological integrity of the bronchial epithelium in mild asthma. *Thorax* 1990;45:12–15.

37. Dunnill MS. The pathology of asthma with specific reference to changes in the bronchial mucosa. *J Clin Pathol* 1960;13:27–33.

38. Montefort S, Roberts JA, Beasley CR, Holgate ST, Roche WR. The site of disruption of the bronchial epithelium in asthmatics and nonasthmatics. *Thorax* 1992;47:499–503.

39. Frigas E, Loegering DA, Gleich GJ. Cytotoxic effects of the guinea pig eosinophil major basic protein on tracheal epithelium. *Lab Invest* 1980;42:35–43.

40. Hers JFP. Disturbances of the ciliated epithelium due to influenza virus. *Am Rev Respir Dis* 1966;93:162–171.

41. Abdi S, Evans MJ, Cox RA, Lubbesmeyer H, herndon DN, Traber DL. Inhalation injury to tracheal epithelium in an ovine model of cotton smoke exposure. Early phase (30 minutes). *Am Rev Respir Dis* 1990;142:1436–1439.

42. Montefort S, Djukanovic R, Holgate ST, Roche WR. Ciliated cell damage in the bronchial epithelium of asthmatics and nonasthmatics. *Clin Exp Allergy* 1993;23:185–189.

43. Sparrow MP, Mitchell HW. The epithelium acts as a barrier modulating the extent of bronchial narrowing produced by substances perfused through the lumen. *Br J Pharmacol* 1991;103:1160–1164.

44. Roche WR, Beasley R, Williams J, Holgate ST. Subepithelial fibrosis in the bronchi of asthmatics. *Lancet* 1989;i:520–524.

45. Brewster CEP, Howarth PH, Djukanovic R, Wilson J, Holgate ST, Roche WR. Myofibroblasts and subepithelial fibrosis in bronchial asthma. *Am J Respir Cell Mol Biol* 1990;3:507–511.

46. Djukanovic R, Lai CK, Wilson JW, et al. Bronchial mucosal manifestations of atopy: a comparison of markers of inflammation between atopic asthmatics, atopic nonasthmatics and healthy controls. *Eur Respir J* 1992;5:538–544.

47. Trigg CJ, Manolitsas ND, Wang J, et al. Placebo-controlled immunopathologic study of four months of inhaled corticosteroids in asthma. *Am J Respir Crit Care Med* 1994;150:17–22.

48. Saetta M, Maestrelli P, Di Stefano A, et al. Effect of cessation of exposure to toluene diisocyanate (TDI) on bronchial mucosa of subjects with TDI-induced asthma. *Am Rev Respir Dis* 1992; 145:169–174.

49. Saetta M, Di Stefano A, Maestrelli P, et al. Airway mucosal inflammation in occupational asthma induced by toluene diisocyanate. *Am Rev Respir Dis* 1992;145:160–168.

50. Azzawi M, Johnston PW, Majumdar S, Kay AB, Jeffery PK. T lymphocytes and activated eosinophils in airway mucosa in fatal asthma and cystic fibrosis. *Am Rev Respir Dis* 1992;145:1477–1482.

51. Djukanovic R, Wilson JW, Britten KM, et al. Quantitation of mast cells and eosinophils in the bronchial mucosa of symptomatic atopic asthmatics and healthy control subjects using immunohistochemistry. *Am Rev Respir Dis* 1990;142:863–871.

52. Kirby JG, Hargreave FE, Gleich GJ, O Byrne PM. Bronchoalveolar cell profiles of asthmatic and nonasthmatic subjects. *Am Rev Respir Dis* 1987;136:379–383.

53. Ädelroth E, Rosenhall L, Johansson S, Linden M, Venge P. Inflammatory cells and eosinophilic activity in asthmatics investigated by bronchoalveolar lavage. *Am Rev Respir Dis* 1990; 142:91–99.

54. Ackerman SJ, Loegering DA, Venge P, et al. Distinctive cationic proteins of the human eosinophil granule: major basic protein, eosinophil cationic protein, and eosinophil-derived neurotoxin. *J Immunol* 1983; 131:2977–2981.

55. Frigas E, Gleich GJ. The eosinophil and the pathophysiology of asthma. *J Allergy Clin Immunol* 1986;77:527–537.

56. Motojima S, Frigas E, Loegering DA, Gleich GJ. Toxicity of eosinophil cationic proteins for guinea pig tracheal epithelium *in vitro*. *Am Rev Respir Dis* 1989;139:801–805.

57. Yukawa T, Read RC, Kroegel C, et al. The effects of activated eosinophils and neutrophils on guinea pig airway epithelium *in vitro*. *Am J Respir Cell Mol Biol* 1990;2:341–353.

58. Bentley AM, Menz G, Storz C, et al. Identification of T lymphocytes, macrophages, and activated eosinophils in the bronchial mucosa in intrinsic asthma. Relationship to symptoms and bronchial responsiveness. *Am Rev Respir Dis* 1992;146:500–506.

59. Bentley AM, Maestrelli P, Saetta M, et al. Activated T lymphocytes and eosinophils in the bronchial mucosa in isocyanate-induced asthma. *J Allergy Clin Immunol* 1992;89:821–829.

60. Azzawi M, Bradley B, Jeffery PK, et al. Identification of activated T lymphocytes and eosinophils in bronchial biopsies in stable atopic asthma. *Am Rev Respir Dis* 1990;142:1407–1413.

61. Heard BE, Nunn AJ, Kay AB. Mast cells in human lungs. *J Pathol* 1989;157:59–63.

62. Ferguson AC, Whitelaw M, Brown H. Correlation of bronchial eosinophil and mast cell activation with bronchial hyperresponsiveness in children with asthma. *J Allergy Clin Immunol* 1992;90:609–613.

63. Gibson PG, Allen CJ, Yang JP, et al. Intraepithelial mast cells in allergic and nonallergic asthma. Assessment using bronchial brushings. *Am Rev Respir Dis* 1993;148:80–86.

64. Pesci A, Foresi A, Bertorelli G, Chetta A, Olivieri D, Olivieri D. Histochemical characteristics and degranulation of mast cells in epithelium and lamina propria of bronchial biopsies from asthmatic and normal subjects. *Am Rev Respir Dis* 1993;147:684–689.

65. Simon RH, Dehart PD, Todd RF. Neutrophil induced injury of rat pulmonay alveolar epithelial cells. *J Clin Invest* 1986;78:1375–1386.

66. Empey DW, Laitinen LA, Jacobs L, Gold WH, Nadel JA. Mechanism of bronchial hyperreactivity in normal and asthmatic subjects after upper respiratory tract infection. *Am Rev Respir Dis* 1976;113:131–139.

67. Laitinen LA, Elkin RB, Empey DW, Mills J, Gold WM, Nadel JA. Changes in bronchial reactivity after administration of the attenuated influenza virus. *Am Rev Respir Dis* 1976;113:194–200.

68. Jacoby DB, Tamaoki J, Borson DB, Nadel JA. Influenza infection increases airway smooth muscle responsiveness to substance P in ferrets by decreasing enkephalinase. *J Appl Physiol* 1988;64:2653–2658.

69. Dusser DJ, Jacoby DB, Djokic TD, Rubinstein I, Borson DB, Nadel JA. Virus induces airway hyperresponsiveness to tachykinins: role of neutral endopeptidase. *J Appl Physiol* 1989;67:1504–1511.

70. Golden JA, Nadel JA, Boushey HA. Bronchial hyperirritability in healthy subjects after exposure to ozone. *Am Rev Respir Dis* 1978; 118:287–294.

71. Holtzman MA, Fabbri LM, O Byrne PM, et al. Importance of airway inflammation for hyperresponsiveness induced by ozone. *Am Rev Respir Dis* 1983;127:686–690.

72. Kehrl HR, Vincent LM, Kowalsky RJ, Horstman DH, O Neil JJ, McCartney WH, Bromberg PA. Ozone expsoure increases respiratory epithelial permeability in humans. *Am Rev Respir Dis* 1987;135:1124–1128.

73. Murlas CG, Roum JH. Sequence of pathologic changes in the airway mucosa of guinea pigs during ozone-induced bronchial hyperreactivity. *Am Rev Respir Dis* 1985;131:314–320.

74. O Byrne PM, Walters EH, Gold BD, et al. Neutrophil depletion inhibits airway hyperresponsiveness induced by ozone exposure. *Am Rev Respir Dis* 1984;130:214–219.

75. Furchgott RF, Vanhouette PM. Endoethelium-derived relaxing and contracting factors. *FASEB J* 1989;3:2007–2018.

76. Flavahan NA, Aarhus LL, Rimele TJ, Vanhoutte PM. Respiratory epithelium inhibits bronchial smooth muscle tone. *J Appl Physiol* 1985; 58:834–838.

77. Barnes PJ, Cuss FM, Palmer JB. The effect of airway epithelium on smooth muscle contractility in bovine trachea. *Br J Pharmacol* 1985; 86:685–691.

78. Hay DWP, Raeburn D, Fedan JS. Regional differences in reactivity and in the influence of the epithelium on canine intrapulmonary bronchial smooth muscle responsiveness. *Eur J Pharmacol* 1987;141:363–370.

79. Stuart-Smith K, Vanhoutte PM. Heterogeneity in the effects of ep-

ithelium removal in the canine bronchial tree. *J Appl Physiol* 1987;63:2510–2515.

80. Goldie RG, Papdimitrou JM, Paterson JW, Rigby PJ, Self HM, Spina D. Influence of the epithelium on responsiveness of guinea-pig isolated trachea to contractile and relaxant agonists. *Br J Pharmacol* 1986;87:5–14.

81. Hay DWP, Raeburn D, Farmer SG, Fleming WW, Fedan JS. Epithelium modulates the reactivity of ovalbumin-sensitized guinea-pig airway smooth muscle. *Life Sci* 1986;38:2461–2468.

82. Frossard N, Muller F. Epithelial modulation of tracheal smooth muscle responses to antigenic stimulation. *J Appl Physiol* 1986;61:1449–1456.

83. Stuart-Smith K, Vanhoutte PM. Epithelium, contractile tone, and responses to relaxing agonists in canine bronchi. *J Appl Physiol* 1990;69:678–685.

84. Raeburn D, Hay DWP, Robinson VA, Farmer SG, Fleming WW, Fedan JS. The effect of verapamil is reduced in isolated airway smooth muscle preparations lacking the epithelium. *Life Sci* 1986;38:809–816.

85. Buckner CK, Fedyna JS, Robertson JL, et al. An examination of the influence of the epithelium on contractile responses to peptidoleukotrienes and blockade by ICI 204,219 in isolated guinea pig trachea and human intralobar airways. *J Pharmacol Exp Ther* 1990;252:77–85.

86. Lev A, Christensen GC, Ryan JP, Wange M, Kelsen SG. Epithelial modulation of trachealis muscle tension is calcium and temperature dependent. *J Appl Physiol* 1989;67:713–719.

87. Hay DWP, Garmer SG, Raeburn D, Robinson VA, Fleming WW, Fedan JS. Airway epithelium modulates the reactivity of guinea-pig respiratory smooth muscle. *Eur J Pharmacol* 1986;129:11–18.

88. Munakata M, Mitzner W. The protective role of the airway epithelium. In: Farmer SG, Hay DWP, eds. *The airway epithelium: physiology, pathophysiology, and pharmacology.* New York: Marcel Dekker, 1991:545–564.

89. Munakata M, Huang I, Mitzner W, Menkes H. Protective role of epithelium in the guinea pig airway. *J Appl Physiol* 1989;66:1547–1552.

90. Fernandes LB, Paterson JW, Goldie RG. Co-axial bioassay of a smooth muscle relaxant factor released from guinea-pig tracheal epithelium. *Br J Pharmacol* 1989;96:117–124.

91. Hall IP, Donaldson J, Hill SJ. Inhibition of histamine-stimulated inositol phospholipid hydrolysis by agents which incrase cyclic AMP levels in bovine tracheal smooth muscle. *Br J Pharmacol* 1989;97:603–613.

92. Munakata M, Masaki Y, Sakuma I, et al. Pharmacological differentiation of epithelium-derived relaxing factor from nitric oxide. *J Appl Physiol* 1990;69:665–670.

93. Palmer RMJ, Ferrige AG, Mancada S. Nitric oxide release accounts for the biological activity of epithelium-derived relaxing factor. *Nature Lond* 1987;327:524–526.

94. Sheng H, Ishii K, Murad F. Generation of an endothelium-derived relaxing factor-like substance in bovine tracheal smooth muscle. *Am J Physiol* 1991;260:L489–L493.

95. Shore SA, Powell WS, Martin JG. Endogenous prostaglandins modulate histamine-induced contraction in canine tracheal smooth muscle. *J Appl Physiol* 1985;58:859–868.

96. White SR, Sigrist KM, Spaethe SM. Bradykinin elicits topography-dependent prostaglandin secretion in canine tracheal epithelial cells. *Am J Respir Cell Mol Biol* 1992;6:375–381.

97. White SR, Sigrist KS, and Spaethe SM. Secretion of prostaglandin mediators by guinea pig tracheal epithelial cells caused by eosinophil major basic protein. *Am J Physiol* 1993;263:L234–L242.

98. Cuthbert MF. Bronchodilator activity of aerosols of prostaglandins E_1 and E_2 in asthmatic subjects. *Proc R Soc Med* 1971;64:15–16.

99. Abela AP, Daniel EE. Neural and myogenic effects of cyclooxygenase products on canine bronchial smooth muscle. *Am J Physiol* 1995;268:L47–L55.

100. Wilkens JH, Becker A, Wilkens H, et al. Bioassay of a tracheal smooth muscle-contracting factor released by respiratory epithelial cells. *Am J Physiol* 1992;263:L137–L144.

101. Butler GB, Adler KB, Evans JN, Morgan DW, Szarek JL. Modulation of rabbit airway smooth muscle respoonsiveness by respiratory epithelium. Involvement of an inhibitory metabolite of arachidonic acid. *Am Rev Respir Dis* 1987;135:1099–1104.

102. Stuart-Smith K, Vanhoutte PM. Arachidonic acid evokes epithelium-dependent relaxations in canine airways. *J Appl Physiol* 1988;65:2170–2180.

103. Barnett K, Jacoby DB, Nadle JA, Lazarus SC. The effects of epithelial cell supernatant on contractions of isolated canine tracheal smooth muscle. *Am Rev Respir Dis* 1988;138:780–783.

104. Holroyde MV. The influence of epithelium on the responsiveness of guinea pig isolated trachea. *Br J Pharmacol* 1986; 87:501–507.

105. Ndukwu IM, Solway J, Arbetter K, Uzendoski K, Leff AR, Mitchell RW. Immune sensitization augments epithelium-dependent spontaneous tone in guinea pig trachealis. *Am J Physiol* 1994;266:L485–L492.

106. Franconi GM, Rubinstein I, Levine EH, Ikeda S, Nadel JA. Mechanical removal of airway epithelium disrupts mast cells and released granules. *Am J Physiol* 1990;259:L372–L377.

107. Miura M, Inoue H, Ichinose M, et al. Increase in luminal mast cell and epithelial damage may account for increased airway responsiveness after viral infection in dogs. *Am Rev Respir Dis* 1989;140:1738–1744.

108. Solway J, Leff AR. Sensory neuropeptides and airway function. *J Appl Physiol* 1991;71:2077–2087.

109. Brofman JD, White SR, Blake JS, Munoz NM, Gleich GJ, Leff AR. Epithelial augmentation of trachealis contraction caused by major basic protein of eosinophils. *J Appl Physiol* 1989;66:1867–1873.

110. White SR, Ohno S, Munoz NM, et al. Direct and augmenting effects on airway smooth muscle contraction from epithelial secretion elicited by the major basic protein of eosinophils. *Am J Physiol* 1990;259:L294–L303.

111. Strek ME, White SR, Munoz NM, et al. Physiological significance of epithelium removal in guinea pig tracheal smooth muscle. *Am Rev Respir Dis* 1993;147:1477–1482.

112. Coyle AJ, Mitzner W, Irvin CG. Cationic proteins alter smooth muscle function by an epithelium-dependent mechanism. *J Appl Physiol* 1993;74:1761–1768.

113. Widdicombe JH. Physiology of airway epithelia. In: SG Farmer, DWP Hay, eds. *The airway epithelium: physiology, pathophysiology, and pharmacology.* New York: Marcel Dekker, 1990:41–64.

114. Wanner A. Mucociliary clearance in the trachea. *Clin Chest Med* 1986;7:247–258.

115. Dulfano MJ, Luk CK. Sputum and ciliary inhibition in asthma. *Thorax* 1982;37:646–651.

116. Tamaoki J, Kondo M, Takizawa T. Adenosine-mediated cyclic AMP-dependent inhibition of ciliary activity in rabbit tracheal epithelium. *Am Rev Respir Dis* 1989;137:899–902.

117. Pavia D, Lopez-Vidriero MT, Clarke SW. Mediators and mucociliary clearance in asthma. *Bull Eur Physiopathol Respir* 1987;23(Suppl 10):89s–94s.

118. Jain B, Rubinstein I, Robbins RA, Leise KL, Sisson JH. Modulation of airway epithelial cell ciliary beat frequency by nitric oxide. *Biochem Biophys Res Comm* 1993;191:83–88.

119. Havez R, Roussel P. Bronchial mucus: physical and biochemical features. In: Weiss EB, Segal MS, eds. *Bronchial asthma: mechanisms and therapeutics.* Boston: Little, Brown and Co., 1976:409–422.

120. Kaliner MA, Shelhamer JH, Borson DB, Patow CA, Marom Z, Nadel JA. Respiratory mucus. In: Kaliner MA, Barnes PJ, eds. *The airways: neural control in health and disease.* New York: Marcel Dekker, 1988:575–593.

121. Borson DB, Corrales R, Varsano S, et al. Enkephalinase inhibitors potentiate substance P-induced secretion of $^{35}SO_4$-macromolecules from ferret trachea. *Exp Lung Res* 1987;12:21–36.

122. Lopez-Vidriero MT, Das I, Smith AP, Picot R, Reid L. Bronchial secretion from normal human airways after inhalation of prostaglandin $F_{2\alpha}$, acetylcholine, histamine and citric acid. *Thorax* 1977;32:734–739.

123. Marom Z, Shelhamer JH, Kaliner M. Effects of arachidonic acid, monohydroxyeicosatetranenoic acid and prostaglandins on the release of mucous glycoproteins from human airways in vitro. *J Clin Invest* 1981;67:1695–1702.

124. Marom Z, Shelhamer JH, Bach MK, Morton DR, Kaliner M. Slow-reacting substances, leukotrienes C_4 and D_4 increase the release of mucus from human airways in vitro. *Am Rev Respir Dis* 1982;126:449–451.

125. Kim KC, Nassir J, Brody JS. Mechanisms of airway goblet cell mucin release: studies with cultured tracheal surface epithelial cells. *Am J Respir Cell Mol Biol* 1989;1:137–143.

126. Rieves RD, Goff J, Wu T, Larivee P, Logun C, Shelhamer JH. Airway epithelial cell mucin release: immunologic quantitation and response

to platelet activating factor. *Am J Respir Cell Mol Biol* 1992;6:158–167.

127. Adler KB, Akley NJ, Glasgow WC. Platelet activating factor provokes release of mucin-like glycoproteins from guinea pig respiratory epithelial cells via a lipoxygenase-dependent mechanism. *Am J Respir Cell Mol Biol* 1992;6:550–556.

128. Messina MS, ORiordan TG, Smaldone GC. Changes in mucociliary clearance during acute exacerbations of asthma. *Am Rev Respir Dis* 1991;143:993–997.

129. Rangachari PK, McWade D. Peptides increase anaion conductance of canine trachea: an effect on tight junctions. *Biochim Biophys Acta* 1986;863:305–308.

130. Boucher RC, Gatzy JT. Regional effects of autonomic agents on ion transport across excised canine airways. *J Appl Physiol* 1982;52:893–901.

131. Dunnill MS. The pathology of asthma. In: Middleton E, Reed CE, Ellis EF, eds. *Allergy principles and practice II.* St. Louis: CV Mosby, 1978:678–686.

132. Hogg JC. The pathology of asthma. *Clin Chest Med* 1984; 5:567–571.

133. Persson CGA, Erjefält IAL. Inflammatory leakage of macromolecules from the vascular compartment into the tracheal lumen. *Acta Physiol Scand* 1986;126:615–616.

134. Persson CGA, Erjefält IAL. Nonneural and neural regulation of plasma exudation in airways. In: Kaliner MA, Barnes PJ, eds. *The airways: neural control in health and disease.* New York: Marcel Dekker 1988:523–550.

135. Simani AG, Inoue S, Hogg JC. Penetration of the respiratory epithelium of guinea pigs following exposure to cigarette smoke. *Lab Invest* 1974;31:75–81.

136. Boucher RC, Johnson J, Inoue S, Hulbert W, Hogg JC. The effect of cigarette smoke on the permeability of guinea pig airways. *Lab Invest* 1980;43:94–100.

137. Bhalla DK, Manniz RC, Kleinman MT, Crocker TT. Relative permeability of nasal, tracheal and bronchoalveolar mucosa to macromolecules in rats exposed to ozone. *J Toxicol Environ Health* 1986;17:269–283.

138. Welsh MJ. Intracellular chloride activities in canine tracheal epithelium. *J Clin Invest* 1983;71:1392–1401.

139. Frizzell RA, Rechkemmer G, Shoemaker RL. Altered regulation of airway epithelial cell chloride channels in cystic fibrosis. *Science* 1986;233:558–560.

140. Persson CGA. Role of plasma exudation in asthmatic airways. *Am Rev Respir Dis* 1986;133:1126–1129.

141. Bennett WD, Ilowite JS. Dual pathway clearance of ^{99m}Tc-DTPA from the bronchial mucosa. *Am Rev Respir Dis* 1989;139:1132–1138.

142. From Ilowite JS, Bennett WD, Sheetz MS, Groth ML, Nierman DM. Permeability of the bronchial mucosa to ^{99m}Tc-DTPA in asthma. *Am Rev Respir Dis* 1988;139:1139–1143.

143. Devalia JL, Godfrey RW, Sapsford RJ, Severs NJ, Jeffery PK, Davies RJ. No effect of histamine on human bronchial epithelial cell permeability and tight junctional integrity *in vitro. Eur Respir J* 1994;7:1958–1965.

144. Ohashi Y, Motojima S, Fukuda T, Makino S. Airway hyperresponsiveness, increased intracellular spaces of bronchial epithelium, and increased infiltration of eosinophils and lymphocytes in bronchial mucosa in asthma. *Am Rev Respir Dis* 1992;145:1469–1476.

145. Cox G, Ohtoshi T, Vancheri C, et al. Promotion of eosinophil survival by human bronchial epithelial cells and its modulation by steroids. *Am J Respir Cell Mol Biol* 1991;4:525–531.

146. Marini M, Soloperto M, Mezzetti M, Fasoli A, Mattoli S. Interleukin-1 binds to specific receptors on human bronchial epithelial cells and upregulates granulocyte-macrophage colony-stimulating factor synthesis and release. *Am J Respir Cell Mol Biol* 1991;4:519–524.

147. Cromwell O, Hamid Q, Corrigan CJ, et al. Expression and generation of interleukin-8, IL-6 and granulocyte-macrophage colony-stimulating factor by bronchial epithelial cells and enhancement by IL-1β and tumour necrosis factor-α. *Immunology* 1992;77:330–337.

148. Wang JH, Trigg CJ, Devalia JL, Jordan S, Davies RJ. Effect of inhaled beclomethasone dipropionate on expression of proinflammatory cytokines and activated eosinophils in the bronchial epithelium of patients with mild asthma. *J Allergy Clin Immunol* 1994; 94:1025–1034.

149. Erger RA, Casale TB. Interleukin-8 is a potent mediator of eosinophil chemotaxis through endothelium and epithelium. *Am J Physiol* 1995; 268:L117–L122.

150. Soloperto M, Mattoso VL, Fasoli A, Mattoli S. A bronchial epithelial cell-derived factor in asthma that promotes eosinophil activation and survival as GM-CSF. *Am J Physiol* 1991;260:L530–L538.

151. Marini M, Soloperto M, Zheng Y, Mezzetti M, Mattoli S. Protective effect of nedocromil sodium on the IL-1-induced release of GM-CSF from cultured human bronchial epithelial cells. *Pulm Pharmacol* 1992;5:61–65.

152. Marini M, Vittori E, Hollemborg J, Mattoli S. Expression of the potent inflammatory cytokines, granulocyte-macrophage-colony-stimulating factor and interleukin-6 and interleukin-8, in bronchial epithelial cells of patients with asthma. *J Allergy Clin Immunol* 1992;89:1001–1009.

153. Sousa AR, Poston RN, Lane SJ, Nakhosteen JA, Lee TH. Detection of GM-CSF in asthmatic bronchial epithelium and decrease by inhaled corticosteroids. *Am Rev Respir Dis* 1993;147:1557–1561.

154. Levine SJ, Larivee P, Logun C, Angus CW, Shelhamer JH. Corticosteroids differentially regulate secretion of IL-6, IL-8, and G-CSF by a human bronchial epithelial cell line. *Am J Physiol* 1993;265:L360–L368.

155. Robbins RA, Shoji S, Linder J, Grossman GL, Allington LA, Klassen LW, Rennard SI. Bronchial epithelial cells release chemotactic activity for lymphocytes. *Am J Physiol* 1989;257:L109–115.

156. Koyama S, Rennard SI, Shoji S, et al. Romberger DJ, Linder J, Ertl R, Robbins RA. Bronchial epithelial cells release chemoattractant activity for monocytes. *Am J Physiol* 1989;257:L130–136.

157. Koyama S, Rennard SI, Leikauf G, et al. Endotoxin stimulates bronchialepithelial cells to release chemotactic factors for neutrophils. *J Immunol* 1991;147:4293–4301.

158. Glanville AR, Tazelaar HD, Theodore J, et al. The distribution of MHC class I and II antigens on bronchial epithelium. *Am Rev Respir Dis* 1989;139:330–334.

159. Look DC, Rapp SR, Keller BT, Holtzman MJ. Selective induction of intercellular adhesion molecule-1 by interferon-γ in human airway epithelial cells. *Am J Physiol* 1992;263:L79–L87.

160. Tosi MF, Stark JM, Smith CW, Hamedani A, Gruenert DC, Infeld MD. Induction of ICAM-1 expression on human airway epithelial cells by inflammatory cytokines: effects on neutrophil-epithelial cell adheison. *Am J Respir Cell Mol Biol* 1992;7:214–221.

161. Bloeman PGM, van den Tweel M, Henricks PAJ, et al. Expression and modulation of adhesion molecules on human bronchial epithelial cells. *Am J Respir Cell Mol Biol* 1993;9:586–593.

162. Wegner CD, Gundel RH, Reilly P, Haynes N, Letts LG, Rothlein R. Intercellular adhesion molecule-1 (ICAM-1) in the pathogenesis of asthma. *Science* 1990;247:456–459.

163. Vignola AM, Campbell AM, Chanez P, et al. HLA-DR and ICAM-1 expression on bronchial epithelial cells in asthma and chronic bronchitis. *Am Rev Respir Dis* 1993;148:689–694.

164. Tosi MF, Stark JM, Hamedani A, Smith CW, Gruenert DC, Huang YT. Intercellular adhesion molecule-1 (ICAM-1)-dependent and ICAM-1-independent adhesive mechanisms between polymorphonuclear leukocytes and human airway epithelial cells infection with parainfluenza virus type 2. *J Immunol* 1992;149:3345–3349.

165. Montefort S, Roche WR, Howarth PH, et al. Intercellular adhesion molecule-1 (ICAM-1) and endothelial leucocyte adhesion molecule-1 (ELAM-1) expression in the bronchial mucosa of normal and asthmatic subjects. *Eur Respir J* 1992;5:815–823.

166. Johnson AR, Ashton J, Schulz WW, Erdös EG. Neutral metalloendopeptidase in human lung tissue and cultured cells. *Am Rev Respir Dis* 1985;132:564–568.

167. Sekizawa K, Tamaoki J, Graf PD, Basbaum CB, Borson DB, Nadel JA. Enkephalinase inhibitor potentiates mammalian tachykinin-induced contraction in ferret trachea. *J Pharmacol Exp Ther* 1987;243:1211–1217.

168. Borson DB, Gruenert DC. Glucocorticoids induce neutral endopeptidase in transformed human tracheal epithelial cells. *Am J Physiol* 1991;260:L83–L89.

169. Kondo M, Tamaoki J, Takizawa T. Neutral endopeptidase inhibitor poentiates the tachykinin-induced increase in ciliary beat frequency in rabbit trachea. *Am Rev Respir Dis* 1990;142:403–406.

170. Devillier P, Advenier C, Drapeau G, Marsac J, Regoli D. Comparison of the effects of epithelium removal and of an enkephalinase inhibitor on the neurokinin-induced contractions of guinea-pig isolated trachea. *Br J Pharmacol* 1988;94:675–684.

171. Djokic TD, Dusser DJ, Borson DB, Nadel JA. Neutral endopeptidase

modulates neurotensin-induced airway contraction. *J Appl Physiol* 1989;66:2338–2343.

172. Maggi CA, Patacchini R, Perretti F, et al. The effect of thiorphan and epithelium removal on contractions and tachykinin release produced by activation of capsaicin-sensitive afferents in the guinea-pig isolated bronchus. *Naunyn-Schmiedebergs Archiv Pharmacol* 1990;341:74–79.

173. Borson DB, Brokaw JJ, Sekizawa K, McDonald DM, Nadel JA. Neutral endopeptidase and neurogenic inflammation in rats with respiratory infections. *J Appl Physiol* 1989;66:2653–2658.

174. Jacoby DB, Tamaoki J, Borson DB, Nadel JA. Influenza infection causes airway hyperresponsiveness by decreasing enkephalinase. *J Appl Physiol* 1988;64:2653–2658.

175. Diamant Z, Timmers MC, van der Veen H, Booms P, Sont JK, Sterk PJ. Effect of an inhaled neutral endopeptidase inhibitor, thiorphan, on airway responsiveness to leukotriene D$_4$ in normal and asthmatic subjects. *Eur Respir J* 1994;7:459–466.

176. Cheung D, Timmers MC, Zwinderman AH, den Hartigh J, Dijkman JH, Sterk PJ. Neutral endopeptidase activity and airway hyperresponsiveness to neurokinin A in asthmatic subjects *in vivo*. *Am Rev Respir Dis* 1993;148:1467–1473.

177. Willis RA. Regeneration and repair: resumed embroyonic growth. *The borderland of embryology and pathology*, 2nd ed. Washington: Butterworths, 1962;495–518.

178. Keenan KP, Combs JW, McDowell EM. Regeneration of hamster tracheal epithelium after mechanical injury. II. Multifocal lesions: stathmokinetic and autoradiographic studies of cell proliferation. *Virchows Arch Cell Pathol* 1982;41:215–229.

179. Keenan KP, Combs JW, McDowell EM. Regeneration of hamster tracheal epithelium after mechanical injury. III. Large and small lesions: comparative stathmokinetic and single pulse and continuous thymidine labeling autoradiographic studies. *Virchows Arch Cell Pathol* 1982;41:231–252.

180. Keenan KP, Combs JW, McDowell EM. Regeneration of hamster tracheal epithelium after mechanical injury. IV. Histochemical, immunocytochemical and ultrastructural studies. *Virchows Arch Cell Pathol* 1983;43:213–240.

181. Zahm J-M, Chevillard M, Puchelle E. Wound repair of human surface respiratory epithelium. *Am J Respir Cell Mol Biol* 1991;5:242–248.

182. Barrow RE, Wang C-Z, Cox RA, Evans MJ. Cellular sequence of tracheal repair in sheep afte smoke inhalation injury. *Lung* 1992;170:331–338.

183. Shimizu T, Nishihara M, Kawaguchi S, Sakakura Y. Expression of phenotypic markers during regeneration of rat tracheal epithelium following mechanical injury. *Am J Respir Cell Mol Biol* 1994;11:85–94.

184. Shimizu T, Nettesheim P, Ramaekers FCS, Randell SH. Expression of cell-type specific markers during rat tracheal epithelial regeneration. *Am J Respir Cell Mol Biol* 1992;7:30–41.

185. Masui T, Wakefield LM, Lechner JF, La Veck MA, Sporn MB, Harris CC. Type β transforming growth factor is the primary differentiation-inducing serum factor for normal human bronchial epithelial cells. *Proc Natl Acad Sci U S A* 1986;83:2438–2442.

186. Shoji S, Rickard KA, Takizawa H, Ertl RF, Linder J, Rennard SI. Lung fibroblasts produce growth stimulatory activity for bronchial epithelial cells. *Am Rev Respir Dis* 1990;141:433–439.

187. Takizawa H, Beckmann JD, Shoji S, et al. Pulmonary macrophages can stimulate cell growth of bovine bronchial epithelial cells. *Am J Respir Cell Mol Biol* 1990;2:245–255.

188. White SR, Hershenson M, Sigrist KM, Zimmermann A, Solway J. Proliferation of guinea pig tracheal epithelial cells induced by calcitonin gene-related peptide. *Am J Respir Cell Molec Biol* 1993;8:592–596.

189. Sanghavi J, Rabe KF, Sigrist KM, Magnusson H, Leff AR, White SR. Migration of human and guinea pig airway epithelial cells induced by calcitonin gene-related peptide. *Am J Resp Cell Molec Biol* 1994;11:181–187.

190. Kim JS, Rabe KF, Magnussen H, Green JM, White SR. Migration and proliferation of guinea pig and human airway epithelial cells in response to tachykinins. *Am J Physiol* 1995;269:L119–L126.

191. Lechner JF, Haugan A, McClendon IA, Pettis EW. Clonal growth of normal adult human bronchial epithelial cells in a serum-free medium. *In Vitro* 1982;18:633–642.

192. Retsch-Bogart A, Stiles BM, Moats-Staats D, Van Scott MR, Boucher RC, D Ercole AJ. Canine tracheal epithelial cells express the Type I insulin-like growth factor receptor adn proliferate in response to insulin-like growth factor I. *Am J Respir Cell Mol Biol* 1990;3:227–234.

193. Jetten AM. Growth and differentiation factors in tracheobronchial epithelium. *Am J Physiol* 1991;260:L361–L373.

194. Whitcutt MJ, Adler KB, Wu R. A biphasic chamber system for maintaining polarity of differentiation of cultured respiratory tract epithelial cells. *In Vitro Cell Devel Biol* 1988;24:420–428.

195. Clark AB, Randell SH, Nettesheim P, Gray TE, Bagnell B, Ostrowski LE. Regulation of ciliated cell differentiation in cultures of rat tracheal epithelial cells. *Am J Respir Cell Mol Biol* 1995;12:329–338.

196. Martin WR, Brown C, Zhang YJ, Wu R. Growth and differentiation of primary tracheal epithelial cells in culture: regulation by extracellular calcium. *J Cell Physiol* 1991;147:138–148.

197. Demoly P, Simony-Lafontaine J, Chanez P, Pujol JL, Lequeux N, Michel F-B, Bousquet J. Cell proliferation in the bronchial mucosa of asthmatics and chronic bronchits. *Am J Respir Crit Care Med* 1994;150:214–217.

Asthma, edited by P.J. Barnes, M.M. Grunstein, A.R. Leff, and A.J. Woolcock.
Lippincott–Raven Publishers, Philadelphia © 1997.

■ 63 ■

Epithelium-Dependent Responsiveness of Airway Smooth Muscle

The Role of Epithelium-Derived Relaxant Factors

Roy G. Goldie and Douglas W.P. Hay

The airway epithelium is critically situated at the interface between the external environment and the internal milieu. Appropriately, the epithelium has a vital barrier function to retard the penetration of inhaled, potentially noxious or stimulatory substances including low molecular weight chemicals as well as proteinaceous macromolecules. This barrier is created via physical, immunologic, and metabolic mechanisms (1,2) (Fig. 1). In each case, the result and ultimate effect can be modulation of the presentation of biologically active molecules to the submucosa and thus modification of responses of tissue elements, including the microvasculature, nerves, and airway smooth muscle, to these penetrating substances. However, in addition to this barrier function, it is now universally recognized that the mammalian airway epithelium is a significant source of biologically active substances, some of which have important effects on the level of airway smooth muscle tone (1). The possibility that the airway epithelium might act as a significant source of spasmolytic substances was brought more sharply into focus after the detection of endothelium-derived relaxant factor in vascular tissue, now identified as nitric oxide (3). This chapter focuses on the influence of the airway epithelium on airway smooth muscle tone and responsiveness to various proinflammatory mediators relevant to the pathogenesis of asthma, with particular reference to epithelium-derived inhibitory mediators.

AIRWAY EPITHELIUM IN ASTHMA

It has been suggested that the fundamental defect in asthma is the inability of the epithelium to control the osmolarity of fluid lining the bronchial mucosa (4). However, O'Byrne et al. (5) showed that whereas asthmatics were markedly more sensitive to inhaled histamine, the permeabilities of their bronchial epithelia were within the normal range. Thus, the data from studies in the human have been conflicting, with some evidence for increased permeability in asthma (6) and other studies failing to observe this (5,7). In experimental animals, ex-

  R. G. Goldie: Department of Pharmacology, University of Western Australia, The Queen Elizabeth II Medical Centre, Nedlands, Western Australia, 6907 Australia.
  D. W. P. Hay: Department of Pulmonary Pharmacology, Division of Inflammation/Respiratory Pharmacology, SmithKline Beecham Pharmaceuticals, King of Prussia, Pennsylvania 19406.

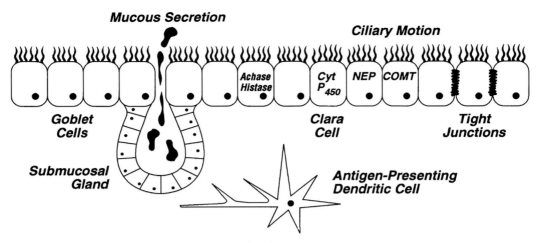

FIG. 1. Barrier functions of airway epithelial cells.

posure of the airways to inflammatory stimuli such as cigarette smoke, which increased epithelium permeability, also increased the responsiveness of the airways to spasmogens (8,9).

Damage and/or desquamation of the epithelium is commonly seen in asthma (10,11), although not all the events resulting in asthma-associated airway epithelial damage have been elucidated. Considerable evidence points to an important role for eosinophils in the pathogenesis of asthma and in the destruction of the bronchial epithelium. Certainly, large numbers of eosinophils are recruited into the airways and epithelium in this disease (12,13) and a correlation between eosinophil number and the changes in pulmonary function has been reported (14). The cytotoxic eosinophil-derived protein, major basic protein (MBP), is thought to be largely responsible for the epithelial damage observed in asthma (15,16). Perhaps importantly, this MBP-induced damage has been associated with increased responsiveness of isolated airway tissues (17,18).

Enhanced access to intra- and subepithelial nerves, inflammatory cells, and vascular and airway smooth muscle to inhaled chemical stimuli including allergens is theoretically increased with epithelial damage, raising the possibility of perturbations of responsiveness of these underlying tissues. In line with this concept, epithelial damage in asthmatic airways has been linked with airway hyperresponsiveness (AHR) to inhaled histamine (15). Importantly, a correlation between the degree of AHR to airway smooth muscle spasmogens and the extent of epithelial damage has been reported (12), although this is not always observed (19). Thus, the pathophysiologic significance of epithelial damage in asthma and other respiratory diseases remains the subject of controversy.

Epithelial desquamation might reasonably be expected to expose sensory afferent nerve fibers in asthmatic airways (20). Stimulation of sensory nerve C-fibers may result in antidromic conduction and release of proinflammatory sensory neuropeptides, which may cause numer-

ous deleterious effects including neurogenic inflammation, enhanced mucous secretion, and bronchoconstriction (21). Furthermore, such damage should permit enhanced access of inhaled stimulants, including allergens, to submucosal target tissues. The consequent release of proinflammatory substances such as leukotrienes (LTs) and bradykinin (BK) may cause direct or reflex bronchoconstriction via vagal or local pathways. In addition, loss of epithelial neutral endopeptidase (NEP), which is a major pathway for peptide metabolism (22), should potentiate the effects of endogenously released tachykinins. Thus, a significantly amplified airway inflammatory response might result. Epithelial damage with associated bronchial hyperresponsiveness is observed in patients with farmer's lung (23) and viral infections (24). Aerosol administration of substances that cause bronchial epithelial damage, including ozone, nitrogen dioxide, or toluene diisocyanate (25,26), also results in bronchial hyperresponsiveness in animals.

Thus, there is widespread support for the notion that damage or dysfunction to the epithelium contributes significantly to the airway hyperreactivity to spasmogens, which is a feature of asthma (27). However, it is important to remember that hyperresponsiveness has not always been detected in association with such damage (19). Despite this, there is general agreement that, by virtue of its location and its biologic characteristics, the epithelium plays a critical role in the processes of airway inflammation characteristic of asthma. Indeed, there is a view that injury to the epithelial cell is a critical early event in airway inflammation (28).

EPITHELIAL PROTECTION OF THE AIRWAY WALL

It is clear from the above that the integrity of the airway epithelium is a significant factor in determining responsiveness of underlying structures including airway smooth muscle, nerves, glands, and blood vessels. The barrier presented by the airway epithelium is created in several ways including physical, immunologic, and metabolic influences (Fig. 1). Each of these can result in the modulation of the concentrations of biologically active molecules arising in the internal milieu from the external environment.

Physical Barriers

Intracellular junctions

Intracellular tight junctions between epithelial cells form the first line of physical protection for underlying cells from external stimuli (29,30). In addition to inhibiting the diffusion of noxious substances into the airway mucosa, this barrier also prevents the leakage of water and solutes from the airway wall into the bronchial lumen. Certainly, there is convincing evidence that the epithelium provides a significant impediment to the access of luminal solutes to underlying tissues including airway smooth muscle (31–35).

Secretion of Mucus

Mucus is produced in healthy airways in sufficient amounts to lubricate the bronchial surface and to entrap inhaled foreign particles. Importantly, bronchial mucus contains proteolytic enzymes that degrade allergens (36). Although in the larger airways submucosal glands provide the bulk of the material secreted to the airway surface (29,37), epithelial serous, goblet, and Clara cells also contribute significantly to airway mucus production (38).

Immunologic Barriers

The epithelium is strategically placed between the external environment and the immune system of the respiratory tract. Allergens that have not been removed by mucociliary clearance may be engulfed by resident antigen-presenting macrophages, which are then in part responsible for delivering antigen to lymphocytes, allowing clearance and/or detoxification of the allergen and the initiation of tissue repair (39). Airway epithelial cells including dendritic cells, which also express class I and class II major histocompatibility complex (MHC) antigens, have an accessory cell function in antigen presentation (40). In this way, the epithelium acts as an immunoregulator relative to the disposition of inhaled antigens.

Metabolic Barriers

The epithelium has a significant capacity to metabolize a range of peptide substances via membrane-bound NEP (41) and thus reduce their active concentrations in airway wall. NEP, which is localized at the surface of airway epithelial cells, can cleave tachykinins such as substance P and other peptides such as BK (42), vasoactive intestinal peptide (43), and endothelin (44). Inhibitors of NEP potentiate the bronchoactive effects of BK (45), neurokinins (46), endothelin (44), atrial natriuretic peptides (47), and vasoactive intestinal peptide (VIP) (41,48) and largely mimic the effects of epithelium removal.

Histamine can be metabolized in airway epithelium via histamine N-methyltransferase, inhibition of which causes enhanced contractile responses to histamine (49), and via histaminase (50). Furthermore, the epithelium may be a major site of extraneuronal uptake and O-methylation of catecholamines such as isoprenaline (51), although the evidence is equivocal. The guinea pig tracheal epithelium has also been described as a site for the uptake and degradation of adenosine (52).

Nonciliated bronchiolar secretory cells (Clara cells) possess enzymes including acid and alkaline phosphatases, nonspecific esterase, hydroxylases, transferases, peroxidases, and catalase, in addition to cytochrome P-450 monoxygenase (53). The metabolism via cytochrome P-450 of cytotoxic agents that enter the respiratory tract from the inspired air or via the bloodstream is a primary function of the Clara cell. This pathway is more active in the Clara cell than in any other pulmonary cell type (53,54).

FUNCTIONAL CONSEQUENCES OF EPITHELIAL DISRUPTION

Airway Smooth Muscle Tone

Orehek et al. (55) were perhaps the first to appreciate that the airway epithelium was a significant source of relaxant/inhibitory substances that could influence the tone of underlying airway smooth muscle. A decade later, the influences of mechanical removal of the epithelium on airway smooth muscle contraction to several agonists and also on relaxant responses to isoproterenol (56) were reported in experiments in canine bronchus. These studies suggested that the airway epithelium was a significant modulator of airway smooth muscle sensitivity to relaxant and spasmogenic substances, possible via the release of an inhibitory mediator. The modulatory effects of the epithelium on isolated tissue responsiveness to spasmogenic and relaxant agonists has subsequently been comprehensively explored and the data extensively reviewed (57,58).

Several mechanisms may be involved, with their contributions varying depending on the specific bronchoactive substance involved. The mechanisms underlying epithelium-dependent modulation of airway smooth muscle responsiveness to various mediators have been deduced from studies examining the effects of mechanical re-

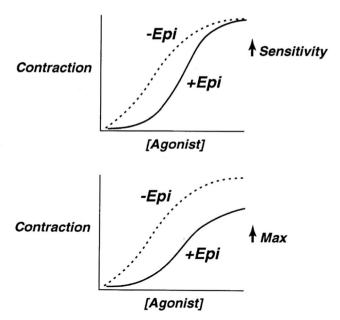

FIG. 2. Potential effects of epithelial cell removal on responsiveness of airway smooth muscle to contractile agonists: increase in sensitivity and/or increase in the maximum *(Max)* response.

moval of the epithelium on responsiveness of isolated airway smooth muscle. The influence of epithelium removal on contractile agonists is generally reflected by either an increase in sensitivity (shift to the left in agonist concentration-response curve) and/or an increase in the maximum response (Fig. 2).

Potassium Ions

K$^+$-induced contraction is not significantly altered by epithelium removal in bovine (59), canine (60), rabbit (61), or guinea pig (62–65) airways.

Muscarinic Cholinoceptor Agonists

Mechanical removal of the epithelium also has been shown to increase significantly the potencies of acetylcholine (ACh), methacholine, and bethanechol by two- to sevenfold in airways from the rat (66), guinea pig (62–68), rabbit (61), dog (56,69), pig (70), cow (59), and human (71–73). Interestingly, the spasmogenic effects of carbachol were not significantly altered by this treatment (62,63,67,72). This does not seem to relate to muscarinic receptor subtype selectivities (68). However, release of epithelium-derived inhibitory factors (EpDIF) in guinea pig trachea appeared to be mediated via M$_3$ muscarinic receptor activation, as is the contractile response (74). Although possible, the differential effect of epithelium removal on cholinergic agonists probably is not due to a greater ep-

ithelial permeability to carbachol than to related agonists that might render it less affected by removal of this tissue. Epithelium-dependent increases in ACh-induced contraction induced by eosinophil-derived MBP also has been documented in dog trachea *in situ*, a phenomenon possibly mediated by an epithelium-derived contractile factor (17) such as endothelin-1 (ET-1), and in guinea pig isolated trachea (18). The presence of epithelium-associated cholinesterase also has been proposed to play a role in the modulatory influence of the epithelium on ACh-induced contraction in guinea pig isolated trachea (75).

Histamine

It is now well established that epithelial ablation results in significant increases in the potency of spasmogens in guinea pig tracheal smooth muscle preparations (63,64, 67). However, whereas in some cases maximum contraction was increased (63,65,76), no effect was observed in others (62,64). Interestingly, these effects are age-dependent, with the greatest increases in histamine potency seen during the early stages of animal maturation (67). Similar epithelium-dependent increases in responsiveness also were observed in bronchial preparations from the guinea pig (76) and dog (56,77).

Braunstein and colleagues (78) concluded that the modulatory influence of the epithelium on responsiveness to histamine in guinea pig trachea was in large part due to the release of relaxant PGE$_2$. However, such release was not observed in a separate study (79). Importantly, human bronchial sensitivity to histamine was also significantly increased after epithelium removal (71,80). However, this was not seen in bronchial preparations from human asthmatic lung, presumably because of disease-associated epithelial damage (71). The epithelium may act as a site of metabolism of histamine via histaminase and modulate histamine-induced contraction (81). The possibility of a non-H$_1$-/non-H$_2$-histamine receptor that mediated the release of a nonprostanoid epithelium-derived inhibitory factor also has been postulated (82).

Leukotrienes

Epithelial stripping also enhances responsiveness of isolated airway preparations to the cysteinyl LTs (CysLTs), although the mechanisms underlying this have not been clarified. Some evidence points to the involvement of both prostanoid and nonprostanoid inhibitory mediators, but species differences thwart attempts to define a unifying mechanism. Indomethacin mimicked the effect of epithelium removal on sensitivity to LTC$_4$ in guinea pig trachea, suggesting that the contractile effect of this substance was modulated by a smooth-muscle inhibitory prostanoid derived from the epithelium, whereas LTD$_4$-induced responses were unaltered by epithelium stripping or indomethacin (83). In contrast, Hisayama et al. (1988) (84) showed that epithelium removal increased LTD$_4$ potency more than sixfold via a cyclo-oxygenase-mediated mechanism. Tachyphylaxis to LTC$_4$, LTD$_4$, and LTE$_4$ in guinea pig isolated trachea was attributed to the release of an inhibitory substance from the epithelium (85).

These data are further confounded by contradictory evidence relating to the release of prostanoids and LTs from isolated airway preparations. For example, LTD$_4$ and histamine caused the release of PGE$_2$ and 6-keto-PGF$_1$ from guinea pig airways. However, this release was not reduced by removal of the epithelium (75). In contrast, no effect of LTD$_4$ on release of PGE$_2$, PGF$_2$, and 6-keto-PGF$_1$ from guinea pig trachea was observed in either the presence or absence of the epithelium (79), suggesting that the modulatory effect of the epithelium involved the release of a nonprostanoid inhibitory factor(s). Importantly, in human isolated bronchial preparations, epithelium removal caused a threefold increase in the spasmogenic potency of LTD$_4$ via an indomethacin-sensitive mechanism. However, removing the epithelium had no influence on bronchial responsiveness to LTC$_4$ or LTE$_4$ (86).

Antigen

Antigen-induced contraction in human and guinea pig airway preparations is apparently mediated exclusively via the release of histamine and LTs (87). Because the epithelium exerts a significant modulatory effect on the actions of these two mediators, it is not surprising that removal of the epithelium increased the sensitivity of ovalbumin-sensitized guinea pig tracheal airway smooth muscle to ovalbumin by six- to eightfold (88,89). However, given the size of ovalbumin, the epithelium also might act as a significant barrier to diffusion. Accordingly, the loss of the protective epithelium may partly explain the enhanced responses to this substance. Co-axial bioassay systems were reported to provide evidence for an epithelium-derived contractile factor that influenced antigen-induced contraction in guinea pig bronchus (90). In a superfusion system, the epithelium did not modulate the response of guinea pig trachea to a high concentration of antigen (91).

Platelet activating Factor

Platelet activating factor (PAF)-induced relaxation of guinea pig isolated trachea may be the result of the release of PGE$_2$ (81,92) from the airway epithelium.

Bradykinin

Whereas bradykinin (BK) is a potent bronchoconstrictor in asthmatics, it does not cause bronchoconstriction in nonasthmatics. Furthermore, BK has little direct spasmo-

genic activity in airway smooth muscle from animal species other than the guinea pig and ferret (93). In ferrets, BK-induced tracheal contraction was not influenced by the epithelium (42), whereas in guinea pigs, this peptide was a relaxant agonist in epithelium-intact trachea and a spasmogen after epithelium removal (94,95). This epithelium-dependent relaxation was mediated by PGE$_2$ (94,95). BK also may modulate indirectly cholinergic neurotransmission in canine airways via the release of PGE$_2$ from the epithelium (96).

Tachykinins

Airway tachykinins include substance P (SP), neurokinin A (NKA), and neurokinin B (NKB). Tachykinin-induced responses in guinea pig trachea are powerfully modified by the epithelium because it provides a major source of NEP and perhaps because of the release of an inhibitory substance(s). Accordingly, epithelial removal has been shown to increase the spasmogenic potency of SP in this tissue by 20- to 150-fold and significantly increased the maximum response (97–99). Inhibitors of NEP such as phosphoramidon mimicked the effects of epithelium removal (97,98,100,101). Indomethacin did not significantly modify this enhancement, although the NEP inhibitor phosphoramidon reduced this from 20- to 150-fold to 18-fold, suggesting that the residual potency increase was due to the effect of a nonprostanoid inhibitory substance (98). Epithelium removal also increased the potency of SP in ferret tracheal (100) and human bronchial preparations, but only by about eight-fold (102). Although inhibition of NEP in human bronchus abolished the effect of epithelium removal on sensitivity to SP, epithelium removal still increased the sensitivity to NKA in the presence of phosphoramidon (102), suggesting that for NKA another inhibitory mechanism also was involved.

Endothelin-1

The endothelins (ETs) also are substrates for NEP (103). The spasmogenic effect of ET-1 in isolated airway smooth muscle (104) was enhanced by removing the epithelium (105), presumably because of the removal of epithelial NEP (106), because this effect was abolished in the presence of phosphoramidon (105). Inhibitors of epithelium-derived prostaglandin production, angiotensin-converting enzyme, endopeptidase, or aminopeptidase had little effect on the potentiating influence of epithelium removal (105).

Nerve-induced Responses

Reports concerning the effects of epithelium removal on the neuronal release of [^{3}H]-ACh in response to electrical field stimulation (EFS) have been conflicting, with some demonstrating increases in release (95) and others showing only small increases (65) or no effect (62). Although epithelium removal had little effect on EFS-induced responses in bovine-isolated trachea (59), this pretreatment did reverse the fade in responses usually seen in dog bronchus, suggesting the absence of an inhibitory modulator of airway tone (56). Similar data in ferret trachea (107) indicated the release of both prostanoid and nonprostanoid inhibitory factors from the epithelium in response to vagus nerve stimulation (107). However, the picture in porcine bronchial smooth muscle preparations is starkly different, because epithelium removal inhibited the frequency-response relationship (70). Interestingly, in guinea pig trachea, removal of epithelium resulted in a small potentiation of excitatory noncholinergic, nonadrenergic (eNANC) responses, but this was probably due to the loss of epithelial NEP (101).

Electrophysiologic and functional analyses suggested the presence of two epithelium-derived factors that modulate neurotransmission and tone in canine airway smooth muscle: an inhibitory hyperpolarizing factor (EpDHF) that is released continuously and another inhibitory substance that appears to be a 5-lipoxygenase product released in response to EFS (108).

Relaxant Agonists

Results from investigations of the influence of the epithelium on *in vitro* airway smooth muscle responses to isoprenaline and related β-adrenoceptor agonists have been contradictory. For example, in guinea pig trachea epithelial stripping had no significant influence on potency, but caused a reduction in maximal relaxant response (E_{max}) (64), as also seen in canine (56,109) and porcine airways (70). Interestingly, in canine bronchial preparations, this effect increased with decreasing airway diameter, suggesting an increasingly important modulatory role for this tissue down the respiratory tract (69). Epithelium removal had no effect or caused a small decrease in isoprenaline potency in bovine tracheal (59) and human bronchial preparations (80). However, these data stand in contrast to reports that the guinea pig tracheal epithelium can act as an extraneuronal uptake compartment for catecholamines such as isoprenaline (51). Inhibition of uptake at this site caused potentiation of relaxant responses to this amine, but predictably had little influence on responsiveness to the noncatecholamine β-agonists terbutaline or salbutamol (51), or on the non-β-adrenoceptor relaxants theophylline, enprophylline (110), and nitroglycerine (64).

Airway smooth muscle relaxant responses to exogenously applied VIP, a peptide that, along with nitric oxide, may be a neurotransmitter or modulate neurotransmission in the inhibitory(i)-NANC nervous system in airways from animal species (111–113), are also potentiated by epithelium removal in the guinea pig (48) and in human bronchus (114). Similarly, airway smooth muscle relaxation to atrial natriuretic peptide (ANP) was markedly potentiated in epithelium-denuded preparations (115). As in the case of the tachykinins and endothelin, these effects were primarily due to the removal of epithelial NEP (115, 116). Importantly, the possibility of the release of an epithelium-derived inhibitory factor arises from data demonstrating a tetrodotoxin-resistant component in the iNANC relaxation to EFS (116).

Clearly, then, epithelium removal has a powerful influence on the sensitivity of underlying airway smooth muscle to various spasmogens. In some cases, this influence is to act primarily as a site of loss of the agonist from the biophase. In others, however, the mechanism of the protection is much less clear. In some cases, agonists may induce the release of inhibitory mediator(s) that have become known as epithelium-derived inhibitory factors (EpDIF).

EPITHELIUM-DERIVED MEDIATORS

The epithelium is a source of a wide range of mediator substances (Fig. 3). No attempt will be made here to discuss all these. Rather, the focus will be on those epithelium-derived substances that are perhaps most likely to alter airway smooth muscle tone directly or indirectly. In the first instance, it is important to recognize that the airway epithelium is a significant source of both potentially spasmogenic and spasmolytic products.

Epithelium-Derived Spasmogens

Lipoxygenase Products

There is convincing evidence that the LTs, particularly the CysLTs, have a significant role to play in bronchial asthma. Certainly, the CysLTs mimic many of the features of the disease. They are approximately 1,000 times more potent than histamine in causing bronchoconstriction in human airways *in vitro* and *in vivo* (117,118). In addition, they potently stimulate mucous secretion from human airways *in vitro* (118) and increase microvascular permeability (119,120). These actions are consistent with airway obstruction resulting from mucous plugging, edema, and airway smooth muscle contraction, which are characteristic of this inflammatory airway disease (121).

The 15-lipoxygenase pathway is predominant in human bronchial epithelium (122,123), whereas the 12-lipoxygenase pathway predominates in bovine epithelium (124). The 12-lipoxygenase pathway is the major route for arachidonic acid conversion to LTs in canine and

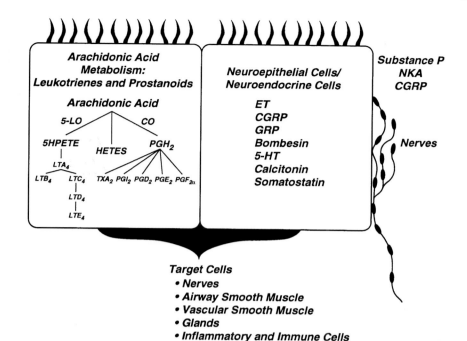

FIG. 3. Mediators released from airway epithelium.

sheep cells (123,125), although low levels of 5-lipoxygenase, which catalyze the synthesis of the CysLTs, LTC$_4$, LTD$_4$, and LTE$_4$, as well as the potent chemotactic factor LTB$_4$, also have been detected in canine (125) and sheep epithelial cells (123).

PAF has been shown to stimulate the release of 15-hydroxyeicosatetraenoic acid (15-HETE) from cultured human bronchial epithelial cells in sufficient quantities to induce contraction of airway smooth muscle (126). In addition, PAF caused the release of significant amounts of LTC$_4$ and LTD$_4$ from rabbit tracheal explants (127). Consistent with the predominance of the 5-lipoxygenase pathway in human epithelium, the 15-HETEs are the major metabolites released cultured human epithelial cells in response to arachidonic acid, PAF, BK, and ACh (126, 128,129).

Cyclooxygenase Products

Arachidonic acid, which relaxed guinea pig (130) and canine (131) airway smooth muscle with an intact epithelium, caused contraction in epithelium-denuded preparations (130). PGE$_2$ and PGF$_2$ are the major arachidonic acid metabolites released from human and animal primary tracheal epithelial cultures (55,132,133). Mechanical disruption of the guinea pig tracheal epithelium also caused the release of both PGE$_2$ and PGF$_2$ (55,133). Importantly, the contractile response of guinea pig tracheal preparations to histamine and serotonin (5-HT) were inhibited in the presence of a cyclooxygenase inhibitor (55,

78). Bioassay of the supernatant from guinea pig cultured tracheal epithelial cells revealed a contractile substance that appeared to be a prostanoid (134). In addition, nerve stimulation appeared to release prostanoid and nonprostanoid inhibitory factors from ferret trachea (135).

Histamine

Mast cells constitute the major storage site for histamine in the airways. These cells are found in the epithelium, mucosa, and submucosa near blood vessels (13). H$_1$-receptor activation mediates histamine-induced bronchospasm, i.e., airway smooth muscle contraction in humans and in most animal species (136,137). In addition, histamine is an important mediator of increased airway microvascular permeability, a response caused by endothelial cell contraction and intercellular gap formation (138,139), leading to the promotion of mucosal edema (140). Whereas histamine H$_2$-receptors can mediate bronchial smooth muscle relaxation in the rat, rabbit, cat, and sheep, this is not seen in the pig, goat, calf, horse, or human (137,141).

H$_3$-receptors also mediate inhibition of cholinergic neurotransmission in human (142) and guinea pig (143) airways and inhibition of excitatory nonadrenergic, noncholinergic (eNANC) neural bronchoconstriction in the guinea pig (144). In addition, these receptors have been reported to inhibit neurogenic airway microvascular leakage (145) and to reduce histamine release from mast cells (146).

Endothelin-1

It is now well established that in addition to vascular endothelium, the endogenous peptide endothelin-1 (ET-1) is synthesized in the bronchial epithelium (147,148). A range of ET-1s pharmacologic effects in the airways suggest a mediator role for this peptide in bronchial asthma. These include the fact that ET-1 is a potent spasmogen in human bronchial smooth muscle (104,149), accelerates the growth of airway smooth muscle cells in culture (150), and stimulates mucous gland secretion (151), responses that are highly relevant to the established pathology of this disease (152). Importantly, levels of ET-like immunoreactive material are significantly elevated in the bronchial epithelium (147) and bronchoalveolar lavage (BAL) fluid of asthmatics (153). Although little immunoreactivity for ET-1 has been detected in basal or ciliated epithelial cells (154), immunoreactive ET has also been shown to be released from human bronchial (155), canine (156), and guinea pig (157) tracheal epithelium. In addition, ET-like immunoreactivity has been demonstrated in bronchiolar epithelial cells *in vivo* in rats and mice and in mucous, serous, and Clara cells (154).

It is noteworthy that low concentrations of ET-1 caused marked potentiation of cholinergic nerve-mediated contraction of airway smooth muscle from the mouse (158) and ET-3 had a similar effect in rabbit bronchus (159). This is potentially a most important amplifier action on this dominant neural bronchoconstrictor mechanism. Presumably, the physiologic role of epithelium-derived ET-1 is primarily in tissue repair and regeneration; this peptide also may be involved in the maintenance of airway smooth muscle tone. However, in asthma, which involves airway inflammation and the production of greater than usual amounts of ET-1, pathologic responses including airway smooth muscle hyperplasia, mucous gland hyperplasia and hypersecretion, and excessive airway smooth muscle contraction may be induced.

Tachykinins

In the pulmonary system, these peptides are found in capsaicin-sensitive peripheral unmyelinated branches of primary afferent neurons, also known as sensory C-fibers, which are located in the airway epithelium, blood vessels associated with several ganglia, mucous glands, and airway smooth muscle (160,161). The NK_2 receptor mediates contraction of isolated airway smooth muscle from several animal species as well as from humans (102,162). In addition, tachykinins such as SP also appear to be responsible for excitatory nonadrenergic, noncholinergic (eNANC) bronchoconstriction (163,164) and induce mucous secretion (21,165). Neurogenically induced airway microvascular permeability increases are also the result of the actions of neurokinins (166,167). These effects are also potentially relevant to the pathology of bronchial asthma, where SP may play a role via an axon reflex, excessively activated as a result of epithelial damage that exposes sensory afferent nerves that can then be activated by proinflammatory substances such as BK or CysLTs (21, 168,169). Furthermore, an epithelium-derived contractile factor has been reported in response to calcitonin gene-related peptide (CGRP) in guinea pig isolated trachea (170). In addition, the epithelium may be a source of CGRP in response to the calcium ionophore A23188 (171).

Epithelium-Derived Relaxants

Cyclooxygenase Products

In 1975, Orehek et al. (55) were the first to demonstrate the potential modulatory influence of the epithelium on the level of tone in airway smooth. They showed that disruption of the mucosal surface of the guinea pig trachea stimulated the release of relaxant prostaglandins, suggesting that such local release might play an important role in the regulation of airway smooth muscle tone (55). It has since been shown that PGF_2, which caused contraction in guinea pig trachea in the absence of basal tone, may be responsible in part for intrinsic airway smooth muscle tone (134,172).

A range of mediators have now been shown to promote the generation and release of epithelium-derived prostaglandins. For example, SP caused relaxation of precontracted rat trachea, a response that is epithelium-dependent and indomethacin-sensitive (172,173). Furthermore, PGE_2 release from canine tracheal epithelium has been reported in response to BK (174). In addition, BK and the calcium ionophore A23187 have been shown to cause PGE_2 release from airway epithelial cultures of the dog (175), rabbit, and rat (176).

Nitric Oxide

Current evidence suggests that nitric oxide (NO) is a primary mediator of iNANC neurotransmission in human airways (172,173,177), although VIP also may be a significant iNANC mediator in animal airways (112). The airway epithelium contains NO synthase (NOS) (178), raising the possibility that NO also may modulate airway smooth muscle tone. This concept is supported by data from the guinea pig showing that ET-1 can cause relaxation of precontracted isolated tracheal smooth muscle, a response that was apparently mediated by epithelium-derived NO (179). Furthermore, inhibition of NOS was shown to cause AHR to histamine in this species (180).

The activity of the inducible form NO synthase can be elevated in the airways by endotoxin (181) and by cytokines including tumor necrosis factor (TNF) (182). This increased expression of NO synthase has been shown to occur in the bronchial epithelium in asthma (182), such that raised levels of NO can be detected in the expired air (183). However, rather than mediating a potentially beneficial bronchodilator response, NO in asthma may be primarily associated with tissue damage (184), and may be a useful marker of bronchial inflammation (183,185).

EPITHELIUM-DERIVED INHIBITORY FACTOR

There appears to be a basal release from the airway epithelium of both relaxant and spasmogenic substances that diffuse to the underlying airway smooth muscle to directly influence tone. In addition, various chemical stimuli can promote the synthesis and release of substances from the epithelium that might subsequently alter the state of airway smooth muscle contraction. This section will address the possibility that the epithelium can release spontaneously and in response to chemical stimulation, factors that can modulate airway smooth muscle responsiveness to agonists. In particular, the case for and against an epithelium-derived inhibitory factor (EpDIF) released by airway spasmogens will be reviewed.

Epithelium-Derived Inhibitory Factor: Fact or Fiction?

As previously discussed, it is established that EpDIF (or EpDRF) exists in the form of known mediators such as PGE$_2$ and NO, which are released spontaneously in response to various chemical stimuli. Spasmogenic mediators also can be derived from the airway epithelium, such as that reported to contract airway smooth muscle (134) and to augment contractile responses to neuronally released ACh (70). Perhaps most importantly, the epithelium also might release a nonprostanoid EpDIF. This was suggested by Flavahan et al. (56) and by Barnes and co-workers (59), who described epithelium-dependent enhancement of histamine-induced airway contraction *in vitro*. Subsequently, a great deal of effort was directed at verifying these data and at identifying the EpDIF. The characterization of EpDIF has proven to be difficult, with the existence of a nonprostanoid EpDIF remaining controversial.

There can be no doubt that epithelial ablation results in modest increases in the potencies and/or maximal effect of various spasmogens of airway smooth muscle (Fig. 3). It is possible that these data are the result of the removal of a critical barrier to agonist diffusion rather than to the absence of an important inhibitory mediator acting as a functional antagonist to contraction. However, if this were so, an increase in the rate of response to agents that are not subject to degradation would be expected, rather than the observed alteration to the sensitivity or magnitude of equilibrium responses. It is also important to note that in isolated airway preparations in which airway smooth muscle tension changes are assessed in a bathing medium, agonists have access to the submucosa from all sides. This reduces the effectiveness of the epithelium as a barrier to agonist diffusion to airway smooth muscle. The argument for a barrier role for the epithelium also does not seem to be appropriate in the case of enhanced contractions to electrical stimulation of intramural cholinergic nerves in epithelium-denuded airway preparations (56,107).

Another powerful argument in support of the existence of a nonprostanoid EpDIF is the fact that epithelial ablation potentiates responses to some but not all airway spasmogens, i.e., the effects of epithelium removal are selective. Thus, contraction of airway preparations to carbachol are not significantly altered by epithelial denudation, whereas the potencies of methacholine and bethanechol have consistently been shown to be significantly increased (64,68). Such a profile is more in line with the stimulation of EpDIF release by only some agonists, rather than with differences in agonist permeation rates or metabolism.

Superfusion Bioassay

Among the most convincing evidence for the existence of a nonprostanoid EpDIF would be that provided by direct superfusion bioassay. However, relatively little evidence has been forthcoming from such studies. Indeed, Holroyde (62) and Undem et al. (89) tried unsuccessfully to detect such a mediator in superfusion cascade systems, although Vanhoutte (186) was able to provide limited preliminary evidence for the release and transfer of an effective epithelium-derived relaxant of canine airway smooth muscle.

Co-axial Bioassay

Currently, the most convincing evidence for a nonprostanoid EpDIF has come from experiments using co-axial bioassay techniques (Fig. 4). However, these involved both vascular and nonvascular smooth muscle (187–190). In these systems, an endothelium-denuded vascular smooth muscle preparation (e.g., rat aorta) was used as the assay tissue, suspended in the long axis for tension measurement within an epithelium-intact guinea pig tracheal tube preparation, which was acting as an EpDIF donor. These assemblies were stimulated with histamine and other agonists that do not contract such vessels in the hope that they might stimulate the release of EpDIF from the airway, causing vascular relaxation (57, 71,189,191). In these cases, apparently clear evidence for the release of an EpDIF was observed in the form of relaxations of the vascular smooth muscle. However, it is important to note that these studies did not provide evidence for an EpDIF that was active in airway smooth

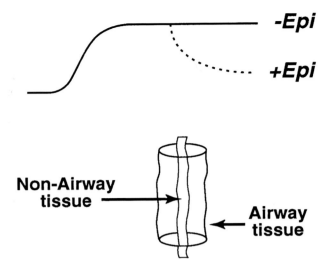

FIG. 4. Co-axial system for examining the effects of epithelium-derived inhibitory substances on nonairway smooth muscle responsiveness (relaxation).

muscle. Indeed, relaxations were not seen in co-axial assemblies that used airway smooth muscle as the assay tissue (191). Thus, whereas these data apparently establish the release of a nonprostanoid inhibitory factor from the airway epithelium, it seems unlikely that it is responsible for the suppression of spasmogen potency seen in epithelium-intact airway preparations.

It is also clear that care must be taken when interpreting the data from co-axial bioassay studies of this kind. A component of the airway epithelium–dependent vascular relaxation seen in co-axial assemblies may be related to luminal hypoxia resulting from the epithelial uptake of oxygen and exacerbated by airway tube constriction, rather than to the release of an inhibitory factor (192). Despite this cautionary note, other pharmacologic and biochemical evidence is at odds with the concept of a significant role for hypoxia in these systems (193,194). For example, not all airway smooth muscle spasmogens induce relaxation of rat aorta in co-axial bioassay experiments (71), suggesting that hypoxia cannot explain all the relaxant activity observed.

Perfused Airway Tube Preparations

Experiments using perfused whole trachea from guinea pigs have provided further indirect evidence for a nonprostanoid EpDIF. Although convincing data for the production and transfer of an EpDIF capable of relaxing airway smooth muscle was lacking from superfusion cascade assays, Munakata and co-workers (195) elegantly demonstrated epithelium-dependent airway smooth muscle relaxation in response to osmotic stimuli in a perfused tracheal preparation, consistent with the release of a nonprostanoid EpDIF.

Several studies have provided evidence in support of a dominant role for the epithelium as a diffusion barrier in the modulation of responsiveness to airway agonists. For example, a significant diffusion barrier role for the epithelium in guinea pig trachea was suggested by studies showing that epithelium removal had a marked effect on responses to mucosally applied ACh or histamine, whereas no response modulation was observed on adventitial application (34). However, the data have not been consistent in studies from different laboratories. Some studies have demonstrated a much greater influence of the epithelium on the potency of luminally (mucosal side) applied agonists than on serosally (adventitial side) applied agonists, suggesting a substantial diffusion barrier role for the epithelium (66,196), whereas others found minimal differences (33). Despite this, a growing body of evidence indicates that the airway epithelium does have a marked diffusion barrier capability against mucosally applied spasmogens in perfused airway tube preparations where the potency of mucosally applied ACh can be increased by 30- to 100-fold after epithelium removal (197–199). It would seem from this that the diffusion barrier role played by the airway epithelium is of considerably greater importance than is the influence of putative EpDIFs, with respect to altering spasmogen potency. However, the lesser potencies of luminally applied than of serosally applied spasmogens may be in part due to EpDIF release preceding contraction on luminal administration. Serosal application would allow contraction to occur largely in the absence of EpDIF release.

Although initial focus was on the potential modulatory effects of EpDIFs on airway smooth muscle, the influence on vascular smooth muscle appears to be more

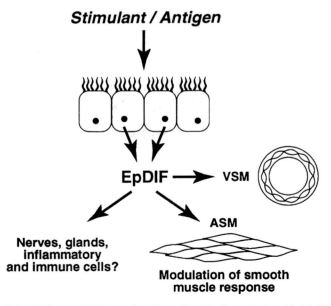

FIG. 5. Potential sites of action of epithelium-derived inhibitory factor (EpDIF).

prominent. Consideration should be given to potential effects of epithelium-derived substances on other effector cells, such as nerves, mucous glands, and immune and inflammatory cells (Fig. 5).

IDENTITY OF EPITHELIUM-DERIVED INHIBITORY FACTOR

As indicated in previous sections, there is evidence for several inhibitory factors derived from the epithelium. These include prostanoid (e.g., PGE_2 and PGI_2) and nonprostanoid EpDIFs and an unidentified EpDHF (Fig. 6). The first is detectable in co-axial bioassay systems and apparently is selective for vascular smooth muscle. This substance may modulate the activity of ingested chemical stimuli at airway smooth muscle by increasing the volume of the airway microvascular sink for their removal (191,200). Indeed, it has been established that a substance is released from the airway epithelium in co-axial assemblies that increases intracellular guanosine 3′,5′-cyclic monophosphate (cGMP) in rat aorta tissue that is acting as the assay preparation (193). Atrial natriuretic peptide (ANP) also stimulates the production of intracellular cGMP, as does NO. However, EpDIF is neither of these substances because, since unlike EpDIF, ANP relaxes airway smooth muscle (116,201) and NO has previously been ruled out as a candidate (71,202). The second might be selective for airway smooth muscle (71,186). However, the identities of these putative substances remain unknown.

CONCLUSIONS

There can be little doubt that damage to the airway epithelium, whether it is deliberately induced in experimental systems or is the result of pathologic events associated with airway disease such as asthma, has a significant influence on the responsiveness and sensitivity of underlying airway smooth muscle. In the case of many airway spasmogens, this is to enhance potency and/or maximal effect. This modulatory influence of the epithelium can occur via various mechanisms. For example, for peptide mediators such as ET-1 and the tachykinins, it is clear that the epithelium modulates tissue response primarily by acting as a site of metabolism for these mediators, via the activity of NEP. However, for cholinergic agonists, histamine, the CysLTs, and others, the loss of epithelial degradative enzymes does not seem to account adequately for the increases in agonist potency and maximal effect commonly observed in a range of model airway systems. This has led to the concept of the release of functionally antagonistic EpDIF(s), which include inhibitory prostanoids. Importantly, tantalizing evidence exists for the release of a nonprostanoid EpDIF, the identity of which remains unknown. Nevertheless, modulatory influences of prostanoid and nonprostanoid EpDIFs are unlikely to appear to be major compared with the significant barrier functions of the epithelium. Thus, the epithelium limits access of airborne allergens and so forth to underlying airway smooth muscle, blood vessels, nerve fibers, and mucous glands that play a critical part in normal and abnormal physiologic and pathophysiologic processes in the lung.

ACKNOWLEDGMENT

Roy G. Goldie is a Senior Principal Research Fellow with the National Health and Medical Research Council in Australia.

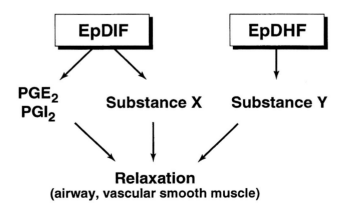

FIG. 6. Potential prostanoid and nonprostanoid epithelium-derived inhibitory substances.

REFERENCES

1. Goldie RG. Control of airway smooth muscle contractility. In: Pauwels R, Advenier C, O'Byrne PM, eds. *Anti-asthmatic drugs.* Basel: Karger, 1996 (*in press*).
2. Goldie RG, Preuss JMH. Epithelial function and airway responsiveness. In: Stewart AG, ed. *Airway remodeling in the pathogenesis of asthma.* Boston: CRC Press Inc, 1996;139–178.
3. Palmer RMJ, Ferridge AG, Moncada S. Nitric oxide release accounts for the biological activity of endothelium-derived rlaxing factor. *Nature* 1987;327:524–526.
4. Hogg JC, Eggleston PA. Is asthma an epithelial disease? *Am Rev Respir Dis* 1984;129:207–208.
5. O'Byrne PM, Dolovich M, Dirks R, Roberts RS, Newhouse MT. Lung epithelial permeability: relation to nonspecific airway responsiveness. *J Appl Physiol* 1984;57:177–183.
6. Ilowite JS, Bennett WD, Sheetz MS, Groth ML, Nierman DM. Permeability of the bronchial mucosa to ^{99m}Tc-DPTA in asthma. *Am Rev Respir Dis* 1989;139:1139–1143.
7. Elwood RK, Kennedy S, Belzberg A, Hogg JC, Paré PD. Respiratory mucosal permeability in asthma. *Am Rev Respir Dis* 1983;128:523–527.
8. Hulbert WC, McLean H, Hogg JC. The effect of acute airway inflammation on bronchial reactivity in guinea pigs. *Am Rev Respir Dis* 1985;132:7–11.
9. Hulbert WC, Walker DC, Jackson A, Hogg JC. Airway permeability to horseradish peroxidase in guinea pigs: the repair phase after injury by cigarette smoke. *Am Rev Respir Dis* 1981;123:320–326.
10. Jeffery PK, Wardlaw AJ, Nelson FC, Collins JV, Kay AB. Bronchial

biopsies in asthma. An ultrastructural, quantitative study and correlation with hyperreactivity. *Am Rev Respir Dis* 1989;140:1745–1753.

11. Laitinen LA, Heino M, Laitinen A, Kava T, Haahtela T. Damage of the airway epithelium and bronchial reactivity in patients with asthma. *Am Rev Respir Dis* 1985;131:599–606.

12. Beasley R, Roche WR, Roberts JA, Holgate ST. Cellular events in the bronchi in mild asthma and after bronchial provocation. *Am Rev Respir Dis* 1989;139:806–817.

13. Cutz E, Levison H, Cooper DM. Ultrastructure of airways in children with asthma. *Histopathology* 1978;2:407–421.

14. Horn BR, Robin ED, Theodore JA, Van Kessel A. Total eosinophil counts in the management of bronchial asthma. *N Engl J Med* 1975; 292:1152–1155.

15. Laitinen LA, Heino M, Laitinen A, Kava T, Haahtela T. Damage of the airway epithelium and bronchial reactivity in patients with asthma. *Am Rev Respir Dis* 1985;131:599–606.

16. Motojima S, Frigas E, Loegering DA, Gleich GJ. Toxicity of eosinophil cationic proteins for guinea pig tracheal epithelium *in vitro. Am Rev Respir Dis* 1989;39:801–805.

17. Brofman JD, White SR, Blake JS, Munoz NM, Gleich GJ, Leff AR. Epithelial augmentation of trachealis contraction caused by major basic protein of eosinophils. *J Appl Physiol* 1989;66:1867–1873.

18. Flavahan NA, Slifman NR, Gleich GJ, Vanhoutte PM. Human eosinophil major basic protein causes hyperreactivity of respiratory smooth muscle. *Am Rev Respir Dis* 1988;138:685–688.

19. Lozewicz S, Wells C, Gomez E, et al. Morphological integrity of the bronchial epithelium in mild asthma. *Thorax* 1990;45:12–15.

20. Sant Ambrogio G. Information arising from the tracheobronchial trees of mammals. *Physiol Rev* 1982;62:531–569.

21. Barnes PJ. Asthma as an axon reflex. *Lancet* 1986;1:242–245.

22. Erdös EG, Skidgel RA. Neutral endopeptidase 24.11 (enkephalinase) and related regulators of peptide hormones. *FASEB J* 1989;3:145–151.

23. Heino M, Monkare S, Haahtela T, Laitinen LA. An electronmicroscopic study of the airways in patients with farmer's lung. *Eur J Respir Dis* 1982;36:52–61.

24. Hers JFPH. Disturbances of the ciliated epithelium due to influenza virus. *Am Rev Respir Dis* 1966;93:162–171.

25. Holtzman MJ, Fabbri LM, O Byrne PM. Importance of airway inflammation for hyperresponsiveness induced by ozone. *Am Rev Respir Dis* 1983;127:686–690.

26. Mapp CE, Polato R, Maestrelli P, Hendrick DJ, Fabbri LM. Time course of the increase in airway responsiveness associated with late asthmatic reactions to toluene diisocyanate in sensitized subjects. *J Allergy Clin Immunol* 1985; 5:568–572.

27. Jeffery PK, Wardlaw AJ, Nelson FC, Collins JV, Kay AB. Bronchial biopsies in asthma. An ultrastructural, quantitative study and correlation with hyperreactivity. *Am Rev Respir Dis*, 1989;140:1745–1753.

28. Holtzman MJ. Inflammation of the airway epithelium and the development of airway hyperresponsiveness. In: Herzog H. Perruchoud AP, eds. *Progress in respiratory research, asthma and bronchial hyperreactivity*. Basel: S Karger, 1985;165–172.

29. Breeze RG, Wheeldon EB. The cells of the pulmonary airways. *Am Rev Respir Dis* 1977;116:705–777.

30. Gumbiner B. Structure, biochemistry and assembly of epithelial tight junctions. *Am J Physiol* 1987;253:C749–C758.

31. Sparrow MP, Mitchell HW. Modulation by the epithelium of the extent of bronchial narrowing produced by substances perfused through the lumen. *Br J Pharmacol* 1991;103:1160–1164.

32. Munakata M, Huang I, Mitzner W, Menkes H. Protective role of epithelium in the guinea pig airway. *J Appl Physiol* 1989;66:1547–1552.

33. Pavlovic D, Fournier M, Aubier M, Pariente R. Epithelial vs. serosal stimulation of tracheal muscle: role of epithelium. *J Appl Physiol* 1989;67:2522–2526.

34. Iriarte CF, Pascual R, Villanueva MM, Román M, Cortijo J, Morcillo EJ. Role of epithelium in agonist-induced contractile responses of guinea pig trachealis: influence of the surface through which drug enters the tissue. *Br J Pharmacol* 1990;101:257– 262.

35. Omari TI Sparrow MP. Epithelial disruption by proteases augments the responsiveness of porcine bronchial segments. *Clin Exp Pharmacol Physiol* 1992;19:785–794.

36. Mayrhofer G. Epithelial disposition of antigen. In: Goldie RG ed. *Immunopharmacology of epithelial barriers*. London: Academic Press Ltd, 1994;19–70.

37. Breeze RG, Turk M. Cellular structure, function and organization in the lower respiratory tract. *Environ Health Perspect* 1984;55:3–24.

38. Basbaum CB, Finkbeiner WE. Mucus-producing cells of the airways. In: Masaro D, ed. *Lung cell biology*. New York: Marcel Dekker, 1989; 37–79.

39. Gundel RH, Letts, LG. Adhesion molecules and the modulation of mucosal inflammation. In: Goldie RG, ed. *Immunopharmacology of epithelial barriers*. London: Academic Press Ltd, 1994;71–84.

40. Sertl K, Takemura T, Tschachler E, Ferrans VJ, Kaliner MA, Shevach EM. Dendritic cells with antigen-presenting capability reside in airway epithelium, lung parenchyma, and visceral pleura. *J Exp Med* 1986;163:436–451.

41. Sekizawa K, Tamaoki J, Graf PD, Basbaum CB, Borson DB, Nadel JA Enkephalinase inhibitor potentiates mammalian tachykinin-induced contraction in ferret trachea. *J Pharmacol Exp Ther* 1987;243:1211–1217.

42. Dusser DJ, Nadel JA, Sekizawa K, Graf PD, Borson DB. Neutral endopeptidase and angiotensin converting enzyme inhibitors potentiate kinin-induced contraction of ferret trachea. *J Pharmacol Exp Ther* 1988;244:531–536.

43. Said SI. Effector actions: influence of neuropeptides on airway smooth muscle. *Am Rev Respir Dis* 1987;136:S52–S58.

44. Hay DWP. guinea pig tracheal epithelium and endothelin. *Eur J Pharmacol* 1989;171:241–245.

45. Frossard N, Stretton CD, Barnes PJ. Modulation of bradykinin responses in airway smooth muscle epithelial forks. *Agents Actions* 1990;31:204–209.

46. DeVillier P, Advenier C, Drapeau G, Marsac J, Regoli D. Comparison of the effects of epithelium removal and of an enkephalinase inhibitor on the neurokinin-induced contractions of guinea pig trachea. *Br J Pharmacol* 1988;94:675–684.

47. Fernandes LB, Preuss JMH, Goldie RG. Epithelial modulation of the relaxant activity of atriopeptides in rat and guinea pig tracheal smooth muscle. *Eur J Pharmacol* 1992;212:187–194.

48. Farmer SG, Togo J. Effect of epithelium removal on relaxation of airway smooth muscle induced by vasoactive intestinal peptide and electrical field stimulation. *Br J Pharmacol* 1990;100:73–78.

49. Yamauchi K, Nakazawa H, Sekizawa K, et al. The regulatory role of histamine-*N*-methyltransferase in allergic reactions in the human airways. *Am Rev Respir Dis* 1993;147:A431.

50. White MV, Slater JE, Kaliner MA. Histamine and asthma. *Am Rev Respir Dis* 1987;135:1165–1176.

51. Farmer SG, Fedan JS, Hay DWP, Raeburn D. The effects of epithelium removal on the sensitivity of guinea pig isolated trachealis to bronchodilator drugs. *Br J Pharmacol* 1986;89:407–414.

52. Advenier C, DeVillier P, Matran R, Naline E. Influence of epithelium on the responsiveness of guinea pig isolated trachea to adenosine. *Br J Pharmacol* 1988;93:295–302.

53. Jones KG, Holland JR, Foureman GL, Bend JR, Fouts JR. Xenobiotic metabolism in Clara cells and alveolar type II cells isolated from lungs of rats treated with -naphthoflavone. *J Pharmacol Exp Ther* 1983;225:316–319.

54. Widdicombe JG, Pack RJ. The Clara cell. *Eur J Respir Dis* 1982;63: 202–220.

55. Orehek J, Douglas JS, Bouhuys A. Contractile responses of the guinea pig trachea *in vitro*: modification by the prostaglandin synthesis inhibiting drugs. *J Pharmacol Exp Ther* 1975;194:554–564.

56. Flavahan NA, Aarhus LL, Rimele TJ, Vanhoutte PM. Respiratory epithelium inhibits bronchial smooth muscle tone. *J Appl Physiol* 1985; 58:834–838.

57. Goldie RG, Fernandes LB, Farmer SG, Hay DWP. Airway epithelium-derived inhibitory factor. *Trends Pharmacol Sci* 1990;11:67–70.

58. Hay DWP, Farmer SG, Goldie RG. Inflammatory mediators and modulation of epithelial/smooth muscle interactions. In: Goldie R, ed. *Immunopharmacology of epithelial barriers*. London: Academic Press, 1994;119–146.

59. Barnes PJ, Cuss FM, Palmer JB. The effect of airway epithelium on smooth muscle contractility in bovine trachea. *Br J Pharmacol* 1985; 86:685–691.

60. Gao Y, Vanhoutte PM. Removal of the epithelium potentiates acetylcholine in depolarizing canine bronchial smooth muscle. *J Appl Physiol* 1988;65:2400–2405.

61. Raeburn D, Hay DWP, Robinson VA, Farmer SG, Fleming WW, Fedan JS. The effect of verapamil is reduced in isolated airways smooth muscle preparations lacking an epithelium. *Life Sci* 1986;38:809–816.

62. Holroyde MC. The influence of epithelium on the responsiveness of guinea pig isolated trachea. *Br J Pharmacol* 1986;87:501–507.

63. Hay DWP, Farmer SG, Raeburn D, Robinson VA, Fleming WW, Fedan JS. Airway epithelium modulates the reactivity of guinea pig respiratory smooth muscle. *Eur J Pharmacol* 1986;129:11–18.

64. Goldie RG, Papadimitriou JM, Paterson JW, Rigby PJ, Self HM, Spina D. Influence of the epithelium on responsiveness of guinea pig isolated trachea to contractile and relaxant agonists. *Br J Pharmacol* 1986;87:5–14.

65. Murlas C. Effects of mucosal removal on guinea pig airway smooth muscle responsiveness. *Clin Sci* 1986;70:571–575.

66. Preuss JMH, Henry PJ, Goldie RG. Influence of age on epithelium-dependent responsiveness of guinea pig and rat tracheal smooth muscle to spasmogens. *Eur J Pharmacol* 1992;228:3–8.

67. Small RC, Good DM, Dixon JS, Kennedy I. The effects of epithelium on the actions of cholinomimetic drugs in opened segments and perfused tubular preparations of guinea pig trachea. *Br J Pharmacol* 1990;100:516–522.

68. Morrison KJ, Vanhoutte PM. Characterization of muscarinic receptors that mediate contraction of guinea pig isolated trachea to choline esters: effect of removing epithelium. *Br J Pharmacol* 1992;106:672–676.

69. Stuart-Smith K, Vanhoutte PM. Heterogeneity in the effects of epithelium removal in the canine bronchial tree. *J Appl Physiol* 1987;63:2150–2115.

70. Stuart-Smith K, Vanhoutte PM. Airway epithelium modulates the responsiveness of porcine bronchial smooth muscle. *J Appl Physiol* 1988;65:721–727.

71. Fernandes LB, Preuss JMH, Paterson JW, Goldie RG. Epithelium-derived inhibitory factor in human bronchus. *Eur J Pharmacol* 1990;187:331–336.

72. Knight DA, Adcock JA, Phillips MJ, Thompson PJ. The effect of epithelium removal on human bronchial smooth muscle responsiveness to acetylcholine and histamine. *Pulm Pharmacol* 1990;3:198–202.

73. Jongejan R, De Jongste J, Raatgeep R, Stijnen T, Bonta I, Kerrebijn K. Effect of epithelial denudation, inflammatory mediators and mast cell activation on the sensitivity of isolated human airways to methacholine. *Eur J Pharmacol* 1991;203:187–194.

74. Eglen RM, Harris GC, Taylor M, Pfister JR, Whiting RL. Characterization of muscarinic receptors mediating release of epithelial derived relaxant factor (EpDRF) in guinea pig isolated trachea. *Naunyn Schmiedebergs Arch Pharmacol* 1991;344:29–35.

75. Koga Y, Satoh S, Sodeyama N, et al. Role of acetylcholinesteras in airway epithelium-mediated inhibition of acetylcholine-induced contraction of guinea pig isolated trachea. *Eur J Pharmacol* 1992;141:141–146.

76. Prié S, Cadieux A, Sirois P. Removal of guinea pig bronchial and tracheal epithelium potentiates the contractions to leukotrienes and histamine. *Eicosanoids* 1990;3:29–37.

77. Manning PJ, Jones GL, Otis J, Daniel EE, O'Byrne PM. The inhibitory influence of tracheal mucosa mounted in close proximity to canine trachealis. *Eur J Pharmacol* 1990;178:85–89.

78. Braunstein G, Labat C, Brunelleschi S, Benveniste J, Marsac J, Brink C. Evidence that the histamine sensitivity and responsiveness of guinea pig isolated trachea are modulated by epithelial prostaglandin E₂. *Br J Pharmacol* 1988;95:300–308.

79. Hay DWP, Muccitelli R, Horstmeyer DL, Raeburn D. Is the epithelium-derived inhibitory factor in guinea pig trachea a prostanoid? *Prostaglandins* 1988;35:625–636.

80. Aizawa H, Miyazaki N, Shigematsu N, Tomooka M. A possible role of airway epithelium in modulating hyperresponsiveness. *Br J Pharmacol* 1988;93:139–145.

81. Lindström EG, Andersson RGG, Granérus G, Grundström N. Is the airway epithelium responsible for histamine metabolism in the trachea of guinea pigs? *Agents Actions* 1991;33:1–2.

82. Güc MO, Ilhan M, Kayaalp SO. Epithelium-dependent relaxation of guinea pig tracheal smooth muscle by histamine: evidence for non-H₁- and non-H₂-histamine receptors. *Arch Int Pharmacodyn* 1988;296:57–65.

83. Hay DWP, Farmer SG, Raeburn D, Muccitelli RM, Wilson KA, Fedan JS. Differential effects of epithelium removal on the responsiveness of guinea pig tracheal smooth muscle to bronchoconstrictors. *Br J Pharmacol* 1987;92:381–388.

84. Hisayama T, Takayanagi I, Nakazato F, Hirano K. Epithelium selectively controls hypersensitization of the response of smooth muscle to leukotriene D₄ by endogenous prostanoid(s) in guinea pig trachea. *Naunyn Schmiedebergs Arch Pharmacol* 1988;337:296–300.

85. Bloomquist E, Kream RM. The mucosa mediates tachyphylaxis to leukotrienes C₄, D₄ and E₄ in guinea pig trachea. *Eur J Pharmacol* 1988;150:185–188.

86. Buckner DK, Fedyna JS, Robertson JL, et al. An examination of the influence of the epithelium on contractile responses to peptidoleukotrienes and blockade by ICI 204,219 in isolated guinea pig trachea and human intralobar airways. *J Pharmacol Exp Ther* 1990;252:77–85.

87. Adams GK, Lichtenstein L. *In vitro* studies of antigen-induced bronchospasm: effect of antihistamine and SRS-A antagonist on response of sensitized guinea pig and human airways to antigen. *J Immunol* 1979;122:555–562.

88. Hay DWP, Raeburn D, Farmer SG, Fleming WW, Fedan JS. Epithelium modulates the reactivity of ovalbumin-sensitized guinea pig airway smooth muscle. *Life Sci* 1986;38:2461–2468.

89. Undem BJ, Raible DG, Adkinson NF, Adams GK III. Effect of removal of epithelium on antigen-induced smooth muscle contraction and mediator release from guinea pig isolated trachea. *J Pharmacol Exp Ther*, 1988;244:659–665.

90. Egilmez Y, Ilhan M. Epithelial modulation of antigen–induced tracheal smooth muscle contractions in actively sensitized guinea pigs. *Arch Int Pharmacodyn* 1992;81:81–92.

91. Grundstrom N, Lindstrom EG, Axelsson KL, Andersson RGG. Epithelial modulation of allergen and drug effects in guinea pig airways. *J Appl Physiol* 1992;72:1953–1959.

92. Brunelleschi S, Haye-Legrand I, Labat C, Norel X, Benveniste J. Platelet activating actor-acether-induced relaxation of guinea pig airway muscle: role of prostaglandin E₂ and the epithelium. *J Pharmacol Exp Ther* 1987;243:356–363.

93. Farmer SG. Role of kinins in airway diseases. *Immunopharmacology* 1991;22:1–20.

94. Bramley AM, Samhoun MN, Piper PJ. The role of the epithelium in modulating the responses of guinea pig trachea induced by bradykinin *in vitro*. *Br J Pharmacol* 1990;99:762–766.

95. Farmer SG, Burch RM, Meeker SN, Wilkins DE. Evidence for a pulmonary bradykinin B₃ receptor. *Mol Pharmacol* 1989;36:1–8.

96. Liu MC, Bleecker ER, Lichtenstein LM, et al. Evidence for elevated levels of histamine, prostaglandin D₂, and other bronchoconstricting prostaglandins in the airways of subjects with mild asthma. *Am Rev Respir Dis* 1990;142:126–132.

97. DeVillier P, Advenier C, Drapeau G, Marsac J, Regoli D. Comparison of the effects of epithelium removal and of an enkephalinase inhibitor on the neurokinin-induced contractions of guinea pig trachea. *Br J Pharmacol* 1988;94:675–684.

98. Fine JM, Gordon T. Sheppard D. Epithelium removal alters responsiveness of guinea pig trachea to substance P. *J Appl Physiol* 1989;66:232–237.

99. Frossard N, Rhoden KJ. Barnes PJ. Influence of epithelium on guinea pig airway responses to tachykinins: role of endopeptidase and cyclooxygenase. *J Pharmacol Exp Ther* 1989;248:292–299.

100. Sekizawa K, Tamaoki J, Graf PD, Basbaum CB, Borson DB, Nadel JA. Enkephalinase inhibitor potentiates mammalian tachykinin-induced contraction in ferret trachea. *J Pharmacol Exp Ther* 1987;243:1211–1217.

101. Djokic TD, Nadel JA, Dusser DJ, Sekizawa K, Graf PD, Borson DB. Inhibitors of neutral endopeptidase potentiate electrically and capsaicin-induced noncholinergic contraction in guinea pig bronchi. *J Pharmacol Exp Ther* 1989;247:7–11.

102. Naline E, DeVillier P, Drapeau G, et al. Characterization of neurokinin effects and receptor selectivity in human isolated bronchi. *Am Rev Respir Dis* 1989;140:679–686.

103. Fagny C, Michel A, Léonard I, Berkenboom G, Fontaine J, Deschodt-Lanckman M. *In vitro* degradation of endothelin-1 by endopeptidase 24.11 (enkephalinase). *Peptides* 1991;12:773–778.

104. Henry PJ, Rigby PJ, Self GJ, Preuss JMH, Goldie RG. Relationship between endothelin-1 binding site densities and constrictor activities in human and animal airway smooth muscle. *Br J Pharmacol* 1990;100:786–792.

105. Hay DWP. guinea pig tracheal epithelium and endothelin. *Eur J Pharmacol* 1989;171:241–245.

106. Johnson AR, Ashton J, Schultz WW, Erdos EG, Neutral metalloendopeptidases in human lung tissue and cultured cells. *Am Rev Respir Dis* 1985;132:564–568.

107. Ullman A. Lofdahl C-G, Svedmyr N, Bernsten L, Skoogh B-E. Mucosal inhibition of cholinergic contractions in ferret trachea can be transferred between organ baths. *Eur Respir J* 1988;1:908–912.

108. Xie Z, Hakoda H, Ito Y. Airway epithelial cells regulate membrane potential, neurotransmission and muscle tone of the dog airway smooth muscle. *J Physiol* (*Lond*) 1992;449:619–639.

109. Stuart-Smith K, Vanhoutte PM. Epithelium, contractile tone and responses to relaxing agonists in canine bronchi. *J Appl Physiol* 1990; 69:678–685.

110. Lundblad KA, Persson CGA. The epithelium and the pharmacology of guinea pig tracheal tone *in vitro*. *Br J Pharmacol*, 1988;93:909–917.

111. Tucker JF, Brave SR, Charalambous L, Hobbs AJ, Gibson A. L-N^G-nitro arginine inhibits nonadrenergic, noncholinergic relaxations of guinea pig isolated tracheal smooth muscle. *Br J Pharmacol* 1990; 100:633–634.

112. Li CG, Rand MJ. Evidence that part of the NANC relaxant responses of guinea pig trachea to electrical field stimulation is mediated by nitric oxide. *Br J Pharmacol* 1991;102:91–94.

113. Belvisi MG, Stretton CD, Yacoub M Barnes PJ. Nitric oxide is the endogenous neurotransmitter of bronchodilator nerves in humans. *Eur J Pharmacol* 1992;210:221–222.

114. Hulsmann AR, Jongejan RC, Raatgeep HR, et al. Epithelium removal and peptidase inhibition enhance relaxation of human airways to vasoactive intestinal peptide. *Am Rev Respir Dis* 1993;147:1483–1486.

115. Fernandes LB, Preuss JMH, Goldie RG. Epithelial modulation of the relaxant activity of atriopeptides in rat and guinea pig tracheal smooth muscle. *Eur J Pharmacol* 1992;212:187–194.

116. Rhoden KJ, Barnes PJ. Epithelial modulation of nonadrenergic, noncholinergic and vasoactive intestinal peptide-induced responses: role of neutral endopeptidase. *Eur J Pharmacol* 1990;171:247–250.

117. Bisgaard H, Groth S, Madsen F. Bronchial hyperreactivity of leukotriene D$_4$ and histamine in exogenous asthma. *Br Med J* 1985;290:1468–1471.

118. Davidson AE, Lee TH, Scanlon PD, et al. Bronchoconstrictor effects of leukotriene E$_4$ in normal and asthmatic subjects. *Am Rev Respir Dis* 1987;135:333–337.

119. Dahlén S-E, Björk J, et al. Leukotrienes promote plasma leakage and leukocyte adhesion in postcapillary venules: *in vivo* effects with relevance to the acute inflammatory response. *Proc Natl Acad Sci USA* 1981;78:3887.

120. Evans TW, Rogers DF, Aursudkij B, Chung KF, Barnes PJ. Regional and time-dependent effects of inflammatory mediators on microvascular permeability in the guinea pig. *Clin Sci* 1989;76:479–485.

121. Dunnill MS. The pathology of asthma with specific reference to changes in the bronchial mucosa. *J Clin Pathol* 1960;13:27–33.

122. Henke D, Danilowicz RM, Curtis JF, Boucher RC, Eling TE. Metabolism of arachidonic acid by human nasal and bronchial epithelial cells. *Arch Biochem Biophys* 1988;267:426–436.

123. Holtzman MJ, Hansbrough JR, Rosen GD, Turk J. Uptake, release, and novel species- dependent oxygenation of arachidonic acid in human and animal airway epithelial cells. *Biochim Biophys Acta* 1988; 963:401–413.

124. Hansbrough JR, Atlas AB, Turk J, Holtzman MJ. Arachidonate 12-lipoxygenase and cyclo-oxygenase: PGE isomerase are predominant pathways for oxygenation in bovine tracheal epithelial cells. *Am J Respir Cell Mol Biol* 1989;1:237–244.

125. Eling TE, Danilowicz RM, Henke DC, Sivarajah K, Yankaskas JR, Boucher RC. Arachidonic acid metabolism by canine tracheal epithelial cells. *J Biol Chem* 1986;261:12841–12849.

126. Salari H, Schellenberg RR. Stimulation of human airway epithelial cells by platelet activating factor (PAF) and arachidonic acid produces 15-hydroxyeicosatetraenoic acid (15-HETE) capable of contracting bronchial smooth muscle. *Pulm Pharmacol* 1991;4:1–7.

127. Adler KB, Schwartz JE, Anderson W, Welton AF. Platelet activating factor stimulates secretion of mucin by explants of rodent airways in organ culture. *Exp Lung Res* 1987;13:25–43.

128. Holtzman MJ. Epithelial cell regulation of arachidonic acid oxygenation. In: Farmer SG, Hay DWP, eds. *The airway epithelium*. New York: Marcel Dekker, 1991;65–115.

129. Salari H, Chan-Yeung M. Release of 15-hydroxyeicosatetraenoic acid (15-HETE) and prostaglandin E$_2$ (PGE$_2$) by cultured human bronchial epithelial cells. *Am J Respir Cell Mol Biol* 1989; 1:245–250.

130. Farmer SG, Hay DWP, Raeburn D, Fedan JS. Relaxation of guinea pig tracheal smooth muscle to arachidonate is converted to contraction following epithelium removal. *Br J Pharmacol* 1987;92:231–236.

131. Stuart-Smith K, Vanhoutte PM. Arachidonic acid evokes epithelium-dependent relaxations in canine airways. *J Appl Physiol* 1988;65: 2170–2180.

132. Leikauf GD, Driscoll KE, Wey HE. Ozone-induced augmentation of eicosanoid metabolism in epithelial cells from bovine trachea. *Am Rev Respir Dis* 1988;137:435–442.

133. Widdicombe JH, Ueki IF, Emery D, Margolskee D, Yergey J, Nadel JA. Release of cyclo-oxygenase products from primary cultures of tracheal epithelia of dog and human. *Am J Physiol* 1989;256:L351–L355.

134. Wilkens JA, Becker A, Wilkens H, et al. Bioassay of a tracheal smooth muscle- constricting factor released by respiratory epithelial cells. *Am J Physiol* 992;263:L137–L141.

135. Ullman A, Lofdahl C-G, Svedmyr N, Skoogh B-E. Nerve stimulation releases mucosa-derived inhibitory factors, both prostanoids and non-prostanoids in isolated ferret trachea. *Am Rev Respir Dis* 1990;141: 748–751.

136. Marin MG, Davis B, Nadel JA. Effect of histamine on electrical and ion transport properties of tracheal epithelium. *J Appl Physiol* 1977; 42:735–738.

137. Chand N, Eyre P. Classification and biological distribution of histamine receptor subtypes. *Agents Actions* 1975;5:277–295.

138. Majno G, Shea SM, Leventhal M. Endothelial contraction induced by histamine-type mediators: An electron microscopic study. *J Cell Biol* 1969;42:647–672.

139. McDonald DM. The ultrastructure and permeability of tracheobronchial blood vessels in health and disease. *Eur Respir J* 1990;3(suppl 12):572s–585s.

140. Persson CGA. Role of plasma exudation in asthmatic airways. *Lancet* 1986;ii:1126–1129.

141. Eiser NM. Hyperreactivity—its relationship to histamine receptors. *Eur J Respir Dis* 1983;64 (suppl 131):99–114.

142. Ichinose M, Barnes PJ. Inhibitory histamine H$_3$-receptors on cholinergic nerves in human airways. *Eur J Pharmacol* 1989;163:383–386.

143. Ichinose M, Stretton CD, Schwartz J-C, Barnes PJ. Histamine H$_3$-receptors inhibit cholinergic neurotransmission in guinea pig airways. *Br J Pharmacol* 1989;97:13–15.

144. Ichinose M, Barnes PJ. Histamine H$_3$-receptors modulate nonadrenergic, noncholinergic neural bronchoconstriction in guinea pig *in vivo*. *Eur J Pharmacol* 1989;174:49–55.

145. Ichinose M, Belvisi MG, Barnes PJ. Histamine H$_3$-receptors inhibit neurogenic microvascular leakage in airways. *J Appl Physiol* 1990;68: 21–25.

146. Ichinose M, Barnes PJ. Histamine H$_3$-receptors modulate antigen-induced bronchoconstriction in guinea pigs. *J Allergy Clin Immunol* 1990;86:491–495.

147. Springall DR, Howarth PH, Counihan H, Djukanovic R, Holgate ST, Polak JM. Endothelin immunoreactivity of airway epithelium in asthmatic patients. *Lancet* 1991;337:697–701.

148. MacCumber MW, Ross CA, Glaser BM, Snyder SH. Endothelin visualization of mRNA s by *in situ* hybridization provides evidence for local action. *Proc Natl Acad Sci USA* 1989;86:7285–7289.

149. Hay DWP, Luttmann MA, Hubbard WC, Undem BJ. Endothelin receptor subtypes in human and guinea pig pulmonary tissues. *Br J Pharmacol* 1993;110:1175–1183.

150. Noveral JP, Rosenberg SM, Anbar RA, Pawlowski NA, Grunstein MM. Role of endothelin-1 in regulating proliferation of cultured rabbit airway smooth muscle cells. *Am J Physiol* 1992;263:L317–L324.

151. Mullol J, Chowdhury BA, White MV. Endothelin in human nasal mucosa. *Am J Respir Cell Mol Biol* 1993;8:393–402.

152. Hay DWP, Henry PJ, Goldie RG. Endothelin and the respiratory system. *Trends Pharmacol Sci* 1993;14:29–32.

153. Sofia M, Mormile M, Faraone SM, Zofra S, Romano L, Carratù L. Increased endothelin-like immunoreactive material on bronchoalveolar lavage fluid from patients with bronchial asthma and patients with interstitial lung disease. *Respiration* 1993;60:89–95.

154. Rozengurt N, Springall DR, Polak JM. Localization of endothelin-like immunoreactivity in airway epithelium of rats and mice. *J Pathol* 1990;160:5–8.

155. Mattoli S, Mezzetti M, Riva G, Allegra L, Fasoli A. Specific binding of endothelin on human bronchial smooth muscle cells in culture and secretion of endothelin-like material from bronchial epithelial cells. *Am J Respir Cell Mol Biol* 1990;3:145–151.

156. Black PN, Ghatei MA, Takahashi K, et al. Formation of endothelin by cultured airway epithelial cells. *FEBS Lett* 1989;255:129–132.

157. Ninomiya H, Uchida Y, Ishii Y, et al. Endotoxin stimulates endothelin release from cultured epithelial cells of guinea pig trachea. *Eur J Pharmacol* 1991;203:299–302.

158. Henry PJ, Goldie RG. Potentiation by endothelin-1 of cholinergic nerve-mediated contractions in mouse trachea via activation of ET_B receptors. Br J Pharmacol 1995;114:563–569.

159. McKay KO, Armour CL, Black JL. Endothelin-3 increases transmission in the rabbit pulmonary parasympathetic nervous system. Cardiovasc Pharmacol 1993;22(suppl 8):S181–S184.

160. Lundberg JM, Hokfelt T, Martling C-R, Saria A, Cuello C. Sensory substance P- immunoreactive nerves in the lower respiratory tract of various mammals including man. Cell Tissue Res 1984;235:251–261.

161. Marom Z, Schelhamer JH, Bach MK, Morton DR, Kaliner MA. Slow reacting substances, leukotrienes C_4 and D_4 increase the release of mucus from human airways in vitro. Am Rev Respir Dis 1982;126:449–451.

162. Advenier C, Naline E, Drapeau G, Regoli D. Relative potencies of neurokinins in guinea pig trachea and human bronchus. Eur J Pharmacol 1987;139:133–137.

163. Lundberg JM, Martling, CR, Saria A. Substance P and capsaicin-induced contraction of human bronchi. Acta Physiol Scand 1983;119:49–53.

164. Maggi CA. Tachykinin receptors in the airways and lung: what should we block? Pharmacol Res 1990;22:527–540.

165. Borson DB, Corrales R, Varsano S, et al. Enkephalinase inhibitors potentiate SP- induced secretion of $^{35}SO_4$-macromolecules from ferret trachea. Exp Lun Res 1986;21:21–36.

166. McDonald DM. Neurogenic inflammation in the respiratory tract: actions of sensory nerve mediators on blood vessels and epithelium of the airway mucosa. Am Rev Respir Dis 1987;136:S65–S72.

167. Brokaw JJ, Hillenbrand CM, White GW, McDonald DM. Mechanism of tachyphylaxis associated with neurogenic plasma extravasation in the rat trachea. Am Rev Respir Dis 1990;141:1434–1440.

168. Payan DG. Neuropeptides and inflammation: the role of substance P. Annu Rev Med 1989;40:341–352.

169. Barnes PJ. Neuropeptides and airway smooth muscle. Pharmacol Ther 1988;36:119–129.

170. Tschirhart E, Bertrand C, Theodorsson E, Landry Y. Evidence for the involvement of calcitonin gene-related peptide in the epithelium-dependent contraction of guinea pig trachea in response to capsaicin. Naunyn-Scmiedeb Arch Pharmacol 1990;342:177–181.

171. Bertrand C, Da Silva A, Landry Y, Theodorsson E, Tschirhart E. An epithelial-dependent contracting factor induced by calcium influx in guinea pig trachea. Pulm Pharmacol 1993;6:69–76.

172. Coleman RA, Kennedy I. Contractile and relaxant actions of prostaglandins on guinea-pig isolated trachea. Br J Pharmacol 1980;68:533–539.

173. DeVillier P, Acker GM, Advenier C, Marsac J, Regoli D, Frossard N. Activation of an epithelial neurokinin NK-1 receptor induces relaxation of rat trachea through release of prostaglandin E_2. J Pharmacol Exp Ther 1992;263:767–772.

174. Leikauf GD, Ueki IF, Nadel JA, Widdicombe JH. Bradykinin stimulates Cl secretion and prostaglandin E_2 release by canine tracheal epithelium. Am J Physiol 1985;248:F48–F55.

175. Barnett K, Jacoby DB, Nadel JA, Lazarus SC. The effects of epithelial cell supernatant on contractions of isolated canine tracheal smooth muscle. Am Rev Respir Dis 1988;138:780–783.

176. Xu GL, Sivarajah K, Wu R, Nettesheim P, Eling T. Biosynthesis of prostaglandins by isolated and cultured airway epithelial cells. Exp Lung Res 1986;10:101–114.

177. Ellis JL, Undem BJ. Inhibition by L-N^G-nitro-L-arginine of nonadrenergic, noncholinergic-mediated relaxations of human isolated central and peripheral airways. Am Rev Respir Dis 1992;146:1543–1547.

178. Kobzik L, Bredt DS, Lowenstein CJ, et al. Nitric oxide synthase in human and rat lung: Immunocytochemical and histochemical localization. Am J Respir Cell Mol Biol 1993;9:371–377.

179. Filep G, Battistini B, Sirois P. Induction by endothelin-1 of epithelium-dependent relaxation of guinea pig trachea: role of nitric oxide. Br J Pharmacol 1993;109:637–644.

180. Nijkamp FP, Van der Linde H, Folkerts G. Nitric oxide sythesis inhibitors induce airway hyperresponsiveness in the guinea pig in vivo and in vitro. Am Rev Respir Dis 1993;148:727–734.

181. Knowles RG, Salter M, Brooks SL, Moncada S. Anti-inflammatory glucocorticoids inhibit the induction by endotoxin of nitric oxide synthase in the lung, liver, and aorta of the rat. Biochem Biophys Res Commun 1990;172:1042–1048.

182. Hamid Q, Springall DR, Riveros-Moreno, V, et al. Induction of nitric oxide synthase in asthma. Lancet 1993;342:1510–1513.

183. Persson MG, Zetterström O, Agrenius,V, Ihre E, Gustafsson LE. Single-breath nitric oxide measurements in asthmatic patients and smokers. Lancet 1994;343:146–147.

184. Mulligan MS, Hevel JM, Marletta MA, Ward PA. Tissue injury caused by deposition of immune complexes in L-arginine-dependent. Proc Natl Acad Sci USA 1991;88:6338–6342.

185. Kharitonov SA, Yates D, Robbins RA, Logan-Sinclair R, Shinebourne EA, Barnes PJ. Increased nitric oxide in exhaled air of asthmatic patients. Lancet 1994;343:133–135.

186. Vanhoutte PM. Epithelium-derived relaxing factor(s) and bronchial reactivity. Am Rev Respir Dis 1988;138:S24–S30.

187. Fernandes LB, Paterson JW, Goldie RG. Co-axial bioassay of an epithelial relaxant factor from the guinea pig trachea. Br J Pharmacol 1989;97:117–124.

188. Fernandes LB, Goldie RG. Pharmacological evaluation of guinea pig tracheal epithelium-derived inhibitory factor (EpDIF). Br J Pharmacol 1990;100:614–618.

189. Güc MO, Ilhan M, Kayaalp SO. The rat anococcygeus muscle is a convenient bioassay organ for the airway epithelium-derived relaxant factor. Eur J Pharmacol 1988;148:405–409.

190. Ilhan M, Sahin I. Tracheal epithelium releases a vascular smooth muscle relaxant factor: demonstration by bioassay. Eur J Pharmacol 1986;131:293–296.

191. Fernandes LB, Goldie RG. Antigen-induced release of airway epithelium-derived inhibitory factor. Am Rev Respir Dis 1991;143:567–571.

192. Gunn LK, Piper PJ. Potential sources of artifact in the co-axial bioassay. Eur J Pharmacol 1991;203:405–412.

193. Hay DWP, Muccitelli RM, Page CP, Spina D. Correlation between airway epithelium-induced relaxation of rat aorta in the co-axial bioassay and cyclic nucleotide levels. Br J Pharmacol 1992;105:954–958.

194. Spina D, Fernandes LB, Preuss, JMH, et al. Evidence that epithelium-dependent relaxation of vascular smooth muscle detected by co-axial bioassays is not attributable to hypoxia. Br J Pharmacol 1992;105:799–804.

195. Munakata M, Mitzner W, Menkes H. Osmotic stimuli induce epithelial-dependent relaxation in the guinea pig trachea. J Appl Physiol 1988;64:466–471.

196. Fedan JS, Nutt ME, Frazer DG. Reactivity of guinea pig isolated trachea to methacholine, histamine and isoproterenol applied serosally versus mucosally. Eur J Pharmacol 1990;190:337–345.

197. Sparrow MP, Mitchell HW. Modulation by the epithelium of the extent of bronchial narrowing produced by substances perfused through the lumen. Br J Pharmacol 1991;103:1160–1164.

198. Fisher JT, Gray PR, Mitchell HW, Sparrow MP. Epithelial modulation of neonatal and fetal porcine bronchial contractile responses. Am J Respir Crit Care Med 1994;149:1304–1310.

199. Mitchell HW, Fisher JT, Sparrow MP. The integrity of the epithelium is a major determinant of the responsiveness of the dog bronchial segment to mucosal provocation. Pulm Pharmacol 1993;6:263–268.

200. Goldie RG. Receptors in asthmatic airways. Am Rev Respir Dis 1990;141:S151–S156.

201. O'Donnell M, Garippa R, Welton AF. Relaxant activity of atriopeptins in isolated guinea pig airway and vascular smooth muscle. Peptides 1985;6:597–601.

202. Munakata M, Masaki Y, Sakuma I. Pharmacological differentiation of epithelium–derived relaxing factor from nitric oxide. J Appl Physiol 1990;69:665–670.

Asthma, edited by P.J. Barnes, M.M. Grunstein,
A.R. Leff, and A.J. Woolcock.
Lippincott–Raven Publishers, Philadelphia © 1997.

■ 64 ■

Plasma Exudation

Carl G. A. Persson

Focus on Gross Functions in Complex *In Vivo*
  Biosystem
Exudation of Plasma as an Airway End Organ
  Response
Exudation Pathways and Mechanisms

Challenge- and Disease-Induced Plasma Exudation
  Responses
Roles of Exuded Plasma
Absorption, Exudation and Epithelial Restitution

The mucosal output in inflammatory airway diseases consists of cells and secretions. In addition, there is a significant output emanating directly from the subepithelial microcirculation. Thus microvascular-epithelial exudation of "bulk" plasma has now been well demonstrated in asthma and rhinitis. Luminal entry of plasma emerges as a specific physiological response that may show the distribution, the intensity, and the time course of multipotential inflammatory processes in the airways. The plasma exudate is also a significant inflammatory factor in its own right, because of its content of peptide mediators, adhesive proteins, proteases, cytokines, immunoglobulins, etc. These plasma-derived effector solutes may, in fact, decide much of the molecular disease milieu *in vivo.* This chapter discusses mechanisms of microvascular-epithelial exudation of plasma in upper and lower airways. The emphasis is on the role of the exudate in mucosal defence, epithelial repair, and airways inflammation.

Focus on Gross Functions in Complex *in vivo* Biosystems

The bulk of novel information on airway epithelium and vascular endothelium now emanates from studies employing reductive biological sciences approaches and cell culture techniques. However exciting and important, the novel molecular and cellular approaches may not always be applied with complete success unless the gross

physiology and pathophysiology of the airway mucosa have first been well assessed. Somewhat conservatively the present discussion therefore will adhere to the experimental strategy of having the proper *in vivo* function established first. The point may be illustrated by an example: One current paradigm is that the airway barrier is abnormally pervious to inhaled molecules in asthma and rhinitis. Accordingly, reductive science approaches now provide data explaining how and by what mechanisms the perviousness is produced. At the same time, however, new functional *in vivo* studies employing increasingly improved physiological methods demonstrate that the absorption rate across the mucosa, if it is at all altered, may actually be decreased in rhinitis and asthma (1). The present focus does not reduce the need for critical comparisons between animal and human findings. Recent concept testing has thus demonstrated that neurogenic inflammation (exudation), which is a major mechanism in guinea-pig and rat airways, is not present in human airways (2).

In airways subjected to inflammatory provocations and in airways where an inflammatory process is going on, the plasma exudation process dramatically alters the composition of proteins, cytokines, and peptide mediators in the lamina propria, in the epithelial basement membrane, in the epithelium, and on the mucosal surface. This microcirculation-plasma-derived molecular milieu (Fig. 1) may affect cellular inflammatory activities in ways which may be difficult to reproduce *in vitro.* The exuded plasma lays down important adhesive proteins such as fibronectin and fibrin(ogen). It provides proteases-antiproteases, binding proteins, and immunoglobulins. The extravasated bulk plasma contains many cytokines in-

C. G. A. Persson: Department of Clinical Pharmacology, University Hospital of Lund, Lund S-221 85 Sweden.

What's in the extravasated plasma ?

Proteins	Adhesive Molecules (fibrinogen, fibronectin, etc.) Proteases - Antiproteases Cytokine Modulating Proteins Immunoglobulins Other
Cytokines	Growth factors (PDGF, IGF, TGF-β, etc.) Interleukins Several cytokines bound, carried, and targeted by α_2-macroglobulin and other plasma proteins
Peptides	Complement Fragments Bradykinins Fibrinolysis Peptides Other

FIG. 1. The plasma exudate contains and generates an abundance of biologically active proteins-peptides that may regulate airway mucosal effector cells in inflammation.

cluding growth factors. Some of the plasma proteins, notably α_2-macroglobulin, are known to bind, carry, and target numerous cytokines. The plasma-derived peptide mediators are not confined to the bradykinins. Fibrinolysis peptides, complement fragments, and many more biologically active molecules are dynamically produced by the extravasated protein systems in contact with airway tissue and surface components. The essential but complex and as yet only partly understood contributions from the microcirculation should probably affect our strategy in exploring the pathophysiology and pharmacology of inflammatory processes. The *in vivo* approach involving tissues with intact microcirculation may still have a prime role in this exploratory research.

Exudation of Plasma as an Airway End Organ Response

The classical signs of inflammation, *rubor, dolor, calor, tumour,* and *functio laesa,* seem of limited help in identifying the active inflammatory process in the airways. *Rubor* may characterise an airway embarrassed by irritants that increase blood flow but do not produce inflammation. Besides, the airway mucosal blood flow is so rich already under baseline conditions that moderate changes in flow may not be critical to airway functions in inflammation. This notion is supported by the observation that topical vasoconstrictors, such as oximetazoline, may not affect the inflammatory stimulus-induced plasma exudation in human nasal airways (3).

Dolor and *calor,* pain and heat, cannot be regarded as characteristic features of the inflammatory condition in asthma and rhinitis. In contrast, *tumour* is clearly impor-

tant. However, what is behind the visible swelling? The airway mucosa may be swollen due to intravascular pooling of blood as in the venous sinuses of the nose. This particular kind of thickening is abrogated by sympathomimetic α-receptor agonists. Long term treatment with topical steroids also inhibits the congestion but this result may reflect the antiinflammatory efficacy of these drugs rather than any direct vasoconstrictor action. The "swelling" that is observed through the bronchoscope may be composed of several factors. Congestion may contribute. Airway remodelling with increased numbers of vessels and cells and an abnormal extracellular matrix may well contribute. Also, simple bronchoconstriction that moves a normal, or thickened mucosa regularly, or irregularly, inwards to reduce the patency of the airway lumen may be quite difficult to distinguish from the other causes of tumefaction.

The most common interpretation of the cause of airway swelling is edema, which simply means that the extravascular tissue holds abnormally large amounts of extravascular fluid. Considerable or sustained extravasation of plasma is normally expected to produce tissue edema. However, the notion that airway edema is a major component of asthma and allergic rhinitis is now more based on hypothetical reasoning coupled with selected histological pictures than on irrefutable quantitative research. The most active microcirculation in airway disease would be the capillary-venular plexus residing in the lamina propria, sometimes going as superficially as to penetrate part of the epithelial basement membrane. The acute mucosal challenge-induced increase in vascular permeability, causing extravasation of plasma from the superficial microcirculation, may not produce mucosal edema but may rather result in luminal entry of "bulk" plasma. Hence, extravasation of plasma in airway tissues may not always be equated with airway edema.

Plasma extravasation and, in the airways, mucosal exudation of plasma deserve attention as breaking points demonstrating that cellular and other mechanisms of inflammation have reached the activity level where tissue end organs become significantly affected. Plasma exudation also differs from many other airway end organ responses by being rather specific to inflammation (3). Bronchial tone, dilatation of venous sinuses, airway secretion, and blood flow are all increased both by inflammation and by simple irritant type of provocations, which also evoke neural reflex activity. The most powerful airway reflexes are cough and sneezes but, again, these reflexes are not exclusive to inflammation, nor are they always induced by inflammation.

The final classical sign, *functio laesa*, is true in the general sense that asthmatic airway inflammation may be a major cause of breathing difficulties. However, in more specific terms this sign seems difficult to reconcile with most cases of asthma and rhinitis where hyper- rather than hypofunction of airway end organs may be prevalent. The increased ability to respond to inhaled stimuli is reflected both by the unexplained phenomenon of nonspecific hyperresponsiveness and by specific hyperresponsiveness of individual mucosal end organs such as the secretory apparatus, the sensory innervation, and the microcirculation (3).

Exudation Pathways and Mechanisms

The acute plasma exudation response to airway mucosal challenges involves a series of events which all occur within minutes after challenge. By indirect, cellular release mechanisms, the inflammatory challenge results in increased mucosal tissue levels of vasoactive agents. Such an agent itself may constitute a directly acting challenge. The vascular permeability-increasing agents act on the venular wall endothelium, which is equipped with a great variety of cell surface receptors. Through receptor stimulation the cell to cell contact is lost at distinct points in the walls of the postcapillary venules. The mechanism of interendothelial gap formation has been widely accepted as a contractile event, but the gaps might also be produced by reduced adhesion along tiny stretches of the endothelial cell to cell junctions. Through these gaps or holes in the venular wall nonsieved plasma is moved by the hydrostatic pressure gradient that exists between the venules (about 20 cm H_2O) and the extravascular tissue. The extravasation is a dramatic event that locally abolishes the colloid osmotic pressure gradient between the microvessels and the tissue. During the first 10–20 seconds after challenge the airway lamina propria is flooded with the plasma exudate. Apparently unhindered, the exudate then passes through the epithelial basement membrane and further up between epithelial cells that normally are separated at the base. At the apical pole circumference the epithelial cells are tightly connected. However, not even the tight junctions of an intact epithelial lining are significant obstacles to the further flux of exudate into the airway lumen. The luminal entry of plasma appears to be a self-sustaining process occurring as long as sufficient amounts of plasma press upon the basolateral aspects of columnar epithelial cells (Fig. 2).

The bulk plasma that is moved to the mucosal surface is not identical to circulating plasma. Promptly after extravasation several protein systems of the blood plasma will be activated, generating a great variety of peptides

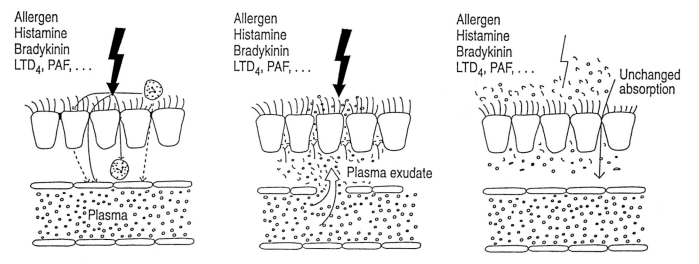

FIG. 2. Challenge with allergen and leukotriene-type mediators and several other proinflammatory factors produces dose-dependent luminal entry of "bulk" plasma, without disrupting the epithelial lining and without increasing the absorption ability of the airway mucosa. Thus, all plasma protein systems, irrespective of molecular size, may appear on the surface of the intact airway mucosa.

and oligoproteins. The extravasated plasma will also have excellent opportunities to interact with interesting cell-derived molecules that are present or released in the lamina propria. For example, several plasma proteins, from the 70000D albumin to the 700000D α_2-macroglobulin, are avid binders of different molecules such as mediators, cytokines, and drugs. The tissue flooding with plasma is not merely a passive lavage. In addition, the extravasated plasma may offer specific piggy-back riding to the airway surface ("lamina propria lavage") (4). In airway disease conditions simple histamine challenges, which produce graded exudations of bulk plasma, may through this action also increase, dose-dependently, airway lavage fluid levels of select cytokines such as IL-6 that are known to be bound by plasma proteins such as α_2-macroglobulin (5). A potentially very effective lamina propria lavage, induced by the plasma exudation process, may need to be considered in studies of disease mechanisms and drug effects involving techniques such as bronchial and nasal lavages and biopsies.

Erjefält et al (6), employing colloidal gold (5 nm in diameter) as plasma tracer, have recently observed that the plasma exudate is moved between all epithelial cells in the area and all around each cell. Hence, the burden on each unit length of cell junctions would be minute also at pronounced rates of exudation of bulk plasma. This possibility tallies with previous observations demonstrating the noninjurious nature of the mucosal exudation process (3,4). A mechanism has also been discovered by which the extravasated plasma may pass through epithelial tight junctions (1). Using intact airway tube preparations mounted in organ baths that allow separate regulation of mucosal and serosal bathing fluids, it has thus been demonstrated that a slightly increased hydrostatic pressure load (<5 cm H_2O) on the basolateral aspects of the airway epithelial lining cells is sufficient for moving macromolecular solutes to the mucosal surface. Indeed, this hydraulic process is reversible and repeatable much in the same way as the *in vivo* exudation evoked by challenge with histamine-type mediators. Furthermore, both *in vitro* and *in vivo* the epithelial junctions evidently yield and close so that luminal entry of macromolecules occurs without being associated with or followed by increased mucosal absorption of polar solutes (Fig. 2). It is somewhat surprising that this noninjurious epithelial mechanism, involving passage of "bulk" plasma, has remained undetected by physiologists who rather have seen luminal entry of plasma as a mechanism of epithelial damage (1). It appears that the plasma exudate itself by its distribution and by its localised hydrostatic pressure influence opens valvelike paracellular pathways for its luminal entry (Fig. 2). The ease by which extravasated plasma enters the airway lumen is underscored by the observation that the regional lymph protein transport may be unchanged at inflammatory stimulus-induced exudation of plasma in the

guinea-pig tracheal mucosa (7). As demonstrated in both nasal and tracheobronchial airways, acute exudation of bulk plasma is associated with an unchanged rate of mucosal absorption of hydrophilic solutes (3,4; Fig. 2). These observations are functional *in vivo* evidence that epithelial tight junctions have a valvelike mechanism that is readily opened by plasma that approaches from beneath. Luminal entry of bulk plasma is now forwarded as a major mucosal defence mechanism that neutralises offending agents on the airway surface even before they penetrate into the tissue (8).

Taken together the experimental data indicate that the active physiological and pharmacological regulation of mucosal exudation of plasma takes place at the level of the endothelial cells of the microvascular wall. This is the site where inflammatory agents produce small, round interendothelial holes initiating the whole airways exudation process. It seems functionally relevant that mediators and drugs shall not act on the epithelial lining cells to selectively regulate the epithelial passage of plasma into the lumen. A tightening effect on the epithelium in this respect would not be a desirable drug action because it would increase the likelihood of edema formation in the airway mucosa.

Challenge- and Disease-Induced Plasma Exudation Responses

A nonspecific contractile and secretory mediator such as acetylcholine or its analogues (methacholine, carbachol, etc.) is without exudative effects in the airways (3,4,8). Furthermore, irritants such as nicotine and capsaicin that evoke strong neurogenic responses are without exudative effects in human nasal airways (2). This latter observation is in sharp contrast to findings in guinea-pig airways, where capsaicin and nicotine produce pronounced exudation responses. Hence, plasma exudation in human airways is more specific to inflammation than in rodent airways, because simple neural reflex mechanisms may not produce this response.

The human nasal mucosa lends itself to airway-specific, well-controlled challenge and lavage studies. To take advantage of these possibilities a nasal pool technique has been developed (9). Using a compressible nasal pool device it is possible to fill the entire ipsilateral nasal cavity with fluid and solutes. A large airway mucosal surface area can thus be exposed to defined concentrations of agents and tracers. After a selected mucosal exposure time the pool fluid may, almost quantitatively, be recovered into the device. Thus the exposed mucosal surface is also gently lavaged by the nasal pool fluid, providing the opportunity to sample mucosal indices selectively from the area of interest. This gentle lavage procedure can be carried out numerous times in sequence without causing undue changes in mucosal function. The technique also allows exposure of the same airway mucosal surface area at repeated provocations. It has not been possible to attain similarly controlled experimental conditions in human tracheobronchial airways. However, many mechanisms of the airway mucosa in health and disease can be examined in the nose and the findings be extrapolated to apply also to the lower airways (3).

Using the nasal pool device Greiff et al. (9) and Svensson et al. (10) have demonstrated graded exudative effects of different mucosal surface concentrations of histamine. Between 20 μg/ml and 2000 μg/ml of this amine produces 5-fold to more than 100-fold increases in lavage fluid levels of plasma proteins (albumin to α_2-macroglobulin). Mediators such as histamine, bradykinin, and leukotriene D_4 produce graded exudative responses over a wide range of concentrations in both guinea-pig and human airways. Histamine, bradykinin, and paf acether are about equally potent when applied on the airway mucosa whereas leukotriene D_4 is about a 100-fold more potent than either of these agents. In addition, select cytokines and proteases may induce plasma exudation in the airways. Presumably, most exudative agents act through activation of appropriate receptors on vascular permeability-regulating endothelial cells.

Allergen challenge in subjects with allergic airway disease may produce both immediate and late phase plasma exudation responses. Similarly, in sensitized guinea-pigs allergen challenge produces dual plasma exudation responses (11). [Neurogenic exudation is not involved in the allergic response even of guinea-pig airways.] If the allergen challenge is given to the whole guinea-pig lung, involving also the peripheral parenchymal tissue, the late phase exudation appears to be sustained for about 20 h. If only the large tracheobronchial airway is challenged, the immediate, airway-specific exudation phase is over in about an hour. Then follows a late airway exudation phase that peaks about 5 h after challenge and then fades off (11).

Differing from allergens, the occupational small molecular weight chemical, toluenediisocyanate (TDI), produces a strong and sustained plasma exudation response also in airways that have not previously been exposed to TDI and thus have not been sensitized to this reactive agent. Within a wide dose range, 3 nl to 30 μl, TDI produces dose-dependent plasma exudation into guinea-pig tracheobronchial airways of previously unexposed guinea-pigs. These doses applied restrictedly on the large tracheobronchial airways of guinea pigs may be compared to the accepted exposure level which corresponds to a daily human body burden of about 15 μl TDI. The acute TDI-induced sustained plasma exudation response in nonsensitised guinea pigs peaks 5 h after challenge and continues for about 15 additional hours.

Guinea pigs that receive repeated challenges with 3 nl of TDI on the large tracheobronchial airways develop an increased inflammatory responsiveness to TDI (12). Thus, challenge with exceedingly low doses of TDI (0.3 nl) in the sensitized animals is associated with pronounced eosinophilia and a marked and sustained exudative response. This TDI-induced plasma exudation response, in contrast to that observed in nonsensitized animals, is inhibited by glucocorticoid pretreatment (12). In patients with occupational asthma it has also been demonstrated that exposure to the occupational agent produces a late phase response that encompasses a plasma exudation process. TDI challenge-induced plasma exudation in patients with occupational asthma due to this chemical is also inhibited by pretreatment with inhaled glucocorticoids (13).

Plasma exudation in inflammatory airway diseases was first demonstrated through determination of plasma proteins in sputum samples obtained in asthma and chronic bronchitis (14). Almost equally early it was observed that steroid treatment significantly reduces the sputum level of different plasma indices (14). Interestingly, the inhibition of exudation seems to occur without concomitant reduction of sputum levels of secretory indices. Indeed, the latter may increase along with reduced sputum volume (14). The relatively poor antisecretory effect of glucocorticosteroids adds to a long list of significant qualitative differences between airway secretory and exudative processes, and supports the notion that the plasma exudation response may reflect airway inflammation better than other physiological end organ responses in the airways.

Albumin is usually the only plasma protein that has been analyzed in the numerous bronchoalveolar lavage (BAL) fluids obtained from asthmatic lungs. However, BAL fluid levels of albumin alone may not always be a useful indicator of the plasma exudation process. Indeed, it has now been demonstrated in studies of the acute response to allergen challenge that BAL fluid albumin may be unchanged whereas large plasma proteins, such as fibrinogen and α_2-macroglobulin, are significantly increased (15,16). Such a result could even be expected because the inflammatory stimulus-induced luminal entry of plasma is almost a bulk flux of proteins with little size-restriction and, differing from albumin, low concentrations are normally present of the much larger plasma proteins. Furthermore, BAL fluid contains material that has accumulated on the surface for variable and unknown periods of time. An additional confounding factor concerns the fact that BAL fluid variably samples both airway and alveolar lining surface material. This latter aspect may pose a general problem in as much as asthma is an airway and not a pulmonary disease. In the nose, where airway-specific challenge and lavage are readily feasible, and where the problem of varying baselines can be eliminated, albumin may well reflect the plasma exudation response (3). Indeed, albumin and α_2 macroglobulin were highly correlated in nasal lavage liquids after allergen challenge in the nose, whereas in corresponding bronchial experiments, involving the same patients, allergen challenge only increased BAL fluid α_2-macroglobulin (16).

Roles of Exuded Plasma

The recent observations on mucosal exudation mechanisms in animal and human airways call for a revision of many of the previously proposed roles of plasma exudation in airway diseases (1,3,4,8). Increased microvascular permeability in the airways may no longer without reservations be equated with airway edema. The presence of plasma proteins in the airway lumen may no longer be interpreted as a sign of epithelial damage. More specifically, just because plasma is exuded into the airway lumen this may no longer tell us anything about the perviousness of the airway mucosa to inhaled molecules. It may also be difficult to conclude about the occurrence of tracheobronchial plasma exudation merely from measurements of BAL fluid levels of albumin; and it may be a complete mistake to conclude that a protein that did increase in BAL fluid must come from a cellular source just because the level of albumin did not exhibit a simultaneous increase. We may further need to know whether plasma exudation has occurred or not to properly interpret the appearance of many cellularly derived indices including cytokines on the mucosal surface; particularly, we may need to distinguish when the indices merely have been carried from the lamina propria to the surface by the exudate.

Even if plasma extravasation in the airways does not always produce mucosal edema, there are several other sequelae to consider. Extravasated plasma may deposit its targeting and carrier proteins as well as its fibrinous macromolecules in the lamina propria, the basement membrane, and both in and on the epithelium. Plasma may thus be an important source providing adhesive protein components to the mucosal extracellular matrix. By continuously supplying these proteins, together with plasma-derived growth factors, and together with important complement fragments, kinins, fibrinolysis peptides, etc., the extravasation process in the airways may be crucial to airway cellular inflammatory processes and to airway remodelling processes. The luminal entry of extravasated plasma is not only a mechanism that reduces the tendency to edema formation in the airways. Plasma-derived fibrin, fibronectin and other proteins in the epithelium and on the mucosal surface may govern an important part of the traffic and the activity of leukocytes in airway inflammation. Plasma-derived mediators and cytokines, a great variety of active oligoproteins and peptides, may, together with the cellular products, be important factors in almost all facets of mucosal inflammation (4,17).

By its physical properties and interactions plasma exudates may further impede the patency of the airway passages in several ways (17). Against a background of stagnated exudate-mucus material in the lumen, a pronounced exudation response in an attack of asthma may cause extremely severe obstruction of the bronchi, also when bronchial smooth muscle contraction is increased only slightly (17).

Absorption, Exudation and Epithelial Restitution

Severe airway infections caused by human influenza virus may be associated with extensive airway epithelial damage and shedding, but the extent of increased mucosal absorptivity under these conditions now remains little studied. It has recently been demonstrated that common cold virus inoculation may produce significant disease symptoms, hyperresponsiveness, and exudation of plasma macromolecules without causing appreciable increases in the human nasal airway absorption permeability. Corona-virus-induced nasal infection is thus associated with plasma exudation responses both at baseline and at challenge with histamine which are significantly greater than the corresponding normal values (18). The hyperresponsiveness to histamine probably reflects true changes in the responsive end-organ (microcirculation) since increased penetration and absorption of topical challenge agents may not apply in common cold (18).

Using the controlled conditions that are offered by the nasal pool technique Greiff et al. (19) have further observed that the nasal absorption rate of a small hydrophilic tracer (Cr ^{52}EDTA) is abnormally slow in subjects with allergic rhinitis. Thus, late into the Swedish birch pollen season, when eosinophilic exudative inflammation would have been present for several weeks, the allergic airway mucosa exhibited an increased functional tightness. In a separate study quite similar findings have now been obtained concerning peptide absorption across the allergic nasal mucosa (20). During the Swedish pollen season rhinitic individuals also develop a significantly increased responsiveness to histamine challenge expressed as abnormally increased plasma exudation (21). Since absorption of histamine would be decreased in these patients, the recorded hyperresponsiveness may be an underestimation of the change that had occurred in the airway microcirculation. It may not be feasible to have perfectly controlled conditions for studies of absorption across a defined bronchial mucosal surface *in vivo* in man. However, in a recent study Halpin et al. (22) made serious attempts to correct for mucociliary transport of the inhaled absorption tracer and could demonstrate that the absorption permeability in asthma may be reduced. It appears that a new paradigm on airway tightness in allergic inflammation is under development.

These clinical observations on reduced absorption permeability in asthma and rhinitis prompt questions about "mediators" of tightness rather than permeability. It has been clearly demonstrated that luminal entry of plasma does not cause epithelial disruption nor is it associated with an increased absorption ability of the airway mucosa (3). Is it then possible that the plasma exudation process under some circumstances may impede airway absorption? Another thought-provoking finding in this context concerns the association between increased epithelial damage and shedding and normal or reduced absorption rates in chronic inflammatory airway disease. A decreased absorption ability would certainly not be compatible with extensively denuded basement membranes in the airways. Perhaps, then, the new absorption data should be taken as support for the possibility that extensive denudation in specimens of asthmatic bronchi may be an artefact of the biopsy procedure rather than a true reflection of the *in situ* condition. A further potentially linked question, and one that may not have received sufficient attention, concerns the epithelial repair or restitution process that would be set in motion as soon as shedding occurs. Can increased knowledge about repair after shedding provide explanations to the well-maintained barrier functions in diseased airways?

Jonas Erjefält et al. (23–25) have recently examined effects induced by and following from gentle epithelial cell removal *in vivo* in guinea-pig trachea. The employed *in vivo* model mimics epithelial shedding by not causing bleeding or damage to the basement membrane. Two important findings are the promptness and the high speed by which epithelial restitution starts and proceeds, respectively. The immediate physiological and cellular *in vivo* responses to denudation are severalfold. The microcirculation responds by exuding bulk plasma and, with little delay, large numbers of neutrophils and are extravasated

(no bleeding occurs) (23–25). Secretion is induced (25). Eosinophil traffic and activation are also induced (24,25). Thus, a plasma-derived fibrin-fibronectin gel increasingly rich in neutrophils and eosinophils soon covers the denuded basement membrane (Fig. 3). This provisional cover is maintained and continuously supplied with plasma until a new tight epithelium has been established. The intact epithelial cells bordering the denuded area also respond immediately after loosing their neighbour cells. Secretory and ciliated cells [sic, ciliated cells do partake as progenitors for the new epithelium], and probably also basal cells, dedifferentiate, flatten and migrate over the membrane (10). The migration rate is particularly fast during the first minutes after denudation. The speed of migration, most likely aided by *in vivo*-specific factors, is so high (~3 μm/min) that shedding, even of clusters of epithelial cells, would result in deepithelialized basement membranes only for quite brief periods of time. Hence, epithelial shedding even to the extent of denudation of limited areas may occur *in vivo* with little consequence to the mucosal barrier functions. Defence and protection during the restitution process would be well catered for by the leukocyte-rich plasma-derived gel. This gel, with its content of plasma-derived migration-promoters such as fibronectin, fibrin and growth factors, is further a highly suitable supramembranal milieu for high speed epithelial restitution. [*In vitro* studies dealing with epithelial repair demonstrate only relatively slow events.] Another conclusion concerns all those physiological and cellular effects that may be evoked by the shedding of airway epithelial cells. Experimental *in vivo* data suggest that plasma exudation, secretory effects, traffic, activation of eosinophils through lysis, neutrophil recruitment and ac-

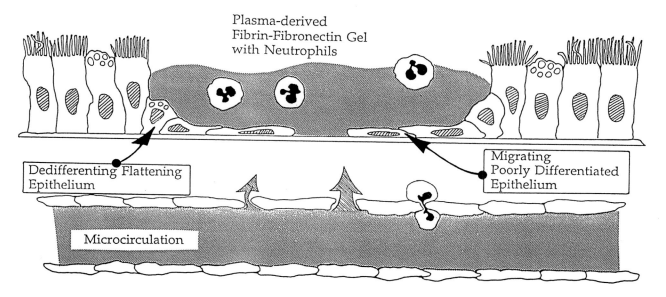

FIG. 3. After denudation epithelial restitution occurs speedily under the provisional cover of a plasma-derived and leukocyte-rich gel. (Drawing by Jonas Erjefält.)

tivation can be caused simply by the shedding of epithelial cells (23–25). Hence, these well-known characteristics of asthmatic airways may now be regarded as potential sequelae to desquamation.

Complete denudation with loss of both columnar and
basal cells may not be the most common kind of shedding. Columnar cells may rather more easily be shed and
thus leave a cobble-stone surface of basal cells behind
(26,27). What happens to the basal cells when they loose
their columnar neighbors? This question is currently being addressed in experiments involving both animal and
human airways (27). It appears that the basal cells
promptly undergo flattening and that they within minutes
establish extensive contact with each other. Airway basal
cells may thus be well suited to keep up the barrier function and cover the basement membrane fully at shedding
of ciliated and secretory cells. Indeed, this newly proposed role of the basal cell may be a major function of
these cells in addition to its role in anchoring of columnar epithelium (26,27). The new flat epithelium that is established after shedding or denudation frequently consists
of cells that have a larger apical surface than the normal
columnar epithelium. As a consequence a reduced junctional length of the epithelium per unit mucosal surface
area would be available for solute absorption. Specula-
tively, this change might explain in part the observations
of reduced absorption in desquamative airway disease.
[The limited barrier defect of epithelial cell removal may
also have to change our view on the role of epithelial
shedding in respiratory defence (1,27)!]

The new findings on basal cell responses and on reepithelialization in a plasma-derived gel *in vivo* after denudation may in part explain why increased absorption
permeability has not been widely demonstrated in allergic and other inflammatory airway diseases where epithelial cells are frequently being shed. Perhaps also the
clues to explain an increased absorption tightness, some
of the pathophysiological effects, and some of the cellular pathology in asthma and rhinitis can be found among
mucosal exudation and epithelial restitution mechanisms
as they evolve under proper *in vivo* conditions.

ACKNOWLEDGMENT

This work was supported by the Swedish Medical Research Council project 8308, the Medical Faculty, University of Lund; Astra Draco, Lund; and the Swedish Association Against Asthma and Allergy. I thank Mai
Broman for the secretarial work.

REFERENCES

1. Persson CGA, Andersson M, Greiff L, Svensson C, Erjefält JS, Sundler F, Wollmer P, Alkner U, Erjefält I, Gustafsson B, Linden M, Nilsson M. Airway Permeability. *Clin Exp Allergy* 1995;25:807–814.
2. Greiff L, Svensson C, Andersson M, Persson CGA. Effects of topical capsaicin in seasonal allergic rhinitis. *Thorax* 1995;50:225–229.
3. Persson CGA, Svensson C, Greiff L, Andersson M, Wollmer P, Alkner U, Erjefält I. The use of the nose to study the inflammatory response of the respiratory tract. Editorial *Thorax* 1992;47:993–1000.
4. Persson CGA. Airway epithelium and microcirculation. *Eur Respir Rev* 1994;4:23,352–362.
5. Persson CGA, Alkner U, Andersson M, Greiff L, Linden M, Svensson C. Histamine-challenge-induced "lamina propria lavage" and mucosal out-put of IL-6 in human airways. *Eur Respir J* 1995;8:125S(abstr).
6. Erjefält JS, Erjefält I, Sundler F, Persson CGA. Epithelial pathways for luminal entry of bulk plasma. *Clin Exp Allergy* 1995;25:187–195.
7. Erjefält I, Luts A, Persson CGA. Appearance of airway absorption and exudation tracers in guinea-pig tracheobronchial lymph nodes. *J Appl Physiol* 1993;74(2):817–824.
8. Persson CGA, Erjefält I, Alkner U, et al. Plasma exudation as a first line respiratory mucosal defence. *Clin Exp Allergy* 1991;21:17–24.
9. Greiff L, Alkner U, Pipkorn U, Persson CGA. The `nasal pool' device applies controlled concentrations of solutes on human nasal airway mucosa and samples its surface exudations/secretions. *Clin Exp Allergy* 1990;20:253–259.
10. Svensson C, Andersson M, Greiff L, Alkner U, Persson CGA. Exudative hyperresponsiveness to histamine in seasonal allergic rhinitis. *Clin Exp Allergy* 1995;25:942–950.
11. Erjefält I, Greiff L, Alkner U, Persson CGA. Allergen-induced biphasic plasma exudation responses in guinea pig large airways. *Am Rev Respir Dis* 1993;148:695–701.
12. Erjefält I, Persson CGA. Increased sensitivity to toluene diisocyanate (TDI) in airways previously exposed to low doses of TDI. *Clin Exp Allergy* 1992;22:854–862.
13. Fabbri LM, Mapp C. Bronchial hyperresponsiveness, airway inflammation and occupational asthma induced by toluene diisocyanate. *Clin Exp Allergy* 1991;21(1):42–47.
14. Persson CGA. Plasma exudation and asthma. *Lung* 1988;166:1–23.
15. Salomonsson P, Grönneberg R, Gilljam H, et al. Bronchial exudation of bulk plasma at allergen challenge in allergic asthma. *Am Rev Respir Dis* 1992;146:1535–1542.
16. Svensson C, Grönneberg R, Andersson M, et al. Allergen challenge-induced exudation of α_2-macroglobulin across human nasal and bronchial microvascular-epithelial barriers. *J Allergy Clin Immunol* 1995;96:239–246.
17. Persson CGA. The role of plasma exudation in asthmatic airways. *Lancet* 1986;2:1126–1129.
18. Greiff L, Andersson M, Åkerlund A, Wollmer P, Svensson C, Alkner U, Persson CGA. Microvascular exudative hyperresponsiveness in human coronavirus-induced common cold. *Thorax* 1994;49:121–127.
19. Greiff L, Wollmer P, Svensson C, Andersson M, Persson CGA. Effect of seasonal allergic rhinitis on airway mucosal absorption of Chromium-51-labelled EDTA. *Thorax* 1993;48:648–650.
20. Greiff L, Lundin S, Svensson C, Andersson M, Erjefält JS, Wollmer P, Persson CGA. Reduced airway absorption in seasonal allergic rhinitis. *Am J Respir Crit Care Med* 1997 (in press).
21. Svensson C, Andersson M, Greiff L, Alkner U, Persson CGA. Exudative hyperresponsiveness to histamine in seasonal allergic rhinitis. *Clin Exp Allergy* 1995;25:942–950.
22. Halpin DMG, Currie D, Jones B, Leigh TR, Evans TW. Permeability of bronchial mucosa to [113en]In-DTPA in asthma and the effects of salmeterol. *Eur Respir J* 1993;6(17):512s.
23. Erjefält JS, Erjefält I, Sundler F, Persson CGA. Microcirculation-derived factors in airway epithelial repair *in vivo*. *Microvascular Research* 1994;48:161–178.
24. Erjefält JS, Erjefält I, Sundler F, Persson CGA. *In vivo* restitution of airway epithelium. *Cell Tissue Res* 1995;281:305–316.
25. Erjefält JS, Sundler F, Persson CGA. Eosinophils, neutrophils and venular gaps in the airway mucosa at epithelial removal-restitution *Am J Crit Care Med* 1996;153:1666–1674.
26. Evans MJ, Plopper CG. The role of basal cells in adhesion of columnar epithelium to airway basement membrane. *Am Rev Respir Dis* 1989;138:481–483.
27. Erjefält JS, Sundler F, Persson CGA. Epithelial barrier formation by airway basal cells. *Thorax* 1997 (in press).

Asthma, edited by P.J. Barnes, M.M. Grunstein, A.R. Leff, and A.J. Woolcock. Lippincott–Raven Publishers, Philadelphia © 1997.

▪ 65 ▪

Airway Wall Thickening

Clive R. Roberts, Mitsushi Okazawa, Barry Wiggs, Peter D. Paré

Structural Changes in the Airway Walls in Asthma
  Subepithelial Collagen Deposition in Asthma
  Mechanisms Underlying Changes in Extracellular
    Matrix Composition in Asthma

Evidence for Increased Extracellular Matrix
  Degradation in Asthma
  Smooth Muscle Proliferation in Asthma
Modeling Airway Function

In this chapter, we review the structural alterations that occur in the airway wall in chronic asthma and discuss how these structural changes in the airways can alter airway function. The details of the structural changes come from morphometric and immuno- and histochemical analyses of the airways of asthmatic individuals. The tissue has been obtained at the time of autopsy after severe fatal attacks of asthma, from autopsy samples of the lungs of patients who had asthma but who died of other causes, and from airway wall biopsies obtained via bronchoscopy in relatively stable asthmatic individuals. Unfortunately, these sources do not provide the full spectrum of pathologic material necessary to describe the morphologic changes in the airway walls as a function of clinical severity, chronicity, or age. Particularly lacking are specimens from patients during acute attacks of allergic bronchoconstriction and from patients who have atopy and abnormal airway responsiveness but no lower respiratory symptoms. In addition, the data derived from biopsies are incomplete because only the submucosal region is normally sampled and no quantitative morphometry of the full thickness of the airway wall can be performed on these samples.

A number of pathologic changes occur in airway walls of asthmatic individuals that would be expected to produce little alteration in the mechanics of the airways, and thus these will not be reviewed here. These changes include the sloughing of the airway epithelium and the proliferation of the mucous glands and goblet cells (1). This is not to say that these alterations are not important; the loss of the epithelium may contribute to symptoms by exposing the epithelial nerve plexus to inhaled irritants and the hyperplasia of mucus-secreting tissues can certainly contribute to airway obstruction. However, these changes are discussed in detail elsewhere in this volume (see Chapters 16 and 17) and we will limit this review to pathologic abnormalities that may have a major effect on airway wall mechanics.

Airway mechanics may be changed because of quantitative changes in airway wall compartments and/or by changes in the biochemical composition or material properties of the various constituents of the airway wall. We will review the data on the quantitative changes in the dimensions and organization of the airway wall compartments as well as the biochemical alterations that have been described. In addition, we will attempt to predict how these structural and biochemical changes might affect the mechanical properties of the airways and, ultimately, their ability to narrow.

C. R. Roberts, B. Wiggs, and P. D. Paré: Department of Medicine, University of British Columbia, St. Paul's Hospital, Vancouver, British Columbia V6Z 1Y6 Canada.

M. Okazawa: Departments of Pathology and Laboratory Medicine, University of British Columbia, St. Paul's Hospital, Vancouver, British Columbia V6Z 1Y6 Canada.

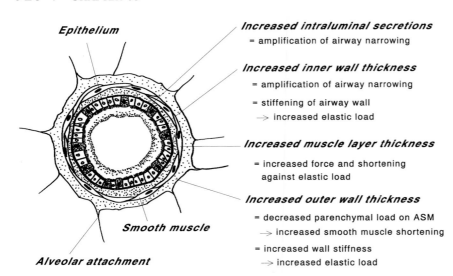

Epithelium

Increased intraluminal secretions
= amplification of airway narrowing

Increased inner wall thickness
= amplification of airway narrowing
= stiffening of airway wall
→ increased elastic load

Increased muscle layer thickness
= increased force and shortening against elastic load

Increased outer wall thickness
= decreased parenchymal load on ASM
→ increased smooth muscle shortening
= increased wall stiffness
→ increased elastic load

Smooth muscle

Alveolar attachment

FIG. 1. Cross-section through a membranous airway. The luminal secretions and the three layers of the airway wall are illustrated, along with the possible functional consequences of thickening of these layers.

STRUCTURAL CHANGES IN THE AIRWAY WALLS IN ASTHMA

Exaggerated airway narrowing constitutes the most fundamental pathophysiologic abnormality in asthma. In normal individuals, high concentrations of bronchoconstricting substances can be inhaled with only mild to moderate airway narrowing; in fact, most normal individuals develop a plateau on the dose-response curve to inhaled pharmacologic agonists, whereas in moderate to severe asthma, a plateau does not develop (2,3). Increased maximal airway narrowing can be caused by structural alterations in the airways. Figure 1 shows a schematic diagram of an intraparenchymal airway cut in cross-section. The wall can be divided into three compartments: the inner wall, consisting of epithelium, basement membrane, lamina propria, and submucosa; the outer wall, consisting of the loose connective tissue between the muscle layer and the surrounding parenchyma; and the smooth muscle layer (4). Increased thickness of the airway wall internal to the smooth muscle layer can amplify the airway narrowing produced by airway smooth muscle shortening. An increased volume of intraluminal secretions can also amplify the effects of smooth muscle shortening in addition to decreasing baseline airway lumenal area. The lung parenchyma that surrounds and attaches to the outside of the airway via alveolar attachments provides an elastic load that impedes airway smooth muscle shortening. The accumulation of material in the adventitial space between the surrounding parenchyma and the smooth muscle will tend to attenuate the afterload provided by these elastic elements so that greater smooth muscle shortening can occur for the same force generated by the muscle (5). Finally, an increased amount of muscle (if it remains phenotypically normal) will increase the force-generating ability of the muscle and allow greater airway smooth muscle shortening for any elastic load. Figure 2 shows the three mechanisms by which structural alterations can cause exaggerated maximal airway narrowing (6).

Although it has been recognized for some time that the airway walls of asthmatic individuals are thickened (7,8), it was not possible to perform a systematic study of the quantitative changes in airway wall dimensions because a yardstick of airway size was not available to allow a valid comparison between control and asthmatic individuals.

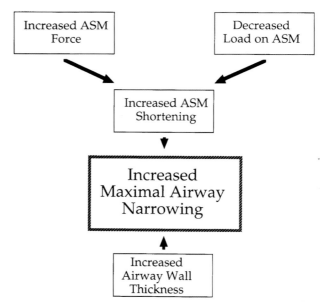

FIG. 2. Three potential mechanisms that could lead to exaggerated maximal airway narrowing. Increased airway narrowing may be caused by increased airway smooth muscle shortening. Increased airway smooth muscle shortening can occur because of decreased airway smooth muscle load or increased airway smooth muscle force. However, increased maximal narrowing can occur without increased shortening if the airway wall is thickened.

TABLE 1. *Relationships between airway wall areas and airway size*[a,b]

		WAinner	WAouter	WAtotal	Amuscle	Asubmucosa
Bosken, et al. (12)						
Obstructed	(n=30[c])	0.101 (0.142)	0.099 (0.148)			
Control	(n=30)	0.095 (0.106)	0.093 (0.099)			
Wiggs, et al. (13)						
Fatal asthma	(n=12)	0.148 (0.062)				
Autopsy control	(n=19)	0.103 (0.055)				
Surgical COPD	(n=30)	0.101 (0.143)				
Surgical control	(n=30)	0.096 (0.104)				
Kuwano, et al. (14)						
Fatal asthma	(n=8)	0.130 (0.007)	0.167 (0.070)		0.068 (0.005)	0.106 (0.015)
Nonfatal asthma	(n=7)	0.103 (0.012)	0.116 (0.047)		0.044 (0.026)	0.092 (-0.004)
COPD	(n=15)	0.065 (0.057)	0.086 (0.084)		0.035 (0.016)	0.056 (0.054)
Control	(n=15)	0.057 (0.083)	0.079 (0.116)		0.020 (0.056)	0.052 (0.067)
Ebina, et al. (15) (coefficients estimated from original author's formulas)						
Asthma	(n=16)				0.033 (0.174)	
Controls	(n=20)				0.018 (0.178)	
Tiddens, et al. (16)						
COPD	(n=59)			0.250 (0.250)		
Reiss, et al. (17) (surgical resection cases divided by methacholine challenge result)						
PC$_{20}$<2	(n=21)	0.087 (0.129)	0.090 (0.141)	0.126 (0.192)		
PC$_{20}$ 2–4	(n=9)	0.059 (0.211)	0.064 (0.190)	0.088 (0.284)		
PC$_{20}$ 4–16	(n=23)	0.084 (0.010)	0.064 (0.126)	0.106 (0.151)		
PC$_{20}$>16	(n=18)	0.078 (0.133)	0.074 (0.126)	0.108 (0.183)		

[a]Data represented as SLOPE (INTERCEPT)
[b]Relationships are linear regression models relating the square root of the noted wall component area and internal perimeter of the airway; where basement membrane perimeter was measured instead of lumenal perimeter, the coefficients are underlined.
[c]All sample sizes reflect number of subjects studied.
COPD, chronic obstructive pulmonary disease.

The demonstration by James et al. (9,10) that the airway basement membrane perimeter is relatively constant after smooth muscle contraction or changes in lung volume has allowed a number of investigators to examine the relationship between airway wall compartment areas and airway size. This is done most easily by examining the relationships between airway internal perimeter (Pi) or basement membrane perimeter (Pbm) and the areas occupied by the respective tissue components. The slopes and intercepts of these relationships can be constructed and compared using valid techniques for pooling data (11). Table 1 shows a summary of these data (12–17).

TABLE 2. *Extracellular Matrix Changes in Asthma and Predicted Functional Consequences*

Structural change (Ref.)	Predicted mechanical effect	Predicted effect on airway function
Collagen deposition in subepithelial matrix (19)	Subepithelial matrix stiffer in compression and tension	Inhibits narrowing
Thickened airway wall internal to the smooth muscle (14)	Geometric amplification of effect of SMC shortening on narrowing; Airway wall encroaches on airspace	Increased narrowing for a given degree of SMC contraction; Chronic airflow obstruction
Thickened adventitia (14)	Altered airway-parenchymal interdependence	
Hyaluronan and versican deposition internal to SMC (33)	Increased resistance to compression	Opposes airway narrowing
Hyaluronan and versican deposition in and around SMC bundles (33)	Preload on SMC due to SMC-associated matrix is increased	Opposes smooth muscle shortening
Elastin degradation (45)	Walls of large airways more flexible; Walls of small airways less patent	Chronic airflow obstruction
Cartilage degradation (33)	Cartilaginous airways more easily deformed by intrathoracic pressure changes and more easily narrowed by SMC contraction	Chronic airflow obstruction; Increased narrowing of bronchi for a given degree of SMC force generation

SMC, smooth muscle cell.

These results confirm that patients with fatal asthma show a marked increase in airway wall thickness that involves all layers of the airway wall. There are less data on patients who have had asthma but who died for other reasons or had a lobectomy. However, the available data suggest that the airway wall dimensions in these individuals are intermediate between the fatal asthmatics and the control or normal individuals (14,18). Thus, an increase in airway wall dimensions does not simply reflect a terminal event in patients with severe asthma.

Abnormal airway wall structure may contribute to altered airway mechanics in asthma, both through geometric effects and through direct changes in tissue biomechanics. In addition, changes in extracellular matrix structure have effects on cellular functions and may themselves modulate the physiologic process of inflammation. We review changes in the extracellular matrix of the airway walls in asthma and consider the likely functional consequences of some of these changes (see Table 2 for summary).

Subepithelial Collagen Deposition in Asthma

Airway wall thickening in asthma involves increased collagen deposition. Roche and co-workers have shown that the thickened subepithelial "basement membrane" in asthma consists of a dense layer rich in fibrillar collagens, under a normal subepithelial basal lamina (19). This distinct collagenous matrix layer is typically doubled in thickness from 5 to 8 mm (normal) to 10 to 15 mm (asthma) and contains types I, III, and V collagen and fibronectin (19) but not basal lamina components (type IV collagen, laminin). This collagenous matrix may be synthesized by its associated myofibroblasts because myofibroblast number correlated with the degree of subepithelial thickening (20). Similar structural changes have been observed in patients with mild asthma, are apparently not reversed by glucocorticoid treatment (21), and have been observed in occupational asthma associated with exposure to a variety of chemicals (22), and with chronic inflammation in the airways caused by cigarette smoking (12). In some individuals with toluene diisocyanate-induced asthma (TDI), cessation of exposure to TDI leads, after 6 to 20 months, to decreased subepithelial collagen thickness and decreased numbers of subepithelial fibroblasts associated with decreased numbers of mast cells and lymphocytes (23). This suggests that these changes are potentially reversible, but the mechanism of this reversal is unknown.

The mechanical effects of changes in abundance of collagen types in the subepithelial matrix are unknown but likely depend on the precise architecture and chemistry of the collagens deposited. Types I, III, and V are the fibril-forming collagens, containing long stretches of triple helix. *In vitro* studies suggest that type V collagen limits the

diameter of collagen fibrils (24,25). The association of proteoglycans including decorin with collagen fibrils also may influence fibril assembly (26). Altered collagen and proteoglycan composition may be one mechanism by which fibril size and hence, tissue mechanical properties are regulated (27). The collagen fibrils in the subepithelial collagen layer in the airways of asthmatics appear to be more densely packed than normal (19) and, although the significance of this is unknown, it is probable that both increased collagen fibril density and thickening of this layer would increase both the tensile stiffness and resistance to deformation of the airway wall, thus tending to oppose smooth muscle contraction and airway narrowing. In recent studies (28) airway distensibility was shown to be decreased in asthmatics; this could be explained by excess collagen deposition in the subepithelial layer.

In addition to collagen, the adhesive glycoprotein fibronectin and the antiadhesive glycoprotein tenascin appear to be deposited in the airway wall in asthmatics (29). These may be synthesized by epithelial cells in response to inflammatory mediators: Fibronectin synthesis by bovine bronchial epithelial cells is stimulated by transforming growth factor-β (TGF-β) (30), and tenascin synthesis by transformed human bronchial epithelial cells is stimulated by tumor necrosis factor-α (TNF-α) and interferon-γ (IFN-γ) (31).

The airway walls contain proteoglycans with their characteristic polysaccharides, the glycosaminoglycans. Specific proteoglycans and glycosaminoglycans of the extracellular matrix influence tissue biomechanics, fluid balance, cellular functions and growth factor, and cytokine biologic activities. Changes in glycosaminoglycan metabolism occur early in a number of animal models of inflammation (32), suggesting that changes in proteoglycan metabolism may contribute to altered extracellular matrix properties in asthma. We have used immunohistochemistry to localize hyaluronan (HA) and the proteoglycans versican and decorin in surgical and postmortem lung samples from persons with normal lung function and persons in whom asthma was the cause of death.

HA and versican were localized in and around the smooth muscle bundles in the airways (33). Decorin was found in areas rich in type I collagen. In airways from asthmatics, staining for all the proteoglycans was particularly prominent around smooth muscle cells and in the submucosa, i.e., between the smooth muscle and the epithelial layer. The matrix of the thickened airway walls stained particularly intensely for versican and hyaluronan, especially between and around the smooth muscle bundles, areas that appear to be "space" after routine formalin fixation and paraffin embedding. These "spaces" appear to be hydrated proteoglycan-rich domains in life (33).

Although the functional correlates of proteoglycan deposition in the airway wall are unknown, hydrated proteoglycans may contribute to the increased volume of the submucosa in asthmatics and may contribute to altered airway mechanics. HA-versican aggregates could influence the compressive stiffness of the airway wall and have an effect on airway interstitial fluid balance, through their osmotic activity. The rationale for this hypothesis is that versican is the closest homolog, in molecular terms, of the cartilage proteoglycan aggrecan, an important determinant of the mechanics of hyaline cartilage (34). The glycosaminoglycans are highly negatively charged at neutral pH. The high concentration of hyaluronan and aggrecan results in an osmotic swelling pressure balanced by tension in the collagenous network of the tissue. It is the reversible redistribution of glycosaminoglycan-bound water that gives cartilage its characteristic mechanical properties in compression. We hypothesize that the versican-hyaluronan complex contributes to compressive stiffness of airway walls in a similar way to the effect of the aggrecan-hyaluronan in cartilage. Versican is also a prominent component of the intima of arterial walls (35), where it is believed to contribute to the resistance of this tissue to compression. The deposition of a versican-HA complex in the submucosal region between the muscle and basement membrane could contribute to exaggerated airway narrowing, as depicted in Figure 2. Conversely, deposition of HA and versican between the smooth muscle and epithelium would be expected to increase tissue turgor and thus to increase the resistance of the airway wall to deformation under loading. In addition, accumulation of a relatively incompressible matrix around smooth muscle cells in the airways might provide a parallel elastic afterload to oppose smooth muscle shortening.

Mechanisms Underlying Changes in Extracellular Matrix Composition in Asthma

A number of growth factors and cytokines released by inflammatory cells, or released by epithelial cells secondary to stimulation in allergic inflammation, have the capacity to drive altered extracellular matrix metabolism by mesenchymal cells in the airway wall. Eosinophil and mast cell numbers are increased in asthma, driven by a T-helper type 2 cell (TH2) response. Both inflammatory cells and stimulated epithelial and mesenchymal cells (including smooth muscle cells) have the capacity to release TGF-β_1, a growth factor that induces matrix deposition, and to release the potent fibroblast mitogens, platelet-derived growth factor (PDGF) and insulinlike growth factor-1 (IGF-1). This combination of mitogens and growth factors is known to induce matrix synthesis in other systems and is a potentially powerful mechanism for remodeling of the architecture of the airway wall in asthma.

A recent study (36) showed that steady-state messenger ribonucleic acid (mRNA) levels for TGF-β_1, as well as the pattern of expression of the latent precursor and mature forms of TG-Fβ_1, were similar in lung tissue from individuals with asthma, a group of individuals with chronic obstructive pulmonary disease (COPD), and a control group of cigarette smokers who had normal lung function. Similarly, there were no clear differences between these same groups of patients in the expression of mRNA for the collagen-associated proteoglycan decorin, a putative regulator of TGF-β_1 biologic activity (37). The precursor protein for TGF-β_1 was detected in epithelial cells, implying epithelial cell synthesis of this growth factor. The fact that abundant mRNA and protein for TGF-β_1 was found in both of the patient groups and the "control" group may reflect a chronic inflammatory process in both the control and COPD groups because members of the control group had a history of smoking, although they did not have significant airway obstruction. Likewise, TGF-β_1 mRNA levels in mononuclear cells from brochoalveolar lavage (BAL) from asthmatics and normals have been shown to be similar (38). Eosinophils also express TGF-β, and their abundance in asthma would be expected to contribute to increased local, if not total, tissue levels of this growth factor. Eosinophils from asthmatics express higher levels of PDGF-B mRNA than normals (39), and this agent is mitogenic for mesenchymal cells including fibroblasts and smooth muscle cells. Aubert et al. (40) examined the presence and distribution of PDGF and PDGF receptor messenger RNA and protein in the lungs and airways of a small group of patients with fatal asthma as well as controls and patients with COPD. PDGF message levels tended to be greater in asthmatics than in normals and lower in COPD than in normals. The PDGF mRNA levels were significantly greater in patients with asthma compared with patients with COPD. In addition, there was a significant association between PDGF mRNA levels and PDGF receptor mRNA levels, suggesting that there is a link between the expression of this growth factor and its receptor.

Human airway epithelial cells have been shown to secrete fibroblast mitogenic activity, at least 50% of which is attributable to IGF-1 (41). This growth factor stimulates collagen production by dermal fibroblasts in vitro (42), suggesting a further mechanism by which epithelial cells might stimulate collagen production and cell proliferation in the underlying matrix.

Corticosteroids have multiple effects but may prevent remodeling both by decreasing influx of inflammatory cells (perhaps without decreasing the amount of mediators such as TGF-β_1 per cell [43]) and by exerting specific inhibitory effects on synthesis of matrix molecules, including collagen (44).

Evidence for Increased Extracellular Matrix Degradation in Asthma

Ultrastructural evidence for elastin degradation in some individuals with asthma has been reported (45). We have observed structural changes in the cartilage in airways of 1 to 5 mm in diameter, consistent with cartilage proteoglycan degradation and cartilage remodeling in each of six fatal asthma cases studied in detail (Fig. 3). These changes may be specific to cartilage proteoglycans and have effects on lung function resulting from softening of airway cartilage. Conversely, the changes in cartilage may be indicators of a much more general process of cleavage of structural elements, with even further-reaching effects. The proteinase(s) responsible for the cartilage changes are unknown, but there are a number of possibilities. Neutrophil elastase, cathepsin G, and lysosomal cysteine proteinases such as cathepsins B and L are able to degrade collagen, elastin, and proteoglycans. Latent cathepsin B is present in the sputum of chronic bronchitics (46). Latent cysteine proteinases can be activated by a number of means, including direct activation by neutrophil proteinases (46) and activation by a cartilage-specific mechanism that is not yet understood (47). Indirect mechanisms for cartilage destruction include interleukin 1–driven resorption of airway cartilage by chondrocytes, mediated by matrix metalloproteinases (48), as has been described in cartilage destruction in inflammatory joint diseases. Proteinases released by mast cells, including tryptase, also may be responsible for degradation of a range of matrix macromolecules in asthma.

Degradation of airway cartilage could contribute to airflow obstruction by decreasing airway wall stiffness, which would decrease maximal expiratory flow rates from the lung. Cartilage degradation also could decrease the force required for the smooth muscle to constrict the airways. Degradation of elastin, as shown by Bousquet

(45), and possibly degradation of other matrix molecules, may have similar effects on airway wall mechanics. Matrix degradation and increased proteoglycan synthesis are associated with tissue swelling during development (49), and proteolysis in the airway wall matrix may facilitate edema in asthma. Mast cell degranulation is associated with edema of the airway wall and an acute decrease in interstitial pressure (50). Proteoglycan synthesis, in concert with matrix degradation, may influence tissue swelling. As discussed above, the force required to deform the matrix constitutes an afterload that must be overcome by smooth muscle during shortening. Degradation of matrix elements could increase the deformability of the airway wall and thus decrease its ability to act as a load on the muscle. Consistent with this hypothesis, *in vitro* studies by Bramley and colleagues (51) suggest that mild proteolysis in the extracellular matrix associated with airway smooth muscle allows increased force generation and shortening by strips of human airway smooth muscle. Degradation of smooth muscle-associated matrix as a consequence of chronic inflammation has been postulated to exacerbate the increased smooth muscle contractility in asthma (51,52).

Because tethering of the parenchyma to both the smooth muscle and perichondrium is believed to limit smooth muscle shortening, we suggest that degradation of collagen connected to smooth muscle bundles is a prerequisite for the uncoupling of airway smooth muscle from parenchymal tethering, which has been suggested by Macklem (5) and others (53) to be an important component of asthma.

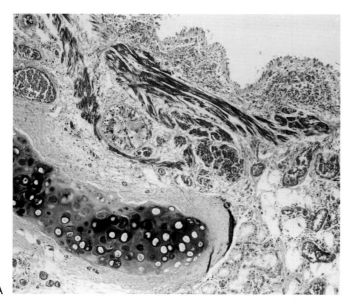
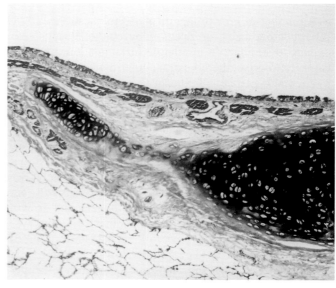

A

B

FIG. 3. Small cartilaginous airway from an individual aged 75 years with a 30-year history of asthma (**A**) and an airway of similar size from a nonasthmatic individual of the same age (**B**) showing increased smooth muscle area, subepithelial collagen deposition, matrix deposition, and cartilage remodeling in the asthmatic.

Smooth Muscle Proliferation in Asthma

A number of studies show that the airway smooth muscle layer is markedly thickened in patients with chronic asthma (54,55). Part of this thickening could have been artifactual, because the airways of asthmatic individuals are often contracted and narrowed by the time of postmortem. However, correction of airway smooth muscle area for basement membrane perimeter indicates that in patients with fatal asthma, peripheral airway smooth muscle area is approximately doubled, whereas in patients who have asthma but die of other causes, lesser degrees of airway smooth muscle thickening are observed (see Table 1). There is evidence that the increase in smooth muscle is due both to hypertrophy of existing airway smooth muscle cells, as well as to hyperplasia. Ebina et al. (15,56) have reported two patterns of airway smooth muscle hypertrophy and hyperplasia. In their type 1 asthmatics, airway smooth muscle mass was increased only in central bronchi where hyperplasia predominated. In type 2 asthmatics, there was increased muscle throughout the tracheobronchial tree; the increased muscle was characterized by hyperplasia as well as hypertrophy, especially in peripheral airways. Thomson et al. (57) suggested that the increase in airway smooth muscle area that has been reported in asthma could have been overestimated. These investigators measured the airway smooth muscle area in the large central airways of five asthmatic individuals and showed no significant difference compared with a matched control group. They used 1.5-mm sections of plastic-embedded tissue and discriminated between smooth muscle cells and their surrounding matrix. They reasoned that the plane of section, the use of thick sections, and a failure to distinguish between smooth muscle cells and their associated extracellular matrix could explain an overestimation of smooth muscle area in other studies. However, Thomson et al. (57) studied only large central cartilaginous airways, and most of the increase in smooth muscle area that has been reported is in peripheral airways.

The increase in airway smooth muscle mass in asthma can have a simple geometric effect on airway narrowing, much like the effect of thickening of the submucosal region of the airway wall, and can narrow the airways as well as amplify the effect of smooth muscle shortening. However, an increase in smooth muscle mass, if associated with a parallel and concomitant increase in force-generating ability of the muscle, will have the additional effect of allowing the airway smooth muscle to shorten excessively against the elastic loads provided by the lung parenchyma and parallel elastic elements. Unfortunately, there have been few studies in which the functional properties of airway smooth muscle from asthmatic individuals have been measured and corrected for the amount of smooth muscle in the preparation. Schellenberg et al. (53) have reported increased maximal isotonic shortening and increased isometric force generation in a single asthmatic bronchial smooth muscle specimen, despite a normal amount of smooth muscle. De Jongste et al. (58) have reported increased maximal force generation in a few samples of central airways of asthmatic individuals; however, they did not correct the force for the smooth muscle mass. Bai (59) found increased force generation and decreased relaxation in the airway smooth muscle obtained from patients with fatal asthma, even after correction for tissue weight. No studies have shown increased airway smooth muscle sensitivity in asthmatic individuals compared with controls.

Although one might expect that an increase in airway smooth muscle mass would be accompanied by an increase in force generation, this is not necessarily the case. Vascular smooth muscle proliferation induced in rabbits by hyperoxia produces an increase in smooth muscle mass, but a decrease in the maximal stress-generating ability of the vascular smooth muscle (60). In vitro, when airway smooth muscle is stimulated to proliferate, the muscle differentiates from a contractile to a more motile phenotype, concomitant with decreased α-smooth muscle actin content and increased γ-actin and nonmuscle myosin content with increasing time in culture (61). Similar dedifferentiation of vascular smooth muscle occurs in vascular remodeling associated with atherosclerosis (62), and it is possible that chronic stimulation by cytokines and growth factors in the inflamed airway walls of asthmatic individuals results in proliferation and dedifferentiation of the airway smooth muscle, making it less contractile.

In summary, structural changes in the airway walls involving extracellular matrix remodeling are prominent features of asthma. These changes likely are driven by mediators released as a consequence of chronic allergic inflammation. It is clear that changes in matrix can influence airway function in asthma. However, it is not clear how each of the many changes that occur in the airway wall contributes to altered airway function in asthma. Collagen deposition in the subepithelial matrix and hyaluronan and versican deposition around and internal to the smooth muscle would be expected to oppose the effect of smooth muscle contraction. Conversely, geometric considerations would result in exaggerated airway narrowing for a given degree of smooth muscle shortening, as the airway wall is thickened by the deposition of these molecules internal to the smooth muscle. Elastin and cartilage degradation in the airway walls would be expected to result in decreased airway wall stiffness and increased airway narrowing for a given amount of force generated by the smooth muscle. Degradation of matrix associated with the smooth muscle may both decrease the stiffness of the parallel elastic component and uncouple smooth muscle from the load provided by lung recoil, allowing exaggerated smooth muscle shortening. Increase in muscle mass may be associated with an increase, decrease, or no change in smooth muscle contractility. If an increase in muscle mass was not associated with any other phenotypic changes it would be expected to contribute to exaggerated airway narrowing.

MODELING AIRWAY FUNCTION

Wiggs et al. (13) and more recently Lambert et al. (6) have attempted to determine which of the structural changes that occur in the airway wall of asthmatic individuals are most important to the development of exaggerated airway narrowing. They developed a computerized model of the tracheobronchial tree in which airway smooth muscle shortening occurred in a dose-response fashion. Airway smooth muscle shortening was allowed to proceed until the force generated by the muscle was equal and opposite to the force occurring in the surrounding lung parenchyma. They assumed that the contractile function and the length-tension relationship of the asthmatic airway smooth muscle was the same as normal, but that the force-generating capacity was increased in proportion to the increase in muscle mass. They found that all three of the structural changes that occur in asthma (increased mucosal thickness, increased muscle thickness, and increased adventitial thickness) contribute to increased maximal airway narrowing in asthma. However, the analysis showed that, of these factors, the increase in airway smooth muscle thickness was the most important abnormality. The increased submucosal and adventitial thickness could increase the maximal airway narrowing by a factor of 2 to 10, whereas the increased muscle thickness has the potential to increase maximal airway narrowing by two orders of magnitude. In this analysis, a number of assumptions were made that remain to be tested. The most important of these was that the increased airway smooth muscle mass that occurs in asthma is accompanied by a parallel increase in the ability of the muscle to generate force (i.e., maximal airway smooth muscle stress remains constant). However, as described above, there is reason to believe that when airway smooth muscle proliferates, there could be a decrease in the contractility of the muscle.

In this analysis, it was also assumed that the only load that the muscle has to overcome to contract is the elastic recoil of the lung. However, it has been recognized recently that the folding of the mucosal membrane that occurs during airway smooth muscle contraction means that there is an additional load that impedes smooth muscle shortening. Excised airways isolated from the surrounding parenchyma do not close. This means that there are elements within the airway wall that maintain airway patency. Okazawa et al. (63) have recently measured the lumenal patency of rabbit airways at zero transpulmonary pressure. The average lumenal area of unconstricted airways at a transpulmonary pressure of 0 was approximately 23% of

the lumenal area at a transpulmonary pressure of 25 cm H_2O. To narrow the airways beyond this equilibrium point, airway smooth muscle is faced with an additional load, that required to deform the mucosal membrane. It might be assumed that this force would be trivial because the application on only slight negative pressure at the airway opening is capable of causing airway closure (at least in some airways) because trapped gas volume is reached at a transpulmonary pressure between 0 and 2 cm H_2O (64). However, trapped gas volume is reached when any airway generation closes and airways proximal and distal to the site of closure may remain patent. In addition, the force required to narrow or close airways during passive deflation of the lung and during active airway smooth muscle constriction may be quite different. When the lung is deflated beyond its equilibrium point with negative pressure, the airways narrow by flattening, as shown in Fig. 3. During airway narrowing produced by active airway smooth muscle contraction, the configuration of the airway is quite different. The mucosal membrane folds as the airway smooth muscle contracts, stiffens, and shortens concentrically. The folded mucosal membrane offers much more resistance to deformation than the "fish mouth" configuration shown in Fig. 4. Lambert (65) was the first to recognize that the magnitude of this load will be related to the number of folds that develop during smooth muscle shortening as well as to the thickness and the mechanical

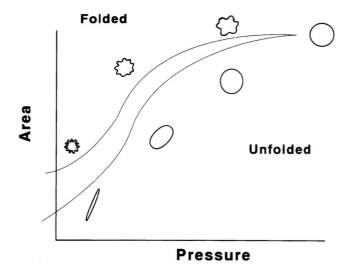

FIG. 4. Pressure-area curves of folded and nonfolded airways. This schematic plot shows theoretical pressure-area curves for an airway narrowed with and without mucosal folds. The least energy configuration is a simple "fish mouth" buckling of the airway wall, as illustrated on the lower, more compliant pressure-area curve. Multilobed buckling requires more force for the same degree of luminal narrowing as shown for the upper, less compliant pressure-area curve. Because the airway smooth muscle becomes stiff during contraction, multiple small folds occur, tending to stiffen the airway and attenuate narrowing.

properties of the tissue. In more recent work, Lambert has described the effect of mucosal buckling on the maximal amount of smooth muscle shortening. By considering the airway wall as a thin-layered material, Lambert shows that as the number of folds in the airway mucosa increases, a greater transmural pressure difference is required to collapse the airway (66). Also, as the number of folds increases, a smaller reduction in luminal cross-sectional area results after smooth muscle constriction.

In a recent theoretical work Wiggs et al. (67) have developed a computational model of the airway, as two concentric cylinders, to analyze geometric and mechanical influences on airway wall buckling. A thicker outer cylinder (layer 1, elastic modulus E1) represented the submucosa and a thinner inner cylinder (layer 2, elastic modulus E2) represented the basement membrane and epithelium. It was assumed that the airways are composed of incompressible material and that the contracting smooth muscle exerts a uniform hoop stress. Finite element analysis showed that multilobed collapse similar to that seen in asthmatic airways occurred only when the ratio E2/E1 was between 8 and 30, i.e., when the inner layer was significantly stiffer than the outer layer. This laminated design was chosen as no other regular structure could be found to exhibit multilobed buckling when loaded in this manner. These results, although based on theoretical models, highlight several interesting factors that should be considered: a) the airway wall is primarily compressed as the smooth muscle shortens. Therefore, compressive tests rather than length-tension style experiments will yield the information required for an understanding of airway mechanics during constriction; b) the relative elastic moduli of successive layers within the airway wall ares a determinant of the folding pattern; and c) organization and relative mechanical properties of the airway wall matrix molecules are important.

This modeling showed that the three factors that contribute to the load that the airway smooth muscle must overcome to shorten are the number of folds, the thickness of the two layers, and the elastic moduli of the two layers. The fewer the folds, the thinner the membrane and the less elastic the membrane, the easier it will be to narrow the lumen. What do we know about these three factors in the airways of normal individuals and asthmatics? There have been no systematic studies of the number of folds that develop in the airways of normal or asthmatic individuals during either passive or active airway narrowing. In addition, there are no studies of the tensile or compressive properties of the airway inner wall, either in normal or asthmatic individuals. If there are no changes in the mechanical properties of the inner wall, then one would predict that thicker airways will impart an increased load because the bending stiffness of a substance increases as the cube of its thickness. Thus, the wall thickening observed in asthma could cause a stiffening of the airway and protect from excessive narrowing. However, as discussed above, it is likely that there are changes in mechanical properties of the airway wall in asthma secondary to altered architecture and increased collagen, proteoglycan, and elastin deposition. It is difficult to predict the nature of these changes. The increased deposition of type I and III collagen in the lamina reticularis might increase the stiffness of the airway, at least in response to tensile stresses. The work of Colebatch et al. (68) and Wilson et al. (28) supports the notion that the airways of asthmatic individuals are less distensible. Theory suggests that this should increase resistance of the wall to buckling. However, there is reason to believe that there could be alterations in the airway wall that make it less elastic and more easily deformable. Bousquet et al. (45) have reported fragmentation of elastic fibers that might decrease airway wall stiffness. Digestion of connective tissue elements by proteases released from mast cells and other inflammatory cells could cause a decrease in the stiffness in the wall despite the increased thickness. The studies of Wiggs et al. (67) illustrated that it is the compressive stiffness of the wall that will have the greatest influence on the ease with which airway smooth muscle can deform and fold the mucosal membrane. It is unclear what the relative roles of the different connective tissue proteins will be in response to compressive stress. These findings lead to an important future direction for airway mechanics research. With newly developed testing devices the soft tissue compressive mechanics of airways in both control and diseased conditions can be investigated. These investigations must consider not only the viscoelastic behavior of the solid tissues but also the hydraulic flow of water through these tissues. With new techniques to determine the fractional content of airway matrix, the mechanical function of these components, and theoretical models, we will be able to develop a more complete description of airway mechanics in normal and diseased conditions.

ACKNOWLEDGMENTS

Our work is supported by the Medical Research Council of Canada and the British Columbia Lung Association.

REFERENCES

1. Jeffery PK. Structural changes in asthma. In: Page C, Black J, eds. *Airways and vascular remodelling*. Cambridge: Academic Press, 1994;3–9.
2. James AL, Lougheed D, Pearce-Pinto G, Ryan G, Musk B. Maximal airway narrowing in a general population. *Am Rev Respir Dis* 1992; 146:895–899.
3. Woolcock A, Salome CM, Yan K. The shape of the dose-response curve to histamine in asthmatic and normal subjects. *Am Rev Respir Dis* 1984;130:71–75.
4. Bai A, Eidel DH, Hogg JC, et al. Proposed nonmenclature for quatifying subdivisions of the bronchial wall. *J Appl Physiol* 1994;77(2): 1011–1014.
5. Macklem PT. Theoretical basis of airway instability. Roger S. Mitchell lecture. *Chest* 1995;107:87S–88S.

6. Lambert RK, Wiggs BR, Kuwano K, Hogg JC, Paré PD. Functional significance of increased airway smooth muscle in asthma and COPD. *J Appl Physiol* 1993;74:2771–2781.

7. Huber HL, Koessler KK. The pathology of bronchial asthma. *Arch Intern Med* 1922;30(6):689–760.

8. Houston JC, de Nevasquez S, Trounce JR. A clinical and pathological study of fatal cases of status asthmaticus. *Thorax* 1953;8:207–213.

9. James AL, Hogg JC, Dunn LA, Paré PD. The use of internal perimeter to compare airway size and to calculate smooth muscle shortening. *Am Rev Respir Dis* 1988;138:136–139.

10. James AL, Paré PD, Hogg JC. Effects of lung volume, bronchoconstriction, and cigarette smoke on morphometric airways dimensions. *J Appl Physiol* 1988;64:913–919.

11. James AL, Paré PD, Hogg JC. The mechanics of airway narrowing in asthma. *Am Rev Respir Dis* 1989;139:242–246.

12. Bosken CH, Wiggs BR, Paré PD, Hogg JC. Small airway dimensions in smokers with obstruction to airflow. *Am Rev Respir Dis* 1990;142:563–570.

13. Wiggs BR, Bosken C, Paré PD, James A, Hogg JC. A model of airway narrowing in asthma and in chronic obstructive pulmonary disease *Am Rev Respir Dis* 1992;145:1251–1258.

14. Kuwano K, Bosken CH, Paré PD, Bai TR, Wiggs BR, Hogg JC. Small airways dimensions in asthma and in chronic obstructive pulmonary disease. *Am Rev Respir Dis* 1993; 148:1220–1225.

15. Ebina M, Yaegashi H, Chiba R, Takahashi T, Motomiya M, Tanemura M. Hyperreactive site in the airway tree of asthmatic patients revealed by thickening of bronchial muscles. *Am Rev Respir Dis* 1990;141:1327–1332.

16. Tiddens HA, Paré PD, Hogg JC, Hop WC, Lambert R, de Jongste JC. Cartilaginous airway dimensions and airflow obstruction in human lungs. *Am J Respir Crit Care Med* 1995;152(1):260–266.

17. Reiss A, Wiggs B, Verburgt L, Wright JL, Hogg JC, Paré PD. Morphologic determinants of airway responsiveness in chronic smokers. *Am J Respir Crit Care Med* (in press).

18. Carroll N, Elliot J, Morton A, James A. The structure of large and small airways in nonfatal and fatal asthma. *Am Rev Respir Dis* 1993;147:405–410.

19. Roche WR, Beasley R, Williams JH, Holgate ST. Subepithelial fibrosis in the bronchi of asthmatics. *Lancet* 1989;522–529.

20. Brewster CEP, Howarth PH, Djukanovic R, Wilson J, Holgate ST, Roche WR. Myofibroblasts and subepithelial fibrosis in bronchial asthma. *Am J Respir Cell Mol Biol* 1990;3:507–511.

21. Jeffery PK, Godfrey RWA, Adelroth E, Nelson F, Rogers A, Johansson S-A. Effects of treatment on airway inflammation and thickening of reticular collagen in asthma: a quantitative light and elctron microscopic study. *Am J Respir Crit Care Med* 1992;145:890–899.

22. Boulet LP, Boulet M, Laviolette M, et al. Airway inflammation after removal from the causal agent in occupational asthma due to high and low molecular weight agents. *Eur Respir J* 1994;7:1567–1575.

23. Saetta M, Maestrelli P, Turato G, et al. Airway wall remodelling after cessation of exposure to isocyanates in sensitized asthmatic subjects. *Am J Respir Crit Care Med* 1995;151:489–494.

24. Adachi E, Hayashi T. *In vitro* formation of fine fibrils with a D-periodic banding pattern from type V collagen. *Collagen Relat Res* 1985;5:225–232.

25. Birk DE, Fitch JM, Babiarz JP, Doane KJ, Linsenmayer TF. Collagen fibrillogenesis *in vitro*; interaction of types I and V collagen regulate fibril diameter. *J Cell Sci* 1990;95:649–657.

26. Vogel KG, Paulsson M, Heinegard D. Specific inhibition of type I and type II collagen fibrillogenesis by the small proteoglycan of tendon. *Biochem J* 1984;223:587–597.

27. Scott JE. Proteoglycan-fibrillar collagen interactions. *Biochem J* 1988;252:313–323.

28. Wilson JW, Li X, Pain MC. The lack of distensibility of asthmatic airways. *Am Rev Respir Dis* 1993;148:806–809.

29. Laitinen LA, Laitinen A. Modulation of bronchial inflammation: corticosteroids and other therapeutic agents. *Am Rev Respir Crit Care Med* 1994;10:S87–S90.

30. Romberger DJ, Beckmann JD, Claasen L, Ertl RF, Rennard SI. Modulation of fibronectin production of bovine bronchial epithelial cells by transforming growth factor-beta. *Am J Respir Cell Mol Biol* 1992;7:149–155.

31. Harkonen E, Virtanen I, Linnala A, Laitinen LL, Kinnula VL Modulation of fibronectin and tenascin production in human bronchial epithelial cells by inflammatory cytokines in vitro. *Am J Respir Cell Mol Biol* 1995;13:109–115.

32. Blackwood RA, Cantor JO, Moret J, Mandl I, Turino GM. Glycosaminoglycan synthesis in endotoxin-induced lung injury. *Proc Soc Exp Biol Med* 1983;174:343–349.

33. Roberts CR, Burke A. Is asthma a fibrotic disease? *Chest* 1995;107:111S–117S.

34. Wight TN, Heinegard DK, Hascall VC. Proteoglycans: structure and function. In: Hay ED, ed. *Cell biology of the extracellular matrix*. New York: Plenum Press, 1991;45–78.

35. Wight TN. Cell biology of arterial proteoglycans. *Arteriosclerosis* 1989;9:1–20.

36. Aubert J-D, Dalal BI, Bai TR, Roberts CR Hayashi S, Hogg JC. Transforming growth factor-β1 gene expression in human airways. *Thorax* 1994;49:225–232.

37. Roberts CR, Burke AK. Unpublished results.

38. Deguchi Y. Spontaneous increase of transforming growth factor beta production by bronchoalveolar mononuclear cells of patients with systemic autoimmune diseases affecting the lung. *Ann Rheum Dis* 1992;51:362–365.

39. Ohno I, Nitta Y, Yamaguchi K, et al. Eosinophils as a potential source of platelet-derived- growth-factor B-chain (PDGF-β) in nasal polyps and bronchial asthma. *Am J Respir Cell Mol Biol* 1995;13:639-647.

40. Aubert J-D., Hayashi S, Hards J, Bai TR, Paré PD, Hogg JC. Platelet-derived growth factor and its receptor in lungs from patients with asthma and chronic airflow obstruction. *Am J Physiol* 1994;266:L655–L663.

41. Cambrey AD, Kwon OJ, Gray AJ, et al. Insulin-like growth factor I is a major fibroblast mitogen produced by primary cultures of human airway epithelial cells. *Clin Sci* 1995;89:611–617.

42. Ghahary A, Shen Y, Nedelec B, Scott P, Tredget E. Enhanced expression of mRNA for insulin-like growth factor 1 in post-burn hypertrophic scar tissue and its fibrogenic role in dermal fibroblasts. *Mol Cell Biochem* 1995;148:25–32.

43. Khalil N, Whitman C, Zuo L, Danielpour D, Greenberg A. Regulation of alveolar macrophage transforming growth factor beta secretion by corticosteroids in bleomycin-induced pulmonary inflammation in the rat. *J Clin Invest* 1993;92:1812–1818.

44. Hamalainen L, Oikarinen J, Kivirikko KI. Synthesis and degradation of type I procollagen in cultured human skin fibroblasts and the effect of cortisol. *J Biol chem* 1985;260:720–725.

45. Bousquet J, Chanez P, Lacoste JY, White R, Vic P, Godard P, Michel FB. Asthma: a disease remodelling the airways. *Allergy* 1992;47: 3–11.

46. Buttle DJ, Abrahamson M, Burnett D, Mort JS, Barrett AJ, Dando PM, Hill SL. Human sputum cathepsin B degrades proteoglycan, is inhibited by α2-macroglobulin and is modulated by neutrophil elastase cleavage of cathepsin B precursor and cystatin C. *Biochem J* 1991;276;325–331.

47. Roberts CR, Opazo-Saez A, Burke A. Cleavage of airway cartilage proteoglycans in papain-induced airflow obstruction: a model for obstructive lung disease. (Unpublished results).

48. Saklatvala J, Sarsfield SJ. How do interleukin 1 and tumour necrosis factor induce degradation of proteoglycan in cartilage? In: Glauert AM, ed. *The control of tissue damage*. New York: Elsevier, 1988;97–108.

49. Toole BP. Proteoglycans and hyaluronan in morphogenesis and differentiation. In: Hay ED, ed. *Cell biology of extracellular matrix*, 2nd ed. New York: Plenum Press, 1991;305–341.

50. Koller ME, Woie K, Reed RK. Increased negativity of interstitial fluid pressure in rat trachea after mast cell degranulation. *J Appl Physiol* 1993;74:2135–2139.

51. Bramley, AM, Thomson RJ, Roberts CR, Schellenberg RR. Hypothesis: excessive bronchoconstriction in asthma is due to decreased airway elastance. *Eur Respir J* 1994;7:337–341.

52. Bramley AJ, Roberts CR, Schellenberg RR. Collagenase increases shortening of human bronchial smooth muscle *in vitro* treatment causes increased contractility of human bronchial smooth muscle *in vitro*. *Am J Respir Crit Care Med* 1995;152:1513–17.

53. Robinson P Okazawa M, Bai T, Paré PD. *In vivo* loads on airway smooth muscle: the role of noncontractile airway structures. *Can J Physiol Pharmacol* 1992;70:602–606.

54. Dunnill MS, Massarella GR, Anderson JA. A comparison of the quantitative anatomy of the bronchi in normal subjects, in status asthmaticus, in chronic bronchitis, and in emphysema. *Thorax* 1969;24:176–179.

55. Heard BE, Hossain S. Hyperplasia of bronchial muscle in asthma. *J Path* 1973;110:319–331.

56. Ebina M, Takahashi T, Chiba T, Motomiya M. Cellular hypertrophy and hyperplasia of airway smooth muscles underlying bronchial asthma. A 3-D morphometric study. *Am Rev Respir Dis* 1993;48:720–726.

57. Thomson RJ, Bramley AM, Schellenberg RR. Airway muscle stereology—implications for increased shortening in asthma. *Am J Respir Crit Care Med* 1996, (in press).

58. de Jongste JC, Mons H, Bonata IL, Kerrebijn KF. In vitro responses of airways from an asthamtic patient. *Eur J Respir Dis* 1987;71:23–29.

59. Bai TR. Abnormalities in airway smooth muscle in fatal asthma. *Am Rev Respir Dis* 1990;141:552–557.

60. Coflesky JT, Jones RC, Reid LM, Evans JN. Mechanical properties and structure of isolated pulmonary arteries remodeled by chronic hyperoxia. *Am Rev Respir Dis* 1987;136:388–394.

61. Halayko AJ, Salari H, Ma H, Stevens NL. Markers of airway smooth muscle cell phenotype. *Am J Physiol* 1996;270:L1040–L1051.

62. Karnovsky MJ, Edelman ER. Heparin/Heparan sulphate regulation of vascular smooth muscle cell behaviour. In: Page C, Black J, eds. *Airways and vascular remodelling*. Cambridge: Academic Press, 1994.

63. Okazawa M. and Paré PD. Pressure-area relationships of membranous airways in rabbits. *Am J Respir Crit Care Med* 1994;149:A770.

64. Handbook of Physiology. Section 3: The respiratory system, vol. III: Mechanics of breathing, pt 1. *Am Physiol Soc* 1986;226–227.

65. Lambert RK. Role of bronchial basement membrane in airway collapse. *J Appl Physiol* 1991;71:666–673.

66. Lambert RK, Codd SL, Alley MR, Pack RJ. Physical determinants of bronchial mucosal foldng. *J Appl Physiol* 1994;77:1206–1216.

67. Wiggs BR. The implications of airway wall buckling in asthmatic airways. *Am J Respir Crit Care Med* 1995;149:A585.

68. Colebatch HJH, Greaves IA, Ng CKY. Pulmonary mechanics in diagnosis. In: de Kock MA, Nadel JA, Lewis CM, eds. *Mechanics of airway obstruction in human respiratory disease*. Cape Town: AA Balkema, 1979.

Asthma, edited by P.J. Barnes, M.M. Grunstein,
A.R. Leff, and A.J. Woolcock.
Lippincott–Raven Publishers, Philadelphia © 1997.

▪ 66 ▪

Bronchial Vessels

Elizabeth M. Wagner

Structure
Regulation
  Mechanical Aspects
  Neural Regulation
  Vasoactive Agonists
Function
  Normal Physiology

Pathophysiology of Asthma
  Airway Smooth Muscle Hyperresponsiveness
  Vascular Engorgement
  Airway Edema
  Mucociliary Clearance

The bronchial vessels are positioned strategically within the airway wall to influence the cellular events that characterize asthma. However, whether their influence minimizes or enhances the symptoms of asthma is controversial. The bronchial circulation provides the systemic arterial perfusion of the lung. This circulatory bed is assumed to provide nutrient flow to, and clearance of metabolites from, all structures of the airway wall. Insofar as airway smooth muscle, nerves, glands, and epithelium are involved in the asthmatic response, adequate perfusion of these airway components links the bronchial circulation to asthma. It is the bronchial endothelium that is important in the recruitment of inflammatory cells to the airway(see Chapters 37 and 38). In addition, changes in the permeability and flow of this vascular bed may alter wall characteristics and lung function.

This chapter provides recent information concerning the normal structure, regulation, and function of the airway circulation and the changes shown to occur with asthma. Several excellent comprehensive reviews of the role of the bronchial circulation in lung health and disease have been published previously (1–4).

STRUCTURE

Although the discovery of the bronchial circulation and a description of its function are generally attributed to Leonardo da Vinci (1452–1519), careful reconstruction of his work shows that Leonardo's drawings were of small pulmonary veins and not bronchial arteries (5). The Dutch Professor of Anatomy and Botany, Frederich Ruysch (1638–1731), provided clear and unambiguous evidence for the existence of the bronchial circulation. In his paper he describes the bronchial circulation by stating (6):

> . . . it is not the quantity but rather the quality of the blood that is maximized in the bronchial artery. Who will deny that the blood which flows through the ventricle of the left heart is more distinguished than the blood from the right ventricle. For this reason I believe that, in order to impose a purpose, this artery is created to supply the lungs with more distinguished, more perfect blood, indeed blood of higher rank.

Figure 1 is reproduced from Ruysch's original scientific article and depicts the branching pattern of the bronchial circulation paralleling the airway tree. The anatomic arrangement of the airway vasculature for humans (7), sheep (8), pigs (9), dogs (10), and rabbits (11) has been described (12). Despite differences in the origin and number of arteries supplying the airways, the vascular arrangement within airways is remarkably consistent across species. Several tracheal arteries originating from

E. M. Wagner: Division of Pulmonary and Critical Care Medicine, The Johns Hopkins University, Baltimore, Maryland 21224.

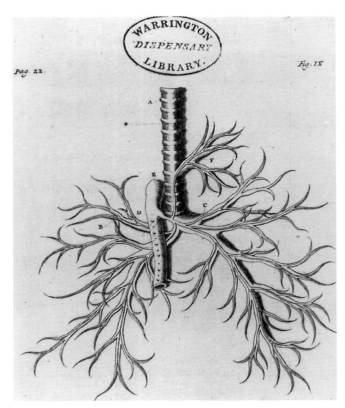

FIG. 1. Bronchial vasculature, as drawn by Frederick Ruysch. (From Mitzner W, Wagner EM. On the purported discovers of the bronchial circulation by Leonardo da Vinci. *J Appl Physiol* 1992;73(3):1196–1201.)

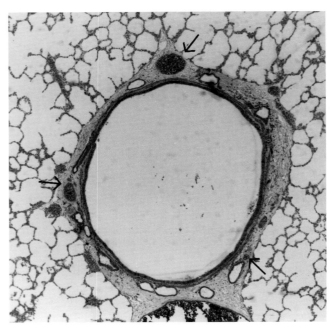

FIG. 2. Histologic section of a 1-mm diameter airway, quick-frozen and stained with toluidine blue. *Arrows* indicate bronchial vessels. (From Blosser S, Mitner W, Wagner EM. Effects of increased bronchial flood flow on airway morphometry, resistance, and reactivity. *J Appl Physiol* 1994; 76(4):1624–1629.)

branches of the carotid arteries, brachiocephalic trunk, and/or directly from the aorta perfuse the length of the trachea. Within the trachea, a mucosal capillary plexus is located internal to the cartilaginous ring and tracheal smooth muscle. An adventitial vascular plexus is situated external to these structures. Blood draining through these capillary beds in the walls of the trachea drain through tracheal veins that ultimately empty into the right heart.

Bronchial arteries originating from intercostal and subclavian arteries or directly from the aorta contact the airway at the level of the carina and supply both extra- and intraparenchymal airways to the level of the terminal bronchioles. Although the arrangement of cartilage changes within the airway wall at the level of the carina, the arrangement of parallel vascular plexuses is preserved throughout the airway tree. The mucosal vascular plexus, comprising primarily capillaries, lies just beneath the epithelial basement membrane and extends to the smooth muscle layer (13). The adventitial vascular plexus comprises capillaries, arterioles, and venules and extends from the smooth muscle layer to the alveolar border (Fig. 2). Communicating vessels course between airway smooth muscle and connect the two vascular networks. Blood flowing through the walls of extraparenchymal air-

ways drains through bronchial veins that empty into the right heart. Within intraparenchymal airways, bronchial veins anastomose with pulmonary veins and drain into the left heart.

Airway smooth muscle is surrounded by the arterioles, capillaries, and venules of the systemic circulation and therefore its metabolic needs depend on this circulation. Several recent studies questioned this assumption and suggested that the pulmonary circulation may actually contribute to airway perfusion (14–16). Using radiolabeled microspheres, these studies have demonstrated a small pulmonary component to large airway perfusion that progressively increases down the airway tree. Because of the recognized difficulty in dissecting completely the parenchymal and connective tissue attachments, these results remain controversial. That conducting airway responsiveness was uninfluenced by the pulmonary circulation was demonstrated in sheep challenged with intravenous methacholine (17). When the bronchial artery was occluded before challenge, airway resistance changes compared with the unoccluded situation were trivial and could be accounted for by tracheal artery delivery of the smooth muscle agonist (17; Fig. 3). In another study, careful histologic assessment of where fluorescent microspheres lodge when injected into the systemic airway circulation versus the pulmonary circulation demonstrated that airway smooth muscle is per-

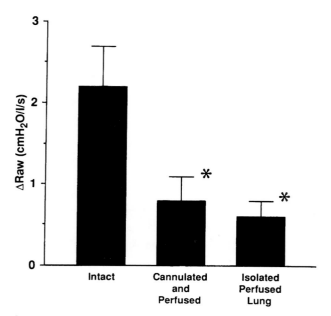

FIG. 3. Change in airway resistance *(Raw)* after intravenous methacholine in vagotomized sheep in the intact preparation, after cannulation and perfusion of the bronchial artery, and in an isolated, perfused lung preparation. Values are means ± SE. *p<0.01 compared with intact condition. (From Wagner EM, Mitzner WA. Contribution of pulmonary versus systemic perfusion of airway smooth muscle. *J Appl Physiol* 1995; 78(2):403–409.)

TABLE 1. *Bronchial vasculature area and number*

	Asthma	Control
Adventitia		
% Vessel area	12.5 ± 7.6[a]	8.1 ± 4.1
Number of vessels/mm^2	71 ± 24	83 ± 30
Submucosa		
% Vessel area	3.3 ± 3.8[a]	0.6 ± 0.9
Number of vessels/mm^2	80 ± 78	28 ± 35

[a]Asthma > control (p<0.01).
Modified from Kuwano K, Bosken CH, Paré PD, Bai TR, Wiggs BR, Hogg JC. Small airways dimensions in asthma and in chronic obstructive pulmonary disease. *Am Rev Respir Dis* 1993;148(5):1220–1225.

matched to the increase in airway tissue. Yet, these new vessels were dilated and occupied a greater fraction of the airway wall. Normal human morphometric data are similar to that of sheep, an experimental animal frequently used to study the airway circulation (21). Vasodilation of both the pulmonary and bronchial vascular beds in sheep with sodium nitroprusside combined with pulmonary hypertension resulted in a doubling of vascular area (22). Morphometric changes in the airway vasculature of asthmatics are likely to have profound effects on the normal physiologic function of the circulation and the airway.

REGULATION

Mechanical Aspects

The mechanical factors that influence flow through the bronchial vasculature are somewhat unique because of extensive pulmonary vascular communications. Ruysch drew comparisons between the circulations of the liver and the lung (6). Although systemic arterial pressure provides the inflow pressure to the bronchial vascular system, it drains predominantly into the low pressure pulmonary vascular bed. Consequently, bronchial vessels are exposed to the mechanical stresses of ventilation both directly because of their location in the airways as well as indirectly through the changes imposed on the pulmonary circulation. An alternate drainage pathway through systemic veins also may be important for blood flow diversion under certain circumstances.

Bronchial blood flow normally bears a direct relationship with the prevailing mean aortic blood pressure. Pressure-flow relationships generated for this vascular bed are surprisingly linear, suggesting no autoregulation, and the vascular bed is fully recruited and distended (23). The zero-flow pressure of this bed is likely to be largely influenced by the pressure at the site of bronchopulmonary anastomoses.

Like several other systemic vascular beds, the bronchial circulation responds to increases in downstream

fused exclusively by the systemic circulation (18). These two studies provide strong evidence for the systemic airway circulation, under normal conditions, to be the exclusive route by which substances reach airway smooth muscle.

Perhaps underemphasized in these anatomic details is the dense vascularity of the airway wall. Electron micrographs underscore the rich vascular supply of airway tissue (19). The highly tortuous nature of arterioles and venules contributes to the density and suggest physiologic functions requiring rapid changes in airway vascular volume. The relative density of bronchial vessels has been determined recently using postmortem or resected lung specimens of human subjects with and without asthma (20; Table 1). The vascular area as a fraction of the airway wall area was increased significantly in the asthmatic airways in both the submucosa and the adventitia compared with the normal control airways. The number of blood vessels in small airways from normal lung in the mucosa was reported to average 28 vessels/mm^2 of tissue and comprise <1% of the airway wall area. For the adventitial region the vascular area comprised 8% of the wall area and averaged 83 vessels/mm^2 of tissue. Although highly variable, the number of vessels/mm^2 was not found to differ in asthmatic airways. Because total airway wall area was shown to increase in asthmatics, these results show that proliferation of blood vessels was

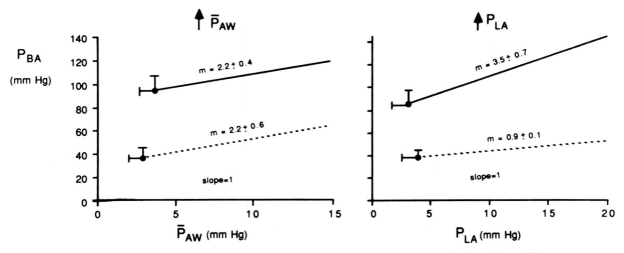

FIG. 4. Effects of increases in airway pressure (P_{AW}) and left atrial pressure (P_{LA}) on bronchial artery pressure at constant bronchial blood flow in sheep. *Solid line* indicates linearized relationship under control conditions and the *dashed line* indicates the relationship after infusion of papaverine into the bronchial artery. Average slope values for the relationships are indicated. (From Wagner EM, Mitzner WA. Effect of left atrial pressure on bronchial vascular hemodynamics. *J Appl Physiol* 1990;69(3): 837–848.)

pressure with active constriction (24). At constant flow in sheep, bronchial artery pressure has been shown to increase 3.5 mm Hg for every mm Hg increase in left atrial pressure. This response could be eliminated with pretreatment of the bronchial bed with a vascular smooth muscle paralytic (24; Fig. 4). This reflex response may be important for limiting airway vascular filtration pressure, especially in cases of left heart failure.

Because changes in lung volume and alveolar pressure exert a major influence on the pulmonary circulation and most bronchial blood drains through the pulmonary bed, it is not surprising that increases in lung volume have a major impact on bronchial vascular resistance. Several studies have documented increases in bronchial vascular resistance with increases in lung volume and airway pressure with the application of positive end-expiratory pressure (PEEP) in dogs (25,26), sheep (23), and humans (27). The increases in vascular resistance were most apparent in the parenchymal airways with tracheal perfusion being largely unaffected (25). It was clear that the changes in blood flow could not be accounted for solely on the basis of a reduction in perfusion pressure gradient, so a reflex mechanism or mediator release was suggested. Subsequent experiments showed that the effects of increases in PEEP were unaltered even when a smooth muscle paralytic was infused into the bronchial circulation (24). These results lead to the conclusion that the changes in vascular resistance with increases in lung volume were likely due to the mechanical distortion of the vasculature (24; Fig. 4). There are no data on the effects of hyperinflation and breathing at increased lung volume

in asthmatic persons on airway perfusion. However, from the experimental studies noted and the effects of PEEP on persons during cardiopulmonary bypass (27), it is likely that significant decreases in airway perfusion might occur because of the mechanical effects of ventilation during exacerbations of asthma.

Neural Regulation

Evaluation of the neural control of the airway vasculature is complicated by the differences in neural and vascular anatomy and physiology between species studied, variable nerve densities in different regions of the tracheobronchial tree, and the coincident changes in airway smooth muscle stimulation and subsequent airway geometry changes that may impact on bronchial vascular dynamics. Information has been derived from histochemical, pharmacologic, and physiologic studies.

Efferent Mechanisms

Adrenergic

Stimulation of sympathetic nerves to the airways decreases both tracheal and bronchial blood flow (28). Infused and inhaled α-adrenergic agonists reduce airway blood flow (28,29) and β-adrenergic agonists increase airway blood flow (29–31). However, α- or β-receptor blockade have little effect on resting airway blood flow (32).

Cholinergic

Stimulation of the vagus nerve and the superior laryngeal nerve result in bronchial and tracheal vascular dilation, respectively (33,34). However, a portion of this vasodilation cannot be blocked by atropine and is due to the co-release of neuropeptides (33,34). Infusion and inhalation of cholinergic agonists elicit increases in tracheal and bronchial blood flow (17,35,36). Cholinergic nerve sectioning has little effect on airway blood flow, suggesting minimal cholinergic regulation of resting vascular tone (32,33).

Nonadrenergic, Noncholinergic

This nervous system lacks a unique anatomic network within the airways but rather co-exists with adrenergic, cholinergic, and sensory fibers. Putative neurotransmitter peptides have been identified in varicosities of nerves surrounding tracheobronchial vessels. Stimulation with capsaicin in the rat (37), dog (38), sheep (39), and pig (34) results in local release of these neurotransmitter peptides and an increase in total and regional airway blood flow. In addition, infusion of the putative neurotransmitters vasoactive intestinal polypeptide, substance P, neurokinin A, neurokinin B, and calcitonin gene-related peptide results in an increase in dog tracheal blood flow (38). In the same study, neuropeptide Y and bombesin were shown to be vasoconstrictors. In addition to altering airway blood flow, capsaicin and several of these neuropeptides cause marked protein and fluid extravasation from the airway vasculature (40,41). Insofar as this neural pathway can be implicated in the pathogensis of asthma, release of these neuropeptides may play a major role in the generation of airway wall edema.

Afferent Mechanisms

Sensory Nerves

Sensory C-fibers are normally stimulated by a variety of respiratory irritants (42). Cigarette smoke (43), hypertonic solutions (44,45), O_3 (46), and water (47) have been shown to increase airway blood flow. A combination of a centrally mediated vagal reflex as well as a neuropeptide-dependent axon reflex has been proposed to account for the increase in blood flow. The relative contribution of these reflex responses to the overall changes in airway blood flow appear to be highly species-dependent.

Carotid Body

Perfusion of carotid body chemoreceptors with hypoxic blood evokes reflex vasodilation of the bronchial vasculature (48). However, chemical stimulation of carotid bodies causes weak vasoconstriction of the tracheal vasculature (49). The precise reflex mechanisms responsible for the blood flow response have not been defined.

Vasoactive Agonists

A growing list of nonneurogenic, vasoactive substances have been identified for the tracheal and bronchial vasculatures (Table 2). Many of the substances

TABLE 2. Vasoactive agents

Tracheal Artery		Bronchial Artery	
Vasoconstrictors	Vasodilators	Vasoconstrictors	Vasodilators
Ascaris suum antigen (old animals) (96)	Ascaris suum antigen (young animals) (52,96)	Endothelin (Wagner, unpublished observation)	Adenosine (97,98)
Systemic hypercarbia (49)	Bradykinin (99)	Systemic hypoxemia—prolonged (100,101)	Ascaris suum antigen (61)
Systemic hypoxemia (102,49)	Histamine (103)		Bradykinin (83)
Vasopressin (52)	Nitroglycerin (52)		Histamine (H_2 receptor) (104,105)
	Platelet activity factor (99)		Nitric oxide (106)
	Prostaglandins $D_2,E_1,F_2\alpha$ (99)		Prostaglandin $F_2\alpha$ (36), I_2 (107)
	Serotonin (108)		Sodium nitroprusside (Wagner, unpublished observation)
			Systemic hypercarbia (100)
			Systemic hypoxemia—immediate (101)

found to be vasoactive also affect airway smooth muscle and nerves. The ultimate blood flow response may be influenced by the changing geometry of the airway because of bronchoconstriction, endothelial cell activation, and overriding neural reflexes. Responsiveness can be further complicated by the experimental preparation used and the route of agonist delivery. Subtle differences have been observed, depending on whether agonists are delivered intravenously, directly to the bronchial artery, or by inhalation challenge (17,29).

FUNCTION

Normal Physiology

The tracheobronchial vascular network likely plays a significant role and supports airway defense, fluid balance, and metabolic function; however, definitive studies demonstrating these functions are lacking. The major physiologic function typically ascribed to the airway circulation is the delivery of nutrients to all cells of the airway wall, nerves coursing through the lung, glands, lymph nodes, and pulmonary vessels. Whether limiting blood flow to these structures will alter airway function and over what time period has not been carefully detailed.

Clearance

A major physiologic function of the airway circulation is that it provides an essential route for clearance of airway smooth muscle agonists and other cellular metabolites. In an animal model specifically designed to measure peripheral lung responses, studies demonstrated that the bronchial circulation affected recovery from an intravenous histamine challenge to a degree equal to that of the pulmonary circulation (50). In support of this finding, in a sheep model, the time constant of recovery from an intrabronchial artery challenge with methacholine could be significantly increased when bronchial blood flow was limited (51; Fig. 5). Extending these observations, additional studies in sheep showed that both the magnitude and the duration of the airway response to an aerosol antigen challenge could be increased or decreased with pharmacologic agents that decrease or increase the airway blood flow, respectively (52). These results confirm that the airway circulation can clear exogenously administered agonists from the airway smooth muscle. In addition, these studies, along with others, show that most agents that cause airway smooth muscle constriction also cause bronchial vascular dilation. This suggests some kind of regulatory function for the clearance capabilities of the airway circulation.

Conditioning Inspired Air

An important function typically ascribed to the airway circulation is the heating and humidification of inspired air. Cold, dry air is heated and humidified as it passes through the airways to the alveoli. As the thermal burden increases, the respiratory air conditioning function of the airway mucosa reaches deeper into the lung. Both the tracheal and bronchial circulation of dogs (53,54) and sheep (55) respond to dry air hyperpnea with marked vasodilation. Increases in airway vascular permeability also have been demonstrated (40). The mechanism of these responses has been proposed to involve neuropeptides and prostaglandins because the vasodilation could be attenu-

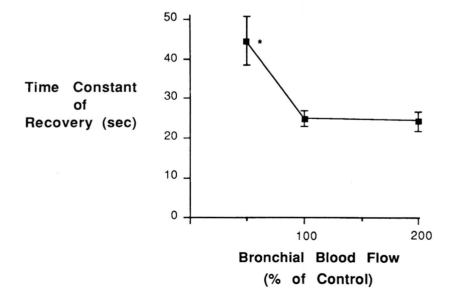

FIG. 5. Time constant of recovery from constant intrabronchial artery methacholine challenge at 50%, 100%, and 200% of control bronchial blood flow (0.7 mL/min/kg). Data are presented as mean values ± SE. *$p<0.01$. (From Wagner EM, Mitzner WA. Bronchial circulatory reversal of methacholine-induced airway constriction. *J Appl Physiol* 1990;69(4):1220–1224.)

ated with lidocaine and indomethacin (56) but not with autonomic blockade (32). The airway circulation is the only source to replenish water lost during dry air challenge, thus preventing mucosal drying and airway desiccation. Airway challenge with hypertonic aerosols have shown both increases in blood flow (45,57) and no change (58). Whether the bronchial circulation contributes significantly to the warming of inspired air has been a topic of debate, because the pulmonary circulation in the lung parenchyma provides a huge heat sink (59). Disruption of pulmonary perfusion but not bronchial perfusion significantly alters airstream temperatures (60).

PATHOPHYSIOLOGY OF ASTHMA

Direct information implicating the bronchial circulation in the pathology of asthma has been difficult to ob-

tain because there are currently no established methods to study the circulation in humans. New techniques to study the airway circulation using gases of different solubilities are being explored in experimental subjects (31). However, current information relies on indirect assessment of the circulation, postmortem evaluation of lung tissue, and animal models of asthma. Models of this disease allow characteristic features to be studied in isolation. However, each of these aspects undoubtedly interacts with others to influence airway patency and normal pulmonary function. Evidence that implicates the bronchial circulation in the pathogenesis of each of the characteristics of the asthmatic airway will be considered.

Airway Smooth Muscle Hyperresponsiveness

As discussed above, the airway circulation is thought to have a major influence on the clearance of endogenous

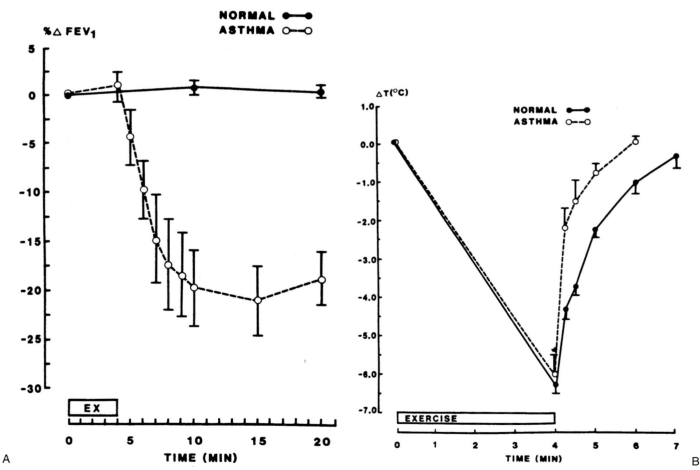

FIG. 6. A: Effect of exercise on changes in FEV₁ in normal and asthmatic individuals. Data are presented as mean values ± SE. (From Gilbert IA, Fouke JM, McFadden ER. Heat and water flux in the intrathoracic airways and exercise-induced asthma. *J Appl Physiol* 1987;63(4):1681–1691.) **B:** Changes in inspiratory airway temperature (ΔT) in trachea during exercise and recovery for normal and asthmatic individuals. Data are presented as mean value ± SE.

metabolites from airway smooth muscle as well as exogenously administered aerosols delivered to the airway. It was initially inferred that this is an important physiologic function of the airway circulation because most bronchoconstrictor substances cause marked vasodilation of both the tracheal and bronchial vascular beds. As described, several studies have documented in normal animals that airway smooth muscle constriction is either enhanced or prolonged when airway perfusion is limited (50–52). Furthermore, Long and colleagues demonstrated that just before the late-phase decline in pulmonary function after antigen challenge in sensitive sheep, there was a significant increase in airway blood flow (61). These results demonstrated that the circulatory response preceded the airway smooth muscle response and provided suggestive evidence for the potential role of this circulation in the recruitment and delivery of substances precipitating the asthmatic response.

Whether airway blood flow is altered in the asthmatic airway and thereby alters smooth muscle responsiveness is unknown. That the number of blood vessels perfusing the airway increases in asthma has been demonstrated (20). However, the characteristics of these vessels need to be determined, as well as their ability to regulate flow in response to inflammatory events.

Vascular Engorgement

The hypothesis that an engorged airway vasculature can contribute significantly to airflow obstruction based on geometric considerations alone has been a topic of recent controversy (62,63). Proposed is that the vascular volume of the airway wall could increase substantially so as to cause direct encroachment on the airway lumen or through the loss of parenchymal tethering, causing lumenal narrowing. Much of the discussion hinges on the observation that asthmatics who experience decrements in pulmonary function after exercise or dry air hyperpnea actually rewarm their airways more rapidly than normal individuals (64; Fig. 6). Airway wall temperature in these studies was assumed to provide an indirect assessment of airway blood flow. These results suggest that airway perfusion is limited during the exercise period and rebounds rapidly with cessation of the challenge. Hyperemia with edema of the airway wall was suggested to account for

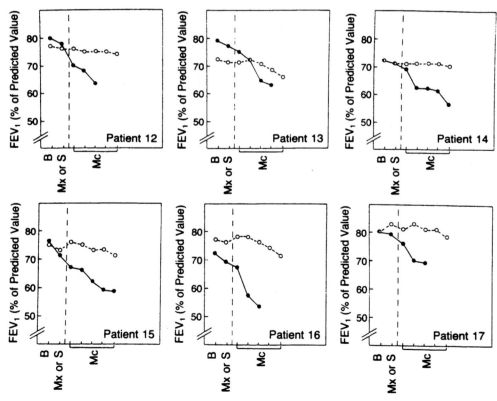

FIG. 7. Effects of methacholine challenge *(Mc: progressive doubling doses)* on FEV₁ after pretreatment with 10 mg inhaled methoxamine hydrochloride *(Mx: open circles)* or saline *(S: closed circles)* in six hyperresponsive patients. *B* indicates baseline value. (From Cabanes LR, Weber SN, Matran R, et al. Bronchial hyperresponsiveness to methacholine in patients with impaired left ventricular function. *N Engl J Med* 1989;320(2):1317–1348.)

the airway obstruction. In another study of exercise challenge in asthmatic persons, pretreatment with an α-agonist presumed to decrease airway perfusion (31,65) significantly attenuated the decrement in pulmonary function typically observed (66). These results were interpreted as the constricted vasculature incapable of rebounding after exercise and thereby preventing engorgement and airflow obstruction.

Further support for the hypothesis that limiting the vascular volume of the airway wall could impact on lumenal patency was provided in patients with congestive heart disease who demonstrated hyperresponsiveness to methacholine (67; Fig. 7). When these patients were pretreated with the α-agonist methoxamine, although their baseline pulmonary function was unaltered, their responsiveness to inhaled methacholine decreased dramatically. These results suggested that the airflow obstruction was mediated at least in part by vascular dilation. When examined all together, these studies in humans provide strong but

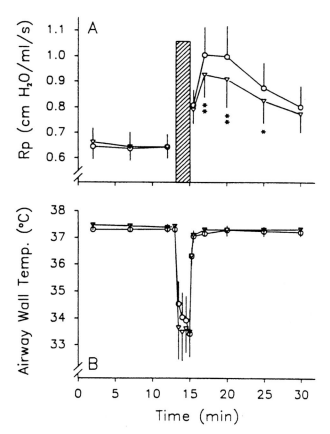

FIG. 8. A: Peripheral lung resistance *(Rp)* measured before and after dry air challenge with either saline *(circles)* or methoxamine *(triangles)* aerosol pretreatment. **B:** Airway wall temperature measured coincident with challenges depicted in A. *******p*<0.01 compared with saline pretreatment. (From Omori C, Mitzner W, Freed A. The effects of α-adrenergic agonists on hyperpnea-induced airway obstruction in dogs. *Am J Respir Crit Care Med* 1995;152:17–23.)

indirect evidence suggesting that decreasing airway vascular volume can attenuate the airflow obstruction observed in persons who demonstrate hyperresponsiveness to certain airway challenges. The evidence is indirect because none of the studies ever attempted to measure bronchial blood flow.

Considerable discrepancy exists when comparing the results obtained by these indirect methods with the direct measurements obtained in animal models. As cited previously, the airway circulation of normal animals responds immediately to cold or dry air hyperventilation with a marked vasodilation during the challenge and a return to normal with cessation of challenge (53,55,56). In these studies, no changes in pulmonary function were reported. However, in a canine model of dry air-induced bronchospasm of peripheral airways, pretreatment with methoxamine had a trivial attenuating effect on the typically observed increase in airway resistance (68; Fig. 8). These studies suggest the asthmatic response to dry-air challenge may be inherently very different from the response in normal animals.

A direct assessment, using physiologic and morphometric techniques, has been performed to determine how bronchial vascular engorgement influences airway dimensions in sheep. No changes in conducting airway resistance were observed when bronchial blood flow was varied from 50% to 500% of control flow (21). Increased vascular area of small airways (0.2–3 mm diameter) was seen with both increased bronchial inflow (300% control flow) and with left-atrial pressure elevation to 15 to 20 mm Hg (69). However, only with increased left atrial pressure was lumenal area decreased (Fig. 9). However, because of the close association of mucosal folds with bronchial mucosal vessels (Fig. 10), it was unclear from these studies whether increased bronchial vascular area was the cause or the effect of mucosal infolding and lumenal narrowing. Additional experiments using this model demonstrated that the lumenal narrowing due to increased left atrial pressure was the result of reflex bronchoconstriction because the response was abolished when smooth muscle tone was eliminated (69). Numerous studies have documented the reflex-mediated increase in airway smooth muscle tone with pulmonary venous congestion (70,71). Lung C-fibers are thought to be stimulated by the mechanical effects of acute pulmonary congestion and edema resulting in vagally mediated bronchoconstriction (72,73). Because of the common drainage pathway of the bronchial and pulmonary vascular beds, activation of this reflex pathway may be the underlying mechanism to account for many of the experimental results obtained in studies of airway vascular engorgement.

Thus, despite the postmortem pathology of an enlarged bronchial vasculature, direct physiologic confirmation of increased vascular volume of the asthmatic airway wall leading to airway narrowing is lacking. Animal models attempting to maximize the vascular volume in the air-

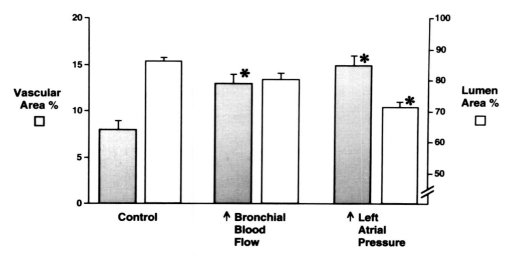

FIG. 9. Changes in vascular area *(shaded bar)* as a percent of wall area and lumen area *(open bar)* as a percent of the maximally dilated airway area for control airways (n=9 sheep), increased bronchial blood flow (1.8 mL/min/kg; n=4), and increased left atrial pressure (n=5). Ten airways (0.2–3.0 mm diameter) were examined/sheep. *$p<0.05$ from control.

way wall have not demonstrated a direct causal effect of systemic vascular engorgement on lumenal dimensions.

Airway Edema

It is well documented that significant airway microvascular extravasation occurs in response to a number of physical and inflammatory stimuli. Dry air (40), cigarette smoke (74), and capsaicin (75) all cause fluid extravasation through stimulation of sensory nerves and the release of neuropeptides, specifically substance P, and neurokinin A and B (76). Inflammatory mediators such as bradykinin, histamine, serotonin (75,76) and platelet activating factor (PAF) (77,78) have all been shown to cause plasma extravasation either directly or through their interactions with sensory nerves. These substances cause a permeability edema whereby tracheal and bronchial endothelial cells of postcapillary venules, which normally are joined by tight junctions, undergo an active change in configuration and allow gaps to form (79). Extravasation is generally quantified by measurement of a tracer that binds to albumin or is of comparable size and later can be extracted from tissue. However, despite the numerous studies identifying the multitude of pharmacologic, neurogenic, and inflammatory cell products that cause fluid

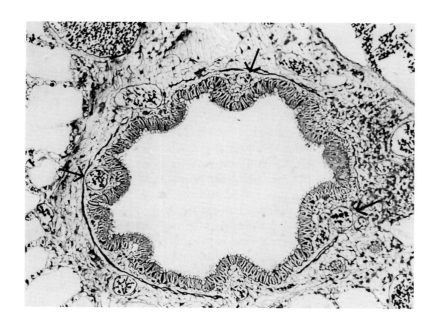

FIG. 10. Histologic section of a 1.5-mm diameter airway quick-frozen and stained with toluidine blue. *Arrows* indicate bronchial vessels in association with mucosal folds. (From Goldman M, Kundson RJ, Mead J, Peterson, Schwaber JR, Wolh ME. A simplified measurement of respiratory resistance by forced oscillation. *J Appl Physiol* 1970;28(1):113–116.)

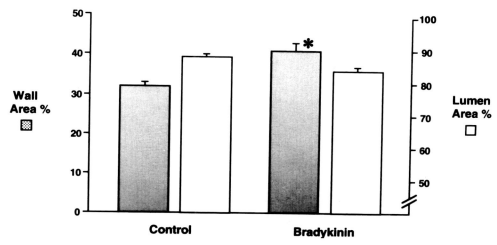

FIG. 11. Changes in wall area *(shaded bar)* as a percent of the total dilated airway area and lumen area *(open bar)* as a percent of the maximally dilated airway area for control airways (*n*=4) and those perfused with intrabronchial artery bradykinin (10^{-6} M). Despite a significant increase in wall area (*$p<0.05$), no change was seen in lumen area.

and protein extravasation, little is known about the relative importance of this process in impairing normal airway function. Several routes for fluid and protein reabsorption exist in the airway. These include reabsorption into capillaries and lymphatics, bulk flow across the epithelium and removal through mucociliary transport (80), and fluid movement to form pulmonary perivascular cuffs. Extravasation is not the same as edema. The question remains as to whether substances that cause fluid transudation cause airway edema. Furthermore, whether wall thickening due to edema plays a major role in airway narrowing is controversial. Like vascular engorgement, airway wall thickening due to edema could cause lumenal narrowing through direct encroachment on the lumen or by a change in the forces of interdependence that link the airway to the surrounding lung parenchyma. Predictions based on morphometric data suggest that wall thickening will have minimal effects under baseline conditions; however, it may play a role in amplifying the response during induced smooth muscle constriction (81).

Experimental evidence demonstrates that significant wall thickening can occur with the inflammatory mediator bradykinin infused directly into the bronchial artery of sheep (82). Unlike asthmatic individuals, normal sheep exhibit no direct smooth muscle constriction with bradykinin challenge (83). Therefore, changes in airway dimensions are due exclusively to the effects of wall thickening. After a continuous 50-min exposure to bradykinin, no changes in conducting airway resistance and trivial changes in small airway dimensions were observed (Fig. 11). In addition, increases in conducting airway resistance measured after methacholine challenge were not altered after bradykinin infusion. Thus, in this model of airway edema, neither baseline airway function nor reactivity altered despite significant wall thickening.

Studies in humans further document that extravasation may take place with little effect on pulmonary function (84). Small airway responsiveness to bradykinin was tested in normal and asthmatic individuals. Despite comparable increases in lavaged protein from the two groups, only in asthmatic individuals was small airway resistance increased.

If airway wall edema exists in asthma, then it is most likely due to the hyperpermeability of the airway circulation. However, another method to study airway wall edema is through the generation of hydrostatic edema. Volume loading with normal saline has been used to cause pulmonary and bronchial vascular engorgement and edema in humans and animals. Rapid saline infusion (30 mL/kg) in normal and asthmatic individuals caused a significant decrease in pulmonary function in both groups, although the decrease in FEV_1 was somewhat greater in asthmatics who started with lower baseline function (85). Whether this response was due to the direct mechanical effect of engorgement and/or edema, or reflex bronchoconstriction due to pulmonary vascular congestion, was not determined. However, in dogs pretreated with atropine, saline loading also had a significant effect on large airway dimensions (86). The results using high-resolution computed tomography (HRCT) to measure sequential changes noninvasively in wall thickness and lumenal area with increasing volume loads are shown in Figure 12. An average 38% increase in wall thickness was elicited by 100 mL/kg of saline, which caused a 27% decrease in airway lumenal area. Blood volume loading to elicit comparable changes in pulmonary artery and wedge pressures as obtained with saline loading resulted in an average 8% increase in wall thickness and a 19% decrease in airway area. The authors concluded that the contribution of bronchial vascular engorgement to airway

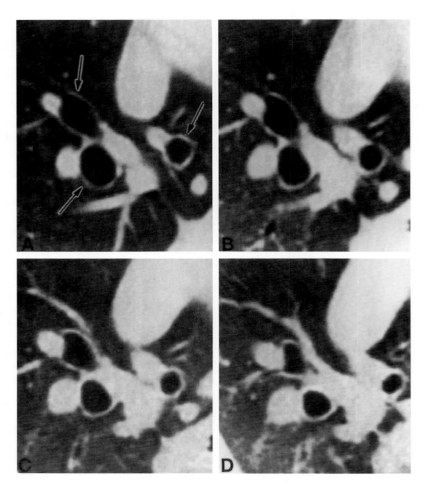

FIG. 12. High-resolution computed tomography scans of matched airways from one dog during normal saline infusion. **A:** *Arrows* indicate baseline state of airway walls and lumen. **B:** Matched airways after 50 mL/kg saline challenge. **C:** Matched airways after 100 mL/kg saline challenge. **D:** Matched airways after 150 mL/kg saline challenge. Note progressive increase in airway wall thickness and decrease in lumen area. (From Brown RH, Zerhouni EA, Mitzner W. Visualization of airway obstruction *in vivo* during pulmonary vascular engorgement and edema. *J Appl Physiol* 1995;78(3):1070–1078.)

narrowing was trivial and the effects of saline were predominantly due to the creation of interstitial edema. However, the degree of obstruction was moderate given the extreme fluid load and, therefore, it is unlikely that airway wall edema is likely to be a primary cause of airflow obstruction in asthma. This technology applied to humans will offer new opportunities to visualize directly airway wall dimensions and determine the importance of these mechanical factors in asthma.

Mucociliary Clearance

Increased amounts of secretions in the tracheobronchial airways is a characteristic feature of asthma (87). The extent to which the airway circulation contributes to excess fluid in the airway lumen has not been determined. Fluid extravasation from the airway circulation as described above has been proposed to provide an important defense mechanism for airways (see Chapter 64). Plasma exudate is suggested to wash away unwanted substances, neutralize allergens, stimulate cough, and increase mucociliary clearance. Increased secretions also may have a protective effect by increasing the mechanical barrier to inhaled substances. However, it has been demonstrated that increased airway liquid can fill airway interstices of lumenal folds, amplifying the degree of lumenal narrowing directly and through the increase in surface forces between the air-liquid interface (88). Furthermore, increased airway liquid may change the viscosity of periciliary fluid and affect the efficiency of mucociliary transport (89).

Mucociliary clearance in chronic, stable asthmatics, as well as in patients with acute exacerbations, has been shown to be significantly decreased compared with normal individuals (90,91). Whether alterations in tracheobronchial blood flow can be implicated in the observed decrease in mucociliary clearance can be only speculated on. Mucociliary clearance in long-term survivors of heart-lung and double lung transplantation (92), as well as in animal models of allo- and autotransplantation, has been shown to be significantly decreased from normal (77,93). Surgical reanastomosis of bronchial arteries was not performed in these studies. These results are provocative and invite speculation that the presumed decrease in airway blood flow may be fundamental to the decrease in mucociliary clearance. However, studies measuring airway blood flow in dogs after left lung transection and

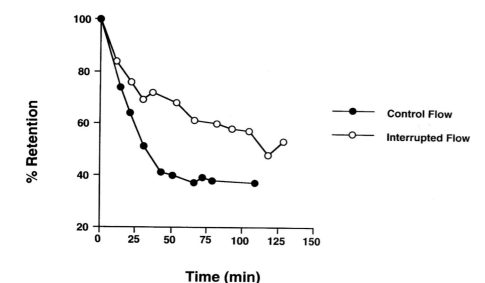

FIG. 13. Time course of particle (2 μm Tc-labeled sulfur colloid) clearance from one sheep with either control or no bronchial blood flow.

anastomosis showed substantial increases in blood flow both proximal and distal to the anastomosis relative to the right lung within 3 days after surgery (94). Thus, a decrease in airway perfusion is unlikely to be responsible for the decreased mucociliary clearance observed after transplantation.

In preliminary studies, the effect of decreased bronchial blood flow on mucociliary clearance was studied directly in sheep. The clearance of (^{99m})Tc-labeled sulfur colloid particles delivered by aerosol to the central airways was determined during control bronchial vascular perfusion and compared with a no-flow condition (Fig. 13). Particle retention was significantly greater under the no-perfusion condition (95). These results suggest a role for the airway circulation in promoting mucociliary clearance. The mechanism responsible for this phenomenon could involve the circulation's role in providing nutrient flow to airway components, temperature regulation, fluid balance, or be the result of an ischemic insult.

CONCLUSIONS

Although morphometric data suggest an increased vascularity of the asthmatic airway, direct measurement of the impact of the circulation on airway function in asthma is lacking. Animal models of the characteristic features of asthma suggest that the airway circulation is unlikely to cause lumenal narrowing through engorgement or edema.

ACKNOWLEDGMENTS

This work was supported by NIH grant HL10342 and an Established Investigator Award of the American Heart Association.

REFERENCES

1. J.B. Butler, ed. *The bronchial circulation.* New York: Marcel Dekker, 1992.
2. American Thoracic Society. Airway circulation. *Am Rev Respir Dis* 1992;146(5):S1–S60.
3. Deffebach ME, Charan NB, Lakshminarayan S, Butler J. The bronchial circulation—small, but a vital attribute of the lung. *Am Rev Respir Dis* 1987;135:463–481.
4. Wanner A. Circulation of the airway mucosa. *J Appl Physiol* 1989; 67(3):917–925.
5. Mitzner W, Wagner EM. On the purported discovery of the bronchial circulation by Leonardo da Vinci. *J Appl Physiol* 1992;73(3):1196–1201.
6. Ruysch F. Observations anatomicae. Observatio XV. In: *Opera omnia anatomico-medico chirurgica.* Amsterdam: Janssonio-Waesbergios, 1721.
7. Kasai T, Chiba S. Macroscopic anatomy of the bronchial arteries. *Anat Anz* 1979;145:166–181.
8. Charan NB, Turk GM, Czartolomny J, Andreazuk T. Systemic arterial blood supply to the trachea and lung in sheep. *J Appl Physiol* 1987; 62(6):2283–2287.
9. Calka W. Vascular supply of the lungs through direct branches of the aorta in domestic pig. *Folia Morphol* 1975;34(2):135–142.
10. Notkovich H. The anatomy of the bronchial arteries of the dog. *J Thorac Surg* 1957;33:242–253.
11. Balding JD, Ogilvie RW, Hoffman CL, Knisely WM. The gross morphology of the arterial supply to the trachea, primary bronchi and esophagus of the rabbit. *Anat Rec* 1964;148:611–614.
12. S. Sisson, J.D. Grossman, R. Getty, eds. *Sisson and Grossman's: The anatomy of the domestic animals,* 5th ed. Philadelphia: WB Saunders Co, 1975.
13. Bai A, Eidelman DH, Hogg JC, et al. Proposed nonmenclature for quantifying subdivsons of the bronchial wall. *J Appl Physiol* 1994; 77(2):1011–1014.
14. Baile EM, Minshall D, Dodek PM, Paré PD. Blood flow to the trachea and bronchi: the pulmonary contribution. *J Appl Physiol* 1994;76(5): 2063–2069.
15. Barman SA, Ardell JL, Parker JC, Perry ML, Taylor AE. Pulmonary and systemic blood flow contributions to upper airways in canine lungs. *Am J Physiol* 1988;255:H1130–1135.
16. Michelassi F, Schuette A, Landa L, Zapol WM, Grillo HC. Pulmonary and systemic contribution to canine tracheobronchial blood flow. *J Surg Sci* 1987;17:105–112.
17. Wagner EM, Mitzner WA. Contribution of pulmonary versus systemic perfusion of airway smooth muscle. *J Appl Physiol* 1995;78(2): 403–409.

18. Bernard SL, Glenny RW, Polissar NL, Luchtel DL, Lakshminarayan S. Distribution of pulmonary and bronchial blood supply to airways measured by fluorescent microspheres. *J Appl Physiol* 1996;80(2):430–436.

19. Charan NB, Turk GM, Dhand R. Gross and subgross anatomy of the bronchial circulation in sheep. *J Appl Physiol* 1984;57:658–664.

20. Kuwano K, Bosken CH, Paré PD, Bai TR, Wiggs BR, Hogg JC. Small airways dimensions in asthma and in chronic obstructive pulmonary disease. *Am Rev Respir Dis* 1993;148(5):1220–1225.

21. Blosser S, Mitner W, Wagner EM. Effects of increased bronchial blood flow on airway morphometry, resistance, and reactivity. *J Appl Physiol* 1994;76(4):1624–1629.

22. Mariassy AT, Gazeroglu H, Wanner A. Morphometry of the subepithelial circulation in sheep airways. *Am Rev Respir Dis* 1991;143:162–166.

23. Wagner E, Mitzner WA, Bleecker ER. Effects of airway pressure on bronchial blood flow. *J Appl Physiol* 1987;62(2):561–566.

24. Wagner EM, Mitzner WA. Effect of left atrial pressure on bronchial vascular hemodynamics. *J Appl Physiol* 1990;69(3):837–848.

25. Baile EM, Albert RK, Kirk W, Lakshaminarayan S, Wiggs BJR, Paré PD. Positive end-expiratory pressure decreases bronchial blood flow in the dog. *J Appl Physiol* 1984;56(5):1289–1293.

26. Cassidy SS, Haynes MS. The effects of ventilation with positive end-expiratory pressure on the bronchial circulation. *Resp Physiol* 1986;66:269–278.

27. Agostoni PG, Arena V, Biglioli P, Doria E, Sala A, Susini G. Increase of alveolar pressure reduces systemic to pulmonary bronchial blood flow in humans. *Chest* 1989;96:1076–1080.

28. Matran R. Neural control of lower airway vasculature. Involvement of classical transmitters and neuropeptides. *Acta Physiol Scand* 1991;601:1–54.

29. Barker JA, Chediak AD, Baier HJ, Wanner A. Tracheal mucosal blood flow responses. *J Appl Physiol* 1988;65(2):829–834.

30. Sanders EA, Gleed RD, Hackett RP, Dobson A. Action of sympathomimetic drugs on the bronchial circulation of the horse. *Exp Physiol* 1991;76:301–304.

31. Onorato DJ, Demirozu MC, Breitenbücher A, Atkins ND, Chediak AD, Wanner A. Airway mucosal blood flow in humans. *Am J Respir Crit Care Med* 1994;149:1132–1137.

32. Baile EM, Osborne S, Paré PD. Effect of autonomic blockade on tracheobronchial blood flow. *J Appl Physiol* 1986;62(2):520–525.

33. Laitinen LA, Laitinen MVA, Widdicombe JG. Parasympathetic nervous control of tracheal vascular resistance in the dog. *J Physiol* 1987;385:135–146.

34. Matran R, Alving K, Martling CR, Lacroix JS, Lundberg JM. Vagally mediated vasodilatation by motor and sensory nerves in the tracheal and bronchial circulation of the pig. *Acta Physiol Scand* 1989;135:29–37.

35. Corfield DR, Hanafi Z, Webber SE, Widdicombe JG. Changes in tracheal mucosal thickness and blood flow in sheep. *J Appl Physiol* 1991;71(4):1282–1288.

36. Lakshminarayanan S, Jindal SK, Butler J. Increases in bronchial blood flow following bronchoconstriction with methacholine and prostaglandin F 2α in dogs. *Chest* 1985;87(5):183S–184S.

37. Piedimonte G, Hoffman JIE, Husseini WK, Hiser WL, Nadel JA. Effect of neuropeptides released from sensory nerves on blood flow in the rat airway microcirculation. *J Appl Physiol* 1987;72(4):1563–1570.

38. Salonen RO, Webber SE, Widdicombe JG. Effects of neuropeptides and capsaicin on the canine tracheal vasculature in vivo. *Br J Pharma* 1988;95:1262–1270.

39. Coleridge HM, Coleridge JCG, Green JF, Parsons GH. Pulmonary C-fiber stimulation by capsaicin evokes reflex cholinergic bronchial vasodilation in sheep. *J Appl Physiol* 1992;72(2):770–778.

40. Garland A, Ray DW, Doerschuk CM, et al. Role of tachykinins in hyperpnea-induced bronchovascular hyperpermeability in guinea pigs. *J Appl Physiol* 1991;70(1):27–35.

41. Lundberg JM, Saria A. Capsaicin-sensitive vagal neurons involved in control of vascular permeability in rat trachea. *Acta Physiol Scand* 1982;115:521–523.

42. Coleridge HM, Coleridge JCG. Pulmonary reflexes: neural mechanisms of pulmonary defense. *Annu Rev Physiol* 1994;56:69–91.

43. Matran R, Alving K, Lundberg JM. Cigarette smoke, nicotine and capsaicin aerosol-induced vasodilatation in pig respiratory mucosa. *Br J Pharma* 1990;100(3):535–541.

44. Pisarri TE, Jonzon A, Coleridge HM, Coleridge JCG. Vagal afferent and reflex responses to changes in surface osmolarity in lower airways of dogs. *J Appl Physiol* 1992;73(6):2305–2313.

45. Prazma J, Coleman CC, Shockley WW, Boucher RC. Tracheal vascular response to hypertonic and hypotonic solutions. *J Appl Physiol* 1994;76(6):2275–2280.

46. Schelege ES, Gunther RA, Parsons GH, Colbert SR, Yousef MAA, Cross CE. Acute ozone exposure increases bronchial blood flow in conscious sheep. *Resp Physiol* 1990;82:325–336.

47. Pisarri TE, Coleridge HM, Coleridge JCG. Reflex bronchial vasodilation in dogs evoked by injection of a small volume of water into a bronchus. *J Appl Physiol* 1993;75(5):2195–2202.

48. Alsberge M, Magno M, Lipschutz M. Carotid body control of bronchial circulation in sheep. *J Appl Physiol* 1988;65(3):1152–1156.

49. Sahin G, Webber SE, Widdicombe JG. Chemical control of tracheal vascular resistance in dogs. *J Appl Physiol* 1987;63(3):988–995.

50. Kelly L, Kolbe J, Mitzner W, Spannhake EW, Bromberger-Barnea B, Menkes H. Bronchial blood flow affects recovery from constriction in dog lung periphery. *J Appl Physiol* 1986;60:1954–1959.

51. Wagner EM, Mitzner WA. Bronchial circulatory reversal of methacholine-induced airway constriction. *J Appl Physiol* 1990;69(4):1220–1224.

52. Csete ME, Chediak AD, Abraham WM, Wanner A. Airway blood flow modifies allergic airway smooth muscle contraction. *Am Rev Respir Dis* 1991;144:59–63.

53. Baile EM, Dahlby RW, Wiggs BR, Paré PD. Role of tracheal and bronchial circulation in respirtory heat exchange. *J Appl Physiol* 1985;58(1):217–222.

54. Salonen RO, Webber SE, Deffebach ME, Widdicombe JG. Tracheal vascular and smooth muscle responses to air temperature and humidity in dogs. *J Appl Physiol* 1991;71(1):50–59.

55. White DA, Parsons GH. Tracheal blood flow during spontaneous and mechanical ventilation of dry gases in sheep. *J Appl Physiol* 1990;69(3):1117–1122.

56. Baile EM, Godden DJ, Paré PD. Mechanism for increase in tracheobronchial blood flow induced by hyperventilation of dry air in dogs. *J Appl Physiol* 1990;68(1):105–112.

57. Wells UM, Hanafi Z, Widdicombe JG. Osmolality alters tracheal blood flow and tracer uptake in anesthetized sheep. *J Appl Physiol* 1994;77(5):2400–2407.

58. Godden DJ, Baile EM, Okazawa M, Paré PD. Hypertonic aerosol inhalation does not alter central airway blood flow in dogs. *J Appl Physiol* 1988;65(5):1990–1994.

59. Hanna LM, Scherer PW. Regional control of local airway heat and water vapor losses. *J Appl Physiol* 1986;61(2):624–632.

60. Solway J, Leff AR, Dreshaj I, et al. Circulatory heat sources for canine respiratory heat exchange. *J Clin Invest* 1986;78:1015–1019.

61. Long WM, Yerger LD, Abraham WM, Lobel C. Late-phase bronchial vascular responses in allergic sheep. *J Appl Physiol* 1990;69(2):584–590.

62. McFadden ER. Hypothesis: exercise-induced asthma as a vascular phenomenon. *Lancet* 1990;335:880–883.

63. Mitzner W, Wagner EM, Brown RH. Is asthma a vascular disorder? *Chest* 1995;107(3):97S–102S.

64. Gilbert IA, Fouke JM, McFadden ER. Heat and water flux in the intrathoracic airways and exercise-induced asthma. *J Appl Physiol* 1987;63(4):1681–1691.

65. Lung MAKY, Wang CC, Cheng KK. Bronchial circulation: An autoperfusion method for assessing its vasomotor activity and the study of alpha- and beta-adrenoceptors in the bronchial artery. *Life Sciences* 1976;19:577–580.

66. Dinh Xuan AT, Chaussain M, Regnard J, Lockhart A. Pretreatment with an inhaled α1-adrenergic agonist, methoxamine, reduces exercise-induced asthma. *Eur Respir J* 1989;2:409–414.

67. Cabanes LR, Weber SN, Matran R, et al. Bronchial hyperresponsiveness to methacholine in patients with impaired left ventricular function. *N Engl J Med* 1989;320(2):1317–1348.

68. Omori C, Mitzner W, Freed A. The effects of α-adrenergic agonists on hyperpnea-induced airway obstructuion in dogs. *Am J Respir Crit Care Med* 1995;152:17–23.

69. Wagner EM, Mitzner W. Effects of bronchial vascular engorgement on airway dimensions. *J Appl Physiol* 1996;81(1):293–301.

70. Jones JG, Lemen R, Graf Pd. Changes in airway calibre following pulmonary venous congestion. *Br J Anaesth* 1978;50:743–752.

71. Kappagoda CT, Man GCW, Ravi K, Teo KK. Reflex tracheal contrac-

tion during pulmonary venous congestion in the dog. *J Physiol* 1988; 402:335–346.

72. Coleridge HM, Coleridge JCG, Schultz HD. Afferent pathways involved in reflex regulation of airway smooth muscle. *Pharmac Ther* 1989;42:1–63.

73. Roberts AM, Bhattacharya J, Schultz HD, Coleridge HM, Coleridge JCG. Stimulation of pulmonary vagal afferent C-fibers by lung edema in dogs. *Circ Res* 1986;58:512–522.

74. Lundberg JM, Martling CR, Saria A. Capsaicin pretreatment abolishes cigarette smoke induced oedema in rat tracheobronchial mucosa. *Eur J Pharmacol* 1983;86:317–318.

75. Saria A, Lundberg JM, Skofitsch G, Lembeck F. Vascular protein leakage in various tissues induced by substance P, capsaicin, bradykinin, serotonin, histamine and by antigen challenge. *Arch Pharmacol* 1983;324:212–218.

76. Rogers DF, Belvisi MG, Aursudkij B, Evans TW, Barnes PJ. Effects of interactions of sensory neuropeptides on airway microvascular leakage in guinea-pigs. *Br J Pharma* 1988;95:1109–1116.

77. Paul A, Marelli D, Shennib H, et al. Mucociliary function in autotransplanted, allotransplanted, and sleeve resected lungs. *J Thorac Cardiovasc Surg* 1989;98:523–528.

78. Tokuyama K, Lötvall JO, Barnes PJ, Fan Chung K. Mechanism of airway narrowing caused by inhaled platelet-activating factor. *Am Rev Respir Dis* 1991;143:1345–1349.

79. McDonald DM. The ultrastructure and permeability of tracheobronchial blood vessels in health and disease. *Eur Respir J* 1990;3(suppl 12):572S–585S.

80. Persson CGA, Erjefält I, Alkner U, et al. Plasma exudation as a first line respiratory mucosal defence. *Clin Exp Allergy* 1991;21:17–24.

81. Wiggs BR, Bosken C, Paré PD, James A, Hogg JC. A model of airway narrowing in asthma and in chronic obstructive pulmonary disease. *Am Rev Respir Dis* 1992;145:1251–1258.

82. Wagner EM, Mitzner W. Effects of airway wall thickening on airway reactivity. *Am J Respir Crit Care Med* 1995;151(4):A132.

83. Parsons GH, Nichol GM, Barnes PJ, Chung KF. Peptide mediator effects on bronchial blood velocity and lung resistance in conscious sheep. *J Appl Physiol* 1992;72(3):1118–1122.

84. Berman AR, Liu MC, Wagner EM, Proud D. Bradykinin (BK) increase peripheral airway resistance in asthmatic, but not in normal, subjects. *Am J Respir Crit Care Med* 1995;151(4):A131.

85. Gilbert IA, Winslow CJ, Lenner KA, Nelson JA, McFadden ER. Vascular volume expansion and thermally induced asthma. *Eur Respir J* 1993;6(2):189–197.

86. Brown RH, Zerhouni EA, Mitzner W. Visualization of airway obstruction *in vivo* during pulmonary vascular engorgement and edema. *J Appl Physiol* 1995;78(3):1070–1078.

87. Wanner A. Clinical aspects of mucociliary transport. *Am Rev Respir Dis* 1977;116:73–125.

88. Yager D, Butler JP, Bastacky J, Israel E, Smith G, Drazen JM. Amplification of airway constriction due to liquid filling of airway interstices. *J Appl Physiol* 1989;66(6):2873–2884.

89. Barnett B, Miller CE. Flow induced by biological mucociliary systems. *Ann N Y Acad Sci* 1966;130(3):891–901.

90. Messina MS, O'Riordan TG, Smaldone GC. Changes in mucociliary clearance during acute exacerbations of asthma. *Am Rev Respir Dis* 1991;143:993–997.

91. O'Riordan TG, Zwang J, Smaldone GC. Mucociliary clearance in adult asthma. *Am Rev Respir Dis* 1992;146:598–603.

92. Herve P, Silbert D, Cerrina J, Simonneau G, Dartevelle P. Impairment of bronchial mucociliary clearance in long-term survivors of heart/lung and double-lung transplantation. *Chest* 1993;103(1): 59–63.

93. Brody JS, Klempfner G, Staum MM, Vidyasagar D, Kuhl DE, Waldhausen JA. Mucociliary clearance after lung denervation and bronchial transection. *J Appl Physiol* 1972;32:160–164.

94. Baile EM, Jasso-Victoria R, Sotres-Vega A, et al. Tracheobronchial blood flow after a modified canine lung autotransplant: effect of omental wrapping. *Transplant Proc* 1992;24(5):2024–2029.

95. Wagner EM, Foster WM. Importance of airway blood flow on particle clearance from the lung. *J Appl Physiol* 1996;81(5) 1878–1883.

96. Webber SE, Salonen RO, Deffebach ME, Widdicombe JG. Effects of antigen on tracheal circulation and smooth muscle in sheep of different ages. *J Appl Physiol* 1989;67(3):1256–1264.

97. Alexander I, Eyre P. P1-purinoceptors mediate relaxation of the bovine bronchial artery. *Eur J Pharma* 1985;107:359–362.

98. Pearse DB, Fessler H, Wagner EM. Polystyrene microspheres dilate the bronchial artery in anesthetized sheep. *Am J Physiol* 1995;269: H1037–H1043.

99. Laitinen LA, Laitinen MA, Widdicombe JG. Dose-related effects of pharmacological mediators on tracheal vascular resistance in dogs. *Br J Pharma* 1987;92:703–709.

100. Baile EM, Paré PD. Response of the bronchial circulation to acute hypoxemia and hypercarbia in the dog. *J Appl Physiol* 1983;55(5):1474–1479.

101. Wagner EM, Mitzner WA. Effect of hypoxia on the bronchial circulation. *J Appl Physiol* 1988;65(4):1627–1633.

102. Elsasser S, Long WM, Baier HJ, Chediak AD, Wanner A. Independent control of mucosal and total airway blood flow during hypoxemia. *J Appl Physiol* 1991;71(1):223–228.

103. Webber SE, Salonen RO, Widdicombe JG. H1- and H2-receptor characterization in the tracheal circulation of sheep. *Br J Pharma* 1988; 95:551–561.

104. Long WM, Sprung CL, Fawal HE, et al. Effects of histamine on bronchial artery blood flow and bronchomotor tone. *J Appl Physiol* 1985; 59(1):254–261.

105. Parsons GH, Villablanca AC, Brock JM, et al. Bronchial vasodilation by histamine in sheep: characterization of receptor subtype. *J Appl Physiol* 1992;72(6):2090–2098.

106. Sasaki F, March R, Verburgt LM, Bai TR, Paré PD, Baile EM. Endogenous nitric oxide influences acetylcholine-induced bronchovascular dilation in sheep. *Am J Respir Crit Care Med* 1994;149(4): A539.

107. Deffebach ME, Agostoni P, Kirk W, Lakshminarayan S. Pulmonary artery infusion of prostacyclin increases lobar bronchial blood flow. *Resp Physiol* 1989;77:147–156.

108. Webber SE, Salonen RO, Widdicombe JG. Receptors mediating the effects of 5-hydroxytryptamine on the tracheal vasculature and smooth muscle. *Br J Pharma* 1990;99:21–26.

109. Goldman M, Kundson RJ, Mead J, Peterson N, Schwaber JR, Wolh ME. A simplified measurement of respiratory resistance by forced oscillation. *J Appl Physiol* 1970;28(1):113–116.

Asthma, edited by P.J. Barnes, M.M. Grunstein,
A.R. Leff, and A.J. Woolcock.
Lippincott–Raven Publishers, Philadelphia © 1997.

▪ 67 ▪

Fibroblasts

William R. Roche

Basement Membranes	**Cellular Interactions in Inflammation**
Myofibroblasts	**Effects of Treatment**

The essential clinical problem in bronchial asthma is that of airways obstruction. Increased airways resistance may be initially reversible, but fixed airways impairment also may develop (1). The redefinition of asthma as a chronic inflammatory disorder of the airways that is manifested clinically as episodic wheezing and altered bronchial reactivity (2) has drawn attention to the role of cellular changes in the bronchial wall in the pathogenesis of the clinical disease state (3). The characteristic eosinophil-rich inflammatory cell infiltration of the airway wall that is associated with bronchial asthma has attracted much attention as being responsible for increased airway resistance, but the documentation of allergic-type inflammation in association with atopy alone (4,5) or with mild asthma in the absence of current symptoms (6) shows the need for careful evaluation of the mechanisms whereby inflammatory cell infiltration of the airways may produce clinical effects.

The search for mechanism of both acute reductions in airway caliber and chronic fixed airway obstruction is increasingly directed toward remodeling of the airway wall. Models have been constructed to explain how inflammation may indirectly produce the physiologic abnormalities that characterize asthma. These abnormalities in airway function in asthma often are divided into two arbitrary categories: the episodic reductions in airway caliber and the underlying abnormalities in baseline airway function and reactivity. This distinction is artificial, and acute events and chronic alterations interact to produce the spectrum of clinical presentations that we know as asthma. The current views on the contribution of the structural cells of the airway wall to the pathogenesis of bronchial asthma accommodate these two categories of physiologic defects. The persistent features of bronchial asthma include increased airway reactivity with loss of the normal plateau in the provocant dose-response curve. There is an increase in bronchial smooth muscle mass in asthma because of the concomitant processes of hyperplasia and hypertrophy (7), but there is no consistent evidence of abnormalities in the response of the individual muscle cells. Physiologic studies have suggested that the asthmatic response to bronchodilators is due to limitation of smooth muscle relaxation (8). This effect could be produced in normal individuals by avoidance of deep inspiration. It is uncertain whether this phenomenon is due to modulation of muscle function by altering resting fiber length or whether this represents the effect of dissociation of the airway wall from the mechanical forces generated by the pulmonary parenchyma.

Wiggs and colleagues (9) used an alternative approach to explain the role of airway remodeling in asthma. A mathematical model of the human tracheobronchial tree allowed the characteristic spirometric response to bronchial provocation in asthma to be reproduced by introducing a small reduction in lung recoil and thickening of the airway walls into the equation. Thickening of the walls of the more peripheral airways was of particular importance in enhancing the effect of smooth muscle contraction. Thus, it would seem likely that an increase in airway wall thickness is at least partly responsible for the altered airway responses to a given dose of histamine or metacholine in asthma.

The effect of smooth muscle contraction on the airflow would be greatly enhanced by airway thickening internal to the smooth muscle because flow depends on the forth

W. R. Roche: Department of University Pathology, Southampton General Hospital, Southampton SO16 6YD United Kingdom.

power of the radius, whereas airway thickening external to the smooth muscle may make the airway refractory to the forces generated by pulmonary elastic recoil, which help maintain patency of the airways. This dissociation of the airway from forces generated by the pulmonary parenchyma may explain the mathematical model and the physiologic observations of the effect of restricted inspiration on the metacholine response curve. Remodeling of the airway is also likely to be the mechanism of the exaggerated decline in pulmonary function associated with asthma (1) and probably contributes to the development of fixed airways obstruction in patients with severe unremitting disease. Thus, any process that contributes to thickening of the walls of the conducting airways may be of considerable clinical importance in determining not only the degree of bronchial hyperreactivity but also its potentially fatal nature.

Bronchial asthma produces structural changes (Fig. 1) in the bronchial epithelium, the epithelial basement membrane and its associated mesenchymal cell population, the subepithelial vasculature, bronchial gland mass, smooth muscle, and extracellular matrix (10). Although there are fewer data available concerning the smaller airways in asthma, all these structures may be involved in changes in the bronchioles except for the bronchial glands, which are confined to the cartilaginous airways. Similarly, the understanding of the composition and clinical importance of the extracellular matrix and fixed cell populations of the

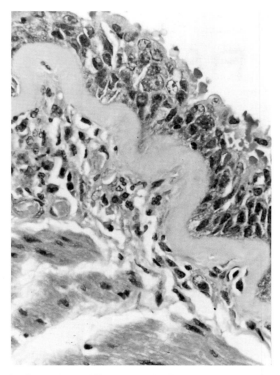

FIG. 1. Subepithelial fibrosis and inflammatory cell infiltration in acute fatal asthma. (H and E staining; magnification ×300.)

bronchi is less developed than the knowledge of the inflammatory cells in asthma. Recent studies have resulted in a revision of the paradigm of the pathogenesis of the tissue changes associated with bronchial asthma (11). The structural cells of the airways are now regarded as playing an important role in the disease state through elaboration of increased extracellular matrix components and interactions with inflammatory cells.

BASEMENT MEMBRANES

Early pathologic studies of asthma fatalities showed a characteristic histologic change of apparent thickening of the bronchial basement membrane (10). The basement membranes beneath epithelia have a number of functions, including the provision of mechanical support for the overlying cells, permeability to nutrients and molecular sieving, anchorage of the epithelial cells and the underlying matrix, and signaling for cellular differentiation, migration, and division (12). The structure of epithelial basement membranes is similar to that of vascular endothelial basement membranes and of the basal lamina of smooth muscle and Schwann cells. Transmission electron microscopy demonstrates three layers in the basement membrane: two apparently homogeneous thin sheets, the lamina lucida immediately beneath the epithelium and the outer lamina densa, and, external to these, fibrillar lamina reticularis, which comprises condensed interstitial components. Understanding of the processes involved in basement membrane alterations in asthma requires that the structural components of the extracellular matrix be reviewed.

The collagens may be divided into two subfamilies: the fibrillar collagens, such as types I, II, III, V, and XI, and the nonfibrillar collagens, including types IV, VI, and VII. These distinctions are based on the ultrastructural appearances of fibrils formed by the staggered assembly of collagen triple helices. The fibrils are formed, after enzymatic cleavage of the C- and N- terminal peptides, by aggregation in the extracellular matrix in intimate contact with the parent cell. This classification has value in distinguishing between the major structural and functional roles of the collagens but cannot be regarded as absolute, as collagens fibrils may be heterogeneous in their composition and nonfibrillar collagens may be closely associated with the formation of collagen fibrils (13).

The nonfibrillar collagens have helical domains of various lengths but retain their terminal peptides, which are available for noncovalent and disulfide-bonded homopolymerization, and the binding of other collagen species, matrix components, and cells. These collagen types are particularly associated with basement membranes, where their greater molecular complexity and physical flexibility contribute to both structural and functional characteristics. Although a quantitatively small component of the interstitial compartment, they also contribute to molecular and cellular adhesive mechanisms in this site. Type IV collagen forms the basic framework of the basement membrane (Fig. 2) by the formation of an open polygonal meshwork composed of collagen fibers polymerized at amino- and carboxy-terminals and by lateral associations (14,15). Collagen VII is confined to the

basement membranes of multilayered epithelia, which probably reflects the greater mechanical forces that these structures experience (16). In keeping with the stratified nature of the overlying bronchial epithelium (17), the bronchial basement membrane is anchored to the underlying connective tissue by collagen VII fibers similar to the arrangement found in skin (18). In contrast, the basement membrane of the single-layered alveolar epithelium is devoid of collagen VII.

Laminin is a large molecular species with multiple binding sites, which is important in the assembly of the basement membrane. This large glycoprotein (molecular mass ~800 kDa) is of asymmetric cruciate shape with one long arm. It is formed from three subunits, one A chain and two smaller B chains, which are joined by disulfide bonds (19). Laminin aggregates into small polymers that in turn form larger complexes in the presence of divalent cations. The bonds between ends of the arms of the molecule allow it to form an open lattice structure. This capacity to form homopolymers may be important in the formation of some basement membranes that are synthesized before collagen IV deposition. Separate sites on the laminin molecule bind heparin sulfate proteoglycans, entactin, and collagen IV. Laminin is also bound by integrin and nonintegrin receptors on cell membranes, which are important in both cell structure and function (20).

The basement membrane contains a heterogeneous group of other glycoproteins with adhesive and other properties. These include fibronectin, a large multispliced molecule that has domains for binding to cell membrane receptors, collagen and heparan sulfate proteoglycans (21), and entactin or nidogen, a sulfated glycoprotein that binds to the central portion of the laminin molecule and to collagen IV. Entactin also has an RDG (arginine-glycine-aspartate) sequence that may allow it to be bound by cell-surface integrin molecules (22).

Basement membranes also contain proteoglycans, which are sugar-protein complexes that differ from glycoproteins in that the sugar molecules form linear chains of repeated disaccharide sequences bound to specific core proteins (23). These molecules have at least four roles in the basement membrane: the cross-linkage of basement membrane molecules including collagen, fibronectin, laminin, and proteoglycans themselves; the determination of the electrical charge of the basement membrane by virtue of their highly anionic glycosaminoglycan chains; transmembrane receptors for cell adhesion and signal transduction; and as a repository for growth factors such as fibroblast growth factor and transforming growth factor-β (TGF-β) (24).

The application of standard tinctorial methods for the detection of basement membrane glycoproteins indicated that the apparent basement membrane thickening in bronchial asthma did not involve the true basement membrane components (25), but the significance of this was not appreciated. This finding was rediscovered by electron mi-

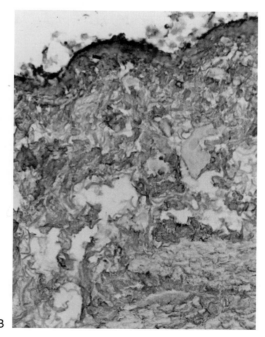

FIG. 2. Extracellular matrix in the bronchial mucosa in asthma. **A:** Collagen IV, which is restricted to epithelial and vascular basement membranes. **B:** Fibronectin in the epithelial basement membrane, lamina reticularis, and interstitium. (Frozen section, immunoperoxidase, magnification ×300.)

croscopic examination of biopsy material obtained from two children with asthma undergoing thoracotomy and from asthma fatalities. This allowed the distinction between the true epithelial basement membrane, comprising the lamina lucida and densa, and the presence of increased fibrillar collagen deposition in the lamina reticularis (26).

The application of electron microscopy and immunohistochemistry to endoscopic bronchial biopsy specimens, from individuals with mild atopic asthma and normal controls, confirmed the thickening of the lamina reticularis beneath the basement membrane (11). In normal individuals this layer measured 4 μm deep, whereas in individuals with mild asthma it extended to approximately twice that depth beneath the epithelium. This is an early event in asthma, occurring in patients with a short clinical history, in mild disease, and in children (26). These appearances are not due to an increase in the basement membrane-specific proteins but are due to the deposition of interstitial collagens III and V, fibronectin (see Fig. 2), and, to a lesser extent, collagen I, beneath the bronchial epithelial basement membrane (11). Collagens type I, III, and V and fibronectin also were detected in the lamina reticularis of normal individuals, suggesting that the alteration in asthma is a quantitative rather than a qualitative change. However, more recent studies have demonstrated the presence of abundant immunoreactivity for the glycoprotein tenascin in association with the lamina reticularis in asthma (27). This glycoprotein is expressed in embryonic organogenesis and in wound healing and is thought to play an important role in the regulation of epithelial-mesenchymal interactions and in modulation of cellular adhesion to the extracellular matrix. The presence of tenascin in asthma may indicate important interaction between the bronchial epithelium and its underlying matrix.

MYOFIBROBLASTS

The recognition of the apparent basement membrane thickening in asthma as the accumulation of interstitial collagens in the lamina reticularis led to the search for the origin of this material. Interstitial fibrillar collagens usually are deposited by fibroblasts and excessive production may occur in response to a range of cytokines (28). The restriction of the fibrotic process to the lamina reticularis of the basement membrane suggested that either there was a specific directional stimulus for collagen deposition by the fibroblasts of the lamina propria or that there was a unique cell population in association with the lamina reticularis. The histologic appearances of an uncommon bowel condition called "collagenous colitis" (29) share some similarities with bronchial asthma. This condition is characterized by a dense band of fibrosis beneath the colonic epithelium and a scattered infiltrate of eosinophil leukocytes. The collagens deposited are types

I and III; this is associated with ultrastructural evidence of activation of a unique fibroblast population (30). These cells have features akin to both smooth muscle cells and fibroblasts and are called "pericryptal myofibroblasts." These cells are present in the intestine of normal individuals and in at least some animals.

The term "myofibroblast" was used initially to describe a cell type found in the granulation tissue of healing wounds (31). The synthetic capacity of the myofibroblast is reflected in the presence of numerous polyribosomes in its cytoplasm. The evidence for the contractile function of these cells includes the ultrastructural detection of arrays of thin filaments with focal densities in the cytoplasm similar to those seen in smooth muscle. These cells also express cytoskeletal filaments, which are normally associated with smooth muscle (32). Individual cells may contain the muscle-specific intermediate filament desmin and the smooth muscle-associated isotype of the contractile protein actin (α-smooth muscle actin) singly or together. The myofibroblasts of wound healing are thought to be derived from resident cells at the site of injury, although the mode of induction of this phenotype is uncertain (33).

The relationship between the induced myofibroblast phenotype and constitutive myofibroblasts is uncertain.

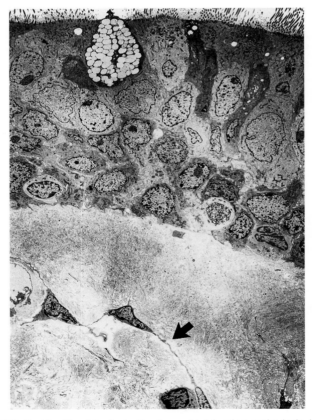

FIG. 3. Myofibroblasts in the bronchial lamina reticularis in asthma *(arrow)*. (Electron Microscopy, uranyl acetate and lead citrate, magnification ×1700.)

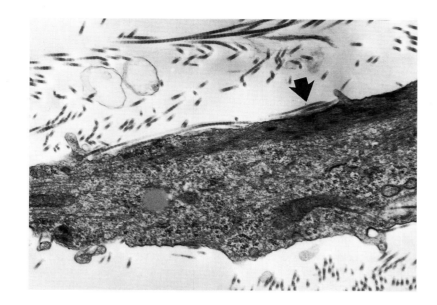

FIG. 4. Electron microscopy showing subplasma-lemmal contractile filaments *(arrow)* in a bronchial myofibroblast. (Electron Microscopy, uranyl acetate and lead citrate; magnification ×20,000.)

These cells apparently maintain their phenotype in the absence of inflammation or wound healing. The pericryptal myofibroblasts of the rabbit intestine form a self-renewing population distinct from the colonic epithelium and other cells of the lamina propria (34). A monoclonal antibody, PR 2D3, raised to rectal tissue scrapings was found to be a marker of these cells in the human colonic mucosa. (35). This antibody appeared to react with a 140-kDa membrane protein, which was shared with smooth muscle cells.

Ultrastructural analysis of bronchial biopsy specimens from normal and asthmatic individuals (Fig. 3) revealed thin cytoplasmic strands running parallel to and beneath the bronchial epithelium (36). Myofibroblasts had not been described previously in this situation, but examination of levels from tissue blocks revealed that the cytoplasmic strands were extensions from cells with elongated, partially crenated nuclei which lay in a horizontal plane beneath the epithelium in a deeper portion of the collagen of the lamina reticularis. The cytoplasm contained ribosomes and thin filaments with focal densities consistent with the ultrastructural appearances of the synthetic and contractile apparatus of myofibroblasts (Fig. 4). The cytoplasmic processes of these cells extend for up to 50 μm on either side of the nucleus and overlap without forming intercellular junctions, thus constituting a discontinuous cytoplasmic network through which inflammatory cells must pass to reach the bronchial epithelium. Other workers subsequently described similar cells in the rat trachea (37); this network of cells may be analogous to the network of pulmonary parenchymal contractile interstitial cells in the alveolar septae (38).

Myofibroblasts are present in the lamina reticularis of the bronchial mucosa of both normal and asthmatic individuals (Fig. 5). Immunohistochemical analysis showed that there was a median of five myofibroblasts per millimeter of epithelial basement membrane in normal individuals and 8/mm in asthmatics. These numbers are consistent with the ultrastructural appearances of elongated sheets of cytoplasm in the region of 100 μm in diameter forming an overlapping myofibroblast layer beneath the bronchial epithelium. The number of myofibroblasts in individual subjects correlated strongly with the depth of collagen beneath the bronchial epithelium, suggesting that the subepithelial myofibroblast is responsible for the synthesis of the interstitial collagens of the lamina reticularis (36).

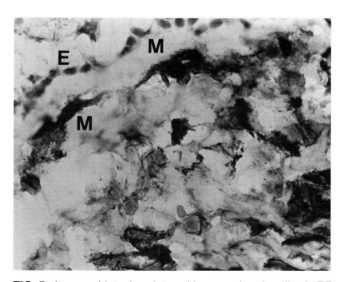

FIG. 5. Immunohistochemistry with monoclonal antibody PR 2D3 showing myofibroblasts *(M)* beneath the bronchial epithelium *(E)* in asthma. (Frozen section, immunoperoxidase; magnification ×900.)

The increase in subepithelial myofibroblast numbers may be a reflection of the range of peptide and other mediators that are released in the bronchial mucosa in asthma. Fibroblast replication may be stimulated by a variety of factors that are potentially active in the bronchial mucosa, including histamine (39), mast cell heparin (40), mast cell tryptase (41), interleukin-1 (IL-1) (42), interleukin-4 (IL-4) (43), platelet-derived growth factor (PDGF) (44), fibroblast growth factor (FGF) (45), and endothelin (46). These may be derived from the inflammatory cell infiltrate or from resident cell populations such as the bronchial epithelium or myofibroblasts themselves, in response to agents released during the inflammatory response.

The increase in subepithelial collagen in asthmatic individuals may be due to increased synthesis, decreased degradation of procollagens in the cytoplasm, or reduced proteolysis of extracellular collagen. A number of potentially fibrogenic cytokines that act to increase collagen synthesis may act in the bronchial mucosa. TGF-β is a potent stimulator of both collagen and fibronectin synthesis by fibroblasts (47) and high levels of TGF-β have been reported in the airways (48). Interleukin-4, which may be derived from T lymphocytes or mast cells, appears to be central to the immunologic abnormalities associated with asthma and also may contribute to deposition of excessive amounts of collagen and fibronectin in the extracellular matrix (49). Mast cells have been shown to contain fibroblast growth factor and may be a biologically important source of this cytokine (50). The relative contribution of individual cytokines to the fibrotic processes in asthma is unknown.

CELLULAR INTERACTIONS IN INFLAMMATION

Fibroblasts have another role in the airway apart from the provision of mechanical support to the tissues. Constitutive cell populations and the extracellular matrix are increasingly recognized as functioning as a source of signals for cellular localization, migration, differentiation, and activation. These signals may result from the interaction of specific cell-surface receptors with components of the matrix or from the exposure of bioactive molecules that are secreted immediately or that have accumulated as complexes with matrix components. Extracellular matrix molecules can reorganize the actin cytoskeleton in fibroblasts that constitutively express β1 integrins, with the formation of focal contacts that link matrix glycoproteins, integrins, actin-binding proteins, and the cytoskeleton (51). Unlike many cell-surface receptors, the integrins do not have intrinsic protein kinase activity. As the intracellular signal transduction of many of the responses that are mediated or modulated by extracellular matrix involve the phosphorylation steps, the integrins must be capable of regulation of kinases. The localization of regulatory protein kinases at the intracellular sites of adhesion plaques may be one mechanism of this response (52). Conversely, intracellular events, such as cell cycle, may modulate the adhesive functions of the cell membrane integrins by phosphorylation of either the α or β chain (53). Phosphorylation of integrins also can be induced by exposure to inflammatory cytokines and can enhance the adhesiveness of cells to the extracellular matrix, although phosphorylation is not universally required for activation of integrin-mediated adhesion.

β-1 integrins are expressed as very late antigen (VLA) cell membrane proteins by T lymphocytes in response to activation signals. This allows the T lymphocyte to bind to cell matrix components; this interaction may stimulate the secretion of cytokines and enhance lymphocyte responsiveness (54). Similarly, the survival and function of eosinophil leukocytes is modulated by the presence of extracellular matrix components, such as fibronectin, acting via cell surface β-1 integrins (55). The secretion of superoxide radicals in response to tumor necrosis factor (TNF), platelet activating factor (PAF), lipopolysaccharide, and substance P has been shown to be inhibited by matrix components (56).

The extracellular matrix also acts as a repository for growth factors, which are mainly bound to proteoglycans. The principal growth factors that are found in the matrix are basic FGF-2 (57) in basement membranes and TGF-β in the interstitium (58). FGF-2 is an angiogenic and highly mitogenic growth factor with activity for a range of epithelial, mesenchymal, and neural cells. It belongs to the heparin-binding family of fibroblast growth factors and its biologic activity is potentiated by heparan sulfate proteoglycans that may protect FGF-2 from proteolytic degradation in the extracellular matrix (59). After the stored FGF-2 in the matrix is released by enzyme action, the free molecule may be bound by cell-surface proteoglycans. The cell-surface proteoglycans alter the conformation of FGF-2 so as to enhance its interaction with high-affinity receptors (60). Similarly, the TGF-β receptors include a transmembrane proteoglycan, β-glycan (61). TGF-β binds to the core protein of β-glycan and also to the core proteins of the small extracellular proteoglycans biglycan and decorin. These interstitial proteoglycans inhibit the biologic activity of TGF-β and may have a therapeutic role in the control of abnormal matrix deposition (62).

The specialized fibroblast population beneath the bronchial epithelium frequently forms membrane appositions of eosinophil leukocytes; this close contact may allow for the stimulation of the eosinophils by both high local concentrations of cytokines and direct cell-cell contact. T lymphocytes and mast cells also come in close contact with myofibroblasts before infiltrating the overlying epithelium. The cytokine repertoire of fibroblasts is large; chemotactic cytokines (63,64) include interleukin-

8 (IL-8), monocyte chemotactic factor, colony-stimulating factors (65) such as granulocyte-macrophage colony-stimulating factor (GM-CSF; which is a potent priming and survival agent for eosinophils), lymphocyte activators such as IL-1 and IL-6 (66,67), stem cell factor for mast cell proliferation, differentiation and migration (68), and scatter factor/hepatocyte growth factor for epithelial cell migration, growth, and morphogenesis (69).

The isolation and cell culture of bronchial myofibroblasts from microdissected bronchial lamina reticularis have allowed for the direct assessment of cytokine secretion by these cells. Myofibroblast-derived cultures secreted stem cell factor constitutively, but the secretion of IL-6, IL-8, and GM-CSF under basal conditions was low, although this was increased by exposure to IL-1 or TNF-α (70). This regulation of cytokine production seemed to be mediated by the regulation of the abundance of specific messenger RNA. The addition of corticosteroids to the cultures reduced GM-CSF secretion in response to TNF-α. This culture system was used similarly for the assessment of eosinophil survival in the presence of myofibroblasts. Co-culture of peripheral blood-derived eosinophils and myofibroblasts caused a marked enhancement of eosinophil survival because of the inhibition of apoptosis. This effect was mainly mediated by increased myofibroblast synthesis and secretion of GM-CSF in response to eosinophil-derived IL-1 and TNF-α, but there also was a small contribution from integrin-mediated interaction between the eosinophils and myofibroblasts (71).

EFFECTS OF TREATMENT

The influence of excessive subepithelial collagen deposition on airway diameter and function is uncertain. Although decreased distensibility of the airway wall has been described *in vivo* in association with asthma (72), it is uncertain as to the relative contribution of components of the wall to this effect. Although the characteristic band of collagen beneath the epithelium of large bronchi may have little effect on airway resistance in the patent airway, the mechanical properties of this layer might lead to airway wall infolding and exaggerate the effects of smooth muscle contraction in asthma. Furthermore, this process extends to small bronchioles where it may contribute to airway thickening that underlies the asthmatic response to inhaled provocants (73).

Studies of individuals who had developed asthma after occupational exposure to toluene diisocyanate (74) confirmed the early appearance of subepithelial fibrosis in asthma. Persons with as little as 3 years' exposure and with symptoms for less than 1 year exhibited subepithelial collagen deposition. Allergen avoidance for 6 months induced a regression toward normal in the collagen thickness, although there was persistence of the bronchial inflammatory cell infiltrate. In contrast, inhaled corticosteroids reduce bronchial inflammation but appear not to affect the extent of subepithelial fibrosis (75). In one study (76) there was a reported reduction in the extent of collagen III deposition beneath the basement membrane in response to inhaled steroids, but the measurements of the thickness of this band were unusually high, with a mean pretreatment thickness of 29.67 μm that fell to 19.8 μm after treatment. These data suggest that either the lamina reticularis was not defined or that the data were skewed by tangential sampling and measurements. Overall, it would appear that the fibrous thickening of the lamina reticularis in asthma is refractory to conventional treatment.

CONCLUSIONS

The structural cells of the airway are recognized as playing a clinically important role in asthma, contributing to both the remodeling of the airways and to the inflammatory processes. Further investigations are required so that therapies aimed at the prevention or reversal of fixed airways obstruction can be devised. The accessibility of the airway wall to inhaled agents should facilitate the application of new treatments based on the biology of the interstitial cells and their surrounding matrix, which may address the current deficiencies in the treatment of what is a chronic inflammatory and fibrosing disorder of the airways.

REFERENCES

1. Peat JK, Woolcock AJ, Culen K. Rate of decline of lung function in subjects with asthma. *Eur J Respir Dis* 1987;70:171–179.
2. Barnes PJ. A new approach to the treatment of asthma. *New Engl J Med* 1989;321:1517–1527.
3. Djukanovic R, Roche WR, Wilson JW, et al. State of the art. Mucosal inflammation in asthma. *Am Rev Respir Dis* 1990;142:434–457.
4. Bradley BL, Azzawi M, Jacobson M, et al. Eosinophils, T-lymphocytes, mast cells, neutrophils and macrophages in bronchial biopsy specimens from atopic subjects with asthma: comparison with biopsy specimens from atopic subjects without asthma and normal control subjects and relationship to bronchial hyperresponsiveness. *J Allergy Clin Immunol* 1991;88:661–674.
5. Djukanovic R, Lai CWK, Wilson JW, et al. Bronchial mucosal manifestations of atopy: a comparison of markers of inflammation between atopic asthmatics, atopic nonasthmatics and healthy controls. *Eur Resp* 1992;5:538–544.
6. Beasley R, Roche WR, Roberts JA, Holgate ST. Cellular events in the bronchi in mild asthma and after bronchial provocation. *Am Rev Respir Dis* 1989;139:806–813.
7. Ebina M, Takakashi T, Chiba T, Motomiya M. Cellular hypertrophy and hyperplasia of airway smooth muscles underlying bronchial asthma. *Am Rev Respir Dis* 1993;148:720–726.
8. Skloot G, Permutt S, Togias A. Airway hyperresponsiveness in asthma: a problem of limited smooth muscle relaxation with inspiration. *J Clin Invest* 1995;96:2393–2403.
9. Wiggs BR, Bosken C, Pare PD, James A, Hogg JC. A model of airway narrowing in asthma and in chronic obstructive pulmonary disease. *Am Rev Respir Dis* 1992;145:1251–1258.
10. Dunnill MS. The pathology of asthma, with special references to changes in the bronchial mucosa. *J Clin Path* 1960;13:27–33.
11. Roche WR, Beasley R, Williams JH, Holgate ST. Subepithelial fibrosis in the bronchi of asthmatics. *Lancet* 1989;I:520–524.

12. Martinez-Hernandez A, Amenta PS. The basement membrane in pathology. *Lab Invest* 1983;48:656–677.

13. Linsenmayer TF, Fitch JM, Birk DE. Heterotypic collagen fibrils and stabilizing collagens. Controlling elements in corneal morphogenesis. *Ann NY Acad Sci* 1990;580:143–160.

14. Abrahamson DR. Structure and development of the glomerular capillary wall and basement membrane. *Am J Physiol* 1987;22:F783–F794.

15. Yurchenco PD. Assembly of basement membrane. *Ann NY Acad Sci* 1990;580:195–213.

16. Montefort S, Roberts JA, Beasley R, Holgate ST, Roche WR. The site of disruption of the bronchial epithelium in asthmatic and nonasthmatic subjects. *Thorax* 1992;47:499–503.

17. Evans MJ, Cox RA, Shami SG, Wilson B, Plopper CG. The role of basal cells in attachment of columnar cells to the basal lamina of the trachea. *Am J Respir Cell Mol Biol* 1989;1:463–469.

18. Wetzels RHW, Robben HCM, Leigh IM, Schaafsura HE, Vooijs GP, Ramaekers FCS. Distribution pattern of type VII collagen in normal and malignant human tissues. *Am J Pathol* 1991;139:451–459.

19. Sasaki M, Kleinman HK, Huber H, Deutzmann R, Yamada Y. Laminin, a multidomain protein: the A chain has a unique globular domain and homology with the basement membrane proteoglycan and the laminin B chains. *J Biol Chem* 1988;263:16536–16544.

20. Beck K, Hunter I, Engel J. Structure and function of laminin: anatomy of a multidomain glycoprotein. *FASEB J* 1990;4:148–160.

21. Hynes RO. Molecular biology of fibronectin. *Annu Rev Cell Biol* 1985; 1:67–90.

22. Mann K, Deutzmann R, Aumailley M, et al. Amino acid sequence of mouse nidogen, a multidomain basement membrane protein with binding activity for laminin, collagen IV and cells. *EMBO J* 1989;8:65–72.

23. Fransson L-A, Carlstedt I, Coster L, Malmstrom A. The functions of the heparan sulphate proteoglycans. *Ciba Fdn Symp* 1986;124:125–142.

24. Yamaguchi Y, Mann DM, Ruoslathi E. Negative regulation of transforming growth factor-β by the proteoglycan decorin. *Nature* 1990; 346:281–284.

25. Crepea SB, Harman JW. Pathology of bronchial asthma;significance of membrane changes in asthma and nonallergic pulmonary disease. *J Allergy* 1955;26:453– 460.

26. Cutz E, Levison H, Cooper D M. Ultrastructure of airways in children with asthma. *Histopathology* 1978;2:407–421.

27. Laitinen LA, Laitinen A. Structural and cellular changes in asthma. *Eur Respir J* 1994;4:384–351.

28. Kovacs EJ. Fibrogenic cytokines: the role of immune mediators in the development of scar tissue. *Immunol Today* 1991;12:17–23.

29. Rams H, Rogers AI, Ghandur-Mnaymeh L. Collagenous colitis. *Ann Intern Med* 1987;106:108–113.

30. Hwang WS, Kelly JK, Shaffer EA, Hershfield NB. Collagenous colitis, a disease of the pericryptal fibroblast sheath. *J Pathol* 1986;149:33–40.

31. Gabbiani G, Ryan GB, Majno G. Presence of modified fibroblasts in granulation tissue and their possible role in wound contraction. *Experientia* 1971;27:549–550.

32. Skalli O, Schurch W, Seemayer T, et al. Myofibroblasts from diverse pathological settings are heterogenous in their content of actin isoforms and intermediate filament proteins. *Lab Invest* 1989;60:275– 285.

33. Sappino AP, Schurch W, Gabbiani G. Differentiation repertoire of fibroblastic cells. Expression of cytoskeletal proteins as a marker of phenotypic modulations. *Lab Invest* 1990;63:144–161.

34. Pascal RP, Kaye GI, Lane N. Colonic pericryptal fibroblast sheath replication, migration and cytodifferentiation of a mesenchymal cell system in adult tissue. I Autoradiographic studies of normal rabbit colon. *Gastroenterology* 1968;54:836–851.

35. Richman PI, Tilly R, Jass JR, Bodmer WF. Colonic pericryptal sheath cells: characterisation of cell type with new monoclonal antibody. *J Clin Pathol* 1987;40:593–600.

36. Brewster CEP, Howarth PH, Djukanovic R, Wilson JW, Holgate ST, Roche WR. Myofibroblasts and subepithelial fibrosis in bronchial asthma. *Am J Resp Cell Mol Biol* 1990;3:507–511.

37. Evans MJ, Guha SC, Cox RA, Moller PC. Attenuated fibroblast sheath around the basement membrane zone in the trachea. *Am J Respir Cell Mol Biol* 1993;8:188–192.

38. Adler KB, Low RB, Leslie KO, Mitchell lJ, Evans JN. Contractile cells in normal and fibrotic lung. *Lab Invest* 1989;60:473–485.

39. Norrby K. Mast cell histamine, a local mitogen acting via H2 receptors in nearby tissue cells. *Virchows Arch [B]* 1980;34:13–20.

40. Roche WR. Mast cells and tumors. The specific enhancement of tumor proliferation in vitro. *Am J Pathol* 1985;119:57–64.

41. Ruoss SJ, Hartmann T, Caughey GH. Mast cell tryptase is a mitogen for cultured fibroblasts. *J Clin Invest* 1991;88:493–499.

42. Rupp EA, Cameron PM, Ranawat CS, Schmidt JA, Bayne EK. Specific bioactivities of monocyte derived interleukin-1à and interleukin-1 are similar to each other on cultured murine thymocytes and on cultured human connective tissue cells. *J Clin Invest* 1986;78:836–839.

43. Monroe JG, Haldar S, Prystowsky MB, Lammie P. Lymphokine regulation of inflammatory processes: interleukin-4 stimulated fibroblast proliferation. *Clin Immunol Immunopath* 1988;49:292–298.

44. Shimokado K, Raines EW, Madtes DK, Barrett TB, Benditt EP, Ross R. A significant part of macrophage-derived growth factor consists of at least two forms of PDGF. *Cell* 1985;43:277–286.

45. Burgess WH, Maciag T. The heparin-binding (fibroblast) growth factor family of proteins. *Annu Rev Biochem* 1989;58:575–606.

46. Simonson MS, Wann S, Mene P, et al. Endothelin stimulates phospholipase C, Na+/H+ exchange, c-*fos* expression, and mitogenesis in rat mesangial cells. *J Clin Invest* 1989;83:708–712.

47. Ignotz RA, Massagn J. Transforming growth factor-β stimulates the expression of fibronectin and collagen and their incorporation into the extracellular matrix. *J Biol Chem* 1986;261:4337–4345.

48. Yamauchi K, Martinet Y, Busset P, Fells GA, Crystal RG. High levels of transforming growth factor-β are present in the epithelial lining of the normal lower respiratory tract. *Am Rev Respir Dis* 1988;137:1360–1363.

49. Gillery P, Fertin C, Nicolas JF, et al. Interleukin-4 stimulates collagen gene expression in human fibroblast monolayer cultures. Potential role in fibrosis. *FEBS Lett* 1992;302:231–234.

50. Qu Z, Lieber JM, Powers MR, et al. Mast cells are a major source of fibroblast growth factor in chronic inflammation and cutaneous hemangioma. *Am J Pathol* 1995;147:564–573.

51. Turner CE, Burridge K. Transmembrane molecular assemblies in cell-extracellular matrix interactions. *Curr Opin Cell Biol* 1991;3:849–853.

52. Schaller MD, Borgman CA, Cobb BS, Vines RR, Reynolds AB, Parsons JT. PP125FAK, a structurally distinctive protein tyrosine kinase associated with focal adhesions. *Proc Natl Acad Sci USA* 1992;89: 5192–5196.

53. Shaw LM, Messier JM, Mercurio AM. The activation dependent adhesion of macrophages to laminin involves cytoskeletal anchoring and phosphorylation of the α6 1 integrin. *J Cell Biol* 1990;110:2167–2174.

54. Yamada A, Nojima Y, Sugita K, Dang NH, Schlossman SF, Morimoto C. Cross-linking of VLA/CD29 molecule has a co-mitogenic effect with anti-CD3 on CD4 cell activation in serum-free culture system. *Eur J Immunol* 1991;21:319–325.

55. Anwar ARF, Moqbel R, Walsh GM, Kay AB, Wardlaw AJ. Adhesion to fibronectin prolongs eosinophil survival. *J Exp Med* 1993;177:839–843.

56. Dri P, Cramer R, Spessotto P, Romano M, Patriarca P. Eosinophil activation on biologic surfaces. Production of O-2 in response to physiologic soluble stimuli is differentially modulated by extracellular matrix components and endothelial cells. *J Immunol* 1991;147:613–620.

57. Folkman J, Klagsbrun M, Sasse J, Wadziniski M, Ingber D, Vodavsky I. A heparin-binding angiogenic protein—basic fibroblastic growth factor—is stored within basement membrane. *Am J Pathol* 1988;130: 393–400.

58. Heine UL, Flanders K, Roberts AB, Munoz EF, Sporn MB. Role of transforming growth factor-β in the development of the mouse embryo. *J Cell Biol* 1987;105:2861–2876.

59. Salsela O, Moscatelli D, Sommer A, Rifkin DB. Endothelial cell-derived heparin sulfate binds basic fibroblast growth factor and protects it from proteolytic degradation. *J Cell Biol* 1988;107:743–751.

60. Prestrelski SJ, Fox FM, Arakawa T. Binding of heparin to basic fibroblast growth factor induces a conformational change. *Arch Biochem Biophys* 1992;293:314–319.

61. Andres JL, Ronnstrand L, Chiefetz S, Massagne J. Purification of the transforming growth factor-β (TGF-β) binding proteoglycan-glycan. *J Biol Chem* 1991;266:23282–23287.

62. Border WA, Noble NA, Yamamoto T, et al. Natural inhibitor of transforming growth factor-β protects against scarring in experimental renal disease. *Nature* 1992;360:361–364.

63. Strieter RM, Phan SH, Showell HJ, et al. Monokine-induced neutrophil chemotactic factor gene expression in human fibroblasts. *J Biol Chem* 1989;264:10621–10626.

64. Yoshimura T, Yuhki N, Moore SK, Appella E, Lerman MI, Leonard EJ.

Human monocyte chemoattractant protein-1 (MCP-1). Full length c-DNA cloning, expression in mitogen-stimulated blood mononuclear leukocytes, and sequence similarity to murine competence gene JE. *FEBS Lett* 1989;244:487–493.

65. Vancheri C, Gauldie J, Bienenstock J, et al. Human lung fibroblast-derived granulocyte-macrophage colony stimulating factor (GM-CSF) mediates eosinophil survival *in vitro*. *Am J Respir Cell Mol Biol* 1989; 1:289–295.

66. Elias JA, Reynolds MM. Interleukin-1 and tumour necrosis factor synergistically stimulate lung fibroblast interleukin-1 production. *Am J Respir Cell Mol Biol* 1990;3:13–20.

67. Elias JA, Trinchieri G, Beck JM, et al. A synergistic interaction of IL-6 and IL-1 mediates the thymocyte-stimulating activity produced by recombinant IL-1–stimulated fibroblasts. *J Immunol* 1989;142:509–514.

68. Nocka K, Buck J, Levi E, Tan J, Besmer P. Candidate ligand for the c-*kit* transmembrane kinase receptor: KL, a fibroblast-derived growth factor stimulates mast cells and erythroid progenitors. *EMBO J* 1990; 9:3287–3294.

69. Montesano R, Matsumoto K, Nakamura T, Orci L. Identification of fibroblast-derived epithelial morphogen as hepatocyte growth factor. *Cell* 1991;67:901–908.

70. Zhang S, Howarth PH, Roche W R. Cytokine production by cell cultures from bronchial subepithelial myofibroblasts. *J Pathol* 1996;180: 45–101.

71. Zhang S, Mohammed Q, Burbidge A, Morland CM, Roche WR. Cell cultures from bronchial subepithelial myofibroblasts enhance eosinophil survival in vitro. *Eur Resp J* 1996;9:1834–1846.

72. Wilson JW, Li X, Pain MCF. The lack of distensibility of asthmatic airways. *Am Rev Respir Dis* 1993;148:806–809.

73. Kuwano K, Bosken CH, Pare PD, Bai TR, Wiggs BR, Hogg JC. Small airways dimensions in asthma and chronic obstructive pulmonary disease. *Am Rev Respir Dis* 1993;148:1220–1225.

74. Saetta M, Maestrelli P, Di Stefano A, et al. Effect of cessation of exposure to toluene diisocyanate (TDI) on bronchial mucosa of subjects with TDI-induced asthma. *Am Rev Respir Dis* 1992;145:169–174.

75. Jeffrey PK, Godfrey RW, Adelroth E, Nelson F, Rogers A, Johansson S-A. Effects of treatment on airway inflammation and thickening of basement membrane reticular collagen in asthma. A quantitative light and electron microscopic study. *Am Rev Respir Dis* 1992;145:890–899.

76. Trigg CJ, Manolitsas ND, Wang J, et al. Placebo-controlled immunopathological study of 4 months inhaled corticosteroids in asthma. *Am J Respir Crit Care Med* 1994;150:17–22.

■ 7 ■

Neural Mechanisms

Asthma, edited by P.J. Barnes, M.M. Grunstein, A.R. Leff, and A.J. Woolcock.
Lippincott–Raven Publishers, Philadelphia © 1997.

▪ 68 ▪

Cholinergic Mechanisms in Asthma

Richard W. Costello and Allison D. Fryer

Innervation of the Airways by Cholinergic Nerves
    Innervation of the Trachea
    Innervation of the Bronchi
    Cholinergic Ganglia
    Muscarinic Receptors in the Airways
Physiologic Function of Cholinergic Nerves in the Airways
    Cholinergic Neuromuscular Junction
    Control of Acetylcholine Release
Cholinergic Mechanisms in Asthma
    Excessive Sensory Nerve Activity
    Excessive Vagal Nerve Center Output

Increased Transmission Through Cholinergic Ganglia
Loss of Function of the Neuronal Muscarinic M_2
    Autoreceptor
Failure to Metabolize Acetylcholine Through
    Impaired Function of the Acetylcholine Enzyme
Importance of Cholinergic Nerves in Asthma
    Nonspecific Hyperresponsiveness
    Allergic Asthma
    Virus-induced Asthma
    Nocturnal Asthma
    Psychogenic Asthma

The vagus nerves carry cholinergic efferent nerve fibers from the central nervous system (CNS) to the lungs, supplying the airway smooth muscle, the submucosal mucus glands, and the bronchial circulation (1). Stimulation of these cholinergic, or parasympathetic nerves, releases acetylcholine (ACh), which causes the airway smooth muscle to contract (2–5), the glandular tissue to secrete mucus (6,7), and the bronchial circulation to dilate (8–10). Under normal resting conditions the cholinergic nerves maintain a baseline tonic contraction of the airway smooth muscle (2,11–14).

There are several key observations suggesting that excessive activity of the cholinergic nerves plays an important role in the pathogenesis of asthma. For example, there is an increase in vagally mediated airway tone in asthmatics compared with normals (14). In addition, excess mucus secretion and increased smooth muscle contraction, the principal clinical features of asthma, can be mimicked by cholinergic nerve stimulation or by giving agents with cholinergic activity (2,15). Furthermore, several clinical studies have demonstrated that blockade of the vagal nerves using anticholinergic drugs effectively reverses bronchospasm in patients with both stable and acute asthma (16–20). The efficacy of anticholinergic agents in the treatment of asthma has been known for more than 150 years. One of the earliest treatments for asthma was inhalation of the smoke from the stramonium plant, the active substance of which is the anticholinergic agent atropine (21). Finally, asthma is characterized by general bilateral bronchoconstriction, which can be mimicked in animal studies by mechanical irritation of the larynx or by the exposure of a segment of lung to either ozone or to an antigen. These effects also are blocked by anticholinergic drugs, demonstrating that they are also mediated via the vagus nerves (22–25).

It has been difficult, however, to measure the exact role that cholinergic nerves play in the development of asthma because, in humans, direct stimulation of these nerves is not feasible. In addition, complete pharmacologic inhibition of these nerves is difficult to achieve. However, as is discussed below, there is considerable evidence that the cholinergic nerves are important in mediating the features of asthma.

R. W. Costello: Department of Medicine, Division of Pulmonary and Critical Care Medicine, The Johns Hopkins University, Baltimore, Maryland, 21205.

A. D. Fryer: Department of Environmental Health Science, Division of Physiology, The Johns Hopkins School of Hygiene and Public Health, The Johns Hopkins University, Baltimore, Maryland 21205.

INNERVATION OF THE AIRWAYS BY CHOLINERGIC NERVES

In humans the vagus nerve carries preganglionic nerve fibers from the vagal nuclei in the medulla to ganglia in the airways. In the airways these nerves relay with postganglionic nerves that innervate the smooth muscle, the pulmonary vasculature, and the airway glands.

Innervation of the Trachea

The vagus nerves originate in the dorsal nucleus of the medulla (nucleus ambiguus) and travel through the neck to the thoracic cavity (26). The upper trachea is supplied by the recurrent laryngeal and pararecurrent laryngeal branches of the vagus nerve; the lower trachea is supplied by branches of the vagus nerve that relay through the cardiac plexus (27,28).

The recurrent laryngeal and pararecurrent laryngeal nerves lie on the dorsal aspect of the trachea between the border of the trachealis muscle and the cartilaginous rings of the trachea (Fig. 1). Branches from these nerves form a plexus of ganglia that are irregularly spaced along the posterior aspect of the trachealis muscle. In both humans and mammals these ganglia contain between 2 and 20 nerve cell bodies. Postganglionic fibers pass from the cell bodies anteriorly to innervate the trachealis muscle and submucosal glands (29–33).

Innervation of the Bronchi

The hilum is the site of the densest cholinergic innervation. At the hilum, about 30% to 35% of the peribronchial nerves are myelinated; this ratio declines further down the bronchial tree (29,34). At the hilum there are between 10 and 15 large nerve bundles located outside the cartilaginous rings of the intrapulmonary airways. These nerve bundles comprise cholinergic nerves from the cardiac plexus and tracheal fibers of the vagus nerve. There are two main types of cholinergic nerve plexus around the intrapulmonary airways: one of these, a peribronchial plexus closely associated with the airways, may be extrachondral or intrachondral, depending on its position relative to the cartilage (35). The other plexus, the periarterial plexus, is associated with the pulmonary vasculature. Approximately 40% of these periarterial fibers are cholinergic in nature and all are nonmyelinated (27,34).

There is evidence that the myelinated and nonmyelinated nerve fibers serve different functions (36). For example, in the guinea pig, the nonmyelinated nerves comprise afferent, sensory fibers and the fibers that mediate parasympathetic nonadrenergic noncholinergic relaxation (37,38). Some of the myelinated nerves are sensory fibers; however, most of the myelinated nerves relay motor contractile action potentials to the ganglia.

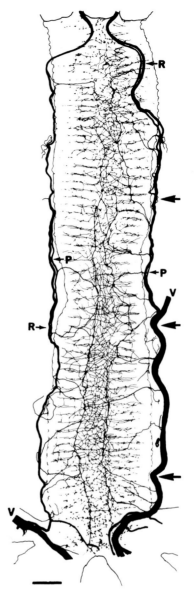

FIG. 1. Tracing of the dorsal aspect of the cholinergic nerves and ganglia of the ferret . The nerves have been stained for acetylcholinesterase activity. The vagus (*V*), the recurrent (*R*), and the pararecurrent (*P*) nerves are shown. Two longitudinal nerve trunks run on the posterior aspect of the trachealis muscle;ganglia are interspersed along these longitudinal nerve trunks. The vagus nerves innervate the superficial muscles, glands, and longitudinal nerve trunks. Branches of the pararecurrent nerve join longitudinal nerve trunks and also innervate the muscle and the glands. (From Baker D, McDonald D, Basbaum C, Mitchell R. The architecture of nerves and ganglia of the ferret trachea as revealed by acetylcholinesterase activity. *J Comp Neurol* 1986;246:513–526.)

In the bronchi, ganglia are found interspersed along the nerve plexus to the level of the small bronchi, as shown in Fig. 2 (30). Most postganglionic efferent cholinergic nerve fibers innervate the bronchial airway smooth muscle and a few fibers innervate the glandular acini (32,33,

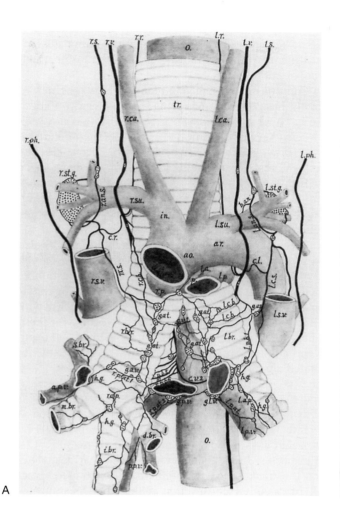
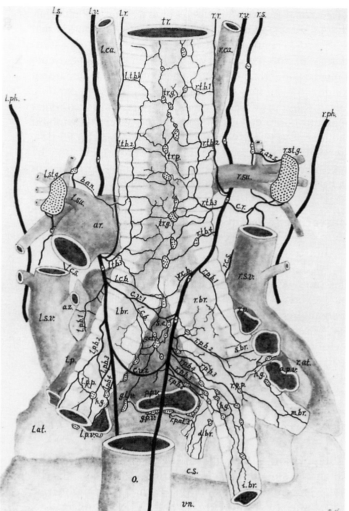

FIG. 2. The anterior (**A**) and posterior aspects (**B**) of the trachea, bronchi, and great vessels of the mouse. The left (*lv*) and right vagus (*rv*) as well as the recurrent (*rr* and *lr*) and superior laryngeal nerves (*rs, ls*) branches, outlined in black, were demonstrated by silver staining. The ganglia are interspersed along the wall of the airway, particularly on the posterior aspect of the trachea and both aspects of the bronchi. The densest neural innervation is at the hilum. (From Honjin R. On the nerve supply of the lung of the mouse with special reference to the structure of the peripheral vegetative and nervous system. *J Comp Neurol* 1956;105:587.)

35,39). Histologic studies cannot demonstrate postganglionic efferent fibers beyond the level of the terminal bronchi (1,35), and functional studies cannot demonstrate an effect of vagal stimulation on the respiratory bronchioles and the alveoli (5).

Cholinergic Ganglia

Neural impulses carried within the parasympathetic nerves pass to the cholinergic ganglia in the airway walls. The preganglionic nerves release ACh, which stimulates nicotinic receptors in the airway ganglia (40). In addition, there are muscarinic receptors in the ganglia (41,42) that may modulate ganglionic transmission (43). The ganglia also receive a significant input of both sympathetic nerves

and nonadrenergic noncholinergic nerves (44,45). In all species studied, the resting electrical properties of the neurons within the cholinergic ganglia are similar (46–49).

Activation of the postganglionic nerves results in nicotinic receptor–mediated, fast excitatory postsynaptic potentials (fEPSPs), as well as muscarinic receptor-mediated slow postsynaptic potentials (sPSPs) (49,50). Cholinergic ganglia in the lungs receive many preganglionic fibers, up to 100 synapses per neuron (51). Cholinergic ganglia contain both tonic and phasic firing neurons that are distinguished based on their response to repeated, subthreshold action potentials. The phasic fibers are more numerous and they accommodate repeated subthreshold tetanic stimulation, whereas tonic neurons repeatedly generate action potentials in response to repeated stimulation (49,52,53).

Electrical field stimulation, which depolarizes postganglionic nerves, induces a smooth muscle contraction that is 56% to 75% greater than that induced by maximal stimulation of the vagus nerve, which involves ganglionic transmission (54,55). These data suggest that the neuronal ganglia play an important role in filtering and integrating stimuli from the CNS. Sympathetic nerves are also found in association with cholinergic ganglia, where they inhibit cholinergic transmission through the ganglia (33,56–58). Sympathetic nerves therefore cause bronchodilation by opposing parasympathetic nerves by removing parasympathetic nerve induced tone (1,13,46,59,60).

Muscarinic Receptors in the Airways

Autoradiographic and *in situ* hybridization studies have demonstrated muscarinic receptors along nerve bundles and within the cholinergic ganglia (41,42). Polymerase chain reaction studies on primary cultures of postganglionic neurons have shown these nerves to possess mRNA for the M_2 receptor (Fryer, unpublished observation). Receptor binding studies and Northern blot analysis have shown that airway smooth muscle contains M_2 and M_3 muscarinic receptors (61,62).

PHYSIOLOGIC FUNCTION OF THE CHOLINERGIC NERVES IN THE AIRWAYS

Stimulation of the vagus nerves causes contraction of the airway smooth muscle, resulting in bronchoconstriction. This bronchoconstricting effect of cholinergic nerves was first shown in 1903 by Dixon and Brodie,

who reported that nicotine caused contraction of isolated cat bronchial smooth muscle (63). In these studies nicotine stimulated receptors in the ganglia to release ACh from postganglionic nerves, which then stimulates M_3 muscarinic receptors on the airway smooth muscle, causing contraction.

In addition to causing contraction, the vagus nerves maintain baseline tone in normal resting airway smooth muscle. This has been shown in animal studies in which the vagus nerves inhibition of, by cooling or cutting, causes bronchodilation (2,4,11,12,64), decreases the functional residual capacity and increases dead space (2,65). In normal humans 80 μg of inhaled ipratropium bromide caused a 40% decrease in airway resistance (Fig. 3) (66), demonstrating that the vagus nerves are important in maintaining airway tone in people.

That the parasympathetic nerves maintain tone is also shown in *in vitro* studies recording neural impulses in the vagi of cats and dogs, which show that even at rest, there is neural activity in the ganglia (8,36,67). The bronchomotor tone varies with respiration and is in phase with the phrenic nerve, indicating a common origin for these two nerves. This common origin allows the rate and depth of ventilation to be coordinated with parasympathetic-mediated airway tone (48).

The degree of bronchoconstriction after electrical stimulation of the vagus nerve is species dependent. At maximal stimulation of the vagus nerves in cats there is a 90% fall in airway conductance (3), in sheep it falls by 44% (2), in dogs by 85% (3), and in rabbits by 30% (12). In all species, bronchoconstriction occurs at a site between the trachea and membranous bronchi. The exact point of maximal constriction within this location ap-

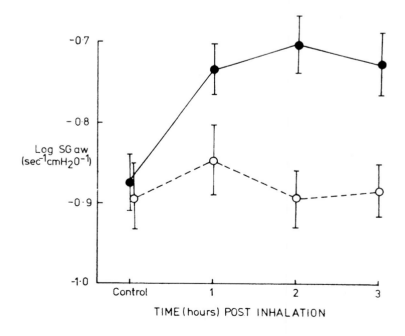

FIG. 3. The change in specific airway conductance at 1, 2, and 3 hr in normal individuals after inhalation of a placebo (*open circles*) and after the inhalation of 80 μg ipratropium bromide (*closed circles*). There is a significant rise in specific airway conductance after inhalation of ipratropium bromide, indicating that there is a baseline vagally induced tone in normal individuals. (From Douglas N, Sudlow M, Flenley D. Effect of an inhaled atropinelike agent on normal airway function. *J Appl Physiol* 1979;46:256–262.)

pears to vary between species and varies slightly between individuals of the same species (66,68,69). In dogs maximal vagally induced bronchoconstriction occurs in bronchi whose internal diameter is between 3 and 8 mm, which is the site of the densest vagal nerve innervation (27,70); however, in some animals bronchoconstriction occurs lower down the airway tree, illustrating that there is a degree of variation within individuals of the same species (69,71,72).

In addition to supplying airway smooth muscle, the parasympathetic nerves also supply the airway mucus glands in humans, sheep, dogs, and ferrets (33,73–75). Mucus production can be induced by mechanical or chemical irritation of the respiratory sensory fibers; atropine can block this effect, indicating that it is reflex-mediated via muscarinic receptors. However, studies using snap-frozen lung tissue have shown that the bronchoconstriction after vagal nerve stimulation is due to smooth muscle contraction rather than to increased mucus secretion in the airways (3). Stimulation of the vagus nerves also causes the bronchial circulation to dilate. Although the resultant increase in blood flow causes the airway wall to become thicker, it does not cause airway narrowing (76).

In summary, the vagus nerves innervate airway smooth muscle, bronchial arteries, and mucus glands. The cholinergic nerves maintain airway tone and cause bronchoconstriction via contraction of the smooth muscle.

Cholinergic Neuromuscular Junction

The airway smooth muscle has been shown to possess both muscarinic M_2 and M_3 receptors. Airway smooth muscle contraction, and thus bronchoconstriction, is mediated by stimulation of M_3 muscarinic receptors by ACh released from cholinergic nerves (77–80). The M_3 receptor is coupled to a pertussis-insensitive G protein that activates phospholipase C, which in turn activates inositol triphosphate production from phosphatidylinositol 4-5 biphosphate (81,82). The role of the M_2 receptors on airway smooth muscle is not well established, although they may limit noradrenaline-induced relaxation of smooth muscle by inhibiting increases in cyclic adenosine monophosphate (cAMP) (83,84). Once released by the parasympathetic nerves, ACh is hydrolyzed into choline and acetate by the enzyme acetylcholinesterase, which is present in the neuromuscular junction.

Control of Acetylcholine Release

The release of ACh from postganglionic nerves is influenced both by neurotransmitters (85–87) and by inflammatory cell products such as prostaglandins (88,89), histamine (90–92), serotonin (93), and leukotrienes (94,95). Many of these agents are found in increased concentrations in the airways of patients with asthma. This is because they are either released by the inflammatory cells recruited into the airways of patients with asthma or, in the case of tachykinins, because there is retarded metabolism due to loss of neutral endopeptidase enzyme activity (96–98). Thus, in patients with asthma, neurotransmitters and inflammatory mediators are likely to have an even greater effect on parasympathetic neural function than in normal individuals.

The most important control over ACh release from postganglionic cholinergic nerves is exerted by ACh itself. ACh acting on neuronal muscarinic M_2 autoreceptors located prejunctionally on postganglionic nerves limits the further release of ACh. Thus, these receptors act as autoreceptors (99–101). The function of the neuronal M_2 autoreceptor can be demonstrated using M_2 receptor antagonists, such as gallamine, which potentiate vagally mediated bronchoconstriction, inducing a 5- to 10-fold increase in bronchoconstriction (Fig. 4). Conversely, the agonist pilocarpine, which stimulates the neuronal receptor, limits, in a dose-dependent manner, the degree of vagally mediated bronchoconstriction to 30% of maximum (see Fig. 7A, below) (102). The presence of an M_2 autoreceptor also has been confirmed by measuring changes in ACh release in the presence of specific M_2 receptor agonists and antagonists using high-performance liquid chromatography (HPLC) (103). Although first described in the airways of guinea pigs, the M_2 receptor has been described in the airways of all species studied including cats (100), dogs (104), rats (105), rabbits (106), horses (107), sheep (108), and humans (103,109,110).

The release of ACh also is influenced by neurotransmitters from both sympathetic and the nonadrenergic noncholinergic nerves (NANC). Tachykinins are polypeptide neurotransmitters released from NANC nerves; they include substance P, neurokinin A, and neurokinin Y. Tachykinins act through three neurokinin receptors termed NK1, NK2, and NK3. In the cholinergic nerves in the lung all the tachykinins facilitate neurotransmission through the ganglia. The subtype of receptor is unknown, but appears to be either an NK1 or NK3 receptor (111, 112). On the postganglionic cholinergic nerves, substance P increases the release of ACh via NK1 receptors (85,87,111,113–116).

Stimulation of the sympathetic nerves inhibits cholinergic neurotransmission. The sympathetic nerves can functionally antagonize the parasympathetic nerves by causing airway smooth muscle relaxation. Because in some species, including humans, the sympathetic nerves do not directly supply the airway smooth muscle, they directly inhibit ACh release from the parasympathetic nerves (1). This has been shown because electrical stimulation of the sympathetic nerves inhibits vagally induced contractions but not exogenous ACh-stimulated contraction (47,117,120). Thus, adrenergic nerves inhibit postganglionic nerves by a prejunctional mechanism. The po-

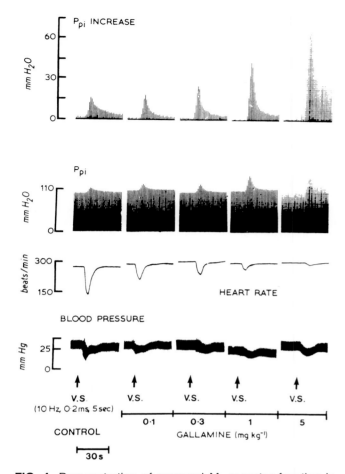

FIG. 4. Demonstration of neuronal M_2 receptor function in anesthetized guinea pigs. Electrical stimulation of both vagus nerves (at *VS, arrows*) causes both bronchoconstriction measured by a rise in pulmonary inflation pressure (*Ppi*) and bradycardia measured as a fall in heart rate. The M_2 receptor antagonist gallamine (0.1–5.0 mg/kg iv) potentiates vagally induced bronchoconstriction and inhibits the fall in heart rate by blocking M_2 receptors in the heart. In contrast, the neuronal M_2 receptor agonist pilocarpine (1–100 µg/kg iv) stimulates the M_2 receptor inhibiting vagally induced bronchoconstriction in a dose-dependent manner (see Fig. 7A). (From Fryer AD, Maclagan J. Muscarinic inhibitory receptors in pulmonary parasympathetic nerves in the guinea-pig. *Br J Pharmacol* 1984;83:973–978.)

tential degree of sympathetic control over the parasympathetic nerves is great because catecholamines can almost completely inhibit vagally induced bronchoconstriction (117). However, the concentration of noradrenaline required to achieve this effect is 10^{-5} M. Although the concentration of noradrenaline in the synapse is unknown, and may reach these levels, circulating catecholamines never reach these levels; thus, their role in the regulation of ACh release is important (118). The prejunctional inhibition is mediated through different adrenergic receptors in different species: In humans and in dogs it is mediated by β_2 receptors, whereas in guinea pigs it is mediated through α_2 receptors (58,119,120).

Thus, ACh release at the neuromuscular junction and the resulting smooth muscle contraction is controlled both by impulses arising in the vagal nerve center of the CNS and by factors produced locally within the airways, including neurotransmitters, prostaglandins, and inflammatory cell products.

CHOLINERGIC MECHANISMS IN ASTHMA

Excessive activity in any part of the vagal nerve reflex can increase efferent cholinergic nerve activity, leading to increased release of ACh and excessive smooth muscle contraction. In theory, therefore, asthmatic symptoms could develop from a) excessive sensory nerve firing that reflexly increases efferent activity, b) increased output from the vagal nucleus in the brain stem, c) increased transmission of efferent nerve signals through cholinergic ganglia, d) increased ACh release from post ganglionic nerves due to a loss of the prejunctional M_2 receptor, or e) loss of function of the acetylcholinesterase enzyme, which metabolizes ACh (Fig. 5). Each of these is discussed in more detail.

Excessive Sensory Nerve Activity

The airway wall contains irritant receptors, nerve endings, that originate in the basement membrane of the lamina propria (Fig. 5, number 1). These irritant sensory nerve fibers can be activated by agents such as cold air, citric acid, and ozone, as well as by inflammatory mediators such as capsaicin, bradykinin, and prostaglandins (60). Together these nerves form the sensory limb of the cholinergic reflex. Activation of these nerves stimulates cholinergic efferent activity because the impulse is orthodromically relayed to the vagal nucleus or is relayed as a local reflex at the cholinergic ganglia (51). In addition, the impulses can be antidromically transmitted directly to the efferent tissue by release of substance P and other tachykinins from these nerves. Airway epithelial cells are damaged in patients by eosinophil products, thus exposing irritant sensory nerve endings (121,122). Similarly, viral infections that damage the epithelium also can expose these irritant receptors (123). The increased activity in these nerves then results in increased efferent cholinergic activity, causing increased smooth muscle tone.

There also is an increase in activity of the afferent nerves after antigen challenge or a viral infection. This increased activity is due to loss of function of the epithelial cell enzyme, neutral endopeptidase, which normally metabolizes sensory nerve tachykinins (97,98,124). Thus, in many types of asthma there is increased activity of the sensory nerves that in turn reflexively increases efferent nerve activity.

The role of the airway sensory nerves in asthma is discussed in Chapter 71.

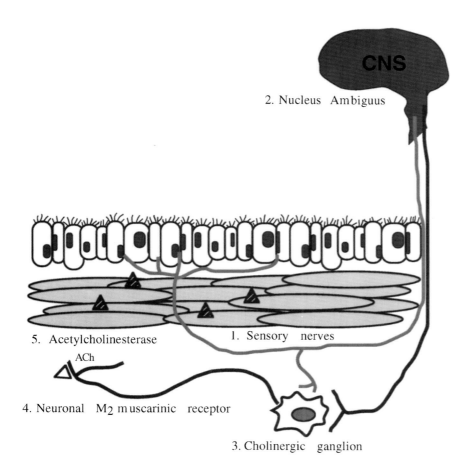

2. Nucleus Ambiguus

5. Acetylcholinesterase

ACh

4. Neuronal M₂ muscarinic receptor

1. Sensory nerves

3. Cholinergic ganglion

FIG. 5. Cholinergic reflex arc. A defect at any of these sites can lead to increased cholinergic nerve activity and increased smooth muscle contractility. The figure shows (*1*) the sensory nerves (*gray line*) relaying to the CNS and antridromically to the airway cholinergic ganglia, (*2*) the nucleus ambiguus, the origin of the vagus nerve (*black line*), and (*3*) the cholinergic ganglia. *4,* The postganglionic cholinergic nerves release ACh (*Ach*) that acts on the neuronal M₂ muscarinic receptors (*white triangle*) and onto M₃ receptors that cause smooth muscle contraction (*black triangles*). *5,* The acetylcholinesterase enzyme hydrolyzes ACh into acetate and choline.

Excessive Vagal Nerve Center Output

There is some indirect evidence that suggests that there may be a generalized increase in neuronal activity and discharge from the vagal nucleus in the CNS of patients with asthma (Fig. 5, number 2). This is demonstrated by the finding of enhanced cardiac reflexes such as an increased Valsalva reflex, more sinus arrhythmia, and a greater diving reflex response in patients with asthma compared with normals (the diving reflex is a bradycardia that occurs after facial immersion in cold water) (125,126). Patients with asthma also have been shown to have a generalized increase in cholinergic activity as demonstrated by greater sweating and pupillary responses compared with normal individuals (127,128). Thus, although there appears to be an increase in central cholinergic activity, these studies identify no definite cause for this increase. Nocturnal asthma and stress-related asthma are two specific forms of asthma in which there is an increase in CNS-mediated vagal nerve activity.

At night, the peak flow rates of normal individuals fall about 8% from daytime values; however, in patients with asthma there may be a 50% fall in peak flow rate (129–131). These changes may be due to an increase in cholinergically mediated airway tone because at the same time there is also a fall in resting heart rate and an in-

crease in the sinus arrhythmia gap, both indicators of increased cardiac vagal activity (132,133). The fall in peak flow rate at night in asthma is also cholinergically mediated because anticholinergic agents can effectively inhibit this fall (134–136). The cause of this nocturnal variation in airway tone is unknown; however, it may reflect a circadian rhythm in the vagal nucleus (137). This is suggested by the finding that shift workers who work at night tend to have a lower peak flow in the daytime when they are sleeping than in the night (137). Alternatively, other factors that demonstrate a circadian rhythm may influence airway tone, such as temperature or plasma epinephrine levels. During the night there is a 0.7°C fall in body temperature. This decrease in temperature may be important because breathing cooled air causes a reflex fall in peak flow rates that may be reversed by breathing warmed humidified air (138). At night, epinephrine levels also fall, which may result in a loss of the modulatory effect of the sympathetic nervous system on cholinergic neurotransmission (139). Inflammatory cell numbers in the airways of patients with asthma also increase at night (140), which may cause an increase in vagally mediated activity, as discussed in further detail below (141).

As discussed above, emotionally stressful events can cause a significant bronchoconstriction in patients with asthma (128,142,143). The mechanisms responsible for suggestion or stress-induced exacerbations are unclear. However, it has been shown that there is increased facial muscle tension in stress, which increases afferent trigeminal nerve activity that in turn leads to bronchoconstriction (144,145).

Increased Transmission Through Cholinergic Ganglia

The cholinergic ganglia in the lungs integrate neural input from peptidenergic and sympathetic nerves as well as from the central nervous system (33,44,45,51,56–58, 60). It is possible, although not yet studied, that in patients with asthma there may be excess transmission through these ganglia because they fail to filter adequately the incoming signals, resulting in increased postganglionic activity (see Fig. 5, number 3).

In animal models, cholinergic neurotransmission through the cholinergic ganglia and, thus the smooth muscle tone, is affected by both neurotransmitters and inflammatory cell products. Tachykinin-containing nerve fibers directly innervate cholinergic ganglia (44,45,146). Tachykinins, in particular substance P, neurokinin B, and neurokinin A, facilitate neurotransmission through cholinergic ganglia in the guinea pig through neurokinin receptors. It is not clear which subtype of receptor is involved, but there is evidence in favor of their being either NK1 or NK3 receptors (111,112). The role of the tachykinins in mediating cholinergic neurotransmission may be important because the enzyme that metabolizes tachykinins, neutral endopeptidase, is impaired in viral infection and in antigen challenge (97,98,124).

Studies on isolated ganglia of antigen sensitized guinea pigs have shown that after application of antigen there is a transient decrease in the resting membrane potential and a transient depolarization of ganglionic neurons (147). In this study the authors also noted that, in the phasic firing neurons, there was a sustained decrease in the accommodative properties of these nerves, that is, there was a greater number of action potentials transmitted by these neurons in response to repeated stimulation (Fig. 6). This change in accommodation lasted for prolonged periods, through the length of the experiments. Such a change could increase the transmission through the ganglia of impulses that may otherwise be filtered out (147,148). Mast cell products applied to the ganglia of nonsensitized guinea pigs mimicked these effects. Prostaglandin D_2 (PGD$_2$) decreased the action potential accommodation properties of phasic firing neurons, whereas histamine application caused a decrease in resting membrane potential through a histamine (H1 type) receptor (149). Mast cells are often found in close association with neuronal tissue in the airways. After antigen challenge, the number of mast cells falls significantly, suggesting that degranulation after antigen challenge could be responsible for these effects (147). Thus, antigen challenge increases the efficiency of the cholinergic ganglia, facilitating neurotransmission and so smooth muscle contraction (150).

Loss of Function of the Neuronal Muscarinic M$_2$ Autoreceptor

As discussed above, there are neuronal muscarinic M$_2$ autoreceptors that limit the release of ACh from postganglionic nerves (Fig. 5, number 4) (99). The function of the M$_2$ muscarinic receptor is assessed, *in vivo*, by studying the effects on vagally induced bronchoconstriction of the M$_2$ receptor agonist, pilocarpine, and antagonist, gallamine. When the receptor is not functional, pilocarpine

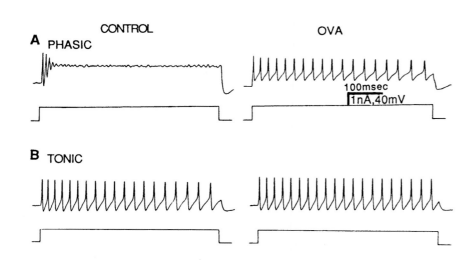

FIG. 6. Antigen challenge causes a loss of accommodation of phasic firing neurons in guinea pig bronchial ganglia. The neurons of antigen-sensitized guinea pigs have been stimulated with suprathreshold current pulses of 500 ms duration before (*left*) and after (*right*) superfusing the ganglia with ovalbumin 10 μg/mL. Normal phasic firing neurons accommodate rapidly to repeated stimulation as demonstrated by the decrease in action potentials with stimulation (*left side,* **A**). Antigen treatment blocks this accommodation in phasic firing neurons. Ovalbumin treatment has relatively little effect on action potential accommodation in tonically firing neurons. (From Myers A, Undem B, Weinrich D. Electrophysiological properties of neurons in guinea pig bronchial parasympathetic ganglia. *Am J Physiol* 1990;259: 403–309.)

no longer attenuates the magnitude of vagally induced bronchoconstriction and gallamine no longer potentiates vagally induced bronchoconstriction. When the neuronal muscarinic receptors are not functional, there is increased ACh release and thus increased smooth muscle contraction in response to vagal nerve firing. Although most studies on loss of neuronal M_2 muscarinic receptor function have been carried out in animals, there is evidence that the neuronal M_2 receptors are dysfunctional in humans with asthma (110,151,152)

In guinea pigs, ozone exposure (2.0 parts per million for 4 hours) causes hyperreactivity, inflammation in the lungs, and loss of neuronal M_2 receptor function, which are all present immediately after exposure. That inflammation, hyperreactivity, and loss of neuronal M_2 receptor function are linked is suggested by their identical time courses of onset and resolution (153). Furthermore, de-

pletion of inflammatory cells, with cyclophosphamide, before ozone exposure, preserved the M_2 receptor function and prevented hyperreactivity after ozone. Thus, inflammatory cells are required for ozone-induced loss of receptor function; however, which inflammatory cell is responsible is still not known (154).

In antigen-challenged guinea pigs, the neuronal M_2 muscarinic receptors are also dysfunctional, as assessed by pilocarpine (Fig. 7). ACh dose-response curves were the same in the control and antigen-challenged animals, indicating that the muscarinic M_3 receptor on airway smooth muscle was functioning normally (155).

In humans with asthma, loss of neuronal M_2 receptor function also has been demonstrated with pilocarpine. Pilocarpine inhibits reflex-mediated bronchoconstriction in nonasthmatic individuals, demonstrating that the receptors are functional in humans. However, pilocarpine has

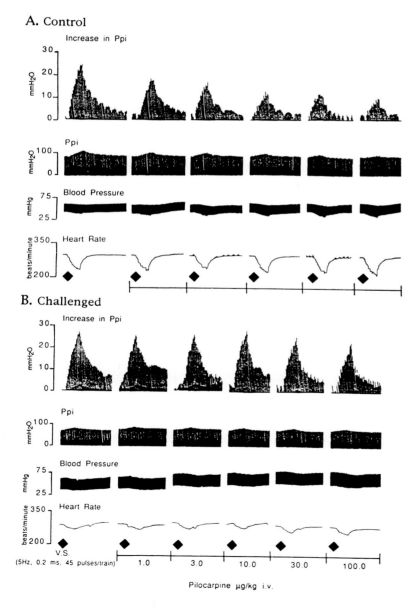

A. Control

B. Challenged

Pilocarpine µg/kg i.v.

FIG. 7. The neuronal M_2 muscarinic receptor is dysfunctional in antigen-challenged guinea pigs. Electrical stimulation of both vagus nerves (at *VS* and *diamonds*) causes both bronchoconstriction measured by a rise in pulmonary inflation pressure (*Ppi*) and bradycardia measured as a fall in heart rate. In control animals the neuronal M_2 receptor agonist pilocarpine (1–100 µg/kg iv) stimulates the M_2 receptor, inhibiting vagally induced bronchoconstriction in a dose-dependent manner (**A**). However, in antigen-challenged animals, pilocarpine does not inhibit vagally induced bronchoconstriction, demonstrating loss of neuronal M_2 receptor function (**B**). (From Fryer A. Muscarinic receptors. In: Busse W, Holgate S, eds. *Asthma and Rhinitis*. Boston: Blackwell Scientific Publications, 1994;691–703.)

no effect on reflex-mediated bronchoconstriction in humans with asthma, demonstrating loss of receptor function (109,151). Thus, the muscarinic M2 receptor is dysfunctional and the M3 receptor is functioning normally in an animal model of allergic asthma and the muscarinic M2 receptor is dysfunctional in patients with asthma.

An influx of inflammatory cells, particularly eosinophils, is seen in the airways of patients with asthma and in animal models of hyperresponsiveness (156; for review see ref. 157). A role for eosinophils in the loss of the M2 receptor function has been suggested by the finding that treatment with either an antibody to the adhesion molecule VLA-4, the ligand recognized by eosinophils and lymphocytes, or an antibody to interleukin 5 before antigen challenge prevented eosinophil influx into the lungs and protected the function of the M2 receptor (158; Fryer, unpublished data). Furthermore, histologic studies have shown that there is an increase in the number of eosinophils around the airway ganglia and nerve fibers of antigen-challenged guinea pigs (Fig. 8) and that there also are eosinophils around the airway nerves of patients dying from an asthma attack (159; Costello, unpublished data).

Eosinophil products may be directly responsible for the loss of receptor function. The eosinophil product major basic protein (MBP) is positively charged, as are many antagonists of M2 muscarinic receptors, such as gallamine (160). In receptor-binding studies, MBP has been shown to be a selective, although allosteric, antagonist for guinea pig and human M2, but not M3, muscarinic receptors (161,162). MBP may have a physiologically relevant role in loss of M2 receptor function because the K_I for MBP at the M2 receptor is 10^{-5} M, which is only minimally higher than the level of MBP found in the sputum of patients with acute asthma (163). Heparin, a polyanionic compound, displaces MBP from the M2 receptor *in vitro* (161). *In vivo*, heparin given intravenously

acutely restores M2 receptor function in antigen-challenged guinea pigs, as shown in Fig. 9 (141). These findings suggest that the M2 receptor becomes dysfunctional after antigen challenge and that positively charged proteins are acting as endogenous antagonists at the M2 receptor. It is likely that eosinophil products, particularly MBP, are responsible for this antagonism of the M2 receptor function.

Viral infection with parainfluenza also causes the M2 receptor to become dysfunctional in guinea pigs and rats (164,165). The mechanism responsible for this loss of receptor function is not known. In studies in which animals were depleted of inflammatory cells by treatment with cyclophosphamide before the infection, the function of the M2 receptor was protected, but only in those animals that had a low viral burden. However, the receptor was still dysfunctional in the absence of inflammatory cells in those animals with a high viral load, suggesting two distinct mechanisms for the loss of receptor function, one independent of inflammatory cells and the other dependent on inflammatory cells (164). It is not clear which inflammatory cell is responsible for the loss of function, although probably it is not a positively charged protein such as MBP because heparin did not restore receptor function as in antigen-challenged guinea pigs (164).

Neuraminidase is an enzyme present on the cell membrane of viruses and in inflammatory cells (166,167). Neuraminidase cleaves sialic acid residues from glycoproteins. The muscarinic M2 receptor has a high concentration of sialic acid residues within the glycoprotein-rich binding domain (168). *In vitro* binding studies have shown that the agonist affinity was significantly decreased by viral infection whereas receptor number and ligand affinity were unchanged (169). Loss of sialic acid from the M2 receptor would decrease ACh binding, resulting in unopposed ACh release.

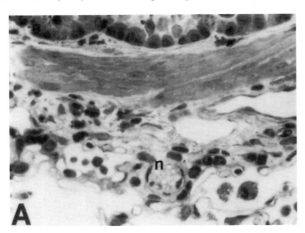 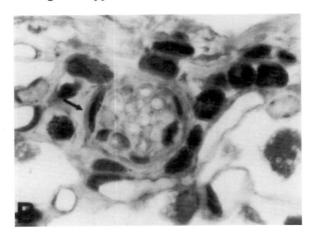

FIG. 8. Eosinophils accumulate around airway nerves of antigen-challenged guinea pigs. One section under low (**A**) and high (**B**) power from the airway wall of an antigen-challenged guinea pig shows a nerve bundle (n). Eosinophils have not only surrounded but have infiltrated the nerve bundles. (From Elbon CL, Jacoby DB, Fryer AD. Pretreatment with an antibody to IL-5 preserves the function of pulmonary M2 muscarinic receptors in antigen challenged guinea-pigs. *Am J Respir Cell Mol Biol* 1995; 12:320–328.)

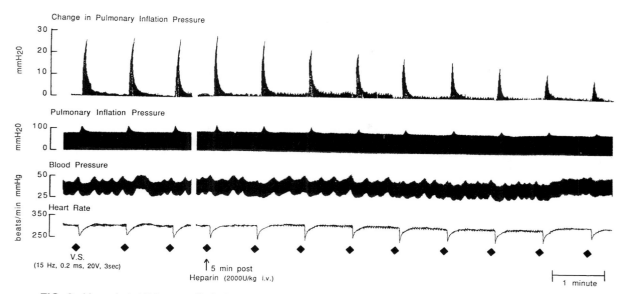

FIG. 9. Heparin inhibits vagally induced bronchoconstriction in sensitized guinea pigs challenged with ovalbumin. Electrical stimulation of both vagus nerves (*Vs* and *black diamonds*) causes bradycardia and bronchoconstriction (measured as a rise in pulmonary inflation pressure). The first three responses to vagal nerve stimulation are in the absence of heparin, whereas the remaining responses are in the presence of heparin (2,000 U/kg iv). Heparin did not alter either baseline inflation pressure or heart rate. (From Fryer AD, Jacoby DB. Function of pulmonary M_2 muscarinic receptors in antigen challenged guinea-pigs is restored by heparin and poly-l-glutamate. *J Clin Invest* 1992;90:2292–2298.)

Although these studies have been performed in the guinea pig, they demonstrate that there is an important interaction between inflammatory cells, in particular eosinophils, and the loss of neuronal M_2 receptor function. Further study is required to see if these interactions also occur in patients with asthma.

Failure to Metabolize Acetylcholine Through Impaired Function of the Acetylcholinesterase Enzyme

ACh released from neuronal cells is hydrolyzed by the enzyme acetylcholinesterase. Loss of acetylcholinesterase activity would be expected to increase ACh levels at the neuromuscular junction and so increase smooth muscle contraction. There is evidence that this enzyme may be less active in the airways of antigen-challenged or ozone-exposed animals (170–173). Mitchell and colleagues showed that ragweed-sensitized and challenged dogs are more responsive to ACh in comparison with nonsensitized littermate controls and that this hyperresponsiveness is blocked by atropine, indicating a cholinergic mechanism (174). These differences were not apparent in the presence of physostigmine, which inhibits acetylcholinesterase activity. The differences between the two groups were not apparent when the muscarinic agonist carbaymlcholine, which is resistant to acetylcholinesterase metabolism, was used in place of ACh (173). These data indicate that the increased responsiveness in sensitized dogs may be due to a loss of acetylcholinesterase activity (175). These data were confirmed in studies of acetylcholinesterase activity using enzyme-linked immunosorbent assay (ELISA) on tracheal and bronchial tissue from ragweed-sensitive dogs (173). The mechanisms responsible for this reduction in the activity of acetylcholinesterase are not known; however, they could not be induced in control tissue by the presence of prostaglandin F_2 (PGF_2-α) or by PGE_2, histamine, serotonin, or leukotriene D_4. An oxidative mechanism may be responsible because there is a loss of acetylcholinesterase activity in the red blood cells after ozone exposure (171).

In support of a loss of acetylcholinesterase activity in the tracheal smooth muscle, ACh levels have been directly measured by high-performance liquid chromatography (HPLC) and are elevated in antigen-challenged mice compared with controls. Whether this increase in ACh reflects a failure of acetylcholinesterase to hydrolyze ACh or reflects increased release of ACh due to the loss of M_2 receptor function still remains to be determined (176,177).

IMPORTANCE OF CHOLINERGIC NERVES IN ASTHMA

The cholinergic nerves probably play an important role in all forms of asthma. When resting airway tone rather than induced bronchoconstriction was measured in asthmatic patients compared with normal controls, there was a significantly higher increase in resting tone in the asthmatics. This increased tone could be completely blocked by ipratropium bromide, demonstrating that it was vagally mediated (14). This study demonstrates that, in asthmatics, there is certainly a degree of increased vagal nerve activity. Much of the controversy surrounding the role of the vagus nerves in asthma probably has arisen because the exact contribution of the vagus nerves to the hyperreactivity characteristic of asthma varies with the type of precipitant, as discussed below (96,178–181). In addition, there are limitations to many of the techniques used to study bronchoconstriction.

In examining the role of cholinergic nerves in patients with asthma, it should be borne in mind that it is not feasible to stimulate the vagus nerves directly or to inhibit the vagus nerves by vagotomy, thus limiting the ability to assess the role of the cholinergic nerves directly. An alternative method of studying vagal nerve function in patients with asthma is to block the vagus nerve pharmacologically. In humans, vagally induced bronchoconstriction may be blocked by muscarinic receptor antagonists, such as atropine, ipratropium bromide, oxitropium bromide, or tiotropium bromide; or by inhibiting ganglionic transmission with hexamethonium. However, there are problems with the interpretation of most studies using anticholinergic drugs.

In many of these studies the effectiveness of the dose of the anticholinergic drug has not been directly tested or has been inferred from cholinergic responses in other organs such as tachycardia or the development of anticholinergic symptoms such as reduced salivation (182,183). In all these studies, innervation of the lung may not be identical to the innervation of another organ, e.g., there are different muscarinic receptor subtypes on the muscle of the heart and lungs (184). Thus, it is not appropriate to draw conclusions based on effects of a drug on an organ other than the lung. Although some studies have tried to demonstrate the effectiveness of anticholinergic agents by showing that they have blocked the bronchoconstriction induced by a cholinergic agent such as ACh, there are problems with this method too (183,185,186,225). In a comparison of vagally induced bronchoconstriction and an equivalent bronchoconstriction induced by inhaled ACh, Holtzmann (187) showed that the dose of inhaled atropine that adequately blocks ACh-induced bronchoconstriction does not inhibit vagally induced bronchoconstriction (Fig. 10). In contrast, intravenous atropine was equally effective in blocking both vagally and ACh-induced bronchoconstriction . Similar results were obtained using cold air–induced bronchoconstriction, which is vagally mediated (188). A much larger dose of inhaled atropine was required to block cold air–induced bronchoconstriction than was required to block methacholine-induced bronchoconstriction (188). Furthermore, in normal humans, when inhaled atropine was compared with intravenous atropine and changes in airway tone measured, intravenous atropine produced a more uniform dilation than did inhaled atropine, which appeared to act centrally only (189,190) Therefore, whereas blockade of exogenous ACh by intravenous atropine indicates adequate blockade of the vagus, the same is not true for inhaled antagonists. Blockade of ACh- or methacholine-induced bronchoconstriction by inhaled atropine or ipratropium bromide does not mean that the vagus nerve also is adequately blocked (187,188). Therefore, many of the pharmacologic studies in humans are difficult to interpret because they have not adequately demonstrated blockade of the vagus nerve.

The different effects of intravenous compared with inhaled atropine or ipratropium bromide on vagally induced bronchoconstriction may be because the distribution of these drugs may be more variable when given by inhalation in comparison with the intravenous route. Inadequate distribution of cholinergic antagonists may be even more likely in persons with asthma, because narrowed airways in these patients may further inhibit adequate distribution (188,190,191).

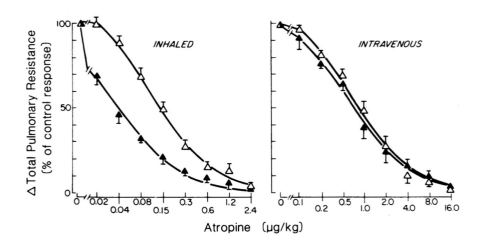

FIG. 10. Electrical stimulation of the vagus nerve (*open triangles*) and inhalation of ACh (*closed triangles*) both cause bronchoconstriction, which was inhibited by atropine. When atropine was given by inhalation doses that inhibited ACh, induced bronchoconstriction did not inhibit vagally induced bronchoconstriction to a similar degree. In contrast, intravenous atropine was equally effective at inhibiting both inhaled ACh and vagally induced bronchoconstriction. Thus, blockade of ACh-induced bronchoconstriction with inhaled atropine does not imply that the vagus nerves also have been blocked. (From Holtzman M, McNamara P, Sheppard D, et al. Intravenous versus inhaled atropine for inhibiting bronchoconstrictor responses in dogs. *J Appl Physiol* 1983;54:134–139.)

There is an additional complication with giving anticholinergic drugs to block vagally induced bronchoconstriction presented by the inhibitory neuronal M_2 muscarinic receptor. At low concentrations, atropine may be preferentially blocking the neuronal M_2 receptor on the pulmonary parasympathetic nerves and so, instead of inhibiting parasympathetic nerve function, atropine may paradoxically increase ACh release, overcoming any postjunctional blockade of the M_3 receptors on airway smooth muscle. Figure 11 illustrates the dose of intravenous atropine required to block vagally induced bronchoconstriction is greater than the dose required to block ACh-induced bronchoconstriction (192). Similar effects of ipratropium bromide on vagally induced bronchoconstriction also have been demonstrated; however, ipratropium actually potentiated vagally induced bronchoconstriction by 100% at doses lower than required to inhibit the postjunctional M_3 receptor (193). Thus, in the presence of a functional M_2 receptor, the effects of any antimuscarinic drug will depend on a balance between blockade of the inhibitory neuronal M_2 receptor and blockade of the postjunctional M_3 receptor.

Although the M_2 receptor is partially dysfunctional in asthma (110,151,152), anticholinergics can still block any remaining functional M_2 receptors, leading to increased ACh release, and thus antagonizing the blockade of the M_3 receptors on the airway smooth muscle. This ability of anticholinergics to potentiate vagally induced bronchoconstriction in the presence of a partially dysfunctional receptor has been demonstrated in animals (155).

A further theoretical consideration in interpreting human studies with anticholinergics is that there are M_1 muscarinic receptors on cholinergic ganglia that facilitate neurotransmission (43). Blockade of these receptors by anticholinergic agents may thus reduce airway tone and release of ACh from postganglionic nerves. Release of ACh from postganglionic nerves by neurotransmitters and inflammatory cell products will, however, remain unaffected. Thus, anticholinergic agents may influence airway tone by blocking M_1 receptors in the ganglia and M_3 receptors on the airway smooth muscle, or enhance ACh release by blocking M_2 receptors on the postganglionic nerves. Therefore, a selective M_3 receptor antagonist is required to define better the role of the cholinergic nerves in asthma. Tiotropium bromide appears to have this property and thus may be a useful candidate for future studies (194).

Finally, in many studies it is assumed that the hyperresponsivness is generalized, i.e., the same degree of hyperresponsivness will be seen with any type of agent, such as methacholine, histamine, and allergen. However, recent studies suggest that this may not be the case, e.g., in comparison with control animals who had similar levels of reactivity to the spasmogens leukotriene LTC_4, histamine, and ACh, ovalbumin-sensitized guinea pigs demonstrated different levels of reactivity to these agents (195,196). This finding may explain the heterogeneous responses to airway challenge. In any one study there are always a few patients with a marked response to the anticholinergics, as well as those with less of a response to the anticholinergics (185,197). When the data are averaged together and compared with data with β-adrenoreceptor agonists, those patients who responded well to the anticholinergics are hidden. The conclusion of these studies appears that the anticholinergics are less effective than the β-agonists, whereas they were in fact very effective for some individuals. Therefore, depending on the individual, the cholinergic nerves may play an important role in that individual's response to an allergen, which accounts for the wide spectrum of effectiveness of anticholinergic agents in patients with asthma.

All studies on the role of the cholinergic nerves in asthma in humans, particularly those using inhaled anticholinergics, must be reinterpreted in light of these confounding problems. In animal models, the role of parasympathetic nerves in the development of airway hyperactivity has been studied using vagal nerve cooling or sectioning. Such techniques overcome the methodologic problems of human studies; the results of these studies have shown a definite role for the cholinergic nerves in the development of airway hyperactivity. Therefore, the role of the cholinergic system in each of the different forms of asthma and equivalent animal models is discussed with an emphasis on the different conclusions of each type. Where applicable, differences between pharmacologic inhibition and direct vagal nerve interruption studies also will be discussed.

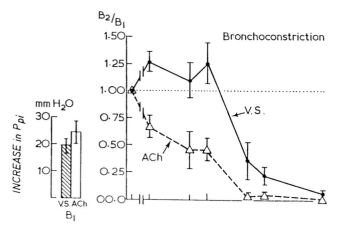

FIG. 11. Atropine (0.1–1.0 µg/kg iv) potentiates vagally induced (*closed circles*) bronchoconstriction because of blockade of the neuronal muscarinic M_2 receptor. Higher doses of atropine (5–100 µg/k iv) inhibits both ACh (*open triangles*) and vagally induced bronchoconstriction due to blockade of the M_3 receptor. Bronchoconstriction is expressed as the ratio of bronchoconstriction before atropine (*B1*) to that after atropine (*B2*). (From Fryer AD, Maclagan J. Pancuronium and gallamine are antagonists for pre- and post-junctional muscarinic receptors in the guinea pig lung. *Naunyn-Schniedeberg's Arch Pharmacol* 1987;335:367–371.)

Nonspecific Hyperresponsivness

A wide array of substances including sulfur dioxide, dust, citric acid, exercise, and cold air can induce bronchoconstriction in patients with asthma. This nonspecific bronchoconstriction is vagally mediated because it can be blocked by giving intravenous atropine, or by giving high, adequate doses of inhaled anticholinergic agents in man (68,182,198–202). In animals, this nonspecific bronchoconstriction can be abolished by cutting the vagus nerves (203,204). That neural reflexes play a role in mediating nonspecific bronchoconstriction is demonstrated by the observations that bronchoconstriction occurs in areas separate from the site of application of the stimulus, e.g., mechanical irritation of the larynx or ozone exposure to one lung can induce a generalized bronchoconstriction that can be blocked with atropine (23,25).

Allergic Asthma

Studies Using Vagal Nerve Interruption in Animal Models

In animals, the vagus nerves play an important role in the development of the increased bronchoconstriction seen in experimental models of allergic hyperresponsiveness. Gold et al. (24), using an allergic dog model, showed that the increase in airway resistance that follows inhaled antigen challenge could be completely inhibited by vagotomy, by intravenous atropine (0.2 mg/kg), or by cooling the vagus nerves. Using a guinea pig model, Koller showed that intravenous atropine (2 mg/kg) partially reversed the increased inspiratory pressures that normally occur after intravenous acute antigen challenge, whereas bilateral vagotomy completely attenuated this response (205). Similar results have been found in many other studies with other species including the dogs (65), guinea pigs (206), rabbits (12), and primates (207,208).

Studies Using Vagal Nerve Interruption in Humans with Asthma

In humans it is far more difficult to block the vagus nerves than in animals. Earlier this century, a few centers performed vagotomy on asthmatic patients who were refractory to other treatments. The results of these studies showed that in many patients there were rapid and sustained improvements in their asthmatic symptoms (209–211). However, these studies were uncontrolled. The improvement could be due to a placebo effect, the removal of the patients from the precipitant, or perhaps better drug compliance while the patients were hospitalized. In many of these procedures the sympathetic and probably also the NANC nerves also were cut, which also may complicate the interpretation of the data. To study the effect of pure vagal nerve blockade, local anesthetics were injected into the base of the skull where the vagus nerve emerges, to paralyze the vagus nerve. There has been no systematic study of the effects of this procedure on pulmonary function; however, asthmatic individuals did show improvement in symptoms, characterized by a decreased ventilatory rate and increased the tidal volume (212,213). Thus, interrupting the vagus nerves appears to improve allergic asthma in humans.

Studies Using Anticholinergic Agents in Animals

Drazen showed that 5 mg/kg of intravenous atropine given before exposure to an antigen completely blocked the acute fall in specific airway conductance after antigen challenge in guinea pigs (214). Using tantalum bronchography, Kessler showed that antigen-induced bronchoconstriction is inhibited by intravenous atropine (0.2 mg/kg) in allergic mongrel dogs (Fig. 12) (215). Similarly, Gold and Dain showed in separate studies that atropine was able to block antigen-induced bronchoconstriction in mongrel dogs allergic to *Ascaric suum*

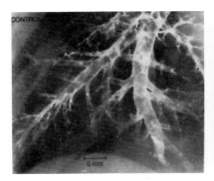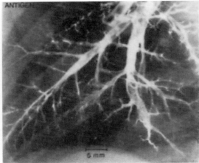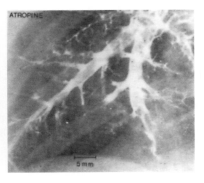

FIG. 12. Atropine inhibits antigen-induced bronchoconstriction in the allergic dog. Tantalum bronchograms of the dog right lower lobe show bronchi between 5 mm and 5 m in diameter. All three images are from the same animal. The figure to the *left* is a baseline image, the *center image* shows antigen-induced bronchoconstriction, and the image to the *right* shows that atropine reverses this bronchoconstriction. (From Kessler G, Austin J, Graf P, Gamsu G, Gold W. Airway constriction in experimental asthma in dogs: tantalum bronchographic studies. *J Appl Physiol* 1975;38:96–99.)

(24,216). It is noteworthy that in all but one of these studies the anticholinergic drugs were given intravenously in relatively high doses (216).

Not all studies have shown that atropine protects against antigen-induced bronchoconstriction. In studies on the Basenji greyhound, pretreatment with atropine had no effect on antigen-induced changes in airway conductance (217). However, the dose of atropine used in this study was quite low (0.2 mg/kg iv) and, although it was effective in attenuating citric acid–induced bronchoconstriction, it may not have been effective in inhibiting the increased vagal output after antigen challenge. In other animal studies, including a primate model, airway hyperresponsivness could not be induced by an acetylcholinesterase inhibitor; neither was there any protective effect of inhaled atropine. It should be noted that in these studies the exact dose of nebulized atropine used is not stated and there was no attempt in these studies to measure the effectiveness of vagal blockade with intravenous atropine (208,218).

Studies Using Anticholinergic Agents in Humans

In human studies, there have been conflicting results concerning the efficacy of inhaled anticholinergic drugs in allergic asthma. Many reports have indicated that anticholinergic agents are effective in inhibiting allergen-induced asthma. Several studies have shown that high doses of intravenous atropine (1.5–2.5 mg) or inhaled atropine (1.5 mg) completely inhibit antigen-induced increases in airway resistance in allergic asthmatics (Fig. 13) (219–221). Similar results also have been obtained using ipratropium bromide and oxitropium bromide (222–224). When given by inhalation, 1.2 mg of atropine attenuated the fall in airway conductance in four of nine patients (225). In this and another similar study, atropine prevented bronchoconstriction induced by low and moderate doses of antigen but not against high doses of antigen in ragweed-sensitive asthmatics (183,225). Unfortunately, neither higher doses of aerosolized atropine nor intravenous atropine were tested in any patients against the high doses of antigen in these studies.

Many studies have concluded that the cholinergic nerves are not important in allergic asthma (183,185, 197,225–227). However, in none of these studies was the effectiveness of vagal nerve blockade adequately tested by using intravenous atropine, because giving an anticholinergic agent by nebulization is inadequate to demonstrate complete vagal nerve blockade, as discussed above. In most of these studies, single, low doses of an inhaled anticholinergic drug were administered without testing higher doses or demonstrating a dose-response effect (183,185,197,225–227). In fact, on close examination of the individual data in these studies, there was a protective effect of anticholinergic agents in some but not all patients after antigen challenge, e.g., 2 of 10 patients (197) re-

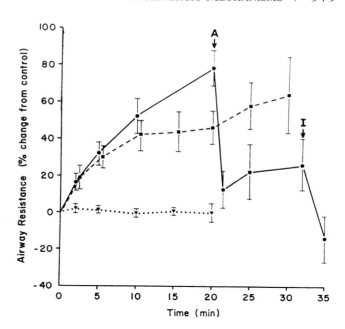

FIG. 13. Intravenous atropine inhibits allergen-induced bronchoconstriction in patients with asthma. The changes in airways resistance are expressed as a percentage of baseline. The effects on airway resistance of a control aerosol (*black triangles*), of an aerosol of antigen (*black circles*) followed by atropine, at A and isoproterenol at I and of 1/10 the original concentration of antigen (*black boxes*), are shown. (From Yu DYC, Galant SP, Gold WM. Inhibition of antigen-induced bronchoconstriction by atropine in asthmatic patients. *J Appl Physiol* 1972;32:823–828.)

sponded, whereas in another study, 5 of 12 responded (185).

Virus-induced Asthma

Viral infections are common precipitants of asthma, in both children, in whom as many as 75% of attacks may be caused by viral infections, and in adults (228–232). A naturally acquired influenza A infection increases sensitivity to carbachol in normal individuals (233). The role of the cholinergic nervous system in the development of the hyperresponsivness seen after viral infection in patients with asthma was suggested by Empey. In this study the authors showed that inhaled atropine protected against histamine-induced hyperresponsivness after a naturally acquired viral infection in normal individuals (234). Also, after a viral infection normal individuals develop bronchoconstriction in response to exercise that can be inhibited by 20 breaths of a 0.2% solution of atropine (235).

After an experimental infection with parainfluenza virus, guinea pigs develop increased smooth muscle responsiveness to histamine. This hyperresponsiveness may be blocked with hexamethonium, indicating that this hyperresponsivness is vagally mediated (236). Vagal nerve stimulation of the trachealis muscle from cats infected with feline herpes virus shows increased contractility in comparison with control noninfected animals. These data suggest that there is an increase in activity in the efferent limb of the cholinergic reflex after a viral infection (237).

Nocturnal Asthma

Asthmatic patients demonstrate a heightened fall in peak flow rates at night compared with nonasthmatic persons. In studies on patients with nocturnal asthma, Morrison showed that high doses of intravenous atropine (30 μg/kg) almost completely attenuated the fall in peak flow at night, indicating that nocturnal asthma is mediated by a cholinergic reflex (136). In other studies, inhaled anticholinergic agents attenuated the fall in peak flow at night in a dose-dependent manner (238). In animal studies, cooling the vagus nerves prevented the expected fall in peak flow during rapid eye movement sleep (239).

Psychogenic Asthma

Emotionally stressful events can cause a significant decrease in pulmonary function (128,142,143; for a review, see ref. 240). In addition, merely inhaling an inert substance believed to cause bronchoconstriction will cause bronchoconstriction (143). Both intravenous atropine and inhaled ipratropium bromide can block suggestion induced and emotionally induced bronchoconstriction, indicating that they are cholinergically mediated (143, 241).

Thus, in all types of asthma in humans and models of airway hyperreactivity in different animal species, bronchial hyperreactivity is abolished by inhibiting the vagus nerves.

CONCLUSIONS

There is good evidence that the cholinergic nervous system plays an important role in all forms of asthma. The mechanisms involved in the increased cholinergic neural activity that result in airway hyperresponsivness are varied. Each limb of the vagal reflex arc may be altered in several different locations by different mechanisms. Recent evidence linking the abnormalities in the cholinergic nerves with inflammatory cell products may be important in understanding some of the mechanisms responsible for increased cholinergic activity in asthma.

ACKNOWLEDGMENTS

The authors wish to thank Kristen Bellmonte and Dr. David Jacoby for their assistance in the preparation of this chapter.

REFERENCES

1. Richardson J. Nerve supply of the lungs. *Am Rev Respir Dis* 1979; 119:785–802.
2. Colebatch H, Halmagyi D. Effect of vagotomy and vagal stimulation on lung mechanics and circulation. *J Appl Physiol* 1963;18:881–887.
3. Olsen C, Colebatch H, Mebel P, Nadel J, Staub N. Motor control of pulmonary airways studied by nerve stimulation. *J Appl Physiol* 1965;20:202–208.
4. Green M, Widdicombe J. The effects of ventilation of dogs with different gas mixtures on airway caliber and lung mechanics. *J Physiol* 1966;186:363–381.
5. Nadel J, Cabezas G, Austin J. *In vivo* roentographic examination of parasympathetic innervation of small airways. Use of powdered tantalanium and fine focal spot X-ray tube. *Invest Radiol* 1971;6:9–17.
6. Brody J, Klempfner G, Staum M, Vidyasagar D, Kuhl D, Waldhausen J. Mucociliary clearance after lung denervation and bronchial transection. *J Appl Physiol* 1972;32:160–164.
7. Gallagher J, Kent P, Passatore M, Phipps R, Richardson P. The composition of tracheal mucous and the nervous control of its secretion in the cat. *Proc R Soc Lond* 1976;192:49–76.
8. Widdicombe J. Regulation of tracheabronchial smooth muscle. *J Physiol* 1966;43:1–37.
9. Paulet G, Le Bars R. Effect of vasomotor innervation on the pulmonary blood mass in dogs. *J Physiol (Paris)* 1969;61:160–161.
10. Phipps R, Richardson P. The nervous and pharmacological control of tracheal mucous secretion in the goose. *J Physiol (Lond)* 1976;258:116–117.
11. Severinghaus J, Stupfel M. Respiratory dead space increase following atropine in man and atropine, vagal or ganglionic blockade and hypothermia in dogs. *J Appl Physiol* 1955;8:81–86.
12. Karczewski W, Widdicombe J. The effect of vagotomy, vagal cooling and efferent vagal stimulation on breathing and lung mechanics of rabbits. *J Physiol (Lond)* 1969;201:259–270.
13. Cabezas G, Kessler G, Yu D. Sympathetic nerve versus parasympathetic nervous regulation of airways in dogs. *J Appl Physiol* 1971;31:651–655.
14. Molfino N, Slutsky A, Julia-Serda G, et al. Assessment of airway tone in asthma. *Am Rev Respir Dis* 1993;148:1238–1243.
15. McKinstry D, Koelle G. Acetylcholine release from cat superior ganglion by carbachol. *J Pharmacol Exp Ther* 1967;157:319–327.
16. Petrie G, Palmer K. Comparison of aerosol ipratropium bromide and salbutamol in chronic bronchitis and asthma. *Br Med J* 1975;1:430–432.
17. Ward M, Fentem P, Roderick Smith W, Davies D. Ipratropium bromide in acute asthma. *Br Med J* 1981;282:598–600.
18. Gross N, Skordoin M. Anticholinergic, antimuscarinic bronchodilators. *Am Rev Respir Dis* 1984;129:856–870.
19. Boushey H. Combination therapy with anticholinergic agents for airflow obstruction. *Postgrad Med J* 1987;63:69–74.
20. Rebuck A, Chapman K, Abboud R, et al. Nebulized anticholinergic and sympathomimetic treatment of asthma and chronic obstructive airways disease in the emergency room. *Am J Med* 1987;82:59–64.
21. Gandevia B. Historical review of parasympatholytic agents in the treatment of respiratory disorders. *Postgrad Med J* 1975;51:13–20.
22. Tomori Z, Widdicombe J. Muscular bronchomotor and cardiovascular reflexes elicited by mechanical stimulation of the respiratory tract. *J Physiol* 1969;200:25–49.
23. Boushey HA, Richardson PS, Widdicombe JG. Reflex effects of laryngeal irritation on the pattern of breathing and total lung resistance. *J Physiol (Lond)* 1972;224:501–513.
24. Gold W, Kessler G, Yu D. Role of the vagus nerves in experimental asthma in allergic dogs. *J Appl Physiol* 1972;33:719–725.
25. Gertner A, Bromberger-Barnea B, Kelly L, Traystman R, Menkes H. Local vagal responses in the lung periphery. *J Appl Physiol* 1984;57:1079–1088.
26. Kalia M. Brainstem localization of vagal preganglionic neurons. *J Auton Nerv Syst* 1981;3:451–481.
27. Richardson J. Nerve supply to the lungs. *Am Rev Respir Dis* 1979; 119:785–802.
28. Baker D, McDonald D, Basbaum C, Mitchell R. The architecture of nerves and ganglia of the ferret trachea as revealed by acetylcholinesterase activity. *J Comp Neurol* 1986;246:513–526.

29. Larsell G, Dow R. The innervation of the human lung. *Am J Anat* 1933;52:125.
30. Honjin R. On the nerve supply of the lung of the mouse with special reference to the structure of the peripheral vegetative and nervous system. *J Comp Neurol* 1956;105:587.
31. Fisher A. The intrinsic innervation of the trachea. *J Anat* 1964;98:117–135.
32. El-Bermani A. Pulmonary nonadrenergic innervation of rat and monkey: a comparative study. *Thorax* 1978;33:167–173.
33. Baker D, Bausbaum C, Herbert D, Mitchell R. Transmission in airway ganglia of ferrets, inhibition by noradrenaline. *Neurosci Lett* 1983;4:139–143.
34. Gaylor J. The intrinsic nervous mechanism of the human lung. *Brain* 1934;57:143.
35. Spencer H, Leof D. The innervation of the human lung. *J Anat* 1964;98:599.
36. Widdicombe J. Action potentials in parasympathetic and sympathetic efferent nerve fibers to the trachea and lungs of dogs and cats. *J Physiol (Lond)* 1966;186:56–88.
37. Canning B, Undem B. Evidence that distinct neural pathways parasympathetic contractions and relaxations of guinea pig trachealis. *J Physiol* 1993;471:25–40.
38. Canning B, Undem B. Relaxation innervation of the guinea pig trachealis: demonstration of capsiacin sensitive and insensitive vagal pathways. *J Physiol* 1993;460:719–739.
39. El-Bermani, Grant M. Acetylcholinesterase positive nerves of the Rhesus monkey bronchial tree. *Thorax* 1975;30:162–166.
40. Coburn R. Peripheral airways ganglia. *Annu Rev Physiol* 1987;49:573–582.
41. van Koppen C, Blankesteijin W, Klassen A, Rodrigues de Miranda J, Beld A, van Ginneken C. Autoradiographic visulization of muscarinic receptors in pulmonary nerves and ganglia. *Neurosci Lett* 1987;83:237–240.
42. van Koppen C, Blankesteijin W, Klassen A, Rodrigues de Miranda J, Beld A, van Ginneken C. Autoradiographic visualization of muscarinic receptors in human bronchi. *J Pharmacol Exp Ther* 1988;244:760–764.
43. Lammer J, Minette P, Mc Cusker M, Barnes P. The role of pirenzipine sensitive (M1) muscarinic receptors in vagally mediated bronchoconstriction in humans. *Am Rev Respir Dis* 1989;139:446–449.
44. Lundberg J, Hokfelt T, Martling C, Saria A, Cuello C. Substance P immunoreactive sensory nerves in the lower respiratory tract of various mammals including man. *Cell Tissue Res* 1984;235:251–261.
45. Kummer W. Ultrastructure of calcitonin gene related peptide immunoreactive nerve fibers in guinea pig peribronchial ganglia. *Reg Peptides* 1992;37:135–142.
46. Baker D, Basbaum C, Herbert D, Mitchell R. Transmission in airway ganglia of ferrets: inhibition by norepinephrine. *Neurosci Lett* 1983;41:139–143.
47. Cameron A, Coburn R. Electrical and anatomic characterization of cells of ferret paratracheal ganglion. *Am J Physiol* 1984;246:450–458.
48. Mitchell R, Herbert D, Baker D, Basbaum C. *In vivo* activity of tracheal parasympathetic ganglion cells innervating tracheal smooth muscle. *Brain Res* 1987;437:157–160.
49. Myers A, Undem B, Weinreich D. Electrophysiological properties of neurons in guinea pig bronchial parasympathetic ganglia. *Am. J Physiol* 1990;259:403–409.
50. Ashe J, Yarosh C. Differential and selective antagonism of the slow-inhibitory postsynaptic potential and slow excitatory postsynaptic potential by gallamine and pirenzipine in the superior cervical ganglia of the rabbit. *Neuropharmacology* 1984;23:1321–1329.
51. Canning B, Undem B. Parasympathetic innervation of airways smooth muscle. In: Raeburn D, Giebycz MA eds. *Airways smooth muscle: structure, innervation and neurotransmission.* Basel: Birkhauser Verlag, 1994;43–78.
52. Granit R, Kernell D, Smith R. Delayed depolarisations and the repetitive response to intracellular stimulation of mammalian motor neurons. *J Physiol* 1963;168:890–910.
53. Knoper S, Bloom J, Halonen M, Kreulen D. Morphological and electrophysiological characteristics of rabbit airways ganglia. *Am Rev Respir Dis* 1988;137:9–13.
54. Undem B, Myers A, Barthlow H, Weinreich D. Vagal innervation of guinea pig bronchial smooth muscle. *J Appl Physiol* 1990;69:1336–1346.
55. Partanen M, Laitinen A, Hervonen A, Toivanen M, Laitinen L. Catecholamine and acetylcholinesterase containing nerves in human lower respiratory tract. *Histochemistry* 1982;76:175–188.
56. Knight D. A light and electron microscopy study of feline intrapulmonary ganglia. *J Anat* 1980;131:413–428.
57. McCaig D. Effects of sympathetic stimulation and applied catecholamine on mechanical and electrical responses to stimulation of the vagus nerve in guinea pig isolated trachea. *Br J Pharmacol* 1987;91:385–394.
58. Rhoden K, Meldrum L, Barnes P. Inhibition of cholinergic neurotransmission in human airways by β2 adrenoreceptors. *J Appl Physiol* 1988;65:700–705.
59. Richardson J. Recent progress in pulmonary innervation. *Am Rev Respir Dis* 1983;128:65–67.
60. Widdicombe J. Innervation of the airways. *Prog Respir Res* 1985;19:8–16.
61. Madison J, Jones C, Tom-Moy M, Brown J. Affinities of pirenzipine for muscarinic cholinergic receptors in membranes isolated from bovine tracheal mucosa and muscle. *Am Rev Respir Dis* 1987;135:719–724.
62. Maeda A, Kubo T, Mishina M, Numa S. Tissue distribution of mRNAs encoding for acetylcholine receptor subtypes. *FEBS Lett* 1988;239:339–342.
63. Dixon WE, Brody TG. Contributions to the physiology of the lungs. Part 1, the bronchial muscles and their innervation and the action of drugs upon them. *J Physiol* 1903;29:97–173.
64. Nadel J, Widdicombe J. Effects of changes in blood gas tensions and carotid sinus pressure on tracheal volume and total lung resistance to airflow. *J Physiol* 1962;163:13–33.
65. Cotton D, Bleecker E, Fischer S, Graf P, Gold W, Nadel J. Rapid, shallow breathing after *Ascaris suum* antigen inhalation: role of vagus nerves. *J Appl Physiol* 1977;42:101–106.
66. Douglas N, Sudlow M, Flenley D. Effect of an inhaled atropinelike agent on normal airway function. *J Appl Physiol* 1979;46:256–262.
67. Widdicombe JG. Action potentials in vagal efferent nerve fibers to the lung of the cat. *Arch Exp Pathol Pharmacol* 1961;241:451.
68. Nadel JA, Salem H, Tamplin B, Tokiwa Y. Mechanism of bronchoconstriction during inhalation of sulfur dioxide. *J Appl Physiol* 1965;20:164–167.
69. Woolcock A, Macklem P, Hogg J, et al. Effect of vagal stimulation on central and peripheral airways in dogs. *J Appl Physiol* 1969;26:806–813.
70. Mann S. The innervation of the mammalian bronchial smooth muscle: the localization of catecholamines and cholinesterases. *Histochem J* 1971;3:319.
71. Macklem P, Woolcock A, Hogg J, Nadel J. Partitioning of pulmonary resistance in the dog. *J Appl Physiol* 1969;26:798–805.
72. Macklem P, Mead J. Resistance of central and peripheral airways measured by a retrograde catheter. *J Appl Physiol* 1977;22:395–401.
73. Bensch K, Gordon G, Miller L. Studies on the bronchial counterpart of the Kulschizy (argentaffin) cell and innervation of bronchial glands. *J Ultrastructural Res* 1965;12:668.
74. Wardell J, Charkin L, Payne B. The canine tracheal pouch. A model for use in respiratory mucous research. *Am Rev Respir Dis* 1970;101:741–754.
75. Mann SP. The innervation of mammalian bronchial smooth muscle. The localisation of catecholamines and cholinesterases. *Histochem J* 1971;3:319–331.
76. Wagner E, Mitzner W. Effects of airway wall thickening on airway reactivity. *Am J Respir Crit Care Med* 1995;151:A132.
77. Roffel A, Elzinga C, Zaagsma J. Muscarinic M3 receptors mediate contraction of human central and peripheral airway smooth muscle. *Pulm Pharm* 1990;3:47–51.
78. Gies J-P, Bertrand C, Vanderheyden P, et al. Characterization of muscarinic receptors in human, guinea pig and rat lung. *J Pharmacol Exp Ther* 1989;250:309–315.
79. Janssen LJ, Daniel EE. Pre- and postjunctional muscarinic receptors in canine bronchi. *Am J Physiol* 1990;259:304–314.
80. Howell R, Laemont K, Gaudette R, Raynor M, Warner A, Noronha-Blob L. Characterization of the airway smooth muscle muscarinic receptor in vivo. *Eur J Pharm* 1991;197:109–112.
81. Wess J, Bonner T, Brann M. Identification of a small intracellular region of the muscarinic M3 receptor as a determinant of selective coupling to PI turnover. *FEBS Lett* 1989;258:133–136.

82. Caulfield M. Muscarinic receptors, characterization, coupling and function. *Pharmacol Therapeut* 1993;58:319–379.

83. Jones C, Madison J, Tom-Moy M, Brown J. Muscarinic cholinergic inhibition of cyclic adenylate cyclase in airway smooth muscle. *Am J Physiol* 1987;253:97–104.

84. Fernandes LB, Fryer AD, Hirshman CA. M_2 muscarinic receptors inhibit isoproterenol-induced relaxation of canine airway smooth muscle. *J Pharmacol Exp Ther* 1992;262:119–126.

85. Tanaka DT, Grunstein MM. Mechanisms of substance P-induced contraction of rabbit airway smooth muscle. *J Appl Physiol* 1984;57:1551–1557.

86. Joos G, Pauwels R, van der Straeten M. The mechanism of tachykinin induced bronchoconstriction . *Am Rev Respir Dis* 1988;137:1038–1044.

87. Colasuardo G, Lander J, Graves J, Larsen GL. Modulation of acetylcholine release in rabbit airways *in vitro*. *Am J Physiol* 1995;268:432–437.

88. Nakanishi H, Yoshida H, Suzuki T. Effects of prostaglandin excitatory transmission in isolated canine tracheal muscle. *Jpn J Pharmacol* 1976;28:883–889.

89. Leff A, Munoz N, Tallet J, Cavigelli M, David A. Augmentation of parasympathetic nerve contraction in tracheal and bronchial airways by PGF2a. *J Appl Physiol* 1985;58:1558–1564.

90. Benson M, Graf P. Bronchial reactivity: interaction between vagal stimulation and inhaled histamine. *J Appl Physiol* 1977;43:643–647.

91. Ichinose M, Barnes P. Inhibitory H3 receptors on cholinergic nerves in human airways. *Eur J Pharmacol* 1989;163:383–386.

92. Ichinose M, Stretton C, Schwartz J, Barnes P. Histamine H3 receptors inhibit cholinergic neurotransmission in guinea pig airways. *Br J Pharmacol* 1989;97:13–15.

93. Takahashi T, Ward J, Tadjkarimi S, Yacoub M, Barnes P, Belvisi M. 5-Hydroxytryptamine facilitates cholinergic bronchoconstriction in human and guinea pig airways. *Am J Respir Crit Care Med* 1995;152:377–380.

94. Tashiro K, Xie Z, Ito Y. Effects of PAF on excitatory neuro transmission in dog airways. *Br J Pharmacol* 1992;107:956–963.

95. Xie Z, Hakoda H, Ito Y. Airway epithelial cells regulate membrane potential, neurotransmission and muscle tone of the dog airway smooth muscle. *J Physiol* 1992;449:619–639.

96. Leff A. Endogenous regulation of bronchomotor tone. *Am Rev Respir Dis* 1988;137:1198–1216.

97. Jacoby DB, Tamaoki J, Borson DB, Nadel JA. Influenza infection causes airway hyperresponsiveness by decreasing enkephalinase. *J Appl Physiol* 1988;64(6):2653–2658.

98. Lilly C, Kobzik L, Hall A, Drazen J. Effects of chronic airway inflammation on the activity and enzymatic inactivation of neuropeptides in guinea pig lungs. *J Clin Invest* 1994;93:2667–2674.

99. Fryer AD, Maclagan J. Muscarinic inhibitory receptors in pulmonary parasympathetic nerves in the guinea-pig. *Br J Pharmacol* 1984;83:973–978.

100. Blaber LC, Fryer AD, Maclagan J. Neuronal muscarinic receptors attenuate vagally-induced contraction of feline bronchial smooth muscle. *Br J Pharmacol* 1985;86:723–28.

101. Faulkner D, Fryer AD, Maclagan J. Post-ganglionic muscarinic receptors in pulmonary parasympathetic nerves in the guinea pig. *Br J Pharmacol* 1986;88:181–188.

102. Fryer AD, Maclagan J. Pancuronium and gallamine are antagonists for pre- and post-junctional muscarinic receptors in the guinea pig lung. *Naunyn-Schmiedeberg's Arch Pharmacol* 1987;335:367–371.

103. Patel H, Barnes P, Takahashi T, Tadjikarimi S, Yacoub M, Belivisi M. Evidence for prejunctional muscarinic autoreceptors in human and guinea pig trachea. *Am J Respir Crit Care Med* 1995;152:872–879.

104. Ito Y, Yoshitomi T. Autoregulation of acetylcholine release from vagus nerves terminals through activation of muscarinic receptors in the dog trachea. *Br J Pharmacol* 1988;93:636–646.

105. Aas P, Maclagan J. Evidence for prejunctional M_2 muscarinic receptors in pulmonary cholinergic nerves of the rat. *Br J Pharmacol* 1990;101:73–76.

106. Eltze M, Galvan M. Involvement of muscarinic M_2 and M_3 , but not M1 and M4 receptors in vagally stimulated contractions of rabbit bronchus/trachea. *Pulm Pharmacol* 1994;7:109–120.

107. Wang Z, Yu M, Robinson N. Prejunctional muscarinic autoreceptors on horse airway cholinergic nerves. *Life Sci* 1995;56:2255–2262.

108. Wagner E, Jacoby D. Airway smooth muscle reflex responses to methocholine. *Am J Respir Crit Care Med* 1996;153;A628.

109. Minette PJ, Lammers JWJ, Dixon CMS, McCusker MT, Barnes PJ. A muscarinic agonist inhibits reflex bronchoconstriction in normal but not asthmatic subjects. *J Appl Physiol* 1989;67:2461–2465.

110. Minette P, Barnes PJ. Prejunctional inhibitory muscarinic receptors on cholinergic nerves in human and guinea-pig airways. *J Appl Physiol* 1988;64:2532–2537.

111. Watson N, Maclagan J, Barnes P. Demonstration of facilitatory role of endogenous tachykinins in cholinergic neurotransmission in guinea pig trachea. *Br J Pharmacol* 1993;107:751–759.

112. Myers A, Undem B. Electrophysiological effects of tachykinins and capsiaicin on guinea-pig bronchial parasympathetic ganglion neurons. *J Physiol* 1993;470:665–679.

113. Sekizawa K, J, Nadel JA, Borson DB. Enkephalinase inhibitor potentiates substance P- and electrically induced contraction in ferret trachea. *J Appl Physiol* 1987;63(4):1401–1405.

114. Joos G, Pauwels R, Van Der Straeton ME. The mechanism of tachykinin-induced bronchoconstriction in the rat. *Am Rev Respir Dis* 1988;137:1038–1044.

115. Black J, Johnson P, Alouan L, Armour C. Neurokinin A with K^+ channel blockade potentiates contraction to electrical stimulation in human bronchus. *Eur J Pharmacol* 1990;180:311–317.

116. Stretton D, Belvisi M, Barnes P. The effect of sensory nerve depletion on cholinergic neurotransmission in guinea pig airways. *J Pharmacol Exp Ther* 1992;260:1073–1080.

117. Vermeire P, Vanhoutte P. Inhibitory effects of catecholamines in isolated canine bronchial smooth muscle. *J Appl Physiol* 1979;46:787–791.

118. Ind P, Causon R, Brown M. Circulating catecholamines in acute asthma. *Br Med J* 1985;290:669–691.

119. Thompson D, Diamond L, Altiere R. Presynaptic alpha receptor modulation of neurally mediated cholinergic excitatory and nonadrenergic noncholinergic inhibitory responses in guinea pig trachea. *J Pharmacol Exp Ther* 1990;254:306–311.

120. Grundstrom N, Anderson R, Wikberg J. Prejunctional alpha 2 adrenoreceptors inhibit contraction of tracheal smooth muscle by inhibiting cholinergic neurotransmission. *Life Sci* 1981;28:2981–2986.

121. Laitinen LA, Heinc M, Laitinen A, Kava T, Haahtela T. Damage of the airway epithelium and bronchial reactivity in patients with asthma. *Am Rev Respir Dis* 1985;131:599–606.

122. Flavahan NA, Slifman NR, Gleich GJ, Vanhoutte PM. Human eosinophil major basic protein causes hyperreactivity of respiratory smooth muscle. Role of the epithelium. *Am Rev Respir Dis* 1988;138:685–688.

123. Walsh JJ, Dietlein LF, Low FN, Burch GE, Mogabgab WJ. Bronchotracheal response in human influenza. *Arch Intern Med* 1960;108 376–388.

124. Dusser DJ, Jacoby DB, Djokic TD, Rubenstein I, Borson DB, Nadel JA. Virus induces airway hyperresponsiveness to tachykinins: role of neutral endopeptidase. *J Appl Physiol* 1989;67:1504–1511.

125. Postma D, Keyzer J, Koeter G, Sluiter H, De Vries K. Influence of the parasympathetic and sympathetic nervous systems on nocturnal bronchial obstructions. *Clin Sci* 1985;69:251–258.

126. Sturani C, Sturani A, Tosi I. Parasympathetic activity assessed by diving reflex and by airway response to methacholine in bronchial asthma and rhinitis. *Respiration* 1985;48:321–328.

127. Kaliner M. The cholinergic nervous system and immediate hypersensitivity. 1. Eccrine seat responses in allergic patients. *J Allergy Clin Immunol* 1976;58:308–315.

128. Smith L, Shelhamer J, Kaliner J. Cholinergic nervous system and immediate hypersensitivity. 2 An analysis of pupillary responses. *J Allergy Clin Immunol* 1980;66:374–378.

129. Gaultier C, Reinberg A, Girard F. Circadian rhythms in lung resistance and dynamic lung compliance. *Respir Physiol* 1977;31:169–182.

130. Connolly C. Diurnal variation in airway obstruction. *Br J Dis Chest* 1979;73:357–366.

131. Hetzel M, Clark T. Comparison of nocturnal and asthmatic circadian rhythms in peak expiatory flow rate. *Thorax* 1980;35:732–738.

132. Baust W, Bohnert B. The regulation of heart rate during sleep. *Exp Brain Res* 1977;7:169–180.

133. Postma D, JJ. K, Koeter G, Sluiter H, de Vries K. Influence of parasympathetic and sympathetic nervous system on nocturnal bronchial obstruction. *Life Sci* 1985;69:251–258.

134. Cox I, Hughes D, Mc Connell K. Ipratropium bromide in patients with nocturnal asthma. *Postgrad Med J* 1984;60:526–528.

135. Coe C, Barnes P. Reduction of nocturnal asthma by an inhaled anticholinergic drug. *Chest* 1986;90:485–488.

136. Morrison J, Pearson S, Dean H. Parasympathetic nervous system in nocturnal asthma. *Br Med J* 1988;296:1427–1429.
137. Martin R, Cicutto L, Ballard R. Factors related to the nocturnal worsening of asthma. *Am Rev Respir Dis* 1990;141:33–38.
138. Chen W, Chai H. Airway cooling and nocturnal asthma. *Chest* 1982;81:675–680.
139. Barnes P, Fitzgerald G, Brown M, Dollery C. Nocturnal asthma and changes in circulating epinephrine, histamine and cortisol. *N Engl J Med* 1980;303:263–267.
140. Kraft M, Djukanovic R, Torvik J, et al. Inflammation in asthma needs to be assessed in distal lung tissue. *Am J Respir Crit Care Med* 1995;150:A386.
141. Fryer AD, Jacoby DB. Function of pulmonary M_2 muscarinic receptors in antigen challenged guinea-pigs is restored by heparin and poly-l-glutamate. *J Clin Invest* 1992;90:2292–2298.
142. Luparello T, Lyons H, Bleeker E, McFadden ER. Influence of suggestion on airway reactivity in asthmatic subjects. *Psychosom Med* 1968;30:536–541.
143. Mc Fadden E, Luparello T, Lyons H, Bleeker E. The mechanism of action of suggestion in the induction of acute asthmatic attacks. *Psychosom Med* 1969;31:134–143.
144. Tomori F, Widdecombe J. Muscular bronchomotor and cardiovascular reflexes elicited by mechanical stimulation of the respiratory tract. *J Physiol* 1969;200:25–49.
145. Schwartz G, Fair P, Salt P, Mandel M, Klerman G. Facial pattering to affective imagery in depressed and non depressed subjects. *Psychosom Med* 1976;38:337–347.
146. Baluk P, Gabella G. Innervation of the guinea pig trachea: a quantitative morphological study of the intrinsic and extrinsic neurons. *J Comp Neurol* 1989;285:117–132.
147. Myers A, Undem B, Weinreich D. Influence of antigen on membrane properties of guinea pig bronchial ganglion neurons. *J Appl Physiol* 1991;71:970–976.
148. Myers A, Undem B. Analysis of preganglionic nerve evoked cholinergic contractions of the guinea pigs bronchus. *J Auton Nerv Syst* 1991; 35:175–184.
149. Myers A, Undem B. Antigen depolarizes guinea pig bronchial parasympathetic ganglion neurons by activation of histamine H1 receptors. *Am J Physiol* 1995;268:879–884.
150. Undem B, Myers A, Weinreich D. Antigen-induced modulation of autonomic and sensory neurons in vitro. *Int Arch Allergy Appl Immunol* 1991;94:319–324.
151. Ayala LE, Ahmed T. Is there loss of a protective muscarinic receptor in asthma? *Chest* 1989;96:1285–1291.
152. Okayama M, Shen T, Midorikawa J, et al. Effect of pilocarpine on propranolol induced bronchoconstriction in asthma. *Am J Respir Crit Care Med* 1994;149:76–80.
153. Schultheis AH, Bassett DJP, Fryer AD. Ozone-induced airway hyperresponsiveness and loss of neuronal M_2 muscarinic receptor function. *J Appl Physiol* 1994;76:1088–1097.
154. Gambone LM, Elbon CL, Fryer AD. Ozone-induced loss of neuronal M_2 muscarinic receptor function is prevented by cyclophosphamide. *J Appl Physiol* 1994;77:1492–1499.
155. Fryer AD, Wills-Karp M. Dysfunction of M_2 muscarinic receptors in pulmonary parasympathetic nerves after antigen challenge in guinea-pigs. *J Appl Physiol* 1991;71:2255–2261.
156. Bousquet J, Chanez P, Lacoste JY, et al. Eosinophilic inflammation in asthma. *N Engl J Med* 1990;323(15):1033–1039.
157. Djukanovic R, Roche W, Wilson J, et al. Mucosal inflammation in asthma. *Am Rev Respir Dis* 1990;142:434–457.
158. Elbon CL, Jacoby DB, Fryer AD. Pretreatment with an antibody to IL-5 preserves the function of pulmonary M_2 muscarinic receptors in antigen challenged guinea-pigs. *Am J Respir Cell Mol Biol* 1995; 12:320–328.
159. Costello RW, Schofield B, Jacoby DB, Fryer AD. Parasympathetic nerves are infiltrated with eosinophils in antigen challenged guinea pigs. *Am J Respir Crit Care Med* 1995;151:A818.
160. Hu J, Wang S, Forray C, El-Fakahany E. Complex allosteric modulation of cardiac muscarinic receptors by protamine: a potential model for putative endogenous ligands. *Mol Pharmacol* 1992;42: 311–324.
161. Jacoby DB, Gleich GJ, Fryer AD. Human eosinophil major basic protein is an endogenous allosteric antagonist at the inhibitory muscarinic M_2 receptor. *J Clin Invest* 1993;91:1314–1318.
162. Jacoby DB, Gleich GJ, Fryer AD. Interaction of human eosinophil

163. Frigas E, Loegering DA, Solley GO, Farrow GM, Gleich GJ. Elevated levels of the eosinophil granule MBP in the sputum of patients with bronchial asthma. *Mayo Clin Proc* 1981;56:345–353.
164. Fryer AD, Jacoby DB. Parainfluenza virus infection damages inhibitory M_2 muscarinic receptors on pulmonary parasympathetic nerves in the guinea pig. *Br J Pharmacol* 1991;102:267–271.
165. Sorkness R, Clough J, Castelman W, Lemanske R. Virus-induced airway obstruction and parasympathetic hyperresponsivness in adult rats. *Am Rev Respir Dis* 1994;150:28–34.
166. Scheid A, Caliguiri LA, Compans RW, Choppin PW. Isolation of paramyxovirus glycoproteins. Association of both hemagglutinating and neuraminidase activities with the larger SV5 glycoprotein. *Virology* 1972;50:640–652.
167. Schauer R. Glycosidases with special reference to the pathophysiological role of sialidases. In: Popper H, Reutter W, Kottgen E, Gudat F, eds. *Structural carbohydrates in the liver.* Boston: MTP Press Ltd, 1983: 83–97.
168. Gies J-P, Landry Y. Sialic acid is selectively involved in the interaction of agonists with M_2 muscarinic acetylcholine receptors. Biochem. *Biophys Res Commun* 1988;150:673–680.
169. Fryer AD, El-Fakahany EE, Jacoby DB. Parainfluenza virus type 1 reduces the affinity of agonists for muscarinic receptors in guinea-pig heart and lung. *Eur J Pharmacol* 1990;181:51–58.
170. Gordon T, Venugopalan CS, Amdur MO, Drazen JM. Ozone induced airway hyperreactivity in the guinea-pig. *J Appl Physiol* 1984;57: 1034–1038.
171. Gordon T, Taylor BF, Amdur MO. Ozone inhibition of tissue cholinesterase in guinea pigs. *Arch Environ Health* 1981;36:284–288.
172. Goldstein BD, Pearson B, Lodi C, Buckley RD, Balchum OJ. The effect of ozone on mouse blood *in vivo. Arch Environ Health* 1968; 16:648–650.
173. Mitchell R, Kelly E, Leff A. Reduced activity of acetylcholinesterase activity in canine tracheal smooth muscle homogenates after active immune sensitization. *Am J Respir Cell Mol Biol* 1991;5:56–62.
174. Mitchell R, Antonissen L, Kroeger E, Stephens N. Effect of atropine on the hyperresponsivness of ragweed sensitized canine tracheal smooth muscle. *J Pharmacol Exp Ther* 1986;236:803–809.
175. Mitchell R, Kroeger E, Kepron W, Stephens N. Local parasympathetic mechanisms for ragweed sensitized canine trachealis hyperresponsivness. *J Pharmacol Exp Ther* 1987;243:907–914.
176. Larsen GL, Fame TM, Renz H, et al. Increased acetylcholine release in tracheas from allergen-exposed IgE-immune mice. *Am J Physiol* 1994;266:263–270.
177. Baker D, Rooney L, Brown J. Inhibiting acetylcholinesterase augments autoregulation of acetylcholine release in murine airways. *Am J Respir Crit Care Med* 1995;151:A112.
178. Widdicombe J. The parasympathetic nervous system in airways disease. *Scand J Respir Dis* 1979;103:38–43.
179. Barnes P. Asthma as an axon reflex. *Lancet* 1986;1:242–245.
180. Shepard D. Physiology of the parasympathetic nervous system of the lung. *Postgrad Med J* 1987;63:21–27.
181. Skoogh B, Ullman A. Modulation of cholinergic neurotransmission to the airways. *Am Rev Respir Dis* 1991;143:1427–1428.
182. O'Byrne P, Thomson N, Morris M, Roberts R, Daniel E, Hargreave F. The protective effect of inhaled chlorpheniramine and atropine on bronchoconstriction stimulated by airway cooling. *Am Rev Respir Dis* 1983;128:611–617.
183. Fish J, Rosenthal R, Summer W, Menkes H, Norman P, Permutt S. The effect of atropine on acute antigen mediated airway constriction in subjects with allergic asthma. *Am Rev Respir Dis* 1977;115:371–379.
184. Hammer R, Giraldo E, Schiavi GB, Monferini E, Ladinsky H. Binding profile of a novel cardioselective muscarine receptor antagonist, AF-DX 116, to membranes of peripheral tissues and brain in the rat. *Life Sci* 1986;38:1653–1662.
185. Cockcroft D, Ruffin R, Hargreave F. Effect of SCH 1000 in allergen induced asthma. *Clin Allergy* 1978;8:361–372.
186. Boulet L, Latimer K, Roberts R, et al. The effect of atropine on allergen induced increases in bronchial responsiveness to histamine. *Am Rev Respir Dis* 1984;130:368–372.
187. Holtzman M, Mc Namara P, Sheppard D, et al. Intravenous versus inhaled atropine for inhibiting bronchoconstrictor responses in dogs. *J Appl Physiol* 1983;54:134–139.
188. Sheppard D, Epstein J, Holtzman M, Boushey H. Effect of route of

delivery of atropine delivery on bronchospasm from cold air and methacholine. *J Appl Physiol* 1983;54:130–133.

189. DeToyer A, Yernault J, Rodenstein D. Effects of vagal blockade on lung mechanics in normal man. *J Appl Physiol* 1979;46:217–226.

190. Weiss W, Mc Fadden E, Ingram R. Parenteral vs. inhaled atropine: density dependence of maximal expiratory flow. *J Appl Physiol* 1982; 53:392–396.

191. Weiner N. Atropine, scopolamine and related antimuscarinic drugs. In: Goodman LS, Gilman A. eds. *The pharmacological basis of therapeutics*, 6th ed. 1980;120–137.

192. Fryer A, Maclagan J. Pancuronium and gallamine are antagonists for pre- and post-junctional muscarinic receptors in the guinea pig lung. *Nauyn-Schmiedeberg's Arch Pharmacol* 1987;335:367–371.

193. Fryer AD, Maclagan J. Ipratropium bromide potentiates bronchoconstriction induced by vagal nerve stimulation in the guinea pig. *Eur J Pharmacol* 1987;139:187–191.

194. Takahashi T, Belivisi M, Patel M, et al. Effect of Ba 679 BR a novel long acting anticholinergic agent on cholinergic neurotransmission in guinea pig and human airways. *Am J Respir Crit Care Med* 1994;150: 1640–1645.

195. Hoshiko K, Morley J. Allergic bronchospasm and airway hyperreactivity in the guinea pig. *Jpn J Pharm* 1993;63:151–157.

196. Morley J. Parasympatholytics in asthma. *Pulm Pharmacol* 1994;7: 159–168.

197. Ruffin R, Cockroft D, Hargreave F. A comparison of the protective effect of fenoterol and SCH 1000 on allergen induced asthma. *J Allergy Clin Immunol* 1978;61:42–47.

198. Simonsson B, Jacobs F, Nadel JA. Role of autonomic nervous system and the cough reflex in the increased responsiveness of airways in patients with obstructive airway disease. *J Clin Invest* 1968;46: 1812–1818.

199. Simonsson B, Skoogh B, Ekstrom-Jodal B. Exercise induced airways constriction. *Thorax* 1972;27:169–180.

200. Gayrard P, Orehek J, Charpin J. The prevention of the bronchoconstrictor effects of deep inspiration or of cigarette smoking in asthmatic patients by SCH 1000. *Postgrad Med J* 1975;51:102.

201. Tinkelman D, Cavanaugh M, Cooper D. Inhibition of exercise induced bronchospasm by atropine. *Am Rev Respir Dis* 1976;114:87–94.

202. Sheppard D, Epstein J, Holtzman MJ, Nadel JA, Boushey HA. Dose-dependent inhibition of cold air-induced bronchoconstriction by atropine. *J Appl Physiol* 1982;53:169–174.

203. Nadel J, Salem H, Tamplin B, Tokiwa Y. Mechanism of bronchoconstriction during inhalation of sulfur dioxide. *J Appl Physiol* 1965;20: 164–167.

204. Widdicombe JG, Kent DC, Nadel JA. Mechanism of bronchoconstriction during inhalation of dust. *J Appl Physiol* 1962;17:613–616.

205. Koller E. Respiratory reflexes during anaphylactic bronchial asthma in guinea pigs. *Experientia* 1969;25:368–369.

206. Mills J, Widdicombe J. Role of the vagus nerves in anaphylaxis and histamine induced bronchoconstriction in guinea pigs. *Br J Pharmacol* 1970;39:724–732.

207. Zimmermann I, Islam M, Lanser K, Ulmer W. Antigen induced airway obstruction and the influence of vagus blockade. *Respiration* 1976;33:95–103.

208. Patterson R, Talbot C, Brandfonbrener M. The use of IgE mediated response as a pharmacological test system: the effect of disodium cromoglycate in respiratory and cutaneous reactions and on the electrocardiograms of rheusus monkeys. *Int Arch Allergy Appl Immunol* 1972;41:592–597.

209. Phillips E, Scott W. The surgical treatment of bronchial asthma. *Arch Surg* 1929;19:1425–1456.

210. Dimitrov-Szokodi D, Husveti A, Balogh G. Lung denervation in the therapy of intractable bronchial asthma. *J Thorac Surg* 1957;33: 166–184.

211. Overholt R. Pulmonary denervation and resection in asthmatic patients. *Ann Allergy* 1959;17:534–545.

212. Guz A, Noble M, Eisele J, Trenchard D. *Breathing: the Hering Breur Centenary Symposium.* London: Churchill, 1970;315–336.

213. Eisele J, Jain S. Circulatory and respiratory changes during unilateral and bilateral cranial nerve 9 and 10 block in two asthmatics. *Clin Sci* 1971;40:117–125.

214. Drazen J, Austen K. Pulmonary response to antigen infusion in the sensitized guinea pig: modification by atropine. *J Appl Physiol* 1975; 39: 916–919.

215. Kessler G, Austin J, Graf P, Gamsu G, Gold W. Airway constriction in experimental asthma in dogs: tantalum bronchographic studies. *J Appl Physiol* 1973;35:703–708.

216. Dain D, Gold W. Mechanical properties of the lungs and experimental asthma in conscious allergic dogs. *J Appl Physiol* 1975;38:96–99.

217. Hirshman C, Downes H. Basenji-Greyhound dog model of asthma: influence of atropine on antigen-induced bronchoconstriction. *J Appl Physiol* 1981;50:761–765.

218. Miller M, Patterson R, Harris K. A comparison of immunological asthma to two types of cholinergic respiratory responses in the rhesus monkey. *J Lab Clin Med* 1976;88:995–1007.

219. Yu DYC, Galant SP, Gold WM. Inhibition of antigen-induced bronchoconstriction by atropine in asthmatic patients. *J Appl Physiol* 1972;32:823–828.

220. Itkin I, Anaand S. The role of atropine as a mediator blocker of induced bronchial obstruction. *J Allergy Clin Immunol* 1970;45: 178–186.

221. Eiser N, Guz A. Effect of atropine on experimentally induced airway obstruction in man. *Bull Eur Physiopath Resp* 1982;18:449–460.

222. Kresten W. Protective effect of metered aerosol SCH 1000 (ipratropium bromide) against bronchoconstriction by allergen inhalation. *Respiration* 1974;31:412–417.

223. Orehek J, Gayard P, Grimaud C, Charpin J. Allergic bronchoconstriction in asthmatics. The effect of a synthetic anticholinergic agent. *Bull Physio Pathol Resp Nancy* 1975;11:193–201.

224. Schultze-Weringhaus G. Anticholinergic versus β-adrenergic therapy in allergic airways obstruction. *Respiration* 1981;41:239–247.

225. Rosenthal R, Norman P, Summer W, Permutt S. Role of the parasympathetic system in antigen induced bronchospasm. *J Appl Physiol* 1977;42:600–606.

226. Cockcroft DW, Ruffin RE, Dolovich J, Hargreave FE. Allergen-induced increases in nonallergic bronchial reactivity. *Clin Allergy* 1977; 7:505–513.

227. Schiller I, Lowell F. The effect of drugs in modifying the response of asthmatic subjects to inhalation of pollen extracts as determined by vital capacity measurements. *Ann Allergy* 1947;5:564–566.

228. Li J, O'Connell E. Viral infections and asthma. *Ann Allergy* 1987; 59:321–328.

229. Patermore P, Johston S, BArdin P. Viruses as the precipitins of asthma symptoms 1 Epidemiology. *Clin Exp Allergy* 1992;22:325–336.

230. Bardin P, Johnston S, Pattermore P. Viruses as precipitants of asthma symptoms. *Clin Exp Allergy* 1992;22:809–822.

231. Sterk P. Virus induced hyperresponsivness in man. *Eur Respir J* 1993; 6:894–902.

232. Johnston S, Pattermore P, Sanderson G, et al. Community study of role of viral infections in exacerbations of asthma in 9–11 year old children. *Br Med J* 1995;310:1225–1229.

233. Hall WJ, Douglas RG, Hyde RW, Roth FK, Cross AS, Speers DM. Pulmonary mechanics after uncomplicated influenza A infection. *Am Rev Respir Dis* 1976;113:141–147.

234. Empey DW, Laitinen LA, Jacobs L, Gold WM, Nadel JA. Mechanisms of bronchial hyperreactivity in normal subjects following upper respiratory tract infection. *Am Rev Respir Dis* 1976;113:523–527.

235. Aquilina AT, Hall WJ, Douglas RG, Utell MJ. Airway reactivity in subjects with viral upper respiratory tract infections: the effects of exercise and cold air. *Am Rev Respir Dis* 1980;122:3–10.

236. Buckner CK, V. S, Dick EC, Busse WW. *In vivo* and *in vitro* studies of the use of the guinea pig as a model for virus-provoked airway hyperreactivity. *Am Rev Respir Dis* 1985;132:305–310.

237. Killingsworth CR, Robinson NE, Adams T, Maes RK, Berney C, Rozanski E. Cholinergic reactivity of tracheal smooth muscle after infection with feline herpesvirus-I. *J Appl Physiol* 1990;69:1953–1960.

238. Catterall J, Rhind G, Shapiro C, Douglas N. Is nocturnal asthma caused by changes in airway cholinergic activity? *Thorax* 1988;43: 720–724.

239. Sullivan C, Zamel N, Kozar L, Murphy E, Phillipson E. Regulation of airway smooth muscle tone in sleeping dogs. *Am Rev Respir Dis* 1979;119:87–99.

240. Isenberg S, Lehrer P, Hochron S. The effects of suggestion and emotional arousal on pulmonary function in asthma: a review and a hypothesis regarding vagal mediation. *Psychosom Med* 1992;54:192–216.

241. Neild JE, Cameron IR. Bronchoconstriction in response to suggestion: Its prevention by an inhaled anticholinergic agent. *Br Med J* 1985;290:674.

242. Fryer AD. *Muscarinic receptors.* In: Busse W, Holgate S, eds. *Asthma and rhinitis.* Boston: Blackwell Scientific Publications, 1994;691–703.

Asthma, edited by P.J. Barnes, M.M. Grunstein,
A.R. Leff, and A.J. Woolcock.
Lippincott–Raven Publishers, Philadelphia © 1997.

■ 69 ■

Role of β₂-Adrenergic Receptors

Tony R. Bai

The English physician Henry Salter reported in 1859 what is probably the first account in modern times of the beneficial effects of activation of beta adrenergic receptors (β-ARs) in asthma when he wrote that "asthma is immediately cured in situations of either sudden alarm or violent fleeting excitements" (1). Endogenous levels of circulating catecholamines, in particular epinephrine, are now known to influence airway caliber in asthmatic patients by stimulating β₂-adrenergic receptors (β₂-ARs) on airway smooth muscle, and possibly cholinergic nerves (2), and it is likely that Salter was describing sympathoadrenal release of epinephrine after emotional triggers. In 1903, epinephrine became available as a pure substance and Bullowa and Kaplan successfully gave injections of it to asthmatic patients (3). Soon after this, epinephrine was shown to relax airway smooth muscle (4). In 1924, ephedrine was introduced to western medicine. Ephedrine, although mainly an α-adrenergic agonist with a β weak agonist activity, and adrenalin (epinephrine) were widely used over the ensuing decades in the treatment of asthma.

In 1941, Konzett isolated isoprenaline (5), the first β-AR agonist devoid of α-adrenergic effect. Ahlquist in 1948 used isoprenaline to partition sympathomimetic effects into α and β based on physiologic responses in isolated tissues (6). β-adrenergic responses are stimulated by isoproterenol more potently than by epinephrine or norepinephrine. Evaluation of a large volume of data generated in the study of β-adrenergic pharmacology enabled Lands in 1967 (7) to suggest a further division of the β-AR response into subtypes termed β₁ and β₂. This distinction was based on the relative potency of the naturally occurring catecholamines, epinephrine and norepinephrine. β₁ responses are equally sensitive to these two agonists; β₂ responses are more potently stimulated by epinephrine. Generally, but not invariably, β₁ responses appear to be initiated by the neurotransmitter norepinephrine in innervated tissues, whereas β₂ responses are triggered by the circulating hormone epinephrine (8). Subsequently, a third subtype, β₃, was defined in nonpulmonary tissues (9).

MOLECULAR BIOLOGY

Before 1974, the β-ARs were known only indirectly as entities that responded to drugs in a selective manner to mediate a variety of physiologically important responses. Then a variety of high-affinity ¹²⁵I-labeled radioligands selective for these receptors were developed that led to experiments using direct binding assays to establish the biochemical properties of the receptor protein. This technique, when coupled with efficient methods for detergent solubilization, formed the basis of receptor purification using affinity chromatography, and when coupled with autoradiographic methods led to the

T.R. Bai: Department of Medicine, University of British Columbia; and Pulmonary Research Laboratory, St. Paul's Hospital, Vancouver, British Columbia V6Z 1Y6 Canada.

cellular localization and quantification of β-ARs on thin sections of tissues (10). Improvements in receptor isolation techniques in the first half of the last decade led to the availability of substantial amounts of purified β₂-AR, which allowed determination of the molecular mass and amino acid sequence of part of the receptor. This new information in turn led to the production of polynucleotide probes and eventually to cloning of the receptor gene and determination of the complete primary sequence of the receptor protein (10–12). The β₂-AR gene lacks introns, maps to chromosome five, and encodes a protein of 413 amino acids, only 54% of which are shared with β₁-AR receptors (12–15). In addition, the gene for the β₃-AR has now been cloned and there is even some pharmacologic evidence for subtypes of β₃-ARs in nonpulmonary tissues (9).

Adrenergic receptors belong to the G protein-linked rhodopsin-related receptor superfamily, one of at least three cell-membrane receptor superfamilies. The current model of this cell membrane-associated receptor indicates seven transmembrane segments connected by alternating intracellular and extracellular loops (Fig. 1). Homology among all the members of the seven transmembrane (serpentine) receptor family is greatest in the transmembrane spanning domains. Genetic and biochemical manipulation of the β₂-AR has identified that the ligand-binding domain is a pocket buried within the membrane bilayer with ago-

nists interacting specifically with amino acids in transmembrane helices III and V (11,12). Antagonists do not bind to the same amino acids.

G proteins are membrane-associated heterotrimers composed of α, β, and γ subunits. Interaction with a receptor causes the release of guanosine diphosphate (GDP) from the α subunit of the G protein, allowing guanosine triphosphate (GTP) to bind and leading to the dissociation of the activated α subunit from the receptor and from the complex. Various G proteins activate or inhibit different effector enzymes, modulating the levels of intracellular second messengers. In the case of the β₂-AR, binding of an agonist to the receptor, coupled to the stimulatory guanine-nucleotide binding protein, G_s, catalyzes the release of GDP from the α subunit of the G protein ($α_s$), allowing the binding of GTP; this in turn leads to the direct activation of adenylyl cyclase by $α_s$-GTP. Adenylyl cyclase catalyzes the formation of the classical second messenger cyclic adenosine monophosphate (cAMP) so that levels of cAMP up to 400-fold over basal can occur within minutes of agonist exposure (10,11,12,16,17). Upon removal of agonist, the activation of adenylyl cyclase persists until the intrinsic GTPase activity of $α_s$ hydrolyzes the bound nucleotide (11,16). Cell relaxation is primarily determined by generation of cAMP and activation of cAMP-dependent kinases, which have several actions including shifting

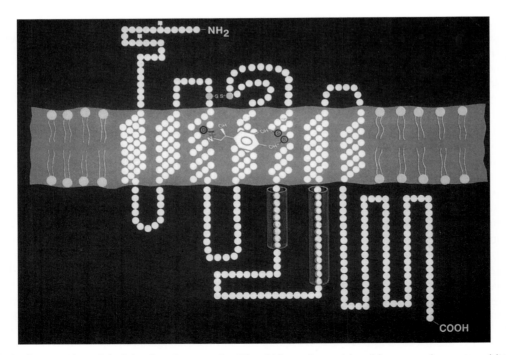

FIG. 1. Structural model of the β₂ adrenoceptor. The 418– amino acid residues are shown as *white circles* with norepinephrine shown in the proposed agonist ligand binding pocket. The cytoplasmic regions predicted to be required for G-protein coupling are shown enclosed in *gray cylinders*. (From Strader CD, Sigal IS, Dixon RA. Mapping the functional domains of the β-adrenergic receptor. *Am J Respir Cell Mol Biol* 1989;1:81–86.)

myosin light-chain kinase to a less active form. However, stimulation of β₂-ARs has other effects. The rise in cAMP leads to calcium re-uptake into the sarcoplasmic reticulum and organelles and calcium extrusion from the cell. cAMP also causes suppression of InsP3 formation. Finally, activation of β₂-ARs stimulates a calcium-activated large conductance potassium channel (Kca) in the cell membrane, which leads to hyperpolarization of the membrane and cell relaxation (18,19). This effect is mediated by a cAMP-dependent protein kinase. Antagonism of β₂-AR-mediated relaxation by muscarinic agonists may occur in part by opposing effects of stimulatory versus inhibitory G proteins at the level of Kca channels (19,20). Such an effect could be clinically important in asthma exacerbations under conditions in which acetylcholine release is increased, because the end result could be decreased efficacy of exogenous β₂ agonists (see below).

The mature messenger ribonucleic acid (mRNA) transcript for the β₂-AR is 2.2 kilobases. Studies of the regulation of gene transcription show that glucocorticoids increase mRNA levels by increasing the rate of gene transcription (21). Isoproterenol decreases mRNA levels by decreasing stability of the mature mRNA (22,23). Gene transcription increases after cytokines such as IL-1β (24). Hamid and co-workers (25) have reported the distribution of β₂-AR mRNA in human lung by *in situ* hybridization and correlated this with receptor autoradiographic distribution. They report striking differences between the density of labeling with the two techniques in different cell types. Pulmonary vascular and airway smooth muscle showed a high intensity of mRNA but only a low density of receptors, and the converse was reported for the alveolar epithelium. These investigators speculate the differences may be due to either a rapid rate of β₂-AR synthesis or high stability of mRNA in the airways; this observation may explain the difficulty in demonstrating desensitization in airway smooth muscle (26,27).

Desensitization

β₂-AR desensitization, i.e., waning of the stimulated response in the face of continuous agonist exposure, can occur by several mechanisms (16). Rapid desensitization is mediated by an alteration in the function of the receptor in that it becomes uncoupled from the stimulatory G protein, Gs. This uncoupling phenomenon involves phosphorylation of the receptor in its terminal intracellular segment by at least two kinases, protein kinase A and a β-AR-associated kinase (BARK), which are activated under different desensitization conditions. The decreased efficiency of coupling of the β₂-AR to Gs leads to decreased adenylyl cyclase activity and hence decreased cAMP levels. Desensitization also can occur by intracellular se-

questration of the receptor complex or by "downregulation." Downregulation refers to agonist-induced decrease in receptor number that occurs upon prolonged exposure to agonists and results in degradation of the receptor, presumably via a lysozymal pathway. Both uncoupling and sequestration (internalization) occur within minutes of exposure to micromolar concentration of β-AR agonists and the process is essentially complete within 30 minutes. Downregulation is evident after only several hours of exposure (16). It has been proposed that the rapid desensitization mechanisms involving phosphorylation of the β-AR (uncoupling) may be operative mainly for non-neural β₂-ARs that respond to circulating concentrations of epinephrine, which are in the nanomolar range (8,10, 28). Downregulation is also mediated by a decrease in mature β₂-AR mRNA caused by a decrease in mRNA stability, rather than a decreased rate of transcription. Phosphorylation, and therefore uncoupling of the β₂-AR, also can be induced by stimulation of adjacent receptors ("receptor cross-talk"), such as cholinergic muscarinic receptors. Activation of muscarinic receptors, in addition to interactions with β₂-ARs via Kca channels (see above), leads to stimulation of phosphatidylinositol pathways with secondary activation of protein kinase C by diacylglycerol, which, in turn, can phosphorylate and uncouple the β-AR (17). Glucorticosteroids have been demonstrated *in vitro* to reverse desensitization (29), and this is probably due to increased β₂-AR gene transcription and possibly increased coupling and may be an important mechanism of action of glucocorticosteroids in the treatment of asthma.

RECEPTOR LOCALIZATION AND PHYSIOLOGIC EFFECTS IN THE HUMAN LUNG

Organ bath and autoradiographic studies have demonstrated that the airway smooth muscle relaxant effect of β-AR agonists is largely via β₂-ARs directly on the muscle surface (28,30,31). This is not unexpected, given that β₁ receptors are found at sites of sympathetic innervation responding to norepinephrine release and there is no direct sympathetic innervation of human airway smooth muscle (28,32). Similarly, the receptors on mucous and serous glands and inflammatory cells are largely of the β₂ type (28,33). β₂ receptors also predominate on epithelium, type I and II pneumocytes, and vascular smooth muscle so that they make up 70% of the β-ARs in the human lung, the other 30% being β₁ on alveolar walls. β₂-ARs are, in general, a low abundance receptor (500–5,000 sites/cell) but the density of receptors increases from the large to small airways and is much greater on alveolar walls than other structures in the lung (31). Although *in vivo* the most obvious and therapeutic effect of β₂-AR stimulation is bronchodilation mediated

TABLE 1. *Physiologic effects of β₂-AR stimulation in human lung*

Airway smooth muscle relaxation
Prejunctional inhibition of acetylcholine release from parasympathetic neurons in airway smooth muscle
Stimulation of mucous and serous cell secretion
Stimulation of chloride ion secretion across the apical membrane of airway epithelial cells
Increase in ciliary beat frequency
Stimulation of surfactant secretion from alveolar type II cells
Inhibition of mediator release from lung mast cells and neutrophils
? reduction in microvascular permeability (animal models)
? increase in bronchial blood flow (animal models)

by airway smooth muscle relaxation, a number of other effects also occur (Table 1).

β-agonists promote secretion from serous cells and, to a lesser extent, mucous cells in mucous glands. Serous cell stimulation produces antibacterial proteins such as lysosomes and lactoferrin. This effect has been demonstrated convincingly *in vitro* only, using human tracheal explants, at relatively high concentrations of β₂-AR (33). However, theoretical calculations of luminal β₂-AR agonist concentrations after inhalation indicate such levels may be achieved *in vivo* (34). Furthermore, β₂-AR agonists increase chloride iron transport through apical membranes of epithelial cells via an increase in cAMP. Sodium follows passively via paracellular channels and water by osmosis. The net effect is to increase periciliary fluid (35,36). The combined effects of stimulation of mucous glands and chloride channels, together with an increase in ciliary beat frequency (35), is to increase mucocilary clearance. Increased clearance has been demonstrated *in vivo* using radiotracer methods, although the clinical relevance of this enhancement in patients with asthma is unknown. Desensitization of β₂-AR function in human epithelial cells has been studied (37). The effect of chronic β₂-AR agonist therapy, as used in asthma, on epithelial cell function is unclear. β₂-AR agonists also stimulate the secretion of surfactant from alveolar type II cells *in vitro*, although the magnitude of the effect is modest (38). In animal models of inflammation, mediators increase microvascular permeability by contracting postcapillary venular endothelial cells so that spaces form between the cells. In such models β₂-AR agonists relax endothelial cells and therefore reduce permeability (39). However, β₂-AR agonists also increase bronchial blood flow by acting as vasodilators of bronchial arterioles (40). The net effect of these two opposing effects on exudation or transudation of fluid into the lumen and wall of inflamed human airways is unclear. A report that the bronchodilatation in acute asthma after nebulized adrenalin is not greater than that after nebulized β-AR agonists that lack an α-adrenergic vasoconstrictor effect suggests that potential alterations

in bronchial blood flow induced by β₂-AR agonists do not adversely affect fluid shifts across the lumen wall (41). Moreover, the lack of additional benefit by adrenalin suggests that the potential decrease in lumen area produced by mucosal bronchodilation induced by β-AR agonists is not an important component of airflow resistance in asthma.

β₂-ARs are present on a variety of inflammatory cells that pass through, or are resident in, the lung. Circulating lymphocytes and neutrophils have low numbers of receptors that appear to be relatively poorly coupled to second messenger pathways in that they are easily downregulated (42). Studies employing circulating lymphocytes or neutrophils as a marker of pulmonary β-AR function, therefore, can be misleading (see below). However, one study showed a strong relationship between β-AR densities in circulating mononuclear leukocytes and in lung tissue obtained at thoracotomy (43). Human alveolar macrophages contain 5,000 β₂-ARs per cell (44). Short-acting β₂-AR agonists do not prevent mediator release from activated human alveolar macrophages (45), but high concentrations of long-acting β₂-AR agonists such as salmeterol may do so (46). There is some evidence that β₂-AR agonists reduce the release of histamine from mast cells and that this is part of their mechanism of action in abating the early response to allergic bronchial challenge, in addition to an action as functional antagonists of the airway smooth muscle contraction induced by release of mediators (28,47). β₂-AR agonists also may inhibit mediator release from basophils (28). Human neutrophils possess 900 to 1,800 β₂-ARs per intact cell and mediator release is inhibited in a dose-dependent manner by isoproterenol (48). In contrast, mediator release from the human eosinophil, although possessing a greater density and affinity of β₂-ARs (5,000 sites per cell), is not inhibited by isoproterenol (49). Both alveolar macrophages and eosinophils are thought to be important effector cells in the pathogenesis of asthma; the lack of influence of β₂-AR agonists on these cell types may explain in part the poor efficacy of these agents as monotherapy in asthma (see below).

β-ARs are present in peribronchial parasympathetic ganglia, which receive direct sympathetic innervation (28), and β₂-ARs also are present on cholinergic nerve terminals in airway smooth muscle and act here to inhibit acetylcholine release (prejunctional inhibition), thereby reducing the cholinergic component of bronchoconstriction (50,51). It is possible that propranolol induces asthma attacks not only by reducing the tonic effect of epinephrine on airway smooth muscle in maintaining airway patency, but also by blocking the effect of epinephrine on cholinergic nerve terminals, leading to the exuberant release of acetylcholine. In support of this hypothesis, cholinergic antagonists have been shown to reverse partially propranolol-induced bronchoconstriction (52).

RECEPTOR EXPRESSION AND FUNCTION IN ASTHMA

The notion that a defective β-AR system or imbalance between α- and β-ARs might be a primary causal abnormality in asthma was first proposed by Szentivanyi in 1968 (53). Currently, however, there is little evidence to suggest that alterations in the properties of β_2-ARs are of critical importance in causality, but considerable evidence that dysfunction may contribute to severity. The usual effectiveness of β_2-AR agonists in the treatment of stable asthma is one obvious argument against a major defect in β-ARs in asthma. There is a large literature in regard to this topic and many of the studies have used circulating leukocyte β_2-AR function as a marker of intrapulmonary β_2-AR function.

Most investigators have focused on β_2-AR function in relation to atopy, allergic inflammation, and/or allergen challenge.

Inflammatory Cells

The published data on β_2-AR function in leukocytes often has been confounded by prior β_2-AR agonist use or elevated circulating catecholamine levels. In other studies, it may be that the abnormalities indicate the atopic state rather than asthma per se. Additionally, leukocyte β-ARs are easily desensitized compared with airway smooth muscle β-ARs (26,27,42). For a detailed review of studies of atopy and asthma using leukocytes, the reader is referred to the review by Insel (42). Illustrative reports include those by Muers (54,55) and Connolly (56). Muers and co-workers observed that bronchial challenge of asthmatics with allergen caused a variety of changes in the β_2-AR-adenylyl cyclase system of lymphocyte membranes, including uncoupling and downregulation as well as nonspecific refractoriness of adenylyl cyclase to nonhormonal stimuli. Connolly and co-workers noted that the density of β-ARs in peripheral blood lymphocytes (β_{max}) and affinity (Kd) were inversely correlated to the severity of asthma, as judged by lung function tests, in drug-naive subjects with normal circulating catecholamine levels. Furthermore, Szefler and co-workers (57) have demonstrated, in asthmatics with nocturnal symptoms, a circadian rhythm in β-AR leukocyte density characterized by a 33% decrease at 4 AM. Leukocyte responses to isoproterenol were impaired in cells sampled at that time, but no such changes were found in individuals free of nocturnal asthma (asthmatic or normal). The usual nocturnal fall in epinephrine occurred 4 hours earlier and these investigators concluded the reduced β_2-AR adrenergic responses were unlikely to be related to epinephrine levels but were more likely due to nocturnal mediator release. However, persons with nocturnal asthma had used more inhaled β_2-AR agonists so that downregulation may have resulted from prior drug treatment.

More studies of adrenergic function in other cell types involved in the inflammatory response of asthma such as airway mucosal mast cells and dendritic cells would be of interest. β_2-AR agonists inhibit antigen-induced release of mast cell mediators from human lung fragments (47) and the infusion of therapeutic concentrations of epinephrine in asthmatics lowers plasma histamine (2,28), suggesting that β_2-ARs on mast cells and related cell types are functional and are capable of influence by circulating β-AR agonists.

Airway Smooth Muscle

Studies of β-ARs using lung tissues from asthmatic patients have yielded conflicting results. Szentivanyi reported that there was decreased ability to synthesize cAMP in response to β-AR stimulation and a decreased number of β-ARs in homogenized membrane preparations of lung tissue from 12 persons with "reversible obstructive lung disease" (including an unknown number of asymptomatic asthmatics [58]). Three groups of investigators have systematically examined β_2-AR-mediated relaxant responses in airway smooth muscle in patients with mild to moderate asthma (59–61). In two of these studies, there was no evidence of abnormal β-AR responsiveness. In the third study, Cerrina and co-workers (59) reported there were decreased relaxant responses in some persons with stable asthma and the decreased response correlated with airway hyperresponsiveness to inhaled histamine *in vivo*, suggesting a possible relationship between β_2-AR function and asthma severity. Ideally, both precontracted airway smooth muscle and muscle under intrinsic tone should be evaluated because subtle defects in the relaxant pathway may not be elicited when tissues are studied only under conditions of intrinsic tone. Van Koppen has provided evidence for this phenomenon in airway smooth muscle from persons with chronic obstructive pulmonary disease (COPD). Without precontraction with methacholine, no differences were seen in β-AR agonist-medicated relaxation. However, after precontraction airways from patients with COPD but not normal airways showed a one-half log-dose decrease in responsiveness (62). Whicker and co-workers (61) studied airway smooth muscle under conditions of intrinsic tone, whereas Svedmyr and co-workers (60) and Cerrina and co-workers (59) precontracted tissues with cholinergic agonists and histamine, respectively.

Although there is conflicting evidence for impairment of β_2-AR-mediated airway smooth muscle relaxation in mild or moderate asthma, the data are more consistent in severe asthma. During exacerbations of asthma, bronchodilation in response to inhaled or parenteral β_2-AR agonists is impaired (63). Although the explanation of this observation is multifactorial, and probably in large part explained by the fact that the obstruction is due to airway wall edema and intraluminal exudate, it is possible that impaired relaxation of smooth muscle plays a part. The results of two systematic studies (30,64,65) have shown impaired β₂-AR-mediated relaxant responses in the airway smooth muscle from patients dying relatively suddenly of asthma outside hospital. In total, 13 asthmatic patients have been compared with 63 control subjects after sudden nonpulmonary deaths. The increase in IC50 (inhibitory concentration of β₂-AR agonist required to relax the muscle by 50% of maximum) in the asthmatic airway tissue ranged from one-half to one log-dose in these studies (Fig. 2). The confounding effect of β₂-AR desensitization by prior drug therapy does not appear to be the only factor involved in the decreased β₂-AR responsiveness, because two persons who died in status asthmaticus and demonstrated decreased *in vitro* β₂-AR responsiveness were not receiving β₂-AR agonist therapy (64). Furthermore, the decreased β₂-AR function noted by Cerrina and co-workers (59) is unlikely to have been due to prior drug treatment, as all β-AR agonists had been withdrawn for 2 weeks before thoracotomy. The relaxant effect of theophylline was unaffected in the studies of fatal asthma cited

above. The cause of this impaired response is unknown, but inflammatory cytokines such as interleukin-1B (IL-1B) induce selective β₂-AR hyporesponsiveness, possibly by activation of phospholipase A₂, which can uncouple the β₂-AR (23,66). Alternatively, other adjacent receptor-mediated events, acting via protein kinase C (cross-talk), may be involved (see below). Furthermore, the β₂-AR-mediated relaxant abnormality may not be unique to asthma, as similar changes have been reported in airway smooth muscle from persons with COPD (62).

To determine if β-AR responsiveness in severe asthma could be explained by a decreased number of cell-surface receptors, we investigated β-AR affinity and density by radioligand binding techniques, including autoradiography, on tissue sections of asthmatic airway smooth muscle adjacent to those tissues shown to be hyporesponsive in the organ bath (67). Comparison was made with normal airways. The results indicated, surprisingly, a threefold increase in the number of receptors compared with that of controls (Figs. 3 and 4). Affinity also was increased in the

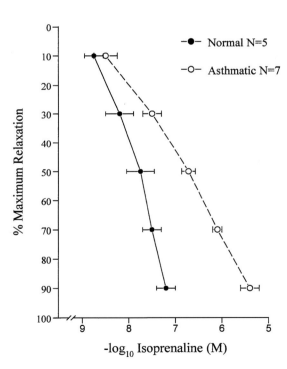

FIG. 2. Mean cumulative isoproterenol concentration-response relationships of tracheal strips (**A**) and bronchial spirals (**B**) from persons with fatal asthma and matched controls. All preparations were precontracted with histamine. Responses were calculated as a percentage of the maximal relaxation produced by isoproterenol in each preparation. Horizontal bars represent standard errors of the mean concentrations producing 10,30,50,70, and 90% of the maximal response. The potency of isoprenaline (IC50) in asthmatics was reduced 5-fold in trachea and 10-fold in bronchi. (From Bai TR. Abnormalities in airway smooth muscle in fatal asthma. *Am Rev Respir Dis* 1990; 141:552–557; and Bai TR. Abnormalities in airway smooth muscle in fatal asthma: a comparison of tracheal and bronchial smooth muscle. *Am Rev Respir Dis* 1991;143:441–443.)

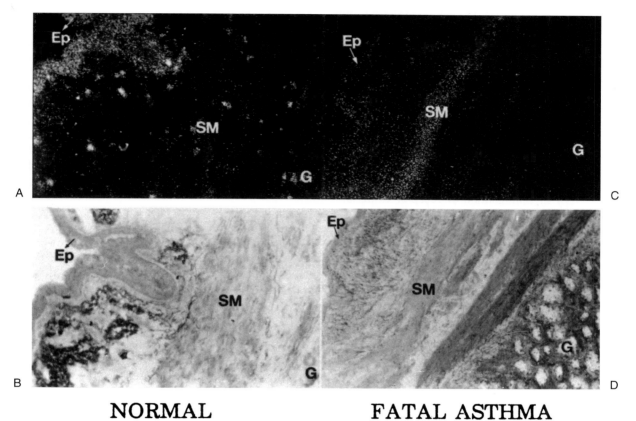

NORMAL   FATAL ASTHMA

FIG. 3. Distribution of β-adrenergic receptors in human nonasthmatic (**A,B**) and asthmatic trachea (**C,D**). B and D are brightfield photomicrographs showing the epithelium (*Ep*), smooth muscle (*SM*), and submucosal glands (*G*) after staining with 1% cresyl fast violet. A and C are darkfield photomicrographs of adjacent sections showing the distribution of autoradiographic grains after incubation with 25pM iodocyanopindolol (*ICYP*). There are fewer grains over the epithelium in asthmatics because of epithelial disruption, but grain density over smooth muscle was increased threefold. (From Bai TR, Mak JC, Barnes PJ. A comparison of beta-adrenergic receptors and *in vitro* relaxant responses to isoproterenol in asthmatic airway smooth muscle. *Am J Respir Cell Mol Biol* 1992;6:647–651.)

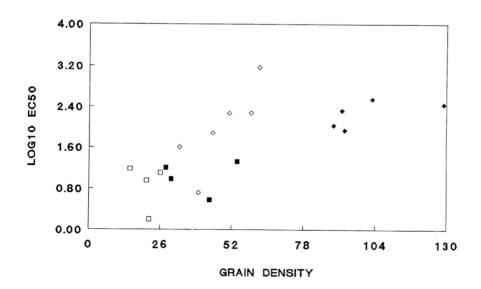

FIG. 4. Relationship between the logarithm of the concentration (*nM*) of isoproterenol to relax airway smooth muscle by 50% of maximum (*EC50*) and β-AR autoradiographic grain density (grains/1,000 μm^2). *Square symbols* are nonasthmatics and *diamonds* are asthmatic. *Shaded symbols* are bronchus and *open symbols* trachea. Surprisingly, the less responsive tissues to isoproterenol possess more β-ARs. (From Bai TR, Mak JC, Barnes PJ. A comparison of beta-adrenergic receptors and *in vitro* relaxant responses to isoproterenol in asthmatic airway smooth muscle. *Am J Respir Cell Mol Biol* 1992;6:647–651.)

asthmatic group. These studies confirm and extend results by Spina and co-workers (68) and Sharma and Jeffery (69) reporting increased and normal numbers of β-ARs, respectively, pointing clearly to a more distal defect in the β2-AR-signaling pathway in asthma. Such studies are clearly in contrast with at least five reports of reduced β-AR density in animal models of allergic airway inflammation (reviewed in refs. 39,68) and the report of Szentivanyi (58). Furthermore, we have recently reported increased levels of β2-AR mRNA in lung homogenates from persons with asthma compared with COPD and normal lungs (71). This increase may be attributable to corticosteroid therapy or upregulation of receptor expression by cytokines and is further evidence that receptor expression is unlikely to be decreased in asthma.

The effects of viral infection on β2-AR function are not well studied, and as viral infection is a common cause of exacerbations in asthma, more research is required. In a murine model, influenza virus caused both an increase in β2-AR number and decreased function (72), similar findings to those reported after severe attacks in human asthma or after *in vitro* treatment of respiratory cells with cytokines.

Association of β2-AR Polymorphisms with Specific Asthma Phenotypes

Six polymorphisms of the β2-AR have been delineated within the coding region (73) (Table 2). The "wild type" β2-AR is the originally cloned receptor and is not necessarily the most prevalent in a given population. The Glu 27 form of the receptor, which is more resistant to agonist-in-

duced downregulation (74), is more common than the wild-type in a UK population (75). The presence of glycine at position 16 of the β2-AR imparts enhanced agonist-promoted downregulation and has been found to be more frequently present in those with severe (73) or nocturnal (76) asthma. The Glu 27 polymorphism is associated with lower airway responsiveness in an asthmatic cohort (75) and has thus been proposed to be of importance in the establishment of the asthmatic phenotype. In support of this proposal, investigators in several of the ongoing large population studies of the genetics of asthma have reported linkage of a microsatellite marker in the region of the β2-AR locus on chromosome 5 to airway responsiveness (77). In addition, Ohe and co-workers (78) have reported linkage of a separate β2-AR restriction fragment length polymorphism (RFLP) to both responses to β2-AR agonists and asthma incidence. This RFLP includes regions outside the coding region, suggesting the possibility of additional abnormalities in the promoter region.

β2-AR Autoantibodies

Several investigators have reported autoantibodies against the β2-AR (79,80). The most recent report indicates immunoglobulin G (IgG) or immunoglobulin M (IgM) antibodies directed against the extracellular or transmembrane regions in 5% of normals and 40% of asthmatics. These antibodies were found to act as either functional antagonists of ligand binding or to promote receptor downregulation, raising the possibility of clinically relevant effects; further studies are needed. Previous negative studies have used nonspecies-specific receptors or both β1 and β2 receptors in assays that might not have allowed for a complete delineation of incidence or functional significance of autoantibodies. The effects of viral infection on the incidence of β2-AR autoantibodies deserves study, as viral infection can induce abnormalities in the β2-AR-adenylyl cyclase system (72).

Influence of β2-AR Agonist Therapy on Receptor Function

β2-AR agonists have been used widely for many years in asthma treatment, but several reports have raised the possibility that regular beta-agonist use is hazardous (81–85). Although some studies have suggested that adverse effects are limited to specific agents such as fenoterol and isoprenaline (81), more recent evidence supports a class effect (84). The possibility that excessive β2-AR agonist use leads to clinically significant desensitization of the β2-AR has been extensively investigated. There is evidence in some studies (86), but not others (87), of a small decrease in peak bronchodilator effect and duration of action in stable mild asthma but not in peak bronchodilator effect in more severe asthmatic patients (88).

TABLE 2. *Polymorphisms and phenotypes of the human β2-AR[a]*

Nucleic acid No.	Nucleic acid	Amino acid No.	Amino acid	Receptor phenotype
46	A	16	Arg	Wild type
	G		Gly	Enhanced downregulation
79	C	27	Gln	Wild type
	G		Glu	Absent downregulation, immature form
491	C	164	Thr	Wild type
	T		Ile	Altered-binding, coupling, sequestration

[a]From Reihaus E, Innis M, MacIntyre N, Liggett SB. Mutations in the gene encoding for the β2-adrenergic receptor in normal and asthmatic subjects. *Am J Respir Cell Biol* 1993; 8:334–339; and Green SA, Turki J, Innis M, Liggett SB. Amino-terminal polymorphisms of the human β2-adrenergic receptor impart distinct agonist-promoted regulatory properties. *Biochemistry* 1994; 33:9414–9419.

Most positive reports have used oral agonists. Duration of bronchodilator action may be a more important variable than peak effect, as suggested by Nelson and co-workers (89), and needs more investigation. Desensitization can be demonstrated more readily in nonasthmatic persons than in asthmatics both in the lung and in nonpulmonary-adrenergic systems (87). Small increases in airway responsiveness have been detected after cessation of regular β₂-AR agonists, which have been hypothesized as being due to desensitization of airway smooth muscle β₂-ARs (82,85). The effect of desensitization of β-ARs on cell types other than smooth muscle requires further study. O'Connor and co-workers (90) have demonstrated the development of tolerance in asthmatics to an indirect bronchoconstrictive stimulus (inhaled cAMP) but not to a direct smooth muscle contractile stimulus (methacholine). This report can be interpreted to indicate the rapid development of desensitization of mast cell β₂-ARs—the probable target cell for cAMP. Other reports imply, after acute or chronic β₂-AR therapy: a) increased airway smooth muscle contractility (91). A theoretical basis does exist for increased smooth muscle contractility after chronic elevation of cAMP (91,92); b) increased IL-4–dependent IgE production (93), which could adversely affect airway inflammation; c) increased contractile vagal reflex activity (94); and d) adverse effects of the inactive (S) enantiomer in racemic mixtures of β₂-AR agonists (94).

CONCLUSIONS

The role of the β₂-AR in both the pathogenesis and treatment of asthma has been a subject of intense speculation and investigation for more than three decades. The physiologic effects of endogenous circulating catecholamines and exogenous adrenergic agonists in the lung are mediated primarily by the β₂-AR, which is present on a variety of cell types. The predominant effect of β₂-AR activation in the human lung is smooth muscle relaxation, although several other effects are well documented. β₂-ARs are present in normal or increased numbers on asthmatic airway smooth muscle. They are uncoupled in severe asthma, leading to functional hyporesponsiveness, probably because of the effects of inflammatory mediators. There is also evidence for dysfunction of β₂-ARs on circulating inflammatory cells after mediator release. There is heterogeneity in the structure of the β₂-AR in the human population; polymorphisms that impart an accelerated agonist-promoted downregulation are overrepresented in steroid-dependent and nocturnal asthma and may contribute to the severity of airway responsiveness. Chronic agonist use also may lead to desensitization of β₂-ARs and contribute to severity. In conclusion, dysfunction of β₂-ARs on airway smooth muscle and inflammatory cells may be of importance in the determination of disease severity in asthma.

ACKNOWLEDGMENTS

The author's research is supported by the B.C. Health Research Foundation, B.C. Lung Association, and Medical Research Council of Canada.

REFERENCES

1. Persson CGA. On the medical history of xanthines and other remedies for asthma: a tribute to H.H. Salter. *Thorax* 1985; 40:881–886.
2. Barnes PJ. Endogenous catecholamines and asthma. *J Allergy Clin Immunol* 1986;77:791–795.
3. Bullowa JGM, Kaplan DM. On the hypodermatic use of adrenalin chloride in the treatment of asthmatic attacks. *Med News* 1903;83:787–790.
4. Kahn RH. Zur physiologie der trachea. *Arch Physiol* 1907;398–426.
5. Konzett H. Neue broncholytische hochwirk same korper der adrenalinreihe. *NS Arch Exp Pathol Pharmakol* 1941;197:27–32.
6. Ahlquist RP. A study of the adrenotrophic receptor. *Am J Physiol* 1948;153:586–599.
7. Lands AM, Arnold A, McAuliffe JP, Ludnena FP, Brown TG. Differentiation of receptor systems activated by sympathomimetic amines. *Nature* 1967;214:597–599.
8. O'Donnell SR, Worstall JC. Functional evidence for differential regulation of beta-adrenoceptor subtypes. *Trends Pharmacol Sci* 1987;8:265–268.
9. Emorine LJ, Marullo S, Briend-Sutren M-M, Patey G, Tate K, Delavier-Klutchko C, Strosberg AD. Molecular characterization of the human 3-adrenergic receptor. *Science* 1989;245:1118–1121.
10. Stadel JM, Lefkowitz RJ. Beta-adrenergic receptors: identification and characterization by radioligand binding studies. In: Perkins JP, ed. *Beta-adrenergic receptors.* Clifton, NJ: Humana Press, 1991;1–41.
11. Fraser CM, Venter JC. Beta-adrenergic receptors—relationship of primary structure, receptor function and regulation. *Am Rev Respir Dis* 1990;141:S22–S30.
12. Strader CD, Sigal IS, Dixon RA. Mapping the functional domains of the β-adrenergic receptor. *Am J Respir Cell Mol Biol* 1989;1:81–86.
13. Chung FZ, Lentes KU, Gocayne J, et al.. Cloning and sequence analysis of the human brain beta-adrenergic receptor. Evolutionary relationship to rodent and avian beta-receptors and porcine muscarinic receptors. *FEBS Lett* 1987;211:200–206.
14. Emorine LJ, Marullo S, Delavier-Klutchko C, Kaveri SV, Durien-Trantmann O, Strosberg AD. Human β₂-adrenergic receptor: expression and promotor characterization. *Proc Natl Acad Sci USA* 1987;84:6995–6999.
15. Kobilca BK, Dixon RA, Frielle T. cDNA for the human β₂-adrenergic receptor: a protein with multiple membrane-spanning domains and encoded by a gene whose chromosomal location is shared with that of the receptor for platelet-derived growth factor. *Proc Natl Acad Sci USA* 1987;84:46–50.
16. Hausdorff WP, Caron MC, Lefkowitz RJ. Turning off the signal: desensitization of β-adrenergic receptor function. *FASEB J* 1990;4:2881–2889.
17. Malbon C. Physiological regulation of transmembrane signalling elements. *Am J Respir Cell Mol Biol* 1989;1:449–450.
18. Jones TR, Charette L, Garcia ML, Kaczorowski GT. Selective inhibition of relaxation of guinea pig trachea by charybdotoxin, a potent Ca²⁺ activated potassium channel inhibitor. *J Pharm Exp Ther* 1990;255:697–706.
19. Kume H, Mikawa K, Takagi K, Kotlikoff MI. Role of G proteins and K_{ca} channels in the muscarinic and β-adrenergic regulation of airway smooth muscle. *Lung Cell Mol Physiol* 1995;12:L221–L229.
20. Watson N, Magnussen H, Rabe KF. Antagonism of β-adrenoceptor-mediated relaxations of human bronchial smooth muscle by carbachol. *Eur J Pharm* 1995;275:307–310.
21. Mak JCW, Nishikawa M, Barnes PJ. Glucocorticosteroids increase 2-adrenergic receptor transcription in human lung. *Am J Physiol* 1995;268:L41–L46
22. Collins S, Caron MG, Lefkowitz RJ. Beta₂-adrenergic receptors in hamster smooth muscle cells are transcriptionally regulated by glucocorticoids. *J Biol Chem* 1988;263:9067–9070.

23. Hadcock JR, Malbon CC. Down-regulation of beta-adrenergic receptors: agonist-induced reduction in receptor mRNA levels. *Proc Natl Acad Sci USA* 1988;85:5021–5025.

24. Anakwe O, Zhou S, Benovic J, Aksoy M, Kelsen SG. Interleukins impair beta-adrenergic receptor adenylate cyclase (β-AR-AC) system function in human airway epithelial cells. *Chest* 1995;107:138S–139S.

25. Hamid QA, Mak JCW, Sheppard MN, Corrin B, Ventor JC, Barnes PJ. Localization of β_2-adrenoceptor messenger RNA in human and rat lung using in situ hybridization: correlation with receptor autoradiography. *Eur J Pharmacol* 1991;206:133–138.

26. Hasegawa M, Townley RG. Difference between lung and spleen susceptibility of β-adrenergic receptors to desensitization by terbutaline. *J Allergy Clin Immunol* 1983;71:230–235.

27. Whicker SD, Black JL. β-receptor desensitization in human airway tissue preparations. *Am Rev Respir Dis* 1991;143(4):A429.

28. Barnes PJ. Neural control of human airways in health and disease. *Am Rev Respir Dis* 1986;134:1289–1314.

29. Davis C, Conolly ME. Tachyphylaxis to β-adrenoceptor agonists in human bronchial smooth muscle: studies *in vitro. Br J Clin Pharmacol* 1980;10:417–421.

30. Bai TR. Abnormalities in airway smooth muscle in fatal asthma. *Am Rev Respir Dis* 1990; 141:552–557.

31. Carstairs JR, Nimmo AJ, Barnes PJ. Autoradiographic visualization of beta-adrenoceptor subtypes in human lung. *Am Rev Respir Dis* 1985; 132:541–547.

32. Daniel EE, Kannan M, Davis C, Posey-Daniel V. Ultrastructural studies of the neuromuscular control of human tracheal and bronchial muscle. *Respir Physiol* 1986;63:109–128.

33. Basbaum CB, Madison JM, Sommerhoff CP, Brown JK, Finkbeiner WE. Receptors on airway gland cells. *Am Rev Respir Dis* 1990;141: S141–S144.

34. Kerrebijn KF. Beta agonists. In: Kaliner MA, Barnes PJ, Persson CGA, eds. *Asthma: its pathology and treatment. Lung biology in health and disease,* vol 49. New York: Marcel Dekker, 1991;526.

35. Wanner A. Autonomic control of mucociliary function. In: Kaliner MA, Barnes PJ, eds. *The airways: neural control in health and disease.* New York: Marcel Dekker, 1988;551–574.

36. Widdicombe JG. Airway mucus. *Eur Respir J* 1989;2:107–115

37. Penn RB, Kelsen SG, Benovic JL. Regulation of β-agonist and prostaglandin E2-mediated adenylyl cyclase activity in human epithelial cells. *Am J Respir Cell Mol Biol* 1994;11:496–505.

38. Mason RJ, Williams MC. Alveolar type II cells. In: Crystal RG, West JB, eds. *The lung: scientific foundations,* vol. 1. New York; Raven Press, 1991;235–246.

39. Persson CGA, Svensjo E. Vascular responses and their suppression: drugs interferring with venular permeability. In: Banta IL, Bray MA, Parnham MJ, eds. *Handbook of inflammation,* vol. 5. Amsterdam: Elsevier, 1985;61–81.

40. Kelly WT, Baile EM, Brancatisano A, Paré PD, Engel LA. The effects of inspiratory resistance, inhaled beta agonist and histamine on canine tracheal blood flow. *Eur Respir J* 1992; 5:1206–1214.

41. Coupe MO, Guly U, Barnes PJ. Comparison of nebulized adrenaline and salbutanol in acute severe asthma. *Clin Sci* 1986;71:80–81.

42. Insel PA. Beta-adrenergic receptors in pathophysiologic states and in clinical medicine. In: Perkins, JP, ed. *The β-adrenergic receptors.* Clifton, NJ: Humana Press, 1991;294–343.

43. Liggett SB, Marker JC, Shah SD, Roper CL, Cryer PE. Direct relationship between mononuclear leukocyte and lung β-adrenergic receptors and apparent reciprocal regulation of extravascular, but not intravascular α and β receptors by the sympathochromaffin system in humans. *J Clin Invest* 1988;82:48–56.

44. Liggett SB. Identification and characterization of a homogeneous population of β_2-adrenergic receptors on human alveolar macrophages. *Am Rev Respir Dis* 1989;139:552–555.

45. Fuller RW, O'Malley G, Baker AJ, MacDermot J. Human alveolar macrophage activation: inhibition by forskolin but not beta adrenoceptor stimulation or phosphodiesterase inhibition. *Pulm Pharmacol* 1988; 1:101–106.

46. Baker AJ, Fuller RW. Comparison of the anti-inflammatory effects of salmeterol on human airway macrophages with those on peripheral monocytes. *Eur Respir J* 1991;4:426s.

47. Butchers PR, Skidmore F, Vardey CJ, Wheeldon AM. Characterization of the receptor mediating the anti-anaphylactic effects of beta-adrenoceptor agonists in human lung tissue *in vitro. Br J Pharmacol* 1980;71: 663–667.

48. Busse WW, Sosman JM. Isoproterenol inhibition of isolated human neutrophil function. *J Allergy Clin Immunol* 1984;73:404–410.

49. Yukawa T, Ukena D, Kroegel C, et al. Betaβ_2-adrenergic recpeotrs on eosinophils—binding and functional studies. *Am Rev Respir Dis* 1990;141:1446–1452.

50. Rhoden KJ, Meldrum LA, Barnes PJ. Inhibition of cholinergic neurotranmission in human airways by β_2 adrenoceptors. *J Appl Physiol* 1988;65:700–705.

51. Bai TR, Lam R, Prasad FYF. Effects of adrenergic agonists and adenosine on cholinergic neurotransmission in human tracheal smooth muscle. *Pulm Pharmacol* 1989;1:193–199.

52. Grieco MH, Pierson. Mechanisms of bronchoconstriction due to β-adrenergic blockage. *J Allergy Clin Immunol* 1971;48:143–152.

53. Szentivanyi A. The beta-adrenergic theory of the atopic abnormality in bronchial asthma. *J Allergy* 1968;42:203–232.

54. Meurs H, Koeter GH, de Vries K, Kauffman HF. The beta-adrenergic system and allergic bronchial asthma: changes in lymphocyte beta-adrenergic receptor number after an allergen induced asthmatic attack. *J Allergy Clin Immunol* 1982;70:272–280.

55. Meurs H, Kaufmann HF, Koeter GH, Timmerman A, de Vries K. Regulation of the beta-receptor-adenylate cyclase system in lymphocytes of allergic patients with asthma: possible role of protein kinase C in allergen-induced nonspecific refractoriness of adenylyl cyclase. *J Allergy Clin Immunol* 1987;80:329–339.

56. Connolly MJ, Crowley JJ, Nielson CP, Charon NB, Vestal RE. Methacholine reactivity and lymphocyte β-receptor density and affinity in drug-naive asthmatics and normals. *Am Rev Respir Dis* 1991;143: A420.

57. Szefler SJ, Ando R, Cicutto LC, Surs W, Hill MR, Martin RJ. Plasma histamine, epinephrine, cortisol, and leukocyte β-adrenergic receptors in nocturnal asthma. *Clin Pharmacol Ther* 1991;49:59–68.

58. Szentivanyi A, Heim O, Schultze P. Changes in adrenoceptor densities in membranes of lung tissue and lymphocytes from patients with atopic disease. *Ann NY Acad Sci* 1979;332:295–298.

59. Cerrina J, Ladurie ML, Labat C, Raffestin B, Bayol A, Brink C. Comparison of human bronchial muscle responses to histamine *in vivo* with histamine and isoproterenol agonists *in vitro. Am Rev Respir Dis* 1986; 134:57–61.

60. Svedmyr NL, Larsson SA, Thiringer GK. Development of resistance in beta-adrenergic receptors of asthmatic patients. *Chest* 1976;69(4): 479–483.

61. Whicker S, Armour C, Black J. Responsiveness of bronchial smooth muscle from asthmatic subjects to contractile and relaxant agonists. *Pulm Pharmacol* 1988;1:25–31.

62. Van Koppen CJ, Miranda JF, Beld AJ, Herwaarden CL, Lammers JJ, Van Ginneken CA. Beta adrenoceptor binding and induced relaxation in airway smooth muscle from patients with chronic airflow obstruction. *Thorax* 1989;44:28–35.

63. Rebuck AS, Read J. Assessment and management of severe asthma. *Am J Med* 1971;51:788–798.

64. Goldie RG, Spina D, Henry PJ, Lulich KM, Paterson JW. *In vitro* responsiveness of human asthmatic bronchus to carbachol, histamine, β-adrenoceptor agonists and theophylline. *Br J Clin Pharmacol* 1986;22: 669–676.

65. Bai TR. Abnormalities in airway smooth muscle in fatal asthma: a comparison of tracheal and bronchial smooth muscle. *Am Rev Respir Dis* 1991;143:441–443.

66. Wills-Karp MJ, Jinot J, Lee J, Hirata F. Interleukin I alters guinea pig tracheal smooth muscle responsiveness to β-adrenergic stimulation. *Eur J Pharmacol* 1990;183(4):A1185.

67. Bai TR, Mak JC, Barnes PJ. A comparison of beta-adrenergic receptors and *in vitro* relaxant responses to isoproterenol in asthmatic airway smooth muscle. *Am J Respir Cell Mol Biol* 1992;6:647–651.

68. Spina D, Rigby PJ, Paterson JW, Goldie RG. Autoradiographic localization of beta-adrenoceptors in asthmatic human lung. *Am Rev Respir Dis* 1989;140:1410–1415.

69. Sharma RK, Jeffery PK. Airway β-adrenoceptor number in cystic fibrosis and asthma. *Clin Sci* 1990;78:409–417.

70. Motojima S, Yukawa T, Fulcade T, Mukino S. Changes in airway responsiveness and β and α_1-adrenergic receptors in the lungs of guinea pigs with experimental asthma. *Allergy* 1989;44:66–69.

71. Bai TR, Zhou D, Aubert J-D, Lizee G, Hayashi S, Bondy GP. Expression of β_2-adrenergic receptor mRNA in peripheral lung in asthma and chronic obstructive pulmonary disease. *Am J Respir Cell Mol Biol* 1993;8:325–333.

72. Henry PJ, Rigby PJ, McKenzie JS, Goldie RG. Effect of respiratory tract viral infection on murine airway beta-adrenoceptor function, distribution and density. *Br J Pharmacol* 1992;104:914–921.

73. Reihsaus E, Innis M, MacIntyre N, Liggett SB. Mutations in the gene encoding for the β_2-adrenergic receptor in normal and asthmatic subjects. *Am J Respir Cell Biol* 1993;8:334–339.

74. Green SA, Turki J, Innis M, Liggett SB. Amino-terminal polymorphisms of the human β_2-adrenergic receptor impart distinct agonist-promoted regulatory properties. *Biochemistry* 1994;33:9414–9419.

75. Hall IP, Wheatley A, Wilding P, Liggett SB. Association of Glu 27 β_2-adrenoceptor polymorphism with lower airway reactivity in asthmatic subjects. *Lancet* 1995;345:1213–1214.

76. Turki J, Pak J, Green SA, Martin RJ, Liggett SB. Genetic polymorphisms of the β_2-adrenergic receptor in nocturnal and nonnocturnal asthma. *J Clin Invest* 1995;95:1635–1641.

77. Postma D, Levitt RC, Panhuysen CIM, Koeter GH, Meyers DA, Blecker ER. Gene mapping studies on atopy, bronchial hyperresponsiveness and asthma. *Eur Respir J* 1994;7:423s.

78. Ohe M, Munakata M, Hizawa N, et al. Beta-2 adrenergic receptor gene restriction fragment length polymorphism and bronchial asthma. *Thorax* 1995;50:353–359.

79. Turki J, Liggett SB. Receptor-specific functional properties of β_2-adrenergic receptor autoantibodies in asthma. *Am J Respir Cell Mol Biol* 1995;12:531–539.

80. Wallukat S, Wollenberger A. Autoantibodies to beta 2-adrenergic receptors with antiadrenergic activity from patients with allergic asthma. *J Allergy Clin Immnuol* 1991;88:581–587.

81. Grainger J, Woodman K, Pearce N, Crane K, Burgess C, Keane A, Beasley R. Prescribed fenoterol and death from asthma in New Zealand 1981–1987: a further case-control study. *Thorax* 1991;46:105–111.

82. Kraan J, Koeter GH, Vandermark TW, et al. Changes in bronchial hyperreactivity induced by four weeks of treatment with anti-asthmatic drugs in patients with allergic asthma: a comparison between budesonide and terbutaline. *J Allergy Clin Immunol* 1985;76:628–636.

83. Sears MR, Taylor DR, Print CG. Regular inhaled beta-agonist treatment in bronchial asthma. *Lancet* 1990;336:1391–1396.

84. Spitzer WO, Suissa S, Ernst P, et al. Asthma death and near-fatal asthma in relation to β-agonist use. *N Engl J Med* 1992;326:501–506.

85. Vathenen AS, Knox AJ, Higgins BG, Britton JR, Tattersfield AE. Rebound increase in bronchial responsiveness after treatment with inhaled terbutaline. *Lancet* 1988;1:554–558.

86. Weber RW, Smith JA, Nelson HS. Aerosolized terbutaline in asthmatics: development of subsensitivity with long-term administration. *J Allergy Clin Immunol* 1982;70:417–422.

87. Harvey JE, Baldwin CJ, Wood PJ, Alberti KG, Tattersfield AE. Airway and metabolic responsiveness to intravenous salbutamol in asthma: effect of regular inhaled salbutamol. *Clin Sci* 1981;60:579–585.

88. Lipworth BJ, Struthers AD, McDevitt DG. Tachyphylaxis to systemic but not to airway responses during prolonged therapy with high dose inhaled salbutamol in asthmatics. *Am Rev Respir Dis* 1989;140:586–592.

89. Nelson HS, Szefler SJ, Martin RJ. Regular inhaled β-adrenergic agonists in the treatment of bronchial asthma: beneficial or detrimental. *Am Rev Respir Dis* 1990;144:249–250.

90. O'Connor BJ, Aikman SL, Barnes PJ. Tolerance to the nonbronchial effects of inhaled β_2-agonists in asthma. *N Engl J Med* 1992;327:1204–1208.

91. Wang Z-L, Bramley AM, McNamara A, Paré PD, Bai TR. Chronic fenoterol exposure increases *in vivo* and *in vitro* airway responses in guinea pigs. *Am J Respir Crit Care Med* 1994;149:960–965.

92. Schacter JB, Wolfe BB. 3-isobutyl-1-methylxanthine increases alpha-1-adrenergic receptor sensitivity and density in DDT1-MF2 smooth muscle cells. *J Pharm Exp Therapeut* 1995;272:215–223.

93. Coqueret O, Dugas B, Menciahuerta JM, Braquet P. Regulation of IgE production from human mononuclear cells by beta-2-adrenoceptor agonists. *Clin Exp Allergy* 1995;25:304–311.

94. Chapman ID, Buchhkit KH, Morley P, Morley J. Active enantiomers may cause adverse effects in asthma. *Trends Pharm Sci* 1992;13:231–232.

Asthma, edited by P.J. Barnes, M.M. Grunstein,
A.R. Leff, and A.J. Woolcock.
Lippincott–Raven Publishers, Philadelphia © 1997.

▪ 70 ▪

Catecholamines

Philip W. Ind

The catecholamines are a generic group of compounds that include the bioactive amines norepinephrine, epinephrine, and dopamine. Catecholamines exert their actions through effects on α- and β-adrenergic receptors that are widely distributed throughout the lung in all species. Their importance in the lung relates to their involvement in the sympathoadrenal system, the control of airway caliber, the pathophysiology of airway diseases, particularly asthma, and its treatment (1), and can be judged by the number of references within this book (see

Chapters 23, 24, 25, 58, 60, 61, 62, 64, 66, 69, 96, 98, 105, 106, 124, 141). Much of the available information is not new but it will be summarized.

STRUCTURE AND BIOSYNTHESIS OF CATECHOLAMINES

Structurally, the catecholamines are derived from the catechol (dihydroxybenzene) nucleus and include an amine group (Fig. 1). In practice, the term usually is reserved for the compounds epinephrine and norepinephrine and their parent compound dopamine (dihydroxyphenylethylamine). The structures are illustrated in Figs. 1 and 2.

Norepinephrine is the principal neurotransmitter of postganglionic sympathetic nerves, whereas epinephrine is secreted by the adrenal medulla and may function as a

P. W. Ind: Department of Respiratory Medicine, Royal Postgraduate Medical School, Hammersmith Hospital, London W12 0HS United Kingdom.

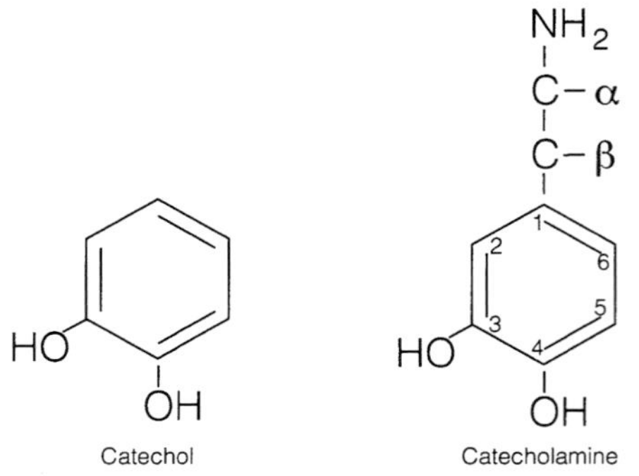

FIG. 1. Catechol nucleus with two -OH groups on positions 3 and 4 of the benzene ring. Catecholamine: amine substituted catechol ring. Norepinephrine α = H-C-H β = OH-C-H. α carbon substitution blocks oxidation by mitochondrial monoamine oxidase (MAO).

circulating hormone. Dopamine has an evolving role as a central neurotransmitter of extrapyramidal and mesolimbic systems.

Catecholamine biosynthesis comprising three steps (Fig. 2) was proposed originally by Blaschko in 1939; the enzymes involved have now been identified, characterized, and cloned (2). The amino acid L-tyrosine, plasma concentration 50 to 80 μM, is taken up into the cytoplasm of sympathetic nerves and chromaffin cells from the circulation by an active transport mechanism (Fig. 3). The percentage of tyrosine used in catecholamine biosynthesis is low, probably <2%.

Tyrosine Hydroxylase

The rate-limiting step of norepinephrine and dopamine biosynthesis is hydroxylation by the mitochondrial mixed function oxidase L-tyrosine hydroxylase (3–5). This enzyme converts L-tyrosine to L-dihydroxyphenylalanine (dopa) with tetrahydrofolic acid and a ferrous salt or tetrahydropteridine or dihydrobiopterin co-factors with a Km of 0.4×10^{-5} M in brain and 2.0×10^{-5} M in adrenals. The enzyme is itself a substrate for cyclic adenosine monophosphate (cAMP)-dependent and Ca^{2+}-calmodulin–sensitive protein kinase and protein kinase C. Phosphorylation is associated with increased hydroxylase activity and nerve stimulation with reduced gene expression. These mechanisms maintain catecholamine content and various catechols produce feedback inhibition of the enzyme.

Dopamine Decarboxylase

The cytoplasmic enzyme L-dopamine decarboxylase [molecular weight (MW) 109,000] acts on all aromatic L-amino acids such as histidine, tryptophan, and phenylalanine in addition to tyrosine and is not confined to catecholamine synthesizing cells (6). It can appropriately be called aromatic L-amino acid decarboxylase. It requires pyridoxal phosphate as a co-factor, has a pH optimum of 7.2, and a Km for dopa and tyrosine of 5×10^{-4} M.

Dopamine-β-Hydroxylase

Dopamine-β-hydroxylase (DBH) is a copper-containing, mixed function oxidase that requires molecular oxygen and ascorbic acid as a co-factor. DBH is found in chromaffin granules or storage vesicles and transforms about 50% of cytoplasmic dopamine (after active uptake into the vesicles) to norepinephrine with a Km of 5×10^{-3} M. It has a MW of 290,000. An antibody to the bovine enzyme has been used to localize the enzyme immunohistochemically. Congenital deficiency has been described (7).

Phenylethanolamine-*N*-methyltransferase

Epinephrine is formed from norepinephrine only in specific adrenal and extramedullary cells and some central neurones by the enzyme phenylethanolamine-*N*-

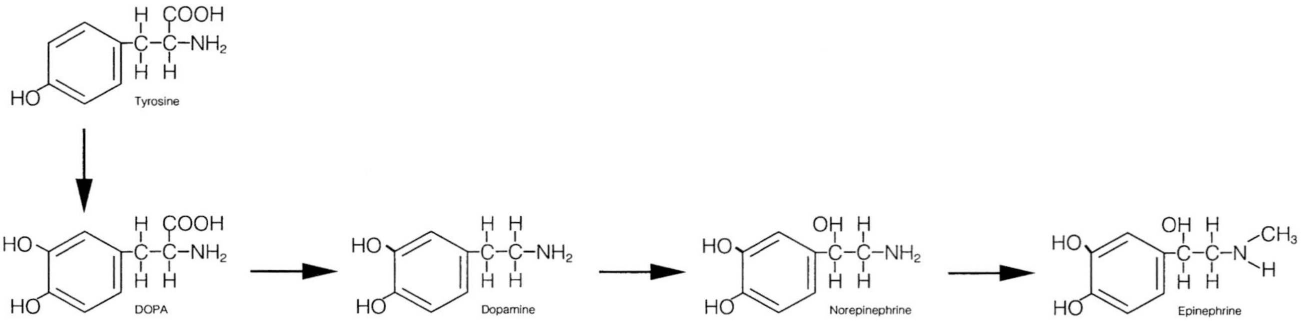

FIG. 2. Biosynthesis of norepinephrine and epinephrine. Conversion of tyrosine to dihydroxyphenylalanine (DOPA) by tyrosine hydroxylase, DOPA to dopamine by dopa decarboxylase, dopamine to norepinephrine by dopamine β-hydroxylase (DBH), and norepinephrine to epinephrine by phenylethanolamine-*N*-methyl transferase (PNMT).

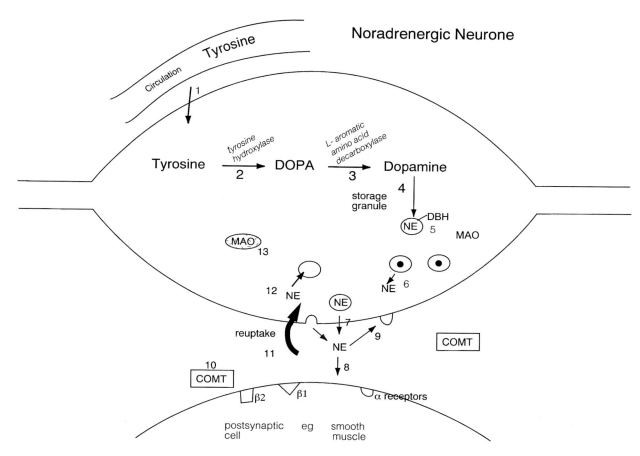

FIG. 3. Diagrammatic representation of a noradrenergic neurone. *1,* tyrosine uptake from the circulation; *2,* conversion of tyrosine to dihydroxyphenylalanine (DOPA) by tyrosine hydroxylase; *3,* conversion of DOPA to dopamine by L-aromatic amino acid decarboxylase; *4,* uptake of dopamine into synaptic vesicle; *5,* dopamine β-hydroxylase (DBH) conversion of dopamine to norepinephrine (*NE*) in chromaffin granule; *6,* release of one pool of NE from granule into cytoplasm; *7,* exocytosis of NE following fusion of vesicle and cell membrane; *8,* diffusion of NE into synaptic cleft; *9,* presynaptic regulation; *10,* catechol-O-methyl transferase (COMT) degradation of NE; *11,* reuptake into noradrenergic neurone; *12,* transport into synaptic vesicle; *13,* mitochondrial monoamine oxidase (MAO). Note that phenylethanolamine-*N*-methyl transferase (PNMT) is present only in adrenal medullary cells.

methyltransferase (PNMT), which has an MW of 30,000 and requires the methyl donor *S*-adenosyl methionine (6). Adrenal corticosteroid concentrations modulate PNMT synthesis as well as tyrosine hydroxylase and DBH activities (8).

STORAGE OF CATECHOLAMINES

Catecholamines, like many other neurotransmitters, are stored in specialized subcellular organelles called synaptic vesicles or storage granules. They are associated with the adenosine nucleotides adenosine triphosphate (ATP), adenosine diphosphate (ADP), and adenosine monophosphate (AMP) in a stoichiometric relationship of 1:4 so that the negative charge of the nucleotides balances the cations of the catecholamines. In addition to lipid and the catecholamines storage granules contain

various soluble proteins including a series of so-called chromogranins, DBH, enkephalins, and neuropeptide Y(NPY). The most important chromogranin is thought to be chromogranin A, which accounts for about 40% of the soluble proteins. It is acidic, rich in glutamine, and has an MW of 77,000. It is thought to constitute the major catecholamine storage pool forming a tetracatecholamine-ATP-chromogranin complex in equilibrium with mobile intragranular and cytoplasmic pools (9).

CATECHOLAMINE RELEASE

Catecholamine release has been studied most from the adrenal medulla; the assumption generally is made that the mechanisms of release from noradrenergic neurones are analogous (10). There is increasing evidence of regulation of release by a variety of local catecholamines through presynaptic receptors but also by adenosine, prostaglandins, and angiotensin II (11).

Excitation-secretion Coupling

Excitation-secretion coupling refers to the events that follow arrival of the action potential leading to catecholamine release from the adrenergic neurone or the adrenal medullary cell. Splanchnic nerve fibers release the preganglionic transmitter acetylcholine, which causes depolarization of the chromaffin cell membrane. This alters calcium permeability so that Ca^{2+} influx occurs, promoting fusion of granular and cell-surface membranes with vesicle docking and exocytotic release of catecholamines to the exterior of the cell (10,12). Catecholamine release is terminated by acetylcholine hydrolysis or diffusion away and by a fall in intracellular Ca^{2+} back to normal levels.

It is generally held that the release of norepinephrine from a noradrenergic nerve also depends on acetylcholine release from the noradrenergic fiber (Rand hypothesis) and similar changes in intracellular Ca^{2+} concentration.

Exocytosis

Exocytosis or reverse micropinocytosis refers to the all-or-none process of discharge of the contents of individual granules, which includes the catecholamine but also all the soluble components including ATP, chromogranins, and DBH in similar molar proportions to those in which they are usually bound (10). The escape of unhydrolyzed ATP and the lack of general cytoplasmic constituents, e.g., lactic dehydrogenase, suggests that it is directly extruded from the inside of the cell. The processes involved in membrane fusion with the cytoplasmic membrane are unclear, but recently many of the participating proteins have been characterized. These include synaptotagmin, synaptobrevin, synaptophysin, and the neurexins and syntaxins. The granule membrane itself is not released (12). There is some evidence of preferential release of newly formed norepinephrine; this supports other evidence of multiple "pools" of norepinephrine. If catecholamine release were exclusively by exocytosis, then high rates of axonal flow from the nerve cell body or protein "re-uptake" or nerve terminal protein synthesis would seem to be required.

CATECHOLAMINE METABOLISM

The two main enzymes involved in catecholamine metabolism are monoamine oxidase (MAO) and catechol-O-methyl transferase (COMT).

Monoamine Oxidase

MAO is a flavoprotein copper-containing enzyme, MW 290,000, that deaminates catecholamines to their corresponding aldehydes (13). It is widely distributed in different forms (A and B) in different tissues of most vertebrates. It is particle bound and present in the outer mitochondrial membrane, but a partial microsomal localization is not excluded. It is extraneuronal as well as intraneuronal, but its main role appears to be in catabolizing free norepinephrine leaking from granules or before incorporation after reuptake.

Catechol-O-methyl transferase

COMT is a cytoplasmic enzyme present in many mammalian tissues, particularly liver, kidney, and brain. It catalyzes the transfer of labile methyl groups from S-adenosyl methionine (SAM) to the metahydroxy group of the catecholamines producing normetanephrine and metanephrine (14). It requires Mg^{2+} and has an MW of about 24,000. Its Km for a catechol substrate varies according to the SAM concentration. COMT probably is mainly extraneuronal, being involved in degradation of circulating catecholamines and in association with extraneuronal uptake (uptake 2).

CATECHOLAMINE UPTAKE

The rapid termination of action of catecholamines is due to re-uptake rather than enzymatic degradation. At physiologic stimulation frequencies (<10 Hz) there is little overflow into the circulation from postganglionic adrenergic nerves. Further, blockade of MAO and COMT does not significantly block this efficient local inactivation. Re-uptake (15) into the sympathetic nerves and subsequently into the granules is the major mechanism involved (uptake 1).

Uptake 1

Intravenous radiolabeled norepinephrine is approximately 40% to 60% inactivated by rapid uptake into tissues, whereas the remainder is metabolized by MAO and COMT. Uptake is correlated directly with the density of sympathetic innervation and the proportion of cardiac output received by the tissue, and is most marked in spleen and heart. Subsequent sympathetic nerve stimulation can re-release labeled norepinephrine. In tissues denervated by surgical, chemical, or immunologic sympathectomy, exogenous catecholamine uptake is severely impaired (16). Uptake 1 is a high-affinity, highly specific, stereoselective, energy-dependent, temperature- and sodium-dependent, saturable process involving Michaelis-Menten kinetics. It is approximately twice as efficient for norepinephrine compared with epinephrine and specific blockers prolong catecholamine action. An active ion transport mechanism is involved and the human norepinephrine transporter has been isolated and cloned (17).

Uptake 2

Uptake 2 refers to a nonsaturable, nonenergy-dependent extraneuronal process (15) that is coupled to COMT. Specific blockers exist. Epinephrine has a higher affinity for uptake 2 than uptake 1 (in contrast to the situation with norepinephrine) and circulating epinephrine may be inactivated principally by this mechanism (15,18).

SYMPATHOADRENAL SYSTEM

The sympathoadrenal system comprises the circulating catecholamines, principally originating from the adrenal medulla and the neuronal components of the sympathetic innervation. Epinephrine has long been used therapeutically as a bronchodilator (19).

β-RECEPTOR BLOCKADE

β-adrenoceptor blocking drugs are widely used in the treatment of hypertension, angina, and postmyocardial infarction. In an uncontrolled study, a long-term effect on ventilatory function was claimed (20). In normal humans in controlled studies β-receptor blockade has no significant effect on airway caliber (21–23). This is in contrast to the situation in animals. β-receptor blockade produces airway narrowing in guinea pigs and dogs with intact vagi (24–26). No significant effect is seen after vagal section (27).

β-adrenoceptor Blockade in Asthma

The problem of bronchoconstriction after β-blocking drugs in asthmatics was recognized soon after their introduction (28). Severe, catastrophic bronchoconstriction can develop after even trivial doses (29) and prove fatal. This observation is the chief basis for the suggestion of increased adrenergic drive to the airways in asthma. It is worth noting that adrenalectomy and adrenergic neurone-blocking or ganglion-blocking drugs have not been reported to cause asthma.

An indirect bronchoconstrictor action of β-receptor blockade has been postulated (30,31), but no evidence of mediator release in propranolol-induced bronchoconstriction was found (although the techniques used may have been too insensitive [32]).

The suggestion (33) that β-receptor blocking drugs cause bronchoconstriction in asthma by antagonism of the inhibitory action of circulating epinephrine on prejunctional β2 receptors on cholinergic nerves in human airways (34) exacerbated by a muscarinic M2 autoreceptor deficiency is ingenious. It proposes that increased acetylcholine release after β-receptor blockade of prejunctional β2 receptors leads to bronchoconstriction via M3 airway smooth muscle receptors, exaggerated by cholinergic hyperresponsiveness. It is argued that this occurs in asthmatics because normal inhibitory prejunctional M2 receptors are deficient (35). It is supported by anticholinergic receptor blockade of propranolol-induced bronchoconstriction (36). However, it still begs the question of whether circulating epinephrine is present in adequate concentrations to exert important regulatory control over β2 receptors on nerves or on airway smooth muscle. The possibility that β2 receptors on NANC or sensory nerves (37,38) or β3 receptors (39,40) are in some way involved remains open.

CIRCULATING PLASMA CATECHOLAMINES

Mathé proposed that the primary defect in asthma might be a failure of secretion of circulating epinephrine on the basis of an apparent deficiency of catecholamine metabolites in urine collections (41,42). Only recently with adequately sensitive and specific radioenzymatic and high performance liquid chromatography (HPLC) assays has it become possible to measure accurately physiologic concentrations of catecholamines (43–46). Dopamine, norepinephrine, and epinephrine are all present in the circulation, but only the latter is thought to be important.

Dopamine is present at low concentrations and infusion to high levels has no significant effect on airway tone (47,48). Plasma norepinephrine represents an index of sympathetic nervous activity as it is derived from neurotransmitter overflow. However, variations in synaptic cleft width, nerve density, cardiac output, tissue extraction, etc., make it at best an indirect measure (43,46). Approximately 50% of norepinephrine detected in plasma from a forearm vein may be derived from forearm tissues. Arterial sampling or plasma measurements across the lungs are ideally required to determine pulmonary sympathetic response. Isotopic studies using radiolabeled norepinephrine have measured clearance and spillover and shown that sympathetic nerve activation may be regionalized and that local activation may not be detected by total body norepinephrine kinetics (44,46).

Plasma Catecholamine Concentrations in Normal Humans

Normal human plasma norepinephrine concentration is between 1 and 5 nmol/L. Studies suggest that up to 10% of plasma norepinephrine may be derived from the lungs presumably released from sympathetic nerves supplying blood vessels (44).

Basal normal human plasma epinephrine concentration is 0.1 to 0.5 nmol/L, but this may increase 5- to 10-fold on heavy exercise (49,50). Under severe pathologic conditions, e.g., life-threatening hypoglycemia, myocardial infarction, or cardiac arrest, levels 30 times higher have been reported (51). Epinephrine has long been regarded as a circulating hormone associated with "fright or flight" (52).

Plasma Catecholamines in Asthma

Plasma concentrations of norepinephrine and epinephrine are normal in persons with stable asthma. There is no relationship to asthma severity as judged by spirometric function (53). Circulating plasma catecholamine concentrations remain in the normal range when bronchoconstriction is induced in asthmatic patients whether by exercise or hyperventilation (54), methacholine (55), histamine inhalation (46,56), antigen challenge (57,58), intravenous histamine (58), or propranolol (59). Even in acute severe asthma when plasma norepinephrine concentration is significantly elevated (related to respiratory muscle activity or stress), plasma epinephrine concentration is unchanged (60–62). In very severe asthma, in the presence of severe acidosis, plasma epinephrine concentrations may be increased (63). It therefore appears that in human asthma a major physiologic mechanism that would be expected to offset bronchoconstriction is not generally activated.

Induced Bronchoconstriction in Animals

The situation in human asthma is distinct from that in experimental animals when circulating epinephrine appears to function as a protective hormone in the face of induced bronchoconstriction. Adrenalectomy and beta-receptor blockade have the same effect in potentiating bronchoconstriction induced by histamine (37,64), bradykinin, or antigen (65). However, measurements of plasma epinephrine concentration in animal models have not been systematic and have generally employed older, less reliable assays.

EXERCISE AND PLASMA CATECHOLAMINES IN ASTHMA

Exercise is a major stimulus to activation of the sympathoadrenal system but also commonly induces bronchoconstriction in asthma. Initial studies (54,66) suggested a blunting of norepinephrine increase and abrogation of the normal trebling of plasma epinephrine concentration in asthmatics undergoing treadmill exercise. This was interpreted as consistent with the concept of a primary deficiency of catecholamines in asthma (41,42). However, subsequent investigations using more severe exercise (50,67–69) have refuted this. Therefore, at most there is a partial defect of initial catecholamine mobilization (rather than an effect on metabolism or clearance) in asthma (70,71). The increase in circulating catecholamine concentrations on heavy exercise occurs independently of whether or not bronchoconstriction is

induced in asthmatics (67), suggesting that this represents physiologic sympathoadrenal activation rather than a homeostatic bronchodilator mechanism.

Diurnal Variation in Plasma Catecholamines and Nocturnal Asthma

The original report of a significant correlation between circulating epinephrine concentrations and peak expiratory flow in nocturnal asthma (72), together with bronchodilatation with intravenous epinephrine (73), was interpreted as favoring a causal relationship. However, equivalent plasma epinephrine concentrations and diurnal variation are seen in normal individuals and it is more likely that this simply represents a coincidence of two circadian rhythms. Nocturnal asthma and overnight fall in peak expiratory flow was documented in a patient who had undergone adrenalectomy and had no detectable circulating epinephrine in her plasma (74). Furthermore, other workers have been unable to show a relationship between nocturnal asthma and plasma epinephrine concentrations (75–77). A recent study over a 3-day period (77) found lower plasma epinephrine concentrations at 22.00 hours in individuals with nocturnal asthma. A reciprocal relationship between the epinephrine concentration and eosinophil count was identified, but the number of patients studied was small. Downregulation of white cell β_2-receptor numbers at 04.00 hours compared with 16.00 hours was reported in individuals with nocturnal asthma (76), but did not correlate with plasma epinephrine; differential over-representation of the susceptible Gly16 β_2-receptor polymorphism may play some part (78). In other studies correction of the overnight reduction in plasma epinephrine with low-dose infusion had no effect on nocturnal asthma (79).

INFUSION OF CATECHOLAMINES

Early on a number of studies infusing catecholamines were carried out to define dose-response characteristics in animals as well as in humans. A variety of cardiovascular and metabolic effects were documented, but we shall concentrate on bronchodilator effects.

EFFECTS OF NOREPINEPHRINE INFUSION

Norepinephrine infusion within the physiologic range (80–84) shows no airway, metabolic, or cardiovascular effects, suggesting that norepinephrine does not function as a circulating hormone (80).

Airway Effects of Epinephrine Infusion in Humans

Although epinephrine has long been used parenterally or by inhalation in asthma therapy (19), there is little in-

TABLE 1. *Dose-response relationships of infused epinephrine in normal and asthmatic persons*

Reference	Epinephrine infusion (ng/kg/min)	Plasma epi achieved (nmol/L)	Number of subjects	Physiologic effect
85	25	1.8	6 N	25% ▲sGaw
	50	2.9		42% ▲sGaw
56	25	1.6	6 N	20% ▲sGaw
				3× ▲PC$_{20}$
81	25	2.1	6 N	30% ▲MEF25
	62.5	4.7		46% ▲MEF25
57	44	1.3	8 A	23% ▲MEF50
	88	4.1		34% ▲MEF50
82	25	1.7	6 A	15% ▲MEF50
	62.5	3.1		110% ▲sGaw
86	16	0.95	10 A	3× ▲PC$_{20}$
	64	3.8		9% ▲FEV$_1$

epi, epinephrine; N, nonasthmatic individual; A, asthmatic individual; sGaw, specific conductance; PC$_{20}$, provocative concentration for 20% fall in FEV$_1$; MEF25, maximum expiratory flow at 25% vital capacity; MEF50, maximum expiratory flow at 50% vital capacity; FEV$_1$, forced expiratory volume.

formation regarding the dose-effect relationships of infused epinephrine. Extrapolation from the lower end of the dose-response curve might allow conclusions regarding the importance of naturally occurring circulating epinephrine concentrations. Published information relating low-dose epinephrine infusion to effects on airway caliber for a number of studies in nonasthmatic and asthmatic individuals are summarized in Table 1.

Minor effects on airway smooth muscle, measured as small changes in sensitive indices of airway caliber or bronchial reactivity to histamine, are found with 5- to 10-fold increments (55–57,73,79,81–86) or greater (57,71, 73) in plasma epinephrine concentration, in the nanomolar range. This suggests that physiologic changes in circulating epinephrine concentration are unlikely to exert significant regulation on airway diameter except in the most severe attacks of asthma. This relates to the *in vitro* effects of epinephrine on human bronchial smooth muscle (87,88) and mast cell preparations (89,90) that occur at concentrations of 10 to 100 nmol/L.

SYMPATHETIC INNERVATION

If circulating catecholamines have only a small role in regulating airway tone, then the effect of β-receptor blockade in patients with asthma suggests an important role of the sympathetic innervation to bronchial smooth muscle. However, considering its potential importance, there is little information available regarding the sympathetic nerve supply to human airways.

Tissue Catecholamine Concentrations

The norepinephrine content of an organ gives an indication of the extent of the sympathetic innervation (91). Pulmonary norepinephrine concentration varies between

0.01 μg/g tissue in pigs to 0.22 in sheep, with 0.04 in humans and other species in between (91,92). Despite this 10-fold variation between the lungs of different animal species (92,93), a considerably greater quantity of norepinephrine and epinephrine is consistently found within the heart, an organ with a much richer adrenergic nerve supply, in each case (Table 2).

Anatomy of Pulmonary Sympathetic Nerves

The sympathetic innervation of the lung is relatively minor compared with the more dominant parasympathetic nervous supply, which originates in the vagus nerve. Preganglionic sympathetic axons exit from the spinal cord in the ventral roots of T1-T6. Postganglionic fibers enter the lung through the hilum after synapsing in the middle and inferior cervical ganglia and in paravertebral ganglia of T1-T4. Sympathetic fibers distribute together with cholinergic nerves in periarterial and peribronchial plexuses to glands, blood vessels, and airway smooth muscle (94–96).

TABLE 2. *Catecholamine content: norepinephrine and epinephrine of lung and heart*

References	Species	Lung Norepi	Lung Epi	Heart Norepi	Heart Epi
91	Human	0.04[a]	0.03	1.04	0.18
93	Rat			0.72	0.04
91		0.02	0.02	0.27	0.05
93	Mouse	0.11			
91		0.03	0.08	0.45	0.10
93	Guinea pig	0.16			
91		0.01	0.04	1.80	0.20
93	Sheep			0.79	0.15
91		0.22	0.09	1.05	0.17

[a]μg/g tissue.
Norepi, norepinephrine; epi, epinephrine.

Histochemical Demonstration of Sympathetic Nerves in Animals

Classical light microscopic histologic studies using methylene blue and silver impregnation techniques demonstrate nervous structures nonspecifically but can result in artifacts and variable results (97). Histochemical fluorescent techniques (97–100) to identify catecholamines have been applied to the respiratory tract, although autofluorescence from elastic tissues may interfere. Noradrenergic nerve fibers were found in substantial numbers in the trachea of most animal species including rat, guinea pig, rabbit, sheep, goat, pig, and calf in early studies (99,100). However, no catecholamine-containing nerves were identified in airways as distal as respiratory bronchioles where, by contrast, cholinergic fibers were readily located. Larger intrapulmonary airways have variable numbers of noradrenergic nerves depending on which species is studied (101,102). The cat has a particularly extensive sympathetic supply, with some fibers extending down to respiratory bronchioles (103,104). Rabbits have few sympathetic fibers in the trachea and none in the bronchi (99). Other species, e.g., goats, pigs, and calves, possess intermediate airway sympathetic innervation. The dog has noradrenergic fibers supplying ganglia and pulmonary vessels but few to the bronchi (105). Guinea pigs have a dense catecholaminergic fiber network in the proximal trachea but much less distally (106, 107); few are found in the bronchi and none supply bronchioles. In the rat a detailed study showed most sympathetic nerves at the hilum were associated with bronchial arteries. Airway smooth muscle at bronchial bifurcations contained a small number of catecholamine-containing varicosities, but most segments of bronchial smooth muscle in between bifurcations had no detectable sympathetic fibers (108,109). In the rhesus monkey (109) most noradrenergic fibers were found to be associated with bronchial arteries, but a few fibers were located in the muscle layer of the first three generations of bronchi and were sometimes continuous with the plexus surrounding bronchial arteries. The monkey has a sparse sympathetic supply compared with most species.

Histochemical Demonstration of Sympathetic Nerves in Humans

There are little histochemical data on human airways. In a small number of individuals few sympathetic nerve fibers were demonstrated in intrapulmonary airways (102, 110,111). The key synthetic enzyme DBH serves as a suitably specific marker of sympathetic nerves (112). Antibodies to neurone-specific enolase and S-100 (a calcium-binding protein that delineates glial cells) have been used to provide a reliable denominator against which specific noradrenergic fibers were compared. The presence of few noradrenergic fibers traversing, let alone terminating on, human bronchial smooth muscle compared with submucosal glands and bronchial vessels was confirmed (112). In another study NPY immunoreactivity was found to co-localize with DBH antibody distribution in sympathetic nerve fibers within human, guinea pig, rat, and cat bronchial smooth muscle extending down to bronchiolar level (113).

Ultrastructural Studies of Sympathetic Nerves

Ultrastructural investigations using electron microscopy identify noradrenergic nerves by small dense-cored granules as distinct from the much more numerous "cholinergic" nerve profiles. Electron microscopy studies in guinea pig airways have confirmed the histochemical findings of a denser innervation proximally with only occasional nerve fibers seen in large bronchi (114). In human tissue few noradrenergic nerves were found in airway smooth muscle compared with those related to airway glands (115–118). Interestingly, some small dense-cored vesicles in axon profiles have been identified on ganglia (119).

SYMPATHETIC NERVE STIMULATION

Physiologic studies of the effects of sympathetic stimulation have been carried out in few intact animals. Electrical stimulation of the thoracic sympathetic supply in cats and dogs partially inhibited cholinergically mediated bronchoconstriction (24,25,27,120). Bronchodilatation was seen in large and small airways. The effect was dependent on the degree of cholinergic tone and was antagonized by β-receptor blockade but not by adrenalectomy, thus implicating sympathetic nerves (25,27). Electrical recording from sympathetic afferents and nerve section experiments suggested the presence of moderate sympathetic bronchodilator tone (121,122). In guinea pigs and dogs vagally mediated bronchoconstriction is increased by intravenous propranolol (25).

In pithed guinea pigs thoracic spinal sympathetic stimulation reverses histamine-induced bronchoconstriction. This effect is antagonized by propranolol and prevented by reserpine pretreatment (123). It has been suggested that this may be due to a secondary effect of norepinephrine overflow released by adjacent sympathetic nerves supplying blood vessels.

Regrowth of sympathetic postganglionic nerve fibers into a previously excised and reimplanted dog lung required nearly 4 years but bronchodilator function was restored (124). Neither reinnervation nor stimulation experiments have been reported for the sympathetic supply to the human lung, but minor effects on lung volume and expiratory flow were reported after upper thoracic sympathectomy for palmar hyperhydrosis (125).

PHARMACOLOGIC STUDIES OF SYMPATHETIC NERVES

Pharmacologic studies have used electrical field stimulation to activate nerves specifically rather than acting directly on smooth muscle. This leads to relaxation of guinea pig trachea but not bronchus (102,126,127), consistent with the site of histochemical demonstration of noradrenergic nerve fibers (107) and the neuronal norepinephrine uptake mechanism (128). Tetrodotoxin and beta-receptor antagonists inhibit relaxation. Cocaine, which blocks neuronal re-uptake of norepinephrine, increases the sensitivity of tracheal smooth muscle to exogenous norepinephrine but not that of peripheral lung strips from guinea pigs (129). Electrical field stimulation of precontracted human bronchial and bronchiolar smooth muscle leads to initial cholinergic contraction succeeded by a marked tetrodotoxin-sensitive (neuronal) but propranolol-resistant (NANC inhibitory) relaxation (102,110,129, 130). Cocaine also is without effect on both bronchi and lung strips, suggesting no significant functional sympathetic innervation to human airway smooth muscle. However, pharmacologic evidence for sympathetic nerves in human bronchial smooth muscle strips has been reported by other workers (131). They showed uptake of radiolabeled norepinephrine with the characteristics of neuronal uptake and demonstrated re-release by field stimulation and by tyramine. The explanation of these apparently contradictory findings remains unclear (132).

In most species of laboratory animals and humans, sympathetic innervation is relatively sparse compared with the parasympathetic supply. However, the functional importance of the adrenergic system as a whole remains incompletely understood. Studies in asthmatics have not been reported.

Indirect Effects of Sympathetic Nerves

Sympathetic nerves may exert indirect effects on bronchial smooth muscle tone by a number of mechanisms. The effect of sympathetic stimulation in dogs depends on the magnitude of vagal tone (24,25,27,120). This raises the possibility that sympathetic nerves may modulate cholinergic neurotransmission. Ultrastructural studies have demonstrated noradrenergic nerves close to cholinergic nerves (118) and ganglia (119) in human tissue, which makes this plausible.

In vitro, exogenous norepinephrine acting via α and β2 receptors inhibits ganglionic transmission in isolated cat and ferret airways (133,134). In canine airways norepinephrine modulates postganglionic nerve release of acetylcholine. Sympathetic nerve stimulation inhibits cholinergic effects in this situation by stimulating presynaptic β1 receptors (135). A similar experiment in human airways demonstrates that β2 agonists inhibit contractions

induced by cholinergic nerve stimulation (34) and by tachykinins (37).

Effect of Tyramine in Asthma

The indirect sympathomimetic agent tyramine has been infused to probe an indirect effect of sympathetic nerves in human asthma. Tyramine releases norepinephrine locally from sympathetic nerves. It produced marked cardiovascular effects in asthmatic persons but had no bronchodilator action, even though the persons responded to β2-receptor stimulation by salbutamol also administered intravenously (136). This constitutes further *in vivo* evidence against a functional sympathetic innervation to bronchial smooth muscle in humans.

CONCLUSIONS

The catecholamines norepinephrine and epinephrine are widely distributed throughout the lung in all species. They exert their actions through effects on α- and β-adrenergic receptors. Norepinephrine is the primary sympathetic neurotransmitter but it does not act as a circulating hormone in humans. Plasma epinephrine concentration is normal in asthma. The importance of circulating epinephrine in regulating airway caliber physiologically and pathophysiologically is uncertain. Plasma epinephrine concentrations fall at night, but the relationship to nocturnal asthma is unclear because correction of the fall does not prevent bronchoconstriction. The sympathoadrenal system is not activated to defend airway caliber except during very heavy exercise or under circumstances of the most severe bronchoconstriction.

The sympathetic innervation of airway smooth muscle varies in its extent in different animal species. Paradoxically, in humans bronchial smooth muscle receives virtually no sympathetic nerve fibers, yet the response of asthmatics to β-adrenergic blockade suggests tonic stimulation, direct or indirect. Further work is required to elucidate the importance of catecholamines in the control of airway caliber in normal humans and in patients with asthma.

REFERENCES

1. Barnes PJ. β-adrenergic receptors and their regulation. State of the art. *Am J Crit Care Med* 1995;152:838–860.
2. Nagatsu T. Genes for human catecholamine-synthesizing enzymes. *Neurosci Res* 1991;12:315–345.
3. Messerano JM, Vuillet PR, Tank AW, Weiner N. The role of tyrosine hydroxylase in the regulation of catecholamine synthesis. In: Trendelenburg U, Weiner N, eds. *Handbook of experimental pharmacology*, vol 90/II. Berlin: Springer-Verlag, 1989;427–469.
4. Zigmond RE, Schwarzchild MA, Rittenhouse AR. Acute regulation of tyrosine hydroxylase by nerve activity and by neurotransmitters via phosphorylation. *Annu Rev Neurosci* 1989;12:415–461.
5. Daubner SC, Lauriano C, Haycock JW, Fitzpatrick PF. Site-directed

mutagenesis of serine 40 of rat tyrosine hydroxylase. Effects of dopamine and cAMP-dependent phosphorylation on enzyme activity. *J Biol Chem* 1992;267:12639–12646.

6. Molinoff PB, Axelrod J. Biochemistry of the catecholamines. *Annu Rev Biochem* 1971;40:465–491.

7. Robertson D, Haile V, Perry SE, Robertson RM, Phillips JA, III, Biaggioni I. Dopamine β-hydroxylase deficiency. A genetic disorder of cardiovascular regulation. *Hypertension* 1991;18:1–8.

8. Viskupic E, Kvetnansky R, Sabban EL, et al. Increase in rat phenylethanolamine N-methyltransferase mRNA level caused by immobilization stress depends on intact pituitary-adrenocortical axis. *J Neurochem* 1994;63:808–814.

9. Winkler H, Apps DK, Fischer-Colbrie R. The molecular function of adrenal chromaffin granules: established facts and unresolved topics. *Neuroscience* 1986;18:283–384.

10. Winkler H. Occurrence and mechanisms of exocytosis in adrenal medulla and sympathetic nerve. In: Trendelenburg U, Weiner N, eds. *Handbook of experimental pharmacology*, vol 90/I. Berlin: Springer-Verlag, 1988;43–118.

11. Langer SZ, Lehman J. Presynaptic receptors on catecholamine neurons. In: Trendelenburg U, Weiner N, eds. *Handbook of experimental pharmacology. Catecholamines I*, vol 90. Berlin: Springer-Verlag, 1988;419–507.

12. Jahn R, Sudhof TC. Synaptic vesicles and exocytosis. *Annu Rev Neurosci* 1994;17:219–246.

13. Axelrod J. Methylation reactions in the formation and metabolism of catecholamines and other biogenic amines. *Pharmacol Rev* 166;18:95–113.

14. Kopin IJ. Metabolic degradation of catecholamines. The relative importance of different pathways under physiological conditions and after administration of drugs. In: Blaschko HKF, Muscholl E, eds. *Handbuch der experimentellen pharmakologie*. Berlin: Springer–Verlag, 1989;33:427–469.

15. Iversen LL. Uptake processes for biogenic amines. In: Iversen LL, Iversen SD, Snyder SH, eds. *Handbook of psychopharmacology*, vol 3. New York: Plenum Press, 1975;381–442.

16. Brownstein MJ, Hoffman BJ. Neurotransmitter transporters. *Rec Prog Horm Res* 1994;49:27–42.

17. Schudiner S. Molecular glimpse of vesicular monoamine transporters. *J Neurochem* 1994;62:2067–2078.

18. Trendelenburg U. A kinetic analysis of the extraneuronal uptake and metabolism of catecholamines. *Rev Physiol Biochem Pharmacol* 1980;87:33–115.

19. Solis-Cohen S. The use of adrenal substance in the treatment of asthma. *JAMA* 1900;34:1164–1166.

20. Northcote RJ, Ballantyne D. Influence of intrinsic sympathomimetic activity on respiratory function during chronic β blockade. *Br Med J* 1986;293:97–101.

21. Zaid G, Beall GN. Bronchial response to β-adrenergic blockade. *N Engl J Med* 1966;275:580–584.

22. Richardson PS, Sterling GM. Effects of β-adrenergic receptor blockade on airway conductance and lung volume in normal and asthmatic subjects. *Br Med J* 1969;3:143–145.

23. Tattersfield AE, Leaver DG, Pride NB. Effect of β-adrenergic blockade and stimulation on normal airways. *J Appl Physiol* 1973;35:613–619.

24. Castro de la Mata R, Penna M, Aviado DM. Reversal of sympathomimetic bronchodilatation after dichloroisoproterenol. *J Pharm Exp Ther* 1962;135:197–203.

25. Woolcock AJ, Macklem PT, Hogg JC, Wilson NJ. Influence of the autonomic nervous system on airway resistance and elastic recoil. *J Appl Physiol* 1969;26:814–818.

26. Drazen JM. Adrenergic influences on histamine-mediated bronchoconstriction in the guinea pig. *J Appl Physiol* 1978;44:340–345.

27. Cabezas GA, Graf PD, Nadel JA. Sympathetic versus parasympathetic nervous regulation of airways in dogs. *J Appl Physiol* 1971;31:651–655.

28. McNeill RS. Effect of a β-adrenergic blocking agent, propranolol, on asthmatics. *Lancet* 1968;ii:1101–1102.

29. Fraunfeder FT, Barker AF. Respiratory effects of timolol. *N Engl J Med* 1984;311:1441.

30. Maclagan J, Ney UM. Investigation of the mechanisms of propranolol induced bronchoconstriction. *Br J Pharmacol* 1979;66:409–418.

31. Terpstra GK, Raaijmakers JAM, Wassink GA. Propranolol-induced bronchoconstriction: a nonspecific side effect of β-adrenergic blocking therapy. *Eur J Pharmacol* 1981;73:107–108.

32. Ind PW, Barnes PJ, Brown MJ, Dollery CT. Plasma histamine concentration during propranolol-induced bronchoconstriction. *Thorax* 1985;40:903–909.

33. Barnes PJ. Muscarinic receptor subtypes: implications for lung disease. *Thorax* 1989;44:161–167.

34. Rhoden KJ, Meldrum LA, Barnes PJ. β-adrenergic modulation of cholinergic neurotransmission. *J Appl Physiol* 1988;65:700–705.

35. Barnes PJ. Muscarinic receptor subtypes in the airways. *Life Sci* 1993;52:521–528.

36. Ind PW, Dixon CMS, Fuller RW, Barnes PJ. Anticholinergic blockade of beta-blocker induced bronchoconstriction. *Am Rev Respir Dis* 1989;139:1390–1394.

37. Kamikawa Y, Shimo Y. Inhibitory effects of catecholamines on cholinergically and noncholinergically mediated contractions of guinea pig isolated bronchial muscle. *J Pharm Pharmacol* 1990;42:131–134.

38. Verleden GM, Belvisi MG, Rabe KF, Miura M, Barnes PJ. β₃-Adrenoceptors inhibit NANC neural bronchoconstrictor responses *in vitro*. *J Appl Physiol* 1993;74:1195–1199.

39. Itabashi S, Aikawa T, Sekizawa K, Sasaki H, Takishima T. Evidence that an atypical β₃-adrenoceptor mediates the prejunctional inhibition of nonadrenergic noncholinergic contraction in guinea pig bronchi. *Eur J Pharmacol* 1992;218:187–190.

40. Martin CAE, Naline E, Manara L, Advenier C. Effects of two β₃-adrenoceptor agonists SR 58611A and BRL 37344 and of salbutamol on cholinergic and NANC neural responses in guinea pig main bronchi *in vitro*. *Br J Pharmacol* 1993;110:1311–1316.

41. Mathe AA, Knapp P. Decreased plasma free fatty acids and urinary epinephrine in bronchial asthma. *N Engl J Med* 1969;281:234–238.

42. Mathe AA. Decreased circulating epinephrine, possible secondary to decreased hypothalamic-adrenal discharge; a supplementary hypothesis of bronchial asthma pathogenesis. *J Psychosom Res* 1971;15:349–359.

43. Brown MJ, Jenner DA, Allison DJ, Dollery CT. Variation in individual organ release of noradrenaline measured by an improved radioenzymatic technique; limitations of peripheral venous measurements in the assessment of sympathetic nervous activity. *Clin Sci Mol Med* 1981;61:585–590.

44. Esler M, Jennings G, Korner P, et al. Total, and organ-specific, noradrenaline plasma kinetics in essential hypertension. *Clin Exp Hypertens* 1984;1:507–521.

45. Jennings G, Leonard P. Plasma catecholamines—analytical challenges and physiological determinations. *Ballieres Clin Endocrinol Metab* 1993;7:307–353.

46. Larsson K, Carlens P, Bevegard S, Hjemdahl P. Sympathoadrenal responses to bronchoconstriction in asthma: an invasive and kinetic study of plasma catecholamines. *Clin Sci* 1995;88:439–446.

47. Thomson NC, Patel KR. Effect of dopamine on airways conductance in normals and extrinsic asthmatics. *Br J Clin Pharmacol* 1978;5:421–424.

48. Michoud MC, Amyot R, Jenneret-Grosjean A. Dopamine effect on bronchomotor tone *in vivo*. *Am Rev Respir Dis* 1984;130:755–758.

49. Cryer PE. Physiology and pathophysiology of the human sympathoadrenal neuroendocrine system. *N Engl J Med* 1980;303:436–440.

50. Berkin KG, Walker G, Inglis GC, Ball SG, Thomson NC. Circulating adrenaline and noradrenaline concentrations during exercise in patients with exercise-induced asthma and normal subjects. *Thorax* 1988;43:295–299.

51. Worstman J, Frank S, Cryer PE. Adrenomedullary response to maximum stress. *Am J Med* 1984;77:779–784.

52. Cannon WB. Studies on the conditions of activity in endocrine organs. Evidence that medulli adrenal secretion is not continuous. *Am J Physiol* 1931;98:447–453.

53. Barnes PJ, Ind PW. Plasma histamine and catecholamines in stable asthmatic subjects. *Clin Sci Mol Med* 1982;62:661–665.

54. Barnes PJ, Brown M, Silverman M, Dollery CT. Circulating catecholamines in exercise and hyperventilation-induced asthma. *Thorax* 1981;36:435–440.

55. Sands MF, Douglas FL, Green J, Banner AS, Robertson GL, Leff AR. Homeostatic regulation of bronchomotor tone by sympathetic activation during bronchoconstriction in normal and asthmatic humans. *Am Rev Respir Dis* 1985;132:993–998.

56. Warren JB, Dalton N, Turner C, Clark TJH. Protective effect of circulating epinephrine within the physiological range on the airway response to inhaled histamine in nonasthmatic subjects. *J Allergy Clin Immunol* 1984;74:683–686.

57. Larsson K, Gronneberg R, Hjemdahl P. Bronchodilatation and inhibition of allergen induced bronchoconstriction by circulating epinephrine in asthmatic subjects. *J Allergy Clin Immunol* 1985;75:586–593.

58. Ind PW, Brown MJ, Barnes PJ. Sympathoadrenal responses in asthma. *Thorax* 1983;38:702.

59. Ind PW, Barnes PJ, Durham SR, Kay AB. Propranolol-induced bronchoconstriction in asthma; β-receptor blockade and mediator release. *Am Rev Respir Dis* 1984;129:10.

60. Ind PW, Causon RC, Brown MJ, Barnes PJ. Circulating catecholamines in acute asthma. *Br Med J* 1985;290:267–269.

61. Dahlof C, Dahlof P, Lundberg JM, Strombom U. Elevated plasma concentration of neuropeptide Y and low level of circulating adrenaline in elderly asthmatics during rest and acute severe asthma. *Pulm Pharmacol* 1988;1:3–6.

62. Parke TR, Steedman DJ, Robertson CE, Little RA, Maycock PF. Plasma catecholamine reponses in acute severe asthma. *Arch Emerg Med* 1992;9:157–161.

63. Clarke B, Ind PW, Causon R, Barnes PJ. Bronchodilator and catecholamine responses to induced hypoglycaemia in acute asthma. *Clin Sci* 1985;69:35P.

64. Colebatch HJH. Adrenergic mechanisms in the effects of histamine in the pulmonary circulation of the cat. *Circ Res* 1970;26:379–396.

65. Collier HOJ, James GWL. Humoral factors affecting pulmonary inflation during acute anaphylaxis in the guinea pig *in vivo*. *Br J Pharm* 1967;30:283–301.

66. Warren JB, Keynes RJ, Brown MJ, Jenner DA, McNichol MW. Blunted sympathoadrenal response to exercise in asthmatic subjects. *Br J Dis Chest* 1982;76:147–150.

67. Larsson K, Hjemdahl P, Martinsson A. Sympathoadrenal reactivity in exercise-induced asthma. *Chest* 1982;82:561–567.

68. Hulks G, Mohammed AF, Jardine AG, Connell JM, Thomson NC. Circulating plasma concentrations of atrial natriuretic peptide and catecholamines in response to maximal exercise in normal and asthmatic subjects. *Thorax* 1991;46:824–828.

69. Gilbert IA, Lenner KA, McFadden ER Jr. Sympathoadrenal response to repetitive exercise in normal and asthmatic subjects. *J Appl Physiol* 1988;64:2667–2674.

70. Barnes PJ. Endogenous catecholamines and asthma. *J Allergy Clin Immunol* 1986;77:791–795.

71. Barnes PJ. Adrenergic regulation of airway function. In: Kaliner MA, Barnes PJ, eds. *The airways: neural control in health and disease.* New York: Dekker, 1988:57–85.

72. Barnes PJ, Fitzgerald G, Brown M, Dollery CT. Nocturnal asthma and changes in circulating epinephrine, histamine and cortisol. *N Engl J Med* 1980;303:263–267.

73. Barnes PJ, Fitzgerald GA, Dollery CT. Circadian vatiation in adrenergic responses in asthmatic subjects. *Clin Sci* 1982;62:349–354.

74. Morice A, Sever P, Ind PW. Adrenaline, bronchoconstriction and asthma. *Br Med J* 1986;293:539–540.

75. Postma DS, Keyzer JJ, Koeter GH, Sluiter HJ, De Vries K. Influence of the parasympathetic and sympathetic nervous system on nocturnal bronchial obstruction. *Clin Sci (Lond)* 1985;69:251–258.

76. Szefler SJ, Ando R, Cicutto LC, Surs W, Hill MR, Martin RJ. Plasma histamine, epinephrine, cortisol and leukocyte β-adrenergic receptors in nocturnal asthma. *Clin Pharmacol Ther* 1991;49:59–68.

77. Bates ME, Clayton M, Calhoun W, et al. Relationship of plasma epinephrine and circulating eosinophils to nocturnal asthma. *Am J Respir Crit Care Med* 1994;149:667–672.

78. Turki J, Pak J, Green SA, Martin RJ, Liggett SB. Genetic polymorphisms of the β2-adrenergic receptor in nocturnal asthma. Evidence that Gly16 correlates with the nocturnal phenotype. *J Clin Invest* 1995;95:1635–1641.

79. Morrison JFJ, Teale C, Pearson SB, et al. Adrenaline and nocturnal asthma. *Br Med J* 1990;301:473–476.

80. Silverberg AB, Shah SD, Hammond MW, Cryer PE. Norepinephrine: hormone and neurotransmitter in man. *Am J Physiol* 1978;234:252–256.

81. Berkin KG, Inglis GC, Ball SG, Thomson NC. Airway responses to low concentrations of adrenaline and noradrenaline in normal subjects. *Q J Exp Physiol* 1985;70:203–209.

82. Berkin KG, Inglis GC, Ball SG, Thomson NC. Effect of low dose adrenaline and noradrenaline infusions on airway calibre in asthmatic patients. *Clin Sci* 1986;70:347–352.

83. Larsson K, Martinsson A, Hjemdahl P. Influence of circulating alpha-adrenoceptor agonists on pulmonary function and cardiovascular variables in patients with exercise induced asthma and healthy subjects. *Thorax* 1986;41:522–528.

84. Larsson K, Hjemdahl P. No influence of circulating norepinephrine on bronchial reactivity to histamine in asthmatic subjects. *Eur J Respir Dis* 1986;69:16–23.

85. Warren JB, Dalton N. A comparison of the bronchodilator and vasodepressor effects of exercise levels of adrenaline in man. *Clin Sci* 1983;64:475–479.

86. Knox AJ, Campos-Gongora H, Wisniewski A, MacDonald IA, Tattersfield AE. Modification of bronchial reactivity by physiological concentrations of plasma adrenaline. *J Appl Physiol* 1992;73:1004–1007.

87. Hawkins DF, Schild HO. The action of drugs on isolated human bronchial chains. *Br J Pharmac* 1951;6:682–690.

88. Goldie RG, Paterson JW, Spina D, Wale JL. Classification of β-adrenoceptors in human isolated bronchus. *Br J Pharmac* 1984;81:611–615.

89. Assem ESK, Schild HO. Inhibition of the anaphylactic mechanism by sympathomimetic amines. *Int Arch Allergy* 1971;40:576–589.

90. Butchers PR, Skidmore IF, Vardey CJ, Wheeldon A. Characterization of the receptor mediating the anti-anaphylactic effects of β-adrenoceptor agonists in human lung tissue *in vitro*. *Br J Pharmac* 1980;71:663–667.

91. Anton AH, Sayre DF. A study of the factors affecting the aluminium oxide-trihydroxyindole procedure for the analysis of catecholamines. *J Pharmacol Exp Ther* 1962;138:360–375.

92. Holtzbauer M, Sharman DF. The distribution of catecholamines in vertebrates. In: Blaschko H, Muscholl E, eds. *Handbook of experimental pharmacology.* New York: Springer-Verlag, 1972;33.

93. Goodall McC. Studies of adrenaline and noradrenaline in mammalian heart and suprarenals. *Acta Physiol Scand* 1951;24(suppl 85):1–51.

94. Larsell G, Dow RS. The innervation of the human lung. *Am J Anat* 1933;52:125–146.

95. Gaylor JB. The intrinsic nervous mechanism of the human lung. *Brain* 1934;57:143–160.

96. Spencer H, Leof D. The innervation of the human lung. *J Anat (Lond)* 1964;98:599–609.

97. Falck B. Observations on the possibilities of the cellular localisation of monoamines by a fluorescence method. *Acta Physiol Scand* 1962;56(suppl197):1–25.

98. Falck B, Owman CH. A detailed methodological description of the fluorescnce method for cellular demonstration of biogenic amines. *Acta Univ Lund* 1965;11:71–123.

99. Mann SP. The innervation of mammalian bronchial smooth muscle: the localization of catecholamines and cholinesterases. *Histochem J* 1971;3:319–331.

100. Malmfors T. Studies on adrenergic nerves. *Acta Physiol Scand* 1965;64(suppl 248):1–93.

101. Richardson JB. Nerve supply to the lungs. *Am Rev Respir Dis* 1979;119:785–802.

102. Doidge JM, Satchell DG. Adrenergic and nonadrenergic inhibitory nerves in mammalian airways. *J Auton Nerv Syst* 1982;5:83–99.

103. Dahlstrom A, Fuxe K, Hokfelt T, Norberg KA. Adrenergic innervation of the bronchial smooth muscle of the cat. *Acta Physiol Scand* 1966;66:507–508.

104. Silva DG, Ross G. Ultrastructural and fluorescence histochemical studies on the innervation of the tracheo-bronchial muscle of normal cats treated with 6-hydroxydopamine. *J Ultrastruct Res* 1974;47:310–328.

105. Suzuki H, Morita K, Kuriyama H. Innervation and properties of the smooth muscle of the dog trachea. *Jpn J Physiol* 1976;26:303–320.

106. O Donnell SR, Saar N. Histochemical localization of adrenergic nerves in the guinea pig trachea. *Br J Pharmacol* 1974;47:707–710.

107. O Donnell SR, Saar N, Wood NJ. The density of adrenergic nerves at various levels in the guinea pig lung. *Clin Exp Pharmacol Physiol* 1978;5:325–332.

108. El-Bermani AI McNary WF, Bradley DE. The distribution of acetylcholinestaerase and catecholamine-containing nerves in the rat lung. *Anat Rec* 1970;167:205–207.

109. El-Bermani AI. Pulmonary noradrenergic innervation of rat and monkey: a comparative study. *Thorax* 1978;33:167–174.

110. Richardson J, Beland J. Nonadrenergic inhibitory nervous system in human airways. *J Appl Physiol* 1976;41:764–771.

111. Partanen M, Laitinen A, Hervonen A, Toivanen M, Laitinen LA. Catecholamine and acetylcholinesterase containing nerves in human lower respiratory tract. *Histochemistry* 1982;76:175–188.

112. Sheppard MN, Kurian SS, Henzen-Logmans SC, et al. Neurone-specific enolase and S-100: new markers for delineating the innervation of the respiratory tract in man and other mammals. *Thorax* 1983;38:333–340.

113. Sheppard MN, Polak JM, Allen JM and Bloom SR. Neuropeptide tyrosine (NPY): a newly discovered peptide is present in the mammalian respiratory tract. *Thorax* 1983;39:326–330.

114. Jones TR, Kannan MS, Daniel EE. Ultrastructural study of guinea pig tracheal smooth muscle and its innervation. *Can J Physiol Pharmacol* 1983;58:974–983.

115. Meyrick B, Reid L. Ultrastructure of cells in human bronchial submucosal glands. *J Anat* 1970;107:281–299.

116. Pack RJ, Richardson PS. The aminergic innervation of the human bronchus: a light and electron microscopic study. *J Anat* 1984;138:493–502.

117. Laitinen A, Partenen M, Harvonen A, Laitinen LA. Electron microscopic study on the innervation of human lower respiratory tract. Evidence of adrenergic nerves. *Eur J Respir Dis* 1985;67:209–215.

118. Daniel EE, Kannan M, Davis C, Pussey-Daniel V. Ultrastructural studies on the neuromuscular control of human tracheal and bronchial smooth muscle. *Respir Physiol* 1986;63:109–128.

119. Richardson J, Fergusson CC. Neuromuscular structure and function in the airways. *Fed Proc* 1979;38:202–208.

120. Daly M, Mount LE. The origin, course and nature of bronchomotor fibers in the cervical sympathetic nerve of the cat. *J Physiol* 1951;113:43–62.

121. Widdicombe JG. Action potentials in parasympathetic and sympathetic efferent fibers to the trachea and lungs of dogs and cats. *J Physiol* 1966;186:56–88.

122. Green M, Widdicombe JG. The effect of ventilation of dogs with different gas mixtures on airway caliber and lung mechanics. *J Physiol* 1966;186:363–381.

123. Ainsworth GA, Garland LG, Payne AN. Modulation of bronchoconstrictor responses to histamine in pure bred guinea pigs by sympathetic nerve stimulation. *Br J Pharmacol* 1981;77:249–254.

124. Lall A, Graf PD, Nadel JA, Edmunds LH. Adrenergic reinnervation of the re-implanted dog lung. *J Appl Physiol* 1973;35:439–442.

125. Molho M, Kurchin A, Ohry A, Bass A, Adar R. Pulmonary abnormalities after upper dorsal sympathectomy. *Am Rev Respir Dis* 1977;116:879–883.

126. Coburn RF, Tomita T. Evidence for nonadrenergic inhibitory nerves in the guinea pig trachealis muscle. *Am J Physiol* 1973;224:1072–1080.

127. Grundstrom N, Andersson RGG, Wikberg JES. Pharmacological characterization of the autonomic innervation of guinea pig tracheobronchial smooth muscle. *Acta Pharmacol Toxicol* 1981;49:150–157.

128. Foster RW, O'Donnell SR. Evidence that adenergic nerves are responsible for active uptake of noradrenaline in guinea pig isolated trachea. *Br J Pharm* 1975;53:109–112.

129. Zaagsma J, van der Heijden PJCM, van der Schaar MWG, Blank CMC. Comparison of functional β-adrenoceptor heterogeneity in central and peripheral airway smooth muscle of guinea pig and man. *J Recept Res* 1983;3:89–106.

130. Davis C, Connolly ME, Greenacre JK. Beta-adrenoceptors in human lung, bronchus and lymphocytes. *Br J Clin Pharmacol* 1980;10:425–432.

131. Davis C, Kannan MS, Jones TR, Daniel EE. Control of human airway smooth muscle: *in vitro* studies. *J Appl Physiol* 1982;53:1080–1087.

132. Zaagsma J, van Amsterdam RGM, Brouwer F, et al. Adrenergic control of airway function. *Am Rev Respir Dis* 1987;136:S45–50.

133. Baker DC, Basbaum CB, Herbert DA, Mitchell RA. Transmission in airway ganglia: inhibition by norepinephrine. *Neurosci Lett* 1983;41:139–143.

134. Skoogh B-E. Transmission through airway ganglia of ferrets. *Eur J Respir Dis* 1983;64(suppl 131):159–170.

135. Danser AHJ, van den Ende R, Lorenz RR, Flavahan NA, Vanhoutte PM. Prejunctional beta$_1$ adrenoceptors inhibit cholinergic neurotransmisson in canine bronchi. *J Appl Physiol* 1987;62:785–790.

136. Ind PW, Scriven AJI, Dollery CT. Use of tyramine to probe pulmonary noradrenaline release in asthma. *Clin Sci Mol Med* 1983;64:9.

Asthma, edited by P.J. Barnes, M.M. Grunstein,
A.R. Leff, and A.J. Woolcock.
Lippincott–Raven Publishers, Philadelphia © 1997.

▪ 71 ▪

Activation of Airway Afferent Nerves

Bradley J. Undem and Margerita M. Riccio

Activation of airway afferent nerve fibers results in reflexes that serve to protect the airways and maintain homeostasis. These reflexes include coughing, sneezing, changes in the depth and rate of breathing, and alterations in the activity of efferent (autonomic) neurons innervating blood vessels, glands, and smooth muscle.

The role played by afferent neurons in airway diseases such as asthma is unclear. Perhaps the most obvious example of afferent stimulation contributing to asthma symptomatology is represented by the sensation of dyspnea and the nonproductive cough that precedes and accompanies a significant percentage of asthmatic episodes. A more hypothetical contention is that central, peripheral, and axonal reflexes contribute directly to the mechanisms of the pathogenesis of airway disease. For example, central and local reflexes may coordinate with the immune system to evoke the inflammation that is considered a hallmark of an asthmatic airway. This remains little more than conjecture, however, until empirical research provides a more complete understanding of the mechanisms by which afferent neurons are activated and of the consequences of this activation. This review focuses on the former: the activation and modulation of tracheobronchial afferent neurons. Relatively little attention is devoted in this chapter to the consequence of afferent nerve stimulation. For excellent reviews of the neuronal reflexes in the airways the reader is referred to refs. 1–3.

CHARACTERIZATION OF AFFERENT FIBERS

Since the studies of Langley, Gaskell, and Dale, there has been a formal characterization scheme for autonomic innervation of visceral tissues (4–7). In the airways the autonomic neurons are characterized as either parasympathetic or sympathetic. Within these subdivisions, fibers are classified as either preganglionic or postganglionic, and finally within these subdivisions the neurons can be characterized based on their transmitter content. No such formal scheme exists for afferent innervation. The most frequent classification scheme for airway afferent neurons has four subclasses: slowly adapting stretch receptors, rapidly adapting stretch receptors (or "irritant receptors"), pulmonary C-fibers, and bronchial C-fibers (8–17). Our understanding of airway afferent biology has been greatly aided by this simple and elegant classification scheme. The utility of such a scheme, however, in some instances may be overshadowed by the confusion it potentially elicits. For example, a logical but false extension of this classification is that C-fibers are nonadapting and are not activated by irritants. Even the term "receptor" may be a bit confusing to those not accustomed to sensory neurobiologic vernacular. Whereas biologists use the term "receptor" strictly to define proteins that bind a specifically defined molecular ligand with high affinity and selectivity, the sensory neurobiologist uses the term

  B.J. Undem: Department of Medicine, The Johns Hopkins University, Baltimore, Maryland 21224.
  M.M. Riccio: Sandoz Research Institute, London SW3 6LY United Kingdom.

more loosely as the afferent neuron per se, or the responding unit of an afferent neuron (i.e., stretch receptor). In any event, the classification of afferent neurons in the airways, as in other tissues, is based on defining anatomic and electrophysiologic properties (Table 1).

Anatomic Properties

The innervation of visceral tissue is predominantly afferent in nature. In the cat, for example, the cervical vagus nerve contains about 30,000 fibers, of which 80% are afferent in nature (18). The innervation of the airways is no exception. The branches from the vagus nerve innervating the bronchial tissue in the cat contain about 6,000 fibers, of which 5,000 are afferent (18). In addition to the vagus nerve, afferent fibers in the peripheral airways also may reach the central nervous system via spinal nerve fibers (19,20). Thus, an airway afferent fiber can be characterized as either a vagal or spinal fiber. The vast majority of physiologic investigations on afferent innervation of the airways has been carried out on vagal afferent fibers.

The cell bodies of vagal afferent fibers in the airways are located in either of two ganglia located along both cervical vagus nerves (21–23). These two ganglia take the form of swellings along the vagus nerves and are referred to as the inferior (nodose) and superior (jugular) vagal ganglia. Thus, airway vagal afferent fibers can be classified as either nodose or jugular fibers. The jugular and nodose ganglia are distinct in origin, although the exact embryologic derivation of the two ganglia is unclear. In rats, for example, these ganglia have been demonstrated to be either of a pure placodal origin (24) or of a pure neural crest origin (25). The physiologic significance of the location of afferent cell bodies is not understood. It is interesting to note, however, that although airway afferent nerves are derived from both ganglia, the cell bodies of neuropeptide-containing airway neurons are present mainly in jugular ganglia. Calcitonin gene-related peptide (CGRP)-containing neurons innervating rat trachea, for example, have their cell bodies located in jugular ganglia but rarely in nodose ganglia (21). Similarly, tachykinin- and CGRP-containing neurons innervating guinea pig airways were derived almost exclusively from jugular ganglia (22). The cell bodies of the spinal afferent neurons innervating the airways are located in the dorsal root ganglia situated along the spinal cord (21–23).

Another anatomic aspect of the afferent fiber used in their characterization is their size and myelination. In the cat, for example, most (72%) afferent neurons contained in the bronchial branches of the vagus have small (<1μm in diameter) axons (18). The axons of the other fibers are myelinated and range in size from 1 to 14μm (18).

As with autonomic neurons, transmitter content can be used to characterize afferent fibers in the airways. Many neurons, especially unmyelinated fibers, contain neuropeptide-laden vesicles (26–29). Afferent fibers have thus been characterized as either tachykinergic (mainly substance P and neurokinin A) or CGRP-containing fibers. Airway afferent fibers containing a variety of other transmitters, including opioid peptides (22) and nitric oxide synthase (NOS) (30), have been identified in the airways.

In cutaneous tissue, microscopic studies on the structure of the nerve endings have provided another anatomic method of characterizing the sensory neurons. Thus, in the skin several anatomically distinct afferent endings have been defined, including Meissner's corpuscles and Ruffini endings (31,32). In the mesentery, anatomically distinct pressure receptors referred to as pacinian corpuscles can readily be identified (33,34). Relatively little progress, however, has been made in morphologically distinguishing different types of afferent terminals in the airways. The vast majority of sensory endings in the airways exist as free endings (35–42) arising from unmyelinated fibers, devoid of distinguishing characteristics that allow for subcategorization. Among the various types of afferent receptors in the airways, the so-called slowly adapting stretch receptor has received the most morphologic attention (35,36,42) and is located in the smooth muscle layer surrounded with multiple layers of basal lamina (43–46). These endings are morphologically similar to other slowly adapting endings, namely, the Ruffini terminals identified in the peridontal ligament of rats (47–49).

Electrophysiologic Properties

Essentially two electrophysiologic characteristics are used routinely to classify afferent neurons in the airways: a) the conduction velocities of their axons, and b) their adaptability to a prolonged stimulus.

In the 1920s Erlanger and Gasser investigated the compound action potential in somatic nerve trunks (50). One end of the nerve was electrically stimulated and the compound potential monitored by placing a recording elec-

TABLE 1. *Criteria used to characterize airway afferent nerve fibers*

Criterion	Examples
Fiber source	Vagal (nodose, jugular);spinal (dorsal root)
Conduction velocity	A-fiber (Aα, Aβ, Aδ); C-fiber
Adaptation	Rapidly adapting receptor (RAR); slowly adapting receptor (SAR)
Activation profile	Mechanosensitive fibers; chemosensitive fibers
Transmitters	Tachykinin-containing; calcitonin gene-related peptide (CGRP)-containing, etc.

trode on the nerve trunk some fixed distance away. Typically, the compound potential consisted of three or four waves distinguished in time (latency from time of stimulation). The group of waves arriving at the recording electrodes first are referred to as A waves and represent the activity of the faster conducting fibers; later a heterogeneous wave appears, referred to as the C wave. The A wave often is seen as a cluster of discrete waves that can be subdivided into A-alpha (Aα), A-beta (Aβ), A-gamma (Aγ), and A-delta (Aδ), with the former conducting at the fastest rate and Aδ the slowest. The C wave represents the slowest group of fibers in the compound action potential. The compound action potential in the recurrent laryngeal nerve (branch of the vagus nerve containing fibers innervating the larynx, trachea and esophagus) of the guinea pig consists of two discrete A waves followed by a heterogeneous C wave (51). The estimated conduction velocities of the fibers conducting in the C wave ranged from 0.4 m/s to about 3 m/s, the Aδ wave reflects fibers conducting at about 10 m/s, and the fastest A wave reflects fibers conducting at about 20 m/s. These values confirm those predicted for the guinea pig recurrent laryngeal nerve on the basis of axon diameter (52). Studies carried out in several species reveal that the conduction velocity of afferent fibers innervating the airways span the spectrum from C-fibers (<2 m/s) to fast conducting A fibers (≈70 m/s) (17).

Adaptability to a sustained stimulation is another electrophysiologic property used to categorize airway afferent fibers (11). During lung inflation there are two phases of stimulation: a dynamic phase in which the stimulation is increasing and a maintained or static phase. All mechanically sensitive afferent neurons respond to the dynamic phase of mechanical stimulation. The response to the static phase, however, can be used to distinguish afferent fiber types. During the static phase, fibers respond with either a relatively constant discharge of action potentials, a gradual decrease discharge frequency, or a rapid decrease in their discharge frequency. The neurons are accordingly referred to as nonadapting fibers, slowly adapting fibers, and rapidly adapting fibers, respectively (Fig. 1) (10,11,45). In some cases, slowly adapting and rapidly adapting fibers are referred to as tonic and phasic fibers, respectively.

ACTIVATION OF AFFERENT NERVES

When evaluating the activation profile of an airway afferent neuron, it should be kept in mind that many airway afferent fibers are polymodal, i.e., capable of being stimulated by several types of stimulation. Thus, for example, it is not uncommon to find neurons that are stimulated in response to both a specific chemical as well as mechanical stimulation. With only a few notable exceptions, the literature on stimulation of airway afferents is derived from *in vivo* studies on various mammals. Thus, one must also keep in mind the significant potential for indirect effects of a stimulus on afferent activation. For example, histamine may directly stimulate a chemosensitive fiber, or it may stimulate an afferent fiber as a consequence of the bronchoconstriction it elicits (see below). With these qualifications in mind, the stimuli that activate airway afferent fibers include mechanical, osmolarity changes, pH changes, and various chemicals (CO_2, autacoids, and xenobiotics). Changes in temperature is another likely stimulus for some airway afferent neurons (especially in the larger airways), but the experimental difficulty in studying this in the tracheobronchial system has left this a relatively unstudied area of research.

Mechanical Activation

Mechanically sensitive fibers are the most commonly studied afferent neurons in the airways. This is a heterogeneous group of fibers ranging in size from small unmyelinated C-fibers to large A-fibers. Anatomically, they exist in every aspect of the airway tree. The amount or rate of adaptation to the mechanical stimulus and the axon conduction velocity are used routinely as conve-

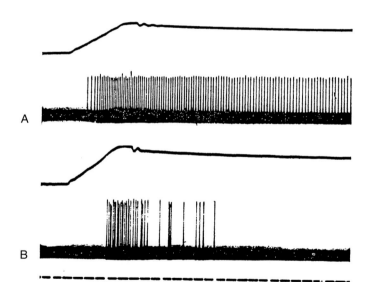

FIG. 1. Response characteristics of two vagal afferent airway fibers to lung inflation in anesthetized cats with chest wall removed. In each panel, *upper line* represents intratracheal pressure (*up* = increased pressure) and *lower panel* is the record of action potential discharge from the afferent fiber. *Dotted line* represents time base in .5 and .1 seconds. In **A**, fiber responds with action potential generation to rising phase (dynamic phase) of lung inflation and continues to discharge on maintained (static phase) inflation. This fiber was termed a slowly adapting fiber. In **B**, however, the fiber began responding to the rising phase of lung inflation but ceased firing within 1 s despite the maintained inflation of the lung and was termed a rapidly adapting fiber. (From Knowlton GC, Larrabee MG. A unitary analysis of pulmonary volume receptors. *Am J Physiol* 1946;147:100–114.)

nient methods of subclassifying mechanically sensitive afferent neurons. Accordingly, mechanosensitive airway afferents are either myelinated (A-fibers) or unmyelinated C-fibers. The former are subclassified further as either slowly adapting or rapidly adapting fibers.

Slowly Adapting Stretch Receptors

Myelinated intrathoracic afferent fibers that elicit a long-lasting discharge of action potentials in response to a maintained lung inflation are referred to as slowly adapting receptors (SARs) (8–10). Afferent fibers with SAR characterists were among the first neurons in any tissue investigated using single-unit electrophysiologic techniques in the pioneering studies of Adrian in the 1920s and 30s (8,53). SARs are found throughout the tracheobronchial tree, but are concentrated in the large conducting airways (43–46). Anatomic studies have identified complex nerve endings situated in the tracheobronchial smooth muscle of several species that are suggested to correspond to the physiologically identified SARs (35–37,42). In the dog, physiologic studies indicate that nearly half the SARs are in the trachea (with most of these in the thoracic region), about 20% were found in the larger bronchi, and 30% were identified in the lower lobe (43,44). As a rule, the SARs found in the intrathoracic airways are stimulated by lung inflation (an increase in transpulmonary pressure), although many continue to discharge, albeit at a much lower frequency, at residual volume. An exception to this can be found in the rat lung, where 20% of the intrathoracic SARs were found to respond either exclusively or predominantly during the deflation phase of the ventilatory cycle (54). The SARs in the extrathoracic trachea of dogs are also activated during expiration (45,55).

The full complement of reflexes initiated by SARs is unknown, but it is clear that they can profoundly influence the respiratory rate. Thus, the evidence firmly supports a role for these fibers in the Hering-Breuer reflex (2,8,56–59), which inhibits inspiratory activity during inflation. Activation of these fibers in the dog lung also has been linked to a decrease in parasympathetic drive to the airway, leading to airway smooth muscle relaxation during lung inflation (60).

Rapidly Adapting Stretch Receptors

Myelinated afferent fibers that respond to mechanical stimulation with a burst of action potentials during the dynamic phase and then rapidly adapt during the static phase of the stimulus are collectively referred to as rapidly adapting receptors (RARs) (10,11). An adaptation index, usually defined as the amount of decay in the discharge frequency of a fiber subjected to a constant stimulus after the maximum activation has been obtained, is used often to quantify the degree of adaptation (see Fig. 1) (11).

Knowlton and Larabee (11) suggested that those stretch receptors with an adaptation index of 80% or greater meet the "rapidly adapting" criterion. It is assumed that the adaptation index is a function of the intrinsic properties of the neuron, not merely a function of its location. Studies on isolated frog lungs, however, have led to the speculation that because of difference in the ratio of tissue viscosity to tissue elasticity, the anatomic location of a nerve ending may significantly impact its discharge characteristics in response to applied mechanical energy (61). One can reason, for example, that depending on the location within a lung, the mechanical energy may decline during the static phase of an inflation. This concept of regional differences in tissue elasticity and viscosity in the airways must be kept in mind when categorizing nerve types as either RAR or SAR.

RARs are located along the entire tracheobronchial tree, but concentrated in the larger airways (62). In contrast with SARs, which are located in the smooth muscle, the RARs are found around the entire circumference of the airway. The conduction velocity of RARs overlap with SARs, but on average are somewhat slower (11,63). In monkeys (64), cats (63), and guinea pigs (65) the average conduction velocity of RARs was about 21, 25, and 20 m/s, respectively. There is considerable variability of the conduction velocities of RARs within a given species. For example, in the cat the conduction velocities ranged from 16 to 37 m/s (63) and in the guinea pig the range was from 3 to 57 m/s (65).

The activity of RARs is typically not coordinated with inspiration or expiration during euphonic breathing. It requires relatively large changes in transmural pressures evoked by either distending or collapsing the airway to stimulate RARs (62,64,66–68). Perhaps because of the superficial localization of many RARs under the epithelium and close to the airway lumen, they are readily stimulated by focal mechanical stimulation. Many RARs are polymodal in their receptivity to stimuli. As discussed below, in addition to mechanical stimulation these fibers respond also to chemical stimulation.

RARs soon became synonymous with the term "irritant receptors" because these endings responded to many noxious agents including dust and histamine (69–71). A precise description of the reflexes initiated by RARs is hindered by the difficulty in selectively stimulating these fibers without concomitant stimulation of C-fiber afferents and other A-fibers. Nevertheless, some of these fibers are generally considered to elicit defensive reflexes including coughing, rapid shallow breathing, bronchoconstriction, and mucous secretion (1–3). Those fibers found in the trachea are thought to stimulate cough reflexes, whereas those in the lower airways the hyperpneic response (72). RARs in the lower airways are activated by a decrease in compliance (73) and can stimulate deep inspirations or sighs (74,75). Because compliance decreases during quiet breathing, it has been suggested that RARs may subserve an important homeostatic function by triggering deep breaths to maintain tidal ventilation as the lungs become stiffer (76).

Mechanically Sensitive C-fibers

The airway C-fibers are subdivided, based on their location, into pulmonary C-fibers (found in the peripheral airways, formally known as juxtacapillary receptors or J-receptors) and bronchial C-fibers found in the larger airways (13,14,16,17,77). Both pulmonary and bronchial C-fibers are mechanically sensitive, although in the dog the latter are less sensitive than the former (12). Spontaneous discharge evoked by artificial breathing is sparse in both pulmonary and bronchial C-fibers (12). Successive increases in tidal volumes (hyperinflation) caused a moderate activation of bronchial endings but a more marked and consistent stimulation of pulmonary C-fibers (12). Lung deflation is an ineffective stimulation of bronchial and pulmonary C-fibers (12,13,16). In rats, as had been noted above with RARs, C-fiber activity is increased when the lung compliance is decreased (54).

Stimulation of C-fibers results in defensive pulmonary reflexes including cough, apnea, rapid shallow breathing, bronchoconstriction, and mucous secretion (1,3,13,78). Jammes and Mei (79) have hypothesized that the baseline cholinergic tone of the airways is secondary to bronchopulmonary C-fiber activation. This intriguing hypothesis is based on their findings that airway smooth muscle tone can be eliminated by surgically removing the right and left nodose ganglia, but keeping the vagal motor pathways intact. This demonstrates that, in their model, the airway smooth muscle cholinergic tone has a peripheral origin. Pharmacologic studies indicate that this peripheral origin is associated with unmyelinated C-fibers. It should be mentioned, however, that others have demonstrated that inspiratory units in the brain, driven by the same pattern generator that drives the phrenic nerve, contribute to the parasympathetic motor control of airway smooth muscle in the cat (80). Substantial evidence supports the view that stimulation of a subset of mechanically sensitive C-fibers is responsible for initiating Head's paradoxical reflex, i.e., the contraction of inspiratory muscle evoked by a large inflation (2,81). Many C-fibers in the airways contain neuropeptides in their peripheral processes, and thus also may cause axonal and peripheral reflexes in the airways (26–29).

Mechanism of Mechanical Activation

The mechanism of mechanical activation of afferent fibers is a multistep process. The initial event is the transmission of mechanical energy through the cells and tissues that surround the nerve ending. This process can be divided into a dynamic component and a static (main-

tained) component. As alluded to earlier, adapting receptors stop responding (or dramatically reduce their frequency of discharge) during the static component of a sustained stimulus. Conceptually, the transmission of energy is followed sequentially by a transducer process that converts the mechanical energy to electrical energy. Ultimately, a process that converts this analog electrical signal (generator potential) to a "digital" frequency-coded electrical signal (action potential) occurs. Mechanical energy to the airway wall can be derived from at least four sources: ventilatory cycle, smooth muscle contraction, changes in interstitial pressure, and focal deformation secondary to deposition of particulate substances.

The increase in transmural pressure that occurs during inspiration and expiration provides sufficient mechanical energy to stimulate SARs, RARs, and C-fibers in the airways. In the structurally simple frog lung, early studies indicated that there was a linear relationship between the lung volume and discharge frequency of mechanically sensitive afferent neurons (82). Taglietti and Casella (83) have noted, however, that a linear relationship does not hold between firing frequency and either lung volume or intrapulmonary pressure. Rather, their study predicted a linear relationship between a derived pulmonary wall tension and discharge frequency.

It is evident that fibers of all sizes respond to mechanical stimulation in the airways, but the threshold for activation varies among the various fiber types. Kaufman and colleagues (84) compared the transpulmonary pressure required to activate the various types of afferent fibers in the airways and found that the most sensitive fibers were the SARs (≈ 6 cm H_2O), the least sensitive were the bronchial C-fibers (≈ 27 cm H_2O), and the RARs and pulmonary C-fibers were intermediate (≈ 13 and 16 cm H_2O, respectively). The peak frequency of stimulation followed the same pattern with frequencies up to 80 Hz reached in the SARs and only about 8 to 10 Hz in the C-fibers. The rate of change in pressure (dynamic phase of the stimulus) can influence the stimulation threshold for mechanically sensitive fibers in the airways. The pressure threshold for both SARs and RARs has been found to decrease as the inflation rate increases (9,85,86).

Another mechanism that may stimulate mechanosensitive afferent fibers is smooth muscle contraction. Smooth muscle contraction can have an indirect effect on mechanically sensitive fiber discharge by increasing the pressure in the airway wall. This is especially true for low threshold receptors. It is possible that the local mechanical deformation set up by smooth muscle contraction also may lead directly to stimulation of mechanosensitive fibers located within the smooth muscle (i.e., SARs). Smooth muscle contraction has been found to modulate SAR activity profoundly in the cat (87).

An increase in interstitial pressure is another potential source of mechanical energy to airway afferent neurons. Several groups have demonstrated that pulmonary congestion and edema are strong stimuli to discharge afferent fibers. Most notable in this regard are the pulmonary C-fibers and RARs; edema has little effect on SARs, and bronchial C-fibers are stimulated only in the severely edematous lung (68,88–91) . Indeed, Paintal (16) suggested an increase in interstitial pressure was the most effective stimulus for J-receptors (pulmonary C-fibers). Inasmuch as the C-fibers and RAR fibers are polymodal, and can be stimulated by means independently of mechanical energy, it would seem likely that factors other than increases in interstitial pressure may contribute to the discharge of afferent neurons during edema. For example, it is conceivable that endogenous factors such as bradykinin and 5-hydroxytryptamine (5-HT) contribute to the overall afferent nerve response to edema and pulmonary congestion (92).

Mechanical energy to airway afferents may be initiated simply from deposition of inhaled particles onto the airway wall. It is a well recognized fact that superficial mechanically sensitive afferent fibers in the larger airways (i.e., many RARs and bronchial C-fibers) can be stimulated by gently touching the mucosal surface with a blunt probe. Using calibrated von Frey hairs, Fox and colleagues (93) found that the C-fibers were less sensitive to touch than the exquisitely sensitive Aδ fibers. Physiologically, this type of mechanical energy may be relevant in stimulating cough reflexes by deposition of inhaled particulate matter on large airways.

Osmolarity and Tonicity

Inhalation of distilled water is a power stimulus for reflex cough and bronchoconstriction (94–97). The mechanism of the afferent nerve stimulation subserving this response is unclear, but likely involves either changes in osmolarity per se or decreases in selected ion concentrations. Eschenbacher and colleagues (96), for example, found that hypo-osmolar solution caused cough and bronchoconstriction, whereas iso-osmolar solutions lacking chloride ions caused cough but not bronchoconstriction. Several studies using single-unit recordings support the reflex studies by demonstrating that separate populations of neurons respond to either hypo-osmolarity or a lack of chloride anion or both (98–103). In a guinea pig isolated tracheal preparation, for example, water stimulated 100% of the C-fibers and Aδ fibers, whereas simply removing chloride ions stimulated about 70% of the C-fibers and 40% of the Aδ fibers (104).

Hypertonic saline solutions stimulate most RARs and C-fibers in the lower airways of dogs (103,105). Application of a 7% saline solution stimulates 100% of the mechanically sensitive Aδ fibers and C-fibers in the guinea pig isolated trachea (104).

The mechanism of stimulation by anosmotic solutions is not known. As discussed above, a lack of chloride appears to be critical in the response of some fibers to water, but many fibers seem to respond to the change in tonicity. The neurons evaluated in these investigations are, for the most part, mechanosensitive fibers. It is therefore possible that the response to water and hypertonic saline is simply a response to the mechanical deformation of the neural membrane caused by the changes in osmolarity. In fact, patch clamp studies have provided numerous examples of opening of mechanosensitive ion channels in various cell types, including neurons, by small changes in osmolarity (106).

Hydrogen Ions

The pH of inflamed joints is lower than that of noninflamed joints (107–109). Because asthma is a condition associated with inflammation, it is perhaps logical to speculate that hydrogen ion concentrations may be elevated in regions of asthmatic airways. Certainly, inhalation of acidic substances such as citric acid results in powerful stimulation of the cough reflex in man and experimental animals (94,110–118).

Hydrogen ions stimulate cutaneous nociceptors (119), a subset of corneal afferents (120), and ischemically sensitive visceral afferents (121). There is relatively little electrophysiologic information, however, on the activation of airway afferent fibers. Decreasing pH from 7 to 5 stimulates afferent fibers in the guinea pig isolated trachea (122). The proton-sensitive fibers were found to be exclusively capsaicin-sensitive C-fibers. Interestingly, capsazepine, a so-called capsaicin receptor antagonist, inhibited the proton-induced discharge from tracheal C-fibers (Fig. 2). This observation was consistent with the observation that acid-induced cough and bronchoconstriction in guinea pigs is antagonized by capsazepine (123,124), and raises the hypothesis that protons release an endogenous activator of capsaicin receptors. Preliminary intracellular studies on the membrane properties of dorsal root ganglion cells indicate that capsaicin and protons may stimulate the same or similar cation conductance pathways (125). In the dorsal root ganglion neurons, however, the proton-induced increase in cation conductance is not blocked by capsazepine (126).

Autacoids

The following section provides an overview of the actions of several autacoids on airway sensory neural pathways and attempts to shed light on what influence these indirect effects have on neural activation. The literature on this subject reveals considerable species heterogeneity and, thus, prudence is warranted when extrapolating to human airway afferents.

The effects of autacoids have been evaluated primarily on RARs and C-fibers. Several autacoids stimulate activity in slowly adapting fibers (SAR), but most often this

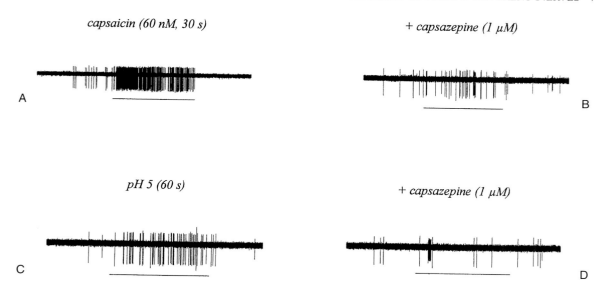

capsaicin (60 nM, 30 s)   *+ capsazepine (1 μM)*

pH 5 (60 s)   *+ capsazepine (1 μM)*

FIG. 2. Capsazepine blocks both capsaicin- and low pH-induced activation of guinea pig tracheal C-fibers *in vitro*. All drugs were selectively perfused over the receptive field of single afferent nerve fibers. **A:** Control response to 30 s application of 60 nM capsaicin (*solid bar*) directly onto the receptive field. **B:** Reapplication of capsaicin to receptive field in the presence of 1 μM capsazepine. **C,D:** Responses of a C-fiber to a 60-s application of pH 5 in the absence (C) and presence (D) of 1 μM capsazepine. (Figure courtesy of Alyson Fox, London.)

appears to be secondary to the bronchoconstrictor effects of the autacoid. Histamine, for example, can stimulate SAR activity (56,127–130), but this effect is correlated in time with the bronchoconstriction and blocked by a bronchodilator such as isoproterenol (128,130).

Histamine

Histamine given by aerosol or injected intravenously stimulates RARs in the airways in several species including guinea pig (65), rabbit (69,71), cat (66,131,132), dog (67,133–136), and monkey (64). The mechanism of activation of RAR fibers by histamine is somewhat controversial. Some studies have demonstrated attenuation of the histamine-induced activation of RARs by isoproterenol, suggesting that histamine's effect on these nerve endings may be secondary to smooth muscle contraction (65,69). In other studies, by contrast, administration of acetylcholine caused a similar degree of bronchoconstriction to histamine in dogs, and produced a markedly weaker excitation of RARs (133–135). Moreover, bronchodilator treatment with isoproterenol failed to inhibit the histamine-induced RAR activity (133). These data suggest that histamine may have a direct stimulatory effect on RAR activity. Another consideration is that histamine indirectly stimulates RAR activity independently of smooth muscle contraction. For example, histamine may cause pulmonary edema, which may in turn activate RARs (137). This issue can be addressed by evaluating the effect of histamine on RAR activity *in vitro*. Bradley

(138) noted that histamine effectively elicited spike discharge from RARs in cat isolated lung preparations. In the guinea pig isolated tracheal preparation, however, histamine failed to evoke spike discharge from myelinated afferents (93). Histamine also has been found to have little effect on RAR activity in rat lungs (54). Considered together, these data indicate that, depending on the species, histamine has a variable effect on RAR activity that may be attributed to both direct and indirect effects.

Histamine can stimulate some (66,131,139,140), but not all (13,16,17) pulmonary C-fibers. It is apparent, however, that, as is the case for RARs, histamine may not stimulate pulmonary C-fibers directly. It was postulated that the histamine-induced stimulation of pulmonary C-fibers is secondary to changes in lung mechanics brought about by smooth muscle constriction (13,17).

Histamine is a more consistent activator of bronchial C-fibers than pulmonary C-fibers (12,13,131). Results from these *in vivo* studies indicate that histamine stimulates bronchial C-fibers independently of mechanical changes in lung function (12). Studies performed *in vitro*, however, demonstrate that histamine failed to cause action potential generation in C-fibers from guinea pig isolated tracheae (93). It is not known whether histamine stimulates C-fibers in the conducting airways of guinea pigs *in vivo*.

Prostaglandins

The concept that prostaglandins stimulate afferent nerves arose from clinical studies that demonstrated side effects of throat irritation and coughing after inhalation with the bronchodilator prostaglandins (PG), prostaglandin E₁ (PGE₁) and E₂ (141,142).

Several prostaglandins stimulate RARs, but in many cases it is unclear if this is a direct or indirect effect secondary to changes in lung mechanics. Relatively large doses of PGE₂, administered into the right atrium, are required to activate RARs in dog lungs (143). PGE₂ mildly stimulated RARs when given by aerosol or left ventricular injection; however, this was attributed to the ventilatory cycle or cardiac influences (144). Right atrial injection of PGF₂α consistently activated RAR fibers, whereas left atrial injection was relatively ineffective in activating these fibers (143). The PGF₂α-induced RAR activation could be attenuated by bronchodilators, suggesting that the effects were secondary to muscle contraction (143). The thromboxane A₂ mimetic, U46619, injected via the vena cava modestly stimulated RAR activity in cat airways (145). This effect also appeared to be related to changes in lung mechanics because activation of RARs correlated with increases in end-inspiratory tracheal airway pressure.

PGE₂ and PGI₂ effectively activated bronchial and pulmonary C-fibers in dogs (143,144). The activation of pulmonary C fibers by prostaglandins was not attenuated by isoproterenol, suggesting that this event occurred independently of secondary changes in smooth muscle tone (143). Right atrial injection of PGF₂α stimulated pulmonary C-fiber activity, but was less effective than PGE₁ and PGE₂ (143).

Two analogs of PGH₂, an intermediary in prostanoid biosynthesis (146,147), called cyclic esters I and II, stimulated both RAR and bronchial C-fiber endings in dogs (148).

5-Hydroxytryptamine

Historically, stimulation of chemosensitive afferent nerve endings was often performed using phenyl diguanide (PDG). It is now apparent, however, that this agent, and the more potent analog phenyl biguanide (PBG), are in fact selective 5-HT₃ receptor agonists (149,150). Therefore, this section deals with the actions of 5-HT on airway afferent nerves, along with those evoked by PDG or PBG.

5-HT agonists have variable effects on RAR activation. When given intravenously to anesthetized dogs, 5-HT stimulated RARs in a manner that appeared to be independent of changes in lung mechanics (135). 5-HT-agonists also have been reported to stimulate airway RARs in rabbits (69) and cats (66), but have been found to be relatively ineffective in activating RARs in monkey (64).

PDG stimulates C-fiber activity in the airways. Indeed, the first extensive description of pulmonary C-fibers (deflation or J-receptors) was made by Paintal (14), who injected PDG into the right atrium. Since then, several other studies have demonstrated a stimulation of pulmonary and bronchial C-fibers by PDG or 5-HT (12–17, 92,140).

Bradykinin

Bradykinin has been found to have little effect on RAR activity in some studies (93,151,152), whereas in other studies stimulation of RAR activity was observed (78,152,153). The activation of RARs was attributed to secondary changes in lung compliance because the discharge of the RARs had a respiratory rhythm and were abolished by hyperinflation (78).

Bradykinin stimulates bronchial C-fibers (78,151,152) and, in higher concentrations, some pulmonary C-fibers (78). *In vitro* single fiber recording from guinea pig tracheal afferents demonstrated that bradykinin activates C-fibers by B₂ receptor stimulation (93).

Activation by Miscellaneous Inhalants

Cigarette smoke in the lungs stimulates RARs (71, 154,155). Nicotine contributes to this response inasmuch as the responses of RARs to high nicotine cigarettes is greater than low nicotine cigarettes (154,155). Moreover, injection of nicotine also stimulates these same nerve endings (155). The actions of cigarette smoke on RARs can be enhanced by pulmonary congestion (155,156).

Cigarette smoke also stimulates pulmonary C-fibers (14,157). Nicotine, as with RAR activation, appears to play a major role in the activation of airway C-fibers by cigarette smoke. Thus, nicotine inhalation mimicked the effect of a single breath of a high-nicotine content cigarette on C-fiber activity (158). Also, high nicotine cigarettes stimulated but low nicotine cigarettes were a weak stimulus for C-fiber stimulation (154) and hexamethonium, a nicotinic receptor antagonist, significantly attenuated the reflex changes in breathing patterns, presumably induced by activation of pulmonary C-fibers by cigarette smoke (157). The activation of C-fibers by cigarette smoke is not blocked by isoproterenol, suggesting that it is unrelated to bronchoconstriction (157).

Carbon dioxide (CO_2) is a relatively ineffective stimulus for afferent fibers in the tracheobronchial tree. As a rule, in fact, myelinated bronchopulmonary afferents are inhibited by increasing CO_2 concentrations (159–162). C-fibers, on the other hand, can be activated by CO_2. Increasing PCO_2 from 19 to 30 mm Hg caused a slight elevation in the discharge from bronchial C-fibers (163). Likewise, Delpierre and colleagues (140) found that a fivefold increase in end-tidal CO_2 concentration caused a doubling of the firing rate of bronchopulmonary C-fibers in the cat airways. Decreasing oxygen concentration did not stimulate C-fibers.

Inhalation of ozone caused activation of bronchial C-fibers independently of secondary changes in lung mechanics, as evidenced by a different time frame of activation compared with falls in lung compliance (164). Pulmonary C-fibers were weakly stimulated by ozone (164). Ozone does not appear to directly stimulate RARs or SARs (164).

Sulphur dioxide (SO_2) causes reflex cholinergic bronchoconstriction, suggesting that it activates airway afferent fibers, and this effect is blocked by cooling the vagus nerve (165,166). Widdicombe noted that SO_2 activated airway afferent fibers located in the mediastinum, but found it to have little effect on RAR and SAR activity (10).

Ammonia vapor, acetone, ether, and alcohol have been reported to stimulate RAR activity (54,64–67). In addition, ether, chloroform, and trichloroethylene stimulated pulmonary C-fibers (15).

Capsaicin

Capsaicin is commonly used to activate visceral and somatic sensory C-fibers (167,168). Capsaicin was shown to evoke a pulmonary chemoreflex characterized by bradycardia, systemic hypotension, and apnea (169–171). This effect initially was attributed to stimulation of baroreceptors located in the pulmonary artery (170), although later investigations revealed that slowly conducting pulmonary endings (C-fibers) within the airways mediated these effects (77). Since these early studies, capsaicin has been viewed as a relatively selective stimulant of C-fiber endings (167,168). Capsaicin effectively activates pulmonary and bronchial C-fibers in several species (12,54,77,92,93). It cannot be considered a specific C-fiber stimulant, however, because there also are reports of a stimulatory effect of capsaicin on RARs, albeit at higher concentrations (66,131).

NEUROMODULATION

Many substances present in the asthmatic airway may modulate the sensitivity of the afferent neurons. This supports the speculation that analogies may be drawn between certain components of the asthma condition and the hyperalgesia associated with inflammation in other tissues (172). The most compelling examples of neuromodulation are observed in experiments in which an inflammatory mediator fails to overtly stimulate action potentials, but influences the electrical membrane properties of the nerve endings such that the nerve discharges action potentials to stimuli that were previously subthreshold (173,174). Afferent fibers that fail to respond even to noxious rotation of a joint, for example, respond to simple flexion after experimental arthritis (175–179). In a similar fashion, afferent fibers that are silent to mechanical distention of the bladder respond to

relatively modest distention pressures after induction of inflammation (180).

It should be mentioned that, in other systems, tissue injury and inflammation have been found to increase in afferent excitability not only at the level of the peripheral endings, but also at the level of the central nervous system. Thus, the classic studies of Sir Thomas Lewis and colleagues regarding the large zone of hyperalgesia after local skin injuries may be due in part to changes in synaptic transmission in the spinal cord (181,182). It is reasonable to speculate that airway inflammation may have substantive effects on the excitability of synaptic transmission in the central nervous system. To our knowledge this is an unstudied area, however, so this review will focus on neuromodulation of the peripheral afferent neurons.

Electrophysiologic Studies

There is little known at the subcellular level about how airway afferent endings transduce the relevant stimulus to frequency-coded action potentials. Based on a large body of knowledge gained from studies of other systems, however, certain fundamental concepts have emerged that are likely to be shared by airway afferents. The stimulus to the afferent ending is transduced, presumably via the opening or closing of ion channels, at a specialized site of the endings (receptive site) into a membrane depolarization (183,184). This change in potential, referred to as a generator potential, is a nonpropagated potential. If the generator potential is of sufficient magnitude, the initiation of a propagated action potential "spike" occurs. The action potential, unlike the generator potential, is driven by the opening of voltage-sensitive sodium channels and thus can be blocked by tetrodotoxin or local anesthetics. In some afferent fibers the site of the generator potential formation and spike initiation are anatomically distinct sites (183,184). The anatomic arrangement of the generator initiation site and the spike initiation site in airway afferents are unknown.

Afferent endings encode the intensity of the stimulus using a frequency code (185). As a rule, there is a graded increase in spike frequency when the stimulus intensity increases. Typically, the discharge frequency is proportional to the $\log_{10}$ of the stimulus intensity. This relationship has been studied in some detail for the crayfish stretch receptor (186) and the photoreceptor of the horseshoe crab (187). In these systems the logarithmic function occurs at the transducer stage. Thus, the generator potential amplitude is a function of the $\log_{10}$ of the stimulus intensity; the discharge frequency is linearly related to the generator potential amplitude.

Airway inflammation can lead to an increase in excitability of airway afferent endings by decreasing the stimulus threshold for spike discharge, increasing the discharge frequency, or by decreasing the adaptation process.

TABLE 2. *Effects of autacoids on some electrophysiologic properties of vagal sensory neurons*

Autacoid	Resting potential	Resistance	AHP$_{fast}$	AHP$_{slow}$	Reference
Serotonin	Depolarize	Decrease	No effect	Inhibit	190,191,193,195,216
Histamine	Depolarize	Increase	No effect	No effect	193,216
Bradykinin	Depolarize	Increase	No effect	Inhibit	193,199,216,217
Prostacyclin	Depolarize	Increase	No effect	Inhibit	193,199
Prostaglandin D$_2$	Depolarize	Increase	No effect	Inhibit	193,196,198
Prostaglandin E$_2$	Depolarize	Increase	No effect	Inhibit	193,198
Thromboxane	No effect	No effect	No effect	No effect	193
Prostaglandin F$_{2\alpha}$	No effect	No effect	No effect	No effect	193,198
Leukotriene C$_4$	Depolarize	Increase	No effect	Inhibit	193
Nicotinic agonist	Depolarize	Decrease	No effect	No effect	195,216

Summary of reported effects on electrophysiologic properties of somal membranes of neurons in vagal sensory ganglia. Not all neurons in the ganglia respond in a consistent fashion; the result reported is the most typical response. Some of the heterogeneity within a ganglia may reflect the different types of neurons represented. For example, serotonin effectively depolarizes C cells, but has relatively little effect on A cells in the rabbit nodose ganglia (195). There are noted species differences in the response to autacoids. For example, whereas prostaglandin D$_2$ potently inhibits the AHP$_{slow}$ in rabbit sensory neurons (196,198), it is without effect on guinea pig nodose neurons (193).

AHP, afterspike hyperpolarization.

Inflammatory mediators may influence each of these steps by altering the ion flow through channels in the membranes of the afferent endings. The peripheral terminals of airway afferent fibers are inaccessible via conventional intra-axonal recording techniques. There is, therefore, no direct information about the characteristics of the ion channels specifically in that portion of the afferent membrane responsible for the generator potential. The membrane properties of cell bodies of the airway afferent neurons, however, can be studied easily using conventional electrophysiologic techniques. Studies on sensory somata have revealed an effect of various inflammatory mediators on ion currents that would be consistent with increasing afferent neuronal excitability (Table 2).

Stimulus Threshold

In a recent study, the mechanical sensitivity of rapidly adapting Aδ-fibers in tracheae isolated from control and immunologically sensitized guinea pigs was examined (Fig. 3) (188). Exposing the tracheae isolated from sensitized guinea pigs to relevant antigen resulted in mast cell activation and inflammatory mediator release (189). Using this model, antigen challenge caused an approximately fourfold decrease in the amount of mechanical force required to initiate action potential formation in single Aδ fibers. Exposing tracheae from nonsensitized animals to the antigen was without effect. The ionic mechanism responsible for decreases in stimulus threshold may be

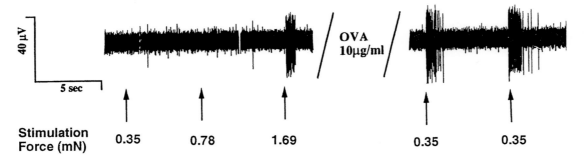

FIG. 3. Antigen-induced increase in mechanical sensitivity of guinea pig tracheal afferent fibers. Representative trace of the effects of ovalbumin (OVA) exposure on mechanical thresholds of single airway-afferent nerve endings from guinea pigs passively sensitized to ovalbumin 24 hours previously. Mechanical responsiveness of the nerve endings before and after ovalbumin was quantified using von Frey filaments, which are calibrated to exert a fixed amount of force. Before ovalbumin exposure, the ending failed to respond to von Frey filaments exerting 0.35 and 0.78 mN of force but was activated by a filament of 1.69 mN. A supramaximal concentration of ovalbumin (10 μg/mL) was then perfused selectively over the airways for 10 min. After ovalbumin exposure, the mechanical threshold of the nerve ending was reduced, responding to a von Frey filament exerting 0.35 mN of force. These data demonstrate that exposing airway afferent nerves to relevant antigen can cause an increase in mechanical responsiveness. Although not illustrated, ovalbumin rarely evoked action potential discharge (1 out of 36).

complex. By increasing the current through channels responsible for the generator potential, inflammatory mediators may increase the amplitude of the generator potential for a given stimulus intensity. This would have the effect of decreasing the stimulus threshold for spike initiation. Serotonin, for example, has been found to depolarize the membrane of vagal sensory neurons by decreasing the membrane resistance to current flow (190–193). Inhibiting resting potassium current may lead to a decrease in spike threshold by causing an ohmic increase in the depolarization for a given level of ionic current across the membrane. Antigenic activation of mast cells or application of inflammatory mediators such as histamine, bradykinin, prostacyclin, prostaglandin D_2 and E_2, and cysteinyl leukotrienes has been found to depolarize the membrane potential of vagal sensory neurons by increasing the resistance to current flow, presumably by inhibiting ion flow through potassium channels (193,194). Inflammatory mediators also may decrease the stimulus threshold in an indirect fashion by affecting the extraneuronal tissue. Edema, for example, may increase the pressure on a mechanically sensitive ending for any given change in lung volume (16).

Discharge Frequency

Modulation of ionic currents that leads to an increase in generator potential amplitude may not only decrease stimulus threshold, as discussed above, but also would be expected to increase the peak discharge frequency. Active membrane properties also may influence stimulation frequency. In virtually all vagal afferent neurons studied, the spike is followed by a brief hyperpolarization of the membrane (193,195,196). This so-called fast afterspike hyperpolarization (AHP_{fast}) is due to a calcium-activated potassium current and may serve to regulate the refractory period of the neuron (196). In a subset of vagal afferent neurons there is another, more slowly developing and long-lasting AHP (AHP_{slow}), that can profoundly affect discharge frequency of visceral afferent neurons (193,195–198). It is perhaps noteworthy to mention in a discussion on neuromodulation that although few mediators seem to affect the AHP_{fast}, several mediators inhibit the AHP_{slow} (see Table 2). The AHP_{slow} in guinea pig nodose neurons can be inhibited by antigenic activation of mast cells, prostacylin, and cysteinyl leukotrienes (193,194). Bradykinin appears to inhibit the AHP_{slow} in these neurons indirectly by stimulating the production of prostacylin (199). In rabbit nodose neurons the AHP_{slow} also is inhibited by low concentrations of PGE_2 and PGD_2 (196).

Single-unit recording of airway afferent fibers have revealed an effect of inflammatory mediators on discharge frequency. Histamine aerosol caused an increase in the peak frequency discharge of C-fibers in dog airways in response to either static lung inflation or capsaicin ad-

ministration (139). In these experiments histamine had no significant effect on baseline action potential activity in the airway C-fibers, but caused greater than a 70% increase in the capsaicin-induced and static lung inflation-induced action potential discharge frequency. In a similar fashion, Zhang and Bonham (155) noted that cigarette smoke increased inspiratory-related firing frequency of RARs. In preliminary studies, Fox and colleagues (200) noted that although prostacylin and platelet-activating factor fail to evoke action potentials in C-fibers in the guinea pig isolated trachea preparation, they increase the discharge frequency elicited by bradykinin.

Adaptation

Inflammation may modulate afferent activity by altering the rate at which the fiber adapts to the stimulus. Extraneural mechanisms may contribute to the adaptation response. For example, a constant mechanical stimulus of a pacinian corpuscle results in a generator potential that rapidly adapts back to resting membrane potential (201). When a constant mechanical stimulus is applied to a denuded pacinian corpuscle in which the extraneuronal capsular lamella has been removed, the generator potential adapts at a much slower rate (201). In addition, using cellular photography techniques, Hubbard (202) demonstrated that during maintained compression of the inner lamellae (i.e., nearest the nerve terminal) of the pacinian corpuscle, there was a transient displacement of these structures followed by a return to their resting state, an event that coincided with the initiation and decay of the generator potential. Thus, it is possible that inflammation may influence adaptation to mechanical stimulation as a consequence of changes in the viscoelastic properties of the airways.

Adaptation also may be regulated electrophysiologically by influencing passive and active electrical properties of the membrane. The ionic mechanisms underlying the adaptation of a generator potential in response to a constant stimulus are not known. It is likely, however, that voltage-dependent rectifying or repolarizing currents are activated during the membrane depolarization. Typically, the adaptation in afferent fibers is based on extracellular recording of action potential discharge. In this case the adaptation may occur at a step beyond the generator potential at the level of action potential generation. As mentioned above, inflammatory mediators may influence adaptation rates by blocking the afterspike hyperpolarizations (193,198). An example of a decrease in the rate of accommodation evoked by an inflammatory mediator can be seen in the work of Lee and Morton (Fig. 4) (139). They found that the spike discharge of a mechanically sensitive C-fiber in response to static lung inflation persists for a longer period of time (adapted more slowly) after dogs were exposed to a histamine aerosol.

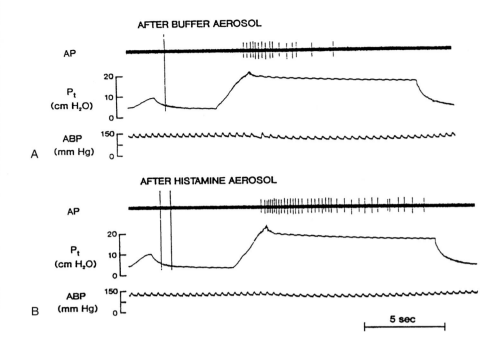

FIG. 4. Representative illustration of the response of a pulmonary C-fiber to static lung inflations 2–5 min after inhalation of buffer (**A**) or histamine (5 breaths, 1% solution; **B**) in anesthetized dogs. In each panel, *upper trace* represents the action potential discharge of a single C-fiber (*AP*), *inner trace* illustrates the tracheal pressure (P_t), and *lower trace* demonstrates the recording of arterial blood pressure (*ABP*). As the lungs were inflated (reflected by an increase in P_t), there was action potential discharge after exposure to buffer (A) and histamine (B) aerosols. There were, however, significantly more action potentials generated for a longer period of time after histamine challenge. These data demonstrate enhanced responsiveness of pulmonary C-fibers to mechanical stimulation after inhalation of histamine aerosol. (Adapted from Lee L-Y, Morton RF. Histamine enhances pulmonary C-fiber responses to capsaicin and lung inflation. *Resp Physiol* 1993;93:83–96.)

Reflex Studies

Electrophysiologic studies predict that certain inflammatory mediators that fail to evoke reflex responses in the airways nevertheless may potentiate the reflex induced by afferent activators. Although there is relatively little work done in this area, studies have demonstrated that both axon-reflex and central reflexes are potentiated in the airways by inflammation.

The release of tachykinins that contribute to the axon reflex in airways often is studied using the guinea pig isolated bronchus preparation. As described elsewhere in this volume, electrical stimulation of the tachykinergic fibers results in an easily quantified bronchial smooth muscle contraction. With this model it was found that a threshold level of antigen augmented the electrically evoked release of tachykinins (203). Inflammatory mediators that appear to be effective in potentiating electrically evoked tachykinin release include histamine (203), cysteinyl leukotrienes (204), and bradykinin (205).

Inflammation may enhance the excitability of afferent fibers leading to an enhancement of central reflex activity. Histamine, for example, has been used to stimulate central reflex activity in guinea pigs (206). A component of the bronchoconstrictor response elicited by histamine in guinea pigs was inhibited by muscarinic receptor antagonists and thus thought to be mediated by central reflex activity. The remaining component of the bronchoconstriction was thought to be due to the direct effect of histamine on bronchial smooth muscle (206). Exposing immunologically sensitized guinea pigs to antigen caused a substantial potentiation in the cholinergic component of the hist-

amine-induced bronchoconstriction (206). The direct component was only marginally affected (206). These findings are consistent with the hypothesis that endogenous autacoids increase the excitability of afferent endings in the airways, resulting in an increased cholinergic reflex activity. Cysteinyl-leukotrienes should be considered as possible candidates for such actions because they are produced during the allergic response and they have been found to potentiate the reflex component of histamine-induced bronchoconstriction (207).

The nose is a useful site to study airway reflex activity in humans. Central reflex activity can be evaluated in the nose by selectively applying a stimulus to one nostril and quantifying the reflex cholinergic response in the contralateral nostril. This model has been used to demonstrate that seasonally allergic persons studied during the relevant allergy season have a significant cholinergic reflex secretory response to bradykinin, whereas when the same individuals are studied out of season, bradykinin fails to evoke reflex cholinergic responses (208). Perennial allergic individuals, who by definition are constantly symptomatic, also display reflex glandular secretion in comparison with nonallergic individuals (208–210). Similar findings are obtained when the stimulus is endothelin (211). In addition to enhanced cholinergic reflexes, a sneezing response to nasal application of bradykinin (208) and endothelin (211) was uncovered during the relevant allergen season. It is tempting to speculate that exposure to allergens results in the production of neuromodulatory autacoids that increase the excitability of nasal afferent fibers. Thus, bradykinin may have caused subthreshold generator potentials in nasal fibers when studied out of season, which became suprathreshold as a result of nasal inflammation.

Neuromodulation by inflammation often is studied in humans with so-called psychophysical experiments. In these studies, the subject quantifies a sensation (most often pain) before and after the application of an autacoid or after an inflammatory insult. This is difficult to assess in the airways because the vast majority of afferent fibers are not sensory fibers in the true sense of the word. Stimulation of airway afferent fibers results in activity in the central nervous system below the level of consciousness. A quantifiable indicator of sensory nerve activation in the airways, however, is cough. Stimulation of rapidly adapting myelinated fibers (and perhaps C-fibers) in the larynx and larger airways results in an irritant sensation that leads to the cough reflex (1,94). It has been found experimentally that patients with upper respiratory viral infections are more sensitive to the tussive effects of citric acid and acetylcholine (115,212). In a similar vein, Mitsuhashi and colleagues (213) found that the cough response to acetic acid was heightened in asthmatic patients. It should be noted that the concept that asthma is associated with an enhanced sensitivity to tussive stimuli is not categorically true. Some studies have found no difference between asthmatic and healthy volunteers with respect to their cough response to citric acid (117,118).

The mechanism by which the cough response is enhanced in certain asthmatics or in patients with upper respiratory tract infections is unknown. It is possible that infection and inflammation lead to a breakdown in the epithelial barrier of the airways, leading to an increase in the accessibility of the afferent endings to inhaled irritants. It is also possible, however, that the neuromodulation of cough fibers by inflammatory mediators contributes to the heightened cough response. Indeed, Choudry and co-workers (214) found that inhalation of PGE_2, but not histamine or bradykinin, caused an increased cough response in persons subsequently exposed to inhaled capsaicin. Similarly, Stone and colleagues (215) demonstrated an enhanced cough response to capsaicin after inhalation of PGE_2 and $PGF_{2\alpha}$, whereas the cough response to inhaled low chloride solution (0.15 M sodium bicarbonate) was enhanced solely by $PGF_{2\alpha}$.

CONCLUSIONS

Afferent nerve fibers represent the majority of neurons innervating the airways. The afferent neurons respond to specific changes in their environment. The response to the environmental change is transmitted to the central nervous system in a "digital" frequency code via propagated action potentials. Through this general mechanism, the airway afferent fibers play a central role in airway defense and homeostasis.

There are many types of afferent fibers in the airways and it is difficult (if not impossible) to devise a clever, unambiguous classification scheme. Typically, the neurons are characterized based on the nature of the stimulus to which they respond, the characteristics of the response to the stimulus, and/or the velocity at which they conduct action potentials along their axon. Activators of airway afferent fibers include changes in mechanical force, osmolarity, changes in pH, carbon dioxide concentration, and various autacoids. The ultimate consequence of afferent stimulation is reflex activity that includes sneezing, coughing, changes in autonomic drive, and alteration in the depth and pattern of breathing.

The immune and nervous systems act in an integrated fashion to defend the airways from noxious substances. Considering the immune and nervous systems as integrated units may be useful in shedding light on the pathophysiology of asthma. On the one hand, immunologic aspects of inflammation, via the production and release of neuromodulatory mediators, can lead to an increase in the excitability of airway afferent neurons, whereas, on the other hand, activation of a subset of afferent fibers may result in axon reflexes that directly contribute to the inflammatory response. Without additional research, however, it remains unproductive to speculate about precise mechanisms by which afferent nerve fiber activation contributes to asthma pathophysiology.

REFERENCES

1. Widdicombe JG, Wells UM. Vagal reflexes. In: Raeburn D, Giembycz M, eds. *Airways smooth muscle: innervation and neurotransmission.* Basel: Birkhauser Verlag, 1994;279–307.
2. Coleridge HM, Coleridge JCG, Schultz HD. Afferent pathways involved in reflex regulation of airway smooth muscle. *Pharmacol Ther* 1989;42:1–63.
3. Coleridge HM, Coleridge JCG. Pulmonary reflexes: Neural mechanisms of pulmonary defense. *Annu Rev Physiol* 1994;56:69–91.
4. Langley JN. *The autonomic nervous system.* Cambridge: W. Heffer & Sons, Ltd, 1921.
5. Kuntz A. *The autonomic nervous system.* Philadelphia: Lea & Febiger, 1953.
6. Gaskell WH. *The involuntary nervous system.* London: Longmans, Green, and Co., 1916.
7. Dale HH. A survey of present knowledge of the chemical regulation of certain functions by natural constituents of the tissues. *Bull Johns Hopkins Hosp* 1933;53:297–347.
8. Adrian ED. Afferent impulses in the vagus and their effect on respiration. *J Physiol* 1933;79:332–358.
9. Davis HL, Fowler WS, Lambert EH. Effect of volume and rate of inflation and deflation on transpulmonary pressure and response of pulmonary stretch receptors. *Am J Physiol* 1956;187:558–566.
10. Widdicombe JG. Receptors in the trachea and bronchi of the cat. *J Physiol* 1954;123:71–104.
11. Knowlton GC, Larrabee MG. A unitary analysis of pulmonary volume receptors. *Am J Physiol* 1946;147:100–114.
12. Coleridge HM, Coleridge JCG. Impulse activity in afferent vagal C-fibers with endings in the intrapulmonary airways of dogs. *Resp Physiol* 1977;29:125–142.
13. Coleridge JCG, Coleridge HM. Afferent vagal C fiber innervation of the lungs and airways and its functional significance. *Rev Physiol Biochem Pharmacol* 1984;99:1–110.

14. Paintal AS. Impulses in vagal afferent fibres from specific pulmonary deflation receptors. The response of these receptors to phenyl diguanide, potato starch, 5-hydroxytryptamine and nicotine, and their role in respiratory and cardiovascular reflexes. *Q J Exp Physiol* 1955; 40:89–111.

15. Paintal AS. The location and excitation of pulmonary deflation receptors by chemical substances. *Q J Exp Physiol* 1957;42:56–71.

16. Paintal AS. Mechanism of stimulation of type J pulmonary receptors. *J Physiol* 1969;203:511–532.

17. Paintal AS. Vagal sensory receptors and their reflex effects. *Physiol Rev* 1973;53(1):159–227.

18. Agostini E, Chinnock JE, De Burgh Daly M, Murray JG. Functional and histological studies of the vagus nerve and its branches to the heart, lungs and abdominal viscera in the cat. *J Physiol* 1957;135: 182–205.

19. Kostreva DR, Zuperku EJ, Hess GL, Coon RL, Kampine JP. Pulmonary afferent activity recorded from sympathetic nerves. *J Appl Physiol* 1975;39(1):37–40.

20. Holmes R, Torrance RW. Afferent fibers of the stellate ganglion. *Q J Exp Physiol* 1959;44:271–281.

21. Springall DR, Cadieux A, Oliveira H, Su H, Royston D, Polak JM. Retrograde tracing shows that CGRP-immunoreactive nerves of rat trachea and lung originate from vagal and dorsal root ganglia. *J Auton Nerv Syst* 1987;20:155–166.

22. Kummer W, Fischer A, Kurkowski R, Heym C. The sensory and sympathetic innervation of guinea-pig lung and trachea as studied by retrograde neuronal tracing and double-labelling immunohistochemistry. *Neuroscience* 1992;49(3):715–737.

23. Dalsgaard C-J, Lundberg JM. Evidence for a spinal afferent innervation of the guinea pig lower respiratory tract as studied by the horseradish peroxidase technique. *Neurosci Lett* 1984;45:117–122.

24. Altman J, Bayer SA. Development of the cranial nerve ganglia and related nuclei in the rat. *Adv Anat Embryol Cell Biol.* 1982;74:1–90.

25. Adelman HB. The development of the neural folds and cranial ganglia of the rat. *J Comp Neurol* 1925;39:19–172.

26. Lundberg JM, Martling C-R, Hökfelt T. (1988). Airways, oral cavity and salivary glands: classical transmitters and peptides in sensory and autonomic motor neurons. In: Björklund A, Hökfelt T, Owman C, eds. *Handbook of chemical neuroanatomy.* Amsterdam: Elsevier, 1988;6: 391–444.

27. Maggi CA, Giachetti A, Dey RD, Said SI. Neuropeptides as regulators of airway function: Vasoactive intestinal peptide and the tachykinins. *Physiol Rev* 1995;75(2):277–322.

28. Barnes PJ, Baraniuk JN, Belvisi MG. Neuropeptides in the respiratory tract. *Am Rev Respir Dis* 1991;144 (pt I, 5):1187–1198.

29. Barnes PJ, Baraniuk JN, Belvisi MG. Neuropeptides in the respiratory tract. *Am Rev Respir Dis* 1991;144 (pt II, 6):1391–1399.

30. Fischer A, Mayer B, Kummer W. Nitric oxide synthase in vagal sensory and sympathetic neurons innervating the guinea-pig trachea. *J Auton Nerv Syst* 1996;56:157–160.

31. Andres KH, von Düring M. Morphology of cutaneous receptors. In: Iggo A, ed. *Handbook of sensory physiology: somatosensory system.* Berlin, Heidelberg, New York: Springer-Verlag, 1973;1–28.

32. Schmidt RF. Somatosensory sensibility. In: Schmidt RF, ed. *Fundamentals of sensory physiology.* Berlin, Heidelberg, New York: Springer-Verlag, 1985;30–67.

33. Quilliam TA, Sato M. The distribution of myelin on nerve fibres from pacinian corpuscles. *J Physiol* 1955;129:167–176.

34. Cauna N, Mannan G. The structure of human digital pacinian corpuscles (Corpuscula lamellosa) and its functional significance. *J Anat* 1958;92:1–20.

35. Baluk P, Gabella G. Afferent nerve endings in the tracheal muscle of guinea pigs and rats. *Anat Embryol* 1991;183:81–87.

36. Yamamoto Y, Hayashi M, Atoji Y, Suzuki Y. Vagal afferent nerve endings in the trachealis muscle of the dog. *Arch Histol Cytol* 1994;57(5):473–480.

37. Larsell O. Nerve terminations in the lung of the rabbit. *J Comp Neurol* 1921;33:105–131.

38. Larsell O, Dow RS. The innervation of the human lung. *Am J Anat* 1933;52:125–146.

39. Elftman AG. The afferent and parasympathetic innervation of the lungs and trachea of the dog. *Am J Anat* 1943;72:1–27.

40. Fischer AWF. The intrinsic innervation of the trachea. *J Anat* 1964; 98(1):117–124.

41. Honjin R. On the nerve supply of the lung of the mouse, with special reference to the structure of the peripheral vegetative nervous system. *J Comp Neurol* 1956;105:587–625.

42. Krauhs JM. Morphology of presumptive slowly adapting receptors in dog trachea. *Anat Rec* 1984;210:73–85.

43. Bartlett DJ Jr, Jeffery P, Sant'Ambrogio G, Wise JCM. Location of stretch receptors in the trachea and bronchi of the dog. *J Physiol* 1976;258:409–420.

44. Miserocchi G, Mortola, J, Sant'Ambrogio G. Localization of pulmonary stretch receptors in the airways of the dog. *J Physiol* 1973;235:775–782.

45. Sant'Ambrogio G. Nervous receptors of the tracheobronchial tree. *Annu Rev Physiol* 1987;49:611–627.

46. Miserocchi G, Sant'Ambrogio G. Distribution of pulmonary stretch receptors in the intrapulmonary airways of the dog. *Resp Physiol* 1974;21:71–75.

47. Byers MR. Sensory innervation of peridontal ligament of rat molars consist of unencapsulated Ruffini-like mechanoreceptors and free nerve endings. *J Comp Neurol* 1985;231:500–518.

48. Maeda T, Sato O, Kobayashi S, Iwanaga T, Fujita T. The ultrastructure of Ruffini endings in the peridontal ligament of rat incisors with special reference to the terminal Schwann cells (K-cells). *Anat Rec* 1989; 223:95–103.

49. Sato O, Maeda T, Kannari K, Kawahara I, Iwanaga T, Takano Y. Innervation of the peridontal ligament in the dog with special reference to the morphology of Ruffini endings. *Arch Histol Cytol* 1992;55(1): 21–30.

50. Erlanger J, Gasser HS. The compound nature of the action current of nerve as disclosed by the cathode ray oscillograph. *Am J Physiol* 1924;70:624–666.

51. Canning BJ, Undem BJ. Evidence that distinct neural pathways mediate parasympathetic contractions and relaxations of guinea-pig trachealis. *J Physiol* 1993;471:25–40.

52. Baluk P, Gabella G. Innervation of the guinea pig trachea: A quantitative morphological study of intrinsic neurons and extrinsic nerves. *J Comp Neurol* 1989;285:117–132.

53. Adrian E D. The impulses produced by sensory nerve endings. *J Physiol* 1926;61:49–72.

54. Bergren DR, Peterson DF. Identification of vagal sensory receptors in the rat lung: are there subtypes of slowly adapting receptors? *J Physiol* 1993;464:681–698.

55. Sant'Ambrogio G, Mortola JP. Behaviour of slowly adapting stretch receptors in the extrathoracic trachea of the dog. *Resp Physiol* 1977;31:377–385.

56. Widdicombe JG. The site of pulmonary stretch receptors in the cat. *J Physiol* 1954;125:336–351.

57. Gaylor JB. The intrinsic nervous mechanism of the human lung. *Brain* 1934;57:143–160.

58. Clark FJ, von Euler C. On the regulation of depth and rate of breathing. *J Physiol* 1972;222:267–295.

59. Widdicombe JG. Regulation of tracheobronchial smooth muscle. *Physiol Rev* 1963;43(1):1–37.

60. Widdicombe JG, Nadel JA. Reflex effects of lung inflation on tracheal volume. *J Appl Physiol* 1963;18:681–686.

61. McKean TA. A linear approximation of the transfer function of pulmonary mechanoreceptors of the frog. *J Appl Physiol* 1969;27(6): 775–781.

62. Mortola J, Sant'Ambrogio G, Clement MG. Localization of irritant receptors in the airways of the dog. *Resp Physiol* 1975;24:107–114.

63. Paintal AS. The conduction velocities of respiratory and cardiovascular afferent fibres in the vagus nerve. *J Physiol* 1953;121:341–359.

64. Ravi K, Singh M, Julka DB. Properties of rapidly adapting receptors of the airways in monkeys (*Macaca mulatta*). *Resp Physiol* 1995;99: 51–62.

65. Bergren DR, Sampson SR. Characterization of intrapulmonary, rapidly adapting receptors of guinea pigs. *Resp Physiol* 1982;47: 83–95.

66. Armstrong DJ, Luck JC. A comparative study of irritant and type J receptors in the cat. *Resp Physiol* 1974;21:47–60.

67. Sampson SR, Vidruk EH. Properties of "irritant" receptors in canine lung. *Resp Physiol* 1975;25:9–22.

68. Sellick H, Widdicombe JG. The activity of lung irritant receptors during pneumothorax, hyperpnoea and pulmonary vascular congestion. *J Physiol* 1969;203:359–381.

69. Mills JE, Sellick H, Widdicombe JG. Activity of lung irritant receptors in pulmonary microembolism, anaphylaxis and drug-induced bronchoconstrictions. *J Physiol* 1969;203:337–357.

70. Mills JE, Widdicombe JG. Role of the vagus nerves in anaphylaxis and histamine-induced bronchoconstrictions in guinea-pigs. *Br J Pharmacol* 1970;39:724–731.

71. Sellick H, Widdicombe J. Stimulation of lung irritant receptors by cigarette smoke, carbon dust, and histamine aerosol. *J Appl Physiol* 1971;31(1):15–19.

72. Coleridge HM, Coleridge JCG. Reflexes evoked from the tracheobronchial tree and lungs. In: Cherniack NS, Widdicombe JG eds. *Handbook of physiology, 3. The respiratory system, vol II, control of breathing*. Bethesda: American Physiological Society, 1986;395–429.

73. Jonzon A, Pisarri TE, Coleridge JCG, Coleridge HM. Rapidly adapting receptor activity in dogs is inversely related to lung compliance. *J Appl Physiol* 1986;61(5):1980–1987.

74. Yu J, Coleridge JCG, Coleridge HM. Influence of lung stiffness on rapidly adapting receptors in rabbits and cats. *Resp Physiol* 1987;68:161–176.

75. Glogowska M, Richardson PS, Widdicombe JG, Winning AJ. The role of the vagus nerves, peripheral chemoreceptors and other afferent pathways in the genesis of augmented breaths in cats and rabbits. *Resp Physiol* 1972;16:179–196.

76. Coleridge JCG, Coleridge HM. Functional role of pulmonary rapidly adapting receptors and lung C fibers. In: Lahiri S, Forster RE II, Davies RO, Pack AI, eds. *Chemoreceptors and reflexes in breathing: cellular and molecular aspects*. New York: Oxford University Press, 1989;287–298.

77. Coleridge HM, Coleridge JCG, Luck JC. Pulmonary afferent fibers of small diameter stimulated by capsaicin and by hyperinflation of the lungs. *J Physiol* 1965;179:248–262.

78. Coleridge HM, Coleridge, JCG, Roberts AM. Rapid shallow breathing evoked by selective stimulation of airway C fibers in dogs. *J Physiol* 1983;340:415–433.

79. Jammes Y, Mei N. Assessment of the pulmonary origin of bronchoconstrictor vagal tone. *J Physiol* 1979;291:305–316.

80. Mitchell RA, Herbert DA, Baker DG. Inspiratory rhythm in airway smooth muscle tone. *J Appl Physiol* 1985;58(3):911–920.

81. Roberts AM, Coleridge HM, Coleridge JCG. Reciprocal action of pulmonary vagal afferents on tracheal smooth muscle tension in dogs. *Resp Physiol* 1988;72:35–46.

82. Bonhoeffer K, Kolatat T. Drukvolumendiagramm und Dehnungsreceptoren der froschlunge. *Pflügers Arch* 1958;265:477–484.

83. Taglietti V, Casella C. Stretch receptors stimulation in frog's lungs. *Pflügers Arch* 1966;292:297–308.

84. Kaufman MP, Iwamoto GA, Ashton JH, Cassidy SS. Responses to inflation of vagal afferents with endings in the lung of dogs. *Circ Res* 1982;51:525–531.

85. Pack AI, DeLaney RG. Response of pulmonary rapidly adapting receptors during lung inflation. *J Appl Physiol* 1983;55(3):955–963.

86. Pack AI, Ogilvie MD, Davies RO, Galante RY. Responses of pulmonary stretch receptors during ramp inflations of the lung. *J Appl Physiol* 1986;61(1):344–352.

87. Richardson CA, Herbert DA, Mitchell R. Modulation of pulmonary stretch receptors and airway resistance by parasympathetic efferents. *J Appl Physiol* 1984;57(6):1842–1849.

88. Marshall R, Widdicombe JG. The activity of pulmonary stretch receptors during congestion of the lungs. *Q J Exp Med* 1958;43:320–330.

89. Roberts AM, Bhattacharya J, Schultz HD, Coleridge HM, Coleridge JCG. Stimulation of pulmonary vagal afferent C-fibers by lung edema in dogs. *Circ Res* 1986;58:512–522.

90. Hargreaves M, Ravi K, Kappagoda CT. Responses of slowly and rapidly adapting receptors in the airways of rabbits to changes in the Starling forces. *J Physiol* 1991;432:81–97.

91. Ravi K, Kappagoda CT. Responses of pulmonary C-fibre and rapidly adapting receptor afferents to pulmonary congestion and edema in dogs. *Can J Physiol Pharmacol* 1992;70:68–76.

92. Anand A, Paintal AS, Whitteridge D. Mechanisms underlying enhanced responses of J receptors of cats to excitants in pulmonary oedema. *J Physiol* 1993;471:535–547.

93. Fox AJ, Barnes PJ, Urban L, Dray A. An *in vitro* study on the properties of single vagal afferents innervating guinea-pig airways. *J Physiol* 1993;469:21–35.

94. Karlsson J-A, Sant'Ambrogio G, Widdicombe J. Afferent neural pathways in cough and reflex bronchoconstriction. *J Appl Physiol* 1988;65(3):1007–1023.

95. Godden DJ, Borland C, Lowry R, Higgenbottam TW. Chemical specificity of coughing in man. *Clin Sci* 1986;70:301–306.

96. Eschenbacher WL, Boushey HA, Sheppard D. Alteration in osmolarity of inhaled aerosols cause bronchoconstriction and cough, but absence of a permeant anion causes cough alone. *Am Rev Respir Dis* 1984;129:211–215.

97. Sheppard D, Rizk NW, Boushey HA, Bethel RA. Mechanism of cough and bronchoconstriction induced by distilled water aerosol. *Am Rev Respir Dis* 1983;127:691–694.

98. Tsubone H, Sant'Ambrogio G, Anderson JW, Orani G. Laryngeal afferent activity and reflexes in the guinea pig. *Resp Physiol* 1991;86:215–231.

99. Anderson JW, Sant'Ambrogio FB, Mathew OP, Sant'Ambrogio G. Water-responsive laryngeal receptors in the dog are not specialized endings. *Resp Physiol* 1990;79:33–44.

100. Boushey HA, Richardson PS, Widdicombe JG, Wise JCM. The response of laryngeal afferent fibres to mechanical and chemical stimuli. *J Physiol* 1974;240:153–175.

101. Boggs DF, Bartlett DJ Jr. Chemical specificity of a laryngeal apneic reflex in puppies. *J Appl Physiol* 1982;53(2):455–462.

102. Lee B-P, Sant'Ambrogio G, Sant'Ambrogio FB. Afferent innervation and receptors of the canine extrathoracic trachea. *Resp Physiol* 1992;90:55–65.

103. Pisarri TE, Jonzon A, Coleridge HM, Coleridge JCG. Vagal afferent and reflex responses to changes in surface osmolarity in lower airways of dogs. *J Appl Physiol* 1992;73(6):2305–2313.

104. Fox AJ, Barnes PJ, Dray A. Stimulation of guinea-pig tracheal afferent fibres by nonisosmotic and low-chloride stimuli and the effect of frusemide. *J Physiol* 1995;482:179–187.

105. Pisarri TE, Jonzon A, Coleridge HM, Coleridge JCG. Intravenous injection of hypertonic NaCl solution stimulates pulmonary C-fibers in dogs. *Am J Physiol* 1991;260:H1522–H1530.

106. Morris CE. Mechanosensitive ion channels. *J Membrane Biol* 1990;113:93–107.

107. McCarty DJ, Phelps MDP, Pyenson J. Crystal-induced inflammation in canine joints. I. An experimental model with quantification of the host response. *J Exp Med* 1966;124:99–114.

108. Joseph NR, Reed I, Homberger E. An *in vivo* study of the pH of synovial fluid in dogs. *Am J Physiol* 1946;146:1–11.

109. Cummings NA, Nordby GL. Measurement of synovial fluid pH in normal and arthritic knees. *Arthritis Rheumatol* 1966;9:47.

110. Allott CP, Evans DP, Marshall PW. A model of irritant-induced bronchoconstriction in the spontaneously breathing guinea pig. *Br J Pharmacol* 1980;71:165–168.

111. Clay TP, Thompson MA. Irritant-induced cough as a model of intrapulmonary airway reactivity. *Lung* 1985;163:183–191.

112. Laude EA, Higgins KS, Morice AH. A comparative study on the effects of citric acid, capsaicin and resiniferotoxin on the cough challenge in guinea pig and man. *Pulm Pharmacol* 1993;6:171–175.

113. Forsberg K, Karlsson JA, Theodorsson E, Lundberg JM, Persson CGA. Cough and bronchoconstriction mediated by capsaicin-sensitive sensory neurons in the guinea-pig. *Pulm Pharmacol* 1988;1:33–39.

114. Silson JE. A new method for evaluating antitussive medications using the citric acid challenge technique. *J New Drugs* 1965;5:94–101.

115. Empey DW, Laitenen LA, Jacobs L, Gold WM, Nadel JA. Mechanisms of bronchial hyperreactivity in normal subjects after upper respiratory tract infection. *Am Rev Respir Dis* 1976;113:131–139.

116. Tatar M, Sant'Ambrogio G, Sant'Ambrogio FB. Laryngeal and tracheobronchial cough in anesthetized dogs. *J Appl Physiol* 1994;76:2672–2679.

117. Bickerman HA, Barach AL. The experimental production of cough in human subjects induced by citric acid aerosols. Preliminary studies on the evaluation of antitussive agents. *Am J Med Sci* 1954;228:156–163.

118. Pounsford JC, Birch MJ, Saunders KB. Effect of bronchodilators on the cough response to inhaled citric acid in normal and asthmatics subjects. *Thorax* 1985;40:662–667.

119. Steen KH, Reeh PW, Anton F, Handwerker HO. Protons selectively induce lasting excitation and sensitization to mechanical stimulation of nociceptors in rat skin, *in vitro*. *J Neuroscience* 1992;12:86–95.

120. Belmonte C, Gallar J, Pozo MA, Rebollo I. Excitation by irritant chemical substances of sensory afferent units in the cat's cornea. *J Physiol* 1991;437:709–725.

121. Stahl GL, Longhurst JC. Ischemically sensitive visceral afferents: importance of H+ derived from lactic acid and hypercapnia. *Am J Physiol* 1992;262:H748–H753.

122. Fox AJ, Urban L, Barnes PJ, Dray A. Effects of capsazepine against capsaicin- and proton-evoked excitation of single airway C-fibers and vagus nerve from the guinea-pig. *Neuroscience* 1995;67:741–752.

123. Lou Y-P, Lundberg JM. Inhibition of low pH evoked activation of airway sensory nerves by capsazepine, a novel capsaicin-receptor antagonist. *Biochem Biophys Res Comm* 1992;189(1):537–544.

124. Satoh H, Lou Y-P, Lundberg JM. Inhibitory effects of capsazepine and SR 48968 on citric acid-induced bronchoconstriction in guinea-pigs. *Eur J Pharmacol* 1993;236:367–372.

125. Bevan S, Forbes CA, Winter J. Protons and capsaicin activate the same ion channels in rat isolated dorsal root ganglion neurones. *J Physiol* 1993;459:401P.

126. Bevan S, Rang HP, Shah K. Capsazepine does not block the proton-induced activation of rat sensory neurones. *Br J Pharmacol* 1992;107:235.

127. Widdicombe JG. Sensory innervation of the lungs and airways. *Progress in Brain Research*, 1986;67:49–64.

128. Matsumoto S, Shimizu T, Kanno T, Yamasaki M, Nagayama T. Effects of histamine on slowly adapting pulmonary stretch receptor activities in vagotomized rabbits. *Jpn J Physiol* 1990;40:737–752.

129. Matsumoto S, Yamasaki M, Kanno T, Nagayama T, Shimizu T. Effects of calcium channel and H_1-receptor blockers on the responses of slowly adapting pulmonary stretch receptors to histamine in vagotomized rabbits. *Lung* 1993;171:1–13.

130. Matsumoto S, Shimizu T. Effects of isoprenaline on the responses of slowly adapting pulmonary stretch receptors to reduced lung compliance and to administered histamine. *Neurosci Letts* 1994;172:47–50.

131. Mohammed SP, Higenbottam TW, Adcock JJ. Effects of aerosol-applied capsaicin, histamine and prostaglandin E_2 on airway sensory receptors of anaesthetized cats. *J Physiol* 1993;469:51–66.

132. Yu J, Roberts AM. Indirect effects of histamine on pulmonary rapidly adapting receptors in cats. *Resp Physiol* 1990;79:101–110.

133. Vidruk EH, Hahn HL, Nadel JA, Sampson SR. Mechanisms by which histamine stimulates rapidly adapting receptors in dog lungs. *J Appl Physiol* 1977;43(3):397–402.

134. Sampson SR. Sensory neurophysiology of airways. *Am Rev Respir Dis* 1977;115:107–115.

135. Dixon M, Jackson, DM, Richards IM. The effects of histamine, acetylcholine and 5-hydroxytryptamine on lung mechanics and irritant receptors in the dog. *J Physiol* 1979;287:393–403.

136. Sampson SR, Vidruk EH. The nature of the receptor mediating stimulant effects of histamine on rapidly adapting vagal afferents in the lungs. *J Physiol* 1979;287:509–518.

137. Ravi K, Teo KK, Kappagoda CT. Action of histamine on the rapidly adapting airway receptors in the dog. *Can J Physiol Pharmacol* 1989;67:1499–1505.

138. Bradley GW. Pulmonary receptor recording *in vitro. Acta Physiol Scand* 1974;91:427–429.

139. Lee L-Y, Morton, RF. Histamine enhances pulmonary C-fiber responses to capsaicin and lung inflation. *Resp Physiol* 1993;93:83–96.

140. Delpierre S, Grimaud CH, Jammes Y, Mei N. Changes in activity of vagal bronchopulmonary C fibres by chemical and physical stimuli in the cat. *J Physiol* 1981;316:61–74.

141. Herxheimer H, Roetscher I. Effects of prostaglandin E_1 on lung function in bronchial asthma. *Eur J Clin Pharmacol* 1971;3:123–125.

142. Kawakami Y, Uchiyama K, Irie T, Murao M. Evaluation of aerosols of prostaglandins E_1 and E_2 as bronchodilators. *Eur J Clin Pharmacol* 1973;6:127–132.

143. Coleridge HM, Coleridge JCG, Ginzel KH, Baker DG, Banzett RB, Morrison MA. Stimulation of "irritant" receptors and afferent C-fibers in the lungs by prostaglandins. *Nature* 1976;264:451–453.

144. Roberts AM, Schultz HD, Green JF, et al. Reflex tracheal contraction evoked in dogs by bronchodilator prostaglandins E_2 and I_2. *J Appl Physiol* 1985;58(6):1823–1831.

145. Karla W, Shams H, Orr JA, Scheid P. Effects of the thromboxane A_2 mimetic, U46,619, on pulmonary vagal afferents in the cat. *Resp Physiol* 1992;87:383–396.

146. Hamberg M, Samuelsson B. Detection and isolation of an endoperoxide intermediate in prostaglandin biosynthesis. *Proc Natl Acad Sci USA* 1973;70(3):899–903.

147. Hamberg M, Svensson J, Wakabayashi T, Samuelsson B. Isolation and structure of two prostaglandin endoperoxides that cause platelet aggregation. Proc Natl Acad Sci USA 1974;71(2):345–349.

148. Ginzel KH, Morrison MA, Baker DG, Coleridge HM, Coleridge JCG. Stimulation of afferent vagal endings in the intrapulmonary airways by prostaglandin endoperoxidase analogues. Prostaglandins 1978;15:131–138.

149. Ireland SJ, Tyers MB. Pharmacological characterization of 5-hydroxytryptamine-induced depolarization of the rat isolated vagus nerve. *Br J Pharmacol* 1987;90:229–238.

150. Kay IS, Armstrong DJ. Phenylbiguanide not phenyldiguanide is used to evoke the pulmonary chemoreflex in anaesthetized rabbits. *Exp Physiol* 1990;75:383–389.

151. Roberts AM, Kaufman MP, Baker DG, Brown JK, Coleridge HM, Coleridge JCG. Reflex tracheal contraction induced by stimulation of bronchial C-fibers in dogs. *J Appl Physiol* 1981;51:485–493.

152. Kaufman MP, Coleridge HM, Coleridge JCG, Baker DG. Bradykinin stimulates afferent vagal C-fibres in intrapulmonary airways of dogs. *J Appl Physiol* 1980;48(3):511–517.

153. Hargreaves M, Ravi K, Senaratne MPJ, Kappagoda CT. Responses of airway rapidly adapting receptors to bradykinin before and after administration of enalapril in rabbits. *Clin Sci* 1992;83:399–407.

154. Kou YR, Lee L-Y. Stimulation of rapidly adapting receptors in canine lungs by a single breath of cigarette smoke. *J Appl Physiol* 1990;68(3):1203–1210.

155. Zhang Z, Bonham AC. Lung congestion augments the responses of cells in the rapidly adapting pathway to cigarette smoke in rabbit. *J Physiol* 1995;484(1):189–200.

156. Ravi K, Kappagoda CT, Bonham AC. Pulmonary congestion enhances responses of lung rapidly adapting receptors to cigarette smoke in rabbit. *J Appl Physiol* 1994;77(6):2633–2640.

157. Lee L-Y, Morton RF. Hexamethonium aerosol prevents pulmonary reflexes induced by cigarette smoke in dogs. *Resp Physiol* 1986;66:303–314.

158. Kou YR, Frazier DT, Lee L-Y. The stimulatory effect of nicotine on vagal pulmonary C-fibers in dogs. *Resp Physiol* 1989;76:347–356.

159. Bystrzycka EK, Nail AB. CO_2 sensitivity of stretch receptors in the marsupial lung. *Respir Physiol* 1980;39: 111–119

160. Kunz AL Kawashiro T, Scheid P. Study of CO_2 sensitive vagal afferents in the cat lung. *Resp Physiol* 1976;27:347–355.

161. Sant'Ambrogio G, Miserocchi G, Mortola J. Transient responses of pulmonary stretch receptors in the dog to inhalation of carbon dioxide. *Resp Physiol* 1974;22:191–197.

162. Mustafa MEKY, Purves MJ. The effect of CO_2 upon discharge from slowly adapting stretch receptors in the lungs of rabbits. *Resp Physiol* 1972;16:197–212.

163. Coleridge HM, Coleridge JCG, Banzett RB. Effect of CO_2 on afferent vagal endings in the canine lung. *Resp Physiol* 1978;34:135–151.

164. Coleridge JCG, Coleridge HM, Schelegle ES, Green JF. Acute inhalation of ozone stimulates bronchial C-fibers and rapidly adapting receptors in dogs. *J Appl Physiol* 1993;74(5):2345–2352.

165. Nadel JA, Salem H, Tamplin B, Tokiwa Y. Mechanism of bronchoconstriction during inhalation of sulfur dioxide. *J Appl Physiol* 1965;20(1):164–167.

166. Coleridge JCG, Coleridge HM. Lower respiratory tract afferents stimulated by inhaled irritants. *Am Rev Respir Dis* 1985;131(suppl):s51–s54.

167. Maggi CA. The pharmacology of the efferent function of sensory nerves. *J Auton Pharmacol* 1991;11:173–208.

168. Holzer P. Capsaicin cellular targets, mechanisms of action, and selectivity for thin sensory neurons. *Pharmacol Rev* 1991;43(2):143–201.

169. Toh CC, Lee TS, Kiang AK. The pharmacological actions of capsaicin and analogues. *Br J Pharmacol* 1955;10:175–182.

170. Porszasz J, Such G, Porszasz-Gibiszer K. Circulatory and respiratory chemoreflexes. I. Analysis of the site of action and receptor types of capsaicine. *Acta Physiol Acad Sci Hung* 1957;12:189–205.

171. Coleridge HM, Coleridge JCG, Kidd C. Role of pulmonary arterial baroreceptors in the effects produced by capsaicin in the dog. *J Physiol* 1964;170:272–285.

172. Adcock JJ, Garland LG. The contribution of sensory reflexes and "hyperalgesia" to airway hyperresponsiveness. In: Page CP, Gardiner PJ,

eds. *Airway hyperresponsiveness—is it really important for asthma?* Blackwell Scientific Press, 1993;234–255.

173. Cervero F. Sensory innervation of the viscera: peripheral basis of visceral pain. *Physiol Rev* 1994;74(1):95–138.

174. Rang HP, Bevan S, Dray A. Chemical activation of nociceptive peripheral neurons. *Br Med Bull* 1991;47(3):534–548.

175. Schaible H-G, Schmidt RF. Responses of fine medial articular nerve afferents to passive movements of knee joint. *J Neurophysiol* 1983; 49(5):1118–1126.

176. Schaible H-G, Schmidt RF. Effects of an experimental arthritis on the sensory properties of fine articular afferent units. *J Neurophysiol* 1985;54(5):1109–1122.

177. Schaible H-G, Schmidt RF. Time course of mechanosensitivity changes in articular afferents during a developing experimental arthritis. *J Neurophysiol* 1988;60:2180–2195.

178. Coggeshall RE, Hong KAP, Langford LA, Schaible H-G, Schmidt RF. Discharge characteristics of fine medial articular afferents at rest and during passive movements of inflamed knee joints. *Brain Res* 1983; 272:185–188.

179. Grigg P, Schaible H-G, Schmidt RF. Mechanical sensitivity of group III and IV afferents from posterior articular nerve in normal and inflamed cat knee. *J Neurophysiol* 1986;55(4):635–643.

180. Häbler H-J, Jänig W, Koltzenburg M. Activation of unmyelinated afferent fibers by mechanical stimuli and inflammation of the urinary bladder in the cat. *J Physiol* 1990;425:545–562.

181. Woolf CJ. Evidence for a central component of post-injury pain hypersensitivity. *Nature* 1983;306:686–688.

182. Woolf CJ. A new strategy for the treatment of inflammatory pain. *Drugs* 1994;47 (suppl 5):1–9.

183. Patton HD. Receptor mechanism. In: Ruch TC, Patton HD, Woodbury JW, Towe AL, eds. *Neurophysiology*. Philadelphia: WB Saunders, 1968;95–112.

184. Fuortes MGF. Generation of responses in receptor. In: Autrum H, Jung R, Loewenstein WR, MacKay DM, Teuber HL. eds. *Handbook of sensory physiology; principles of receptor physiology*. New York: Springer-Verlag, 1971;243–268.

185. Adrian ED, Zotterman Y. The impulses produced by sensory nerve endings. Part 3. Impulses set up by touch and pressure. *J Physiol* 1926;61:465–483.

186. Terzuolo CA, Washizu Y. Relation between stimulus strength, generator potential and impulse frequency in stretch receptor of crustacea. *J Neurophysiol* 1962;25:56–66.

187. Fuortes MGF. Electric activity of cells in the eye of Limulus. *Am J Ophthal* 1958;46:210–223.

188. Riccio MM, Myers AC, Undem BJ. Immunomodulation of afferent neurons in guinea-pig isolated airway. *J Physiol* 1996;491: 499–509.

189. Undem BJ, Pickett WC, Adams GK. Antigen-induced sulfidopeptide leukotriene release from the guinea-pig perfused trachea. *Eur J Pharmacol* 1987;42:31–37.

190. Higashi H. 5-Hydroxytryptamine receptors on visceral primary afferent neurones in the nodose ganglion of the rabbit. *Nature* 1977; 267:448–450.

191. Higashi H, Nishi S. 5-Hydroxytryptamine receptors of visceral primary afferent neurones on rabbit nodose ganglia. *J Physiol* 1982;323: 543–567.

192. Christian EP, Taylor GE Weinreich D. Serotonin increases excitability of rabbit C-fiber neurons by two distinct mechanisms. *J Appl Physiol* 1989;67:584–591.

193. Undem BJ, Weinreich D. Electrophysiological properties and chemosensitivity of guinea pig nodose ganglion neurons *in vitro*. *J Auton Nervous Syst* 1993;44:17–34.

194. Undem BJ, Hubbard W, Weinreich D. Immunologically induced neuromodulation of guinea pig nodose ganglion neurons. *J Auton Nerv Syst* 1993;44:35–44.

195. Stansfield CE, Wallis DI. Properties of visceral primary afferent neu-

196. Fowler JC, Greene R, Weinreich D. Two calcium-sensitive spike afterhyperpolarizations in visceral sensory neurones of the rabbit. *J Physiol* 1985;365:59–75.

197. Higashi H, Morita K, North RA. Calcium-dependent after-potentials in visceral afferent neurones of the rabbit. *J Physiol* 1984;355:479–492.

198. Weinreich D, Wonderlin WF. Inhibition of calcium-dependent spike after-hyperpolarization increases excitability of rabbit visceral sensory neurones. *J Physiol* 1987;394:415–427.

199. Weinreich D, Koschorke GM, Undem BJ, Taylor GE. Prevention of the excitatory actions of bradykinin by inhibition of PGI_2 formation in nodose neurones of the guinea-pig. *J Physiol* 1995;483:735–746.

200. Fox AJ, Dray A, Barnes PJ. The activity of prostaglandins and platelet activating factor on single airway sensory fibres of the guinea-pig *in vitro*. *Am J Respir Crit Care Med* 1995;151(4):110.

201. Mendelson M, Loewenstein WR. Mechanism of receptor adaptation. *Science*, 1964;144:554–555.

202. Hubbard SJ. A study of rapid mechanical events in a mechanoreceptor. *J Physiol* 1958;141:198–218.

203. Ellis JL, Undem BJ. Antigen-induced enhancement of noncholinergic contractile responses to vagus nerve and electrical field stimulation in guinea pig isolated trachea. *J Pharmacol Exp Ther* 1992;262:646–653.

204. Ellis JL, Undem BJ. Role of peptidoleukotrienes in capsaicin-sensitive sensory fibre-mediated responses in guinea-pig airways. *J Physiol* 1991;436:469–484.

205. Miura M, Belvisi MG, Barnes PJ. Effect of bradykinin on airway neural responses *in vitro*. *J Appl Physiol* 1992;73:1537–1541.

206. Santing RE, Pasman Y, Olymulder CG, Roffel AF, Meurs H, Zaagsma J. Contribution of a cholinergic reflex mechanism to allergen-induced bronchial hyperreactivity in permanently instrumented, unrestrained guinea-pigs. *Br J Pharmacol* 1995;114:414–418.

207. Stewart AG, Thompson DC, Fennessy MR. Involvement of capsaicin-sensitive afferent neurones in a vagal-dependent interaction between leukotriene D_4 and histamine on bronchomotor tone. *Agents Actions* 1984;15:500–508.

208. Riccio MM, Proud D. Evidence that enhanced nasal reactivity to bradykinin in allergic individuals is mediated by neural reflexes. *J Allergy Clin Immunol* 1996;97:1252–1263.

209. Baraniuk JN, Silver PB, Kaliner MA, Barnes PJ. Perennial rhinitis subjects have altered vascular, glandular, and neural responses to bradykinin nasal provocation. *Int Arch Allergy Immunol* 1994;103: 202–208.

210. Baraniuk JN, Silver PB, Kaliner MA, Barnes PJ. Effects of ipratropium bromide on bradykinin nasal provocation in chronic allergic rhinitis. *Clin Exp Allergy* 1994;24:724–729.

211. Riccio MM, Reynolds CJ, Hay DW, Proud D. Effects of Intranasal administration of endothelin-1 to allergic and nonallergic individuals. *Am J Respir Crit Care Med* 1995;152:1757–1764.

212. Tiffeneau, R. The acetylcholine cough test. *Dis Chest* 1957;31: 404–422.

213. Mitsuhashi MH, Mochizuki K, Tokuyama K, Morikawa A, Kuroume T. Hyperresponsiveness of cough receptors in patients with bronchial asthma. *Pediatrics* 1985;75:855–858.

214. Choudry M, Fuller RW, Pride NB. Sensitivity of the human cough reflex: effect of inflammatory mediators Prostaglandin E_2, bradykinin and histamine. *Am Rev Respir Dis* 1989;140:137–141.

215. Stone R, Barnes PJ, Fuller RW. Contrasting effects of prostaglandins E_2 and $F_{2\alpha}$ on sensitivity of the human cough reflex. *J Appl Physiol* 1992;73:649–653.

216. Higashi H, Ueda N, Nishi S, Gallagher JP, Shinnick-Gallagher P. Chemoreceptors for serotonin (5-HT), acetylcholine (ACh), Bradykinin (BK), histamine (H) and γ-aminobutyric acid (GABA) on rabbit visceral afferent neurons. *Brain Res Bull* 1982;8:23–32.

217. Weinreich D. Bradykinin inhibits a slow spike afterhyperpolarization in visceral sensory neurons. *Eur J Pharmacol* 1986;132:61–63.

rons in the nodose ganglion of the rabbit. *J Neurophysiol* 1995;54(2): 245–260.

Asthma, edited by P.J. Barnes, M.M. Grunstein,
A.R. Leff, and A.J. Woolcock.
Lippincott–Raven Publishers, Philadelphia © 1997.

▪ 72 ▪

Bronchodilator Nerves

Maria G. Belvisi

<table>
<tr><td>

Inhibitory (Relaxant) Mechanisms
  Amphibians and Reptiles
  Birds
  Guinea Pig
  Rabbit
  Dog
  Cat
  Sheep
  Pig
  Cow
  Horse
  Nonhuman Primates
  Human
Tetrodotoxin-insensitive Relaxations
Adrenergic Mechanisms
  Sympathetic Innervation
  Indirect Effects of Sympathetic
    Nerves
  Circulating Catecholamines
  β-Adrenoceptor Function
  α-Adrenoceptor Function
NANC Mechanisms

</td><td>

Putative Transmitters
  Purines
  Vasoactive Intestinal Peptide
  Guinea Pig
  Cat
  Human
  Vasoactive Intestinal Peptide as a Neuromodulator
  Nitric Oxide
  Nitric Oxide Synthases
  Nitric Oxide as a Neurotransmitter
  Nitric Oxide as the i-NANC Transmitter in the Airways
  Guinea Pig
  Cat
  Pig
  Rabbit
  Horse
  Ferret
  Human
  Distribution of NANC Responses in the Respiratory
    Tract
  Functional Significance of the i-NANC Response
  NANC Inhibitory Pathways in Disease

</td></tr>
</table>

Autonomic nerves regulate several aspects of airway function including the control of airway smooth muscle tone (1). Neural control of airway smooth muscle is complex because, in addition to cholinergic and adrenergic innervation, there is a nonadrenergic noncholinergic (NANC) innervation. The existence of an NANC nervous system in the gastrointestinal tract, which controls gut motility, sphincters, and secretions, had previously been established in vertebrates from fish to humans (2). The airways develop embryologically from the foregut, so the existence of NANC nerves in the respiratory tract was not an unexpected finding.

On the whole, most experiments in the literature describing patterns of innervation in the airways have centered on developing *in vitro* systems of measuring smooth muscle relaxation. In this manner the effects of electrical field stimulation (EFS), which stimulates all nerves in a preparation, on isometric tension development by the trachealis or bronchial smooth muscle have been determined in the presence and absence of various drugs. From these experiments it was elucidated that the smooth muscle of mammalian airways receives a dual contractile and relaxant innervation (3,4). In general, neural relaxation of airway smooth muscle is achieved via activation of adrenergic and NANC neural pathways (5). However, the

M.G. Belvisi: Department of Thoracic Medicine, Imperial College of Medicine at the National Heart and Lung Institute, London SW3 6LY United Kingdom.

sympathetic innervation to airway smooth muscle is species-dependent and may be sparse or even absent (6). Moreover, in humans, sympathetic nerves innervate bronchial blood vessels, submucosal glands, and parasympathetic ganglia, and there are few, if any, nerve fibers supplying the airways smooth muscle (7). Therefore, at least in human airways, the major neural bronchodilator pathway is the NANC system. Because changes in bronchial smooth muscle tone can occur rapidly in inflammatory airway diseases such as asthma, it has been suggested that this could be due to a defect in the autonomic control of the airways smooth muscle (8). This could manifest itself as an increase in the constrictor and a decrease in the dilator control of the airways. Therefore, if the NANC dilator innervation is dysfunctional in inflammatory conditions, its absence may lead to exaggerated bronchoconstriction (4).

Studies in animals have provided valuable information on the neural control of the respiratory tract; many of these studies have taken place on dogs, cats, and rodents, with few studies performed on human airways until the last few years. These experiments have highlighted an obvious variability in the innervation of the lung among species of animals, and any extrapolation between species in terms of either their physiologic responses or the anatomic distribution of the nerves should be viewed with caution. In this chapter I will illustrate the intraspecies and regional differences in the relaxant innervation and the possible physiologic and morphologic changes that may be seen in the relaxant innervation to the respiratory tract under pathophysiologic conditions.

INHIBITORY (RELAXANT) MECHANISMS

Amphibians and Reptiles

The first studies investigating the inhibitory bronchodilator neural system in the lung were carried out in amphibians and reptiles (9,10). The lungs of the lizard and the toad have been studied using pharmacologic and histochemical techniques. These studies provided evidence that suggested the existence of an inhibitory system with preganglionic fibers present in the vagus and ganglion cells within the lung. In contrast with other species, it seems that the predominant inhibitory pathway in the lizard was the adrenergic fibers because norepinephrine evoked bronchodilation and adrenergic blocking agents significantly reduced, but did not abolish, nerve-mediated relaxation (10). This residual response was later confirmed to be nonadrenergic in nature because it was not blocked in tissues pretreated with 6-hydroxydopamine (11–13). In addition, morphologic studies in amphibians demonstrated the existence of large opaque vesicles (80–200 nm in diameter) within autonomic nerve terminals in the respiratory tract suggestive of the NANC inhibitory system (11).

Birds

Most studies on the neural innervation in birds have been carried out on the domestic chicken. Physiologic studies have been carried out on the major bronchus of the chicken in vitro. Electrical field stimulation (EFS) of this preparation in vitro elicited a primary response that was relaxant in nature. However, although adrenergic agonists, either administered to the animal (14) or added to airway smooth muscle in vitro, evoked relaxations, ultrastructural studies have failed to demonstrate axon profiles characteristic of adrenergic nerves (15). Furthermore, the relaxant response obtained in response to EFS was not blocked by propranolol (16). Interestingly, the chicken bronchus produced only a contraction (atropine-sensitive) when the muscle was relaxed before the EFS stimulus (16). Therefore, from these studies it was suggested that the major bronchus of the chicken is controlled by NANC inhibitory fibers that dominate the cholinergic constrictor response, a situation that is the reverse of that found in most species, including human (17).

After the above-mentioned studies on amphibians, reptiles, and birds, the presence of the NANC inhibitory system also was detected in mammalian airways, where it was first demonstrated in the guinea pig (18–22).

Guinea pig

The guinea pig has been used extensively in pharmacologic studies involving the mechanisms contributing to neural relaxation of the airways. Most studies suggest that parasympathetic, adrenergic, and NANC nerves innervate guinea pig airway smooth muscle, with the cholinergic system being dominant. The adrenergic inhibitory nerves have been demonstrated physiologically to be more frequent in the proximal portions of the trachea (19). This has been confirmed by morphologic studies, which have demonstrated the proximal localization of the adrenergic nerves, and also showed a complete lack of adrenergic fibers in the distal airways (22). It was presumed that this lack of adrenergic dilator fibers in the distal airways would be compensated for by an increased NANC innervation to the lower airways, but functional data did not support this hypothesis. However, in contrast with the findings of Coburn and Tomita (19), other studies have shown that the relative contribution of the two inhibitory neural inputs to the total relaxation response appeared to be similar in all regions of the guinea pig trachea (23). Furthermore, this study also demonstrated that both adrenergic and NANC inhibitory responses were frequency-dependent and that adrenergic nerves were activated at lower frequencies than NANC nerves.

The first evidence to suggest the existence of NANC inhibitory nerves in guinea pig airways came from studies of electrical field–stimulated tracheal smooth muscle

(19,20,21,24). Coburn and Tomita (19) demonstrated a biphasic response to EFS that consisted of an initial contraction followed by a relaxation. The contractile response was prevented by atropine, whereas the relaxation response was not affected by muscarinic receptor antagonists and only partially inhibited by β-adrenoceptor blockade, with bretylium or by reserpine pretreatment, establishing the existence of a NANC response in this species. The existence of NANC inhibitory nerves in guinea pig trachea also were described in studies in which luminal pressure changes were measured in a tracheal tube preparation after transmural stimulation. Neurally evoked contractile responses were inhibited by atropine and inhibitory responses were reduced, but not abolished, by propranolol, guanethidine (adrenergic neurone blocker), or pretreatment of the animals with 6-hydroxydopamine (which depletes catecholamines). These relaxations were blocked by tetrodotoxin (TTX), indicating that these NANC responses were neural in origin (20,21).

Other investigators studied the inhibitory innervation of an *in situ* cervical tracheal tube preparation in which vagal and sympathetic nerves could be selectively stimulated. In addition, the preparation allowed for stimulation of the cervical trachea directly via transmural electrodes. These studies suggested that adrenergic relaxations (elicited via sympathetic nerve stimulation) accounted for 60% to 80% and NANC relaxations (elicited by vagal nerve stimulation) accounted for the residual (20–40%) of the relaxation response elicited via transmural stimulation (25). These data also confirmed an earlier study that suggested that the NANC inhibitory system in the guinea pig trachea receives preganglionic innervation from the vagus nerve (26). In contrast, other investigators found that the NANC nerves are the major inhibitory neural input to airway smooth muscle and that these responses were more evident at higher frequencies of stimulation (27). Importantly, the NANC relaxant response also has been demonstrated *in vivo* in this species (28).

The precise anatomic pathways of the NANC innervation have not been determined and there may be species differences. However, most information has been gathered from studies undertaken in guinea pig airways. The guinea pig trachea receives inhibitor/NANC (i-NANC) innervation from at least two extrinsic sources (29). These two vagal pathways that serve the rostral portion of the guinea pig trachea include a hexamethonium-sensitive relaxant innervation with preganglionic fibers carried by the recurrent laryngeal nerves and capsaicin-sensitive vagal pathways carried by the superior laryngeal nerves. These pathways traverse through ganglia associated with the esophagus (29). Autonomic neurones often contain multiple transmitter substances. This co-transmission probably is a mechanism via which nerves can achieve precise control over a target organ. This has given rise to the common assumption that the i-NANC transmitter substance is co-localized with acetylcholine (ACh) (and possibly vasoactive intestinal peptide) in postganglionic parasympathetic neurones. However, Canning and Undem (29) have suggested that the cholinergic contractile response and the i-NANC relaxation response of guinea pig trachea are differentially sensitive to esophageal removal. Therefore, it is now in doubt as to whether the i-NANC transmitter and ACh are in fact co-localized.

Rabbit

NANC relaxant responses, evoked by EFS, also can be demonstrated in rabbit tracheal smooth muscle but not in bronchial smooth muscle or lung parenchymal strips (30,31). In the same studies, rat tracheal smooth muscle did not exhibit NANC inhibitory responses to EFS.

Dog

Most studies in the dog have been carried out in isolated tracheal or bronchial strips *in vitro* in the presence and absence of adrenergic receptor antagonists. On the whole, these studies suggest that the principle inhibitory innervation in dog airways is adrenergic and that the NANC nerves are either absent or have no significant functional role in regulating airway tone in this species (32–34).

Cat

Neural relaxation responses have been demonstrated in isolated segments of cat trachea and bronchi precontracted with 5-hydroxytryptamine (5-HT; 35). These experiments suggested that both adrenergic and NANC nerves contributed to the relaxant response evoked by EFS. Moreover, experiments performed in the cat were among the first to demonstrate that the NANC inhibitory system could be demonstrated *in vivo* (36,37) by stimulation of efferent vagal nerves. This response can be inhibited by the ganglion blocker hexamethonium, indicating that nerves containing the NANC transmitter have a preganglionic parasympathetic origin (36). Inhalation of capsaicin or mechanical stimulation of the larynx induces a similar bronchodilator response in cats after pretreatment with atropine and propranolol, indicating that reflex activation of these pathways is possible (38,39).

Sheep

The autonomic innervation of sheep airway smooth muscle also has been studied by examining responses to EFS in isolated segments of the airway *in vitro* in the presence of adrenoceptor blockade. These studies suggested that sheep airways are innervated by both sympathetic and NANC inhibitory nerves, with the adrenergic nerve population being more pronounced in the trachea compared with the bronchi (40).

Pig

Initially, experimental evidence pointed to the absence of NANC nerves in porcine airways. In these experiments the ganglion stimulant, 1; 1-dimethyl-4-phenylpiperazine (DMPP), evoked frequency-related relaxations in the cat trachea *in vivo* that were blocked completely by propranolol. In addition, supramaximal bilateral vagal nerve stimulation failed to elicit airway smooth muscle relaxation after administration of propranolol (41). Therefore, these authors concluded that NANC inhibitory nerves are not present in porcine airways. However, more recently, NANC relaxation responses have been demonstrated after EFS in porcine tracheal smooth muscle (42).

Cow

In the bovine trachea, where there is little resting tone, it is difficult to demonstrate a neural inhibitory response in an already relaxed preparation. Therefore, experiments in which investigators have examined a NANC inhibitory response *in vitro* usually have used preparations that have high tone. In these experiments Cameron et al. (43) demonstrated the existence of NANC inhibitory nerves in isolated bovine trachea.

Horse

In equine tracheal smooth muscle that has been pretreated with indomethacin, atropine, and phentolamine, EFS evoked a frequency-dependent relaxation response (44). After the addition of propranolol to the tissue baths, EFS still caused a frequency-dependent relaxation but the magnitude of the relaxation was less at each frequency in the trachea. These observations suggest the presence of both sympathetic and NANC inhibitory innervation in trachea of horses with an equal importance of each inhibitory system at this level. This response was mainly limited to the trachea and central bronchi, with no detectable nerve supply to the peripheral bronchi (45). Interestingly, this response is absent in the third generation airways of horses with recurrent obstructive disease (heaves) (44).

Nonhuman Primates

The baboon (46) and rhesus monkey (47) also have an NANC inhibitory system as the major inhibitory pathway in the relaxation of airway smooth muscle. In this way primates are very similar to humans with cholinergic excitatory constrictor nerves and NANC inhibitory nerves

with no evidence for the existence of adrenergic nerves functioning in the control of airway smooth muscle tone. Therefore, because the pattern of innervation in nonhuman primates seems to be identical to that in humans, they may be the species of preference for studying any abnormalities. Previously, most investigators have studied neural control in the guinea pig that, in addition to the NANC system, also has an adrenergic system (48,49), or the dog, which lacks NANC innervation to the airway smooth muscle (33,50).

Human

The existence of an NANC system was first reported by Richardson and Béland (17). These workers demonstrated that EFS of isolated tracheal or bronchial strips evoked a biphasic response that consisted of a cholinergic contractile response and a relaxant response, in the presence of atropine, that was unaffected by propranolol and partially blocked by TTX. These findings were later confirmed by other workers (27,31,51,52). Moreover, these responses can be elicited in both large and small airways in humans down to an internal diameter of 0.5 mm (53,54). Furthermore, these NANC relaxant responses also have been described *in vivo* in human by reflex stimulation of the larynx (55–57). These studies involve stimulation of the laryngeal afferent pathways with capsaicin or mechanical irritation. Capsaicin inhalation induces a transient bronchoconstrictor response in normal subjects (58) but, after cholinergic inhibition with ipratropium bromide and β-adrenoceptor blockade with propranolol, capsaicin causes a bronchodilator response in the presence of increased bronchomotor tone induced by leukotriene D_4 (56). This bronchodilator response is transient (<2 min) and does not totally reverse the bronchoconstrictor effect of LTD_4. This is in contrast with studies in cats (36,59), in which the bronchodilator effect lasted for several minutes; this may suggest the involvement of different transmitter substances mediating the i-NANC response in the two species. This bronchodilator response appeared to be neural in origin as capsaicin-induced bronchodilator responses were blocked by local anesthesia of the airway mucosa (56). In similar experiments Ichinose et al. (57) demonstrated a bronchodilator response to capsaicin inhalation in normal subjects after muscarinic and β-adrenoceptor blockade in airways constricted with prostaglandin $F_2\alpha$. Again, this NANC dilator response appeared to be transient and, as described for cat airways, *in vivo* the response was blocked by hexamethonium. Interestingly, localization studies using fluorescence histochemical techniques have failed to reveal the presence of adrenergic nerves in tracheal or bronchial smooth muscle. Therefore, it seems that the NANC system provides the primary inhibitory control over human airways that, like baboon and monkey airways, seem to lack functional adrenergic innervation.

However, contradictory results have been obtained by Hutás et al. (60), who demonstrated that β-adrenoceptor blockade, without atropine, partially or completely blocked the neural relaxant response. These findings lead to the suggestion that the relaxant response before atropine was mainly due to the activation of adrenergic nerves and that NANC relaxation responses are evident only after muscarinic receptor blockade.

TETRODOTOXIN-INSENSITIVE RELAXATIONS

To determine whether responses obtained as a result of EFS are due to activation of neural or muscular structures, investigators rely on the ability of TTX, a fast sodium channel blocker, to selectively inhibit nerve conduction. However, TTX-resistant relaxation responses have been observed in response to EFS *in vitro* in many species (17,27,51,52). TTX-resistant responses have been reported in guinea pig (19), cat (35), and baboon (46) and appear to depend on the pulse duration of the stimulus. Interestingly, TTX-resistant relaxations are evoked most readily in species that possess only NANC inhibitory nerves. For example TTX-insensitive relaxation amounts to almost 30% of the maximal inhibitory response in baboon airways (46) and appears to be the major inhibitory response to EFS in human airways (27,51). In contrast, TTX abolished EFS-induced relaxation in dog airways that do not possess a NANC inhibitory innervation (33).

In human airways, frequency-dependent NANC relaxations have been detected in TTX-treated trachea (51) and bronchi (27) that were almost equal in magnitude to those seen in untreated tissues. More recently, Ward et al. (54) demonstrated a reduction in neural and nonneural i-NANC relaxation in distal regions of the human tracheobronchial tree. However, in this and other studies a nonneural component of the NANC response was evident only at higher stimulation frequencies (>5 Hz) in the human trachea (54,61) and bronchi (53).

The mechanism underlying TTX-insensitive relaxation is unclear. Richardson and Béland (17) suggested poor access of TTX to NANC nerve terminals. However, TTX completely abolished cholinergic responses, which may indicate that this is not the reason. Other investigators have suggested that these relaxations may be due to direct effects of EFS on smooth muscle membrane potentials (19), whereas Middendorf and Russell (46) suggested that nonneural mechanisms may involve mediator release from TTX-insensitive secondary cell types. However, all these proposed mechanisms for nonneural NANC relaxations in human airways are purely speculative and therefore require further investigation because TTX-insensitive NANC relaxations are a substantial part of the i-NANC response. More importantly, it is important to determine whether TTX-resistant NANC relaxations have any physiologically relevant role in the regulation of bronchomotor tone.

ADRENERGIC MECHANISMS

The adrenergic system in the airways encompasses the sympathetic nervous system and the adrenal medulla. Norepinephrine is the neurotransmitter of sympathetic nerves, whereas epinephrine is secreted by the adrenal medulla and may function as a circulating hormone to activate airway α- and β-adrenoceptors evoking smooth muscle relaxation.

Because epinephrine has long been used therapeutically for the treatment of acute severe asthma (62) and selective β2-adrenoceptor agonists remain the most effective and most widely prescribed bronchodilator drugs, it has been suggested that there might be a defect in adrenergic mechanisms in asthma.

Sympathetic innervation

Compared with the dominant parasympathetic nervous system that originates from the vagus nerve, the sympathetic innervation of the human lung is relatively minor. The sympathetic supply originates from the spinal cord in the ventral roots of thoracic segments T1-T6. Postganglionic fibers synapse in the middle and inferior cervical ganglia and in paravertebral ganglia of segments T1-T4. Postganglionic fibers run from the ganglia to the lung and enter at the hilum to form a close association with the cholinergic nerves that form a dense plexus around the vessels and airways (16). However, the content of norepinephrine in human lung is low when compared with other organs such as the heart, indicating that there are probably few sympathetic nerves (8). However, there seems to be considerable species differences in the sympathetic innervation of the airways. As indicated above, guinea pig, cat, and dog airways have considerable sympathetic innervation, whereas primates have a sparse sympathetic innervation of the airways (8). However, in human airways, adrenergic nerve fibers have been found in close association with submucosal glands and bronchial arteries with few, if any, fibers innervating airway smooth muscle (63). These results seem to correlate with functional studies that have demonstrated that neurally mediated relaxation evoked by EFS can be inhibited by β-antagonists in dogs and guinea pigs but not in human airways (8).

Further evidence against a functional sympathetic innervation to bronchial smooth muscle in humans *in vivo* has been obtained using the indirect sympathomimetic agent tyramine. This substance is known to act by releasing norepinephrine locally from sympathetic nerves. However, tyramine, when infused into normal subjects, has profound cardiovascular effects but has no bronchodilator effect in patients with mild asthma, even though the same patients responded to β2-adrenoceptor stimulation by salbutamol administered by the same route

(64). This suggests that sympathetic nerves do not influence the resting bronchomotor tone in humans.

Indirect Effects of Sympathetic Nerves

Although noradrenergic nerves do not directly control airways smooth tone, they may influence cholinergic neurotransmission via activation of prejunctional α- or β-adrenoceptors (1). In fact, even in species that lack a direct sympathetic supply to the airways smooth muscle, cholinergic and noradrenergic varicosities lie in close apposition, which has led to the suggestion that there may be cross-talk between both nervous systems (65). For example, the effect of sympathetic stimulation in dogs depends on the magnitude of vagal bronchomotor tone, suggesting that sympathetic nerves may have a modulatory influence on cholinergic neurotransmission (66).

Circulating Catecholamines

β-Agonists are potent relaxants of human airway smooth muscle *in vitro* (51) and without any direct functional sympathetic innervation circulating epinephrine may be the important endogenous ligand for activating adrenoceptors on airway smooth muscle. Studies in animals have demonstrated that β-adrenoceptor blockers potentiate bronchoconstrictor responses to histamine (67, 68) and to antigen in sensitized animals (69). This exaggerated constrictor response is most likely due to inhibition of circulating catecholamines that normally subserve a protective, bronchodilator role in the airways. Furthermore, circulating catecholamines also may act to combat the bronchial hyperreactivity characteristic of asthmatic airways, inasmuch as β-adrenoceptor blockers cause bronchoconstriction in asthmatic patients but not in normal subjects (70,71). One suggestion as to the mechanism behind this β-blocker-induced bronchoconstriction is that antagonism of the inhibitory action of circulating epinephrine on prejunctional β2-adrenoceptors on cholinergic nerves in human airways (72) results in increased airway tone that can be exacerbated in asthmatic airways because of a possible dysfunction of the muscarinic autoreceptors (73). The implication from these data is that the adrenergic drive to the airways is an important mechanism to counteract bronchoconstriction.

β-Adrenoceptor Function

β-Adrenoceptors have been localized to many cell types within the lung of many species, including humans (74–76). β-Receptors are found in the smooth muscle of all airways from trachea to bronchioles. This correlates with functional studies that describe a potent relaxant action of β-agonists on human airway smooth muscle at all

airway levels (51,77–80). Functional studies in canine airway smooth muscle *in vitro* have demonstrated that relaxation in response to exogenous β-agonists is mediated by β2-receptors, whereas relaxation to sympathetic nerve stimulation is mediated by β1-receptors (81). Experiments like this have led to the hypothesis that β1-receptors are regulated by sympathetic nerves ("innervated receptors"), whereas β2-receptors are regulated by circulating epinephrine ("hormonal receptors").

Functional studies *in vitro* have suggested that relaxation of human central and peripheral airways is mediated only by β2-receptors (77,78). This is not an unexpected finding given the absence of significant sympathetic innervation to human airway smooth muscle. Furthermore, β1-receptor selective agonists have no bronchodilator function in asthmatic subjects despite significant cardiac effects (82). Interestingly, it has been suggested that β-receptors are abnormal in asthma. Thus, some studies have suggested that airways from patients who have died from asthma have an impaired relaxation in response to isoprenaline, suggesting a dysfunction of the β-adrenoceptor on the airway smooth muscle (83,84). However, surprisingly, autoradiographic studies have demonstrated an increase, rather than a decrease, in β-receptors on airway smooth muscle in these patients who have died from asthma (85). This inverse relationship between reduced responsiveness to isoprenaline and the number and affinity of β-receptors indicates that the dysfunction may be due to uncoupling of airway smooth muscle β-receptors in fatal asthma.

In addition to the direct relaxant action of catecholamines on β-receptors on airway smooth muscle, they also may activate β-receptors on parasympathetic nerve endings to modulate cholinergic neurotransmission and thereby reduce cholinergic constrictor responses. Many studies have provided evidence that activation of β-adrenoceptors on cholinergic nerve terminals can inhibit ACh release and thereby reduce constrictor responses evoked by cholinergic nerve stimulation. Generally, this conclusion has been based on indirect evidence obtained from mechanical experiments in which changes in airway smooth muscle tone were measured. Thus, β-adrenoceptor agonists inhibit nerve-induced contractions of canine (86–90) and human airway smooth muscle (72,91) after EFS of the parasympathetic supply more effectively than the tension generated by exogenous ACh. Although these data indicate that the preferential action of β-adrenoceptor agonists is to inhibit cholinergic neurotransmission, they are difficult to interpret unambiguously because β-adrenoceptor agonists also are potent relaxants of airways smooth muscle, making it difficult to differentiate a prejunctional inhibitory action of these compounds on ACh release from a direct suppressive effect at the level of the airway smooth muscle. Alternatively, other studies in guinea pig airways have demonstrated that the EC50 value for inhibition of nerve-induced contractions was similar to that obtained for the suppression of contractile responses evoked by exogenous ACh applied directly to the tissue, which may indicate that, in contrast with other species, isoprenaline inhibits EFS-induced contractile responses by interacting with β-adrenoceptors located postjunctionally on the airways smooth muscle (92–94).

The β-adrenoceptor subtype that modulates cholinergic neurotransmission is apparently species-dependent. Thus, whereas activation of $β_1$-receptors by norepinephrine or after EFS of the sympathetic nerves inhibits cholinergic contractile responses in canine airways (87), the selective $β_2$-agonist, procaterol, evokes the same response (89), suggesting that receptors of both the $β_1$- and $β_2$ subtype co-exist prejunctionally on the cholinergic nerves that innervate this species (90). In contrast, current evidence suggests that the inhibition of cholinergic neurotransmission in human airways is mediated solely via $β_2$-adrenoceptors (72,91). The discrepancies in prejunctional adrenoceptor subtype between species may be related to the catecholamine that is seen predominantly by the β-receptors. This interpretation would be consistent with the hypothesis that $β_1$-receptors are activated by norepinephrine released from noradrenergic nerves (which are abundant in canine airways), whereas $β_2$-receptors are activated by circulating epinephrine.

In some studies, the problem of obtaining indirect evidence from functional studies on the modulation of cholinergic neurotransmission has been circumvented by measuring directly the output of ACh after EFS of the parasympathetic supply. In canine trachea, for example, norepinephrine has no effect on ACh release evoked by EFS (95), whereas more recent experiments have demonstrated that activation of prejunctional β-adrenoceptors inhibits cholinergic neurotransmission in rat and guinea pig airways (96) (Fig. 1). Paradoxically, other studies have suggested that β-agonists facilitate rather than inhibit ACh release from airway parasympathetic nerves when transmitter output is measured directly from guinea pig (97) and equine trachea (98,99) (Fig. 1). However, these results were not predicted by functional experiments demonstrating the inhibitory effect of β-agonists on contractile responses evoked by endogenously released and exogenous ACh. The marked discrepancy between pre- and postjunctional measures of neurotransmitter release is surprising and indicates that despite the facilitation of neurotransmission, isoprenaline acts primarily at a postjunctional level to prevent contraction of airway smooth muscle, which masks the more subtle enhancement of ACh output. Alternatively, this paradox could reflect a modulatory action of isoprenaline on ACh release from nerves that synapse with effector cells other than the airway smooth muscle, such as submucosal glands and tracheobronchial vessels. However, the ability of β-adrenoceptor agonists to facilitate cholinergic neurotransmission in parasympathetic nerve endings is entirely consistent with what has already been in motor nerves (100,101).

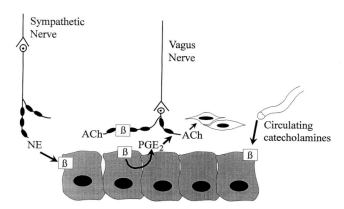

FIG. 1. Direct and indirect actions of β-adrenoceptor activation on acetylcholine (*ACh*) release and consequently cholinergic transmission in guinea pig trachea. In this manner the varicosities of postganglionic parasympathetic and sympathetic airway nerves are localized close to the airway mucosa and the airway smooth muscle. β-Adrenoceptors located on airway parasympathetic cholinergic nerve terminals can be activated by norepinephrine (*NE*) released from sympathetic nerves or circulating epinephrine resulting in an increase in ACh release. Alternatively, β-adrenoceptors located on the epithelium may be activated by neuronally released NE and by circulating catecholamines. Upon stimulation, prostaglandins are liberated from the epithelium, which can inhibit the release of ACh from cholinergic nerve terminals. (Adapted from Wessler I, Reinheimer T, Brunn G, Anderson GP, Maclagan J, Racké K. β-Adrenoceptors mediate inhibition of [³H]-acetylcholine release from the isolated rat and guinea-pig trachea: role of the airway mucosa and prostaglandins. *Br J Pharmacol* 1994;113:1221–1230.)

The finding that isoprenaline facilitated EFS-evoked ACh release from guinea pig trachea is in contrast with data recently reported by other investigators. In particular, Wessler et al. (96) found that isoprenaline inhibited, rather than enhanced, the EFS-induced output of ACh from parasympathetic nerves that innervate both rat and guinea pig airways. Significantly, however, the inhibition of neurotransmitter release by isoprenaline was not apparent in epithelium-denuded preparations or when cyclo-oxygenase was inhibited (96). Because β-adrenoceptor agonists enhance phospholipase A_2 activity in guinea pig lung (102,103) and generate PGD_2 and PGE_2 from airway epithelial cells, Wessler et al. (96) concluded that stimulation of β-adrenoceptors on airway epithelial cells leads to the liberation of prostanoids that then act to inhibit EFS-evoked ACh release (Fig. 1). This is a plausible theory and satisfactorily explains the differences between the two studies. Indeed, the inhibitory influence of endogenously released PGE_2 on the release of ACh is substantiated by another study that demonstrated that PGE_2 evoked a concentration-dependent inhibition of cholinergic neurotransmission from guinea pig trachea (105). These data also agree with data demonstrating an inhibitory action of PGE_2 on EFS-evoked ACh release (97) and on contractile responses evoked by EFS of cholinergic nerves in other species (104–109), although a direct inhibitory effect of PGE$_2$ on the smooth muscle also is likely to contribute to this response.

In contrast with the results obtained in guinea pig airways, isoprenaline failed to detectably affect EFS-evoked ACh release from human trachea even though it has been reported previously that EFS-induced cholinergic contractions are more potently inhibited by β-adrenoceptor agonists than are contractions evoked by exogenous ACh (72,91). The reason underlying the discrepancy between the mechanical and ACh release studies is unclear, but may simply reflect a lack of functional prejunctional β-adrenoceptors on parasympathetic nerves innervating human airways. Therefore, these data imply that changes in EFS-induced contractile responses in airways smooth muscle are an unreliable measure of neurotransmitter output. In addition, it is important to emphasize, however, that these data also could suggest that the methods employed to measure ACh release are not sufficiently sensitive to detect changes in neurotransmitter output in human airways.

α-Adrenoceptor Function

Relatively few α-adrenoceptors have been demonstrated in the lung. α-Receptors that mediate bronchoconstriction have been demonstrated in the airways of several species (110,111), although α-adrenergic responses can be demonstrated only under certain experimental conditions. For example, no α-adrenergic contraction can be demonstrated in canine airways *in vitro* unless there is a high degree of β-adrenergic blockade (112). In addition, if canine airways are pretreated with histamine or 5-HT, a marked contractile response to α-agonists or sympathetic nerve stimulation is found (111), suggesting that these mediators enhance α-adrenergic responsiveness.

In human airways there is considerable doubt as to the role of α-adrenoceptors in the regulation of tone and it has proved difficult to demonstrate their presence functionally or by autoradiography (113). Moreover, α-adrenoceptor–blocking drugs do not appear to be effective bronchodilator agents. However, it may be possible that the major role of α-receptors is not regulation of airway tone but control of airway blood flow.

NONADRENERGIC NONCHOLINERGIC MECHANISMS

The first conclusive evidence that pointed to the existence of a NANC relaxant response in airway smooth muscle came with the development of potent adrenergic receptor antagonists. Neural relaxation responses evoked by EFS in guinea pig trachea were not altered in the presence of the muscarinic antagonist atropine and were inhibited only partially by propranolol (19). This response had stimulus characteristics similar to NANC inhibitory

nerves described in other tissues such as the gut. Subsequently, NANC bronchodilator (i-NANC) responses have been demonstrated in airways smooth muscle *in vitro* by EFS in man, guinea pig cat, ferret, sheep, horse, mouse, cow, and pig (114). i-NANC relaxations also can be demonstrated *in situ* (25) or *in vivo* by electrical stimulation of the cervical vagus nerve (36,37) and by reflex stimulation of the larynx (55–57). The relaxant response is abolished by TTX and therefore is assumed to be neural in origin. In several species, both adrenergic and i-NANC pathways co-exist, but in human airways, the i-NANC response is the only neural bronchodilator mechanism (47). In contrast, the dog (32–34) and rat (30) airways appear to lack a functional i-NANC relaxant response. However, the neural relaxant response is not always consistent throughout the airways in either the density of innervation or receptor population (31). In human airways the i-NANC relaxant response is greatly reduced in the peripheral compared with central airways (4,54).

Although identification of the mediators of this i-NANC response has been the subject of much research, the identity of the putative neurotransmitter(s) has remained obscure until recently. Several candidates have been proposed to be mediators involved in the i-NANC response. γ-Aminobutyric acid (GABA), opiates, and the prostaglandins were thought to be unlikely candidates for the role of i-NANC transmitter. GABA failed to mimic the effects of nerve stimulation, and naloxone (opioid receptor antagonist) and indomethacin (an inhibitor of prostaglandin production) failed to reduce or abolish the inhibitory response in bovine trachea (43). More promising candidates have included adenosine-5-triphosphate (ATP), vasoactive intestinal peptide (VIP), and, more recently, nitric oxide (NO). The reason these specific mediators were investigated to assess their involvement in the i-NANC relaxant response in the airways was because they also have been implicated in NANC neural relaxation responses of the gastrointestinal and genitourinary tracts (115). This chapter discusses the evidence for and against the involvement of these mediators in neurally mediated relaxation of airways smooth muscle in a variety of species.

PUTATIVE NEUROTRANSMITTERS

Purines

Purines have been implicated as neurotransmitters in the gastrointestinal and genitourinary tracts. Evidence for a role of purines in i-NANC responses in the airways began with the observation that adenosine uptake-blocking drugs potentiated responses to adenosine, ATP, and the neural relaxant response in guinea pig trachea (21,116) and exogenous adenosine caused relaxation of guinea pig tracheal strips (30). In addition, adenosine deaminase, which breaks down adenosine, blocked both responses to exogenous adenosine and NANC relaxant effects in guinea pig airways (117).

However, in contrast, there also is evidence against a role for purines as mediators of the i-NANC relaxant response. Previous studies were unable to detect the large opaque vesicles that are thought to be characteristic of the nerve varicosities in purinergic nerves (43). Adenosine, aerosolized or injected, failed to alter the tonic bronchoconstriction in the cat in vivo (59). The purine uptake inhibitor, dipyridamole, failed to enhance the i-NANC relaxant response in guinea pig trachea (118), human bronchus (51), cat trachea (119), and cat airways in vivo (59) and bovine trachea (43). In addition, desensitization with adenosine failed to inhibit NANC relaxant responses in the cat trachea (119). More conclusive evidence using adenosine receptor antagonists indicates that purines may not play an important role in NANC relaxant responses. It has been demonstrated that adenosine receptor antagonists do not block the NANC relaxant response in vitro in guinea pig (118–122) and bovine trachea (43) and human trachea and bronchus (51). Moreover, adenosine receptor antagonists also were inactive against NANC bronchodilator responses in the cat in vivo (59). These data suggest that adenosine does not play a role in the NANC relaxation response in the airways.

Furthermore, ATP relaxes cat and guinea pig airway smooth muscle (24,119), although when ATP was administered to the cat in vivo no relaxation response was observed (59). On the contrary, reactive blue 2, the P2y receptor antagonist, had no effect on i-NANC relaxant responses in guinea pig (118) and human trachea (61), suggesting that ATP is not a mediator of the NANC relaxant response.

Vasoactive Intestinal Peptide

Vasoactive intestinal peptide (VIP) is a 28–amino acid peptide, with a wide distribution in the peripheral nervous system, that was among the first peptides to be detected in the respiratory tract (123). VIP-immunoreactive nerves are distributed widely throughout the respiratory tract. In the trachea and bronchi, VIP-containing nerve fibers are found in a subepithelial layer and in the submucosa. They occur around blood vessels, glandular acini, and within smooth muscle bundles (124–126). VIP-immunoreactive nerve fibers innervating airway smooth muscle have been demonstrated in many species including humans (5,124,125,127–133). VIP-immunoreactive fibers have been demonstrated in many species to originate from intrapulmonary ganglia (125,128,132, 134) and in some cases from nonnoradrenergic cell bodies in the stellate ganglion (133). However, surprisingly, there have been some reports that guinea pig tracheal ganglia do not contain VIP (133,135).

VIP is a potent relaxant of airways smooth muscle in vitro, an effect that is not altered by propranolol or indomethacin (52,61,119,136,137), although in some studies VIP produced little (51) or no (138) relaxant activity. In vivo, inhaled VIP is a bronchodilator and attenuates histamine-induced bronchoconstriction in animals (139). In humans inhaled VIP has no bronchodilator effect and provides only slight protection against histamine-induced bronchoconstriction, possibly because it is degraded by enzymes resident in the epithelium (140), although in one study VIP appeared to have a good bronchodilator effect when given by infusion to atopic asthmatic subjects (141).

Several lines of evidence have implicated VIP as a neurotransmitter of i-NANC bronchodilator nerves in the airways, but this seems to be species dependent (3,4). The first report that suggested VIP could be the NANC neurotransmitter in the airways was from the work of Matsuzaki et al. (142), who demonstrated a TTX-sensitive release of VIP from guinea pig trachea during EFS, the amount of which seemed to correlate with the magnitude of the relaxation evoked. Furthermore, preincubation of tissue with VIP antiserum reduced the i-NANC responses obtained, although in these studies the specificity of the antibodies used was not investigated. Moreover, VIP has been shown to stimulate cyclic adenosine 3'5'-monophosphate (cAMP) production in the guinea pig trachea (143) and similarly cAMP release has been documented during relaxation responses evoked by EFS in this tissue (142). Furthermore, VIP can mimic the i-NANC relaxant response in bovine tracheal smooth muscle, has been found in the tracheal smooth muscle in amounts similar to those reported for whole lung, and has been detected in the effluent during stimulation of i-NANC nerves in bovine trachea (43). However, the role of endogenously released VIP is uncertain because there are no potent and selective antagonists available. Two VIP antagonists have been described: [AC-Tyr^1, D-Phe^2]-GRF (1-29)-NH$_2$ was found to be a VIP antagonist in rat pancreatic membranes (144), and [4-Cl-D-Phe^6, Leu^{17}]-VIP, a VIP antagonist both of guinea pig pancreatic amylase secretion, and in colonic epithelial tumor cells (145). In contrast, these antagonists had no effect on i-NANC relaxation responses to EFS in guinea pig trachea in vitro and surprisingly they also were without effect on relaxation responses to VIP and peptide histidine isoleucine (PHI) (118).

Without a suitable antagonist for VIP, experiments have been performed to elucidate its role in neurotransmission using antibodies against VIP, desensitization of VIP receptors, and nonspecific peptidases such as α-chymotrypsin, which are known to degrade VIP. On the basis of experiments of this type, VIP has been suggested as a candidate for the role of the neurotransmitter involved in i-NANC bronchodilator responses in the airways of several species.

Guinea Pig

More recently, experiments have been performed with VIP antiserum; these produced approximately 50% reduction in the magnitude of the i-NANC response evoked by EFS in the guinea pig trachea (118,146), suggesting that VIP may be involved as a neurotransmitter of the i-NANC relaxant response in this species. In addition, several studies have investigated the effect of specific desensitization to VIP. Ellis and Farmer (118) found that the i-NANC response in guinea pig trachea was reduced by about 40%; these data agreed with studies involving desensitization of responses to VIP in the *in situ* guinea pig tracheal pouch preparation (147). However, even after desensitization or pretreatment of tissues with VIP antibody, a major component of the i-NANC response was still evident, suggesting that VIP may be involved in this response but not ruling out the possibility of the involvement of other transmitter substances.

Additional positive evidence for the role of VIP in i-NANC neurotransmission in guinea pig airways comes from experiments using the nonspecific peptidase α-chymotrypsin, which breaks down VIP and inhibits NANC relaxant responses (146,148,149). Furthermore, VIP produces relaxation of airways smooth muscle by activating adenylyl cyclase and increasing cAMP. Cyclic AMP hydrolysis by phosphodiesterases can be inhibited by the PDE3 inhibitor SK&F 94120, which potentiates the bronchodilator response to VIP; the same inhibitor also enhances NANC relaxant responses (150). Alternatively, the fact that NANC relaxation was not affected in guinea pig trachea that was already relaxed with maximally effective concentrations of exogenously applied VIP seems to argue against a role for VIP in the NANC dilator response

Peptide histidine isoleucine, which resembles VIP by having 13 of 28 amino acid residues in identical positions, may be co-localized with VIP in guinea pig trachea (128). PHI and other peptides similar in structure to VIP also may contribute to the NANC relaxant response. Indeed, antiserum to PHI generated a small inhibition of the NANC response (118).

Cat

The evidence presented in favor of VIP being involved in i-NANC neurotransmission is less convincing in all other species studied. VIP is a potent relaxant of cat isolated tracheal and bronchial smooth muscle (136) and causes bronchodilation in the cat *in vivo* (151). Moreover, Ito and Takeda (119) have demonstrated that VIP desensitization reduced the NANC relaxant response in feline airways. In addition, Hakoda and Ito (152) demonstrated that overnight incubation with VIP antiserum or immunization with VIP-BSA conjugate markedly reduced the tracheal relaxation in response to EFS when constrictor

tone had been established in the preparation with 5-HT (153). These results would seem to indicate that VIP is at least partly responsible for the NANC relaxant response in cat airways. However, in contrast, there is evidence arguing against a role for VIP as the i-NANC transmitter in cat airways. First, although α-chymotrypsin abolished responses to exogenous VIP in cat trachea (154), there was no effect on the NANC relaxant response (155). Second, both VIP desensitization and VIP antiserum did not affect NANC dilator responses in cat airways (156).

Interestingly, recent evidence suggests that in cat trachea EFS, in the presence of atropine and guanethidine, elicited a monophasic NANC relaxation. By contrast, NANC relaxation elicited in the peripheral airway was biphasic, which comprised an initial fast component followed by a second slower component (157). This secondary component of the NANC response in the peripheral airways was greatly attenuated by α-chymotrypsin. Hence, these results suggest that at least two neurotransmitters, VIP and another transmitter (NO, see below), are involved in i-NANC neurotransmission and that the contribution of these two transmitter substances to the NANC response differs in the central and peripheral airway of the cat (157).

Human

VIP also has a relaxant effect on human airway smooth muscle *in vitro* (52,61,137,138) and it has been suggested that VIP may be the neurotransmitter responsible for i-NANC relaxant responses. However, phosphoramidon, an inhibitor of neutral endopeptidase, significantly potentiated relaxations to low concentrations of VIP with no effect on i-NANC responses (61). In addition, relaxations evoked by VIP were abolished by α-chymotrypsin but i-NANC responses were unaffected in human tracheal and bronchial smooth muscle (53,61,137,158). These data support the view that VIP does not mediate any component of the NANC relaxant response in human airways. This is somewhat surprising because it has been demonstrated that there are large numbers of VIP-immunoreactive nerves in human airway smooth muscle (129) and VIP has been localized in intrinsic parasympathetic ganglia in the trachea (Fig. 2); however, it may be that VIP is more involved in pulmonary vasodilation than in bronchodilation (although this still does not explain the presence of VIP-immunoreactive nerve fibers within human airway smooth muscle). However, the presence of VIP in airway nerves within smooth muscle is not proof that it will function as a neurotransmitter involved in the control of airway tone. This point is probably best illustrated by the fact that VIP-immunoreactive nerve fibers have been observed in relation to bronchial smooth muscle in the dog (125), a species that has no NANC relaxant innervation. However, the role of VIP in nerves within airway

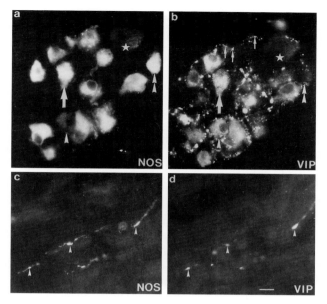

FIG. 2. Localization of NOS and VIP in human airway innervation. **a,b:** Intrinsic ganglion in the trachea with several neurones displaying NOS-immunoreactivity (*IR*) (*double arrowhead*) or VIP-IR (*arrowhead*). Most neurones contain NOS and VIP-IR (*large arrow*). Asterisk on a neurone negative for NOS and VIP. Note the VIP-containing nerve fibers (*small arrows*) in B that do not contain NOS (A). **c,d:** Nerve fiber in the tracheal smooth muscle displaying NOS- and VIP-IR (arrowheads). Scale bar: 5 μm. (Photograph provided by Dr. A. Fischer and Prof. W. Kummer, Justus-Liebig-Universität Giessen, Germany and reproduced from Belvisi MG, Bai TR. Inhibitory nonadrenergic noncholinergic innervation of airways smooth muscle: role of nitric oxide. In: Raeburn D, Giemybycz MA, eds. *Airways smooth muscle: structure, innervation and neurotransmission.* Basel: Birkhauser Verlag, 1994;157–187.)

smooth muscle may not be as a transmitter involved in mediating relaxation. In fact, in addition to its spasmolytic action, VIP also has been shown to modulate other functions such as smooth muscle cell proliferation (159). This possible antiproliferative effect of VIP released from NANC nerves within airway smooth muscle may be important in the pathogenesis of asthma, where a loss of VIP immunoreactivity has been documented (160). Alternatively, the absence of effects of endogenously released VIP from human airways could be due to the release of tryptase, which has been shown to inhibit the bronchodilator action of VIP *in vitro* (161), from activated mast cells in human airways. Another factor to consider is that, in general, studies investigating the role of transmitter substances in the i-NANC response are using specimens *in vitro* that may have been harvested several hours before the experiment takes place. In this case the peptides at the nerve terminals may be depleted and, depending on the preparation and the nerves that contain the peptide, may not be replenished because of the absence of the cell body. However, the role of VIP in neurally evoked

relaxation will remain elusive until definitive studies evaluating the effect of selective VIP receptor antagonists on NANC relaxations are performed.

Vasoactive Intestinal Peptide as a Neuromodulator

The role of endogenously released VIP is uncertain because there are no selective antagonists of the VIP receptors in the airways currently available. However, α-chymotrypsin enhances cholinergic contractile responses to EFS in guinea pig trachea by between 31% and 38%, with no effect on contractile responses to exogenous ACh. This suggests that endogenous VIP may modulate cholinergic neurotransmission through a prejunctional action on cholinergic nerves to inhibit ACh release or by functional antagonism of ACh at the level of the airway smooth muscle, or both (162,163). The most likely explanation for these results is that the percentage enhancement of cholinergic responses produced by α-chymotrypsin is related to the percentage inhibition of the i-NANC bronchodilator response produced by α-chymotrypsin (i.e., Ellis and Farmer [148] found that the i-NANC neural response was inhibited by approximately 35%; Tucker et al. [149] by 41%; Li and Rand [146] by 36%). Interestingly, Watson et al. (164) have demonstrated that although α-chymotrypsin facilitated contractions of the guinea pig trachea in a vagally innervated tracheal tube preparation induced by transmural stimulation, there was no effect on contractile responses induced by preganglionic stimulation. These results suggest that stimulation of preganglionic vagal nerve fibers does not result in the release of VIP; alternatively, VIP can be released in these preparations by stimulation of the intrinsic nerves via transmural stimulation. These data agree with other studies described earlier suggesting that preganglionic inhibitory NANC fibers enter the trachea from a source other than the main vagal nerve trunks.

Alternatively, α-chymotrypsin had no effect on the excitatory NANC (e-NANC) constrictor response, which is due to the release of tachykinins (substance P, neurokinin A) from sensory nerve endings evoked by EFS in guinea pig bronchi (162). These data are surprising because exogenous VIP inhibits e-NANC responses in guinea pig bronchi at concentrations that have no effect on contractile responses to exogenous substance P (165). One explanation for the apparent difference between the modulatory effects of exogenous and endogenous VIP on e-NANC responses could be related to the innervation of the tracheobronchial tree of the guinea pig. Guinea pig tracheal, but not bronchial, smooth muscle exhibits i-NANC relaxation responses to EFS (121), so α-chymotrypsin may have no effect on e-NANC neural responses in guinea pig bronchi because VIP may not be released in these airways. In contrast, α-chymotrypsin potentiated NANC bronchoconstriction induced by vagal stimulation in the guinea pig *in vivo* (166). These results suggest that, at least *in vivo* when there is stimulation of upper and lower airways, endogenous VIP is involved in the regulation of neurogenic bronchoconstriction.

In contrast with data obtained in guinea pig airways, α-chymotrypsin, at a concentration shown to inhibit VIP-induced neural responses in guinea pig trachea (146,148, 149) and abolish relaxant responses to exogenous VIP in human trachea (61), had no effect on cholinergic contractile responses to EFS in human airways (4). This suggests that endogenous VIP does not modulate cholinergic neurotransmission in human trachea, exposing a marked difference between human and guinea pig airways. However, to establish directly whether VIP acts prejunctionally to inhibit transmitter release from cholinergic nerves, it would be necessary to examine the effect of VIP (endogenous and exogenous) on ACh release directly.

Nitric Oxide

The release of NO by mammalian cells was first demonstrated by Furchgott and Zawadzki (167). In these early experiments it was shown that the endothelium released a relaxing factor when stimulated by ACh. Subsequently, this factor was characterized by its short half-life (1–100 s), its destruction by superoxide anions, and its activation of soluble guanylyl cyclase. Similarities between the actions of this factor and the nitrovasodilators led to its identification as NO (168). Since these early studies numerous mammalian cells have been shown to release NO under different conditions.

Indeed, endogenously produced NO may play an integral role in many physiologic and pathophysiologic events in the lung (169). It seems to be involved in the neural NANC bronchodilator system in human airways, in vasodilator mechanisms, and in the regulation of airway and pulmonary blood flow, and is known to be produced as a consequence of the inflammatory process.

Nitric Oxide Synthases

NO formed from L-arginine by NO synthase (NOS) is released from a wide variety of cells (170). Several isoforms of NOS have now been isolated, purified, cloned, and expressed (171) (Table 1). The isoform present in endothelial cells is a 135-kDa protein located in the membrane fraction (172), whereas neuronal or brain NOS is a 155-kDa protein located in the soluble fraction (173–175). Bacterial lipopolysaccharide (LPS) or cytokines induce macrophages, vascular smooth muscle cells, endothelial cells, neutrophils, pulmonary epithelial cells (176,177), and other cells to express a different isoform of NOS (iNOS) (170,171). Constitutive and inducible NOS isoforms have the same co-factor requirements for reduced nicotinamide adenine dinucleotide phosphate (NADPH)

TABLE 1. *Isoforms of nitric oxide synthase*

Isoform	Mr	Location	Co-factor requirement
eNOS	135	Particulate	Ca^{2+}, calmodulin, BH_4, FAD, FMN, NADPH
nNOS	155	Soluble	Ca^{2+}, calmodulin, BH_4, FAD, FMN, NADPH
iNOS	135	Soluble	Calmodulin, BH_4, FAD, FMN, NADPH

Characterization of the different isoforms of nitric oxide synthase (NOS), endothelial NOS (eNOS), neuronal NOS (nNOS), and inducible NOS (iNOS). Mr is the apparent molecular mass of the purified enzyme.

and tetrahydrobiopterin, and contain/require flavin adenine dinucleotide (FAD)/flavin mononucleotide (FMN) (171); however, they differ in that, in general, the constitutive enzymes are calcium-dependent, whereas inducible NOS is calcium-independent (see Table 1).

All isoforms of NOS are inhibited by guanidine nitrogen-substituted L-arginine analogues such as NG monomethyl-L-arginine (L-NMMA) and NG nitro-L-arginine (L-NNA). These compounds have been used as tools to demonstrate the role of NO in numerous physiologic and pathophysiologic events.

Nitric Oxide as a Neurotransmitter in the Airways

There is now a substantial body of evidence involving the use of NOS inhibitors that suggests that NO is involved in (i-NANC) neurotransmission in various organs e.g., reproductive organs, gut, and bladder (178). These findings originated from the fact that NO mediated the effects of nitrovasodilator drugs and that endothelium-derived relaxing factor (EDRF) was NO or an NO-yielding substance. Further evidence to suggest a role for NO as a neurotransmitter is that constitutive NOS (in this case neuronal NOS) has been localized to peripheral nerves (179) and the enzyme could be activated by calcium influx into the nerve terminal on depolarization. However, neuronal NOS does not seem to be stored in synaptic vesicles as are classic neurotransmitters such as ACh but, at least in the gut, seems to be free in the cytoplasm (180) (Fig. 3).

Nitric Oxide as the i-NANC Transmitter in the Airways

In the airways, NOS inhibitors have been shown to inhibit the i-NANC neural relaxation response evoked by EFS in guinea pig trachea *in vitro* by approximately 50% (146,149), suggesting a role for NO in neurotransmission. Similar results have been observed in human, cat, pig, and horse airways (4,181,182) although, in contrast with guinea pig airways, the inhibition evoked by NOS inhibitors was almost complete. Experimental evidence suggests that certain substances (hydroquinone, superox-

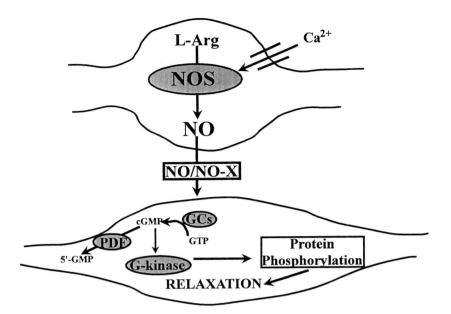

FIG. 3. Putative role of nitric oxide (*NO*) as a neurotransmitter. After EFS and depolarization of the nerve, there is an influx of Ca^{2+} into the nerve terminal. The elevated Ca^{2+} activates neuronal nitric oxide synthase (*NOS*) directly, which results in the synthesis of NO. NO, or NO bound to a carrier molecule (*NO-X*), passes through the synapse and activates soluble guanylyl cyclase, thereby causing an increase in the synthesis of cGMP in the target cell (in this case smooth muscle). Increased levels of cGMP will lead to the activation of G-kinase, and after protein phosphorylation steps that have not yet been determined lead to smooth muscle relaxation. Subsequently, increased levels of cGMP can be hydrolyzed by phosphodiesterase isoenzymes.

ide anions) reduce relaxations to exogenous NO but not to i-NANC nerve stimulation. Therefore, it is still in doubt as to whether it is NO itself that is released as the NANC transmitter or NO attached to a carrier molecule (e.g., released as a nitrosothiol) (see Fig. 3).

Guinea Pig

The peptidase-resistant component of the i-NANC relaxation response to EFS, evoked in precontracted tissue, is attenuated in a concentration-dependent manner by L-NNA and L-NAME (137,146,149). The inhibition observed was approximately 89%, but this was of relaxations elicited by low stimulation frequencies (4 Hz) (149). However, in some reports, L-NAME completely abolished i-NANC relaxation responses at lower frequencies of stimulation (1 Hz) (146). In addition, L-NAME was more potent than L-NMMA in reducing i-NANC relaxations. The reason for this potency difference is not clear, but it may be that L-NMMA is less effective because it also can act as a substrate for NOS (183) or that it is due to an effect other than inhibition of the enzyme. In fact, L-NMMA, but not L-NAME, recently has been shown to inhibit the endothelial cell L-arginine transporter (184) and so may inhibit its own transport into the cell. The effect of these NOS inhibitors is stereoselective because D-NNA and D-NMMA are without effect (146,149). The inhibitory effects of L-NNA and L-NMMA are reversed partially by L-arginine but not D-arginine (137,146,149). There are several reasons why reversal by L-arginine is only partial. L-NAME and L-arginine may have different abilities to access intact cells. These enantiomer-specific effects are similar to those that have been observed in

other tissues that exhibit i-NANC relaxant responses such as the anococcygeus muscle (185,186). NOS inhibitors do not affect responses to sodium nitroprusside or isoprenaline, more evidence suggesting that a component of the i-NANC relaxation response in guinea pig trachea is mediated by NO or a NO-related compound.

Interestingly, there is some evidence in other organs, e.g., gastrointestinal tract, that VIP stimulates the release of NO from gastric muscle cells, so that NO acts as an indirect transmitter of relaxation (187). However, in the airways, L-NOARG and L-NAME had no effect on relaxation responses to VIP (137,146,149). Therefore, it is unlikely that NO is released as a secondary event by the release of VIP from airway nerves.

More evidence implicating NO in the neural control of airway tone comes from immunohistochemical studies describing the presence of the enzyme NOS in nerve fibers that project to the airways. In the guinea pig, the origin of NOS-containing nerves has been demonstrated by NOS-immunoreactivity and NADPH-diaphorase staining to be extrinsic ganglia (jugular, nodose, stellate ganglia) with no positive staining in the intrinsic parasympathetic ganglia (188).

The release of the NANC transmitter in guinea pig trachea is Ca^{2+}-dependent because relaxant responses to NANC stimulation are reduced or abolished at low frequencies of stimulation by ω-conotoxin, which inhibits Ca^{2+} influx through neuronal N-type channels (146,189). With respect to the classic neurotransmitters, this could suggest that exocytotic release of transmitter is taking place. However, this may not be the case for NO because constitutive NOS contained in neurones is a Ca^{2+}-dependent enzyme and therefore the Ca^{2+} entry may be purely to activate the enzyme within the nerve terminals (see Fig. 3).

Cat

In the cat trachea, the NOS inhibitor L-NAME completely inhibited i-NANC responses as measured as changes in isometric force of contraction, evoked by EFS in tissues precontracted with 5-HT (156). A tenfold greater concentration of L-arginine, the substrate for NOS, reversed this inhibitory response. These results suggest that the i-NANC response evoked by EFS in cat trachea is mediated primarily by NO.

In contrast, other workers have demonstrated that NOS inhibitors failed to affect i-NANC relaxation responses evoked by EFS of cat intrapulmonary bronchi precontracted with 5-HT at concentrations that abolished ACh-induced vascular relaxation in cat femoral artery and thoracic aorta (190). In addition, NOS inhibitors had no effect on i-NANC responses evoked by vagal stimulation in mechanically ventilated cats in which airways tone had been elevated by 5-HT (190). These results, in contrast with Fisher et al. (156), do not appear to support a role for NO as a mediator of the i-NANC response in cat airways.

More recently data have been presented that suggest that at least two neurotransmitters are involved in i-NANC neurotransmission (191). These workers have demonstrated that EFS applied to the tracheal smooth muscle during contraction induced by 5-HT in the presence of atropine and guanethidine elicited a monophasic NANC relaxation. By contrast, NANC relaxation elicited in peripheral airway was biphasic, comprising an initial fast component that was blocked by L-NAME followed by a second slow component that was not affected by L-NAME (157). These results indicate that at least two neurotransmitters, possibly NO or NO-containing compounds and VIP, are involved in NANC neurotransmission, and the distribution of the two components differs in the central and peripheral airways.

Pig

In pig tracheal smooth muscle, which has been precontracted with carbachol and in which isometric force of contraction is monitored, EFS evokes a frequency-dependent relaxation response that is NANC in origin (42). This i-NANC response is inhibited completely by NOS inhibitors and reversed by L-arginine in a stereospecific manner (181). In addition, in the presence of a NOS inhibitor, VIP, the nicotinic cholinoceptor agonist dimethylphenylpiperazinium bromide (DMPP) and isoprenaline relaxed carbachol-induced tone in pig trachea, implying that none of the aforementioned agents relax tracheal smooth muscle via a mechanism involving NO. These results seem to indicate that NO may be a transmitter involved in i-NANC neurotransmission in pig trachea. In fact, nerves immunoreactive for constitutive NOS have been localized in the bronchial wall of the pig adjacent to blood vessels, submucosa, and smooth muscle (3).

Rabbit

i-NANC relaxant responses, evoked by EFS, also can be demonstrated in rabbit smooth muscle, but not in bronchial smooth muscle or in lung parenchymal strips (31,192).

Horse

In equine tracheal smooth muscle that has been pretreated with indomethacin, atropine, phentolamine, and propranolol, EFS evoked a frequency-dependent i-NANC relaxation response in vitro (44). This i-NANC relaxant innervation is limited mainly to the trachea and main bronchi. Interestingly, this response is absent in the third generation airways of horses with recurrent obstructive disease (heaves). Recently it has been demonstrated that the i-NANC relaxation response is abolished completely by inhibitors of NOS, suggesting that the i-NANC response is mediated by NO (45).

Ferret

NOS and VIP have been localized in a subpopulation of neurones within the plexus of the ferret trachea. The nerve cell bodies were located in specific ganglia and in the nerve fibers associated with tracheal smooth muscle and blood vessel walls (134). However, there is no functional evidence, as yet, for an i-NANC relaxant response.

Human

There is a prominent i-NANC response in human airways in vitro that is blocked in a concentration-dependent manner by the NOS inhibitor L-NAME (61,158) (Fig. 4). This would seem to indicate that NO is the only demonstrable mediator involved in the i-NANC response in human tracheal smooth muscle. In these experiments L-NAME had no significant effect on relaxation response curves to sodium nitroprusside (SNP) in human tracheal and bronchial smooth muscle, demonstrating that L-NAME inhibits NOS and does not act via blockade of NO-dependent responses or by inhibition of any responses that are cyclic GMP-dependent (61,137). L-NAME also was without effect on relaxation responses to VIP and isoprenaline (137), which is in agreement with the data described for guinea pig airways. D-NAME was ineffective at producing inhibition of the i-NANC response and the inhibitory effect of L-NAME was partially reversed by L-arginine but not D-arginine (61,158) (see Fig. 4). These enantiomer-specific effects are similar to those described in guinea pig trachea (146,149).

i-NANC relaxant responses also may be evoked by EFS in human peripheral bronchioles (0.5–2 mm inner diameter) and central airways (5–12 mm inner diameter)

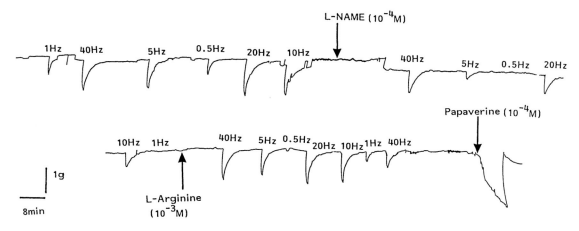

FIG. 4. i-NANC responses to electrical field stimulation (EFS) in human tracheal smooth muscle *in vitro* (40 V, 0.5 ms, 0.5–40 Hz for 30 s) and the inhibitory effect of L-N^G-nitroarginine methyl ester (L-NAME) (10^{-4} M) added 15 min before nerve stimulation was repeated. The inhibitory effect of L-NAME was reversed by addition of L-arginine (10^{-3} M) 10 min before repeating the EFS. Responses are expressed as a percentage of the maximal response to papaverine (10^{-4} M). (From Belvisi MG, Bai TR. Inhibitory nonadrenergic noncholinergic innervation of airways smooth muscle: role of nitric oxide. In: Raeburn D, Giemybycz MA, eds. *Airways smooth muscle: structure, innervation and neurotransmission*, Basel: Birkhauser Verlag, 1994;157–187.)

(53,137). Ellis and Undem (53) have suggested that the i-NANC innervation is quantitatively similar between central and peripheral airways. However, these authors did not compare i-NANC responses evoked by EFS in trachea and main bronchi. Other investigators have suggested that the i-NANC response diminishes as the size of the airway decreases (52). NOS inhibitors seem to inhibit i-NANC relaxant responses to EFS in human bronchial smooth muscle *in vitro* (53,137) and 3-morpholinosydnonimine (SIN-1), an NO donor, relaxes both central and peripheral airways (53), suggesting that i-NANC responses may be mediated by NO. Ellis and Undem (53) have demonstrated that there was almost complete inhibition by L-NNA of the TTX-sensitive portion of the i-NANC relaxant response in human peripheral and central airways precontracted with histamine (3 μM). This study is in agreement with studies on i-NANC responses of human tracheal smooth muscle (61). In contrast, Bai and Bramley (137) found that L-NAME inhibited only approximately 50% of the neurally mediated airways smooth muscle relaxation in human bronchi (137). This study seems to suggest that a large TTX-sensitive residual relaxation persists after NOS inhibition in human bronchi. However, in this later study, the tissues were precontracted with methacholine before i-NANC responses were elicited and therefore atropine was not added to the bathing medium during the course of the experiment. The omission of atropine from the experiment could lead to a certain amount of functional antagonism being produced that may have reduced the magnitude of the inhibitory effect. Alternatively, in these experiments, ACh release from cholinergic nerve terminals could be acting at muscarinic cholinoceptors to release other neurotransmitters/mediators that also may be able to relax human airways smooth muscle. Finally, differences between studies may just simply reflect differences in tissue viability, the age group studied, the medical history of the patient, or the time from organ removal to the start of the experiment.

NO activates soluble guanylyl cyclase after binding to its heme moiety to initiate a three-dimensional change in the shape of the enzyme, which increases activity and consequently the production of cyclic guanosine 3'5'-monophosphate (cGMP). The rise in cGMP can initiate a whole series of events including relaxation of smooth muscle (193), but the mechanism by which this happens is unknown. However, it appears that neurally mediated NANC relaxations in human trachea are associated with a concomitant selective elevation of cGMP, but not cAMP levels, which is inhibited by L-NAME (194). This confirms the hypothesis that the L-arginine-NO-cGMP pathway, and not VIP, is responsible for mediating the NANC relaxant response in this tissue.

It is not certain from where the NO is formed or the location of the NOS enzyme. However, the NO released on EFS does not appear to be localized in the epithelium because its removal has no effect on the i-NANC response evoked by EFS, at least in guinea pig airways (164,195). Recently, in human trachea obtained at autopsy, neuronal NOS immunoreactivity has been described in nerve fibers originating from intrinsic neurones (196) and in some cases is co-localized with VIP (see Fig. 2). In addition, the density of neuronal NOS immunoreactivity is reduced from proximal to distal airways; this correlates with the functional data, demonstrating a reduced i-NANC relaxation response in peripheral compared with central airways (54). Therefore, in view of the extensive array of studies describing the localization of neuronal NOS in neurones within the airways of several species (134,188,196,197), and its correlation with functional data, it is more likely that NO is released from nerves to evoke an i-NANC relaxant response rather than another neurotransmitter substance inducing the release of NO from another cell type, e.g., endothelial, epithelial, or airway smooth muscle cells.

Distribution of NANC Responses in the Respiratory Tract

In human airways *in vitro* NANC responses evoked by EFS were progressively reduced from main airways (trachea/main bronchi) through peripheral airways (3–10 mm) to distal airways (<3 mm) (54). This functional decrease was associated with a decrease in the NOS-immunoreactive nerve density, suggesting that the NANC neural relaxations are reduced going down the tracheobronchial tree apparently because of a decrease in the

density of the nitrergic innervation (54) (Fig. 5). In contrast, Ellis and Undem (53) found no significant difference between i-NANC relaxations in human central (5–12 mm internal diameter) compared with peripheral (0.5–2 mm internal diameter). However, responses in the smaller airways were not compared with those in the larger airways (trachea),where the differences may have been more profound.

The reduction in NANC responses down the human tracheobronchial tree observed by Ward et al. (54) in human airways are also consistent with a number of studies in other species. In feline airways both *in vivo* (36) and *in vitro* (136), the i-NANC response is reduced in distal bronchi. Similar results were found for the NO-mediated i-NANC response in equine airways (44,182). In guinea pig airways i-NANC responses were obtained in trachea but not bronchial smooth muscle (121). Undem et al. (198), however, showed that when the noncholinergic contractions were inhibited by capsaicin desensitization and the tone raised with histamine, NANC relaxations could be elicited by EFS in the mainstem bronchi. This is supported by anatomic studies demonstrating the existence of NOS-positive nerves in the peripheral bronchi of the guinea pig (196). However, the NANC relaxant re-

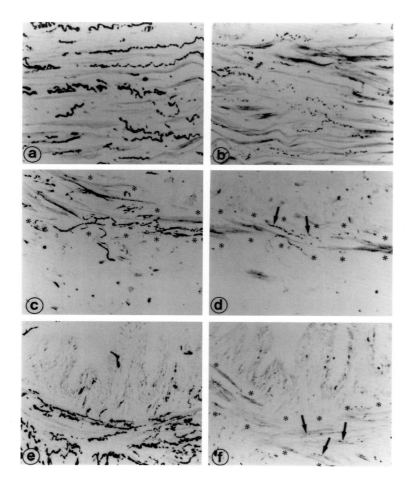

FIG. 5. Nerve immunostaining at three levels of the human tracheobronchial tree. Nerves stained for PGP 9.5 (**a,c,e**) aand NOS (**b,d,f**) are shown in equivalent areas of serial sections from main (a,b), promixal (c,d), and distal airways (e,f). Smooth muscle is recognizable by slight background staining, appearing in most of panels a and b and as a thinner band in panels c through f (edges defined by *asterisks*). A dense plexus of nerves is seen in the muscle at all airway levels, NOS staining appearing as fine varicose fibers (*arrows*) that become sparse in more distal airways (original magnification ×240). (From Ward JK, Barnes PJ, Springall DR, et al. Distribution of human i-NANC bronchodilator and nitric oxide-immunoreactive nerves. *Am J Respir Cell Mol Biol* 1995;13:175–184.)

sponse to EFS in the guinea pig trachea is still more prominent in the cervical compared with the thoracic trachea (199). Reduced i-NANC responses also have been demonstrated in rabbit, monkey (31), and bovine (200) distal bronchi.

Therefore, results obtained in several mammalian species all seem to support the theory that i-NANC nerves exhibit their primary influence on airways located in the conducting airways rather than the gas exchange regions of the lung. However, the functional significance of this pattern of innervation is unclear.

Functional Significance of the i-NANC Response

The exact role of the NANC relaxant response in health and disease has not been defined; however, there are several theories that have been put forward to explain the purpose of this phenomenon: (a) probably the most obvious explanation is that the NANC inhibitory system may play an important physiologic role in the regulation of bronchomotor tone (4); (b) alternatively, Coburn and Tomita (19) hypothesized that it may be important in the control of the cough reflex; and (c) a more heretical explanation that has been put forward is that the NANC relaxant response is an innocuous response remaining from a primitive inhibitory system that has been conserved through the evolutionary process (201).

NANC Inhibitory Pathways in Disease

The i-NANC bronchodilator nerves are the only neural relaxant pathway in human airways; therefore, it is important to determine whether there is any defect in the ability of these nerves to function in diseased airways. In fact, it has been suggested that a defective function of the NANC nerves may contribute to bronchoconstriction and bronchial hyperresponsiveness in asthma (202). On the basis of experiments performed in animals it seemed as though this hypothesis could be true, inasmuch as i-NANC nerve stimulation potently inhibited antigen-induced bronchoconstriction and the increase in arterial plasma histamine in cats (203), suggesting that the transmitter substances responsible for the i-NANC dilator response prevent the release of mediators such as histamine from activated sensitized mast cells (204). Furthermore, the same workers also demonstrated that the bronchodilator action of VIP and the neural relaxation response were reduced after allergen exposure and that the protease inhibitor leupeptin abolished the allergen-induced i-NANC dysfunction in sensitized cats (205). These results would seem to indicate that NANC relaxation is less effective in sensitized animals because of the degradation of the putative NANC neurotransmitter, such as VIP, by proteases released during the allergic response. VIP and related peptides are degraded by mast cell pro-

teases such as tryptase and chymase (206). This possible increase in mast cell proteases found in allergic conditions may contribute to bronchial hyperresponsiveness and to the decreased VIP immunoreactivity seen in nerves in asthmatic airways (160), as mast cells often are found in close association with nerves (207). However, these observations may be more relevant in structures (e.g., human pulmonary vessels rather than airways) and species (guinea pig and cat airways) that receive an i-NANC innervation mediated by a neuropeptide susceptible to peptidases such as VIP.

However, in human airways in vitro i-NANC responses do not appear to be impaired in airways of patients with chronic airflow limitation (208). Moreover, airways from mild asthmatic patients have been found to have a normal i-NANC response (209). In addition, airways from patients who died during severe asthma attacks showed similar NANC inhibitory responses to control airways from nonasthmatic individuals (210). In agreement with the in vitro data, other investigators demonstrated that the degree of bronchodilator response observed in mild asthmatic patients was of similar duration and magnitude as that seen in nonasthmatic persons, suggesting that the NANC bronchodilator system was functioning in mild asthmatics (55,202).

A reduction in VIP immunoreactivity recently has been reported in the airways of asthmatic patients with severe disease (160). This loss of VIP may be due to the presence of human tryptase secreted from airway mast cells. However, more recently, preliminary data have emerged suggesting no difference in VIP immunoreactivity in nerves from biopsy samples from nonasthmatics and mild asthmatics (211). If VIP were the neurotransmitter of i-NANC nerves in human airways, these data may suggest that there could be a decrease in the i-NANC dilator response in asthma according to the severity of the disease. However, as yet, there are no conclusive data implicating a role for VIP in i-NANC neurotransmission, at least in the nerves innervating the airway smooth muscle, in human airways (Fig. 6).

In contrast with asthmatic airways, i-NANC responses were significantly reduced in tissues from patients with cystic fibrosis compared with i-NANC responses in normal donor tissue (212). It is possible that nitrergic neurotransmission is impaired in inflammatory diseases of the airways, as production of superoxide anions by inflammatory cells, such as neutrophils and eosinophils, would lead to a rapid degradation of neurally released NO (Fig. 6). This abnormality in the airway i-NANC innervation of cystic patients may lead to exaggerated bronchoconstrictor responses (Fig. 6). Because the "nitrergic" innervation appears to be dysfunctional in some inflammatory diseases it was tempting to suggest that NO functions as an endogenous braking mechanism in the airways and that its absence therefore may lead to exaggerated bronchoconstriction. We investigated the ef-

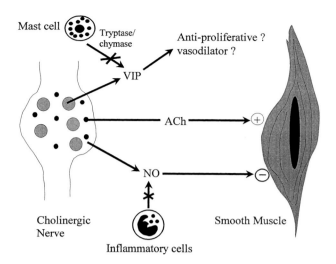

FIG. 6. Release of multiple transmitter substances [acetylcholine, vasoactive intestinal peptide (VIP), nitric oxide (NO)] from airway nerves. VIP and NO may be stored together and co-released on nerve stimulation to act as a functional brake for cholinergic nerve–induced bronchoconstriction by counteracting the constrictor action of ACh on airway smooth muscle. There was no neural control of airway tone (at least in human airway) exerted because of the release of VIP. This may be because, in human airways, VIP may be broken down by mast cell tryptase and chymase or it may be that VIP-containing nerves are more important for controlling the proliferative actions of airway smooth muscle. Alternatively, it could be that VIP has a role as a neural vasodilator. In human airways, where nitrergic neurotransmission is dominant, mediators such as superoxide anions from activated inflammatory cells may rapidly degrade NO, leading to unopposed cholinergic bronchoconstriction.

fect of NOS inhibition (i.e., effectively removing i-NANC relaxation responses) on cholinergic constrictor responses evoked by EFS in human donor tissue from trachea to peripheral airways. L-NAME produced a concentration-dependent enhancement of cholinergic neural constrictor responses to EFS with no effect on cumulative concentration-response curves to ACh in guinea pig and human airways (162,163,214). In human airways, L-NAME evoked maximal enhancement of cholinergic contractile responses in main airways and this became smaller in segmental and subsegmental airways, suggesting that the NO-mediated i-NANC response was less prominent in lower airways (214); recently we have demonstrated this to be the case (54). The mechanism of this modulation was determined by studying the effects of endogenously released NO on ACh release evoked by EFS from strips of human tracheal smooth muscle that had been denuded of epithelium. Overflow of ^{3}H, evoked by EFS, in tissues previously loaded with [^{3}H]-choline, which seems to be a good marker for measurement of neuronally evoked ACh release, is not affected by NOS inhibitors (214). Therefore, it seems that endogenous NO

does not modulate cholinergic contractile responses by prejunctional inhibition of ACh release from the nerve terminal. In conclusion, it would appear that NO probably is modulating cholinergic neurotransmission postjunctionally by functional antagonism of ACh at the level of the airway smooth muscle that could, in theory, oppose cholinergic bronchoconstriction.

CONCLUSIONS

In this chapter I have illustrated the species differences in the neural control of the relaxation of airway smooth muscle. This serves to remind us of the problems that might be encountered when studying neural relaxation responses in animal airways and extrapolating the findings to the human condition.

In terms of the criteria for defining whether a substance is a neurotransmitter, it seems that NO differs radically from the classic neurotransmitters such as ACh and norepinephrine. However, the criteria that are satisfied by NO for neurotransmitter status in the airways are as follows: (a) the enzyme involved in the synthesis of NO from L-arginine has now been localized in neurones in the airways; (b) exogenously administered NO itself or alternatively nitrodilators have been shown to relax airway smooth muscle and therefore NO is able to mimic the effects of i-NANC nerve stimulation; and (c) inhibition of NO formation with a NOS inhibitor results in the attenuation of the nerve evoked relaxation of airway smooth muscle. However, this is where the similarity to classic neurotransmitter substances seems to end. The most difficult concept to reconcile, in terms of the classic ideas of neurotransmission, is the absence of a conventional stimulus-secretion coupling mechanism as the release of NO does not appear to involve vesicular, quantal release of neurotransmitter.

However, although this substance seems an unlikely candidate, in that it is a gas that is not stored in synaptic vesicles or released by exocytosis, and that does not act at typical cell membrane-associated receptors, NO may prove to have a more widespread and fundamental role than most classic neurotransmitters. The discovery of NO as a transmitter substance revolutionizes the classic pharmacologic basis for neurotransmission and may lead to the identification of other equally unlikely candidates.

In conclusion, the NANC bronchodilator mechanism has been identified as the predominant system in the neural control of human airway smooth muscle relaxation. However, the precise physiologic or pathophysiologic role of this system remains to be defined. The identification of a disruption in this pathway in tissue from patients with airway inflammation is interesting, but the mechanism behind this dysfunction and the consequences of this are unknown and warrant further study.

ACKNOWLEDGMENT

MGB is supported by a Wellcome Trust Fellowship.

REFERENCES

1. Barnes PJ. Modulation of neurotransmission in airways. *Physiol Rev* 1992;72:699–729.
2. Burnstock G. Purinergic nerves. *Pharmacol Rev* 1972;24:247–324.
3. Belvisi MG, Bai TR. Inhibitory nonadrenergic noncholinergic innervation of airways smooth muscle: role of nitric oxide. In: Raeburn D, Giemybycz MA, eds. *Airways smooth muscle: structure, innervation and neurotransmission*, Basel: Birkhauser Verlag, 1994;157–187.
4. Belvisi MG, Ward JK, Mitchell JA, Barnes PJ. Nitric oxide as a neurotransmitter in human airways, *Arch Int Pharmacodyn Thér* 1995; 329:97–110.
5. Ellis JL, Undem BJ. Pharmacology of nonadrenergic, noncholinergic nerves in airway smooth muscle. *Pulm Pharmacol* 1994;7:205–223.
6. Mann SP. The innervation of mammalian bronchial smooth muscle, the localisation of catecholamines and cholinesterases. *Histochem J* 1971;3:319–331.
7. Richardson J, Béland J. Nonadrenergic inhibitory nervous system in human airways. *J Appl Physiol* 1976;41:764–771.
8. Barnes PJ. Neural control in health and disease. *Am Rev Respir Dis* 1986;134:1289–1314.
9. Burnstock G, Wood MJ. Innervation of the lungs of the sleepy lizard (*Trachysaurus regosus*). II. Physiology and pharmacology. *Comp Biochem Physiol* 1967;22:815–831.
10. Wood MJ, Burnstock G. Innervation of the lungs of the toad (*Bufo marinus*). I. Physiology and Pharmacology, *Comp Biochem Physiol* 1967;22:755–766.
11. Robinson PM, Mclean JR, Burnstock G. Ultrastructural identification of nonadrenergic inhibitory nerve fibres. *J Pharmacol Exp Ther* 1971;179:149–160.
12. Berger PJ. Autonomic innervation of the visceral and vascular smooth muscle of the lizard lung. *Comp Gen Pharmacol* 1973;4:1–10.
13. Burnstock G. Comparative studies of purinergic nerves. *J Exp Zool* 1975;194:103–134.
14. Fedde MR, Burger RE, Kitchell R. The influence of the vagus nerve on respiration. *Poult Sci* 1961;40:1401–1407
15. Cook RD, King AS. Observations on the ultrastructure of the smooth muscle and its innervation in the avian lung. *J Anat* 1969;105:202–208.
16. Richardson JB. Nerve supply to the lungs. *Am Rev Respir Dis* 1979;119:785–802.
17. Richardson JB, Béland J. Nonadrenergic inhibitory nervous system in human airways. *J Appl Physiol* 1976;41:764–771.
18. Bando TX, Shindo N, Shimo Y. Nonadrenergic inhibitory nerves in tracheal smooth muscle of guinea pig. *Proc J Physiol Soc Jpn* 1973;35:508–509.
19. Coburn RF, Tomita T. Evidence for nonadrenergic inhibitory nerves in the guinea pig trachealis muscle. *Am J Physiol* 1973;224:1072–1080.
20. Coleman RA. Evidence for a nonadrenergic inhibitory nervous pathway in guinea-pig trachea. *Br J Pharmacol* 1973;48:360–361.
21. Coleman RA, Levy GP. A nonadrenergic inhibitory nervous pathway in guinea-pig trachea. *Br J Pharmacol* 1974;52:167–174.
22. O'Donnell SR, Saar N. Histochemical localization of adrenergic nerves in the guinea-pig trachea. *Br J Pharmacol* 1973;47:707–710.
23. Kalenburg S, Satchell DG. The inhibitory innervation of the guinea-pig trachea: a study of its adrenergic and nonadrenergic components. *Clin Exp Pharmacol Physiol* 1979;6:53–64.
24. Richardson JB, Bouchard T. Demonstration of a nonadrenergic inhibitory nervous system in the trachea of the guinea-pig. *J Allergy Clin Immunol* 1975;56:473–480.
25. Yip P, Palambini B, Coburn RF. Inhibitory innervation of the guinea-pig trachealis muscle. *J Appl Physiol* 1981;50:373–382.
26. Hammarström M, Sjöstrand NO. Pathways for excitatory and inhibitory innervation to the guinea-pig tracheal smooth muscle. *Experimentia* 1979;35:64–65.
27. Taylor JF, Paré PD, Schellenburg RR. Cholinergic and nonadrenergic mechanisms in human and guinea-pig airways. *J Appl Physiol* 1984;56:958–965.
28. Chesrown SE, Venugoplan CS, Gold WM, Drazen JM. *In vivo* demonstration of nonadrenergic inhibitory innervation of the guinea-pig trachea. *J Clin Invest* 1980;65:314–320.
29. Canning BJ, Undem BJ. Relaxant innervation of the guinea-pig trachealis: demonstration of capsaicin-sensitive and insensitive vagal pathways. *J Physiol* 1993;460:719–739.
30. Satchell D. Nonadrenergic noncholinergic nerves in mammalian airways: their function and the role of purines. *Comp Biochem Physiol* 1982;72:189–196.
31. Doidge JM, Satchell DG. Adrenergic and nonadrenergic inhibitory nerves in mammalian airways. *J Autonomic Nervous System* 1982;5: 83–99.
32. Suzuki H, Morita K, Kuriyama H. Innervation and properties of the smooth muscle of the dog trachea. *Jpn J Physiol* 1976;26:303–320.
33. Russell J. Noradrenergic inhibitory innervation of canine airways. *J Appl Physiol* 1980;48:16–22.
34. Kannan MS, Daniel EE. Structural and functional study of control of canine tracheal smooth muscle. *Am J Physiol* 1980;238:C27–C33.
35. Altiere RJ, Szarek JL, Diamond L. Neural control of relaxation in cat airways smooth muscle. *J Appl Physiol* 1984;57:1536–1544.
36. Diamond L, O Donnell M. A nonadrenergic vagal inhibitory pathway to feline airway. *Science* 1980;208:185–188.
37. Irvin CG, Boileau R, Tremblay J, Martin RR, Macklem PT. Bronchodilatation: Noncholinergic, nonadrenergic mediator demonstrated *in vivo* in the cat. *Science* 1980;207:791–792.
38. Szarek JL, Gillespie MN, Altiere RJ, Diamond L. Reflex activation of the nonadrenergic noncholinergic inhibitory system in feline airway. *Am Rev Respir Dis* 1986;133:159–162.
39. Inoue H, Ichinose M, Miura M, Katsumata U, Takishima T. Sensory receptors and reflex pathways of nonadrenergic inhibitory nervous system in feline airway. *Am Rev Respir Dis* 1989;139:1175–1178.
40. Sheller JR, Brigham, KL. Bronchomotor responses of isolated sheep airways to electrical field stimulation. *J Appl Physiol* 1982;53: 1088–1093.
41. Leff AR, Munoz NM, Tallet J, David AC, Cavigelli MA, Garrity ER. Autonomic response characteristics of porcine airway smooth muscle *in vivo*. *J Appl Physiol* 1985;58:1176–1188.
42. Kannan MS, Johnson DE. Functional innervation of pig tracheal smooth muscle:neural and nonneural mechanisms of relaxation. *J Pharmacol Exp Ther* 1992;260:1180–1184.
43. Cameron AR, Johnston CF, Kirkpatrick CT, Kirkpatrick MCA. The quest for the inhibitory neurotransmitter in bovine tracheal smooth muscle. *Q J Exp Physiol* 1983;68:413–426.
44. Broadstone RV, Leblanc PH, Derksen FJ, Robinson NE. *In vitro* responses of airway smooth muscle from horses with recurrent airway obstruction. *Pulm Pharmacol* 1991;4:191–202.
45. Yu M, Wang Z, Robinson NE, Leblanc PH. Inhibitory nerve distribution and mediation of NANC relaxation by nitric oxide in horse airways. *J Appl Physiol* 1994;76:339–344.
46. Middendorf WF, Russell JA. Innervation of airway smooth muscle in the baboon: evidence for a nonadrenergic inhibitory system. *J Appl Physiol Respir Environ Exercise Physiol* 1980;48:947–956.
47. Richardson JB. Nonadrenergic inhibitory innervation of the lung. *Lung* 1981;159:315–322.
48. Rikimaru A, Sudoh M. Innervation of the smooth muscle of the guinea-pig trachea. *Jpn J Smooth Muscle Res* 1971;7:35–44.
49. Foster RW, O'Donnell, SR. Evidence that adrenergic nerves are responsible for the active uptake of norepinephrine in the guinea-pig isolated trachea. *Br J Pharmacol* 1975;53:109–112.
50. Ind PW. Role of the sympathetic nervous system and endogenous catecholamines in the regulation of airways smooth muscle tone. In: Raeburn D, Giembycz MA, eds. *Airway smooth muscle: structure, innervation and neurotransmission*. Basel: Birkhauser Verlag, 1994; 29–41.
51. Davis C, Kannan MS, Jones TR, Daniel EE. Control of human airway smooth muscle: *in vitro* studies. *J Appl Physiol* 1982;53:1080–1087.
52. Palmer JBD, Cuss FMC, Barnes PJ. VIP and PHM and their role in nonadrenergic inhibitory responses in isolated human airways. *J Appl Physiol* 1986;61:1322–1328.
53. Ellis JL, Undem BJ. Inhibition by L-NG-nitro-L-arginine of nonadrenergic noncholinergic relaxations of human isolated central and peripheral airways. *Am Rev Respir Dis* 146:1543–1547.
54. Ward JK, Barnes PJ, Springall DR, et al. Distribution of human i-NANC bronchodilator and nitric oxide-immunoreactive nerves. *Am J Respir Cell Mol Biol* 1995;13:175–184.

55. Michoud MC, Jeanneret-Grosjean A, Couture J Amyot R. Reflex decrease of histamine-induced bronchoconstriction after laryngeal stimulation in humans. *Am Rev Respir Dis* 1988;136:616–622.

56. Lammers J-W, Minette M, McCusker M, Chung KF, Barnes PJ. Nonadrenergic bronchodilator mechanisms in normal human subjects *in vivo*. *J Appl Physiol* 1988;64:1817–1822.

57. Ichinose M, Inoue H, Miura M, Takishima T. Nonadrenergic bronchodilation in normal subjects. *Am Rev Respir Dis* 1988;138:31–34.

58. Fuller RW, Dixon CMS, Barnes PJ. The bronchoconstrictor response to inhaled capsaicin in humans. *J Appl Physiol* 1985;85:1080–1085.

59. Irvin CG, Martin RR, Macklem PT. Nonpurinergic nature and efficacy of nonadrenergic bronchodilation. *J Appl Physiol* 1982;52:562–569.

60. Hutás I, Hadházy P, Debreczeni L, Vizi ES. Relaxation of human isolated bronchial smooth muscle. *Lung* 1981;159:153–161.

61. Belvisi MG, Stretton CD, Miura M, et al. Inhibitory NANC nerves in human tracheal smooth muscle: a quest for the neurotransmitter. *J Appl Physiol* 1992;73:2505–2510.

62. Solis-Cohen S. The use of adrenal substance in the treatment of asthma. *J Am Med Assoc* 1900;34:1164–1166.

63. Pack RJ, Richardson PS. The aminergic innervation of the human bronchus: a light and electron microscopic study. *J Anat* 1984;138:493–502.

64. Ind PW, Scriven AJI, Dollery CT. Use of tyramine to probe pulmonary norepinephrine release in asthma. *Clin Sci Mol Med* 1983;65:9.

65. Jones TR, Kannan MS, Daniel EE. Ultrastructural study of guinea-pig tracheal smooth muscle and its innervation. *Can J Physiol Pharmacol* 1980;58:974–983.

66. Cabezas GA, Graf PD, Nadel JA. Sympathetic versus parasympathetic nervous regulation of airways in dogs. *J Appl Physiol* 1971;31:651–655.

67. Drazen JM. Adrenergic influences on histamine-mediated bronchoconstriction in the guinea-pig. *J Appl Physiol* 1978;44:340–345.

68. Leff AR, Munoz NM, Hendrix SG. Sympathetic inhibition of histamine-induced contraction of canine trachealis *in vivo*. *J Appl Physiol* 1982;53:21–29.

69. Piper PJ, Collier HOJ, Vane JR. Release of catecholamines in the guinea-pig by substances involved in anaphylaxis in the guinea-pig *in vivo*. *Br J Pharmacol* 1967;30:283–301.

70. McNeill RS. Effect of a β-adrenergic blocking agent propranolol, on asthmatics. *Lancet* 1964;2:1101–1102.

71. Richardson PS, Sterling GM. Effects of β-adrenergic receptor blockade on airway conductance and lung volume in normal and asthmatic subjects. *Br Med J* 1969;3:143–145.

72. Rhoden KJ, Meldrum LA, Barnes PJ. Inhibition of cholinergic neurotransmission in human airways by β2-adrenoceptors. *J Applied Physiol* 1988;65:700–705.

73. Barnes PJ. Muscarinic receptor subtypes: implications for lung disease. *Thorax* 1989;44:161–167.

74. Rugg EL, Barnett DB, Nahorski SR. Coexistence of β1 and β2 adrenoceptors in mamalian lung: evidence from direct binding studies. *Mol Pharmacol* 1978;14:996–1005.

75. Barnes PJ, Karliner JS, Dollery CT. Human lung adrenoceptors studied by radioligand binding. *Clin Sci* 1980:58:457–461.

76. Engel G. Subclasses of beta-adrenoceptor. A quantitative estimation of beta1 and beta2 adrenoceptors in guinea-pig and human lung. *Post Grad Med J* 1981;57:77–83.

77. Goldie RG, Paterson JW, Wale JL. Pharmacological responses of human and porcine lung parenchyma, bronchus and pulmonary artery. *Br J Pharmacol* 1982;76:515–521.

78. Zaagsma J, van der Heijden PJCM, van der Schaar MWG, Blank CMC. Comparison of functional β-adrenoceptor heterogeneity in central and peripheral airway smooth muscle of guinea-pig and man. *J Recept Res* 1983;3:89–106.

79. Finney MJB, Karlsson J-A, Persson CGA. Effects of bronchoconstrictors and bronchodilators on a novel human small airway preparation. *Br J Pharmacol* 1985;85:29–36.

80. Guillot C, Fornaris M, Badier M, Orehek J. Spontaneous and provoked resistance to isoproterenol in isolated human bronchi. *J Allergy Clin Immunol* 1984;74:713–718.

81. Barnes PJ, Nadel JA, Skoogh B-E, Roberts JM. Characterisation of β-adrenoceptor subtypes in canine airway smooth muscle by radioligand binding and physiologic responses. *J Pharmacol Exp Ther* 1983;225:456–461.

82. Löfdahl C-G, Svedmyr N. Effects of prenalterol in asthmatic patients. *Eur J Clin Pharmacol* 1982;23:297–303.

83. Goldie RG, Spina D, Henry PJ, Lulich KM, Paterson JW. *In vitro* responsiveness of human asthmatic bronchus to carbachol, histamine, β-adrenoceptor agonists and theophylline. *Br J Clin Pharmacol* 1986;22:669–676.

84. Bai TR. Abnormalities in airway smooth muscle in fatal asthma: a comparison between trachea and bronchus. *Am Rev Respir Dis* 1991;143:441–443.

85. Bai TR, Mak JCW, Barnes PJ. A comparison of β-adrenergic receptors and *in vitro* relaxant responses to isoproterenol in asthmatic airway smooth muscle. *Am J Respir Cell Mol Biol* 1992;6:647–651.

86. Vermeire PA, Vanhoutte PM. Inhibitory effects of catecholamines in isolated canine bronchial smooth muscle. *J Appl Physiol* 1979;46:787–791.

87. Ito Y, Tajima K. Dual effects of catecholamines on pre- and post-junctional membranes in the dog trachea. *Br J Pharmacol* 1982;75:433–440.

88. Danser AHJ, Van den Ende R, Lorenz RR, Flavahan NA, Vanhoutte PM. Pre-junctional β1-adrenoceptors inhibit cholinergic transmission in canine bronchi. *J Appl Physiol* 1987;62:785–790.

89. Ito Y. Pre- and post-junctional actions of procaterol, a β2-adrenoceptor stimulant, on dog tracheal tissue. *Br J Pharmacol* 1988;95:268–274.

90. Janssen LJ, Daniel EE. Characterisation of the pre-junctional beta-adrenoceptors in canine bronchial smooth muscle. *J Pharmacol Exp Ther* 1990;254:741–749.

91. Aizawa H, Inoue H, Ikeda T, Hirose T, Ito Y. Effects of procaterol, beta2-adrenoceptor stimulant, on neuroeffector transmission in human bronchial tissue. *Respiration* 1991;58:3–166.

92. Kamikawa Y, Shimo Y. Inhibitory effects of sympathomimetic drugs on cholinergically mediated contractions of guinea-pig isolated tracheal muscle. *J Pharmacy Pharmacol* 1986;38:742–747.

93. Martin CA, Naline E, Manara L, Advenier C. Effects of two β3-adrenoceptor agonists, SR58611 A and BRL 37344, and of salbutamol on cholinergic and NANC neural contraction in guinea-pig main bronchi *in vitro*. *Br J Pharmacol* 1993;110:1311–1316.

94. Ten Berg REJ, Weening EC, Roffel AF, Zaagsma J. β2- but not β3-adrenoceptors mediate pre-junctional inhibition of nonadrenergic noncholinergic contraction of guinea-pig main bronchi. *Eur J Pharmacol* 1995;275:199–206.

95. Martin JG, Collier B. Acetylcholine release from canine isolated airway is not modulated by noradrenaline. *J Applied Physiol* 1986;61:1025–1030.

96. Wessler I, Reinheimer T, Brunn G, Anderson GP, Maclagan J, Racké K. β-Adrenoceptors mediate inhibition of [³H]-acetylcholine release from the isolated rat and guinea-pig trachea: role of the airway mucosa and prostaglandins. *Br J Pharmacol* 1994;113:1221–1230.

97. Belvisi MG, Patel HJ, Takahashi T, Barnes PJ, Giembycz MA. Paradoxical facilitation of acetylcholine release from parasympathetic nerves innervating guinea-pig trachea by isoprendaline. *Br J Pharmacol* 1996;117:1413–1420.

98. Zang XY, Olszewski MA, Robinson NE. β2-Adrenoceptor activation augments acetylcholine release from tracheal parasympathetic nerves. *Am J Physiol* 1995;268:L950–L956.

99. Zang XY, Robinson NE, Wang ZW, Yu MC. Catecholamine affects acetylcholine release in trachea: α2-mediated inhibition and β2-mediated augmentation. *Am J Physiol* 1995;12:L368–L373.

100. Wessler I, Anachutz S. β-Adrenoceptor stimulation enhances transmitter output from rat phrenic nerve. *Br J Pharmacol* 1988;94:669-674.

101. Wessler I, Holzer G, Szarma E. Stimulation of β1-adrenoceptors enhances electrically evoked [³H]acetylcholine release from rat phrenic nerve. *Clin Pharmacol Physiol* 1990;17:23–32.

102. Blackwell GJ, Flower RJ, Nijkamp FP, Vane JR. Phospholipase A2 activity of guinea-pig isolated perfused lungs: stimulation and inhibition by anti-inflammatory steroids. *Br J Pharmacol* 1978;62:79–89.

103. Suzuki K, Sugiyama S, Takagi K, Satake T, Ozawa T. The role of phospholipase in β-agonist induced down regulation in guinea-pig lungs. *Biochem Med Metab Biol* 1987;37:157–166.

104. Nakanishi H, Yashida H, Suzuki T. Inhibitory effects of prostaglandins on excitatory transmission in isolated canine tracheal muscle. *Jpn J Pharmacol* 1978;28:883–889.

105. Jones TR, Hamilton JT, Lefcoe NM. Pharmacologic modulations of cholinergic neurotransmission in guinea-pig trachea *in vitro*. *Can J Physiol Pharmacol* 1980;58:974–983.

106. Walters EH, O Byrne PM, Fabbri LM, Graf PD, Holtzman MJ, Nadel JA. Control of neurotransmission by prostaglandins in canine trachealis smooth muscle. *J Appl Physiol* 1984;57:129–184.

107. Inoue T, Ito Y, Takeda K. Prostaglandin-induced inhibition of acetylcholine from neuronal elements of dog tracheal tissue. *J Physiol* 1984;349:553–570.

108. Deckers IA, Rampart M, Bult H, Herman AG. Evidence for the involvement of prostaglandins in modulation of acetylcholine release from canine bronchial tissue. *Eur J Pharmacol* 1989;167:415–418.

109. DeLisle S, Biggs D, Wang A, Martin JG. Effects of prostaglandin E2 on ganglionic transmission in the guinea-pig trachea. *Respiration Physiol* 1992;87:131–139.

110. Simonsson BG, Svedmyr N, Skoogh BE, Anderson R, Bergh NP. *In vivo* and *in vitro* studies on α-adrenoceptors in human airways. Potentiation with bacterial endotoxin. *Scand J Respir Dis* 1972;53:227–236.

111. Kneussl MP, Richardson JB. α-adrenergic receptors in human and canine tracheal and bronchial smooth muscle. *J Appl Physiol* 1978;45:307–311.

112. Leff AR, Tallet J, Munoz NM, Shoulberg N. Physiological antagonism caused by adrenergic stimulation of canine tracheal smooth muscle. *J Appl Physiol* 1986;60:216–224.

113. Spina D, Rigby PJ, Paterson JW, Goldie RG. α-adrenoceptor function and autoradiographic distribution in human asthmatic lung. *Br J Pharmacol* 1989;97:701–708.

114. Barnes PJ, Baraniuk JN, Belvisi MG. Neuropeptides in the respiratory tract. *Am Rev Respir Dis* 1991;144:1187–1198.

115. Burnstock G, Campbell G, Satchell DG, et al. Evidence that adenosine triphosphate or a related nucleotide is the transmitter substance released by nonadrenergic inhibitory nerves in the gut. *Br J Pharmacol* 1970;40:668–675.

116. Coleman RA. The effects of some purine derivatives on the guinea-pig trachea and their interaction with drugs that block adenosine uptake. *Br J Pharmacol* 1976;57:51–57.

117. Satchell D. Adenosine deaminase antagonises inhibitory responses to adenosine and nonadrenergic, noncholinergic inhibitory nerve stimulation in isolated preparations of guinea-pig trachea. *Br J Pharmacol* 1984;83:323–325.

118. Ellis JL, Farmer SG. The effects of vasoactive intestinal (VIP) antagonists, and VIP and peptide histidine isoleucine antisera on nonadrenergic, noncholinergic relaxations of tracheal smooth muscle. *Br J Pharmacol* 1989;96:513–520.

119. Ito Y, Takeda K. Nonadrenergic inhibitory nerves and putative neurotransmitters in the smooth muscle of cat trachea. *J Physiol (Lond)* 1982;330:497–511.

120. Coleman RA. Purine antagonists in the identification of adenosine-receptors in guinea-pig trachea and the role of purines in nonadrenergic inhibitory neurotransmission. *Br J Pharmacol* 1980;69:359–366.

121. Grundstrom N, Andersson RGG, Wikberg JES. Pharmacological characterisation of the autonomous innervation of guinea-pig tracheobronchial smooth muscle. *Acta Pharmacol Scand* 1981;49:150–157.

122. Karlsson JA, Persson CGA. Neither vasoactive intestinal peptide (VIP) nor purine derivatives may mediate nonadrenergic tracheal inhibition. *Acta Physiol Scand* 1984;122:589–598.

123. Sundler F, Ekblad E, Grunditz T, Håkanson R, Uddman R. Vasoactive intestinal peptide in the peripheral nervous system. *Ann N Y Acad Sci* 1988;527:143–167.

124. Uddman R, Alumets J, Densert O, Håkånson R, Sundler F. Occurrence and distribution of VIP nerves in the nasal mucosa and tracheobronchial wall. *Acta Otolaryngol* 1978;86:443–448.

125. Dey, RD, Shannon WA, Said SI. Localisation of VIP-immunoreactive nerves in airways and pulmonary vessels of dogs, cats and human subjects. *Cell Tissue Res* 1981;220:231–238.

126. Luts A, Sundler F. Peptide-containing nerve fibres in the respiratory tract of the ferret. *Cell Tissue Res* 1989;258:259–267.

127. Ghatei MA, Sheppard MN, O Shaughnessy DJ et al. Regulatory peptides in the mammalian respiratory tract. *Endocrinology* 1982;111:1248–1254.

128. Lundberg JM, Fahrenkrug J, Hökfelt T. Co-existence of peptide histidine isoleucine (PHI) and VIP in nerves regulating blood flow and bronchial smooth muscle tone in various mammals including man. *Peptides* 1984;5:593–598.

129. Laitinen A, Partanen M, Hervonen A, Pelto-Huikko M, Laitinen LA. VIP-like immunoreactive nerves in human respiratory tract. *Histochemistry* 1985;82:313–319.

130. Uddman R, Sundler F. Neuropeptides in the airways: a review. *Am Rev Respir Dis* 1987;136:S3–8.

131. Dey RD, Hoffpauir J, Said SI. Co-localisation of vasoactive intestinal peptide- and substance P-containing nerves in cat bronchi. *Neuroscience* 1988;24:275–281.

132. Dey RD, AltemusJB, Michalkiewicz M. Distribution of vasoactive intestinal peptide- and substance P-containing nerves originating from neurons of airway ganglia in cat bronchi. *J Comp Neurol* 1991;304:330–340.

133. Bowden JJ, Gibbins IL. Vasoactive intestinal peptide and neuropeptide Y co-exist in nonnoradrenergic sympathetic neurons to guinea-pig trachea. *J Auton Nerv Sys* 1992;38:1–20.

134. Dey RD, Mayer B, Said SI. Colocalisation of vasoactive intestinal peptide and nitric oxide synthase in neurons of the ferret trachea. *Neuroscience* 1993;54:839–843.

135. Kummer W, Fischer A, Kurkowski R, et al. The sensory and sympathetic innervation of guinea-pig lung and trachea as studied by retrograde neuronal tracing and double-labelling immunohistochemistry. *Neuroscience* 1992;49:715–737.

136. Altiere RJ, Diamond L. Comparison of vasoactive intestinal peptide and isoproterenol relaxant effects in isolated cat airways. *J Appl Physiol* 1984;56:986–992.

137. Bai TR, Bramley AM. Effect of an inhibitor of nitric oxide synthase on neural relaxation of human bronchi. *Am J Physiol* 1993;8:L425–L430.

138. Raffestin B, Cerrina J, Boullet C, Labat C, Benveniste J, Brink C. Response and sensitivity of isolated human pulmonary muscle preparations to pharmacological agents. *J Pharmacol Exp Ther* 1985;233:186–194.

139. Said SI. Vasoactive peptides in the lung, with special reference to vasoactive intestinal peptide. *Exp Lung Res* 1982;3:343–348.

140. Barnes PJ, Dixon CMS. The effect of inhaled vasoactive intestinal peptide on bronchial hyperreactivity in man. *Am Rev Respir Dis* 1984;130:162–166.

141. Morice A, Unwin RJ, Sever PS. Vasoactive intestinal peptide causes bronchodilation and protects against histamine induced bronchoconstriction in asthmatic subjects. *Lancet* 1983;2:1225–1227.

142. Matsuzaki Y, Hamasaki Y, Said SI. Vasoactive intestinal peptide: a possible transmitter of nonadrenergic relaxation of guinea-pig airways. *Science* 1980;210:1252–1253.

143. Fransden EK, Krishna Y, Said SI. Vasoactive intestinal peptide promotes cyclic adenosine 3'5'-monophosphate accumulation in guinea-pig trachea. *Br J Pharmacol* 1978;62:367–369.

144. Waelbroeck M, Robberecht P, Coy DH, Camus J-C, De Neef P, Christophe J. Interaction of growth hormone-releasing factor (GRF) and 14 GRF analogues with vasoactive intestinal peptide (VIP) receptors of rat pancreas. Discovery of [AC-Tyr^1, D-Phe^2]-GRF(1-29)-NH$_2$ as a VIP antagonist. *Endocrinology* 1985;116:2643–2649.

145. Pandol SJ, Dharmsathaphorn K, Schoeffield MS, Vale W, Rivier J. Vasoative intestinal peptide receptor antagonist [4-Cl-D-Phe^6, Leu^{17}]-VIP. *Am J Physiol* 1986;250:G553–G557.

146. Li CG, Rand MJ. Evidence that part of the NANC relaxant response of guinea-pig trachea to electrical field stimulation is mediated by nitric oxide. *Br J Pharmacol* 1991;102:91–94.

147. Venugopalan CS, Said SI, Drazen JM. Effect of vasoactive intestinal peptide on vagally mediated tracheal pouch relaxation. *Respir Physiol* 1984;56:205–216.

148. Ellis JL, Farmer SG. Effect of peptidases on nonadrenergic, noncholinergic inhibitory responses of tracheal smooth muscle: a comparison with effects on VIP and PHI-induced relaxation. *Br J Pharmacol* 1989;96:521–526.

149. Tucker JF, Brave SR, Charalambous L, Hobbs A, Gibson AJ. L-NG-nitro arginine inhibits nonadrenergic, noncholinergic relaxations of guinea-pig tracheal smooth muscle. *Br J Pharmacol* 1990;100:663–664.

150. Rhoden KJ, Barnes PJ. Potentiation of nonadrenergic neural relaxation in guinea-pig airway by a cAMP phosphodiesterase inhibitor. *J Pharmacol Exp Ther* 1990;252:396–402.

151. Diamond L, Szarek JL, MN, Altiere RJ. *In vivo* bronchodilator activity of vasoactive intestinal peptide. *Am Rev Respir Dis* 1983;128:827–832.

152. Xie ZQ, Hirose T, Hakoda H, Ito Y. Effects of vasoactive intestinal

polypeptide antagonists on cholinergic neurotransmission in dog and cat trachea. *Br J Pharmacol* 1991;104:938–944.

153. Hakoda H, Xie ZQ, Aizawa H, Inoue H, Hirata M, Ito Y. Effects of immunisation against VIP on neurotransmission in cat trachea. *Am J Physiol* 1991;261:L341–L348.

154. Altiere RJ, Diamond L. Relaxation of cat tracheobronchial and pulmonary arterial smooth muscle by vasoactive intestinal peptide: lack of influence of peptidase inhibitors. *Br J Pharmacol* 1984;82:321–328.

155. Altiere RJ, Diamond L. Effect of α-chymotrypsin on the nonadrenergic noncholinergic inhibitory system in cat airways. *Eur J Pharmacol* 1985;114:75–78.

156. Fisher JT, Anderson JW, Waldron MA. Nonadrenergic noncholinergic neurotransmitter of feline trachealis: VIP or nitric oxide. *J Appl Physiol* 1993;74:31–39.

157. Takahashi N, Tanaka H, Abdullah N, Jing L, Inoue R, Ito Y. Regional difference in the distribution of L-NAME-sensitive and -insensitive NANC relaxations in cat airway. *J Physiol* 1995;488:709–720.

158. Belvisi MG, Stretton CD, Yacoub MH, Barnes PJ. Nitric oxide is the endogenous neurotransmitter of bronchodilator nerves in humans. *Eur J Pharmacol* 1992;210:221–222.

159. Maruno K, Said SI. Inhibition of human airway smooth muscle cell proliferation by vasoactive intestinal peptide (VIP). *Am Rev Respir Dis* 1993;147:A253.

160. Ollerenshaw Jarvis D, Woolcock A, Sullivan C, Scheibner T. Absence of immunoreactive vasoactive intestinal polypeptide in tissue from the lungs of patients with asthma. *N Engl J Med* 1989;320:1244–1248.

161. Caughey GH. Role of mast cell tryptase and chymase in airway function. *Am J Physiol* 1989;257:L39–L46.

162. Belvisi MG, Miura M, Stretton CD, Barnes PJ. Endogenous vasoactive intestinal peptide and nitric oxide modulate cholinergic neurotransmission in guinea-pig trachea. *Eur J Pharmacol* 1993;231:97–102.

163. Brave SR, Hobbs AJ, Gibson A, Tucker JF. The influence of L-NG-nitro-arginine on field stimulation-induced contractions and acetylcholine release in guinea-pig isolated smooth muscle. *Biochem Biophys Res Commun* 1991;179:1017–1022.

164. Watson NJ, Maclagan J, Barnes PJ. Vagal control of guinea-pig tracheal smooth muscle: lack of involvement of VIP or nitric oxide. *J Appl Physiol* 1993;74:1964–1971.

165. Stretton CD, Belvisi MG, Barnes PJ. Modulation of neural bronchoconstrictor responses in the guinea-pig respiratory tract by vasoactive intestinal peptide. *Neuropeptides* 1991;18:149–157.

166. Lei Y-H, Barnes PJ, Rogers DF. Regulation of NANC neural bronchoconstriction *in vivo* in the guinea-pig: involvement of nitric oxide, vasoactive intestinal peptide and soluble guanylyl cyclase. *Br J Pharmacol* 1993;108:228–235.

167. Furchgott RF, Zawadzki JV. The obligatory role of endothelial cells in the relaxation of arterial smooth muscle by acetylcholine. *Nature (Lond)* 1980;288:373–376.

168. Palmer RMJ, Ferrige AG, Moncada S. Nitric oxide release accounts for the biological activity of endothelium-derived relaxant factor. *Nature* 1987;327:524–526.

169. Barnes PJ, Belvisi MG. Nitric oxide and lung disease. *Thorax* 1993;48:1034–1043.

170. Nathan CF. Nitric oxide as a secretory product of mammalian cells. *FASEB J* 1992;6:3051–3064.

171. Forstermann U, Schmidt HHHW, Pollock JS, et al. Isoforms of nitric oxide synthase: characterisation and purification from different cell types. *Biochem Pharmacol* 1991;42:1849–1857.

172. Pollock JS, Forstermann U, Mitchell JA et al. Purification and characterisation of particulate endothelium-derived relaxant factor synthase from cultured and native aortic endothelial cells. *Proc Natl Acad Sci (USA)* 1991;88:10480–10484.

173. Bredt DS, Snyder SH. Isolation of nitric oxide synthetase, a calmodulin-requiring enzyme. *Proc Natl Acad Sci (USA)* 1990;87:682–685.

174. Schmidt HHHW, Pollock JS, Nakane M, Gorsky LD, Forstermann U, Murad F. Purification of a soluble isoform of guanylyl cyclase-activating-factor synthase. *Proc Natl Acad Sci* 1991;88:365–369.

175. Mitchell JA, Sheng H, Forstermann U, Murad F. Characterisation of NO synthase in nonadrenergic noncholinergic nerve containing anoccocygeus. *Br J Pharmacol* 1991;104:289–291.

176. Hamid Q, Springall DR, Riveros-Moreno V. et al. Induction of nitric oxide synthase in asthma. *Lancet* 1993;342:1510–1513.

177. Robbins RA, Barnes PJ, Springall DR, et al. Expression of inducible nitric oxide synthase in human bronchial epithelial cells. *Biochem Biophys Res Commun* 1994;203:209–218.

178. Rand MJ. Nitrergic transmission: nitric oxide a mediator of nonadrenergic, noncholinergic neuroeffector transmission. *Clin Exp Pharmacol Physiol* 1992;19:147–169.

179. Bredt DS, Hwang PM, Snyder SH. Localisation of nitric oxide synthase indicating a neural role for nitric oxide. *Nature* 1990;347:768–770.

180. Llewellyn-Smith IJ, Song ZM, Costa M, Bredt DS, Snyder SH. Ultrastructural localization of nitric oxide synthase immunoreactivity in guinea-pig enteric neurons. *Brain Res* 1992; 577:337–3342.

181. Kannan MS, Johnson DE. Nitric oxide mediates the neural nonadrenergic, noncholinergic relaxation of pig tracheal smooth muscle. *Am J Physiol* 1992;262:L511–L514.

182. Yu M, Robinson NE, Wang Z. Regional distribution of nitroxidergic and adrenergic nerves in equine airway smooth muscle. *Am Rev Respir Dis* 1993;147:A286.

183. Hecker M, Mitchell JA, Harris HJ, Katsura M, Thiemermann C, Vane JR. Endothelial cells metabolize N^G-monomethyl-L-arginine to L-citrulline and subsequently to L-arginine. *Biochem Biophys Res Commun* 1990;167:1037–1043.

184. Bogle RG, Moncada S, Pearson JD, Mann GE. Identification of inhibitors of nitric oxide synthase that do not interact with the endothelial cell L-arginine transporter. *Br J Pharmacol* 1993;105:768–770.

185. Li CG, Rand MJ. Evidence for a role of nitric oxide in the NANC-mediated relaxations in rat anococcygeus muscle. *Clin Exp Physiol Pharmacol* 1989;16:933–938.

186. Li CG, Rand MJ. Nitric oxide and vasoactive intestinal polypeptide mediate nonadrenergic, noncholinergic inhibitory transmission to smooth muscle of the rat gastric fundus. *Eur J Pharmacol* 1990;191:303–309.

187. Grider JJ, Murthy KS, Jin JG, Makhlouf GM. Stimulation of nitric oxide from muscle cells by VIP: pre-junctional enhancement of VIP release. *Am J Physiol* 1992;262:G774–G778.

188. Fischer A, Mundel P, Mayer B, Preissler U, Philippin B, Kummer W. Nitric oxide synthase in guinea-pig lower airway innervation. *Neurosci Letts* 1993;149:157–160.

189. De Luca A, Li CG, Rand MJ, Reid JJ, Thaina P, Wong-Dusting HK. Effects of ω conotoxin GVIA on autonomic neuroeffector transmission in various tissues. *Br J Pharmacol* 1990;101:437–447.

190. Diamond L, Lantta J, Thompson D, Altiere RJ. Nitric oxide synthase inhibitors fail to affect cat airway nonadrenergic noncholinergic inhibitory (NANCI) responses. *Am Rev Respir Dis* 1992;145:A382.

191. Jing L, Inoue R, Tashiro K, Takahashi S, Ito Y. Role of nitric oxide in inhibitory and modulation of excitatory neuroeffector transmission in cat airway. *J Physiol* 1995;481:225–237.

192. Fame TM, Loader JE, Graves J, Colasurdo GN, Larsen GL. Decrease in the airways nonadrenergic, noncholinergic inhibitory system in allergen sensitised rabbit. *Am Rev Respir Dis* 1993;147:A285.

193. Rapoport RM, Murad F. Agonist induced endothelium-dependent relaxation in rat thoracic aorta may be mediated through cGMP. *Circ Res* 1983;52:352–357.

194. Ward JK, Barnes PJ, Tadjkarimi S, Yacoub MH, Belvisi MG. Neural relaxation in human tracheal smooth muscle (HTSM) is mediated by an increase in cGMP: further evidence for the role of nitric oxide. *J Physiol* 1995;483:525–536.

195. Rhoden KJ, Barnes PJ. Epithelial modulation of NANC and VIP-induced responses: role of neutral endopeptidase. *Eur J Pharmacol* 1989;171:247–250.

196. Fischer A, Hoffman B, Hauser-Kronberger C, Mayer B, Kummer W. Nitric oxide synthase in the innervation of the human respiratory tract. *Am Rev Respir Dis* 1993;147:A662.

197. Hassall CJS, Saffrey MJ, Burnstock G. NADPH-diaphorase activity by guinea-pig paratracheal neurones. *NeuroReport* 1993;4:49–52.

198. Undem BJ, Myers AC, Barthlow H et al. Vagal innervation of the guinea-pig bronchus. *J Appl Physiol* 1990;69:1336–1346.

199. Ellis JL, Undem BJ. Nonadrenergic, noncholinergic contractions in the electrically field stimulated guinea-pig trachea. *Br J Pharmacol* 1990;101:875–880.

200. Palmer JBD, Sampson AP, Barnes PJ. Cholinergic and nonadrenergic inhibitory responses in bovine airways: distribution and functional association. *Am Rev Respir Dis* 1985;A283.

201. Diamond L, Altiere RJ. Airway nonadrenergic noncholinergic inhibitory nervous system. In: Kaliner M, Barnes PJ, eds. *Lung biology*

in health and disease. *The airways: neural control in health and disease.* New York: Marcel Dekker, 1989;343–394.

202. Lammers J-WJ, Barnes PJ, Chung KF. Nonadrenergic, noncholinergic airway inhibitory nerves. *Eur Respir J* 1992;5:239–246.

203. Miura M, Inoue H, Ichinose M, Kimura K, Katsumata U, Takishima T. Effect of nonadrenergic, noncholinergic inhibitory nerve stimulation on the allergic reaction in cat airways. *Am Rev Respir Dis* 1990; 141:29–32.

204. Undem BJ, Dick EC, Buckner CK. Inhibition by vasoactive intestinal peptide of antigen-induced histamine release from guinea-pig minced lung. *Eur J Pharmacol* 1983;88:247–250.

205. Miura M, Kimura K, Takahashi T, Inoue H, Takishima T. Possible mechanisms of the antigen-induced dysfunction of nonadrenergic, noncholinergic inhibitory nervous system. *Am Rev Respir Dis* 1990; 141:A387.

206. Tam EK, Caughey, GH. Degradation of airway neuropeptides by human lung typtase. *Am J Respir Cell Mol Biol* 1990;3:27–32.

207. Kakuta Y, Stead RH, Perdue MH, Marshall JS, Bienenstock J. Microanatomical relationship of mast cells and nerves in rat lung and trachea. *Am Rev Respir Dis* 1989;139:A118.

208. Taylor SM, Paré, Armour CL, Hogg JC, Schellenburg RR. Airway reactivity in chronic obstructive pulmonary disease. Failure of *in vivo* methacholine responsiveness to correlate with cholinergic, adrenergic, or nonadrenergic responses *in vitro*. *Am Rev Respir Dis* 1985;132: 30–35.

209. Belvisi MG, Ward JK, Tadjkarimi S, Yacoub MH, Barnes PJ. Inhibitory NANC nerves in human airways: differences in disease and after extrinsic denervation. *Am Rev Respir Dis* 1993;147:A286.

210. Bai TR. Abnormalities in airway smooth muscle in fatal asthma. *Am Rev Respir Dis* 1990;141:552–557.

211. Howarth P, Britten KM, Djukanovic RJ. et al. Neuropeptide containing nerves in human airways *in vivo*: a comparative study of atopic asthma, atopic nonasthma, and nonatopic nonasthma. *Thorax* 1990; 45:786–787.

212. Belvisi MG, Ward JK, Springall DR. et al. Nitrergic innervation in the airways of patients with cystic fibrosis. *Am J Respir Med Crit Care Med* 1994;149:A675.

213. Belvisi MG, Stretton CD, Barnes PJ. Nitric oxide as an endogenous modulator of cholinergic neurotransmission in guinea-pig airways. *Eur J Pharmacol* 1991;198:219–221.

214. Ward JK, Belvisi, MG, Fox AJ, et al. Modulation of cholinergic bronchoconstrictor responses by endogenous nitric oxide and vasoactive intestinal peptide in human airways *in vitro*. *J Clin Invest* 1993;92: 736–742.

Asthma, edited by P.J. Barnes, M.M. Grunstein, A.R. Leff, and A.J. Woolcock.
Lippincott–Raven Publishers, Philadelphia © 1997.

▪ 73 ▪

Sensory Neuropeptides

Peter J. Barnes and Maria G. Belvisi

Experimental Approaches
Tachykinins
  Localization
  Effects on Airways
Metabolism
Calcitonin Gene-related Peptide
  Localization
  Airway Effects
Neurogenic Inflammation in Airways
  Neurogenic Airway Inflammation in
    Animal Models

Capsaicin Depletion Studies
Inhibition of Neuropeptide Metabolism
Antagonists
Inhibition of Sensory Neuropeptide Release
Neurogenic Inflammation in Asthma
  Sensory Nerves in Human Airways
  Sensory Nerve Activation
  Studies with NEP Inhibitors
  Tachykinin Responsiveness
  Modulation of Neurogenic Inflammation

The peptides substance P (SP), neurokinin A (NKA), and calcitonin gene-related peptide (CGRP) are localized to a population of sensory neurons in the respiratory tract (1–3). These peptides have potent effects on bronchomotor tone, airway secretions, bronchial circulation, and inflammatory and immune cells. Although some clues to the physiologic and pathophysiologic role of these peptides are provided by their localization and functional effects, the most useful information is provided by depletion studies using capsaicin, and increasingly by the use of potent and specific receptor antagonists. Many of the inflammatory and functional effects of sensory neuropeptides are relevant to asthma and there is compelling evidence for the involvement of neuropeptides in the pathophysiology and symptomatology of asthma (4). Here we discuss effects of sensory neuropeptides that are relevant to the pathophysiology of asthma.

EXPERIMENTAL APPROACHES

Several approaches have been used to investigate the role of sensory neuropeptides in airways. The effects of exogenous sensory neuropeptides on various target cells relevant to asthma *in vitro* and their effects on airway function *in vivo* have been studied widely in animals and humans (2). This approach is valuable in revealing the potential effects of a particular peptide, but it is not possible to know exactly what the local concentration of a particular peptide might be. Furthermore, there are striking differences between species. Even data in normal human airways may not be relevant to the situation in the diseased airway, where there might be alterations in neuropeptide receptor expression and metabolic breakdown.

A more informative approach is to investigate the action of specific blockers or enhancers, or to study depletion of the relevant peptide because this can reveal the role of the endogenous neuropeptide. Again, it is possible that the disease state may alter the synthesis, release, or metabolism of a particular peptide or its receptors and therefore produce changes in the effects of blocking drugs. It is only recently that potent specific tachykinin receptor blockers have become available; these will prove to be increasingly important tools in the investigation of the role of neuropeptides in disease.

Several animal models of asthma have been investigated, but none of these closely mimic the chronic eosinophilic inflammation characteristic of asthma and they have been poorly predictive of drugs that will have clinical efficacy. The only certain way to evaluate the role

P. J. Barnes and M. G. Belvisi: Department of Thoracic Medicine, Imperial College of Medicine at The National Heart and Lung Institute, London, SW3 6LY United Kingdom.

of neuropeptides in asthma is to study the effect of specific antagonists or inhibitors in patients with asthma. Specific neuropeptide antagonists suitable for clinical use are now developed and studies are already underway in asthma. Again there may be pitfalls in this approach, as it is usual practice to select patients with mild asthma for such studies. It is possible that neuropeptides are relevant only in certain types of asthma or in more severe and intractable disease. Furthermore, it may be difficult to evaluate the effects of neuropeptides on airway function in clinical studies if their main action is on mucosal inflammation, mucous secretion, or airway blood flow, because techniques to evaluate these responses are difficult in patients.

TACHYKININS

Localization

SP and NKA, but not neurokinin B, are localized to sensory nerves in the airways of several species. SP-immunoreactive nerves are abundant in rodent airways, but are very sparse in human airways (5–7). Rapid enzymatic degradation of SP in airways, and the fact that SP concentrations may decrease with age and possibly after cigarette smoking, could explain the difficulty in demonstrating this peptide in some studies. SP-immunoreactive nerves in the airway are found beneath and within the airway epithelium, around blood vessels, and, to a lesser extent, within airway smooth muscle. SP-immunoreactive nerve fibers also innervate parasympathetic ganglia, suggesting a sensory input that may modulate ganglionic transmission and so result in ganglionic reflexes.

SP in the airways is localized predominantly to capsaicin-sensitive unmyelinated nerves in the airways, but chronic administration of capsaicin only partially depletes the lung of tachykinins, indicating the presence of a population of capsaicin-resistant SP-immunoreactive nerves, as in the gastrointestinal tract (8,9). Similar capsaicin denervation studies are not possible in human airways, but after extrinsic denervation by heart-lung transplantation there appears to be a loss of SP-immunoreactive nerves in the submucosa (10).

Effects on Airways

Tachykinins have many different effects on the airways that may be relevant to asthma; these effects are mediated via NK_1- (preferentially activated by SP) and NK_2-receptors (preferentially activated by NKA), whereas there is little evidence of NK_3-receptors (Table 1).

Airway Smooth Muscle

Tachykinins constrict smooth muscle of human airways *in vitro* via NK_2-receptors (11,12). The contractile response to NKA is significantly greater in smaller human bronchi than in more proximal airways, indicating that tachykinins may have a more important constrictor effect in peripheral airways (13), whereas cholinergic constriction tends to be more pronounced in proximal airways. This is consistent with the autoradiographic distribution of tachykinin receptors that are distributed to small and large airways. *In vivo*, SP does not cause bronchoconstriction or cough, either by intravenous infusion (14,15) or by inhalation (14,16), whereas NKA causes bronchoconstriction after both intravenous administration (15) and after inhalation in asthmatic individuals (16). Inhalation of SP increased airway responsiveness to methacholine in asthmatics, an effect that has been ascribed to airway edema (17). Mechanical removal of airway epithelium potentiates the bronchoconstrictor response to tachykinins (18,19), largely because the ectoenzyme neutral endopeptidase 24.11 (NEP), which is a key enzyme in the degradation of tachykinins in airways, is strongly expressed on epithelial cells (Fig. 1).

TABLE 1. *Effects of tachykinins on airways*

Target cell	Effect	Receptor
Airway smooth muscle	Constrict (peripheral>central)	NK_2 (+NK_1 in guinea pig)
Bronchial vessels	Vasodilatation	NK_2 + NK_1 (via NO release)
	Plasma exudation	NK_1
	Angiogenesis?	?
Submucosal glands	Increased secretion	NK_1
Airway epithelium	Increased ion transport	NK_1
	Increased ciliary beating	NK_1
	Release of prostanoids	NK_1
	Increased mucous secretion (goblet cells)	NK_1
Nerves	Increased acetylcholine release	NK_2
	Increased ganglionic transmission	NK_1, NK_3
Macrophages	Increased mediator release	NK_2
Fibroblasts	Increased collagen secretion	NK_1 + NK_2
T lymphocytes	Increased cytokine release	?

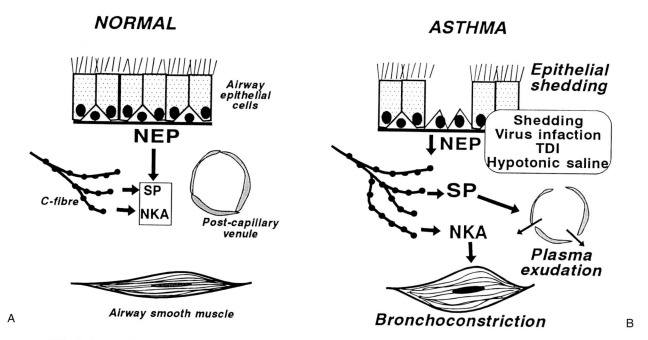

FIG. 1. Interaction of tachykinins with airway epithelium. When epithelium is intact neutral endopeptidase (*NEP*) degrades substance P (*SP*) and neurokinin A (*NKA*) released from sensory nerves (**A**). In asthmatic airways when epithelium is shed or NEP downregulated, any tachykinins released will have an exaggerated effect (**B**).

Airway Secretions

SP stimulates mucous secretion from submucosal glands in ferret and human airways *in vitro* (20,21) and is a potent stimulant to goblet cell secretion in guinea pig airways (22). Indeed, SP is likely to mediate the increase in goblet cell discharge after vagus nerve stimulation and exposure to cigarette smoke (23,24).

Stimulation of the vagus nerve in rodents causes microvascular leakage, which is prevented by prior treatment with capsaicin or by a tachykinin antagonist, indicating that release of tachykinins from sensory nerves mediates this effect. Among the tachykinins, SP is most potent at causing leakage in guinea-pig airways (25) and NK$_1$-receptors have been localized to postcapillary venules in the airway submucosa (26). Inhaled SP also causes microvascular leakage in guinea pigs and its effect on the microvasculature is more marked than its effect on airway smooth muscle (27). It is difficult to measure airway microvascular leakage in human airways, but SP causes a weal in human skin when injected intradermally, indicating the capacity to cause microvascular leak in human postcapillary venules; NKA is less potent, indicating that an NK$_1$-receptor mediates this effect (28).

Vascular effects

Tachykinins have potent effects on airway blood flow. Indeed, the effect of tachykinins on airway blood flow may be the most important physiologic and pathophysiologic role of tachykinins in airways. In canine and porcine trachea both SP and NKA cause a marked increase in blood flow (29,30). Tachykinins also dilate canine bronchial vessels *in vitro,* probably via an endothelium-dependent mechanism (31). Tachykinins also regulate bronchial blood flow in pig; stimulation of the vagus nerve causes a vasodilatation mediated by the release of sensory neuropeptides, and it is likely that CGRP as well as tachykinins are involved (30).

Effects on Nerves

In guinea pig trachea tachykinins also potentiate cholinergic neurotransmission at postganglionic nerve terminals, and an NK$_2$-receptor appears to be involved (32). There is also potentiation at ganglionic level (33,34), which appears to be mediated via an NK$_1$-receptor (34). There is also evidence that NK$_3$-receptors are involved (35). Endogenous tachykinins also may facilitate cholinergic neurotransmission because capsaicin pretreatment results in a significant reduction in cholinergic neural responses both *in vitro* and *in vivo* (36,37). However, in human airways there is no evidence for a facilitatory effect on cholinergic neurotransmission (38), although such an effect has been reported in the presence of potassium channel blockers (39).

In conscious guinea pigs very low concentrations of inhaled SP are reported to cause cough; this effect is potentiated by NEP inhibition (40). Citric acid-induced cough is blocked by a nonpeptide NK$_2$-receptor antagonist (SR 48968), suggesting the involvement of NK$_2$-receptors, although these may be centrally located (41).

Immunologic Effects

Tachykinins also may interact with inflammatory and immune cells (42,43), although whether this is of pathophysiologic significance remains to be determined. There is likely to be increasing research in the area of neuroimmune interaction and in some species there is already evidence for neuropeptide innervation of bronchus-associated lymphoid tissue (44). SP degranulates certain types of mast cells, such as those in human skin, although this is not mediated via a tachykinin receptor (45). There is no evidence that tachykinins degranulate lung mast cells (46). SP has a degranulating effect on eosinophils (47); again, the degranulation is related to high concentrations of peptide and, as for mast cells, is not mediated via a tachykinin receptor. At lower concentrations tachykinins have been reported to enhance eosinophil chemotaxis (48). Tachykinins may activate alveolar macrophages (49) and monocytes to release inflammatory cytokines, such as interleukin-6 (IL-6) (50). Topical application of SP to human nasal mucosa results in increased expression of several cytokines, suggesting that SP may have important chronic immune effects (51), and these deserve further study. Tachykinins and vagus nerve stimulation also cause transient vascular adhesion of neutrophils in the airway circulation (52) and in human skin (53).

Structural Effects

SP stimulates proliferation of blood vessels (angiogenesis) (54) and therefore may be involved in the new vessel formation found in asthmatic airways (55). SP and NKA also stimulate the proliferation and chemotaxis of human lung fibroblasts, suggesting that tachykinins may contribute to the fibrotic process in chronic asthma (56). These effects appear to be mediated by both NK$_1$- and NK$_2$-receptors.

METABOLISM

Tachykinins are subject to degradation by at least two enzymes: angiotensin-converting enzyme (ACE) and NEP (57). ACE is predominantly localized to vascular endothelial cells and therefore breaks down intravascular peptides. ACE inhibitors, such as captopril, enhance bronchoconstriction because of intravenous SP (58,59), but not inhaled SP (60). NKA is not a good substrate for ACE, however. NEP appears to be the most important enzyme for the breakdown of tachykinins in tissues. Inhibition of NEP by phosphoramidon or thiorphan markedly potentiates bronchoconstriction in vitro in animal (61) and human airways (62) and after inhalation in vivo (60). NEP inhibition also potentiates mucous secretion in response to tachykinins in human airways (20). NEP inhibition enhances excitatory nonadrenergic noncholinergic (e-NANC) and capsaicin-induced bronchoconstriction, because of the release of tachykinins from airway sensory nerves (18,63).

The activity of NEP in the airways appears to be an important factor in determining the effects of tachykinins; any factors that inhibit the enzyme or its expression may be associated with increased effects of exogenous or endogenously released tachykinins. Several of the stimuli known to induce bronchoconstrictor responses in asthmatic patients have been found to reduce the activity of airway NEP (57).

CALCITONIN GENE-RELATED PEPTIDE

Localization

CGRP-immunoreactive nerves are abundant in the respiratory tract of several species. CGRP is co-stored and co-localized with SP in afferent nerves (64). CGRP has been extracted from and is localized to human airways (7,65). CGRP-immunoreactive nerve fibers appear to be more abundant than SP fibers, possibly because CGRP has greater stability, and is also present in some nerves that do not contain SP. CGRP is found in trigeminal, nodose-jugular, and dorsal root ganglia (66) and also has been detected in neuroendocrine cells of the lower airways.

Airway Effects

CGRP is a potent vasodilator that has long-lasting effects. CGRP is an effective dilator of human pulmonary vessels in vitro and acts directly on receptors on vascular smooth muscle (67). It also potently dilates bronchial vessels in vitro (67) and produces a marked and long-lasting increase in airway blood flow in anesthetized dogs (68) and conscious sheep in vivo (69). Receptor mapping studies have demonstrated that CGRP receptors are localized predominantly to bronchial vessels rather than to smooth muscle or epithelium in human airways (70). It is possible that CGRP may be the predominant mediator of arterial vasodilatation and increased blood flow in response to sensory nerve stimulation in the bronchi (30). CGRP may be an important mediator of airway hyperemia in asthma.

By contrast, CGRP has no direct effect of airway microvascular leak (25). In the skin, CGRP potentiates the leakage produced by SP, presumably by increasing the blood delivery to the sites of plasma extravasation in the postcapillary venules (71) (Fig. 2). This does not occur in guinea pig airways when CGRP and SP are co-adminis-

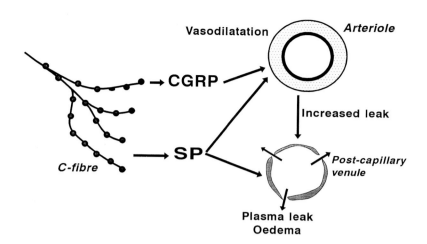

FIG. 2. Effect of sensory neuropeptides in airway vessels. Substance P causes vasodilatation and plasma exudation, whereas calcitonin gene-related peptide causes vasodilatation of arterioles, which may theoretically increase plasma extravasation by increasing blood delivery to leaky post-capillary venules.

tered, possibly because blood flow in the airways is already high (25), although an increased leakage response has been reported in rat airways (72). It is possible that potentiation of leak may occur when the two peptides are released together from sensory nerves.

CGRP causes constriction of human bronchi *in vitro* (65). This is surprising because CGRP normally activates adenylyl cyclase, an event usually associated with bronchodilatation. Receptor mapping studies suggest few, if any, CGRP receptors over airway smooth muscle in human or guinea pig airways; this suggests that the paradoxical bronchoconstrictor response reported in human airways may be mediated indirectly. In guinea pig airways, CGRP has no consistent effect on tone (73). The variable effects of CGRP on airways may be explained by the fact that it may release other mediators that have effects on tone. Thus, CGRP may release both nitric oxide (NO) and endothelin in airways (74).

CGRP has a weak inhibitory effect on cholinergically stimulated mucous secretion in ferret trachea (75) and on goblet cell discharge in guinea pig airways (22). This is probably related to the low density of CGRP receptors on mucous secretory cells, but does not preclude the possibility that CGRP might increase mucous secretion *in vivo* by increasing blood flow to submucosal glands.

CGRP injection into human skin causes a persistent flare, but biopsies have revealed an infiltration of eosinophils (76). CGRP itself does not appear to be chemotactic for eosinophils, but proteolytic fragments of the peptide are active (77), suggesting that CGRP released into the tissues may lead to eosinophilic infiltration.

CGRP inhibits the proliferative response of T lymphocytes to mitogens and specific receptors have been demonstrated on these cells (78). CGRP also inhibits macrophage secretion and the capacity of macrophages to activate T lymphocytes (79). This suggests that CGRP has potential anti-inflammatory actions in the airways. CGRP also induces proliferation of guinea pig airway epithelial cells and therefore may be involved in healing the airway after epithelial shedding in asthma (80).

NEUROGENIC INFLAMMATION IN AIRWAYS

In rodents there is now considerable evidence for neurogenic inflammation in the airways because of the antidromic release of neuropeptides from nociceptive nerves or C-fibers via an axon reflex (81–83); it is possible that it may contribute to the inflammatory response in asthma (84,85) (Fig. 3).

Neurogenic Airway Inflammation in Animal Models

There are several lines of evidence, which may have relevance to asthma, that neurogenic inflammation may be important in animal models. These models usually have been in rodents, where tachykinin effects are pronounced and may not be predictive of the role of tachykinins in human airways, however. There are four main experimental approaches that have been used to assess the role of sensory neuropeptides in animal models of asthma: studies of depletion with capsaicin depletion, enhancement with inhibitors of NEP, tachykinin receptor antagonists, and inhibitors of sensory neuropeptide release.

Capsaicin Depletion Studies

Capsaicin pretreatment depletes neuropeptides from C-fibers, either in neonatal animals (which results in degeneration of C-fibers) or acute treatment in adult animals (resulting in depletion of sensory neuropeptides). In rat trachea capsaicin pretreatment inhibits the microvascular leakage induced by irritant gases, such as cigarette smoke (86), and inhibits goblet cell discharge and microvascular leak induced by cigarette smoke in guinea pigs (24). Capsaicin-sensitive nerves also may contribute to the bronchoconstriction and microvascular leak induced by isocapnic hyperventilation (87), hypocapnia (88), inhaled sodium metabisulfite (89), nebulized hypertonic saline (90), and toluene diisocyanate (91) in rodents. In guinea pigs, capsaicin pretreatment has little or no effect on the acute bron-

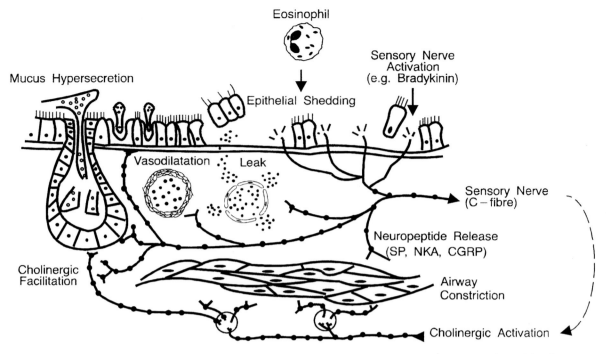

FIG. 3. Possible neurogenic inflammation in asthmatic airways via retrograde release of peptides from sensory nerves via an axon reflex. Substance P (*SP*) causes vasodilatation, plasma exudation, and mucous secretion, whereas neurokinin A (*NKA*) causes bronchoconstriction and enhanced cholinergic reflexes and calcitonin gene-related peptide (*CGRP*) vasodilatation.

choconstrictor or plasma exudation response to allergen inhalation in sensitized animals (92). Administration of capsaicin increases airway responsiveness in guinea pigs to cholinergic agonists; this effect is prevented by prior treatment with capsaicin, suggesting that capsaicin-sensitive nerves release products that increase airway responsiveness (93). Similarly, in a virus model of airway hyperresponsiveness in guinea pigs capsaicin pretreatment completely blocks the virus-induced hyperresponsiveness (94). In pigs capsaicin pretreatment inhibits the vasodilator response to allergen (which may be mediated by the release of CGRP) (95). In allergic sheep capsaicin pretreatment prevents the airway hyperresponsiveness to both allergen and cholinergic agonists (96). In a model of chronic allergen exposure in guinea pigs capsaicin pretreatment results in complete inhibition of airway hyperresponsiveness, without any change in the eosinophil inflammatory response (97), and prevents the increased responsiveness to ovalbumin *in vitro* (98). In rabbits neonatal capsaicin treatment inhibits the airway hyperresponsiveness associated with neonatal allergen sensitization, although this does not appear to be associated with any change in content of sensory neuropeptides in lung tissue (99). This suggests that capsaicin-sensitive nerves may play a role in chronic inflammatory responses to allergen.

There has been speculation that mast cells in the airways might be influenced by capsaicin-sensitive nerves.

Histologic studies have demonstrated a close proximity between mast cells and sensory nerves in airways (100). There is also evidence that antidromic stimulation of the vagus nerve leads to mast-cell mediator release in canine airways (101). Furthermore, allergen exposure has effects on ion transport in guinea pig airways that are dependent on capsaicin-sensitive nerves (102).

Inhibition of Neuropeptide Metabolism

The activity of NEP may be an important determinant of the extent of neurogenic inflammation in airways; inhibition of NEP in rodent by thiorphan or phosphoramidon has been shown to enhance neurogenic inflammation in various rodent models. NEP is not specific to tachykinins and is involved in the metabolism of other bronchoactive peptides, including kinins and endothelins. Certain virus infections enhance e-NANC responses in guinea pigs (103) and mycoplasma infection enhances neurogenic microvascular leakage in rats (82), an effect mediated by inhibition of NEP activity. Influenza virus infection of ferret trachea *in vitro* and of guinea pigs *in vivo* inhibits the activity of epithelial NEP and markedly enhances the bronchoconstrictor responses to tachykinins (104). Similarly, Sendai virus infection potentiates neurogenic inflammation in rat trachea (105). This may explain why respiratory tract virus infections are so deleterious to patients with asthma. Hypertonic saline also impairs epithelial NEP function, leading to exaggerated tachykinin responses (90), and cigarette smoke exposure has a similar effect that can be explained by an oxidizing effect on the enzyme (106). Toluene diisocyanate, albeit at rather high doses, also reduces NEP activity; this may be a mechanism contributing to the airway hyperresponsiveness that may follow exposure to this chemical (107). Inhalation of IL-1β is associated with increased responsiveness to bradykinin; this may be due to inhibition of NEP expression (108). Thus, many of the agents that lead to exacerbations of asthma appear to reduce the activity of NEP at the airway surface, thus leading to exaggerated responses to tachykinins (and other peptides) and so to increased airway inflammation.

Antagonists

Specific antagonists of tachykinin receptors have now been developed to provide a more specific tool to investigate the role of tachykinins in animal models. Several highly potent and stable peptide and nonpeptide tachykinin antagonists have been developed that are highly selective for either NK$_1$- or NK$_2$-receptors (109). The NK$_1$-receptor antagonist CP 96,345 is able to block the plasma exudation response to vagus nerve stimulation and to cigarette smoke in guinea pig airways (110,111) without affecting the bronchoconstrictor response, which is blocked by the NK$_2$-antagonist SR 48,968 (12). Similar results have been obtained with the potent NK$_1$-selective antagonist FK-888 (112). CP 96,345 also blocks hyperpnea- and bradykinin-induced plasma exudation in guinea pigs (113, 114), but has no effect on the acute plasma exudation induced by allergen in sensitized animals (114). These specific antagonists are useful new tools in probing the involvement of tachykinins in disease, and will be invaluable in clinical studies in the future.

Inhibition of Sensory Neuropeptide Release

Several agonists act on prejunctional receptors on airway sensory nerves to inhibit the release of neuropeptides and neurogenic inflammation (115) (Fig. 4). Opioids are the most effective inhibitory agonists, acting via prejunctional μ-receptors and have been shown to inhibit cigarette smoke-induced discharge from goblet cells in guinea pig airways *in vivo* (116) and to inhibit ozone-induced hyperreactivity in guinea pigs, which appears to be mediated via sensory nerves (117). Several other agonists also are effective and may act by opening a common calcium-activated large conductance potassium channel in sensory nerves (118). Openers of other potassium channels, which achieve the same hyperpolarization of the sensory nerve, also are effective in blocking neurogenic inflammation in rodents (119) and have been shown to

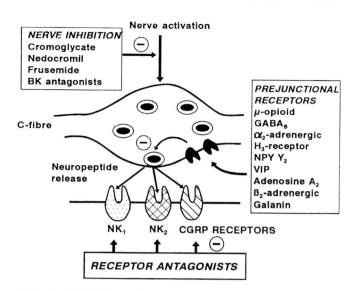

FIG. 4. Modulation of neurogenic inflammation in airway sensory nerves.

block cigarette smoke-induced goblet cell secretion in guinea pigs (120).

NEUROGENIC INFLAMMATION IN ASTHMA

Although it was proposed several years ago that neurogenic inflammation and peptides released from sensory nerves might be important as an amplifying mechanism in asthmatic inflammation (84), there is little evidence to date to support this idea, despite the extensive work in rodent models (121,122). This is partly because it has proved difficult to apply the same approaches to human volunteers. There is evidence both in favor and against neurogenic inflammation and a role for sensory neuropeptides in asthmatic inflammation (Table 2).

Sensory Nerves in Human Airways

In comparison with rodent airways, SP- and CGRP-immunoreactive nerves are sparse in human airways. Quantitative studies indicate that SP-immunoreactive fibers constitute only 1% of the total number of intraepithelial fibers, whereas in guinea pig they make up 60% of the fibers (123). This raises the possibility that sensory nerves in humans may contain some unidentified transmitter that may be involved in neurogenic inflammation. Chronic inflammation may lead to changes in the pattern of innervation through the release of neurotrophic factors from inflammatory cells. Thus, in chronic arthritis and inflammatory bowel disease there is an increase in the density of SP-immunoreactive nerves (124,125). A striking increase in SP-like immunoreactive nerves has been reported in the airway of patients with fatal asthma (126). This increased density of nerves is particularly noticeable

TABLE 2. *Evidence for and against a role of sensory neuropeptides in asthma*

For	Against
Increased SP-immunoreactive nerves (severe/fatal asthma)	No increase in SP-immunoreactivity
Increased response to tachykinins	Poor response to exogenous SP
Increased airway responsiveness after SP inhalation	Capsaicin inhalation causes only transient bronchoconstriction
Increased SP concentrations (BAL, sputum)	NEP inhibitors have similar effect in nonasthmatic and asthmatic subjects
Increased NK$_1$-receptor expression	Modulators of neuropeptide release (opioids, H$_3$-agonists) ineffective
SP antagonist inhibits bradykinin responses	Tachykinin antagonists not effective in asthma?
NEP expression reduced in asthma?	

SP, peptide substance P; BAL, bronchoalveolar lavage; NEP, neutral endopeptidase.

in the submucosa. Whether this apparent increase is due to proliferation of sensory nerves or to increased synthesis of tachykinins has not been established. However, other studies have failed to confirm an increase in SP in lungs from patients with asthma (127). After nasal challenge with allergen an increase in SP in nasal lavage fluid has been reported (128). Recently elevated concentrations of SP in bronchoalveolar lavage of patients with asthma have been reported, with a further rise after allergen challenge (129), suggesting that there may be an increase in SP in the airways of asthmatic patients. Similarly, SP has been detected in the sputum of asthmatic patients after hypertonic saline inhalation (130). SP also increases in the bronchoalveolar lavage of nonasthmatic volunteers exposed to ozone, possible because of a reduction in NEP activity (131).

Cultured sensory neurons are stimulated by nerve growth factor (NGF), which markedly increases the transcription of preprotachykinin A (PPT-A) gene, the major precursor peptide for tachykinins (132). Similarly, adjuvant-induced inflammation in rat spinal cord increases the gene expression of PPT-A (133). Preliminary studies suggest that allergen challenge is associated with a doubling in PPT-A messenger ribonucleic acid (mRNA)-positive neurons in nodose ganglia of guinea pigs and an increase in SP-immunoreactivity in the lungs (134). However, bronchial biopsies of mild asthmatic patients have not revealed any evidence of increased SP-immunoreactive nerves (135). This may indicate that the increased innervation (126) may be a feature of either prolonged or severe asthma and indicates the need for more studies.

Sensory Nerve Activation

Sensory nerves may be activated in airway disease. In asthmatic airways the epithelium is often shed, thereby exposing sensory nerve endings. Sensory nerves in asthmatic airways may be "hyperalgesic" as a result of exposure to inflammatory mediators such as prostaglandins and certain cytokines (such as IL-1β and tumor necrosis factor (TNF)-α (136). Hyperalgesic nerves may then be activated more readily by other mediators, such as kinins.

Capsaicin induces bronchoconstriction and plasma exudation in guinea pigs (8) and increases airway blood flow in pigs (95). In humans, capsaicin inhalation causes cough and a transient bronchoconstriction, which is inhibited by cholinergic blockade and is probably due to a laryngeal reflex (137,138). This suggests that neuropeptide release does not occur in human airways, although it is possible that insufficient capsaicin reaches the lower respiratory tract because the dose is limited by coughing. In patients with asthma, there is no evidence that capsaicin induces a greater degree of bronchoconstriction than in normal individuals (137).

Bradykinin is a potent bronchoconstrictor in asthmatic patients and also induces coughing and a sensation of chest tightness, which closely mimics a naturally occurring asthma attack (see Chapter 43). Yet, it is a weak constrictor of human airways *in vitro*, suggesting that its potent constrictor effect is mediated indirectly. Bradykinin is a potent activator of bronchial C-fibers in dogs (139) and releases sensory neuropeptides from perfused rodent lungs (140). In guinea pigs bradykinin instilled into the airways causes bronchoconstriction, which is reduced significantly by a cholinergic antagonist (as in asthmatic patients [141]), and also by capsaicin pretreatment (142). The plasma leakage induced by inhaled bradykinin is inhibited by an NK$_1$-antagonist and bronchoconstriction by an NK$_2$-antagonist (114,143). This indicates that bradykinin activates sensory nerves in the airways and that part of the airway response is mediated by release of constrictor peptides from capsaicin-sensitive nerves. In asthmatic patients an inhaled nonselective tachykinin antagonist, FK-224, recently has been shown to reduce the bronchoconstrictor response to inhaled bradykinin and also to block the cough response in those persons who coughed in response to bradykinin (144).

Studies with NEP Inhibitors

In rodents inhibition of NEP with thiorphan or phosphoramidon results in striking potentiation of tachykinin and sensory nerve-induced effects and has been used as an approach to explore the potential for neurogenic inflammation in disease (57). Intravenous acetorphan, which is hydrolyzed to thiorphan, was administered to asthmatics and, although there was potentiation of the weal and flare response to intradermal SP, there was no effect on baseline airway caliber or on bronchoconstriction induced by a "neurogenic" trigger sodium metabisulfite (145). The lack of effect could be due to inadequate inhibition of NEP in the airways, and particularly at the level of the epithelium. Nebulized thiorphan has been shown to potentiate the bronchoconstrictor response to inhaled NKA in nonasthmatics and asthmatics (146,147), but there was no effect on baseline lung function in asthmatic patients (147), indicating that there is unlikely to be any basal release of tachykinins. NEP is strongly expressed in the human airway (148), but there is no evidence based on immunocytochemical staining or *in situ* hybridization that it is defective in asthmatic airways (Baraniuk J, Barnes PJ: unpublished observations); the fact that after inhaled thiorphan the bronchoconstrictor response to inhaled NKA is further enhanced in asthmatic subjects, provides supportive functional data that NEP function may not be impaired, at least in mild asthma (147). Of course, it is possible that NEP may become dysfunctional after viral infections or exposure to oxidants and thus contribute to asthma exacerbations.

Tachykinin Responsiveness

In inflammatory bowel disease there is evidence for a marked upregulation of tachykinin receptors, particularly in the vasculature, suggesting that chronic inflammation may lead to changes in tachykinin receptor expression (149,150). In patients with allergic rhinitis an increased vascular response to nasally applied SP is observed (151). There is evidence that NK_1-receptor gene expression may be increased in the lungs of asthmatic patients (152). This might be due to increased transcription in response to activation of transcription factors, such as AP-1, which are activated in human lung by cytokines such as TNF-α (153). A consensus sequence both for AP-1 binding has been identified upstream of the NK_1-receptor gene (154). Corticosteroids conversely reduce NK_1-receptor gene expression (155), presumably via an inhibitory effect on AP-1 activation.

Modulation of Neurogenic Inflammation

Apart from tachykinin receptor antagonists, neurogenic inflammation may be modulated either by preventing activation of sensory nerves or preventing the release of neuropeptides. Both approaches may be tried in asthmatic patients, using currently available drugs, although these approaches are not as specific as tachykinin antagonists because the drugs used have additional effects.

Activation of sensory nerves may be inhibited by local anesthetics, but it has proved difficult to achieve adequate

local anesthesia of the respiratory tract. Inhalation of local anesthetics, such as lidocaine, has not been found to have consistent inhibitory effects on various airway challenges, and indeed even may promote bronchoconstriction in some patients with asthma (156). This paradoxical bronchoconstriction may be due to the greater anesthesia of laryngeal afferents that are linked to a tonic nonadrenergic bronchodilator reflex (157,158). Other drugs may inhibit the activation of airway sensory nerves. Cromolyn sodium and nedocromil sodium may have direct effects on airway C-fibers (159,160), and this might contribute to their antiasthma effect. Nedocromil sodium is highly effective against bradykinin-induced and sulfur dioxide-induced bronchoconstriction in asthmatic patients (159, 161), which is believed to be mediated by activation of sensory nerves in the airways. In addition, nedocromil sodium, and to a much lesser extent cromolyn sodium, inhibit the e-NANC neural bronchoconstriction due to tachykinin release from sensory nerves in guinea pig bronchi *in vitro,* indicating an effect on release of sensory neuropeptides as well as on activation (162). The loop diuretic furosemide (frusemide) given by nebulization behaves in a similar fashion to nedocromil sodium and inhibits metabisulfite-induced bronchoconstriction in asthmatic patients (163) as well as e-NANC and cholinergic bronchoconstriction in guinea pig airways *in vitro* (164). In addition, nebulized furosemide also inhibits certain types of cough (165), providing further evidence for an effect on sensory nerves.

Many drugs act on prejunctional receptors to inhibit the release of neuropeptides, as discussed above. Opioids are the most effective inhibitors, but an inhaled μ-opioid agonist, the pentapeptide BW 443C, was found to be ineffective in inhibiting metabisulfite-induced bronchoconstriction, which is believed to act via neural mechanisms (166). One problem with BW443C is that it may be degraded by NEP in the airway epithelium and therefore may not reach a high enough concentration in the vicinity of the airway sensory nerves. Another agent that has a prejunctional modulatory effect in guinea pigs is the H_3-receptor agonist α-methyl histamine (167). However, inhalation of α-methyl histamine had no effect on either resting tone or metabisulfite-induced bronchoconstriction in asthmatic patients (168).

REFERENCES

1. Uddman R, Hakanson R, Luts A. Distribution of neuropeptides in airways. In: Barnes PJ, ed. *Autonomic control of the respiratory system.* London: Harvard Academic, 1997;7:21–38.
2. Barnes PJ, Baraniuk J, Belvisi MG. Neuropeptides in the respiratory tract. *Am Rev Respir Dis* 1991;144:1187–1198 (part I), 1391–1399 (part II).
3. Kaliner M, Barnes PJ, Kunkel GHH, Baraniul J, eds. *Neuropeptides in respiratory medicine.* New York: Marcel Dekker, 1994.
4. Barnes PJ. Neuropeptides and asthma. *Am Rev Respir Dis* 1991;143: S28–32.
5. Martling CR, Theodorsson-Norheim E, Lundberg JM. Occurrence

and effects of multiple tachykinins: substance P, neurokinin A, and neuropeptide K in human lower airways. *Life Sci* 1987;40:1633–1643.

6. Laitinen LA, Laitinen A, Panula PA, Partanen M, Tervo K, Tervo T. Immunohistochemical demonstration of substance P in the lower respiratory tract of rabbit and not of man. *Thorax* 1983;38:531–536.

7. Komatsu T, Yamamoto M, Shimokata K, Nagura H. Distribution of substance-P-immunoreactive and calcitonin gene-related peptide-immunoreactive nerves in normal human lungs. *Int Arch Allergy Appl Immunol* 1991;95:23–28.

8. Lundberg JM, Saria A, Lundblad L et al. Bioactive peptides in capsaicin-sensitiive C-fiber afferents of the airways: functional and pathophysiological implications. In: Kaliner MA, Barnes PJ, eds. *The airways: neural control in health and disease* New York: Marcel Dekker, 1988:417–430.

9. Dey RD, Altemus JB, Michalkiewicz M. Distribution of vasoactive intestinal peptide- and substance P-containing nerves originating from neurons of airway ganglia in cat bronchi. *J Comp Neurol* 1991;304:330–340.

10. Springall DR, Polak JM, Howard L, et al. Persistence of intrinsic neurones and possible phenotypic changes after extrinsic denervation of human respiratory tract by heart-lung transplantation. *Am Rev Respir Dis* 1990;141:1538–1546.

11. Naline E, Devillier P, Drapeau G, Totly L, Bakdach H, Regoli D, Advenier C. Characterization of neurokinin effects on receptor selectivity in human isolated bronchi. *Am Rev Respir Dis* 1989;140:679–686.

12. Advenier C, Naline E, Toty L, et al. Effects on the isolated human bronchus of SR 48968, a potent and selective nonpeptide antagonist of the neurokinin A (NK$_2$) receptors. *Am Rev Respir Dis* 1992;146:1177–1181.

13. Frossard N, Barnes PJ. Effects of tachykinins on small human airways. *Neuropeptides* 1991;19:157–162.

14. Fuller RW, Maxwell DL, Dixon CMS, et al. The effects of substance P on cardiovascular and respiratory function in human subjects. *J Appl Physiol* 1987;62:1473–1479.

15. Evans TW, Dixon CM, Clarke B, Conradson TB, Barnes PJ. Comparison of neurokinin A and substance P on cardiovascular and airway function in man. *Br J Pharmacol* 1988;25:273–275.

16. Joos G, Pauwels R, van der Straeten ME. Effect of inhaled substance P and neurokinin A in the airways of normal and asthmatic subjects. *Thorax* 1987;42:779–783.

17. Cheung D, van der Veen H, den Hartig J, Dijkman JH, Sterk PJ. Effects of inhaled substance P on airway responsiveness to methacholine in asthmatic subjects. *J Appl Physiol* 1994;77:1325–1332.

18. Frossard N, Rhoden KJ, Barnes PJ. Influence of epithelium on guinea pig airway responses to tachykinins: role of endopeptidase and cyclooxygenase. *J Pharmacol Exp Ther* 1989;248:292–298.

19. Devillier P, Advenier C, Drapeau G, Marsac J, Regoli D. Comparison of the effects of epithelium removal and of an enkephalinase inhibitor on the neurokinin-induced contractions of guinea pig isolated trachea. *Br J Pharmacol* 1988;94:675–684.

20. Rogers DF, Aursudkij B, Barnes PJ. Effects of tachykinins on mucus secretion on human bronchi *in vitro*. *Eur J Pharmacol* 1989;174:283–286.

21. Ramnarine SI, Hirayama Y, Barnes PJ, Rogers DF. "Sensory-efferent" neural control of mucus secretion: characterization using tachykinin receptor antagonists in ferret trachea *in vitro*. *Br J Pharmacol* 1994;113:1183–1190.

22. Kuo H, Rhode JAL, Tokuyama K, Barnes PJ, Rogers DF. Capsaicin and sensory neuropeptide stimulation of goblet cell secretion in guinea pig trachea. *J Physiol* 1990;431:629–641.

23. Tokuyama K, Kuo H, Rohde JAL, Barnes PJ, Rogers DF. Neural control of goblet cell secretion in guinea pig airways. *Am J Physiol* 1990;259:L108–L115.

24. Kuo H, Barnes PJ, Rogers DF. Cigarette smoke-induced airway goblet cell secretion: dose dependent differential nerve activation. *Am J Physiol* 1992;7:L161–L167.

25. Rogers DF, Belvisi MG, Aursudkij B, Evans TW, Barnes PJ. Effects and interactions of sensory neuropeptides on airway microvascular leakage in guinea pigs. *Br J Pharmacol* 1988;95:1109–1116.

26. Sertl K, Wiedermann CJ, Kowalski ML, et al. Substance P: the relationship between receptor distribution in rat lung and the capacity of substance P to stimulate vascular permeability. *Am Rev Respir Dis* 1988;138:151–159.

27. Lötvall JO, Lemen RJ, Hui KP, Barnes PJ, Chung KF. Airflow ob-

struction after substance P aerosol: contribution of airway and pulmonary edema. *J Appl Physiol* 1990;69:1473–1478.

28. Fuller RW, Conradson T, Dixon CMS, Crossman DC, Barnes PJ. Sensory neuropeptide effects in human skin. *Br J Pharmacol* 1987;92:781–788.

29. Salonen RO, Webber SE, Widdicombe JG. Effects of neuropeptides and capsaicin on the canine tracheal vasculature *in vivo*. *Br J Pharmacol* 1988;95:1262–1270.

30. Matran R, Alving K, Martling CR, Lacroix JS, Lundberg JM. Effects of neuropeptides and capsaicin on tracheobronchial blood flow in the pig. *Acta Physiol Scand* 1989;135:335–342.

31. McCormack DG, Salonen RO, Barnes PJ. Effect of sensory neuropeptides on canine bronchial and pulmonary vessels *in vitro*. *Life Sci* 1989;45:2405–2412.

32. Hall AK, Barnes PJ, Meldrum LA, Maclagan J. Facilitation by tachykinins of neurotransmission in guinea-pig pulmonary parasympathetic nerves. *Br J Pharmacol* 1989;97:274–280.

33. Undem BJ, Myers AC, Barthlow H, Weinreich D. Vagal innervation of guinea pig bronchial smooth muscle. *J Appl Physiol* 1991;69:1336–1346.

34. Watson N, Maclagan J, Barnes PJ. Endogenous tachykinins facilitate transmission through parasympathetic ganglia in guinea-pig trachea. *Br J Pharmacol* 1993;109:751–759.

35. Myers AC, Undem BJ. Electrophysiological effects of tachykinins and capsaicin on guinea-pig parasympathetic ganglia. *J Physiol* 1993;470:665–679.

36. Martling C, Saria A, Andersson P, Lundberg JM. Capsaicin pretreatment inhibits vagal cholinergic and noncholinergic control of pulmonary mechanisms in guinea pig. *Naunyn Schmiedeberg Arch Pharm* 1984;325:343–348.

37. Stretton CD, Belvisi MG, Barnes PJ. The effect of sensory nerve depletion on cholinergic neurotransmission in guinea pig airways. *J Pharmacol Exp Ther* 1992;260:1073–1080.

38. Belvisi MG, Patacchini R, Barnes PJ, Maggi CA. Facilitatory effects of selective agonists for tachykinin receptors on cholinergic neurotransmission: evidence for species differences. *Br J Pharmacol* 1994;111:103–110.

39. Black JL, Johnson PR, Alouvan L, Armour CL. Neurokinin A with K$^+$ channel blockade potentiates contraction to electrical stimulation in human bronchus. *Eur J Pharmacol* 1990;180:311–317.

40. Kohrogi H, Graf PPD, Sekizawa K, Borson DB, Nadel JA. Neutral endopeptidase inhibitors potentiate substance P and capsaicin-induced cough in awake guinea pigs. *J Clin Invest* 1988;82:2063–2070.

41. Advenier C, Girard V, Naline E, Vilain P, Emons-Alt X. Antitussive effect of SR 48968, a nonpeptide tachykinin NK$_2$ receptor antagonist. *Eur J Pharmacol* 1992;250:169–171.

42. McGillis JP, Organist ML, Payan DG. Substance P and immunoregulation. *Fed Proc* 1987;14:120–123.

43. Daniele RP, Barnes PJ, Goetzl EJ, Nadel J, O'Dorisio S, Kiley J, Jacobs T. Neuroimmune interactions in the lung. *Am Rev Respir Dis* 1992;145:1230–1235.

44. Nohr D, Weihe E. The neuroimmune link in the bronchus-associated lymphoid tissue (BALT) of cat and rat: peptides and neural markers. *Brain Behav Immun* 1991;5:84–101.

45. Lowman MA, Benyon RC, Church MK. Characterization of neuropeptide-induced histamine release from human dispersed skin mast cells. *Br J Pharmacol* 1988;95:121–130.

46. Ali H, Leung KBI, Pearce FL, Hayes NA, Foreman JC. Comparison of histamine releasing activity of substance P on mast cells and basophils from different species and tissues. *Int Arch Allergy* 1986;79:121–124.

47. Kroegel C, Giembycz MA, Barnes PJ. Characterization of eosinophil activation by peptides. Differential effects of substance P, mellitin, and f-met-leu-phe. *J Immunol* 1990;145:2581–2587.

48. Numao T, Agrawal DK. Neuropeptides modulate human eosinophil chemotaxis. *J Immunol* 1992;149:3309–3315.

49. Brunelleschi S, Vanni L, Ledda F, Giotti A, Maggi CA, Fantozzi R. Tachykinins activate guinea pig alveolar macrophages: involvement of NK$_2$ and NK$_1$ receptors. *Br J Pharmacol* 1990;100:417–420.

50. Lotz M, Vaughn JH, Carson DM. Effect of neuropeptides on production of inflammatory cytokines by human monocytes. *Science* 1988;241:1218–1221.

51. Okamoto Y, Shirotori K, Kudo K, Ishikawa K, Ito E, Togawa K. Cytokine expression after the topical administration of substance P to human nasal mucosa. *J Immunol* 1995;151:4391–4398.

52. Umeno E, Nadel JA, Huang HT, McDonald DM. Inhibition of neutral endopeptidase potentiates neurogenic inflammation in the rat trachea. *J Appl Physiol* 1989;66:2647–2652.

53. Smith CH, Barker JNWH, Morris RW, McDonald DM, Lee TH. Neuropeptides induce rapid expression of endothelial cell adhesion moleculaes and elicit granulocytic infiltration in human skin. *J Immunol* 1993;151:3274–3282.

54. Fan T, Hu DE, Guard S, Gresham GA, Watling KJ. Stimulation of angiogenesis by substance P and interleukin-1 in the rat and its inhibition by NK₁ or interleukin-1 receptor antagonists. *Br J Pharmacol* 1993;110:43–49.

55. Kuwano K, Boskev CH, Paré PD, Bai TR, Wiggs BR, Hogg JC. Small airways dimensions in asthma and chronic obstructive pulmonary disease. *Am Rev Respir Dis* 1993;148:1220–1225.

56. Harrison NK, Dawes KE, Kwon OJ, Barnes PJ, Laurent GJ, Chung KF. Effects of neuropeptides in human lung fibroblast proliferation and chemotaxis. *Am J Physiol* 1995;12:L278–283.

57. Nadel JA. Neutral endopeptidase modulates neurogenic inflammation. *Eur Resp J* 1991;4:745–754.

58. Shore SA, Stimler-Gerard NP, Coats SR, Drazen JM. Substance P induced bronchoconstriction in guinea pig. Enhancement by inhibitors of neutral metalloendopeptidase and angiotensin converting enzyme. *Am Rev Respir Dis* 1988;137:331–336.

59. Martins MA, Shore SA, Gerard NP, Gerald C, Drazen JM. Peptidase modulation of the pulmonary effects of tachykinins in tracheal superfused guinea pig lungs. *J Clin Invest* 1990;85:170–176.

60. Lötvall JO, Skoogh B, Barnes PJ, Chung KF. Effects of aerosolized substance P on lung resistance in guinea pigs: a comparison between inhibition of neutral endopeptidase and angiotensin-converting enzyme. *Br J Pharmacol* 1990;100:69–72.

61. Sekizawa K, Tamaoki J, Graf PD, Basbaum CB, Borson DB, Nadel JA. Enkephalinase inhibitors potentiate mammalian tachykinin-induced contraction in ferret trachea. *J Pharmacol Exp Ther* 1987;243:1211–1217.

62. Black JL, Johnson PRA, Armour CL. Potentiation of the contractile effects of neuropeptides in human bronchus by an enkephalinase inhibitor. *Pulm Pharmacol* 1988;1:21–23.

63. Djokic TD, Nadel JA, Dusser DJ, Sekizawa K, Graf PD, Borson DB. Inhibitors of neutral endopeptidase potentiate electrically and capsaicin-induced noncholinergic contraction in guinea pig bronchi. *J Pharmacol Exp Ther* 1989;248:7–11.

64. Martling CR. Sensory nerves containing tachykinins and CGRP in the lower airways: funcitonal implications for bronchoconstriction, vasodilation, and protein extavasation. *Acta Physiol Scand* 1987;(Suppl 563):1–57.

65. Palmer JBD, Cuss FMC, Mulderry PK, et al. Calcitonin gene-related peptide is localized to human airway nerves and potently constricts human airway smooth muscle. *Br J Pharmacol* 1987;91:95–101.

66. Uddman R, Luts A, Sundler F. Occurrence and distribution of calcitonin gene related peptide in the mammalian respiratory tract and middle ear. *Cell Tissue Res* 1985;214:551–555.

67. McCormack DG, Mak JCW, Coupe MO, Barnes PJ. Calcitonin gene-related peptide vasodilation of human pulmonary vessels: receptor mapping and functional studies. *J Appl Physiol* 1989;67:1265–1270.

68. Salonen RO, Webber SE, Widdicombe JG. Effects of neuropeptides and capsaicin on the canine tracheal vasculature *in vivo. Br J Pharmacol* 1988;95:1262–1270.

69. Parsons GH, Nichol GM, Barnes PJ, Chung KF. Peptide mediator effects on bronchial blood velocity and lung resistance in conscious sheep. *J Appl Physiol* 1992;72:1118–1122.

70. Mak JCW, Barnes PJ. Autoradiographic localization of calcitonin gene-related peptide binding sites in human and guinea pig lung. *Peptides* 1988;9:957–964.

71. Khalil Z, Andrews PV, Helme RD. VIP modulates substance P induced plasma extravasation *in vivo. Eur J Pharmacol* 1988;151:281–287.

72. Brockaw JJ, White GW. Calcitonin gene-related peptide potentiates substance P-induced plasma extravasation in the rat trachea. *Lung* 1992;170:89–93.

73. Martling CR, Saria A, Fischer JA, Hokfelt T, Lundberg JM. Calcitonin gene related peptide and the lung: neuronal coexistence and vasodilatory effect. *Regulatory Peptides* 1988;20:125–139.

74. Ninomiya H, Uchida Y, Endo T, et al. The effects of calcitonin gene-related peptide on tracheal smooth muscle of guinea pigs *in vitro. Br J Pharmacol* 1996;119:1341–1346.

75. Webber SG, Lim JCS, Widdicombe JG. The effects of calcitonin gene related peptide on submucosal gland secretion and epithilial albumin transport on ferret trachea *in vitro. Br J Pharmacol* 1991;102:79–84.

76. Pietrowski W, Foreman JC. Some effects of calcitonin gene related peptide in human skin and on histamine release. *Br J Dermatol* 1986;114:37–46.

77. Haynes LW, Manley C. Chemotactic response of guinea pig polymorphonucleocytes *in vivo* to rat calcitonin gene related peptide and proteolytic fragments. *J Physiol* 1988;43:79P.

78. Umeda Y, Arisawa H. Characterization of the calcitonin gene related peptide receptor in mouse T lymphocytes. *Neuropeptides* 1989;14:237–242.

79. Nong YH, Titus RG, Riberio JM, Remold HG. Peptides encoded by the calcitonin gene inhibit macrophage function. *J Immunol* 1989;143:45–49.

80. White SR, Hershenson MB, Sigrist KS, Zimmerman A, Solway J. Proliferation of guinea pig tracheal epithelial cells induced by calcitonin gene-related peptide. *Am J Respir Cell Mol Biol* 1993;8:592–596.

81. Barnes PJ. Neurogenic inflammation in airways and its modulation. *Arch Int Pharmacodyn* 1990;303:67–82.

82. McDonald DM. Neurogenic inflammation in the respiratory tract: actions of sensory nerve mediators on blood vessels and epithelium of the airway mucosa. *Am Rev Respir Dis* 1987;136:S65–S72.

83. Solway J, Leff AR. Sensory neuropeptides and airway function. *J Appl Physiol* 1991;71:2077–2087.

84. Barnes PJ. Asthma as an axon reflex. *Lancet* 1986;i:242–245.

85. Barnes PJ. Sensory nerves, neuropeptides and asthma. *Ann NY Acad Sci* 1991;629:359–370.

86. Lundberg JM, Saria A. Capsaicin-induced desensitization of the airway mucosa to cigarette smoke, mechanical and chemical irritants. *Nature* 1983;302:251–253.

87. Ray DW, Hernandez C, Leff AR, Drazen JM, Solway J. Tachykinins mediate bronchoconstriction elicited by isocapnic hyperpnea in guinea pigs. *J Appl Physiol* 1989;66:1108–1112.

88. Reynolds AM, McEvoy RD. Tachykinins mediate hypocapnia-induced bronchoconstriction in guinea pigs. *J Appl Physiol* 1989;67:2454–2460.

89. Sakamoto T, Elwood W, Barnes PJ, Chung KF. Pharmacological modulation of inhaled metabisulphite-induced airway microvascular leakage and bronchoconstriction in guinea pig. *Br J Pharmacol* 1992;107:481–488.

90. Umeno E, McDonald DM, Nadel JA. Hypertonic saline increases vascular permeability in the rat trachea by producing neurogenic inflammation. *J Clin Invest* 1990;85:1905–1908.

91. Thompson JE, Scypinski LA, Gordon T, Sheppard D. Tachykinins mediate the acute increase in airway responsiveness by toluene diisocyanate in guinea-pigs. *Am Rev Respir Dis* 1987;136:43–49.

92. Lötvall JO, Hui KP, Löfdahl C, Barnes PJ, Chung KF. Capsaicin pretreatment does not inhibit early allergen-induced airway microvascular leakage in guinea pig. *Allergy* 1991;46:105–108.

93. Hsiue T, Garland A, Ray DW, Hershenson MB, Leff AR, Solway J. Endogenous sensory neuropeptide release enhances non specific airway responsiveness in guinea pigs. *Am Rev Respir Dis* 1992;146:148–153.

94. Adenius ARC, Folkerts G, van der Linde HJ, Nijkamp FP. Potentiation by viral respiratory infection of ovalbumin-induced guinea-pig tracheal hyperresponsiveness: role for tachykinins. *Br J Pharmacol* 1995;115:1048–1052.

95. Iving K, Matran R, Lacroix JS, Lundberg JM. Allergen challenge induces vasodilation in pig bronchial circulation via a capsaicin sensitive mechanism. *Acta Physiol Scand* 1988;134:571–572.

96. Braham WM, Ahmed A, Cortes A, Delehunt JC. C-fiber desensitization prevents hyperresponsiveness to cholinergic and antigenic stimuli after antigen challenge in allergic sheep. *Am Rev Respir Dis* 1993;147:A478

97. Atsuse T, Thomson RJ, Chen X, Salari H, Schellenberg RR. Capsaicin inhibits airway hyperresponsiveness, but not airway lipoxygenase activity nor eosinophilia following repeated aerosolized antigen in guinea pigs. *Am Rev Respir Dis* 1991;144:368–372.

98. Adenius ARC, Nijkamp FP. Capsaicin pretreatment of guinea pigs *in vivo* prevents ovalbumin-induced tracheal hyperreactivity *in vitro. Eur J Pharmacol* 1993;235:127–131.

99. Riccio MM, Manzini S, Page CP. The effect of neonatal capsaicin in the development of bronchial hyperresponsiveness in allergic rabbits. *Eur J Pharmacol* 1993;232:89–97.

100. Bienenstock J, Perdue M, Blennerhassett M, et al. Inflammatory cells and epithelium: mast cell/nerve interactions in lung *in vitro* and *in vivo*. *Am Rev Respir Dis* 1988;138:S31–S34.

101. Leff AR, Stimler NP, Munoz NM, Shioya T, Tallet J, Dame C. Augmentation of respiratory mast cell secretion of histamine caused by vagal nerve stimulation during antigen challenge. *J Immunol* 1982; 136:1066–1073.

102. Sestini P, Bienenstock J, Crowe SE, et al. Ion transport in rat tracheal ganglion *in vitro*. Role of capsaicin-sensitive nerves in allergic reactions. *Am Rev Respir Dis* 1990;141:393–3397.

103. Saban R, Dick EC, Fishlever RI, Buckner CK. Enhancement of parainfluenze 3 infection of contractile responses to substance P and capsaicin in airway smooth msucle from guinea pig. *Am Rev Respir Dis* 1987;136:586–591.

104. Jacoby DB, Tamaoki J, Borson DB, Nadel JA. Influenza infection increases airway smooth muscle responsiveness to substance P in ferrets by decreasing enkephalinase. *J Appl Physiol* 1988;64:2653–2658.

105. Piedimonte G, Nadel JA, Umeno E, McDonald DM. Sendai virus infection potentiates neurogenic inflammation in the rat trachea. *J Appl Physiol* 1990;68:754–760.

106. Dusser DJ, Djoric TD, Borson DB, Nadel JA. Cigarette smoke induces bronchoconstrictor hyperresponsiveness to substance P and inactivates airway neutral endopeptidase in the guinea pig. *J Clin Invest* 1989;84:900–906.

107. Sheppard D, Thompson JE, Scypinski L, Dusser DJ, Nadel JA, Borson DB. Toluene diisocyanate increases airway responsiveness to substance P and decreases airway neutral endopeptidase. *J Clin Invest* 1988;81:1111–1115.

108. Tsukagoshi H, Sakamoto T, Xu W, Barnes PJ, Chung KF. Effect of interleukin-1β on airway hyperresponsiveness and inflammation in sensitized and nonsensitized Brown-Norway rats. *J Allergy Clin Immunol* 1994;93:464–469.

109. Watling KJ. Non peptide antagonists heralded a new era in tachykinin research. *Trends Pharmacol Sci* 1992;13:266–269.

110. Lei Y, Barnes PJ, Rogers DF. Inhibition of neurogenic plasma exudation in guinea pig airways by CP-96,345, a new nonpeptide NK$_1$-receptor antagonist. *Br J Pharmacol* 1992;105:261–262.

111. Delay-Goyet P, Lundberg JM. Cigarette smoke-induced airway oedema is blocked by the NK$_1$-antagonist CP-96,345. *Eur J Pharmacol* 1991;203:157–158.

112. Hirayama Y, Lei YH, Barnes PJ, Rogers DF. Effects of two novel tachykinin antagonists FK 224 and FK 888 on neurogenic plasma exudation, bronchoconstriction and systemic hypotension in guinea pigs *in vivo*. *Br J Pharmacol* 1993;108:844–851.

113. Solway J, Kao BM, Jordan JE, et al. Tachykinin receptor antagonists inhibit hypernea-induced bronchoconstriction in guinea pigs. *J Clin Invest* 1993;92:315–323.

114. Sakamoto T, Barnes PJ, Chung KF. Effect of CP-96,345, a nonpeptide NK$_1$-receptor antagonist against substance P-, bradykinin-, and allergen-induced airway microvascular leak and bronchoconstriction in the guinea pig. *Eur J Pharmacol* 1993;231:31–38.

115. Barnes PJ, Belvisi MG, Rogers DF. Modulation of neurogenic inflammation: novel approaches to inflammatory diseases. *Trends Pharmacol Sci* 1990;11:185–189.

116. Kuo H, Rohde J, Barnes PJ, Rogers DF. Differential effects of opioids on cigarette smoke, capsaicin and electrically-induced goblet cell secretion in guinea pig trachea. *Br J Pharmacol* 1992;105:361–366.

117. Yeadon M, Wilkinson D, Darley-Usmar V, O'Leary VJ, Payne AN. Mechanisms contributing to ozone-induced bronchial hyperreactivity in guinea pigs. *Pulm Pharmacol* 1992;5:39–50.

118. Stretton CD, Miura M, Belvisi MG, Barnes PJ. Calcium-activated potassium channels mediate prejunctional inhibition of peripheral sensory nerves. *Proc Natl Acad Sci USA* 1992;89:1325–1329.

119. Ichinose M, Barnes PJ. A potassium channel activator modulates both noncholinergic and cholinergic neurotransmission in guinea pig airways. *J Pharmacol Exp Ther* 1990;252:1207–1212.

120. Kuo H, Rohde JAL, Barnes PJ, Rogers DF. K+ channel activator inhibition of neurogenic goblet cell secretion in guinea pig trachea. *Eur J Pharmacol* 1992;221:385–388.

121. Barnes PJ. Neuropeptides in asthma. In: Kaliner MA, Barnes PJ, Kunkel GHH, Baraniuk JN, eds. *Neuropeptides in respiratory medicine*. New York: Marcel Dekker, 1994;285–311.

122. Joos GF, Germonpre PR, Pauwels RA. Neurogenic inflammation in human airways: Is it important? *Thorax* 1995;50:217–219.

123. Bowden J, Gibbins IL. Relative density of substance P-immunoreactive nerve fibres in the tracheal epithelium of a range of species. *FASEB J* 1992;6:A1276

124. Levine JD, Dardick SJ, Roizan MF, Helms C, Basbaum AI. Contribution of sensory afferents and sympathetic efferents to joint injury in experimental arthritis. *J Neurosci* 1986;6:3423–3429.

125. Holzer P. Local effector functions of capsaicin-senstive sensory nerve endings: involvement of tachykinins, calcitonin gene related peptide, and other neuropeptides. *Neuroscience* 1988;24:739–768.

126. Ollerenshaw SL, Jarvis D, Sullivan CE, Woolcock AJ. Substance P immunoreactive nerves in airways from asthmatics and nonasthmatics. *Eur Resp J* 1991;4:673–682.

127. Lilly CM, Bai TR, Shore SA, Hall AE, Drazen JM. Neuropeptide content of lungs from asthmatic and nonasthmatic patients. *Am J Respir Crit Care Med* 1995;151:548–553.

128. Mossiman BL, White MV, Hohman RJ, Goldrich MS, Kaliner MA. Substance P, calcitonin gene-related peptide and vasoactive intestinal peptide increase nasal secretions after allergen challenge in atopic patients. *J Allergy Clin Immunol* 1993;92:95–104.

129. Nieber K, Baumgarten CR, Rathsack R, Furkert J, Oehame P, Kunkel G. Substance P and b-endorphin-like immunoreactivity in lavage fluids of subjects with and without asthma. *J Allergy Clin Immunol* 1992;90:646–652.

130. Tomaki M, Ichinose M, Miura M, et al. Elevated substance P content in induced sputum from patients with asthma and patients with chronic bronchitis. *Am J Respir Crit Care Med* 1995;151:613–617.

131. Hazbun ME, Hamilton R, Holian A, Eschenbacher WL. Ozone-induced increases in substance P and 8 epi-prostaglandin F$_{2a}$ in the airways of human subjects. *Am J Resp Cell Mol Biol* 1993;9:568–572.

132. Lindsay RM, Harmar AJ. Nerve growth factor regulates expression of neuropeptide genes in sensory neurons. *Nature* 1989;337:362–364.

133. Minami M, Kuraishi Y, Kawamura M, Yamaguchi T, Masu Y, Nakanishi S. Enhancement of preprotachykinin A gene expression by adjuvant-induced inflammation in the rat spinal cord: possible inducement of substance P-containing spinal neurons in nociceptor. *Neurosci Lett* 1989;98:105–110.

134. Fischer A, Philippin B, Saria A, McGregor G, Kummer W. Neuronal plasticity in sensitized and challenged guinea pigs: neuropeptides and neuropeptide gene expression. *Am J Resp Crit Care Med* 1994;149:A890

135. Howarth PH, Djukanovic R, Wilson JW, Holgate ST, Springall DR, Polak JM. Mucosal nerves in endobronchial biopsies in asthma and nonasthma. *Int Arch Allergy Appl Immunol* 1991;94:330–333.

136. Cunha FQ, Poole S, Lorenzetti BB, Ferreira SH. The pivotal role of tumour necrosis factor a in the development of inflammatory hyperalgesia. *Br J Pharmacol* 1992;107:660-664.

137. Fuller RW, Dixon CMS, Barnes PJ. The bronchoconstrictor response to inhaled capsaicin in humans. *J Appl Physiol* 1985;85:1080–1084.

138. Midgren B, Hansson L, Karlsson JA, Simonsson BG, Persson CGA. Capsaicin-induced cough in humans. *Am Rev Respir Dis* 1992;146:347–351.

139. Kaufman MP, Coleridge HM, Coleridge JCG, Baker DG. Bradykinin stimulates afferent vagal C-fibres in intrapulmonary airways of dogs. *J Appl Physiol* 1980;48:511–517.

140. Saria A, Martling CR, Yan Z, Theodorsson-Norheim E, Gamse R, Lundberg JM. Release of multiple tachykinins from capsaicin-sensitive nerves in the lung by bradykinin, histamine, dimethylphenyl-piperainium, and vagal nerve stimulation. *Am Rev Respir Dis* 1988; 137:1330–1335.

141. Fuller RW, Dixon CMS, Cuss FMC, Barnes PJ. Bradykinin-induced bronchoconstriction in man: mode of action. *Am Rev Respir Dis* 1987; 135:176–180.

142. Ichinose M, Belvisi MG, Barnes PJ. Bradykinin-induced bronchoconstriction in guinea-pig *in vivo*: role of neural mechanisms. *J Pharmacol Exp Ther* 1990;253:1207–1212.

143. Sakamoto T, Tsukagoshi H, Barnes PJ, Chung KF. Role played by NK$_2$ receptors and cyclooxygenase activation in bradykinin B$_2$ receptor-mediated airway effects in guinea pigs. *Ag Act* 1993;111:117.

144. Ichinose M, Nakajima N, Takahashi T, Yamauchi H, Inoue H, Takishima T. Protection against bradykinin-induced bronchoconstriction in asthmatic patients by a neurokinin receptor antagonist. *Lancet* 1992;340:1248–1251.

145. Nichol GM, O'Connor BJ, Le Compte JM, Chung KF, Barnes PJ.

Effect of neutral endopeptidase inhibitor on airway function and bronchial responsiveness in asthmatic subjects. *Eur J Clin Pharmacol* 1992;42:495–498.

146. Cheung D, Bel EH, den Hartigh J, Dijkman JH, Sterk PJ. An effect of an inhaled neutral endopeptidase inhibitor, thiorphan, on airway responses to neurokinin A in normal humans *in vivo. Am Rev Respir Dis* 1992;145:1275–1280.

147. Cheung D, Timmers MC, Bel EH, den Hartigh J, Dijuman JH, Sterk PJ. An isolated neutral endopeptidase inhibitor, thiorphan, enhances airway narrowing to neurokin A in asthmatic subjects *in vivo. Am Rev Respir Dis* 1992;195:A682.

148. Baraniuk JN, Mak J, Letarte M, Davis R, Twort C, Barnes PJ. Neutral endopeptidase mRNA expression in airways. *Am Rev Respir Dis* 1991;143:A40.

149. Mantyh CR, Gates TS, Zimmerman RP, et al. Receptor binding sites for substance P but not substane K or neuromedin K are expressed in high concentrations by arterioles, venules and lymph nodes in surgical specimens obtained from patients with ulcerative colitis and Crohn's disease. *Proc Natl Acad Sci USA* 1988;85:3235–3259.

150. Mantyh PW. Substance P and the inflammatory and immune response. *Ann NY Acad Sci* 1991;632:263–271.

151. Devillier P, Dessanges JF, Rakotashanaka F, Ghaem A, Boushey HA, Lockhart A. Nasal response to substance P and methacholine with and without allergic rhinitis. *Eur Respir J* 1988;1:356–361.

152. Adcock IM, Peters M, Gelder C, Shirasaki H, Brown CR, Barnes PJ. Increased tachykinin receptor gene expression in asthmatic lung and its modulation by steroids. *J Mol Endocrinol* 1993;11:1–7.

153. Adcock IM, Shirasaki H, Gelder CM, Peters MJ, Barnes PJ. The effects of glucocorticoids on phorbol ester and cytokine stimulated transcription factor activation in human lungs. *Life Sci* 1994;55:1147–1153.

154. Nakanishi S. Mammalian tachykinin receptors. *Ann Rev Neurosci* 1991;14:123–136.

155. Ihara H, Nakanishi S. Selective inhibition of expression of the substance P receptor mRNA in pancreatic acinar AR42J cells by glucocorticoids. *J Biol Chem* 1990;36:22,441–22,445.

156. McAlpine LG, Thomson NC. Lidocaine-induced bronchoconstriction in asthmatic patients. Relation to histamine airway responsiveness and effect of preservative. *Chest* 1989;96:1012–1015.

157. Lammers J, Minette P, McCusker M, Chung KF, Barnes PJ. Nonadrenergic bronchodilator mechanisms in normal human subjects *in vivo. J Appl Physiol* 1988;64:1817–1822.

158. Lammers J-WJ, Minette P, McCusker M, Chung KF, Barnes PJ. Capsaicin-induced bronchodilatation in mild asthmatic subjects: possible role of nonadrenergic inhibitory system. *J Appl Physiol* 1989;67:856–861.

159. Dixon N, Jackson DM, Richards IM. The effect of sodium cromoglycate on lung irritant receptors and left ventricular receptors in anasthetized dogs. *Br J Pharmacol* 1979;67:569–574.

160. Jackson DM, Norris AA, Eady RP. Nedocromil sodium and sensory nerves in the dog lung. *Pulm Pharmacol* 1989;2:179–184.

161. Dixon CMS, Fuller RW, Barnes PJ. The effect of nedocromil sodium on sulphur dioxide induced bronchoconstriction. *Thorax* 1987;42:462–465.

162. Verleden GM, Belvisi MG, Stretton CD, Barnes PJ. Nedocromil sodium modulates nonadrenergic noncholinergic bronchoconstrictor nerves in guinea-pig airways *in vitro. Am Rev Respir Dis* 1991;143:114–118.

163. Nichol GM, Alton EWFW, Nix A, Geddes DM, Chung KF, Barnes PJ. Effect of inhaled furosemide on metabisulfite- and methacholine induced bronchoconstriction and nasal potential difference in asthmatic subjects. *Am Rev Respir Dis* 1990;142:576–580.

164. Elwood W, Lotvall JO, Barnes PJ, Chung KF. Loop diuretics inhibit cholinergic and noncholinergic nerves in guinea pig airways. *Am Rev Respir Dis* 1991;143:1340–1344.

165. Ventresca GP, Nichol GM, Barnes PJ, Chung KF. Inhaled furosemide inhibits cough induced by low chloride content solutions but not by capsaicin. *Am Rev Respir Dis* 1990;142:143–146.

166. O'Connor BJ, Chen-Wordsell M, Barnes PJ, Chung KF. Effect of an inhaled opioid peptide on airway responses to sodium metabisulphite in asthma. *Thorax* 1991;46:294P.

167. Ichinose M, Belvisi MG, Barnes PJ. Histamine H$_3$-receptors inhibit neurogenic microvascular leakage in airways. *J Appl Physiol* 1990;68:21–25.

168. O'Connor BJ, Lecomte JM, Barnes PJ. Effect of an inhaled H$_3$-receptor agonist on airway responses to sodium metabisulphite in asthma. *Br J Clin Pharmacol* 1993;35:55–57.

Asthma, edited by P.J. Barnes, M.M. Grunstein,
A.R. Leff, and A.J. Woolcock.
Lippincott–Raven Publishers, Philadelphia © 1997.

▪ 74 ▪

Other Regulatory Peptides

Peter J. Barnes

Co-transmission
Vasoactive Intestinal Peptide
  Localization
  Receptors
  Effects on Airway Smooth Muscle
  Effects on Airway Secretion
  Vascular Effects
  Neuromodulatory Effects
  Anti-inflammatory Actions
  Vasoactive Intestinal Peptide as an i-NANC
    Transmitter
  Co-transmission with Acetylcholine
  Possible Abnormalities in Asthma
Vasoactive Intestinal Peptide-related Peptides
  Peptide Histidine Isoleucine
  Helodermin
  Pituitary Adenylate Cyclase-activating Peptide

Neuropeptide Y
  Localization
  Effects on Airway Tone
  Vascular Effects
  Effects on Secretion
Gastrin-releasing Peptide
  Localization
  Airway Effects
Cholecystokinin
Somatostatin
Galanin
Adrenomedullin
Enkephalins
Neurotensin
Atrial Natriuretic Peptide
Corticotrophin-releasing Factor

Many neuropeptides are localized to sensory, parasympathetic, and sympathetic neurons in the airways (1,2)(Table 1). Many of these peptides have potent effects on bronchomotor tone, airway secretions, bronchial circulation, and inflammatory and immune cells. The precise physiologic roles of each peptide is still not known, but some clues are provided by their localization and functional effects. The precise physiologic and pathologic role of each peptide will be revealed only by the development of potent and specific inhibitors; there recently have been important advances in the development of both peptide and nonpeptide receptor antagonists. Sensory neuropeptides (substance P, neurokinin A, and calcitonin gene-related peptide) are discussed in Chapter 73. This chapter reviews other peptides that have been localized to the respiratory tract and discusses their possible pathophysiologic role in asthma (3). These neuropeptides function as neurotransmitters of nonadrenergic noncholinergic (NANC) neural mechanisms and act as co-transmitters in classic autonomic nerves of the airway.

CO-TRANSMISSION

Although NANC nerves were envisaged originally as an anatomically separate nervous system, it is now more likely that NANC neural effects are mediated by the release of neurotransmitters from classical autonomic nerves (Fig. 1). Thus, inhibitor NANC (i-NANC) responses in airway smooth muscle are likely to be mediated by the release of co-transmitters, such as nitric oxide (NO) and vasoactive intestinal peptide (VIP), from parasympathetic nerves that classically release acetylcholine (ACh) (see Chapter 72). NANC vasoconstrictor responses are mediated by the release of neuropeptide Y

P.J. Barnes: Department of Thoracic Medicine, Imperial College of Medicine at the National Heart and Lung Institute, London SW3 6LY, United Kingdom.

TABLE 1. *Regulatory peptides in the respiratory tract*

Peptide	Localization
Vasoactive intestinal peptide	
Peptide histidine isoleucine/methionine	
Peptide histidine valine-42	Parasympathetic nerves
Helodermin	(Afferent nerves)
Helospectins I and II	
PACAP-27	
Galanin	
Substance P	
Neurokinin A	
Neuropeptide K	Afferent nerves
Calcitonin gene–related peptide	
Gastrin-releasing peptide	
Neuropeptide Y	Sympathetic nerves
Somatostatin	
Enkephalin	Afferent/uncertain nerves
Cholecystokinin octapeptide	
Atrial natriuretic peptide	
Adrenomedullin	Circulating factors ?
Corticotrophin-releasing factor	

(NPY) from sympathetic nerves. Excitatory NANC (e-NANC) bronchoconstrictor responses are mediated by the release of tachykinins from unmyelinated sensory nerves (as discussed below). The physiologic relevance of co-transmission is likely to be related to the "fine tuning" of classic autonomic nerves; in disease states co-transmission may play a greater role.

Co-existence of several peptides within the same nerve is commonly described in the peripheral nervous system, and multiple combinations are possible, giving rise to the concept of "chemical coding" of nerve fibers. VIP and the related peptide histidine isoleucine (PHI) usually coexist because they are derived from the same precursor peptide coded by a single gene. Galanin is often present together with VIP in cholinergic neurons. In sensory nerves substance P, neurokinin A (NKA), and calcitonin

gene-related peptide (CGRP) often coexist, but some sensory nerves also may contain galanin and VIP (1). Similarly, sympathetic nerves that contain NPY also may contain somatostatin, galanin, VIP, and enkephalin. Thus, there is a complex distribution of neuropeptides in the innervation of the airways, with the same peptides occurring in different types of nerve. The physiologic significance of this complexity is not clear, but it seems likely that there may be functional interactions between the multiple neuropeptides released and the classic transmitters that allow complex integration and regulation of functions in the airway.

Neuropeptides often are released by high frequency firing and therefore may be co-released only with classic neurotransmitters with certain patterns of neural activation. Little is known about the optimal conditions for neuropeptide release, but it seems likely that release may be favored by certain physiologic and pathophysiologic conditions. Furthermore, little is known about the effect of repeated neural activation on the synthesis and release of neuropeptides, but it is possible that in certain diseases, when chronic nerve irritation may occur, there may be increased neuropeptide gene expression, synthesis, and release.

VASOACTIVE INTESTINAL PEPTIDE

VIP is a 28-amino acid peptide that is localized to several types of nerve in the respiratory tract of several species, including humans. VIP has potent effects on airway and pulmonary vascular tone and on airway secretion, which suggests that it may have an important regulatory role.

Localization

VIP has been isolated from lung extracts of several species, including humans, and is one of the most abundant of the neuropeptides found in lung. VIP-like immunoreactivity is localized to nerves and local ganglia within the airways (1,4). VIP immunoreactivity is present in ganglion cells in the posterior trachea and around intrapulmonary bronchi, diminishing in frequency as the airways become smaller. Although VIP-immunoreactive neurons occur within parasympathetic ganglia, isolated ganglion cells also are seen. VIP-immunoreactive nerves are widely distributed throughout the respiratory tract. There is a rich VIP-ergic innervation in the proximal airways, but the density of innervation diminishes peripherally so that few VIP-ergic fibers are found in bronchioles. The pattern of distribution largely follows that of cholinergic nerves in airways, consistent with the co-localization of VIP and ACh in human airways (5). VIP-ergic nerves are found within airway smooth muscle, around bronchial vessels, and surrounding submucosal glands.

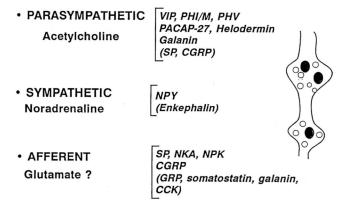

- **PARASYMPATHETIC**
  Acetylcholine
  VIP, PHI/M, PHV
  PACAP-27, Helodermin
  Galanin
  (SP, CGRP)

- **SYMPATHETIC**
  Noradrenaline
  NPY
  (Enkephalin)

- **AFFERENT**
  Glutamate ?
  SP, NKA, NPK
  CGRP
  (GRP, somatostatin, galanin, CCK)

FIG. 1. Peptidergic co-transmission in airway nerves. Classic autonomic nerves release multiple neuropeptides.

VIP also may be localized to some sensory nerves, including subepithelial nerves in the airways, which may arise in the jugular and nodose ganglia (4). VIP, at least in some species, also may be localized to sympathetic nerves (6).

Receptors

VIP receptors have been identified in the lung of several species by receptor binding techniques using [^{125}I]VIP (7). Binding of VIP to its receptor activates adenylyl cyclase and stimulates cyclic adenosine monophosphate (cAMP) formation. The actions of VIP are therefore similar to those of β-adrenoceptor agonists and any differences in response of different tissues to VIP or β-agonists depends on the relative densities or coupling of their respective receptors. Autoradiographic mapping of VIP receptors demonstrates a high density in airway smooth muscle of large, but not small, airways (8). VIP receptors are also found in high density in airway epithelium and submucosal glands. VIP receptors have now been cloned and two forms are recognized: a form that mediates the classic responses to VIP and another form that is expressed in certain immune cells (9).

Effects on Airway Smooth Muscle

VIP relaxes human airway smooth muscle *in vitro* and is more potent than isoproterenol (10). Because there is a rich VIP-ergic innervation of human bronchi, this suggests that VIP may be an important regulator of bronchial tone and may be involved in counteracting the bronchoconstriction of asthma. Human bronchi are potently relaxed by VIP, whereas bronchioles barely respond at all (Fig. 2). This response is consistent with the distribution of VIP-receptors, which are localized to smooth muscle of proximal but not distal airways (8). This peripheral diminution of VIP receptors also is consistent with the distribution of VIP-immunoreactive nerves that diminish markedly as airways become smaller (4). These studies suggest that VIP, although regulating the caliber of large airways, is unlikely to influence small airways.

Intravenous VIP causes bronchodilatation *in vivo* in feline airways (11). In asthmatic patients, however, inhaled VIP has no bronchodilator effect, and only a small protective effect against inhaled histamine, although a β-adrenergic agonist in the same subjects is markedly effective (12). This lack of potency of inhaled VIP may be explained by the epithelium, because this possesses proteolytic enzymes and may present a barrier to diffusion. Infused VIP has no bronchodilator effect in nonasthmatic persons who readily bronchodilate with isoproterenol (13). However, infusion of VIP produces flushing, marked hypotension and reflex tachycardia. These cardiovascular responses limit the dose that can be given by infusion and, as VIP has a more potent relaxant effect on vessels than on airway smooth muscle, thus prevents administration of a sufficient bronchodilating dose. Infused VIP causes bronchodilatation in asthmatic persons, but the effect is trivial (14) and might be explained by the reflex sympathoadrenal activation secondary to the profound cardiovascular effects. VIP therefore has relatively limited therapeutic potential in asthma. Recently a stable analog of VIP has been developed as a novel bronchodilator (15).

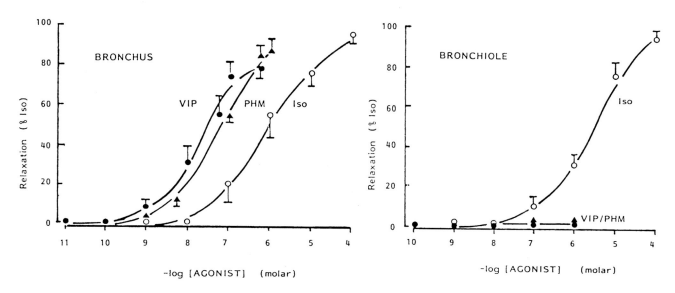

FIG. 2. Effect of vasoactive intestinal peptide (*VIP*), peptide histidine methionine (*PHM*) and isoproterenol (*Iso*) on human airways *in vitro*.

Effects on Airway Secretion

VIP-immunoreactive nerves are closely associated with airway submucosal glands and form a dense network around the gland acini. VIP potently stimulates mucous secretion, measured by ^{35}S-labeled glycoprotein secretion, in ferret airway *in vitro*, being significantly more potent than isoproterenol [16]. VIP receptors have been localized to human submucosal glands, suggesting that VIP-ergic nerves may regulate mucus secretion in human airways [8]. VIP has an inhibitory effect on glycoprotein secretion from human tracheal explants [17], although agonists that stimulate cAMP formation would be expected to stimulate secretion. More recently, the effects of VIP on mucous secretion have been found to be more complex and may depend on the drive to gland secretion. Mucous secretion stimulated by cholinergic agonists is inhibited in ferret trachea but stimulated in cat trachea, whereas secretion stimulated with the β-adrenergic agonist phenylephrine is augmented [18].

VIP is a potent stimulant of chloride ion transport and therefore water secretion in dog tracheal epithelium [19], suggesting that VIP may be a regulator of airway water secretion and therefore mucociliary clearance. The high density of VIP receptors on epithelial cells of human airways suggests that VIP may regulate ion transport and other epithelial functions in human airways [8], but this has not been explored in detail.

Vascular Effects

VIP is a potent vasodilator in systemic vessels (Fig. 3). It increases airways blood flow in dogs and pigs and is more potent on tracheal than on bronchial vessels [20]. There is convincing evidence that VIP is a mediator of NANC vasodilatation in trachea, whereas in more peripheral airways other neuropeptides are involved [21]. Because VIP is likely to have a greater effect on bronchial vessels than on airway smooth muscle, it may provide a mechanism for increasing blood flow to contracted smooth muscle. Thus, if VIP is released from cholinergic nerves, it may improve smooth muscle perfusion during cholinergic contraction. Perhaps the apparent protective effect of inhaled VIP against histamine-induced bronchoconstriction in humans [22], despite a lack of effect on bronchomotor tone, may be explained by an increase in bronchial blood flow that would more rapidly remove inhaled histamine from sites of deposition in the airways.

Neuromodulatory Effects

VIP is localized to nerves that surround airway ganglia, suggesting a possible neuromodulatory effect on cholinergic neurotransmission. VIP appears to modulate cholinergic neurotransmission in parasympathetic ganglia [23] and postganglionic nerves [24,25] because it has a greater inhibitory effect on neurally induced bronchoconstriction than on an equivalent contractile response induced by exogenous ACh. VIP also modulates the release of peptides from sensory nerves in guinea pig bronchi *in vitro* [24].

Anti-inflammatory Actions

VIP inhibits release of mediators from pulmonary mast cells [26] and may have several other anti-inflammatory

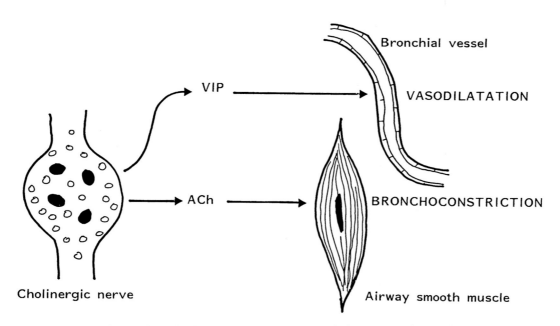

FIG 3. Effect of VIP on bronchial vessels and airway smooth muscle.

actions in airways. VIP inhibits the release of prostanoids from perfused guinea pig lung, suggesting that it may have anti-inflammatory effects (27). VIP may interact with T lymphocytes and has the potential to act as a local immunomodulator in airways (28).

Vasoactive Intestinal Peptide as an i-NANC Transmitter

Several lines of evidence have implicated VIP as a neurotransmitter of i-NANC nerves in airways (see Chapter 72). VIP is rapidly broken down into inactive fragments by trypsin and α-chymotrypsin and also by mast cell tryptase (29). Incubation of guinea pig trachea with α-chymotrypsin, under conditions that completely block responses to exogenous VIP, results in a significant reduction in i-NANC response (30). However, inhibition is incomplete, indicating that some other transmitter (now known to be NO) is involved. However, in human airways the i-NANC response is unaffected by α-chymotrypsin, suggesting that VIP is not important in i-NANC responses in human airways (31).

Co-transmission with Acetylcholine

VIP coexists with ACh in airway cholinergic nerves. VIP may be released from cholinergic nerves only with high frequency firing and may serve to increase the blood flow to exocrine glands under conditions of excessive stimulation. VIP also appears to co-exist with ACh in airways (5), and it seems likely that there is a functional relationship between VIP and cholinergic neural control. It is possible that excessive stimulation of cholinergic nerves and certain patterns of firing result in VIP release.

VIP acts as a functional antagonist to ACh-induced bronchoconstriction, but also inhibits the release of ACh from parasympathetic nerves in the airways, therefore providing a "double braking" system to cholinergic reflex bronchoconstriction (24,25) (Fig. 4). Conversely, α-chymotrypsin, which degrades VIP, potentiates cholinergic nerve-induced contractions in guinea pig airways (32), but this has not been observed in human airways (33). Thus, in guinea pig airways VIP and NO both contribute to the braking system, whereas in human airways only NO appears to be involved (Fig. 4). If this mechanism were to be deficient with either reduced release or increased breakdown of VIP, then an exaggerated bronchoconstrictor response may result.

Possible Abnormalities in Asthma

Whether dysfunction of VIP-ergic innervation contributes to asthma is uncertain. A striking absence of VIP-immunoreactive nerves has been described in the lungs of patients with asthma in tissues largely obtained at postmortem (34). The loss of VIP immunoreactivity from all tissues including pulmonary vessels is so complete that it seems unlikely to represent a fundamental absence of VIP-immunoreactive nerves in asthma. More likely is the possibility that enzymes, such as mast cell tryptase, are released from inflammatory cells in asthma and that these rapidly degrade VIP when sections are cut (35). Biopsies taken from patients with mild asthma suggest that VIP-immunoreactive nerves appear normal in asthma (36) and assays of lung tissue from asthmatic patients show no evidence for a reduced content of VIP (37). VIP antibodies, which would neutralize the effects of VIP, also have been described in the plasma of asthmatic patients (38). They are found with the same prevalence in nonasthmatic pa-

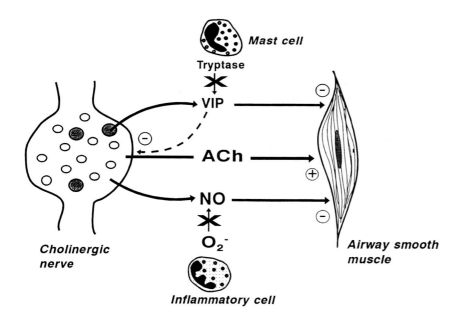

FIG. 4. VIP and nitric oxide (*NO*) may be co-released from cholinergic nerves and act as functional antagonists of cholinergic bronchoconstriction. In addition, they may act prejunctionally to inhibit ACh release. In asthma, enzymes such as tryptase released from airway mast cells may rapidly degrade VIP, and oxygen free radicals, such as superoxide anions (O_2-), from inflammatory cells may inactivate NO, thus leading to exaggerated cholinergic neural bronchoconstriction.

tients, so that their significance is doubtful. Although it seems unlikely that there would be any primary abnormality in VIP innervation in the airways of patients with asthma, it is possible that a secondary abnormality may arise as a result of the inflammatory process in the airway. Recently, low plasma concentrations of VIP have been described during exacerbations of asthma, but the significance of this observation is difficult to evaluate because the source of VIP in plasma is unknown (39).

Mast cell tryptase is particularly active in degrading VIP (29). Tryptase released from mast cells in the asthmatic airway may then more rapidly degrade VIP and related peptides released from airway cholinergic nerves. In sensitized guinea pigs exposed to allergen, a reduction in i-NANC responses has been reported (40). This is presumably due to the release of enzymes or oxygen-free radicals from inflammatory cells in the airways. However, there is no convincing evidence supporting a functional role for VIP in regulation of airway smooth muscle caliber in humans, and it seems more likely that VIP plays a role in the regulation of airway blood flow. VIP may therefore contribute to the increased blood flow in asthmatic airways, and in this respect may be regarded as potentially proinflammatory.

VASOACTIVE INTESTINAL PEPTIDE–RELATED PEPTIDES

Several other peptides have now been identified in the mammalian nervous system that are similar in structure and effect to VIP.

Peptide Histidine Isoleucine

PHI and its human equivalent, peptide histidine methionine (PHM), have a marked structural similarity to VIP, with 50% amino acid sequence homology. PHI and PHM are encoded by the same gene as VIP and both peptides are synthesized in the same prohormone (41). It is therefore not surprising to find that PHI has a similar immunocytochemical distribution in lung to VIP, and that PHI-IR nerves supply airway smooth muscle (especially larger airways), bronchial and pulmonary vessels, submucosal glands, and airway ganglia (42–44). The amount of PHI is similar to the amount of VIP in respiratory tract (44). Like VIP, PHI stimulates adenylyl cyclase and appears to activate the same receptor as VIP (7).

There are some differences between VIP and PHI, because PHI is less potent as an airway vasodilator (20,45) and more potent as a stimulant of secretion than VIP (46). Like VIP, PHI potentiates cholinergic and inhibits β-adrenergic stimulation of mucous secretion in vitro (46). In human bronchi in vitro, PHM is a potent relaxant and is equipotent to VIP (10).

Peptide Histidine Valine

Peptide histidine valine (PHV-42) is an N-terminally extended precursor of VIP. PHV is a potent bronchodilator of guinea pig airways in vitro (47), but when infused in asthmatic patients has no demonstrable bronchodilator effect (48). It is not clear whether this peptide is released from airway nerves.

Helodermin

Helodermin is a 35-amino acid peptide of similar structure to VIP that has been isolated from the salivary gland venom of the Gila monster lizard. Helodermin-IR has been localized to airway nerves and the peptide has similar effects to VIP, but has a longer duration of action (49). Helodermin is a potent relaxant of airway smooth muscle in vitro, and helodermin-IR has been reported in trachea (50). Helodermin appears to activate a high-affinity form of the VIP receptor (7). Helospectins I and II are two closely related peptides that have recently been localized to nerves within the respiratory tract (50,51) and both peptides potently relax guinea pig airways (50).

Pituitary Adenylate Cyclase–activating Peptide

PACAP, a 38–amino acid peptide isolated from sheep hypothalamus, and PACAP-27, a truncated fragment, have marked sequence homology with VIP and have been demonstrated in the peripheral nervous system (52). PACAP-IR has a similar distribution to VIP in airways of several species, and may be localized to cholinergic and also to capsaicin-sensitive afferent nerves (51). The effects of PACAP-27 are similar to those of VIP. PACAP relaxes guinea pig tracheal and bronchial smooth muscle in vitro (53) and is approximately 3 times less potent than VIP (54). PACAP, like VIP, also inhibits the release of inflammatory mediators from chopped lung tissue (54). There appears to be a particularly high density of receptors for PACAP in lung tissue (55).

NEUROPEPTIDE Y

NPY is a 36–amino acid peptide that is a co-transmitter with norepinephrine in adrenergic nerves and usually amplifies its effects (56).

Localization

The distribution of NPY follows the distribution of adrenergic nerves and is predominantly to nasal vessels, and bronchial vessels and glands, with less marked innervation of airway smooth muscle (1,57–59). After extrinsic denervation in heart-lung transplantation recipients, there is an apparent increase in NPY-IR nerves, suggesting that there may normally be some descending inhibitory influence to the expression of this peptide (60). In rodents, depletion of sensory neuropeptides with capsaicin is associated with an increase in adrenergic nerves, indicating that there may be a reciprocal interaction between sensory and adrenergic innervation in lung (61). NPY also may be found within parasympathetic ganglia, where it co-exists with VIP, because sympathectomy does not completely deplete NPY. This suggests that there is a population of NPY-IR fibers in the respiratory tract that are not sympathetic in origin.

Effects on Airway Tone

NPY has no direct effect on airway smooth muscle of guinea pig (62), but may cause bronchoconstriction via release of prostaglandins (63). NPY has a modulatory effect on cholinergic transmission of postganglionic cholinergic nerves (62). This appears to be a direct effect on prejunctional NPY-receptors, rather than secondary to any effect on β-adrenoceptors. Prejunctional and postjunctional NPY receptors may differ, with prejunctional Y_2-receptors acting to inhibit adenylyl cyclase, whereas postjunctional Y_1-receptors stimulate phosphoinositide hydrolysis (64). NPY also has a modulatory effect on e-NANC bronchoconstriction both *in vitro* and *in vivo,* and this effect is surprisingly long lasting (62,65).

Vascular Effects

NPY binding sites are present on arterial smooth muscle and arteriosinusoidal anastamoses in human nasal mucosa (59). These also are the sites of the highest densities of NPY nerve fibers. NPY is a potent vasoconstrictor in some vascular beds, acting predominantly on the resistance arterioles. NPY causes a long-lasting reduction in tracheal blood flow in anesthetized dogs (66), but has no direct effect on canine bronchial vessels *in vitro* (67), suggesting a preferential effect on resistance vessels in the airway. NPY also causes long-lasting vasoconstriction in the nose and is released with sympathetic nerve stimulation, particularly at higher frequencies (68,69). NPY may constrict resistance vessels, reducing mucosal blood flow and microvascular leak through the reduction in the perfusion of permeable postcapillary venules. This mechanism has been demonstrated in the airways for epinephrine (70).

Effects on Secretion

NPY has no direct effect on secretion from ferret airways, although it has complex effects on stimulated secretion. NPY enhances both cholinergic and adrenergic stim-

ulation of mucous secretion, but inhibits stimulated serous cell secretion (46). NPY has no effect on mucin secretion from human nasal mucosal explants *in vitro* (59).

GASTRIN-RELEASING PEPTIDE

Gastrin-releasing peptide (GRP) is a 27–amino acid peptide and is the mammalian form of the amphibian peptide bombesin (71). Other shorter peptides that share the active C-terminal sequence have also been described. These peptides interact with specific receptors and initiate phosphoinositide metabolism and elevation of *c-myc* and *c-fos* mRNA levels (71,72).

Localization

GRP/bombesin-IR is localized to neuroendocrine cells in human and animal lower airways (71,73,74). Bombesin-IR peptides have been recovered from the bronchoalveolar lavage fluid from smokers (75). GRP-containing nerve fibers have been demonstrated around blood vessels and submucosal glands in the airways of several species (76). GRP has also been identified in trigeminal sensory nerves that innervate the nasal mucosa of humans and animals (77). The distribution of GRP-containing nerves in nasal arterial and venous vessels and glands is identical to that of SP, NKA, and CGRP (78). GRP/bombesin binding sites in nasal and bronchial epithelium are present on epithelial cells and submucosal glands (77,79).

Airway Effects

GRP and bombesin-like peptides may play important roles in lung maturation. GRP mRNA production in lungs is increased on the day before birth and then declines (80). Bombesin-like immunoreactivity decreases with maturation (81). A marked reduction in bombesin-IR has been described in the lungs of infants who have died of fetal respiratory distress syndrome (81). Bombesin has a trophic effect on several cell types and may be important in epithelial growth (72,82). Bombesin is secreted by certain small cell bronchial carcinomas and may have an autocrine effect on tumor growth (71).

Bombesin is a potent bronchoconstrictor in guinea pigs *in vivo* (83,84). However, *in vitro* it has no effect on either proximal airways or on lung strips, indicating that it produces bronchoconstriction indirectly. The bronchoconstrictor response is not blocked by an antihistamine, cyclo-oxygenase inhibitor, lipoxygenase inhibitor, platelet-activating factor antagonist, or serotonin antagonist, indicating that mediator release is unlikely, nor is it inhibited by capsaicin pretreatment or by cholinergic antagonists, suggesting that neural reflex mechanisms are not involved. The bronchoconstrictor response is inhibited by a bombesin receptor antagonist, BIM 26159, indicating that bombesin/GRP receptors are involved (84). Bombesin reduces tracheal blood flow in dogs, indicating a vasoconstrictor action (66).

GRP and bombesin are potent stimulants of airway mucous secretion in human and cat airways *in vitro* (77,79) and guinea pig nasal mucosa *in vivo* (85). GRP stimulated both serous cell lactoferrin and mucous glycoconjugate secretion from human nasal mucosa. *In vivo*, topical application of bombesin results in increased secretion from mucous and serous cells of the nose (86).

CHOLECYSTOKININ

Cholecystokinin octapeptide (CCK$_8$) has been identified in low concentrations in lungs and airways of several species (87). It may be localized to sensory nerves (88), although there are now suspicions that the visualized immunoreactivity reflects cross-reactivity with CGRP (89).

CCK$_8$ is a potent constrictor of guinea pig and human airways *in vitro* (90). The bronchoconstrictor response is potentiated by epithelial removal and by phosphoramidon, suggesting that it is degraded by epithelial neutral endopeptidase (NEP). The bronchoconstrictor effect of CCK$_8$ is also potentiated in guinea pigs sensitized and exposed to inhaled allergen, possibly because allergen exposure reduces epithelial NEP function. CCK$_8$ acts directly on airway smooth muscle and is potently inhibited by the specific CCK antagonist L363,851, indicating that CCK$_A$-receptors (peripheral type) are involved (90). CCK$_8$ has no apparent effect on cholinergic neurotransmission either at the level of parasympathetic ganglia or at postganglionic nerve terminals (90). Although few CCK-immunoreactive nerves are present in airways, they may still have a significant effect on airway tone if these particular neural fibers are activated selectively.

SOMATOSTATIN

Somatostatin has been localized to some afferent nerves (91,92), but the concentration detectable in lung is low (1,87). Somatostatin has no direct action on airway smooth muscle *in vitro*, but appears to potentiate cholinergic neurotransmission in ferret airways (93). Although somatostatin has a modulatory effect on neurogenic inflammation in the rat foot pad (94), no modulation of e-NANC nerves in airways is apparent (Stretton CD, Barnes PJ, unpublished observations).

GALANIN

Galanin is a 29-amino acid peptide named after its N-terminal glycine and C-terminal alanine (95). Galanin is widely distributed in the respiratory tract innervation of several species. It is co-localized with VIP in cholinergic nerves of airways and is present in parasympathetic ganglia (96,97). It is also co-localized with SP/CGRP in sensory nerves and dorsal root, nodose, and trigeminal ganglia (1). Galanin has no direct effect on airway tone or on cholinergic neurotransmission in guinea pigs (98), but modulates e-NANC neurotransmission (98,99). It has no effect on airway blood flow in dogs (66), and its physiologic role in airways remains a mystery.

ADRENOMEDULLIN

Adrenomedullin (AM) is a 52-amino acid vasodilator peptide recently isolated from human pheochromocytoma, which has analogies to CGRP. AM mRNA and immunoreactivity are expressed in several tissues, including lung (100). AM is a potent and long-lasting bronchodilator in guinea pig trachea (101). The role of AM in the control of airway tone is not known, and it is not certain whether it is released from airway nerves.

ENKEPHALINS

Leucine-enkephalin has been localized to neuroendocrine cells in airways (73) and [Met]enkephalin-Arg^6-Gly^7-Leu^8-IR nerves have been described in guinea pig and rat lungs (88,102), with a similar distribution to VIP (103). The anatomic origins and functional roles of the endogenous opioids are not clear because the opioid antagonist naloxone has no effect on neurally mediated airway effects (104,105). However, it is possible that these opioid pathways may be selectively activated from brain stem centers under certain conditions. Exogenous opioids potently modulate neuropeptide release from sensory nerves in airways (104–107) via μ-opioid receptors and may also modulate cholinergic neurotransmission via μ- or δ-opioid receptors (108).

NEUROTENSIN

Neurotensin is a 13-amino acid peptide that was initially isolated from the hypothalamus, but is also localized to epithelial cells and nerves in the gut (109). Its distribution in airways has not been reported. Neurotensin is a relatively potent constrictor of rat bronchi *in vitro*, and also increases the contractile responses to cholinergic nerve stimulation, indicating that there may be facilitatory prejunctional receptors on airway cholinergic nerves in this species (110). Neurotensin also degranulates certain types of mast cell, although this may be related to its basic N-terminal sequence. Neurotensin is a substrate for NEP, and its bronchoconstrictor effects are potentiated by

66. Salonen RO, Webber SE, Widdicombe JG. Effects of neuropeptides and capsaicin on the canine tracheal vasculature *in vivo*. *Br J Pharmacol* 1988;95:1262–1270.

67. McCormack DG, Salonen RO, Barnes PJ. Effect of sensory neuropeptides on canine bronchial and pulmonary vessels *in vitro*. *Life Sci* 1989;45:2405–2412.

68. Lacroix JS. Adrenergic and nonadrenergic mechanisms in sympathetic vascular control of the nasal mucosa. *Acta Physiol Scand* 1989;136(suppl 581):1–63.

69. Baraniuk JN, Silver PB, Kaliner MA, Barnes PJ. Neuropeptide Y is a vasoconstrictor in human nasal mucosa. *J Appl Physiol* 1992;73:1867–1872.

70. Boschetto P, Roberts NM, Rogers DF, Barnes PJ. The effect of antiasthma drugs on microvascular leak in guinea pig airways. *Am Rev Respir Dis* 1989;139:416–421.

71. Miller YE. Bombesin-like peptides: from frog skin to human lung. *Am J Respir Cell Mol Biol* 1990;3:189–190.

72. Rozengurt E, Sinnett-Smith J. Bombesin stimulation of fibroblast mitogenesis: specific receptors, signal transduction and early events. *Phil Trans R Soc Lond* 1990;B327:209–221.

73. Cutz E. Neuroendocrine cells of the lung—an overview of morphological characteristics and development. *Exp Lung Res* 1982;3:185–208.

74. Polak JM, Bloom SR. Regulatory peptides of the gastrointestinal and respiratory tracts. *Arch Int Phamacodyn* 1986;280:16–49.

75. Aguayro SM, Kane MA, King TE, Schwartz MI, Grauer L, Miller YE. Increased levels of bombesin-like peptides in the lower respiratory tract of asymptomatic smokers. *J Clin Invest* 1989;84:1105–1113.

76. Uddman R, Moghimzadeh E, Sundler F. Occurrence and distribution of GRP-immunoreactive nerve fibres in the respiratory tract. *Arch Otorhinolaryngol* 1984;239:145–151.

77. Baraniuk JN, Lundgren JD, Goff J, et al. Gastrin releasing peptide (GRP) in human nasal mucosa. *J Clin Invest* 1990;85:998–1005.

78. Baraniuk JN. Neural control of nasal secretion. *Pulm Pharmacol* 1990;4:20–31.

79. Lundgren JD, Ostrowski N, Baraniuk JN, Shelhamer JH, Kaliner MA. Gastrin releasing peptide stimulates glycoconjugate release from feline tracheal explants. *Am J Physiol* 1990;258:L68–L74.

80. Spindel ER, Sunday ME, Hofler H. Transient elevation of mRNAs encoding gastrin releasing peptide (GRP), a putative pulmonary growth factor, in human fetal lung. *J Clin Invest* 1987;80:1172

81. Ghatei MA, Sheppard MN, Henzen-Logman S, Blank MA, Polak JM, Bloom SR. Bombesin and vasoactive intestinal peptide in the developing lung: marked changes in acute respiratory distress syndrome. *J Clin Endocrinol Metab* 1983;57:1226–1232.

82. Sunday ME, Kaplan LM, Motoyama E, Chin WW, Spindel ER. Gastrin releasing peptide (mammalian bombesin) gene expression in health and disease. *Lab Invest* 1988;59:5–24.

83. Impicciatore M, Bertaccini G. The bronchconstrictor action of the tetradecapeptide bombesin in the guinea pig. *J Pharm Pharmacol* 1973;25:812–815.

84. Belvisi MG, Stretton CD, Barnes PJ. Bombesin-induced bronchoconstriction in the guinea pig: mode of action. *J Pharmacol Exp Ther* 1991;258:36–41.

85. Gawin A, Baraniuk JN, Lundgren JD, Kaliner MA. The effects of gastrin releasing peptide (GRP) and analogues on guinea pig nasal mucosa. *Am Rev Respir Dis* 1990;141:A173

86. Baraniuk JN, Silver PB, Lundgren JP, Cole P, Kaliner MA, Barnes PJ. Bombesin stimulates mucous cell and serous cell secretion in human nasal provocation tests. *Am J Physiol* 1992;262:L48–L52.

87. Ghatei MA, Sheppard M, O'Shaunessy DJ, et al. Regulatory peptides in the mammalian respiratory tract. *Endocrinology* 1982;111:1248–1254.

88. Gibbins IL, Furness JB, Costa M. Pathway specific patterns of coexistence of substance P, calcitonin gene related peptide, cholecystokinin, and dynorphin in neurons of the dorsal root ganglion of the guinea pig. *Cell Tissue Res* 1987;248:417–432.

89. Ju G, Hökfelt T, Fischer JA, Frey JF, Rehfeld JF, Dockery GJ. Does cholecystokinin-like immunoreactivity in rat primary sensory neurons represent calcitonin gene related peptide? *Neurosci Lett* 1986;68:305.

90. Stretton CD, Barnes PJ. Cholecystokinin octapeptide constricts guinea-pig and human airways. *Br J Pharmacol* 1989;97:675–682.

91. Holzer P. Local effector functions of capsaicin-senstive sensory nerve endings: involvement of tachykinins, calcitonin gene related peptide, and other neuropeptides. *Neuroscience* 1988;24:739–768.

92. Maggi CA, Meli A. The sensory efferent function of capsaicin sensitive sensory nerves. *Gen Pharmacol* 1988;19:1–43.

93. Sekizawa K, Graf PD, Nadel JA. Somatostatin potentiates cholinergic neurotransmission in ferret trachea. *J Appl Physiol* 1989;67:2397–2400.

94. Lembeck F, Donnerer J, Bartho L. Inhibition of neurogenic vasodilation and plasma extravasation by substance P antagonists, somatostatin and [D-Met2, Pro5]-enkephalinamide. *Eur J Pharmacol* 1982;85:171–176.

95. Rokaeus A. Galanin: a newly isolated biologically active peptide. *Trends Neurol Sci* 1987;10:158–164.

96. Dey RD, Mitchell HW, Coburn RF. Organization and development of peptide-containing neurons in the airways. *Am J Respir Cell Mol Biol* 1990;3:187–188.

97. Cheung A, Polak JM, Bauer FE, et al. The distribution of galanin immunoreactivity in the respiratory tract of pig, guinea pig, rat, and dog. *Thorax* 1985;40:889–896.

98. Takahashi T, Belvisi MG, Barnes PJ. Modulation of neurotransmission in guinea-pig airways by galanin and the effect of a new antagonist galantide. *Neuropeptides* 1994;26:245–251.

99. Guiliani S, Amann R, Papini AM, Maggi CA, Meli A. Modulatory action of galanin on responses due to antidromic activation of peripheral terminals of capsaicin sensitive sensory nerves. *Eur J Pharmacol* 1989;163:91–96.

100. Ichiki Y, Kitamura K, Kangawa K, Kawamoto M, Matsuo H, Eto T. Distribution and characterization of immunoreactive adrenomedulin in human tissue and plasma. *FEBS Letts* 1994;338:6–10.

101. Kanazawa H, Kurihara N, Hirata K, Kudo S, Kawaguchi T, Takeda T. Adrenomedullin, a newly discovered hypotensive peptide, is a potent bronchodilator. *Biochem Biophys Res Commun* 1994;205:251–254.

102. Jancso G, Hökfelt T, Lundberg JM, et al. Immunohistochemical studies on the effect of capsaicin on spinal and medullary peptide and monoamine neurons using antisera to substance P, gastrin/CCK, somatostatin, VIP, enkephalin, neurotensin, and 5-hydroxytryptamine. *J Neurocytol* 1981;10:963–975.

103. Shimosegawa T, Foda HD, Said SI. [Met]enkephalin-Arg6-Gly7-Leu8-immunoreactive nerves in guinea pig and rat lungs: distribution,origin, and coexistence with vasoactive intestinal polypeptide immunoreactivity. *Neuroscience* 1990;36:737–750.

104. Belvisi MG, Rogers DF, Barnes PJ. Neurogenic plasma extravasation: inhibition by morphine in guinea pig airways *in vivo*. *J Appl Physiol* 1989;66:268–272.

105. Belvisi MG, Chung KF, Jackson DM, Barnes PJ. Opioid modulation of noncholinergic neural bronchoconstriction in guinea-pig *in vivo*. *Br J Pharmacol* 1988;95:413–418.

106. Frossard N, Barnes PJ. m-Opioid receptors modulate noncholinergic constrictor nerves in guinea-pig airways. *Eur J Pharmacol* 1987;141:519–521.

107. Bartho L, Amann R, Saria A, Szolcsanyi J, Lembeck F. Peripheral effects of opioid drugs in capsaicin-sensitive neurones of the guinea pig bronchus and rabbit ear. *Naunyn Schmiedeberg Arch Pharm* 1987;336:316–320.

108. Russell JA, Simons EJ. Modulation of cholinergic neurotransmission in airways by enkephalin. *J Appl Physiol* 1985;58:853–858.

109. Schultzberg M, Hokfelt T, Nilsson G, et al. Distribution of peptide- and catecholamine-containing neurons in the gastrointestinal tract of rat and guinea pig: immunohistochemical studies with antisera to substance P, vasoactive intestinal polypeptide, enkephalins, somatostatin, gastrin/cholecystokinin, neurotensin and dopamine-b-hydroxylase. *Neuroscience* 1980;5:689–744.

110. Aas P, Helle KB. Neurotensin receptors in rat bronchi. *Reg Peptides* 1982;3:405–413.

111. Djokic TD, Dusser DJ, Borson DB, Nadel JA. Neutral endopeptidase modulates neurotensin-induced airway contraction. *J Appl Physiol* 1989;66:2338–2343.

112. Gutowska J, Nemer M. Structure, expression and function of atrial natriuretic factor in extra atrial tissues. *Endocr Rev* 1989;10:519–536.

113. Nally JE, Clayton RA, Thomson NC, McGrath JC. The interaction of a-human atrial natriuretic peptide (ANP) with salbutamol, sodium nitroprusside and isosorbide dinitrite in human bronchial smooth muscle. *Br J Pharmacol* 1995;113:1328–1332.

114. Hulks G, Jardine AG, Connell JMC, Thomson NC. Bronchodilator ef-

fect of atrial natriuretic peptide in asthma. *Br Med J* 1989;292: 1081–1082.

115. Angus RM, Mecallaum MJA, Hulks G, Thomson NC. Bronchodilator, cardiovascular and cyclic guanylyl monophosphate response to high dose infused atrial natriuretic peptide in asthma. *Am Rev Respir Dis* 1993;147:1122–1125.

116. Hulks G, Thomson NC. High dose inhaled atrial natriuretic peptide is a bronchodilator in asthmatic subjects. *Eur Respir J* 1994;7: 1593–1597.

117. Angus RM, Millar EA, Chalmers GW, Thomson NC. Effect of inhaled atrial natriuretic pepetide and a neutranl endopeptidase inhibitor on histamine-induced bronchoconstriction. *Am J Respir Crit Care Med* 1995;151:2003–2005.

118. Suga S, Nakao K, Hosoda K. Receptor selectivity of natriuretic peptide family: atrial natriuretic peptide, brain natriuretic peptide and C-type natriuretic peptide. *Endocrinology* 1992;229–239.

119. Fluge T, Hoyman HG, Hohlfeld J, Heinrich U, Fabel H, Wagner TO, Forssman WG. Type A natriuretic peptides exhibit different bronchoprotective effects in rats. *Eur J Pharmacol* 1994;271:395–402.

120. Wei ET, Kiang JC. Inhibition of protein extravasation from the trachea by corticotrophin-releasing factor. *Eur J Pharmacol* 1987;140:63–67.

121. Yoshihara S, Ricciardolo FLM, Geppetti P, et al. Corticotrophin-releasing factor inhibits antigen-induced plasma extravasation in airways. *Eur J Pharmacol* 1995;280:113–118.

122. Daniele RP, Barnes PJ, Goetzl EJ, et al. Neuroimmune interactions in the lung. *Am Rev Respir Dis* 1992;145:1230–1235.

phosphoramidon in guinea pig (111). The effects of neurotensin on human airways have not yet been reported.

ATRIAL NATRIURETIC PEPTIDE

Human atrial natriuretic peptide (ANP) is a 28-amino acid peptide synthesized in atria and isolated lung tissue (112) and is expressed in vascular smooth muscle cells. It may function as a circulating hormone and is a potent vasodilator substance *in vitro* and *in vivo*. Its relaxant effect is through stimulation of particulate guanylyl cyclase to increase the intracellular concentration of cyclic guanosine monophosphate (cGMP). *In vitro*, ANP counteracts methacholine-induced constriction of human bronchi and appears to act synergistically with β_2-agonists (113). *In vivo*-infused ANP causes bronchodilatation in asthmatic patients (114,115) and protects against methacholine-induced bronchoconstriction (115). Inhaled ANP is less effective, although high concentrations bronchodilate asthmatic patients (116). ANP is degraded by NEP and the NEP inhibitor thiorphan markedly potentiates the effects of inhaled ANP (117). Other members of the natriuretic family include brain and C-type natriuretic peptides (BNP, CNP) derived from different genes, which have similar effects (118). All three natriuretic peptides are expressed in vascular smooth muscle and therefore may have an influence on airway tone via the circulation. The renal natriuretic peptide urodilatin also relaxes airway smooth muscle and is more effective than ANP in protecting against ACh-induced bronchoconstriction (119).

CORTICOTROPHIN-RELEASING FACTOR

Corticotrophin releasing factor (CRF) is a 41-amino acid peptide that controls the pituitary-adrenal axis. It is co-localized with other neuropeptides in capsaicin-sensitive nerves in the brain. CRF inhibits plasma extravasation in the airways (120,121), but its physiologic role in the airways remains uncertain.

CONCLUSIONS

The presence of so many neuropeptides in the respiratory tract raises questions about their physiologic role. Neuropeptides appear to be co-transmitters in classic autonomic nerves and may be regarded as modulators of autonomic effects, perhaps acting to "fine tune" airway functions and to modulate the release of other neurotransmitters. Although much of the research on neuropeptides in the airways previously concentrated on their effects on airway smooth muscle, it is now clear that the most potent effects of many of the relevant peptides are on airway vasculature and secretions, and that neuropeptides may have an important role in regulating the mucosal surface of the airways. The effect of neuropeptides on mucosal immunity is also highly relevant to their potential role in asthma, and there are complex interactions between neuropeptides and the immune system (122). The lack of understanding of the physiologic role of individual peptides is largely due to the lack of specific antagonists that can be given safely to humans. Whether neuropeptides contribute to the pathophysiology of asthma has not been elucidated, although there are indications that increased effects of some peptides or defective function of other peptides may have effects on the inflammatory process and symptoms.

REFERENCES

1. Uddman R, Sundler F. Neuropeptides in the airways: a review. *Am Rev Respir Dis* 1987;136:S3–S8.
2. Barnes PJ, Baraniuk J, Belvisi MG. Neuropeptides in the respiratory tract. *Am Rev Respir Dis* 1991;144:1187–1198 (part 1), 1391–1399 (part 2).
3. Barnes PJ. Neuropeptides and asthma. *Am Rev Respir Dis* 1991;143:S28–32.
4. Lundberg JM, Fahrenkrug J, Hokfelt T, et al. Coexistence of peptide histidine isoleucine (PHI) and VIP in nerves regulating blood flow and bronchial smooth muscle tone in various mammals including man. *Peptides* 1984;5:593–606.
5. Laitinen A, Partanen M, Hervonen A, Peto-Juikko M, Laitinen LA. VIP-like immunoreactive nerves in human respiratory tract. Light and electron microscopic study. *Histochemistry* 1985;82:313–319.
6. Dey RD, Altemus JB, Michalkiewicz M. Distribution of vasoactive intestinal peptide- and substance P-containing nerves originating from neurons of airway ganglia in cat bronchi. *J Comp Neurol* 1991;304:330–340.
7. Robberecht P, Waelbroeck M., deNeef P, Camus JC, Coy DH, Christophe J. Pharmacological characterization of VIP receptors in human lung membranes. *Peptides* 1988;9:339–345.
8. Carstairs JR, Barnes PJ. Visualization of vasoactive intestinal peptide receptors in human and guinea pig lung. *J Pharmacol Exp Ther* 1986;239:249–255.
9. Speedharan SP, Robichen A, Peterson KE, Goetzl EJ. Cloning and expression of the human vasoactive intestinal peptide receptor. *Proc Natl Acad Sci USA* 1991;88:4986–4990.
10. Palmer JBD, Cuss FMC, Barnes PJ. VIP and PHM and their role in nonadrenergic inhibitory responses in isolated human airways. *J Appl Physiol* 1986;61:1322–1328.
11. Diamond L, Szarek JL, Gillespie MN, Altiere RJ. *In vivo* bronchodilatory activity of vasoactive intestinal peptide in the cat. *Am Rev Respir Dis* 1991;128:827–832.
12. Barnes PJ, Brown MJ. Venous plasma histamine in exercise and hyperventilation-induced asthma in man. *Clin Sci* 1981;61:159–162.
13. Palmer JBD, Cuss FMC, Warren JB, Barnes PJ. The effect of infused vasoactive intestinal peptide on airway function in normal subjects. *Thorax* 1986;41:663–666.
14. Morice A, Unwin RJ, Sever PS. Vasoactive intestinal peptide causes bronchodilation and protects against histamine-induced bronchoconstriction in asthmatic subjects. *Lancet* 1983;2:1225–1226.
15. O'Donnell M, Garippa RJ, Rinaldi N, et al. Ro25-1553: a novel long-acting vasoactive intestinal peptide agonist. Part 1: *in vitro* and *in vivo* bronchodilator studies. *J Pharmacol Exp Ther* 1994;270:1282–1288.
16. Peatfield AC, Barnes PJ, Bratcher C, Nadel JA, Davis B. Vasoactive intestinal peptide stimulates tracheal submucosal gland secretion in ferret. *Am Rev Respir Dis* 1983;128:89–93.
17. Coles SJ, Said SI, Reid LM. Inhibition by vasoactive intestinal peptide of glycoconjugate and lysozyme secretion by human airways *in vitro. Am Rev Respir Dis* 1981;124:531–536.
18. Webber SE, Lim JCS, Widdicombe JG. CGRP and methacholine-induced mucus secretion and epithelial albumin transport. *Eur Resp J* 1009;3(suppl):280S.

19. Nathanson I, Widdicombe JH, Barnes PJ. Effect of vasoactive intestinal peptide on ion transport across dog tracheal epithelium. *J Appl Physiol* 1983;55:1844–1848.
20. Widdicombe JG. The NANC system and airway vasculature. *Arch Int Pharmacodyn* 1990;303:83–90.
21. Matran R, Alving K, Martling CR, Lacroix JS, Lundberg JM. Effects of neuropeptides and capsaicin on tracheobronchial blood flow in the pig. *Acta Physiol Scand* 1989;135:335–342.
22. Barnes PJ, Dixon CMS. The effect of inhaled vasoactive intestinal peptide on bronchial hyperreactivity in man. *Am Rev Respir Dis* 1984;130:162–166.
23. Martin JG, Wang A, Zacour M, Biggs DF. The effects of vasoactive intestinal polypeptide on cholinergic neurotransmission in isolated innervated guinea pig tracheal preparations. *Respir Physiol* 1990;79:111–122.
24. Stretton CD, Belvisi MG, Barnes PJ. Modulation of neural bronchoconstrictor responses in the guinea pig respiratory tract by vasoactive intestinal peptide. *Neuropeptides* 1991;18:149–157.
25. Hakoda H, Ito Y. Modulation of cholinergic neurotransmission by the peptide VIP, VIP antiserum and VIP antagonists in dog and cat trachea. *J Physiol* 1990;428:133–154.
26. Undem BJ, Dick EC, Buckner CK. Inhibition by vasoactive intestinal peptide of antigen-induced histamine release from guinea pig minced lung. *Eur J Pharmacol* 1983;88:247–250.
27. Conroy DM, Samhoun MN, Piper PJ. Vasoactive intestinal peptide and helodermin inhibit the release of cyclo-oxygenase products induced by leukotriene D$_4$ and bradykinin from guinea-pig perfused lung. *Eur J Pharmacol* 1992;218:43–50.
28. O'Dorisio MS, Shannaon BT, Fleshman DJ, Campolito LB. Identification of high affinity receptors for vasoactive intestinal peptide on human lymphocytes of B cell lineage. *J Immunol* 1989;142:3533–3536.
29. Caughey GH, Leidig F, Viro NF, Nadel JA. Substance P and vasoactive intestinal peptide degradation by mast cell tryptase and chymase. *J Pharmacol Exp Ther* 1988;244:133–137.
30. Ellis JL, Framer SG. Effects of peptidases on nonadrenergic, noncholinergic inhibitory responses of tracheal smooth muscle; a comparison with effects on VIP- and PHI-induced relaxation. *Br J Pharmacol* 1989;96:521–526.
31. Belvisi MG, Stretton CD, Miura M, et al. Inhibitory NANC nerves in human tracheal smooth muscle: a quest for the neurotransmitter. *J Appl Physiol* 1992;73:2505–2510.
32. Belvisi MG, Miura M, Stretton CD, Barnes PJ. Endogenous vasoactive intestinal peptide and nitric oxide modulate cholinergic neurotransmission in guinea pig trachea. *Eur J Pharmacol* 1993;231:97–102.
33. Ward JK, Belvisi MG, Fox AJ, Miura M, Tadjkarimi S, Yacoub MH, Barnes PJ. Modulation of cholinergic neural bronchoconstriction by endogenous nitric oxide and vasoactive intestinal peptide in human airways *in vitro*. *J Clin Invest* 1993;92:736–743.
34. Ollerenshaw S, Jarvis D, Woolcock A, Sullivan C, Scheibner T. Absence of immunoreactive vasoactive intestinal polypeptide in tissue from the lungs of patients with asthma. *N Engl J Med* 1989;320:1244–1248.
35. Barnes PJ. Vasoactive intestinal peptide and asthma. *New Engl J Med* 1989;321:1128–1129.
36. Howarth PH, Britten KM, Djukanovic RJ, Wilson JW, Holgate ST, Springall DR, Polak JM. Neuropeptide containing nerves in human airways *in vivo*: a comparative study of atopic asthma, atopic nonasthma and nonatopic nonasthma. *Thorax* 1990;45:786–787 (abstr).
37. Lilly CM, Bai TR, Shore SA, Hall AE, Drazen JM. Neuropeptide content of lungs from asthmatic and nonasthmatic patients. *Am J Respir Crit Care Med* 1995;151:548–553.
38. Paul S, Said SI, Thompson AB, et al. Characterization of autoantibodies to vasoactive intestinal peptide in asthma. *J Neuroimmunol* 1989;23:133–142.
39. Cardell LO, Uddman R, Edvinsson L. Low plasma concentration of VIP and elevated levels of other neuropeptides during exacerbations of asthma. *Eur Respir J* 1994;7:2169–2173.
40. Miura M, Ichinose M, Kimura K, et al. Dysfunction of nonadrenergic noncholinergic inhibitory system after antigen inhalation in actively sensitized cat airways. *Am Rev Respir Dis* 1992;145:70–74.
41. Tatemoto K. PHI—a new brain-gut peptide. *Peptides* 1984;5:151–154.
42. Lindh B, Lundberg JM, Hokfelt T. NPY-, galanin-, VIP/PHI-, CGRP-
43. Lundberg JM, Fahrenberg J, Hokfelt T. Coexistence of peptide HI (PHI) and VIP in nerves regulating blood flow and bronchial smooth muscle in various animals, including man. *Peptides* 1984;5:593–606.
44. Christofides NO, Yiangou Y, Piper PJ, et al. Distribution of peptide histidine isoleucine in the mammalian respiratory tract and some aspects of its pharmacology. *Endocrinology* 1984;115:1958–1963.
45. Laitinen LA, Laitinen A, Salonen RO, Widdicombe JG. Vascular actions of airway neuropeptides. *Am Rev Respir Dis* 1987;136:559–564.
46. Webber SE. The effects of peptide histidine isoleucine and neuropeptide Y on mucous volume output from ferret trachea. *Br J Pharmacol* 1988;55:40–54.
47. Yiangou Y, DiMarzo V, Spokes RA, Panico M, Morris HR, Bloom SR. Isolation, characterization, and pharmacological actions of peptide histidine valine 42, a novel prepro-vasoactive intestinal peptide derived peptide. *J Biol Chem* 1987;262:14010–14013.
48. Chilvers ER, Dixon CMS, Yiangou Y, Bloom SR, Ind PW. Effect of peptide histidine valine on cardiovascular and respiratory funtion in normal subjects. *Thorax* 1988;43:750–755.
49. Foda HD, Higuchi J, Said SI. Helodermin, a VIP-like pepetide, is a potent and long-acting vasodilator. *Am Rev Respir Dis* 1990;141:A486.
50. Cardell LO, Sundler F, Uddman R. Helospectin/helodermin-like peptides in guinea pig lung: distribution and dilatory effects. *Reg Peptides* 1993;45:435–443.
51. Uddman R, Luts A. Pituitary adenylate cyclase activity peptide (PACAP), a new vasoactive intestinal peptide (VIP)-like peptide in the respiratory tract. *Cell Tissue Res* 1991;265:197–201.
52. Miyata A, Jiang L, Dahl RD, et al. Isolation of a neuropeptide corresponding to the N-terminal 27 residues of the pituitary adenylate cyclase activating polypeptide with 38 residues (PACAP38). *Biochem Biophys Res Commun* 1990;170:643–648.
53. Araki N, Takagi K. Relaxant effect of pituitary adenylate cyclase-activating polypeptide on guinea-pig tracheal smooth muscle. *Eur J Pharmacol* 1992;216:113–117.
54. Conroy DM, St Pierre S, Sirois P. Relaxant effects of pituitary adenylate cyclase activating peptide (PACAP) on epithelium-intact and denuded guinea pig trachea: a comparison with vasoactive intestinal peptide. *Neuropeptides* 1995;29:121–127.
55. Gottschall PE, Tatsumo I, Miyata A, Arimura A. Characterization and distribution of binding sites for the hypothalamic peptide pituitary adenylate cyclase activating polypeptide. *Endocrinology* 1990;127 272–277.
56. Potter EK. Neuropeptide Y as an autonomic neurotransmitter. *Pharmac Ther* 1988;37:251–273.
57. Sheppard MN, Polak JM, Allen JM, Bloom SR. Neuropeptide tyosine (NPY), a newly discovered peptide, is present in the mammalian respiratory tract. *Thorax* 1984;39:326–330.
58. Uddman R, Sundler F. Innervation of the upper airways. *Clin Chest Med* 1986;7:201–209.
59. Baraniuk JN, Castellino S, Goff J, et al. Neuropeptide Y (NPY) in human nasal mucosa. *Am J Respir Cell Mol Biol* 1990;3:165–173.
60. Springall DR, Polak JM, Howard L, et al. Persistence of intrinsic neurones and possible phenotypic changes after extrinsic denervation of human respiratory tract by heart-lung transplantation. *Am Rev Respir Dis* 1990;141:1538–1546.
61. van Ranst L, Lauweryns JM. Effects of long-term sensory vs. sympathetic denervation of the distribution of calcitonin gene-related peptide and tyrosine hydroxylase immunoreactivity in the rat lung. *J Neuroimmunol* 1990;29:131–138.
62. Stretton CD, Barnes PJ. Modulation of cholinergic neurotransmission in guinea pig trachea by neuropeptide Y. *Br J Pharmacol* 1988;93:672–678.
63. Cadieux A, Benchekroun MT, St. Pierre S, Fournier A. Bronchoconstrictive action of neuropeptide Y (NPY) on isolated guinea pig airways. *Neuropeptides* 1989;13:215–219.
64. Håkanson R, Wahlestadt C. Neuropeptide Y acts via prejunctional (Y2) and postjunctional (Y1) receptors. *Neuroscience* 1987;22:S679.
65. Matran R, Martling C-R, Lundberg JM. Inhibition of cholinergic and nonadrenergic,noncholinergic bronchoconstriction in the guinea-pig mediated by neuropeptide Y and α2-adrenoceptors and opiate receptors. *Eur J Pharmacol* 1989;163:15–23.

Subject Index

Note: Page numbers followed by f indicate figures; those followed by t indicate tables.